Pharmacology and drug therapy in nursing

Pharmacology and drug therapy in nursing

3RD EDITION

Morton J. Rodman, B.S., Ph.D.

Professor of Pharmacology
Department of Pharmacology and Toxicology
College of Pharmacy, Rutgers
The State University of New Jersey

Amy M. Karch, R.N., M.S.

Assistant Professor of Nursing (Cardiovascular)/Clinician II
University of Rochester School of Nursing
Rochester, New York

Eleanor H. Boyd, B.A., Ph.D.

Formerly Assistant Professor of Pharmacology and
    Toxicology and of Nursing
University of Rochester School of Medicine and Dentistry
University of Rochester School of Nursing
Rochester, New York

Dorothy W. Smith, R.N., Ed.D.

Professor of Nursing
College of Nursing, Rutgers
The State University of New Jersey

A DAVID T. MILLER BOOK

**J.B. Lippincott
Company**
Philadelphia

London
Mexico City
New York
St. Louis
São Paulo
Sydney

Sponsoring editor:
David T. Miller/Joyce Mkitarian

Manuscript editor:
Mary K. Smith

Indexer:
Ann Cassar

Art director:
Tracy Baldwin

Designer:
Chris Myers

Design Coordinator:
Susan Caldwell

Production supervisor:
Kathleen P. Dunn

Production assistant:
Elizabeth Anne O'Donnell

Compositor:
TAPSCO, Inc.

Printer/Binder:
The Murray Printing Company

3rd Edition

1 3 5 6 4 2

Library of Congress Cataloging in Publication Data

Main entry under title:
Pharmacology and drug therapy in nursing.

   Rev. ed. of: Pharmacology and drug therapy in
nursing   /Morton J. Rodman and Dorothy W. Smith.   2nd ed.
c1979.
   "A David T. Miller book."
   Includes bibliographies and index.
   1. Pharmacology.   2. Chemotherapy.   3. Drugs.
4. Nursing.   I. Rodman, Morton J. II. Rodman, Morton J.
Pharmacology and drug therapy in nursing.   [DNLM:
1. Drug Therapy—nurses' instruction.   2. Pharmacology—
nurses' instruction.   QV 4 P53615]
RM300.P519 1985   615'.1'024613   84-28907

ISBN 0-397-54356-5

It is an honor for us, the two new authors (AMK and EHB), to become associated with this textbook, which we have held in highest esteem and have used for many years in our teaching of both undergraduate and graduate level nursing students. In preparing this revised third edition of the book, we have given highest priority to maintaining the standards of accuracy and readability established by Drs. Rodman and Smith in the first two editions.

The profession of nursing has changed greatly since the first edition of *Pharmacology and Drug Therapy in Nursing* appeared in 1968. Scientific and technological advances, increased public awareness of new drugs and medical procedures, and an increase in consumerism, combined with new nurse practice acts and advances in the unique science of nursing, have resulted in expanded and more comprehensive responsibilities for the practicing nurse. Today's nurse is called on to be skilled in all aspects of the nursing process: total patient assessment; accurate nursing diagnoses; appropriate interventions, including direct patient care as well as the increasingly important intervention of patient teaching; and continual evaluation of the total patient situation and reformulation of the nursing care plan. Changes in this new edition were designed to address these latest professional concerns.

Drug therapy is a complex and integral aspect of health care today. The thousands of drugs available and the complexity of their actions make the rote memorization of pharmacology totally impossible. Building on the excellent scientific foundation established by the original authors, this new edition attempts to explain the principles of drug therapy and the actions of the basic classes of drugs in a manner that will allow the student to develop an understanding of the basic concepts *and incorporate them into the expanded use of the nursing process.* To facilitate the often difficult transition of information from basic pharmacology to clinical application, each class of drugs is presented with a nursing process table to serve as a guide to the application of basic pharmacologic information to each aspect of the nursing process—assessment, diagnosis, intervention, and evaluation. Patient teaching guides are also presented for each class of drugs. These guides not only list concepts to include in patient teaching, but they are also examples of *how* to present those concepts to the patient. These guides can serve as direct resources to practicing nurses as they assume even more primary responsibility for patient education.

We have added information both on the calculation of dosage and preparation of solutions and on the techniques of administering drugs by various routes. Special consideration has also been given to clinically important drug–drug and drug–food interactions.

In addition, we have added illustrations, many of which our students have found helpful in understanding particular concepts, and we have changed many aspects of the overall organization of the book, so that the material is presented in the order which we have found to be optimal for teaching an undergraduate nursing pharmacology course. In selecting the chemotherapeutic agents as the first group of drugs to be discussed, our intention is to give the student time to become familiar with and apply the principles of pharmacology, which have been presented in the first section, without being distracted by the often complex drug effects on organ systems that occur with other drug classes. It has also proven desirable to present autonomic pharmacology (and with it, the pharmacology of the rest of the peripheral nervous system) early in the book, since this knowledge is basic to the understanding of so many therapeutic and toxic effects of drugs in other classes.

To facilitate the teaching of this material by those instructors who do not wish to present topics in this order, we have retained from the earlier editions the practice of using extensive cross-references. We have also retained the Drug Digests at the end of each chapter, a feature that has been greatly appreciated by students through the years. As in previous editions, a plus sign following the name of a drug in the narrative indicates that detailed information about that drug's actions and uses, adverse effects, cautions and contraindications, as well as dosage and administration, is available in a Drug Digest at the end of the chapter.

The great increase in understanding of the immune system, its responses to stressors, and the ways drugs can interact with this system has necessitated a separate chapter (Chapter 36) to summarize briefly the state of knowledge in this rapidly growing field and to introduce terms and concepts that are used in describing drug effects on this system.

We would like to conclude with the final paragraph from the preface to the second edition of this book. "As teachers, we have made special efforts to teach—that is, to offer explanations and reasons for statements made about the status of drug therapy in various clinical situations. In this way, and by trying to write in a style more readable than the term 'textbook' ordinarily denotes, we hope to capture the student's attention and interest." If, in our additions to this book, our efforts to teach and to stimulate student interest are anywhere near as successful as those of Dr. Rodman and Dr. Smith, we shall indeed have succeeded admirably.

Amy M. Karch, R.N., M.S.
Eleanor H. Boyd, B.A., PH.D.

We are grateful to the many people who have helped us make this edition of the book a reality. These include

our students, who have sharpened our teaching skills by their combined years of listening to us and letting us know when we made the point and when we failed;

David T. Miller, Vice President and Editor, Nursing Division, J. B. Lippincott Company, who first approached us with the possibility of our revising this book, who has been supportive throughout the undertaking, and who, along with Joyce Mkitarian, Development Editor, has maintained confidence in us even when our own confidence lagged;

Mary K. Smith, manuscript editor, who has so admirably coordinated manuscript, proofs, and our many changes therein, and who somehow managed to maintain order in all of the confusion;

all of the other people at J. B. Lippincott who have suggested changes, caught our errors, and worked diligently to bring this book into existence;

JoAnn Belle–Isle for her expertise and assistance in preparing the practice problems for dosage and solution;

Carol Root, our typist, who learned to read our handwriting when sometimes even we could not do so, for her endless hours of work preparing the manuscript, the countless little things done to make the job tolerable, and her wonderful supply of enthusiasm, encouragement, and smiles;

the University of Rochester School of Nursing for giving us the first opportunity to work together and for support during the preparation of the manuscript;

our husbands, Dr. Fred E. Karch and Dr. Eugene S. Boyd, who encouraged us in this undertaking, put up with our frustration and fatigue and with long hours of our absence, and were readily available to share their wisdom and knowledge and to discuss with us material from their areas of pharmacologic expertise.

Finally, EHB would like to thank Dr. Louis Lasagna, formerly Chairman, Department of Pharmacology and Toxicology at the University of Rochester School of Medicine and Dentistry, currently Dean of the Sackler School of Graduate Biomedical Sciences, Tufts University, who first gave her the opportunity to teach nursing students and first suggested the possibility of authorship in the field of nursing pharmacology; and AMK would like to thank Timothy, Mark, Cortney, and Kathryn for giving up so much, and for all that they tolerated so that the book could be done on time, while providing so much sunshine and encouragement.

Acknowledgments

Contents

Contents

Contents

Contents

Contents

The authors and editors of this book have expended considerable time and effort to insure that the facts and opinions offered in the text and tables of this book are in accordance with official standards and with the consensus of foremost authorities at the time of publication.

However, drug therapy is a very dynamic branch of medicine, marked by the continual marketing of new drugs and the discontinuation and withdrawal (often without notice) of older drug products. In addition, the Food and Drug Administration constantly orders changes in the labeling of even well-established drug products, on the basis of ongoing studies of their safety and efficacy. For this reason, no claims are made that statements made here concerning the current status of these drugs will continue to reflect the stated view or that the data presented in tabular form are, or will remain, complete and correct in every detail.

The most important aspect of this problem lies in the area of dosage recommendations. Every effort has been made to check that the statements made in the tables are, within the limits of space, precisely correct. However, dosage schedules are frequently ordered changed in accordance with accumulating clinical experiences.

For this reason, we urge that *before administering any drug, you check the manufacturer's latest dosage recommendations* as presented in the package insert which accompanies each unit of every drug product.

Section 1

Introduction
to pharmacology
and drug
therapy
in nursing

1 This introductory section will provide the foundation for the study of the many different classes of drugs that are used in treating patients. By understanding the basic principles of the science of pharmacology, and how these principles can be applied within the science of nursing, the nurse will be prepared to deal with the hundreds of individual drugs that are encountered in daily practice.

Chapter 1 will begin by indicating how drugs were discovered in the past and by describing the processes by which drug products are developed and tested today. The purpose in doing this is not to present a detailed historical and technical discussion of these topics. Rather, it is to introduce certain terms and concepts that should be learned early in the study of this subject to facilitate later learning. In addition, advice will be offered here in regard to methods of studying about drugs and to developing those attitudes that will help to increase the nurse's knowledge of drug actions and their application to the treatment of patients.

Chapters 2 and 3 will examine the incorporation of pharmacologic principles into the nursing process. The relevance of the study of pharmacology will be discussed in all steps of the nursing process—assessment, diagnosis, intervention, and evaluation. A framework for the incorporation of drug therapy into all aspects of the nursing process will then be introduced.

Once the relevance of the study of pharmacology has been demonstrated, Chapter 4 will examine in some depth certain fundamentals of drug action that have been derived from modern scientific studies of the interactions between body chemicals and the molecules of drugs entering the living system. Although regarding drug and tissue interactions in this way may, at first, seem far removed from using drugs in actual clinical situations, the greater understanding of drug action that can be developed by considering such basic concepts will provide the basis for effective application of this knowledge in the clinical situation.

Because the use of drugs is a two-edged sword, the potential adverse effects of drugs must always be considered, as well as their therapeutic effects. Thus, the several major classes of adverse drug effects will be described (Chap. 5), and the factors involved in managing their effects will be discussed.

By understanding all these basic concepts, and by applying them to daily clinical practice, the nurse will be prepared to deal with drug therapy in a manner that will allow the patient to gain maximum benefit from it with minimal danger.

Chapter 1

An
orientation
to drugs

1

Definition and scope of pharmacology

You are about to embark on the study of drugs, a subject of considerable importance in the present-day practice of nursing. In this chapter, the information that is needed about drugs before administering them to patients will be discussed, along with how to go about acquiring pharmacologic knowledge both as a student and as a practicing nurse.

First, the definition of pharmacology and the principles of pharmacology that will be important for clinical practice will be examined.

Pharmacology is, in the broadest sense, the branch of knowledge that has to do with those chemicals that have biologic effects. Actual clinical practice is concerned only with the biologic and medical aspects of the subject. In this text, then, pharmacology will be considered to be the study of the *actions of chemicals on living organisms.*＊

In the clinical setting, the main concern is what chemicals can do, for better or worse, when they come into contact with human tissues. Thus, nurses are concerned primarily with *pharmacotherapeutics*, the branch of pharmacology that deals with drugs—chemicals that are used in medicine for the treatment, prevention, and diagnosis of disease. This area is sometimes called *clinical pharmacology*, because it deals with the effects of the drugs that are used medically for treating *human patients.*

In addition, it is important to study some aspects of still another offshoot of pharmacology. This is *toxicology*, the study of poisons—chemical substances that are harmful to health or are injurious to life. Because overdoses of drugs are often toxic, it is important to learn the signs and symptoms of adverse drug actions and the measures to be taken to counteract the poisonous effects of drugs.

This book, then, deals mainly with the actions of drugs on humans and with the application of such knowledge to problems that arise in treating patients. However, because of the rapid advances and changes that are being made in drug therapy today, it is also important to know something about the experimental science on which drug treatment is based. This science is called *pharmacodynamics*, and it deals with the interactions between the chemical components of living systems and the foreign chemicals, including drugs, that enter living organisms.

Two types of events occur as a result of such interactions: (1) the drug brings about changes in the body's biochemistry and physiology—functional changes that constitute the drug's *effects;* and (2) the body deals with the drug by subjecting it to various biochemical and physicochemical processes. This affects the movements of the drug within the body, and even results in alteration of its chemical structure and finally in its elimination from the body.

Studies of the latter type of events have recently assumed greater importance because of technical advances in analytic chemistry that now make it possible to detect and trace the movements of minute amounts of drugs within the body. This branch of pharmacology, called *pharmacokinetics*, allows scientists to follow the fate of many drugs from the time they enter the body and are absorbed into the bloodstream until they, or the chemical by-products produced by biochemical reactions, are eliminated.

The technical details of how pharmacologists study the actions of drugs that affect the functioning of living tissues are beyond the scope of this book, as are the analytic methods by which the scientific practitioners of pharmacokinetics study the absorption, distribution, biotransformation, and excretion of drugs. However, the practicing nurse should have a general understanding of

＊ The science of pharmacology also encompasses such subjects as (1) *pharmacy*, the study of the preparation, compounding, and dispensing of medicines; and (2) *pharmacognosy*, the study of the sources of drugs derived from plants and animals and of the chemical and physical properties of such substances.

how drugs were discovered in the past and how new drugs are developed and scientifically evaluated today. These two topics will be discussed in the following two sections.

Historical development of pharmacology

Although experimental pharmacodynamics is one of the youngest of the medical sciences, pharmacotherapeutics is one of the most ancient branches of knowledge. This is known not only from the discovery of Sumerian clay tablets dating back beyond 2000 BC and Egyptian papyri from about 1500 BC, but also from the activities of present-day primitive peoples living in Stone Age-type cultures—Australian aborigines, for example, and Papua New Guinea natives.

People everywhere found potent natural chemicals as they foraged for food among the plants of the field. Gradually, they learned which fruits, roots, berries, and barks were safe to eat and which had discomforting effects on body function. Through this slow system of trial and error, and by observing which growing things animals ate and which they avoided, a great deal of knowledge was acquired and passed along as part of the peoples' folklore.

Primitive pharmacology
The type of natural product first used internally for medical purposes was probably a cathartic, because laxative chemicals are frequently found in nature in the form of purgative plants and mineral salts. Such substances were likely used for religious purposes, because it seemed reasonable that something that cleansed the bowel might also drive out the evil spirits that were thought to be defiling a sick person.

Thus, drugs were first used for their mystical or magic powers rather than for their physiologic effects; and, indeed, it is true today that a drug's effects are not limited to what it does to body function directly. People still respond not only physiologically but also psychologically to the taking of a drug—a point that can sometimes be used to advantage in administering medicines. The nature of this psychologic response is not fully understood, but it is related to the patient's hopes and expectations and to his anxieties and fears concerning the effects of the drug he is getting. This is often referred to as the *placebo* effect of medications.

Ancient, medieval, and modern medicines
Through experience, and by trial and error—the method called *empiricism*—a number of natural substances of plant, animal, and mineral origin that seemed to have been proved useful for relief of symptoms came into use and were handed down, first through oral tradition and later in the form of pharmacopeias, or books of drug preparations.

Many medicines discovered empirically by the ancient Egyptians, Hebrews, and Greeks are still in use today, as are substances employed as medicines by the Arabs of the Middle Ages and by the Indians whom Europeans met in their voyages of exploration that ushered in the Modern Era.

The famous Ebers Papyrus, an Egyptian compilation of drug lore dating from around 1500 BC, refers to the use of opium, castor oil, and squill, among many other medicines. The ancient Greek physician Dioscorides mentioned *Colchicum* in his encyclopedic work on materia medica. The herbals of the medieval monasteries included belladonna; and the Swiss physician Paracelsus introduced mercury for treating syphilis in the 16th century. The North American Indians used the cathartic properties of cascara bark, and *Cinchona*, the quinine-containing fever bark, was a standard remedy for malaria and other ills among the Indians of South America.

Although a few of the remedies handed down in this way were effective, the vast majority of them were actually quite worthless. Most illnesses, of course, clear up spontaneously as a result of the body's own ability to heal itself; yet, as often happens even today during poorly controlled clinical trials, medicines that happened to be administered simultaneously were credited with the cure. Uncritical acceptance of such seeming successes led to the retention of countless worthless substances in the medicinal compendia. Even though a few enlightened skeptics tried to rid the pharmacopeias of the relics and rubbish that had accumulated over the centuries, Dr. Oliver Wendell Holmes could still say, as late as 1860, that "if the whole materia medica . . . were sunk to the bottom of the sea, it would be all the better for mankind and all the worse for the fishes."

Pharmacology becomes a science
This sort of therapeutic nihilism—the view that all drug treatment is worthless—was never shared by patients, whose need for help bred a simple faith in the efficacy of medicines. In addition, some doctors trained in the basic medical sciences that began to develop during the 19th century came to feel that *rational* therapy was, indeed, possible if it could be based on knowledge of normal physiology and of the pathologic processes underlying the disease to be treated.

At about this time, chemical science began to make the first of its remarkable advances. Early in the 19th century, chemists became skilled in the extraction and isolation of the active pure principles from crude drugs of vegetable and animal origin. The isolation, in about 1805, of morphine, the active alkaloid of opium, by a young German pharmacist, Friedrich Sertürner, was followed in the next few years by the extraction of strychnine, quinine, emetine, and other potent plant principles in pure form.

The availability of these potent biologically active chemicals with constant physical properties that could be relied on stimulated the development of studies using the methods of experimental physiology. As a result, the first pharmacodynamic studies conceived and carried out in the *quantitative* manner characteristic of modern medical science were reported at this time. Thus, the French physiologist and pioneer pharmacologist François Magendie, in his work with strychnine, was able to determine exactly how much drug was needed to cause a particular effect in most of his experimental animals. Today, the first thing the pharmacologist tries to do in studying a biologically active chemical is to establish its *dose–response relationships*—that is, exactly how much of the pure drug it takes to bring about its various effects.

Further advances in pharmacology were related to the rise of organic synthetic chemistry. One of the first drugs to be produced synthetically was the anesthetic ether. Later, in the 19th century, the search for quinine substitutes led to the synthesis of the salicylates; and a chemist trying to find a safer form of these drugs discovered that he could improve the original molecule by treating it with acetic acid to get aspirin.

This procedure—preparing whole families of drugs related in chemical structure to a natural or synthetic chemical known to possess biological activity—opened up a new field of pharmacologic study called *biochemorphology,* the study of the relationships between chemical structure and biological activity. Such *structure–activity relationships* studies have resulted in the development of many classes of modern drugs, as will be seen in the following section.

Other areas of biology and chemistry are also making important technical contributions today to the study of what happens to drugs while in the body. Isotopically labeled drugs can be followed as they are absorbed, distributed, biotransformed, and excreted. Chromatographic, spectrophotometric, and, most recently, radioimmunoassay techniques are being applied to determine the presence of drugs in microgram and nanogram amounts in blood plasma and in other body fluids.* The level of the drug can then be correlated with the patient's clinical responses to help maintain the therapeutically desired effect and to avoid overdosage and toxicity.

Most recently, pharmacologists have employed the methods of enzyme chemistry and molecular biology to learn *where* a drug is acting and exactly *how* its molecules interact with the macromolecules of living cells. The study of the exact mechanisms by which drugs act to affect the

functioning of body cells and systems is still in its infancy. However, it is hoped that this still largely theoretic area of study will lead some day to the development of drugs that will selectively kill viruses and cancer cells without harming normal human cells at all. Intimate knowledge of the cellular actions of drugs is useful even now for increasing our understanding of fundamental life processes.

Development and evaluation of drugs

The preceding section described in a general way how pharmacologists work to establish the pharmacodynamic properties of drugs. Once a substance has been shown to be biologically active, pharmacologists perform studies mainly of four types:

1. Determination of the *dose–response relationships* of the drug—that is, *how much* of the agent it takes to produce various effects
2. Investigation of its *structure–activity relationships* (SAR)—that is, the extent to which the drug's actions resemble and differ from those of compounds of closely related chemical structure
3. Determination of the drug's *metabolic fate* in the body—that is, how the body handles the foreign chemical from the time it enters the body and is absorbed into the system, until it, or the metabolites into which it has been transformed, are excreted
4. Investigation of the drug's *site and mechanism of action*—that is, just *where* in the body the drug acts to exert its various effects and just *how* it affects the metabolism of the reactive cells through the interaction of its molecules with those of the responsive tissues

This section will discuss in somewhat more detail certain aspects of studies of the first two types listed above, with emphasis on the terms and concepts that are most pertinent to the clinical uses of drugs. The studies of the third and fourth types will be discussed in Chapter 4—again in terms of clinical significance.

Few people realize how many years of scientific study are required before a newly discovered chemical may be marketed for medical use. The processes by which new drugs are discovered, developed, and tested for efficacy and toxicity are long and difficult. These procedures will be discussed briefly because, by becoming aware of what is necessary to determine a drug's safety and true

---

* A microgram is one millionth of a gram, and a nanogram is one billionth of a gram.

value, the need for all the precautions required in administering drugs to patients will be better understood.

Sources of drugs

As noted earlier, both primitive witch doctors and modern physicians use certain *natural substances* in treating disease. Plant and animal parts and minerals dug from the ground are still sources of drugs today, as they were in the earliest days of pharmacotherapeutics. In addition, for only the past century or so pharmacologists have been able to draw on a fourth source of drugs—the laboratories of the organic chemists who *synthesize* substances that never before existed. Each of these sources of drugs will be examined more closely, because knowing something about where drugs originate will add to the understanding of the dosage forms of drugs—the pharmaceutical formulations that will finally be administered to the patient.

Plant constituents

Until early in the last century, physicians generally used crude botanic drugs or liquid extracts of their active constituents. Preparations of this kind—extracts, fluidextracts, and tinctures, for example—are called *galenicals* (after the Greek physician *Galen,* who practiced in Rome in the second century AD). Even though some products of this type are still available, the most common clinical use is of the purified crystalline chemicals that modern chemists have succeeded in isolating from plants.* Among the most important classes of vegetable drug constituents are the alkaloids and the glycosides.

Alkaloids are nitrogenous chemicals that can be extracted from various parts of many plants, and are usually quite active pharmacologically. Pure medicinal alkaloids can be depended on to produce a rapid, powerful action; however, the danger from overdosage is also greater from these constituents than from the galenic preparations or crude drugs that contain them. Alkaloids can be recognized by a name ending in *ine*—for example, morphine, atropine, pilocarpine, and strychnine. These are not, however, the only drugs with names that end in this suffix. The names of certain other natural and synthetic substances such as the adrenal hormone epinephrine and local anesthetics such as procaine bear this ending. Despite their potency and their relationship to plant products such as ephedrine and cocaine, though, these substances cannot be classed correctly as alkaloids.

Glycosides are active plant principles containing a sugar such as glucose in the molecule. Actually, it is the noncarbohydrate portion of the molecule, or aglycone (genin), that accounts for its pharmacologic activity. However, in the case of the digitalis glycosides (medically, the most important of the drugs of this class), the sugar portion of the molecule is very important because it permits the aglycone to penetrate into cardiac muscle cells and to exert its stimulating effect on myocardial function. The glycoside digitoxin is a thousand times more potent in this respect than the powdered digitalis leaf. Interestingly, it is now cheaper for a heart patient to be maintained on this purified crystalline glycoside than on the crude drug itself. The names of the official glycosides usually end in *in,* such as digoxin and digitoxin.

Plants also yield oils, gums, resins, and tannins, which are still used in medicine. Among the *fixed oils* are olive, cottonseed, and castor oils; the *volatile oils* include aromatic flavoring essences such as peppermint, spearmint, and clove. *Gums* are exudative plant secretions that form thick mucilaginous masses when mixed with water. Some, such as psyllium seed and agar, are used internally as laxatives; others, such as tragacanth and acacia, are often used externally in soothing lotions or as pharmaceutic suspending agents. *Resins* include substances such as the rosin found in pine tree sap. Some are pharmacologically active local irritants with minor uses in medicine as laxatives and caustics. *Tannins* are phenol derivatives found widely in the vegetable kingdom. They are used mainly in industry to tan hides; in medicine, this ability to precipitate protein has led to their employment as astringents and for forming protective coverings over burn surfaces.

Animal sources

The organs of animals—and, indeed, those of humans—were once used in medicine on a mystical basis. Today, some of the most potent drugs are obtained by extraction from animal tissues for use as substitutes for human glandular secretions that may be lacking. The hormone insulin, which is used in treating diabetes, is an active principle from animal pancreas; corticotropin (ACTH) is isolated from the pituitary glands of animals that are slaughtered for food. The thyroid glands of animals are dried, defatted, and powdered for use in replacement, or substitution, therapy of hypothyroid patients. Recently, the pituitary glands of human corpses have been employed for extracting the human growth hormone (HGH), which is more effective than animal-derived somatotropin for treatment of certain types of dwarfism.

Inorganic chemicals

Some elements such as sulfur and iodine and the salts of metals such as iron have long been used in medicine. The salts of silver and mercury are still employed as antiseptics and disinfectants. Clays such as kaolin and attapulgite are ingredients of certain products for treating

---

* *Digitalis* and *opium tinctures,* containing the active constituents of the plant dissolved in alcohol, and fluidextracts and powdered extracts of *belladonna,* containing the active constituents of that plant in concentrated but not completely pure form, are still sometimes employed by those who somehow prefer these preparations rather than the more reliable pure plant principles.

diarrhea, and aluminum hydroxide and the phosphate salt of that metal are used for counteracting excessive amounts of hydrochloric acid in the upper gastrointestinal tract. Magnesium hydroxide also is used in digestive disorders as both an antacid and a laxative, and salts of the same mineral—the sulfate and the citrate—are employed as saline cathartics. Most recently, the radioactive isotopes of inorganic substances such as gold, phosphorus, and iodine have come into use in the diagnosis and treatment of disease.

Synthetic organic chemicals

More than half a million carbon-containing chemicals that do not exist in nature at all have come from the laboratories of synthetic organic chemists, since Wohler's discovery early in the last century that scientists might make what was previously believed to be formed only by living organisms (animals and plants). Only a small fraction of all these synthetic chemicals possess medically significant biologic activity, and an even smaller proportion are both safe and effective enough to be used in the treatment of disease. Such chemicals become drugs only after they have undergone intensive study, first in animals and later in humans, to prove that they are safe and effective enough to be used in modern medical practice.

Sources of new drugs

Drugs were once found by a random search for active substances among the plants, minerals, and animals of the countryside. Today, scientists are still searching for new drugs in plant and animal tissues and in the soil. The main difference from the earlier approach lies in their use of systematic methods for uncovering specific kinds of actions caused by chemicals coming into contact with living tissues.

The biologic methods called *screening tests* are relatively simple inexpensive procedures for determining quickly whether or not substances of natural or synthetic origin have any activity of the particular kind that is being sought. Such screening procedures are sometimes applied to thousands of chemicals in programs designed to find drugs for treatment of various diseases. During World War II, for example, when the Japanese cut off the sources of quinine, scientists set up a "crash" program to find substitutes for quinine: they screened thousands of new and old chemicals and discovered a few valuable new antimalarial drugs. Later, the thousands of soil samples from all over the world that were screened for antibiotic activity produced a handful of useful antimicrobial agents, including chloramphenicol, chlortetracycline, and streptomycin. Currently, vast numbers of chemicals are being screened for antineoplastic activity.

Once the presence of a particular action has been recognized in a crude extract, the relative amount of such activity can be determined in a roughly quantitative way by procedures called *biologic assays*, because they use animals or microorganisms rather than chemical or physical tests. As increasingly pure and potent plant or animal tissue extracts are obtained, their activity is compared with that of a preparation of known strength. This so-called reference standard is used as a measure of the amount of activity present only until the hormone, antibiotic, vitamin, or plant principle becomes available in pure form and can be standardized by chemical assay.

Such screening and bioassay techniques, which were the basis for the early discovery of some potent drugs of natural origin, are again being applied to crude drugs used by the inhabitants of various lands. Among the alkaloids extracted from anciently employed plants and made available in pure form relatively recently are reserpine, the tranquilizing and blood pressure-reducing drug obtained from *Rauwolfia serpentina*, a plant used in India for thousands of years; vinblastine, an antileukemic chemical extracted from a species of the decorative flowering periwinkle plant; and *d*-tubocurarine, the pure active principle of a crude curare extract ("tube curare") that South American Indians have used as arrow poisons since prehistoric times.

The same methods have been used as a guide to the extraction and purification of vitamins from foods and hormones from animal glands. However, these substances are sometimes present in quantities so minute that scientists must seek other sources to lower the cost. This was the case with cortisone, an adrenocortical hormone present in amounts so small that it was impossible to extract enough to determine what uses it might have in human patients. Therefore, once its chemical structure was determined, efforts were made to synthesize this steroid hormone. Finally, by starting with simpler steroids and laboriously building the complicated cortisone molecule from them, enough was prepared to permit clinical testing in patients with severe arthritis.

Recent advances in recombinant DNA biology have led to another source of organic compounds. By reordering genetic information, scientists have been able to develop bacteria that produce an insulin useful for human therapy. Although its production is still costly, the potential benefits of such a process have far-reaching implications.

Structure—activity relationship studies

The discovery of the remarkable anti-arthritic power of cortisone and the recognition of its useful anti-inflammatory activity in many other illnesses set off a search for even better corticosteroid compounds. The procedures employed in the discovery of the newer synthetic corticosteroids serve as an example of another experimental approach to the development of new drugs. This involves attempts to modify the chemical structure of a compound of known activity in ways that produce a closely related chemical with improved properties.

It may seem strange that chemists should be able to make chemicals that never existed before and yet are capable of acting more powerfully than hormones and other body chemicals produced during millions of years of evolution. However, this proved to be true with various synthetic corticosteroids, such as prednisolone, triamcinolone, and betamethasone. These substances are as effective as the natural adrenocortical hormones cortisone and hydrocortisone, even when administered in much smaller doses. The synthetically tailored molecules are also free of certain undesirable actions of the natural hormone molecules.

Many other classes of drugs have come into being as a result of attempts to produce new compounds that would be better in some respect than a *prototype*—a chemical of a particular configuration that produces a therapeutically desirable effect. The very many "chemical cousins" built by making slight changes in the molecular structure of the prototype are called its *congeners* or *analogues.* Among the classes of drugs derived in this way are the local anesthetics, the antihistaminics, the anticholinergics, and, more recently, the phenothiazine-type tranquilizers and the benzothiazide-type diuretics.

Starting with a "lead" compound of known activity, the organic chemist can often produce dozens or even hundreds of derivatives by tinkering with the structure of the basic molecule in various ways. These are then screened for activity by pharmacologists in the hope that some relatively small change in chemical structure will have resulted in the synthesis of a new compound that is an improvement over those that were previously available.

Sometimes, a small change in structure—the addition of a chlorine atom at a particular point in the molecule, for example—may give the new congener significant advantages over the parent compound. For example, the new drug may be effective when taken by mouth, whereas the prototype may have had to be given by painful injections (the synthetic progestins have this advantage over the natural female hormone progesterone).

Sometimes, a new analogue may bring about the clinically desired effect when administered in much smaller doses than the prototype drug—perhaps because the new molecule fits more specifically into sites in the reactive cells. Altering the architecture of a prototype molecule to obtain compounds of increased potency is not, in itself, necessarily desirable, and the fact that the new drug can be administered in a smaller dose does not in itself make it superior to the parent compound. Thus, it is doubtful that the prototype benzothiazide diuretic chlorothiazide is less useful than various newer congener compounds, even though its milligram dosage may be about a hundred times larger than that of the more potent

"improved" compounds produced by the molecule-manipulating chemists. This is because the *ratios* between the amounts of all these drugs required to produce *the desired effect* (*i.e.,* removal of excess sodium from the body by way of the kidneys) and the amounts that cause an *undesired effect* (*i.e.,* loss of excessive quantities of potassium) are essentially similar in all these chemically related substances.

Sometimes, however, a slight change made in the molecule of a prototype drug does more than merely lower the dose needed to produce the desired action. It may, for example, lead to a reduction in some undesired or toxic effect. This occurs when the tailoring of the molecule allows it somehow to seek out the target cells for therapeutic activity while avoiding other tissues. Such *selectivity* or *specificity* of action is one of the properties most sought in modifying the molecular structure of natural and synthetic prototype drugs. Yet, there are few clear-cut rules for rationally predicting which modifications will produce new compounds of greater selectivity. Thus, the search for better drugs by these methods is still mainly a matter of trial and error.

Preclinical pharmacologic evaluation

Only a tiny minority of chemicals that display biologic activity in a screening program are ever marketed as drugs (Fig. 1-1). According to one survey, fewer than 2,000 of over 100,000 compounds screened by the pharmaceutical industry in 1 year were cleared for trial in human patients. Fewer than 50 of these chemicals eventually became medicines. Most of the active compounds that failed to become drugs were discarded because the doses required to produce a therapeutically desirable effect were too close to those that produced toxicity in preliminary laboratory tests in animals.

Once screening has revealed that a chemical is capable of producing a particular effect, it is often subjected to a battery of other tests in animals to determine its entire *spectrum of activity. No drug has only a single action;* it is essential to learn, at an early stage, *all* of a drug's varied actions and how much of the drug is required to produce each of its different effects. For example, a drug discovered in a search for antihistaminic activity may also have anticholinergic–antispasmodic effects on smooth muscle; it may possess a local anesthetic action that blocks nerve impulse conduction in peripheral nerves; and, often, it may cause drowsiness by depressing the central nervous system.

A drug that produces its desirable primary action only at dose levels very close to those that cause various secondary effects (side-effects) of a type likely to cause discomfort would probably be judged not likely to prove clinically useful. Thus, a drug may be able to protect laboratory animals from the ill effects of inhaled histamine but, if it did so only at dose levels that made the animals drowsy, it would probably be discarded, because it would

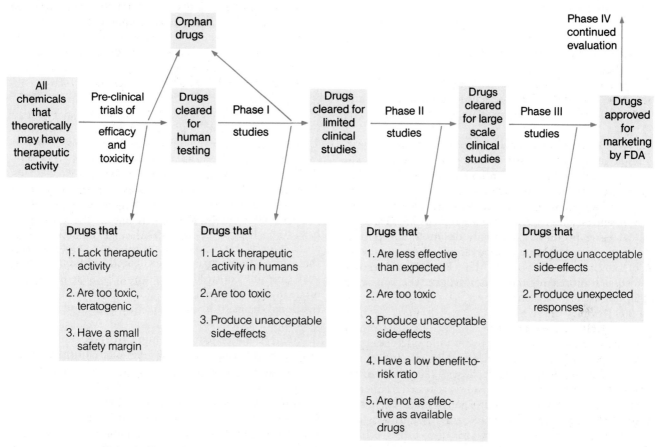

Figure 1-1. Phases of drug development.

be less useful than some of the already available antihista-minic drugs that are relatively free of this adverse side-effect.

On the other hand, if the new drug's *pharmacologic profile* appears interesting and its *dose–response relationships* seem favorable in comparison to certain standard drugs already in clinical use, it may be put through several series of *toxicity tests*. These tests, which are designed to predict whether the drug can be safely administered to human subjects, are carried out in groups of small animals such as mice, rats, and rabbits.

Groups of animals are used to reduce the chance of error resulting from differences in the way individual animals respond to drugs. This is necessary because no two animals (or people) react to drugs in the same way. Even when the animals are litter mates of the same sex and weight, they may differ from one another physiologically and biochemically in ways that are not readily apparent. Such biochemical or physiologic individuality may profoundly influence the ways in which the bodies of related animals handle a drug or the ways in which their tissues respond to the same dose of the drug. Thus, drugs are tested in *groups* of animals to minimize mistakes

in evaluation of a drug that stem from *individual variations* among animals of the same species.

Consideration of these facts leads to an understanding of why tests in animals (and ultimately in humans) are necessary to learn the therapeutic benefits and toxic effects caused by a potential new drug. Animal testing is costly and time-consuming for the pharmaceutical companies that discover and develop most new drugs. The profit motive and humane considerations for experimental animals are strong arguments for using the minimum number of animals needed to obtain information about the therapeutic and toxic effects of a potential new drug before humans are exposed to it. Computer models have been suggested as replacements for animal tests to eliminate the sickness and pain sometimes produced in the animals used in these tests. Unfortunately, computer models are only as good as the data included in the computer program, and knowledge of the relevant variables to be included in such a program is far too limited to be useful. Even with extensive animal testing, an occasional drug is approved for use in humans that proves to have disastrous consequences (for example, thalidomide; see below).

Acute toxicity tests

Several species of animals receive a range of doses of the test drug and are observed for pharmacologic effects and for symptoms of toxicity. The data obtained by the laboratory pharmacologist in such tests serve as a guide to the clinical pharmacologist who wants to know what the drug is likely to do in human patients. The ratio between the dose of a drug that produces a desirable effect and that causing toxic effects is an estimate of the drug's *safety margin.**

The test drug's *relative safety* in comparison to already available standard drugs—that is, its *therapeutic index*—is a factor used in considering whether it should be discarded or studied further. Most chemicals that are found to have a particular effect in pharmacodynamic screening tests fail to pass the acute toxicity studies. That is, the drug produces potentially desirable effects only when given in doses that are too close to those that cause acute toxic reactions, or the test chemical proves less effective or more toxic than other drugs of the same class that are already marketed.

Chronic toxicity tests

If a drug seems to have a relatively wide safety margin, long-term studies are initiated, in which several species of animals receive large daily doses. The animals are closely observed for long periods and are tested frequently to determine the state of vital organ systems, including the liver, kidneys, blood, and bone marrow. Adverse laboratory reports in such chronic toxicity studies usually prevent a drug from going on to further trials in humans unless it seems potentially useful for treating a previously incurable disease.

Information is also obtained by gross and microscopic pathologic studies of the tissues of dead animals. The drug's effects on the fertility of female animals and on the fetuses of pregnant females are also carefully observed. At the same time, studies of the drug's metabolism are conducted to determine how rapidly and completely it is absorbed by various routes of administration, and how it is distributed in the body and finally broken down and excreted. (Such studies furnish information concerning how frequently the drug should be administered and by which routes it should be given to obtain the most rapid or long-lasting effects.)

If the results of all these preclinical trials indicate that the compound is reasonably safe, potentially useful in the treatment of one or more clinical conditions, and possibly superior to presently available drugs, it may be cleared for clinical trial in humans. The physicians who are to act as clinical investigators are then supplied with a brochure containing detailed data of all aspects of the preclinical studies, as a guide for planning their clinical trials.

Clinical evaluation of drugs

Drugs are tested in humans only after the preclinical toxicity tests in animals have shown them to be reasonably safe. Yet, the occurrence of unforeseen toxicity in humans always exists, as was demonstrated by the thalidomide disaster of 1962. Hundreds of pregnant women who took this seemingly harmless sedative drug gave birth to dreadfully deformed babies. This tragedy, which occurred largely outside of the United States, served to spur passage of new legislation regulating investigational drugs—the Kefauver–Harris amendments to the Federal Food, Drug and Cosmetic Act, which became effective in 1963. Under these regulations, drugs are evaluated in humans under very carefully controlled conditions. Because nurses are often involved in caring for patients who receive investigational drugs, it is important to understand the basic philosophic principles underlying the evaluation of so-called investigational drugs in humans. Some of the terms, concepts, and premises employed in such clinical research will be reviewed.

Evaluations of the effects of drugs on humans are generally conducted in three stages, which differ mainly in the number of patients and physicians involved and in the type of data collected. The purposes of all three phases of clinical investigation are essentially the same: first, to prove that the drug is reasonably *safe* for most patients under conditions of clinical use; and second, to demonstrate that the drug is in fact *useful* in one way or another in treating patients suffering from an actual illness. The Food and Drug Administration (FDA) now demands proof of *efficacy* as well as safety before a new drug may be marketed.

A *phase I* or *pilot study*, which is conducted in a limited number of people, usually by a single very well-qualified clinical investigator, is intended to determine the human dosage range of the drug based on how well it is tolerated by humans. These tests are designed to eliminate errors that may have gone undetected in the tests carried out in animals.

Species variation in response to drugs is a common occurrence. It is often the result of differences in the way animals of other species may metabolize a drug. Thus, for example, a drug that may have caused no ill effects in animals of a particular species may still prove toxic to humans because the livers of the animals contained enzymes (lacking in the human liver) that could rapidly destroy the drug before it reached toxic levels in the tissues.

Occasionally the reverse is true, and a drug that may have caused a dangerous reaction in only a single

---

* This ratio is expressed as a number that is derived from the dose that produces a specific toxic effect (TD) or lethal effect (LD) in half (50%) of the laboratory animals tested compared with the dose that is effective (ED) in producing a potentially useful or desired effect. Thus, the therapeutic index, or TI, equals the TD_{50}/ED_{50} or the LD_{50}/ED_{50}.

animal species may prove harmless to the human volunteers who agree to take it. The most recent example of this occurred during the testing of probucol (Lorelco), a drug introduced in 1977 for reducing elevated serum cholesterol levels in patients with primary hypercholesterolemia. Beagle dogs that were being treated with probucol during a 2-year chronic toxicity study suffered fatal cardiac arrhythmias when they were subjected to certain tests. However, because this toxic effect did not occur in four other animal species, it was administered cautiously to humans and turned out to be entirely safe. Apparently, probucol is uniquely toxic to the canine species, and the target organ for the drug's toxicity is the dog's heart.

In addition, species differences may have obscured the presence of a *desirable* action. This is caused, in part, by the difficulty of duplicating human disease states in laboratory animals. It is, for example, especially difficult to tell from animal studies how a drug is likely to affect the mental state of humans. Thus, the phenothiazine-type tranquilizers were not shown to affect psychotic symptoms favorably until they were actually tried in mental patients rather than in experimental animals.

Safety in human studies

Most investigational drugs are first tried out in healthy human volunteers to select a safe starting dose. Sometimes a physician begins by giving the drug to sick patients in a dose much smaller than that which had caused toxic effects in animals. The dose is raised gradually in first one subject and then in others, until either a toxic effect or a therapeutic response is seen.

In almost all such cases, the patient knows that he is participating in an experiment and has given his consent to the procedure. The clinical investigator usually gives the subject a full explanation of the purpose of the experiment and makes it clear to him that there is an element of uncertainty involved concerning the drug's potential usefulness and toxicity; this procedure is called *informed consent,* and it is an integral requirement of human investigational studies. This ethical and moral obligation has recently been codified in guidelines for clinical investigation set by the Food and Drug Administration. However, controversy continues in regard to just how fully the experimenter must inform the patient about what drug effects may be expected, and whether this information may actually lead to the occurrence of these effects.

A *phase II* clinical drug study is an expanded version of the first cautious tests. It is conducted by several physicians who are specialists both in drug investigations and in the illness that the drug is designed to treat. These physicians watch their patients for signs of both improvement and possible toxicity. They are especially alert for signs of toxicity of the same type seen in animals during the preclinical trials, but they also sometimes spot unusual reactions that require halting of the test.

Before the drug is administered, the patients undergo a whole battery of laboratory tests. Most important are tests of liver and kidney function and the status of the blood-forming organs. Such studies are repeated at regular intervals over the months of phase II testing. If abnormalities appear, the clinical investigators have to decide whether the drug's value to the patient is worth the risk of continuing treatment.

Drugs that cause reactions involving the bone marrow and skin or affecting hepatic or renal function often have to be withdrawn. There are, however, some circumstances in which drugs may continue to be employed clinically despite the occasional development of such reactions in some patients during long-term therapy. For example, few of the drugs introduced recently for preventing epileptic seizures are free of potentially dangerous long-term effects on vital organ systems. Yet, clinical investigators have recommended their acceptance and the FDA has cleared them for marketing (and only rarely called for their withdrawal) because they feel that the risk of therapy with these drugs is worth taking in epileptic patients who may be helped by these drugs but who might otherwise become invalids or even have to be institutionalized.

Similarly, in fatal or life-threatening diseases, the investigators often decide that the benefits to be gained by continued administration of a potentially dangerous drug outweigh its hazards. This decision involves an assessment of what is called the *benefit-to-risk ratio* of the drug. Most compounds used in cancer chemotherapy, for instance, have very narrow safety margins, but they are cleared for use in leukemia and in other neoplastic diseases despite clinical tests that reveal the risk of bone marrow damage and hematopoietic and gastrointestinal tract toxicity.

On the other hand, drugs that are intended for use in relatively minor ailments are withdrawn if this phase of clinical testing reveals evidence of toxicity. This is especially true when safe and effective drugs of the same class are already available. Thus, if an analgesic–antipyretic being tested showed even the smallest incidence of blood dyscrasias, it would very likely be promptly discarded because the risk of causing dangerous depression of bone marrow function in even one patient would not be warranted by the drug's ability to relieve a headache or reduce a fever. This is especially true when a comparatively safe drug such as aspirin is available for the same purposes. (That is why aminopyrine is prescribed infrequently in this country.)

Phase III clinical testing is carried out only after enough pharmacokinetic and toxicity data have been obtained to determine safe dosage and safe frequency of administration schedules. The clinical investigators are supplied with a brochure containing information about all known reactions to the drug and the precautions required for its safe use in the controlled therapeutic trials that they intend to perform. The investigative drug is then made available to dozens or scores of practicing physicians who use it in treating hundreds or even thousands of patients suffering from the various clinical conditions for which it is thought the drug may be indicated.

During this phase of the study, the patient must be evaluated carefully for side-effects. If the patient's safety or comfort seems to be compromised, the drug may have to be withdrawn and the experiment brought to an abrupt end.

The patient should be encouraged to report any signs or symptoms that occur. Any discomfort might represent a toxic effect of the drug, and should be evaluated. The physician can determine whether the patient's complaints are caused by the test drug or by the disease. If the symptoms are, indeed, drug-induced, the physician may order the drug discontinued; if, on the other hand, the symptoms are part of the patient's illness, this will need to be explained to the patient. The clinical investigator, in reporting the patient's reactions, will not attribute these reactions unfairly to the drug that is on trial.

Toxic effects so severe as to seem prohibitive sometimes occur during therapeutic trials. Yet, if the patient's condition is a serious one and the drug produces definite improvement, its continued use may be considered warranted despite its evident dangers. Some of the most valuable existing drugs, such as digitalis, which often causes cardiotoxicity, and d-tubocurarine and succinylcholine, which commonly cause respiratory muscle paralysis, can be safely employed provided that cardiac and respiratory functions are properly monitored. Thus, potentially valuable investigative drugs are not discarded when measures are available for detecting and counteracting toxicity at an early stage.

Similarly, just as colchicine often causes diarrhea when given in the doses required for control of an acute gout attack, the clinical trials of a new drug that causes discomforting side-effects may be continued when it shows superior promise. Thus, trials of the anticancer drugs carmustine and lomustine were continued for several years despite the fact that they frequently cause nausea and vomiting, and the drugs finally received FDA approval in 1977. Of course, members of the medical team are obligated to employ all possible measures to relieve such disabling and sometimes dangerous side-effects.

Efficacy evaluation

Determining the therapeutic usefulness of a new drug in human patients is often a formidable task. Many of the difficulties that arise in attempting to evaluate a drug's efficacy stem from the very humanity of the people involved—the patient, the physician, and the nurses. Indeed, the concern of physicians and nurses with the patient's welfare is one of the main complications that sometimes prevent scientific evaluation of a drug.

In some studies, the effects of the drug can be measured objectively. Thus, the efficacy of a diuretic drug may be determined by collecting and measuring the patient's urine output and by noting the loss of body weight as edema fluid leaves his tissues. The effects of other drugs can be judged by recording changes in body temperature, blood sugar levels, or electrocardiographic readings. On the other hand, difficulties arise when the patient's *subjective response* is the sole basis for deciding if a drug has been effective for relieving pain, itching, nausea, nervousness or mental depression, or other symptoms.

In such cases, conscious and unconscious psychological forces often operate in ways that make it difficult to determine a drug's true pharmacologic activity and therapeutic value. All of us are subject to suggestion to some extent. However, some patients (known as *positive placebo reactors*) are unusually susceptible to the positive symbolic implications of receiving medications. These patients tend to report that they feel better even when they have received only a *placebo*—a "blank" or "dummy" medication. Others, called *negative placebo reactors,* may complain of adverse side-effects even when they have actually received no active drug.

One technique often used by clinical investigators for reducing unconscious bias is the *double-blind* study. This is a procedure in which neither the patient nor the physicians or nurses who check the patient's responses to medication know what the patient is actually receiving. That is, both are kept in the dark as to whether the capsule or other dosage form being administered is the drug being tested, a standard drug of known activity, or a placebo. The identity of the coded contents of each dose is known only to another member of the research team, who is often the pharmacist or another physician or nurse. This technique is intended to keep the physicians or nurses from unconsciously communicating their attitudes about the new drug to the patient, who is often very responsive to positive or negative suggestion about his therapy.

Ordinarily, in administering medications to patients, a nurse tries to take advantage of placebo responses by offering patients subtle positive suggestions, which are often as potent as the drug's own pharmacodynamic effects in helping to relieve symptoms and in making patients feel better. However, when assisting in the clinical evaluation of an *investigational* drug, it is important to make every effort to avoid influencing the patient's attitude toward the test drug. This is especially important during the final phase of broad clinical trials, when it is often not feasible to employ the double-blind method of evaluation.

A protocol is developed by the investigational team to determine what information patients receive, what signs and symptoms are monitored, and how the patients can be assured and comforted when they have doubts about their participation in the study. Such a protocol helps to ensure that patients are adequately informed, and that no member of the investigational team will be placed in a situation that might allow personal bias or feelings to influence the patient's response.

Postrelease studies

Even after a drug has been permitted to be marketed, much may still be learned about its potential toxicity and usefulness. Thus, manufacturers of drugs that have been approved for general use must continue to furnish additional information (phase IV evaluation) that accumulates during its general clinical use in the years after its release. Occasionally, toxicity has been encountered only when the drug was being used on hundreds of thousands of patients. The manufacturer and the FDA are then faced with deciding whether to withdraw the approved drug from the market, or whether the risk to a small minority of patients is warranted by the benefits gained by the majority of patients.

Often the manufacturer of a drug that has come under fire because of reports of life-threatening toxicity, such as previously undiscovered liver damage, voluntarily withdraws the drug. Occasionally, the manufacturer may contend that the drug's benefit-to-risk ratio warrants its use in at least some segment of the patient population. After holding hearings on the matter, the FDA may alter its withdrawal order—as it did, for example, in the case of tranylcypromine, an antidepressant drug that was withdrawn and then reinstated for use with certain restrictions in severely depressed and suicidal patients.

Serendipity

Alert observation of the way patients respond to new drugs has sometimes led to the discovery of new uses for such agents. The ability to recognize and exploit an accidental observation is called *serendipity,* and is a phenomenon that has led to the discovery of new and useful drugs as well as to other scientific advances.

The antidepressant action of iproniazid—the first of the powerful modern drugs for treating depression—was first recognized in patients receiving the drug as a treatment for tuberculosis. The tranquilizing effect of chlorpromazine, the first phenothiazine tranquilizer, was first noted in patients receiving the drug as an adjunct administered before and after anesthesia. The antihistaminic drug dimenhydrinate was found useful against motion sickness by allergists who were giving it to patients with hay fever. And, certain observed side-effects of the early sulfonamide anti-infective drugs—an increased urine flow and a drop in blood sugar in a few patients being treated for infections—provided the clues that resulted eventually in the development of two entirely new classes of drugs: the sulfonamide-type diuretics, such as acetazolamide and its successors, and the oral hypoglycemic drugs used against diabetes, such as tolbutamide and its sulfonylurea relatives.

Legal regulation and drug standards

Federal regulations

In the preceding discussion of how modern drugs are developed and how their safety and efficacy are evaluated, the main concern has been to convey the meanings of certain terms and concepts involved in drug development. The legislation through which the federal government is empowered to regulate and control the manner in which drugs are manufactured and marketed is another important aspect of drug development (Table 1-1).

Food and Drug Administration (FDA)

This agency of the Department of Health and Human Services is charged with the enforcement of a body of law that has gradually developed during this century in recognition of the fact that the manufacture and sale of drugs requires close regulation to protect the public's health. The legislation under which this regulatory agency operates is primarily the *Federal Food, Drug and Cosmetic Act of 1938* and its various amendments. The many detailed provisions of this law will not be discussed; however, a brief history of how such legislation developed may illustrate the need for ensuring that all drugs meet high standards of strength and safety.

The earliest federal legislation regulating the quality of medicines was the *Pure Food and Drug Act of 1906.* Its passage followed a 25-year fight to give the government some control over the then totally unrestricted sale of drugs, many of them worthless or dangerous. The law was intended primarily to prevent the marketing of adulterated drugs, and a later amendment concerning the labeling of medications was designed to eliminate false and misleading claims concerning therapeutic usefulness.

Although it corrected various flagrant abuses, the law of 1906 really did little to ensure the *safety* of drug products, and bills that were intended to do so made little headway during the next generation. It required a tragic accident in 1937 to arouse public pressure on Congress for the passage of new legislation to guarantee greater safety of prescription drug products. The Elixir of Sulfanilamide incident, which took over 100 lives, occurred when a drug manufacturer seeking a solvent for the then new anti-infective chemical, sulfanilamide, selected diethylene glycol. This substance proved to be an excellent vehicle for the drug but, because its pharmacologic effects had not been tested in animals, its toxicity was unknown until the reports of illness and death in patients taking the product began to pour in.

The *Federal Food, Drug and Cosmetic Act of 1938,* which was then passed, made it mandatory for manufacturers to perform toxicity tests in laboratory animals before seeking FDA approval to market any drug. The law provided procedures by which that agency could keep a

Table 1–1. Federal legislation affecting the clinical use of drugs

Year enacted	Law	Impact
1906	Pure Food and Drug Act	Prevented the marketing of adulterated drugs; required labeling to eliminate false or misleading claims
1938	Federal Food, Drug and Cosmetic Act of 1938	Mandated tests for drug toxicity and provided means for recall of drugs; established procedures for introducing new drugs; gave FDA the power of enforcement
1951	Durham–Humphrey Amendment	Tightened control of certain drugs; specified drugs to be labeled "may not be distributed without a prescription"
1962	Kefauver–Harris Act	Tightened control over the quality of drugs; gave FDA regulatory power over the procedure of drug investigations; stated that efficacy as well as safety of drugs had to be established
1970	Controlled Substances Act	Defined drug abuse and classified drugs as to their potential for abuse; provided strict controls over the distribution, storage, and use of these drugs
1983	Orphan Drug Act	Provided incentives for the development of orphan drugs for treatment of rare diseases

drug from being marketed, or order its recall, if its scientists decided that the drug's safety had not been adequately tested, or if they felt that the drug was too dangerous for use in the clinical situations for which it was intended.

Public alarm and revulsion resulting from the thalidomide incident mentioned previously led to legislation that made important changes in the Food, Drug and Cosmetic Act of 1938. The Drug Amendments of 1962 (the Kefauver–Harris Act) tightened control over the quality of all marketed drugs. Among other provisions, these amendments give the FDA the authority to regulate the procedures by which new drugs are investigated. They also require that drugs be proved *effective* as well as *safe* before marketing.

Investigational use of drugs in humans

Before any new drug can be tested in humans, the pharmaceutical company must submit all available information about it to the FDA. The form that must be filed—an Investigational New Drug Exemption, or IND—supplies the results of all the preclinical studies that were carried out in animals. The IND also offers an outline of the plan for conducting the phase I study of the clinical pharmacology. The manufacturer also agrees to submit periodic reports of the progress of the proposed clinical studies.

Following completion of all three phases of the extensive clinical studies on the new drug, the manufacturer must submit a New Drug Application, or NDA. Only about one compound out of ten that reach the start of phase I clinical testing is ever finally approved by the FDA. Most such drug products are discarded in the early stages of their clinical trials because they have proved too toxic for humans or relatively ineffective compared to drugs already available. Drug manufacturers compile an NDA only for the rare drug that they are convinced is at least as safe and effective as any similar drug used in treating a particular condition. This is understandable in view of the enormous cost of developing and marketing a new drug product in the 1980s—an estimated fifty million dollars for each product.

Scientists of the FDA then evaluate the evidence submitted in support of the NDA, which usually consists of many massive volumes of raw data and a lengthy summary. By law, the NDA review process must be completed within 180 days. If the new drug application is considered complete, the drug is then approved for marketing. Applications judged incomplete are returned to the manufacturer, who must then develop the data that are lacking and supply them to the FDA in a completed application.

Even after a new drug has been approved for marketing, the manufacturer is required to submit periodic reports about it to the FDA. In addition to information from continuing clinical studies that are completed in later months and years, prompt reports are required whenever unexpected adverse reactions come to the manufacturer's attention. Immediate reports must also be made of any incidents of contamination or mix-ups that occur during the course of the drug's manufacture or distribution.

An example of this was the Tylenol scare of 1982. Some capsules of this over-the-counter drug were found to contain cyanide when several people in the Chicago area died after taking the drug. All the Tylenol was recalled nationwide, and investigation revealed that the drug had been tampered with after it left the factory. This incident led to the requirement of tamper-proof packaging to prevent the occurrence of such incidents.

The FDA can suspend its approval of an NDA at any time and thus prevent its marketing. Ordinarily, such prior approval is withdrawn only after hearings have been held at which the manufacturer is given the opportunity to present further evidence indicating that the product is safe and effective. However, a provision of the Food, Drug and Cosmetic Act permits the Secretary of Health and Human Services to order a drug be taken off the market immediately if he considers it an "imminent hazard to public health."

This provision was invoked for the first time in 1977 to halt the further marketing of phenformin, a drug that had been introduced in 1959 for treating diabetes. From the time it was first approved, this drug was known to be capable of causing a potentially fatal metabolic disorder in some diabetic patients. However, it took almost two decades to accumulate enough evidence to convince the FDA's Bureau of Drugs that drug-induced deaths from lactic acidosis occurred often enough to warrant revocation of the drug's NDA.

Drug efficacy study

Among the powers granted to the FDA by the Drug Amendments of 1962 was the right to regulate the *effectiveness* (as well as the safety) not only of new drugs but also of *all* drugs marketed since passage of the act in 1938. This meant that products that had been approved between 1938 and 1962, after being tested for safety only, now had to also be evaluated for effectiveness. To carry out the task of evaluating several thousand such drug products, the FDA turned to the National Academy of Sciences–National Research Council (NAS–NRC).

The Academy recruited hundreds of scientists and divided their studies among 30 panels. Operating under guidelines developed by the NRC, these panels tried to evaluate the extent to which the claims made for more than 4,000 older formulations were justified by the weight of scientific evidence. More than 16,000 claims made for these products have been evaluated since 1967 and rated in one of six categories, ranging from "effective" to "ineffective."

Manufacturers of products rated less than effective in this Drug Efficacy Study Implementation (DESI) were required to eliminate questionable claims or to develop substantiating scientific data for them. In 1971, the FDA required that each remaining product still judged only "probably" or "possibly" effective must reveal those ratings in a prominently displayed box in the labeling.

Such a status will be only temporary until additional evidence leads to the drug's being ruled effective or to its being removed from the market. Thus, patients will finally be assured that every drug that is ordered for them is one that has been judged effective for the purpose for which it is being prescribed.

Recent laws related to drug abuse prevention

Public concern with the dangers of self-medication, drug abuse, and drug addiction has been expressed in ever-increasing demands for laws to regulate drug distribution. The Harrison Narcotic Act of 1914 was the first federal act devised to control traffic in narcotic drugs. Later, federal marihuana regulations were formulated. The Food, Drug and Cosmetic Act of 1938 was also amended in efforts to bring about better regulation, first of habit-forming hypnotic drugs (the Durham–Humphrey Amendment of 1951) and later of other so-called dangerous drugs, including stimulants (the Drug Abuse Control Amendments of 1965).

As a result of the continuing spread of drug abuse to the point of almost epidemic proportions late in the 1960s, Congress enacted the *Comprehensive Drug Abuse Prevention and Control Act of 1970*. Title II of this law, called the *Controlled Substances Act*, deals with control and enforcement aspects. In effect, it replaces more than 50 former federal laws regulating narcotics and other dangerous drugs. The old Harrison Narcotic Act of 1914 and the Drug Abuse Amendments of 1965, for example, have now been repealed and replaced by this new legislation. Unlike the Harrison Act, which took the form of a tax measure, the new federal Controlled Substances Act (CSA) is intended to control drug traffic by requiring the registration of all persons in the chain of drug production and distribution.

The responsibility for enforcing the CSA is shared by two governmental agencies: the FDA and the Drug Enforcement Agency (DEA) in the Department of Justice. Regulations issued when the act became effective in 1971 set up five schedules of controlled substances, known as schedules I, II, III, IV, and V. Drugs are listed in these categories in accordance mainly with the extent of their abuse potential and medical usefulness.

Schedule I includes drugs with a high potential for abuse, such as heroin, drugs such as LSD and other hallucinogens, and marihuana. These drugs have no currently accepted medical use in this country, and possession of them is illegal.

Schedule II lists drugs that do have medical use but are considered dangerous because their abuse may lead to severe dependence. Various narcotics (natural and synthetic opiates such as morphine and methadone) are in this category, as are such stimulants as cocaine and the amphetamines, and the commonly abused central nervous system depressants amobarbital, pentobarbital, and secobarbital. Schedule II drugs are under very strict control. No prescription can be refilled, and physicians must have a special license (DEA number) to prescribe these drugs. Physicians and institutions that administer these drugs are required to keep careful records of the use of these drugs. These drugs are routinely kept under lock and key, and are counted regularly to keep strict control over their whereabouts.

Schedule III contains drugs deemed to have less potential for abuse than those in schedules I and II. These include products that contain only limited quantities of the narcotic, codeine, and paregoric.

Schedule IV presently lists several minor tranquilizers, such as meprobamate and chlordiazepoxide, and hypnotics (*e.g.*, chloral hydrate) believed to have less abuse potential than the barbiturates listed in schedule II.

Schedule V is made up of mixtures of limited quantities of narcotic drugs in combination with various non-narcotic medicinal ingredients (*e.g.*, diphenoxylate combined with atropine sulfate) and another antidiarrheal drug, loperamide, that was introduced in 1977 after tests revealed only very slight opiate-type properties.

Inasmuch as the drugs listed within each schedule are subject to periodic relisting—for example, the amphetamines were reclassified from schedule III to schedule II in 1971—it would be pointless to offer the latest published lists here, or to attempt to cover in this text any further aspects of this comprehensive drug control law.

The nurse must be familiar with those provisions of this law that apply to professional practice. In addition, it is important to learn the local city and state regulations concerning the administration of narcotic and other drugs covered by the Controlled Substances Act. Not only do the states—and sometimes even municipalities—have legislation that differs in some respect from the federal act, but various hospitals have set up their own rules and procedures for handling and accounting for narcotics. In every case, the law that primarily applies is the strictest one.

Other regulations and agencies

Federal regulations control not only narcotics but also antibiotics, biologicals, and the advertising of drugs. All antibiotics must meet standards of purity and potency set by the FDA. However, biologicals are regulated by a division of the Public Health Service—the *Division of Biological Standards* of the *National Institutes of Health*. This agency sets the control requirements that must be met by each lot of such biologic products as vaccines, antitoxins, immune serums, immunologic diagnostic aids, and blood derivatives.

The *Federal Trade Commission* (FTC) has jurisdiction over the advertising of non-prescription drugs, among other commodities. Under the Wheeler–Lea Act of 1938 the FTC is charged with protecting the public from false advertising and from deceptive practices. The agency also formerly exerted some control over adver-

tisements directed at the medical profession, but such jurisdiction is now largely in the hands of the FDA as a result of the Kefauver–Harris Amendments of 1962. Some authorities on the subject of drug advertising feel that the interests of the general public would be better served if the promotion of products advertised for purchase without a prescription were subject to the greater power of the FDA. Many who are disturbed by radio and television advertising of drugs and the tendency to sacrifice full disclosure of factual information for less than completely honest statements feel that further controls would be desirable.

The FTC has frequently been criticized for its failure to put a stop to advertising claims for home remedies that are, at the very least, misleading. The agency has, in fact, at times conducted vigorous, although often futile, campaigns against such abuses. In one attempt to prevent a company from claiming that its cathartic promoted the flow of "golden" liver bile, the Commission fought a 15-year battle against a battery of company lawyers who always managed to find legal loopholes for nullifying the agency's "cease and desist" orders.

The recent activity of various consumer groups, spurred on by the Tylenol disaster of 1982, is having a significant impact on truthfulness in advertising. In the long run, however, it will be public education that will bring about more exacting and informative advertising standards.

Drug standards

Many of the standards that the FDA now maintains were originally set by scientists employed by the drug industry and by others outside of government. The need for standards for quality of drugs has long been recognized, and physicians, pharmacists, and others have long made up compendia of the most useful drugs and formulations, which were intended to ensure uniformity and purity of these products. The very first federal regulation passed in 1906 recognized two of these compendia—the *United States Pharmacopeia* (the *USP*) and the *National Formulary* (the *NF*)—as official standards (the term "official," indicating the pharmacopeial status of a drug, means that the standards set for that drug have the force of federal law).

The *USP* was first published in 1820 as a guide for apothecaries, who then sometimes still collected the plants from which vegetable medicinal products were prepared, and for physicians, who at that time often did their own compounding. Later, as pharmacists came to rely on chemical and pharmaceutical manufacturers to supply the new synthetic drugs and purified plant principles, the scientists employed by these companies developed the analytic tests and biologic assays that served as the basic objective standards of drug quality.

Today, representatives from medical and pharmacy schools and state associations, and from various professional and scientific groups, including the American Medical Association, the American Pharmaceutical Association, and the American Chemical Society, serve on a Committee of Revision of the *USP*, which works to develop and publish specifications for modern potent drugs.

Under the supervision of this Committee, the *USP* is now revised and published at 5-year intervals. The present pharmacopeia is the 20th revision. *USP XX*, like earlier editions, contains monographs dealing with drugs chosen because of their demonstrated usefulness in the diagnosis and treatment of disease or because they are considered so-called pharmaceutic necessities (substances that aid in the manufacture of the therapeutically valuable medications).

The *USP* is the most authoritative source of information in regard to safe dosage ranges for the important drugs discussed in its pages. Most of the dosage details listed in the tables of this book comes from the *USP* and from the other official compendium, the *National Formulary* (*NF*). The *NF,* now in its 15th edition, merged with the *USP* in 1980; the two books are published in one volume. The *NF* includes information on drugs compounded from several ingredients, as well as drugs that had been dropped from the *USP*.

Nomenclature of drugs

The Drug Amendments of 1962 made it mandatory that the monographs of the *USP* and the *NF* provide only one *official name* for each drug. This attempt to reduce the proliferation of confusing names that all too often have been applied to a particular drug in the past is a step in the right direction, because the same drug often has a chemical name, a code name while in an investigational status, and various synonyms or "trivial" common names and proprietary or trade names.

The FDA has now been given the authority to designate a single, simple official name for any drug that does not have one; however, it has, in practice, permitted this task to be taken over in almost every case by a special committee on nomenclature, called the *USAN Council* (USAN stands for United States Adopted Name). This group, which is made up of representatives from the *USP* Convention, the American Pharmaceutical Association, and the American Medical Association, selects suitable *nonproprietary (generic) names* for new drugs. These will later be adopted automatically as the *USP* or *NF* titles of any compound that becomes officially recognized.

The use of the generic name is desirable for teaching purposes because it aids communication and reduces confusion. Thus, this name is used to designate the drugs discussed in this book wherever possible. However, respect for the realities of the present state of affairs makes it necessary to refer in many cases to the *proprietary* or *trade* name of certain drugs. Thus, when a drug is far

better known by its manufacturer's trademark designation than by its *non*proprietary, official, generic, or USAN name, that name will, of necessity, be used. (The manufacturer's name is always capitalized, whereas generic names begin with a lower case letter.)

Sometimes, an older name that has been discarded in favor of a newly coined official designation refuses to die; in this case, the older name will be listed parenthetically as a synonym. However, in the labeling of prescription drug packages, only the established generic name may appear in addition to the manufacturer's *trademark,* or *brand name,* and the drug's chemical designation.

Orphan drugs

There are certain drugs that have been discovered and that could be used to treat a wide variety of diseases, but that are not available for use by the patients who could benefit from them. These drugs are referred to as *orphans* because, although they have been discovered, no one has *adopted* them for development through the many and costly stages of clinical trials.

The reasons for the lack of development of these drugs are as varied as the drugs themselves. Some are naturally occurring compounds, which cannot be protected by patent laws; several are useful for treating relatively rare diseases, making their future market very limited; others have a potentially high risk, making insurance costs very high. Overall, the problem is a financial one. The cost of developing a new drug is extremely high, as discussed earlier, and a pharmaceutical company or private foundation needs to be assured of an adequate return on its investment. For the thousands of patients suffering from diseases that could be effectively treated by known orphan drugs, but who cannot get these drugs, the situation is intolerable.

In 1983, the Orphan Drug Act was signed into law. This law provides for substantial tax credits as incentives to those who develop these orphan drugs. Such credits amount to a return of 73 cents on each dollar spent toward the cost of developing an orphan drug. Small drug companies can receive 12 million dollars in grants over a 3-year period for research and development of such drugs. Although this legislation represents a very positive step, the drugs that will actually be developed as a result of the passage of this law remains a matter of speculation.

Over-the-counter drugs

Another group of drugs, called *over-the-counter* (OTC) drugs, is available to the American public for the self-medication of various symptoms. These drugs have been deemed safe enough for use without a prescription from a health-care provider. The FDA maintains control over the safety, efficacy, and advertising of these drugs. There are so many OTC drugs that have been used for so long that full review of all the drugs available is still an ongoing process.

OTC drugs allow the public to treat cold symptoms, aches and pains, gastrointestinal upsets, constipation, overweight, and sleep disorders, as well as other complaints, without professional help. The public can also purchase vitamins, minerals, and an assortment of nutritional supplements for supposed deficiencies. Advertising campaigns in the mass media have resulted in an unbelievably high intake of OTC drugs by the American public. Many believe that there is "a pill for everything," and will attempt to find medication for treating every minor complaint.

For the most part, OTC drugs are quite safe when used as directed. Most are low-dose medications, which may exert more of a placebo effect than a true therapeutic effect. One danger of the availability of so many OTC drugs is that people tend to self-diagnose and self-medicate, delaying appropriate medical supervision. In some situations the delay could be serious, as in the case of treating a rectal cancer as self-diagnosed hemorrhoids and not receiving medical intervention in time. Similarly, the use of OTC drugs could mask important signs and symptoms that might be useful or even essential in making an accurate medical diagnosis.

Another danger of OTC drugs in clinical practice is the misuse of these compounds. Patients often don't regard these drugs as medications, and frequently fail to report their use to health-care professionals who are taking a drug history. Because of this, potential drug–drug interactions with prescription drugs or drug–disease interactions with specific clinical conditions could be overlooked or misdiagnosed, leading to potentially dangerous situations for the patient. People are also not as careful in the use of OTC drugs as they are with prescription medications. Dosage recommendations are often exceeded, leading to the accumulation of toxic levels of the drug. Because many OTC preparations contain varying combinations of the same drugs, those who take several preparations for different complaints may develop toxic levels of the drugs with no awareness of the possible problem.

An essential aspect of all patient education is the inclusion of information about OTC drugs to avoid and drugs that may be safely substituted. Patient recognition of the benefits and dangers of OTC drugs is necessary to ensure the safe and effective use of these medications. Throughout this book, therefore, patient teaching guides will include pertinent teaching points about OTC drugs and their potential interactions with each class of drug discussed.

Introduction to the study of pharmacology

Approaches to learning

Pharmacology is, admittedly, not an easy subject to learn. It requires attending to a great deal of very detailed information. The number of potent new drugs introduced into clinical practice continues to be greater than the number of older drugs being discarded. Thus, the subject seems to grow ever greater in scope and complexity, so some suggestions regarding how best to study pharmacology may be helpful.

By approaching the study of drugs with the feeling that it is an exciting and rewarding aspect of the world of patient care, it is possible to master the principles of pharmacology that the nurse should know and be able to apply in patient care. Clinical practice affords ample opportunities to see all the theoretic concepts of pharmacology at work, and using drugs in patient care is one of the best ways of learning about clinical pharmacology.

The study of a drug such as digitalis becomes more meaningful by seeing how its cardiac actions make the difference between a dyspneic, edematous exhausted woman and one who can return home able to care for her family once more. The factual details concerning the pharmacology of morphine also become easier to retain by observing how this drug assuages the agony of a severely injured accident victim in a seemingly miraculous fashion. The term "miracle drug" is often reserved for certain recently discovered agents that open up ways of controlling conditions not previously treatable, but some of the tried and true drugs handed down through the generations are often just as dramatic in their effects.

Despite the intrinsic interest of observing how the actions of drugs help to improve the condition of sick patients, it would be wrong to imply that the task of learning the details of drug action is ever an easy one. Some aspects of any discipline are tedious, and learning the details calls for concentration and perseverance. Thus, it is important to employ a systematic approach.

One way of systematizing the study of pharmacology is to concentrate first on the most important and well-established drugs in each class. For example, by learning the main facts about the *prototype* agents digitalis, morphine, atropine, and epinephrine, it becomes easier to understand most of the other drugs that are classed as cardiovascular drugs, analgesics, and autonomic nervous system mimetics and blockers. It is relatively easy to learn the main facts about new drugs if the basic pharmacology of the older agents is understood.

If each new drug encountered is thought of in terms of its significant *similarities to* and *differences from* the *prototypes* of each major drug category, mastery of this important but difficult subject will begin. If, instead, every agent encountered is viewed as an isolated entity, the mass of unrelated details will be overwhelming and frustrating.

When learning about the prototype drugs in each major class, a good way to begin is to learn each drug's *primary* and *secondary pharmacologic actions.* By knowing what a drug does to alter normal physiologic function, it is often easy to guess how it may have a favorable effect on a pathologically functioning organ. Thus, it becomes easier to remember rationally that the drug is indicated in the treatment of a particular clinical disorder.

Similarly, knowledge of some of the secondary actions of a drug helps in understanding why side-effects of certain types are likely to occur, even when ordinary doses are administered. In addition, this type of information provides an awareness of the factors that are most likely to cause a patient to react poorly to the drug— that is, those conditions in which the use of a given drug may be *contraindicated* or require special precautions. Knowledge of a drug's actions also helps in predicting the likely signs and symptoms of a toxic reaction to massive overdosage and the antidotal drugs and other measures that may be necessary.

No one can ever memorize all the factual data about all the drugs encountered in practice. Understanding the concepts and principles involved for each class of drug will lay the foundation for providing effective drug therapy in a particular situation. Numerous resources are available for checking all the details when administering drugs to patients.

Look it up when in doubt is an essential rule for any nurse, no matter how experienced in drug therapy. It is essential to have up-to-date reference materials available on the unit and to seek the assistance of other members of the health-care team when any doubts arise about any particular drug. There is no substitute for having the necessary reference books available concerning the drugs used in clinical practice.

Sources of further information

Many different types of books and journals are available to provide information on dosages and on therapeutic and side-effects of drugs. Those discussed briefly below should prove useful for meeting varied needs for facts about drugs and their proper use in therapeutics.

Package inserts

The essential data on any drug product can be found in the insert that accompanies every packaged unit. These inserts contain material on all clinically significant aspects of a drug's desirable and adverse effects, including information on its dosage and methods of administration. Because the contents of these brochures have been approved by the FDA, some of the statements in them reflect excessive bureaucratic caution rather than the realities of clinical situations.

Reference books

The *Physicians' Desk Reference* (*PDR;* Medical Economics Company) is an annually published compendium that car-ries information on about 2500 drug products. Many of the product descriptions are actually identical with the package insert, and therefore follow the language of the FDA-approved labeling word for word. Comprehensive discussions of some other products that have been prepared by the manufacturer's medical department or by its medical director or consultants are also included. *PDR* is conveniently arranged and cross-indexed for quick reference on individual products, and supplements are supplied during the year. However, *PDR* offers no discussions on the various general classes of drugs, as do the following three compendia.

AMA Drug Evaluations is now in its fourth edition (1980; American Medical Association). The first edition of this publication, which appeared in 1971, replaced *New Drugs,* a less comprehensive book published previously by the former Council on Drugs. The present Department of Drugs in cooperation with the American Society for Clinical Pharmacology and Therapeutics continues the effort to furnish authoritative and unbiased information on drugs to those in medical, nursing, and pharmacy practice. This newer book contains not only detailed evaluative monographs on over 1300 individual drugs and compounds, but also discussions of groups of related drugs and a section of general information. It offers several separate indexes to help make specific information more readily accessible.

The *American Hospital Formulary Service* is comprised of a two-volume book and four to six supplements that are added during each year, available by subscription from the American Society of Hospital Pharmacists. The service offers both individual drug monographs on single generic drugs and more comprehensive general statements on groups of drugs with similar actions and uses. The drug descriptions are presented in sections organized on the basis of pharmacologic and therapeutic properties, and the drugs are indexed by trade name, generic name, and therapeutic class. Insertion of each supplement into the ring-bound set permits easy updating with new important information.

Drug Facts and Comparisons (JB Lippincott; annual) is a reference book that provides a broad range of drug information. It is organized by drug class, making comparisons of drug products relatively easy. Patient education points are included with each class of drugs.

Journals

As indicated, some of the sources listed above furnish periodic supplements that help keep drug information up to date. However, to stay abreast of the latest developments in drug therapy it is necessary to read various current journals. The *American Journal of Nursing* (*AJN*) carries information on new drugs and on the use of older agents in almost every issue. Recently, the *AJN* began to include a monthly newsletter, *Nurses' Drug Alert* (Powers, New York), as part of its journal format. This newsletter contains current information about new drugs, drug reactions, and clinical situations. *Nurses' Drug Alert* is also available by itself in monthly issues. *RN* magazine contains a monthly feature on drugs and drug therapy. The biweekly *Medical Letter* provides unbiased evaluations of the effectiveness and potential toxicity of drugs that are currently important in terms of the extent to which they are being prescribed and promoted.

Textbooks

Goodman and Gilman's The Pharmacological Basis of Therapeutics (6th edition, 1980; Macmillan) is the classic textbook for studying pharmacology. The book contains an in-depth review of the pharmacokinetics and pharmacodynamics of drugs, so it is a quite complete and scientific reference.

Meyler's Side Effects of Drugs Annual (Excerpta Medica) is an annual review of all reported adverse drug reactions and interactions. It is a helpful reference for indicating the actual frequency of drug side-effects.

Medical Pharmacology: Principles and Concepts (11th edition, 1984; CV Mosby) by Andres Goth reinforces much of the material in *Goodman and Gilman's* text at a more basic level.

Clinical Pharmacology, Basic Principles in Therapeutics (2nd edition, 1978; Macmillan), by Melmon and Morrelli, is a more detailed presentation of pharmacology with clinical emphasis.

Conclusion

The following chapters of this section should give the discerning reader some insight into the wide scope of modern pharmacology. Many of the generalizations and specific examples deal with aspects of the subject that are of the most immediate practical importance to clinical practice—that is, what drugs do when they are administered to sick people to bring about therapeutic benefits.

However, it is important to understand the actions of drugs in situations other than those involving the treatment of disease. As indicated in Chapter 4, drugs are of value to biologists who often use drug molecules as tools for determining the nature of still unknown biochemical and physiologic processes.

The social significance of drugs and other biologically active chemicals should also be obvious from the general discussions concerning such subjects as drug toxicity (Chap. 5). An understanding of the effects that toxic chemicals released into our environment may have on the health of all people is of extreme significance to vast segments of the population other than patients who are being treated with prescribed medications. Pharmacology is a growing, changing, and exciting science, with wide implications not only for clinical practice but also for daily life.

References

Blackwell B: For the first time in man. Clin Pharmacol Ther 13:812, 1971

Brahams D: Clinical trials and the consent of the patient. Practitioner 226:1889, 1982

Burger A: Approaches to drug discovery. N Engl J Med 270:1098, 1964

DiPalma JR: DESI ratings, a revolution in the making. RN 36:51, 1973

Dowling HF: What's in a name? JAMA 173:1580, 1960

Gilgore SG: Clinical pharmacology. Researching a new drug in man. Drug Cosmet Ind May, 1969

Greiner T: Subjective bias of the clinical pharmacologist. JAMA 181:92, 1962

Hayes AH: Food and drug regulation after 75 years. JAMA 246:1223, 1981

Irwin S: Drug screening and evaluative procedures. Science 136:123, 1962

Jerome JB: Current status of nonproprietary nomenclature for drugs. JAMA 185:256, 1963

Karch FE (ed): Orphan Drugs. New York, Marcel Dekker 1982

Kennedy D: A calm look at "drug lag." JAMA 239:423, 1978

Kirwan JR: Clinical trials: Why not do them properly? Ann Rheum Dis 41:551, 1982

Kohlstaedt KG: Introduction to clinical investigation. JAMA 187:344, 1964

Leake CD: The scientific study of pharmacology. Science 134:2069, 1961

Mazzullo J: The nonpharmacological basis of therapeutics. Clinic Pharmacol Ther 13:157, 1972

Miller LC: Doctors, drugs, and names. JAMA 177:14, 1961

Modell W: Safety in new drugs. JAMA 190:141, 1964

Peck HM: Adequacy of the preclinical safety evaluation. JAMA 187:341, 1964

Starr I: The testing of new drugs and other therapeutic agents. JAMA 177:14, 1961

Temple RJ et al: Adverse effects of newly marketed drugs. N Engl J Med 300:1046, 1979

Zubrod CG: Clinical trials in cancer patients. Controlled Clin Trials 3:209, 1982

Chapter 2

The nursing process and drug therapy: assessment and diagnosis

2

Nursing and its expanding role

Nursing is a unique and complex science, traditionally defined as taking care of people. Although nursing has long been considered to be a caring and nurturing art, involved with ministering to the needs of the sick and with relieving suffering, this concept is no longer adequate.

Many factors have contributed to the need for an expanded role for the nursing profession. The mobility of the population, the separation of families, changing concepts of the individual's responsibility for aging parents, the increase in the proportion of the population who are elderly and living with some chronic infirmity that limits their activity and ability to function independently, and the recent tremendous increases in the cost of health care, combined with an economic recession, have all created problems for the health-care delivery system, as well as voids that can be and are being filled by qualified nurses who are ready to assume an expanded role. At the same time as these sociologic and economic changes have occurred, scientific and technologic advances have made it possible to offer new diagnostic techniques and new therapies, drug and nondrug, for diseases that only a short time ago were rapidly terminal. These advances have contributed to the lengthening of life, to the rising costs of health care, and therefore to the problems of delivering quality health care effectively. Nonetheless, a better educated populace, made aware of the latest advances in the diagnosis and treatment of disease by the media, especially television, want these latest advances for themselves and their families.

Nursing as a profession exists because it performs a necessary service for society. This entails caring directly for people; providing physical, emotional, and intellectual support as the situation demands; and teaching people how to assume responsibility for their own health needs effectively. The nurse, then, must be not only a helping and caring person, but also a scientist and teacher who is knowledgeable about the functions of the human body and the impact of disease, chemicals, and other stressors on it.

The practice of nursing today must be based on a broad foundation in the sciences. It must draw on the disciplines of anatomy, physiology, the biologies, the chemistries, nutrition, pharmacology, psychology, sociology, and education. Nursing encompasses a unique body of knowledge: how people respond to stressors, and how they may be helped to achieve a state of equilibrium—physical, emotional, and social—in their lives.

It is especially in the area of drug therapy that the practice of nursing requires a broad knowledge base in the sciences. Many modern drugs have the potential not only to restore function but also to produce serious, life-threatening adverse effects that directly or indirectly involve various organ systems. For optimum patient benefit with least risk, the nurse must understand normal organ system function, the mechanisms by which this can be altered by drugs, and the signs and symptoms that indicate the occurrence of these changes.

Nursing practice and the law

The actual practice of nursing is regulated by state and local laws that are often redefined by individual institutional and agency policies. In the 1970s, many new nurse practice acts were enacted across the United States. These attempted to redefine the practice of nursing to meet the needs of society for an expanded role for the nurse in the delivery of health care. Of relevance to the field of nursing pharmacology, consideration was given to allowing some nurses to prescribe drugs (as well as to administer drugs directly into a vein), tasks that had previously been limited to physicians, dentists, and others by the practice acts of the various professions. Many states now have laws that specify the conditions under which nurses may actually prescribe as well as administer drugs.

States vary in the specifics of their nurse practice acts. Nurses need to be aware of the legal implications of nursing practice in their state, particularly as these relate to drug therapy. Institutions establish their own policies to govern the practice of nursing within their jurisdiction. In regard to drug therapy, these policies establish the responsibility and authority of each group of health-care professionals (physicians, pharmacists, and nurses) in matters of drug dispensing, delivery, administration, and record keeping. Professional nursing organizations, by their standards of quality nursing practice and ethical standards, provide a third source of control over the nurse's role in drug therapy.

Nursing practice and drug therapy

Although nursing theorists have not arrived at a single definition of nursing, most nursing theories contain certain key elements in common that can be used as a basis for establishing the role of nursing in drug therapy. It is generally agreed that nursing is involved with the patient as a whole person—that is, with the patient's physical, emotional, intellectual, spiritual, and social needs. Nursing considers the patient's response to disease, treatment, and change in life style caused by either one or both. In drug therapy, this means that the nurse is responsible for the total response of the patient to the drug(s). That is, the nurse must assess the patient's response to the disease and to drug therapy to maximize therapeutic benefit and minimize discomfort and toxicity. As appropriate to the patient's physical and mental status, the nurse must do the following: teach the patient or family to make these assessments; help the patient to cope with the disease and with the effects of the drug therapy; and help the patient to face the consequences both of the disease and the therapy realistically, and to incorporate these consequences into daily life, even if this requires changes from normal activity or financial, social, or emotional changes.

Effective and safe drug therapy requires the cooperation of the entire health-care team. Each health-care professional has his own area of expertise, legal responsibility, and authority, with some areas of overlap, so that the health-care system functions with checks and balances. Physicians provide the diagnostic and medical aspects of care. Pharmacists provide for the dispensing of the drug prescribed. In addition, they are alert for prescribing errors, and may monitor a patient's prescriptions for drug–drug interactions, but, generally they do not know the patient's history or disease status. In a large institution, clinical pharmacologists may provide consultation on the effects of drugs given. It is the nurse, though, who provides direct care to the patient, sees and administers the drugs, knows about the patient's diseases, eval-

uates the patient for the drug's effectiveness, and monitors the patient for potential interactions—and who, therefore, is in a unique position among all health-care team members to anticipate and initially detect the signs of an adverse reaction to a drug or an unanticipated response.

Despite individual differences, a review of the various regulations regarding nursing practice and drug therapy reveals that usually the nurse is considered legally and ethically responsible for the following:

1. To evaluate the drug being given as appropriate—that is, to ensure that the correct drug is administered for a particular patient and particular disease, and in the correct dosage, by the correct route of administration, and at the correct time
2. To administer the drug appropriately, or to provide for its administration
3. To assess the patient for therapeutic and adverse effects, including drug–drug interactions, drug–food interactions, and drug–body interactions
4. To be alert to changes in the results of the patient's laboratory diagnostic tests that could be caused by drugs the patient is taking
5. To be alert to changes in the patient's signs and symptoms that could be misinterpreted as caused by the disease when, in fact, they are caused by the drug; conversely, to be alert to a drug masking important signs and symptoms of disease
6. To provide comfort measures to help the patient to cope with any adverse effects of the drug
7. To provide health teaching and counseling to ensure that the patient will receive the greatest benefit from the drug with the least danger

The nursing process

The nursing process is the decision-making or problem-solving method that has been developed to implement the science of nursing. Unlike the physical sciences, in which repetition of an experiment produces a fairly predictable outcome every time, nursing, as a biologic and clinical science, is continually confounded by biologic variation and by the human element. No two people are exactly the same, and therefore no two people respond in exactly the same way to diseases, stressors, or even drug therapy. Thus, effective and safe clinical treatment has to be individualized to meet each patient's needs; each patient must be assessed and treated individually.

There is really no such thing as "standard treatment" that is both safe and effective.

The nursing process evolved to deal with the overwhelming task of applying the broad store of scientific knowledge on which nursing practice is based to each individual patient. The nursing process is a format for systematically approaching each clinical situation; it consists of four steps: assessment, diagnosis, intervention, and evaluation. These steps have been given other names in some texts but, for the purposes of describing the nursing process in relation to drug therapy, these are the four steps that will be used. The application of the nursing process results in the collection and analysis of information about the total patient, the definition of information needed to direct specific nursing activities, the implementation of these activities, and the continual evaluation of the overall situation. As the end product of this process, the patient is provided with the best scientifically based holistic care possible.

Assessment

The first step of the nursing process is the systematic and organized collection of data about the patient. Because the nurse is responsible for the provision of holistic care, this data base must include information regarding physical, intellectual, emotional, social, and environmental factors. In clinical practice, this step never ends; it is an ongoing, continual process. The patient is rarely in a steady state but rather is in a dynamic state, adjusting to new physical, emotional, and environmental stressors, which can influence the response to drug therapy.

Nursing diagnosis

The analysis of all the data collected results in the formulation of a nursing diagnosis (for examples of specific nursing diagnoses, see Table 2-1). This is a statement of the patient's potential, or actual, health problems; it directs nursing care activities and interventions and helps to determine the priorities of the patient's needs.

Table 2—1. Nursing diagnoses*

1. Airway clearance, ineffective
2. Bowel elimination, alteration in: constipation
3. Bowel elimination, alteration in: diarrhea
4. Bowel elimination, alteration in: incontinence
5. Breathing patterns, ineffective
6. Cardiac output, alteration in: decreased
7. Comfort, alteration in: pain
8. Communication, impaired verbal
9. Coping, ineffective individual
10. Coping, ineffective family: disabling
11. Coping, ineffective family: compromised
12. Coping, family: potential for growth
13. Diversional activity, deficit
14. Fear
15. Fluid volume, deficit, actual
16. Fluid volume, deficit, potential
17. Gas exchange, impaired
18. Grieving, anticipatory
19. Grieving, dysfunctional
20. Home maintenance management, impaired
21. Injury, potential for (specify)
22. Knowledge deficit (specify)
23. Mobility, impaired physical
24. Noncompliance (specify)
25. Nutrition, alteration in: less than body requirements
26. Nutrition, alteration in: more than body requirements

27. Nutrition, alteration in: potential for more than body requirements
28. Parenting, alteration in: actual
29. Parenting, alteration in: potential
30. Rape trauma syndrome
31. Self-care deficit (specify level): feeding, bathing–hygiene, dressing–grooming, toileting
32. Self-concept, disturbance in
33. Sensory–perceptual alteration
34. Sexual dysfunction
35. Skin integrity, impairment of: actual
36. Skin integrity, impairment of: potential
37. Sleep pattern disturbance
38. Spiritual distress (distress of the human spirit)
39. Thought processes, alteration in
40. Tissue perfusion, alteration in
41. Urinary elimination, alteration in patterns
42. Violence, potential for

Diagnoses to be developed

43. Cognitive dissonance
44. Family dynamics, alterations in
45. Fluid volume excess, potential
46. Memory deficit
47. Rest–activity pattern, ineffective
48. Role disturbance
49. Social isolation

* Accepted by the American Nurses' Association at the Fourth National Conference for the Classification of Nursing Diagnosis, April 9–13, 1980. St. Louis, Missouri.

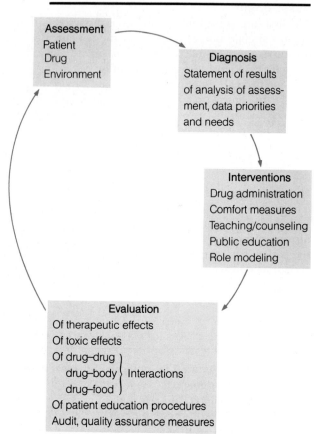

Figure 2-1. The nursing process in drug therapy: a continual, ongoing process.

Intervention

The interventions used in patient care are derived from the patient's needs, as determined by the nursing diagnosis. They are usually expressed as the nursing care plan. In drug therapy, some interventions are almost always considered as part of the nursing care plan. These are the correct and accurate administration of prescribed drugs; the provision of comfort measures to help the patient cope with and adapt to the effects of the drugs; and patient and family teaching and counseling to ensure that the patient is well informed and can participate in and make decisions about his own care. In more general terms, the nurse also intervenes with the public by acting as a role model and by helping to educate the public about drugs and drug use.

Evaluation

Once the interventions have been instituted, the situation must be evaluated to determine how effective the overall plan has been in meeting the patient's needs. It is during this phase that the anticipated and unanticipated effects of drug therapy are encountered and must be identified. The nurse must evaluate the patient's response to drug therapy for the desired therapeutic effects, as well as for

any toxic effects. The patient's overall situation must be evaluated for drug–drug, drug–body, and drug–food interactions that could affect the therapeutic response. The patient must be further evaluated for the occurrence of drug–body interactions that could alter or invalidate the results of laboratory diagnostic tests or confuse the assessment of the disease. The effectiveness of patient teaching procedures must be evaluated to ensure that the desired outcomes are being achieved. The evaluation process should lead to a new analysis of the patient care plan and to a formulation of new approaches to the situation. The overall process of patient care evaluation is called the *nursing audit*. It can be concurrent (*i.e.,* doing quality assurance monitoring while the patient is under direct care) or retrospective (*i.e.,* looking at trends in care as reflected in medical records). This part of the evaluation process considers procedures, techniques, and gaps in practice policies.

As intimidating and complex as this whole process may seem at first to the student, in clinical practice the process should occur almost instantly. The experienced nurse incorporates it into every contact with the patient, often so completely that conscious awareness of its use is lost. For example, a clinician may discover a patient unconscious in his room. Almost instantly, a physical assessment is made: no pulse, no respirations, pupils dilated. The data are analyzed to arrive at a nursing diagnosis: alteration in cardiac output—decreased (see Table 2-1). Interventions are begun: an airway is established, cardiopulmonary resuscitation is started. The situation is evaluated moment to moment to determine the effect of the interventions, to reestablish priorities, and to organize appropriate additional interventions. All these actions occur almost instantly and appear to be almost reflex. In reality, however, they are all part of a learned scientific approach to the clinical situation.

The nursing process and drug therapy

Drug therapy is such a complex, integral, and important part of health care today that the principles of drug therapy need to be incorporated into every patient care plan. The thousands of drugs available and the hundreds of thousands of possible reactions that could occur make the rote memorization of pharmacology totally impossible. The nurse needs to understand the principles of drug therapy and the actions of the basic classes of drugs fully, and then to incorporate these basic concepts into the nursing process.

To provide a useful guide for the incorporation of pharmacology and therapeutics into routine clinical practice, the rest of this chapter and all of Chapter 3 will examine each step of the nursing process as it applies to drug therapy. Figure 2-1 presents the key points in applying the nursing process to drug therapy.

Assessment in relation to drug therapy

Patient assessment

Evaluation of the patient is the first element in the assessment process. Table 2-2 lists the essential factors in patient assessment (described below). Patient assessment is a systematic and concise collection of data about an individual patient. Each nurse develops a unique approach to the organization of the assessment, one that is most functional and useful to that nurse's particular area and type of practice. The assessment consists of two main parts—past history and physical assessment. Both parts of the assessment process should be well organized to enable the nurse to obtain all necessary information without repetition, and with as little stress to the patient as possible. The scientific bases of nursing should always be considered during the assessment process, because they provide rationality and validity for the nursing diagnosis and interventions.

Past history

Sources of information. *The patient* is the most valuable source of data. Even if the data are not precise, they provide insight into the patient's attitudes, perceptions, and beliefs, all of which have a great influence on the patient's compliance with drug therapy and on educational needs. *The medical record* provides the official version of the patient's health and medication history. However, it is important to remember that any one medical record may not contain all the details of a patient's care. Most people seek professional health care from several sources, the records of which are often not contained in one medical record. *The patient's family or significant others* sometimes need to be consulted to obtain details or insight into the patient's health status or drug therapy.

The assessment of past history is usually done using an assessment tool, often a patient history form.

The tool should elicit holistic information—that is, it should consider all aspects of the patient as a person: not only the patient's physical state, but also his emotional state and level of functioning in society. Such a tool should provide a thorough knowledge base for the next steps in the nursing process, be flexible enough to allow updating so that the assessment can provide an everchanging reflection of the patient's progress and "state of health," and allow for continuity in care.

Points to include. Regardless of what type of assessment tool the nurse adapts to clinical practice, certain key points about the patient's drug therapy should always be included (see below). Although ideally each patient's detailed medication history should be included in the chart, the time constraints of clinical practice usually make this impractical. The most realistic approach to the accurate assessment of a patient on drug therapy is the incorporation of these critical concepts into the general patient assessment tool.

Contraindications. The patient should be evaluated for the presence of contraindications—that is, chronic or persistent conditions that could be exacerbated by drug therapy. A patient with congestive heart failure, for example, should not receive a drug such as propranolol (Inderal) that could cause heart failure or make the condition worse. Contraindications are specific for certain drugs. They should be noted on the patient's chart in red to alert any nurse or physician to their presence.

The patient should also be evaluated for chronic conditions that would make it desirable to administer certain drugs in a lower dosage than normal. Of particular concern are liver and kidney disorders, because these organs are the usual sites of drug metabolism and excretion and disorders of these organs could cause drugs to build up in the body, leading to serious drug toxicity (see Chap. 3).

Table 2–2. Patient assessment in drug therapy

Past history	Physical assessment
Chronic conditions—may be contraindications to use of the drug or indicate need for reduced dosage	Weight and height
Drug use—prescription drugs: identity, dose, frequency; OTC drugs: identity, dose, frequency; street drugs; alcohol; nicotine; caffeine (coffee, soft drinks)	Age
Allergies—drug and reaction; food and reaction; animal and reaction	Physical parameters related to disease state, drug effects
Level of education	
Level of understanding of disease and therapy	
Social supports	
Financial supports	
Pattern of health care	

Drug use. The use of any drugs should be noted to avert the possibility of drug–drug interactions. The patient should be asked what *prescription drugs* are being taken, including the dose and frequency. It is important to ask about all prescription drugs; frequently, birth control pills or drugs ordered by dentists are omitted. If the names or dosages of the drugs aren't known, the patient can bring in the bottles so that the nurse can read the label or match the capsules, tablets, and so forth to the illustrations in the *PDR* identification guide.

Over-the-counter (OTC) drugs should also be noted. Information on OTC drugs is often very difficult to elicit because most people do not consider these to be medications. It is sometimes helpful to query the patient specifically about several classes of OTC drugs—that is, to ask directly if such drugs as laxatives, cold pills, sleeping aids, vitamins, and headache remedies are being taken. Try to ascertain the specific drug preparation and dosage. OTC drugs are frequently involved in drug–drug or drug–disease interactions, and they may also mask signs and symptoms that are needed for accurate patient assessment.

The use of such drugs as *alcohol, caffeine, and nicotine* also needs to be evaluated. These drugs can greatly influence the body's response to some other drugs, both directly and indirectly—for example, by influencing the metabolism of the other drug. These substances are so routinely used in society that their use, like that of OTC drugs, may be overlooked.

The use of *street drugs* should also be explored. Because this area is a very sensitive one, a good nurse–patient relationship is crucial to obtaining accurate information.

Drug allergies. Any report of drug allergy should also be noted in red on the patient's chart as a contraindication to therapy with that drug or with others that could cross react. It is very important, when discussing drug allergy with a patient, to ascertain exactly what the patient has experienced during an "allergic reaction." For example, a man reported that he was allergic to the diuretic furosemide (Lasix). On further questioning, the patient revealed that the "allergy" consisted of being up all night going to the bathroom, and that he had taken the diuretic before going to bed. Frequently, patients report an allergy to a drug when they are, in fact, just annoyed by the side-effects of the drug. It is very important to know this information when a condition requires the use of a drug to which the patient is reportedly allergic. Food, animal, or other allergies should also be noted. This information will alert the physician or nurse to the patient who has a tendency toward allergies, and who may therefore also experience an allergic reaction to a drug. In addition, some drug preparations use as binders or bases substances that either are allergens or contain food or animal substances that can act as allergens. If the patient's allergy to these substances is known, a drug preparation that is devoid of these substances can frequently be chosen.

Other information that should be obtained before instituting drug therapy includes the patient's level of education, general level of understanding of the disease and the health care involved, social and financial supports, and the pattern of previous health care (that is, does the patient seek health care routinely or only in emergency situations?). This information can be helpful in developing a teaching program and in finding ways of helping the patient to cope with the drug and adapting his life style to the drug therapy.

Physical assessment. Before beginning drug therapy, it is essential to assess the patient's physical condition thoroughly. This predrug assessment serves as a baseline to which future assessments can be compared to determine the effects of drug therapy. The specific parameters that should be assessed will depend on the disease process being treated and on the expected therapeutic and adverse effects of the drug therapy. In general, the patient's height and weight should be recorded. These factors contribute to the overall effects of drug therapy. Patients at the extremes of underweight and overweight are most likely to benefit from a change from the standard dosage recommended by the drug manufacturer. Some drugs have so low a margin of safety that avoidance of toxicity requires the dose to be calculated on the basis of the individual patient's size. The patient's age is also important. Young children and the elderly sometimes have different drug distribution, metabolism, and excretion than the "norm," and will require adjustments in drug dosage. In this book the specific physical parameters that should be assessed before instituting drug therapy will be described for each class of drugs.

Because of the structure of the health-care system in this country, the nurse is the person who has the greatest direct contact with the patient. In the hospital, community health center, or clinic setting, the nurse has the greatest opportunity to assess, minute by minute or over the long term, changes in the patient's condition, including changes caused by drug therapy. The need for accuracy in this physical assessment, therefore, cannot be stressed enough.

Drug assessment

This is the second essential element in the assessment process. Drug assessment includes evaluation of the drug order and drug dosage and consideration of the anticipated effects of the drug.

Evaluation of medication order

Medication orders and prescriptions. Orders for medication originate with a physician or other licensed practitioner. State law and institutional policy will determine who can write orders for medications. In the hospital, orders may be written on the patient's chart or in a special medication book. Patients seen in the office or at home receive prescriptions that they then have filled at a local pharmacy.

No medication should ever be administered without an appropriate order. Ordinarily, all orders are written but, in an emergency, medication may be ordered by telephone and later signed by the physician who ordered it. This process is called a verbal order and, although perfectly acceptable in some circumstances, it can present a real problem. It is legally imperative that the verbal order be signed as soon as possible. The order should also be carefully written as the order is given, and then reread to clarify the details. If there is any doubt about the appropriateness of the order, it should be refused. Verbal orders should be avoided whenever possible. It is important to remember that, no matter who has given the drug order, the nurse or physician who administers the drug is totally responsible.

Prescriptions are written in a traditional form (Fig. 2-2). A traditional prescription contains eight components:

1. The date—federal drug control laws require specific limits to be indicated on the length of time that prescriptions are valid.
2. Full name and address, and often a patient identification number. Many physicians also write the age of the patient in this section. This alerts other members of the health-care team to potential age-related particular needs of the patient and, in an outpatient setting, makes it more difficult for someone to use another person's prescription.

3. Superscription—this is the symbol R_x, an abbreviation for the Latin *recipe,* which means "take thou."
4. Inscription—this is the main body of the prescription. It lists the drug name, dosage form, and amount of the dose.
5. The subscription—this includes the directions to the pharmacist for preparation of the drug and the amount that should be dispensed.
6. The signature, or *Sig* (as it appears on prescription forms). These are the directions for the label, or the directions to the patient. This includes instructions for time and frequency of the dose, storage information, and so forth.
7. Refill information—federal law also regulates the number and frequency of refills that are allowed, and these should be specified in the prescription.
8. The prescriber's signature—this is an essential aspect of the prescription. It must be followed by the licensed title of the physician; it is often followed by a DEA number and, in many states, it is written (signed) on one line if the drug must be dispensed as written, or on another line if a generic substitution is allowed.

It is important for the nurse to be familiar with prescription formats, even if not involved with writing

---

Downtown Health Service
800 Western Lane
Philadelphia, NY 16606
Telephone: 555-6606

1. January 12, 1985

2. Andrew Brown, 2 years
82 Circle A.
Philadelphia, NY 16606

3. R_x

4. Gantrisin, suspension,

5. 500 mg/5 cc–300 cc

6. Sig: 1 teaspoonful b.i.d. × 1 month for prophylaxis, otitis media
Shake well, refrigerate, drink lots of H_2O.

7. Refill _____ times
Nonrefill ____X____

8. _____   _____
   Substitution permissible   Dispense as written

Figure 2-2. A drug prescription: (*1*) date; (*2*) patient identification; (*3*) superscription; (*4*) inscription; (*5*) subscription; (*6*) signature or label; (*7*) refill information; (*8*) prescriber's signature and title.

medication orders. Understanding what drug is ordered and how it is ordered are parts of safe clinical nursing practice. The nurse is also often asked by patients to interpret the "hieroglyphics" on prescription forms.

Institutional medication orders. If the patient is institutionalized for health care, the medication orders are usually written directly on the patient's chart or on special medication order forms. Each institution has its own mechanisms for getting the order to the pharmacy. Often this involves transcribing the orders onto special forms or keying them into a computer. Whatever method is used, the nurse is ultimately responsible for ensuring that the whole procedure is carried through without error. Institutional medication orders can be for the following: *one-time doses; one-time doses to be given immediately* (stat orders); *one-time doses to be given only if needed* (SOS orders); *doses to be repeated at given time intervals; prn* or "whenever necessary" orders—usually for pain, laxative, or sleeping medications; *standing orders*—specific drugs that are routinely used in a particular setting (*e.g.*, drugs used in labor and delivery, ICUs, CCUs, or emergency departments are often covered by standing or blanket orders), and *protocols*—orders that outline drugs and dosages to be given in certain situations (*e.g.*, sliding scale insulin to be given for particular blood sugar levels). Each institution has regulations governing how long an order is valid and how often orders must be reevaluated and reviewed. It is very important to make sure that medication orders are current.

Evaluation of appropriateness. Once the medication order is obtained, it should be assessed for appropriateness. As more drugs become available, it becomes even more important for everyone responsible to scrutinize each drug order carefully. For instance, if a drug order is interpreted as Amodrine, an antiasthma drug, but the prescriber actually intended the order to be for Amonidrin, an expectorant, the patient could be treated with the wrong drug for a "flulike" cough. There are so many drugs whose names are similar in spelling but whose actions are very different that it is very important to make sure that the drug fits the problem. Never hesitate to question an order that seems inappropriate.

The dosage of the drug should also be evaluated for appropriateness for the patient's age and size. The *PDR* or any of various quick reference books can be used to check this information. If certain drugs are used continually in a particular setting, the usual dosages should be posted in a convenient area for quick reference.

Drug orders are often written with one or more abbreviations. There are standard abbreviations for the words and phrases most commonly used in medication orders (Table 2-3). In addition, each institution and practice area often develops some abbreviations of its own. Any unfamiliar abbreviations should be clarified.

Finally, the medication order should be evaluated as to the appropriateness of the route of administration. Patients who cannot take anything by mouth cannot take oral medications. Patients who have intravenous lines might benefit from intravenous medications rather than from repeated intramuscular injections. These factors must be considered in regard to the overall patient situation.

Environmental assessment

The third element to be assessed before instituting drug therapy is the environment (Table 2-4). This has two components: the conditions of the surroundings as they affect the patient both physically and emotionally, and the drug distribution systems used to supply drugs to the patient.

Patient's surroundings. The patient's surroundings can be very important in the actual effect of drug therapy. Frequently, alterations in the patient's environment will alleviate the need for drug therapy or will make the drug therapy more effective. Important environmental factors include room temperature and lighting, comfort measures and counseling, and family involvement.

Drug distribution system. The second component of the environment, the drug distribution system, should be assessed whether the patient is in the community, at a health-care facility, or at home. This assessment should consider the facilities for storing and administering drugs. If the drug needs to be refrigerated, is refrigeration available? If the drug is a liquid that needs to be measured, is equipment available and is the patient, or someone else, capable of doing this? Can the patient see well enough to measure his own medication? Are the patient's hands steady enough not to spill a liquid drug? Can the patient's arthritic hands open a bottle? These subjects should also be included in teaching and counseling protocols.

Various modern systems that help to get medications to patients more efficiently and with less chance for error have come into use in institutions. These involve closer liaison between the patient care unit and pharmacy personnel, the use of prepacked unit doses of medication, and even machine-operated automated systems.

Unit–dose medication system. This system can provide prepackaged individual doses of all drugs, including not only tablets and capsules but also liquids for oral administration and prefilled syringes for direct use in making injections. Many frequently employed drugs are now available as strip-packed or blister-packed capsules or tablets, suppository pack units, or cartridge injection systems. The injectables are dispensed in the form of sterile syringe and needle units that are disposable. In addition to their convenience, these are free of contamination by infectious organisms. Narcotics and barbiturates now come packaged in ways that make it easier to keep stock records. (One such injectable system, called Tubex, employs a tamper-resistant package, trade-named

Table 2–3. Some abbreviations commonly employed in prescription orders

Abbreviation	Latin derivation	Meaning	Abbreviation	Latin derivation	Meaning
aa	*ana*	of each	OD	*oculus dexter*	right eye
ac	*ante cibum*	before meals	oh	*omni hora*	every hour
ad lib	*ad libitum*	as freely, or as often, as is desired	OS	*oculus sinister*	left eye
			os	*os*	mouth
Aq (dest)	*aqua (destillata)*	water (distilled)	pc	*post cibum*	after meals
bid	*bis in die*	twice a day	Pil	*pilula*	pill
c̄	*cum*	with	po	*per os*	orally
Caps	*capsula*	capsule	prn	*pro re nata*	literally, as the occasion arises; occasionally; when it seems to be desirable or necessary
Chart	*chartula*	a medicated powder in a paper wrapping			
Comp	*compositus*	compond			
dil	*dilue*	dilute			
dis	*dispensare*	dispense	q or qq	*quaque*	every
DTD	*datur talis dosis (no.)*	give as many doses (as indicated by the number)	qh or qqh	*quaque hora*	every hour
			qd or qqd	*quaque die*	every day
			qid	*quater in die*	four times a day
elix	*elixir*	elixir	qs	*quantum satis*	a sufficient amount
et	*et*	and	℞	*recipe*	take
ext	*extractum*	extract	s̄	*sine*	without
F, or ft	*Fac or fiat*	make; let be made	S or Sig	*signa* or *signetur*	write (on the label)
Flext	*fluidextractum*	fluidextract	SOS	*si opus sit*	if needed
g	*gramma*	gram	sol	*solutio*	solution
gr	*granum*	grain	sp	*spiritus*	spirit
gt	*gutta*	a drop	ss	*semis*	half
H	*hora*	hour	stat	*statim*	immediately
hs	*hora somni*	at bedtime	Syr	*syrupus*	syrup
M	*misce*	mix	tab	*tabella*	tablet
No	*numerus*	number	tid	*ter in die*	three times a day
Noct	*nocte*	at night	tinct	*tinctura*	tincture
non rep	*non repetatur*	do not repeat	ung	*unguentum*	ointment
o	*omnis*	every	Ut dict	*ut dictum*	as directed
od	*omni die*	every day	Vin	*vinum*	wine

Tamp-R-Tel, for such products.) Commercial unit doses are relatively expensive, but many medications can be put up by the pharmacist at a lower cost per unit dose. Such premeasured and prelabeled packages are not only convenient, but are also helpful for avoiding medication mistakes.

Pouring medications. Institutions that do not supply drugs in unit dose form have medication rooms or

Table 2–4. Assessment of the drug and environment

Assessing the drug	Assessing the environment
Appropriate drug for patient	Patient environment: lighting; temperature; comfort measures; counseling; family involvement
Appropriate dosage for patient	Drug delivery system: drug available; dispensing facilities available; storage facilities available; home resources for assistance
Appropriate route for patient	
Order is complete and meets legal requirements	
Order is current	

medication closets in which the nurse will "pour" the drugs ordered from large stock supplies. There is greater chance for error in this approach because the drug ordered has to be matched to one of many bottles of drugs in the medication closet, and the individual patient's cups of pills must then be kept in some sort of order between pouring and administration.

Self-medication by the patient. In some health-care facilities, or if a patient is at home, the medication is supplied in a container from the pharmacy. The label of the container should contain the patient's name, name of the drug, dosage of the drug, and instructions for taking and storing the drug. In the institutional setting, if the patient self-administers the drug, the nurse is still responsible for ensuring that the drug is taken as ordered.

In assessing the particular delivery system in use, the availability of the drug and appropriate storage and dispensing facilities should be ensured.

Nursing diagnosis in relation to drug therapy

This is the second step in the nursing process. Figure 2-3 illustrates how this step fits into the overall nursing process. Once all the assessment data have been collected, a clinical judgment or diagnosis is made. The diagnosis is a statement of the patient's status. It is arrived at through the synthesis and analysis of all the data acquired in the assessment. Although many members of the health-care team may assess the same factors, the analysis and use of the information vary with the profession. A physician arrives at a medical diagnosis that directs the medical treatment of the patient. The nurse arrives at a nursing diagnosis that, in turn, directs the nursing care of that patient.

Although most nurses will agree that nursing diagnoses have been made for 30 to 40 years, the actual taxonomy or classification system of nursing diagnoses is still relatively new. The First National Conference on Nursing Diagnoses was held in St. Louis in 1973. Since that initial attempt to put official and acceptable labels on the diagnoses made as a result of a nursing assessment, hundreds of nurses in practice, research, and education have participated in national and regional conferences and in research to establish an acceptable nomenclature. The American Nurses' Association (ANA) has approved a list of nursing diagnoses (Table 2-1). No firm concrete nomenclature has been universally accepted but nurses and student nurses are using nursing diagnoses, the ANA list, or other terms to direct nursing care in practice and to provide a means of communicating to other health-care professionals. The concept of nursing diagnoses is a very important aspect of the scientific use of the nursing process.

Throughout this book, the ANA-approved diagnoses will be used where appropriate. The diagnoses listed will then reflect actual or potential alterations in patient functioning. It is important to remember that the nursing diagnosis is a statement of total patient status, of which drug therapy is only one small part. Coupled with the incompleteness of the current list of nursing diagnoses, this may make some nursing diagnoses seem too far-reaching or not totally appropriate. For each class of drugs discussed, the nursing diagnoses reflecting *potential alteration of function* related to that particular drug's actions will be listed. For example guanethidine (Ismelin) is a drug used to treat hypertension. Frequent side-effects of the drug include postural or orthostatic hypotension, dizziness and weakness, diarrhea, bradycardia, and sexual impotence. Knowing that these are potential alterations in patient functioning when the patient is receiving guanethidine, the following nursing diagnoses could be considered: potential alteration in cardiac output, decreased (would be assessed by blood pressure changes, heart rate, signs of cerebral anoxia); potential for injury (*i.e.,* weakness, dizziness—related to changes in cerebral blood flow with position); potential alteration in bowel elimination (diarrhea—as evidenced by the occurrence of frequent loose stools); potential alteration in patterns of sexuality (as assessed by the occurrence of sexual impotence); and potential lack of knowledge about drug therapy (a diagnosis that would probably apply to all patients on drug therapy). These are intended to be suggested diagnoses that should be considered; the actual nursing diagnoses established for a patient will incorporate all the data about the patient and the physical and emotional status. As the

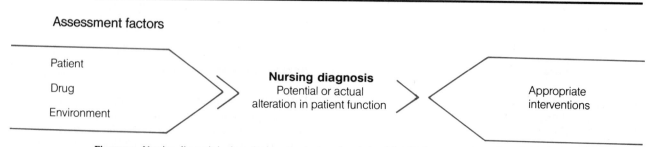

Assessment factors

Patient

Drug

Environment

Nursing diagnosis
Potential or actual
alteration in patient function

Appropriate
interventions

Figure 2-3. Nursing diagnosis in drug therapy. Synthesis and analysis of data lead to a statement of potential or actual alterations in patient function, which directs appropriate nursing interventions.

classification of nursing diagnoses is further developed and refined, the specific diagnoses appropriate for drug therapy will become more exact.

References

Bell SK: Guidelines for taking a complete drug history. Nursing 80 10:11, 1980

Carlson S: A practical approach to the nursing process. Am J Nurs 72:1589, 1972

Carrieri UK, Sitzman Z: Components of the nursing process. Nurs Clin North Am 6:115, 1971

Geiger J: The endlessly revolving door. Am J Nurs 69:573, 1969

Gordon M: Nursing Diagnoses: Process and Application. New York, McGraw–Hill, 1982

Kim MJ, Maritz DA: Classification of Nursing Diagnoses. New York, McGraw-Hill, 1982

Kneedler J: Nursing process is a continuous cycle. Assoc Operating Room Nurs J 20:245, 1974

Lunney M: Nursing diagnosis: Refining the system. Am J Nurs 82:456, 1982

Riehe J, Roy C: Conceptual Models for Nursing Practice. New York, Appleton–Century–Crofts, 1980

Shafer J: The interrelatedness of decision making and the nursing process. Am J Nurs 74:1852, 1974

Swinyard E: Principles of prescription order writing. In Gilman AG, Goodman LS, Gilman A (eds): Goodman and Gilman's Pharmacological Basis of Therapeutics, 6th ed, pp 1660–1673. New York, Macmillan, 1980

Chapter 3

The nursing process and drug therapy: intervention and evaluation

3

Intervention

The assessment and diagnosis phases of the nursing process flow directly into the phases of intervention and evaluation. Although each patient's nursing care plan will be unique and individual, based on the assessment of each patient's total situation and on the nursing diagnoses that result, there are three types of interventions that will frequently be involved with the drug therapy aspect of patient care: drug administration, provision of comfort measures, and patient teaching. Because these are such important concepts of total drug therapy, each intervention will be discussed in some detail.

Drug administration

In most of the world, most drugs are taken in the home setting. However, when drugs are taken within healthcare institutions, it is inevitably within the realm of nursing to provide for the administration of drugs to the patients. Because of the immense responsibility of providing the right drug to the right patient at the right time, this job is very often one of the most time-consuming aspects of patient care. The specific details of drug administration will vary from institution to institution, but certain concepts are universal. In administering a drug, the nurse must consider the route of administration, delivery of the correct dose, timing of administration, and recording of the administration.

Routes of administration

The manner in which a drug is administered is one of the most important factors influencing its action. Depending on how a dose of a drug is given, it may produce a profound effect or none at all. Thus, when a solution of magnesium sulfate (Epsom salt) is taken by mouth, it acts only within the intestine to exert a cathartic effect; when the same magnesium salt is injected intramuscularly,

its molecules reach the central nervous system and produce deep depression.

The path by which a drug is introduced into the body influences primarily the rate and completeness of its absorption into the bloodstream. This, in turn, plays a primary part in determining how quickly the drug begins to act and the intensity with which it acts. In addition to influencing the speed of *onset* and the degree of *intensity* of a drug's action, the dosage form and manner of administration also often influence the *duration,* or length of action.

The main *routes* by which drugs are administered so that they can enter the systemic circulation and exert their effects on the distant tissues that can react to them will be reviewed. At the same time, some information about the *dosage forms* in which drugs are available will be offered (Table 3-1). The basics of correct administration of drugs by the various routes will also be included.

Oral administration. The best way to give drugs, whenever possible, is by mouth. This is the simplest, safest, and least expensive way to get a drug into the patient's body and on its way into the bloodstream and other tissues. Thus, except for some poorly absorbable substances such as insulin and other polypeptide hormones and certain highly ionized antibiotics, most drugs are available in dosage forms suitable for oral administration.

Solid oral dosage forms. Drugs are available for oral administration in many solid and liquid dosage forms. *Tablets* made by compressing powdered or granulated drugs into a compact, readily swallowed form are currently the most common type. A well-made tablet breaks up quickly in the stomach into a finely divided powder that is readily absorbed.

This is so significant in determining a drug's bioavailability that tests have been devised to determine the dissolution rate of solid oral dosage forms, and tablet batches must meet official standards based on the results of such tests. The ability of tablets to disintegrate and

Table 3–1. Routes of administration and dosage forms of drugs

Oral

Solid dosages

Tablets: compressed powder, granules
Capsules: gelatin-covered; enteric-coated–delays
   dissolution; timed release–slow release of granules
Powders

Liquid dosages

Syrups: solutions with water and sugar (*Note:* caution
   with diabetics)
Elixirs: hydroalcoholic liquids (*Note:* caution with
   diabetics and alcoholics)
Emulsions: oil and water mixtures
Gels–magmas: viscous suspensions of mineral
   precipitates
Aromatic waters: aqueous solutions of volatile
   substances
Tinctures: solutions of drug in alcohol
Fluidextracts: concentrated liquid preparations of
   vegetable drugs
Extracts: concentrated preparations with the
   hydroalcoholic solvent evaporated

Parenteral

Intradermal: within the dermis of the skin
Subcutaneous: within the subcutaneous layer of the
   skin; hypodermoclysis—prolonged, slow,
   subcutaneous injection
Intramuscular: within the muscle
Intravenous: directly into a vein
Intrathecal: directly into the subarachnoid space
Intraspinal: directly into the spinal fluid
Intra-articular: directly into a joint
Intralesional: directly into a lesion
Intra-arterial: directly into an artery

Application to mucous membranes

Rectal: suppository or enema
Inhalation: droplets, vapor, gas, dust dispensed from
   specialized devices
Mouth and throat: sprays, swabs, sublingual tablets,
   buccal tablets
Nasal: sprays, drops
Vaginal: suppository, douche, foam, cream

Topical administration

Skin (dermal): lotions, liniments, ointments,
   compresses, creams, patches,
Ophthalmic (eye): drops, ointments, irrigations,
Otic (ear): drops, irrigations

dissolve depends not only on the nature of the active drug but also on the binders, diluents, and other inactive materials, or excipients, that go into the manufacture of compressed tablets. In regard to disintegration and absorption, tablets are much more reliable than *pills,* which often dried out during storage and were then likely to pass through the entire GI tract without ever dissolving. Pills are now largely passé, even though people still persist in calling tablets "pills."

Capsules made of gelatin that dissolves in stomach acids are another common oral dosage form. They come in various sizes and colors, and usually bear the initials of the pharmaceutical manufacturer and an identifying code number. Unlike tablets, capsules are not coated with sugar or chocolate to disguise the taste of drugs or to improve their palatability. However, they are sometimes covered with substances that keep the gelatin protected from gastric acids but that do dissolve in the alkaline secretions of the duodenum.

Enteric-coated tablets or capsules are intended to delay the release of drugs that might cause nausea or vomiting if they come in contact with the stomach lining in high concentrations. The coating is insoluble in stomach acids but, once the tablet passes into the upper part of the intestine, it dissolves in the alkaline secretions there. Occasionally, however, the enteric coating may fail to dissolve, and the drug may then pass out of the intestinal tract without being absorbed.

Prolonged-action tablets and capsules also have a delayed action. However, the purpose here is not to protect the stomach from irritation but to produce a long-sustained drug action and thus reduce the number of doses that the patient has to remember to take. A patient is much more likely to get the benefits of prescribed drug therapy when he needs to take only two rather than four to six doses a day, according to several studies of the factors that determine patient compliance.

These so-called sustained-action or timed-release products are available in various physical forms based on different biopharmaceutic principles of release and absorption. Some of the contents of the capsule or tablet are released almost immediately and absorbed to bring about quick action. The remainder of the material is released gradually as the capsule gives up its contents for absorption over a period of several hours. Thus, drugs are sometimes prescribed in the form of Spansules, Gradumets, or other sustained-release medications that need be taken only once very 12 hours or so. An important point to remember is that these products—unlike regular tablets that are sometimes crushed and mixed with jelly or jam for children—should never be tampered with in any way. Pouring out the pellets and breaking them up could result in rapid absorption of an overdose.

Powders also are relatively rare today and are limited mainly to products for relief of gastrointestinal distress. Such bulky effervescent antacids and laxatives are currently being made available more frequently as large tablets that form a bubbling solution, which is apparently just as effective and psychologically satisfying as the older form.

Lozenges, or *troches,* are flattened disks that are intended to be held in the mouth until dissolved. They contain demulcent, or soothing, substances that are supposed to relieve a sore throat through local action. Also characteristic of these relatives of the common cough drop is their high content of sugar or other sweetener, flavors, and colors.

Liquid oral dosage forms. Several types of liquid preparations are available for oral use. These contain drugs dissolved or suspended in water, alcohol, or hydroalcoholic vehicles.* Some of these, such as syrups, elixirs, and aromatic waters, are intended to present medicinal substances in more palatable form; others—for example, tinctures and fluidextracts—are made by extracting the active ingredients from ground-up medicinal plants by treating the crude drug with water and alcohol to obtain strong concentrates while leaving behind the inert plant residues.

Syrups are solutions of sugar in water to which flavors of various types are usually added. Children like to take syrupy liquids and are less likely to balk when bitter, salt, or insipid substances are disguised in one of the official syrups—the fruit flavors cherry and orange, licorice, chocolate (cocoa syrup), and aromatics such as eriodictyon or tolu balsam syrups. Their use is often preferable to the practice of putting drugs in milk or in fruit juice to disguise the disagreeable taste. Although doing this with salty drugs such as potassium iodide, ammonium chloride, or sodium bromide usually works with adults, children may later refuse to eat or drink foods that they have come to associate with an "off" taste or odor. It is, of course, better for the child to enjoy the taste of medicine that he must take instead of gagging on it and struggling against efforts to give it to him. However, it is not desirable to put too much emphasis on flavor or to fool a child into taking medication by calling it "candy." It should not be surprising if the child then eats the entire contents of the bottle—and becomes ill. Similarly, television commercials for cough syrups, which put excessive emphasis on palatability, do a disservice ("Gee, Mom, it tastes just like the syrup you put on ice cream"). It is hardly an accident if a child so conditioned downs the entire contents of a common cold product containing salicylates and antihistamine drugs and is poisoned by a product promoted in this way. Another clinical effect of syrups is that their high sugar level can cause problems for diabetic patients. An order for a drug in syrup form for a diabetic patient should be questioned.

Elixirs are hydroalcoholic liquids flavored with volatile oils and slightly sweetened. Adults often prefer

these clear liquids—the cough preparation elixir of terpin hydrate and codeine is an example—to cough mixtures with a heavy viscous syrup base. However, children may find the 15% to 25% or so alcohol content too strong. Thus, it would be best to dilute the dose of an elixir with water before asking a child to take it. Small quantities of water will not precipitate the drug or volatile oils out of the alcohol-based solution. However, when greater dilutions are ordered that *could* upset the delicately adjusted hydroalcoholic balance, the pharmacist uses a combination of low-strength and high-strength hydroalcoholic solutions—isoalcoholic elixir—to adjust the amount of alcohol needed to keep the different drugs in solution. Again, alcohol-based drugs can cause problems with blood sugar control in diabetic patients and should be used with caution in these patients. Patients who are known alcoholics or who are on disulfiram (Antabuse) to help prevent the drinking of alcohol may also have problems taking elixirs; the use of elixirs should probably be avoided in these patients.

Emulsions are mixtures of oil and water made by the artful introduction of certain pharmaceutic agents that keep the oil particles dispersed in tiny droplets throughout the aqueous phase of the emulsion. Like homogenized milk, which is also an emulsion, these pharmaceutic forms can be readily diluted with water if so desired, just prior to administration. The advantage of these products lies in the increased palatability that they give to oily liquids such as mineral oil and cod liver oil—substances that are therefore commonly made available as emulsions.

Gels and *magmas* are more or less viscous suspensions of mineral precipitates in water. The antacid aluminum hydroxide is available as a gel made palatable with sweetening and flavoring substances. Magnesium hydroxide is made available as a magma (milk of magnesia). Preparations of both types, like other mixtures of suspended solids, should be well shaken before use, because the finely divided particles tend to settle out on standing, leaving a layer of clear watery liquid on top. The use of disposable medicine cups is especially desirable in administering such suspensions. Many such preparations come in efficient unit-dose packaging.

Aromatic waters are aqueous solutions saturated with various volatile substances, such as cinnamon oil, spearmint oil, and peppermint. The amount of the oil that dissolves in water is relatively low compared to the quantities contained in alcoholic solutions. However, the flavoring is often adequate as an aid in disguising certain salty substances dissolved in the watery vehicle. Other substances such as iodine and potassium iodide dissolve so readily in water that they are sometimes made available in highly concentrated aqueous solutions containing large amounts of the drug in doses of only a few drops (*e.g,* strong iodine solution and saturated solution of potassium iodide).

---

* An *alcoholic vehicle* is a strongly alcoholic solution capable of dissolving substances such as volatile oils and other principles not soluble in aqueous solutions.

Tinctures are usually made by extracting the useful principles of plants with solvents containing alcohol. Tinctures of therapeutically potent drugs such as opium and belladonna have a drug strength of 10%. That is, 10 ml of a tincture contains the active constituents extracted from 1 g of drug. Thus, for example, if 1 g of opium contains 100 mg of morphine, that amount of the active constituent would be contained in 10 ml of tincture of opium. Similarly, belladonna tincture contains about 30 mg of active constituents such as atropine and hyoscine in 100 ml—the same amount of these alkaloids contained in 10 g of the coarsely powdered leaf from which the tincture is prepared.

Less potent drugs are made into tinctures that contain the active principles of 20 g of drug in every 100 ml. Compound tinctures such as paregoric (camphorated tincture of opium) and compound tincture of benzoin contain amounts of the various active constituents that vary in accordance with traditionally established formulations. (Alcoholic solutions of some nonvegetable chemicals also are called tinctures—*e.g.*, tincture of iodine.)

Fluidextracts are much more concentrated liquid preparations of vegetable drugs. The strength of the alcoholic solution is such that each milliliter contains the active constituents of 1 g of the drug from which it is made. Thus, fluidextract of belladonna contains in 10 ml the 30 mg of extractives that are found in 10 g of powdered belladonna leaf (or in 100 ml of the tincture).

Extracts are concentrated preparations made by evaporating the hydroalcoholic extractive solvents until a syrupy liquid, plastic mass, or dry powder is left. The strength of extracts is adjusted so that they are usually several times stronger than the crude drug itself. Thus, for example, belladonna extracts contain between three and four times the active constituents of the leaf itself.

The patient should be encouraged to drink plenty of fluid after taking oral medication to ensure that it gets to the stomach and into solution. If the drug is being instilled into a feeding tube, remember that water should be given before and after administering the medication. This will ensure that the medication is dissolved adequately for proper absorption.

One of the most important parameters to consider when administering oral medications is the patient's ability to swallow. If a patient has difficulty swallowing, several procedures may help to initiate the swallowing reflex: placing the medication way back on the tongue; applying ice to the tongue and lips before administering the drug; and applying ice to the sternal notch or to the back of the neck (or to both). In some cases, the medication may need to be crushed and administered in soft cold foods—for example jello or applesauce—if considerations of drug–food interactions do not contraindicate this. Soft foods such as these have a consistency that is easy to swallow. Enteric-coated tablets and capsules, and capsules containing timed-release granules, should not be crushed because crushing destroys the special properties of the preparation. If a patient is severely nauseated or has a great deal of difficulty in swallowing and might be at risk for aspirating the medication, a decision has to be made about the route ordered. In such cases, parenteral administration might be necessary.

Parenteral administration. The term "parenteral" means by any route other than the enteral, or gastrointestinal, tract. Taken literally, the term includes methods that involve getting a drug into the bloodstream—for example, by way of the lungs or through the mucous membranes of the mouth. However, as ordinarily used, parenteral routes refer only to various ways by which drugs are given as *injections.*

Injection. Injection of drugs is preferred when it is important that all the drug be absorbed as rapidly and completely as possible or at a steady, controlled rate. It is also the route of choice if the patient is unconscious, cannot swallow, or is extremely nauseated. However, despite the efficiency with which high blood levels of a drug can be quickly attained and also sometimes maintained for prolonged periods, parenteral administration has various drawbacks and disadvantages. Injectable medications that come in sterile ampules, vials, or plastic syringes are relatively expensive compared to oral dosage forms and, of course, the patient usually also has to bear the expense of paying for the skilled person needed to make the injection.

Injection of drugs requires skill and special care because parenteral administration is more hazardous than oral dosage forms. This is mainly the result of the rapidity and efficiency with which drugs are absorbed from most injection sites. The effect of overdosage resulting from an error in calculating and measuring the dose or in administering it is much more likely to prove disastrous when the drug is given parenterally. Once the drug is injected, it is usually difficult—and, in some situations, impossible—to keep it from being fully absorbed and from producing all of its effects, including adverse ones.

Injections may be painful, cause local tissue damage, or permit the entrance of infectious microorganisms. However, all these difficulties can be kept to a minimum by the use of proper equipment and procedures. For example, an injection need not hurt if the needle is sharp and is inserted and withdrawn quickly except, of course, when the injected solution is itself irritating to the tissues. Similarly, infection is unlikely when the medication is furnished in sterile form, the patient's skin is properly cleansed, and the sterility of needles and syringes is ensured.

Parenteral administration employs various routes. Some—such as the subcutaneous, intramuscular, intraperitoneal, and intravenous routes—are used when a drug's systemic actions are desired; others—for example, intracutaneous and intrasynovial injections—are employed for achieving local effects with minimal generalized activity. Some significant aspects of the more commonly employed parenteral methods of administering drugs will now be discussed. Table 3-2 summarizes the equipment needed for different commonly used parenteral routes of administration and clinical aspects to consider.

Medications that are injected have to be sterile and in liquid form. To prevent excessive irritation and damage to the tissues, the drug is usually in a solution that is adjusted to near physiologic pH and osmolality. The drug is injected from a sterile syringe through a sterile needle. The needles vary in diameter (gauge) and length. Generally, the larger the number of the gauge, the smaller the diameter or thickness of the needle. Needle gauges commonly used clinically vary from 14 (the largest size) to 28 (a very tiny needle), and the needles vary in length from ⅜ inch to 4 inches. The gauge and length that should be used are determined by the viscosity and other properties of the drug being injected and by the desired site of drug deposition. Needles are usually made of metal. In some cases a plastic cannula is threaded through the needle to maintain an intravenous line over a long period of time.

One part of the syringe is a hollow cylindric barrel that attaches to the needle; the other part is a plunger used to push the fluid through the needle. In most institutions glass syringes that needed to be washed and sterilized after each use have been replaced by disposable plastic syringes that are sterilized and sealed in a paper envelope. To maintain that sterility, it is essential to open the envelope according to the instructions on it and to handle the syringe only by the outside of the barrel and by the flared back of the plunger. Pushing the tip of the syringe through the envelope or putting fingers on the plunger causes contamination.

To withdraw the solution from the vial or ampule, the needle is immersed in the solution and the plunger is pulled back to draw out the medication by suction. To withdraw a drug solution from a vacuum-sealed bottle, it is first necessary to inject a volume of air equal to or slightly greater than the volume of drug solution to be withdrawn. The solution can then be readily withdrawn from the inverted bottle. Air, which is usually drawn up with the drug solution, must be expelled before injecting the drug.

Intravenous solutions use a bottle or bag connected by a length of tubing to the needle or cannula. Aseptic technique must be used in establishing intravenous lines and, if they are in use for an appreciable length of time, the insertion site must be checked and dressed frequently to decrease the chance of infection at the injection site. Specialized setups are used for special procedures such as hyperalimentation or blood administration. It is important to remember that any time the skin is broken, a possible route for infection is established. Before giving any drug parenterally, the site should be cleansed, usually by using an alcohol swab in a rotating motion from the inside of the target area to the outside. Cleansing the skin helps to decrease the bacteria in the area and is an essential precaution for decreasing the risk of infection.

Intradermal injections. These are made directly below the surface of the skin, superficial to the subcutaneous tissues (Fig. 3-1). These injections are usually used for sensitivity tests—for example, allergy tests or tuber-

Table 3–2. Injection equipment for parenteral medication

Type of injection	Needle		Syringe	Clinical points
	Gauge	Length		
Intradermal	26	⅜ in.	Tuberculin	Area must be marked or mapped if several tests are done
Subcutaneous	25	½ in.	Tuberculin, insulin	Angle of insertion depends on size of patient; sites must be rotated
Intramuscular	20–23	1–3 in.	2–5 ml	Needle gauge depends on consistency of drug; rapid insertion and slow injection help to decrease pain
Intravenous				
Fluid	20, 21		Bottle or IV bag with tubing	Regular careful assessment and cleansing of injection site;
Blood	16, 18		Bottle or bag with appropriate tubing	regular changing of equipment and needle placement

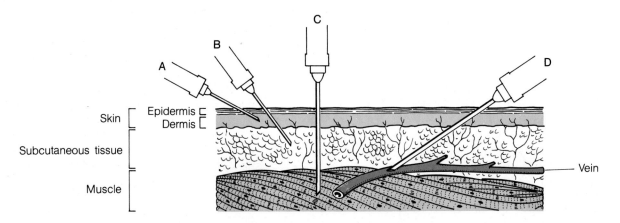

Figure 3-1. Needle insertion for parenteral medication. (*A*) Intradermal injection: a 26-gauge, ⅜-inch long needle is inserted at a 10° to 15° angle. (*B*) Subcutaneous injection: a 25-gauge, ½-inch long needle is inserted at an angle that depends on the size of the patient. (*C*) Intramuscular injection: a 20-gauge to 23-gauge, 1-inch to 3-inch long needle is inserted into the relaxed muscle with a dart-throwing type of hand movement. (*D*) Intravenous injection: the diameter and length of the needle used depend on the substance to be injected and on the site of injection (see text).

culin tests. A very fine 26-gauge ⅜-inch needle on a tuberculin syringe is used for these injections (see Table 3-2). The needle is inserted directly beneath the skin, and the injection produces a wheal or fluid-filled bump that can be seen beneath the skin at the injection site. Because of the nature of these types of injections, the site should be carefully cleansed and marked in some way to allow the reaction to be "read" in 24 to 48 hours. If several injections are made, the skin of the back or forearm is the usual site, and a map of the sites is made in the patient's record. Equipment for performing tuberculin tests now comes in the form of a stamp—a six-pointed needle with tuberculin solution on each tip that is gently pressed into the skin to deposit the solution. This is a quicker and more efficient manner of giving tuberculin tests.

Subcutaneous (hypodermic) injections. These are made into the loose connective tissue underneath the skin (both the above Latin and the Greek-derived terms mean exactly that; Fig. 3-1). Soluble drugs deposited at sites such as the outer surface of the arm or the front of the thigh are ordinarily rapidly absorbed into the blood, and the drug's effects come on promptly. However, if the patient is in shock, or has very poor peripheral circulation, this route is undesirable because the sluggish circulation slows the drug's absorption. The drug solution is best delivered directly into the bloodstream by intravenous (IV) injection in such situations.

Not all drugs are suited to subcutaneous injection. Because no more than 2 ml can ordinarily be deposited at such sites, the drugs given in this way must be highly soluble and potent enough to be effective in small volume. (Epinephrine, morphine, heparin, and insulin are commonly administered in this manner.) The sub-

cutaneous tissues contain nerve endings that transmit pain impulses when the injected solutions are irritating. Sometimes sterile abscesses develop as a result of chemical irritation, and the tissues may become necrotic and slough off.

The usual subcutaneous injection uses a 25-gauge ½-inch-long needle and a tuberculin or thin-barreled 1-ml to 2-ml syringe (see Table 3-2). In giving these injections, an area of the body with enough subcutaneous tissue to "pinch up" is usually selected—the abdomen, upper thigh, or upper arm is generally the best site (Fig. 3-2). The needle is inserted at a 45° angle, the plunger is drawn back to ensure that the needle has not penetrated a vessel and, if no blood returns, the medication is injected. If the patient has a large amount of adipose tissue, a more acute angle of insertion may be needed. In such patients a 90° angle of insertion may be necessary to reach the subcutaneous tissue. When repeated subcutaneous injections must be made—for example, of heparin or insulin—the injection sites must be rotated or changed each time to decrease the risk of abscess or of fibroid formation. Insulin can now be delivered subcutaneously with an external infusion pump that senses glucose levels and delivers a preset amount of insulin when indicated by the patient's blood glucose levels.

Hypodermoclysis. This form of subcutaneous injection permits the slow administration of large amounts of fluids, such as isotonic saline and glucose solutions. A larger bore needle is inserted into the loose tissues to the outer sides of the upper body or into the anterior aspect of the thigh, or elsewhere, and the fluid is slowly infused. Aseptic technique must be carefully observed in these patients because of the large needle used and because of

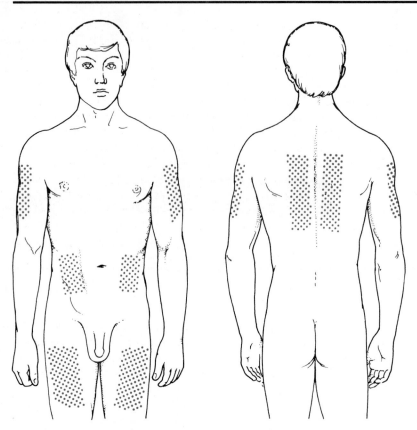

Figure 3-2. Sites on the body at which subcutaneous injections can be given.

its continued presence in the tissues. This procedure helps to counteract thirst in a dehydrated patient unable to take fluids by mouth; however, the amount of fluid that can be administered is self-limited by the pressure of the infused fluid upon the vessels that must absorb it.

Occasionally, the spread of such locally injected fluid is facilitated by adding the enzyme *hyaluronidase* to the hypodermoclysis solution. This enzyme helps to break down one of the main components of the intracellular connective tissues and thus opens up more space for fluid diffusion. These temporary enzyme-induced changes in the intracellular subcutaneous ground substances aid the dispersal of the fluid from the injection site and therefore lessen painful tissue tension. This is particularly useful for infants and young children, but care is required to avoid too rapid absorption with resulting overload of the circulatory system.

Delayed absorption. The rate of absorption from subcutaneous injection sites can sometimes be slowed when a more prolonged action is desired. Addition of the vasoconstrictor epinephrine to local anesthetic solutions, for example, keeps the drug at the desired site of action and reduces the likelihood of systemic toxicity from too rapid absorption. Substances such as insulin may be suspended in a protein colloid solution, and heparin and corticotropin may be administered in gelatin solutions, to reduce the rate of absorption and thus prolong their action. Application of an ice bag above the site of subcutaneous injection slows absorption still further, as does application of a tourniquet in cases in which an adverse reaction occurs.

Intramuscular injections. These are made with a longer heavier needle that penetrates past the subcutaneous tissues and permits the drug solution or suspension to be deposited deep between the layers of muscle masses (Fig. 3-1). A 20-, 21-, 22-, or 23-gauge needle, 1 to 3 inches long, is usually used, depending on the solution being given and on the patient's physical state (see Table 3-2). Watery drug solutions are spread over a larger area than when injected subcutaneously, and absorption is even more rapid than by the latter route. On the other hand, finely divided suspensions of insoluble substances are only very slowly absorbed when deposited in an intramuscular depot (*repository* or *depot* injections). Thus, this route is employed for administering the long-acting esters of sex hormones and corticosteroid drugs or poorly soluble salts, such as benzathine penicillin G and procaine penicillin G, which are absorbed over periods of days or even exert their antibacterial effects for weeks.

Intramuscular (IM) injections can be of a volume

of 1 ml to 5 ml. The IM injection site contains fewer sensory nerve endings than the subcutaneous sites, so that IM injections tend to be less painful. However, with irritating substances, a small amount of the local anesthetics procaine or lidocaine is often added to the injection solution. Irritation is less likely to lead to tissue necrosis deep in the muscle than when irritants are placed under the skin. The danger of inadvertent intravenous injection is greater, though, when the needle is placed deep down into these more vascular muscular tissues. Thus it is essential—especially with oily suspensions of insoluble particles—to ascertain that the needle has not entered a blood vessel by pulling up the plunger after inserting the needle. If blood is aspirated and appears in the syringe, the needle is withdrawn and the injection is given at another site.

Care is also required to avoid injury to nerves when injections are made into the deltoid muscles of the arm, the gluteal muscles of the buttocks, or the vastus lateralis muscles of the thigh. The latter is the safest injection site for infants, because the muscle mass of the gluteal region does not become well developed until about the age of 3 years. Even in older children, the risk of damaging the sciatic nerve makes the buttocks an undesirable injection site. Thus, to avoid possible leg muscle paralysis, the ventrogluteal area is preferred for children as it now often is for adults.

Figure 3-3 presents examples of the various IM injection sites. To minimize pain, the muscle to be injected should be as relaxed as possible. This can best be achieved by positioning the patient so there is the least amount of strain on the muscle to be used. The skin over the site

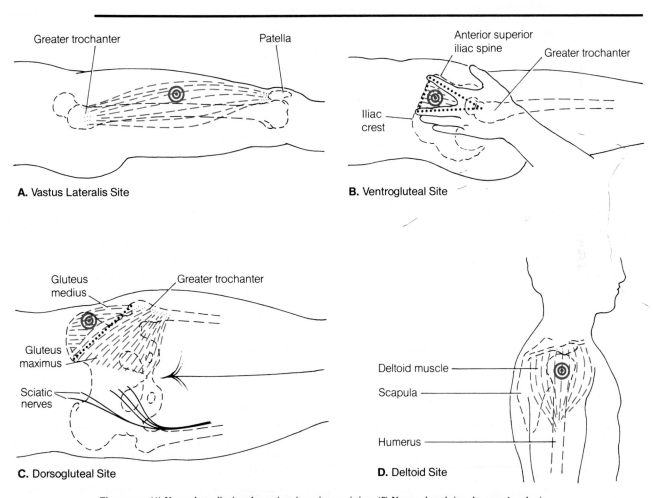

Figure 3-3. (A) Vastus lateralis site: the patient is supine or sitting. (B) Ventrogluteal site: the nurse's palm is placed on the greater trochanter and the index finger is placed on the anterior superior iliac spine; the injection is made into the middle of the triangle formed by the nurse's fingers and the iliac crest. (C) Dorsogluteal site: to avoid the sciatic nerve and accompanying blood vessels, an injection site is chosen above and lateral to a line drawn from the greater trochanter to the posterior superior iliac spine. (D) Deltoid site: the middeltoid area is located by forming a rectangle, the top of which is at the level of the lower edge of the acromion, and the bottom of which is at the level of the axilla; the sides are one-third and two-thirds of the way around the outer aspect of the patient's arm.

is cleansed to prevent the introduction of bacteria; the needle is inserted as quickly as possible, much like throwing a dart; the plunger is pulled back to check for blood; the plunger is pushed in—a slow push will allow the tissue to adjust to a large volume and will help to decrease pain; and the needle is withdrawn and the area is briskly rubbed to increase blood flow to the area to facilitate absorption.

IM injections, or "shots," are often anticipated with fear by children and adults. The treatment can be painful and the patient should be alerted to that possibility. Giving the injection with a swift insertion of the needle and a rather slow push on the plunger can help to decrease the pain. Something to divert the patient's attention is also often helpful. Telling the patient to take a very deep breath and hold it, just as the injection is given, is often enough to distract the patient, and frequently the patient will not even be aware of the injection.

Z-track injections. Some medications, such as iron, are so irritating or staining to the tissues that regular IM injection technique is not adequate. In this situation the skin is prepped and pulled very tightly to one side, the needle is inserted into the muscle, and the drug is injected as the needle is withdrawn slowly and the skin released. This procedure allows the various overlapping layers of tissue to slide back into position in a Z formation, thus sealing off the injected material (Fig. 3-4).

Intravenous injection. This bypasses all barriers to drug absorption. As a result this is the most rapidly effective and, at the same time, the most dangerous route of administration, because once a drug is placed directly into the bloodstream it cannot be recalled, nor can its action be slowed by tourniquets or other means. Thus, every effort must be made to avoid errors and to detect early signs of adverse reactions. This route is usually reserved for the emergency administration of potent drugs

when very rapid action is required. Bolus doses of lidocaine, for example, are injected rapidly by vein to control dangerous cardiac dysrhythmias, and these are then followed by prolonged IV infusion to prevent recurrences.

The procedure for delivering drugs by IV injection involves the use of a tourniquet to trap blood in a vein and to distend it, insertion of the needle into the distended vein, withdrawal of blood to ensure needle placement, release of the tourniquet to allow blood flow within the vein, and then slow injection of the medication directly into the vein (Fig. 3-1).

Sometimes substances that would be very irritating to subcutaneous and intramuscular tissues (highly alkaline sulfonamide sodium salt solutions, for example) are given by slow IV injection, because they do not harm the inner lining of the veins. Care is taken to avoid leakage of such solutions into the surrounding tissues because pain, sterile abscesses, and necrotic sloughing can develop if highly irritating substances or potent local vasoconstrictors such as norepinephrine extravasate.

Infusions of large amounts of fluid are often made by venoclysis to overcome dehydration and to supply nutritive substances if patients are unable to take fluids or foods orally. The technique of inserting the needle into the vein under sterile conditions is similar to that used when small quantities of drug solutions are injected. In this case, however, the rate of flow must be adjusted, and it should be kept at a speed that will avoid overloading the patient's circulation and, at the same time, ensure an adequate delivery of fluids and electrolytes.

The patient's blood volume can be assessed through evaluation of the jugular venous pressure (JVP), skin and mucous membrane hydration, urinary output, and blood pressure and pulses. The IV injection site will need regular monitoring for signs of infection or phlebitis, the formation of clots in the needle or tubing, and dis-

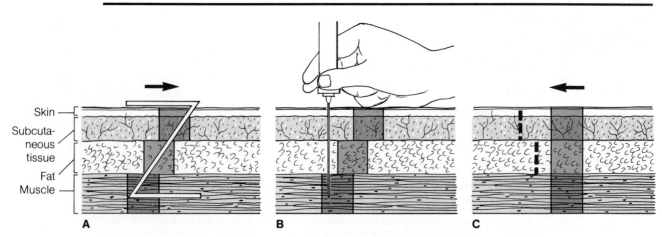

Skin
Subcutaneous tissue
Fat
Muscle

A   **B**   **C**

Figure 3-4. Z-track technique for intramuscular injection. (*A*) The tissue is tensed laterally at the injection site before the needle is inserted, which pulls the skin, subcutaneous tissue, and fat planes into a Z formation. (*B*) After the tissue has been displaced, the needle is thrust straight into the muscle mass. (*C*) After injection, tissues are released while the needle is withdrawn; as each tissue plane slides by the other, the track is sealed.

placement of the needle from the vein and tissue infiltration.

The vein used and the gauge of needle chosen will depend on the solution to be delivered. Blood products require needles with large lumens to prevent mechanical injury to blood cells, while aqueous solutions used to maintain access to a vein (KVO, or "Keep Vein Open") require only small needles (see Table 3-2).

The rate of delivery of fluid has to be set and constantly checked. When using a gravity feed system, some nurses put a long piece of tape marked for each hour on the IV bottle or bag to indicate how much solution should have been infused in a given time period, thus providing a fast and simple check. Infusion pumps— called for example, IVACs or IMEDs—are used in many institutions. These electrical machines sense the number of drops delivered and actively push fluid through IV tubing at a given rate. Many of these pumps are provided with alarms to alert the nurse if a problem develops in the delivery of a predetermined amount of solution.

Other injection sites. Several types of injections are intended to achieve high local concentrations of certain drugs while minimizing their systemic absorption. The following are some examples.

Intrathecal or *intraspinal* injections are made by physicians trained in these special techniques. Spinal anesthesia is achieved by careful placement of a local anesthetic solution in the subarachnoid space. Similarly, anti-infective drugs are sometimes injected intrathecally in the treatment of meningitis to attain a high local concentration of an antibiotic or sulfonamide that does not readily penetrate the subdural and other meningeal spaces by way of the bloodstream.

Intra-articular and *intralesional* injections are employed mainly to attain high local concentrations of corticosteroid drugs within inflamed joints and skin lesions with less danger of causing systemic steroid toxicity. It is important for the physician to employ aseptic procedures to avoid joint infections. Patients must be warned not to overuse the injected joint when their pain is relieved, because this may lead to deterioration of the joint.

Antineoplastic drugs are sometimes given directly into the tumor or into its arterial supply to concentrate the effect of the drug where it is most needed. Pumps are sometimes used to deliver these substances into the liver, spine, joints, kidney, or other organ with an identified malignancy.

Application to mucous membranes. Drugs are often applied to the mucous membranes of the mouth and throat, the nose and other parts of the respiratory tract, the eyes, and the genitourinary and gastrointestinal tracts. In the case of the nose and eyes, such applications are usually intended to have only a local effect. On the other hand, drugs are sometimes brought into contact with the mucosa of the mouth and rectum as a means of getting them into the bloodstream when swallowing the

agents is undesirable or impossible. The dosage forms that are administered either for absorption into the systemic circulation through a mucosal surface or for a topical or local effect at the site of contact of the drug with a mucous membrane are both discussed.

Rectal administration. Drugs in the form of enema solutions and glycerinated gelatin or cocoa butter-based suppositories are commonly employed for local effects as well as for getting drugs into the systemic circulation when the oral route cannot or should not be used. Such situations may occur if the patient is comatose, the drug is destroyed by GI enzymes, the patient cannot swallow, or the stomach is severely diseased.

The best time for administering drugs rectally is immediately after the patient has moved his bowels. The lower tract may be emptied by administering an evacuant enema or by the use of suppositories that act locally to set off the defecation reflex. After the lower bowel has been cleansed, the suppository or the retention enema containing the dose of the drug for systemic absorption and action is inserted, and the patient is kept lying down for at least 20 minutes in the case of a suppository and about 30 minutes for an enema. If the patient gets up too soon, the unmelted suppository may be evacuated or the unabsorbed enema fluid may be expelled. The patient should lie still and breathe deeply to help prevent loss of the medication.

One drug commonly administered rectally is aminophylline, a substance that often causes gastric distress when given by mouth. It must be noted, however, that this drug—like the organic mercurial suppositories, which are also given in this way—may cause rectal irritation in some patients. Solutions are less likely to cause local irritation and inflammation because they are absorbed more rapidly and completely than is the material erratically released from suppository bases. On the other hand, the amount of fluid that can be retained is relatively small, and the more rapidly absorbed drug may have too fleeting an action.

Rectal administration of depressant drugs is sometimes employed to put children to sleep prior to general anesthesia with other agents. Thiopental sodium, for example, is available as a rectal suspension for producing preanesthetic hypnosis or basal narcosis, and is administered by the use of a disposable plastic syringe and applicator. Antiemetic drugs such as prochlorperazine (Compazine) are commonly administered as rectal suppositories, because the vomiting patient may not be able to retain these drugs when they are given by mouth.

Inhalation. Drugs are often administered by inhalation into the deeper respiratory tract passages, either to produce high local concentrations of the drug or to produce systemic drug effects. Locally active drugs include the mucolytic detergents, enzymes, and other substances employed as aerosols (or instilled as solutions) to liquefy thick secretions obstructing the bronchi, and bronchodilator drugs such as epinephrine and isoproterenol. Unfortunately, the actions of these drugs are not always limited to the respiratory tract. Epinephrine and isoproterenol can both be absorbed into the systemic circulation by this route—isoproterenol can cause serious cardiac irregularities, and epinephrine also has unwanted systemic effects, including a tendency to make patients jittery and tremulous. Drugs that are intended to pass through the thin lining of the lung surfaces include not only oxygen and volatile general anesthetics, such as ether, but also the coronary vasodilator drug, amyl nitrite, whose vapor is inhaled by angina pectoris patients, and ergotamine, which has sometimes been given by this route to abort a migraine headache. The tremendous surface area of the lungs makes the inhalation route of administration one of the fastest ways to get drugs with appropriate physicochemical properties into the systemic circulation.

Many drugs used in the treatment of chronic lung diseases are delivered through inhalation therapy. Positive pressure inhalators are often used to disperse small droplets of the drug deep into the lungs. Patients often self-administer their drugs using a hand-held inhaler. Each brand of inhaler works slightly differently, and the patient needs instruction in the proper use of the inhaler prescribed to ensure that the correct amount of the drug is delivered with each use.

Mouth and throat. The mucous membranes of the mouth and throat are often treated with local applications of antiseptic, anesthetic, and astringent drugs. The public is subjected to much misleading advertising for nonprescription mouth washes, gargles, throat lozenges or troches, and medicated chewing gums. Much of the folklore of mouth and throat therapy must be discounted. However, oral hygiene is a very important part of patient care. The most effective oral hygiene is generally done with a tooth brush, dental floss, and clear water, used consistently.

The throat is sometimes sprayed with local anesthetics during surgical or diagnostic procedures. In this way, sensory receptors are deadened to avoid gagging and thus permit passage of instruments such as endotracheal tubes, laryngoscopes, and bronchoscopes. Topically applied anesthetics may be absorbed systemically in amounts that can prove toxic; thus, amounts of solution being employed in this way should be carefully recorded to ensure that safe amounts are not exceeded.

Sublingual tablets. These are placed under the tongue, where they dissolve rapidly and are absorbed by way of the venous capillaries. This prevents drugs from being destroyed by gastric digestive juices or by the enzymes of the liver, when the drug is carried there from the upper gastrointestinal tract by the portal system. *Nitroglycerin* is the most important drug administered in this manner. Taken in this way by a person who is suffering the chest pains of angina pectoris, this drug's effects begin to come on within 1 minute, and the patient ordinarily

experiences quick relief. However, patients taking sublingual tablets must be instructed in how to use them properly. The tablet should never be chewed, but should be placed under the tongue until it dissolves. The patient will experience a "fizzing" or tingling sensation under the tongue. If no sensation is experienced, the drug may be outdated or may be ineffective for some other reason.

Buccal tablets. Patients taking these tablets, which are held in the mouth to attain effects by way of the systemic circulation, must also be shown how to employ them correctly. Like sublingual tablets, these must not be chewed or swallowed. Buccal tablets are best placed next to the upper molar teeth, and the patient is instructed to avoid disturbing them after placement in the parabuccal space. As with sublingual tablets, the patient avoids eating, chewing, drinking, or smoking, lest the tablet be swallowed and destroyed instead of being absorbed by way of the mucosa of the buccal pouch between gums and cheek. The polypeptide hormone *oxytocin* is sometimes administered in this manner in obstetrics.

Nasal administration. The nasal mucosa is commonly treated with drug solutions applied as sprays, nose drops, and tampons. Among the drugs applied in this way are decongestants for opening blocked nasal passages and hemostatics to stop nosebleeds. Here, too, the public is often led to expect too much from such topical application, with the result that nonprescription preparations are misused in ways that can prove harmful. The nurse should be familiar with the correct procedure for instilling drops into the nose so that they do not pass into the throat, where they may be swallowed or absorbed systemically. Systemic absorption of the drugs contained in nasal medications can have adverse effects on the cardiovascular and central nervous systems.

Nose drops are administered directly into the nose with the patient's head tilted back. The position is maintained for a few seconds and then the patient is encouraged to lean forward, with the head down, which helps to spread the medication over the mucosa. In contrast to nose drops, most nasal sprays are designed to be used with the head in the upright position. Tilting the head backward can cause the drug to run into the throat, from where it may be absorbed into the systemic circulation.

Drugs may also be purposely applied to the nasal mucosa to produce systemic effects. *Oxytocin* and *vasopressin*, another polypeptide hormone of the posterior pituitary gland, are sometimes administered this way, because they would be digested and inactivated if taken by mouth. Patients with diabetes insipidus, for example, often take vasopressin in the form of snuff. Similarly, the synthetic form of oxytocin is now available as a spray that is absorbed into the systemic circulation when applied intranasally. Among drug abusers, cocaine users often sniff the drug, and early experimenters with heroin sometimes begin by "snorting" it. People experimenting with the hallucinogenic effects of various household substances have been known to sniff the vapors of glue, lighter fluid, paint thinner, and other such volatile substances.

Genitourinary tract. Medication applied to the genitourinary tract is usually intended for local effect, but drugs can reach the systemic circulation by being absorbed from the urethral or vaginal mucosa. Dangerously high plasma concentrations of local anesthetics, for example, have been reached when solutions were instilled into a traumatized urethra prior to passage of a sound or cystoscope. Urethral suppositories containing soothing substances are sometimes employed after dilatation or other painful procedures. Vaginal suppositories containing estrogens combined with anti-infective drugs are applied in cases of vaginitis, and irrigating solutions, or douches, are sometimes instilled to cleanse and to acidify the vaginal mucosa. Contraceptive creams and foams are often prescribed for vaginal instillation.

Vaginal medications are available as suppositories, to be inserted directly into the vagina with an applicator or a gloved hand; as douche solutions, either in a unit-dose disposable applicator or in a solution to be administered as irrigation using a vaginal probe and an irrigation unit; or as creams, gels, or foams, to be inserted using a specially designed applicator. Vaginal instillation of suppositories, creams, and gels is more successful if the patient remains lying down for a period of time after administration. Such patients should be advised to wear a pad to prevent the staining of clothes or bed linen if medication drains out.

Topical administration

Dermal (skin) medications. Drugs are not ordinarily absorbed through the skin. However, measurable amounts of nitroglycerin reach the bloodstream when an ointment containing this drug is rubbed into the skin. Poisoning from organic phosphates has occurred when workers applying these insecticides have neglected to put on protective garments, and dermal absorption of the liquid alkaloid nicotine has also caused poisoning. Although small amounts of salicylates may be absorbed through the skin, not enough reach the systemic circulation to produce an antirheumatic action. The advertising for some creams that are rubbed on the skin to relieve arthritic pain suggests that their active ingredients are absorbed into the joints. However, whatever effects such products may have (in addition to those that are psychological) are limited mainly to the local skin areas to which they are applied.

The skin is treated locally with liquid lotions and liniments and with semisolid ointments and pastes containing oily bases such as petrolatum or lanolin, or with water-miscible bases such as surface-active, or wetting, agents. The dermatologist chooses the dosage form and bases that are best suited for application to the particular area and skin condition that require treatment.

Lotions and ointments are best applied in small amounts to avoid both waste and messiness. Applications are made gently, by patting rather than rubbing, to avoid damaging irritated, inflamed areas. A firm stroke is desirable, because too lightly dabbing the pruritic skin tends to increase itchiness. If the preparation is one that stains clothing, the patient should be warned about it and advised to avoid having the medication come into contact with clothing or, if this is not possible, to wear old clothes during the treatment period. Ointments should be removed from jars with a tongue blade and never with the fingers to avoid contaminating the remainder of the contents.

Compresses are moist dressings made by soaking sterile towels in plain water or in solutions of chemicals such as potassium permanganate or aluminum acetate that exert astringent and drying effects when the cloths are wrung out and applied to oozing skin lesions. Poultices are mainly home remedies made by mixing absorptive substances such as bread crumbs, linseed meal, or kaolin with boiling water or glycerin. The moist mass is then spread on inflamed skin areas to keep constant heat on the affected part.

The fact that the skin acts as a barrier is an advantage when corticosteroid drugs are applied to the skin to relieve the symptoms of local inflammation. Applied as ointments, creams, lotions, and aerosols, these steroid drugs relieve itching, oozing, and other discomfort without causing their characteristic systemic toxicity. However, when corticosteroid preparations are applied to large areas of skin, particularly when occlusive dressings are used, appreciable amounts of the steroid may be absorbed.

The nurse who is applying a topical medication repeatedly over an extended period of time should take precautions to avoid personal skin absorption of the medication. It is best to avoid skin contact by using a glove, tongue blade, or dressing gauze to apply the medication.

Some medications can now be applied topically using *dermal patches* that provide a slow sustained release of the medication. Nitroglycerin patches are available for angina patients, and scopolamine, a drug used to prevent motion sickness, can be applied using a patch that slowly releases the drug over a 3-day period.

Ophthalmic (eye) medications. Drugs are instilled directly into the eye for diagnostic tests, treatment of irritation and infections, removal of irritating foreign particles, and therapy of ophthalmic disorders such as glaucoma. Because the eyes are so susceptible to infection, extreme care should be taken to avoid any contamination of the eyes during drug administration. The ointment or solution being used should be kept sterile, aseptic technique should be used, and different applicators should be used for each eye, where appropriate, to avoid cross contamination.

To instill eye drops, the patient tilts the head back while the nurse exposes the lower conjunctival sac by applying gentle pulling pressure at a point slightly below the lower lid. The drops are instilled into the area between the eyeball and the lower lid and, after a moment, the patient gently closes the eye. Squeezing the eye shut will force the medication out of the eye. If the drug being administered is one with possible toxic systemic effects, pressure should be exerted and maintained on the inner canthus of the eye during and for a short time after administration of the drug. This pressure will prevent the drug from entering the nasolacrimal duct and from being absorbed into the systemic circulation.

Ophthalmic ointments are applied in much the same way. Once the conjunctival sac is exposed, a thin line of ointment is applied along the inner edge of the eye lid. The eye is then closed and the area is gently rubbed with a cotton swab to distribute the ointment throughout the area.

Otic (ear) medications. Medication is instilled directly into the ear canal for antibiotic, antifungal, antiinflammatory, and local anesthetic effects. The solutions should be as close to body temperature as possible before instillation, because extremes of temperature can cause an overstimulation of the auditory nerve, resulting in a sensation of vertigo. The patient should be lying down on one side with the ear to be treated uppermost, and should stay in this position for a short time following administration of the drug to prolong the length of time the medication remains in the ear canal.

Calculating drug dosage

The correct dosage of a drug for a particular patient should be determined by consideration of the patient's age, weight, physical state, and other drugs that the patient is receiving. Frequently, the dose that is ordered is not a dose that is available and, to convert the dosage form available into the prescribed dose, mathematical calculations have to be made.

Systems of measurement. Prescriptions may be written in the metric, apothecary, or household system of measurement. In some instances, prescriptions may even contain a combination of measurements from two or more systems. The system that is used depends, for the most part, on the preference of whoever is ordering the drug. Drugs are conventionally supplied worldwide in metric system dosages. The conversion of the amount of drug ordered into the available measurement form is the responsibility of the pharmacist or of the person administering the drug. The nurse who administers the drug should recalculate any drug dosage that is provided in a form different from that ordered. This provides one more safety check in the system and legally covers the nurse to ensure safe drug administration. Table 3-3 presents the basic units of each measuring system.

Metric system. In this system the basic measure of mass is the *gram* (g); the basic measure of capacity is the *liter*. These basic units are multiplied by 10 or by 1/10 to arrive at larger or smaller units. Appropriate Latin or Greek prefixes specify the multiples, making calculations within the metric system easy, once the basics are learned. The clinically important prefixes, which should be memorized, are also shown in Table 3-3 (*kilo* = 1,000 times; *centi* = 1/100th [0.01]; *milli* = 1/1,000th [0.001]; and *micro* = 1/1,000,000th, [0.000001]).

Both the gram and the liter are related to the basic measure of length in the metric system, the *meter*

Table 3–3. Basic units of the three systems of measurement

System	Measures of mass	Measures of volume
Metric	gram (g) 1 milligram (mg) = 0.001 g 1 microgram (μg) = 0.000001 g 1 kilogram (kg) = 1000 g	liter 1 milliliter (ml) = 0.001 liter 1 ml = 1 cubic centimeter (cc) = 1 cm^3
Apothecary	grain (gr) 60 grains (gr) = 1 dram (dr)* 8 drams (dr) = 1 ounce (oz)*	minim (min) 60 minims (min) = 1 fluidram (f dr)* 8 fluidrams (f dr) = 1 fluidounce (f oz)*
Household	pound (lb) 1 pound (lb) = 16 ounces	pint (pt) 2 pints (pt) = 1 quart (qt) 4 quarts (qt) = 1 gallon (gal) 16 ounces (oz) = 1 pint (pt) = 2 cups (C) 32 tablespoons (tbsp) = 1 pint (pt) 3 teaspoons (tsp) = 1 tablespoon (tbsp) 60 drops (qtt) = 1 teaspoon (tsp)

* Sometimes the apothecary system uses special symbols to abbreviate units: drams (ʒ), ounces (℥), fluidrams (fʒ), and fluidounces (f℥).

(*m*—hence, the name "metric" for the entire system). (One meter is approximately equal to 39 inches in the system of linear measure more familiar to most Americans.) The liter is essentially equal to the volume contained in a cube 0.1 m on a side. The milliliter (*ml;* 0.001 liter) is essentially equal to the volume contained in a cube 1 centimeter (*cm;* 0.01 m) on a side. One milliliter (ml) and one cubic centimeter (cc, or cm³) are thus essentially equal. The word "essentially" has been used to qualify some of the equivalencies above because the liter and milliliter are actually very slightly greater than the capacities of the cubes described above. In clinical practice, these slight differences do not need to be taken into account: 1 ml = 1 cm³ = 1 cc. The gram, the basic measure of mass, is the weight of 1 ml or 1 cm³ of water at standard conditions of temperature and pressure.

Apothecary system. This is an old system of measurement that is now rarely used, but that should be understood when encountered. Some older physicians who are used to this system continue to write prescriptions using it. The basic measure of mass is the *grain* (gr); the basic measure of capacity is the *minim* (min). Interestingly, these two measures are related. The grain was based on the weight of a single grain of wheat; the minim was based on the volume of water that would weigh one grain. Larger units of measure have different names, as shown in Table 3-3.

Household system. This is the system of measuring mass and volume used in most American households. Recipes in American cookbooks use this system, and most households have appropriate devices available for making these measurements. The basic measure of mass is the *pound* (lb), but measures of capacity are expressed as drops, teaspoons, tablespoons, cups, pints, quarts, and gallons (Table 3-3). It is convenient for a patient who is to self-administer a liquid drug at home to be given instructions in terms of household measures. However, a problem could arise because the silverware teaspoon or tablespoon, or the teacup, that may be used could differ considerably in capacity from the standard or "measuring" teaspoon or cup that the prescriber assumes will be used. For example, a silverware teaspoon may hold anywhere from ¾ to 1½ measuring teaspoonsful. To avoid under- or overdosing, patients need to be instructed to use proper, standardized measuring devices.

Table 3-4 lists some of the accepted equivalents between the three systems. Memorizing the whole table would be a very cumbersome task, but the most commonly used equivalents should be learned and will no doubt become very well known with use. As with any other aspect of drug therapy, if there are any doubts, always check the facts with an appropriate reference book.

Conversions from one system to another. The simplest way to convert measurements from one system to another is to set up a proportion equation. Put the ratio containing the two known equivalent amounts on

Table 3–4. Accepted conversions between systems of measurement

Metric	Household	Apothecary
Mass		
1 kg	2.2 lb	
454 g	1.0 lb	
1 g = 1000 mg		15 gr (gr xv)*
60 mg		1 gr (gr i)*
30 mg		½ gr (gr ss)*
Volume		
1 liter = 1000 ml	Approximately 1 qt	
240 ml	1 C	8 f oz (f℥ viii)*
30 ml	2 tbsp	1 f oz (f℥ i)*
15–16 ml	1 tbsp = 3 tsp	4 f dr (f℥ iv)*
8 ml	2 tsp	2 f dr (f℥ ii)*
4–5 ml	1 tsp = 60 drops	1 f dr (f℥ i)*
1 ml		15–16 min (min xv or xvi)*
0.06 ml		1 min (min i)*

* In the apothecary system, units are usually placed before the quantity, and the quantity is expressed in small Roman numerals. The quantity ½ is expressed as ss, an abbreviation for the Latin *semis*, one-half.

one side of the equation, and put the ratio containing the amount you wish to convert and its unknown equivalent on the other side. (There are other valid ways of setting up this equation, but only one method is shown here.)

For example, you would like to convert 6 f oz (apothecary system of measure) to the metric system of measure. Checking the table of conversions (Table 3-4), you see that 1 f oz is equivalent to 30 ml. Write these equivalents as a ratio on the left side of the equation, then write as a ratio on the right side of the equation the amount you wish to convert (6 f oz) and its unknown equivalent (?):

$$\frac{1\ f\ oz}{30\ ml} = \frac{6\ f\ oz}{?}$$

Because fluidounces are in the numerator—that is, "on top" on the left side of the equation—fluidounces must also be in the numerator on the right side of the equation. The above equation may be read as: "One f oz is to 30 ml as 6 f oz are to how many milliliters?" That is, because 1 f oz is equivalent to 30 ml, how many milliliters would be found in 6 f oz? The first step in finding the answer is to cross multiply:

$$\frac{1 \text{ f oz}}{30 \text{ ml}} \times \frac{6 \text{ f oz}}{?}$$

$$30 \text{ ml} \times 6 \text{ f oz} = 1 \text{ f oz} \times ?$$

You can also write this as

$$(30 \text{ ml})(6 \text{ f oz}) = (1 \text{ f oz})(?)$$

Multiplying the numbers, you obtain

$$(180)(\text{ml})(\text{f oz}) = (1)(\text{f oz})(?)$$

Rearranging terms, to let the unknown stand alone on one side of the equation, gives

$$? = \frac{(180)(\text{ml})(\cancel{\text{f oz}})}{(1)(\cancel{\text{f oz}})}$$

Whenever possible, cancel out numbers as well as units of measure. In the above equation, cancelling leaves

$$? = 180 \text{ ml}$$

By cancelling out the units of measure, you are left with the appropriate amount and unit of measure. The answer is that 6 f oz are equivalent to 180 ml.

Another example may help to clarify the process. You must convert 32 gr (apothecary system) to the metric system and express it in milligrams. From the conversion table, you find that 1 gr is equivalent to 60 mg. In solving equations with one unknown, called "?" in the first example above, the unknown is more commonly expressed as "x" rather than as "?". Hence,

$$\frac{1 \text{ gr}}{60 \text{ mg}} = \frac{32 \text{ gr}}{x}$$

$$(x)(1 \text{ gr}) = (32 \text{ gr})(60 \text{ mg})$$

$$(x)(1 \text{ gr}) = (1920)(\text{gr})(\text{mg})$$

$$x = \frac{(1920)(\cancel{\text{gr}})(\text{mg})}{(1)(\cancel{\text{gr}})}$$

$$x = 1920 \text{ mg}$$

The answer is that 32 gr are equivalent to 1920 mg.

Being able to follow these examples is inadequate preparation for the nursing intervention of drug administration. You must be able to do these calculations on your own. (You may practice calculating conversions with the conversion problems shown in Appendix A, Practice Problems in Dosage and Solutions.)

Oral dosage problems

Solid dosage forms. Frequently, tablets or capsules for oral administration are not available in the exact dose ordered. In these cases, the nurse who is administering the drug must calculate the number of tablets or capsules that are needed to make up the desired dose. Another proportion equation can be used. Again, the ratio containing the two known equivalent amounts is put on one side of the equation, and the ratio containing the unknown is put on the other side. In this case, the known equivalents are the amount of drug available in one tablet or capsule; the unknown amount is the number of tablets to give for the prescribed dose:

$$\frac{\text{amount of drug available}}{\text{one tablet}} = \frac{\text{amount of drug prescribed}}{\text{number of tablets to give}}$$

Because "amount of drug" is in the numerator on the left side of the equation, "amount of drug" must also be in the numerator on the right side of the equation.

For example, an order is written for 10 gr of aspirin. The tablets available each contain 5 gr. How many tablets should you give?

$$\frac{5 \text{ gr}}{1 \text{ tablet}} = \frac{10 \text{ gr}}{x}$$

Cross multiplying gives

$$(5 \text{ gr})(x) = (10 \text{ gr})(1 \text{ tablet})$$

Cancelling numbers and units of measure, after rearranging, gives

$$x = \frac{(\cancel{10 \text{ gr}})^2 (1 \text{ tablet})}{(\cancel{5 \text{ gr}})_1}$$

$$x = 2 \text{ tablets}$$

The desired dose of 10 gr is contained in two tablets, so you should give two tablets.

Sometimes calculations involving more than one equation are necessary. For example, an order is written for the antimicrobial drug, sulfisoxazole (Gantrisin), 2 g. The tablets available each contain 5 gr. How many tablets should you give? The first step is a conversion calculation, because the dose ordered and the amount of drug in each of the tablets available are in two different systems of measure. You could either convert the desired dose from the metric to the apothecary system, or convert the amount of drug in the tablets from the apothecary to the metric system. In the latter case, you would need to calculate the number of grams of Gantrisin in each 5-gr tablet, and you would proceed as follows:

From Table 3-4, you learn that 1 gram is equivalent to 15 grains; thus,*

$$\frac{1 \text{ gram}}{15 \text{ grains}} = \frac{x}{5 \text{ grains}}$$

Cross multiplying gives

$$(15 \text{ grains})(x) = (1 \text{ gram})(5 \text{ grains})$$

$$x = \frac{(1 \text{ gram})(\overset{1}{\cancel{5}} \text{ grains})}{(\underset{3}{\cancel{15}})(\text{grains})}$$

$$x = \tfrac{1}{3} \text{ gram}$$

That is, each tablet contains ⅓ gram of Gantrisin.

The next step is to calculate how many tablets are needed for the prescribed dose of 2 grams. You must write and solve a second equation:

$$\frac{\tfrac{1}{3} \text{ gram}}{1 \text{ tablet}} = \frac{2 \text{ gram}}{x}$$

$$\frac{x \text{ gram}}{3} = (2)(\text{gram})(1)(\text{tablet})$$

$$x \,(\text{gram}) = (3)(2)(\text{gram})(\text{tablet})$$

$$x = \frac{6 \,(\text{gram})(\text{tablet})}{(\text{gram})}$$

$$x = 6 \text{ tablets}$$

The desired dose of 2 g of Gantrisin is contained in six tablets. You should give six tablets—and that's a lot to ask a patient to swallow!

Practice in calculating drug doses on your own is also necessary. You can find some practice problems in Appendix A, Practice Problems in Dosage and Solutions.

Practical considerations. One point to consider when calculating the desired number of capsules or tablets is that sometimes the answer will be a fraction—for example, ½ tablet. Many tablets are manufactured with a scoring line or indentation through the middle to facilitate halving the tablet. If, however, the desired amount turns out to be ⅓ or ¼ of a tablet, there is a problem: it is impossible to cut a tablet into these fractional parts accurately. The tablet will break apart and some parts will turn to powder, making it impossible to tell how much of the tablet is being administered. Breaking the tablet up also changes the way that it is dissolved and absorbed

in the stomach, so the actual dosage the patient receives cannot be known exactly. Capsules cannot be divided at all. If, therefore, the desired dosage works out to be a fraction of a capsule, or a fraction other than ½ tablet, the pharmacist should be consulted to determine if the drug is available in another dosage form. Otherwise, whoever wrote the order must be consulted to determine if a different dose or drug may be substituted.

Liquid dosage forms. Oral drugs are also supplied in various liquid forms, either as solutions or suspensions. Liquid oral dosage forms are routinely used for pediatric patients or for those who have difficulty swallowing tablets or capsules. They are also used for drugs that cannot be prepared in tablet or capsule form. The principles used to calculate the number of tablets to give may also be used to calculate the volume of liquid drug to give. That is, a proportion equation is set up, with the ratio containing the known equivalents on the left side of the equation and the ratio containing the unknown on the right. The ratio on the left is an expression of the concentration of the drug available, which is given on the label of the bottle:

$$\frac{\text{amount of drug available}}{\text{volume available}} = \frac{\text{amount of drug prescribed}}{\text{volume to give}}$$

Because "amount of drug" is in the numerator on the left, "amount of drug" must also be in the numerator on the right.

For example, an order is written for 250 mg of sulfisoxazole (Gantrisin), the antimicrobial drug ordered in oral tablet form in the previous example. The label on the bottle states that the solution contains 125 mg/5 ml. To calculate the dose, you set up the following equation:

$$\frac{125 \text{ mg}}{5 \text{ ml}} = \frac{250 \text{ mg}}{x}$$

where x is the volume (in milliliters) to give.

$$x(125 \text{ mg}) = (5 \text{ ml})(250 \text{ mg})$$

$$x = \frac{(5 \text{ ml})(\overset{2}{\cancel{250}} \text{ mg})}{(\cancel{125})(\text{mg})}$$

$$x = 10 \text{ ml}$$

Thus, you should give the patient 10 ml of Gantrisin.

Parenteral medications. All drugs administered parenterally must be in liquid form. The nurse responsible for administering the drug will need to calculate the correct dose of the drug and to determine the volume that needs to be given. The same basic calculation is performed

---

* When working with two different units of measure that have similar abbreviations, such as grams (g) and grains (gr) in this example, you can avoid dangerous confusion by writing out the units of measure.

as for calculating oral liquid dosage above—that is, the following equation can be used:

$$\frac{\text{amount of drug available}}{\text{volume available}} = \frac{\text{amount of drug prescribed}}{\text{volume of drug to give}}$$

For example, an order is written for 75.0 mg of meperidine (Demerol, a pain relief medication, called pethidine in much of the world outside the United States), IM. The vial states Demerol, 1.0 ml = 50.0 mg.

$$\frac{50.0 \text{ mg}}{1 \text{ ml}} = \frac{75.0 \text{ mg}}{x}$$

$$x(50.0 \text{ mg}) = (1 \text{ ml})(75.0 \text{ mg})$$

$$x = \frac{(1 \text{ ml})(\overset{3}{\cancel{75.0 \text{ mg}}})}{(\underset{2}{\cancel{50.0 \text{ mg}}})}$$

$$x = \frac{3 \text{ ml}}{2}$$

$$x = 1.5 \text{ ml}$$

You would inject 1.5 ml Demerol solution IM to carry out the drug order.

Intravenous solutions. Intravenous (IV) therapy is used to provide a constant infusion of fluids, electrolytes, nutrients, or drugs into a vein. These substances must be delivered at a prescribed rate, usually a given number of milliliters per hour. When a gravity-feed apparatus is used for IV therapy, the nurse who is responsible needs to calculate the drop rate from the bottle that will deliver the solution to the patient at the prescribed rate. The easiest formula to use to calculate this drop rate is

drops per minute

$$= \frac{(\text{ml of solution prescribed/hr}) \times (\text{drops/ml})}{60 \text{ min/hr}}$$

The number of drops/ml, called the "drop factor," is determined by the IV equipment being used. Most institutions provide a macrodrip set that delivers large drops, often 10 drops to 15 drops/ml, and a microdrip set that delivers 60 drops/ml. The latter is used to meter low rates of flow accurately. It is imperative to determine (from the packaging) the drop factor for the IV set you will use, and to calculate the flow rate using this drop factor. For example, an order is written for a patient to receive 400 ml of D-5-W (dextrose 5% in water) over a 4-hour period. This is equal to 100 ml/hour. The IV equipment is a macrodrip set with a drop factor of 15.

Therefore,

$$x = \frac{(100 \text{ ml}/1 \text{ hr}) \times (15 \text{ drops/ml})}{60 \text{ min/hr}}$$

In the above equation, x is the number of drops per minute, the rate that you will set by adjusting the valve below the bottle on the IV equipment you are using.

$$x = \frac{\dfrac{(100 \text{ ml})}{\text{hr}} \times \dfrac{(15 \text{ drops})}{\text{ml}}}{\dfrac{60 \text{ min}}{\text{hr}}}$$

$$x = \frac{\dfrac{1500 \text{ drops}}{\text{hr}}}{\dfrac{60 \text{ min}}{\text{hr}}}$$

To divide fractions, the divisor $\left(\text{denominator, or "what's on the bottom"—here, } \dfrac{60 \text{ min}}{\text{hr}}\right)$ is inverted and multiplied.

$$x = \frac{\overset{25}{\cancel{1500}} \text{ drops}}{\cancel{\text{hr}}} \times \frac{\cancel{\text{hr}}}{\underset{1}{\cancel{60} \text{ min}}}$$

$$x = 25 \text{ drops/min}$$

You will deliver the correct amount of D-5-W to the patient if you set the equipment to deliver 25 drops/minute and maintain this rate of flow for 4 hours.

Often, drugs are administered into an already established IV line (Fig. 3-5). This can be accomplished in several different ways, depending on the type of IV set that has been used for the established IV line. Secondary intravenous chambers are chambers in the tubing between the bottle and patient into which medication can be injected (using sterile technique) with a needle and syringe. The medication is then flushed into the vein by the solution in the secondary chamber (Fig. 3-5A). Other IV setups have a Y connection in the tubing between the bottle and patient. One arm of the Y is connected to the original IV bottle; the other arm can be connected to a secondary or "piggybacked" bottle that contains medication. Flow from the original or primary bottle is shut off while the solution in the piggybacked bottle runs in (Fig. 3-5B). The rate of infusion from the secondary chamber or piggybacked bottle is determined in the same way as IV infusion rates calculated above. For example,

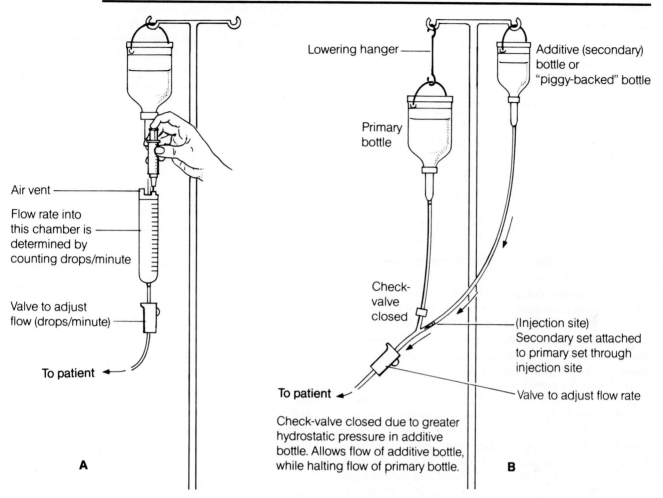

Figure 3-5. Administration of medication into an already established intravenous line. (*A*) The drug is injected into a secondary chamber located between the bottle of solution and the patient. (*B*) The drug is administered from a secondary or ''piggy-backed'' bottle into an established intravenous line.

an order is written for a patient to receive 50 ml of a particular antibiotic IV over a 30-minute period. The secondary chamber (piggybacked bottle) has a microdrip setup with a drop factor of 60 drops/ml:

$$x = \frac{50 \text{ ml}/0.5 \text{ hr} \times 60 \text{ drops/ml}}{60 \text{ min/hr}}$$

$$x = \frac{\dfrac{50 \text{ ml}}{0.5 \text{ hr}} \times \dfrac{60 \text{ drops}}{\text{ml}}}{\dfrac{60 \text{ min}}{\text{hr}}}$$

$$x = \frac{\dfrac{3000 \text{ drops}}{0.5 \text{ hr}}}{\dfrac{60 \text{ min}}{\text{hr}}}$$

$$x = \frac{\overset{100}{\underset{3000}{\cancel{\underset{6000}{\cancel{3000}}}}} \text{ drops}}{0.5 \text{ hr}} \times \frac{\text{hr}}{60 \text{ min}}$$

$$x = 100 \text{ drops/min}$$

The correct amount of antibiotic will be delivered if you set the IV bottle to deliver 100 drops/minute and continue the flow for 30 minutes. (Practice problems can be found in Appendix A, Practice Problems in Dosage and Solutions.)

Drugs ordered in units. Heparin, insulin, tetanus toxoid, and penicillin are commonly used drugs that are measured in units instead of in one of the systems of measure described previously. Units are handled in the same way as other measures. For example, an order is written for 5000 units of heparin, subcutaneous (SC). The heparin is stocked in vials of 20,000 units/ml. You need to calculate how much to give. You can set up an equation here as you did for calculating the amount of liquid drugs to give:

$$\frac{\text{amount of drug available}}{\text{volume available}} = \frac{\text{amount of drug prescribed}}{\text{volume to give}}$$

$$\frac{20,000 \text{ units}}{1 \text{ ml}} = \frac{5,000 \text{ units}}{x}$$

$$x(20,000 \text{ units}) = (1 \text{ ml})(5,000 \text{ units})$$

$$x = \frac{(1 \text{ ml})(\cancel{5,000} \text{ units})}{\underset{4}{(\cancel{20,000} \text{ units})}}$$

$$x = \frac{1 \text{ ml}}{4} \text{ , or } 0.25 \text{ ml}$$

You would administer 0.25 ml to deliver the 5000 units of heparin prescribed.

Pediatric dosage. Children require different doses of drugs than adults. The "standard" drug dosage found in package inserts, in the *PDR,* and in textbooks is appropriate only for adult patients, and is frequently described as the "usual, or average, adult dosage." It is based on the pharmacokinetics of the drug in the adult body and on the responses of adult organ systems to the drug. A child's body may handle a drug very differently from an adult's: drug distribution, metabolism, and excretion may differ (see Chap. 4). The responses of organ systems to a drug may also differ. Often, children require a drug dose much lower than the adult dose; rarely, children require a larger dose. For ethical and medicolegal reasons, clinical trials of drugs are not conducted in children. Therefore, new drugs are marketed with minimal, if any, information about appropriate pediatric dosage, yet drug therapy is an important part of intervention in the nursing care of children. In certain cases there has been enough experience with the administration of a particular drug to children so that safe and effective pediatric dosages are known and can be found in sources of drug information, such as the *PDR,* or in specialized references, such as the *Pediatric Dosage Handbook* (American Pharmaceutical Association, Washington), *Manual of Pediatric Therapeutics* (Little Brown & Company, Boston), *Pediatric Therapy* by Harry C. Shirkey (C. V. Mosby, St. Louis), and *Current Pediatric Therapy,* edited by Sidney S. Gellis and Benjamin M. Kagan (W. B. Saunders, Philadelphia).

Sometimes these sources recommend a dose based on the body weight of the child (the pediatric population is not homogeneous as to body weight, or to any other variable that can influence a child's response to a drug). The dose may be based on the child's body weight in pounds or in kilograms. It may be necessary to convert the child's body weight from one system of measure to the other before calculating drug dose. Remember that 1 kg = 2.2 lb.

Often, however, a decision about pediatric dosage has to be made without such specific information. Several methods have been developed for estimating the pediatric dose of drugs. These methods determine pediatric dose by factoring the average adult dose according to the child's age, weight, or surface area. Thus, Fried's rule states that

infant's dose (under 1 year old)

$$= \frac{\text{infant's age (in months)}}{150 \text{ months}} \times \text{average adult dose}$$

This rule assumes that an adult dose would be appropriate for a child of 12½ years (150 months).

Young's rule states that

child's dose (1–12 years)

$$= \frac{\text{child's age (in years)}}{\text{child's age (in years)} + 12} \times \text{average adult dose}$$

and Clark's rule states that

$$\text{child's dose} = \frac{\text{weight of child (lb)}}{150 \text{ lb}} \times \text{average adult dose}$$

Clark's rule assumes that the adult dose is based on an adult body weight of 150 lb (70 kg), and that the appropriate child's dose would be proportionately less, depending on the child's body weight.

The surface area rule states that

$$\text{child's dose} = \frac{\text{surface area of child (in square meters)}}{1.73}$$

$$\times \text{average adult dose}$$

The surface area of the child is determined from a nomogram, which is entered with the child's height and body weight (Fig. 3-6).

When working with small pediatric doses of potent drugs, an error of even 1 mg can be critical. The nurse who works with children should be totally familiar with at least one of these conversions, and should check all pediatric drug orders using it.

For example, a 3-year-old child weighing 30 lb is to receive a therapeutic dose of aspirin. The usual adult dose is 5 gr. How much would you give the child? Using Young's rule,

$$\text{child's dose} = \frac{3 \text{ years}}{(3 + 12) \text{ years}} \times 5 \text{ gr}$$

$$\text{child's dose} = \frac{\overset{1}{\cancel{3 \text{ years}}}}{\underset{5}{\cancel{15 \text{ years}}}} \times \overset{1}{\cancel{5}} \text{ gr} = 1 \text{ gr}$$

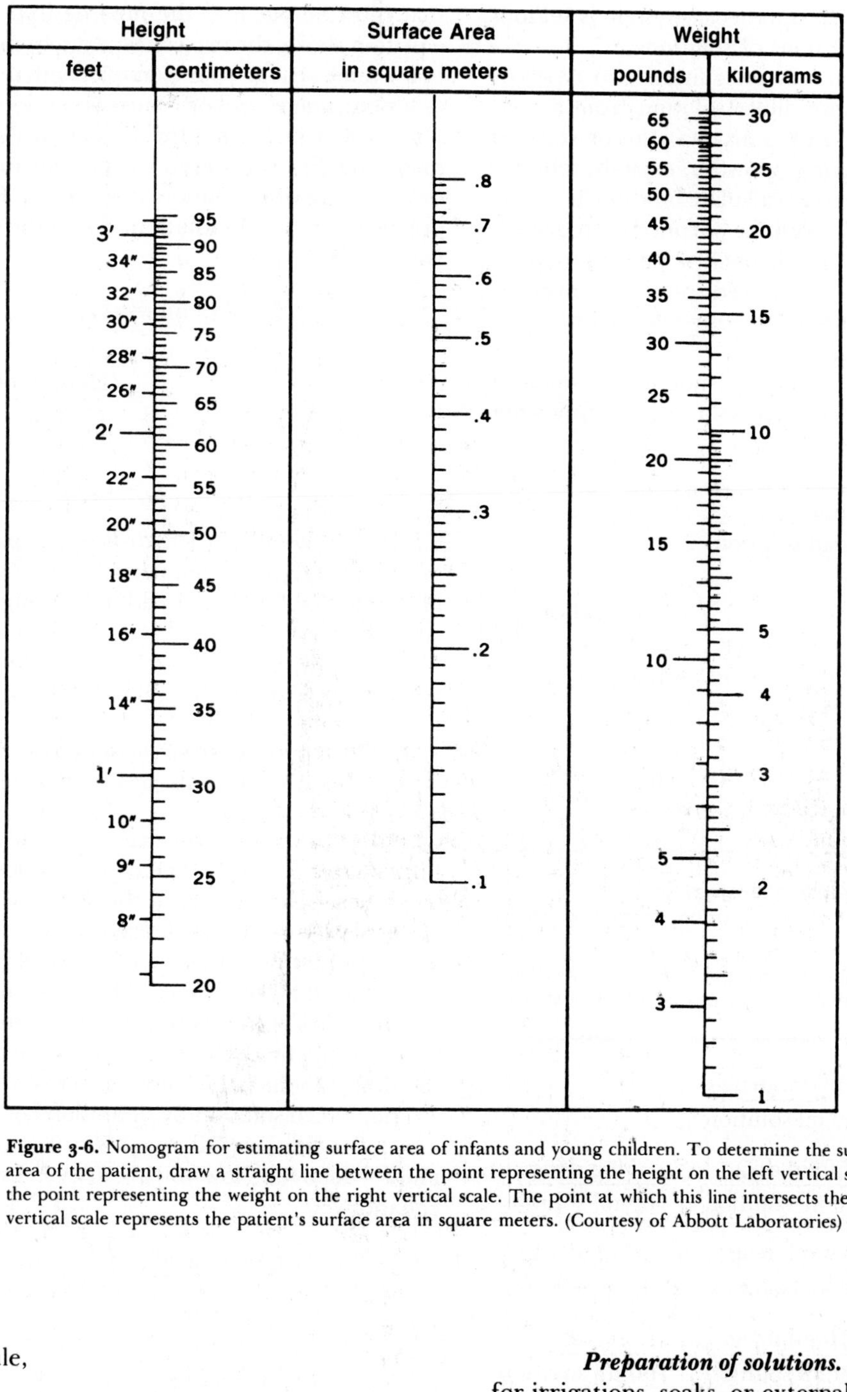

Height		Surface Area	Weight	
feet	centimeters	in square meters	pounds	kilograms

Figure 3-6. Nomogram for estimating surface area of infants and young children. To determine the surface area of the patient, draw a straight line between the point representing the height on the left vertical scale to the point representing the weight on the right vertical scale. The point at which this line intersects the middle vertical scale represents the patient's surface area in square meters. (Courtesy of Abbott Laboratories)

Using Clark's rule,

$$\text{child's dose} = \frac{\overset{1}{\cancel{30 \text{ lb}}}}{\underset{5}{\cancel{150 \text{ lb}}}} \times \overset{1}{\cancel{5}} \text{ gr}$$

child's dose = 1 gr

(For practice problems, see Appendix A, Practice Problems in Dosage and Solutions.)

Preparation of solutions. A solution is often used for irrigations, soaks, or external treatments. A solution is made by dissolving a substance, either a liquid or a solid, in a liquid, called a solvent. The strength or concentration of a solution is expressed as a ratio or as a percentage. For instance, a 1:100 or 1% solution contains one part of drug per 100 parts of solution. This could be 1 g of dry drug or 1 ml of liquid drug dissolved in a volume of appropriate solvent sufficient to make 100 ml of solution (Table 3-5). In the apothecary system, a 1:100 or 1% solution

51

would contain 1 gr of dry drug or 1 min of liquid drug in 100 min of solution. The apothecary system is seldom used to express concentrations of solutions.

The nurse commonly encounters two types of problems: to make a more dilute solution from a concentrated stock solution, and to make a solution starting with a dry form of drug (*e.g.*, powder, crystals, tablets). In each case the problem is to calculate how much "starting material"—that is, the volume of concentrated stock solution or weight of drug—that will be needed to make the required volume of the desired solution. Solvent is then added to this amount of starting material to make up the desired volume of solution.

If the problem is to make a more dilute solution from a more concentrated stock solution, the following equation can be used:

$$\begin{pmatrix} \text{concentration of} \\ \text{desired solution} \end{pmatrix} \begin{pmatrix} \text{volume of} \\ \text{desired solution} \end{pmatrix}$$

$$= \begin{pmatrix} \text{concentration} \\ \text{of available} \\ \text{solution} \end{pmatrix} x$$

Table 3–5. Equivalent expressions of the concentration of solutions

	Concentration expressed as		
Ratio	Percentage	Volume of liquid drug in 100 ml of solution	Weight of dry drug in 100 ml of solution
1:1	100%	$\dfrac{100 \text{ ml drug}}{100 \text{ ml solution}}$	
1:2	50%	$\dfrac{50 \text{ ml drug}}{100 \text{ ml solution}}$	$\dfrac{50 \text{ g drug}}{100 \text{ ml solution}}$
1:4	25%	$\dfrac{25 \text{ ml drug}}{100 \text{ ml solution}}$	$\dfrac{25 \text{ g drug}}{100 \text{ ml solution}}$
1:10	10%	$\dfrac{10 \text{ ml drug}}{100 \text{ ml solution}}$	$\dfrac{10 \text{ g drug}}{100 \text{ ml solution}}$
1:20	5%	$\dfrac{5 \text{ ml drug}}{100 \text{ ml solution}}$	$\dfrac{5 \text{ g drug}}{100 \text{ ml solution}}$
1:100	1%	$\dfrac{1 \text{ ml drug}}{100 \text{ ml solution}}$	$\dfrac{1 \text{ g drug}}{100 \text{ ml solution}}$
1:1000	0.1%	$\dfrac{0.1 \text{ ml drug}}{100 \text{ ml solution}}$	$\dfrac{0.1 \text{ g drug}}{100 \text{ ml solution}}$

where x = volume of available or on-hand stock solution that must be put into the final desired solution. In the equation above, the two concentrations must be expressed in the same system—for example, both must be expressed as a percentage, or both must be expressed as a ratio.

Let us assume that a soak of 1% hydrogen peroxide solution is ordered for a small wound. A 3% hydrogen peroxide solution is in stock. How would you prepare 30 ml of 1% solution? Using the above equation, you write,

$$(1\%)(30 \text{ ml}) = (3\%)x$$

$$x = \frac{(1\%)(\overset{10}{\cancel{30}} \text{ ml})}{\underset{1}{(\cancel{3\%})}}$$

$$x = 10 \text{ ml}$$

To prepare 30 ml of 1% hydrogen peroxide from a stock solution of 3% hydrogen peroxide, you would take 10 ml of the stock solution and add to it enough water to make 30 ml of solution.

If the problem is to make a solution starting with a dry form of drug, the following equation can be used:

$$\begin{pmatrix} \text{concentration of} \\ \text{desired solution} \end{pmatrix} \begin{pmatrix} \text{volume of} \\ \text{desired solution} \end{pmatrix} = x$$

where x = the weight of drug that must be put into the final solution desired. The concentration of solution desired must be expressed in the same units of measure as the volume of solution desired.

For example, an order is written for 1 liter of 1:20 solution of boric acid. The floor stock is boric acid crystals. How would you prepare the solution? The first step is to express the concentration of the desired solution in units of measure, rather than as a ratio. A 1:20 solution by definition contains 1 g of drug in 20 ml of solution (Table 3-5). You want 1 liter of solution; 1 liter = 1000 ml. Now you are are ready to use the above equation:

$$\frac{(1 \text{ g boric acid})}{\underset{1}{(\cancel{20} \text{ ml})}} \overset{50}{(\cancel{1000} \text{ ml})} = x$$

$$x = 50 \text{ g}$$

To prepare 1 liter of 1:20 boric acid solution, you would weigh out 50 g of boric acid crystals and add sufficient sterile water to make 1 liter of solution. (For practice problems, see Appendix A, Practice Problems in Dosage and Solutions.)

Timing of drug administration

When an order or prescription is written for a drug, the frequency of administration must be indicated—for example, once a day (qd) or twice a day (bid), or every 4 hours (q4h) or every 6 hours (q6h). Most institutions establish a policy as to when drugs are administered that takes into consideration the time when daily drug orders are written, the work loads of the personnel involved, and the routines of the department. These policies often state such times as 10 AM for all qd medications, and so forth. The nurse responsible for administering drugs in an institution is responsible for following policy, but must also take into consideration the drugs that are being given. For most satisfactory results, many drugs are given on an empty stomach to ensure adequate absorption and therapeutic effect; these drugs should be given 1 hour before or 2 hours after meals. This type of consideration should have priority, even if the timing of drug administration does not fit well into the routine of the unit.

Other drugs should be given with meals or food to decrease gastric irritation or to facilitate absorption. Two drugs that are known to interact cannot be given together—for instance, tetracycline antibiotics are not absorbed into the systemic circulation if they are taken with various antacids that bind them. Drugs whose anticipated side-effects may endanger an ambulatory patient's safety (e.g., drowsiness, hypotension) are best given when the patient will be in bed for a while, but drugs that cause diuresis are best given when the patient is up and about, can get to a bathroom, and will not have sleep disrupted. Juggling the timing of drug administration can be a real challenge in an institution because of the number of personnel and the policies involved. Effective drug therapy, however, requires that the nurse administering the drugs assess the drugs adequately to ensure that the timing of the administration is optimal. The intervention section of each chapter will include important aspects of the timing of drug delivery for each class of drug.

Patients who are taking medications at home need extensive teaching about the importance of proper timing of taking their medications. All too often patients solve the problem of trying to remember to take all the drugs prescribed by taking them all in one batch or by always taking them with meals, which can block a drug's therapeutic effects. The section on patient education (see below) contains suggestions of ways to teach patients to manage the timing of their drugs. Throughout the text, the patient education section of each chapter will include information on timing drugs.

Recording

Recording the administration of all medications is an essential aspect of drug therapy. Methods of putting information down on the patient's record vary from place to place. In general, however, it is necessary to see that each dose and the time of its administration are recorded along with an indication of who gave it. This provides a legal statement about the drug administered as well as a

ready reference for the drug history. How the patient responded to medication is an important point of information for charting. If the patient did not receive the medication that was ordered, this must be noted, along with an explanation of why the medication was withheld. This is important both medically and legally. If a prn medication is given, the bases for the decision to give the medication should be charted, as should the patient's response. Drugs given to treat specific clinical signs should be charted with the assessment of that parameter—for example, the blood pressure of a patient receiving an antihypertensive medication should be recorded with the drug data at the time of administration of the drug. If a drug is discontinued, the reasoning for the discontinuance should be charted.

Various measures are now used for reducing the amount of time spent in recording medications. If, for example, the same medicine is administered four times daily, only the time of each dose need be charted in some institutions, and the name of the drug need not be entered each time.

Thus, to perform the intervention of drug administration efficiently, the nurse, having assessed the patient and the environment and made one or more nursing diagnoses, will deliver the correct drug by the correct route, in the correct dose, at the correct time, and will chart this action in the patient's medical record.

Provision of comfort measures

A crucial aspect of drug therapy that falls almost totally within the realm of nursing practice is the provision of comfort measures to help the patient deal with his response to the drug therapy. This can entail direct interventions that decrease the impact of the anticipated side-effects of the drug and promote patient safety, or indirect interventions that help the patient to adapt his life style to cope with the drug's effects.

The placebo effect of medications has already been discussed at some length. Research has shown that the environment in which drugs are given and the attitude of the nurse administering the drugs have a great influence on the patient's response to the drug. A positive and supportive attitude often imparts the message to the patient that the drug therapy will help. Attempting to use nondrug measures of relief before giving a prn medication gives a message to patients that there are ways other than medication for dealing with discomfort or with a particular problem. The nurse administering medications has the responsibility and opportunity to use therapeutic interventions that augment the effect of the drug therapy.

No drug is so specific that it produces only one effect. Whenever a patient takes a drug to treat a particular problem, that drug may have effects in addition to the desired therapeutic effect. These other effects are referred to as the side-effects of the drug. Coping with and adjusting to the side-effects of drugs is often one of the most difficult aspects of drug therapy for patients. By knowing the actions of the drug being given, the nurse can usually anticipate the predictable side-effects of the drugs and can prepare the patient to deal with them before they occur.

The specific comfort measures needed for each patient will depend on the particular drug or drugs being given, and on the total assessment of the patient. These comfort measures should be incorporated into the total patient care plan. Throughout this book, specific comfort measures will be listed for each class of drugs, based on the actions of the drugs. For example, patients who receive certain antihypertensive drugs often experience postural hypotension, fainting, dizzy spells, and sexual impotence. The nurse therefore should anticipate a need to provide for patient safety, help the patient to learn to change position slowly, provide sexual counseling and support, and help the patient to adjust to the problem of dizziness or lack of fine motor control, perhaps by changing occupation or other activities. The specific comfort measures to be incorporated into the actual care of a particular patient, will, of course, depend on the total assessment of the patient and on the individual response to the drug therapy.

Patient education

The third and final group of interventions that will be addressed in this book is that of patient teaching. Every patient who enters the health-care system and receives treatment has the right to know what is wrong, what is being prescribed and why, and what can be anticipated from the disease and the treatment. This information is given to the patient through formal or informal patient education sessions. As societal demands for quality health care increase, and as other health-care providers have less time to spend with the patient and have more technical tasks to perform, the nurse is becoming the member of the health-care team who assumes the responsibility for providing patient education. The laws of several states now recognize this, and include patient teaching as an essential component of nursing.

The objectives of patient teaching are the following: to allow the patient to participate fully in decisions about his own care, without being forced to accept the values of the health-care professional; to cooperate with health-care providers; and to integrate the experience of his illness and its treatment into his own life style. In most cases the patient alone has the power to heal by complying with suggested therapy; nursing can only offer supports. Patient teaching has been proven to be a legitimate support that leads to increased compliance with medical regimens. For example, a man with hypertension is more likely to make the decisions to change diet and life style, and to take medication that causes him to feel uncomfortable, if he understands the rationale for so doing and believes that it will actually influence his state of health.

Many studies have been undertaken in the past 10 years to determine the effects of patient teaching on compliance with medical regimens and on rehabilitation and recovery. The results of almost all these studies are the same: the patients who receive organized, well-planned, teaching programs do better than patients who receive this information in less deliberate ways or not at all. Surprisingly, the patients' specific knowledge about disease or drug therapy does not seem to change as a result of teaching. Rather, it seems that educational programs are influential in making the patient believe that he has control over the situation, and in giving him the message that he is important and is expected to do well, because the health teacher has invested time and energy in the teaching process and has worked to develop his trust and to encourage him. This may, again, be part of the powerful "placebo" effect of any intervention.

Drug therapy for any given patient has essential "facts" connected with it that the patient must know—for example, dose and timing—because these are essential for patient compliance to the prescribed therapy. Therefore, the nursing care of any patient on drug therapy must incorporate basic principles of teaching and learning.

The age of the patient can be a key to understanding of his development and abilities, factors that always need to be considered in the teaching plan. Other factors that need to be considered in the teaching plan are the following:

1. *The patient's readiness to learn.* Teaching is best done when the patient can devote time and attention to the material being presented. A patient in pain or one about to undergo a procedure or anticipating immediate discharge is not likely to be motivated to learn. Although it frequently does happen, trying to teach the patient about his drug therapy as he leaves the institution is not conducive to learning or retaining the material you are presenting.
2. *The learning environment.* Learning is a difficult task. In a room full of distractions—for example, noise, visitors, lunch trays—it is often impossible. Teaching requires a quiet environment in which concentration is possible. It requires a teacher that the patient respects and trusts. Adults learn best if they have the opportunity to direct, to some extent, the resources and objectives used in learning.

3. *The appropriateness of the content.*
Information has to be presented using terminology that the patient can understand. This is often a very difficult task, because health-care professionals forget that the terms and phrases that are familiar to them are foreign to lay people. It has also been found that, when a patient is under stress or feels a threat to health and body, he has a lower level of comprehension than usual. Explanations are best made by incorporating the information to be learned into personal experiences and past knowledge—such as using analogies and applying the information directly to the patient's situation. Patients learn direct information better than vague, broad statements—for example, "Take this pill at 10 AM, 2 PM, and 6 PM" has more impact and a better chance for retention than "Take this pill three times a day."

It has also been shown that information is better retained when several senses are engaged by the teaching process—that is, if oral discussion is combined with visual aids or with "hands-on" experience with equipment. Such aids also serve as memory devices when the patient is at home. Finally, adults are especially task-oriented, dealing better with information that helps them to solve specific life problems. Factual information that results in better coping and adapting to therapy should, therefore, be a major consideration in developing content.

4. *Evaluation of teaching and follow-up.* The teaching process cannot begin and end with a teaching session. The information needs to be covered repeatedly, over time, to facilitate retention. The patient should also be tested on what has been presented—for example, by being asked to repeat what has been discussed or demonstrated, so that misconceptions can be clarified and the teaching style and format evaluated.

The patient's readiness to learn and environmental situation are assessed as a general part of the nursing process. The intervention of patient teaching is based on the information obtained in this assessment. The patient's total educational needs will, most likely, include information about the illness, prognosis, therapy, diet, and follow-up care, as well as on basic preventive measures he should take. When the patient is on drug therapy, certain key points should always be included in teaching sessions, although the details will vary with the drugs being used:

1. The *name, dose,* and *action* of the drug (in lay terms). This information used to be withheld from patients, but it is now known that it is essential for patients to know this. Most people seek care from more than one health-care provider, and many people travel or move frequently. In such situations, patient care is very difficult unless the patient knows these facts.

2. *Timing of administration.* It is best to teach specific information about when to take the drug. This can be especially important if the drug is known to have drug–food or drug–drug interactions that prohibit its use with meals, specific foods, or specific drugs. Teaching the patient about timing is also important if the drug has an action that could be a problem at particular times in the day (*e.g.,* diuretics are best taken at a time when the patient has easy access to a bathroom, and should be avoided just before bedtime).

Another area of patient teaching that requires some imagination and inventiveness is the awesome task of teaching patients on multiple medications how to follow through on taking their medications in the home setting. Many approaches have been used in this area: making a poster for the patient and gluing actual pills onto the hours at which the drugs are taken; preparing a calendar with boxes to check each day as the drugs are taken; and using the holes in empty egg cartons to represent days and prefilling the days a week at a time. Commercially prepared pill boxes are available to set up medications a week at a time; some pills are now available from the manufacturer in weekly to monthly dispensers. Helping patients to incorporate many drugs with different timing into their life styles is a major challenge to the nurse.

3. *Special storage and preparation instructions.* Some drugs need special handling—for instance, to be stored at specific temperatures or in light-resistant bottles, and some solutions need to be shaken or warmed. This information needs to be listed for the patient.

4. *Specific OTC drugs to avoid.* In many instances this point is of major importance. Because many people do not consider over-the-counter (OTC) remedies as drugs, the use of OTC drugs is often not even considered, but many of them do contain

ingredients that interact with those in prescription medications.

5. *Special comfort measures to use with the drug.* Techniques for avoiding or minimizing uncomfortable side-effects should also be listed for the patient. Examples include wearing sunglasses if the pupils are dilated by the drug and bowel training techniques if constipation is a frequent problem.

6. *Safety points.* The need to keep all medications out of the reach of children is a safety point that cannot be stressed enough. Needless poisonings of young children occur every year because medications are not stored out of their reach. The patient should also be reminded that the use of all drugs should be reported to any physician or dentist who might provide concurrent treatment.

7. *Specific points about drug toxicity.* Some of the most common signs and symptoms of drug toxicity should be listed for the patient. The patient should simply be advised to notify the appropriate nurse or physician if any of a list of signs or symptoms are experienced.

Debate continues over whether or not patients should be informed about potential toxic effects. Some health-care professionals believe that teaching the patient these signs and symptoms increases the likelihood of their occurrence. Others feel that the patient has the right to know about these potential problems, and that there is no increase in occurrence in informed patients. In this text, a middle-of-the-road posture will be assumed. The most common toxic effects, and not all possible ones, will be presented in the patient teaching guides. It is felt that this information gives the patient some control over and participation in his health care. It also encourages responsibility for self care and prevention of problems or, at least, for early recognition of toxic responses.

8. *Problems to anticipate with sudden cessation of drug therapy.* Therapy with many drugs used today cannot be stopped suddenly without some adverse effects. If the patient is receiving one of these drugs, the adverse effects consequent on cessation need to be explained. The patient is the one who will be reponsible for buying, taking, and maintaining the supply of drugs in the home setting. The importance of continued therapy needs to be pointed out and explained.

Because many patients take more than one drug at a time, because facts can be confusing, and because the points included in drug teaching are so important for total patient health care, it is a very good idea to give the patient the drug information in writing after the teaching session. Patient teaching cards are available from many sources for use with various drugs but, if these are not available, it is easy to design your own. Throughout this book, each class of drugs will be presented with a sample patient teaching guide that can be adapted for use in the clinical setting. Although the importance of patient teaching is heavily stressed today, the "how to" of patient teaching remains a new frontier in health care. The guides presented in this book will provide one example of how to teach patients about drug therapy (see format in Table 3-6).

The nurse should always remember that patients learn from the attitudes of those they respect and from what they observe, as well as from what they hear. The nurse is a constant role model for the approach to and use of drugs. The attitude expressed while administering drugs and while teaching patients may well have a greater influence on long-term patient compliance than the conveyance of any specific facts. The nurse, in a similar manner, serves as a role model for the general public and is in the position to offer public education on the use and effects of drugs in our society.

Evaluation

The fourth step of the nursing process is that of evaluation. It cannot be considered as the final step because evaluation is a continual process that usually leads to changes in assessment, nursing diagnosis, or the interventions being used in patient care.

Once the patient care plan has been put into operation, the patient's situation must be evaluated to determine how effective the overall plan has been in meeting the patient's needs. The nurse must evaluate the patient's response to drug therapy for desired therapeutic effects as well as for any toxic effects. It is at this time that both anticipated and unanticipated effects of drug therapy are encountered and must be identified and dealt with, if necessary. If the patient experiences the desired therapeutic effects of the drug without adverse effects, the administration of the drug and provision of comfort measures can continue in the same manner. If the patient is not experiencing the desired therapeutic effects or if he exhibits toxic effects, the overall patient situation must be evaluated for possible drug–drug, drug–food, or drug–body interactions that could alter the therapeutic effectiveness and toxicity of the drug. In such cases, one of two interacting drugs may have to be changed or at least given at different times, certain foods may need to be

Table 3–6. Sample patient teaching guide

Patient teaching guide: ___(class)___ Drugs

(Brief description of the way the drug works in concrete lay terminology will be presented.)

Instructions:

1. The name of your drug is _____ .

2. The dose of the drug ordered for you is _____ .

3. Special storage needs of the drug include _____ .

4. The drug should be taken __ time(s) a day. The best time to take your drug is _____ , _____ , _____ , etc.

5. The drug should (not) be taken with meals, because food will affect the way the drug is absorbed.

6. Some special activities that should be considered while taking the drug are _____ , _____ , _____ , etc.

7. Tell any physician, nurse, or dentist who takes care of you that you are taking this drug.

8. Keep this and all medications out of the reach of children.

Notify your nurse or physician if any of the following occur:

1. (Specific problems commonly encountered with drug toxicity will be listed.)

2. Abrupt stoppage of this drug should be avoided. Suddenly stopping the drug can cause _____ .

---

avoided when the drug is given, or the drug dose being used may have to be adjusted to achieve optimal drug benefits with minimal toxicity for the patient. Once the adjustments have been made, the situation will need to be evaluated again.

If, on evaluation, the patient is found to be experiencing a great deal of discomfort from the side-effects of the drug, appropriate comfort measures need to be instituted or, in severe cases, the drug dose may have to be adjusted or the drug itself changed. In some situations, the benefit-to-risk ratio of the drug will need to be carefully considered and, if the drug is ultimately the drug of choice, the patient will need support and counseling to cope with the adverse effects of drug therapy.

The patient will also need to be evaluated for the possible occurrence of drug–body interactions that could alter or invalidate the results of diagnostic laboratory tests or confuse the signs and symptoms of the disease. This aspect of evaluation should be done when the patient has a sudden change of laboratory values or, in some cases, an isolated and otherwise unexplained abnormal finding. For example, morphine, a drug used for pain, causes an increase in levels of blood CPK (creatine phosphokinase), an enzyme used to determine muscle damage. The astute nurse should also be aware that a drug can alter physical findings so that they are no longer diagnostic guides for progress of the disease. For example, a cardiac patient on propranolol (Inderal) may complain of chest pain but may not exhibit the usual signs of pain—for example, increased heart rate, increased blood pressure, dilated pupils, sweating—because these autonomic responses to pain are blocked by the drug. The nurse needs to evaluate the patient situation for such drug interactions with disease signs and symptoms.

Table 3–7. Guide to the use of the nursing process in drug therapy

Assessment	Diagnoses	Interventions	Evaluation
Past history (*contraindications*)	Potential alterations in function that can be anticipated	Administration points (foods, timing, storage)	Therapeutic effects; toxic effects
Medication history (potential drug interactions)		Comfort measures	Drug–drug, drug–body, drug–food interactions
Physical assessment (baseline data needed to assess drug effects)		Teaching points (see Table 3–6)	Adverse side-effects; Effectiveness of patient teaching

The effectiveness of the patient teaching procedures must also be evaluated. This can be done by asking the patient to explain what each drug is for, when it should be taken, and what toxic effects should be monitored. This evaluation procedure may be carried out informally with the patient and family, but it must be carried out in some form. All too often, the patient does not understand what it is the nurse thinks has been clearly conveyed. Patient teaching should be recorded in the medical record: the patient's understanding of the therapy and the details of drug administration are essential factors in assessing patient compliance and in ensuring continuity in patient teaching interventions. This crucial information is too frequently omitted.

The evaluation process leads to new interventions, new approaches to the drug therapy, and a reassessment of the patient situation. Through this process, each patient is assured of individualized, optimal drug therapy.

The formal, all-encompassing evaluation of patient care is called the nursing audit. This is a procedure for providing quality assurance measures and constant surveillance of the patient care being given. Concurrent audits review the patient, the environment, and the medical record while the patient is still under direct care and corrective actions can be taken to ensure quality. Retrospective audits review medical records to obtain a picture of the general trend of the quality of care offered to a large number of patients over time. The results of such audits evaluate the procedures being used in drug therapy, the equipment and charting practices, and the needs of the staff for in-service training and updating. This overall evaluation process is essential in all settings for reaching the optimum level of patient care.

In summary, the application of the nursing process in drug therapy involves assessment of the whole patient situation, diagnosis of potential problems, interventions that include drug administration, the provision of comfort measures, and patient teaching, and evaluation of the overall situation, which leads in turn to new assessments, interventions, and diagnoses. All the factual details of pharmacology can never be memorized. The nurse needs to learn the general concepts of the science of pharmacology, to understand the basic actions of the different classes of drugs, and then to apply these through the use of the nursing process (Table 3-7).

References

Bell SK: Guidelines for taking a complete drug history. Nursing 80 10:10, 1980

Geever LN: Administering drugs through the skin. Nursing 82 12:88, 1982

Geolot P, McKinney N: Administering parenteral drugs. Am J Nurs 75:788, 1975

Gilman AG, Goodman LS, Gilman A (eds): Goodman and Gilman's The Pharmacological Basis of Therapeutics, 6th ed. New York, Macmillan, 1980

Karch AM: Concurrent Nursing Audit: Quality Assurance in Action. Thorofare, NJ, Charles B. Slack, Inc., 1979

Newton DW, Newton M: Route, site and technique: Three key decisions. Nursing 79 9:18, 1979

Redman BK: The Process of Patient Teaching in Nursing. St. Louis, C.V. Mosby, 1976

Redman BK: Issues and Concepts in Patient Education. New York, Appleton–Century–Crofts, 1981

Sackett DL, Haynes RB: Compliance with Therapeutic Regimens. Baltimore, The Johns Hopkins University Press, 1976

Shepherd MJ, Swearington PL: Z track injections. Am J Nurs 84:746, 1984

Weaver ME, Koehler VJ: Programmed Mathematics of Drugs and Solutions. Philadelphia, J.B. Lippincott, 1979

Youngman DE: Improving patient compliance with a self-medication teaching program. Nursing 81 11:60, 1981

Chapter 4

The interactions of drugs and body tissues

4

The first three chapters have tried to establish the role of nursing in providing effective and safe drug therapy. This chapter begins the study of the science of pharmacology. As the earlier chapters have tried to demonstrate, the scientific concepts of pharmacology are very relevant to the safe and effective clinical practice of nursing; this should help to make the study of pharmacology exciting to the student of nursing.

Drugs and living systems

The living body and each of its cells are the site of countless chemical reactions that go on continuously and endlessly. When a drug enters a living system, its millions and millions of molecules immediately begin to react with those of the system's cells. Some of the drug molecules react with those of the living tissues in ways that change the functioning of the cells—that is, they produce pharmacologic effects. However, most of the foreign molecules are inactivated by the body's biochemical reactions and are eliminated from the system—that is, the drug is metabolized and excreted.

In this chapter, what happens to drugs after they are administered to patients will be discussed. In very broad and general terms, the following will be covered:

1. How body cells respond to the presence of drugs that can alter their functioning
2. How the body handles drugs to detoxify and remove them
3. How very many factors can influence both the responsiveness of the reacting target tissues to drugs and the ways in which drugs are eliminated and their actions are terminated

The experimental sciences *pharmacodynamics* and *pharmacokinetics,* which have to do with the collection of data concerning the fate of drugs in the body and the statistical analysis and graphing of these data, may seem to have little relevance to clinical practice. It is true that the techniques of monitoring a drug's metabolism and of treating the resulting data mathematically so that they can be visualized graphically in the form of *dose–response* and *time–action curves* are of little immediate concern to most practicing nurses. However, the nurse who has some understanding of these complex processes is often able to give better patient care by making more meaningful observations of the patient's response to drug therapy.

Knowledge of what happens to drugs while they are in the body helps, for example, to account for the fact that different patients often react very differently to the same dose of a drug. In fact, the same patient may react in quite different ways when he receives the identical dose of a drug at different times. Such variability in response to the administration of a drug can best be understood and dealt with in ways that benefit the patient when we are aware of the *principles*—though not necessarily the technical methodology—of experimental clinical pharmacology.

The nurse who understands these principles will be better able to carry out the responsibilities involved in the patient's pharmacotherapy. That is, in observing how the patient responds to a drug that has been administered, the nurse is more likely to be able to account for any unusual reactions and to take steps to prevent other adverse effects from occurring when later doses are given. The nurse will also be better able to teach patients and their families why it is essential to follow the directions for taking medication during long-term maintenance therapy. If the nurse can apply to clinical practice the kind of seemingly impractical theory that will be presented in some parts of this chapter, the nurse will also be better able to communicate with the other members of the health-care team who are participating in the patient's drug therapy regimen.

Responses of reactive cells to drugs

The drugs that are used as therapeutic agents act in many ways to bring about their desired effects. Some drugs simply act like natural substances that are essential to the body's proper biochemical and physiologic activities. Thus, for example, when a person is deficient in a hormone of one or another of the endocrine glands, the deficiency can be counteracted by administering substances obtained from animal glands, such as insulin, or prepared synthetically, such as levothyroxine and certain adrenocorticosteroids. Such *substitution* or *replacement therapy* in exactly the amounts needed to maintain normal physiologic function can be life-saving. Similarly, the administration of iron or vitamin B_{12} to an anemic patient can bring the level of circulating erythrocytes back to normal. Other drugs produce their therapeutically desirable effects by acting as *chemotherapeutic agents* to interfere with the functioning of cell populations foreign to the body, such as invading microorganisms. The term "chemotherapy," which was originally employed to describe the use of chemicals in the treatment of infectious diseases, is now often used to indicate also the action of drugs employed for selectively destroying cancer cells.

Actually, however, instead of substituting for a missing essential metabolite or eradicating potentially harmful foreign invaders and neoplastic cells, most drugs act by interfering with the functioning of the patient's own cells, tissues, and organs—that is, by their *pharmacodynamic* actions and effects. In that sense, all drugs can be considered to be poisons. Fortunately, however, drugs can be used in ways that interfere mainly with pathophysiologic rather than normal function.

The terms "stimulation" and "depression" are often used to indicate that drugs may either speed up or slow down the rate at which cells and organ systems are functioning. Stimulation refers to a drug-induced increase in the activity of reactive cells, with a resulting improvement of the functions over which they exert control. Depression refers to a reduction in cellular activity that is brought about by drug action. Actually, the interactions between drugs and living tissues are much more complicated than the casual use of these terms suggests.

A drug's primary action may, for instance, increase the rate of some cellular biochemical step. Yet, the end result of such "stimulation" may be the slowing of a particular function of the organ. Thus, the injection of acetylcholine activates special receptors in cardiac cells, but the effect produced by this stimulation of cellular activity is a slowing of the heart. Similarly, a drug may act to depress a normal process such as nerve impulse transmission. Yet, the end result of this drug-induced

inhibition of activity may be an increase in the functioning of the organ or physiologic system. Thus, the nerve impulse blocking action of atropine on certain cardiac cells results in an acceleration of the heart rate. Similarly, within the central nervous system, a nerve cell depressant drug—such as a general anesthetic—may actually intensify some cell-controlled functions, so that the patient may show signs of excitement at a certain stage of anesthesia induction and recovery. Drugs may also stimulate some functions while depressing others. Thus, morphine may depress the so-called cough center in the medulla, while stimulating nearby neurons in a manner that sets off vomiting.

Consequently, although drugs will sometimes be referred to as stimulants or depressants—of the central nervous system, for example—attempts will be made to indicate more specifically not merely what a drug does, but *where* and *how* it acts to produce therapeutically useful and clinically important toxic effects. Instead of merely saying that a drug does something—causes a fall in blood pressure, for example, or relieves pain—its actions will be explored at somewhat deeper levels. So, when the nurse has a deeper understanding of precisely where and how a drug is acting, more intelligent care will be offered to the patient, and a greater sense of satisfaction will be gained from clinical practice. Thus, the following generalizations about the locus and mechanism of drug action are offered as background for the more specific discussions of these aspects of the action of individual drugs that will be discussed later.

Sites and mechanisms of drug action

Locus of drug action

To bring about their actions and the changes in function that follow, most drugs must first be absorbed into the systemic circulation and then be carried to the tissues that are capable of responding to them. The drugs must reach a critical, or threshold, concentration at this site to begin producing increased or decreased biochemical or physiologic activity in the reactive tissues.

A pathologic state may be altered by drugs that act at any of several different sites. For example, drugs can reduce high blood pressure by acting either at central nervous system sites or peripherally at sites in the heart or blood vessels. Thus, one drug may act at the vasomotor center, another at the sympathetic ganglia, a third at the sympathetic nerve endings, and still another in the smooth muscles of the blood vessels or in the myocardium. The end result of the actions of all these drugs is the same—a drop in blood pressure.

Similarly, pain may be relieved by any of several different classes of drugs, each of which acts at a different site. The pain caused by the spasm of smooth muscle may be made to vanish by administering an antispasmodic drug that causes the muscle to relax. Pain also disappears when the peripheral nerve fibers that carry sensory impulses toward the central nervous system are blocked by injecting a local anesthetic drug. Other agents—analgesics and general anesthetics—can reduce awareness of pain through their actions on groups of nerve cells in the brain.

Knowledge of a drug's exact sites of action has practical value in various ways. Drugs with different sites of action are sometimes combined to gain their additive effects in producing a particular therapeutically desirable action. Thus, in treating a patient with hypertension, a combination of two or more drugs that lower blood pressure by actions at different sites may be ordered. The sum of the actions of relatively small doses of several drugs is often greater than the action that could be produced by a large dose of one drug acting at a single site, and the side-effects of each may be diminished.

Mechanisms of drug action

Once the action of a drug has been localized, attempts are sometimes made to determine the nature of the affinity between drug molecules and cellular constituents that account for the functional changes in cellular activity. Scientists try to learn whether the drug acts on the surface of the cell to alter the characteristics of the cell membrane, or whether it penetrates into the cell to react with constituents in some intracellular structure, such as the nucleus, mitochondria, or microsomes. They may even try to pinpoint the drug's action at a particular enzyme system or seek to understand the nature of the physical and chemical forces that drive an active group of atoms in the drug molecule toward a complementary chemical grouping on the surface of an enzyme molecule or other cell constituent.

In most cases the exact mechanisms whereby drugs produce their pharmacologic effects are not known. However, as scientists learn more about molecular biology, they become better able to explain just how drug molecules interact with the macromolecules of cells to affect cellular metabolism and function. In this text, the manner of action of various potent drugs, particularly those that affect the functioning of organs that receive impulses from the autonomic nervous system, will be discussed in some detail. At this point, current theories of how drugs act at the cellular and molecular level will be discussed.

Theories of drug action

Most potent drugs are chemically specialized to combine and react with cellular components. This is how they produce their effects. However, there is no one theory capable of explaining all the different ways in which drugs

act. Broadly speaking, it may be said that drugs act in the following ways:

1. By combining with cellular constituents called *receptors*
2. By interacting with cellular *enzyme systems*
3. By affecting the *physicochemical properties* of the outer cell membrane and of intracellular structures in ways still not well understood

Each of these modes of action will be briefly reviewed.

Receptor theory

Many potent drugs are believed to act by combining with chemical groups, on the cell surface or within the cell, for which they possess a *specific affinity*. Such a specific cellular reagent is called a *receptor* or the *receptive substance*. In no case is the exact chemical nature of a cellular receptor known. However, it is believed that receptors contain chemical groups that attract drug molecules with a shape that permits them to approach the receptor surface and to fit into it. When the foreign chemical key fits this cellular lock in the same way as do natural body chemicals, the drug may be able to set off the same chain of biochemical reactions as the natural chemical, thus resulting in increased cellular activity.

For example, the natural body chemical acetylcholine combines with receptors in the membranes of muscle and nerve cells that are chemically specialized to receive it. This binding of acetylcholine with the cholinoceptive substance then sets off changes that may, for example, make muscle cells contract or trigger nerve cell signals. Certain synthetic drugs that resemble acetylcholine chemically can fit the same cellular receptors. As a result, these foreign chemicals interact with the receptors to bring about functional changes similar to the ones that occur naturally. Drugs that have a chemical affinity for a receptor and form a complex with it of a type that produces a functional change are called *agonists*.

Not all drugs with chemical structures that fit cellular receptors can act as agonists. A foreign chemical may be bound to tissue components for which its molecules have a chemical affinity without initiating any pharmacologic action. The drug–receptor complex formed in such cases is *not* capable of setting off the sequence of biochemical events that result in a pharmacologic effect. Such a drug may, in fact, act as an *antagonist* to a natural agonist.

If, for example, a chemical such as atropine or curare, which is capable of attaching itself to a cholinergic receptor, forms a complex that *lacks intrinsic activity*, the natural agonist, acetylcholine, may be unable to initiate the series of steps responsible for normal cellular activity.

That is, the atropine or curare molecules *compete* with acetylcholine for the cellular receptor sites. If these bulky molecules occupy the receptors, they block acetylcholine's access to these cellular sites and thus interfere with the normal activity of the muscle, gland, or nerve cells. Although such *competitive antagonists* of acetylcholine as atropine and curare do not produce the type of activity that results when the natural chemical combines with cellular receptors, these drugs are, of course, anything but "inactive." On the contrary, by interfering with the normal agonist–receptor reactions, these blocking drugs produce powerful pharmacologic effects—that is, changes from normal physiologic functions.

A third group of drugs have weak agonist activity but also can interfere with the normal agonist–receptor reactions. These drugs are referred to as *partial agonists.* Examples include the narcotic analgesic, pentazocine (Talwin), and a drug used in diagnosing hypertension, saralasin (Sarenin).

Drug–enzyme interactions

Many drugs are believed to act by affecting the functioning of cellular enzyme systems. Enzymes are the protein molecules that catalyze, or facilitate, all the chemical reactions constantly going on within living cells. Each cellular enzyme catalyzes only one type of chemical reaction; that is, an enzyme is capable of reacting with only one specific molecule or with a very few chemically related molecules. These molecules are called the enzyme's *substrate.* Thus, a drug that affects the functioning of an enzyme does so because its molecular configuration resembles in some respect the enzyme's normal substrate.

Many principles of drug–receptor reactions apply also to drug–enzyme interactions. Just as the receptor surface possesses chemical groups specialized to receive the molecules of agonists that possess a complementary shape or configuration, the surface of each enzyme has special *active sites* or *centers* that are designed to receive certain atomic groupings of the substrate molecule. The enzyme–substrate complex formed by the binding of these complementary chemical groups is broken in a tiny fraction of a second, but not before the substrate has been converted into new chemical products. These new products in turn form the substrates for still other enzymes in the series of continuing chemical reactions by which the cell produces its energy and synthesizes its own substance. The freed enzyme molecule is ready to react with still another molecule of substrate within thousandths of a second. The enzyme series thus forms a chain reaction of activity.

Many drugs produce their effects by inhibiting the activity of an enzyme and by preventing formation of the enzyme–substrate complex. For example, a foreign chemical may have a structure similar in some respects to that of the natural substrate of an enzyme. Thus, the drug molecule can approach the enzyme surface and form a complex with the active centers. However, the enzyme cannot work on the foreign chemical in exactly the way it acts on its natural substrate. As a result, the products needed for normal cellular activity are not formed, and the cell fails to function properly.

Selective toxicity

Ideally, chemotherapeutic agents should have a selectively toxic effect on an enzymatic reaction that is essential to the life of an infective pathogen or parasite, or of neoplastic cells. Penicillin is a rare example of a drug that interferes with a life process unique to bacteria—the enzymatically catalyzed biosynthesis of a bacterial cell wall component—without, at the same time, adversely affecting any enzymatic or other cellular component essential for the functioning of human cells and tissues. More commonly, as in the case of anticancer drugs, the tissues of the patient also may be poisoned because they employ enzymatic reactions essentially similar to those of the neoplastic tissues. However, cancer cells, which grow more rapidly, require more of the essential metabolites for survival, growth, and reproduction than do normal, healthy cells. Consequently, leukemic and other neoplastic cells are selectively poisoned, and the patient's disease can be kept under control, for a while at least, with only minimal toxicity to his own tissues.

Many adverse effects of the anticancer drugs are a result of the death of rapidly growing normal cells, such as cells of hair follicles, the gastrointestinal tract, and bone marrow. Scientists continue to seek biochemical differences between cancerous cells and normal tissues to exploit this principle of selective toxicity more effectively.

Similarly, in the case of antibacterial drugs, it is sometimes possible to inhibit a specific metabolic step in a series of steps that leads to the production of an essential substance common to both bacteria and humans without interfering with human cellular function. Bacterial cells can, for example, be deprived by sulfonamide drugs of a natural nutritive substance that they require for the biosynthesis of another substance that human cells do not need to manufacture. These drugs do so because they possess a chemical structure similar to that of the metabolite essential for bacterial nutrition.

The antibacterial sulfonamide drugs are believed to act by competing for bacterial enzyme systems that normally take up the vitamin *p*-aminobenzoic acid (PABA). Although the sulfonamide molecule closely resembles PABA, the bacterial cells cannot use it in the series of enzymatic steps by which the bacteria make folic acid, a substance essential for their growth and reproduction. Human cells obtain folic acid directly from foods, and so they are not affected by the ability of sulfonamide drugs to interfere with the earlier step by which the precursor component is biosynthesized. Thus, the sulfonamides exert selective toxicity on bacterial species that require an essential metabolite that is not as vitally important to human cells.

Competitive and noncompetitive antagonism

The actions of drugs that compete with natural substrates for enzymatic sites, and the actions of drugs that compete with agonists for receptor sites, can often be counteracted by administering the substrate or agonist in large enough amounts. For example, poisoning by anticoagulant drugs that act by competitively inhibiting liver enzyme systems that require vitamin K can often be treated by administering massive amounts of that vitamin. Vitamin K is said to be an *antidote* in such cases. Similarly, poisoning by atropine or curare, competitive antagonists of the agonist acetylcholine, can be overcome by administering drugs that raise the local level of acetylcholine at the partially blocked receptor sites.

Drugs may also inhibit enzymes and receptors in a *noncompetitive* manner. These drugs do not compete with the substrate for a specific enzyme center or with an agonist for the same receptor; instead, these drugs inhibit the enzyme or block the receptor site by binding in a different way, perhaps even to a different site, that somehow reduces the affinity of the enzyme or the receptor for the substrate or agonist (Fig. 4-1).

Noncompetitive inhibitors or antagonists can often bind *irreversibly* to their sites of action. In such cases, the drug that has suppressed the activity of an enzyme *cannot* be displaced from the active sites of the enzyme surface by any amount of the natural substrate. Various poisons become so firmly bound to the active sites of cellular enzymes that the natural substrate can never make the necessary attachments required for carrying on normal cellular activity. Thus, the function normally performed by that enzyme is interfered with, until—if the poisoned person or animal survives—new enzyme units are biosynthesized. This happens, for example, in poisoning by nerve gases of the organic phosphate class.

This does not mean, however, that the effects of such poisoning are irreversible. Often, specific chemical antidotes are capable of breaking the bond between the active groups on the enzyme surface and the poison molecule. For example, poisoning by certain organic phosphates that combine irreversibly with the enzyme acetylcholinesterase can be counteracted by the antidotal chemical *pralidoxime* (PAM; Protopam), which pries the poisonous organic phosphate molecules loose from their tight attachment to the active sites of the enzyme. The enzyme is then once more able to take up and destroy its natural substrate, acetylcholine, which had been piling up to toxic levels in the patient's tissues. Similarly, in poisoning by arsenic and heavy metals such as mercury, it may be possible to remove the molecules from the

enzyme system components to which they are bound by administering the antidotal drug *dimercaprol* (British Anti-Lewisite; BAL).

Chemical antagonism

Binding of drugs to chemical groups that are components of enzyme systems is the mechanism by which the heavy metals interfere with cellular function, and metal binding by drugs that have a greater chemical affinity for the poisonous heavy metal is the mechanism by which the antidote works.

Arsenic, for example, poisons many cellular enzymes simultaneously by combining with sulfhydryl ($-SH$) groups common to all these catalysts. Dimercaprol, the arsenic antidote mentioned above, contains sulfhydryl groups that have an even greater affinity for the poison, which is then removed from the enzyme systems. Metal binding also plays a specific part in the poisoning of certain other enzymes that require tiny traces of metal ions to function properly.

The highly active poison cyanide, for example, inactivates the enzyme cytochrome oxidase, which plays a key part in the series of reactions by which all cells use oxygen to burn foodstuffs for the production of energy. Cyanide ions do their deadly work by combining with iron atoms at the active sites on the surface of this enzyme. When cyanide binds these iron atoms that control the activity of this important enzyme, the cells cannot utilize the oxygen brought to them by the blood, and death follows within minutes.

Other metal-binding drugs act primarily not as poisons such as cyanide but as poison antidotes such as dimercaprol. A chemical called *calcium disodium edetate* (EDTA) acts, for example, to tie up and remove lead. Similarly, a substance called *penicillamine* may be administered to combine with and carry away excess copper ions, and *deferoxamine* is employed to bind and eliminate an excess of iron.

Physicochemical activity

Many drugs produce their effects by seeking out cellular components for which they have a particular chemical affinity. That is, their molecules possess groups of atoms that fit into specific sites on the surfaces of cellular receptors or enzymes. However, not all drug molecules act by combining with cellular molecules for which they have a special chemical affinity. Some drugs alter cellular function by their physical properties rather than by any specific interaction with biologic macromolecules.

Alcohol and the general anesthetics, for example, are thought to act on the cells of the central nervous system by affecting the physical properties of their membranes. Ether and other volatile substances are inhaled and carried from the lungs to the brain, where they dissolve in the lipids of the nerve cell membranes.

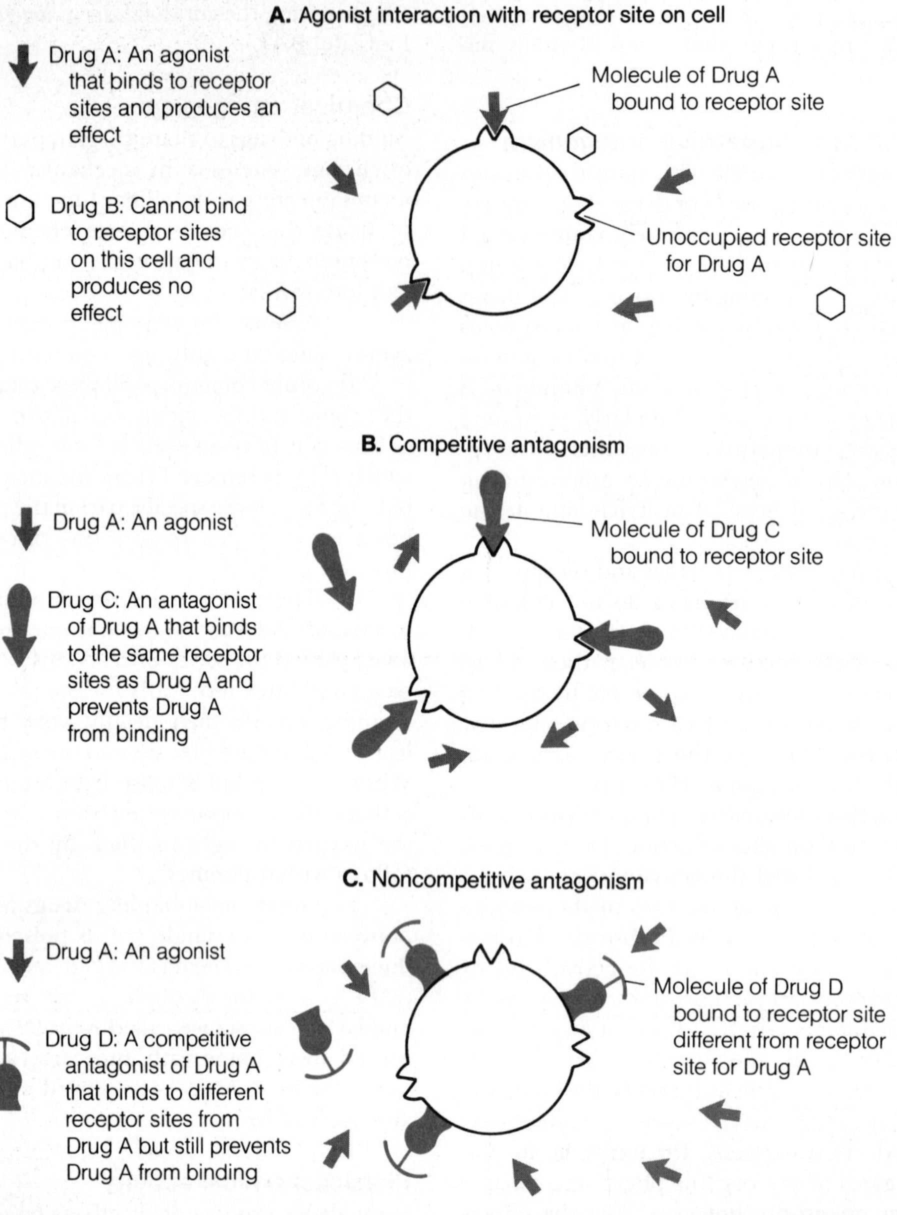

A. Agonist interaction with receptor site on cell

Drug A: An agonist that binds to receptor sites and produces an effect

Drug B: Cannot bind to receptor sites on this cell and produces no effect

Molecule of Drug A bound to receptor site

Unoccupied receptor site for Drug A

B. Competitive antagonism

Drug A: An agonist

Drug C: An antagonist of Drug A that binds to the same receptor sites as Drug A and prevents Drug A from binding

Molecule of Drug C bound to receptor site

C. Noncompetitive antagonism

Drug A: An agonist

Drug D: A competitive antagonist of Drug A that binds to different receptor sites from Drug A but still prevents Drug A from binding

Molecule of Drug D bound to receptor site different from receptor site for Drug A

Figure 4-1. Receptor theory of drug action. (*A*) Agonist interaction with receptor site on cell: molecules of drug A react with specific receptor sites on cells of effector organs and change the cell's activity. (*B*) Competitive antagonism: drug A and drug C have an affinity for the same receptor sites and compete for these sites; drug C has a greater affinity, occupies more of the sites, and antagonizes drug A. (*C*) Noncompetitive antagonism: drug D reacts with a receptor site that is different from the receptor site for drug A, but still somehow prevents drug A from binding with its receptor sites. Drugs that act by inhibiting enzymes can be pictured as acting similarly to the receptor site antagonists illustrated in *B* and *C*, above. Enzyme inhibitors block the binding of molecules of normal substrate to active sites on the enzyme.

This physical effect could affect neuronal function in any of several ways. For example, solution of the drug molecules in the membrane might change the permeability characteristics of the membrane. This, in turn, would affect the flow of ions in and out of the cell and thus alter the polarity on which nerve impulse generation and conduction depend (see Chap. 13). The nerve cell membranes could not then carry on their normal cycles of depolarization and repolarization. The exact mechanism by which general anesthetics produce their effects is still the subject of speculation.

The handling of drugs by the body (pharmacokinetics)

Pharmacologists study not only what an administered drug does to alter body functions, but also how the body deals with the foreign chemical, both to transport it from the site of administration and to inactivate it and remove all traces of it from the system (Figs. 4-2 and 4-3). The latter type of study is called *pharmacokinetics.* The data obtained from such studies—first in several species of animals and later in human subjects—help to tell biochemical and clinical pharmacologists when to expect the *onset* of a drug's activity, when its *intensity* is likely to reach a peak, and how long its effects will last—that is, the probable *duration* of the drug's action. Clinically, such information helps to determine the *dose* of the drug to be administered, the *dosage form* and *route of administration,* and the *frequency* with which the drug must be repeated to maintain its desired effects.

Pharmacokinetic principles are also increasingly being applied today to aid in developing drug dosage regimens for treating individual patients. That is, employing data obtained by monitoring a particular patient's plasma concentrations of an administered drug, nurses and physicians, in consultation with clinical pharmacists, can often work out the dosage schedules of potent drugs that are best suited to safe and effective pharmacotherapy.

Critical concentration

Before a drug can act to produce its effects on physiologic functions, it must reach a certain concentration in the fluids bathing the tissues that respond to the drug. That is, the molecules of the chemical must make their way from the point at which they enter the body to the vicinity of those tissues with which they react. When the systemically active drug has reached a certain minimal level in

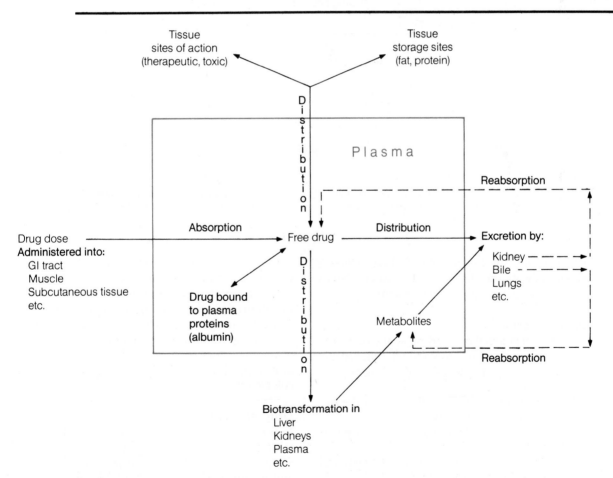

Figure 4-2. The processes by which a drug is handled in the body. Dashed lines indicate that some portion of a drug and its metabolites may be reabsorbed from the excretory organs.

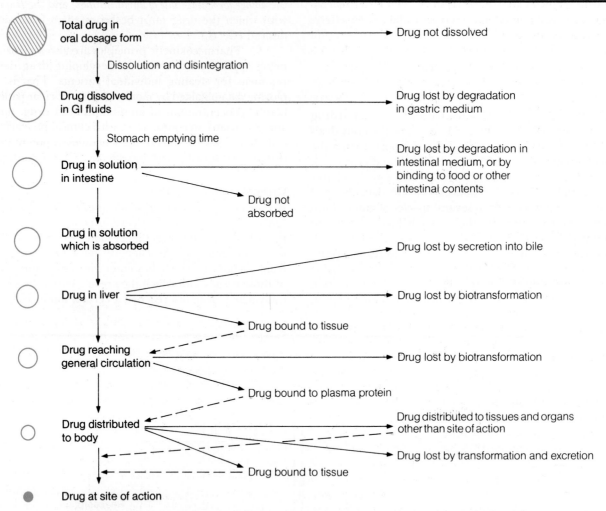

Figure 4-3. Factors modifying the quantity of drug reaching a site of action after a single oral dose. (Redrawn after Levine RR: *Pharmacology: Drug Actions and Reactions*, 3rd ed. Boston, Little, Brown & Co., 1983.)

the reactive tissues, the functioning of these tissues is changed—usually in the direction of greater activity (stimulation) or reduced activity (depression).

Dynamic equilibrium

The concentration attained by the drug at any time after its administration depends on a constantly shifting balance between the rate and extent to which the drug is

1. Absorbed into the body fluids from the site of its entry into the body
2. Transported or distributed to distant points in the body
3. Detoxified, inactivated, or transformed into breakdown products
4. Excreted or eliminated from the body by various routes

The following are some examples of how a drug's concentration in the tissues and, consequently, its pharmacologic effects, can be altered by factors that influence the absorption, distribution, biotransformation, and excretion of drugs. These clinical examples will show how various factors operate to determine the concentration of the drug that reaches the tissues capable of reacting to it to produce the desired (or the undesired) pharmacologic effects.

Drug absorption

In the process of making their way from the site of entry to the site of action, drugs must pass many barriers. They are also subjected to mechanisms that tend to destroy and eliminate these foreign substances from the body. The first factors that must be considered are those that affect the drug's absorption. The term "absorption" refers to what happens to a drug from the time it enters the body until it enters the circulating fluids. Thus, a drug that is taken by mouth is absorbed into the venous and lymphatic circulations by making its way through the mucous membranes lining the upper part of the gastrointestinal tract. A drug that is injected subcutaneously or intramuscularly must be able to move from these local sites into the bloodstream. On the other hand, when a drug is injected intravenously and enters the bloodstream immediately, there is no need to consider any factors related to absorption but only what happens to the drug thereafter.

Oral absorption

The oral route of administration is the one most commonly employed, because it is the most convenient, safest, and cheapest way to get a drug into the patient's system. Most drug molecules are readily absorbed from the mucosal surface of the gastrointestinal tract. Drugs that cannot pass into the bloodstream intact and in adequate amounts must be given by parenteral injection. Injection of such substances ensures their more rapid and complete absorption, but it also increases the danger of accidental overdosage and possible infection.

Orally administered drugs are most readily absorbed from the small intestine, the inner lining of which is covered with millions of villi that, with their network of capillaries, offer a vast mucosal surface area through which the drug molecules can pass into the systemic circulation. Thus, although some substances such as the salicylates (aspirin) and alcohol begin to be absorbed almost immediately from the mucosa of the stomach, most drugs are more rapidly and completely absorbed when the stomach quickly empties its contents into the duodenum.

First-pass effect. After absorption all drugs given orally are carried by the circulation directly to the liver, where they may be largely inactivated before they ever reach the systemic circulation for distribution to the desired site. The term "first-pass effect" refers to the combined inactivation of an orally administered drug by enzymes in the epithelial lining of the gastrointestinal tract and by enzymes in the liver. Inactivation at these sites sometimes makes it necessary to give a higher dose of a drug when it is administered orally than when it is given parenterally.

Drugs and food. Because the stomach empties more slowly when filled with food, orally administered drugs are more rapidly absorbed when taken between meals. One hour before meals or 2 hours after meals is the ideal timing for most oral medications. In addition to delaying gastric emptying, protein and other food components often bind the drug molecules. Although this tends to reduce irritation of the gastrointestinal mucosa by drugs such as the iron salts used in the treatment

of anemia, binding to proteins and other food constituents also often ties up drug molecules in complexes that cannot readily pass through the mucosal lining of the intestine. Thus, for example, most tetracycline-type antibiotics must not be administered orally with milk, milk products, or antacids containing calcium salts, because the complexes formed with calcium cannot be absorbed and less of the drug reaches the systemic site of infection.

Similarly, the higher acidity and peptic activity of the gastric contents during digestion of a meal may destroy most of the dose of drugs that are unstable in such circumstances. For example, most oral penicillin G products are best given between meals to prevent their destruction and to increase the chances of the antibiotic's reaching effective antibacterial levels in the infected tissues. Other drugs are wrapped in special enteric coatings to help them escape digestion in the upper gastrointestinal tract or to keep them from causing irritation and vomiting. Some substances must be administered parenterally because they are inactivated by digestive secretions before they can be absorbed. The hormones insulin and corticotropin, for example, are protein molecules that are digested when taken orally, and the anticoagulant drug heparin, a natural polysaccharide, must also be given by injection rather than orally.

Physicochemical factors. Some substances are both readily dissolved in the stomach and resistant to digestion, yet they are often inadequately absorbed because of physicochemical properties that make it difficult for their molecules to penetrate the mucosa of the intestinal tract. This mucous membrane is made up of epithelial cells that let some substances pass through readily and prevent others from penetrating. The membranes of these cells, like those of *all* cells, are made up of a sort of "sandwich" of lipids, or fatty substances, bounded by protein on both sides. Small water-soluble drug molecules may pass through tiny pores in the cell membrane. Larger molecules must, however, diffuse through the nonporous portion that makes up the largest part of the membrane surface.

Substances that are *soluble in lipids* (alcohol, for example) readily pass through the mucosal surface of the stomach and intestine, but substances that are low in lipid solubility, such as certain antibiotics, are less likely to be absorbed when taken by mouth. Thus, when neomycin (Neobiotic), an aminoglycoside-type antibiotic (see Chap. 8) is administered orally, its molecules do not penetrate the intestinal mucosa in amounts that permit them to reach effective anti-infective concentrations in the blood and tissues. Instead, they accumulate in the lumen of the lower bowel, and the high concentration that this antibiotic drug attains there makes it useful for "sterilizing" the gut, for example, before bowel surgery.

Similarly, certain other aminoglycoside-type antibiotics, such as gentamicin (Garamycin) and kanamycin

(Kantrex), must be given by injection for treating severe urinary tract infections, septicemia, tuberculosis, or other systemic infections, because the poor solubility of their ions in lipids make their passage through the intestinal mucosa difficult. (Drugs that are *highly ionized*—that is, present mostly in the form of electrically charged particles—tend to be repelled by the cell membranes of the intestinal mucosa and by other cell membranes also.)

Other highly ionized drugs include the skeletal muscle relaxant curare, which must be given by injection because it cannot be absorbed through the membranes of the gastrointestinal mucosa. Its quaternary ammonium grouping is responsible for its poor oral absorption. Other quaternary ammonium compounds employed in the management of peptic ulcer and hypertension are also irregularly and incompletely absorbed. Although such compounds are available in oral dosage forms that are partially absorbed from the gastrointestinal tract, their physicochemical properties have proved to be a drawback.

The absorption of most drugs, which are weak acids or bases, is also dependent in part on the *p*H of the gastrointestinal contents. The *p*H is a factor that helps to determine what proportion of the drug's particles will be present in the nonionized form that moves easily through the mucosal membranes rather than in the ionized form that penetrates poorly. Aspirin, a weak acid, stays mainly in the nonionized form in acid gastric juices. Thus, some of it begins to be absorbed from the stomach as soon as its particles dissolve. When aspirin is combined with alkaline buffers, more of the aspirin becomes ionized and less of it is absorbed from the stomach. However, alkalinizing the gastric contents increases the rate at which the stomach empties into the duodenum. Because drugs are very rapidly absorbed from the large surface area of the small intestine, the total amount of aspirin absorbed is actually increased by alkalinization. Actually, aspirin is so readily absorbed from both the stomach and the duodenum—whether given alone or combined with alkaline buffers—that all the television commercials that claim faster absorption for one type of product or another are essentially pointless. Patients should be advised that in reality one aspirin preparation is not likely to be better than any other, and purchase of a buffered preparation is not likely to be a beneficial or economical investment. The placebo effect of a given brand name, however, should not be overlooked.

It is important to remember the factors that influence drug absorption when evaluating a patient's response to a drug. If a patient has been adequately maintained on a specific dose of a drug and suddenly loses the desired effect of the drug, the absorption of the drug may have changed. For example, a patient's congestive heart failure has been adequately controlled by a given dosage of digoxin. For no apparent reason, the patient develops the signs and symptoms of congestive heart failure. Careful evaluation of the situation reveals that the patient had recently begun taking the medication with a snack of ice cream. The cold milk product stimulated gastric acid and mucus production and delayed gastric emptying just enough to increase the breakdown of the digoxin and to lower the levels of drug absorbed, and the patient no longer has a high enough serum digoxin level to control the heart failure. The situation is remedied once the patient resumes taking the medication on an empty stomach.

Bioavailability and bioequivalence. Pharmaceutic products may contain the same drug in the same dose, yet the amount of the drug that is absorbed into the bloodstream from these different products may vary considerably. This, in turn, tends to lead to differences in the concentration that the drug reaches at its site of action. Consequently, two chemically equivalent products can sometimes exert different degrees of therapeutic effectiveness. The term "bioavailability" is used to indicate the extent to which an active ingredient is absorbed into the systemic circulation; the term "bioequivalence" is employed in applying this concept to comparisons of the therapeutic efficacy of chemically equivalent drug products.

Studies have shown that some chemically equivalent products differ significantly in their therapeutic effectiveness. This can be extremely important when the drug that is presented in different product formulations is a highly potent and, thus, potentially toxic agent. On the other hand, many drug products that differ considerably in cost have been shown to be essentially similar in their bioavailability and bioequivalence. These concepts may not have great significance in the case of some not very potent drugs insofar as differences in the therapeutic effects of different pharmaceutic formulations of these drugs are concerned.

The question of whether different brands of the same drug product can be substituted for one another without significantly affecting the patient's response is extremely controversial. The reason for this is related to socioeconomic issues that involve the cost of health care for patients, as well as their health. Consumer groups, for instance, claim that all chemically equivalent drug products—whether available by a widely advertised brand name or by a little known generic name—are essentially similar. Thus, they suggest that the patients who are compelled to purchase the usually more expensive brand name products most commonly prescribed are paying excessive amounts for medication. Such activities by consumer groups have resulted in the enactment of generic drug laws in many states. These laws require pharmacists to fill prescriptions with a generic form of the prescribed drug unless the prescription is signed in a manner indicating that such substitution is not acceptable.

However, situations have arisen in which patients taking some brands of a potent drug—digoxin, for example—were shown to be in danger either of poisoning by overdosage or of failing to receive adequate therapy. In such cases, it would certainly seem desirable for brand name products of recognized quality to be prescribed, rather than to be concerned with cost alone. Of course, the only real way to resolve such questions of quality is through the actual testing of all batches of such drug products to determine whether or not they meet accepted standards of bioavailability and bioequivalence.

Such testing procedures are, indeed, being perfected by specialists in pharmacokinetics and biopharmaceutics, who are studying the factors that influence the absorption of drugs and other aspects of their fate in the human body. Despite the availability of sophisticated methods of studying bioavailability and pharmacokinetics, though, current manufacturing and testing practices do not always really ensure bioequivalence. Handbooks of bioequivalent drugs are sometimes useful in providing control over the quality of the generic products. However, many generic drugs do not carry with them the proven reliability of brand name products.

Parenteral absorption

The speed of absorption of a drug in aqueous solution from an injection site depends, in part, on the blood supply of the injection site. Thus, drugs are absorbed from muscles, which are abundantly supplied with blood vessels, more rapidly than from subcutaneous tissues, with their relatively poor blood supply. In general, therefore, the intramuscular route would be preferred in an emergency when more rapid onset of action is desired. On the other hand, when it is desirable for the drug to act more slowly but with a steadily sustained effect—for example, when epinephrine is used in treating bronchial asthma—the route of choice may be a subcutaneous depot site.

Of course, the absorption of drugs from injection sites can be retarded or accelerated by other means. For example, massaging the area into which epinephrine was injected can force more of the drug into an asthmatic patient's bloodstream if breathing becomes difficult. On the other hand, a drug may be administered in a pharmaceutic dosage form that delays its absorption. Because a drug is eliminated from the body only after it has entered the bloodstream and has been carried to the detoxifying and excretory organs, the length of the drug's activity can sometimes be considerably prolonged by measures that slow its passage into the circulation.

Repository dosage forms. One way to slow a parenterally administered drug's absorption and to increase the duration of its action is to suspend it in a colloidal or fatty substance from which it is only slowly released. The antidiabetic hormone insulin, for example, requires much less frequent injection when it is suspended in protamine. Patients who require anticoagulant drug therapy can be kept heparinized around the clock with relatively few injections of a gelatin suspension of heparin into an intramuscular depot. The duration of action of corticotropin (ACTH) can be similarly extended.

Drugs that are so rapidly absorbed and eliminated that they require inconveniently frequent and possibly painful injections are sometimes converted into relatively insoluble salts and esters. Penicillin G, for example, is available in the form of its benzathine and procaine salts. When aqueous suspensions of these substances are deposited deep in a muscular site, the antibiotic dissolves only gradually in tissue fluids, and is consequently absorbed slowly into the circulation. Thus, this dosage form serves as a muscular depot that keeps penicillin in the blood and tissues for long periods by slowly and steadily replacing the portion of the circulating antibiotic that is being excreted by the patient's kidneys.

The hormones testosterone and estradiol are now available as relatively insoluble esters. Dissolved in a suitable vegetable oil, these substances provide long-lasting hormonal activity. The patient is spared the pain and expense of the frequent injections that were required when the rapidly absorbed and quickly metabolized pure hormone form was employed. (It is imperative to take every precaution with oily solutions or suspensions of particulate material to avoid intravascular injection, which might cause formation of a fat embolism.)

Intravenous administration. When a drug solution is injected directly into a vein, its absorption is instantaneous. Sometimes (although not always) its onset of action is also all but immediate. This has both advantages and dangers. Administering morphine by vein is, for example, preferable to subcutaneous injection when a patient is in shock, because absorption of the drug from under the skin may be very undependable when the patient's peripheral circulation is poor. On the other hand, the instantaneous presence of high blood and brain levels of a too rapidly administered IV dose of morphine may result in deeper depression of the patient's circulation and respiration. Such a severe response could not be counteracted by applying a tourniquet or ice packs to slow absorption, as is possible in the case of most other parenteral injections.

Because of its potential dangers, intravenous injections are usually made slowly to avoid having the drug reach the brain, heart, or other vital organ in so high a concentration that it exerts too powerful an effect. The patient is observed closely before the plunger is pressed to inject each new increment of the drug to detect any signs of adverse effects that might make it necessary to discontinue the injection. Slow administration is also desirable when the IV solution is known to be irritating, because this permits the drug to be diluted by the blood to a less concentrated level.

Drug distribution

The term "distribution" refers to the ways in which drugs are transported by body fluids to their sites of action, metabolism, and excretion. The presence of a drug in the bloodstream does not necessarily mean that it produces immediate effects. Once the drug has been absorbed into the circulation, it must still make its way from the blood into the fluids that bathe the reactive tissues. Many complex physicochemical factors determine whether or not a particular drug can reach an effective concentration in the tissues and exert its effects on the cells.

Among the factors that determine a drug's distribution are the degree of its ionization and its solubility in lipids. As indicated previously, such physicochemical factors influence a drug's ability to pass through all biologic membranes. This aspect involves not only the absorption of drugs from the gastrointestinal tract but also their transport from the blood into the extravascular fluid compartment and from there into the cells of other body tissues, including the brain.

Also of significance in determining the initial and subsequent distribution of a drug is the relative amount of blood that is perfusing different tissues. Thus, for example, tissues that receive a large proportion of the cardiac output—the heart muscle itself, the brain, liver, and kidneys—are the first to receive high concentrations of a drug that is being carried by the bloodstream. Drugs accumulate only later in such tissues as muscle, fat, and bone that receive less blood per unit of time.

Binding to plasma proteins

Drugs that are absorbed into the bloodstream become attached to the plasma proteins—particularly plasma albumin—to varying degrees. This drug–protein complex cannot diffuse through the capillary membranes and into the tissues. However, some drug molecules are constantly being freed from their protein binding sites. The free drug then passes from the blood to its sites of action, metabolic breakdown, and excretion. The free, or active, drug molecules can then interact with cellular receptors to produce the drug's actions and effects. Other molecules of the drug become bound in tissues that do not respond with a pharmacologic action—so-called silent sites. Finally, of course, freedom to move about in an unbound form exposes the drug's molecules to destruction and elimination.

Once it has reached an effective concentration in the reactive tissues, a drug that is transported with most of its molecules tied tightly to plasma proteins often has a long duration of action. This is because the drug molecules diffuse to the organs of detoxification and excretion only very slowly, and a drug that does not leave the bloodstream cannot be destroyed by enzymes in such tissues as the liver, nor can it be excreted by the kidneys. Thus, the antimicrobial drug suramin, used to treat trypanosomiasis (sleeping sickness), can be effectively given at intervals as long as several days to several weeks. Its long-lasting antimicrobial action results from the fact that a large proportion of each dose is bound to plasma pro-

teins and is released only slowly from this circulating storage depot.

Sometimes two drugs may compete for the same *plasma binding sites.* If one drug displaces the other, the freed molecules then diffuse into the tissues at an abnormally rapid rate and may thus tend to reach toxic concentrations. This is of particular significance with potent drugs that are organic acids, including the coumarin-type anticoagulants, such as warfarin (Coumadin), and anti-inflammatory agents, such as phenylbutazone (Butazolidin). The possible consequences of some such drug interactions, and some examples of the possible effects of the displacement of one potent drug from its plasma binding sites by another, are described below.

The blood–brain barrier

The blood–brain barrier is a functional barrier provided by the endothelial cells of brain capillaries and by glial cells in close proximity to those capillaries. Many drugs that would readily penetrate the tissue of other organs cannot penetrate brain tissue to an appreciable extent. Neurotransmitters and some antibiotics are among the clinically important substances that do not penetrate the blood–brain barrier effectively. Like other cells, the cells of this blood–brain barrier most readily let in lipid-soluble nonionized substances and bar the entrance of molecules that are strongly ionized and poorly soluble in fat. Thus, thiopental (Pentothal), a drug of very high lipid solubility, passes promptly from the blood into the brain, and the relatively high concentration that it immediately attains there produces sleep within seconds. On the other hand, other less lipid-soluble barbiturates, such as phenobarbital (Luminal) or barbital (Veronal), may take 30 to 45 minutes to bring about the same degree of central nervous system depression, even when they are injected directly into the bloodstream.

Redistribution. Drugs ordinarily do not remain in the tissues to which they are first transported. Thus, a drug such as thiopental, which first accumulates in the brain because of that organ's rich blood supply, does not ordinarily stay there very long but is redistributed to the much larger mass of body tissues for which it has an equal (or even greater) physicochemical affinity. After a very short time, the drug molecules are carried by the circulation to the rest of the body, the level of thiopental in the nervous system falls below that needed to keep the patient asleep, and the patient quickly awakens.

Where does the drug go when it leaves the brain? It is carried to the fat depots, skeletal muscles, connective tissues, skin, and bones. These regions do not have as rapid a rate of blood flow as the brain and, thus, do not get as much of the lipid-soluble drug immediately after its injection as does the nervous system. Eventually, however, most of the drug makes its way to this greater mass of tissue and accumulates there.

Because the drug is still present in the body in

an active form, some of its molecules continue to move from fat and muscles back into the bloodstream, which then carries them to the brain. Ordinarily, the drug's concentration in the nervous system stays well below the level needed to put the patient back to sleep. In some circumstances, however, the so-called ultrashort-acting barbiturates may keep the patient asleep for an unexpectedly long time—for example, when a patient has received large amounts of thiopental by continuous intravenous infusion to keep him unconscious during a lengthy surgical procedure. Eventually, the depots of fat and muscle become completely saturated with the barbiturate that they receive directly and by redistribution from the brain. The excess spills over into the blood and is carried back to the brain to accumulate there once more, and the brain levels can then be reduced only by the metabolism and excretion of the drug by the body.

Other sites of distribution and storage

Many drugs readily diffuse from the circulation of a pregnant woman into the blood and tissues of the embryo or fetus by way of the circulation. This can expose the unborn infant to teratogenic and other pharmacologic effects of drugs taken by the mother. For this reason, drugs should be avoided at all stages of pregnancy, and should be used only when the benefits of treating the mother clearly outweigh the potential risks to the fetus. In fact, all women of childbearing age should consider the possibility that an embryo formed from a still undetected pregnancy may be damaged by drugs, including caffeine, nicotine, alcohol, and all over-the-counter drugs that they are taking.

Some drugs are bound to bony tissues in ways that ordinarily cause no effects. However, some drugs— antibiotics of the tetracycline class, for example—may interfere with the growth of bones when they accumulate in the skeletal tissues of young children or of the fetus (when carried there by crossing the placenta). Distribution of these drugs to the unerupted teeth of unborn infants or of young children may lead to later discolorations of the tooth enamel. This mainly affects the first, or deciduous teeth, but administration of these drugs to children during early childhood may also cause brownish pigmentation to appear later in the permanent teeth.

Biotransformation of drugs (drug metabolism)

The bodies of humans and of other animals possess mechanisms for converting foreign molecules into harmless substances. These chemical alterations are brought about by enzyme systems in the blood and in all body cells, particularly those of the liver. The enzyme systems capable of catalyzing these chemical reactions have, of course, been developed over the ages by evolutionary processes.

It may seem strange that the body should have the means for dealing with newly synthesized drugs in the same manner in which it protected itself against foreign compounds taken in with foods in ages past. Actually,

almost all biochemical reactions in which drugs and chemicals are transformed to harmless substances are based on a relatively few broad, general processes. These biochemical reactions, which occur with all kinds of chemical compounds, may be classified into four main types: *oxidation, reduction, hydrolysis,* and *conjugation,* or *synthesis.* The nature of these reactions will not be discussed in detail; however, it should be noted that all these metabolic transformations usually result in the formation of new chemicals that are *less active* pharmacologically than the parent compound and *more readily eliminated* by the kidneys. (See Excretion of Drugs, below.) It should also be noted that the process of drug metabolism sometimes produces compounds equal to the parent compound in pharmacologic activity. In addition, drug metabolism sometimes produces compounds that are responsible for adverse effects. For example, some sulfanomides are converted in the body to water-insoluble compounds that can precipitate out in the urine and cause kidney damage.

Liver enzyme systems

The liver is the single most important site for the metabolic biotransformation of pharmacologically active drug molecules into pharmacologically inactive fragments that can be excreted by the kidneys. The most important of the liver's drug metabolizing enzymes are located in an intracellular structure called the endoplasmic reticulum, a network of canals that runs through the hepatic cells. This is frequently referred to as the hepatic microsomal system because, when liver tissue is minced and centrifuged, the enzymes are found packed in tiny fragments called microsomes.

People vary greatly in their inborn ability to metabolize drugs both by their hepatic microsomal enzyme system and by the actions of other enzymes. In addition, the ability of liver cells to break drugs down to inactive metabolites is affected by many factors, including the patient's age, the presence of hepatic pathology, and even the presence of other drugs.

Enzyme induction

When patients take certain drugs regularly, the drugs stimulate an increase in the activity of the microsomal enzymes that catalyze their metabolism. This leads to an increased rate of destruction of these drugs and of other drugs that are also inactivated by the same kinds of enzymatically catalyzed reactions. Such enzyme induction is often important in changing the response of patients to various drugs that they are taking.

It has been found, for example, that the chronic administration of phenobarbital (Luminal) and of other barbiturates induces the biosynthesis of hepatic microsomal drug-metabolizing enzymes. This is thought to account, in part, for the fact that patients who are taking barbiturates require larger doses to attain the same effects after a while (*i.e., tolerance* develops to barbiturates). Also

71

of clinical significance is the fact that barbiturate-stimulated enzyme induction leads to an increased rate of biotransformation of such *other* drugs as the coumarin-type anticoagulants, dicumarol and warfarin. This is one example of a drug–drug interaction that is important to remember when evaluating a patient's response to drug therapy.

The significance of this phenomenon is discussed further below in the section of this chapter that deals in more detail with the various specific factors that influence the effects of drugs.

Excretion of drugs

The body eliminates drugs and their metabolites by many routes. Drugs may be excreted through the sweat glands onto the skin surface; they may appear in saliva, bile, or even mother's milk. The volatile general anesthetics and some other drugs and their metabolites are eliminated largely by the lungs. The gases cyclopropane and nitrous oxide, for example, are exhaled after returning intact to the alveoli from the central nervous system; and alcohol excreted in the breath can be measured chemically by using breathalyzer tests for indirect determination of blood–alcohol concentrations.

The kidneys are the organs that play the most important part in the elimination of drugs. The molecules of the unchanged drug or of its metabolites are first filtered through the glomeruli. Some drugs are dealt with by still another renal excretory mechanism: tubular secretion, a process in which substances are transported from the blood directly into the renal tubular fluid. Penicillin, for example, is rapidly eliminated because it is both filtered by the glomeruli and secreted by the renal tubules without undergoing tubular reabsorption.

With most other drugs, however, the process of tubular reabsorption is important in delaying drug excretion. This occurs because the drug molecules that were filtered by the glomeruli into the tubular fluid diffuse back into the plasma through the membranes of the epithelial cells that line the renal tubules. Interestingly, the metabolites of most drugs are less readily reabsorbed and more rapidly excreted than their parent compounds. This is so because the biotransformation of these drugs by the liver converts them into compounds that are more highly ionized and less lipid-soluble—physicochemical properties that reduce a drug's ability to penetrate cell membranes. Thus, the metabolite molecules that appear in the glomerular filtrate do not readily make their way through the tubular cell membranes and back into the blood, but are largely carried off in the urine and excreted.

Reabsorption of drug molecules by the renal tubules may be reduced artificially to speed their elimination. In poisoning by aspirin or barbiturates, for example, the patient's urine is alkalinized by injecting sodium bicarbonate intravenously to raise the number of ionized drug particles in the glomerular filtrate. This, in turn, reduces the amount of the drug that returns to the blood and increases the amount excreted by the kidneys. As a result, the patient recovers more readily from poisoning by these drugs.

This is but one means of treating a patient who is poisoned by these drugs. Figure 4-2 diagrams the processes described in this section (such as absorption and distribution), and Figure 4-3 shows that, because of these processes, only a small part of the dose of an orally administered drug may actually arrive at the desired site of action.

Factors influencing the effects of drugs

The inexperienced nurse, administering drugs to patients for the first time and observing how they respond, soon learns that the dose that was given does not always produce the desired effect. In some patients the drug's effects are unexpectedly great, while in others little, if any, response is shown to the same dose. In fact, the same patient may respond in quite different ways when an identical dose is given under differing conditions.

Recently, investigators have begun to discover the real reasons for differences in the ways in which patients respond to drugs. Some of these factors are physiologic, pathologic, and biochemical; others are now known to be genetic and immunologic in nature. Psychologic factors also play a part in the response of humans to drugs, particularly to psychopharmacologic agents. This topic will be explored by discussing the following:

1. The factors that influence the functional response of cells to drugs
2. The factors that depend on individual differences in the way drugs are metabolically biotransformed and excreted. These factors, of course, influence the concentration that drugs can reach in the reactive tissues.

Many factors that make one person very sensitive to a dose of a drug to which others may be very resistant are relatively obscure. All that should be done is to start with the usual dose for the "average" patient and to alter the amount administered if this dosage proves to be too little or too much for the particular patient being treated. Ideally, it is desirable to adjust the dosage to fit the individual patient at the time that the original drug order is written and, to the extent that knowledge of the patient permits, this should be done routinely. Table 4-1 summarizes the considerations described in the sections below.

Body weight

Most commonly, the patient's body weight is taken into consideration in determining whether to reduce or to raise the usual dose of a potent drug, because there is a definite relationship between the mass of administered chemical and the mass of body tissues and fluids through which it is distributed and diluted. Generally speaking, the greater a person's body weight, the smaller the amount of the administered dose likely to arrive at the reactive target tissues; the less the person weighs, the greater the portion of the dose reaching the reactive cells and, of course, the more powerful the effect.

The dosage of certain potent drugs is often calculated and administered on the basis of the ratio of milligrams of the drug to pounds or kilograms of the patient's body weight. Most formulas for adjusting adult dosage of a drug for a child use the child's body weight rather than age. Actually, however, the fraction of the adult dose most suitable for a child is most accurately calculated on the basis of *body surface area* (BSA), obtained from nomograms, and then stated in terms of milligrams or grams per square meter (see Chap. 3).

Age

The age of a patient will often affect the response to drugs. This is of greatest significance for those at the extremes of life—that is, newborn infants (neonates) and the very elderly. In most cases, the much more intense effect that drugs produce in such patients can be traced to deficiencies in their ability to transform drugs to inactive metabolites or in the capacity of their kidneys to eliminate drugs and their still active metabolites. Sometimes, however, the unexpected responses of children and the elderly to drugs result from differences to drugs at the cellular level.

No formula of any kind can be relied on in calculating dosage for a premature infant or even for a full-term newborn less than 1 week old. This is because these infants differ from older infants, children, and adults in their ability to eliminate administered drugs. For example, very young infants lack the liver enzyme system for breaking down the antibiotic *chloramphenicol,* and very small doses of that drug have caused toxicity and death when administered during the first week of life.

The excessive susceptibility of some elderly patients to *digoxin* stems most often from the reduced capacity of their kidneys to excrete this potent heart-stimulating drug. Thus, treatment of elderly patients is often begun with smaller doses than those used in younger adults. Dosage for each patient is then adjusted on the basis of blood levels of the drug or on the basis of tests of renal function—for example, blood urea nitrogen and serum creatinine levels—that indicate the capacity of the kidneys to clear the drug from the body. This helps to keep the drug from accumulating to toxic levels with continued daily maintenance doses.

Elderly patients and young children also differ in their responses to drugs that affect central nervous system function. Older patients often become confused and disoriented when they receive an ordinary dose of

Table 4–1. Factors affecting the response of the body to a drug

Weight
Age
Sex
Physiologic factors: diurnal rhythm, acid–base balance, electrolyte balance
Pathology: kidney disease, liver disease, peripheral vascular disease, low blood pressure
Genetic factors: sensitivity to drug, resistance to drug, idiosyncratic reaction
Immunologic factors: allergy
Psychological factors: placebo effect, compliance, health beliefs
Environmental factors: temperature
Tolerance
Cumulation of drug: toxicity

a sleep-producing drug. Similarly, children seem more prone to suffer drug-induced convulsions than do adults. High overdoses of certain antihistaminic drugs that are used to treat allergies would only make adults drowsy, whereas they sometimes set off seizures in youngsters. Drugs such as the salicylates (aspirin and chemically related drugs) also have unexpectedly strong effects on the nervous systems of children. Those who are feverish and dehydrated are especially prone to suffer from salicylate poisoning.

Sex

The sex of a patient sometimes affects the response to a drug. For example, women are said to be more susceptible to the excitatory effects sometimes seen when morphine is administered. Of course, an important consideration when drugs are ordered for women of childbearing age is the possibility of pregnancy and the possibility of an adverse effect on the fetus or uterus. As indicated previously, the administration of medication to women who may be in the early weeks of pregnancy carries some risk of causing damage to the developing fetus.

The tissues of the uterus vary in their responsiveness to certain drugs, depending on the physiologic state of the smooth muscle cells. During the early months of pregnancy, oxytocic drugs such as the ergot alkaloids and posterior pituitary hormone oxytocin exert little or no effect on the uterus. However, as pregnancy advances, this organ undergoes changes that make it increasingly sensitive to drugs that stimulate uterine contractions. Finally, at term, quite small doses of these drugs can elicit powerful uterine contractions.

Drugs given by intramuscular (IM) injection are absorbed at different rates in men and women. The muscles of women have a higher fat content and poorer blood supply than the muscles of men. Drugs are normally absorbed at a slower rate in women; thus, the effects of drugs appear later after IM injection and persist longer in women than is usually expected in men.

The phase of a woman's menstrual cycle and the concomitantly changing hormone levels in her body may also affect her response to a drug. For instance, when the estrogen and progesterone levels are elevated, the woman's immune response is suppressed. Antibiotics given to a woman at the time in her cycle when these hormones are at high levels may not be as effective as when given at other times, because her body's ability to deal with bacterial invasion is below normal levels.

Physiologic factors

The physiologic state of the cells and systems of the patient plays an important part in determining the response to drugs at different times. Thus, a hypnotic or sleep-producing drug is much less effective in the morning than at night, presumably because the body's diurnal rhythms make the nervous system more resistant to depressant drugs early in the day. Of course, as with drug tolerance of all types, increased resistance to hypnotics is limited, and a patient can be put to sleep by increasing the dose of the drug.

Diurnal rhythm is also often important in the administration of *adrenocorticosteroid* drugs. To minimize toxicity during long-term maintenance therapy, such steroid drugs are often ordered to be administered in the early morning. This imitates the body's own pattern of adrenal steroid production and secretion. By administering these drugs when the adrenal glands are secreting similar steroids at their maximal morning rate, their potential long-term adverse effects on the pituitary gland and other tissues are minimized.

The response of patients to drugs is often different when such physiologic factors as acid–base and water or electrolyte balance are distorted. Patients taking most diuretic drugs may become temporarily refractory to further treatment if they develop metabolic alkalosis as a result of excess loss of chloride and potassium ions. On the other hand, the diuretic effect of acetazolamide (Diamox) is diminished by metabolic acidosis induced by excessive loss of bicarbonate and sodium ions.

Pathologic factors

Patients often respond to drugs in an unusual way because of the presence of underlying pathology. As indicated earlier, diseases of the liver and kidneys that interfere with the detoxification and excretion of drugs can cause ordinary doses to accumulate to toxic levels in the body's tissues. In addition, other pathologic states sometimes alter the responsiveness of various tissues in ways that can lead to toxic reactions or to resistance to drug therapy.

Unexpectedly severe drug reactions sometimes develop in patients with pathology of their drug-metabolizing and excreting organs. For example, a patient with a severely damaged liver is not a good candidate for basal anesthesia with a barbiturate such as thiopental (Pentothal). Lack of the liver enzymes that ordinarily destroy this drug may lead to abnormally high blood and brain drug levels of long duration. Thus, in patients with unsuspected partial hepatic insufficiency, the use of this usually ultrashort-acting barbiturate may cause unexpectedly deep and prolonged unconsciousness or death from respiratory failure.

In addition, the brain cells of patients with severe liver damage may be unusually sensitive to small doses of depressant drugs. Even small sedative doses of barbiturates, or of morphine, for example, may cause a patient with cirrhosis of the liver to lapse into hepatic coma. Similarly, in patients with bronchial asthma and other obstructive lung diseases, cells of the respiratory center are extremely sensitive to low doses of these depressant drugs. Thus, caution is required in administering sedative or narcotic analgesic drugs to such patients, because respiratory failure may result.

Drugs that are ordinarily excreted by the kidneys can cause unusual reactions when administered in seemingly safe doses to patients with renal insufficiency. The drug, which the kidneys cannot transfer to the urine, stays in the blood and tissues at unexpectedly high levels. If further doses are administered, the drug can accumulate to toxic levels. Thus, it is desirable to test the patient's renal function periodically or to determine the levels of drug in the plasma, and to administer the drug in lower doses and at less frequent intervals when the tests indicate that the patient's kidneys have not cleared the drug from the system in a normal manner.

Antibiotics such as gentamicin and kanamycin, for example, require renal excretion. In patients with impaired renal function, these drugs may accumulate, first in the kidney tissues and later in other organs, including both branches of the eighth cranial nerve. This may then lead to further kidney damage from the nephrotoxic effects of these drugs. In addition, continued accumulation of unexcreted drug in the auditory and vestibular nerves (the eighth cranial nerve) may cause deafness and loss of equilibrium, even though only seemingly safe doses had been injected at what was thought to be proper intervals.

Patients suffering from more than one disorder sometimes prove excessively sensitive or resistant to a drug that is administered to treat one of their ailments. A person suffering from hyperthyroidism, for example, is especially sensitive to epinephrine and other adrenergic drugs. Thus, if these drugs are administered for another medical disorder, they may make such a patient tachycardic. On the other hand, hyperthyroid patients are relatively resistant to doses of digitalis that would be able to slow the rapidly beating heart of a patient with normal thyroid function. Similarly, hyperthyroid patients tend to resist the depressant effects of morphine on the respiratory center. Patients with *hypo*thyroidism tend to respond to these drugs in the opposite way. Thus, for example, even small doses of digitalis tend to slow the heart of a thyroid-deficient patient profoundly.

A patient who requires a cholinergic drug to promote postoperative bowel motility may suffer breathing difficulties if he also has a history of bronchial asthma. It is important to be aware of the presence of pathologic processes other than the disease for which the patient is receiving a drug. Remember that these pathologic processes may predispose the patient to adverse reactions to certain drugs and that, therefore, these drugs may be contraindicated. The patient must be carefully observed for development of any sign of adverse effects that might make it necessary to discontinue the medication or reduce its dosage.

Sometimes patients respond differently to drugs depending on whether pain, fever, or other symptoms of underlying disease are present. Thus, a person with fever will often respond to aspirin with a drop in temperature of a degree or two, whereas a patient with normal temperature will show no change in that parameter when this analgesic–antipyretic is given. Similarly, in a patient with congestive heart failure, digitalis increases the cardiac output, whereas this heart stimulant fails to increase the strength and efficiency of a more normally dynamic heart and may, indeed, cause a reduction in its output.

The presence of severe pain tends to increase a patient's resistance to pain relief by opiates, and an extremely anxious patient can prove resistant to very large doses of sedative drugs. Therefore, if analgesics or sedatives have been ordered on a prn basis, it is better to administer these drugs soon after the symptoms arise than to wait until the pain is severe or the patient is agitated; in both instances, very much larger doses will be required.

Patients who are in severe pain can resist the respiratory depression produced by morphine more readily than when their pain is only moderately severe. Thus, if the source of a patient's pain is suddenly removed—as when a biliary or kidney stone is passed—a morphinized patient's respiration may become slower or shallower than it was while the pain persisted.

Pharmacogenetic factors

Genetic factors sometimes account for differences in the response of patients receiving similar doses of the same drug. People in some families, for example, have a greater ability to break down the antituberculosis drug isoniazid (INH) than do people with a different genetic background. These "rapid inactivators" require higher daily doses of this drug to maintain its anti-infective effect. Those who lack the gene for producing the drug-metabolizing enzyme system inactivate isoniazid so slowly that the ad-

ministration of even ordinary doses at the usual intervals soon causes the drug to accumulate to toxic levels in peripheral nerves and cause neuritis.

Genetic factors have also been shown to lead to a lack of other drug-metabolizing enzymes and thus to unusual responses to various drugs. For example, some members of a few families are born with an abnormal plasma cholinesterase, or pseudocholinesterase; this enzyme normally catalyzes the hydrolytic breakdown of various esters, including the drugs procaine (Novocain) and succinylcholine (Anectine). Ordinarily, the latter drug, which is injected by vein to relax skeletal muscles during anesthesia, is rapidly detoxified. However, patients who have abnormal pseudocholinesterase have suffered prolonged paralysis of the respiratory muscles after administration of relatively small amounts of succinylcholine. The abnormally slow metabolic activity of the altered, or atypical, plasma pseudocholinesterase enzyme permits the undestroyed drug to exert its effects on the muscles of respiration for long periods. The patient then requires mechanical oxygenation during the period of prolonged apnea that results. An inborn lack of various enzymes also accounts for the extreme susceptibility of some people to certain other drugs (see Chap. 5, Drug Idiosyncrasy).

Immunologic factors

Immunologic factors cause some people to react in ways that are totally different from what is expected, based on a drug's pharmacologic actions. The presence of drug molecules stimulates the patient's immune mechanisms to produce protective antibodies. Later, when the person again receives the same drug, an immune reaction occurs that can result in many types of changes in physiologic function. The signs and symptoms of illness that result are varied, ranging from immediate breathing and circulatory difficulties to gradual development of skin, joint, and even blood disorders (see Chap. 5, Drug Allergy).

Psychological, emotional, and environmental factors

Nonspecific, or nonpharmacologic, factors often also play an important part in the way people respond to drugs. People often respond even to the administration of a pharmacologically inert material, or *placebo*. A person's response to active drugs is also often influenced by the underlying personality structure and by hopes, fears, or expectations. This is particularly true of drugs that affect the mood and thought processes, so-called *psychotropic drugs*. Thus, whether a person taking LSD finds the experience pleasurable or panic-provoking (a "bad trip") often depends upon the mental set. Patients who are being treated for mental and emotional illnesses should be carefully observed to see how they respond to the tranquilizing and mood-elevating agents that they are taking and the patient and environment should be carefully evaluated for factors that could be influencing the response.

The patient's personality is also a factor in determining whether a prescribed drug will be taken properly or at all. Thus, to ensure that the patient will follow instructions for taking the medication, it is important for those involved in his health care to understand the patient's mental processes and to try to help him by tailoring the language of their directions to his specific capacity to comply with them. The environment in which the patient is taught how to take the medication is also important. Studies suggest that patient compliance with medication instructions is greatest when patients are taught while still in the hospital what they will have to do when they get home.

Environmental factors also often influence the effects of drugs. For example, the circumstances or setting in which a person takes a drug is often as important as the mental attitude or set in determining behavioral responses to psychotropic drugs. For instance, a person drinking alcoholic beverages or smoking marihuana may merely get drowsy if drinking or smoking alone. On the other hand, the same amount of alcohol or marihuana taken when with a group of friends may make the person giddy, gay, and outgoing. The nature of the environment also affects responses to drugs by altering the patient's physiology. Heat tends to dilate blood vessels, for example. Thus, it is often desirable to reduce the dose of vasodilator drugs given during hot weather. Patients taking antihypertensive agents may suffer an unexpectedly sharp drop in blood pressure from their usual dose when they take it at the start of a heat wave or following a winter plane trip to a subtropical resort.

Tolerance

Another often important factor that influences the way people respond to drugs is the phenomenon called tolerance or reduced responsiveness. Some strains of animals possess an inborn resistance to the actions of certain drugs (see Chap. 1, Preclinical Pharmacologic Evaluation) and some people are born with an unusual ability to withstand the presence of particular drugs in the body. Such *congenital tolerance* is usually the result of an increased capacity to inactivate drugs by hepatic and other drug-metabolizing enzymes.

Tolerance to the actions of drugs may also be *acquired* when a person continues to take certain drugs over a period of time. In such situations, a dose of the drug that had produced a particular pharmacologic effect no longer does so or, if the effect occurs, it lasts only a relatively short time. The patient then requires larger doses of the drug than were taken at first to obtain the effects of the drug desired for therapeutic purposes. One reason why resistance develops in this way is that the continued presence of the drug in the body stimulates the synthesis of increased amounts of drug-detoxifying

enzymes in the patient's liver. Phenobarbital (Luminal), for example, induces production of the liver enzymes that catalyze its own destruction. After a while, the patient must take higher doses of this sedative–hypnotic to become drowsy or calm than were needed when it was first used. However, tolerance of this type is limited, and death from respiratory failure will result when a person who has acquired resistance to barbiturates exceeds the upper limits of his ability to tolerate them.

Actually, however, an increased ability to degrade drugs and to dispose of them before they can reach effective concentrations in the reactive tissues is not the only—or even the most important—way in which people acquire tolerance to drugs. Such *disposal* or *metabolic* tolerance, which depends on *pharmacokinetic* factors, is often less significant than *pharmacodynamic* or *tissue tolerance,* which results when the reactive tissues develop the ability to continue functioning more or less normally even in the presence of abnormally high concentrations of the drug. In most cases the real reasons for such tissue tolerance are still obscure.

A dramatic example of increased adaptability of reacting cells to the presence of a drug is the remarkable degree of resistance to opiates often acquired by nervous system cells. Addicts often become capable of taking heroin in doses many times the amount that would kill a nontolerant person. Unfortunately, this phenomenon also occurs in patients who require morphine and other potent pain-relieving drugs for long periods. As a result, the dosage must be continually increased to keep the patient's pain under control.

Attempts are made to delay the development of cellular, or tissue, tolerance in such patients by giving them only small doses of narcotic analgesics in combination with nonaddicting agents. Dosage of these tolerance-producing drugs is raised only gradually, and they are given on an irregular dosage schedule. The drugs are discontinued temporarily whenever the patient's condition improves and the pain eases. Tolerance diminishes in such circumstances and can even be lost if the period of drug abstinence is long enough.

Cross tolerance is a phenomenon that develops with different drugs acting at the same cellular sites to produce similar pharmacologic effects. Thus, a person who acquires tolerance to the vasodilator effects of nitroglycerin is also relatively resistant to other nitrate and nitrite vasodilators. Addicts tolerant to heroin also withstand the effects of morphine and of other opiate and opioid drugs. Alcoholic patients often prove resistant to ether and other general anesthetics that depress the central nervous system in much the same way as alcohol.

Physical dependence is a phenomenon that often—but not always—accompanies the development of tolerance. In such cases, the cells of the central nervous system are not only adapted to the presence of the drug but also they cannot function normally when the level of the drug is lowered. Thus, the presence of the drug—opiates, barbiturates, or alcohol, for example—is required to preserve normal equilibrium and, when the drug is withdrawn, the abnormal activities of the neuronal cells result in a characteristic abstinence or withdrawal syndrome.

Cumulation of drugs

Another important factor that influences the effect of any administered drug is the presence of residues of previously administered doses of the same drug in the body. When a drug is taken in several successive doses at intervals too short to allow elimination of earlier doses, it tends to accumulate in the body. The increased concentration of the drug at its site of action then results in a more intense pharmacologic effect; the duration of the drug's action will be prolonged, because the body's drug-metabolizing and excreting processes require a longer time to remove the accumulated drug.

The tendency of drugs to produce cumulative effects when taken in at a greater rate than they can be cleared from the body accounts for overdosage from administration of too frequent multiple doses. A familiar example of this occurs when a person takes several drinks of an alcoholic beverage in a relatively short period of time. Because the drinker absorbs more alcohol than the body can metabolize, the level of alcohol in the blood and brain rises steadily. As each new increment of alcohol is added to what has already reached the nervous system, the total effect is much greater than that produced by any single drink, and alcoholic intoxication results.

A primary objective of drug therapy is to attain an effective concentration of the drug in the reactive tissues and then to maintain this level by administering the drug repeatedly at appropriate intervals and doses. This goal is most rationally reached by applying to each patient what is known about the pharmacokinetic properties of the drugs that are being employed in the treatment. That is, the patient's dosage schedule is adjusted in accordance with data about each drug's rates of absorption, distribution and redistribution, metabolic inactivation, and excretion. These data, when applied to the particular patient together with monitoring of specific responses, help to guide the establishment of the best therapeutic regimen.

Applications of pharmacokinetics

Although the example given above of how alcohol accumulates to toxic levels is one that is familiar, the body handles alcohol in a way that differs from its handling of most drugs in one important respect. Alcohol is metabolized at a steady rate that remains the same whether the amount in the body is large or small—that is, the amount of alcohol eliminated per unit of time remains about the same no matter how much is in the body. With most other drugs, the rate of elimination is proportional to the amount in the body—the *amount* of drug eliminated is *not* constant; instead, a *constant fraction* of the total amount of drug in the body at any time is being eliminated.

In practice, this means that if several doses of a drug are taken at regular intervals that cause the drug to accumulate in the body, the amount of drug removed from the body in the intervals between doses also becomes greater. Inevitably, a point is finally reached at which the amount of the drug that is cleared between two doses is equal to the amount taken in with the previous dose. After that, the drug's concentration in the body stays the same (within certain limits) when the same schedule of doses and intervals is maintained.

Half-life

The time it takes for a drug to reach this *steady state* or *plateau level* depends on the rate of the processes by which it is eliminated. This is expressed in terms of the drug's biologic, or elimination, half-life, or $t\frac{1}{2}$—the time it takes for the amount of drug in the body to decrease to one-half of the peak previously attained. This index of the rate at which different drugs are eliminated varies widely (Fig. 4-4A). Penicillin, for example, normally has a short half-life, because it is rapidly excreted by the kidneys. The anticoagulant drug dicumarol (Coumadin) has a long half-life, because it is only slowly released from its plasma protein binding sites.

When a drug's half-life is known, dosage schedules can be calculated both for patients who possess the capacity to clear the drug from the body normally and for those with impaired excretory functions. For example, digoxin, a drug that is eliminated mainly by the kidneys in amounts proportional to the total amount in the body, normally has a half-life of 36 hours ($1\frac{1}{2}$ days). A patient with normal kidney function can be digitalized—that is, attain a steady state plateau of the drug—in about 1 week (slightly more than four half-lives) of regular daily dosing. In a patient with impaired renal function, the drug's half-life would be greatly prolonged, as would the time required to reach a steady state. To avoid accumulation to toxic levels, digoxin must then be given at intervals based on the drug's half-life in the patient with kidney damage, or it must be given in doses much smaller than those employed in patients with normal kidney function.

Loading and maintenance doses

In emergencies it is often necessary to raise a drug's concentration in the reactive tissues quickly to a fully effective level. To do so, the drug is administered initially in doses that exceed the body's ability to eliminate it. Such a so-called *loading dose* is potentially dangerous, so it is usually administered within a short time in several smaller doses, and the patient's response to each fraction is carefully monitored before each new increment is administered.

After a steady state level is attained, daily dosage

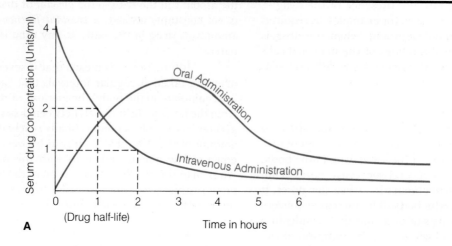

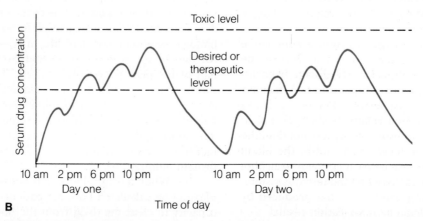

Figure 4-4. Influence of biologic half-life, route of administration, and dosage regimen on serum drug levels. (*A*) Influence of route of administration on time course of drug levels following a single dose of a drug. The dashed lines indicate how the biologic half-life of the drug may be determined from the curve of drug concentration after an IV dose. At time zero, immediately after the injection, there were 4 units of drug in each milliliter of serum. The drug concentration fell to half this amount, 2 units/ml, after 1 hour, the drug's biologic half-life. (*B*) Influence of dosage regimen on serum drug levels (drug given qid, 10-2-6-10). The drug accumulates as successive doses are given throughout each day; the drug is being given at a rate greater than the patient's body can eliminate it. This dosage regimen has been chosen so that the patient will have a therapeutic level of the drug for a significant portion of the day, yet never have a toxic level of the drug.

is reduced to a much smaller amount that is intended to make up for the portion of drug eliminated each day—the *maintenance dose.* Often, *digoxin* (Lanoxin) is administered to previously undigitalized patients by starting them off on maintenance doses to reduce the risk of overdosage. With *digitoxin* (Crystodigin; Purodigin), a drug that has a much longer half-life—about 1 week—it is not usually practical to try to digitalize patients in this way. Thus, loading doses of digitoxin are commonly employed to produce steady state plateau concentrations much more quickly than the more than 3 weeks of maintenance dose therapy that would be required to reach the same plateau level.

Figure 4-4*A* illustrates the difference in time course and maximum serum drug concentration when the same drug is given in the same dose intravenously as compared to orally. Figure 4-4*B* shows how a drug can

accumulate in the body when the rate of dosing exceeds the rate of drug elimination (metabolism and excretion). It also shows that the information obtained from pharmacokinetic studies can be used to establish a dosage regimen that maintains therapeutic levels of a drug for a significant proportion of the day, avoids toxic levels, and is practical to administer. When a therapeutic level of a drug must be continuously sustained, especially if the toxic and therapeutic levels are close together, the drug must be given by continuous intravenous infusion.

Drug–drug interactions: the combined effects of drugs

An important factor influencing the effect that a drug may produce is the presence in the body of another drug at the same time. That is, when one drug is given together with a second drug, its effects may differ from those that occur when it is administered alone. The effect produced by the action of the first drug may be either *increased* or *decreased* by the concurrent administration of the second drug or by the continuing effects of another drug that had been taken some time previously.

Definitions of terms

The various terms that describe the combined effects of drugs are used in different ways by different writers. Some use the terms so loosely that important distinctions become blurred. For example, the writers who prepare promotional copy for pharmaceutical manufacturers of drug mixtures sometimes seem to misuse some terms in ways that tend to make the mixture appear more effective than it really is. On the other hand, some laboratory scientists in the field of experimental pharmacodynamics often give the terms special meanings that are not readily applicable to clinical situations. In this textbook, the terms used in describing various clinically significant drug–drug interactions will have the meanings referred to in the following general discussion of the combined effects of drugs.

Synergism (from the Greek *syn*, together + *erg*, work) refers to the effects of combined drugs, in which the presence of one drug tends to *increase* the intensity or prolong the duration of an effect caused by another drug. The greater effect of the synergistic combination may be brought about in one of two general ways:

1. By two drugs, *both* of which produce *similar* effects. Thus, for example, if a dose of drug A exerts *x* effect and it is given together with a dose of drug B that also has *x* effect, the two together may produce a $3x$ effect, or a $5x$ effect, rather than the expected $2x$ effect
2. By two drugs, only *one* of which produces a particular effect. For example, drug A that has *x* effect may be combined with drug B that exerts o effect. Yet, the two together produce a $2x$ (or $3x$, and so forth) effect rather than the predicted $1x$ effect

The first type of synergistic effect is best seen when two drugs produce the *same type of effect* but do so by exerting their actions at *different sites* and by *different mechanisms*. For example, combining two drugs that can each cause a fall in blood pressure in different ways will produce a greater drop in a patient's high blood pressure through this type of double action than if either drug were given alone.

Another example of a similar type of synergism may be seen when the narcotic analgesic codeine is combined with the antipyretic–analgesic aspirin. Codeine probably exerts its pain-relieving effect by acting at central

nervous system sites; aspirin probably acts in the tissue from which pain impulses are emanating. Because these two drugs have different mechanisms of action, the combination may relieve pain more effectively than when either type of analgesic is given alone. Thus, adding codeine to aspirin is said to be synergistic, or *supra-additive*, while the combination of aspirin and phenacetin, another antipyretic–analgesic, is merely *additive*. (The term *addition*, or *simple summation*, refers to situations in which the combined effect of two drugs is equal to the sum of the effects of each—*i.e.*, $x + x = 2x$—rather than $3x$ or more, as is the case in supra-additive synergism.)

Potentiation is a term that is best reserved for describing the second general type of synergism mentioned above—that is, drug interactions in which only one of two drugs exerts the action that is made greater by the presence of the second drug. The term "potentiation" is best employed to describe those combined drug effects in which the effects of an *active* drug are intensified by the presence of an *inactive* drug that acts in some way to interfere with the metabolic breakdown or elimination of the active drug. Some adverse drug interactions discussed below in the section on clinical applications are examples of potentiation that sometimes occur unexpectedly in patients who are taking two or more drugs at the same time.

Antagonism is a term used to describe situations in which two active drugs given together produce an effect that is *less intense* than when either drug is given alone. This can occur when two drugs affect the same physiologic system in opposing ways, so that the effects of each drug tend to cancel each other out. Antagonism may also occur when two drugs combine chemically in the body to neutralize one another. In some clinical situations the simultaneous administration of two drugs can cause one of the drugs to produce an effect of less than the desired degree of intensity. Sometimes a second drug is given deliberately to antagonize the toxic effects of a drug that was taken earlier (see Chap. 5, Antidotes).

Clinical applications

Drugs may be administered together intentionally as mixtures that are thought to have a more desirable therapeutic effect when taken in combination than when administered alone. On the other hand, patients who take several medications concurrently sometimes suffer unexpected and undesired effects. Some aspects of both situations in which it is important to understand the effects that drugs may have when combined with one another will be discussed.

Drug mixtures. Sometimes two or more drugs are deliberately combined. One reason for doing this is to reduce the side-effects that may occur when a full dose of a single effective drug is administered. In the management of grand mal epilepsy, for instance, patients are often unable to tolerate fully effective doses of pheno-

Table 4–2. Examples of drug–drug interactions that result in altered absorption from the gastrointestinal tract

Interacting drugs (drug A with drug B)	Nature of interaction	Resulting effectiveness of drug B	Clinical manifestations of interaction	Appropriate nursing action
Antacids with				
Coumarin-type oral anticoagulants (dicumarol, warfarin)	↓ Absorption of drug B	↓	↓ Anticoagulant effect	Schedule drug B 2 hr after antacid
Certain antibacterial drugs: sulfonamides, nalidixic acid, nitrofurantoin	↓ Absorption of drug B	↓	↓ Antibacterial effect	Schedule drug B 2 hr after antacid
Tetracycline-type antibiotics	Drug B bound by drug A → ↓ absorption of drug B	↓	↓ Antibacterial effect	Schedule drug B 2 hr after antacid
Enteric-coated drugs	Premature disintegration of coating	↓	↓ Therapeutic effect; nausea and vomiting may result from liberation of some drugs in stomach	Schedule drug B 2 hr after antacid
Mineral oil with				
Fat-soluble vitamins (A, D, E, K)	↓ Absorption of drug B	↓	↓ Therapeutic effect (chronic use of mineral oil → hypovitaminosis, including bleeding caused by hypovitaminosis K)	Schedule drug B 2 hr after mineral oil and avoid chronic use of mineral oil
Coumarin-type oral anticoagulants	↓ Absorption of drug B (anticoagulant) caused by laxative effect of drug A	↓	↓ Anticoagulant effect (but ↓ absorption of vitamin K can ↑ anticoagulant effect)	Schedule drug A and drug B separately
Cholestyramine with				
Thyroxine and other thyroid preparations	Drug B bound to drug A → ↓ absorption of drug B (thyroid preparation)	↓	Hypothyroidism	Schedule drug B 1 hr before or 4–6 hr after drug A
Vitamins A, D, K	↓ Absorption of drug B (vitamins)	↓	Hypovitaminosis	Schedule drug B 1 hr before or 4–6 hr after drug A
Coumarin-type anticoagulants	↓ Absorption of drug B	↓	↓ Anticoagulant effect	Schedule drug B 1 hr before or 4–6 hr after drug A

Table 4–2. Examples of drug–drug interactions that result in altered absorption from the gastrointestinal tract (continued)

Interacting drugs (drug A with drug B)	Nature of interaction	Resulting effectiveness of drug B	Clinical manifestations of interaction	Appropriate nursing action
Chlorothiazide (Diuril)-type diuretics	↓ Absorption of drug B	↓	↓ Diuretic effect	Schedule drug B 1 hr before or 4–6 hr after drug A
Phenylbutazone (Butazolidin)	↓ Absorption of drug B	↓	↓ Analgesia and ↓ anti-inflammatory effect	Schedule drug B 1 hr before or 4–6 hr after drug A
Other acidic drugs	↓ Absorption of drug B	↓	Depends on drug B	Schedule drug B 1 hr before or 4–6 hr after drug A
Fecal softeners (*e.g.*, dioctyl sodium sulfosuccinate, DSS; Colace) with				
Mineral oil	Surfactant activity may permit systemic absorption of mineral oil		Mineral oil emboli; foreign body reactions in liver, lymph nodes, spleen	Schedule drug A and drug B separately

barbital (Luminal) or of phenytoin (Dilantin). That is, a full dose of phenobarbital may make the patient too drowsy, and full doses of phenytoin may make the patient walk unsteadily or cause stomach upset.

The neurologist may then try to treat the epileptic patient by ordering both drugs together in fractions of the full therapeutic dose of each. The dose of each antiseizure agent may be adjusted until a mixture of the two with optimal therapeutic effects is established. The additive antiepileptic effects of the two drugs may then keep the patient free of seizures but, because the side-effects of the two drugs are different, the smaller doses of each drug may cause neither type of adverse reaction. If drowsiness still tends to occur, a third drug may be added to the mixture—a psychomotor stimulant such as caffeine or an amphetamine to antagonize the central depression.

Ready-made combinations. The prescribing of manufactured dosage forms containing combinations of drugs has come under attack from several quarters. The FDA has called some combination products "ineffective" and has required that they be withdrawn from the market. Many drug mixtures still on the market are, indeed, irrational. Obviously, if any of the ingredients fails to contribute to the total therapeutic effect, the patient for whom it is prescribed is not receiving the benefits intended. Not only is the patient paying for a drug that is not needed, but its presence may produce unnecessary toxic effects.

Even when all the drugs that are mixed together in a single dosage form do what they are supposed to do, there may be disadvantages in some fixed dose combinations. The dosage ratios in which the several components are combined may not be suited to the needs of many patients. Thus, because fixed dose combinations fail to offer the flexibility of tailoring the dosage of each drug and the timing of its administration to each individual patient, most fixed combination prescription drug products are now not recommended.

Nonetheless, the administration of several drugs combined in doses that are appropriate for most people sometimes has certain important advantages over administering the several drugs separately. Certainly, patients find it more convenient to take several drugs combined in a single capsule or tablet than to take the same set of drugs from different bottles. A prescription for a combination product is also usually less expensive than several of the same drugs purchased separately and, if a patient tends to get confused in following directions, it may even be safer to take a single combination product than several separate drugs.

Unintended drug–drug interactions. It has been recognized that patients who are taking several potent drugs simultaneously may react in ways that were not intended when the drugs were ordered. In some cases the presence of one drug may prevent a patient from benefiting from treatment with another drug by antagonizing its therapeutic effect. In other cases, which are more frequent and potentially more serious, one drug potentiates the action of another. This can cause an unexpected toxic effect to develop in patients taking what had previously been considered to be a safe dose of a potent drug. According to one study, a hospitalized patient may receive a dozen different drugs during the hospital stay. The probability of the occurrence of an undesirable drug–drug interaction when the patient takes several drugs simultaneously is very high. Actually, although the more than 700 specific drug substances available have the potential for more than 55 million drug–drug interactions, there are very few clinically important drug–drug interactions.

All medical personnel have a professional responsibility to prevent drug–drug interactions that may endanger the patient or deprive him of desired therapeutic effects. Nurses are being urged to check the medication record and to ask the patient whether any drugs prescribed by someone else or bought without a prescription are being taken. Pharmacists are being called on to maintain records on every patient indicating every medication that they may be taking, including both prescription drugs and over-the-counter products. Nurses have the continual responsibility of observing the responses of patients whom they know to be on multiple drug therapy. They must also be aware of which drugs are most likely to interact in ways that result in unintended reactions. Although booklets are now available that contain long lists of reported drug–drug interactions, the best way to be prepared to prevent adverse drug effects is to *understand the basic mechanisms* involved, rather than merely to refer to lists.

Reasons for drug–drug interactions

The most common way in which one drug causes a second drug to produce unexpected effects is by influencing its pharmacokinetics. That is, when one drug affects the processes by which the other is *absorbed, distributed, biotransformed,* and *excreted,* the *concentration* that the second drug reaches in the body will be different from what is ordinarily attained when the same dose of the second drug is administered alone. As a result, the pharmacologic response to the drug may be either less than expected or markedly more intense and long-lasting than was anticipated by whoever ordered the drug to be given in that particular dose and at those intervals.

Absorption. Drugs ordered for peptic ulcer patients who are under treatment with high doses of antacids intended to neutralize gastric acidity may be poorly absorbed into the systemic circulation (Table 4-2). This, of course, results in a reduction of the intended therapeutic effects of the drugs that are taken together with the antacid. Patients taking anticoagulants may not be fully protected against blood-clotting episodes if they take high doses of sodium bicarbonate for relief of stomach hy-

peracidity or heartburn. Patients taking most tetracycline-type antibiotics should be told not to take antacids or milk simultaneously, because calcium, magnesium, and aluminum ions tend to combine with the antibiotic in the gastrointestinal tract to form a poorly absorbable complex. This could delay the patient's recovery from the infection that is being treated.

Distribution. As previously indicated, when some drugs are absorbed into the bloodstream, most of their molecules attach themselves to plasma proteins. The portion that is being transported in the bound form is not pharmacologically active; only those molecules that are free can diffuse into the tissues and exert their effects. The presence of a second drug in the blood can intensify the activity of some strongly bound drugs by displacing their molecules from plasma proteins, thus increasing the amount of drug that is free to leave the blood and to reach the reactive tissues.

This increased availability of free drug is brought about because the second drug competes for the plasma-binding sites and displaces the first drug, which is then free to diffuse to its site of action. If the displaced drug is a highly potent one, the added amount of active drug can lead to toxic effects. For example, a cancer patient taking methotrexate in prescribed doses may become poisoned simply by taking a salicylate drug such as aspirin. This happens because the extra methotrexate displaced by the salicylate may destroy the narrow margin between this drug's therapeutic effects (the destruction of cancer cells) and its toxic effects on normal cells.

The effects of the coumarin-type anticoagulant drugs dicumarol and warfarin (Coumadin) can also be dangerously potentiated by various drugs that displace them from plasma proteins (Table 4-3). Over 95% of any dose of these potent drugs is transported in the bound form; only the less than 5% that is free has effects on blood clotting. But, if another drug—the anti-inflammatory agent phenylbutazone (Butazolidin) for example—displaces some of the bound anticoagulant, enough extra drug may be freed to bring about unexpected bleeding in a patient who had previously been well stabilized on the anticoagulant drug dosage.

Metabolism. The effects of drugs that are inactivated by the drug-metabolizing enzymes of the liver may be either increased or decreased by the presence of other drugs that affect the functioning of these enzymes. The activity of the hepatic enzymes may be inhibited by some drugs; other drugs may stimulate their biosynthesis (see Enzyme Induction, above). In one case the metabolism of certain other drugs taken at the same time is interfered with, so that these drugs are less readily inactivated; in the other instance, induction of the enzymes leads to more rapid metabolism of other drugs that are being taken concurrently. In both situations, the drug–drug interactions lead to pharmacologic effects different in intensity from what may have been expected.

Table 4–3. Examples of drug–drug interactions resulting from changes in a drug's distribution or transport

Interacting drugs (drug A with drug B)	Nature of interaction	Resulting effectiveness of drug B	Clinical manifestations of interaction	Appropriate nursing action
Anti-inflammatory drugs such as phenylbutazone (Butazolidin); indomethacin (Indocin); salicylates; oral hypoglycemic agents (Diabinese); sulfonamides; other acidic drugs with				
Coumarin-type anticoagulants	↓ Plasma protein binding of drug B (anticoagulant)	↑	Bleeding	↓ Dose of anticoagulant and monitor
Salicylates (aspirin); phenylbutazone; sulfonamides; phenytoin (Dilantin); tetracyclines with				
Methotrexate (Amethopterin)	↓ Plasma protein binding of drug B (methotrexate)	↑	↑ Toxicity of methotrexate, especially to GI tract and bone marrow	Avoid the combinations
Valproic acid (Depakene) with				
Phenytoin (Dilantin)	↓ Plasma protein binding of drug B (phenytoin)	↑	Sedation; nystagmus; ataxia	Monitor and adjust dosage of phenytoin

Phenytoin (Dilantin), for example, is a drug that is ordinarily detoxified by a liver enzyme system that catalyzes a hydroxylation-type reaction (Table 4-4). An epileptic patient who has been stabilized on a certain safe dosage of this drug may later be found to be suffering from tuberculosis as well. If such a patient is then placed on treatment with the first-line antituberculosis drug isoniazid (INH), signs of phenytoin toxicity may soon be shown. This has been traced to the fact that the antituberculosis drug inhibits the enzymatic breakdown of the anti-epileptic drug. If the patient continues to take this drug in the usual dose, its concentration in the brain may rise to toxic levels, and adverse effects caused by the potentiation of the drug's central effects may occur.

As already indicated, phenobarbital and other barbiturates can stimulate the biosynthesis of the enzymes responsible for their own metabolic breakdown. This not only leads to tolerance to the barbiturates themselves, but it also increases the rate of inactivation of various other drugs, including drugs such as warfarin that are used clinically to prevent blood clotting. Thus, a patient who had been stabilized on a therapeutic dose of an anticoagulant drug may fail to benefit fully from the medication if he also begins to take a barbiturate or various other sedatives and tranquilizers. That is, because of the increased rate at which the anticoagulant may now be metabolized, the previously effective dose may no longer be adequate for protecting the patient from suffering episodes of intravascular blood clotting.

The phenomenon of drug-induced enzyme induction has also been found to lead to dangerous drug interactions of still another type. For example, a patient who has suffered a heart attack may be treated simultaneously with barbiturates or with certain other sedatives such as meprobamate (Equanil; Miltown) or chloral hydrate and with an anticoagulant such as warfarin. Presence of the sedative may stimulate the synthesis of detoxifying enzymes to such an extent that much higher than ordinary doses of the anticoagulant drug are required to reduce the patient's clotting components to a therapeutically desirable level. Later, the sedative drug may be discontinued but the patient may be kept on the same dose of anticoagulant. Elimination of the sedative drug allows the level of liver enzymes to drop back to normal. Because this, of course, reduces the body's ability to metabolize the anticoagulant drug, it can then accumulate to toxic levels. Fatal hemorrhages have resulted from this type of drug–drug interaction.

Excretion. As previously discussed, some drugs depend on the kidneys for their elimination; other drugs

Table 4—4. Examples of drug–drug interactions resulting from changes in drug metabolism

Interacting drugs (drug A with drug B)	Nature of interaction	Resulting effectiveness of drug B	Clinical manifestations of interaction	Appropriate nursing action
Barbiturates and glutethimide (Doriden); phenytoin (Dilantin) with				
Coumarin-type oral anticoagulants	↑ Metabolism of drug B (anticoagulant)	↓	↓ Anticoagulant effect	↑ Dose of anticoagulant and monitor
Coumarin-type oral anticoagulants with				
Oral hypoglycemic drugs such as chlorpropamide (Diabinese)	↓ Metabolism of drug B (hypoglycemic agent)	↑	Hypoglycemic reactions	↓ Dose of hypoglycemic agent and monitor
Coumarin-type oral anticoagulants; chloramphenicol (Chloromycetin); phenylbutazone (Butazolidin); isoniazid (INH); sulfonamides; disulfiram (Antabuse); cimetidine (Tagamet) with				
Phenytoin (Dilantin)	↓ Metabolism of drug B (phenytoin)	↑	Sedation; nystagmus; ataxia	↓ Dose of phenytoin and monitor
Cigarette smoke and phenobarbital with				
Theophylline	↑ Metabolism of drug B (theophylline)	↓	Bronchoconstriction	↑ Dose of theophylline and monitor
Allopurinol (Zyloprim) with				
Mercaptopurine (Purinethol)	↓ Metabolism of drug B (mercaptopurine)	↑	Severe bone marrow depression	↓ Dose of mercaptopurine and monitor

exert their pharmacologic effects by altering renal function. In both cases, interactions may result between two drugs because of the altered renal effects of one or both of the drugs when given in combination. Diuretic drugs given with digitalis to aid in eliminating sodium may also cause loss of potassium ions and so precipitate digitalis intoxication. On the other hand, administering the drug probenecid (Benemid) together with penicillin tends to prevent the renal excretion of penicillin by the kidney tubules in a way that causes *not* increased toxicity but potentiation of the antibacterial effect of the antibiotic as a result of the relatively high levels that it then reaches in the tissues (Table 4-5).

Probenecid is also sometimes involved in less desirable drug–drug interactions. Its ability to aid gout patients by increasing the elimination of plasma uric acid is interfered with by the simultaneous administration of aspirin, a drug that tends to antagonize the effect of pro-

benecid on the renal excretion of uric acid. Thus, to avoid this therapeutic incompatibility that prevents the gout patient from obtaining the desired benefits of his antigout medication, a *non*salicylate analgesic is selected for relief of the patient's joint pain.

A common and potentially dangerous drug–drug interaction occurs at the renal level between digoxin and quinidine, both of which are given to treat cardiac problems. The quinidine seems to block the renal excretion of digoxin, allowing the serum levels of digoxin to increase to toxic levels. These high levels of digoxin can cause potentially fatal arrhythmias in cardiac patients.

Clinical significance

Because two drugs are known to interact in ways that tend to potentiate or antagonize each other does not necessarily mean that the two can never be administered together. A patient who needs to take two medications

Table 4–5. Examples of drug–drug interactions resulting from interference with excretion

Interacting drugs (drug A with drug B)	Nature of interaction	Resulting effectiveness of drug B	Clinical manifestations of interaction	Appropriate nursing action
Aspirin with				
Probenecid (Benemid)	↓ Renal tubular secretion of probenecid → ↓ ability of probenecid to block tubular reabsorption of uric acid → ↑ plasma uric acid levels	↓	↑ Gout symptoms	Use acetaminophen or some other nonsalicylate analgesic in patients on probenecid
Probenecid with				
Sulfonamides	↓ Renal excretion of drug B	↑	↑ Risk of sulfonamide toxicity	↓ Dose and monitor
Oral hypoglycemics (Diabinese)	↓ Renal excretion of drug B	↑	Hypoglycemia	↓ Dose and monitor
Indomethacin (Indocin)	↓ Renal excretion of drug B	↑	↑ Risk of GI and other adverse effects of indomethacin	↓ Dose and monitor
Furosemide (Lasix), ethacrynic acid (Edecrin) and other diuretics with				
Lithium	↓ Renal excretion of drug B (lithium)	↑	Lithium toxicity	Avoid the combination
Quinidine with				
Digoxin (Lanoxin)	↓ Renal excretion of drug B (digoxin)	↑	Digoxin toxicity; cardiac arrhythmias	↓ Dose of digoxin and monitor

concurrently need not be deprived of the benefits of one of them. Both drugs may be ordered, but doses of each will need to be adjusted very carefully. That is, as long as the possibility of an unfavorable interaction is known, it can be avoided by reducing the dose of a drug that may be potentiated or by raising the dose of a drug that may be antagonized. The key point is the need for remaining alert to the possibility of drug–drug interactions during multiple drug therapy. Clinically important drug–drug interactions are especially likely to occur between drugs that have relatively small margins of safety—that is, between drugs whose therapeutic and toxic levels are close together.

Before administering drugs, the nurse should evaluate the overall situation for the occurrence of known drug–drug interactions. When evaluating and teaching patients who are on more than one drug, several key points should be included to avoid the problems of drug–drug interactions.

Dosage. If two drugs interact in the body, the doses of the drugs have to be carefully adjusted and balanced to counteract the effects of the interaction and to provide the patient with the optimal therapeutic benefit. The patient has to understand that the precise dose of each drug is crucial to the therapy. Missing the dose of one drug or running out of one drug can have detrimental effects. If a patient has been maintained on interacting drugs and one is discontinued, the nurse or physician must be very careful to readjust the dose of the other drug to compensate for the loss of the interacting influence.

OTC drugs. Many over-the-counter (OTC) medications contain drugs that are known to cause drug–drug interactions. Patients need to be advised to avoid self-medication with OTC drugs when they are taking drugs with relatively low margins of safety. When evaluating unanticipated responses to drugs, the nurse should question the patient carefully regarding the possible use of OTC drugs.

Scheduling. If drugs are taken at different times, drug–drug interactions can often be avoided. If it is important that the patient take two drugs at different times to avoid drug–drug interactions, it is essential that the patient understand this timing and the reason for it. Otherwise, the patient is likely to take all medications at one time for the sake of convenience.

Monitoring toxic effects. The nurse and patient should be aware of and alert for the most common side-effects of drugs that may be involved in drug–drug interactions. Detecting any undesired effects when they first occur can lead to early readjustment of doses and to minimal discomfort and risk for the patient.

Summary

This chapter has attempted to illustrate by practical examples some of the current concepts of how drugs and other foreign chemicals interact with the chemical constituents of the cells of the human body. Although these aspects of biochemical and molecular pharmacology may seem extremely complex and irrelevant to clinical practice, this knowledge will help to broaden and deepen the nurse's growing understanding of how drugs achieve their therapeutic effect, and to improve the nurse's clinical judgment.

References

Anderson R: Drug prescribing for patients in renal failure. Hosp Pract 18:145, 1983

Beckman DA, Brent RL: Mechanisms of teratogenesis. Ann Rev Pharmacol Toxical 24:483, 1984

Carr CJ: Food and drug interactions. Ann Rev Pharmacol Toxicol 22:19, 1982

Døssing M: Changes in hepatic microsomal enzyme function in workers exposed to mixture of chemicals. Clin Pharmacol Ther 32:340, 1982

Drug interactions update. Medical Letter 26:11–14, Feb 3, 1984

Goldman P: Rate-controlled drug delivery. N Engl J Med 307:286, 1982

Grabiniski P et al: Plasma levels and analgesia following deltoid and gluteal injections of methadone and morphine. J Clin Pharmacol 23:48, 1983

Karch AM: Mixing drugs may be hazardous to your patient's health. J Prac Nurs 29:18, 1979

Karch FE, Karch AM: Clinically important drug interactions, 1979. Nurses Drug Alert 3:25, March, 1979

Levine RR: Pharmacology: Drug Actions and Reactions, 3rd ed. Boston, Little, Brown, 1983

Medical Letter: The Medical Letter Handbook of Drug Interactions. New Rochelle, 1983

Orr ML: Drugs and renal disease. Am J Nurs 81:969, 1981

Overstreet DH, Yamamura HI: Receptor alterations and drug tolerance. Life Sci 25:1865, 1979

Pantuck EJ et al: Stimulatory effect of brussel sprouts and cabbage on human drug metabolism. Clin Pharmacol Ther 25:88, 1979

Snyder SH: Receptors, neurotransmitters and drug responses. N Engl J Med 300:465, 1979

Tobey LE et al: Antimicrobial drug interactions. Am J Nurs 75:1470, 1975

Vesell ES: Pharmacogenetics. N Engl J Med 287:904, 1972

Weintraub M: The therapeutic window: When more is much, much less. Drug Therapy 9:163, 1979

Chapter 5

The toxic effects of drugs and chemicals

5

All drugs are potentially poisonous. Even after chemicals have been carefully screened and tested for toxicity in animals, the drug products containing them often cause unexpectedly severe reactions when administered to patients under clinical conditions. Many different factors can make some patients react adversely to a dose of a drug that is harmless to most people. This chapter will describe in more detail various types of toxic effects of drugs and other chemicals.

Broadly speaking, the undesirable effects of drugs fall into two classes:

1. Adverse effects that are the result of a drug's known pharmacologic effects. Toxic effects of this kind can occur in any patient, provided that the dose is high enough. These *dose-related* effects can be brought about by relatively small doses in the minority of patients who are hypersusceptible to one or another of the drug's primary or secondary pharmacologic effects. However, massive overdosage can cause drug poisoning in *all* patients.
2. Adverse effects that are *not* related to a drug's expected pharmacologic effects. These effects, which cannot be predicted on the basis of animal and human toxicity tests, are the result of something peculiar to a particular patient's tissue reactivity. *Drug allergy,* or hypersensitivity-type reactions of an immunologic nature, come under this category, as do *idiosyncratic reactions* related to pharmacogenetic factors.

Adverse drug reactions that occur during ordinary drug therapy will be discussed next. Acute toxicity caused by accidental or deliberate intake of massive amounts of drugs and other chemicals will be discussed separately later in this chapter. Another type of chronic toxicity, that which develops in drug abusers and leads to drug dependence, addiction, and its complications, will be discussed separately in the chapter on drug abuse (Chap. 53).

Adverse drug reactions

The exact extent of drug-induced illness is uncertain. Reports range from as high as 5% of all hospital admissions to as low as 0.5%. Similarly, there are wide discrepancies in different studies as to the number of hospital patients who react adversely to medications that they receive during treatment. Some studies suggest that between 15% and 30% of patients suffer a drug reaction of one kind or another, and the number of drug-related deaths in hospitalized patients, although disputed, is significant.

In any case, there is no doubt that the problem of coping with the adverse effects of drugs has never been as serious as it is today. The many newly synthesized chemicals that are now being introduced as therapeutic and diagnostic agents can cause a much greater variety of reactions than those that occurred with medicines from natural sources. Such reactions are also often much more severe than those caused by the relatively weak medicines that were once used to treat patients. Thus, the same actively potent drugs that have brought such benefits to so many people in this golden age of drug therapy are often the very ones that are also responsible for the rising tide of adverse reactions.

The nurse should be aware that every drug that is used in therapy can cause adverse effects in some patients. Thus, the nurse must constantly be alert to detect the signs of drug reactions of different types. Patients and their families need to be taught what to look for when patients are taking drugs at home. Thus, throughout this book, the signs and symptoms of toxicity that the nurse should look for with each class of drugs that is being discussed will be emphasized. Here, some general principles of drug toxicity detection and prevention will be presented along with some examples of situations that illustrate various types of toxicity.

Pharmacologic, or predictable, toxicity

Primary actions

One of the most common occurrences when drugs are being administered is the development of adverse effects from simple overdosage. In such cases the patient suffers from effects that are merely an *extension of the desired action* of the compound. Thus, a patient taking a dose of phenobarbital that was intended only to reduce nervous tension may become excessively drowsy and find that ordinary activities cannot be performed. More serious, but still similar in principle, is the case of the patient receiving an anticoagulant drug in a dose that produces the intended effect to a greater degree than was expected. Instead of lowering the clotting factors in the blood only to the point at which the chances of clot formation are reduced, the drug's action may lead to development of spontaneous bleeding.

Such excessive reactions to a drug's main action can usually be avoided by adjusting the dosage carefully to the needs of each individual patient instead of having the patient take the "usual" or "average" dose. Thus, when the nurse evaluates the patient's response to drug therapy and finds that the patient is reacting in the expected way but more strongly than intended, a reduction in dosage or an increase in the intervals between doses would be ordered. If, for example, it is noted that a hypertensive patient taking a blood pressure-reducing drug becomes weak, dizzy, and faint on arising, the drug's dosage will usually be adjusted in a manner intended to limit the drug-induced fall in pressure. Similarly, when certain abnormalities are detected in the pulse of a heart failure patient receiving digitalis, the dosage will be lowered to a level that will produce the desired cardiac effects and not the toxic ones.

Secondary actions

Drugs rarely possess a single specific action but can usually produce a wide variety of effects in addition to the primary one. Many of these multiple actions are uncovered during the initial screening tests, on the basis of which the pharmacologist determines the drug's profile of pharmacologic activity. Fortunately for most patients, it is usually possible to find a dose that brings about the desired effect without producing undesired secondary reactions. Sometimes, however, this is not possible, and the occurrence of a side-effect is almost inevitable when a patient receives an ordinary therapeutic dose of the drug.

For example, a patient being treated for allergy with an antihistaminic drug may become drowsy because the dose of the drug required for controlling allergic symptoms may also depress parts of the brain. If the patient reports this, the physician may discontinue the drug and try another antihistaminic agent or prescribe a small dose of central stimulant in an attempt to counteract the depressant effects. Interestingly, some antihistaminic drugs are actually employed for treating insomnia. Thus, the very action that is considered undesirable in one patient may be the one for which a drug is employed in another. Currently a new group of antihistaminic drugs that lacks sedative properties is under investigation for use in the United States and is in use elsewhere.

Hypersusceptibility

Patients are often excessively responsive to either the primary or the secondary pharmacologic actions of therapeutic agents. Various clinical situations in which patients proved to be hypersusceptible to the primary actions of various drugs were discussed in Chapter 4. Given an initial dose that produces the therapeutically desired effect in most patients, these patients respond with too great an effect and require reduced dosage if treatment is to be continued.

The most common cause of such reactions is the presence of some pathologic condition other than the one being treated. For example, patients with liver and kidney disease are hypersusceptible to the actions of drugs that depend on healthy hepatic and renal functions for their elimination from the body. Thus, many drugs are administered only with great caution, and others are contraindicated, because of the dangerous reactions that can occur when an unmetabolized or unexcreted drug accumulates to toxic levels. This is a frequent consideration in elderly patients or in others with disorders of these vital organs.

Other illnesses may make it unsafe to administer certain drugs because their ordinary actions may produce adverse effects in those patients who are particularly susceptible to them. These predisposing conditions are contraindications to the use of specific drugs. Thus, a hyperthyroid patient may react excessively to the stimulating effects of an adrenergic drug such as epinephrine or ephedrine, and an ordinary dose of morphine may produce excessive depression in a hypothyroid patient. Similarly, the use of many other potent drugs may be contraindicated in the presence of pre-existing disease, because the effect produced in most patients cannot be safely attained in those with certain types of illnesses.

Some patients may be more susceptible to one of a drug's secondary actions than they are to its therapeutic action. Thus, atropine and similar natural and synthetic anticholinergic drugs used for treating peptic ulcer are contraindicated in certain patients, who may suffer severely from one or another of several secondary effects when these agents are administered in doses intended only to reduce gastric acid secretion and to relax gastrointestinal smooth muscle spasm. These drugs may, for instance, precipitate an attack of glaucoma when administered to patients especially susceptible to this condition, even though they cause only some annoying but bearable blurring of vision in most people. Similarly, atropine and other drugs of this class are contraindicated in elderly men with an enlarged prostate gland, because a secondary action that most people are hardly aware of may lead to bladder paralysis and urinary retention, requiring catheterization.

The important point about side-effects that stem from a drug's primary and secondary pharmacologic actions is that they are largely predictable and can therefore be prevented or, at least, minimized. Thus, if the physician and nurse are aware of a drug's fundamental actions and apply their knowledge to the case of the particular patient being treated, severe side-effects of this type need never occur.

In the weighing of potential benefit against potential risk the primary responsibility belongs, of course, to whoever is writing the drug order. For example, in a patient with a history of asthma, the nurse or physician may avoid treating postoperative abdominal distention or urinary retention with a smooth muscle stimulant such as bethanechol (Urecholine), because muscle-contracting drugs of this class may constrict the patient's bronchial tubes and interfere excessively with the respiratory exchanges. If all the risks have been weighed, and it is decided to employ a drug despite its potentially adverse pharmacologic effects, the patient must be closely watched to detect early laboratory and clinical signs of the onset of toxicity.

Drug allergy and idiosyncrasy

Some adverse drug reactions have little to do with a drug's ordinary pharmacologic effects. They occur as the result of a patient's extreme sensitivity to certain types of chemical substances. Reactions that do not develop the first time a patient takes a drug but only on later exposures to it are usually the result of drug *allergy*. Patients who prove abnormally sensitive to small doses of a drug the very first time it is administered are often said to suffer from drug *idiosyncrasy*.

Both types of ill effects have in common the fact that they are not seen in experimental animals during preclinical studies of a drug's potential toxicity. They are also not likely to be detected during the early phases of a drug's clinical evaluation, but only after the drug has been taken by large numbers of people. This is because only a minority of exposed people develop drug allergy,

and the number of idiosyncratic persons is very much smaller. Thus, these reactions are not readily predictable unless the patient has a prior history of a particular drug allergy or idiosyncrasy.

Drug allergy

The term "allergic" refers to immunologically based reactions of the body to the presence of various "foreign" substances. In brief, the body's immunologic system responds to the presence of large foreign molecules (mainly proteins) called *antigens* by producing specific immunoglobulins called *antibodies*. The person whose body responds in this way on first exposure to the foreign macromolecule is said to be *sensitized* to it. If this hypersensitive person is later exposed to the same antigen, an antigen–antibody reaction occurs that can indirectly cause damage to body tissues.

Most drugs are small molecules that do not themselves stimulate the production of antibodies. However, drugs do cause allergic reactions by bringing about changes in such body macromolecules as proteins and, sometimes, in polysaccharides and polynucleotides. Actually, it is usually not the administered drug itself that does so but one or another of the drug's breakdown products, or metabolites.

These more chemically reactive metabolites, called *haptens* or *partial antigens,* combine with carrier macromolecules to form a complex that can stimulate the biosynthesis of antibodies (Fig. 5-1). These then become attached to body tissues and, when the drug-sensitized person is again exposed to the drug or its metabolites, a reaction occurs between these haptens and the preformed antibodies. This reaction causes various types of tissue damage, leading to the many signs and symptoms of drug allergy.

Types of allergic reactions

In the past, allergic drug reactions were classified as immediate or delayed on the basis of how quickly or slowly the clinical signs and symptoms began to appear after a sensitized person was re-exposed to the drug that acted as a hapten. Now that more is known about the immunologic basis for different types of drug allergy, it seems more suitable to classify such hypersensitivity reactions in terms of their underlying immunologic mechanisms. Thus, one common classification subdivides allergic drug reactions into the following four main types.

Type I: Anaphylactic, or immediate, type. This type involves formation of a specific class of antibodies, called *reagins,* that belong to the immunoglobulin E (IgE) group. These antibodies become fixed to the surface of certain types of blood and tissue cells of the drug-sensitized person. On later re-exposure to the hapten, which combines with the antibodies that are bound to the target tissue cells, a reaction takes place that releases several

Initial exposure   Subsequent exposure

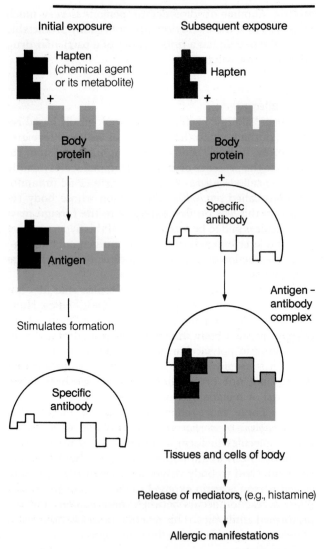

Figure 5-1. Mechanism of the allergic response. In the initial exposure, the drug (hapten) combines with a body protein to form the antigen, which then stimulates the formation of specific antibodies. The present concept of the immunopathogenesis of histamine release from mast cells on subsequent exposure to the hapten involves the following sequence of events: (1) the specific antibodies bind at one end to mast cells, leaving antigen-binding sites free to react; (2) the antigen binds to antibody at antigen-binding sites; and (3) the antigen–antibody complex triggers the release of histamine. (Redrawn after Levine RR: Pharmacology: Drug Actions and Reactions, 3rd ed. Boston, Little, Brown & Co., 1983)

natural substances or chemicals. These pharmacologically active chemicals bring about the signs and symptoms of type I reactions.

Type II: Cytotoxic-type reactions. In this type of reaction, the antibodies that were formed in response to previous exposure to the drug are circulating in the serum. When the administered antigens localize on cell surfaces, the antibodies react with them to form a cell-damaging antigen–antibody complex (see Hemolytic Anemia, below).

Type III: Serum sickness-type reactions. In these reactions the soluble antigen–antibody complexes circulate within the blood vessels and cause damage to various tissues. Serum sickness is an example of this type of allergic reaction that occurs about 1 week or more after exposure to the antigen, which may be either an injected foreign protein or a small molecule drug.

Type IV: Delayed allergic reactions (tuberculin type). These develop several hours after exposure to the allergen, which reacts with preformed antibodies that are bound to sensitized lymphocytes. Poison ivy and other forms of contact dermatitis are examples of this type of allergic drug reaction.

Signs and symptoms

The most dramatic drug reactions are those of the immediate and anaphylactic type, which develop within minutes of exposure to a chemical to which the person has previously been sensitized. The antigen–antibody reaction is believed to result in the release of active chemical substances, such as *histamine,* from the tissues themselves. These chemical mediators that are suddenly set free from a bound form act on the smooth muscles of small blood vessels to cause vasodilatation, and they act on smooth muscle and secretory glands of other organs, such as the bronchi.

Allergic reactions of this type may be relatively mild, or they may be severe enough to be rapidly fatal. The less severe reactions may be manifested by the appearance of raised, itchy wheals, or by swellings in the skin (urticaria, or "hives"). The anaphylactic-type reactions can lead to swift circulatory collapse or to asphyxia from swelling of the larynx and blockage of bronchial passages. Small doses of otherwise safe drugs such as aspirin and penicillin have caused death within a few minutes. The degree of severity does not depend on the drug that set off the allergic reaction but on how strongly sensitized the person was when the drug was given on the second, or later, occasion.

Serum sickness-type reactions are marked by the delayed development of an itchy rash, high fever, swollen lymph nodes and joints, edema of the face and limbs, and other discomforting signs and symptoms. This reaction was first seen clinically when patients received injections of antitoxins contained in the serum of horses. Although caution is still required in patients who are about to receive antitoxins of animal origin for treating tetanus, diphtheria, rubella, and other diseases, so-called serum sickness occurs much more commonly today as a delayed reaction to various types of drugs, including the sulfonamides and penicillin.

Specific organ damage often occurs as a result of drug allergy. That is, damage may be localized in the skin or in specific formed elements of the blood. Such localization in a single organ or tissue—liver, kidneys, or eyes, for example—is thought to result from accumulation of the sensitizing drug at one or another of these sites. The reason for such local accumulation of the antigenic substance is probably the fact that the tissue contains drug-degrading enzymes that produce chemically reactive metabolites—haptens—that then combine with local tissue proteins.

Often immunologic reactions of this type cannot be differentiated from nonimmunologic reactions that cause similar clinical responses. Thus, before discussing various adverse reactions to drugs that involve specific organs and tissues, such as the skin, blood vessels, blood and bone marrow, liver, kidney, and ocular tissues, the type of adverse drug reactions that have been termed "idiosyncrasies" will be described. Examples of tissue-damaging drug reactions that may be either immunologic (allergic) or nonimmunologic in origin will then be discussed.

Drug idiosyncrasy

This term, which is sometimes used to describe abnormal reactions to drugs, is not easy to define. It does not refer to drug reactions that result from a patient's allergic *hypersensitivity*, nor does it describe the result of dose-related hypersusceptibility to a drug's ordinary pharmacologic actions. The term is not correctly employed to excuse catastrophic drug reactions that were really the result of the improper administration of a drug with resulting sudden overdosage-type toxicity.

Unpredictable reactions of this type are probably best limited to those that have a pharmacogenetic basis. As indicated in Chapter 4, some people are born with hereditary defects that result in abnormal responses when they are exposed to ordinary doses of various drugs. Recently, the specific genetic flaws that account for idiosyncratic abnormalities have been determined in detail for some drugs. In most cases, the unusual responses of persons in certain families have been traced to a deficiency or an excess of an enzyme involved in the metabolism of the drug to which they display an idiosyncrasy.

Types of idiosyncratic reactions
Drug-induced hemolysis. Some people, for example, are prone to suffer a breakdown of large numbers of the circulating erythrocytes, red blood cells, when they receive small doses of certain drugs that do not ordinarily cause the hemolysis of red blood cells. Such sensitivity was first noted in black soldiers who were given the antimalarial drug primaquine when they were returning to the United States after service in the Korean

conflict. About 5% to 10% of black men are now known to be susceptible to such drug-induced hemolytic anemia.

However, the same idiosyncrasy also occurs in other racial and ethnic groups, and it is not limited to that one antimalarial drug. Thus, for example, some white people of Mediterranean origin suffer the same reaction from eating fava beans, which contain a chemical compound that breaks down their red blood cells. The erythrocytes of all such people, black or white, are also sensitive to small doses of such commonly administered drugs as the analgesics phenacetin and aspirin, sulfonamide-type antibacterials, and the antiarrhythmic agent quinidine.

This type of drug toxicity has been traced to a defective gene that leads to a deficiency of the enzyme glucose-6-phosphate dehydrogenase (G-6-PD) in the red blood cells. A lack of this enzyme leads in turn to too little reduced glutathione, a substance needed to protect the integrity of the red cell membranes against oxidizing forces. Thus, the erythrocytes cannot resist hemolysis by small amounts of drugs of different chemical and pharmacologic classes that can convert reduced glutathione to its oxidized form.

Other idiosyncrasies. Another example of idiosyncrasy is seen in the tendency of some people to suffer acute attacks of porphyria following administration of small doses of barbiturates.* These persons have a hereditary abnormality related to biosynthesis of a constituent of hemoglobin. Barbiturates are thought to cause increased production of porphyrin by stimulating the production of an enzyme that regulates its biosynthesis (see Chap. 4, Enzyme Induction). As a result, genetically prone people with latent porphyria may suffer an attack marked by toxic psychosis, peripheral neuritis, and abdominal colic.

A less well-understood idiosyncrasy occurs in some patients after inhalation of a general anesthetic such as halothane (Fluothane). The condition, called malignant hyperthermia, is marked by high fever and skeletal muscle rigidity. This potentially fatal disorder occurs in certain families, but the exact genetic defect that is the basis of susceptibility to this reaction is still uncertain. Apparently, membranes within muscle cells of these people release abnormal amounts of calcium ions when exposed to various chemicals, thus greatly increasing muscular heat production.† This rare reaction has also been reported in patients who receive the skeletal muscle relaxant succinylcholine (Anectine). The hereditary defect here is apparently different from that which leads to prolonged apnea from small doses of this drug (see Chap. 4, Pharmacogenetic Factors).

Tests
Several simple screening tests have been devised for detecting some drug idiosyncrasies. For example, the susceptibility of a person's red blood cells to destruction by

---

* Porphyria is a metabolic disorder characterized by an increase in the formation of porphyrins, chemicals used in synthesizing hemoglobin and other respiratory pigments.
† Dantrolene sodium (dantrolene), a directly acting skeletal muscle relaxant that reduces the release of calcium ions from certain sites within skeletal muscle cells, has proven effective for preventing and treating this reaction, which has a high mortality rate in susceptible people.

oxidant drugs can be determined by taking a small blood sample and checking the reaction of erythrocytes when a potent hemolysis-producing chemical is added. Checking the same level of the enzyme creatinine phosphokinase may help to identify patients prone to develop malignant hyperthermia. Patients can also be screened for the presence of an atypical cholinesterase enzyme prior to the administration of succinylcholine.

Drug-induced tissue and organ damage

Drugs can act directly or indirectly to cause many types of adverse effects in various tissues, structures, and organs (Table 5-1). Some significant points about drug-induced injuries of various types will be briefly reviewed. These account for the precautions that are often required in the administration of drugs of many classes. The possible occurrence of such reactions also accounts for the fact that the use of some drugs is contraindicated in patients with a particular history.

Dermatologic reactions (drug eruptions)

The skin is the organ most commonly involved in allergic drug reactions, and often it may also show signs that offer a clue to the presence of systemic, or generalized, drug toxicity. Drugs that are taken internally and carried to the skin by way of the blood can cause eruptions similar to those seen in dermatoses (skin disorders) of almost every type. Most common are the urticarial reactions ("hives") observed with penicillin and hormones that are made up of amino acids. However, drugs may also cause rashes resembling those of measles (morbilliform eruptions), acne, psoriasis, pemphigus, eczema, and other dermatologic disorders.

Table 5–1. Types of drug-induced tissue and organ damage

Skin: hives, rash, lesions
Blood dyscrasias: anemia, thrombocytopenia, leukopenia, pancytopenia
Liver injury: hepatitis, enzyme changes
Kidney damage: glomerulonephritis, acute or chronic renal failure
Ocular damage: blurring of vision, corneal damage, blindness
Auditory damage: dizziness, "ringing" in ears, loss of hearing, loss of balance
CNS: confusion, delirium, insomnia, drowsiness, hyper- or hyporeflexia
Teratogenicity: fetal death, fetal structural abnormalities, fetal functional abnormalities

People who already have skin difficulties sometimes seem predisposed to react to certain drugs in specific ways. Thus, youngsters with acne tend to be most susceptible to the acneiform eruptions induced by bromides, iodides and the male sex hormone. People with atopic dermatitis are prone to respond to procaine or to penicillin with eczematous reactions marked by redness, blistering, weeping, and crusting of the skin.

Most of the common erythematous skin reactions are minor and tend to subside soon after the drug is stopped. However, some drug-induced dermatologic disorders may be life-threatening and long-lasting. For example, exfoliative dermatitis and erythema multiforme exudativum (Stevens–Johnson syndrome) are two severe and often fatal skin reactions that sometimes occur during administration of long-acting sulfonamides and certain other drugs. Patients taking these drugs must be closely observed so that the drug can be immediately withdrawn at the first sign of certain characteristic skin lesions. Even then, these disorders may continue to progress; patients with such severe skin reactions and accompanying systemic illness require skilled care.

Blood dyscrasias

Abnormalities of the formed elements of the blood—erythrocytes, leukocytes, thrombocytes, and platelets—are among the most serious adverse reactions caused by drugs. Registries of drug-induced *blood dyscrasias* have been established to which nurses are encouraged to report such cases of hematotoxicosis. Nurses must teach patients who are taking certain drugs to watch for early signs and symptoms of blood disorders. To facilitate this process, some pertinent points about the types of blood dyscrasias most commonly encountered will be summarized.

Hemolytic anemia

The most common cause of drug-induced destruction of erythrocytes is the inborn lack of the enzyme glucose-6-phosphate dehydrogenase (G-6-PD) in the patient's red cells. However, hemolysis may also occur as a result of various types of allergic reactions to drugs. In either case, the patient may develop not only signs and symptoms of anemia but also potentially fatal kidney complications, including uremia.

Cytotoxic red cell reactions occur as the result of type II immunologic mechanisms. In some cases, the drug coats the surface of the erythrocyte and reacts with a circulating drug-induced gamma globulin antibody (IgG). This occurs when penicillin-induced hemolytic anemia develops in patients who have been receiving very high doses of the antibiotic. In other situations, this immunoglobulin coats the red cell and reacts with the circulating drug or its hapten metabolite. In either case, presence of a potentially dangerous situation can be detected by a positive reaction in a blood test called the Coombs' test.

Many patients who are treated for 6 months or more with methyldopa (Aldomet), an antihypertensive drug, also develop a positive Coombs' test. However, clinical hemolytic anemia occurs in only a small proportion of these patients. Unfortunately, because it is not possible to predict which patients will eventually suffer red blood cell breakdown, blood counts must be performed periodically during continued treatment to detect early signs of methyldopa-induced hemolysis, which would make it necessary to stop further therapy with this drug.

In actual practice, the nurse may be the first to note signs and symptoms of a hemolytic reaction—complaints of weakness, back pain, and the passage of dark urine. If any of these signs and symptoms occur, the patient's hemoglobin levels should be checked and the drug withdrawn, if necessary.

Thrombocytopenia

This is a deficiency of blood platelets, which develops occasionally during treatment with various types of drugs. Unless the condition is quickly detected and the drug promptly discontinued, serious bleeding, and even death from brain hemorrhage, may result. The most common drugs causing this disorder are quinidine, meprobamate (Equanil), chlorothiazide (Diuril), and anti-infective drugs, such as the sulfonamides, rifampin, and chloramphenicol. Patients taking most of these drugs tend to develop antibodies that then react with drug molecules bound to the surface of the platelet. This leads to a loss of these blood cells as the result of their clumping together (agglutination) or their disintegration (lysis).

Sometimes, in *non*allergic cases, it is not possible to detect antibodies. Among such cases, thrombocytopenia that results from damage to the bone marrow elements that produce the platelets is most dangerous. Certain drugs used in treating epilepsy and diabetes have caused irreversible damage of this kind. Patients are watched for signs of the development of purpura, such as a loss of blood and fluid into the tissues. Most cases of drug-induced purpura respond rapidly when the condition is detected and the drug is discontinued.

Leukopenia

This is a drug-induced reduction in the total number of circulating white blood cells, and is the most common of the drug-induced hematologic adverse reactions. The condition in its acute form—*agranulocytosis*—is characterized by a sharp drop in the total leukocyte count and by an almost complete absence of granulocytes. As a result, patients are deprived of one of the body's main defense mechanisms against infection. Thus, the condition is often first detected when the patient comes down with a severe infection.

Aminopyrine is the drug most commonly associated with this type of blood dyscrasia. This drug has virtually disappeared from use in the United States, where

analgesics with less potential for harm than this one are preferred. However, the related drug, phenylbutazone (Butazolidin), is relatively widely used for treating rheumatic disorders that have proved resistant to salicylate therapy. When this drug or other agents often associated with agranulocytosis—chlorpromazine or propylthiouracil (PTU), for example—are used, frequent white blood cell and differential counts should be done.

When a patient is put on long-term treatment with a drug that has reportedly caused this and other blood dyscrasias, the patient is asked to return to the clinic frequently for blood tests. Often, differential blood counts help to detect drops in the various types of cells. Discontinuing the drug may then help to keep the patient's bone marrow from being damaged irreversibly. Sometimes, however, clinical signs and symptoms appear in the interval between blood tests. Thus, patients with chronic conditions should be taught what signs and symptoms to look for.

For example, it should be explained to a patient taking the anti-inflammatory agent phenylbutazone, which can cause agranulocytosis, that the appearance of a severe sore throat and fever may signal the onset of this disorder. The patient is told to report such signs to the physician or nurse at once. Similarly, the parents of a child receiving the anticonvulsant drug trimethadione (Tridione) for petit mal epilepsy should be told what signs of illness to watch for during long-term use.

Once the condition is detected, the offending drug is immediately withdrawn, and any infection that may be present is vigorously treated with antibiotics. Patients are told to inform any physician or nurse whom they may later consult of their sensitivity to the drug in question, because taking even a single small dose years later may set off a similar reaction.

Aplastic anemia

This is one of the most serious of the blood disorders that may be induced by drugs. More than half of the patients who develop this condition die in spite of all treatment efforts. The condition is characterized by damage to the bone marrow, with the result that the blood cell-forming tissue is largely replaced by fatty tissue. As a result, there is a reduction in *all* the formed elements of the circulating blood (pancytopenia). The patient becomes pale and weak and is subject to episodes of bleeding and infection.

Among the drugs reported to have produced this condition are chloramphenicol, phenylbutazone, trimethadione, and certain sulfonamides and their derivatives. The manner in which these and other chemicals damage the bone marrow is unknown. The fact that the vast majority of patients who receive these drugs do not develop this blood dyscrasia indicates that the reaction is idiosyncratic. Although immunologic mechanisms have recently been demonstrated in some cases, there is still no test to help predict which patients are likely to develop drug-induced aplastic anemia.

These drugs are now ordered only when it is felt that their usefulness for treating certain serious illnesses far outweighs the chance—however slight, statistically—that the particular patient may be one of the very small minority to develop aplastic anemia. When such drugs are being employed over prolonged periods, frequent blood tests are ordered to detect the earliest signs of hematologic abnormalities. Patients are warned to report signs of illness such as sore throat, weakness, pallor, and bleeding. Early detection through such signs and by the results of blood tests permits the immediate discontinuation of therapy with the potentially dangerous drug before irreversible bone marrow aplasia sets in.

Liver injury

The liver is the first organ to receive orally administered substances after they are absorbed from the duodenum. This makes it prone to injury by toxic chemicals such as arsenic, phosphorus, or chloroform and other halogenated hydrocarbons that may be ingested. These and any newly discovered synthetic chemicals that are capable of causing direct damage to the liver are readily revealed to do so by preclinical toxicity test procedures in experimental animals (see Chap. 1). Thus, such laboratory screening prevents inherently hepatotoxic chemicals from proceeding to the clinical phases of testing required before drugs are approved for use in patient therapy.

Nonetheless, substances have been introduced as drugs that were later shown to cause liver injury in some patients treated with them. Such substances adversely affected liver function in only a small number of the many patients treated. This, along with the fact that jaundice and other signs and symptoms developed with low doses that had no such effects on the vast majority of patients, suggests that drug-induced injury is caused by idiosyncrasy, or possibly by drug allergy—that is, the immunologic hypersensitivity of the patient. However, this has been hard to prove, and it has not been possible to predict in advance which patients would react adversely.

Drug-induced liver injury that occurs clinically takes two main forms. One type of toxicity affects the liver parenchyma itself—that is, the mass of functioning cells. The other involves primarily the channels within the liver by which bile moves from the cells to the gallbladder. The first type is the more serious because it can lead to hepatic necrosis and liver failure that is fatal in about 10% of cases. In cases of the second type, recovery usually occurs shortly after the drug is withdrawn.

Most drugs that were found to cause severe liver cell damage after having passed all the usual tests in laboratory animals and in hundreds of human subjects during clinical trials have had to be withdrawn from further use in therapy. Even though only a very small proportion of tens or hundreds of thousands of treated patients were adversely affected, injury to this vital organ has such serious consequences that the risks of continuing to use these drugs in therapy outweighed their possible beneficial effects. However, some drugs such as the general anesthetic halothane and the broad-spectrum antibiotic tetracycline are considered so valuable that they have been retained despite the possibility of parenchymal hepatotoxicity.

In the case of such drugs, it is advisable to avoid administration to patients with a history of hepatic disease, and liver function tests should be done before and during therapy. Patients are observed for such signs as fever and jaundice, or for nausea, vomiting, and abdominal pain, signals that may appear before jaundice becomes evident. It may also be desirable to check the patient's kidney function if the drug—tetracycline, for example—is one that requires renal excretion; if its elimination is impaired, ordinary doses of an otherwise safe drug may accumulate to toxic levels in the liver.

Liver toxicity of the type that involves the bile channels, or canaliculi, leads to development of cholestasis, a condition that resembles extrahepatic biliary obstruction. Most cases are believed to be the result of a hypersensitivity-type reaction that causes the thin walls of the channels to swell and block the flow of bile. As the unexcreted bile backs up into the blood and is deposited in the skin and other tissues, it can cause pruritus (itching), fever, and cholestatic jaundice. Among the drugs that occasionally cause this hepatic reaction are the antipsychotic drug chlorpromazine, the male sex hormone derivative methyltestosterone, and the antibiotics troleandomycin and erythromycin estolate. Patients taking these drugs should be observed for the signs mentioned above and for complaints of malaise, nausea and vomiting, and abdominal colic.

Kidney damage

The kidneys are vulnerable to various types of injury by the chemicals that they excrete and by others that are carried in the blood that flows through their tissues. Nephrotoxicity is particularly likely to occur in people who already have renal lesions. It has been caused by the nephrotoxic aminoglycoside antibiotics, streptomycin and kanamycin, and by the loop diuretics, furosemide and ethacrynic acid. In some such cases, the poorly excreted drug may accumulate in the body and cause other toxic effects, especially in nerve tissues, including both branches of the eighth cranial nerve. (Such secondary neurotoxic damage to the auditory and vestibular branches is called ototoxicity.)

The abuse of products containing analgesics such as phenacetin and aspirin for long periods has led to development of chronic interstitial nephritis with necrosis of the renal papillae. This is most probably the result of direct toxicity caused by accumulation of the drugs and their metabolites. However, allergic hypersensitivity may also play a part in some cases of phenacetin-induced necrosis; and as already indicated, phenacetin-induced hemolysis of red blood cells may lead to mechanical damage by released hemoglobin and result in acute kidney failure.

Various antibiotics are potentially nephrotoxic, including polymyxin B, colistin, and those of the aminoglycoside class such as kanamycin, neomycin and, to a lesser extent, newer antibiotics of this type such as amikacin, gentamicin, and tobramycin. This can be a serious problem in patients with already poor kidney function who often require treatment for complicating infections by the gram-negative bacteria against which these drugs are especially effective. Consequently, modified dosage schedules have been devised for treating patients with severe renal disease.

The objective of treatment in such cases is to reach and then maintain effective antibacterial blood levels quickly without letting the drug's concentration rise to toxic levels. To do so, an initial loading dose (see Chap. 4) is first administered, and the therapeutic concentration attained in this way is then maintained by administering additional doses at appropriate intervals. The dose and frequency of administration are determined by what can be learned about the drug's half-life in the patient with impaired renal function.

The patient's blood urea nitrogen (BUN) and creatinine clearance capabilities are also used as a guide to therapy, because these values have been found to correlate well with the half-lives of many drugs. The serum levels tend to rise to varying degrees in patients with kidney function that has been reduced to less than 25% of normal by renal disease. Depending on the results of these tests and on direct monitoring of the blood levels of the potentially nephrotoxic–ototoxic antibacterial drugs, either of the following may be ordered: the administration of normal doses at intervals much longer than normal; or greatly reduced doses that are to be administered at more or less ordinary fixed intervals. (Of course, these calculations are not made based solely on formulas employing laboratory data; the patient's clinical responses to each administered dose must also be followed closely.)

Ocular toxicity

The delicate structures of the eye are subject to direct and indirect injury by drugs taken in therapeutic doses. Among the most common occurrences are the disturbances in color vision reported by some patients taking digitalis glycosides for heart failure, and the blurring of vision that occurs in patients taking atropine and similar drugs that affect the function of the iris and ciliary body muscles. Both these ocular effects are promptly reversible when these drugs are discontinued, but patients with narrow angle glaucoma may suffer an acute attack after treatment with atropinelike drugs that raise intraocular pressure.

More serious are the effects that some drugs have on the cornea, lens, retina, and optic nerve when administered for prolonged periods in moderately high doses. The antimalarial drug chloroquine, which is also used to treat patients with systemic lupus erythematosus (SLE), and the antipsychotic phenothiazine drugs chlorpromazine and thioridazine (Mellaril) can cause corneal and retinal changes. Corticosteroid drugs have caused clouding of the lens by favoring the development of posterior subcapsular cataracts in some patients.

The adverse effects of chloroquine on the cornea are reversible, but drug-induced retinopathy may result in permanent visual loss. Thus, patients taking this drug for prolonged periods for rheumatoid arthritis or for SLE must have ophthalmologic examinations performed before beginning treatment and periodically during the course of treatment. The drug must be immediately discontinued if signs of retinal damage are discovered.

The ocular changes brought about by phenothiazines usually occur only in patients taking moderately high doses for prolonged periods. Chlorpromazine use occasionally leads to development of granular deposits of the drug in the lens and cornea. Rarely, this has led to impaired vision, which may improve after the drug is discontinued. Thioridazine therapy has led to deposits of pigment in the retina, which can be seen when the fundus of the eye is examined. The patient's vision may gradually return after this drug is withdrawn, even though the pigmentary changes may be permanent.

Teratogenicity

Drugs that reach the developing embryo and fetus during the critical periods when the organs are being formed can cause congenital defects. Thus, the possibility of a drug's doing damage to a developing fetus when it is taken by a pregnant woman must be considered. The fact that drugs taken by the mother may pass across the placenta to affect the unborn child was brought home most forcibly by the maiming of hundreds of infants whose mothers took *thalidomide*, a seemingly harmless sedative–hypnotic. Most physicians or nurses are now cautious about prescribing any drugs for pregnant women or even for women of childbearing age who may have become pregnant and not yet know it. Women who may be pregnant should be warned not to treat themselves with nonprescription medicines. Of course, the risks of *not* treating a pregnant woman who has a dangerous disorder may be greater than the risk of potential harm to the fetus. In such cases, the use of most drugs during pregnancy is justified. The pregnant woman must, however, be informed of the risks and be given the opportunity to deal with these risks as she desires.

Drugs administered late in the fetal period do not cause obvious structural deformities. However, they can cause toxic effects on the fetus or neonate similar to those seen in an adult who takes an overdose. This is particularly true when narcotic analgesics are given to the mother during labor and in the infants of narcotic addicts. The long-term effects of these drugs on the developing human's physical, intellectual, and emotional functioning have not been well established.

Poisoning by drugs and chemicals

Poisons are sometimes defined as chemical substances capable of causing harm in living systems with which they come into contact in even very small amounts. Actually, almost any chemical, including all drugs, can be poisonous if improperly employed and if enough is taken. Thus, many medicines that are therapeutically useful in ordinary doses are also poisonous when overdoses are administered.

In this book, aspects of the toxicity of the various drugs that commonly cause poisoning when people accidentally or deliberately take doses much greater than those used therapeutically will be reviewed. Aspirin, for example, is a very safe drug when people take only a couple of tablets for a headache, yet young children who eat many tablets from a bottle that they find in the medicine cabinet frequently die from the resulting severe salicylate intoxication. Barbiturates are safe drugs when taken in sedative doses but can cause death when a dozen or more capsules are taken at once in a suicide attempt. Other medications, including cold remedies containing antihistamines, have caused accidental poisoning in children, and depressed patients who have ingested all the tablets of tranquilizer or antidepressant drug prescriptions at once have sometimes succeeded in killing themselves with medication that was intended to help them.

Other chemicals that are not meant to be taken internally as medicines are also a cause of accidental poisoning. These include not only rat poisons, weed destroyers, and insecticides, but also many other household products not usually thought of as poisons. Furniture polishes, for example, may contain kerosene and similar toxic petroleum distillates that can cause serious lung damage and death. Other organic solvents in paint thinners, varnish removers, and related products are also dangerous. Disinfectants and drain cleaners containing lye and other caustic substances can cause destruction of the esophagus, stomach perforation, and fatal shock when swallowed. Bleaches, detergents, and even cosmetics often contain chemicals that can be harmful when ingested by youngsters who drink liquids left where they can easily be reached. The signs, symptoms, and emergency treatment of poisoning caused by ingestion of such products are listed in Table 5-2.

Incidence
Poisoning by drugs and chemicals is one of the most common medical emergencies. More efficient collection of epidemiologic data in recent years has revealed that more than 5 million cases occur annually in this country, and over 13,000 people die after accidentally or deliberately taking poison. Until recently, this total regularly included about 1,000 children under 5 years of age.

Fortunately, this figure has been falling for several years. This may be because the long efforts of such groups as the American Association of Poison Control Centers and the American Academy of Pediatrics to prevent poisoning by educating the public are beginning to have a significant effect. In addition, diagnostic and treatment measures have become better standardized through the efforts of various organizations, including the Emergency Department Nurses Association and the American College of Emergency Physicians. Better communication of the most effective measures for managing such cases has helped more victims of poisoning to survive.

In the remainder of this chapter, the general aspects of the diagnosis, treatment, and prevention of poisoning that apply to all types of drugs and chemicals will be discussed.

Diagnosis
Diagnosis of poisoning is a difficult task. The signs and symptoms of poisoning are essentially the same as those seen in other disorders, and the combinations of toxic effects produced by many drugs resemble syndromes seen in various diseases. Thus, drug-induced convulsions may not differ from status epilepticus, and coma caused by a depressant drug may not be easily differentiated from the same state that develops as a result of disease.

In the emergency room setting important facts about what was ingested, the circumstances of the ingestion, and presenting signs and symptoms are noted. This often aids in early detection of a case of poisoning and results in more rapid and effective treatment.

Laboratory screening tests are useful in some situations to help determine whether a patient—one who is comatose, for example—has been poisoned at all and, if so, what substance is responsible. Such tests are usually performed on samples of urine, blood, and vomited or suctioned stomach contents. General supportive measures should always be instituted without awaiting the results of such tests.

Thus, if a patient is admitted in a comatose condition with labored breathing, it is more important to support respiration than to determine whether an overdose of a barbiturate or of a narcotic has been taken. (In the latter case, an injection of the specific narcotic antagonist naloxone (Narcan) may be both diagnostic *and* therapeutic.)

Treatment
The management of poisoning emergencies involves several general steps:

(Text continues on p. 100)

Table 5–2. Poisoning by common chemicals*

Poison and sources	Assessment factors	Emergency treatment
Acids (corrosive)		
Hydrochloric Sulfuric Nitric Phosphoric (toilet bowl cleaners)	1. Burns about mouth and throat 2. Abdominal pain, nausea, vomiting 3. Circulatory collapse: ↓ BP, ↑ P, cold and clammy 4. Respiratory tract edema, asphyxia 5. Long-term effects: respiratory strictures, stenoses	1. *Do not use emetics or lavage.* 2. Give milk of magnesia, aluminum hydroxide gel, or dilute soap solution. 3. Have victim drink large quantities of water. 4. Give demulcents such as milk, egg whites, or olive oil. 5. Flood external skin burns with large amounts of water, followed by application of sodium bicarbonate paste. 6. Flush eye burns with water, possibly after use of topical anesthetic.
Alkali (caustic)		
"Lye": sodium hydroxide, potassium hydroxide, caustic soda, alkaline carbonates (drain cleaners, paint removers, Clinitest urine tablets, stove grease removers, solid household bleaches)	1. Burns about the mouth and throat; throat edematous, white, then turning brown 2. Burning pain in esophagus and stomach; mucoid, then bloody vomitus 3. Circulatory collapse indicated by cold clammy skin and by ↑ P, ↓ BP 4. Death may result rapidly from shock or asphyxia, or occur later from shock as a result of perforation of viscera or from more slowly developing respiratory tract infections	1. *Do not induce emesis or employ gastric lavage.* 2. Have patient drink large quantities of water or milk to dilute the alkali. 3. Give demulcents, including olive oil and egg white. 4. Wash external burns with large amounts of water or with dilute vinegar. 5. Give potent analgesics, IV fluids, and electrolytes, antibiotics, and corticosteroids, as appropriate.
Arsenic compounds		
Arsenic trioxide Arsenic pentoxide Sodium arsenite Sodium arsenate (weed killers, rat poison, insecticides, paints)	1. Burning, cramping abdominal pain; difficulty swallowing; severe, watery or bloody diarrhea 2. Signs of dehydration 3. Complaints of metallic taste; garliclike odor on breath 4. Death may result from cardiovascular collapse, or from fluid and electrolyte imbalances 5. Chronic effects: headache, dizziness, delirium, coma, convulsions	1. Use emetics, gastric lavage, and saline cathartics. 2. Give milk; give penicillamine orally. 3. Administer dimercaprol (BAL) intramuscularly. 4. Give IV fluids and electrolytes to correct dehydration and deficiencies and to counteract shock.

(continued)

Table 5–2. Poisoning by common chemicals* (continued)

Poison and sources	Assessment factors	Emergency treatment
Aromatic hydrocarbons		
Benzene Toluene Xylene (solvents, paint removers, insecticide solutions, glue)	1. Inflammatory reaction at site of local skin contact 2. Nausea, vomiting, increased salivation; if swallowed, patient reports a burning sensation on swallowing 3. Acute inhalation exposure results in signs and symptoms of alcohol intoxication; continued inhalation results in coma, hyperactive reflexes, death 4. Chronic exposure: bone marrow suppression ($\downarrow$ WBC, $\downarrow$ RBC, $\downarrow$ platelets)	1. Wash skin and eyes thoroughly. 2. Use gastric lavage; instill mineral oil or saline cathartic into stomach. 3. Institute supportive measures to maintain respirations and fluid balance. 4. Do not give epinephrine, alcohol, or vegetable fats.
Bleaches (household)		
Liquid: sodium hypochlorite (Clorox)—releases hypochlorous acid in acidic gastric juice (*Caution:* combining liquid bleach with acidic toilet bowl cleaners may produce dangerous chlorine gas) Solid: sodium perborate	1. Vomiting; complaints of upper GI burning 2. Tearing, red eyes; irritation of nose and throat 3. Gastrointestinal signs and symptoms; shock; CNS effects leading to convulsions and coma	1. Give milk to dilute; antacids may also be given. 2. Wash areas exposed to local contact. 3. Supportive and protective measures.
Camphor		
(Liniment, camphorated oil, moth repellents)	1. Nausea, vomiting—vomitus smells like camphor 2. CNS signs: headache, dizziness, confusion, restlessness, delirium 3. Grand mal seizures, coma, respiratory failure, death	1. Use gastric lavage or induce vomiting if CNS excitement has not occurred. 2. Sedate with IV barbiturates.
Carbon monoxide—CO combines with hemoglobin to form carboxyhemoglobin, which cannot carry oxygen to tissues		
(Automobile exhaust; exhaust from heaters, stoves; fumes from burning of certain synthetic materials)	1. Headache in varying degrees, depending on dose 2. CNS effects: confusion, ataxia, loss of consciousness, coma 3. Skin: cherry-red color	1. Provide fresh air or pure oxygen, if possible (hyperbaric O_2 is very effective). 2. Provide respiratory support if needed.

Table 5–2. Poisoning by common chemicals* (continued)

Poison and sources	Assessment factors	Emergency treatment
Carbon tetrachloride (Dry cleaning stain remover, industrial degreasers, some home fire extinguishers)	1. Nausea, vomiting, abdominal pain 2. CNS effects: headache, confusion, dizziness, drowsiness, visual changes, coma, respiratory failure 3. Chronic effects: liver failure; anorexia, nausea, vomiting, jaundice; renal failure: oliguria, anuria, albuminuria, edema, weight gain	1. Provide fresh air if inhaled; use gastric lavage or induce vomiting if ingested; flush with soap and water if skin contact has occurred. 2. Provide oxygen to help protect liver from anoxia. 3. Provide support and prophylaxis for liver and kidney complications.
Cyanides (Exterminator's fumigants, salts used in metal polishes and in photography, electroplating, metallurgy)	1. Rapid respiratory failure and death 2. CNS signs and symptoms of hypoxia, if minute doses; headache, dizziness, respiratory difficulty, tremors to convulsions	1. Give artificial respiration; positive pressure oxygen. 2. Have patient inhale amyl nitrite (smelling salts) or give IV sodium nitrite, both of which form methemoglobin, which in turn will combine with cyanide. 3. Inject sodium thiosulfate to convert cyanide to thiocyanate, a safer substance. 4. Provide for whole blood transfusion, in extreme cases.
Fluorides Sodium fluoride Sodium fluorsilicate (insecticides, roach powders) (*Note:* fluoridated water supplies are *not* toxic)	1. Abdominal pain and cramps; nausea, vomiting, diarrhea 2. Dehydration; shock: weak, rapid pulse; pallor; weakness 3. Muscular effects: tremors, partial paralysis, spasms, convulsions 4. Death from shock or respiratory or cardiac failure	1. Give milk or fluid with calcium salts. 2. IV calcium salts may be used to treat muscle spasms. 3. Give parenteral fluids to counteract dehydration and to prevent shock.
Nicotine (Black Leaf 40, tobacco products)	1. Abdominal pain, nausea, vomiting, diarrhea 2. CNS effects: headache, dizziness, weakness, visual disturbances, confusion 3. Cardiovascular effects: ↑ BP, arrhythmias 4. In severe cases, shock, respiratory failure, convulsions, loss of reflexes, respiratory paralysis, death	1. Use gastric lavage with potassium permanganate 1:5000; give universal antidote in water. 2. Wash skin to prevent absorption. 3. Provide respiratory support and give diazepam if convulsions occur.

(continued)

Table 5–2. Poisoning by common chemicals* (continued)

Poison and sources	Assessment factors	Emergency treatment
Petroleum distillates		
Kerosene Gasoline Other oils (fuels, furniture waxes, paint thinners, cleaning fluids)	1. Nausea, vomiting, complaints of GI burning; coughing and choking if inhaled 2. CNS effects: drowsiness, stupor, coma 3. Rapidly developing pulmonary edema: rales, dyspnea, cyanosis; fever, tachycardia; death occurs frequently	1. *Do not induce emesis.* 2. Use careful gastric lavage with water and sodium bicarbonate solution. 3. Use olive oil, mineral oil, or saline cathartic to prevent absorption. 4. Provide supportive treatment: give oxygen, steroids, antibiotics; do not use epinephrine.
Phenol (carbolic acid)		
(Disinfectants: if used appropriately, in small doses, should not be toxic to skin)	1. White burns of skin, mucous membranes 2. Upper GI burning, nausea, vomiting, diarrhea 3. Cardiovascular effects: weak pulse, arrhythmias, pale, cyanotic skin, shallow respirations, shock 4. CNS effects: excitement followed by depression 5. Death from respiratory failure; chronic kidney damage: oliguria, dark urine	1. Give olive oil or vegetable oils as a solvent; use gastric lavage, milk, eggs 2. Wash skin with water if there are contact burns. 3. Provide supportive measures and protection.
Turpentine		
(Varnish and paint solvent; disinfectants; cleansing solutions)	1. Upper GI and abdominal pain; nausea, vomiting, diarrhea 2. Choking, coughing if inhaled 3. CNS effects: excitement followed by depression 4. Kidney damage: albuminuria, hematuria, urine smells like violets	1. Lavage stomach with water or sodium bicarbonate solution. 2. Instill milk or mineral oil to allay GI irritation. 3. Force fluids to prevent kidney damage. 4. Provide supportive and protective measures.

* Poisoning by these chemicals is not discussed elsewhere in this text. See index for references to discussions of poisoning by drugs and chemicals not mentioned here.

1. Remove ingested poisons from the gastrointestinal tract or wash chemicals from the skin and eyes before they can do extensive local damage or be absorbed into the bloodstream and tissues.
2. Administer chemical and pharmacologic antidotes that combine with the poison in the gastrointestinal tract or block its effects in body tissues.
3. Apply supportive measures to keep the patient's vital functions operating. This also includes treating complications and speeding the excretion of absorbed poisons.

Removal of ingested poisons

Vomiting. This is the most rapidly effective way to remove poisons from the stomach soon after they have been swallowed. Thus, no time should be lost in inducing a patient to vomit, except in the following circumstances:

1. When caustic alkali or corrosive mineral acids have been ingested
2. When a volatile petroleum distillate (kerosenelike substance) has been swallowed
3. When the patient is semicomatose or shows signs of impending convulsive seizures

In such instances, vomiting can do more harm than good. Corrosive substances can do further damage to the esophagus and mouth if regurgitated. Volatile petroleum distillates are readily aspirated into the lungs and, when this happens, a fulminant and often untreatable pneumonia often develops rapidly. The semicomatose or convulsing patient is also prone to aspirate vomitus into the lungs.

Vomiting may be induced in several ways. Sometimes simply encouraging the patient to take a glass or two of water or milk and then touching the back of the throat with a finger, spoon handle, or other blunt object may be enough to set off the gag and vomiting reflexes.

Syrup of ipecac is an effective emetic that the FDA now permits people to buy in 1-ounce bottles without a prescription to have available at home. Whoever has ingested the toxic substance takes half an ounce of ipecac with a glass or two of water. This may be repeated if vomiting has not occurred in 15 minutes. However, no more than 2 ounces should be taken because the alkaloids of ipecac may themselves be toxic if absorbed. (The more concentrated fluidextract of ipecac should *never* be used, because it contains 14 times as much emetine as the syrup and is poisonous when taken by mistake.)

Apomorphine, an opium alkaloid, is a rapid-acting emetic that may be employed when the patient has not yet vomited. Injected subcutaneously, 5 mg often causes copious vomiting within 5 minutes. This clears the stomach completely and sometimes even brings up still unabsorbed material from the upper intestine. However, apomorphine may not be effective for producing vomiting in patients who have taken an overdose of phenothiazine-type antipsychotic agents, because these drugs depress the central emetic mechanism site that is ordinarily stimulated by apomorphine.

Apomorphine is itself a depressant of other central areas, including the respiratory center, so it is not recommended when the patient is already somewhat stuporous. Repeated doses of apomorphine that do not produce the desired vomiting may leave the patient deeply depressed. Narcotic antagonists of the type that are used to treat opiate overdosage can readily counteract this adverse effect of apomorphine. In fact, some authorities recommend the routine administration of the narcotic antagonist *levallorphan* (Lorfan) following apomorphine administration, even when the patient shows no signs of drowsiness or stupor.

Gastric lavage. This is often employed in hospital emergency rooms for emptying the stomach. A catheter or plastic tube is passed gently down into the patient's stomach by way of the mouth (in young children), or through a nostril (in older children and adults). A syringe is then attached and the stomach contents are withdrawn by suction.

The stomach tube may be left in place after the lavage fluid—usually tap water or saline solution—has been introduced and syringed out repeatedly. It may then be used for administration of any of various other substances. These include demulcent fluids for soothing local irritation, concentrated solutions of saline cathartics such as sodium sulfate for speeding the removal from the intestinal tract of any toxic material that may already have passed the pyloric sphincter, and specific chemical antidotes designed to neutralize, precipitate, oxidize, or otherwise alter the poison to a relatively harmless form.

The contraindications for gastric lavage are similar to those described above for emetics, except that the likelihood of aspiration pneumonia may be less when a stomach tube is skillfully employed in comatose patients and in those who have swallowed kerosene or products containing petroleum distillates. Care and skill are required to avoid possible aspiration of the lavage fluid or of stomach contents into the patient's lungs.

Antidotes

Chemical antidotes. Chemical antidotes (Table 5-3) are various substances that interact chemically with poisons. They may be put into the stomach to neutralize poisons and to prevent their systemic absorption. Some, such as dilute vinegar or citrus fruit juices, act specifically to neutralize alkali, just as magnesium oxide neutralizes only acids. Other chemical antidotes antagonize a wide range of organic and inorganic poisonous substances.

The most effective material for inactivating most poisons while they are still in the gastrointestinal tract is *activated charcoal*, a fine black powder that offers a large surface area for the physical adsorption of many substances, ranging from metallic salts such as mercury bichloride to alkaloids such as strychnine to organic acids such as aspirin. One or 2 tbsp are mixed with water to make a paste, which is then diluted further to make a glassful of a black soupy mixture. The patient may have to be persuaded to swallow this liquid, which looks unappetizing but is actually tasteless and odorless. It is very important to get the patient's cooperation, because early administration of this harmless and effective substance prevents poisons from entering the blood and reaching the tissues. Once within the system, poisons are much more difficult to antagonize with specific chemical antidotes.

Among other antidotes that act chemically within the gastrointestinal tract are the following: potassium permanganate, which in dilutions of 1:10,000 to 1:5,000 oxidizes various alkaloids and other organic poisons;

Table 5–3. Drugs for treating poisoning

Drugs for use against unabsorbed poisons

Acetic acid (diluted vinegar)—neutralizes alkali
Activated charcoal—adsorbs most chemicals
Ammonium acetate—neutralizes formaldehyde
Ammonium hydroxide—neutralizes formaldehyde
Apomorphine HCl—emetic
Calcium salts (chloride, gluconate, lactate)—neutralize fluorides and oxalic acid
Copper sulfate—neutralizes phosphorus
Ipecac syrup—emetic
Iodine tincture—neutralizes some metals and alkaloids
Magnesium oxide and hydroxide (milk of magnesia)—neutralize acids, including acid from bleach; also demulcent and cathartic
Magnesium sulfate (Epsom salt)—cathartic
Milk, diluted dairy or evaporated—demulcent, diluent, precipitant
Olive oil—demulcent, laxative
Petrolatum, liquid—demulcent, solvent
Potassium permanganate—oxidizes alkaloids
Sodium bicarbonate—neutralizes ferrous sulfate and other iron salts; externally only to neutralize acids
Sodium chloride (normal saline solution)—neutralizes silver nitrate
Sodium sulfate—cathartic
Sodium thiosulfate—neutralizes iodine
Starch solution—neutralizes iodine
Tannic acid—neutralizes metals, alkaloids, other organic substances
Universal antidote (activated charcoal, magnesium oxide, tannic acid)—neutralizes most poisons (theoretically; practically, activated charcoal alone is preferred)

Drugs for use against systemically absorbed poisons

Anticonvulsants and skeletal muscle relaxants

Amobarbital sodium (Amytal)
Benztropine mesylate (Cogentin)—for use against dyskinetic spasms caused by phenothiazines and other neuroleptic drugs
Calcium gluconate—for use in hypocalcemic tetany, seizures and black widow spider bites
Diazepam (Valium)
Diphenhydramine (Benadryl)—for use in drug-induced dystonia
Methocarbamol (Robaxin)
Methohexital (Brevital)
Orphenadrine citrate (Norflex)

Anticonvulsants and skeletal muscle relaxants (continued)

Paraldehyde
Pentobarbital sodium (Nembutal)
Phenobarbital sodium (Luminal)
Phenytoin (Dilantin)
Succinylcholine chloride (Anectine; Sucostrin)
Thiopental sodium (Pentothal)

Chelating agents for use in heavy metal poisoning

Calcium disodium edetate (Calcium Disodium Versenate)
Deferoxamine (Desferal)
Dimercaprol (BAL)
Penicillamine (Cuprimine)

Cyanide poison antidotes

Amyl nitrite
Sodium nitrite
Sodium thiosulfate

Narcotic antagonists

Levallorphan (Lorfan)
Naloxone (Narcan)

Miscellaneous specific antidotes

N-acetyl-L-cysteine (Mucomyst)—prevents liver damage after acetaminophen overdose
Atropine sulfate—antagonizes anticholinesterase drugs, organic phosphate ester-type insecticides, nerve gases
Chlorpromazine (Thorazine)—antagonizes amphetamine psychosis and LSD "trips"
Ethyl alcohol—antagonizes methyl alcohol
Methylene blue—antagonizes methemoglobinemia caused by nitrites and aniline derivatives
Phytonadione (vitamin K_1)—counteracts bleeding caused by overdosage of oral anticoagulants of the coumarin and indandione classes
Physostigmine salts—antagonize central as well as peripheral effects of atropine and tricyclic antidepressants
Pilocarpine salts—antagonize peripheral effects of atropine
Pralidoxime chloride (Protopam)—antagonizes organic phosphate ester insecticides
Protamine sulfate—counteracts hemorrhages caused by heparin overdosage

Table 5–3. Drugs for treating poisoning (continued)

Drugs for supportive therapy*

Cardiac drugs

Atropine sulfate
Digoxin (Lanoxin and others)
Dobutamine HCl (Dobutrex)
Epinephrine (Adrenalin)
Glyceryl trinitrate (Nitroglycerin)
Isoproterenol HCl (Isuprel)
Lidocaine (Xylocaine)
Procainamide HCl (Pronestyl)
Quinidine HCl

Vasopressor drugs

Dopamine HCl (Intropin)
Levarterenol bitartrate (Levophed)
Metaraminol bitartrate (Aramine)
Methoxamine HCl (Vasoxyl)
Phenylephrine HCl (Neo-Synephrine)

Soluble corticosteroids

Dexamethasone sodium phosphate (Decadron
  phosphate; Hexadrol phosphate)
Hydrocortisone sodium succinate (Solu-Cortef)
Methylprednisolone sodium succinate (Solu-Medrol)
Prednisolone sodium phosphate (Hydeltrasol)

Diuretic drugs

Ethacrynic acid (Edecrin)
Furosemide (Lasix)
Mannitol (Osmitrol)
Urea (Ureaphil)

Analgesics

Codeine sulfate or phosphate
Meperidine (Demerol)
Morphine sulfate

Fluid and electrolyte replenishers

Dextrose injection
Fructose injection
Potassium chloride injection
Sodium chloride injection

Systemic and urinary alkalinizers

Sodium bicarbonate injection
Sodium citrate
Sodium lactate injection
Tromethamine (THAM; Tris buffer)

Dialysis solutions

Dianeal with dextrose

Plasma substitutes and expanders

Dextran 40 (Gentran 40; LMD, Rheomacrodex)
Dextran 70 (Gentran 75; Macrodex)
Normal human serum albumin (Albuminar)
Plasma protein fraction (Plasmanate)

Miscellaneous

Antibiotics
Antihistamines
General and local anesthetics
Nutrients
Vitamins

* This is only a small sampling of the types of substances most commonly employed in poisonings to support vital
functions and to counteract complications.

sodium chloride, which precipitates soluble silver salts as insoluble silver chloride; and copper sulfate, which coats phosphorus particles with inactive copper phosphide. Calcium salts help to bind oxalates and fluorides, ammonium acetate neutralizes formaldehyde, and sodium bicarbonate solution converts corrosive, soluble iron salts to the less soluble and less irritating iron salt ferrous carbonate.

In addition, certain foods make excellent poison precipitants. Milk and raw egg whites contain proteins that combine with mercury, arsenic, and other heavy metals to form insoluble and inactive albuminates. Starch is an especially effective precipitant of iodine when tincture of iodine has been swallowed. These substances also have a soothing demulcent action on the irritated gastrointestinal mucosa.

Chemicals are also sometimes employed externally to neutralize toxic chemicals contaminating the skin and eyes. However, prolonged washing with large amounts of running water is the most important measure so, in such cases, valuable time should not be wasted in locating or preparing special solutions. Sometimes, however, special solvents may be preferred for removing certain chemicals—for example, fixed oils such as olive oil and castor oil remove phenol more readily than water does. Later a paste of sodium bicarbonate can be applied to skin burned by acid, or a dressing soaked in dilute vinegar may be placed over any area contaminated by caustic alkali. The pain of eye burns may be relieved by topical anesthetics, and a corticosteroid ophthalmic solution or ointment can be instilled into an injured eye.

Systemically acting antidotes. Systemically acting antidotes are drugs used to counteract the actions of poisons that have already been absorbed into the systemic circulation and have begun to exert their toxic effects on various tissues. Some of these drugs are referred to as *physiologic antidotes* because they alter tissue function in a manner directly opposed to the action of the poison. Thus, if a person is suffering from strychnine poisoning, which is marked by excessive stimulation of the central nervous system, the symptoms of nervous hyperexcitability may often be best counteracted by administration of diazepam (Valium) or of a parenteral barbiturate to produce depression of the overstimulated nerve cells, thus helping to prevent or to counteract convulsive spasms and the complication of continued seizures.

Among the few other specific *pharmacologic antidotes* that are available, the most effective when employed early enough are the narcotic antagonists naloxone (Narcan) and levallorphan (Lorfan). The use of these antidotes and of others, such as atropine in the management of poisoning by organic phosphate-type insecticides and nerve gases, will be taken up at the appropriate points in the text—that is, in the discussions of the toxic effects of overdosage by individual drugs.

Other systemic antidotes also act only after absorption but differ from the physiologic and pharmacologic antidotes in that they counteract the poisonous chemical itself, instead of antagonizing its effects. These are the *chemical antidotes*—drugs that act by combining with and thus inactivating toxic chemicals that have entered the tissues. They are similar to the chemical antidotes discussed earlier, except that the chemical reactions take place in tissues other than the gastrointestinal tract. Specific antidotes of either the chemical or physiologic type are relatively few. Some specific chemical antidotes and the treatment of poisoning not presented elsewhere in the text will be discussed here.

Antidotes for heavy metal poisoning. The so-called heavy metals, including lead, arsenic, mercury, copper, and gold, are all toxic to living tissues. They are thought to exert their various adverse biologic effects through their ability to tie up chemicals in living tissue that must

be free in order for cells to function normally. When these substances (sulfhydryl [−SH] or thiol groups, carboxyls, phosphoryls, and others) are bound by these metals, certain cellular enzyme systems are inactivated, cellular functions fail and, finally, the cells die.

Numerous effective drugs are now available for counteracting heavy metal toxicity. These drugs act by breaking the bond between the metal and the vital cellular constituents. Administered early enough, these antidotal chemicals can prevent the development of the very many severe signs and symptoms of heavy metal toxicity. The poisonous metallic ions are clasped by the antidote molecules and carried out of the body before they can harm the tissues. (These metal-binding antidotal chemicals are called *chelating agents*—a name derived from the Greek *chele,* which means claw.)

Chelating agents can bind the molecules of heavy metals and thus prevent these poisons from damaging body cells and tissues. The complex formed in this way is *nontoxic* and can be excreted by the kidneys. *Dimercaprol+* (BAL; British Anti-Lewisite) is effective for antagonizing arsenic, mercury, gold, and other poisonous metallic salts. *Calcium disodium edetate+* (EDTA; Calcium Disodium Versenate) can be lifesaving when administered intravenously to bind lead in the tissues of a child with acute encephalitis caused by this metal. Other specific antidotes of this kind include the iron-chelating chemical *deferoxamine* (Desferal) and *penicillamine* (Cuprimine), a substance capable of combining with copper, lead, mercury, and other metals that may be present in excessive quantities in body tissues.

Lead poisoning is the most commonly encountered heavy metal toxicosis. Lead encephalopathy is an especially severe form of poisoning. The metal-induced brain damage causes convulsions, coma and, in about 25% or more of the victims, death. The condition most often develops in children, who eat flakes of paint containing white lead. When toxic levels of the poorly excreted metal accumulate in the tissues, symptoms are seen that range from gastrointestinal upset to muscle weakness ("lead palsy") to the fatal convulsions mentioned earlier.

Modern treatment of lead poisoning is based on the use of the chelating agent, calcium disodium edetate. Administered by vein, this antidote gives up its calcium and takes on the free lead ions in the tissues, for which it has a higher affinity. The metal mobilized in this manner is then removed from the body by way of the kidneys without doing damage to these or other organs. Unfortunately, this antidotal treatment often fails to halt the explosive course of acute lead encephalopathy in children. Thus, early detection of the presence of lead in the tissues, followed by removal of the child from the dangerous environment, is the most important preventive measure against lead poisoning.

Arsenic, especially in the form of the nearly tasteless arsenic trioxide, was a poison traditionally employed in criminal homicides in the Middle Ages and even into this century. The development of chemical methods for detecting its presence in body tissues has discouraged the use of arsenic compounds as a means of committing murder. However, arsenic compounds are commonly employed as weed killers and pesticides. Thus, arsenic still causes often fatal poisoning of children or adults who gain access to and ingest such dangerous products.

Accidental ingestion of even small amounts of sodium arsenite or other inorganic arsenic compounds causes severe gastroenteritis after a brief latent period. This leads to severe loss of fluids and electrolytes, circulatory collapse, and death in about 24 hours. Occasionally, absorption of the drug into the central nervous system results in a more rapidly fatal outcome after a period of convulsions and coma.

Poisoning by arsenic can be counteracted by the early administration of dimercaprol. Dimercaprol, also known as British Anti-Lewisite, or BAL, was developed by British scientists during World War II for use against the arsenic chemical warfare gas, lewisite, which it was feared that the Germans might employ. It was synthesized and studied because of the belief that arsenic toxicity was the result of reactions of the metalloid with cellular sulfhydryl (—SH) groups. Dimercaprol, a dithiol, furnishes sulfhydryl groups, which grasp arsenical compounds and thus prevent them from inactivating essential sulfhydryl enzyme systems in the tissues.

In addition to the prompt injection of dimercaprol, supportive measures such as correction of dehydration and treatment of shock may also be required. First aid immediately after ingestion requires the use of gastric lavage, followed by a freshly prepared solution of ferric hydroxide or sodium thiosulfate and, finally, by a saline cathartic such as sodium sulfate. In the absence of these chemical antidotes, induction of emesis and administration of milk are indicated until the patient can receive more active medical treatment.

Mercury in the form of mercuric chloride (corrosive sublimate) was once a common cause of acute poisoning. Although the use of this substance as a disinfectant has declined, poisoning by other forms of mercury is still often reported—for example, from ingestion of fish caught in lakes contaminated with mercury. Acute poisoning by ingestion of soluble mercury salts is marked by immediate burning pain in the mouth, throat, esophagus, and stomach. The patient may die of circulatory collapse after a few hours of continuous vomiting and severe bloody diarrhea. Prompt gastric lavage with a solution of egg white or of the reducing agent sodium formaldehydesulfoxylate may help to inactivate and remove the corrosive mercuric salts. In the absence of these substances, a mixture of egg whites and milk may be given to help to precipitate the mercury in the upper gastrointestinal tract; the patient may then be made to drink a dilute solution of sodium bicarbonate.

Patients who survive the shock state may still develop signs of systemic mercury poisoning in a day or two. The kidneys are most commonly involved, with damage resulting in renal tubular necrosis. This can lead to anuria, azotemia, and death, unless the patient's renal insufficiency can be successfully managed by supportive measures until tubular regeneration and recovery occur in about 2 weeks. (The organic mercurial compounds employed as diuretics rarely cause severe toxicity. Metallic mercury, or quicksilver, such as that which is sometimes spilled from broken mercury thermometers or manometers, is also potentially hazardous.)

To prevent kidney damage, dimercaprol must be administered promptly and repeatedly. Good results have also reportedly been obtained with another chelating agent, penicillamine (Cuprimine). This penicillin derivative, which is *not* an antibiotic, is also employed in the treatment of Wilson's disease, or hepatolenticular degeneration, a condition caused by a metabolic defect that permits the accumulation of copper in certain tissues. The degenerative changes of this disorder may be delayed by a dietary regimen low in copper and by the administration of penicillamine capsules for chelating this metal. Penicillamine is also used to treat arthritis.

Other chemical antidotes. Two types of poisons that act by interfering with the transport of oxygen to the tissues (carbon monoxide) or by the use of oxygen by the tissues (cyanide) are also treated with chemical antidotes. Poisoning from inhalation of gas containing carbon monoxide (CO) is said to occur more frequently than all other types of poisoning combined. Its treatment by the inhalation of pure oxygen is intended to displace CO from the hemoglobin molecule, so that oxygen can again be carried by the blood to all the body tissues, including those of the brain.

The cyanide ion (CN^-) keeps poisoned tissues from using oxygen in the series of cellular oxidation–reduction reactions essential to life. Treatment of cyanide poisoning depends on the rapid administration of systemically acting chemical antidotes such as amyl or sodium nitrite and sodium thiosulfate. These bring about the production of substances that bind the cyanide ion before it can fatally interfere with cellular respiration.

General supportive measures

Support of vital functions is especially important in poisoning, because the poison may not only adversely affect the patient's respiratory and circulatory systems but may also interfere with its own elimination by way of the liver and kidneys. Some supportive measures must be applied immediately—artificial respiration and treatment for shock, for example—but others are often carried out long after the poison has been removed from the body and emergency antidotal drugs have been administered. Supportive care is sometimes required for days and weeks. Often, the quality of this supportive nursing care determines whether the patient will survive or develop fatal complications.

The actual medical and nursing measures employed in poisoning cases are the same as those used in caring for other critically ill patients. Thus, only a brief review of some general measures relevant to the management of most patients who have been made seriously ill by systemically absorbed poisons will be presented. More detailed discussions of the management of poisoning by individual agents such as barbiturates, opiates, antidepressant drugs, and anticholinesterase-type insecticides are taken up elsewhere (see Index).

Respiratory function. Drugs that depress or overstimulate the central nervous system often cause respiratory difficulties, but overdosage with any drug can lead to interference with normal respiration. Thus, it is important to detect early signs of respiratory tract obstruction (*e.g.*, wheezes, rales, high-pitched respirations) and to correct the causes before complications develop. The patient's airway must always be kept open, if need be, by such measures as tilting the patient's head backward, pulling the lower jaw forward, and clearing clogging secretions from the mouth and throat. Such procedures as endotracheal intubation, gentle suctioning of the oropharynx, and preparation for tracheotomy may be necessary. Signs and symptoms of hypoxia, such as early restlessness and confusion that, along with lethargy, often appear well before the onset of cyanosis, should be constantly watched for. Artificial respiration and oxygen inhalation are commonly employed when the patient's own breathing is inefficient and hypoxia is developing. In an extreme emergency, mouth-to-mouth and manual techniques may be lifesaving. More commonly, the observation and care of a patient whose lungs are being rhythmically inflated by a mechanical resuscitator are necessary.

Patients with prolonged drug-induced respiratory depression run the risk of contracting hypostatic pneumonia and other infections. Preventive measures should be employed with these patients. Patients deeply depressed by barbiturates, for example, should have their position in bed changed frequently to counteract the adverse effects of stasis on pulmonary function. Those whose cough reflex is sluggish should be assisted to cough to expel mucus from the lungs. The patient's exposure to infection should be kept at a minimum. Among the drugs employed in pneumonia and pulmonary edema are antibiotics and detergents or other agents for reducing surface tension in the tracheobronchial tree.

Cardiovascular function. Circulatory function must be maintained in poisoned patients not only to keep vital organs functioning as effectively as possible, but because inadequate circulation delays the elimination of the poison and reduces the effectiveness of parenterally administered antidotal drugs. Administration of intravenous fluids to counteract shock is a very important aspect of circulatory system support. The patient's blood pressure should be checked frequently, and necessary measures should be taken to ensure that the intravenous fluid is flowing at the proper rate.

In addition to replacement fluids such as whole blood, plasma, isotonic saline solution, and synthetic plasma expanders, vasopressor drugs are often employed to counteract hypotension. The patient who is receiving an infusion of the potent vasopressors levarterenol (Levophed), phenylephrine (Neo-Synephrine), metaraminol (Aramine), or dopamine (Intropin) should receive constant monitoring of blood pressure to determine response to the drug. The rate of infusion must be adjusted to keep the patient's blood pressure from rising too high, because this can adversely affect cardiac function. Any failure of the patient's blood pressure to respond can be dealt with by other means, such as the administration of a soluble corticosteroid drug (hydrocortisone sodium succinate, Solu-Cortef), or the correction of acidosis, a condition that sometimes makes shock patients resistant to adrenergic vasopressor drug therapy.

Cardiac complications that develop during poisoning may require emergency supportive measures. One of the main responsibilities in such cases is to see that the various types of potent drugs for treating heart failure and cardiac irregularities or arrest are readily available, including isoproterenol, epinephrine, dobutamine, atropine, digitalis, and lidocaine. These drugs, along with most of the equipment needed in acute situations, are usually available on emergency carts that are regularly checked for readiness. Other equipment, such as electrical defibrillators, must be kept in good condition and available for treating poisoning by drugs and chemicals that interfere with cardiac function, such as the tricyclic antidepressants that are often used in suicide attempts by emotionally depressed patients.

Renal function. Kidney function may fail either because of damage to renal tubular cells by certain poisons such as mercury or following prolonged circulatory collapse. During the period of recovery of normal kidney function, the nurse has many responsibilities in the management of oliguria. Measuring the patient's fluid intake and daily urinary output, providing encouragement to sip small amounts of fluid, and supervising the intravenous infusions of fluid and electrolytes are all necessary interventions.

Often, whether renal failure is present or not, hemodialysis, peritoneal dialysis, forced diuresis, or other measures to remove certain poisons from the blood and tissues at a greater rate than the kidneys can eliminate them may be used. Hemodialysis and peritoneal dialysis are two procedures employed to help rid the body of high concentrations of salicylates (*e.g.*, in aspirin and oil of wintergreen poisoning), barbiturates, and similar central nervous system depressant drugs.

Actually, when the patient's kidneys are functioning adequately and can eliminate the drugs or their metabolites, water diuresis is the simplest and safest way to hasten excretion of the poison, provided that adequate care is taken to avoid fluid overload. In some circumstances, injections of the osmotic diuretics mannitol and urea (Ureaphil) may be beneficial; in others, the potent loop diuretics furosemide (Lasix) and ethacrynic acid (Edecrin) may be preferred. Careful regular assessment is important for the successful management of such patients and of those who must receive diuretic drugs and large amounts of replacement fluids containing potassium, sodium, and other electrolytes for maintaining acid–base balance when acidosis or alkalosis threatens.

Hepatic function. Liver function may be interfered with or even fail as a result of direct damage by hepatotoxic agents such as the halogenated hydrocarbons carbon tetrachloride and chloroform and other organic solvents, or as a result of poisoning by phosphorus or by the toxin of the poisonous mushroom *Amanita phalloides.* Once the poison is removed from the body and more immediately dangerous drug effects are counteracted, the main treatment may consist of measures to keep the patient alive while liver tissue is being regenerated.

The patient must be encouraged to eat the diet prescribed despite persistent anorexia. Diets high in calories, carbohydrates, and protein are considered more important than any drugs in the management of patients with acute liver damage. High doses of many vitamins are often administered, and an antiemetic phenothiazine tranquilizer-type drug may occasionally be administered to control nausea, vomiting, and restlessness. More potent central depressants such as barbiturates and opiates are ordinarily avoided, because these drugs may precipitate hepatic coma in patients with severe liver damage.

Fever, convulsions, coma. Other complications of poisoning in which skilled care is necessary include infection, which must be quickly detected and promptly treated. *Fever* that may be drug-induced or secondary to infection must be detected by monitoring the patient's temperature. Hyperpyrexia may then be treated by physical measures, such as warm water sponging, application of cool wet towels or cool water enemas, or the administration of an antipyretic drug such as aspirin. (In *hypopyrexia* and shock states, attempts may be made to *raise* body temperature by keeping the patient covered with blankets or by the use of heat applied externally, not directly but by a heat cradle.)

Drug-induced coma must be carefully evaluated by checking the patient's reflexes to determine the depth or grade of neurologic depression. The patient's temperature, pulse, respiration, and blood pressure are regularly noted. No attempts are ordinarily made to rouse the patient by administering central nervous system stimulants. Instead, supportive measures are aimed at maintaining the patient's physiologic functions, as described above.

Drug-induced convulsions may occur as the result of the direct action of central stimulants such as strychnine or cocaine, or seizures may be caused by poor oxygenation of brain tissues during coma caused by drugs that deeply depress the central nervous system and the respiratory center. In addition to the use of antiepileptic and anti-convulsant drugs such as diazepam (Valium) and barbiturates, as mentioned above, other measures are necessary to protect the patient. These include the use of padded side rails to prevent injury, insertion of a mouth gag or tongue clamp to maintain an airway and to prevent the patient from biting the tongue, and inhalation of oxygen to counteract hypoxia that occurs during convulsive apnea.

Other supportive measures

These are concerned with maintaining the patient's comfort and well-being. Here, too, nursing care is of major significance in hastening the patient's recovery from poisoning. For example, patients suffering from drug-induced delirium or from one of the withdrawal syndromes following chronic depressant drug toxicity must be kept from hurting themselves during delirium. They are assisted in orienting themselves in regard to where they are and what is being done to help them. Other poisoned patients may require more than the usual amount of mouth and skin care following contact with irritant chemicals. Comatose patients require changes in position to prevent decubitus ulcer formation, and they require eye care to prevent corneal exposure and permanent injury. Patients in pain require not only analgesic drugs but measures such as massage, changes of position, and physical support when they must be moved.

Prevention of poisoning

Treatment of a poisoned patient is often difficult, even for experienced and skilled personnel with the most modern equipment and facilities. Thus, it is more important to prevent poisoning accidents from happening in the first place. Studies carried out by various medical groups and governmental agencies have gathered information concerning the causes of household poisoning. Federal laws concerning the packaging and labeling of chemical products have helped to reduce the number of cases to some extent. However, the most important preventive measure of all is to educate the public concerning the safe handling and storage of drugs and other chemicals in the home.

The nurse is in a unique position to teach people how to avoid accidents of this type. Public health and school nurses have an especially important part to play. The school nurse can educate parents by teaching their school age children. The instructions given to children about handling and storing potential poisons properly can keep their preschool brothers and sisters from being exposed to this danger. Follow-up visits to homes in which poisoning accidents have occurred will usually reveal even more uncorrected hazards. Suggestions can be made to the mother that may keep another accident from happening. In some situations, the visiting nurse may wish to enlist the services of a medical social worker or even request psychiatric consultation for members of an accident-prone family.

The following (Patient Teaching Guide: Poison Prevention) presents some key teaching points that should be incorporated into education programs for all patients and the public.

Patient teaching guide: Poison prevention

1. Keep all drugs and household chemicals out of the reach of children. Cleaning materials should be in locked or latched cupboards above children's reach. Medicine should be kept in tight cabinets.

2. Keep all chemicals in their original containers, which now often have special childproof safety closures.
    Pouring chemicals into old food or drink containers often results in tragedy.

3. Read the label before using any medicine or chemical specialty product. Failure to follow instructions often results in accidental poisoning.

4. Take medication only under safe conditions.
    Never take drugs in the dark; mistakes are often made. Children watching adults take medications will often imitate them. Children should never be encouraged to take medicine as "candy."

5. Destroy all old medications instead of just discarding them.
    Children, or adults, may pick up and ingest discarded medications, leading to toxic overdoses. Saving drugs to use for a future illness, or to lend to friends, may result in the use of outdated and wrong medications, as well as to poisoning, and may lead to delay in seeking appropriate medical care.

First aid instructions

Serious consequences can sometimes be prevented following ingestion of a drug or chemical by furnishing first aid information to people who telephone in an emergency. Actually, the best advice is that they take the victim to the nearest hospital emergency ward or health-care facility.

When the nature of the ingested substance is known, the person may be told whether or not to induce vomiting and how best to do so or, if the question concerns contamination of the skin and eyes with chemicals, the person should be urged to wash these areas immediately with copious quantities of tap water. Of course, the patient should be brought in for further medical attention after first aid has been administered. The caller should be advised to save the container of the product and to bring it, or the suspected poison itself, to the hospital or health-care office.

Identification

Identifying the substance that has been ingested often helps to differentiate a harmless ingestion that requires no treatment from a dangerous incident that calls for immediate action. In the case of drug products, com-munity or hospital pharmacists can almost always furnish factual information that will help in the identification of drug products that have been accidentally ingested. The pharmacist may do so by referring to the *Identification Guide for Solid Dosage Forms* made available by the American Medical Association or by consulting the section in the *PDR* in which pictures of many common capsules and tablets are shown. Other useful compendia of drug data include the *American Drug Index*, the *United States Dispensatory*, and the *Modern Drug Encyclopedia*.

Poison information centers

No member of the health-care team can know all there is to know about the prevention and treatment of poisoning. Thus, special centers—usually located in the health departments of large cities or states or in medical and pharmacy schools—function as sources of information in poisoning emergencies. They are often called Poison Control Centers. Often they can be reached 24 hours a day for answers to the questions most commonly asked in a poison emergency: "What is in it?" "How toxic is it?" "What's the best treatment?" Treatment centers and hospital emergency rooms also are often called on to furnish such information. Available reference materials and other sources from which the answers to such questions may be found should be readily accessible to all members of the health-care team.

Other sources of information

A large number of books are available dealing with such subjects as toxicology, pharmacology, and the chemical contents of various types of household products (see References). Two comprehensive compendia have proved especially useful as sources of information in poison emergencies: the massive card file prepared by the National Clearinghouse for Poison Control Centers, and *Clinical Toxicology of Commercial Products (CTCP)* by Gosselin and colleagues (5th ed, Williams & Wilkins, 1984).

Both are sources of the types of information that is most frequently needed: the chemical contents of a specific trade-named product; how hazardous its ingestion is likely to prove; the signs and symptoms to look for; and first aid and more comprehensive treatment measures that should be employed. The Clearinghouse File consists of a constantly expanding set of alphabetized cards of two types—*white cards,* which deal with the management of cases in which any one of thousands of specific products may have been ingested, and *orange cards,* which outline in greater detail the procedures for treating poisoning by the most toxic chemical ingredients of some of these products. The compendium, *CTCP,* by Gosselin furnishes similar information in its seven sections, together with an illustrative chart on how to use the text in the most efficient manner for acquiring the data that may be needed in a poisoning emergency.

Occasional cases cannot be readily dealt with by consulting such sources. Such calls are relayed to regional information centers that have the facilities for tracing specialized data. Sometimes, long-distance calls are made to the manufacturers of the ingested products or to expert consultants who may possess vital specialized information, and can often furnish the information needed in managing poisoning by plants, venomous animals, foods, and pharmaceuticals. The Center for Disease Control (CDC) in Atlanta, Georgia is often the source for hard-to-find data and rare antidotes.

Poison treatment centers

In addition to the centers mentioned above, which function mainly to disseminate information, some services located in general hospitals and medical centers offer facilities for the treatment of victims of accidental poisoning. They are organized to offer not only immediate first aid measures but also medical and surgical specialty services that require advanced technical equipment and extensive laboratory facilities. The telephone numbers of local, state, and regional poison control centers of both types should be posted in emergency facilities. There are now over 600 such centers located in every state, all coordinated by state departments of public health.

For a summary, see Guide to the Nursing Process: Poisoning.

Guide to the nursing process: poisoning

Assessment	Diagnoses	Interventions	Evaluation
Past history: underlying medical conditions	Potential alteration in cardiac output	Maintain airway and vital signs	Monitor vital signs
Drug history: substance ingested, inhaled, contacted; amount; time of exposure; measures taken for relief; presenting complaints	Potential alteration in gas exchange	Remove ingested substance: gastric lavage, induce vomiting, flush surface area, force liquids, dialysis, diuresis	Monitor signs of renal or hepatic toxicity
	Potential alteration in skin integrity		Evaluate effectiveness of attempts to remove substance
	Potential alteration in fluid volume	Administer specific antidotes	Evaluate patient comfort level
	Knowledge deficit	Supportive measures	Evaluate response to antidotes
		Comfort measures	Evaluate effectiveness of teaching
Physical Assessment		Patient and family teaching	
Cardiovascular: blood pressure, pulse, perfusion			
Respiratory: rate, rhythm, depth, adventitious sounds			

(continued)

Assessment	Diagnoses	Interventions	Evaluation
GI: bowel sounds, mucous membranes, GI tract Renal: output, amount, character Skin: color, temperature, specific lesions Neurologic: mental status, pupils, reflexes			

Case study

Presentation

Mrs. K, a 26-year-old mother of two, rushed her 3-year-old son, Billy, into the local emergency room following an incident that involved Billy's 5-year-old sister playing doctor and "treating" Billy with what turned out to be children's aspirin. Mrs. K brought with her a bottle of 1-gr children's aspirin, from which 8 to 12 tablets were missing. Mrs. K did not know if Billy had actually ingested any of the tablets. Billy appears to be a happy, active 3-year-old—P, 96; R, 12; T, 98.6° F; alert, oriented. The potential ingestion would have occurred 20 to 30 minutes before admission. What action should be taken?

Discussion

Billy shows no signs or symptoms of aspirin toxicity. Despite this, poison control cards show that if 8 to 12 tablets were actually ingested, Billy could face severe salicylate poisoning. Vomiting should be induced, probably using ipecac syrup. The patient should then be carefully observed for results of emesis—contents, and so forth—and for the appearance of any signs or symptoms of salicylate poisoning—such as fever, hyperactivity, increased respiration. Mrs. K should be assured that she took the correct action, regardless of the results of the induction of vomiting. Safety and preventive measures can be taught once the situation has calmed down and the patient and Mrs. K are receptive. The proper storage of medications, the importance of never taking medications for fun or for trivial reasons, and never taking medications from anyone but adults can be stressed. Mrs. K can also be advised to purchase 1-oz containers of ipecac syrup to keep in the house for such emergencies, and taught how to induce vomiting through pharyngeal stimulation if this is not feasible. Again, assure the patient and his mother that seeking professional care was the best action in this instance and, if any such ingestion should ever occur again, the same steps should be taken.

Drug digests

Calcium disodium edetate USP (Calcium Disodium Versenate)

Actions and indications. This chemical combines with various metallic ions, including lead, to form a nonionized complex called a chelate. This complex is water-soluble and can be removed from the body by way of the patient's kidneys, provided that they are functioning normally.

This chelating agent is used mainly to treat lead poisoning and acute lead encephalopathy. When administered by vein, this antidotal drug mobilizes lead as it leaves the tissues and enters the extracellular fluids. The level of lead in the urine begins to rise within 6 hours and reaches a peak excretory rate in 24 to 48 hours.

An oral form of this drug is available for use following parenteral therapy and in patients with abnormally high lead levels who show no symptoms of poisoning. It has also been used for prophylaxis in industrial workers but is not recommended now for that purpose.

Adverse effects, cautions, and contraindications. This chemical can cause acute necrosis of the renal tubules. Thus, it is used cautiously in patients with kidney disease and is contraindicated in severe renal diseases. Caution is also necessary in patients with a history of healed or active tuberculosis. Injection is sometimes followed by general malaise, chills, fever, and muscle cramps. Histaminelike reactions, including lacrimation, sneezing, and nasal congestion, sometimes occur. The oral form may cause some gastrointestinal irritation, but more serious is the possibility that if lead is present in the GI tract, this drug may increase its systemic absorption and result in a possible increase in toxic symptoms. Thus, use of the oral form is not desirable in cases of acute lead poisoning.

Dosage and administration. For intravenous use, the 1.0-g ampule is diluted with 250 ml to 500 ml of isotonic saline or dextrose solution and administered as an IV infusion over a 1-hour period. This is repeated later the same day for 5 days. After a 2-day rest period, a second course of up to 5 days may be given if necessary. Dosage for children should not exceed 1.0 g/day for every 30 lb of body weight.

Oral dosage is 4 g/day administered in divided doses or, for children, 1g/35 lb of body weight.

Dimercaprol USP (BAL; British Anti-Lewisite)

Actions and indications. This antidote to poisoning by heavy metals acts by combining with the metallic ions to form a *nontoxic* chelate called a mercaptide, which is then excreted by the kidneys. It is particularly effective in poisoning by mercury and arsenic, provided that it is administered promptly, before severe kidney damage has developed. It has recently proved effective for increasing the rate of removal of lead when administered in combination with calcium disodium edetate, thus lessening brain damage in children with acute lead encephalopathy.

BAL has also helped to prevent hemorrhagic encephalitis following overdoses of arsenical chemotherapy. It counteracts various adverse reactions to the gold salts used in treating rheumatoid arthritis, including especially gold dermatitis. It may be helpful for reducing tissue levels of copper when combined with penicillamine in treating Wilson's disease (hepatolenticular degeneration).

Adverse effects, cautions, and contraindications. BAL should be discontinued if acute kidney damage from the metallic poison develops, because it cannot reverse the renal tubular damage. Continued use of this drug could then result in its reaching tissue levels high enough to cause toxicity, including convulsions and coma. It should *not* be used in treating iron poisoning, because the complex that is formed can cause kidney damage. Ordinary doses of BAL do not produce severe toxic effects. However, treatment may be accompanied by various discomforting symptoms, including pain at the injection site, salivation, lacrimation, nausea, and vomiting. The drug sometimes also causes transient tingling in the hands and feet, a burning sensation in the mouth, and a sense of tightness in the chest.

Dosage and administration. BAL is administered only by deep intramuscular injection in doses of 2.5 mg/kg of body weight. This dose is repeated every 4 hours for the first 2 days. Later, it is administered only twice a day for 10 days, or until the patient appears completely recovered. The sites of intramuscular injection should be rotated, and the patient's urine should be alkalinized to prevent the chelate from dissociating during renal excretion, with possible resulting kidney damage.

References

Anderson RJ: Drug prescribing in patients in renal failure. Hosp Pract 18:145, 1983

Arena JM: Poisoning: Toxicology, Symptoms and Treatment, 3rd ed. Springfield, IL, Charles C Thomas, 1973

Bayer MY, Rumack BH: Poisoning and Overdose. Rockville, Maryland, Aspen Systems, 1983

Bennett WM: Drug therapy in renal failure: Dosing guidelines for adults. Ann Intern Med 93:62, 286, 1980

Bennett WM et al: Guide to drug usage in adult patients with impaired kidney function. JAMA 223:991, 1973

DiPalma JR: Preventing drug reactions. Am Fam Physician 12:154, 1975

Doull J et al (eds): Toxicology: The Basic Science of Poisons, 2nd ed. New York, Macmillan Publishing, 1980

Gosselin RE et al: Clinical Toxicology of Commercial Products, 5th ed. Baltimore, Williams & Wilkins, 1984

Horoshak I: What to do in a poison emergency. RN 40:44, 1977

Hrizo RW: My family's fight with malignant hyperthermia. RN 40:21, 1977

Karch FE, Lasagna, L: Adverse drug reactions: Critical Review. JAMA 234:1236, 1975

Lawrence RA, Haggerty RJ: Household agents and their potential toxicity. Mod Treat 8:511, 1971

Mennear JH: The poisoning emergency. Am J Nurs 7:842, 1977

Miller RK: Drugs during pregnancy: Therapeutic dilemma. Ration Drug Ther 15:1, 1981

Papadopoulous C: Cardiovascular drugs and sexuality. Arch Int Med 140:1341, 1980

Parker CW: Drug allergy. N Engl J Med 292:511, 732, 957, 1975

Prescott LF, Critchley JAJH: The treatment of acetaminophen poisoning. Ann Rev Pharmacol Toxicol 23:87, 1983

Roxe DM: Toxic nephropathy due to drugs. Ration Drug Ther 9:1, 1975

Sibert JR, Craft AW, Jackson RH: Child-resistant packaging and accidental child poisoning. Lancet 2:89, 1977

Section 2

Chemotherapeutic agents: anti-infective and antineoplastic drugs

2 This section introduces the first group of specific drugs to be discussed in this text, *anti-infective drugs,* which comprise one, albeit large, group of *chemotherapeutic agents.* These drugs are designed to act selectively on foreign organisms that have invaded and infected the body of a host. Ideally, anti-infective drugs should be specifically toxic to the infecting organisms, but have no effects on the cells of the host; unfortunately, this ideal is almost never attained, and knowledge of the toxic and adverse side-effects produced by these drugs, and how to deal with these effects, are important aspects of learning about the pharmacology of these drugs.

Drugs used to treat cancer constitute the other group of chemotherapeutic agents to be discussed in this section. The principles of cancer chemotherapy are similar to those of the therapy of infectious diseases: ideally, the drugs used to treat cancer should be selectively toxic to tumor cells, but this goal is reached even less frequently with drugs used to treat cancer than with drugs used to treat infectious diseases.

The introductory chapter of this section will not discuss any specific class of anti-infective agents or individual drugs, but will set the scene for the study of such drugs and their use against specific infections in subsequent chapters. First some aspects of the history of systemic infection treatment with drugs will be reviewed. Then certain essential terms and underlying concepts that serve as the basis for the proper use of drugs in the clinical management of infection will be defined and examined. Finally, the general principles that are applied in selecting the most effective and safest drugs for treating individual infections will be described and the pitfalls that must be avoided in achieving the objective of such treatment will be pointed out: cure of the patient's infection with few or no drug-induced adverse effects.

Although the nurse usually does not select the drugs employed to treat specific infections, monitoring the patient's responses to such therapy is an important part of the nursing process. Thus, understanding the principles that serve as the basis of proper employment of anti-infective agents is important for the nurse, because when these drugs are misused—as they often are—the patient is not only deprived of their valuable and even lifesaving properties, but may also suffer needlessly from disabling and even fatal drug reactions.

The chapters in this section that describe specific anti-infective drugs are organized according to the infecting organisms; the treatment of infections caused by the smallest organisms, viruses, is described first, followed by a description of the treatment of infections caused by unicellar organisms (bacteria, protozoa), fungi, and finally multicellular parasites (*e.g.*, helminths). The last chapter in the section discusses the other group of chemotherapeutic drugs, those used against malignant tumors and other cancers—that is, against cells of the host's own body that are no longer under normal control mechanisms.

Chapter 6

General principles of anti-infective therapy

6

History

Chemicals have been used to treat infectious diseases for many centuries, and the occasional curative properties of soils, plants, and other materials containing living molds and bacteria also were recognized by primitive peoples. For example, mercury was used to treat syphilis from the time of the first recorded outbreak of that disease in Europe about 1500 AD, and ancient Chinese medical manuscripts recommend application of moldy soybean curds to boils, carbuncles, and infected wounds.

However, anti-infective drug treatment of systemic infections was put on a rational scientific basis only with the work of Paul Ehrlich, early in this century. Before his pioneer research, many chemicals were known that eliminated pathogenic organisms when applied topically as antiseptics and disinfectants (see Chap. 43). However, such substances were too toxic for internal administration aimed at eliminating microorganisms that had established themselves deep within the tissues of the host.

Ehrlich reasoned that it might be possible to prepare synthetic chemicals that would act selectively on parasitic cells without injuring the person being treated. He felt that drugs might be devised that would have a specific affinity for chemicals present in the microbial cells but absent from human tissues. When injected just once into the infected patient, such a drug would seek out the bacterial invaders and kill them all without harming their host.

In pursuit of this goal, Ehrlich synthesized hundreds of chemicals and tested them on laboratory animals injected with pathogenic organisms. His first synthetic anti-infective compound proved as toxic to the tissues of the animals as it was to such infecting pathogens as the protozoan that causes trypanosomiasis and the spirochete responsible for syphilis. However, in the course of his work with organic arsenic compounds, he continued

to prepare anti-infective chemicals with higher degrees of selective toxicity for the microbes in comparison to their animal hosts. His 606th drug of this class, *arsphenamine*, finally proved safe enough for effective use in treating human patients with syphilis, as was the 909th compound, *neoarsphenamine.*

Ehrlich's work laid the foundation for other successes in the use of chemicals to fight systemic infection. Other scientists employing his concepts and methods during the next 25 years developed drugs for treating diseases caused by invaders other than bacteria, such as malaria, amebiasis, and other protozoal diseases. However, no drugs safe enough for treating bacterial infections were found during this time, and patients who could not be protected by biologic products such as vaccines and antitoxins continued to die of many common bacterial diseases.

Finally, in 1935, Domagk reported that *Prontosil*, one of a series of sulfonamide dyes that had been synthesized early in the century, could protect mice against infection by streptococci. *Sulfanilamide,* introduced in the following year, proved effective for treating systemic infections by streptococci, staphylococci, pneumococci, and meningococci. Many sulfanilamide derivatives were introduced during the rest of the decade for treating these and other bacterial infections.

These successes in antibacterial chemotherapy led not only to the synthesis of other chemical classes effective against bacteria but also to the study of *natural* substances known to possess antimicrobial activity. The first of these antibiotics, *penicillin*, had been discovered by Fleming in 1928, but the work that led to its clinical introduction in the early 1940s was not done until after the successful clinical use of the sulfonamides stimulated an intensive reinvestigation of the properties of filtrates of *Penicillium* mold cultures. Other scientists, including Waxman and his group at Rutgers University in this country, then discovered streptomycin, neomycin, and other natural products of soil microorganisms called actinomycetes.

The search for effective synthetic and natural antimicrobial agents continues today, because—contrary to the early high expectations—microbial diseases have not been eradicated. Their treatment is, in fact, often more difficult than when only the sulfonamides, penicillin, and streptomycin were available following the end of World War II in the mid-1940s. One reason for this has been the emergence of microorganisms capable of resisting antimicrobial therapy (see below). Up to now, fortunately, the discovery of new anti-infective drugs and the development of more effective derivatives of older drugs have helped to maintain control of microbial infections. However, authorities in the management of infection periodically express concern over the possibility that the indiscriminate and unwise use of these valuable drugs may lead to a disastrous reduction in their effectiveness against infectious diseases.

Terms and concepts

Antibiotics, according to the original definition, are chemical compounds produced by living microorganisms that can inhibit the growth of other microorganisms or even kill them. The term has now come to be used more loosely, and often it refers to *synthetic* antimicrobial drugs. The terms "microbe" and "microorganism" refer to bacteria, protozoa, fungi, and even viruses.

Synthetic anti-infective drugs differ from the naturally derived antibiotics only in their origin. Basically, both types of antimicrobials bring about their therapeutic effects in the same ways. All possess properties that help their molecules react with microbial cell molecules in ways that interfere with the normal metabolic or biosynthetic processes of the microorganism.

Chemotherapy is a term that applies to the use of both natural and synthetic chemicals in a manner intended to interfere with the functioning of foreign cell populations. Originally, this term was applied only to chemicals employed to treat infectious disease. Now the term has been further broadened to include not only anti-infective agents but also the antineoplastic drugs employed in treating cancer and leukemia (see Chap. 12).

Selective toxicity is a concept employed in seeking safe and effective chemotherapeutic agents. It refers to the ability of such chemicals to strike selectively at foreign cells in ways that harm them without—ideally, at least—doing significant damage to the cells of the host. This is the result of the affinity that such molecules have for the microbial cell constituents to which they bind—for example, ribosomes, nucleic acids, and specific enzymes—and of their relative lack of reactivity with the macromolecules of the host.

Mechanisms

The ways in which certain anti-infective agents exert their selective toxicity will be briefly discussed when properties of the individual drugs are taken up in the following chapters of this section. The following examples of the manner of action of several representative drugs on cellular and subcellular constituents can, for the present, serve as a brief summary of anti-infective drug mechanisms:

1. *Penicillin* inhibits biosynthesis of bacterial cell walls.
2. *Sulfonamides* and *trimethoprim* are antimetabolites that prevent microbial cells from utilizing substances essential to their growth, development, and reproduction.
3. Many drugs interfere with one or another of the several steps of protein synthesis. *Aminoglycoside* antibiotics such as *streptomycin* and *gentamicin* bind to bacterial ribosomes in a way that results in a misreading of the genetic code. The *tetracyclines, chloramphenicol, clindamycin,* and *erythromycin* all also act to inhibit protein synthesis in various other ways.
4. *Polymyxin*-type antibiotics alter the permeability of bacterial cell membranes in a way that lets essential metabolites leak out. *Amphotericin* and *nystatin* have a somewhat similar effect on the membranes of fungal cells.

Antimicrobial spectrum

The currently available anti-infective drugs vary in their degree of effectiveness against different microorganisms. Some are so selective in their inhibitory effects on specialized metabolic processes that their effectiveness is limited to a relatively few microorganisms. Thus, the antifungal antibiotics are said to possess a *narrow spectrum* of activity. At the other extreme are the *broad-spectrum* antibiotics—agents that interfere with a biochemical reaction common to many microorganisms, including not only bacteria of the gram-positive and gram-negative types, but also *non*bacterial microbes such as rickettsiae and even large viruses.

Degrees of activity

Anti-infective agents vary considerably in their potency. Some are so active that they exert a *bactericidal* action against sensitive organisms when present in the environment in extremely low concentrations. *Penicillin,* for example, kills actively multiplying streptococci when as little as 1 µg of the antibiotic comes into contact with 2 or 3 oz of culture medium. Other substances are, at best, only *bacteriostatic.* That is, they merely inhibit the growth of previously multiplying microorganisms without actually killing them. However, provided that the patient's own immune system is operating efficiently, bacteriostatic drugs, such as the sulfonamides and tetracyclines, can be very useful. For some antibacterial drugs, the terms "bacteriostatic" and "bactericidal" are relative, not absolute—that is, the drug is bacteriostatic in low concentrations, but in high concentrations, which may cause host toxicity, the drug is bactericidal.

Host defenses

Effective chemotherapy of infections with both bacteriostatic and bactericidal drugs requires the activity of the patient's own immune system. These antimicrobial defenses, which ordinarily eliminate most pathogens before they can progress far enough to cause clinical infection, include production of immune antibodies, phagocytosis by leukocytes and other cells, and proliferation of sensitized lymphocytes that then attack the invaders (see Chap. 36). When the patient's defenses have been impaired by disease or by the effects of drugs that suppress his immune responses, it may not be possible to combat infection successfully by antimicrobial drug therapy alone.

Among the diseases that most commonly compromise the patient's defenses against infection are neoplasms such as Hodgkin's disease and other lymphomas, leukemia, and cancers, diabetes, and various debilitating disorders that interfere with nutrition and thus alter the ability of the patient's body to produce the elements necessary for the immune response. Drugs that interfere with host defense mechanisms include those used in cancer chemotherapy such as the cytotoxic alkylating agents and antimetabolites, the corticosteroids employed in the management of collagen diseases and in many other disorders including some neoplasms, and the immunosuppressive drugs used following organ transplants, including azathioprine as well as certain antineoplastic agents and the corticosteroid drugs. These drugs actively destroy or inactivate various essential elements involved in the immune response.

Microbial resistance

As indicated in the above discussion of the antimicrobial spectrum concept, some drugs have little or no effect on various species of microorganisms. Such organisms are said to possess a *natural* or *intrinsic resistance* to these drugs, which prevents the chemicals from interfering with any of their vital processes. Clinically, such intrinsic resistance is rarely a problem because other drugs are usually available with antibacterial activity to which the pathogens are sensitive. Much more serious is the fact that many types of bacteria, which were at first sensitive to certain drugs, have developed the ability to withstand the drugs' effects. This type of *acquired resistance* is, of course, a serious clinical problem because the once effective drug becomes useless for treating infections caused by resistant strains of the previously sensitive species.

Biochemical mechanisms of resistance

The biochemical mechanisms by which microorganisms are intrinsically resistant or develop resistance to antimicrobial drugs include the following:

1. Production by the microbes of an enzyme that inactivates the antimicrobial drug
2. Changes in the permeability of the microbes to the antimicrobial drug, *or*
3. Changes in the drug transport system of the microbes (both mechanisms 2 *and* 3 result in the exclusion of the drug from access to drug-sensitive sites)
4. Production by the microbes of a chemical antagonist to the antimicrobial drug
5. Changes in the drug-binding site on a ribosomal protein that prevent the antimicrobial drug from binding

The specific mechanisms of resistance are related to some extent to the drug's mechanism of action. A specific example of one mechanism of resistance is the production by some strains of bacteria of penicillinase, an enzyme that inactivates many types of penicillin drugs. A detailed understanding of this mechanism allowed researchers to design penicillin molecules that were not inactivated by the enzyme. Research into the mechanisms of microbial susceptibility and resistance to antimicrobial drugs is vitally important to the development of new antimicrobial drugs that will be effective against resistant strains of microbes.

Mechanisms by which resistance is acquired

How do microorganisms acquire resistance to antimicrobial drugs and what can be done to delay the development of resistance? Antimicrobial drugs are now known to act in several ways that favor the emergence of resistant strains. The most common mechanism depends on the drug's selectively eliminating the most sensitive cells of the infecting population. That is, as the drug acts to eliminate the members of a species that are sensitive to its action, the few bacterial cells that are intrinsically resistant to the drug multiply until they comprise the majority of the species population. These resistant cells are "selected out" by the action of the drug on susceptible cells that formerly competed with the resistant ones (*e.g.*, for nutrients). The originally resistant cells are *mutants*, variant organisms that differ from others of the same species. Drugs do not cause such mutations, but a drug may act as a *selective force* that favors the emergence of mutants, until this once tiny resistant minority gradually becomes the dominant strain—one that causes infections that are no longer susceptible to treatment with that anti-infective drug.

Scientists have recognized several other mechanisms by which individual drug-sensitive microorganisms can quickly become resistant to anti-infective agents. All these methods of acquiring resistance involve the transfer of genetic material responsible for resistance from drug-resistant bacteria to drug-sensitive organisms by cell-to-cell contact. The bacteria that acquire resistance in this way then transmit this heritable trait to their offspring, so that the entire population then becomes resistant.

One mechanism of acquired drug resistance—the result of a form of sexual mating between bacteria of different species, called *conjugation*—has caused particular concern among public health authorities. One reason for this is that harmless inhabitants of the intestinal tract may transfer their drug resistance trait to pathogenic species. Another danger is that the pathogens that receive this genetic information, or *R factor,* can become resistant to many different antimicrobial drugs at once as the result of a single such transfer.

Clinical significance

This type of *infectious multiple drug resistance* has raised the threat that in theory, at least, such diseases as bacillary dysentery, typhoid fever, and cholera might become resistant to control by any of the drugs now available. It has also been suggested that strains of staphylococci resistant to the antibiotics that now control them might emerge suddenly, particularly in hospitals that continually employ large quantities of such drugs. To avoid the possibility of epidemics against which present drugs would be useless, public health epidemiologists often warn that these drugs must be used with more care than is now usually the case in medical practice and in animal husbandry.

Preventing resistance

Because exposure of microbes to antimicrobial drugs tends to favor their developing resistance, these drugs should not be used indiscriminately or unnecessarily. They should not, for example, be used for treating colds or other infections caused by viruses. Anti-infective drugs should, instead, be reserved for treating patients whose illnesses have been proved to be caused by a specific microorganism that is susceptible to the drug (see Treatment of Systemic Infections, below). The agent should then be used in high enough doses and for long enough periods to eradicate even the more resistant pathogenic mutants that may be present, because administration of low doses may let these organisms live and rapidly become the dominant strain, not only in the patient who is being treated, but also in the entire community or hospital environment. This is a real problem in clinical practice. Many people stop taking their antibiotics when they start to feel better and others treat themselves with "leftover" antibiotics when they don't feel well. Such practices, which are very common, tend to favor the emergence of resistant strains. Hospitals should also reserve potent new antibiotics for use in patients severely ill with serious infections that do

not respond to established drugs, because the new drugs can quickly lose their value when widely used for treating infections that could be readily controlled by other drugs already available.

Treatment of systemic infections

The many antimicrobial drugs now available can quickly clear up most infections that might once have caused lengthy illnesses, organ-damaging complications, and death. However, patients sometimes fail to gain all the benefits of modern chemotherapy. Some may even be made worse by the drug-induced adverse effects that are added to the discomfort caused by their underlying illness. Thus, it is important to be aware of the factors that can help to ensure effective and safe treatment of infection.

Drug selection

The physician tries to determine the cause of illness and selects the drug or drug combination best suited for the specific infection and the individual patient. First, of course, it is necessary to rule out other possible causes for the patient's signs and symptoms. Fever, redness, and swelling—common signs of infection—may be caused by *non*infectious disease processes. A persistent rise in temperature may, for example, be the first sign of a still "silent" malignant growth, such as an intra-abdominal carcinoma or lymphoma. A hot, red swollen digit, joint, or extremity may be caused by an acute gout attack or other inflammatory joint disorder rather than by infection.

Identification of the pathogen

This is the first step in rational antimicrobial therapy, once the physician has determined that the patient is suffering from an infection. The most certain source of such information is the laboratory's report of the results of bacteriologic culture. Thus, specimens for bacterial culture should be obtained before beginning drug treatment of any potentially serious infection. Often, however—particularly when it is not desirable to delay treatment while waiting for a detailed bacteriologic diagnosis—enough information for a working diagnosis can be collected from quicker, less costly tests. Often, a Gram smear of pus, urine or other exudative discharges or body fluids will reveal the probable pathogen, particularly when these findings are combined with what has been learned from the patient's history and from the presenting signs and symptoms.

Sensitivity testing

This is the most certain way to select a drug that will be effective against the organism responsible for the infection. However, such laboratory tests are not always necessary, and the physician often orders a drug that experience has proved to be effective against the pathogen that is presumed—on the basis of microscopic findings or clinical signs and symptoms—to be the probable cause of the patient's infection. For example, when clinical signs and quick laboratory evidence indicate that a respiratory infection is probably caused by a β-hemolytic streptococcus or the pneumococcus, or that a venereal disease is the result of infection by the gonococcus or *Treponema pallidum*, the spirochetal cause of syphilis, no further testing is needed to determine the organism's sensitivity to drugs. Penicillin or one of its substitutes is prescribed routinely, because these pathogens have remained highly sensitive to these antibiotics.

On the other hand, when the infection is caused by a pathogenic species known to produce many drug-resistant strains, it is essential to use sensitivity tests to guide drug selection. For example, many strains of staphylococci or of various gram-negative bacilli such as *Escherichia coli* or *Pseudomonas* are now resistant to drugs to which these species were once uniformly sensitive. Thus, in urinary tract and other infections by these species, it is necessary to determine which drugs are actually capable of controlling the specific strain responsible for each infection.

Drug combinations

Therapy with two or more effective anti-infective agents is sometimes superior to treatment with a single drug. On the other hand, two drugs given together may be no more effective than one drug alone, particularly when the drugs are combined in a fixed dosage mixture. Occasionally, the therapeutic effectiveness of a combination of drugs may actually prove inferior to that of a single well-selected drug. Thus, the administration of antimicrobial drug combinations is best limited to the few clinical situations in which such therapy has definitely been proved effective for treating or preventing certain types of infections. Combinations of several drugs should never be ordered and administered as a sort of "shotgun" approach to therapy—that is, with the idea that if one drug does not work, another will.

Emergency treatment of certain serious infections before the causative organism is known is sometimes best begun with a combination of two drugs, both of which are known to be effective against the pathogens that experience suggests are most likely to be involved in the particular clinical circumstances. If, for example, the presence of septicemia is suspected, the immediate administration of full therapeutic doses of both an aminoglycoside-type antibiotic such as gentamicin and a penicillin-type drug such as ampicillin or carbenicillin may be ordered (Chap. 8).

These combinations are employed because the various organisms responsible for septicemic infections are known to be almost always sensitive to one or both of these drug classes and many are, in fact, more sensitive to a combination than to either drug alone. Although treatment is begun without delay because of the seriousness of septicemia and septic shock, cultures are, of course, taken first so that the specific organism can be identified and its sensitivity to drugs determined. Then, if tests indicate that the pathogenic strain is fully susceptible to one of the drugs, the other may be withdrawn or, if some other drug proves even more effective against the pathogen, the combination is withdrawn and treatment is continued with maximal tolerated doses of the drug that testing indicated was most likely to prove effective.

Synergism between two antimicrobial drugs is also known to occur in certain other specific infections. For example, cases of bacterial endocarditis caused by enterococcal organisms are best treated with a combination of penicillin and streptomycin rather than with either drug alone, and brucellosis is probably best treated by combining a tetracycline with streptomycin.

Antagonism between antibiotics is also possible. Thus, for example, it has long been known that penicillin alone is much more effective for treating pneumococcal meningitis than is a combination of penicillin with a broad-spectrum tetracycline compound such as oxytetracycline. This may be because penicillin exerts it bactericidal action against rapidly dividing bacteria. The addition of the bacteriostatic tetracycline, which slows bacterial cell division, reduces the effectiveness of the penicillin component of the combination.

Mixed bacterial infections caused by two or more organisms, each of which is sensitive to entirely different drugs, respond best to treatment with a properly selected combination of antimicrobial agents. Perforation of the intestine may, for example, contaminate the abdominal cavity with organisms that require a combination of antibiotics to prevent or treat peritonitis. Other mixed infections that require combinations of chemotherapeutic agents occur in some chronic conditions involving the respiratory and urinary tracts.

Prevention of resistance is another reason for administering two or more antimicrobial agents simultaneously. Resistant strains emerge more slowly when a chronic infection is treated by two drugs, both of which are effective against the pathogenic species. In treating tuberculosis, for example, it is customary to administer two tuberculostatic drugs together, because this has been found to delay the emergence of resistant strains of the causative mycobacterium. This occurs because the minority of tuberculosis organisms that might survive the attack of one drug alone and then form a family of bacterial cells resistant to that drug are controlled by the second drug, thus preventing development of a new drug-resistant strain.

On the other hand, some mixtures of antimicrobial drugs may actually favor the emergence of resistant strains. This is most likely to occur with commercial products containing a combination of drugs, one of which is present in too small a dose to be fully effective. The antimicrobial drug that is present in an inadequate concentration kills off only the most sensitive pathogens, while it leaves the more resistant microorganisms alive. Those organisms that might not have survived a full dose of the drug then serve as the source of a strain more resistant to the drug than was the previous bacterial population.

Most *fixed-dose combinations* of the type mentioned above have been removed from the market at the insistence of the Food and Drug Administration. Most of those remaining have a DESI rating of "ineffective," and so they are also likely to be withdrawn before long.* Thus, when it is desirable to treat an infection with two or more antimicrobial agents, each drug ordered will have to be selected and administered in fully adequate doses. An exception to the current trend against fixed dosage combinations is the product co-trimoxazole (Bactrim; Septra) containing sulfamethoxazole and trimethoprim that has proved effective for treating urinary tract and other infections.

Other factors

The sensitivity of the pathogen to the drug or drug combination is not the only factor that must be considered in selecting the most appropriate agent for treating each patient's infection. Additional parameters include choice of the most appropriate dose, route of administration, and dosage schedule. This, in turn, often depends on the severity of the infection. Oral dosage is usually reserved for mild to moderate infections, except when there is some doubt that the drug will be adequately absorbed by that route because the patient is vomiting, or for some other reason.

In such instances, and in all *severe* systemic infections, parenteral routes are employed. However, injections are stopped and the patient is switched to oral forms of the antimicrobial drug as soon as the infection seems under control. This is done to minimize the pain caused by some intramuscular injections and to avoid local hemorrhage in patients who have a tendency to bleed readily. Similarly, although intravenous administration is the surest way to obtain the high blood and tissue levels of the drug needed in serious life-threatening infections such as bacteremia and bacterial endocarditis, intermittent IV injections or continuous infusions by this route may have to be discontinued if the patient begins

to suffer from severe phlebitis. Patients with meningitis may require intrathecal administration to attain adequate concentration of the drug in the spinal fluid.

The *length of treatment* is also very important in avoiding relapses or the development of resistance or adverse reactions. Once an anti-infective drug is selected and administered, it should be continued until such signs of infection as fever and abnormally high white blood counts are absent for at least several days to a week or more. Thus, most bacterial pneumonias require 7 to 10 days of treatment, and staphylococcal pneumonia must often be treated continuously for a month or more to avoid recurrences.

Patients with a sore throat that stems from a streptococcus infection sometimes become symptom-free following a single injection of penicillin or just a day or two of oral drug treatment. Nevertheless, the patient should be urged to continue penicillin treatment for a full 10 days to avoid relapses. Such recurrences of streptococcal pharyngitis can sometimes result in rheumatic fever or in glomerulonephritis that leads to cardiac or kidney damage.

Cases of miliary tuberculosis or of tuberculous meningitis may require therapy for as long as 2 years, often with a combination of drugs. Although this favors the emergence of resistant organisms, this risk is warranted in such cases. In other conditions, however, excessively prolonged antibiotic treatment is undesirable because of the danger of drug-induced tissue toxicity, allergic reactions, and secondary superinfections caused by the emergence of resistant strains (see below).

Adverse reactions to anti-infective agents

All the available antimicrobial agents can cause adverse effects of one type or another. These fall into the following three general classes:

1. *Direct toxic effects* on such organs as the gastrointestinal tract, kidneys, and liver, or the auditory, optic, and other peripheral nerves
2. *Allergic reactions* and other types of hypersensitivity affecting the skin and other organs and structures, including the bone marrow and circulating blood; anaphylactic reactions can occur
3. *Superinfections* as a result of drug-induced overgrowths by resistant bacterial strains or fungal organisms

Direct tissue toxicity

This is the result of the drugs' pharmacologic effects on the tissues. Usually overdosage is involved, because ex-

---

* This is a rating established by the 1962 Kefauver–Harris amendment to the Food, Drug and Cosmetic Act. Proof of safety and efficacy of all drugs released before 1962 is required by law; the investigations underlying this are called the Drug Efficacy Study Implementation, DESI. As drugs are investigated, they are given a DESI rating.

cessive amounts of a drug may cause local irritation of the gastrointestinal mucosa or at the sites of intramuscular, intravenous, or intrathecal injection. Sometimes, however, such dose-related reactions may occur even when ordinary doses are administered, particularly when the drugs accumulate in such tissues as the auditory and other nerves because of failure of the body's mechanisms for detoxifying or excreting the drugs.

Kidney damage

This is a particularly dangerous form of direct toxicity. Some antimicrobials that are eliminated in the urine in unchanged form exert no adverse effects on renal tissue. The penicillins and erythromycin, for example, are safe in this respect even in newborn babies, elderly patients, and those with impaired kidney function. However, other antibiotics, including the polymyxins, amphotericin B, cephaloridine, and the aminoglycosides, may exert nephrotoxic effects in some circumstances. When such drugs are employed—particularly by parenteral administration—it is especially important to monitor the patient's kidney function for signs of drug-induced renal impairment. If elimination of the drug is delayed and its blood level tends to rise, continued treatment may require dosage reduction and lengthening of the intervals between injections.

Neurotoxicity

Damage to nerve tissue or interference with its function occurs when some systemically administered drugs accumulate to high levels or when drugs are applied locally in excessively high concentrations. The aminoglycoside antibiotics, for example, are capable of causing impairment of eighth cranial nerve function. Sometimes, as is the case with streptomycin, vestibular branch function is affected most, and the patient complains mainly of dizziness and vertigo; with kanamycin and neomycin, the main neurotoxic effects are on the auditory nerve, and hearing impairment results. The aminoglycosides and polymyxins may also affect peripheral motor nerve function, particularly in anesthetized patients who have also received a neuromuscular blocking agent. This can lead to muscle weakness and arrest of respiration. Penicillin G can cause convulsive seizures when very high concentrations come in contact with the tissues of the central nervous system. Optic neuritis has sometimes been reported in patients receiving chloramphenicol for long periods.

Hepatic and gastrointestinal toxicity

Direct liver damage from antimicrobial drugs is relatively rare. Tetracyclines have sometimes caused hepatitis when high doses were administered parenterally to pregnant women with impaired kidney function. Antibiotics such as chloramphenicol and lincomycin that are metabolized in the liver or that tend to concentrate there must be administered with caution to patients with impaired liver function. The same applies to erythromycin estolate and to other antibiotics known to have adverse hepatic effects in some patients who have an idiosyncrasy to them. Many antimicrobials cause nausea, vomiting, and diarrhea, but the most serious damage to the intestinal mucosa has been reported after oral administration of lincomycin and clindamycin, which cause a drug-induced colitis.

Hypersensitivity-type reactions

Allergic reactions of the immediate and delayed types have been reported to occur with almost every type of antimicrobial drugs in atopic and other persons who have become hypersensitive to a particular agent. These are particularly common with penicillin-type antibiotics. Patients who take these valuable antibiotics for self-treatment of trivial infections may become sensitized to them. Then, if they later develop a severe infection, these patients may not be able to receive the required penicillin treatment. Thus, it is important to warn patients against casual self-medication with anti-infective drugs left over from an earlier illness or prescribed for a friend or another member of the family.

Other reactions of a *non*allergic nature sometimes occur in patients receiving antimicrobial chemicals to which they are abnormally sensitive. In some cases, such as the aplastic anemia that occasionally occurs with chloramphenicol, the reason for the idiosyncratic reaction is still obscure. In others, such as the hemolytic anemia sometimes seen during treatment with sulfonamides, some patients are now known to have an inherited defect in their ability to cope with the presence of the foreign chemicals—for example, a deficiency of the enzyme glucose-6-phosphate dehydrogenase (G-6-PD).

Superinfections

One difficulty from the widespread indiscriminate use of antibiotics is that the drugs may induce dangerous changes in the patient's own bacterial flora. That is, by eliminating susceptible organisms in the intestinal, respiratory, or genitourinary tract, the drug permits pathogens in these areas, which were previously kept under control by the natural antibiotic activity of their competitors, to grow rapidly and without restraint. As a result of the overgrowth of resistant staphylococci, yeasts, and fungi, or strains of *Proteus* and *Pseudomonas,* the patient may suffer a *superinfection* more serious by far than the infection that the drug was intended to treat.

Overgrowth of organisms that invade the tissues can occur during treatment with any anti-infective drug, but such superinfections are most common with broad-spectrum antibiotics such as the tetracyclines. These complications also occur most commonly during long-term treatment of debilitated patients, including those who are also receiving corticosteroids, and cytotoxic and immunosuppressive drugs. In patients known to be prone to develop superinfection, it is desirable to take frequent cultures of material from the genitourinary, gastrointestinal, and upper respiratory tracts. If these reveal an overgrowth of a pathogen such as a resistant staphylococcus or *Pseudomonas,* the antimicrobial drug that has been routinely administered is promptly withdrawn. The superinfection is then treated with a drug to which it is susceptible.

Prevention of infection

Antimicrobial drugs are often used to prevent infection in people who have been exposed to pathogens or who are thought to need special protection against disease. In some situations, chemoprophylaxis has proved quite effective and is recommended as a rational procedure. In other cases, the administration of anti-infective drugs is not only considered of no value, but it is believed likely to increase the chances of an infection developing. Often their use tends to cause superinfections by drug-resistant species and strains. In still other situations, the question of whether or not to use drugs for prophylaxis is still unsettled and controversial. The status of drug use for infection prophylaxis will be indicated in several types of clinical situations.

Successful chemoprophylaxis is most likely when the aim is to prevent implantation and invasion by a single specific pathogen that is known to be highly sensitive to the antimicrobial drug that is employed for this purpose. One example is the use of penicillin G in therapeutic doses for preventing gonorrhea in people who have been exposed to this disease by sexual contact. Penicillin G is also highly effective against group A streptococci, and thus may be useful for long-term prophylaxis against recurrences of rheumatic fever in children who have had an acute attack of this disorder. The same antibiotic is also recommended for preventing bacterial endocarditis in patients with a history of rheumatic or congenital heart disease or prior cardiac surgery who are exposed to *Streptococcus viridans* during dental extractions or other procedures that cause oral bleeding, and at the time of tonsillectomy or other oropharyngeal operations.

Contraindications to prophylactic antimicrobials include their use in patients with acute virus infections. Claims have been made for the value of commercial combination products containing antibiotics and sulfonamides that were supposed to prevent secondary bacterial complications in patients with the common cold. There is, however, no evidence that the routine use of antimicrobial drugs is of any value for this purpose in patients with colds, influenza, or other viral diseases, including measles, mumps, chickenpox, or infectious mononucleosis. Chemoprophylaxis with systemically administered drugs is also considered undesirable for preventing infection in burn patients because of its tendency to cause superinfections. Use of antimicrobials for preventing recurrent urinary tract infections in patients with kidney stones or other organic obstructions is also considered unwise, because it is likely to lead to development of drug-resistant strains of uropathogens.

Controversial areas include the questions of when to employ antimicrobial drugs in patients who have suffered severe trauma, in those undergoing intestinal and other surgical procedures in which bacterial contamination is likely, and in sufferers from chronic obstructive respiratory disorders. Some of these patients may possibly profit from the judicious use of anti-infective drugs for brief periods. In other cases, drugs will not prevent infections, and some patients may even be made more susceptible than if treatment had not been employed at all.

The administration of drugs for preventing infections should never take the place of strict adherence to physical procedures for preventing the spread of infection. For a time after the introduction of systemic anti-infective drugs, there was a trend toward relaxation of the standards set in the preantibiotic area. Fortunately, once it became clear that antibiotics were no substitute for strict aseptic technique, there was a return to traditional mechanical methods for avoiding bacterial contamination. Thus, for example, although oral chemoprophylactic agents may have a place in the preoperative preparation of patients for gastrointestinal tract surgery, such measures as physical cleansing of the bowel, proper surgical technique, and topical antisepsis are also essential.

Additional clinical considerations

The improper administration of anti-infective drugs can result in therapeutic failure and lead to such other undesirable consequences as emergence of resistant microbial strains and development of drug hypersensitivity or toxicity in the patient. Antimicrobial therapy is a difficult task in clinical practice. Patients with colds or the "flu" feel sick and want to be treated with medication. Many people self-medicate with borrowed or leftover antibiotics in the mistaken belief that they can both help themselves feel better and avoid a trip to a health-care professional. Patient teaching is a crucial aspect of antimicrobial therapy. The patient needs to know why the drug is being used, as well as why *no* drug would be effective in some cases. The patient also needs to know the dangers of not

Table 6–1. Clinical considerations related to the use of antimicrobial drugs

Consideration	Intervention
Do not use antibacterials for inappropriate infections (*e.g.,* viral).	Do not overuse antimicrobials for minor or inappropriate infections (*e.g.,* colds).
Do not use antimicrobials to treat infections when causative organism is resistant.	When a culture shows an organism to be resistant to an antibiotic, the drug should be stopped immediately and an antimicrobial to which the organism is sensitive should be started.
Do not undertreat with antimicrobials.	The full course of antimicrobial therapy is needed to eradicate bacteria in all stages of development. Patients *must* be taught to complete the full course of treatment.
Culture infected area before beginning treatment with antimicrobials.	To avoid interference with cultures, patients must be taught not to self-medicate with leftover medications. A culture should be done at the initial patient contact to verify the diagnosis.
Use appropriate adjunctive measures to eradicate the source of infection.	Draining of abscesses, removal of stones or other foreign objects, acidification or alkalinization of urine, and avoidance of exposure to the organism may be needed.

finishing the course of therapy, as well as the risks of self-medication. Nurses and physicians also need to be reminded about the potential problems involved with such misuse of anti-infective drugs.

Bacterial cultures should always be taken prior to the administration of the antimicrobial medication, and sensitivity testing to various drugs should also be ordered. This ensures that the organism has been properly identified and that the most effective drug is being used. In some cases of serious infection, such as bacteremia, treatment is begun immediately after the culture is taken. After the results are known, changes in drug therapy may be necessary.

Administration of anti-infective drugs alone may sometimes prove inadequate. Surgery is sometimes required to drain abscesses, eradicate deep infections, or remove foreign bodies. Some anti-infectives used to treat urinary infections require the use of measures to acidify or alkalinize the urine to maximize the effects of the drugs. Table 6-1 summarizes the clinical considerations of antimicrobial drug therapy.

Drugs for treating specific infections

Table 6-2 summarizes the current status of the drugs employed in the management of infections caused by various kinds of pathogenic microorganisms. This table indicates the antimicrobial drug for each organism that is considered the drug of choice according to the consensus of current authoritative opinion. It should be remembered that there are situations in which another drug will have to be used—for example, when a patient is allergic to the first-line drug or otherwise unable to tolerate it, or when the patient fails to respond to the drug of choice. The recommendations made here may not always apply to all infections caused by the specific pathogen that has been identified as the etiologic agent in a particular case. Most important in this regard is the fact that the specific strain of a pathogenic species isolated from an infected patient may prove to be relatively resistant to the drug listed here as the preferred agent. This is so because pathogens of the same species may vary in their sensitivity to antimicrobial drugs, depending on the part of the country or of the world in which the infection occurs, and often also on whether the infection develops in the community or in a hospital environment.

Thus, in practice, an agent can be considered the drug of first choice only when laboratory susceptibility tests have proved that the strain of the invading pathogen is actually sensitive to it, and the patient to be treated is shown not to be hypersensitive to the first-line drug or otherwise unable to tolerate it. From time to time, *The Medical Letter* publishes an updated table similar to Table 6-2; it also lists common alternative drugs that have proven to be successful in treating these pathogens.

Table 6–2. Antimicrobial drug treatment by specific pathogen

Pathogenic microorganisms	Type of infection	Drug of choice
Gram-positive cocci		
Staphylococcus aureus 1. Nonpenicillinase-producing strains	1. Surgical wounds; burns; pneumonia; otitis; endocarditis; osteomyelitis; bacteremia	1. penicillin G or penicillin V
2. Penicillinase-producing strains	2. Same as 1	2. Cloxacillin or dicloxacillin; methicillin; nafcillin; oxacillin
Streptococcus pyogenes (groups A, C, G)	Upper respiratory infections; otitis; scarlet fever; pneumonia	Penicillin G or V
Streptococcus viridans group	Endocarditis; bacteremia	Penicillin G with or without streptomycin
Streptococcus: Enterococcus group	Endocarditis; peritonitis; bacteremia	Penicillin G or ampicillin with or without gentamicin or streptomycin
Streptococcus bovis	Urinary tract infections; endocarditis, bacteremia	Penicillin G
Streptococcus (Diplococcus) pneumoniae	Pneumonia; meningitis; otitis; endocarditis	Penicillin G or V
Gram-negative cocci		
Neisseria gonorrhoeae (gonococcus)	Gonorrheal urethritis; salpingitis; vaginitis; endocarditis; arthritis	Tetracycline or amoxicillin; penicillin G with or without probenecid
Neisseria meningitidis (meningococcus)	Meningitis; bacteremia Carrier state	Penicillin G Rifampin
Gram-positive bacilli		
Clostridium perfringens	Gas gangrene	Penicillin G
Clostridium tetani	Tetanus	Penicillin G
Corynebacterium diphtheriae	Pharyngitis; laryngitis; tracheitis; pneumonia	Erythromycin
Gram-negative bacilli		
Bacteroides	Genital infections; abscesses; endocarditis	Penicillin G, clindamycin or chloramphenicol
Bordetella pertussis	Whooping cough	Erythromycin; co-trimoxazole
Enterobacter aerogenes	Urinary tract infections; systemic infections	Gentamicin, tobramycin, or netilmicin
Escherichia coli	Urinary tract infections; systemic infections	Gentamicin, tobramycin, or netilmicin
Hemophilus influenzae	Meningitis; epiglottitis; other serious infections Other infections	Chloramphenicol plus ampicillin Ampicillin or amoxicillin
Klebsiella pneumoniae	Pneumonia; urinary tract infections; osteomyelitis	Gentamicin, tobramycin, or netilmicin

Table 6–2. Antimicrobial drug treatment by specific pathogen (continued)

Pathogenic microorganisms	Type of infection	Drug of choice
Proteus mirabilis	Urinary tract infections; systemic infections	Ampicillin
Proteus (other species)	Urinary tract infections	Gentamicin, tobramycin, or netilmicin
Pseudomonas aeruginosa	Urinary tract infections	Carbenicillin or ticarcillin
	Systemic, respiratory or skin infections	Tobramycin or gentamicin with carbenicillin or another broad-spectrum penicillin
Salmonella typhi	Typhoid fever	Chloramphenicol
Salmonella (other species)	Gastroenteritis; bacteremia	Ampicillin or amoxicillin; chloramphenicol; co-trimoxazole
Serratia	Systemic infections	Gentamicin or amikacin
Shigella	Gastroenteritis	Co-trimoxazole; chloramphenicol
Acid-fast bacilli		
Mycobacterium leprae	Leprosy (Hansen's disease)	Dapsone with rifampin with or without clofazimine
Mycobacterium tuberculosis	Pulmonary and other types of tuberculosis infections	Isoniazid with rifampin
Spirochetes		
Leptospira	Weil's disease	Penicillin G; a tetracycline
Treponema pallidum	Syphilis	Penicillin G; a tetracycline
Treponema pertenue	Yaws	Penicillin G; a tetracycline
Rickettsia	Typhus; Rocky Mountain spotted fever; Brill's disease, etc.	A tetracycline; chloramphenicol
Mycoplasma		
Mycoplasma pneumoniae	Pneumonia	Erythromycin or tetracycline
Ureaplasma urealyticum	Nonspecific urethritis	Erythromycin; tetracycline
Fungi		
Aspergillus	Mycotic lesions of skin, bone; systemic mycotic infections	Amphotericin B
Candida species	Candidiasis of skin, mucous membranes	Amphotericin B with or without flucytosine; ketoconazole; nystatin
Dermatophytes (tinea)	Tinea infections of skin, hair, nails	Clotrimazole, miconazole, or tolnaftate (all topical)
Histoplasma capsulatum	Histoplasmosis	Amphotericin B
Viruses		
Herpes simplex	Keratitis	Trifluridine; vidarabine; idoxuridine
	Encephalitis	Vidarabine; acyclovir
Influenza A_2	Influenza	Amantadine

References

Bauer AW et al: Antibiotic susceptibility by a standardized single disc method. Am J Clin Pathol 45:493, 1966

Benveniste R, Davies J: Mechanisms of antibiotic resistance in bacteria. Ann Rev Biochem 42:471, 1973

Caldwell JR, Cluff LE: Adverse reactions to antimicrobial agents. JAMA 230:77, 1974

The choice of antimicrobial drugs. Med Lett Drugs Ther 26:19–26, 1984

Hash JH: Antibiotic mechanisms. Ann Rev Pharmacol 12:35, 1972

Medical Letter on Drugs and Therapy: Handbook of Antimicrobial Therapy, rev ed. New Rochelle, NY, 1984

Sande MA, Mandell GL: Antimicrobial agents: General considerations. In Gilman AG, Goodman LS, Gilman A (eds): Goodman & Gilman's The Pharmacological Basis of Therapeutics, 6th ed, pp 1080–1105. New York, Macmillan, 1980

Simmons HE, Stolley PD: This is medical progress? Trends and consequences of antibiotic use in the United States. JAMA 227:1023, 1974

Watanabe T: Infectious drug resistance in bacteria. N Engl J Med 275:888, 1966

Weinstein L: Some principles of antibiotic therapy. Ration Drug Ther 11:1, 1977

Whitehead JEM: Bacterial resistance. Changing patterns among common pathogens. Br Med J 2:224, 1973

Chapter 7

The chemotherapy of viral infections

7

Viral infection treatment is the last frontier of chemotherapy. Virus particles that invade mammalian cells are difficult to attack chemically without also damaging the tissues of the host. Up to now, few antiviral drugs have been introduced, and these have only limited effectiveness. Thus, in contrast to the next chapter, which describes the chemotherapy of bacterial infections, this chapter will be very short.

A great deal of research is going on, however, based on recent advances in molecular biology. A sudden breakthrough could occur at any time in the area of antiviral chemotherapy.

General considerations of antiviral chemotherapy

Current status
Viruses in the external environment can be readily destroyed by direct contact with many inorganic and organic chemicals, such as chlorine, iodine, phenol, and formaldehyde. However, disinfectants of this type are too toxic for internal use. Thus, from the time of their first successes in devising drugs for antimicrobial chemotherapy, scientists have been searching for safe and effective antiviral drugs.

Unfortunately, unlike the case in the chemotherapy of bacterial and parasitic infections, few therapeutically useful drugs have been found for fighting virus infections. Those currently available have proved effective against only a few specific viruses and in only a limited number of clinical infections. However, research based on a better understanding of viral and host cell interactions may lead to development of drugs that will be safer and more widely useful than those now available.

To understand the reasons for the relative lack of success up to now and to prepare for the hoped for future progress require knowledge of the nature of viruses and the way in which they function in infecting the cells of mammalian hosts, including those of humans.

Viruses and virus infection
Viruses are tiny organisms too small to be seen by even the most powerful optical microscopes. Each virus particle, or virion, is a submicroscopic package made up of a nucleic acid core surrounded by a coat of protein. The nucleic acid in various viruses is either DNA or RNA. These viral genomes can reproduce similar molecules only within the living cells that they invade, and only after they have first been stripped of their protein coat by the action of host cell enzymes.

Viral infection of the host's cells occurs in three main stages. First, the virus particles make their way to the tissues for which they have a particular affinity and, after attaching themselves to the cell surfaces, the viruses penetrate into the interior of the cell where they release their nucleic acid into the cytoplasm. Next, the naked viral nucleic acid makes a duplicate molecule and supervises the synthesis of proteins used for producing viral enzymes and structural components. Such replication and synthetic processes are the result of interactions with the host cell's functional mechanisms. Finally, the new nucleic acid genome and the viral protein are put together to form a new virus particle, and this newly assembled virion is released from the cell. By the end of this infective process, the parasitized host cells are often dead, while viral progeny swarm from the dying cells to attack millions of cells in the invaded tissues.

Mechanisms of antiviral drug actions
To be effective against viruses, drugs must interfere with one or another of the various steps in this three-stage cycle. A drug might, for example, prevent the virus from entering the cell. It could do so by blocking attachment

of the virus particle to receptors on the surface of the host cell, or the chemical could keep the attached virus from penetrating the cell membrane. Even after the virus has entered the cell its activity could be inhibited by a drug that prevents viral nucleic acid from being uncoated, or drugs might interfere with the processes by which the freed nucleic acid duplicates itself and makes the viral protein molecules. Antiviral drugs could also interfere with the final assembly of the new virion or prevent its release from the cell.

In practice, these theoretic infection-inhibiting actions are not readily accomplished without injury to host cells. The viral core that is set free in the cellular cytoplasm takes command of the host cell's mechanism for producing energy and making protein and converts these processes to its own use. Thus, any drug capable of preventing viral nucleic acid from replicating itself and synthesizing viral protein is also likely to interfere with the metabolic machinery of the cell that the virus has taken over. As a result, drugs that stop the intracellular activity of the virus also tend to be toxic to host cells. In any case, by the time a patient shows signs and symptoms of a virus infection, the disease process is already far advanced, and the patient's body has already reacted with defense mechanisms of its own that are protective but also sometimes disabling.

Antiviral drugs

The prophylactic use of *vaccines* to produce active immunity against viral infections, such as measles, mumps, and polio, will be described in Chapter 55, along with the use of *immune sera* to produce passive immunity. This chapter describes the following drugs, which are currently available in the United States for treating viral infections: amantadine (a drug also used to treat Parkinson's disease), and the pyrimidine and purine derivatives (acyclovir, idoxuridine, trifluridine, and vidarabine; Tables 7-1 and 7-2).

Amantadine

The mechanism of antiviral action of this drug is not completely understood, but the drug appears to interfere with the penetration of the virus into the host cell and with the subsequent uncoating of the virus. Amantadine (Symmetrel) is used in the prevention and treatment of influenza caused by influenza A viruses, but is ineffective against influenza B viruses. Initially it was recommended only for prophylactic use—that is, for preventing infection in patients who might be exposed to this type of influenza and who were at high risk of severe illness from an influenza infection. This is still an important use, but the drug has also been found useful in decreasing the severity of influenza A infections. Clinical improvement may occur because the new virus particles that are being released from already parasitized cells are prevented from entering additional cells.

Amantadine may be used to treat people of any age, but it is often reserved for elderly patients and others who have a high risk of severe illness from an influenza infection, such as patients with any chronic diseases. In such cases vaccination before exposure is the prophylactic measure of choice but, if this is contraindicated or not

Table 7–1. Routes of administration and uses of antiviral drugs

Drug	Use	Routes of administration		
		Systemic	Topical	Ophthalmic
Amantadine (Symmetrel)	Prophylaxis and treatment of influenza A infections	Oral only		
Acyclovir (Acycloguanosine; Zovirax)	Treatment of skin and mucous membrane HSV infections	IV only	Ointment	
Idoxuridine (Dendrid; Herplex; Stoxil)	Treatment of HSV keratitis			Ophthalmic ointment and solution
Trifluridine (trifluorothymidine; Viroptic)	Treatment of HSV keratitis			Ophthalmic solution
Vidarabine (adenine arabinoside; Ara-A; Vira-A)	Treatment of HSV encephalitis and keratitis	IV only		Ophthalmic ointment

Table 7–2. Usual adult dosage of antiviral drugs

Drug	Dosage
Amantadine HCl	Prophylaxis: 200 mg once a day or 100 mg twice a day, orally, for at least 10 days after exposure, and up to 90 days if vaccination is impossible and exposure is repeated Treatment: Same daily dosage as above, continued for 24–48 hr after disappearance of symptoms
Vidarabine	15 mg/kg/day for 10 days by *slow* IV infusion at constant rate over 12–24 hr (maximum concentration is 450 mg/liter)
Acyclovir (parenteral)	15 mg/kg/day, administered by IV infusion as follows: 5 mg/kg at constant rate over 1 hr, every 8 hr, for 5–7 days
Acyclovir ointment	Cover the lesion with ointment every 3 hr, 6 times a day, for 7 days

feasible, amantadine should be given. Patients already exposed to the virus can be given amantadine in conjunction with the inactivated influenza A virus vaccine; in such cases amantadine can prevent infection until antibodies develop. There is no evidence of adverse or antagonistic interactions between amantadine and the vaccine.

Adverse effects from the use of this drug are reported more often with the higher doses indicated for treating Parkinson's disease. However, adverse reactions can occur at lower doses in sensitive patients. These include atropinelike (anticholinergic) symptoms—for example, dry mouth, blurred vision, constipation, and urinary retention. The dosage of atropinelike drugs, or of drugs with atropinelike side-effects taken concomitantly, may need to be reduced. Serious CNS reactions include depression and psychosis. Rarely, convulsions occur, but seizure activity is more likely to occur in patients with a past history of seizures. Congestive heart failure (CHF) has occurred, as have hypotensive episodes. Ninety percent of a dose of amantadine is excreted unchanged by the kidneys, placing patients with impaired renal function at risk for developing toxic levels of the drug. Because protection against influenza is particularly important for elderly patients, and renal function is often decreased in these patients, the possible need for dosage reduction to avoid toxicity should be kept in mind.

Pyrimidine and purine derivatives

Four antiviral drugs that are chemically similar to one or another of the bases thymine, cytosine, guanine, and adenine, the building blocks of the nucleic acids DNA and RNA, are available in the United States. Their mechanisms of action are not completely understood, but each is believed to be incorporated into viral nucleic acids in place of the natural base that it resembles in its chemical structure. The false nucleic acid thus formed cannot be used for making new virus particles.

All four of these drugs are effective in treating infections caused by herpes simplex viruses (HSV) types 1 and 2. These infections are currently the only indications for their use, although acyclovir has been shown to be active against other viruses. Acyclovir (Zovirax) and vidarabine (Vira-A) are the only drugs of this group that are given systemically. Idoxuridine (Dendrid; Herplex; Stoxil) and trifluridine (Viroptic) are used in the form of ophthalmic ointments or solutions to treat herpes simplex keratitis. (The use of these drugs to treat this serious corneal infection is discussed more fully in Chapt. 42.) Acyclovir is also available for topical use.

Acyclovir (Zovirax) is given intravenously to treat initial and recurrent mucosal and cutaneous herpex simplex 1 and 2 infections in patients whose immune systems are depressed by drugs or disease. It is also given intravenously to treat *serious* initial herpes genitalis infections. The ointment form is used topically to treat nonlife-threatening mucocutaneous HSV infections in immune-deficient patients. The ointment has been shown to shorten the course of *initial* genital herpes infections in patients whose immune systems are normal, but no evidence of clinical benefit was found when the drugs were used to treat *recurrent* genital or labial infections. (Labial or lip infections caused by HSV are often called "cold sores.") The ointment is absorbed only minimally through the skin and does not cause systemic toxicity. However, intravenous administration can cause inflammation or phlebitis at the injection site, and about 1% of patients show encephalopathic changes (lethargy, tremors, confusion, seizures, or coma). The drug can precipitate in renal tubules, so the patient must be kept well-hydrated and be regularly evaluated for renal function status. The drug is excreted unchanged by the kidneys, so patients with renal disease may need a decreased dosage to avoid toxicity.

Vidarabine (Vira-A), a purine derivative related to the antineoplastic drug *cytarabine* (Cytosar; see Chap. 12), is used in the treatment of the serious brain infection herpes simplex encephalitis, which most commonly afflicts cancer patients whose immune defenses have been lowered by their disease and by the cytotoxic chemotherapeutic agents employed in treating it. When this infection is promptly diagnosed and treated with intravenously administered vidarabine, the death rate is said to be reduced from about 70% to below 30%.

Adverse effects of vidarabine include anorexia, nausea, vomiting, and diarrhea. CNS effects include tremor, dizziness, and psychosis; fatal metabolic encephalopathy has been reported. Hematologic disturbances can occur.

Vidarabine is poorly soluble in body fluids and aqueous media and should be given only intravenously, because absorption from an IM or SC injection site would be very poor. Its low solubility also necessitates the administration intravenously of considerable fluid volume to achieve therapeutic drug dosage. This can lead to fluid overload in susceptible patients, such as those with cerebral edema or impaired renal function. These patients need careful monitoring when they receive this drug. The drug is metabolized by the liver and excreted mostly by the kidneys. Patients with liver or kidney disease must therefore be monitored closely for toxic effects. Results of animal studies have shown the drug to be carcinogenic and mutagenic. Thus, the toxic potential of this drug is such that if brain biopsy results turn out to be negative for HSV, administration of the drug should be discontinued immediately.

Other antiviral drugs: methisazone

Methisazone (Marboran), a drug of different chemical structure and still uncertain manner of action, acts against various DNA-containing viruses including adenoviruses that cause respiratory infections and poxviruses such as variola (smallpox) and vaccinia (cowpox). It was first used successfully during a smallpox epidemic in India, where it helped to protect people who had been vaccinated too recently to build up enough antibodies to the virus to which they had been exposed. The drug was not effective when given too late in the incubation period of the virus, nor was it useful for treating smallpox cases that had reached the clinical stage. Methisazone was also considered helpful for treating certain complications that sometimes occur following smallpox vaccination with vaccinia virus. Such complications as eczema vaccinatum, vaccinia gangrenosa, and postvaccinial encephalitis used to cause more illness and deaths in this country than the disease that inoculation with vaccinia virus was intended to prevent.

Methisazone has never been available in the United States, although it is available in some other countries. Because smallpox has essentially been eradicated, and because vaccination against smallpox is no longer given, methisazone can no longer be considered a very important drug clinically.

Future prospects

The goal of research in this field has been to find drugs capable of destroying virus invaders of human cells without damaging the cells themselves. To achieve such selective toxicity to viruses, scientists have first had to discover differences between the replicative cycles and metabolic processes of the viruses and the cells that they invade. These differences can then be exploited by the use of chemical compounds that attack the stages in viral replication that are not shared by the infected cells.

Some scientists are confident that recent advances and others that are expected to follow during the next decade will revolutionize the treatment of viral diseases in much the same way that the discoveries of the 1930s and 1940s did in the case of bacterial infections. Several drugs that are claimed to be superior in their selective toxicity to those available up to now are currently undergoing clinical trials. These are said to be safer and more effective against a wider variety of viruses than the few drugs in clinical use at the present time.

Ribavirin

One drug undergoing trials, *ribavirin* (Virazol), is a nucleotide analogue that is believed to inhibit the synthesis of viral nucleoproteins without disrupting the biosynthesis of similar substances in the virus-invaded cells. This drug is said to be effective in various viral respiratory and liver infections such as influenza and infectious hepatitis. It is also active against several viruses of the herpes family, including those that cause herpes keratitis, mucocutaneous herpes, herpes genitalis, and herpes zoster, or shingles.

This drug has proved most effective when applied topically in some of these infections. It is also claimed that because of its selective toxicity for viral processes, it causes relatively few side-effects when taken internally. Rapidly dividing embryonic cells may, however, be adversely affected in ways that can lead to birth defects, so this drug cannot be used to treat viral infections during early pregnancy. Ribavirin is available in several Latin American countries.

Other approaches

Other drugs that are being employed experimentally do not strike directly at invading viruses. Instead, these substances are intended to stimulate greater activity by two types of natural defenses against virus infections: the immune system responsible for the production of *antiviral antibodies;* and the production of a class of carbohydrate-containing proteins that are collectively called *interferon.*

Two investigational drugs, *levamisole* and *inosiplex* (Isoprinosine), are claimed to increase the activity of the body's immune system. Levamisole has been used as an anthelmintic. The recent discovery that it stimulates the immune system has led to its investigational use in patients with various viral infections and cancers, as well as arthritis and autoimmune disease. In humans, it stimulates primarily cell-mediated immunity. It is apparently effective as an immunostimulant only in immunocompromised patients. At present, however, the most effective way to produce antiviral antibodies is by the administration of specific viral vaccines. These immunobiologic products are discussed in Chapter 55. In addition, several vaccines are being investigated for the prevention of herpes simplex virus infections.

Interferon offers a more general defense against virus infections than does the production of virus-specific antibodies. These defensive molecules, which are produced and released by virus-invaded cells even before the body's immune defenses produce antibodies, are effective against various viruses. They act to keep the virus particles from replicating in the body tissue to which the particles spread from the first invaded cells.

Until recently attempts to obtain, purify, and administer interferon for treating viral infection did not prove practical. Interferon obtained from laboratory animal species of the lower orders is not effective against virus infections in human patients. Thus, the interferon had to be harvested from human cells or from those of related primate species. The large amounts of interferon needed for treating a virus infection were prohibitively expensive. Work is now underway to manufacture the large amounts of interferon needed using the new techniques of recombinant DNA. An interferon-based ointment for mucocutaneous HSV infections is also under development.

Interferon inducer drugs are also under investigation. These include *statolon,* a substance extracted from fungi, and *poly I:C,* one of a series of synthetic polymers that resemble RNA. So far these and other tested substances have not proved sufficiently safe or effective for routine use in treating viral infections. However, some clinical test results suggest that drugs of this type may some day prove useful for treating respiratory viral infections, including the common cold, which is caused by so many different types of viruses that prevention by vaccination has not proved practical.

Additional clinical considerations

Because there is still very little drug therapy available for treating viruses, some specific clinical points should be considered when dealing with viruses. Avoidance of the viral infection is the best approach. This includes avoiding crowded public areas during the peak respiratory virus season, eradicating insect and animal vectors (*e.g.,* mosquitoes, ticks, rodents), and avoiding direct contact with others who are known to have viral diseases. High-risk patients should be vaccinated against viral infection before exposure to the virus. This is often done in the autumn before the peak winter flu season.

The use of amantadine for prophylaxis against and treatment of type A influenza viruses is relatively new drug therapy, but it has already decreased the discomfort involved with viral infections and the often serious complications that can occur. This is especially important for elderly patients and patients with chronic diseases who can suffer severe complications from such viral diseases.

Nurses need to be on the alert for exacerbations of specific medical conditions as a result of the effects of amantadine. These conditions include congestive heart failure, liver disease, renal failure, seizure problems, and psychoses. Patients taking CNS stimulant drugs concomitantly also need careful observation.

Care must be taken when applying acyclovir ointment to viral lesions. The patient who self-administers the drug should be instructed to use a finger cot or rubber glove to prevent autoinoculation of other body parts or the spread of the virus to other people. Vidarabine should never be given IM or SC because of its low solubility and poor absorption, which will result in ineffective drug levels and local tissue toxicity. Before acyclovir solution is administered IV, the vial must be checked for crystal formation. The solution is not stable, and should be used within 24 hours.

As with many drugs, the safety of the use of these drugs during pregnancy and lactation has not been established.

There are several specific *drug–drug interactions* that should be considered when using antiviral drugs. *Probenecid* (Benemid) can slow the excretion of *acyclovir.* If a patient is on probenecid, the systemic (IV) dosage of acyclovir may need to be decreased to avoid toxicity. *Allopurinol* (Zyloprim), a drug used to decrease serum uric acid levels in patients with gout and in patients on certain antineoplastic drugs, can interfere with the metabolism of *vidarabine.* Dosage of systemic (IV) vidarabine may need to be reduced in patients who are also on allopurinol. *Anticholinergic drugs* in combination with *amantadine* may cause atropinelike side-effects. In such cases, the dose of the anticholinergics should be reduced to a point at which the side-effects are controlled.

The patient teaching guide summarizes education points for the patient receiving amantadine. The guide to the nursing process with antiviral drugs summarizes the clinical aspects of amantadine therapy.

Patient teaching guide: amantadine

The drug that has been prescribed for you is called an antiviral drug. It works by destroying specific virus activity in the body. It has been ordered to treat the Influenza A virus. It is important to remember that it works specifically against this virus, and cannot be used to self-medicate other viral disorders.

Instructions:

1. The name of your drug is amantadine.

2. The dose of the drug that has been ordered for you is _____ .

3. The drug should be taken _____ time(s) a day. The best time to take your drug is _____ _____ _____ .

4. Some effects that might occur, which you should be aware of, include the following:

Drowsiness, blurred vision	Take precautions if driving or working with dangerous machinery.
Dizziness, lightheadedness	This is frequently caused by a fall in blood pressure; take care to avoid sudden changes in position, which can cause this fall in blood pressure.
Irritability, mood changes	It may help to know that this is a result of the drug's effects; if it becomes too much of a problem, the drug may need to be changed.

5. Avoid the use of over-the-counter medications, especially antihistamines or cold remedies, because these medications contain ingredients that can aggravate the side-effects of amantadine. If you need one of these medications, contact your nurse or physician.

6. Tell any physician, nurse, or dentist who takes care of you that you are taking this drug.

7. Keep this and all medications out of the reach of children.

Notify your nurse or physician if any of the following occur:

Dizziness or light-headedness

Swelling of fingers or ankles

Shortness of breath

Difficulty urinating

Tremors, slurred speech, difficulty walking

Guide to the nursing process: amantadine

Assessment	Nursing diagnoses	Interventions	Evaluation
Past history Medical conditions that are *contraindications:* • Seizures • Liver disease • Eczematoid rash • Psychoses • Congestive heart failure • Renal disease • Pregnancy • Lactation **Medication history** • Allergies, reactions • Current use of anticholinergics **Physical assessment** • Neurologic: orientation, vision, speech, reflexes • Cardiovascular: BP, orthostatic BP, P, auscultation, perfusion, edema • Respiratory: R, adventitious sounds • Renal: output, BUN, serum creatinine	Potential sensory–perceptual alteration Potential disturbance in self-concept related to potential neurologic changes Potential alteration in cardiac output Knowledge deficit regarding drug therapy	Preparation and safe administration of drug Patient teaching regarding drug therapy Comfort and safety measures: • Safe environment • Assist patient to avoid sudden moves Support and encouragement to deal with mood changes, neurologic alterations	Monitor response to drug: • Prevention of viral disease • Improvement in viral signs and symptoms Monitor for adverse effects of drug: • CHF • Neurologic effects • Psychoses • Orthostatic BP changes Monitor for exacerbation of previous medical conditions Monitor for drug–drug interactions: • Amantadine with anticholinergics or levodopa Monitor effectiveness of patient teaching Monitor effectiveness of comfort and safety measures Monitor effectiveness of support measures

Case study

Presentation IG, a 72-year-old white woman, with a long history of rheumatic valve disease and congestive heart failure (CHF), arrives for a regularly scheduled office visit with complaints of aching joints, lethargy, and fever of 1-day duration. It is nearly "flu" season, and IG did not receive the flu vaccine this year because she was traveling until just recently. Considering the patient and the situation, what clinical actions are indicated?

Discussion A careful and thorough patient history should be the first step in the nursing process. The nurse will need details about drug therapy the patient is on, dietary changes, the exact progression and details of the presenting signs and symptoms, other signs or symptoms that have been developing at the same time, measures that have been taken to alleviate the discomforts described, and the activities of the patient in the last few weeks, with special interest in any exposures to other people who might have had the flu. Although the initial presentation of IG at "flu" season should make the nurse very suspicious of a viral infection, the patient's past history necessitates consideration of other possibilities (*e.g.*, worsening valve disease, rheumatic involvement).

The physical assessment will substantiate the history and provide an evaluation of the patient's cardiac status as well as general well-being. If the assessment reveals that the patient most likely has been exposed to influenza A virus and is exhibiting signs of early viral infection, amantadine would probably be the drug of choice. A prophylactic 6- to 8-week course of amantadine therapy might well be ordered along with the viral vaccine. The patient should be encouraged to rest, to push fluids as much as is permitted with her CHF, and to take aspirin or another anti-inflammatory agent to relieve the fever and aches of the viral infection (unless she is already taking one of these drugs). The nurse, being aware of the possible-side effects of amantadine, will need to reinforce teaching about CHF and the medical regimen the patient has been maintained on; special emphasis should be placed on the signs and symptoms to watch for and to report. With this information reinforced, the patient should be alert to any CHF that is precipitated by the amantadine therapy. Because of the patient's age, special consideration should also be given to the various safety measures that have been covered. The patient should also be asked to be alert for any change in urinary function, and to report it to the nurse. A follow-up visit in 1 to 2 weeks would be important for evaluating the effectiveness of the drug, as well as for monitoring any adverse effects that might be occurring.

Overall education of patients such as IG should include the advisability of vaccination against the flu each year, avoidance of crowded public areas during peak flu season, and special efforts to maintain nutritional and exercise status during these high-risk periods.

References

Cesario TC: The clinical implications of human interferon. Med Clin North Am 67:1147, 1983

Corey L et al: Trial of topical acyclovir in genital herpes simplex infections. N Engl J Med 306:1313, 1982

Dolon R et al: A controlled trial of amantadine and rimantadine in the prophylaxis of influenza A infection. N Engl J Med 307:580, 1982

Douglas RG: Antiviral drugs, 1983. Med Clin North Am 67:1163, 1983

Hirsch MS, Swartz MN: Antiviral agents. N Engl J Med 302:903, 949, 1983

Intravenous acyclovir (Zovirax). Med Lett Drugs Ther 25:34, 1983

Mindel A et al: Intravenous acyclovir treatment for primary genital herpes. Lancet 1:697, 1982

Sande MA, Mandell GL: Miscellaneous antibacterial agents; antifungal and antiviral agents. In Gilman AG, Goodman LS, Gilman A (eds): Goodman & Gilman's The Pharmacological Basis of Therapeutics, 6th ed, pp 1222–1248, New York, Macmillan, 1980

Saral R et al: Acyclovir prophylaxis of herpes simplex virus infections. N Engl J Med 305:63, 1981

Serota FT et al: Acyclovir treatment of herpes zoster infections. JAMA 247:2132, 1982

Smith RA et al: Antiviral mechanism of action. Ann Rev Pharmacol Toxicol 20:259, 1980

Topical acyclovir for herpes simplex. Med Lett Drugs Ther 24:55, 1982

Whitley RJ et al: Vidarabine: Preliminary review of its pharmacological properties and therapeutic use. Drugs 20:267, 1980

Chapter 8

The chemotherapy of bacterial infections

8

Historical introduction

This chapter describes the drugs that are used mainly to treat systemic bacterial infections. Attempts to treat such diseases with chemicals date back to the 16th century when the Swiss physician and alchemist, Paracelsus, advocated the use of mercury to treat syphilis. Later, after salts of mercury and other heavy metals proved effective when applied externally as antiseptics and disinfectants, they were administered to animals with experimental systemic infections. However, when taken internally, these and other inorganic chemicals proved as likely to kill the animals as they were to wipe out the microbial invaders of their tissues.

During the first two decades of this century, Paul Ehrlich and his successors synthesized new compounds in which such toxic metals as mercury, arsenic, and bismuth were tied up into complex organic molecules. Tried first for treating experimental infections and later used clinically, these organometallic compounds proved safer for animals and humans (see Chap. 6). Introduced during the 1920s, synthetic chemicals of this type were clinically useful in malaria and other parasitic diseases and for syphilis treatment. Some, containing arsenic and antimony, are still used today for treating diseases caused by protozoa and other parasites (see Chaps. 10 and 11).

Despite these advances, most serious *bacterial* infections continued to take a heavy toll until the mid-1930s. The *sulfonamides* were then found to be effective against pathogens responsible for many common bacterial infections. Clinical successes with these drugs stimulated scientists to study the antibacterial properties of other synthetic chemicals. The *sulfones,* for example, were studied for their effects on the tubercle bacillus, the cause of tuberculosis, one of mankind's greatest killers. These drugs, although effective in experimental tuberculosis, were not clinically successful. The sulfones did, however,

prove effective against a related bacillus, the organism responsible for leprosy, a disease as incurable until then as it was when described by writers of the Bible.

In the late 1930s and early 1940s, *penicillin,* an antibacterial substance synthesized by molds, was discovered and became available for clinical use. Further work with natural and synthetic anti-infective drugs led to the discoveries of streptomycin (in the late 1940s) and of isoniazid (in the early 1950s), the first agents effective against tuberculosis. Soon scores of antibacterial agents, pouring out of the laboratories, brought many other bacterial infections under control.

This chapter will describe the sulfonamides, the penicillins, and the other synthetic and naturally occurring antibacterial drugs. Each type of drug will be described in regard to its antibacterial spectrum, its use in the treatment of infectious disease, its potential toxicity, and the precautions that must be employed to ensure its safe clinical use. The chapter will conclude with a discussion of drugs used mainly or only to treat some specific diseases (tuberculosis and leprosy), and drugs used only to treat urinary tract infections.

The sulfonamides

History and current status
Early in this century German chemists synthesized a series of dyes containing a chemical grouping called a sulfonamide. However, the biologic properties of these dyes were not studied until almost 25 years later. One of these chemicals, a compound called *Prontosil,* was then shown to be able to save mice from an otherwise invariably fatal experimental infection with streptococci. This substance also proved effective for treating human patients seriously ill with streptococcal and staphylococcal infections.

Table 8–1. Sulfonamide preparations

Generic or official name	Trade name	Usual dosage; adults*	
		Initially	Maintenance
Oral drugs			
Sulfacytine	Renoquid	500 mg	250 mg qid
Sulfadiazine USP		2 g–4 g	1 g q 4 hr
Sulfamethizole USP	Thiosulfil	0.5 g–1 g	0.5–1 g tid or qid
Sulfamethoxazole USP	Gantanol	2 g	1 g bid or tid
Sulfapyridine		0.5 g	0.5 g qid
Sulfasalazine USP	Azulfidine	250 mg–500 mg qid for several days	1 g qid
Sulfisoxazole USP	Gantrisin; SK-Soxazole	2 g–4 g	1 g four to six times daily
Sulfisoxazole acetyl USP	Gantrisin	For children: 75 mg/kg; for adults: 2 g–4 g	For children: 150 mg/kg/day divided into four to six doses; for adults: 4–8 g/day divided into four to six doses
Sulfisoxazole acetyl emulsion	Lipo Gantrisin	For children: 60–75 mg/kg; for adults: 4 g–5 g	For children: 60–75 mg/kg bid; for adults: 4 g–5 g bid
Parenteral drug			
Sulfisoxazole diolamine USP	Gantrisin Diolamine	50 mg/kg	100 mg/kg/day divided into two to four doses
Topical preparations—burns			
Mafenide acetate cream USP	Sulfamylon cream		Apply in a $^1/_{16}$-inch thick layer once or twice a day
Silver sulfadiazine	Silvadene cream		Apply in a $^1/_{16}$-inch thick layer once or twice a day
Ophthalmic preparations			
Sulfacetamide sodium USP	Bleph; Isopto Cetamide; Sodium Sulamyd		1–2 drops of solution every 1–2 hr; or apply ointment tid and hs
Sulfisoxazole diolamine USP	Gantrisin		1–2 drops of solution every 1–2 hr; or apply ointment tid and hs
Sulfonamide combinations			
Trisulfapyrimidines USP	Neotrizine; Triple Sulfa; Sultrin; Terfonyl	2 g–4 g orally	2–4 g/day divided into three to six doses
Sulfathiazole, sulfacetamide, sulfabenzamide	Sultrin		1 tablet or applicatorful intravaginally bid

Table 8–1. Sulfonamide preparations (continued)

Generic or official name	Trade name	Usual dosage; adults*	
		Initially	Maintenance
Sulfonamide combinations with other drugs			
Sulfamethoxazole and trimethoprim USP (co-trimoxazole)	Bactrim; Septra		Orally: 160 mg trimethoprim and 800 mg sulfamethoxazole q 12 hr; also available for IV administration
Sulfadoxine and pyrimethamine	Fansidar		500 mg sulfadoxine and 25 mg pyrimethamine once a week for malaria prophylaxis
Sulfisoxazole (500 mg), phenazopyridine HCl (50 mg) tablets	Azo Gantrisin	4–6 tablets orally	2 tablets orally qid for up to 3 days
Sulfamethoxazole (500 mg) & phenazopyridine HCl (100 mg) tablets	Azo Gantanol	4 tablets orally	2 tablets orally bid for up to 3 days

* Pediatric dosage is given only for those preparations intended particularly to be given to children.

Further research by French scientists showed that the antibacterial activity of this prototype sulfonamide depended on its being broken down in the body to a simpler molecular fragment called *sulfanilamide.* Clinical trials in the late 1930s with a synthetically prepared form of this substance proved its effectiveness against several types of severe bacterial infections including pneumonia, meningitis, and septicemia.

The dramatic reduction in illness and deaths from bacterial infections brought about by sulfanilamide therapy stimulated chemists to synthesize and test over 5000 sulfonamide derivatives. Some of these proved safer and more effective than the original drugs of this class. Many sulfonamides were marketed and proved very useful, even lifesaving, in the early 1940s, before penicillin and other antibiotics were available. Many of these preparations were taken off the market as safer and more efficacious drugs became available. However, some sulfonamides still are important in therapy, and a number of these preparations are still used (Table 8-1).

Sulfisoxazole (Gantrisin) is frequently used for treating urinary tract infections. *Sulfacetamide sodium* is used topically to treat eye infections. *Mafenide*, a sulfonamide despite its name, and *silver sulfadiazine* are used topically to prevent and treat bacterial infections of burned skin. Some sulfonamides are used alone or as adjuncts in treating nonbacterial infections, such as malaria, toxoplasmosis, and trachoma. Two have uses unrelated, or probably unrelated, to their antimicrobial activity: *sulfapyridine* is used in dermatology to treat dermatitis herpetiformis, and *sulfasalazine* is used to treat ulcerative colitis.

Antimicrobial spectrum. As indicated in detail in Table 8-2, the sulfonamides are effective against a wide range of pathogenic microorganisms. Among the susceptible organisms are various gram-positive and gram-negative bacterial species, certain chlamydial ("large virus") organisms, and some protozoa. These drugs are not effective against true fungi or true viruses.

Problems in the use of sulfonamides. A major reason for the reduced usefulness of the sulfonamides is the emergence of resistant strains of bacterial species that were once sensitive to these drugs. Resistance to sulfonamides has resulted mainly from their prophylactic administration in subtherapeutic doses. Thus, the sulfonamides at first produced dramatic cures in cases of gonorrhea. Later, after the sulfonamides had been widely used for the prophylaxis of venereal disease during World War II, most gonorrheal infections encountered in many areas were no longer susceptible to sulfonamide treatment. Apparently the low-dose regimens employed for preventing this disease had fostered the survival of sul-

Table 8–2. Antimicrobial spectrum and therapeutic uses of sulfonamides

Microbial susceptibility*	Therapeutic effectiveness
Gram-positive cocci	
Streptococcus pyogenes, group A β-hemolytic type	No longer used for treating an active infection by this organism, but may be used for prophylaxis against pharyngitis and recurrences of rheumatic fever in patients allergic to penicillin
Staphylococcus aureus	Occasionally effective in urinary tract infections caused by susceptible strains of these organisms
Gram-negative cocci	
Meningococcus	IV administration of sulfadiazine sodium or of sulfisoxazole diolamine may be very effective in meningitis infections caused by susceptible strains. An oral sulfonamide may also be administered to the patient's contacts, particularly if a sensitive group A strain is the known cause of infection
Gram-positive bacilli	
Nocardia asteroides (formerly considered as a fungus)	Effective against lung and brain lesions of this bacterial infection
Gram-negative bacilli	
Escherichia coli	Acute urinary tract infections caused by most strains of this organism are still very susceptible to treatment with sulfonamides. The drugs are also effective in chronic bacteriuria for suppressing this pathogen
Proteus mirabilis	May be effective in urinary tract infections caused by this and by other *Proteus* species
Klebsiella and *Enterobacter* (*Aerobacter*) species	Only occasionally effective in urinary tract infections caused by strains shown to be susceptible by laboratory studies
Hemophilus influenzae	Sometimes effective for acute and chronic otitis media and respiratory infections caused by this organism when combined with penicillin or erythromycin
H. ducreyi	Chancroid, a venereal disease, is quite responsive to treatment with sulfonamides
Chlamydia	
Chlamydia trachomatis (trachoma agent)	Effective in this eye disease when taken orally and applied topically
Inclusion conjunctivitis agent (blenorrhea)	Topical application of ophthalmic preparations of sulfacetamide sodium or of sulfisoxazole diolamine may be effective in this eye disease

Table 8–2. Antimicrobial spectrum and therapeutic uses of sulfonamides (continued)

Microbial susceptibility*	Therapeutic effectiveness
Protozoa	
Toxoplasma gondii	An effective adjunct to pyrimethamine in treating toxoplasmosis
Plasmodium falciparum	An effective adjunct to quinine and other antimalarial drugs in chloroquine-resistant cases of malaria
Uses unrelated, or probably unrelated, to antimicrobial spectrum	
	Dermatitis herpetiformis (sulfapyridine)
	Ulcerative colitis (sulfasalazine)

* Many strains of previously susceptible species are now resistant to sulfonamides. Thus, these drugs are now best used for treating certain serious infections only after the causative organism has been proved sensitive to sulfonamides in laboratory tests.

fonamide-resistant strains of the gonococcus. Similarly, the routine use of sulfonamides to protect army recruits from respiratory infections soon produced sulfonamide-resistant strains of staphylococci, and the continued careless use of sulfa drugs seems even to have resulted in some resistance among the once very sensitive meningococci.

To reduce the likelihood of bacteria developing resistance, and for other reasons, a sulfonamide is sometimes combined with another type of antimicrobial drug. For example, when sulfamethoxazole is combined with trimethoprim, bacterial resistance develops more slowly than with either drug alone, giving the drug combination and the host's defenses more time to eradicate the infection.

A second problem in the use of the early sulfonamides was their insolubility and the insolubility of their acetylated metabolites in the urine. To prevent their crystallizing out and causing renal tubular damage, it was often necessary to alkalinize the urine by administering sodium bicarbonate or other alkalinizing drugs simultaneously, and to reduce the urinary concentration of the sulfonamides and metabolites by having the patient force fluids. Newer sulfonamides and their metabolites are more acid-soluble, but patients taking all sulfonamides, especially *sulfadiazine* and *sulfapyridine,* should still be encouraged to keep up a high fluid intake. Concomitant administration of sodium bicarbonate is also recommended when sulfadiazine and sulfapyridine are given.

Another solution to the problem of low urinary solubility was the use of combinations of sulfonamides (trisulfapyrimidines, or "triple sulfas"; Table 8-1). These combinations were devised in an attempt to achieve high enough drug concentrations to be therapeutic, yet prevent

any one drug from reaching a high enough concentration in the urine for it to crystallize and cause renal damage.

Despite these problems and despite the decline in the clinical indications for sulfonamide therapy, these drugs have properties that account for their continued importance in some clinical situations. The sulfonamides are widely distributed throughout all tissues, including the brain, ocular fluids, and joints, where some antibiotics penetrate poorly.

The more recently introduced sulfonamides have little direct tissue toxicity and are less costly than most other antibacterial agents. A sulfonamide can often still be substituted for the antibiotic drug of choice when the latter cannot be tolerated—for example, if the patient is allergic to penicillin—and when tests have proved that the pathogen is sensitive to sulfonamides. In addition, even in some infections that are best treated by various antibiotics, the addition of a sulfonamide to the patient's regimen often produces a better result than administration of the antibiotic alone. Finally, in a few important infections, sulfonamides are still considered to be the most effective treatment.

Mechanism of antimicrobial action

Understanding the mechanism of antimicrobial action of these drugs is now not only of theoretic importance, but also serves to explain the most significant recent advance in sulfonamide therapy: the increased activity of one of these sulfa drugs (sulfamethoxazole) against various clinical infections when it is administered in combination with the *non*sulfonamide drug trimethoprim (see above).

The most important way in which sulfonamides exert their bacteriostatic effect on susceptible organisms is by preventing bacterial cells from taking up and using para-aminobenzoic acid (PABA). This, in turn, prevents the bacteria from biosynthesizing folic acid, a substance that serves as a coenzyme in further chemical reactions that lead finally to the synthesis of DNA and other nucleic acids. Thus, when these drugs inhibit PABA uptake and folic acid synthesis, the bacterial cells cannot grow and reproduce themselves by dividing into daughter cells.

Competitive antagonism (see Chap. 4) of PABA by sulfonamides occurs because the sulfa drug molecule closely resembles the structure of the essential metabolite in its molecular configuration. However, although the drug molecule fits into the place ordinarily occupied by PABA, the biochemical compound formed in this way cannot perform the metabolic functions of the folic acid that the bacterial cell would have formed had the sulfonamide not been present. As a result of its lack of folate, the bacterium fails to make the macromolecular precursors of the nucleic acids needed for growth and reproduction. Knowing the mechanism of sulfonamide action helps several clinically practical points about these drugs to be understood, such as why resistance develops and how sulfonamide antagonism and synergism occur.

Resistance to sulfonamides is seen in bacteria that can take up folic acid directly from the medium in which they are growing. Thus, because these bacteria do not need to biosynthesize folic acid from PABA, they are unaffected by the presence of sulfa drug molecules in their environment. The wide use of sulfonamides that wipe out the susceptible majority of a bacterial species but leave unharmed the few insensitive cells has favored the emergence of resistant strains of previously susceptible species. A similar difference in the biochemical requirements of human and bacterial cells accounts for the relative safety of the sulfonamides. That is, human cells take up and use dietary folic acid directly, and so do not need PABA in order to make folate. Thus, these drugs exert *selective toxicity* only on bacterial cells.

Antagonism of sulfonamides may occur when large amounts of PABA or of the end products of the reactions in which it plays a part become available to bacteria. In purulent infections, for example, the pus and other products of tissue necrosis may supply enough of these substances to counteract the action of sulfonamides on the growth of bacteria in the tissues. Similarly, many local anesthetics contain PABA in their molecules. Thus, these drugs, if used in large amounts, may antagonize the antibacterial effectiveness of sulfonamides given concurrently. Enough PABA may be released from the anesthetic drug molecules to maintain bacterial growth, even in the presence of sulfa molecules in the tissues.

Synergism of sulfonamides with other drugs that tend to cause a microbial folate deficiency can produce more effective antibacterial activity. For example, a product called *co-trimoxazole* (Bactrim; Septra), which contains *sulfamethoxazole* in combination with *trimethoprim*, has been shown to have supra-additive activity against microorganisms sensitive to these drugs and even against some strains that are resistant to sulfonamides alone. The basis for such synergism is the fact that trimethoprim—although it is not a sulfonamide—also helps to create a lack of metabolically active folate. It does so in a manner different from the sulfonamides. That is, it acts at a point in the pathway beyond PABA uptake, the step that is inhibited by sulfonamides. By interfering with a second step in the series of reactions, trimethoprim increases the activity of the sulfa drug and expands its antibacterial spectrum.

Pharmacokinetics

The sulfonamides are readily absorbed after oral administration but food can interfere with their absorption, so they should be taken on an empty stomach. They are widely distributed in body fluids and are bound to plasma proteins in varying degrees. They are metabolized in the liver to compounds that lack antimicrobial activity, and the parent compounds and metabolites are excreted mostly by glomerular filtration in the kidney. One of the most important ways for the liver to metabolize and inactivate sulfonamides is by the process of acetylation. Thus, patients who are genetically slow acetylators may be at greater risk for developing sulfonamide toxicity.

The sulfonamides differ greatly in the extent to which they are bound to plasma proteins. This in turn affects their rate of excretion and their duration of action. Some sulfonamides (*e.g.*, sulfacytine, sulfadiazine, sulfisoxazole) are very rapidly excreted and must be given four to six times a day; others (sulfamethoxazole) are excreted more slowly. Formerly, some ultralong-acting sulfonamides were available for administration only once a day or once every other day. These drugs had the advantage of convenience, but the treatment of toxic reactions was difficult because of their long half-lives.

Current clinical indications

Although the place of sulfonamides in treating infections is now relatively limited, these drugs are still very useful in certain clinical conditions and for properly selected patients. The role of sulfonamide therapy in the infections for which these drugs are still employed will be discussed in terms of their usefulness in comparison with other available anti-infective agents.

Urinary tract infections (UTI). The sulfonamides are still important in the management of acute and chronic infections by susceptible gram-negative uropathogens. Most acute uncomplicated bladder infections are caused by sulfa-sensitive strains of *Escherichia coli*. Thus, the sulfonamides are rapidly effective for such cases of acute cystitis and in those caused by sensitive strains of other enteric bacillary species, such as *Proteus mirabilis* and species of *Klebsiella* and *Enterobacter*.

However, if the patient's symptoms are not relieved within a couple of days, and especially if the infection seems to have spread to the kidneys, sulfonamides are discontinued. The patient is then started on another drug selected by laboratory determination of the identity of the specific pathogenic strain and by the degree of its sensitivity to various anti-infective agents. Often this is an antibiotic such as ampicillin or a cephalosporin, because such bactericidal agents are preferred for eradicating pathogens that have invaded the kidneys to cause acute pyelonephritis.

The sulfonamides preferred for treating *acute* UTI are such short-acting agents as sulfisoxazole (Gantrisin) and sulfamethizole (Thiosulfil). The main advantage of these drugs and of others such as sulfacytine (Renoquid) is their high solubility in urine. Thus, although urinary concentrations high enough to be bactericidal are often reached during their rapid excretion, these drugs—unlike the earlier sulfonamides—do not tend to precipitate out of the urine to form crystals capable of damaging delicate kidney tissue. Nevertheless, patients should be advised to drink plenty of fluids while taking any sulfonamide.

A disadvantage of these short-acting sulfas is the frequency with which they must be administered. Patients often fail to follow their regimen when they are required to take a drug four or more times daily. Some, in fact, may discontinue treatment entirely when their discomforting symptoms subside after a few days. It is important to explain to the patient that all the tablets ordered for each day and for the full ten-day treatment period should be taken to bring the infection under quick control and to prevent a late flare-up. Patient compliance is even more important in the management of *chronic* UTI.

Recently, the intermediate-acting sulfonamide sulfamethoxazole (Gantanol) combined with trimethoprim (Proloprim; Trimpex—a drug used alone to treat urinary tract infections) in the product co-trimoxazole (Bactrim; Septra) has been advocated for preventing recurrent, as well as acute, UTI in highly susceptible patients. Two tablets—or only a single double-strength tablet—administered twice daily is effective for suppressing chronic infections caused by strains of *E. coli* and of *Proteus, Klebsiella,* or *Enterobacter* that sensitivity tests have shown to be susceptible to this drug combination. An advantage of adding the nonsulfonamide trimethoprim is that the emergence of sulfonamide-resistant strains is delayed, because this synergistic combination keeps bacteria resistant to the sulfonamide alone from surviving to form dominant families.

Respiratory tract infections. Although the sulfonamides were the first antibacterial drugs found to be effective for treating pneumococcal pneumonia, these drugs are rarely used today for this or for other respiratory infections. These are now treated with anti-infective agents known to be more effective against such common gram-positive invaders as the pneumococcus, streptococcus, and staphylococcus. Recently, however, the sulfamethoxazole–trimethoprim combination co-trimoxazole has been recommended for treating acute flare-ups of infection in patients with chronic bronchitis.

Streptococcal pharyngitis is also better treated with other antibacterial agents, such as penicillin or erythromycin, rather than with sulfonamides. However, the sulfas are as effective as penicillin for *preventing* streptococcal infections of the throat. Thus, penicillin-sensitive patients with a history of rheumatic fever sometimes take daily doses of sulfisoxazole or sulfadiazine to prevent recurrences. Chemoprophylaxis of this kind has proved to be effective, free of side-effects in patients not hypersensitive to sulfonamides, and not likely to lead to overgrowths of resistant pathogens in the upper respiratory tract.

Acute otitis media. Sulfadiazine, sulfisoxazole, sulfamethoxazole, and triple sulfas are used, as are penicillin or erythromycin, to treat otitis media caused by sensitive strains of *Hemophilus influenzae.* Co-trimoxazole is also used to treat acute otitis media in children.

Intestinal tract disorders. Bacillary dysentery (shigellosis) is now rarely treated with a single sulfonamide, because most strains of *Shigella* have become resistant to sulfonamides. However, the combination of sulfamethoxazole and trimethoprim (co-trimoxazole) is now the drug of choice in treating infections caused by sensitive strains of *Shigella.* Co-trimoxazole may also be an effective alternative to ampicillin or chloramphenicol in some cases of salmonellosis, in which it may help to relieve not only the enterocolitis but also the systemic effects of a disease such as typhoid fever. The combination is also effective for eliminating *Salmonella* in some typhoid carriers.

Ulcerative colitis, regional enteritis, and Crohn's disease are sometimes benefited by oral administration of sulfasalazine (Azulfidine), a drug that is converted in the colon to sulfapyridine and aminosalicylic acid. It is uncertain whether the improvement seen in some mild to moderate cases and the prevention of relapses during prolonged administration of this drug are the result of antibacterial activity or of an anti-inflammatory–immunosuppressive effect caused by the salicylic acid component of the drug. Although this drug and its active breakdown products reach high local concentrations in the wall of the large intestine, a significant amount is also absorbed systemically from the small intestine before the drug reaches the lower tract.

Meningitis. Most strains of meningococci are now resistant to sulfonamides but are still sensitive to penicillin G and, when meningitis is caused by *H. influenzae,* as it often is in children, the infection is best treated with ampicillin or chloramphenicol. However, in some situations, meningitis that is caused by a microorganism shown to be sensitive to sulfonamides may be managed with intravenously administered soluble derivatives, such as sulfisoxazole diolamine or sulfadiazine sodium. These drugs readily penetrate the inflamed meninges to reach therapeutically effective levels in the cerebrospinal fluid. Later, if able to swallow, the patient is switched to oral sulfonamides supplemented sometimes by streptomycin or by other antibiotics to which the pathogenic strain has also proved sensitive. Oral sulfadiazine is also sometimes ordered for those who have been in close contact with a patient infected by a sulfonamide-sensitive meningococcus.

Venereal diseases. Many strains of the gonococcus are now resistant to sulfonamides. However, chancroid, a venereal disease caused by *H. ducreyi*, often responds to therapy with sulfadiazine or sulfisoxazole, as does lymphogranuloma venereum, a chlamydial infection.

Other chlamydial infections. The eye diseases trachoma and inclusion conjunctivitis, for example, also respond to sulfonamide therapy, particularly when these drugs are administered both orally and topically (*i.e.,* in the eye). Generally a tetracycline (for trachoma) or erythromycin (for inclusion conjunctivitis) is the drug of choice. Sulfacetamide sodium and sulfisoxazole diolamine are also effective when applied topically in these and other eye infections, including conjunctivitis, corneal ulcers, and blepharitis, an eyelid inflammation.

Systemic mycoses. Sulfonamides have been employed in the past to treat such systemic fungal infections as *blastomycosis* and *histoplasmosis*. Although long-continued administration keeps some cases in remission, these diseases can be cured only by amphotericin B. However, sulfonamides are often lifesaving in *nocardiosis*, a dangerous disease caused by a filamentous bacterium that has some features of a fungus. Successful treatment requires administration of very high doses of sulfisoxazole, sulfadiazine, or trisulfapyrimidines. Co-trimoxazole is also used. Sometimes improvement occurs more rapidly when these drugs are supplemented by ampicillin or other anti-infective agents.

Protozoan infections. Sulfonamides administered in combination with various other drugs are sometimes useful in several protozoan diseases. *Malaria* caused by *Plasmodium falciparum* strains resistant to chloroquine is controlled by treatment with quinine and pyrimethamine combined with sulfadiazine, sulfisoxazole, sulfamethoxazole, or trisulfapyrimidines. More recently, a preparation (Fansidar) combining pyrimethamine and sulfadoxine, another sulfonamide, has been recommended for prophylaxis against chloroquine-resistant *P. falciparum; toxoplasmosis* caused by the protozoan organism *Toxoplasma gondii* has also been effectively controlled by a combination of sulfadiazine with pyrimethamine. These drugs and co-trimoxazole, the sulfamethoxazole–trimethoprim combination (Bactrim; Septra), are also useful for treating *pneumocystosis*, an acute respiratory infection caused by *Pneumocystis carinii*, an organism that is probably a protozoan. To avoid bone marrow toxicity as a result of a possible folate deficiency caused by the combined effects of these drugs, patients also receive daily doses of folinic acid.

Burns and skin disorders. Sulfonamides are rarely applied topically to the skin, because their use in this way commonly causes allergic sensitization. Application to purulent skin lesions is relatively ineffective, in any case, because PABA present in pus and tissue debris tends to antagonize the antibacterial action of most sulfonamides. However, certain sulfonamide creams are employed in the management of severe burns to prevent local sepsis and the subsequent septicemia that causes most fatalities. Their use in patients with extensive second- and third-degree burns has reduced the death rate from this common complication.

Mafenide acetate (Sulfamylon), the first sulfonamide used in this way, was found to retain its antibacterial activity even in the presence of pus, serum, and necrotic tissue. The water-soluble cream is applied by hand with a sterile glove after tissue debris has been removed surgically from the burn surface. It then penetrates into the wound tissues and releases the sulfonamide, which inhibits growth of both gram-positive organisms such as staph and strep and gram-negative bacilli such as *Pseudomonas aeruginosa*. The wound is not covered by a dressing but is kept exposed except for a $\frac{1}{16}$-inch layer of the cream until after the burn eschar separates. The application of this medication is extremely painful, and the patient will often require sedation or potent analgesics before its use.

Silver sulfadiazine (Silvadene cream) is said to have several advantages over mafenide. It does not cause the stinging pain that occurs when mafenide cream is applied to the burned area, and it has a lower incidence of allergic hypersensitivity. This drug is also said not to cause metabolic acidosis, a serious complication sometimes seen when mafenide is applied in patients with burns over 50% of the body surface and particularly when pulmonary dysfunction has also developed. For these reasons this agent has replaced the first sulfonamide for topical antimicrobial burn therapy in most burn centers.

Dermatitis herpetiformis, a skin disease of uncertain origin, is relieved by sulfapyridine for reasons that are as obscure as the cause of the disease itself. This drug, one of the first sulfonamides, has been replaced in infection treatment by safer drugs, but in this condition it seems superior to other sulfas. It often stops itching, burning, and blistering of the skin within a few days.

Vaginitis caused by the organism *Hemophilus vaginalis* responds to topical sulfonamide therapy. One topical product available as a cream and vaginal tablet contains a combination of three drugs of this class that are not usually administered for their systemic effects: sulfacetamide, sulfathiazole, and sulfabenzamide.

Adverse effects

Most patients receiving sulfonamides suffer no ill effects or only transient headache and gastrointestinal disturbances such as nausea, vomiting, and abdominal discomfort. However, serious side-effects of many types have been reported, and patients sensitized to these drugs or with idiosyncrasies of various types have suffered fatal reactions (also see Summary at the end of this section). Thus, although modern sulfonamides are safer than the first to be introduced, patients must be watched carefully for signs of drug-related toxicity. These may involve almost every organ and system, including the kidneys, liver, hematopoietic system, central nervous system, and skin.

Renal damage. Complications of this type occur mainly when crystals of a sulfonamide drug or of one of its metabolites precipitate out of the urine in the kidneys. *Crystalluria* here or elsewhere in the urinary tract can cause blockage in the kidney tubules, ureters, or bladder. This and local irritation may be manifested by hematuria and may lead to severe functional deficiency, resulting in oliguria, anuria, and fatal uremia. Thus, patients receiving sulfonamides should have frequent urinalyses, including microscopic examination of the urine for crystals and calculi.

Crystalluria is less likely to occur with the use of current sulfonamides that are highly soluble in acid urine. Sulfisoxazole, sulfamethizole, and trisulfapyrimidines, a mixture of three sulfonamides including sulfadiazine, cause a low incidence of crystalluria. As explained earlier, each drug in the trisulfapyrimidines is present in only about one-third of its full therapeutic dose, but the total of the three drugs exerts full antibacterial activity. A therapeutic dose of the mixture, however, is only about one-third as likely to cause crystalluria as an equally effective full dose of any single drug in the mixture.

Nevertheless, despite the relative safety of these drugs, it is still necessary to see that patients drink an amount of fluid that will produce enough urine to keep the excreted drugs in solution—at least 1200 ml of urine daily. Thus, patients should be encouraged to drink plenty of fluids, and the amount of urine eliminated should be measured and recorded. When the patient's urine volume is unusually low and highly acid, a teaspoonful of sodium bicarbonate or some other systemic alkalinizer may have to be taken with each dose of sulfa drug to raise its solubility in the urine.

Blood and bone marrow disorders. Blood dyscrasis of various types have been reported. Thus, although these are rare, patients must be watched for such clinical signs and symptoms as sore throat, purpura, paleness, or jaundice, because these may indicate possible agranulocytosis, thrombocytopenia, or aplastic anemia, and complete blood counts should be performed weekly during prolonged sulfonamide therapy. Some clinics also screen patients routinely to see whether their red blood cells possess normal amounts of the enzyme glucose-6-phosphate dehydrogenase (G-6-PD), because sulfonamides are one of the classes of drugs that can cause acute hemolytic anemia in people whose red cells are deficient in this protective enzyme (see Chap. 5).

Allergic reactions. Patients previously sensitized to sulfonamides may suffer immediate (anaphylactoid) or delayed reactions manifested by minor or extremely severe signs and symptoms. Drug fever, joint pains, and skin eruptions of various types may develop, including signs of the Stevens–Johnson syndrome (a form of erythema multiforme). If signs of this disorder such as skin and mucosal blisters with bleeding centers (bull's eye le-

sions) develop, the drug should be immediately discontinued, because death can occur as a result of damage to the respiratory tract and to other organs. Because these drugs can cause photosensitivity reactions, patients taking them should be cautioned against prolonged exposure to sunlight.

Rarely, a sulfonamide hypersensitivity reaction may affect various vital organs, including the heart, blood vessels, liver, lungs, and kidneys. Thus, for example, a patient may occasionally die of toxic nephrosis without having had crystalluria prior to development of anuria, azotemia, and uremia. Hepatitis of a hypersensitivity type was reported with the early sulfas. Lung lesions have been found occasionally during sulfonamide therapy, and the drugs have induced asthma attacks in hypersensitive patients.

Other reactions of various types have also been reported. Occasionally, patients show signs of central and peripheral nervous system malfunction, including ataxia, dizziness, and vertigo; drowsiness and fatigue or insomnia and confusion; mental depression and acute psychosis; and peripheral neuritis. Rarely, goiter production and hypothyroidism have been reported as a result of a goitrogenic effect.

Additional clinical considerations

The important clinical concerns involved with avoiding the side-effects of the sulfonamides have been described. A few other clinical considerations should also be mentioned. If sulfonamides are to be given IV, they must be given slowly to avoid serious side-effects. Sulfasalazine causes oligospermia and infertility in men. It seems that these problems resolve spontaneously after the drug is stopped, and the patient should be reassured and offered the opportunity to discuss his feelings about this effect. If a patient is to be on prolonged sulfonamide therapy, periodic testing is advisable to permit early detection of adverse effects. Testing should include liver function tests, kidney function tests (blood urea nitrogen—BUN; creatinine), complete blood count, and urinalysis. As with many other drugs, caution should be used if giving the drug to pregnant or nursing women or to infants.

Drug–drug interactions. The sulfonamides can be displaced by or can displace other protein-bound drugs from the protein carrier. These drugs include *tolbutamide* (which can be displaced and cause hypoglycemia), *warfarin* (which also can be displaced and cause excessive anticoagulation), *methotrexate, phenylbutazone, salicylates, probenecid,* and *phenytoin.* A patient on any of these drugs and a sulfonamide should be observed carefully to prevent toxicity from the sulfonamide or the other drug.

Sulfasalazine is known to interact with several drugs. Sulfasalazine decreases the bioavailability of *digoxin,* and patients may need an increase in digoxin dose to maintain adequate digitalization. *Folic acid* absorption is decreased by sulfasalazine, and the patient may need supplemental folic acid. *Antibiotics* will decrease the distribution of sulfasalazine, possibly because of the decrease in normal intestinal flora. *Ferrous sulfate* may decrease the blood levels of sulfasalazine; the clinical significance of this is unclear.

The patient teaching guide summarizes points that should be covered when teaching a patient on sulfonamides. The guide to the nursing process with sulfonamide drugs summarizes the clinical application of the nursing process to sulfonamide therapy.

Summary of sulfonamide toxicity

Urinary tract disorders
> Crystalluria: pain, obstruction, hematuria, oliguria, anuria, azotemia, uremia

Sensitization reactions
> Stevens–Johnson syndrome: blisters on skin, mucous membranes; respiratory tract complications
>
> Skin: eruptions, exfoliative dermatitis, petechiae, purpura, photosensitivity
>
> Drug fever: headache, chills, malaise

Blood and bone marrow disorders
> Acute hemolytic anemia, thrombocytopenia, agranulocytosis, aplastic anemia

Gastrointestinal side-effects
> Anorexia, nausea, vomiting, diarrhea, abdominal pain, jaundice, hepatomegaly, hepatitis

Neurologic and psychiatric complications
> Confusion, depression, drowsiness, ataxia, vertigo, peripheral neuritis

Patient teaching guide: The sulfonamides

The drug that has been prescribed for you is an anti-infective drug from the sulfonamide (sulfa) family. It has specific antibacterial properties and has been prescribed to treat _____ . It is important to remember that these drugs are specific in their action and should not be used to self-medicate for any other problem.

Instructions:

1. The name of your drug is _____ .

2. The dosage of the drug ordered for you is _____ .

3. The drug should be taken _____ time(s) a day. The best time to take your drug is _____ , _____ , _____ . The drug should not be taken with meals, because this will interfere with its absorption. The drug should be taken 1 hour before or 2 hours after meals. (*Sulfasalazine* may be taken with food if GI upset occurs.)

4. Some side-effects of this drug that you should be aware of include:

Kidney problems	Force fluids—drink as much as you can tolerate to help to flush the drug through your kidneys.
Sensitivity to sunlight	Protect your skin against sunburn by using sunscreens or protective clothing; wear sunglasses to protect the eyes.
Orange-yellow coloring of urine (and skin; sulfasalazine)	Do not be concerned; the color will disappear when the drug course is finished.

5. Tell any physician, nurse, or dentist who takes care of you that you are taking this drug.

6. Keep this and all medications out of the reach of children.

(continued)

7. Finish the full course of your prescription. You may begin to feel better in a few days, but you must take the whole prescription to clear up the infection.

Notify your nurse or physician if any of the following occur:

Wheezing, difficulty breathing
Unusual bruising or bleeding
Pain or burning while urinating
Blood in the urine
Sore throat, fever or chills, pallor

Guide to the nursing process: the sulfonamides

Assessment	Nursing diagnosis	Interventions	Evaluation
Past history (underlying problems that may be *contraindications*): • Porphyria • Renal failure • Hepatic failure • Urinary or GI obstruction (sulfasalazine) • Pregnancy • Lactation • *Allergies:* sulfonylureas, thiazides, salicylates (sulfasalazine) Medication history: other drugs being taken **Physical assessment** Neurologic: orientation, sensation Cardiovascular: BP, P, cardiac output Respiratory: rate, adventitious sounds GI: bowel sounds, liver palpation, output, liver enzymes Renal: BUN, output, urinalysis Skin: integrity, lesions	Potential alteration in urinary elimination patterns Potential alteration in breathing patterns Knowledge deficit regarding drug therapy Potential male reproductive dysfunction (sulfasalazine)	Preparation and safe administration of drug Patient teaching regarding drug course, side-effects, precautions Provide comfort measures as appropriate: • Discussion and support for potential infertility with sulfasalazine • Protection from sunlight • Force fluids	Monitor response to drug: resolution of infection Monitor for adverse effects to drug: • Urinalysis • Periodic tests of liver and kidney function • Observe for asthma, hypersensitivity reactions Monitor for the occurrence of drug–drug interactions—because so many drugs interact, the loss of effectiveness or development of toxicity of any other drug should be scrutinized for drug–drug interactions Monitor for drug–laboratory test interaction: false-positive urine glucose test (Benedict's test), interference with Urobilistix test Evaluate effectiveness of comfort and support measures Evaluate effectiveness of patient teaching

Table 8–3. Penicillin preparations

Generic or official name	Trade name	Penicillinase-resistant	Acid-stable	Route of administration	Dosage
Penicillin G preparations					
Penicillin G potassium tablets or injection USP	Pentids; Pfizerpen G; SK-Penicillin	No	No	IM, IV, oral	400,000 U orally, or IM q 6 hr; or IV: 10 million U to 20 million U daily
Penicillin G sodium for injection USP		No	No	IM, IV	400,000 U IM qid or IV 10 million U daily
Penicillin G benzathine tablets or suspension USP	Bicillin L-A; Permapen	No	No	IM, oral	400,000 U–600,000 U orally q 4–6 hr, or 1.2 million U IM at various intervals, up to 1 month in rheumatic fever prophylaxis
Penicillin G procaine suspension USP	Crysticillin; Duracillin; Wycillin	No	No	IM	300,000 U–600,000 U q 12–24 hr
Penicillin G benzathine and procaine	Bicillin C-R	No	No	IM	600,000 U–1,200,000 U every 2–3 days or 2.4 million U once
Acid-stable penicillins					
Penicillin V potassium USP (phenoxymethyl penicillin)	Betapen VK; Pen-Vee K; SK-Penicillin VK; Pfizer-pen VK; V-cillin K	No	Yes	Oral	250 mg–500 mg (400,000 U–800,000 U) qid
Penicillinase-resistant penicillins					
Cloxacillin sodium USP	Cloxapen; Tegopen	Yes	Yes	Oral	250 mg–500 mg q 6 hr
Dicloxacillin sodium USP	Dycill; Dynapen; Pathocil; Veracillin	Yes	Yes	Oral	125 mg orally q 6 hr; or 250 mg for more severe infections
Methicillin sodium USP	Celbenin; Staphcillin	Yes	No	IM, IV	1 g–1.5 g q 4–6 hr
Nafcillin sodium USP	Nafcil; Unipen	Yes	Yes	IM, IV, oral	250 mg–1000 mg q 4–6 hr
Oxacillin sodium USP	Bactocill; Prostaphlin	Yes	Yes	IM, IV, oral	500 mg q 4–6 hr for 5 or more days
Ampicillins					
Amoxicillin USP	Amoxil; Larotid; Polymox; Sumox; Trimox; Utimox; Wymox	No	Yes	Oral	250 mg–500 mg q 8 hr

Table 8–3. Penicillin preparations (continued)

Generic or official name	Trade name	Penicillinase-resistant	Acid-stable	Route of administration	Dosage
Ampicillin USP and ampicillin sodium, parenteral	Amcill; Omnipen; Pfizer-pen-A; Polycillin; Principen; SK-Ampicillin; Totacillin	No	Yes	IM, IV, oral	250 mg–500 mg q 6 hr
Bacampicillin HCl	Spectrobid	No	Yes	Oral	400 mg–800 mg q 12 hr
Cyclacillin	Cyclapen-W	No	Yes	Oral	250 mg–500 mg q 6 hr
Hetacillin	Versapen; Versapen K	No	Yes	Oral	225 mg–450 mg qid
Extended-spectrum penicillins					
Azlocillin sodium	Azlin	No		IV	100–300 mg/kg/day in 4–6 divided doses (maximum daily dose = 24 g)
Carbenicillin disodium	Geopen; Pyopen	No		IM, IV	50–500 mg/kg/day continually or in divided doses (maximum daily dose = 40 g)
Carbenicillin indanyl sodium	Geocillin	No	Yes	Oral	382–764 mg qid
Mezlocillin sodium	Mezlin	No		IM, IV	100–350 mg/kg/day in divided doses (maximum daily dose = 24 g)
Piperacillin sodium	Pipracil	No		IM, IV	100–300 mg/kg/day in divided doses (maximum daily dose = 24 g; maximum dose IM at one site = 2 g)
Ticarcillin disodium	Ticar	No		IM, IV	150–300 mg/kg/day in divided doses every 4–6 hr

The penicillins

Penicillin, the first antibiotic introduced for clinical use, is still one of the most useful of all antimicrobial agents. Because the first form of penicillin to become available had properties that limited its usefulness, a great effort was made to reduce these drawbacks. As a result of such research, scientists have succeeded in developing various new pharmaceutic and chemical forms that are superior in some respect to the original penicillin. Although all these products are called *penicillin*, they differ from one another in significant ways that make one form preferable to another in different clinical situations (Table 8-3).

History and sources of penicillin

The antibacterial activity of biosynthetic products obtained from certain strains of *Penicillium* molds was first noted by Sir Alexander Fleming in 1928. Although he tried to use filtrates from cultures of these fungi for treating infected wounds, these first penicillin broths proved too weak to affect the pathogens. Fleming's discovery remained a laboratory curiosity until 1939, when a group working at Oxford under the direction of Florey succeeded in making crude but potent extracts from broth cultures of *P. notatum.*

The potential importance of this material, which proved potent but nontoxic in infected experimental animals, was quickly appreciated. In 1940 efforts to prepare penicillin in clinically usable quantities were intensified because of the obvious value of such a systemically safe and effective anti-infective agent for treating the wounded of World War II. By 1943, as a result of government-supported research in the United States, penicillin was being employed for treating infections in American military personnel.

Chemistry. The development of a deep fermentation process for producing penicillin on a large scale made it possible to obtain huge amounts of the antibiotic at low cost during the postwar years. Study of its molecular structure then revealed that there were several natural penicillins. All contained the same basic β-lactam nucleus but differed in their attached side chains. The natural penicillin with a *benzyl* side chain proved most active and benzylpenicillin, or *penicillin G,* is today the only one still in common use.

Penicillin G is a very useful antibiotic but, because of various problems that detract from its effectiveness, several other types of penicillins have been developed. Some of these are modifications of penicillin G itself. For example, penicillin G *procaine*[+] and penicillin G *benzathine*[+] are insoluble salts available as suspensions for intramuscular injection. These pharmaceutic preparations are intended to prolong the duration of action of penicillin G, which in the form of its potassium and sodium salts is often too rapidly excreted by the kidneys.

Semisynthetic penicillin products. Many chemical modifications have also been made in attempts to develop new products free of the drawbacks of penicillin G. At first new chemical congeners were made by adding substances to the mold culture during fermentation. These precursors were then incorporated as side chains while the penicillin molecule was being biosynthesized. For example, *penicillin V*[+], which contains a phenoxymethyl side chain in place of the benzyl group of penicillin G, is an artificially modified penicillin made in this way.

Now, however, new semisynthetic penicillins are usually prepared by first employing an enzyme to split the natural side chain from the nucleus of a penicillin prepared by fermentation. Then this penicillin nucleus, 6-aminopenicillanic acid, is treated chemically to attach a new side chain to the natural core. The number of new penicillins that can be made in this way is theoretically unlimited. In practice, however, only a few have been found to possess clinical advantages that warranted their introduction as new products. The following are examples of semisynthetic penicillins that offer advantages over penicillin G:

1. Penicillin G is readily broken down and inactivated by stomach acids. Acid-stable compounds such as *penicillin V* may be preferred for oral administration in some cases. Table 8-3 indicates the penicillin preparations that are acid-stable.
2. Penicillin G is also inactivated by penicillinase, an enyme produced by some strains of staphylococci and other bacteria. Penicillinase-resistant semisynthetic penicillins, including *methicillin*[+], *oxacillin*[+], and derivatives of the latter, are now available for more effective treatment of infections by penicillinase-producing pathogens. Table 8-3 indicates the preparations of penicillin that are resistant to penicillinase.
3. Penicillin G has a relatively narrow antibacterial spectrum and is not active against gram-negative bacilli except in extremely high concentrations. Semisynthetic penicillins, including *ampicillin*[+] and *carbenicillin*[+] and related antibiotics, all have a broader antibacterial spectrum that includes many species and strains of gram-negative rods. Table 8-3 lists the ampicillin derivatives of penicillin and other extended-spectrum preparations.

Although these chemically modified penicillins possess properties that make them very valuable in certain specific situations, none can be considered to be the ideal penicillin. Despite claims to the contrary in the past, for example, none of the semisynthetic penicillins is free of the sensitizing property of natural penicillin. Thus, any person with a history of allergy to penicillin G must be considered as potentially cross-sensitive to all its congeners. There is even evidence that the newer compounds are capable of causing some types of toxic effects not previously reported with penicillin G.

Penicillin G is the most widely useful of the many penicillin products now available. It is the prototype penicillin, and therefore will be described in some detail. The major semisynthetic penicillins will then be compared to it, and significant differences will be indicated.

Penicillin G

Administration

Scientists have long been concerned with the development of penicillin preparations that would make possible the most efficient use of this valuable antibiotic. To accomplish this they have carefully studied how the body handles penicillin. From what they have learned of how this antibiotic, as administered by various routes, is absorbed, distributed to different tissues, and finally eliminated, they have been able to devise products suited for use in various clinical situations.

To be effective in any type of infection, antibiotics have to reach blood and tissue levels capable of inhibiting the bacteria or killing them. Many organisms are still so highly sensitive to penicillin G that the minimal inhibitory concentration (MIC) is often very low and can be readily reached when the antibiotic is taken orally. Severe infections caused by bacteria that are less sensitive to penicillin require higher blood levels. In such cases, and when the infecting organisms are in tissues not readily penetrated by the antibiotic, parenteral administration of an aqueous solution of penicillin G is preferred. For maintaining somewhat lower but longer-lasting blood levels of this antibiotic, it may be injected intramuscularly in the form of a slowly absorbed suspension.

Oral absorption. The most convenient, inexpensive, and pain-free way to administer penicillin is by mouth. Allergic reactions are also least likely when this antibiotic is given by mouth. However, a drawback of oral administration of penicillin G or of its potassium and other salts is that their absorption from the gastrointestinal tract, although rapid, is rather erratic and unpredictable. This is because much of any oral dose is destroyed by acidic gastric juice before it can reach its site of maximal absorption in the duodenum. What fails to be absorbed into the bloodstream in the upper intestine is broken down by bacteria in the colon, except for a very small amount that is eliminated unchanged in the feces.

Other oral penicillins that are more completely absorbed than penicillin G are now available (see below, and Table 8-3). These usually somewhat more expensive products, such as penicillin V, have not replaced oral penicillin G potassium for treating most mild to moderate infections caused by penicillin-sensitive bacteria. The less costly penicillin G can be given in amounts large enough to make up for the loss of much of any dose by stomach acid degradation. Similarly, although attaining equal plasma concentrations requires four or five times more oral penicillin G than when it is given by injection, its relatively low cost makes up for this seeming waste. (As noted, however, the parenteral route is required for treating severe infections.)

To minimize their inactivation by gastric acid and to prevent delay in absorption, penicillin G tablets and solutions are best taken on an empty stomach. Thus, oral penicillin G should be given at least 2 or 3 hours after the patient has eaten or at least 1 hour before meals.

Parenteral absorption. Parenteral administration of potassium or sodium salt solutions of penicillin G is required for serious infections. These are rapidly absorbed from intramuscular injection sites to reach peak plasma levels in less than half an hour. In certain life-threatening infections massive amounts may be injected intravenously to maintain high concentrations of penicillin G in the infected tissues. However, unless it is infused continuously, high tissue levels are difficult to maintain because of the speed of its elimination by the kidneys.

Repository forms. Special preparations of penicillin G have been developed for prolonging its stay in the body and thus minimizing the number of injections needed. These are suspensions of poorly soluble salts of penicillin G (penicillin G procaine suspension+ and penicillin G benzathine suspension+). They are injected deep into a muscle—never intravenously or subcutaneously—to form a depot from which the drug is only slowly absorbed into the blood. Peak levels are always lower than with potassium penicillin G but high enough to inhibit susceptible bacteria. Once bactericidal levels are reached, the therapeutic concentration continues to be maintained for relatively long periods—several days or weeks, depending on the dose of the repository preparation in the muscle reservoir.

Distribution

As penicillin G is absorbed into the blood, a large part of it is bound to plasma proteins. This serves as a circulating depot from which the antibiotic is released into the watery fluids that bathe various body tissues. The extent to which it accumulates in the different tissues determines its effectiveness for treating infections at various sites. Pencillin G does not, for example, penetrate very well into infected eyes; on the other hand, it readily reaches bactericidal concentrations in the fluid of infected joints. This is why the drug has to be injected directly under the conjunctiva in treating intraocular infections but it is injected intramuscularly rather than locally in septic arthritis or in osteomyelitis caused by susceptible pathogenic cocci.

Penicillin G does not penetrate the meninges very well, except in the presence of inflammation or of very high (toxic) blood levels. However, even in meningitis, the level attained in the spinal fluid is usually only a small fraction of the drug's plasma concentration. For this reason, some physicians inject the drug directly into the subarachnoid space to achieve high spinal fluid levels immediately. However, others who prefer to avoid possibly dangerous intrathecal injections give penicillin G intravenously or intramuscularly. Enough of the antibiotic passes through the inflamed meninges to kill pathogens that are highly sensitive to this antibiotic.

Excretion

Penicillin is cleared from the plasma by glomerular filtration and renal tubular secretion. Penicillin G is excreted almost entirely in unchanged form; thus, normal renal function is crucial for preventing accumulation of penicillin in the body.

The efficiency with which penicillin is normally excreted—which would be very useful if penicillin were a poison—posed a difficult problem for physicians trying to keep the drug at effective levels in the days when penicillin was in very short supply. Sometimes the scientists even tried to recover penicillin from the patient's own urine for reuse! They later worked at developing drugs that would delay the rapid renal excretion of penicillin when administered together with the antibiotic. Among the drugs that do this is *probenecid* (Benemid). Its molecules compete with those of penicillin for the tubular transport system that transfers the antibiotic from the blood to the tubular fluid. To the extent that the probenecid molecules occupy this mechanism, the penicillin molecules are blocked from these sites of excretory activity. As a result, the penicillin remains in the blood and tissues at higher levels for longer periods. This type of combined probenecid–penicillin therapy has sometimes proved useful for potentiating the activity of penicillin in treating infections that require high tissue concentrations of penicillin G—for example, subacute bacterial endocarditis and acute gonorrhea. Probenecid is also sometimes given with a repository form of penicillin in one-shot therapy.

Mechanism of action

Penicillin produces its bactericidal effects by interfering with the ability of susceptible bacteria to build their cell walls when they are dividing. The bacterial cell wall, which protects the organism from osmotic forces in its internal environment, is a complex structure. It contains a rigid framework made up of macromolecules of a mucopeptide called *peptidoglycan*. The penicillins (and certain other antibiotics such as the cephalosporins) prevent bacterial cells from biosynthesizing this substance. When the peptide cross linkages of this molecule are lacking, the developing cell walls cannot be completed.

The bacterial cell with an incomplete wall is a very fragile "L form," or protoplast, that then swells and bursts open from its own internal osmotic pressure, which is very high in contrast to the hypotonic environment of all body tissue fluids (except urine). This action of penicillin, which is specific for bacteria—especially gram-positive cocci—does not occur in mammalian cells, because these have only a limiting cytoplasmic membrane rather than the rigid cell walls of bacteria. This *selective toxicity* of penicillin for a biochemical process of bacteria that is not required by their human hosts accounts for its lack of direct toxicity on human cells. Thus the penicillins, which exert their toxic action only against microbial cells, come closest of all antimicrobial agents to being the ideal chemotherapeutic agent.

Antibacterial spectrum

Although penicillin G is effective against fewer types of bacteria than some other antibiotics, including certain semisynthetic penicillins, its activity against organisms that are sensitive to it is greater than that of other drugs (Table 8-4). The pathogens that are susceptible to penicillin G are the cause of some of the most common and serious infections that afflict mankind. These etiologic agents have, with a few important exceptions, remained highly sensitive to this antibiotic, so it has remained a very valuable anti-infective agent.

Penicillin G is still, for example, highly effective against such *gram-positive cocci* as the streptococcus and pneumococcus, although many resistant staphylococcal strains have now emerged. The *gram-negative cocci* that cause meningitis and gonorrhea are still sensitive, even though some strains now require higher concentrations than before. Although gram-negative bacilli are better attacked with other antibiotics, various *gram-positive bacilli*, including species of *Listeria* and those of *Clostridium* responsible for tetanus and gas gangrene, are responsive to penicillin G. Spirochetes, including *Treponema pallidum*, the microbial cause of syphilis, remain highly sensitive to this antibiotic. Pathogenic fungi are *not* affected, but actinomycetes, filamentous microorganisms that have sometimes been misclassified as fungi, are responsive to penicillin G, which is the drug of choice for treating actinomycosis.

Therapeutic indications

Streptococcal infections. Streptococci are pyogenic pathogens that cause such diseases as acute pharyngitis and tonsillitis, scarlet fever, and endocarditis. They grow in characteristic chainlike patterns and spread rapidly through the tissues by releasing liquefying enzymes that also produce a serous runny pus. (This differs from the thick viscous pus of staphylococcal infections.) Two of the main types of disease producers, the group A β-hemolytic and α-hemolytic streptococci, are highly sensitive to very low blood levels of penicillin G when they are rapidly dividing and making new cell walls. This accounts for the continued effectiveness of penicillin in the prevention and treatment of streptococcal pharyngitis and bacterial endocarditis.

Acute pharyngitis. Sore throat and fever, like most upper respiratory infections, are symptoms that are most commonly caused by viruses that are unaffected by any available antibiotic. However, when this syndrome is the result of throat tissue invasion by *Streptococcus pyogenes* (the group A β-hemolytic streptococcus that is also the cause of scarlet fever), the signs and symptoms are often promptly improved by treatment with an oral or parenteral penicillin preparation. Even low tissue concentrations of penicillins will eliminate this pathogen in a few days and prevent suppurative complications. The present practice of administering penicillin after taking a throat culture accounts for the relative rarity today of such once common complications as streptococcal mastoiditis, otitis media, and pneumonia.

Table 8–4. Antibacterial spectrum of the penicillins*

Penicillin G†; Penicillin V

Gram-positive cocci

Staphylococcus aureus (*non*penicillinase-producing strains)
Streptococcus pyogenes (groups A, B, C, and G)
Streptococcus viridans group
Streptococcus faecalis (enterococcus)
Streptococcus—anaerobic species such as *Peptostreptococcus*
Streptococcus bovis
Streptococcus (*Diplococcus*) *pneumoniae*

Gram-negative cocci

Neisseria gonorrhoeae (gonococcus)
Neisseria meningitidis (meningococcus)

Gram-positive bacilli

Bacillus anthracis (anthrax)
Clostridium perfringens (gas gangrene)
Clostridium tetani (tetanus)
Corynebacterium diphtheriae (diphtheria)
Listeria monocytogenes

Gram-negative bacilli

Bacteroides (all species except for many strains of *B. fragilis*)
Fusobacterium nucleatum (fusiform bacillus)
Pasteurella multocida
Spirillum minor ⎱ etiologic agents of
Streptobacillus moniliformis ⎰ rat-bite fevers

Spirochetes

Treponema pallidum (syphilis)
Treponema pertenue (yaws)
Borrelia recurrentis (relapsing fever)
Leptospira icterohaemorrhagiae (Weil's disease)

Actinomycetes

Actinomyces israelii

Penicillinase-resistant penicillins‡ (see Table 8–3)

Staphylococcus aureus (penicillinase-producing)

Broad- (or extended-) spectrum penicillins§ (see Table 8–3)

Ampicillin, amoxicillin, hetacillin, bacampicillin, cyclacillin

Gram-negative bacilli, including the following:

Escherichia coli
Hemophilus influenzae
Proteus mirabilis
Salmonella typhosa and other *Salmonella* species
Shigella flexneri

Carbenicillin disodium, carbenicillin indanyl sodium, mezlocillin, piperacillin, ticarcillin

Gram-negative bacilli, including the following:

Pseudomonas aeruginosa
Proteus species (indole-positive)

* Susceptibility of all infecting strains should be tested in the laboratory to determine whether the actual etiologic agent is sensitive or resistant to penicillins. The listing of a species as sensitive *in vitro* does not necessarily mean that penicillin is commonly employed clinically for infections caused by that organism, nor does it necessarily mean that penicillin is the drug of choice.
† Penicillin G, particularly in its parenteral forms, is considered the most effective of these penicillins, and it is preferred for severe infections caused by susceptible strains. Penicillin V is now often preferred for oral treatment of less severe infections.
‡ Penicillins of this type are also effective against the *non*penicillinase-producing gram-positive cocci and other organisms, but a penicillin G preparation is usually preferred for such infections. Cloxacillin and dicloxacillin are preferred for oral use; for parenteral use, methicillin, nafcillin, and oxacillin are employed.
§ Although these penicillins are often also effective against the same organisms as penicillins G and V, they are ordinarily reserved for infections in which the latter penicillins are not effective to avoid development of resistant strains of those species that are sensitive *only* to the penicillins of this subgroup.

If the throat culture taken before the start of treatment reveals the presence of streptococci, the medication must be continued for 10 days to eradicate the organism completely. This is because the bactericidal effect of penicillin occurs only when the streptococci are dividing rapidly. Bacterial organisms that are not in their growth phase during the first few days are not killed. Thus, if penicillin is stopped too soon, these survivors may begin to multiply rapidly and cause a recurrence of the infection.

Frequent recurrences can lead to development of rheumatic fever and carditis or glomerular nephritis. To avoid this risk of serious complications, the patient must comply with instructions to take the penicillin tablets as prescribed for the full 10 days. Too often, however, patients stop taking their medication when their symptoms clear up after a few days. If there is reason to doubt that the patient will comply with the medication order, or if a follow-up culture after 7 or 10 days reveals streptococci, a repository penicillin may be injected. For example, a single injection of 1.2 million units of penicillin G benzathine (Bicillin; Permapen) will provide low but effective blood levels for at least 2 weeks and ensure bacteriologic cure as well as clinical improvement. This penicillin product is also employed for long-term prophylaxis against streptococcal reinfection of patients with a history of rheumatic fever to prevent possible development of rheumatic heart disease.

Subacute bacterial endocarditis. Most cases of this heart infection, which once killed almost all of its victims, can be cured today by proper treatment with bactericidal antibiotics, including the penicillins. The disease develops most often when certain types of bacteria reach the blood of people with heart disease and invade already abnormal surfaces on the heart valves. Such implantation can be prevented by prophylactic antibiotics. Penicillin G should be administered to patients with heart valve disease before dental procedures such as tooth extraction, periodontal (gum) surgery, or even simple scaling. A single injection of penicillin G procaine preoperatively, followed by several daily doses of penicillin G after the procedure, is considered to be adequate for this purpose.

Two types of streptococci, the α-hemolytic *Streptococcus viridans* and the nonhemolytic group D *Streptococcus faecalis,* or enterococcus, are among the most common causes of endocarditis. Most *S. viridans* strains are still highly sensitive to penicillin G, and infections can be cured by large doses of that antibiotic alone. Enterococcal endocarditis is more difficult to treat, and combinations of penicillin G with synergistic aminoglycoside antibiotics such as streptomycin or gentamicin are required.

Antibiotics cannot readily penetrate fibrinous material encrusted on scarred diseased heart valves. To reach the bacterial invaders penicillin G must be administered in very high intravenous doses for several weeks. In such cases special IV techniques must be used to prevent bacterial contamination of the IV catheter and thrombophlebitis. Other antibiotics are also effective, but penicillin is so superior that it is often employed even in patients with a history of allergy to it. Here, too, special precautions are required, such as the use of small doses initially and the use of antihistamines and corticosteroids for control of delayed reactions (see below).

Staphylococcal infections. Infections by staphylococci vary greatly in severity. Some skin infections by

Staphylococcus aureus require no antimicrobial drug treatment and are best managed by local application of heat, incision, and drainage. Other systemic infections such as staphylococcal pneumonia must be promptly diagnosed and treated with large doses of antibiotics for long periods. Penicillin G is still a very useful drug for treating serious infections by staphylococci that are susceptible to its action. However, it is now never used alone for starting treatment of a serious staph infection, and treatment with penicillin G alone is initiated only after the laboratory has reported that the infecting staphylococcal strain is more sensitive to it than to other penicillins now available.

The reason for this is that so many staphylococcal strains have emerged that are now resistant to penicillin G. This is especially true in hospitals, in which fewer than 10% of isolated strains are sensitive to penicillin G, but the number of resistant staph strains in communities is also rising. These resistant organisms produce an enzyme capable of destroying the penicillin molecule by breaking open the β-lactam ring in its structure that is responsible for its antibacterial activity. Thus, it is now necessary to begin treatment of any suspected staph infection with one of the newer semisynthetic penicillins that can resist inactivation by the bacterial enzyme penicillinase or by β-lactamase. For this reason, further discussion of staphylococcal disease treatment will be deferred until the semisynthetic penicillinase-resistant penicillins have been described.

Pneumococcal pneumonia. Infections of the lungs and other organs by the pneumococcus can be readily controlled by intramuscular administration of penicillin G procaine. When treatment is begun early in acute lobar pneumonia, the patient's fever often breaks dramatically within 48 hours. However, treatment must be continued for a week to prevent relapses or complications, particularly in elderly or disease-debilitated patients and in infants. If pneumococcal meningitis develops as a complication, massive doses of penicillin G administered intravenously at frequent intervals may be required, or the drug may have to be injected intrathecally to reach spinal fluid concentrations capable of eradicating the pneumococcus.

Meningococcal meningitis. This disease occurs most commonly among adolescents or young adults infected during epidemics. It is sometimes best treated by intravenous administration of penicillin G, but, because these infections are now often caused by *Hemophilus influenzae,* some authorities prefer to use ampicillin or even chloramphenicol (see below). Penicillin should *not,* however, be used for prophylaxis of those exposed to the meningococcus during an epidemic. Sulfonamides such as sulfadiazine are preferred for this purpose, providing the infective strain is susceptible.

Gonorrhea. The emergence of resistant strains has led to a need for larger doses of penicillin G, but the drug is still considered to be the most effective antimicrobial agent for treating some types of this venereal disease. Current recommendations call for injection of 4.8 million units of an aqueous preparation of penicillin G procaine. This large dose is injected into two or more intramuscular sites to ensure a rapid rise to peak plasma levels. The effect of penicillin is potentiated and prolonged by prior administration of a 1-g oral dose of probenecid about half an hour before the injections. As indicated elsewhere, this drug delays the renal excretion of penicillin and raises its tissue concentrations.

Although a single treatment of this type is effective in most uncomplicated cases of acute gonorrhea, much more intensive therapy may be required in cases complicated by spread of the gonococcus to other pelvic tissues or to the joints, bloodstream, or heart. Ophthalmia neonatorum also responds readily to penicillin G.

Syphilis. This venereal disease is very responsive early in its course to treatment with parenteral penicillin G preparations. The penicillin G benzathine preparation may be administered in a single dose of 2.4 million units, with half of each dose being injected into each buttock. Although the blood levels attained in this way are not considered adequate for treating gonorrhea, the much more sensitive spirochete that causes syphilis is completely eradicated.

Other regimens for primary, secondary, and latent syphilis employ the other repository product, penicillin G procaine, which reaches higher plasma and tissue levels. A disadvantage of this form is that it is more rapidly excreted than the benzathine preparation and thus has a shorter duration of action. The patient may therefore be required to return for daily injections of penicillin G procaine during a 15-day treatment course. The patient with no signs or symptoms may need careful teaching and much encouragement to comply with this course of therapy. Some authorities consider this preparation to be the treatment of choice for neurosyphilis because of the higher plasma and spinal fluid levels that it attains.

Semisynthetic penicillins

As indicated earlier, penicillin G has certain limitations: its instability in gastric acid; its susceptibility to inactivation by penicillinase enzymes produced by some pathogenic bacteria; and its relatively narrow antimicrobial spectrum. Researchers have developed semisynthetic penicillins that do not have some of these limitations.

Acid-stable penicillins

A number of oral penicillins are now available that are more resistant to stomach acids than penicillin G (Table 8-3). In *penicillin V* (Pen-Vee K; V-Cillin K) the benzyl side chain has been replaced by a phenoxymethyl group. This is said to result in plasma levels two to five times higher than with oral penicillin G, because more of any orally administered dose of these drugs escapes destruction and is absorbed into the bloodstream. Penicillin V has essentially the same antibacterial spectrum as penicillin G (Table 8-4), and can be used to treat the same types of mild to moderate infections for which oral penicillin G is indicated. It *cannot* be used against infections caused by penicillinase-producing staphylococci or by other bacteria that produce β-lactamase. (Other acid-resistant penicillins that *are* also resistant to penicillinase are discussed in the next section.)

Penicillinase-resistant penicillins for staphylococcal infections

Staphylococci that get past the body's outer defenses can cause very severe systemic infections. Bacteria of this type can do great harm when they get into the bloodstream and are borne to the heart, brain, kidneys, or other organs. Abscesses caused by staphylococci are difficult to treat because penicillin and other antibiotics do not readily penetrate into the necrotic tissue and accumulating pus in which the staphylococci continue to multiply. Thus, medical treatment is best begun while tissue necrosis is still minimal.

As soon as a serious staph infection is suspected, a penicillinase-resistant penicillin should be ordered. Virtually all strains of staphylococci are susceptible to a penicillinase-resistant penicillin.

Thus, the first drug administered in most such cases is one of the penicillinase-resistant penicillins available in injectable form such as *methicillin* (Staphcillin), *oxacillin* (Prostaphlin), *nafcillin* (Unipen), *cloxacillin* (Cloxapen; Tegopen), or *dicloxacillin* (Dycill; Dynapen). All are equally effective against penicillin G-resistant staphylococci when given in large intramuscular or intravenous doses.

Aqueous penicillin G injections have often also been administered together with one of these semisynthetic penicillins until the results of identity and sensitivity tests have come back from the laboratory. The reason for this is that the penicillinase-resistant penicillins are less active than penicillin G against the *non*penicillinase-producing staphylococci and such other gram-positive pyogenic cocci as the streptococcus and pneumococcus.

Of course, if the laboratory reports that the infecting organism is *not* a penicillinase-producing staph but a gram-positive organism sensitive to the more effective and less expensive penicillin G, the patient is switched to that antibiotic. On the other hand, penicillin G is withdrawn and treatment is continued with only the other antistaphylococcal drug of the original combination when the organism is identified as a penicillinase-producing staph. Patients may also be switched to an oral form of nafcillin or oxacillin, or to one of the relatives of the latter, such as cloxacillin (Tegopen) or dicloxacillin (Dynapen). This spares the patient the local pain caused by continuing injections for the 4 weeks or more of treatment usually required in severe staph infections. The use of an oral penicillinase-resistant penicillin is now also recommended for initiating treatment of *all* gram-positive infections of mild to moderate severity.

Ampicillins

One of the limitations of penicillin G has been its relatively narrow antibacterial spectrum. This natural penicillin is remarkably active against the most common gram-positive and gram-negative *cocci,* but it has only relatively weak activity against gram-negative *rods.* Certain semisynthetic penicillins prepared by substituting new side chains for the benzyl group of penicillin G provide much greater antibacterial activity against gram-negative bacilli (Table 8-3).

Ampicillin, a congener in which an α-aminobenzyl group is the substituent, is active not only against gram-positive organisms but is also much more effective than penicillin G in infections caused by such gram-negative species as *Hemophilus influenzae, Escherichia coli, Salmonella, Shigella,* and the indole-negative *Proteus mirabilis.* It is not resistant to breakdown by penicillinase and thus it should not be employed when an infection by resistant staphylococci or some other penicillinase-producing pathogens is suspected, and for which methicillin, nafcillin, or oxacillin and its derivatives are indicated. Also, when the laboratory identifies the causative organism as a gram-positive species sensitive to penicillin G *alone,* ampicillin should *not* be employed. The main reason for this is that the wide use of a broader spectrum penicillin, when penicillin G would do as well or better, speeds the emergence of resistant gram-negative species. This has already begun to make ampicillin (as well as carbenicillin; see below) ineffective for treating some infections caused by pathogenic species against which it was once active. In addition, antibiotic-induced diarrhea and other adverse effects occur more commonly with ampicillin than with penicillins G or V, and ampicillin is generally more expensive.

Ampicillin itself is available for parenteral as well as oral administration. The other antibiotics that are closely related to ampicillin are given only orally (Table 8-3).

Amoxicillin (Amoxil; Larotid), which is more rapidly and completely absorbed than ampicillin when taken by mouth, may have two types of advantages. First, because this antibiotic reaches higher blood levels and is excreted in the urine in larger amounts for longer periods, it may be more effective for treating certain systemic and urinary tract infections. Second, because less of this antibiotic reaches the lower intestine, it may be less likely to alter the bacterial flora of the bowel. This would lessen the likelihood of antibiotic-induced diarrhea and tend to reduce the rate at which antibiotic-resistant enteric bacterial strains emerge.

Bacampicillin (Spectrobid) is also more readily absorbed and produces higher blood levels than ampicillin. It is effective when given only twice a day. Like amoxicillin and *cyclacillin* (Cyclapen-W), it may cause less diarrhea. After absorption, bacampicillin and *hetacillin* (Versapen) are metabolized to ampicillin. Thus, their antimicrobial spectrum, like that of the other drugs in this group, is similar to that of ampicillin.

Clinical indications for ampicillin and related antibiotics. Ampicillin (Amcill; Omnipen) is useful for treating many of the same infections as penicillin G (Table 8-4). However, as discussed above, the broader spectrum penicillins should not be used to treat infections that would respond to penicillin G.

Pediatric infections. Because of its activity against the pathogens that most commonly cause serious infections in young children, ampicillin has proved particularly useful for beginning treatment of infants and children under 3 years of age. It is especially effective against *Hemophilus influenzae,* a gram-negative inhabitant of the nose and throat of youngsters between the ages of 3 months and 3 years and a common invader of the middle ear. Thus, it is most useful for treating acute otitis media and its most serious complication, meningitis, when the cause of these infections is *H. influenzae.*

Ampicillin is also effective against such other causes of childhood acute otitis media as the pneumococcus and streptococcus, including *Streptococcus faecalis,* a penicillin G-resistant enterococcus. It is active against the meningococcus, which, along with pneumococci and streptococci, is among the causes of meningitis in these youngsters and in adolescents and others. This antibiotic is even effective against the most common causes of meningitis in infants under 3 months of age: *E. coli* and *Salmonella.* Thus, ampicillin is the most useful single antibiotic with which to begin treatment after cultures have been taken but before the infecting organism is known. Of course, after the specific organism is identified and its antimicrobial sensitivity is determined, ampicillin may be discontinued, and treatment with the most appropriate agent may be begun.

Because ampicillin-resistant strains of *H. influenzae* have begun to appear in some geographic areas, some authorities recommend that ampicillin be used only after tests have shown that the infecting strain responsible for bacterial meningitis is actually sensitive to it. The development of resistance among other gram-negative organisms, including those most commonly involved in urinary tract infections, *E. coli* and *P. mirabilis,* has also made ampicillin less useful than it was when first used for treating bladder and kidney infections and bacterial diarrhea (see below).

Gastrointestinal infections. Ampicillin may nonetheless be useful for treating intestinal infections by strains of *Shigella* and *Salmonella* that are still sensitive to it. In shigellosis, or bacillary dysentery, oral ampicillin therapy is especially effective for preventing diarrhea-induced dehydration and electrolyte imbalance in children. It may also be administered in milder cases of salmonellosis, although some authorities think that such treatment of enterocolitis may not be desirable, because it may increase the likelihood of the patient's becoming a carrier after the symptoms are relieved. Typhoid fever and other severe salmonella infections in which the organisms enter the bloodstream and spread to other parts of the body are generally best treated with parenteral chloramphenicol, except when chloramphenicol-resistant strains of bacteria are the causative agents; ampicillin is then the drug of choice, and oral ampicillin may be employed for treating patients who continue to carry *Salmonella typhi* until the organism no longer appears in the stool.

Extended-spectrum penicillins: carbenicillin-type antibiotics

Carbenicillin disodium (Geopen; Pyopen), which contains an α-aminocarboxybenzyl group in place of the benzyl side chain of penicillin G, is not only effective against the same gram-negative bacilli as the ampicillins, but it is also the first penicillin active against *Pseudomonas aeruginosa* strains and such indole-positive *Proteus* species as *P. vulgaris, P. morgani,* and *P. rettgeri,* which are resistant to ampicillin. Carbenicillin has a broader antibacterial range than any other available penicillin. However, to prevent the development of bacterial resistance, it should be reserved mainly for the treatment of serious infections by *Pseudomonas aeruginosa* and indole-positive *Proteus* strains—pathogens that are not responsive to treatment with other penicillins.

Carbenicillin has properties that make it particularly useful for treating patients hospitalized for treatment of urinary tract infections by uropathogens that are resistant to ampicillin, the sulfonamides, and the other more commonly employed antibiotic and chemotherapeutic agents. Unlike the only other antibiotics effective in similar resistant kidney and bladder infections, carbenicillin does not have any adverse effects on renal function. This gives it an important advantage over the only antibiotics previously available for this purpose, the polymyxins and the aminoglycoside antibiotics. Carbenicillin also has the advantage of being excreted unchanged by the kidneys in amounts that make a highly concentrated solution in the urine.

Carbenicillin is also useful for treating pseudomonal septicemia and other systemic infections by these and other gram-negative bacteria. It is best given parenterally in combination with an aminoglycoside antibiotic such as gentamicin[+], because these two types of drugs have synergistic antibacterial effects on susceptible strains of *Pseudomonas aeruginosa.* In fact, many authorities believe that carbenicillin and the other penicillins in this group should never be used alone to treat any serious infection. When carbenicillin or any other drug of this group is given concomitantly with an aminoglycoside antibiotic, the two antibiotic solutions should not be mixed together, because they may chemically inactivate one another.

Carbenicillin indanyl sodium (Geocillin) is a derivative of carbenicillin that, unlike the parent compound, is stable in gastric acid. When taken by mouth it is readily absorbed and then converted to carbenicillin, which is rapidly excreted by the kidney to reach exceptionally high levels in the urine. This is a safe, effective, and convenient antibiotic for treating patients who suffer recurrent UTI caused by uropathogens resistant to other antimicrobial agents. However, if it is ordered too frequently, this oral form of the antibiotic may increase the rate at which resistant strains emerge. This, in turn, could result in the parenteral form of carbenicillin becoming less useful for the treatment of life-threatening septicemia and other severe systemic infections.

Four other drugs that are similar to carbenicillin have been introduced more recently. *Ticarcillin disodium* (Ticar) was the first of these, followed by *mezlocillin sodium* (Mezlin), *piperacillin sodium* (Pipracil) and, most recently *azlocillin sodium* (Azlin). The wholesale cost of each successive drug introduced is greater than the cost of earlier drugs in the series, and many see little advantage of any of the newer preparations over carbenicillin. These drugs have generally been promoted as having greater activity than carbenicillin against *Pseudomonas aeruginosa,* but evidence of clinical advantage is lacking. Maximum daily doses of the three newest drugs of the series, mezlocillin, piperacillin, and azlocillin, contain less sodium than the maximum daily dose of ticarcillin, which in turn contains less sodium than carbenicillin. Thus, these drugs may offer an advantage for the patient whose sodium intake should be restricted.

Adverse effects of the penicillins

The penicillins can cause all of the three general types of antibiotic-induced adverse effects discussed in Chapter 6: direct tissue toxicity, superinfections, and hypersensitivity reactions. Adverse effects of the first two types are much less common and less hazardous with penicillin than with most other classes of antibiotics. However, hypersensitization probably occurs more often with penicillin than with any other kind of drug. This antibiotic class is also the most common cause of fatal anaphylactoid drug reactions.

Hypersensitivity reactions

Incidence. According to the results of epidemiologic studies, about 5% of the population is now thought to be hypersensitive to penicillin. When actually exposed to the antibiotic, as few as 1% or as many as 10% may suffer adverse allergic reactions or immune responses.

As this indicates, the proportion of patients who react adversely varies in different studies. The nature of the reactions also varies in terms of the signs and symptoms reported and the degree of their severity. Just about every possible type of hypersensitivity reaction has been reported, including all the signs and symptoms of the immediate and delayed types of drug reactions described in Chapter 5.

The most common manifestations of penicillin hypersensitivity are skin eruptions such as urticaria (hives) and exanthematous rashes of every type. These are often only mildly discomforting and may not even require the patient's penicillin regimen to be stopped. On the other extreme are penicillin reactions so severe that death occurs within minutes after the drug is administered. Fatalities are relatively rare in terms of statistical rates—only about two deaths for every 100,000 patients treated with penicillins. However, penicillin is so widely employed that, even at this low rate, an estimated 300 Americans die each year of the anaphylactic complications of penicillin.

Sensitivity tests. If a patient has a known sensitivity to penicillin but penicillin is the drug of choice for the particular problem, skin tests can be performed in which a dilute solution of penicillin or of one of its metabolites may be scratched onto the skin or injected intradermally. If, for example, scratching a small amount of penicillin into the skin surface causes a vivid red flare and local wheal to develop, the patient can be expected to have a severe systemic reaction if treated with the antibiotic. In fact, because the degree of the reaction is not related to the dose, some highly sensitive people have sometimes suffered a severe generalized reaction as a result of the scratch test itself. Thus, a kit containing supplies for counteracting anaphylactoid reactions (see Chap. 39) should always be available when skin tests are being performed. Skin testing itself can cause a patient to become sensitized, so this testing procedure should not be undertaken without careful weighing of the consequences.

Even when the scratch test is negative, allergic reactions to larger doses can still occur. Thus, further testing is done by infiltrating the superficial skin layers with a small quantity of dilute penicillin solution. If the intradermal bleb does not enlarge and become surrounded by a reddened area, it is usually considered safe to proceed. However, because false negative test results are common, scientists have been seeking safer and more reliable tests for detecting patients allergic to penicillin.

A more specific diagnostic test is now available that employs a major degradation product, benzylpenicilloyl, combined with an amino acid derivative. This hapten of penicillin, when conjugated with the carrier, becomes a specific antigen capable of reacting with specific penicillin antibodies in the skin. Intradermal injection of *benzylpenicilloyl pólysine* (Pre-Pen) is said to be several times more reliable than penicillin itself for detecting those who are likely to have an allergic reaction when treated with therapeutic doses of the antibiotic. However, neither this nor other tests that are being developed can offer complete assurance that an allergic reaction to penicillin will not occur.

For this reason, clinical judgment must be used to determine whether the risk of employing penicillin is warranted by the probable benefits. Occasionally, penicillin is employed for treating a life-threatening infection, even though the patient has a history of hypersensitivity to it. In some forms of endocarditis, for example, penicillin is so superior to other antibiotics that its use is considered necessary, even for patients allergic to it. In such cases the physician may try to desensitize the patient by beginning with small doses that are then raised gradually to the very large amounts needed in bacterial endocarditis. During this dangerous procedure drugs for treating immediate and delayed reactions must be kept available. (The treatment of anaphylactic reactions to penicillin is the same as that for reactions to other substances that cause the release of histamine and other chemical mediators. The use of epinephrine, antihistamines, corticosteroids and other drugs for this purpose is discussed in Chapter 39.)

Product comparisons. Hypersensitivity reactions can occur with any type of penicillin. Severe reactions are less likely to develop when penicillin is taken orally than when it is injected in aqueous solution or as a repository suspension such as penicillin G procaine. Patients have sometimes died, however, after ingestion of just a few penicillin tablets. Ampicillin may cause fewer urticarial and anaphylactoid reactions than penicillin G. However, delayed reactions marked by a measleslike (morbilliform) or a maculopapular skin rash are more common with ampicillin. Repository penicillins also tend to cause delayed reactions of the serum sickness type with fever and joint pains, as well as skin eruptions.

Direct tissue toxicity

Penicillin has remarkably few direct effects on human tissues. This may be because the antibiotic is so specific in its antibacterial action. That is, it exerts selective toxicity on bacterial cell walls by interfering with metabolic processes that do not occur in human cells. Another factor may be that most penicillins are rapidly excreted by the kidneys without being broken down to possibly toxic byproducts.

Despite this lack of direct pharmacologic effects, penicillins that accumulate in high local concentrations that are irritating to tissue can cause various adverse effects. The intramuscular injection of carbenicillin, for example, sometimes causes local pain and inflammation. Intravenous injections of penicillins should be made slowly in dilute solution to avoid high local concentrations that may irritate the vein and cause phlebitis or thrombophlebitis. The high blood concentrations needed in treating severe infections may sometimes cause muscle twitching and even generalized convulsions. Neuroscientists studying epilepsy and antiepileptic drugs have used penicillin preparations experimentally to produce seizures in animals.

Patients with kidney disease have occasionally developed signs of tubular damage following large doses of penicillin for long periods. This may occur more often with such semisynthetic penicillins as methicillin, oxacillin, and carbenicillin. Blood counts are recommended because of occasional development of transient reduction of blood cell levels in patients treated with methicillin. Some patients receiving nafcillin, carbenicillin, and the other extended-spectrum penicillins have had bleeding episodes that required discontinuation of therapy. The high sodium content of the large doses of carbenicillin that must be administered may lead to sodium retention and potassium loss, with undesirable effects on patients with heart disease. Similarly, the large load of potassium taken in with high doses of potassium penicillin salts may upset electrolyte balance and cause hyperkalemia in some cases; fatalities have resulted.

Superinfections

Infection by overgrowths of resistant microorganisms is not a serious problem with penicillin G. Occasional oral, vaginal, or rectal moniliasis may be reported. The penicillins with a broader antibacterial spectrum are more likely to cause superinfections by overgrowths of resistant gram-negative bacteria. Carbenicillin, for example, may cause the emergence of resistant strains of *Klebsiella* and *Serratia* species during treatment of *Pseudomonas* infections in elderly debilitated patients or in those being treated for cancer with cytotoxic drugs that reduce their natural defense mechanisms.

In summary, the penicillins are relatively safe antibiotics, except for patients who are hypersensitive to them and possibly for some patients who have to receive very high doses, particularly of certain of the semisynthetic penicillins. Fortunately for those who cannot tolerate penicillin, a number of alternative antibiotics are available that can be substituted for it to treat both severe and mild infections.

Additional clinical considerations

Although the adverse effects of the penicillins are relatively few, as has been mentioned, hypersensitivity reactions to the penicillins are fairly common and are potentially dangerous. The best way to prevent hypersensitivity reactions is by obtaining a patient history that carefully screens for known allergies and adverse drug reactions. Except in life-threatening infections, in which

a penicillin would provide unique and lifesaving therapeutic benefits, allergy to penicillins or to cephalosporins constitutes a contraindication to the use of any penicillin. In addition, procaine penicillin should be avoided in patients allergic to procaine. Certain oral preparations of penicillin G potassium (*e.g.,* Pentids) and penicillin G benzathine (*e.g.,* Bicillin) contain tartrazine and should be avoided in patients allergic to that substance. Allergy to tartrazine is frequently seen in patients who are allergic to aspirin, so tartrazine-free preparations are preferable in patients allergic to aspirin. In taking the history, the nurse should also ask the patient about other allergies, because patients who are prone to allergic responses should be carefully monitored for penicillin hypersensitivity.

Because the penicillins are excreted through the kidneys, any difficulties in renal function can lead to penicillin accumulation and toxicity. This is often a problem with elderly patients and infants, whose renal function is marginal. Keeping this in mind with these patients, reduced doses of penicillin or a penicillin that is metabolized or excreted in the bile should be ordered; nafcillin, oxacillin, cloxacillin, and piperacillin are examples of penicillins that do not accumulate in patients with impaired renal function.

Patients with potential electrolyte problems need to be monitored carefully if penicillins high in sodium or potassium content are used. Continuous IV infusions of potassium penicillin G have been reported to cause serious potassium poisoning. Sodium salts of penicillin can cause serious problems in patients with congestive heart failure or hypertension when the sodium causes increased circulating fluid volume.

Penicillins cross the placenta and are excreted in breast milk. Although clinical testing has not established any direct links between fetal or infant problems and the administration of penicillin to the mother, it is probably advisable to avoid the use of these and any drugs during pregnancy and lactation.

Drug–drug and drug–laboratory test interactions. Carbenicillin and the *aminoglycoside antibiotics* (see below) should not be mixed together in a syringe or in an IV bottle. These drugs will interact to inactivate the aminoglycoside drug. Concomitant therapy with bacteriostatic drugs, such as the *tetracyclines,* and penicillins may reduce the efficacy of the penicillin, because penicillin inhibits cell wall synthesis only in actively dividing bacterial populations. Ampicillin and penicillin V may decrease the effectiveness of *oral contraceptives,* leading to breakthrough bleeding or to unwanted pregnancies. The exact mechanism of this interaction is unclear, although it may be the result of a decreased amount of the contraceptive drug being absorbed because of the antibiotic-induced loss of normal intestinal flora, which in some way may facilitate the absorption of the oral contraceptives.

The penicillins have been found to cause false-positive *urine glucose test* results by certain methods. If a patient is on penicillin and a urine glucose test is necessary, the Clinistix or Tes-Tape methods should be used.

The patient teaching guide presents key points for patient education about penicillin therapy. The guide to the nursing process with penicillins summarizes the applications of the nursing process to penicillin therapy.

Patient teaching guide: The penicillins

The drug that has been prescribed for you is an antibiotic of the family of penicillins. The penicillins are used to help to destroy specific bacteria that are causing infections in the body. They are effective against only certain bacteria; they are not effective against viruses, cold germs, or other bacteria. To clear up a bacterial infection, the penicillins have to act on the bacteria over a period of time, so it is very important to complete the full course of your penicillin to avoid recurrence of the infection. Your penicillin has been prescribed to treat _____ .

Instructions:

1. The name of the drug ordered for you is _____ .

2. The dose of the drug ordered for you is _____ .

3. The drug should be taken _____ time(s) a day. It is best to space the drug throughout the day. The best times to take your drug are _____ , _____ , _____ .

4. The drug should be taken on an empty stomach with a full glass of water. One hour before meals or 2 to 3 hours after meals is best. Do not use fruit juices, soft drinks, or milk to take the drug, because these may interfere with its effectiveness (except for bacampicillin, amoxicillin, and penicillin V).

5. Side-effects of the drug that you should be aware of include:

   Stomach upset
   Diarrhea
   Change in taste
   Change in color of tongue

   All these are a result of the drug's activities, and will go away when the drug is stopped.

6. Tell any physician, nurse, or dentist who takes care of you that you are taking this drug.

7. Keep this and all medications out of the reach of children.

8. Do not use this medication to self-treat any other infection; do not give this medication to others or use similar medications borrowed from others.

9. Be sure to complete the full course of your prescription. Take all the prescription that has been ordered for you.

Notify your nurse or physician if any of the following occur:

   Hives
   Rash
   Fever
   Difficulty breathing
   Severe diarrhea

Guide to the nursing process: the penicillins

Assessment	Nursing diagnoses	Interventions	Evaluation
Past history (*contraindications*): Renal failure Pregnancy Lactation *Allergies:* penicillin, cephalosporins, procaine, tartrazine, others; reactions Medication history: current drugs (*Cautions:* oral contraceptives, other antibiotics) **Physical assessment** General: assess infected area Respiratory: rate, adventitious sounds GI: bowel sounds, output, liver function tests Renal: urinalysis, BUN, electrolytes Skin: lesions, temperature	Potential alteration in bowel elimination Potential alteration in respiratory function Knowledge deficit regarding drug therapy	Culture infected area Preparation and safe administration of drug Patient teaching: Drug Dosage Administration Side-effects Warning signs Support and encouragement to comply with drug therapy	Monitor for effectiveness of drug: resolution of infection Monitor for adverse effects of drug (sensitivity reactions): GI reactions Changes in liver function tests Coagulation tests Changes in urinalysis Monitor electrolytes Monitor drug–drug interactions: Decreased effect of *oral contraceptives* Decreased effect with *other antibiotics* Evaluate effectiveness of teaching program Evaluate effectiveness of support offered

Alternatives to penicillin

The penicillins now available can control most of the common bacterial infections that arise in the community. Ordinarily, potentially more toxic antibiotics, such as the aminoglycosides, polymyxins, vancomycin, and chloramphenicol are reserved mainly for treating serious infections caused by the resistant pathogenic strains that tend to emerge in the hospital environment.

Certain other antibiotics may be grouped together on the basis of the similarity of their antibacterial spectrum to that of the penicillins (Table 8-5). Some of these agents—such as erythromycin—are similar to penicillin G and V in their effectiveness against gram-positive cocci such as strep, staph, and pneumococci. Others—the cephalosporins, for instance—resemble ampicillin in their effectiveness against such gram-negative bacilli as *E. coli* and *Proteus mirabilis,* as well as against the penicillin G-sensitive gram-positive pathogens.

The most important indication for use of these

alternative antibiotics is in the treatment of patients who are allergic to penicillin who have an infection caused by a pathogen that is sensitive to one of the other drugs. These antibiotics are, however, also substituted for penicillins when the results of bacteriologic tests identify the infecting organism as a species or strain more sensitive to the alternative antibiotic than to the penicillin with which treatment may have been initiated.

Thus, for example, erythromycin may be employed when the organism responsible for a respiratory infection is revealed by laboratory data or clinical observation to be *Mycoplasma pneumoniae* or *Legionella pneumophila,* which causes Legionnaires' disease. The patient may be switched to a cephalosporin if the infecting organism is identified as a *Klebsiella pneumoniae* strain most susceptible to this class of antibiotics. Clindamycin[+] may be indicated if special culturing shows that the infecting organism is an anaerobic species resistant to penicillin.

Some clinically significant generalizations about this and other alternatives to penicillin will now be made

Table 8–5. Antibiotics used as alternatives to the penicillins

Generic or official name	Trade name	Route of administration	Usual adult dosage
Cephalosporins			
First generation			
Cefadroxil	Duricef; Ultracef	Oral	1–2 g/day, in divided doses, q 12–24 hr
Cefazolin sodium	Ancef; Kefzol	IM, IV	1–6 g/day, in divided doses, q 6–8 hr
Cephalexin monohydrate	Keflex	Oral	1–4 g/day, in divided doses, q 6 hr
Cephalothin sodium USP	Keflin	IM, IV	2–12 g/day, in divided doses, q 4–6 hr
Cephapirin sodium	Cefadyl	IM, IV	2–12 g/day, in divided doses, q 4–6 hr
Cephradine	Anspor; Velosef	IM, IV, oral	2–8 g/day, in divided doses, q 4–6 hr, IM or IV; 1–4 g/day, in divided doses, q 6 hr, oral
Second generation			
Cefaclor	Ceclor	Oral	0.75–4 g/day, in divided doses, q 8 hr
Cefamandole nafate	Mandol	IM, IV	1.5–12 g/day, in divided doses, q 4–8 hr
Cefoxitin sodium	Mefoxin	IM, IV	3–12 g/day, in divided doses, q 4–8 hr
Cefuroxime sodium	Zinacef	IM, IV	750 mg–1.5 g q 8 hr
Third generation			
Cefoperazone sodium	Cefobid	IM, IV	2–12 g/day, in divided doses, q 6–8 hr
Cefotaxime sodium	Claforan	IM, IV	2–12 g/day, in divided doses, q 4–6 hr
Ceftizoxime sodium	Cefizox	IM, IV	1–2 g q 8–12 hr
Moxalactam disodium	Moxam	IM, IV	2–12 g/day, in divided doses, q 6–8 hr
Macrolide antibiotics			
Erythromycin			
Erythromycin base USP	E-Mycin; Eryc; Ery-Tab; Ilotycin	Oral	250 mg q 6 hr
Erythromycin estolate USP	Ilosone	Oral	250 mg q 6 hr
Erythromycin ethylsuccinate USP	E-Mycin E; E.E.S.; Pediamycin; Wyamycin-E	Oral	400 mg q 6 hr
Erythromycin gluceptate USP	Ilotycin Gluceptate	IV	15–20 mg/kg/day, by continuous infusion or in divided doses, q 6 hr
Erythromycin lactobionate USP	Erythrocin Lactobionate-IV; Erythrocin Piggyback	IV	15–20 mg/kg/day, by continuous infusion or in divided doses, q 6 hr
Erythromycin stearate USP	Bristamycin; Erypar; Erythrocin Stearate; Ethril '500'; Pfizer-E; SK-Erythromycin; Wyamycin S	Oral	250 mg, q 6 hr

Table 8–5. Antibiotics used as alternatives to the penicillins (continued)

Generic or official name	Trade name	Route of administration	Usual adult dosage
Troleandomycin			
Troleandomycin; triacetyloleandomycin	TAO	Oral	250 mg–500 mg, q 4 hr
Clindamycin			
Clindamycin HCl USP, clindamycin palmitate HCl USP	Cleocin HCl	Oral	150 mg–300 mg, q 6 hr
Clindamycin phosphate USP	Cleocin phosphate	IV	600–1200 mg/day in two to four divided doses
Miscellaneous			
Spectinomycin HCl USP	Trobicin	IM	2 g in a single injection
Vancomycin HCl USP	Vancocin	IV, oral	500 mg, q 6 hr, or 1000 mg, q 12 hr, IV or oral

here, and detailed information about some representative antibiotics of this group can be found in the individual Drug Digests at the end of this chapter.

The cephalosporins

Antibiotics of the cephalosporin family were introduced in the 1960s. They are similar to the penicillins in chemical structure and in their mechanism of action: they inhibit the synthesis of cell wall by bacteria. They are bacteriostatic or bactericidal, depending on the dose, organism, and concentration of drug in the tissue. They are very rarely the drug of choice for treating an infection, and they have caused hypersensitivity reactions in some patients allergic to penicillins (5%–15% of such patients are probably allergic to cephalosporins also). Therefore, it cannot be assumed that they are an absolutely safe alternative to penicillin in penicillin-allergic patients. The early cephalosporins were inactivated by β-lactamase enzymes produced by some bacteria (penicillinase is one form of β-lactamase). Newer cephalosporins are more resistant to inactivation by these enzymes.

The cephalosporins can be classified into three "generations" of drugs (Table 8-5). The drugs within each group have a similar antibacterial spectrum but, going from first- to third-generation drugs, a loss of activity against gram-positive bacteria and an increase in activity against gram-negative organisms and against antibiotic-resistant organisms can be seen. Cost of the drugs

generally increases also. "First-generation" cephalosporins have been available the longest; their antimicrobial spectrum includes many gram-positive cocci—for example, *E. coli*, *Klebsiella pneumoniae*, and *Proteus mirabilis*. The "second-generation" cephalosporins have a broader spectrum of activity against gram-negative bacteria; the "third-generation" cephalosporins are less active than those of the first generation against gram-positive cocci, but are more active against gram-negative enteric bacilli. The third-generation drugs are active against some hospital-acquired infections caused by strains of bacteria that are resistant to many other antibiotics. However, strains of bacteria previously sensitive to second- and third-generation cephalosporins have developed resistance to them. Thus, use of these drugs should be limited to the treatment of infections against which other antibiotics are ineffective. Penicillins are generally safer and cheaper than cephalosporins and should be used whenever possible.

Pharmacokinetics

The oral preparations of cephalosporins are well absorbed from the gastrointestinal tract. Although absorption may be delayed by the presence of food, the total amount of drug absorbed is not influenced. To lessen the likelihood of causing GI upset, these drugs should be taken with food or milk. Only four of the fourteen cephalosporins now marketed in the United States are available for oral use.

The cephalosporins are widely distributed in body fluids and tissues, including bone (especially inflamed bone). They cross the placenta and are secreted in the milk of nursing mothers. Although the first- and second-generation drugs do not cross the blood–brain barrier very well, even when the meninges are inflamed, the third-generation drugs do penetrate well in patients with meningitis; *cefotaxime sodium* (Claforan) or *moxalactam disodium* (Moxam) is the drug of choice for treating enteric gram-negative bacillary meningitis.

Except for *cefoperazone sodium* (Cefobid), most cephalosporins are excreted unchanged by the kidneys. In patients whose renal function is compromised, the dosage of most cephalosporins may need to be reduced. Because these drugs are nephrotoxic, the monitoring of renal function is one of the important aspects of safe therapy with these drugs. Cefoperazone differs from other cephalosporins in its excretion, being excreted mainly in the bile; normal dosage of this drug does not cause accumulation in patients with renal insufficiency but the drug does accumulate in patients with impaired hepatic function. Thus, such patients may need a reduced dosage.

Therapeutic uses

Two third-generation cephalosporins, cefotaxime and moxalactam, are drugs of choice for treating enteric gram-negative bacillary meningitis in adults, but an aminoglycoside (see below) plus an extended-spectrum penicillin (ticarcillin or piperacillin) are used for *Pseudomonas*-caused meningitis. Only the third-generation cephalosporins are active against *P. aeruginosa*, and strains of this organism that are resistant to the three oldest cephalosporins of this group (cefoperazone, cefotaxime, and moxalactam) have been reported.

First-generation cephalosporins are used to treat staphylococcal infections, including staphylococcal pneumonia, and to treat pneumococcal pneumonia in patients allergic to penicillin. *Cefamandole nafate* (Mandol), a second-generation cephalosporin, and the third-generation drugs, are effective in pneumonia caused by *H. influenzae*, and the third-generation drugs are very effective in treating pneumonia caused by *E. coli* or *K. pneumoniae*. A cephalosporin is sometimes used with an aminoglycoside in the initial treatment of suspected sepsis.

The oral cephalosporins are sometimes used to treat UTI that have not responded to sulfonamides, ampicillin, or tetracyclines, all of which are less expensive than cephalosporins. *Cefoxitin sodium* (Mefoxin) and the third-generation cephalosporins, especially moxalactam, are effective in abdominal and pelvic infections, and these drugs can be used instead of spectinomycin (see below) to treat penicillinase-producing *Neisseria gonorrhoea*.

As stated above, cephalosporins penetrate inflamed bone well, and the first-generation drugs are used,

especially in penicillin-allergic patients, to treat staphylococcal osteomyelitis. Newer cephalosporins are used to treat osteomyelitis caused by gram-negative bacteria.

Adverse reactions

The most common side-effects are GI disturbances and hypersensitivity reactions. The orally administered drugs cause nausea, vomiting, and diarrhea in about one-third of the patients taking them. Cefoperazone, although it is not given orally, may cause a higher incidence of diarrhea because of its biliary excretion. The oral drugs should be given with food or a glass of milk to minimize the adverse GI effects. Colitis, including pseudomembranous colitis, a very serious condition that has caused fatalities in patients taking other broad-spectrum antibiotics, has also been reported. A patient who develops diarrhea should be carefully evaluated, and consideration should be given to discontinuing the drug or changing to a different antibiotic. Pseudomembranous colitis has been attributed to superinfection, especially with *Clostridium* strains. Superinfections with bacteria and *Candida* can occur during cephalosporin therapy.

Hypersensitivity reactions are most common in patients with a history of allergic reactions (asthma, hay fever, hives); they may be mild or life-threatening. As mentioned before, cross sensitivity often occurs with penicillin.

The intramuscular administration of the cephalosporins, especially of *cephalothin sodium* (Keflin) and cefoxitin, usually causes pain and inflammation. Subcutaneous administration has caused sterile abscesses; thus, injections need to be made deep into the muscle. Intravenous administration has caused phlebitis and thrombophlebitis.

The cephalosporins also cause renal toxicity, as do the aminoglycosides (see below), with which they are often given. Because renal excretion is the primary means by which both of these groups of antibiotics are cleared from the body (except for cefoperazone), renal function should be monitored carefully and dosage should be reduced in patients with compromised renal function.

Side-effects related to the CNS include headache, dizziness, and paresthesias. *Cefazolin sodium* (Ancef; Kefzol), like some of the penicillins, has caused tonic–clonic convulsions, especially after high doses and in patients with renal failure.

Serious bleeding resulting from prothrombin deficiency or platelet dysfunction has been reported with one of the second-generation cephalosporins, cefamandole, and with two of the four third-generation cephalosporins, cefoperazone and, especially, moxalactam. This hypoprothrombinemia occurred usually in elderly or debilitated patients with deficient vitamin K stores, and was promptly reversed by administration of vitamin K.

Patients taking cefamandole, moxalactam, and

cefoperazone have reported a disulfiram-like reaction when they ingested alcohol (see Chap. 53). Concurrent administration of bacteriostatic drugs may decrease the effectiveness of cephalosporins. Concurrent use of probenecid may cause toxic levels of the cephalosporin to accumulate, because the two drugs compete for renal tubular secretion sites. Concurrent use of nephrotoxic drugs (*e.g.*, aminoglycosides) will increase the chance of nephrotoxicity developing, as will concomitant use of the loop diuretics (See Chap. 27).

In summary, the cephalosporins are relatively safe and very effective against a wide variety of pathogenic bacteria, but they are the drugs of choice in only a few instances. Their use should be restricted to the treatment of infections resistant to older antibiotics, or to the treatment of susceptible infections in patients who cannot tolerate first-choice antibiotics. The patient teaching guide and guide to the nursing process with cephalosporins summarize the clinical application of the nursing process to cephalosporin drug therapy.

Patient teaching guide: the cephalosporins

The drug that has been prescribed for you belongs to the class of drugs called antibiotics. Your drug is called a cephalosporin. The cephalosporins work to destroy specific bacteria that are causing infections in the body. They are active only against specific bacteria; they are not useful in treating other bacterial or virus infections or "colds." Because of the way that the cephalosporins destroy bacteria, they have to be taken over a period of time to rid the body of the bacteria. It is very important to take *all* of your prescription to avoid recurrence of the infection. Your cephalosporin was prescribed to treat _____ .

Instructions:

1. The name of the drug ordered for you is _____ .

2. The dose of the drug ordered for you is _____ .

3. The drug should be taken _____ times a day. The best time to take your drug is _____ , _____ , _____ .

4. The drug can be taken with meals. If the drug causes an upset stomach, it is best to take it with food.

5. Some side-effects of the drug that you should be aware of include:

   Stomach upset | Take the drug with meals.

   Sore mouth or tongue | Perform frequent mouth care, avoid foods at extremes of temperature, and avoid spicy foods.

   Diarrhea | Stay near bathroom facilities for a few hours after taking the drug.

   Sensitivity to alcohol | Avoid the use of alcoholic beverages (when taking cefamandole, moxalactam, and cefoperazone).

6. Tell any physician, nurse, or dentist who takes care of you that you are taking this drug.

7. Keep this and all medications out of the reach of children.

(continued)

8. Do not use this medication to self-treat any other infection; do not give this medication to others or use similar medications borrowed from others.

9. Be sure to complete the full course of your prescription. Take all the prescription that has been ordered for you.

Notify your nurse or physician if any of the following occur:

Severe abdominal cramps or pain
Severe or bloody diarrhea
Rash or hives
Difficulty breathing
Unusual weakness, tiredness

Guide to the nursing process: the cephalosporins

Assessment	Nursing diagnosis	Interventions	Evaluation
Past history (*contraindications*): Renal failure Pregnancy Lactation *Allergies:* penicillin, cephalosporins, others; reactions Medication history: current drugs (*Cautions:* bacteriostatic agents, probenecid, nephrotoxic agents, loop diuretics, alcoholic beverages) **Physical assessment** General: infected area Respiratory: rate, adventitious sounds GI: bowel sounds, output, liver function Renal: urinalysis, BUN, electrolytes Skin: lesions	Potential alteration in bowel function Potential alteration in respiratory function Knowledge deficit regarding drug therapy	Culture infected area Preparation and safe administration of drug Patient teaching: Drug Dosage Administration Side-effects Warning signs Support and encouragement to comply with drug therapy	Monitor for effectiveness of drug: resolution of infection Monitor for adverse effects of drug (sensitivity reactions): GI reactions: colitis Liver function changes Renal function changes Superinfections Monitor drug–drug interactions: ↓ Effect with *bacteriostatic* drugs ↑ Toxicity with *probenecid* *Alcohol* intolerance Evaluate effectiveness of teaching program Evaluate effectiveness of support offered

---

The macrolide antibiotics: erythromycin and troleandomycin

Antimicrobial activity, therapeutic uses, toxicity

Erythromycin (E-Mycin; Erythrocin; Ilotycin) is an antibiotic of the macrolide class that exerts its antibacterial effect by interfering with the ability of microorganisms to biosynthesize protein (Table 8-5). Depending on the dose employed and the sensitivity of the infecting organism, it may be either bacteriostatic or bactericidal. It is used mainly in the management of patients who are hypersensitive to penicillin, which is usually the drug of choice in most infections for which erythromycin is employed. However, this antibiotic is effective against some microorganisms that are resistant to penicillins, including *Mycoplasma pneumoniae*, *Entamoeba histolytica*, and *Legionella pneumophila*, the organism that causes Legionnaires' disease. It is the drug of choice in treating Legionnaires' disease and is sometimes given with rifampin (see below) in this disease. It is also the drug of first choice for halting toxin production by *Corynebacterium* in patients with diptheria, and for prophylaxis against whooping cough in contacts of patients who are in the communicable stage of this disease. Erythromycin can also eliminate the *Bordetella* bacteria, which cause whooping cough, from the nasopharynx of infected patients, thus minimizing the likelihood of spread of the disease.

Erythromycin is similar to penicillin G in its effectiveness against the common gram-positive and gram-negative cocci. Thus it may, for example, be substituted in the long-term prevention of streptococcal pharyngitis in children with a history of rheumatic fever, or in the short-term prophylaxis against streptococcal endocarditis in similar patients before mouth and throat operations.

Other patients who are allergic to penicillin may receive erythromycin for the treatment of gonorrhea or primary syphilis. The soluble gluceptate or lactobionate salts may be administered by slow IV infusion (never by IV bolus injection) in treating pneumococcal pneumonia in this and other severe illnesses caused by organisms susceptible to erythromycin.

This antibiotic is most commonly administered by mouth before meals in buffered forms with acid-resistant coatings that protect it from being inactivated. The estolate ester and the ethylsuccinate form of erythromycin may be administered with meals because their absorption is unaffected, or even enhanced, by food.

The erythromycins are excreted in the bile. Patients with compromised liver function may need reduced dosage. Furthermore, the erythromycins, especially the estolate form, can cause hepatotoxicity, with or without jaundice. This distressing condition usually has its onset after about 2 weeks or so of treatment, with symptoms similar to those of a gallbladder attack. Such early symptoms as abdominal cramps, nausea, and vomiting, which precede the development of jaundice, should be promptly reported. The reaction seems to be a form of hypersensitivity resulting from sensitization to the drug. Overall, adverse reactions to erythromycin are uncommon. Other signs of toxicity reported include pseudomembranous colitis, reversible hearing loss, and psychiatric effects (uncontrollable crying, fear, and confusion). Nausea, vomiting, diarrhea, and abdominal cramps can occur after oral doses.

Troleandomycin (TAO) is an antibiotic that is similar to erythromycin. However, it is recommended for use only against bacterial strains that prove insensitive to the other agents. This is because of the drug's tendency to disrupt liver function and, occasionally, to cause cholestatic jaundice. This is not likely to occur, however, when the drug is used for no more than 10 days to 2 weeks, as in the treatment of β-hemolytic streptococcal infections. Large doses are employed for control of the rare case of acute gonococcal urethritis that fails to respond to treatment with ordinarily more effective and safer drugs.

Additional clinical considerations

The adverse effects of these drugs are relatively few. As with other antibiotics it is important to avoid hypersensitivity reactions by carefully screening the patient for the possibilities of allergic response. Sensitivity to tartrazine (often seen in patients with aspirin allergies) can cause an allergic response; it is used in the oral erythromycin preparation called Ethril '500'. Caution must also be used to screen for hepatic problems; patients on long-term therapy should undergo frequent liver function testing and physical assessment for any signs of liver failure. As with other antibiotics superinfection by resistant bacteria or fungi can occur. Patients should be warned of this possibility so that the antibiotic can be withdrawn or other appropriate therapy can be started. Both of these drugs are known to cross the placenta and are excreted in breast milk. The effects of these drugs on the developing fetus and on the infant are not known completely, but these drugs should be avoided if at all possible during pregnancy and lactation.

Drug–drug and drug–laboratory test interactions. Concurrent use of erythromycin or troleandomycin and *theophylline* can result in increased theophylline levels and in potential theophylline toxicity. The dose of theophylline will have to be lowered to achieve adequate response without toxicity. Use of erythromycin and *digoxin* can lead to increased blood levels of digoxin and to potential digoxin toxicity. The dosage of digoxin should be lowered during the concomitant therapy. Concurrent use of erythromycin and carbamazepine (*Tegretol*) can cause increased carbamazepine levels and therefore toxicity. Concurrent use of troleandomycin and *ergotamine drugs* has been reported to cause severe ischemic attacks, and the combination should be avoided. *Urinary catecholamines* cannot be accurately determined fluorometrically while a patient is on erythromycin.

The patient teaching guide and the guide to the nursing process with macrolide antibiotics summarize the clinical application of the nursing process to such drug therapy.

Patient teaching guide: the macrolide antibiotics

The drug that has been prescribed for you belongs to a family of drugs called the macrolide antibiotics. These drugs destroy specific bacteria and do not work against any other bacteria, viruses, or "cold" germs. Because of the way that these drugs work, they must be taken over a period of time. It is very important to complete the full course of your prescription to prevent a recurrence of the infection. Your antibiotic was prescribed to treat _____ .

Instructions:

1. The name of the drug ordered for you is _____ .

2. The dose of the drug ordered for you is _____ .

3. The drug should be taken _____ times a day. It is best to take the drug throughout the day so that it can work continually. The best times to take your drug are _____ , _____ , _____ .

4. The drug (if an erythromycin) should be taken with food (erythromycin estolate or ethyl succinate), or on an empty stomach (other erythromycins), and with a full glass of water, *not* fruit juice. This will decrease the stomach upset that the drug can cause. (If troleandomycin is used, the drug should be taken on an empty stomach—1 hour before or 2 hours after meals).

5. Some side-effects of the drug that you should be aware of include:

Stomach upset, cramping Mild diarrhea Mild nausea	Taking the drug with food, if appropriate will help. None of these side-effects should continue after the course of drug therapy is over.

6. Tell any physician, nurse, or dentist who is taking care of you that you are taking this drug.

7. Keep this and all medications out of reach of children.

8. Do not use this medication to self-treat any other infection; do not give this medication to others or use similar medications borrowed from others.

9. Be sure to complete the full course of your prescription. Take all the prescription that has been ordered for you.

Notify your nurse or physician if any of the following occur:

Severe or watery diarrhea
Severe nausea or vomiting
Abdominal pain
Dark-colored urine
Yellowing of skin or eyes
Skin rash or itching

Guide to the nursing process: the macrolide antibiotics

Assessment	Nursing diagnosis	Interventions	Evaluation
Past history (*contraindications*): Hepatic failure Pregnancy Lactation *Allergies:* erythromycin, tartrazine, others; reactions Medication history: current drugs (*Cautions:* theophylline, digoxin, carbamazepine, ergotamines) **Physical assessment** General: site of infection Respiratory: rate, adventitious sounds GI: bowel sounds, output, liver function Renal: urinalysis Skin: color, lesions	Potential alteration in comfort (GI upset) Potential alteration in bowel function Potential alteration in respiratory function Knowledge deficit regarding drug therapy	Culture infected area Preparation and safe administration of drug Patient Teaching: Drug Dosage Administration Side-effects Warning signs Support and encouragement to comply with drug therapy	Monitor for effectiveness of drug: resolution of infection Monitor for adverse effects of drug (sensitivity reactions): GI upset Change in liver function Jaundice Superinfections Monitor for drug–drug interactions: Toxicity of *theophylline* Toxicity of *digoxin* Toxicity of *carbamazepine* Severe ischemic attacks with *ergotamines* Inaccurate urine catecholamine test results Evaluate effectiveness of teaching program Evaluate effectiveness of support offered

Clindamycin and lincomycin

Antimicrobial spectrum and therapeutic uses

These chemically related antibiotics are effective against the same gram-positive cocci as penicillin and so they have been used for treating patients allergic to penicillin who have infections caused by streptococci, pneumococci, and susceptible staphylococci. They exert bacteriostatic or bactericidal effects by inhibiting bacterial protein synthesis. However, because of their potential toxicity, they are not a first choice for any infection, and erythromycin is preferred for treating most penicillin-sensitive patients. These drugs are best reserved for treatment of infections by microorganisms that are relatively resistant to other antimicrobial agents, including methicillin-resistant staphylococci.

These antibiotics are particularly effective for treating infections by anaerobic bacteria, including *Bacteroides fragilis,* a gram-negative bacillus that is resistant

to penicillin. Organisms of this type sometimes cause peritonitis and abscesses when they spill into the abdominal cavity following rupture of the appendix or other visceral organs. They are involved in postpartum and postabortal sepsis and in other infections of the female pelvis and genital tract. Anaerobes entering the bloodstream from such tissue sources can cause septicemic infections with a high mortality rate.

In all such situations, *clindamycin* (Cleocin) is employed only after the causative organism has been identified by special bacteriologic studies and has been shown to be highly sensitive to this antibiotic (Table 8-5). It is not, for example, effective against such organisms as *Streptococcus faecalis* (enterococcus), or against the gram-negative cocci that cause gonorrhea and meningitis. Clindamycin and lincomycin (Lincocin) should not be used, in any case, for treating meningitis even when the infecting organism is sensitive to them, because they diffuse poorly into the cerebrospinal fluid as compared to other available antibiotics. For example, even though clinda-mycin is effective against *Bacteroides,* chloramphenicol is preferred for treating brain abscesses or meningitis caused by this anaerobic species.

Adverse effects

Clindamycin was introduced with the claim that it caused diarrhea less frequently than its parent compound, lin-comycin. This may be true, but the incidence of adverse gastrointestinal effects has been high enough to limit the use of clindamycin mainly to the relatively few types of infections in which the bacteria are not sensitive to safer antibiotics, such as penicillin, erythromycin, or the tet-racyclines. The most serious complication has been drug-induced bowel damage resembling the condition called pseudomembranous colitis. The incidence of colitis has not been high, but death has occurred in some cases. It is believed to be caused by an enterotoxin produced by antibiotic-resistant strains of *Clostridium.*

Patients who develop persistent diarrhea (five or more movements daily) should not continue to be treated with clindamycin, particularly if blood or mucus is seen in the stool. Diarrhea may continue for weeks after the drug is discontinued but yet it should not be treated with diphenoxylate (Lomotil), paregoric, or other antiperis-taltic agents, because such treatment tends to prolong the colitislike condition or make it worse. Corticosteroid drugs administered by retention enema or by mouth may help to suppress the drug-induced colon inflammation. Vancomycin (see below) has been lifesaving in patients with antibiotic-induced colitis caused by *Clostridium difficile.*

In summary, the potential toxicity of clindamycin and lincomycin limits their clinical usefulness in com-parison to other antibiotics effective against the same bac-teria. However, these antibiotics can be lifesaving in severe infections caused by bacteria resistant to other anti-in-fective agents—particularly anaerobes such as *Bacteroides fragilis* and methicillin-resistant staphylococcal strains. Some believe that lincomycin should never be used be-cause of its dangerous toxicity, and because clindamycin is more active and somewhat less toxic.

The clinical use of these drugs involves many of the problems and cautions of other antibiotics. Because these drugs are so toxic, whenever they are used, the manufacturer's insert should be consulted before use and complete support equipment should be available.

Miscellaneous alternatives

Spectinomycin

Spectinomycin (Trobicin) inhibits protein synthesis in sus-ceptible gram-negative bacteria, including *Neisseria gon-orrhoeae.* It is used in single-dose treatment of urogenital and anal gonorrhea in men and women who are allergic to penicillin, or who have infections caused by penicillin-resistant strains of *N. gonorrhoeae.* Few adverse reactions occur with the single-dose therapy.

Vancomycin: special uses and toxicity

Vancomycin (Vancocin) is an antibiotic that has occasionally proved lifesaving when injected by vein in penicillin-sen-sitive patients who were seriously ill with severe staph-ylococcal pneumonia, septicemia, or other infections re-sistant to safer drugs. It has been used in the treatment and prevention of bacterial endocarditis in patients al-lergic to penicillin.

Although it is not absorbed when taken orally, it is administered by mouth for its local effects in treating staphylococcal enterocolitis. Streptococci of the entero-coccal group are also sometimes sensitive to vancomycin. As mentioned above, it has been lifesaving in patients with antibiotic-related pseudomembranous colitis caused by *Clostridium* species. Its antibacterial action is a result of its interference with bacterial cell wall synthesis.

Vancomycin is very irritating and must be well diluted to minimize thrombophlebitis. Kidney function must be monitored because this drug is nephrotoxic and is cleared from the body mainly by renal excretion. It should not be administered to patients with poor kidney function because its accumulation in the blood and in auditory nerve tissue can cause deafness, particularly in patients with some previous loss of hearing.

In summary, this toxic antibiotic is reserved mainly for treating serious gram-positive coccal infections caused by pathogenic strains more sensitive to it than to other safer agents, or when the patient is allergic to penicillin and to other more effective and less toxic antibiotics. It should not be given with other neurotoxic or nephrotoxic antibiotics (*e.g.,* cephalosporins and aminoglycosides; see below).

Infrequently used alternatives

Novobiocin (Albamycin) is another drug effective against the common gram-positive organisms. It is rarely em-ployed, however, because it causes more side-effects than most of the other penicillin substitutes, and it has a very narrow antibacterial spectrum. Many believe it has no rational place in drug therapy.

The tetracyclines

History and development

The success of penicillin and streptomycin (an amino-glycoside antibiotic; see below), the first clinically available antibiotics, sent scientists back to the soil in a search for other natural substances with antibiotic activity. Two such substances, *chlortetracycline* (Aureomycin; now available only for topical use; see Chap. 43) and *oxytetracycline* (Ter-ramycin) were isolated from molds found in soil samples.

Table 8–6. The tetracyclines and chloramphenicol

Generic or official name	Trade name	Route of administration	Usual adult dosage
Tetracyclines			
Demeclocycline HCl USP	Declomycin	Oral	600 mg/day, in divided doses, bid or qid
Doxycycline hyclate, USP and doxycycline monohydrate	Doxychel; Vibramycin	IV, oral	200 mg (100 mg, q 12 hr) on the first day, followed by 100 mg/day as single dose, or as 50 mg, q 12 hr
Methacycline HCl USP	Rondomycin	Oral	600 mg/day, bid or qid
Minocycline HCl USP.	Minocin	IV, oral	200 mg initially, followed by 100 mg every 12 hr
Oxytetracycline HCl USP	Oxamycin; Terramycin	IM, IV, oral	250 mg once a day, IM; 250 mg–500 mg, q 12 hr, IV; or 1 g–2 g/day, in divided doses, bid or qid
Tetracycline HCl USP	Achromycin; Panmycin; SK-Tetracycline; Sumycin; Tetracyn	IM, IV, oral	250 mg once a day, IM; 250 mg–500 mg bid, IV; or 1–2 g/day, in divided doses, bid or qid oral
Tetracycline phosphate complex USP	Tetrex	Oral	1 g–2 g/day, in divided doses, bid or qid
Chloramphenicol preparations			
Chloramphenicol USP	Chloromycetin; Mychel	Oral	50–100 mg/kg/day, in divided doses, q 6 hr
Chloramphenicol palmitate USP	Chloromycetin Palmitate	Oral	50–100 mg/kg/day, in divided doses, q 6 hr
Chloramphenicol sodium succinate USP	Chloromycetin Sodium Succinate; Mychel-S	IV	50–100 mg/kg/day, in divided doses, q 6 hr

Intensive study of the molecular structure of these natural antibiotics and of the structure–activity relationships of similar molecules led to the development of *tetracycline*[+] (Achromycin) and other semisynthetic derivatives (Table 8-6). These antibiotics possessed a much broader spectrum of antimicrobial activity than those discovered earlier. They proved active not only against bacteria of both gram-positive and gram-negative types, but also against such microorganisms as rickettsia, mycoplasma, and chlamydia, the etiologic agents of various diseases that resist treatment with other antibiotics (see Table 8-7). The tetracyclines are bacteriostatic and act by inhibiting protein synthesis in sensitive bacteria.

The most recently introduced drugs of this class, *doxycycline*[+] (Vibramycin) and *minocycline* (Minocin) are the result of research aimed at developing derivatives that would be more rapidly and completely absorbed, penetrate more readily into infected tissues, and remain there to exert an antibacterial effect for longer periods. Another research objective, the development of new tetracycline-type antibiotics that would be active against tetracycline-resistant bacteria, does *not* seem to have been attained despite such claims that have been made for minocycline.

Pharmacokinetics

The tetracyclines are well absorbed after oral administration, but food, iron preparations, and antacids containing divalent and trivalent cations (Ca^{2+}, Mg^{2+}, and A^{3+} salts) can interfere with their absorption. Food interferes little with the absorption of doxycycline and minocycline, and they are usually given with food to reduce gastric irritation.

Table 8–7. Antimicrobial spectrum of the tetracyclines*

Gram-positive cocci

Streptococcus (anaerobic type)
Streptococcus pyogenes (group A β-hemolytic type)
Streptococcus viridans (α-hemolytic type)
Streptococcus faecalis (enterococcus group)
Staphylococcus aureus
Streptococcus (Diplococcus) pneumoniae

Gram-negative cocci

Gonococcus (*Neisseria gonorrhoeae*)
Meningococcus (*Neisseria meningitidis*)

Gram-positive bacilli

Bacillus anthracis
Clostridium tetani
Listeria monocytogenes

Gram-negative bacilli

Escherichia coli
Enterobacter (Aerobacter) aerogenes
Hemophilus influenzae
H. ducreyi (chanchroid)
Bordetella (Hemophilus) pertussis (whooping cough)
Calymmatobacterium granulomatis (granuloma inguinale)
Klebsiella pneumoniae
Shigella species
Yersinia (Pasteurella) pestis (bubonic plague)
Brucella species (brucellosis)

Bacteroides species (lung and other abscesses; bacteremia)
Leptothrix buccalis (Vincent's infection)
Vibrio cholerae (comma) (cholera)

Spirochetes

Treponema pallidum (syphilis)
Treponema pertenue (yaws)
Borrelia recurrentis (relapsing fever)

Rickettsia

Species responsible for typhus, murine typhus, scrub typhus, tick typhus, Rocky Mountain spotted fever, Q fever, and other infections

Chlamydia

Agents responsible for psittacosis, lymphogranuloma venereum, trachoma, and inclusion conjunctivitis

Mycoplasma

Mycoplasma pneumoniae (Eaton agent; PPLO; the agent responsible for primary atypical "viral" pneumonia)
Mycoplasma hominus (*e.g.*, nonspecific urethritis)

Actinomyces

Actinomyces israeli and *A. bovis*—the causes of actinomycosis

* Although infections caused by these and other organisms are often responsive to treatment with the broad-spectrum antibiotics of this class, many strains have become resistant to the tetracyclines. Thus, these drugs are indicated for treating clinical infections by these pathogens only after the results of culturing and bacteriologic testing indicate that the responsible organism is sensitive to them.

The tetracyclines are generally concentrated in the bile and are excreted unchanged in the urine and feces. Tetracyclines should generally not be given to anuric patients, and the dosage should be reduced in patients with decreased renal function to avoid accumulation of the drug. Doxycycline is an exception: it is inactivated and secreted into the intestinal lumen for elimination with the feces.

Doxycycline and minocycline are the most highly lipid-soluble and, of all the tetracyclines, penetrate best into such structures as the brain and the eye; oxytetracycline is the least lipid-soluble. These drugs readily cross the placenta and are excreted in the milk of lactating women. They have an affinity for developing teeth and bones and are contraindicated in the last two trimesters of pregnancy and in children under 8 years of age (see Adverse Effects, below).

Therapeutic uses
Despite their wide range of antimicrobial activity, relatively low toxicity, and effectiveness when taken orally, the tetracyclines are today only rarely the best antibiotic for treating most of the common bacterial infections. More important in this regard than the fact that they are bacteriostatic rather than bactericidal are problems related to the emergence of tetracycline-resistant bacteria.

Thus, for example, a high proportion of streptococcal strains are now resistant, as are an increasing number of pneumococci and other gram-positive organisms. Although minocycline is said to be more active against staphylococci resistant to other tetracyclines in laboratory studies, this has not been proved true in the treatment of clinical infections.

Respiratory infections. Drugs of this class can be used for treating infections by the common gram-positive cocci, particularly in patients who are hypersensitive to penicillin. However, the infecting microorganism must be shown by laboratory bacteriologic testing to be susceptible to treatment with tetracyclines. Other antibiotics are now usually preferred for treating streptococcal pharyngitis, pneumococcal pneumonia, and other respiratory tract infections. The tetracyclines are still recommended for prophylaxis against acute respiratory infections in patients with chronic bronchitis and other obstructive lung diseases. However, the prolonged use of these broad-spectrum antibiotics in such patients may lead to the emergence of resistant microorganisms, some of which—such as fungi—may become invasive and cause possibly fatal superinfections (see Adverse Effects, below).

The tetracyclines are, however, more effective than most other antibiotics for treating respiratory infection caused by *Mycoplasma pneumoniae*, the microorganism responsible for so-called primary atypical, or "viral," pneumonia. This organism is not a true virus, and neither the tetracyclines nor any other antibiotics now available are active against the viruses that are responsible for very many respiratory infections. Thus, these anti-infective agents should not be taken indiscriminately for treating trivial colds or influenza uncomplicated by secondary bacterial infections.

Urinary tract and venereal infections. The tetracyclines are less active than they once were against strains of common gram-negative uropathogens such as *E. coli.* They should not be employed until the infective organism isolated from the urine has been shown to be sensitive to tetracyclines. These drugs may then be useful for treating ampicillin-sensitive patients with acute or chronic UTI, such as cystitis and pyelonephritis.

Antibiotics of this class are also useful alternatives to penicillin for treating gonorrhea and syphilis. The newer agents *doxycycline* and *minocycline* are said to be effective in acute gonorrheal infection following administration of a single oral dose. However, treatment for several days followed by posttreatment cultures provides more certain control. Similarly, in syphilis, daily dosage is best continued for 10 days to 2 weeks in patients who do not tolerate penicillin.

The tetracyclines are also effective against other pathogens responsible for venereal diseases, including the gram-negative bacilli that cause chancroid and granuloma inguinale. Another venereal infection, lymphogranuloma venereum, also responds to tetracycline treatment, which is more effective for this disease than any other antibiotic when administered alone or with sulfonamide drugs. (The causative organism is an agent of a group that was once referred to as "large viruses" but is now called chlamydiae.) Tetracyclines are also highly active against the chlamydiae responsible for such diseases as psittacosis, or parrot fever, and the chronic eye infections trachoma and inclusion conjunctivitis.

Rickettsial diseases. Rocky Mountain spotted fever is remarkably responsive to treatment with tetracyclines. The rickettsiostatic effect of these antibiotics also makes them very useful for treating typhus-type infections. These dangerous diseases are best treated promptly with high doses of doxycycline or other tetracyclines, administered preferably by a parenteral route at first. In most patients who are treated early enough, fever and other symptoms are relieved within 2 or 3 days, but treatment with oral tetracyclines is continued for a few days after temperature becomes normal.

Bacillary infections. The tetracyclines are still considered among the most effective agents for treating such bacillary infections as brucellosis and cholera, even though the emergence of resistant strains of other gram-negative rods has reduced their effectiveness in other infections caused by organisms of this type.

Other uses. Demeclocycline has been used to manage a syndrome of inappropriate secretion of antidiuretic hormone (ADH). Doxycycline has been used to prevent "traveler's diarrhea." The use of tetracyclines in the management of amebiasis, acne, and ocular infections is discussed elsewhere (see Index).

Adverse effects

The tetracyclines are relatively safe antibiotics. However, they can cause a wide range of reactions that are the result of local irritation, hypersensitivity, or overgrowths of nonsusceptible organisms (superinfections). In some circumstances severe systemic toxicity can occur, particularly in patients whose impaired kidney function permits accumulation of the drugs of this class that require renal secretion.

Gastrointestinal irritation. The most common complaint of some patients after the first few oral doses is abdominal discomfort with nausea, vomiting, and sometimes diarrhea. Symptoms of this type are sometimes said to occur less often with the newer tetracyclines that are administered in smaller daily doses than the prototypes of this class. Another advantage claimed for doxycycline and minocycline is that to allay gastric distress they can be given with milk and a snack without interfering with their absorption. (Taking most tetracyclines with milk or other dairy products containing calcium is considered undesirable because the antibiotic may be bound into an unabsorbable form.) However, antacids containing large amounts of aluminum, magnesium, or calcium should not be employed, because these medications do impair absorption of all oral tetracyclines.

Effects on developing teeth and bones. Tetracyclines tend to be tied up with calcium in bones and teeth. The chemical term for this reaction is *chelation.* The deposition of tetracyclines in developing teeth can cause permanent discoloration and interfere with normal calcification. The yellow, brown, or gray stain occurs most commonly when babies have been given tetracycline during development of the first teeth. Women treated with tetracyclines during pregnancy may bear children whose teeth erupt discolored. Ordinarily only the deciduous teeth are affected, but long-term treatment with large doses during early childhood may lead to discoloration of the permanent teeth also. Similar tetracycline deposits in the bone-forming tissues may retard the rate of fetal skeletal system development or may slow bone growth in young children temporarily. Thus, the prolonged or repeated use of tetracyclines in such patients should be avoided.

Skin reactions. Various types of eruptions including urticaria, angioedema, and measleslike rashes have occurred as a result of hypersensitivity to tetracycline, but reactions of this type are less common than with the penicillins. Photosensitivity may develop in patients taking *demeclocycline* and other tetracyclines but not, so far, with *minocycline.* However, patients taking *any* of these drugs should be advised to keep covered or to stay out of direct sunlight. If skin redness begins to develop, the drug should be discontinued to avoid development of more severe signs and symptoms of sunburn. Patients with a history of photosensitivity are most likely to have such phototoxic reactions.

Hypersensitivity reactions. In addition to skin rashes and hives, the tetracyclines have caused anaphylaxis and serum sickness-like reactions. An unusual manifestation of hypersensitivity is elevated intracranial pressure with headache, vomiting, and visual disturbances.

Direct tissue toxicity. The tetracyclines can cause fatty degeneration of the liver when administered in large doses, especially in patients whose kidneys are not functioning properly. Fatalities have been reported in pregnant women who received 3 to 6 g parenterally for severe infections. Failure to excrete repeated doses of the antibiotic led to its accumulation in the liver in hepatotoxic quantities. It is now suggested that patients with renal impairment receive only a fraction of the full therapeutic dose, and that the levels of tetracycline in the plasma of patients on prolonged high doses be determined periodically.

An unusual, but reversible, reaction resembling Fanconi's syndrome has been reported. The signs and symptoms, which stem mainly from impairment of kidney tubule function, include acidosis, aminoaciduria, proteinuria, and glycosuria. The patient's illness has been traced to tetracycline products that were outdated or degraded as a result of improper storage. The nurse who is administering tetracyclines should thus be especially careful to check the expiration date. It is important on receiving tetracycline products from the pharmacy both to be sure that the package expiration date has not passed and to store the container where its contents will not be subjected to excessively high heat and humidity.

Minocycline has caused vestibular disturbances and demeclocycline has caused nephrogenic diabetes insipidus, neither of which is typical of the side effects of tetracyclines as a group.

Superinfections. Overgrowths with organisms resistant to tetracyclines occur more commonly than with narrow-spectrum antibiotics such as penicillin G. Diarrhea that develops during the later days of treatment may be caused, not by direct drug-induced irritation, but by an overgrowth of staphylococci following suppression of the other intestinal organisms by the broad-spectrum antibiotic. Staphylococcal enterocolitis caused by the emergence of tetracycline-resistant staph may be marked by mild diarrhea or by much more severe symptoms. Severe diarrhea may also be a manifestation of pseudomembranous colitis, the sometimes fatal condition caused by antibiotic-resistant strains of *Clostridium difficile.*

Whenever severe diarrhea occurs during therapy with a tetracycline, the drug should be discontinued and the patient's fluid–electrolyte status determined. Fluid–electrolyte imbalance should be corrected. Oral administration of the antibiotic *vancomycin* is effective therapy for both staphylococcal enterocolitis and pseudomembranous colitis caused by clostridia (see above). Patients diagnosed as having staphylococcal enterocolitis, whose staphylococcal infection has spread systemically, may also require treatment with a penicillinase-resistant penicillin such as *methicillin* or *nafcillin,* if the organism is sensitive to one of these drugs.

Overgrowths of the yeastlike fungal organism, *Candida albicans,* may occur not only in the intestine but also on the skin and on the mucous surfaces of the mouth and vagina. Some tetracycline products contain small amounts of antifungal antibiotics such as amphotericin and nystatin for prophylaxis against the development of intestinal moniliasis. It is doubtful, however, that such combinations are effective for preventing monilial diarrhea. Rather than using these drugs routinely for prophylactic purposes, it is preferable to employ them by oral administration in the relatively few cases in which a broad-spectrum antibiotic actually induces symptoms of intestinal candidiasis.

The addition of the poorly absorbed antifungal drugs to oral tetracycline products will not prevent candidal organisms from causing inflammatory superinfections of the mouth, anus, or vagina of susceptible patients. (Candidiasis during antibiotic therapy is most likely to occur in diabetic or debilitated patients, during pregnancy, and during corticosteroid drug therapy.) However, if drug-induced anal or vulvovaginal pruritus actually occurs, these antifungal antibiotics may be applied topically in the form of creams, ointments, powders, or vaginal tablets (see Chap. 43). Washing the perineum several times daily is also said to reduce antibiotic drug-induced anogenital pruritus.

In summary, the tetracyclines are antibiotics of relatively low toxicity and broad antibacterial spectrum. Because of the emergence of resistant strains of gram-positive cocci and gram-negative bacilli, the tetracyclines are not now the antibiotics of choice for initiating treatment of most common respiratory or urinary tract infections. However, if tests indicate that the infecting bacterial strain is sensitive to tetracyclines, these drugs can be effectively employed, particularly in patients allergic to ampicillin and other penicillins. The tetracyclines are still the drugs of choice for treating many rickettsial, mycoplasmal, and chlamydial infections, and some bacillary infections.

Additional clinical considerations

To re-emphasize, the use of tetracyclines during pregnancy, lactation, or early childhood is contraindicated because of their effects on developing teeth and bones. Although the hypersensitivity reactions to tetracyclines are not as frequent as reactions to the penicillins, care should be taken to avoid the possibility of an allergic response through careful patient screening. Tartrazine

is used in the preparation of some tetracyclines (certain oral preparations—*e.g.,* Panmycin) and patients with known allergy to tartrazine or aspirin should be given a different preparation.

Drug–drug interactions. The tetracyclines increase the bioavailability of *digoxin* if both drugs are given together. The effect may last for months after the tetracycline has been stopped. Because of this, if tetracycline is given to a patient on digoxin, the digoxin dose will need to be decreased and the patient evaluated over a long period of time for effectiveness of digoxin. *Barbiturates, carbamazepine,* and *phenytoin* increase the metabolism of doxycycline by hepatic enzymes. If doxycycline is given to a patient on one of these drugs, the dosage will need to be increased. The general anesthetic *methoxyflurane* is more likely to cause renal toxicity in a patient on tetracycline; anesthesia with methoxyflurane should be avoided. *Antacids* and *iron preparations* inhibit tetracycline absorption and decrease its effectiveness. Concomitant use of tetracyclines and *oral contraceptives* can decrease the effectiveness of the steroid preparation and lead to breakthrough bleeding or to unwanted pregnancy. Tetracyclines depress prothrombin activity in the body, so if a patient is also on *oral anticoagulants* the dose will need to be decreased to avoid possible bleeding. Concurrent use of *theophylline* and tetracycline may increase the incidence of adverse GI effects relative to those caused by either drug alone.

The patient teaching guide and guide to the use of the nursing process with tetracyclines summarize the clinical application of the nursing process to tetracycline therapy.

Patient teaching guide: the tetracyclines

The drug that has been prescribed for you is an antibiotic of the family of tetracyclines. These drugs work to destroy bacteria that are causing infections in the body. They are active against specific bacteria and do not destroy other bacteria, viruses, or "cold" germs. Because of the way that these drugs work, they must be taken over a period of time. It is very important to complete the full course of your prescription to prevent a recurrence of the infection. Your antibiotic has been prescribed to treat _____ .

Instructions:

1. The name of the drug ordered for you is _____ .

2. The dosage of the drug ordered for you is _____ .

3. The drug must be taken _____ times a day. It is best to take the drug throughout the day so that it can work continually. The best times to take your drug are _____ , _____ , _____ .

(continued)

4. The drug should be taken on an empty stomach, at least 1 hour before or 2 hours after meals. Never take the drug with milk or milk products, iron preparations, or any type of antacid. It is best to take the drug with a full glass of water. (Doxycycline and minocycline may be taken with food or milk.)

5. *Never* take any outdated tetracycline product. Finish your prescription as ordered. If any old tetracycline is found, destroy it immediately. If you are on prolonged tetracycline therapy, store your drug supply in a cool dry place.

6. Some side-effects of the drug that you should be aware of include:

Stomach upset, burning, nausea	These will pass when the course of drug therapy is finished.
Superinfections: monilial infections of mouth, vagina	Frequent washing of these areas will help; medication is available.
Sensitivity of the skin to sunlight	Wear protective clothing and avoid prolonged exposure to the sun while on this drug.
Dizziness or lightheadedness	Take extra care when changing positions; do not drive or operate dangerous machinery if you experience these effects.

7. Tell any physician, nurse, or dentist who is taking care of you that you are taking this drug.

8. Keep this and all medications out of the reach of children.

9. Do not use this medication to self-treat any other infection; do not give this medication to others and do not use similar medications borrowed from others.

10. Be sure to complete the full course of your prescription. Take all the prescription that has been ordered for you.

Notify your nurse or physician if any of the following occur:

Severe cramps, vomiting
Severe or watery diarrhea
Rash or itching
Difficulty breathing
Extreme thirst or frequent and copious urination
Dark urine or light-colored stools
Yellowing of skin or eyes

Guide to the nursing process: the tetracyclines

Assessment	Nursing diagnosis	Interventions	Evaluation
Past history (*contraindications*): Renal failure Pregnancy Lactation *Allergies:* tetracyclines, tartrazine, others; reactions Medication history: current drugs (*Cautions:* digoxin, barbiturates, carbamazepine, phenytoin, methoxyflurane, oral contraceptives, oral anticoagulants, theophylline, antacids) **Physical Assessment** General: site of infection Respiratory: rate, adventitious sounds GI: bowel sounds, output, liver function Renal: urinalysis, BUN Skin: color, lesions	Potential alteration in comfort (GI upset) Potential alteration in bowel function Potential alteration in respiratory function Potential alteration in skin integrity Knowledge deficit regarding drug therapy	Culture infected area Preparation and safe administration of drug: No outdated drugs No drugs given with milk products, antacids, foods Patient teaching regarding: Drug Dosage Administration Side-effects Warning signs Comfort measures: Protection from sunlight Frequent hygiene of vaginal or oral areas if superinfections occur Encourage to comply with drug therapy	Monitor for effectiveness of drug: resolution of infection Monitor for adverse effects of drug: Sensitivities GI reactions Photosensitivity Superinfections Liver changes BUN ↑ Monitor for drug–drug interactions: Toxicity of *digoxin* Failure of *oral contraceptives* ↑ effects of *oral anticoagulants* ↓ tetracycline effectiveness with: *antacids, barbiturates, phenytoin, carbamazepine, iron preparations* Renal toxicity with *methoxyflurane* GI toxicity with *theophylline* Evaluate effectiveness of patient teaching measures Evaluate effectiveness of comfort and support measures

Chloramphenicol

Current status

Chloramphenicol[+] (Chloromycetin), a drug introduced in 1948—the same year as tetracycline—has an antimicrobial spectrum as broad as that of the tetracyclines (Table 8-6). In practice, however, its clinical usefulness is limited by its potentially lethal toxicity. It is recommended for use only when bacteriologic tests indicate that it is the most active antimicrobial drug available against the in- fecting organism. In such cases it should be employed with frequent blood studies to detect early signs of bone marrow depression, and it should be discontinued as soon as laboratory or clinical signs of toxicity occur. When reserved for treating serious infections for which it is obviously the best drug available and when used in ac- cordance with recommended guidelines, chloramphenicol can be a very valuable drug with relatively few adverse effects in the vast majority of patients. Chloramphenicol is bacteriostatic. It inhibits the growth of susceptible strains of bacteria by preventing protein synthesis.

Pharmacokinetics

Chloramphenicol is readily absorbed after oral administration and is widely distributed in the body, penetrating the brain even in the absence of inflammation of the meninges. It also crosses the placenta and enters breast milk.

The drug is metabolically inactivated in the liver by enzymes that are not developed in neonates at birth (see Adverse Effects, below). The metabolites and a small amount of the unchanged parent drug are excreted in the urine. Patients with compromised liver function need a reduced dosage to prevent toxic drug accumulation.

Therapeutic uses

Salmonella infections. Chloramphenicol is considered the drug of choice for control of acute symptoms of typhoid fever and of other systemic salmonelloses. However, here, as in all other infections in which this drug is used, the infecting strain must be isolated and shown to be sensitive to chloramphenicol. In fact, chloramphenicol must be shown to be more active than ampicillin and other safer drugs. Administered orally or by vein to patients with salmonella bacteremia, this drug causes rapid disappearance of the pathogen from the blood. The patient's temperature becomes normal within a few days, although intestinal symptoms may continue for a longer period. Ampicillin is preferred for treating typhoid carriers.

Meningitis. Chloramphenicol is an excellent alternative to penicillins in patients allergic to penicillin G or to ampicillin. It is effective against the organisms most commonly responsible for meningitis, including *Hemophilus influenzae*, as well as against less frequently encountered pathogens such as *Klebsiella* and *Listeria* species. This drug has the additional advantage of diffusing readily into the cerebrospinal fluid. However, in patients who are *not* allergic to penicillin and in whom the infecting organism is sensitive to penicillin G or to ampicillin, the chloramphenicol with which treatment may have been begun is withdrawn and further therapy is continued with the safer antibiotic.

Anaerobic bacterial infections. Chloramphenicol is one of the few antimicrobials effective against *Bacteroides fragilis* and other enteric anaerobes. It may be lifesaving in peritonitis, postabortal sepsis, and septicemia caused by these organisms. However, if the infecting organism also proves sensitive to clindamycin, that somewhat safer antibiotic should be employed.

Rickettsial and chlamydial infections. Chloramphenicol is active against the organisms that cause typhus-type infections and those of the lymphogranuloma–psittacosis group. Thus it is an effective alternative to the tetracyclines in patients who cannot tolerate the ordinarily safer antibiotics of that class. It is, for example, the preferred drug for pregnant women with poor kidney function who may not excrete tetracyclines and so run the risk of liver damage by drugs of that broad-spectrum class.

Miscellaneous infections. Chloramphenicol is among the desirable alternatives to drugs of choice for treating many serious infections by gram-negative bacilli. Among the diseases in which it may be lifesaving when the infecting strain is resistant to the ordinarily more effective drug or when the ordinarily safer drug is not well tolerated are tularemia, brucellosis, bubonic plague, cholera, and melioidosis.

In cases of acute pyelonephritis caused by strains of bacilli resistant to safer antibiotics, chloramphenicol may also prove lifesaving. A special advantage here is that this drug can be given to patients with impaired renal function without danger that it will accumulate to toxic levels. The reason for this is that, although free active chloramphenicol is excreted by the kidneys, the drug does not depend on the renal route for elimination because it is mainly inactivated by liver enzymes.

Adverse effects

Blood dyscrasias. The main danger with this drug is that it can cause bone marrow depression. The most common symptom of this is anemia marked by a reduction in reticulocytes, the precursors of red blood cells. The reticulocytopenia that develops during treatment is related to the amount of drug administered. This condition is reversible in about 2 weeks after the drug is discontinued. Thus, blood studies are done at 2-day intervals during therapy to detect reticulocytopenia, changes in early erythroid cell forms, anemia, leukopenia, and thrombocytopenia.

A second type of bone marrow disorder induced by this drug is much more serious because it can result in an irreversible depression of the ability to produce all types of blood cells—pancytopenia, or aplastic anemia. This blood dyscrasia is not dose-related, and it may develop weeks or months after even a short course of chloramphenicol therapy. Thus, though blood studies are done during the treatment period, these do not necessarily help to detect this disorder, and withdrawal of the drug may not help to prevent bone marrow hypoplasia or aplasia.

Fortunately, this usually fatal form occurs only in a small proportion of patients treated with chloramphenicol—estimates range from about 1 in 25,000 to 1 in 40,000 patients treated. Thus, the risk of using this drug for treating a serious infection for which it appears to be the best choice is outweighed for most seriously ill patients by the benefits of treatment, which are often dramatic. On the other hand, chloramphenicol must never be used—as it once was—for treating trivial infections such as the common cold. This antibiotic is, like all others, not active against viruses, and is thus worthless against viral respiratory infections, including influenza. It should also not be used to treat or prevent primary or secondary bacterial infections of the throat such as streptococcal pharyngitis, for which penicillin is so safe and effective and for which so many safer alternatives to penicillin are available.

Gray baby syndrome. Toxicity of another type has been observed in premature infants and in other newborns who required chloramphenicol treatment for severe infections developing shortly after birth. This condition has been called the "gray syndrome" because the babies often became cyanotic and ashen gray in color. This drug-induced syndrome is characterized by abdominal distention, diarrhea, respiratory irregularities, and peripheral vascular collapse.

This severe illness, which has a high mortality rate, is believed to result from the newborn infant's inability to detoxify and eliminate chloramphenicol. That is, newborn infants, particularly those born prematurely, do not possess the liver enzyme mechanisms for converting chloramphenicol to an inactive compound that can readily be excreted by the kidneys. As a result, if infants are given ordinary doses calculated on a weight basis, the drug accumulates in the tissues and reaches toxic levels. Thus, all premature babies and full-term infants under 2 weeks old should receive only half the usual dose (see Drug Digest) and should be observed very closely during all treatment with chloramphenicol so that the drug may be withdrawn in favor of another active antibiotic at the first sign of drug-induced toxicity.

Neurotoxicity. Occasionally patients on long-term therapy develop signs and symptoms of central and peripheral nerve disorders, including headache, mild depression, mental confusion, and neuritis. Most serious is an optic neuritis that may lead to atrophy of optic nerve fibers. Thus, although long-term chloramphenicol is very effective for preventing flare-ups of respiratory infection in children with cystic fibrosis, it is better to employ tetracyclines, ampicillin, or other antimicrobial agents for this purpose whenever possible.

Hypersensitivity and superinfections. Allergic skin reactions occur much less often than with penicillin and most other antibiotics. However, skin eruptions and other signs of hypersensitivity are sometimes seen. Similarly, although superinfections are less common than with tetracyclines, this broad-spectrum antibiotic can cause the emergence of resistant bacteria and fungi. Invasion of the mouth, throat, and colon tissues by these microorganisms may account for such symptoms as pruritus and

diarrhea and such disorders as glossitis, stomatitis, and enterocolitis.

In summary, chloramphenicol can be lifesaving when reserved for use in serious infections caused by organisms against which it is shown to be highly active. However, because of possible fatal blood dyscrasias, it should not be used when other safer antimicrobial agents are also effective. It should never be used for treating minor infections or without performing sensitivity tests.

Additional clinical considerations

The extreme caution that must be used when giving chloramphenicol cannot be emphasized enough. The drug should never be used for trivial or inappropriate infections. Culture and sensitivity tests should always be done before beginning treatment with chloramphenicol, and appropriate measures should be taken if chloramphenicol has been started and the sensitivity test results are negative. Chloramphenicol is prescribed frequently by veterinarians for pets but its effects in animals are not as dangerous as its effects in humans.

Chloramphenicol sodium succinate is intended only for IV use. It should never be given IM, because it is ineffective if given by this route.

Drug–drug interactions. Chloramphenicol inhibits the hepatic metabolism of *dicumarol, phenytoin, phenobarbital, tolbutamide,* and *chlorpropramide.* Consequently the serum levels of these drugs may increase to toxic levels. When given concurrently with chloramphenicol the dosage of these drugs will need to be decreased. The metabolic activation of *cyclophosphamide,* an antineoplastic drug, is also inhibited. If chloramphenicol must be given during treatment of a cancer patient with cyclophosphamide, this fact should be kept in mind. *Acetaminophen* may increase the effects of chloramphenicol, and the dosage of chloramphenicol will need to be decreased to avoid toxicity. The response of the bone marrow to *iron salts* and to *vitamin B_{12}* may be decreased by chloramphenicol. *Penicillin* and chloramphenicol interact to decrease the effectiveness of penicillin and to increase the half-life of chloramphenicol. If these two drugs are given concurrently, extreme caution must be taken to adjust the dosage of each drug appropriately.

The patient teaching guide and guide to the nursing process with chloramphenicol summarize the clinical application of the nursing process to chloramphenicol therapy.

Patient teaching guide: chloramphenicol

The drug that has been prescribed for you is an antibiotic called chloramphenicol. This drug works to destroy specific bacteria that are causing infections in the body. It is active against specific bacteria and does not destroy other bacteria, viruses, or "cold" germs. This drug has many serious side-effects, but its effects against bacteria

(continued)

are very necessary for your problem. It is very important to complete the full course of your prescription. Your antibiotic has been prescribed to treat _____ .

Instructions:

1. The name of the drug ordered for you is _____ .

2. The dosage of the drug ordered for you is _____ .

3. The drug must be taken _____ times a day. It is best to take the drug throughout the day so that it can work continually. The best times to take your drug are _____ , _____ , _____ .

4. The drug should be taken on an empty stomach, 1 hour before or 2 hours after meals is best. The drug should be taken with a full glass of water. (If GI upset is very uncomfortable, the drug can be taken with food.)

5. Some side-effects of the drug that you should be aware of include:

Nausea, vomiting	If severe, the drug can be taken with food.
Diarrhea	This will clear up when the drug is stopped.
Headache, confusion	Aspirin may be used to help the headache—take safety precautions if confusion occurs.
Superinfection (monilial)	Frequent hygiene care of infected area will help. If severe, medications are available.

6. Avoid the use of any over-the-counter preparation that contains acetaminophen (*e.g.,* Tylenol).

7. Tell any physician, nurse, or dentist who is taking care of you that you are taking this drug.

8. Keep this and all medications out of the reach of children.

9. Be sure to complete the full course of your prescription. Take all of the prescription that has been ordered for you.

10. *Never* use any leftover medication to self-treat any other infection; do not give this medication to others and do not use similar medications borrowed from others.

Notify your nurse or physician if any of the following occur:

Sore throat, fever, pale skin,
unusual bleeding, or bruising (even
if these occur several weeks after
drug therapy)
Numbness, tingling, or pain in the
extremities
Pregnancy

Guide to the nursing process: chloramphenicol

Assessment	Nursing diagnoses	Interventions	Evaluation
Past history (*contraindications*): Renal failure Hepatic failure G-6-PD deficiency Intermittent porphyria Pregnancy Lactation *Allergies:* chloramphenicol, others; reactions Medication history: current drugs (*Cautions:* dicumarol, phenytoin, phenobarbital, tolbutamide, chlorpropramide, cyclophosphamide, acetaminophen, iron salts, vitamin B$_{12}$, penicillin)	Potential alteration in comfort (GI upset) Potential alteration in bowel elimination Potential alteration in respiratory function Potential alteration in tissue perfusion (clotting and blood dyscrasia) Knowledge deficit regarding drug therapy	Culture infected area Preparation and safe administration of drug Patient teaching regarding: Drug Dosage Administration Side-effects Warning signs Comfort measures: Drug with food Hygiene Headache therapy Safety precautions Encouragement to comply with drug therapy	Monitor for effectiveness of drug: resolution of infection Monitor for adverse effects of drug: Blood screening Liver function tests Superinfections GI effects CNS effects Renal function tests Monitor for drug–drug interactions: ↑ effects of dicumarol, phenytoin phenobarbital tolbutamide chlorpropramide ↓ effects of penicillin cyclophosphamide ↑ toxicity of chloramphenicol with: acetaminophen penicillin Evaluate effectiveness of patient teaching measures Evaluate effectiveness of support measures
Physical Assessment General: site of infection CNS: orientation, reflexes, sensation Respiratory: rate, adventitious sounds GI: bowel sounds, output, liver function Renal: urinalysis, BUN Blood: CBC Skin: color, lesions			

Drugs of the aminoglycoside group share not only the similarity in molecular structure from which their name is derived but also biophysical properties that account for the ways in which they are handled by the body (Table 8-8). These pharmacokinetic factors, in turn, determine the manner in which these antimicrobial agents are best administered in the various clinical situations in which they are employed. All drugs of this class also have a similar antibacterial spectrum and cause the same kinds of toxic effects.

Clinical status

Despite their similar chemical, pharmacokinetic, and antibacterial properties, these drugs are not equally useful as therapeutic agents. *Streptomycin*, the first drug of this class, is now used mainly in the treatment of tuberculosis, and its application for this purpose is discussed later in this chapter. Because of its toxicity, *neomycin*[+], another early derivative, is now almost never administered parenterally for treating serious systemic infections. It is, instead, commonly applied topically for treating or preventing skin infections. It is also administered orally for its local effects in the gastrointestinal tract, as discussed

Table 8–8. Aminoglycoside antibiotics

Generic or official name	Trade name	Route of administration	Usual adult dosage
Amikacin sulfate	Amikin	IM, IV	15 mg/kg/day in divided doses, q 8–12 hr
Gentamicin sulfate USP	Apogen; Bristagen Garamycin Jenamicin	IM, IV (Intrathecally) (Topically)	3–5 mg/kg/day in divided doses, q 8 hr IM, IV
Kanamycin sulfate USP	Kantrex; Klebcil	IM, IV, oral	15 mg/kg/day in divided doses, q 12 hr, IM, IV; 8 g–12 g/day, in divided doses, orally, for managing hepatic coma
Neomycin sulfate USP	Mycifradin Sulfate; Neobiotic	IM, oral (Topically)	15 mg/kg/day, in divided doses, q 6 hr, IM; 4 g–12 g/day, in divided doses, orally, for managing hepatic coma
Netilmicin sulfate	Netromycin	IM, IV	3–4 mg/kg/day, in divided doses, q 12 hr
Paromomycin sulfate USP	Humatin	Oral	25–75 mg/kg/day, in divided doses, tid for amebiasis; 4 g/day in divided doses for managing hepatic coma
Streptomycin sulfate USP		IM	1–2 g/day, in divided doses, bid
Tobramycin sulfate	Nebcin	IM, IV	3 mg/kg/day, in divided doses, q 8 hr

below. *Paromomycin,* which is available only in tablet form, is used mainly for treating intestinal amebiasis (see Chap. 11) and also for treating hepatic coma (see below).

Kanamycin[+] was for many years the drug most often selected to begin treatment of a severe systemic infection when the specific bacterial cause had not yet been identified but was suspected to be a gram-negative enteric bacillus. Now, however, because of the emergence of kanamycin-resistant strains of formerly susceptible species and the increasing incidence of infections by *Pseudomonas* species, which have never been sensitive to this antibiotic, it is not ordinarily the first drug of this class to be tried in such cases. Kanamycin is also given orally to treat hepatic coma.

At present, *gentamicin*[+] is considered the drug of choice for "covering" suspected infection by a wide spectrum of enteric and nonenteric gram-negative aerobic pathogens. *Tobramycin, amikacin,* and *netilmicin,* the most recently introduced drugs of this class, are reserved for short-term therapy of patients with serious bacterial infections sensitive to these drugs. Amikacin and netilmicin are sometimes effective in treating infections that are resistant to both gentamicin and tobramycin.

Antibacterial spectrum

Aminoglycosides are highly active against gram-positive and gram-negative bacteria. However, they are rarely used clinically for treating infections caused by gram-positive organisms, because other less toxic and more effective antimicrobial drugs are available. The main clin-

ical use of these drugs is in severe infections caused by gram-negative aerobic bacteria, including *E. coli,* the *Klebsiella–Enterobacter–Serratia* group, and various *Proteus* species. Gentamicin, unlike kanamycin, is also active against *Pseudomonas aeruginosa;* and tobramycin is said to be even more effective against various *Pseudomonas* and *Proteus* species. Because resistance to these drugs tends to develop readily, it is always desirable to have the laboratory determine whether or not the infecting organism is actually sensitive to the antibiotic with which treatment is initiated before continuing to use it.

Mechanisms of action and of resistance

Action. Drugs of this chemical class exert their bacteriostatic and bactericidal effects by interfering with protein biosynthesis. The drug molecules make their way into bacterial cells and bind to a specific site on the ribosome, the cell structure responsible for processing genetically coded information. This leads to misreading of the code, so that amino acids are no longer linked together correctly to form the proper peptide chains. As a result, the protein molecules required for maintaining the structure of the bacterial cell and its metabolic activity cannot be formed.

Resistance. Bacterial species that are naturally resistant to the aminoglycosides may not let the drug molecules enter the cell or attach themselves to the ribosome. Bacterial strains of originally susceptible species that acquire resistance may do so in any of several ways. They may, for example, become capable of producing enzymes that destroy the antibiotic drug molecules. Resistance of this type is often rapidly acquired through the transfer of R factor (see Chap. 6) from naturally resistant microorganisms to strains of gram-negative bacilli that were previously sensitive to drugs of this class.

Synergism. Some aminoglycosides, such as gentamicin and tobramycin, are made more active clinically when given in combination with a penicillin or cephalosporin family antibiotic. Carbenicillin, for example, tends to enlarge openings in the cell wall of *Pseudomonas* bacilli. This makes it easier for gentamicin molecules to reach their intracellular site of action—a mechanism that may account for the synergistic effects of these drugs when they are administered together in the treatment of pseudomonal septicemia. In turn, aminoglycosides tend to increase the bactericidal effectiveness of penicillin on enterococci, possibly by weakening the structure of the cell walls of these bacteria and thus making them more susceptible to the action of penicillin. This may also account for the fact that a combination of streptomycin and penicillin G is more effective for treating endocarditis caused by enterococci and other streptococci than is either drug given alone.

Therapeutic uses

Parenteral administration. The injectable forms of these drugs are very valuable for treating life-threatening systemic infections such as gram-negative bacteremia, peritonitis, and meningitis. They are also effective in lung infections caused by *Klebsiella pneumoniae* and in other gram-negative bacterial pneumonias. Infections of the urinary tract by strains of enteric bacilli resistant to less toxic antibiotics often respond to treatment with aminoglycoside antibiotics, particularly when obstruction to urinary flow is corrected.

The use of streptomycin in tuberculosis and in enterococcal meningitis has already been mentioned. Other drugs of this class are also occasionally employed for these purposes. Kanamycin is, for example, sometimes combined with other chemotherapeutic antituberculosis agents for the treatment of patients reinfected by strains of the organism that have become resistant to the first-line drugs previously employed. Similarly, in streptococcal endocarditis, gentamicin may be combined with penicillin G, or it may be administered with carbenicillin to treat pseudomonal endocarditis. Aminoglycosides are not ordinarily used in staphylococcal or in other gram-positive infections. However, gentamicin is sometimes successful against infection by penicillinase-producing staphylococci resistant to methicillin or to other penicillinase-resistant penicillins.

Oral administration. These drugs are all poorly absorbed from the gastrointestinal tract, and are not administered orally to treat systemic infections. Kanamycin, neomycin, and paromomycin are given orally to kill ammonia-forming bacteria in the GI tract and thus to lower blood ammonia levels in patients with hepatic coma. These drugs are also sometimes given orally before and after bowel surgery to suppress intestinal bacteria.

Intrathecal administration. Gentamicin is sometimes given intrathecally to treat serious central nervous system infections caused by sensitive strains of *Pseudomonas.* These drugs do not normally penetrate the blood–brain barrier in appreciable amounts, but cerebrospinal fluid concentrations are greater when the meninges are inflamed.

Topical application. These antibiotics are often applied topically for control of skin infections. However, in severe burns, bacteremic sepsis is best prevented by parenteral administration, and topical use is not recommended on account of the rapidity with which resistant strains develop in this situation. Certain drugs of the aminoglycoside class, however, are widely employed in the form of ointments and creams for management of dermatologic and ophthalmic disorders. Gentamicin, for example, is available in topical form for treating bacterial infections of the skin caused by susceptible staphylococcal, streptococcal, and pseduomonal strains, and by other bacterial invaders.

Neomycin is also applied topically—usually in combination with polymyxin and bacitracin—for treating pyodermas such as impetigo and furunculosis (boils) and secondary skin infections in patients with poison ivy, acne, eczema, and other dermatoses. Combinations of these antibiotics are also available as solutions for topical application to the outer surface of the eye in ocular infections and for use in irrigating the urinary bladder to prevent bacteriuria in patients with an indwelling catheter. The antibacterial effectiveness of these and other topically applied antimicrobial agents is uncertain.

Adverse effects. The aminoglycosides cause two main types of tissue toxicity: ototoxicity, or inner ear nerve damage; and nephrotoxicity, or kidney damage. These effects are claimed to be less likely to occur with the more recently introduced drugs such as gentamicin than with streptomycin or neomycin. However, with all drugs of this class, it is important to follow dosage recommendations carefully, because the margin between therapeutic and toxic doses is narrow. Patients must be monitored for early signs of changes in auditory and vestibular nerve and renal function.

Nephrotoxicity. The aminoglycosides depend almost entirely on the kidneys for clearance from the body. They are excreted almost completely unchanged by glomerular filtration. Thus, patients with renal impairment need a reduced dosage to prevent drug accumulation. Ideally, blood levels of the drug are determined and dosage is adjusted so as not to exceed maximum safe levels. The dosage may also be based on the patient's creatinine clearance rate. All these drugs are also toxic to the kidneys. Thus, scrupulous attention to the patient's kidney function during therapy is critical. Maintaining the patient in a well-hydrated state can help to reduce the renal tubular concentration of these drugs and to lessen the chance of renal toxicity occurring.

Ototoxicity. The accumulation of an aminoglycoside antibiotic in the two branches of the eighth cranial nerve—the auditory and vestibular portions—can lead to temporary or irreversible changes in their sensory functions. This can even occur with orally administered drugs when the kidneys do not adequately excrete the small amounts of neomycin or kanamycin that are absorbed, and occasionally enough can accumulate following topical application to cause damage in patients with reduced renal excretory function. The likelihood of hearing loss and disturbances in balance is, of course, higher in patients receiving drugs by injection for treating a severe infection.

These patients should not be deprived of life-saving antibiotic drug treatment because of the threat of drug-induced neurotoxicity. The danger of permanent nerve damage can be reduced by observing the patient for early signs and symptoms and then adjusting the dosage and frequency of drug administration. The patient may complain of a persistent ringing or roaring in the ears or of headache, dizziness, and vertigo. Most such symptoms do not ordinarily persist for more than a few days after a short treatment course is terminated. More lasting effects occur mainly in patients who continue to take these drugs for several weeks or more without adequate supervision. During long-term therapy, audiometric examinations and tests of labyrinthine function should be carried out periodically to detect and prevent permanent changes in hearing and coordination, including deafness and ataxia. Serious eighth nerve damage is more likely to occur when the aminoglycosides are given with the loop diuretics—ethacrynic acid (Edecrin), furosemide (Lasix), and bumetanide (Bumex)—or with other neurotoxic or nephrotoxic drugs such as the cephalosporins, cisplatin (an anticancer drug), and amphotericin B (an antifungal drug). Because these drugs cross the placenta, they should be given during pregnancy only when the benefits clearly outweigh the risks. Children with permanent deafness have been born to mothers who received streptomycin during pregnancy.

Other adverse effects. The aminoglycoside antibiotics can sometimes cause paralysis of skeletal muscles, including those involved in breathing. This is most likely to occur in patients with myasthenia gravis or Parkinson's

disease, or in patients who are also receiving neuromuscular blocking drugs for muscle relaxation during surgery. Respiratory failure has also been reported following instillation of antibiotic solutions into the abdominal cavity to prevent postoperative infection from fecal contamination. Apnea can be counteracted by administration of neostigmine or calcium salts.

Oral administration of neomycin or kanamycin for their effects on the bacterial flora of the colon commonly leads to diarrhea. Less often, neomycin may interfere with fat absorption, with resulting steatorrhea and other signs of a syndrome similar to sprue. Malabsorption of vitamins, minerals, and electrolytes has also been reported, particularly in liver-diseased patients receiving large daily doses. However, these adverse effects are unlikely in patients taking small doses for only short periods.

The incidence of allergic hypersensitization from topically applied neomycin has been rising in recent years. Skin rashes have been reported in 5% or more of patients treated topically with this drug or following injection of other aminoglycosides.

Additional clinical considerations

Proper preparation and administration of these drugs is often difficult. Systemic doses of most of these drugs are based on body weight; thus, body weight needs to be known before therapy is begun. Obese patients present a special therapeutic dilemma: the manufacturer's inserts contain formulas for calculating lean body weight and these should be used but, in addition, remember that for each drug, there is a maximum safe daily dose that should not be exceeded, even for very obese patients. Parenteral drugs should be prepared according to each manufacturer's guidelines for mixing and storing solutions, and conditions to ensure stability should be provided. Do not mix aminoglycosides in IV solution with penicillins or cephalosporins because mutual inactivation of the drugs can occur. Because these two types of antibiotics are synergistic they are often used in combination, but appropriate spacing of the doses must be provided for. Patients with impaired (elderly patients) or immature (neonates) renal function will require decreased dosage.

The patient teaching guide and guide to the nursing process summarize the application of the nursing process to aminoglycoside therapy.

Patient teaching guide: the aminoglycosides

The drug that has been prescribed for you is an antibiotic of the group called aminoglycosides. These drugs destroy specific bacteria that are causing infections in the body. They are active against specific bacteria only and are not effective against other bacteria, viruses or "cold" germs.*

(continued)

Instructions:

1. The name of your drug is _____ .

2. The dosage of your drug is _____ .

3. Your drug should be given at _____ , _____ , _____ .

4. Some side-effects of the drug that you should be aware of include:

Ringing in the ears, headache, dizziness	These effects are reversible; safety precautions should be taken if necessary.
Nausea, vomiting, loss of appetite	These effects will pass; small, frequent meals may help, as will frequent mouth care.

Notify your nurse or physician if any of the following occur:

Pain at injection sites
Severe headache, dizziness
Changes in urine pattern
Difficulty breathing
Rash or skin lesions

* Because these drugs are frequently given parenterally, the patient teaching guide will refer to parenteral administration. Frequently, drug teaching is minimal with patients who are receiving parenteral drugs because they do not assume primary responsibility for their own therapy. These patients, however, need and have the right to know what is being given to them. If oral drugs are used, similar application can be made following examples in other patient teaching guides.

Guide to the nursing process: the aminoglycosides

Assessment	Nursing diagnoses	Interventions	Evaluation
Past history (*contraindications*): Renal failure Myasthenia gravis Pregnancy Lactation *Allergies:* aminoglycosides, others; reactions Medication history: current drugs (*Cautions:* other aminoglycosides, amphotericin B, bacitracin, cisplatin, cephalothin,	Potential alteration in bowel function Potential alteration in sensory–perceptual function (ototoxicity) Potential alteration in fluid volume (secondary to nephrotoxicity) Potential alteration in respiratory function Knowledge deficit regarding drug therapy	Culture infected area Preparation and safe administration of drug Provision of comfort measures: Hygiene measures Safety measures Small, frequent meals Patient teaching regarding: Drug dosage Administration Side-effects Warning signs Support and encouragement to	Monitor for effectiveness of drug: resolution of infection Monitor for adverse effects: Ototoxicity Nephrotoxicity CNS changes GI reactions Superinfections Sensitivity reactions Monitor drug–drug interactions: ↑ toxic effects with: amphotericin B bacitracin

(continued)

Assessment	Nursing diagnoses	Interventions	Evaluation
vancomycin, methoxyflurane, loop diuretics, succinylcholine, penicillin)		comply with drug therapy	cisplatin cephalothin vancomycin methoxyflurane loop diuretics succinylcholine ↓ effects if mixed *in vitro* with penicillin
Physical Assessment General: site of infection Neurologic: orientation, reflexes, eighth cranial nerve tests Respiratory: rate, adventitious sounds GI: bowel sounds, liver function Renal: urinalysis, BUN, electrolytes Skin: color, lesions			Evaluate effectiveness of comfort measures Evaluate effectiveness of patient teaching Evaluate effect of support and encouragement

Miscellaneous antibacterial antibiotics

The drugs described in this section have relatively limited use in treating systemic infections. The main reason for this is that other safer antimicrobial drugs are now available for treating the infections for which these narrow-spectrum antibiotics might be effective. Most of these antibiotics are used mainly for their local antibacterial effects on the skin and on the mucous membranes of the eye and gastrointestinal tract.

The polymyxins

This group of antibiotic substances includes *polymyxin B sulfate*[+] (Aerosporin) and *colistin,* which is available in two forms—colistin sulfate for oral use and colistimethate sodium for intramuscular and intravenous injection (Table 8-9). Both are active against gram-negative bacteria and are used in their injectable forms for treating UTI caused by strains of *Pseudomonas aeruginosa* and by other bacilli that are resistant to less toxic antimicrobial agents. Colistimethate sodium (Coly-Mycin M Parenteral) is pre-

Table 8–9. Miscellaneous antibacterial antibiotics

Generic or official name	Trade name	Route of administration	Usual adult dosage
Bacitracin intramuscular USP		IM—infants only (Topically)	IM: 900 U/kg/day, in divided doses, bid or tid for infants < 2.5 kg; 1000 U/kg/day, in divided doses, bid or tid for infants > 2.5 kg
The polymyxins			
Colistimethate sodium USP	Coly-Mycin M Parenteral	IM, IV	2.5–5 mg/kg/day, in two to four divided doses (300 mg maximum daily dose)
Colistin sulfate USP; polymyxin E	Coly-Mycin S Oral Suspension	Oral–children	5–15 mg/kg/day in three divided doses
Polymyxin B sulfate, parenteral	Aerosporin	IV; not recommended for IM use (Intrathecally) (Topically)	15,000–25,000 U/kg/day, in divided doses, q 12 hr, IV; 25,000–30,000 U/kg/day, in divided doses, q 4–6 hr, IM

ferred for intramuscular injection because this salt, which releases polymyxin E in the tissues, causes much less local muscle pain than polymyxin B.

However, the main difficulty with both these drugs is that they can cause severe kidney damage, particularly in patients whose renal function is already impaired. Because of this and other types of toxicity, the polymyxins have been largely replaced in the treatment of pseudomonal UTI by gentamicin or ticarcillin and carbenicillin. They are reserved for treating kidney and lung infections and meningitis caused by pseudomonal strains and other bacilli resistant to these less toxic antibiotics.

The polymyxins are also available in preparations for topical application to the skin and external auditory canal and to the eye (see Chaps. 42 and 43 for further discussion). Colistin sulfate is administered to infants and children as an oral suspension for treating infectious diarrhea and gastroenteritis. For details concerning precautions to avoid toxicity, see the Drug Digest for polymyxin B sulfate. (These precautions apply also for the injectable form of colistin, colistimethate sodium.)

Bacitracin and bacitracin zinc

These antibiotics (Table 8-9), which are active mainly against gram-positive cocci, are most commonly employed in combination with polymyxin B and neomycin for topical treatment of skin infections (see Chap. 43). Bacitracin is now almost never injected for treating systemic infections caused by penicillinase-producing staphylococci because it is nephrotoxic, and safer antistaphylococcal antibiotics such as the penicillinase-resistant penicillins and the cephalosporins are now available. In the few infections caused by methicillin-resistant staphylococci, the antibiotics gentamicin or vancomycin are almost always effective and are less toxic than intramuscularly administered bacitracin.

Drugs for specific disorders

Urinary tract infections

Acute urinary tract infections are second in frequency only to respiratory tract infections. Some people—particularly women of childbearing age—are subject to frequent bladder and kidney infections. Acute pyelonephritis is painful, discomforting, and inconvenient, but in the absence of any organic abnormality of the urinary tract no widespread kidney damage ordinarily occurs. However, recurrent acute infections in patients with uncorrected abnormalities that block normal urine flow can cause kidney tissue destruction. The resulting chronic pyelonephritis or renal medullary (papillary) necrosis can interfere severely with kidney function and lead finally to renal failure. Children with congenital obstructive disease of the urinary tract are also likely to suffer frequent

kidney infections that can result in severe tissue damage and scarring.

Therapeutic indications

The main aim of treatment in ordinary urethral, bladder, and kidney infections is not merely relief of symptoms but the complete eradication of the causative uropathogen. Thus, it is not enough for anti-infective drug therapy to relieve the frequency, urgency, and burning pain on urination in cystitis, or the systemic signs (chills and fever) and the back and flank pain or tenderness of acute pyelonephritis. More significant is drug-induced *sterilization* of the urine and urinary tract tissues, because failure to do so may lead to relapses or to recurrent infections with increasingly resistant strains of uropathogens.

Urinary tract antiseptics

Many of the antibacterial agents already described are used to treat UTIs. These drugs include the following: the sulfonamides, sulfisoxazole and sulfamethoxazole, both of which are often combined with *phenazopyridine HCl*, a urinary tract analgesic that colors the urine red; co-trimoxazole, the sulfamethoxazole–trimethoprim combination; the penicillin drugs ampicillin, amoxicillin, carbenicillin, and ticarcillin; many of the cephalosporins; the tetracyclines; and many of the aminoglycosides.

In addition to these drugs, all of which are used to treat systemic bacterial infections, several other drugs that have antibacterial effects are used only to treat UTI (Table 8-10). These drugs do not reach antibacterial levels in the bloodstream or in tissues other than the kidney. They are commonly referred to as urinary tract antiseptics, and they are used most often to suppress chronic UTI.

Cinoxacin (Cinobac) is a new drug in this group. It is very similar to the older drug, *nalidixic acid* (NegGram). Both drugs are bactericidal and act by inhibiting the DNA replication of sensitive bacteria. They are effective in UTIs caused by many gram-negative organisms, and bacterial resistance develops in only a low percentage of patients. Both drugs are well absorbed orally and are excreted mainly in the urine. Dosage needs to be reduced in patients with impaired renal function.

Experimentally, both drugs have produced damage to the cartilage in weight-bearing joints of animals. They are therefore not recommended for use in prepubertal children. The most common adverse effects of both drugs are gastrointestinal disturbances: nausea, vomiting, and diarrhea. Nalidixic acid has occasionally caused serious central nervous system toxicity, including elevated intracranial pressure and convulsions. It has also caused liver toxicity. Because of its potential for causing severe adverse effects, many authorities prefer to use drugs other than nalidixic acid to treat UTIs.

Methenamine and two salts of methenamine, *methenamine mandelate* (Mandelamine) and *methenamine hip-*

Table 8–10. Urinary tract antiseptics

Generic or official name	Trade name	Route of administration	Usual adult dosage
Cinoxacin	Cinobac Pulvules	Oral	1 g/day in two to four divided doses
Methenamine USP		Oral	1 g qid
Methenamine hippurate	Hiprex; Urex	Oral	1 g bid
Methenamine mandelate USP	Mandelamine	Oral	1 g qid, pc and hs
Methylene blue USP	Urolene Blue	Oral	60 mg–130 mg tid
Nalidixic Acid USP	NegGram	Oral	1 g qid
Nitrofurantoin USP	Furadantin; Ivadantin; Macrodantin	IV, oral	180 mg bid, IV, for patients weighing more than 120 lb; 3 mg/lb/day in two divided doses, IV, for patients weighing less than 120 lb; or 50 mg–100 mg qid, oral

purate (Hiprex; Urex), which break down to methenamine, are also used as urinary tract antiseptics (Table 8-10). The salts of methenamine liberate the organic acids to which they are bound—mandelic acid and hippuric acid, which are weakly bacteriostatic when excreted in the urine. However, the main antibacterial effect of these drugs results from the release of *formaldehyde* from the methenamine component of the compound. Because this formation of formaldehyde occurs only in acidic urine, the patient sometimes has to supplement these drugs with an added urinary acidifier such as ascorbic acid, sodium acid phosphate, or ammonium chloride.

Drinking cranberry juice, which forms urinary hippuric acid, is also sometimes suggested for maintaining the patient's urine at an acidic *p*H. Such adjunctive measures for acidifying the urine and for ensuring the release of enough free formaldehyde to suppress bacterial growth in the urine are especially necessary in infections caused by certain *Proteus* species. Infection by these and other bacteria that produce urease, an enzyme that splits urea into ammonia, make it particularly difficult to maintain a sufficiently acidic urine to ensure that these methenamine salts will exert their full antibacterial activity. Administration of an inhibitor of urease, acetohydroxamic acid (Lithostat), has also recently been advocated to help keep the urine acidic during suppressive therapy of *Proteus*-infected urine. Such drug-induced enzyme inhibition also helps to prevent the precipitation of stone-forming substances in the urine of these patients.

The methenamine urinary tract antiseptics are quite nontoxic, especially in comparison to the other effective drugs in this group. They occasionally cause GI disturbances, which are minimized when the drugs are taken with food, and sometimes cause dysuria (painful urination).

Methylene blue is a mild urinary tract antiseptic used for cystitis and urethritis. It colors the urine (and feces) blue green. Gastrointestinal disturbances and dysuria may occur, and hemolysis has occurred in patients with G-6-PD deficiency.

Nitrofurantoin (Furadantin; Macrodantin) is not as effective as the sulfonamides or ampicillin and other bactericidal antibiotics when used for treating acute UTI. However, it is often valuable in chronic infections caused by uropathogenic strains that have acquired resistance to the more potent antibacterial agents. The large daily doses needed for treating acute infections tend to cause gastrointestinal upset. It also frequently causes pulmonary reactions, and a number of other serious adverse effects (blood dyscrasias, peripheral neuropathy, hepatotoxicity, a lupuslike syndrome, increased intracranial pressure) have occurred. The preparation for intravenous use (Ivadantin) is new, and many feel it should not be used because of its potential to cause adverse effects without clear-cut benefit relative to that of other available drugs.

Other drugs

Drugs with little or no anti-infective activity are also often used in the management of patients with UTI. These are used to relieve the discomfort and pain that occur in cystitis as a result of local irritation of the bladder mucosa and reflex spasm of bladder smooth muscle.

Phenazopyridine, for example, is an azo dye that is often combined with sulfonamides and other urinary antibacterial agents. Although this substance has weak antibacterial activity, it is not used for its antiseptic effect. Instead, when excreted in the urine, the drug is said to have a soothing topical anesthetic effect. This tends to relieve the local bladder irritation and to lessen both the burning pain and reflex contractions that are set off by sensory stimuli, which account for the urgency and frequency that keep the patient awake and restless.

Anticholinergic drugs such as atropine and other natural or synthetic belladonna alkaloids are also often prescribed. By blocking the motor portion of the bladder reflex arc, atropinelike drugs are said to reduce the frequency of bladder contractions and to delay the patient's desire to void. Because of the many side-effects of these drugs (see Chap. 16), it would be desirable to have available safer drugs capable of exerting the desired antispasmodic action on the bladder.

The most recent addition to the many drugs claimed to cause fewer side-effects than atropine is *oxybutynin* (Ditropan). This antispasmodic is claimed to be useful for patients with neurogenic bladder, who are of course prone to have frequent UTIs. However, when used in doses capable of relieving painful bladder contractions, oxybutynin can cause side-effects resembling those of atropine and other anticholinergic drugs.

Additional clinical considerations

Many drugs used to treat UTIs are discussed with other general families of antibiotics. The clinical application of this type of drug therapy needs to be combined with overall consideration of the cause of the chronic UTI and of the preventive measures that can be taken. The patient teaching guide considers some of these measures.

There are some special considerations to keep in mind with the use of the urinary antiseptic *methenamine*. For example, the drug should not be used if a patient has renal insufficiency or is dehydrated, and patients with severe hepatic insufficiency should not be treated with this drug because of the increased dangers from the ammonia released by it. Some *mandelamine* suspensions are prepared with a vegetable oil base; use of this particular preparation has potential dangers for elderly patients or for patients who have difficulty swallowing and could aspirate the solution.

Drug–drug interactions. *Sulfonamides* can form an insoluble precipitate with formaldehyde in the urine. *Drugs that alkalinize the urine* can decrease the effect of methenamine, which requires an acidic urine to be effective. Urine-alkalinizing drugs include sodium bicarbonate and acetazolamide.

The use of the nursing process with patients suffering from urinary tract infections depends very much on the disease process, and the drug therapy is but a small part of the overall regimen.

Patient teaching guide: methenamine

The drug that has been prescribed for you is a urinary tract antiseptic called methenamine. This drug works to treat urinary tract infection by destroying bacteria and by helping to develop an environment that is not conducive to bacteria growth.

Instructions:

1. The drug that has been ordered for you is _____ .

2. The dosage of the drug is _____ .

3. The drug should be taken _____ times a day. The drug should be spaced throughout the day so that it can work continually. The best times to take your drug are _____ , _____ , _____ .

4. If the drug causes GI upset, it may be taken with food. It is important to *avoid* foods that alkalinize the urine—for example, citrus juices, milk—because they decrease the effectiveness of the drug. Cranberry juice is one juice that can be used. Fluids should be pushed as much as possible (8 to 10 glasses a day) to help to treat the infection.

5. Do not take any over-the-counter (OTC) drugs that might contain sodium bicarbonate (*e.g.,* antacids, baking soda). If you question the use of any OTC drug, call your nurse or physician.

6. Some side-effects of the drug that you should be aware of include:

Stomach upset, nausea   Take drug with food.

(continued)

Painful urination

If this occurs, report to your nurse or physician; the dose may need to be decreased.

7. Tell any physician, nurse, or dentist who is taking care of you that you are on this drug.

8. Keep this and all medications out of the reach of children.

9. Take the full course of your prescription. Do not use this drug to self-treat any other infection.

10. There are several other activities that could help to decrease urinary tract infections that should be considered:

Avoid bubble baths.
Women should always wipe from *front* to *back.*
Void whenever you feel the urge; try not to wait. If possible, always void after sexual intercourse to clear the urethra.

Notify your nurse or physician if any of the following occur:

Skin rash or itching
Severe GI upset
GI upset that prevents adequate
   fluid intake
Very painful urination
Pregnancy

Tuberculosis

Cause and current status

Tuberculosis is an infection caused mainly by the acid-fast bacillus *Mycobacterium tuberculosis.* These bacilli are inhaled in droplets from coughs of infected persons. Bacterial colonies grow in the lungs and invade their tissues, setting off an intense inflammatory response that can lead to tissue necrosis and development of open cavities. Sometimes the bacilli spread to extrapulmonary sites by way of the blood and lymph. This can lead to tuberculosis infection of the kidneys, bones, central nervous system, and other tissues.

Tuberculosis has long been one of the most prevalent of the infectious diseases that afflict humans. Bones found in archeologic diggings show evidence of tuberculous damage, thus indicating the presence of the disease even among prehistoric peoples. The earliest Egyptian and Greek medical writers described the course and clinical features of the pulmonary form of this disease. During the last century pulmonary tuberculosis—or consumption, as it was called because of the wasting away of its victims—still remained the greatest killer of young men and women in their twenties and thirties.

In this country there has been a steady decrease in new cases of active tuberculosis. This may be because of generally good sanitation and living conditions—factors that help to reduce the spread of infection. However, the disease is still a serious problem among poor people, particularly those who live in substandard inner city housing, and whose resistance to bacterial invasion has been reduced by inadequate nutrition. In 1981, over 27,000 new cases of tuberculosis were reported in the United States, and close to 1,800 deaths occurred. It is likely that there are many more cases of active tuberculosis than those that are diagnosed and reported. Thus, it is important to discover these cases before they become an active reservoir for further spread of the infection. These people and those with whom they come into contact could then be cured by treatment with the excellent chemotherapeutic agents now available for the treatment and prevention of tuberculosis.

In this section the current chemotherapy of tuberculosis will be discussed with emphasis on the general principles of treatment and on the individual drugs now available.

Chemotherapy

The outlook for people who become infected with tuberculosis today is vastly different from what it was before drugs effective against the tubercle bacillus became available. This is reflected not only in the greatly reduced mortality rate from this disease, but also by the relative ease with which most patients can now be managed. For example, the vast majority of patients with newly diagnosed pulmonary tuberculosis need no longer be confined to special sanatoriums for long periods, nor need most patients with advanced disease undergo extensive lung surgery.

Drug therapy is best begun in a general hospital with x-ray and other facilities for determining the extent of the patient's disease and the susceptibility of the infecting tubercle bacilli to various drugs. However, after several weeks of rest, during which drugs are administered and the response to chemotherapy is observed, the patient is released from the hospital to go home and even to return to work. Medication must be continued daily, or even four times a day, depending on the drug regimen, and the patient must be followed closely while on this regimen for up to 2 years.

Modern chemotherapy of tuberculosis is so effective that cures are now possible in almost all cases. Unfortunately, actual results are not as good as they could be. Although drugs usually bring about rapid clinical improvement in active pulmonary tuberculosis, they do not eradicate all the bacteria in large lung lesions. The organisms left alive there can cause relapses unless drug treatment is continued long enough to let the body's own defense mechanisms bring the infection under final control. Thus, the disease will not be cured if the patient does not take the drug faithfully for the prolonged period required for natural healing of tuberculosis lesions. If the patient discontinues the drug or if the body's own defenses are not fully effective, drug-resistant strains of tubercle bacilli tend to develop. Successful control of the disease then becomes increasingly difficult.

Resistance. Almost all tubercle bacilli isolated from lung lesions of patients who have not had previous drug treatment are susceptible to the antituberculosis drugs available. However, as these drug-sensitive tubercle bacilli die off during the long-continued treatment, mutant microorganisms resistant to these drugs may gradually emerge as the predominant strain populating the lesions. After 4 to 6 months of treatment, any bacilli still remaining in the sputum are likely to be resistant to the drugs that have failed to eliminate them.

Combined therapy. To reduce the emergence of drug-resistant strains, antituberculosis drugs are administered in combinations of two or three chemotherapeutic agents. The reason for this is that the small minority of microorganisms that are resistant to each drug are likely to be killed by an added drug that acts by a different mechanism. Thus, the bacteria resistant to each drug die before they can form families that can become predominant. Another reason for employing drugs in combination is that therapy with moderate doses of two or three drugs is likely to prove more effective and less toxic than large doses of only one drug.

Antituberculosis drugs

The currently available drugs are broadly classified as primary or first-line, second-line, and third-line therapeutic agents (Table 8-11). Drugs are grouped in this way mainly on the basis of their antimicrobial effectiveness and their safety. Thus, new cases are treated with combinations of first-line drugs, because these inhibit susceptible bacteria when administered in low to moderate doses that are not likely to cause toxic reactions during prolonged treatment. The second- and third-line drugs are ordinarily reserved for use when the infecting organisms are thought to have become resistant to one or more of the agents with which treatment was begun. The main difficulty with these second- and third-choice drugs is that they are likely to prove much more toxic than the primary agents. They are also often less effective, and bacterial resistance to them tends to develop rapidly in some cases.

First-line drugs. Isoniazid+ (INH) is bactericidal, killing actively growing tubercle bacilli by interfering with lipid and nucleic acid synthesis. INH is the single most effective drug for treating tuberculosis. It is also used alone prophylactically in certain people (infants and those who are immunosuppressed) who have been exposed to tuberculosis and in some tuberculin-positive people without signs or symptoms of disease.

After rapid absorption from the intestine, INH is distributed throughout the body and reaches effective concentrations in all infected tissues, including the central nervous system, as well as the lungs. Its ability to penetrate caseous (cheesy) lung lesions makes it particularly useful in pulmonary disease, and its easy diffusion into cerebrospinal fluid accounts for its usefulness in tuberculous meningitis.

Less than 2% of bacilli isolated from patients who have never received this drug show primary resistance to it. Resistant strains do emerge during treatment with INH, so it must be administered with at least one other drug (usually rifampin; see below) in the management of active tuberculosis cases. However, this drug should not be discontinued when resistance is suspected because the drug's presence in a combination adds to the effectiveness of the other primary drugs.

People vary in their ability to metabolize, or acetylate, INH. About 50% of Americans are so-called *slow acetylators* of INH. In such patients, ordinary doses readily reach high levels in the plasma and tissues. Although this accounts for the drug's effectiveness in such cases, it can also lead to toxic reactions, particularly in patients with poor kidney function. On the other hand, it may be difficult to maintain effective tissue concentrations with ordinary doses in patients who are *rapid acetylators* of this drug. In such cases, it may be necessary to increase the daily dosage to almost twice the usual amount.

Ordinary doses of INH do not cause direct tissue toxicity or hypersensitivity reactions in most patients.

Table 8–11. Antituberculosis drugs

Generic or official name	Trade name	Route of administration	Usual adult dosage
First-line drugs			
Isoniazid; isonicotinic acid hydrazide; INH	Laniazid; Nydrazid; Teebaconin	Oral	5–10 mg/kg once daily
Rifampin	Rifadin; Rimactane	Oral	10 mg/kg once daily
Second-line drugs			
Ethambutol	Myambutol	Oral	15–25 mg/kg once daily
Pyrazinamide		Oral	20–35 mg/kg once daily
Streptomycin sulfate		IM	15–25 mg/kg once daily
Third-line drugs			
Para-aminosalicylate sodium (PAS)	PAS Sodium; Teebacin	Oral	200 mg/kg/day in four equal doses every 6 hr
Ethionamide	Trecator-SC	Oral	7–15 mg/kg/day in four equal doses every 6 hr
Cycloserine	Seromycin	Oral	10–15 mg/kg/day in four equal doses every 6 hr
Capreomycin	Capastat	IM	15 mg/kg once daily

Measures to avoid adverse effects must be employed routinely, however, to avoid potentially serious hepatitis and neuritis. The likelihood of liver damage is low in children, but patients over 35 years old, and especially those who consume significant amounts of alcohol, must be monitored for early signs of hepatic dysfunction. The drug is discontinued if clinical or laboratory evidence indicates possible liver cell injury. Other adverse effects include blood dyscrasias, depression, agitation, and skin reactions.

INH tends to produce a deficiency of the B-complex vitamin pyridoxine (vitamin B_6). This may account for the peripheral neuritis that commonly occurs and for the convulsions sometimes seen during INH treatment. These reactions rarely occur in patients who take a prophylactic dose of pyridoxine daily during INH treatment. Such vitamin supplementation is especially desirable in alcoholic patients and in those who are slow acetylators of INH or who require high doses of the drug for severe infections of the central nervous system.

Clinically significant drug–drug interactions may occur between INH and *phenytoin* (Dilantin), *carbamazepine* (Tegretol), and *benzodiazepines* (diazepam; Valium), necessitating a reduction in dosage of these drugs. In ad-

dition, INH may act to inhibit the enzymes *monoamine oxidase* (MAO) and *diamine oxidase*. Inhibition of MAO can lead to exaggerated responses to tyramine, an amino acid found in many foods (see Chap. 46 for a discussion of this drug–food interaction in regard to antidepressant drugs that are MAO inhibitors). Inhibition of diamine oxidase can lead to exaggerated responses to histamine, which is found in some fish (*e.g.*, tuna), sauerkraut, and yeast extracts.

Rifampin[+] (Rifadin; Rimactane) is the other first-line drug used for treating tuberculosis. It, too, is bactericidal, interfering with nucleic acid metabolism of the mycobacteria. It is used in two- and three-drug combinations with INH. In general, the more advanced and serious cases of the disease are treated with three drugs, or a third drug is added when resistance to one of the first two drugs develops. Rifampin is also now recommended as prophylaxis against *Hemophilus influenzae* B for those exposed to patients with positive *H. influenzae* B cultures or *H. influenzae* B meningitis, and it is used as prophylaxis in contacts of patients with meningitis caused by sulfonamide-resistant strains of *Neisseria meningitidis*.

In the treatment of tuberculosis, two-drug combinations of rifampin and INH (Rifamate) are available. This one capsule/day drug regimen is claimed to be ideal for outpatient use, because the less often a patient needs to remember to take a drug, the more probable is the patient's compliance.

Rifampin, like INH, causes liver dysfunction, particularly when combined with INH or other hepatotoxic drugs. Other adverse effects include the following: GI disturbances; rarely, but more often with intermittent therapy, a flulike syndrome, sometimes with hematologic disturbances and renal failure; and an acute organic brain syndrome. It can color skin, urine, tears, and soft contact lenses orange.

Clinically significant drug–drug interactions occur with a number of drugs whose metabolism is enhanced. These include *oral coumarin-type anticoagulants; metroprolol tartrate* (Lopressor); *propranolol hydrochloride* (Inderal); *quinidine; clofibrate* (Atromid-S); *oral hypoglycemics; oral contraceptives;* and *corticosteroids.* The dosage of all these drugs may need to be increased when rifampin therapy is initiated. Patients who are being maintained on *methadone* may need an increase in dosage to prevent withdrawal symptoms.

Second-line drugs. These drugs are always used in combination with at least one other antituberculosis drug.

Ethambutol[+] (Myambutol) exerts its bacteriostatic effects by interfering with bacterial cell metabolism. Like the first-line drugs, it is well absorbed orally. It should be taken with food to minimize GI upsets. It sometimes causes an optic neuritis, and the patient's vision should be evaluated before therapy is begun and at monthly intervals during therapy. Changes in color perception may be the first symptom of toxicity. The visual changes are usually reversible if diagnosed early and if ethambutol is withdrawn. The drug may also cause confusion and may precipitate attacks of gout. The dosage should be reduced in patients with impaired kidney function.

Pyrazinamide is a highly active synthetic chemotherapeutic agent whose mechanism of action is little understood. It is effective orally and is mostly metabolized in the liver. It is contraindicated in severe liver disease and is itself hepatotoxic, so that liver function should be monitored before and during therapy (every 2 to 4 weeks). It may precipitate gouty arthritis.

Streptomycin[+] is an antibiotic that was the first drug to prove effective in tuberculosis. Bacteria were found to develop resistance to it rapidly, but this drawback was overcome when para-aminosalicylate sodium (PAS), isoniazid, and later rifampin, became available for combination therapy. A continuing limitation has been the toxicity of streptomycin to the eighth cranial nerve. The adverse effects on vestibular and auditory function (see above, Aminoglycoside Antibiotics) may be reduced by administering this drug only twice weekly instead of every day once the worst phase of the acute illness has been brought under control. The need to administer streptomycin parenterally (IM) is a consideration in the decision to add this drug to an antituberculosis drug regimen.

Streptomycin is now often reserved for use in cases marked by large cavities in the lungs or as part of a triple-drug regimen for *extra*pulmonary tuberculosis. In such advanced cases of cavitary tuberculosis and in tuberculous meningitis and miliary, or disseminated, disease, this antibiotic is always combined with isoniazid and often also with rifampin or ethambutol. Otherwise, resistance to streptomycin develops very rapidly. Resistance also often results when streptomycin is administered intermittently. Thus, when it is used together with isoniazid, daily injections of streptomycin are now recommended as long as the patient's sputum remains positive.

Third-line drugs. *Para-aminosalicylate sodium* (PAS) was once a mainstay of antituberculosis therapy. However, it causes a high incidence of distressing GI disturbances (*e.g.,* nausea, vomiting, diarrhea, abdominal pain) and this, combined with the need to take doses four times/day, led to low patient compliance. It is now used mainly to delay the development of resistance to other antituberculosis drugs with which it is administered. In addition to GI disturbances, PAS may cause blood dyscrasias, liver damage, crystalluria (minimized by keeping the urine at a neutral or alkaline *p*H), and thyroid enlargement. It may inhibit the absorption of rifampin; doses of the two drugs should be administered 8 to 12 hours apart. It may also inhibit the absorption of both oral folic acid and vitamin B_{12}. The sodium content of this drug may cause problems in patients with known or impending congestive heart failure.

Ethionamide (Trecator-SC) is administered orally and may be taken with food to minimize GI disturbances, which occur frequently. It is cleared from the body by metabolism in the liver and may cause liver damage. Liver function tests should be performed periodically. It has caused central nervous system toxicity, including psychosis and convulsions, and visual changes and gynecomastia. It can increase the hypoglycemia produced by oral hypoglycemic drugs. It is recommended that pyridoxine (vitamin B_6) be given concomitantly with ethionamide.

Cycloserine (Seromycin) is an antibiotic that inhibits bacterial cell wall synthesis and is effective against a broad spectrum of bacteria. However, it is used clinically only in difficult cases of tuberculosis and in some stubborn UTIs caused by *E. coli* and those of the *Aerobacter* group that do not respond to sulfonamides and other safer anti-infective agents. The main limitation of this drug is its tendency to cause toxic central nervous system effects when administered in adequate doses for treating tuberculosis.

Patients receiving cycloserine must be observed for early signs of central toxicity including headache, drowsiness, and confusion. Tremors may precede convulsive seizures, and a period of increasing anxiety and disorientation may be followed by a psychotic episode of mental depression. The drug is contraindicated in tubercular patients who also have epilepsy or a history of psychosis or chronic alcoholism. The central nervous system toxicity may be increased by concomitant therapy with INH and ethionamide. Pyridoxine and antiepileptic drugs may control the convulsions.

Capreomycin (Capastat) must be administered by deep intramuscular injection to minimize pain and to prevent sterile abscess development. Like other polypeptide-type antibiotics, it is potentially toxic to the kidneys and to the eighth cranial nerve. Thus, tests of hearing, balance, and renal function are made before and during treatment. Despite these drawbacks, this new tuberculostatic drug is valuable when used with other antituberculosis drugs in cases no longer controllable by first-line drugs to which the tubercle bacilli have developed resistance.

Additional clinical considerations

The patient with tuberculosis presents a complex clinical picture. The drug therapy is intricately intertwined with all aspects of the disease. Because of the encompassing nature of tuberculosis and tuberculosis therapy, the patient teaching points and key points of the nursing process as it applies to antituberculosis drugs are best incorporated into a discussion of the patient's general therapy. Some of the main points that should be considered are listed below.

INH. This drug can cause GI upset and, if it becomes severe, the drug can be taken with food. Because of the tyramine interaction discussed earlier, certain foods should be avoided—for example, Chianti wine, cheddar cheese—and the patient should be aware of the signs and symptoms of problems (*e.g.*, headache, hypertension). Other signs and symptoms that the patient should be aware of include the histamine interaction (headache, flushing, sweating, palpitations), vitamin B_6 deficiency

(tingling, weakness, fatigue), and hepatic failure or hepatitis (nausea, vomiting, yellowing of eyes or skin, darkening of urine).

Rifampin. This drug should be taken on an empty stomach. The drug turns the body's secretions orange, which means that the saliva, urine, stools, tears, and sweat will be orange. Soft contact lenses may even be stained orange. The stain will wash out of clothing, diapers, and off the skin. The patient should report any "flu" symptoms (fever, chills, weakness, nausea, vomiting) and should be alert for signs of hepatic toxicity. Hepatic toxicity of INH and rifampin is increased if the drugs are used together. Rifampin induces liver enzyme systems and thus increases the metabolism of many drugs, making them less effective. The manufacturer's insert should be consulted before any drug is given with rifampin.

Ethambutol. This drug can be given with food to counteract the GI upset. The patient should report any changes in vision (*e.g.*, red–green color blindness, blurring).

PAS. This drug can be taken with food to counteract the GI upset. Patients should be warned that the powdered and tablet forms are unstable when in contact with heat, water, and sunlight. They should check the drug and should not use PAS that is brownish or purplish in color. *Probenecid* prevents the excretion of PAS, which can lead to PAS toxicity. Because PAS may inhibit the absorption of rifampin, the two drugs should be administered 8 to 12 hours apart. The patient should report any fever, sore throat, or increased bleeding or bruising.

With all these drugs, the importance of following the prescription must be stressed. The patient needs to understand the importance of the drug therapy, the crucial aspects of timing and of not discontinuing therapy, as well as the importance of follow-up medical care. The patient and family will also need encouragement and support to cope with the diagnosis and with the prolonged treatment regimen.

Summary of toxic effects of antituberculosis drugs

Aminosalicylic acid and its salts

   Gastrointestinal upset: nausea, vomiting, diarrhea
   Hypersensitivity reactions: skin eruptions, fever, sore throat, blood dyscrasias
   Rarely, liver damage and goiter

Capreomycin

   Nephrotoxicity: rise in BUN level and changes in other tests of kidney function
   Ototoxicity: some hearing loss, ringing in the ears, vertigo
   Liver function test abnormalities
   Hypersensitivity reactions: fever, skin eruptions

Cycloserine

   CNS toxicity: convulsions, headache, drowsiness, confusion, disorientation, hallucinations, coma
   Peripheral neuropathy: paresthesia, paresis

Ethambutol

   Optic neuritis: loss of visual acuity, peripheral vision, color discrimination
   Peripheral neuropathy: numbness and tingling
   Hypersensitivity: pruritic skin rashes

(continued)

Ethionamide

Gastrointestinal: anorexia, unpleasant metallic taste, epigastric burning and discomfort, nausea, vomiting, diarrhea

Peripheral neuropathy, including rare optic neuritis

CNS and endocrine abnormalities: depression, amenorrhea, impotence

Isoniazid

Peripheral neuropathy: numbness, tingling, burning pain, muscle weakness, rarely optic neuritis

CNS effects: hallucinations, mental depression, convulsive seizures

Liver damage: jaundice, abnormalities in liver function tests

Autonomic blockage: postural hypotension, difficulty in micturition

Pyrazinamide

Hepatotoxicity: liver function test abnormalities, jaundice

Hyperuricemia: gout symptoms

Hypersensitivity: fever, joint pains

Rifampin

Liver dysfunction: test abnormalities, high serum bilirubin level, jaundice

Gastrointestinal: anorexia, epigastric distress, nausea, vomiting, cramps, diarrhea

Blood: thrombocytopenia, leukopenia

Streptomycin

Eighth nerve damage: vertigo, headache, tinnitus, deafness

Hypersensitivity reactions: skin eruptions, anaphylactoid shock

Blood dyscrasias: occasional agranulocytosis, thrombocytopenia, aplastic anemia

Leprosy (Hansen's Disease)

Leprosy is a chronic disease caused by an acid-fast bacillus, *Mycobacterium leprae*, a microorganism related to the tubercle bacillus. These rods multiply only very slowly in the body and not at all in culture media. Thus, no vaccine is available. The bacteria invade the skin and certain peripheral nerves but, in some forms of the disease, the damaging results of the body's chronic inflammatory responses can be seen in many other systems, including the eyes and respiratory tract.

The skin lesions of leprosy are often disfiguring, and nerve damage may lead to muscle wasting and limb deformities. The facial disfigurement often seen in the lepromatous form of the disease probably accounts for the prejudice that people have had against its victims. In times past, lepers were often cast out of the community because of public loathing and fear of the infection. In the Middle Ages, when the disease was widespread in Europe, the church set up special hospitals, or lazarettos, to care for lepers. Prejudice and fear still exist today, and patients are often still segregated in special hospitals or leprosariums, even though the infectiousness of this disease is relatively low.

Chemotherapy

Prospects for control of this disease changed dramatically with the introduction in the 1940s of a drug group called *sulfones* (Table 8-12). These chemical relatives of the sulfonamides are still the best treatment for leprosy; and the first agent of this class, *dapsone*[+] (DDS) is still the drug of choice. *Acedapsone* (Hansolar), a repository drug that is investigational in the United States, is another leprostatic sulfone. Other drugs now available for use in

the occasional patient who cannot tolerate dapsone and its derivatives, or in whom resistant strains of bacilli develop, include *clofazimine* (Lamprene), a drug that is also investigational in the United States.

Clinical improvement is seen after several months of treatment with oral doses of dapsone, but several years may be required for skin lesions to disappear. Because living bacteria have been isolated after many years, low-dose drug treatment of lepromatous-type leprosy is best continued for the rest of the patient's life to avoid relapses. Sulfone resistance may occur during long-term therapy, especially when low doses are taken only irregularly. The new lesions that then arise may respond to treatment with *non*sulfone compounds such as clofazimine. The antituberculosis drugs *rifampin* and *ethionamide* (Trecator-SC; see above), and the investigational drug *prothionamide*, are

Table 8–12. Leprostatic chemotherapeutic agents: sulfones*

Generic or official name	Usual adult dosage
Dapsone USP (DDS)	10-mg–25-mg initial oral doses are increased gradually up to 300 mg several times/week

* Other drugs of the sulfone class are investigational in the United States and available from the United States Public Health Service Hospital, Carville, Louisiana.

also sometimes useful in such cases. The investigational drugs are available from the United States Public Health Service Hospital at Carville, Louisiana. The treatment of leprosy is so complex that the specialists at this hospital should always be consulted for assistance with diagnosis and therapy.

Adverse effects

Reactions to treatment with sulfones vary from minor, readily controlled side-effects to signs of severe toxicity that require discontinuing the drug. Early gastrointestinal upset can be avoided by beginning treatment with small oral doses that are administered only once weekly at first and then raised gradually over many weeks to as much as five doses/week. Patients taking higher doses are watched for signs of hemolytic anemia, particularly if tests indicate that their red blood cells are deficient in the protective enzyme G-6-PD. Methemoglobinemia and manifestations of drug allergy may also develop in some cases.

Lepromatous lepra reactions. Many patients receiving sulfones develop *erythema nodosum,* a sudden acute flare-up of the disease that is thought to be induced by the therapeutic effect of these drugs. Painful red lesions may rise over the patient's entire body, and there may be fever, malaise, and occasionally exacerbation of neuritis, iritis, orchitis, and other signs and symptoms of lepromatous leprosy that had been controlled by previous drug treatment. This is thought to be the result of an immune reaction, not to the drug itself but to antigenic material derived from the dead bacteria.

In severe reactions of this type sulfone drugs are discontinued, and any of several other drugs may be used for symptomatic control of the reaction. *Corticosteroids* such as prednisone, administered in large doses that are then gradually reduced and soon withdrawn entirely, are often effective for suppressing erythema nodosum reactions. *Thalidomide* is also claimed to be effective, but it cannot be given to women of childbearing age because

of its possible adverse effects on the fetus if an early unrecognized pregnancy has occurred (see Chap. 5).

Prognosis

The prognosis for most properly managed leprosy patients is now very good. Drug therapy prevents death from respiratory infection and nephritis, which were once common complications. Blindness and deformities can also be prevented by chemotherapy, as can permanent scarring, when drug treatment is begun early in the course of the disease. Patients already deformed can be helped by surgical procedures and by rehabilitative physiotherapy. Patients with limbs that have no feeling because of sensory nerve damage must be taught to prevent skin injury and infection, because damage to their digits and extremities may make amputations necessary. Education of the public as well as of the patient can also help make life easier for those with Hansen's disease.

Additional clinical considerations

It is somewhat unusual to encounter a patient being treated for Hansen's disease. The drug therapy for this disease must be closely incorporated with total patient care. The patient will require a great deal of support and encouragement to cope with the impact and possible disfigurement of this disease. Those on the clinical staff who are unfamiliar with the disease will also need encouragement to deal with the patient. Some particulars of drug therapy that should be incorporated include the following:

1. Take the drug with food to avoid GI upset.
2. Be aware of the possibility of dermatologic reactions.
3. Report any serious GI or neurologic changes.
4. Follow the prolonged prescription for the drug because it is very important for the success of therapy.

Case Study

Presentation I

GS, a compulsive, organized married woman, began graduate school with plans to start a family in 2 years at the completion of her graduate program. GS had successfully used low-dose oral contraceptives or birth control pills (BCP) for 4 years and had planned to continue this method of birth control. A few weeks into the fall semester, GS developed severe sinusitis that cultured out as a *Klebsiella* strain that was sensitive to tetracycline. GS was treated with a standard 5-day course of tetracycline, at the end of which the sinusitis had resolved. In mid-January, GS was seen in the clinic for a number of complaints, which turned out to be caused by a pregnancy. Uterine size was consistent with a 12-week gestational size. GS denied any lapse in BCP use. What happened to GS? What measures are now appropriate for GS?

Discussion

Low-dose birth control pills work by providing a constant level of estrogens and progestins in the body that signal the hypothalamus to stop the release of the gonadotropic-releasing hormone (GnRH), thus preventing ovulation and the normal cycling of the female sex hormones (see Chap. 23). The low levels of these hormones also cause minimal endometrial development and set up an environment that would not be conducive to implantation and pregnancy if ovulation should actually occur. Several antimicrobials, including rifampin, ampicillin, chloramphenicol, and the tetracyclines, have been associated with BCP failure, as evidenced by breakthrough bleeding and unwanted pregnancies. The exact cause of the BCP failure is not completely understood, but it is thought to be related to the loss of normal intestinal bacterial flora as a result of the antibiotic therapy. The normal flora are responsible for the breakdown and absorption of the steroids; in their absence, it seems, the hormones are lost in the feces and there is a resultant decrease in serum hormone levels. The 5-day course of antibiotic therapy could have caused a loss of normal bacterial flora for several days, with a resultant drop in blood hormone levels. This drop probably constituted a sufficient loss of the negative feedback control on the hypothalamus to allow the release of GnRH, which in turn stimulated release of the follicle-stimulating and luteinizing hormones and eventually led to ovulation. The 12-week gestational size of the uterus would support this idea.

Understanding the cause of the BCP failure may help GS to cope with the pregnancy, but her total situation must be considered for adequate care. Considering her compulsive, organized life-style, this surprise pregnancy may be especially difficult to deal with. The nurse will need to assess GS's support systems, her feelings about the pregnancy, her stress level in relation to school, and her ability to cope with this change. Because stress predisposes people to a myriad of physical problems, a total physical examination should be done to determine GS's baseline physical status. Specific patient teaching needs will include an explanation of the drug–drug interaction that has occurred and the teaching protocol needed for pregnancy. In this case, GS will also need to know the possible risks to the fetus involved with taking BCPs throughout the first trimester of pregnancy. Some studies report teratogenic effects involving the neural tube and reproductive organ development related to BCP use during early pregnancy. GS will need to know this and consider the options available to her: testing to determine if fetal problems exist; carrying the pregnancy to term; or terminating the pregnancy. Whatever GS decides, she will need a great deal of support and encouragement throughout her medical care. All those involved with this case should learn again the importance of careful patient teaching whenever a patient receives a drug. The consequences of such drug–drug interactions can be avoided.

Presentation 2

Jill, a 6-year-old girl, has a history of repeated urinary tract infections. She is seen in Pediatric Clinic with presenting complaints of dysuria, frequency, urgency, and a low-grade fever. A urine sample is sent for culture and sensitivity testing. Jill is started on methenamine, 500 mg qid, and referred, with her mother, to the nurse for patient teaching. What key points should be considered?

Discussion

Because Jill has a history of recurrent bladder infections, patient teaching should incorporate preventive measures as well as key points about drug therapy. Girls and women are more susceptible to bladder infections because of the short urethra leading to the bladder. Keeping this in mind, several points can be covered with Jill and her mother: she should avoid bubble baths (the effervescent bubbles can help bacteria enter the bladder); she should wear cotton panties (cotton absorbs fluid and helps to draw fluid and thence bacteria away from the body); she should avoid tight jeans or pants (a closed, warm, dark environment can favor bacterial proliferation); and she should always wipe herself from front to back, away from the urethra (wiping back to front brings *Escherichia coli* and other intestinal bacteria into the area of the urethra). Certain dietary measures can help the activity of the drug therapy and can also help to establish growth. Jill should drink plenty of fluids (8 to 10 glasses a day) to flush the bladder regularly, and avoid the ingestion of alkaline ash foods, such as citrus juice, milk, and milk products (acidifying the urine by eliminating dietary alkaline substances helps the drug therapy, and bacteria do not survive well in acidic environments); cranberry juice may help to acidify the urine and satisfy any desire for drinking juice.

In regard to methenamine therapy, Jill's mother will need to understand the importance of Jill's completing the full course of therapy—that is, the entire prescription should be used, even if Jill feels much better in a few days. Methenamine should also be given around the clock for best results. A schedule should be worked out to determine the timing that best accommodates Jill's daily activities. The patient and her mother should know that the drug can be taken with food if stomach upset occurs. They should also be told to call the nurse if a rash, extreme GI upset, or very painful urination occurs.

For greatest effectiveness, the teaching facts along with a telephone number to call if needed should be written down for easy reference. The patient should be scheduled for a follow-up visit for evaluation of the drug therapy and the teaching program. Careful patient teaching involving all the measures mentioned can augment the drug therapy. Hopefully, such an approach can prevent further bladder infections for this child.

Drug digests

Ampicillin USP (Amcill; Omnipen)

Actions and indications. This semisynthetic penicillin possesses a relatively wide spectrum of antibacterial activity that includes not only the common gram-positive organisms but also such gram-negative bacilli as *Hemophilus influenzae, Escherichia coli, Proteus mirabilis,* and many strains of *Shigella* and *Salmonella* species, including *Salmonella typhosa,* the cause of typhoid fever.

Ampicillin is a frequent first choice for initiating treatment of acute otitis media in young children, because it is active against the most common gram-positive and gram-negative bacterial causes of middle ear infections and their most common complication, meningitis, in that age group. It is also commonly employed in urinary tract infections. However, because of the appearance of ampicillin-resistant strains of the gram-negative species responsible for the respiratory, urinary, and GI tract infections for which it is most frequently employed, it is essential to show that the infective strain is actually susceptible to this antibiotic.

Adverse effects, cautions, and contraindications. Hypersensitivity reactions ranging from urticaria and other skin rashes to fatal anaphylactoid reactions are possible. Thus, particular caution is required in patients with a history of allergy or of previous allergic reactions to any penicillin product, even though the incidence of urticarial and anaphylactoid reactions is claimed to be lower for ampicillin than for penicillin G products. Erythematous macropapular and morbilliform (measleslike) rashes of the delayed reaction type are said to occur more often with ampicillin than with penicillin G.

Although serious allergic reactions occur more commonly following parenteral administration of ampicillin, the oral dosage forms are more likely to cause adverse gastrointestinal reactions as a result of the overgrowth of nonsusceptible organisms. This may be manifested in the mouth by stomatitis and glossitis, including so-called black or "hairy" tongue. Nausea, vomiting, and diarrhea may also result from such superinfection.

Dosage and administration. Oral doses of 250 mg to 500 mg are administered every 6 hours to adults with mild to moderate infections; and children receive 25 to 50 mg/kg/day in similar infections. For serious infections such as bacterial meningitis or septicemia, adults and children receive 150 to 200 mg/kg/day divided into equal doses administered IV or IM every 3 or 4 hours, after an initial period in which IV drip is employed.

Carbenicillin disodium (Geopen; Pyopen)

Actions and indications. This penicillin has a broader spectrum than others, because its antibacterial spectrum includes not only the gram-positive and gram-negative organisms that are sensitive to penicillin G and ampicillin, but also *Pseudomonas aeruginosa* and indole-positive *Proteus* species not susceptible to other penicillins. Despite its extended spectrum, this antibiotic is best reserved for treating only severe systemic infections such as septicemia, or genitourinary and respiratory tract infections in which the infecting organisms are not sensitive to the other penicillins.

The main reason for this limitation is that strains resistant to this valuable antibiotic tend to emerge during its use. Among the resistant organisms that may cause superinfections are *Klebsiella* and *Serratia* species and penicillinase-producing staphylococci. Sensitivity tests should be done during therapy with this antibiotic to detect the development of resistance in previously susceptible strains during therapy.

Adverse effects, cautions, and contraindications. The main types of adverse reactions to this antibiotic are the result of hypersensitivity to penicillin. Because of the possibility of severe anaphylactoid reactions, this drug is ordinarily contraindicated in patients with a history of penicillin hypersensitivity or of allergy to various other drugs and substances. Pain at the intramuscular injection site and venous irritation and phlebitis from intravenous infusion have been reported. The high blood levels required for antipseudomonal effectiveness may sometimes cause nervous tissue irritability with possible muscular twitching or convulsions.

Some patients with impaired kidney function have developed episodes of bleeding when treated with high doses of carbenicillin. Consequently, clotting time and prothrombin time tests should be done during treatment of uremic and other such patients to detect coagulation abnormalities before actual hemorrhagic manifestations appear.

Because of the high sodium content of this salt and the large doses that are often necessary, patients in whom sodium restriction is required should be checked for clinical signs of sodium retention that may adversely affect cardiovascular function. Laboratory determinations should be made periodically, not only of serum sodium levels but also of potassium levels, because hypokalemia may also occur.

Dosage and administration. In serious systemic pseudomonal infections, including septicemia, as much as 400 to 500 mg/kg (30 g–40 g) may be administered by continuous IV drip or in divided doses, injected as slowly as possible to avoid venous irritation. As little as 1 g or 2 g every 6 hours may be administered intramuscularly in uncomplicated urinary tract infections. In acute uncomplicated gonorrhea, a single 4-g dose is injected—one-half the total dose at each of two different IM sites. This may be preceded by a 1-g oral dose of probenecid 30 minutes before. When gentamicin is also administered, the two solutions must not be mixed.

Cephalothin sodium USP (Keflin)

Actions and indications. This prototype of the injectable cephalosporin antibiotics possesses a broad antibacterial spectrum that includes both penicillin-sensitive and penicillinase-producing staphylococci among other gram-positive cocci, as well as such common gram-negative enteric bacilli as *E. coli*, *Proteus mirabilis*, and *Klebsiella*. (It is not active against such other gram-negative rods as *Pseudomonas* species or indole-producing *Proteus* species, or *Serratia*, nor is it effective for treating infections caused by the enterococcus *Streptococcus faecalis*.)

Cephalothin is widely employed in the treatment of serious infections by susceptible organisms, such as respiratory and urinary tract, skin, and soft tissue infections and septicemia. Actually, however, like other drugs of this antibiotic class, it is only rarely the drug of choice in any infection, except when the pathogen is identified as a highly susceptible strain of *Klebsiella pneumoniae*.

Except in patients who are hypersensitive to penicillin, for example, penicillin G, ampi-

cillin, or one of the penicillinase-resistant antistaphylococcal penicillins is preferred for treating infections caused by gram-positive cocci or by such gram-negative enteric bacilli as *E. coli*, *P. mirabilis*, or *Hemophilus influenzae*. An aminoglycoside antibiotic alone or in combination with carbenicillin or penicillin G is preferred in infections caused by the cephalothin-resistant gram-negative rods mentioned above.

Adverse effects, cautions, and contraindications. Hypersensitivity reactions occur in about 5% of patients and are most likely to develop in patients previously sensitized to penicillin. Eruptions of both the urticarial and macropapular types may be seen, but these alone do not necessarily require discontinuation of the drug in severely ill patients with infections that are responding to treatment. Severe anaphylactic reactions are rare. However, if one occurs, no further doses are administered, and the patient is treated with antagonistic agents that are kept readily available, including epinephrine.

Large doses (or ordinary doses in patients with impaired kidney function) sometimes cause neutropenia and thrombocytopenia, or a positive direct Coombs' test that may be followed by hemolytic anemia.

Intramuscular injection may cause pain and tenderness with possible induration or development of sterile abscess and tissue sloughing. Intravenous infusion for several days may lead to thrombophlebitis.

Dosage and administration. The usual adult dosage is between 500 mg and 1 g every 4 to 6 hours, but as much as 2 g every 4 hours may be required for severe infections. In patients with marked renal impairment, an initial loading dose of 1 g to 2 g may be followed every 6 hours by 500 mg to 1 g. Infants and children receive a total daily dose of 40 to 80 mg/lb in divided doses.

Intravenous doses may be given intermittently or by continuous infusion of a solution prepared by dilution with sterile water, normal saline solution or 5% dextrose.

Chloramphenicol USP and its palmitate and sodium succinate esters (Chloromycetin)

Actions and indications. This antibiotic has a broad spectrum of antimicrobial activity, but its clinical usefulness is limited by its potentially lethal toxicity. It may be employed to begin treatment of certain infections in which it is known to be highly effective. However, treatment should be continued only if sensitivity tests indicate that this drug is more active than other safer anti-infective drugs against the organism responsible for the patient's illness.

Among the infections for which chloramphenicol may be used to initiate therapy and in which it may continue to be employed if no equally effective drug of less potential toxicity is available are the following: typhoid fever and other systemic salmonella infections; Rocky Mountain spotted fever and other rickettsial infections such as typhus fever; chlamydial infections such as psittacosis and lymphogranuloma venereum; meningitis caused by *Hemophilus influenzae*; other gram-negative bacillary infections such as brucellosis, bubonic plague, and tularemia; or serious urinary tract infections, especially when

complicated by bacteremia.

Adverse effects, cautions, and contraindications. The most serious adverse effect is bone marrow depression that may lead to two general types of blood dyscrasias. The most common of these is characterized mainly by a reduction in reticulocytes and in changes in the form of early erythroid cells. Blood studies should be done every 2 days during treatment so that the drug may be discontinued if such changes are detected. This disorder is reversible and responds to the withdrawal of the drug.

The second type of disorder is irreversible and may develop weeks or months after treatment has been completed. The most common result of this relatively rare hypersensitivity reaction is fatal pancytopenia, but sometimes only anemia, leukopenia, or thrombopenia may occur. Although such reductions in red or white cells and platelets may be detected by blood studies or clinical signs and symptoms, withdrawal of the drug may not prevent development of bone marrow aplasia and aplastic anemia.

A toxic reaction called the "gray baby syndrome" has occurred in newborn and, particularly, premature infants. This disorder, which is marked by pallor and cyanosis, can lead to fatal vasomotor collapse and respiratory failure within a few hours. If this drug is used at all in infants under 2 weeks to 1 month old, the serum levels should be measured frequently to maintain safe concentrations. Caution is also required in administering the drug late in pregnancy or during labor, because it passes the placental barrier.

Dosage and administration. The total daily dose is 50 mg/kg administered in four divided doses at 6-hour intervals. Occasionally, severe infections may require up to 100 mg/kg per day administered orally or by slow intravenous injection of the sodium succinate ester.

For newborn infants a total of only 25 mg/kg/day is divided into four equal doses and administered at 6-hour intervals. This may be raised to a total daily dose of 50 mg/kg in full-term infants after the first 2 weeks of life.

Clindamycin HCl USP and other salts and esters (Cleocin HCl)

Actions and indications. This antibiotic may be used as an alternative to penicillins in the treatment of gram-positive coccal infections. Although the less toxic antibiotic erythromycin is the preferred penicillin substitute, this agent has also been employed in penicillin-sensitive patients to treat streptococcal pharyngitis and other upper and lower respiratory tract infections caused by streptococci, pneumococci, and staphylococci. Cases of chronic osteomyelitis caused by staphylococcal strains resistant to other antibiotics have sometimes responded very well to treatment with this anti-infective agent. Clindamycin is particularly effective against various types of anaerobic microorganisms, including species of *Bacteroides, Fusobacterium,* and *Actinomyces.* It has proved useful for treating pneumonia and other lower respiratory tract infections such as pneumonitis, empyema, and lung abscesses caused by penicillin-resistant anaerobes such as *Bacteroides fragilis.* This antibiotic may also be very useful for control of peritonitis and other intra-abdominal infections caused by gastrointestinal anaerobes and in female pelvic or genital tract infections caused by such organisms. It can be lifesaving in septicemia caused by anaerobic gram-negative bacilli.

Adverse effects, cautions, and contraindications. The most common adverse effects are abdominal pain, nausea, vomiting, and diarrhea. If diarrhea persists and blood or mucus appears in the stool, the drug should be discontinued because fatal colitis has occurred. It is contraindicated in patients with a history of a similar reaction to the related antibiotic lincomycin. Caution is required in patients with a history of allergy or severe kidney or liver disease. Jaundice and abnormalities in liver function tests have been reported, but no cases of irreversible damage to organs or tissues other than the mucosa of the colon have occurred.

The clindamycin phosphate solution employed for parenteral administration may be irritating. Pain, induration, and sterile abscesses may be minimized by injecting the solution deep into the muscle and using no more than 600 mg in any one injection. To prevent possible thrombophlebitis the solution is diluted and injected intravenously over a period of 10 minutes to about 1 hour, and indwelling catheters should not be employed for a prolonged period.

Dosage and administration. Oral dosage for adults is 150 mg to 300 mg every 6 hours and, for severe infections, 300 mg to 450 mg at the same intervals. The oral dose of clindamycin palmitate in children is 8 to 12 mg/kg/day in mild infections, 13 to 16 mg/kg/day for moderately severe infections, and 17 to 25 mg/kg/day for severe infections. These total daily doses are divided into three or four equal doses.

Parenteral administration of clindamycin phosphate varies from 600 mg a day divided into two equal doses to 1200 mg to 2700 mg a day divided into four equal doses. However, doses as high as 4.8 g daily have been administered by vein to adults with life-threatening infections.

Dapsone USP (DDS)

Actions and indications. The most important use of this prototype sulfone derivative is as a leprostatic agent in the control of leprosy, or Hansen's disease. Administered over long periods, this drug gradually brings about variable degrees of improvement in most leprous patients. New lesions do not develop during treatment, and healing of skin nodules is adequate enough to make possible the return of some patients to their communities.

Adverse effects, cautions, and contraindications. Toxicity is related to dosage and the subsequent blood levels of the drug. Side-effects of low doses affect mainly the gastrointestinal tract—anorexia, nausea, and vomiting—and the central nervous system—headache, nervousness, and sleeplessness. More serious are effects on the circulating red blood cells, resulting in hemolysis, particularly in those with a deficiency of the protective enzyme glucose-6-phosphate dehydrogenase (G-6-PD). These untoward effects are less likely to occur if dosage is built up gradually, and if blood levels of the drug are checked periodically to avoid accumulation of the slowly excreted drug to toxic levels.

The drug must be discontinued and corticosteroids administered if acute lepra reaction develops.

Dosage and administration. Initially the drug is administered in oral doses of 25 mg to 50 mg twice a week for 4 or 5 weeks. It is then increased by 100 mg at monthly intervals until a maximum dose of 400 mg two times a week is reached. Doses of 100 mg to 200 mg daily are occasionally employed to suppress acute flare-ups of dermatitis herpetiformis.

Doxycycline hyclate USP (Vibramycin)

Actions and indications. This tetracycline derivative has the same antimicrobial spectrum of effectiveness as other antibiotics of this chemical class. That is, it has a broad spectrum that includes not only gram-positive and gram-negative bacteria, but also *Rickettsia, Mycoplasma, Chlamydia*—the agents that cause psittacosis, lymphogranuloma venereum, and trachoma—spirochetes, and amebae. Thus, like other tetracyclines, it is useful for treatment of very varied infectious diseases, including some for which it is especially valuable, such as Rocky Mountain spotted fever, Q fever, and typhus fever; mycoplasmal ("atypical viral") pneumonia; chanchroid; cholera; brucellosis; and bacteroides bacteremia and brain or other abscesses.

Doxycycline differs from other tetracyclines in certain aspects of its pharmacokinetic factors in ways that have clinical significance. It is, for example, more slowly absorbed and excreted than most others and is about 90% bound to plasma proteins. The resulting long length of its half-life permits its use in smaller doses and at longer intervals of administration. (See below for other significant differences of this tetracycline.)

Adverse effects, cautions, and contraindications. This compound is similar to other tetracyclines in its systemic toxicity, including hypersensitivity reactions, photosensitivity effects in patients exposed to direct sunlight, and discoloration of teeth. However, because of its almost complete absorption from the upper intestinal tract, lower bowel side-effects including diarrhea as a result of irritation or changes in the intestinal microbial flora occur less frequently than with other tetracyclines. This drug also seems safer for patients with poor renal function, because little is excreted by the kidneys, and so the drug does not accumulate to toxic levels in the liver and elsewhere in patients with renal insufficiency or failure.

Dosage and administration. This drug, unlike other oral tetracyclines, may be taken with milk, because its absorption is not influenced by the calcium content of dairy products or by the simultaneous ingestion of other foods. The usual oral adult dose is 200 mg on the first day (divided into two 100-mg doses at 12-hour intervals). This is followed by a maintenance dose of 100 mg daily (administered as a single oral dose or as two 50-mg doses at 12-hour intervals).

The usual adult dose of the injectable form is 200 mg on the first day and later daily doses of 100 mg to 200 mg, depending on the severity of the infection. These are administered intravenously in one or two daily infusions, each of which lasts 1 to 4 hours, depending on the dose. Care is required to keep the irritating solution from entering the tissues adjacent to the vein, and the drug should not be administered intramuscularly or subcutaneously. Patients should be put on oral therapy as soon as possible, because prolonged intravenous use may lead to thrombophlebitis.

Erythromycin USP and its salts and esters (Erythrocin; Ilotycin)

Actions and indications. This antibiotic has an antibacterial spectrum similar to that of penicillin and is used mainly as an alternative for treating infections caused by susceptible pathogens in patients allergic to penicillin. It is especially effective against gram-positive cocci, such as streptococci, pneumococci, and staphylococci of both the penicillin G-sensitive and G-resistant types. (However, because of the emergence of increasing numbers of staphylococcal strains resistant to this antibiotic, it should be used only when susceptibility of the organism has been proved by sensitivity tests.)

Among the infections for which erythromycin is employed are the following: streptococcal pharyngitis (treatment and prevention); pneumococcal pneumonia and meningitis; subacute bacterial endocarditis and especially for prophylaxis against α-hemolytic infections prior to dental procedures and mouth or throat operations in patients with a history of congenital or rheumatic heart disease.

It is also used as an alternative to penicillin in women with acute gonorrheal inflammation of pelvic organs and in patients with primary syphilis. It may be effective in cases of primary atypical pneumonia caused by *Mycoplasma pneumoniae*. It is sometimes used for treating intestinal amebiasis. Some urinary tract infections caused by gram-negative bacilli respond to treatment with this antibiotic when the urine is kept alkaline by administration of sodium bicarbonate. It is the drug of choice in treating pneumonia caused by *Legionella pneumophila* (Legionnaires' disease); it is often given with rifampin in these cases.

Adverse effects, cautions, and contraindications. The most common side-effects are those affecting the gastrointestinal tract—abdominal discomfort and cramps, and occasional nausea, vomiting, and diarrhea. The estolate ester of erythromycin and, less often, the other drug forms, may occasionally cause an allergic hepatitis of the cholestatic type marked by jaundice, fever, and abdominal

pain resembling acute cholecystitis. Caution is required in patients with a history of liver disease and impaired hepatic function. Occasional allergic skin eruptions and more severe hypersensitivity reactions have been reported. Overgrowths of resistant bacteria and fungi may develop during prolonged treatment; if superinfection occurs, treatment is discontinued.

Dosage and administration. Adult oral dosage of erythromycin base is 250 mg every 6 hours, but this may be raised to 4 g or more per day depending on the severity of the infection. Erythromycin gluceptate and lactobionate are administered intravenously in doses of 15 to 20 mg/kg/day, in divided doses every 6 hours in more severe infections or when large oral doses are not tolerated. Erythromycin lactobionate is administered for acute gonorrhea in 500 mg intravenous doses every 6 hours for the first 3 days and then followed by the erythromycin base in doses of 250 mg every 6 hours for 7 more days.

Ethambutol HCl USP (Myambutol)

Actions and indications. This tuberculostatic drug is administered both with such standard drugs as isoniazid and rifampin in the initial treatment of primary tuberculosis and—for retreatment of relapsing chronic cases—together with one of the second-line drugs that had not been previously employed. This drug is not administered alone, because resistance to it develops rapidly.

Adverse effects, cautions, and contraindications. The most serious adverse effect of high dosage for long periods is the possible development of optic neuritis. Patients must

have their vision thoroughly examined before treatment is begun and at intervals of 1 month or less during therapy to detect decreases in visual acuity. If such tests show significant progressive changes, the drug must be discontinued. Recovery then takes place over a period of several weeks or months.

Other side-effects include gastrointestinal disturbances, headache, dizziness, and mental confusion, and allergic skin eruptions, joint pains, or anaphylactoid reactions. Abnormalities may be noted in liver function

tests, and serum uric acid levels may rise. The drug is not recommended for use in children under 13 years old, and it is given only in reduced dosage to patients with kidney impairment.

Dosage and administration. A single oral dose of 15 mg/kg is taken daily together with isoniazid in initiating treatment. The retreatment dosage is 25 mg/kg daily, taken together with one or more drugs not previously employed to which the organism has been shown to be susceptible.

Gentamicin sulfate USP (Garamycin)

Actions and indications. This aminoglycoside-group antibiotic has bactericidal activity against various gram-negative bacilli and gram-positive cocci, including some resistant staphylococcal strains. However, it is used mainly for treating serious urinary tract infections, septicemia, and meningitis caused by susceptible strains of *Pseudomonas aeruginosa*, *Proteus* species, *Escherichia coli*, and species of the *Klebsiella–Enterobacter–Serratia* group. It is often administered together with carbenicillin, with which it is synergistic against *Pseudomonas;* and it may be given together with ampicillin for the same reason to treat endocarditis caused by susceptible strains of the enterococcus *Streptococcus faecalis*.

Gentamicin may also be applied topically to treat such primary skin infections as impetigo, ecthyma, and furunculosis. It may also control secondary infections of the skin in various allergic and other dermatoses such as eczema, contact dermatitis including poison ivy, seborrheic dermatitis, and other dermatoses that may have become infected because of scratching. It has also been used in treating infected decubital ulcers and superficial burn sepsis.

Adverse effects, cautions, and contraindications. Like other drugs of the aminoglycoside group, gentamicin may cause adverse effects on the kidneys and on eighth cranial nerve function. The ototoxicity is manifested mainly by changes in vestibular branch functioning such as dizziness and vertigo. However, the auditory branch may also be affected, as indicated by ringing or buzzing in the ears or partial loss of hearing.

Neurotoxicity of this kind is most likely to occur in patients with impaired renal function who excrete the drug too slowly in comparison with the frequency at which it is being administered. This drug may itself cause nephrotoxicity, as indicated by rises in BUN, nonprotein nitrogen (NPN), and serum creatinine levels, or by the appearance of cells and casts in the urine and the occurrence of oliguria. It should not be administered together with other potentially nephrotoxic antibiotics such as cephaloridine or the polymyxins or with potent diuretics such as ethacrynic acid and other drugs that are potentially ototoxic.

Although the topical form of gentamicin is sometimes used to treat bacterial superin-

fections in patients with fungal skin diseases, use of this drug may itself lead to overgrowths of fungi and other nonsusceptible microbial pathogens. Its use topically in hospitalized burn patients may lead to the emergence of resistant bacterial strains that could later cause systemic infections for which gentamicin injections would then be ineffective.

Dosage and administration. The usual daily dose is 3 mg/kg administered intravenously or intramuscularly in three equal doses at 8-hour intervals in patients with normal kidney function. This may be adjusted upward to 5 mg/kg daily during life-threatening infections or downward in patients with renal impairment. The frequency of administrations may be changed from every 8 to every 12, 18, 24, 36, or 48 hours depending on the BUN or creatinine clearance rate of the patient with impaired kidney function.

A cream or ointment is applied topically after removal of crusts or incision and drainage of skin abscesses three or four times daily. An ophthalmic ointment is applied two or three times daily and an ophthalmic solution is instilled more frequently.

Isoniazid USP (INH; Nydrazid)

Actions and indications. This is the single most effective chemotherapeutic agent for treating and preventing tuberculosis. For use in active tuberculosis treatment it is ordinarily combined with such other antituberculosis drugs as rifampin or rifampin and a second- or third-line drug, because this helps to prevent or delay development of resistance.

This tuberculostatic agent is also employed prophylactically for treating those who are considered likely to develop tuberculosis. People in such high-risk groups include the following: (1) those living with a patient who has active tuberculosis (i.e., household contacts); (2) those who have recently developed a positive tuberculin test (i.e., recent converters); (3) other positive tuberculin reactors, such as those under 20 years of age, those with chest x-ray abnormalities, and those in certain special clinical situations; (4) those with presently inactive tuberculosis who have never received adequate chemotherapy.

Adverse effects, cautions, and contraindications. This drug is generally well tolerated. However, serious reactions can occur in patients who take high doses, in those in whom accumulation may occur as a result of congenitally slow acetylation of this drug, and in patients who prove hypersensitive to it. Hepatitis is an occasional reaction that is considered to be the result of hypersensitivity. Patients must be checked at monthly intervals for symptoms (nausea, vomiting, and epigastric distress) and signs (jaundice, bilirubinuria, and liver test abnormalities) that suggest possible liver damage. The drug should then be discontinued and the patient's course followed closely. Further use of this drug is contraindicated if a severe drug-induced hypersensitivity reaction actually develops. Otherwise, treatment may be begun again with small doses.

Other reported reactions include hematologic, dermatologic, metabolic and endocrine effects, and a syndrome resembling systemic lupus erythematosus. Nervous system reactions include peripheral neuropathy and convulsions, particularly in malnourished patients. (Administration of pyridoxine in such cases and in adolescent patients is recommended.) Caution is required in patients with a history of convulsive disorders, diabetes, active liver disease, and severe kidney dysfunction.

Dosage and administration. Usual adult dosage is 5 mg/kg/day in single or divided oral doses up to a total of 300 mg. Children receive between 10 and 30 mg/kg daily, depending on the severity of the infection. For prophylaxis, children receive 10 mg/kg/day up to a total dose of 300 mg daily.

Kanamycin sulfate USP (Kantrex)

Actions and indications. This antibiotic is active against strains of gram-negative bacilli such as species of the *Klebsiella–Enterobacter–Serratia* group, the *Mima–Herellea* group, and others; it is also active against some strains of gram-positive cocci, including *Staphylococcus aureus*.

The injectable form is used in the short-term treatment of serious systemic infections including Friedländer's pneumonia, gram-negative infections of the urinary tract, and septicemia. The oral form acts locally within the gastrointestinal tract to control infections caused by enteropathogens, including diarrhea-inducing strains of *E. coli*. It is also used to suppress intestinal bacteria as an adjunct to other therapeutic measures in the management of hepatic coma, and for sterilizing the bowel prior to surgery.

Adverse effects, cautions, and contraindications. This drug is not used parenterally for prolonged periods because of its potential for damaging the auditory nerve and causing deafness. Even when used for 5 days or more, it is desirable to monitor the patient's hearing with audiograms. If these show loss of high-frequency perception, treatment is stopped. Ototoxicity of this type is most likely to occur in patients with impaired kidney function, and the drug is itself potentially nephrotoxic.

The risk of hearing loss is increased when this drug is administered together with other ototoxic drugs (such as the diuretic ethacrynic acid) or nephrotoxic antibiotics such as the polymyxins and gentamicin.

Dosage and administration. The usual total daily dose for adults is 1.0 g IM, and no more than 1.5 g should be administered. This is usually given in four injections at intervals of 6 hours. The IV route is only rarely used, and the drug is administered intraperitoneally only if peritonitis is present or possible. Oral administration of 1.0 g every 4 hours is usual, but as much as 8 g to 12 g may be given daily in cases of hepatic coma.

Methenamine mandelate USP (Mandelamine)

Actions and indications. This compound breaks down in the urinary tract to two components, mandelic acid and methenamine, both of which act as urinary antiseptics in an acidic urine. Methenamine is then converted to formaldehyde, which exerts a bactericidal effect on both gram-positive and gram-negative bacteria, including *E. coli* and certain staphylococci and streptococci.

This drug is used mainly in chronic infections to suppress bacteriuria in patients with recurring cystitis, pyelonephritis, or pyelitis. It is *not* effective against acute kidney infections that cause such systemic symptoms as chills and fever. Organisms originally sensitive do not develop resistance.

Adverse effects, cautions, and contraindications. Irritation caused by gastric distress is minimized by administering this drug after meals or in enteric-coated form. Skin rash is a relatively rare sign of hypersensitivity. High doses cause occasional painful urination (dysuria).

This drug is not toxic to the kidneys but is contraindicated in patients with renal insufficiency. It should not be administered when the patient's urine cannot be acidified.

Dosage and administration. One gram is administered orally after each meal and at bedtime for adults and fractions of this 4-g total are taken by children. The patient's urine is tested to determine whether acidifying agents such as ammonium chloride or ascorbic acid are needed to keep the urinary pH at the necessary 5.5 or below. (Such supplementation is particularly required to control infections by bacterial strains that split urea to form ammonia.)

Methicillin sodium USP (Staphcillin)

Actions and indications. This semisynthetic penicillin is highly effective against strains of staphylococci that produce penicillinase, an enzyme that inactivates natural penicillin G and V. It is less effective than the latter penicillins in infections caused by other organisms, including streptococci, pneumococci, and *non*penicillinase-producing staphylococci and, consequently, should not be used in such cases. Among the resistant staph infections that often do respond to this antibiotic are lobar or bronchial pneumonia and lung abscesses, septicemia, endocarditis, osteomyelitis, and infections of the skin and soft tissues.

Adverse effects, cautions, and contraindications. Hypersensitivity reactions of the type common to all penicillins have been reported. These range from minor skin rashes to fatal anaphylactoid reactions. Staphylococci and other organisms resistant to methicillin have caused serious superinfections. This drug has occasionally caused bone marrow depression and nephritis. The latter disorder may lead to sodium retention.

Dosage and administration. Methicillin is unstable in stomach acids and poorly absorbed from the intestine, so it must be administered parenterally. It is injected IM fairly frequently (every 4 to 6 hours) in relatively large doses (1 g to 1.5 g). Because IM injections are somewhat painful, the IV route is often preferred, in which case 1 g is injected slowly in the form of a freshly prepared dilute solution (50 ml in 5 minutes) every 6 hours.

Neomycin sulfate USP (Mycifradin)

Actions and indications. This antibiotic is effective against many gram-positive and gram-negative bacteria, but because of its potential toxicity, it is only very rarely used for treating systemic (urinary tract) infections caused by susceptible strains of gram-negative bacilli.

Because it is poorly absorbed from the gastrointestinal tract and tends to accumulate there before finally being eliminated in the feces, neomycin is often administered by mouth to suppress the normal bacterial flora of the bowel. Among the clinical conditions in which this is considered desirable is hepatic coma, in which the drug-induced reduction in ammonia-producing intestinal bacteria is believed to bring about improved brain cell function. Oral administration is also employed to treat infectious diarrhea caused by enteropathogenic *E. coli*. It is also used as an adjunct to mechanical cleansing of the large bowel in the preoperative preparation of the patient for abdominal surgery.

Neomycin is also applied topically in combination with other antibiotics and sometimes with corticosteroids as an adjunct in treating localized skin infections or for preventing infection of cuts, abrasions, burns, and decubital ulcers. Its efficacy for this purpose and for the treatment of infected atopic, contact, or seborrheic dermatitis is uncertain. This antibiotic is also applied topically in the form of a solution for irrigating the urinary bladder of patients with indwelling catheters to help prevent bacteriuria and possible gram-negative bacillary bacteremia.

Adverse effects, cautions, and contraindications. The most common side-effects of oral administration are nausea, vomiting, and diarrhea. Rarely, a reversible malabsorption syndrome has been reported. Occasionally, overgrowths of resistant strains of *Enterobacter*, staphylococci, or yeastlike fungi may cause superinfections. The antibiotic should not be given by mouth to patients with intestinal obstruction or with large ulcerative lesions because of possible systemic absorption.

The drug should be used only with extreme caution in patients with impaired kidney function, because even the small amounts absorbed from the gastrointestinal tract or from skin surfaces may accumulate to toxic levels. The tissues most severely affected in such circumstances, and especially when neomycin is injected, are those of the eighth cranial nerve and of the kidneys themselves. This could lead to irreversible deafness and to renal damage.

Topical administration of neomycin has in recent years been causing hypersensitivity reactions in an increasing number of patients. This is manifested mainly by skin rashes, but more serious is the development of cross sensitivity to other aminoglycoside antibiotics, which might prevent their use in serious systemic infections.

Dosage and administration. Oral doses of 4 g to 12 g a day are administered for 5 or 6 days in hepatic coma management. In infectious diarrhea 3 g is the daily dose. For preoperative preparation the drug is administered after a saline cathartic in a dose of 1 g every hour for four doses, followed by 1 g every 4 hours for the rest of the 24-hour preparation period.

Nitrofurantoin USP (Furadantin; Macrodantin)

Actions and indications. This antibacterial agent is used for treating urinary infections such as cystitis, pyelitis, and pyelonephritis. When excreted in the urine, it exerts bacteriostatic or even bactericidal effects on susceptible gram-negative and gram-positive bacteria, including some strains resistant to sulfonamides and other urinary antiseptics. Among these uropathogens are *E. coli*, enterococci, *Staphylococcus aureus*, and some strains of *Pseudomonas*, *Proteus*, and the *Klebsiella–Aerobacter* group. Organisms that prove sensitive do not ordinarily develop resistance.

Adverse effects, cautions, and contraindications. The most common side-effects are nausea and vomiting. Other minor discomforts include headache, dizziness, and drowsiness. Various types of skin eruptions may occur as a result of hypersensitivity, including urticarial, eczematous, erythematous, or macropapular rashes. Serious pulmonary toxicity, blood dyscrasias, a lupuslike syndrome, and increased intracranial pressure have also occurred.

This drug is highly soluble in urine, and crystalluria does not occur. However, it must not be administered to patients with severely damaged kidneys, because it is ineffective in such cases and may accumulate to toxic levels in nervous tissue. Severe peripheral polyneuropathy has occurred in such cases. Hemolytic anemia may occur in those who lack the protective enzyme G-6-PD and in very young infants with immature enzyme systems. The drug is contraindicated in such cases and in pregnant patients at term. Its safety earlier in pregnancy is not established.

Dosage and administration. Oral doses of 50 mg to 100 mg are taken qid with food for at least 1 week. The parenteral form is injected IM or IV in doses of 180 mg for individuals weighing over 120 lb, or 3 mg/lb for those weighing less.

Oxacillin sodium USP (Prostaphlin)

Actions and indications. This semisynthetic penicillin is useful against infections caused by staphylococcal strains resistant to penicillin G or V. Its molecule resists destruction not only by bacterial penicillinase but also by stomach acids. Thus, it is effective orally as well as parenterally. Although it may be used to begin treatment in various skin, soft tissue, and respiratory infections believed to be caused by resistant staph organisms, it should be discontinued in favor of penicillin G if sensitivity tests prove the organism to be susceptible to treatment with that natural penicillin.

Adverse effects, cautions, and contraindications. Allergic reactions typical of other penicillin products have occurred with this drug, especially in patients with a history of previous hypersensitivity to penicillin. The drug should be discontinued if such reactions, or the development of superinfections by nonsusceptible microorganisms, are seen to develop.

Dosage and administration. The injectable form is preferred for use in serious infections. However, once the infection is brought under control, the oral form, which is effective for mild to moderate infections, may be employed. The oral form should be taken on an empty stomach, 1 or 2 hours before meals, for maximal absorption. Oral dosage of 500 mg every 4 to 6 hours is recommended for mild staph infections, and 1 g for more severe infections. For staphylococcal septicemia or other deep-seated infections, doses as high as 500 mg to 1000 mg may be administered by intramuscular or slow intravenous injection.

Para-aminosalicylate sodium USP (PAS)

Actions and indications. This drug is effective in the treatment of tuberculosis when administered in combination with other drugs, usually isoniazid and another first-line or a second-line antituberculosis drug. Although its own tuberculostatic effect is relatively weak, it adds to the effectiveness of the other drugs and slows the rate at which drug-resistant strains tend to emerge.

Adverse effects, cautions, and contraindications. The main side-effects are the result of irritation of the gastrointestinal tract and include anorexia, nausea, vomiting, cramps, and diarrhea. These may be reduced by administering the drug in divided doses after meals or with antacid-absorbing drugs. Its use in patients with peptic ulcer is contraindicated, and it is withdrawn if gastric bleeding or other indications of developing ulceration occur.

The main types of hypersensitivity reactions reported may involve the skin and blood-forming organs. Sudden development of prolonged high fever, headache, and skin eruptions may require withdrawal of the drug to prevent more serious reactions, including fatal blood dyscrasias and liver damage. Goiter and signs of hypothyroidism developing during prolonged treatment may require administration of thyroid supplements.

Dosage and administration. A daily dose of 8 g to 12 g is usually administered in four equally divided doses after meals.

Penicillin G benzathine suspension USP (Bicillin; Permapen)

Actions and indications. This dosage form of penicillin G is administered only by deep intramuscular injection of an aqueous suspension. It is only very slowly absorbed into the bloodstream from the repository, or depot, in the muscle. After hydrolytic conversion to penicillin G, it produces long-lasting bactericidal effects on the same spectrum of microorganisms as the parent antibiotic. These include gram-positive cocci such as group A and other streptococci, pneumococci, and nonpenicillinase-producing staphylococci. It is also effective against the gonococcus and spirochetes, including *Treponema pallidum*, the etiologic agent of syphilis.

The use of this repository form of penicillin G is indicated mainly in the treatment and prophylaxis of infections caused by organisms so sensitive to penicillin that they will be killed by the relatively low but very prolonged blood and tissue levels that are attained. These include streptococcal pharyngitis and other mild to moderate upper respiratory tract infections, but *not* gonorrhea.

This preparation is also used for long-term prophylaxis against recurrences of rheumatic fever, acute glomerulonephritis, and chorea, particularly in patients with a history of rheumatic heart disease.

Adverse effects, cautions, and contraindications. The most common type of adverse reactions are the result of hypersensitivity to penicillin. These are mostly skin eruptions of the urticarial and maculopapular types. However, because of the possibility of severe, possibly fatal anaphylactic reactions, this antibiotic is contraindicated in patients who have had previous reactions to penicillin, and all patients must be questioned concerning their history of sensitivity to this and other drugs and other allergens. Superinfections may occur during long-term therapy as a result of overgrowths of fungi and of other organisms not susceptible to penicillin G.

Dosage and administration. Care is required to avoid injecting this suspension into a blood vessel. If blood enters the syringe on aspiration, remove the needle and inject at another deep intramuscular site in the upper outer quadrant of the buttock or elsewhere. For treating staphylococcal pharyngitis, adults receive a single injection of 1.2 million U, and older children 900,000 U. For prophylaxis against recurrences of rheumatic fever or glomerulonephritis 600,000 U may be administered every 2 weeks or 1.2 million U every 4 weeks.

For primary, secondary or latent syphilis, a single dose of 2.4 million U is employed. Tertiary (late) syphilis and neurosyphilis require three such doses repeated at intervals of 1 week.

Penicillin G potassium USP (Pentids)

Actions and indications. This form of penicillin is the first choice for treating and preventing infections by susceptible pathogens, because it is more effective and less expensive than the semisynthetic derivatives. Its antibacterial spectrum includes gram-positive and gram-negative cocci, certain gram-positive bacilli, and spirochetes.

Penicillin G is used for prophylaxis and treatment of streptococcal pharyngitis, pneumococcal respiratory tract and meningeal infections, and infections by *non*penicillinase-producing strains of staphylococci. It is also effective for treating meningococcal infections, gonorrhea and syphilis, tetanus, and diphtheria.

Adverse effects, cautions, and contraindications. Penicillin causes little direct tissue toxicity except when it is injected into the spinal canal in too high concentration. Such intrathecal injection can cause central nervous system stimulation and convulsions. The administration of very large IV doses of the potassium salt may also cause convulsions and hyperkalemia, particularly in patients with kidney damage.

Allergic reactions are common and potentially very serious. Thus, all patients must be questioned concerning any previous reactions to penicillin, the use of which is contraindicated in those with a history of hypersensitivity to it. The drug is ordinarily discontinued if skin reactions develop during treatment. Caution is required in patients with a history of asthma or other significant allergies.

Dosage and administration. Oral doses for adults range between 600,000 U and 1.6 million U daily, in most cases. Children may receive 400,000 U daily for prophylaxis. IM or IV doses of 5 to 20 million U or more may be administered daily for treating severe infections.

Penicillin G procaine suspension, sterile USP (Crysticillin; Duracillin; Wycillin)

Actions and indications. This preparation of penicillin in combination with the local anesthetic procaine is only slowly absorbed into the systemic circulation when deposited in depot sites by intramuscular injection. Thus, both the aqueous suspension and the oily aluminum stearate suspension produce long-lasting plasma-tissue levels of the antibiotic (15 to 20 hours).

These concentrations are adequate for treating moderately severe infections. However, when high penicillin levels must be maintained in the treatment of severe infections such as bacteremia, meningitis, pericarditis, and peritonitis, aqueous penicillin G itself (rather than this poorly soluble procaine derivative) should be injected IM or IV during the acute stages. This form of penicillin G is recommended for the 1-day treatment of uncomplicated gonorrheal infections and for prophylaxis against gonorrhea. Follow-up treatment may be required if clinical signs and laboratory test results indicate that the infection is still present. For such severe complications of gonorrhea as septic arthritis or endocarditis, intensive treatment with aqueous penicillin G (*not* this procaine preparation) should be employed.

Adverse effects, cautions, and contraindications. Hypersensitivity reactions similar to those with other penicillin G preparations may occur. Some patients are also sensitive to the procaine component.

Dosage and administration. Because of its procaine content, IM injections are almost entirely pain-free but, because of the presence of suspending agents, it is particularly important to aspirate to be sure that the needle has not accidentally entered a vein.

Dosage varies with the sensitivity of the organism and severity of the infection. In syphilis, for example, doses of 1.2 to 2.4 million U repeated at 3-day intervals are employed; in gonorrhea, a single 4.8 million-U dose is given. For prophylaxis against bacterial endocarditis, doses of 300,000 U to 600,000 U are administered on the day before dental or oropharyngeal operations and for 2 days after these procedures. (On the operative day, aqueous penicillin G is employed.)

Penicillin V potassium USP (Pen-Vee K; V-Cillin K)

Actions and indications. The substitution of a phenoxymethyl side chain for the benzyl group of penicillin G increases the ability of this compound to resist inactivation by gastric acid. Consequently, this penicillin is more rapidly and reliably absorbed from the gastrointestinal tract to reach blood levels that are two to five times as high as those attained with oral administration of penicillin G.

The clinical significance of the greater acid stability of this penicillin analogue is uncertain. In most of the mild to moderate infections caused by penicillin-sensitive microorganisms in which this drug is employed, penicillin G is just as effective and much less expensive. In severe infections parenteral penicillins are preferred to the oral dosage form of either penicillin G or V. A possible advantage of this more predictably absorbed penicillin may be in situations that require prolonged high blood levels of penicillin but in which daily injection of a penicillin is inconvenient or otherwise undesirable. Under such circumstances high oral doses of this penicillin may be substituted for frequent parenteral administration. An example of this is the use of penicillin V for keeping bacterial endocarditis under control and especially for preventing this infection in patients with rheumatic or congenital heart valve damage. Administration prior to dental procedures and minor surgery or instrumentation of the upper respiratory tract, such as tonsillectomy, is an example.

Adverse effects, cautions, and contraindications. An advantage claimed for this penicillin over parenterally administered penicillins is that severe anaphylactoid reactions are less likely to occur after its administration to penicillin-hypersensitive patients. However, fatal anaphylactoid reactions *have* occurred occasionally even after ingestion of oral penicillins. Other adverse effects of all penicillins can also occur with penicillin V, but those relatively rare untoward responses that are reported mainly after high and prolonged parenteral administration of penicillin, such as nephropathy, neurotoxicity, hemolytic anemia and other blood cell disorders, are less likely to occur with this and other oral forms of penicillin.

Dosage and administration. Dosage depends upon the severity of the infection, the response of the patient to therapy, and the degree to which the infecting pathogen is sensitive to penicillin. Adult doses range from about 200,000 U to 500,000 U every 6 to 8 hours for treatment of such common gram-positive coccal infections as streptococcal pharyngitis and other staphylococcal and pneumococcal infections.

Treatment for children under 12 years old is based on body weight. Dosage for infants is between 15 and 50 mg/kg. For prophylaxis against rheumatic fever recurrences, about 250,000 U is taken twice daily every day. Prior to performance of procedures in the mouth and throat, 500,000 U of this penicillin is administered on the day of the procedure and every 6 hours for 2 days after it. (One hour before the procedure, an intramuscular injection of aqueous penicillin G is made to ensure high blood levels.)

Polymyxin B sulfate USP (Aerosporin)

Actions and indications. This antibiotic is active against a wide range of gram-negative bacilli but *not* against gram-negative or gram-positive cocci. It is injected mainly for treating urinary tract infections caused by susceptible strains of *Pseudomonas aeruginosa*. It may also be useful in pseudomonal meningitis and septicemia and in these and lung infections caused by other gram-negative species when the infecting strain proves resistant to safer antimicrobial agents.

Polymyxin is also applied topically—usually in combination with such other antibiotics as bacitracin and neomycin—for treatment of skin, eye and external ear infections.

Adverse effects, cautions, and contraindications. The main adverse effects of this antibiotic are nephrotoxicity and neurotoxicity. Patients should be hospitalized so that their renal function can be checked before and during treatment. If cellular casts and protein appear in the urine, and especially if azotemia and oliguria develop, the drug should be discontinued. It should not be given together with other potentially nephrotoxic and neurotoxic drugs such as the aminoglycoside group antibiotics.

Signs and symptoms of neurotoxicity include dizziness, drowsiness, ataxia, blurring of vision, numbness, and tingling around the mouth and in the feet and hands. Overdoses may cause respiratory muscle paralysis, especially in patients receiving such neuromuscular blocking agents as tubocurarine, succinylcholine, and ether anesthesia.

Dosage and administration. The dose administered by continuous intravenous drip is 15,000 to 25,000 U/kg/day. The dose by intramuscular injection (which is not recommended for routine use because it can cause severe pain) is 25,000 to 30,000 U/kg/day, divided and administered at intervals of 4 to 6 hours. The dose for intrathecal injection is 50,000 U once daily for 3 or 4 days, and then the same dose every other day for at least 2 weeks after the cerebrospinal fluid becomes normal. This drug may also be injected subconjunctivally in amounts up to 10,000 U daily. It is applied topically to the eye in solution and to the skin in the form of ointments, creams, and ear drops.

Rifampin (Rifadin; Rimactane)

Actions and indications. This antibiotic is used mainly as a primary drug in the treatment of pulmonary tuberculosis, but it may also prove effective in cases of infection that have spread to extrapulmonary sites. It is always used in combination with another tuberculostatic drug such as isoniazid or ethambutol, because resistant tubercle bacilli may emerge rapidly when it is used alone.

A number of other pathogens are susceptible to this antibiotic, but it is used at present only to treat asymptomatic carriers of meningococci. It is *not* used to treat meningitis infections but only to eliminate meningococci from the nose and throat of the carrier in situations in which the risk of spreading meningococcal meningitis is high.

Adverse effects, cautions, and contraindications. This drug is said to cause fewer side-effects than most other antituberculosis drugs. These include gastrointestinal disturbances, headache, drowsiness and dizziness, skin eruptions, thrombocytopenia and leukopenia, and fever. Patients should be cautioned that their saliva, skin, urine, tears, and so forth may be stained orange. The color will come out; clothing should be washed immediately.

Caution is required in patients with liver disease and in those taking anticoagulant drugs. Jaundice and transient liver test abnormalities may occur and tests should be continued periodically during treatment to detect any further hepatotoxicity. Daily prothrombin time tests should be performed while readjusting anticoagulant drug dosage to the higher levels that may be required during treatment with rifampin.

Dosage and administration. A single dose of 600 mg is administered orally 1 hour before or 2 hours after a meal. Children receive 10 to 20 mg/kg but no more than 600 mg daily.

Streptomycin USP

Actions and indications. This antibiotic is now a second-line antituberculosis agent. It is commonly administered together with isoniazid and ethambutol. These drugs help to reduce the rapid rate at which resistant organisms develop and emerge when streptomycin is employed alone.

Various other infections respond to treatment with this antibiotic alone or in combination with other anti-infective drugs. It is particularly useful against the *Pasteurella* species that cause plaque and tularemia. It is combined with penicillin for treating enterococcal infections of the urinary tract. A combination with chloramphenicol is effective for *Klebsiella pneumoniae* infections. It may be combined with a sulfonamide to treat nocardiosis.

Adverse effects, cautions, and contraindications. The most common side-effect is the development of vertigo as a result of damage to the vestibular portion of the eighth cranial nerve. Disturbances in hearing may also result from dysfunction of the auditory nerve.

The optic nerve and other peripheral nerves may also be adversely affected occasionally. Allergic reactions, including skin eruptions, may occur both in patients and in personnel handling and administering the antibiotic. Blood dyscrasias develop occasionally. Kidney damage is uncommon with ordinary doses of the drug but may occur in patients with impaired kidney function who do not

excrete it well.

Dosage and administration. Streptomycin is usually administered by deep IM injection in daily doses of 1 g to 2 g divided into two equal parts at 12-hour intervals. It is administered intermittently in dosage schedules that vary in accordance with the severity and location of the infection.

Sulfacetamide sodium USP (Sulamyd Sodium)

Actions and indications. This sulfonamide penetrates readily into ocular tissues when applied topically. It is used for treating eye infections caused by susceptible strains of various gram-positive and gram-negative bacteria.

Among the external eye infections in which it is employed are blepharitis (lid styes), conjunctivitive and corneal inflammation, and ulceration (keratitis). It is also applied top-

ically in trachoma as an adjunct to systemic sulfonamide drug therapy.

Adverse effects, cautions, and contraindications. This drug is contraindicated in patients with a history of hypersensitivity to sulfonamides. Its use should be discontinued if signs of a sensitivity reaction develop. Patients are observed for signs of overgrowth of nonsusceptible organisms such as fungi.

Dosage and administration. The 10% oint-

ment is applied qid and at bedtime as an adjunct to treatment with the solution forms. One or two drops of a 10% solution containing methylcellulose 0.5% are instilled into the lower conjunctival sac every 2 or 3 hours during the day. One drop of the 30% solution is instilled every 2 hours for treating acute conjunctivitis or corneal ulcer. Two drops are applied in trachoma in conjunction with systemic sulfonamides.

Sulfadiazine USP

Actions and indications. This sulfonamide is administered alone or combined with sulfamethazine and sulfamerazine in the combination called trisulfapyrimidines. It is used for treating acute urinary infections such as cystitis, urethritis, pyelitis, pyelonephritis, and prostatitis caused by susceptible strains of *E. coli* and other uropathogens.

This, like other sulfonamides, is also used for prophylaxis and treatment of meningococcal meningitis caused by group A strains of meningococci and for prevention of rheumatic fever (group A hemolytic

streptococci) in patients sensitive to penicillin. Among relatively rare infections for which it is useful are toxoplasmosis (in combination with pyrimethamine), chloroquine-resistant strains of *Plasmodium falciparum* malaria (in combination with quinine), nocardiosis, trachoma, and chancroid.

Adverse effects, cautions, and contraindications. This drug must be administered with adequate quantities of fluid to avoid crystalluria. It is discontinued if hematuria develops and is contraindicated in patients with kidney failure or severe liver damage.

It should not be administered during late pregnancy, to premature infants, or to newborn babies under 2 months old because of possible development of kernicterus in the very young child. Patients should be watched for signs of allergic reactions characteristic of sulfonamides.

Dosage and administration. The usual initial dose administered orally to adults is 2 g to 4 g; doses of 1 g to 1.5 g are then administered every 4 to 6 hours. Children's dose is 100 to 150 mg/kg followed by one-sixth of the first dose every 4 hours.

Sulfisoxazole USP (Gantrisin); sulfisozazole diolamine USP (Gantrisin Diolamine); acetyl sulfisoxazole USP (Lipo Gantrisin)

Actions and indications. This soluble, short-acting sulfonamide exerts a bacteriostatic antibacterial effect on susceptible strains of a broad spectrum of pathogenic microorganisms. Thus, it is potentially useful for treating a wide variety of infections. However, in actual clinical practice, it is only relatively rarely the preferred anti-infective agent because of the availability of antibiotic drugs of greater safety and effectiveness.

This sulfonamide is commonly employed in the treatment of acute, chronic, and recurrent urinary tract infections such as cystitis, pyelitis, and pyelonephritis caused by such organisms as *E. coli, Proteus vulgaris,* and *Proteus mirabilis.* However, the usefulness of this drug and other sulfonamides is often limited by the frequent emergence of resistant strains of these and such other uropathogens as *Staphylococcus aureus* and species of the *Klebsiella–Aerobacter* group.

This and other sulfonamides are employed for prophylaxis against infections by group A β-hemolytic streptococci in patients who

do not tolerate penicillin. However, it should *not* be used for *treating* established streptococcal infections, because it does *not* eradicate the organism in such circumstances. Thus, its use *in treatment* rather than prophylaxis will *not* prevent later development of rheumatic carditis or glomerulonephritis.

The parenteral form of this drug has been employed in treating meningitis caused by susceptible strains of meningococci and *Hemophilus influenzae* and (combined with penicillin) in acute otitis media caused by the latter pathogen. A cream is used in the treatment of infections caused by *H. vaginalis.*

Adverse effects, cautions, and contraindications. Allergic reactions and blood dyscrasias may occur in hypersensitive persons, and the drug is contraindicated in such cases. Among the most dangerous of such reactions are exfoliative dermatitis, erythema multiforme (Stevens–Johnson syndrome), anaphylactoid reactions, agranulocytosis, hemolytic anemia, thrombocytopenia, and aplastic anemia.

More common and less serious reactions include nausea, vomiting, epigastric distress, and headache. Caution is required in patients with impaired hepatic and kidney function. Patients should drink adequate amounts of fluid to prevent formation of urinary crystals or stones. Its use is avoided late in pregnancy and during early infancy.

Dosage and administration. Sulfisoxazole is administered orally to adults in a loading dose of 2 g to 4 g, which is then followed by 1 g to 2 g every 4 to 6 hours. Children's dosage of acetyl sulfisoxazole is 60 to 75 mg/kg initially followed by two similar doses during the course of the day.

Sulfisoxazole diolamine is administered parenterally in a loading dose of 50 mg/kg, followed by daily doses of 100 mg/kg that are divided and administered bid to qid. A 4% ophthalmic solution is instilled in the eye. A 10% vaginal cream is employed in the morning and when retiring.

Tetracycline HCl USP (Achromycin)

Actions and indications. This broad-spectrum antibiotic is effective against a wide variety of microorganisms including gram-positive and gram-negative cocci and bacilli, spirochetes, rickettsiae, and other pathogenic

agents. However, many strains have become resistant to it. Thus, it is desirable to culture the organism in each infection and to determine its actual susceptibility to the antibiotic.

Tetracycline is rarely the most effective anti-infective drug, despite the frequency with which it is prescribed. It is most commonly employed as an alternative to penicillin for patients who are hypersensitive to that first choice antibiotic. However, tetracycline is considered superior for treating rickettsial infections such as Rocky Mountain spotted fever, Q fever, and typhus. It is also effective in atypical pneumonia caused by *Mycoplasma pneumoniae*, and in infections by the agents that cause trachoma, psittacosis, and various relatively rare as well as common venereal diseases.

Adverse effects, cautions, and contraindications. Tetracycline is an antibiotic of relatively low toxicity. Gastrointestinal side-effects including epigastric distress, nausea, vomiting, and diarrhea are the most common. Overgrowths of fungal organisms such as *Candida* may occur and cause superinfections of the mouth and anogenital region. Relatively rare staphylococcal superinfections of the GI tract may cause serious illness and death.

Patients exposed to sunlight may sometimes suffer a photosensitivity reaction resembling sunburn. The drug may cause permanent discoloration and abnormal calcification of the teeth of children when taken during the period of tooth development. It may also do so when administered to the mother during the latter half of pregnancy. Animal studies indicate that tetracyclines passing to the fetus by way of the placenta may retard development of the skeleton.

Accumulation of this drug in the tissues of patients with damaged kidneys may lead to liver damage. Dosage should be reduced for patients with renal insufficiency.

Dosage and administration. The usual daily oral dose for adults is 1 g to 2 g divided into two or four doses. Children's dosage is 10 to 20 mg/lb of body weight. The drug is best administered between meals, because some foods interfere with its absorption.

References

Abraham EP: The beta-lactam antibiotics. Sci Am 244:76 (June) 1981

Antimicrobial prophylaxis for surgery. Med Lett Drugs Ther 25:113, 1983

Bartlett JG: Anti-anaerobic antibacterial agents. Lancet 2:478, 1982

Bartlett JG: Chloramphenicol. Med Clin North Am 66:91, 1982

Bierman CW et al: Reactions associated with ampicillin therapy. JAMA 220:1098, 1972

Binford CH et al: Leprosy. JAMA 247:2283, 1982

Brewin A et al: High-dose penicillin therapy and pneumococcal pneumonia. JAMA 230:409, 1974

Brumfitt W, Pursell R: Trimethoprim–sulfamethoxazole in the treatment of bacteriuria in women. J Infect Dis 128 (Suppl):S657, 1973

Cefuroxime sodium (Zinacef). Med Lett Drugs Ther 26:15, 1984

Cunha BA et al: Tetracyclines. Med Clin North Am 66:293, 1982

Curry FJ: Prophylactic effect of isoniazid in young tuberculin reactors. N Engl J Med 277:563, 1967

Drugs for tuberculosis. Med Lett Drugs Ther 24:17, 1982

Eliopoulos GM et al: Azlocillin, mezlocillin and piperacillin: New broad spectrum penicillins. Ann Intern Med 97:740, 1982

Fekety R: Vancomycin. Med Clin North Am 66:175, 1982

Flick MR, Cluff LE: *Pseudomonas* bacteremia. Review of 108 cases. Am J Med 60:501, 1976

Fox WA, Mitchison DA: Short-course chemotherapy for pulmonary tuberculosis. Am Rev Respir Dis 111:325, 1975

Glassroth J et al: Tuberculosis in the 1980s. N Engl J Med 302:1441, 1980

Gutman L et al: Bacterial L-forms in relapsing urinary tract infection. Lancet 1:464, 1967

Handbook of Antimicrobial Therapy, rev ed. New Rochelle, New York, Med Lett Drugs Ther, 1984

Harding GKM, Ronald AR: A controlled study of antimicrobial prophylaxis of recurrent urinary infections in women. N Engl J Med 291:597, 1974

Houk VN: Rifampin: Its role in the treatment of tuberculosis. Chest (special issue) 61:518, 1972

Kovnat P et al: Antibiotics and the kidney. Med Clin North Am 57:1045, 1973

Kucers A: Chloramphenicol, erythromycin, vancomycin, tetracyclines. Lancet 2:435, 1982

Kunin CM et al: Use of antibiotics: A brief exposition of the problem and some tentative solutions. Ann Intern Med 79:555, 1982

Lau WK, Young LS: Co-trimoxazole treatment of Pneumocystis carinii pneumonia in adults. N Engl J Med 295:716, 1976

LeFrock JL et al: Clindamycin. Med Clin North Am 66:103, 1982

Maddey WC, Boitnott JK: Isoniazid hepatitis. Ann Intern Med 79:1, 1973

Mandell GL, Sande MA: Drugs used in the chemotherapy of tuberculosis and leprosy. In Gilman AG, Goodman LS, Gilman A (eds): Goodman and Gilman's The Pharmacological Basis of Therapeutics, 6th ed, pp 1200–1221. New York, Macmillan, 1980

Mandell GL, Sande MA: Penicillins and cephalosporins. In Gilman AG, Goodman LS, Gilman A (eds): Goodman and Gilman's The Pharmacological Basis of Therapeutics, 6th ed, pp 1126–1161. New York, Macmillan, 1980

Mandell GL, Sande MA: Sulfonamides, trimethoprim–sulfamethoxazole, and urinary tract antiseptics. In Gilman AG, Goodman LS, Gilman A (eds): Goodman and Gilman's The Pharmacological Basis of Therapeutics, 6th ed, pp 1106–1125. New York, Macmillan, 1980

Millikan LE: Sulfones: A review of approved and investigational indications. Hosp Form 17:102, 1982

Mitchell JR et al: Isoniazid liver injury: Clinical spectrum, pathology, and probable pathogenesis. Ann Intern Med 84:181, 1976

Neu HC: Clinical uses of cephalosporins. Lancet 1:252, 1982

Neu CH: The *in vitro* activity, human pharmacology, and clinical effectiveness of new β-lactam antibiotics. Ann Rev Pharmacol Toxicol 22:599, 1982

Phillips I: Aminoglycosides. Lancet 2:311, 1982

Pollock AA et al: Amikacin therapy for serious gram-negative infections. JAMA 237:562, 1977

Prevention of bacterial endocarditis. Med Lett Drugs Ther 26:3, 1984

Rubin R, Swartz MN: Trimethoprim-sulfamethoxazole. N Engl J Med 303:426, 1980

Sande MA, Mandell GL: The aminoglycosides. In Gilman AG, Goodman LS, Gilman A (eds): Goodman and Gilman's The Pharmacological Basis of Therapeutics, 6th ed, pp 1162–1180. New York, Macmillan, 1980

Sande MA, Mandell GL: Miscellaneous antibacterial agents; antifungal and antiviral agents. In Gilman AG, Goodman LS, Gilman A (eds): Goodman and Gilman's The Pharmacological Basis of Therapeutics, 6th ed, pp 1222–1248. New York, Macmillan, 1980

Sande MA, Mandell GL: Tetracyclines and chloramphenicol. In Gilman AG, Goodman LS, Gilman A (eds): Goodman and Gilman's The Pharmacological Basis of Therapeutics, 6th ed, pp 1181–1199. New York, Macmillan, 1980

Smith CR et al: Controlled comparison of amikacin and gentamicin. N Engl J Med 296:349, 1977

Strominger JL: The actions of penicillins and other antibiotics on bacterial cell wall synthesis. Johns Hopkins Med J 133:63, 1973

Symposium on Trimethoprim–Sulfamethoxazole. J Infect Dis 128 (Suppl.):S425, 1973

The choice of antimicrobial drugs. Med Lett Drugs Ther 26:19, 1984

The treatment of sexually transmitted diseases. Med Lett Drugs Ther 26:5, 1984

Turck M: Alternative antibiotics for the penicillin-sensitive patient. Hosp Pract 18:77, 1981

Turck M: Therapeutic principles in the treatment of urinary tract infections and pyelonephritis. Adv Intern Med 18:141, 1973

Wink D: Bacterial meningitis in children. Am J Nurs 84:456, 1984

Winslow EJ et al: Hemodynamic studies and results of therapy in 50 patients with bacteremic shock. Am J Med 54:421, 1973

Chapter 9

The chemotherapy of fungal infections

9

Fungi can cause infections that range from relatively minor annoyances, such as mild cases of "athlete's foot" (*tinea pedis*), to severe life-threatening systemic infections. The minor dermatologic and vaginal fungal infections are often effectively and safely treated with topical drugs; the life-threatening systemic infections are usually treated with intravenous drugs. This chapter describes the drugs that are administered systemically (orally or IV) to treat fungal infections. (Some of these are also available in topical or vaginal preparations, which are described, along with other topical antifungal drugs, in Chapter 43, Drugs Used in Dermatology.)

Antifungal drugs

Four drugs are available to treat systemic fungal infections (mycoses), the dangerous diseases that occur when fungi are spread by the blood to various vital organs. These drugs are *amphotericin B, flucytosine, ketoconazole,* and *miconazole.* Another antifungal drug, *griseofulvin,* is useful when taken orally for treating dermatomycoses—infections of the skin, hair, and nails caused by ringworm-type fungi. A sixth antifungal drug, *nystatin,* is used mainly to control the yeastlike fungus, *Candida albicans;* it is used topically for *Candida* infections of the skin, mucous membranes, and vagina, and is given orally for *Candida* infections of the intestinal tract.

Agents for treatment of systemic infections

Amphotericin B[+] (Fungizone) was the first truly effective and dependable drug for treating the so-called disseminated mycoses (Table 9-1). These are diseases in which certain fungi enter the body by way of the mouth, lungs, or skin and spread to various internal organs including the brain, bones, and heart. *Histoplasmosis* is one such

condition that is seen with increasing frequency in this country. Inhaled in the dust from pigeon or chicken dung, the fungal organism often causes a pulmonary infection resembling tuberculosis. Other fungi—the causes of *blastomycosis, coccidiomycosis,* and *cryptococcosis,* for instance—are even more dangerous because of their rapid spread to the meninges and elsewhere as a generalized infection.

Amphotericin B is potentially a very toxic drug. Although it has a broad antifungal spectrum, its use should be limited to patients with progressive and potentially fatal fungal infections. It is usually given only to hospitalized patients who can be closely monitored for adverse reactions, some of which are shown by most patients. The most common reactions are fever, sometimes with shaking chills; headache and generalized pain; renal impairment; nausea, vomiting, and abdominal pain; and anemia. Severe reactions may be lessened by giving aspirin, antihistamines, and antiemetics. Less common but still serious reactions include cardiac arrhythmias and arrest, convulsions, hearing loss, agranulocytosis, hemorrhagic gastroenteritis, and renal and hepatic failure. Other nephrotoxic drugs should not be given concomitantly. Because it causes hypokalemia, amphotericin B can potentiate the effects of cardiac glycosides and neuromuscular junction blocking drugs.

Amphotericin B is given by slow IV infusion. Because it does not penetrate the cerebrospinal fluid well, it is sometimes given intrathecally or into the cerebral ventricles to treat fungal meningitis. It is also used topically to treat mucocutaneous *Candida* infections.

Despite the problems associated with its systemic use, amphotericin B, when administered with great care to hospitalized patients, has changed the previously poor prognosis for patients with systemic fungal infections.

Some patients with certain serious mycotic infections who failed to improve with amphotericin B treatment have responded when a newer antifungal agent

207

Table 9–1. Antifungal drugs

Generic or official name	Trade name	Route of administration	Usual adult dosage
Amphotericin B USP	Fungizone	IV	0.25 mg/kg body weight/day infused over 6 hr; dose may be increased if necessary and tolerated, to a maximum of 1.5 mg/kg body weight/day
		Intrathecal; intraventricular	0.1 mg initially; may increase to 0.5 mg q 48–72 hr
Flucytosine (5-FC; 5-fluorocytosine)	Ancobon	Oral	50–150 mg/kg body weight/day in divided doses, q 6 hr
Griseofulvin USP	Fulvicin-U/F; Grifulvin V; Grisactin	Oral	0.5–1 g in divided doses
Ketoconazole	Nizoral	Oral	200 mg once a day; may increase to 400 mg/day
Miconazole	Monistat	IV; intrathecal	200–1200 mg tid 20 mg/dose
Nystatin USP	Mycostatin; Nilstat	Oral	0.5–1 million U tid

called *flucytosine* (Ancobon) was added to the regimen. This drug, which is a chemical relative of the cancer chemotherapeutic agents fluorouracil and floxuridine (see Chap. 12), has also been employed alone in patients who are unable to tolerate amphotericin B. Its main disadvantage is that fungi rapidly develop resistance to it when it is used alone. It helps patients with pulmonary infections caused by susceptible strains of *Cryptococcus* who have relapsed following amphotericin B therapy. It has also proved effective in some cases of cryptococcal meningitis and in septicemia, endocarditis, and urinary tract infections caused by *Candida*.

Flucytosine has the advantage of being orally administered. It is a relatively safe drug when compared to amphotericin B and to the anticancer agents to which it is chemically related. However, it must be employed with extreme caution in patients with impaired kidney function, because failure of the drug to be excreted can lead to its accumulating and causing complications. (Because amphotericin B may cause decreased kidney function, patients who are being changed to flucytosine therapy must have their renal function closely monitored.) Caution is also required in patients whose bone marrow may be depressed by prior treatment with cytotoxic drugs or radiation, because anemia, leukopenia, and thrombopenia have sometimes occurred from flucytosine.

Miconazole (Monistat) is also reserved for the treatment of severe systemic fungal infections. Like amphotericin B, it has a broad antifungal spectrum, and is usually given intravenously. It may be given intrathecally as well as IV to treat fungal meningitis, and it may be used as a bladder irrigation as well as IV to treat urinary tract infections. Initial treatment should always be performed in the hospital with a physician present, using a test dose of 200 mg. Severe reactions have occurred, including cardiac and respiratory arrest, with the first dose. Pruritus is a major side-effect. Other adverse effects include phlebitis, chills, rash, nausea, and vomiting. The effect of oral anticoagulants (coumarin-type drugs) is increased by miconazole, and the dose of these drugs may need to be reduced. Miconazole and amphotericin B are mutually antagonistic; the antifungal effect of the two together is less than that of either administered alone. Miconazole is also used topically to treat vaginal fungal infections.

Ketoconazole (Nizoral) is the newest antifungal drug. It has a broad antifungal spectrum and is used in various systemic fungal infections. It does not penetrate the cerebrospinal fluid well, and is therefore not used to treat fungal meningitis. It is orally effective, although precautions need to be taken to prevent alkalinization of the gastric contents when it is given; it needs an acidic medium for dissolution. Antacids, anticholinergic (atropinelike) drugs, and histamine H_2 receptor blockers (*e.g.*, cimetidine [Tagamet] and ranitidine [Zantac]) should be given at least 2 hours after administration of ketoconazole. It has low toxicity, although nausea and vomiting are frequent. Pruritus, headache, and dizziness also occur occasionally, and hepatitis occurs rarely. Its oral effectiveness and low toxicity are advantages for the therapy of systemic fungal infections, but clinical improvement is slow to occur, limiting its usefulness in severe infections.

Agents for treatment of *Candida* infections

Nystatin[+] (Mycostatin) is similar to amphotericin B chemically and in its manner of action, but it is too toxic to be administered parenterally to treat systemically disseminated mycoses. Instead, it is applied topically and taken orally to treat *Candida* infections of the skin, intestinal tract, and mucous membranes of the mouth (thrush) and vaginal tract. Cutaneous candidiasis responds readily to local application of nystatin (or of amphotericin B), provided that measures are taken to keep the patient's skin dry (see Chap. 43). Vaginal infections also ordinarily clear up when nystatin tablets or miconazole (Monistat) cream are inserted with an applicator once daily for 1 or 2 weeks. A cream or ointment containing one of these anticandidal antibiotics may also be effective for relief of pruritus vulvae.

Nystatin and amphotericin B are also often added to oral tetracycline antibiotics with the intention of preventing fungal infections caused by overgrowths of *Candida* species when the broad-spectrum antibiotic alters the normal microbial flora of the intestine. These fixed-dose antibiotics are now considered ineffective for this prophylactic purpose. However, taking oral nystatin tablets separately when specifically indicated can be effective for control of intestinal overgrowths of *Candida albicans.* (Intestinal candidiasis occurs most often in patients who are predisposed to develop such infections because they are suffering from diseases that lower their defenses against infection, or are taking drugs that do so.)

Griseofulvin for treatment of dermatophytoses

Griseofulvin[+] (Fulvicin P/G; Fulvicin-U/F; Grifulvin V; Grisactin) is an antifungal antibiotic that is used for purposes entirely different from those of the other agents. It is not effective against *Candida* or the other fungi that cause localized or systemic infections. It acts, instead, against various *dermatophytes,* fungi of the genera *Microsporum, Trichophyton,* and *Epidermophyton,* which cause the most common fungal infections of the skin, hair, and nails such as athlete's foot, ringworm, and barber's itch.

Although such superficial infections are seldom serious, they sometimes cause intolerable itching and are often disfiguring. They are ordinarily controlled by topical applications of creams, ointments, and other preparations containing combinations of antifungal and keratolytic chemicals (see Chap. 43).

Several new antifungal chemicals appear to be very effective for relief of itching and other symptoms. However, they do not prevent some types of superficial fungal infections from recurring. This is because the tiny parasitic plants burrow down to the base of the keratin layer where some survive an attack from above by topically applied medications. Thus, even when the keratolytic drugs dissolve the dead keratin cells, the newly forming skin, hair, and nails carry bits of fungi that being to grow again.

Griseofulvin has offered dermatologists an entirely new approach to the treatment of such chronic fungal infections. The drug is rarely applied topically, because apparently it penetrates the skin poorly from above. It is instead taken by mouth in tablet form or as an oral suspension. After its absorption into the blood from the intestine the antibiotic is deposited in the living cells, which are converted to keratin when they die. The drug's continued presence in the keratin layer acts as a barrier to the further growth of fungi already established there. Then, as new cells grow out, they push the fungus-infected tissues before them until they are naturally shed or can be clipped.

The time required for treatment with griseofulvin varies, depending on various factors including the location and severity of the fungal infection. Tinea capitis (ringworm of the scalp) and tinea pedis (athlete's foot) require only about 4 weeks for complete eradication of the fungal invader; tinea unguium (onychomycosis; ringworm of the nails) may need 6 months to a year of treatment.

Fortunately for patients on long-term therapy, griseofulvin has given little indication of toxicity. Although minor side-effects, including headache and gastrointestinal irritation, are the cause of occasional complaints, more serious toxicity has not been reported. Patients taking the drug over a period of many months may be given blood and liver function tests periodically, and should be instructed to report the occurrence of sore throat, fever, or other unusual symptoms. They should also, of course, be instructed in the measures required to prevent their becoming reinfected.

Additional clinical considerations

Just as the spectrum of fungal infections ranges from minor irritations to potentially fatal systemic infections, the clinical problems involving antifungal drug therapy range from relatively little toxicity and few problems (Griseofulvin) to possibly severe toxicity (amphotericin B). Special clinical considerations pertain to each range of drug.

The *amphotericin B* solution must be prepared with great care, using aseptic technique to avoid contamination. The solution can be refrigerated for up to 24 hours, but it must be protected from light exposure. When infusing this drug IV, it must be given very slowly to minimize potentially severe toxicity. Ampotericin B can cause renal toxicity and, therefore, should not be combined with other nephrotoxic agents.

Miconazole must also be given by very slow IV

infusion; there have been reports of cardiac arrest following rapid injection. *Flucytosine* use must be accompanied by frequent monitoring of hepatic, renal, and hematologic functioning. Nausea, vomiting, and diarrhea are frequent adverse effects of this drug. The patient can be taught to take one or two capsules at a time over a 10 to 15-minute period (slow dosing), which may decrease or eliminate the GI upset. *Ketoconazole* must have an acidic gastric environment for proper absorption. Because of this, anything that alkalinizes the stomach contents (*e.g.*, food, milk products, antacids, certain drugs) should not be taken concurrently with the ketoconazole. The ketoconazole dose should be administered at least 2 hours before any of these other agents are used. The use of any of these agents in pregnancy or lactation is contraindicated—with some of these drugs, adverse fetal effects have been reported; with others, there is no documented evidence of safety. In all cases of fungal infection, the patient should be carefully evaluated for the underlying cause of the problem, such as source of infection, lack of natural defenses, and debilitated state.

The guide to the nursing process summarizes the application of the nursing process to therapy with antifungal drugs. The patient teaching guide offers key points to consider with a patient taking oral antifungal agents.

Patient teaching guide: oral antifungal agents

The drug that has been prescribed for you is an antifungal drug. It works in the body to destroy fungi that have invaded the body. Because of the way that these drugs work, they must be taken over a period of time. It is very important to take all the medication that has been prescribed for you.

Instructions:

1. The drug that has been ordered for you is _____ .

2. The dosage of the drug is _____ .

3. The drug should be taken _____ times a day. The best time to take your drug is _____ , _____ , _____ .

4. (Ketoconazole must be taken 2 hours before ingesting meals, milk products, antacids, or any other drugs. Flucytosine can be taken slowly over a 10- to 15-minute period, a few capsules at a time to help to decrease the stomach upset.)

5. Some side-effects of the drug that you should be aware of include the following:

Stomach upset, nausea, vomiting, diarrhea	If appropriate, take slowly or with meals.
Headache, dizziness	Aspirin may help; take precautions if you experience dizziness—avoid such activities as driving or operating dangerous equipment.

6. Tell any physician, nurse, or dentist who is taking care of you that you are on this drug.

7. Keep this and all medication out of the reach of children.

8. Take the full course of your prescription. Never use this medication to self-treat any other infection or give it to any other person.

(continued)

Notify your nurse or physician if any of the following occur:

Severe vomiting, abdominal pain
Fever, chills
Yellowing skin or eyes
Dark urine
Pale stools
Skin rash

Guide to the nursing process: antifungal drugs

Assessment	Nursing diagnoses	Interventions	Evaluation
Past history—underlying medical conditions (*contraindications*): Renal failure Hepatic failure Bone marrow depression Pregnancy Lactation Allergies: *these agents,* others; reactions Medication history: current drugs (*Cautions:* Antacids; ketoconazole: H_2 blockers, anticholinergics; amphotericin B: steroids; miconazole: coumarins)	Potential alteration in comfort (GI pain; headache) Potential alteration in bowel elimination Potential alteration in tissue perfusion (secondary to renal or liver failure, bone marrow depression) Knowledge deficit regarding drug therapy	Safe preparation, storage, and administration of drug Comfort measures: Small frequent meals Hygiene measures; Safety measures if CNS effects occur Pain relief Antiemetics, etc. Patient teaching regarding: drug Drug dosage Administration Comfort Warnings Support and encouragement for therapy and disease Life support measures, if indicated	Evaluate the effectiveness of the drug: resolution of infection Evaluate for adverse effects: Renal function Liver enzymes Hematologic tests GI symptoms Fever Pain Cardiac effects Evaluate effectiveness of patient teaching Evaluate effectiveness of support and encouragement— coping, compliance Monitor vital functioning, if indicated

Physical assessment
Neurologic: orientation, reflexes
Cardiovascular: baseline EKG, pulse
Respiratory: rate, adventitious sounds
GI: liver function tests, bowel sounds
Renal: BUN, creatinine, urinalysis
Tests: CBC

Case Study

Presentation

PP, an ambitious young model, has been on very strict diets for a long period of time. At times her dieting is close to starvation. In the last 16 months she has been treated for various bacterial infections (*e.g.*, pneumonia, cystitis) with a series of antibiotics. She presents in the clinic with complaints of abdominal pain, difficulty in swallowing, and a sore throat. In appearance she is an extremely pale and thin young woman, who looks older than her stated age (19 years). Her mouth was found to be moist and the mucosa covered with small white colonies that extended down the pharynx. A vaginal examination revealed similar colonies. Cultures were done, and it was determined that she had mucocutaneous candidiasis. She was started on ketoconazole (Nizoral) and asked to return to the clinic in 10 days for a follow-up evaluation. What measures should be taken with PP before she leaves the clinic?

Discussion

Because of PP's appearance, a complete physical exam should be done before beginning drug therapy. The nurse will need to know PP's baseline functioning and to determine any underlying problems that may exist. Poor nutrition and total starvation have characteristic deficiencies that predispose people to opportunistic infections and prevent their bodies from protecting themselves adequately through the inflammatory and immune responses. Of particular importance with this drug therapy is the fact that liver changes often occur with poor nutrition; this can cause deficient drug metabolism and lead to toxicity. An intense patient education program should be started with PP. She will need support to accept her diagnosis and to adapt to drug therapy and nutritional changes. She should have an opportunity to ventilate her feelings. She will need to understand the possible causes of her fungal infection—poor nutrition plus the loss of normal flora secondary to antibiotic therapy—as well as her drug therapy—the dosage, special precautions for administration, side-effects, and warning signs to monitor. PP may benefit from nutritional counseling or referral to a dietician for thorough nutritional teaching. She should be monitored carefully for adverse effects of the drug, and should have regular follow-up care to monitor the drug's actions and her progress. The resolution of this fungal infection may well occur only as the result of prolonged drug and nutritional therapy. This will have tremendous impact on PP's life style, and she will need a great deal of support and encouragement to make the changes that will be required to comply. The nurse involved in her care will need to work with her and develop an approach to her care that is acceptable and tolerable, but that will still allow the best possible chance for eradication of the fungal infection.

Drug digests

Amphotericin B USP (Fungizone)

Actions and indications. Administered parenterally, this antifungal antibiotic is effective for treatment of most serious systemic fungal infections. Among the disseminated mycotic infections that often respond to treatment with this drug are blastomycosis, coccidiomycosis, cryptococcosis, histoplasmosis, and candidiasis.

It is also effective against candidiasis when applied topically to the skin and nails, or to the mucous membranes of the mouth. Taken internally in oral dosage forms, amphotericin B is sometimes employed to prevent the overgrowth of intestinal fungi that occurs during treatment with tetracyclines and other broad-spectrum antibiotics.

Adverse effects, cautions, and contraindications. The topical application of this antibiotic causes little irritation and few allergic reactions. However, toxic effects are frequent during intravenous administration, and efforts must be made to minimize toxicity. For example, administration of this drug in the lowest effective dose together with antipyretic, antihistamine, and antiemetic drugs may help to reduce reactions.

Patients' renal function must be carefully monitored to detect increases in blood urea nitrogen (BUN) and nonprotein nitrogen (NPN) levels. If these levels rise, the drug is discontinued for a time. Kidney excretion of the antibiotic is increased by alkalinizing the urine.

Dosage and administration. Dosage is adjusted individually, but should not ordinarily be more than 1 mg/kg/day or 1.5 mg/kg every other day. Solutions for slow intravenous infusion must be freshly prepared and protected from light.

Griseofulvin USP (Fulvicin-U/F; Grifulvin V; Grisactin)

Actions and indications. This antifungal antibiotic is effective for treating tinea (ringworm) infections of the skin. Taken orally, it is absorbed into the bloodstream and deposited in new skin and nail keratin, which can then resist invasion by species of *Trichophyton, Microsporum,* and *Epidermophyton.* Among the infections that respond to treatment are tinea pedis (athlete's foot), tinea capitis (scalp ringworm), tinea cruris (groin ringworm), and tinea unguium (onychomycosis, a fungal disease of the nails).

Adverse effects, cautions, and contraindi- cations. Skin rashes of the hypersensitivity type sometimes occur, as do photosensitivity-type reactions in some patients exposed to sunlight. Because this drug is not effective against *Candida,* overgrowths of *Monilia* may cause oral thrush. Gastrointestinal distress with nausea, vomiting, and diarrhea, and central effects such as headache, dizziness, and mental confusion may occur. This drug is contraindicated in patients with acute porphyria or liver damage.

Drug interactions with warfarin-type anticoagulants may result in reduced responsiveness to the anticoagulants, which then require an upward adjustment of their dosage. The effectiveness of griseofulvin may be reduced when barbiturates are taken at the same time. Thus, dosage of the antibiotic may have to be raised.

Dosage and administration. Daily oral doses of 0.5 g or 1 g are taken after meals. The length of treatment may vary from several weeks in skin infections to several months for nail infections. The adjunctive use of topically applied antifungal chemicals is also often desirable.

Nystatin USP (Mycostatin; Nilstat)

Actions and indications. This antifungal antibiotic is effective against candidal infections (moniliasis) when it is applied topically to the skin or to the mucous membranes of the mouth (in thrush) or of the vagina. It is also often taken orally to prevent superinfections by overgrowths of intestinal fungi in patients who are being treated with tetracyclines or other broad-spectrum antibacterial drugs.

It is doubtful that the small amounts of this antibiotic contained in commercial fixed dosage combinations can serve a useful prophylactic purpose. However, the adminis- tration of adequate oral doses may be desirable for preventing intestinal moniliasis during antibacterial treatment of diabetics and other high-risk patients, such as those receiving corticosteroids for systemic lupus or antineoplastic drugs for leukemia, lymphoma, and so forth.

Adverse effects, cautions, and contraindications. Large oral doses sometimes cause epigastric distress and diarrhea. However, the drug is not absorbed and does not cause systemic toxicity. Topical application rarely causes irritation or hypersensitivity-type reactions.

Dosage and administration. This drug may be administered orally in doses of 0.5 million to 1 million U tid daily for suppression of yeastlike intestinal fungi. Tablets may be deposited in the vagina by applicator in doses of 100,000 U to 200,000 U daily. Other dosage forms for topical application include an oral suspension that is dropped into the mouth four times daily to treat thrush in infants and children; a dusting powder for fungal infections of the feet; and a cream and ointment that are applied twice daily to cutaneous areas affected by candidiasis.

Reference

Cantanzaro A et al: Ketoconazole for treatment of disseminated coccidioidomycosis. Ann Intern Med 96:436, 1982

Cohen J: Antifungal chemotherapy. Lancet 2:532, 1982

Drugs for treatment of systemic fungal infections. Med Lett Drugs Ther 26:35–38, 1984

Heel RC et al: Ketoconazole: Review of therapeutic efficacy in superficial and systemic fungal infections. Drugs 23:1, 1982

Medoff G et al: Antifungal agents useful in therapy of systemic fungal infections. Ann Rev Pharmacol Toxicol 23:303, 1983

New topical antifungal drugs. Med Lett Drugs Ther 25:98–100, 1983

Sande MA, Mandell GL: Antimicrobial agents: Miscellaneous antibacterial agents; antifungal and antiviral agents. In Gilman AG, Goodman LS, Gilman A (eds): Goodman & Gilman's The Pharmacological Basis of Therapeutics, 6th ed, pp 1222–1248. New York, Macmillan, 1980

Chapter 10

The chemotherapy of malaria and other protozoan infections

10

Parasitic diseases caused by infestation with protozoan organisms and worms of various types are among the most common of all ailments. In the tropical areas in which these types of illnesses are most prevalent, many people suffer several such infestations at the same time. Although parasitic infections are relatively rare here, travelers returning from abroad sometimes bring back parasites with which they were infected on their trips to parts of Africa, Asia, South America, and elsewhere. Of course, climate is only one of several factors that favor transmission of parasites. These types of diseases are most likely to break out wherever people live in overcrowded and unsanitary conditions. Thus, for example, parasitic infections caused by ingestion of contaminated food and drink can occur readily in countries with a temperate climate when there is a breakdown of sanitation.

This chapter deals mainly with drugs used against infections by the mosquito-borne protozoa that cause human *malaria*. It will also discuss drugs used in the treatment of two other diseases, *trypanosomiasis* and *leishmaniasis,* that are also caused by protozoa transmitted to humans by insects. Some of the same drugs are also effective for treating *pneumocystosis,* an often fatal respiratory infection by organisms that are probably protozoa capable of invading the lungs of patients with poor immunologic defense mechanisms.

The following chapter is generally concerned with the drug treatment of parasitic diseases that are transmitted not by insects but by the ingestion of food and drink containing protozoa or the eggs, larvae, or other forms of worms. Many effective chemotherapeutic agents are now available for treating protozoan and helminthic infections. However, the most important disease control measures are those aimed at breaking the chain by which parasites are transmitted to humans. Programs of mass chemoprophylaxis, although of some help here, are less significant than improved sanitation measures, reduction of overpopulation and overcrowding, and control of insects and other vectors.

Malaria

Malaria is a parasitic disease that has killed hundreds of millions of people and changed the course of history. Even today, when great advances have been made in the control of malaria, millions of people are infected in the many lands in which this mosquito-borne disease is still endemic. The continued prevalence of malaria in many parts of the globe indicates the need to sustain a vigorous attack on the malaria parasite and on its insect vector, the *Anopheles* mosquito. Strains of mosquitoes that have developed resistance to DDT and other insecticides have appeared. Similarly, malaria parasites insensitive to antimalarial drugs now cause disease in various parts of the world.

Biologic nature of malaria

Types of malaria

Four species of protozoa of the genus *Plasmodium* cause malaria in humans. The two that are of prime importance are *Plasmodium vivax,* the cause of benign tertian malaria, and *Plasmodium falciparum,* the cause of malignant tertian malaria. The term "tertian" refers to the fact that the attacks of chills and fever tend typically to recur every third day. The term *benign* indicates only that *P. vivax* infection is less severe than *P. falciparum* infection, and is less likely to kill quickly. The malignant disease, although relatively easy to cure in most cases with modern drugs, may start explosively and end fatally, with its victims following a rapidly progressive downhill course. The drugs used in the control of malaria have variable effects on the different stages of the parasite as well as on the different species and strains. Thus, to understand how the drugs act and how this determines their clinical uses and limitations, it is necessary to know something about the life cycle of plasmodial organisms. The following brief review will emphasize the terms and concepts necessary for the later discussion of the several classes of drugs and their clinical uses.

Life cycle of the plasmodium

The parasites that cause clinical malaria spend part of their lives in the female *Anopheles* mosquito and part in the human host (Fig. 10-1). The mosquito that bites an infected person and sucks up a drop of blood ingests *gametocytes,* which are sexual (male and female) forms of

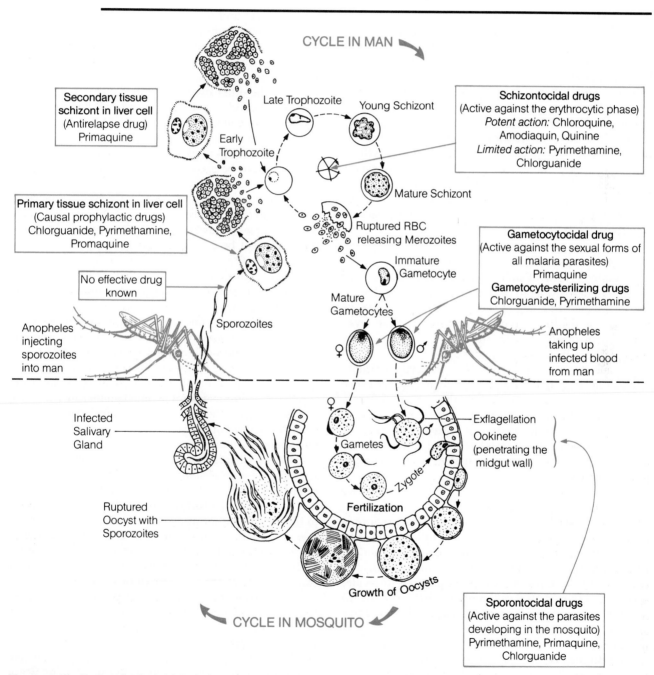

CYCLE IN MAN

Secondary tissue
schizont in liver cell
(Antirelapse drug)
Primaquine

Late Trophozoite   Young Schizont

Early
Trophozoite

Schizontocidal drugs
(Active against the erythrocytic phase)
Potent action: Chloroquine,
Amodiaquin, Quinine
Limited action: Pyrimethamine,
Chlorguanide

Mature Schizont

Primary tissue schizont in liver cell
(Causal prophylactic drugs)
Chlorguanide, Pyrimethamine,
Promaquine

Ruptured RBC
releasing Merozoites

No effective drug
known

Immature
Gametocyte

Gametocytocidal drug
(Active against the sexual forms of
all malaria parasites)
Primaquine
Gametocyte-sterilizing drugs
Chlorguanide, Pyrimethamine

Mature
Gametocytes

Anopheles
injecting
sporozoites
into man

Sporozoites

♀   ♂

Anopheles
taking up
infected blood
from man

Infected
Salivary
Gland

Gametes

Exflagellation
Ookinete
(penetrating the
midgut wall)

Zygote

Ruptured
Oocyst with
Sporozoites

Fertilization

Growth of Oocysts

Sporontocidal drugs
(Active against the parasites
developing in the mosquito)
Pyrimethamine, Primaquine,
Chlorguanide

CYCLE IN MOSQUITO

Figure 10-1. Classification of antimalarial drugs in relation to different stages in the life cycle of the parasite. Two of the drugs shown here (amodiaquin and chlorguanide) are no longer commonly available in the United States. (Adapted from Bruce–Chwatt LJ: WHO Bull, No. 27:287, 1962)

the plasmodial parasite. These gametocytes mate in the mosquito's stomach, and the product of this mating (the zygote) goes through several stages and finally forms *sporozoites* (spore animals) that make their way to the mosquito's salivary glands.

The next person bitten by the mosquito gets an injection of thousands of these sporozoites. These do not linger very long in the bloodstream but, instead, lodge in the liver and other tissues, where they undergo *asexual cell division* and reproduction.

During the next week to 10 days, these *primary tissue schizonts* grow and multiply by simple division within the liver cells. Finally, *merozoites* are formed by malarial schizonts and burst forth when the liver cells that had been parasitized are ruptured. Most of the merozoites enter the circulation and invade red blood cells.

After a period of development and asexual division within the first blood cells to be invaded, a new batch of merozoites bursts forth from the ruptured red cells. These liberated spores invade still more erythrocytes, and repeat the process of division. After several such cycles, the number of organisms is so great and the number of parasitized red cells so large that the patient begins to suffer from the symptoms of an acute attack of malaria.

Clinical course

The sudden release of swarms of malaria parasites from millions of destroyed red cells sets off the chills and fever that mark the beginning of the clinical attack. The chill is caused by the breakup of the erythrocytes; the fever is the result of a pyrogenic effect of the freed foreign protein and cellular debris (toxins).

Each time a new mass of erythrocytic schizonts bursts, releasing toxins into the circulation (about every 48 hours in the tertian malarias), the patient suffers a paroxysm of chills and fever. In *P. vivax* malaria such attacks continue for a long time if untreated. Even after the body's defense mechanisms have brought the infection more or less under control, the patient is subject to periodic relapses.

Relapses

Relapses occur in *P. vivax* malaria because some schizonts make their way back into the liver and other tissue cells. Then these so-called *exoerythrocytic forms,* or secondary tissue schizonts, periodically send forth more invaders of red cells. As these plasmodial spores proceed to divide, invade, and then destroy still more erythrocytes, the infected person suffers yet another attack. Relapses of this type can occur periodically for years if the person goes untreated.

In the case of *P. falciparum* malaria, no such secondary exoerythrocytic schizonts persist in the tissues. Thus, provided that the patient survives the first series of attacks, no further relapses will be suffered. However,

this form of malaria is often fatal, because the parasite-damaged red cells tend to clog the patient's capillaries and thus cut off the circulation in vital organs.

Chemotherapy

The currently most important antimalarial drugs are *chloroquine*[+], *primaquine*[+], and *pyrimethamine*[+]. These and *quinine*[+], a drug that for centuries was the only available agent for treating malaria, are discussed in detail in the Drug Digests in terms of their actions, uses, adverse effects, dosage, and administration. The increasing incidence of chloroquine-resistant strains of *P. falciparum* has made the combination drug form Fansidar (*sulfadoxine* plus *pyrimethamine*), which constitutes effective prophylaxis and treatment for these strains, of increasing importance.

The other drugs listed in Table 10-1 will not be discussed individually. However, some of their properties and their place in malaria therapy will be apparent from the following discussion.

The drugs used in the treatment and prevention of malaria can be classified in several ways: (1) in terms of their chemical structure; (2) in terms of the forms of the plasmodial parasite against which they are most effective; and (3) in terms of their clinical uses. Only some brief examples (below) of the first two types of drug classifications will be presented. However, because of the practical significance of considering the drugs in that way, the chief discussion of this topic will deal with the circumstances in which the several classes of drugs are employed clinically.

Chemically, one important group of drugs is derived from 4-aminoquinoline. These include chloroquine and hydroxychloroquine. Another chemical group, the 8-aminoquinolines, is now represented only by primaquine. Similarly, the only diaminopyrimidine employed at present against malaria is pyrimethamine; another drug of this class, trimethoprim, is now used mainly for treating urinary tract and other bacterial infections, often in combination (co-trimoxazole) with a sulfonamide, sulfamethoxazole (see Chap. 8). Quinacrine is an acridine derivative, and quinine is an alkaloid derived from the bark of the cinchona tree.

Plasmodial forms differ in their responsiveness to the various antimalarial drugs. Only the *sporozoites* are *in*sensitive to drugs during their brief stay in the patient's bloodstream before they enter the liver. Most sensitive to drug action are the *erythrocytic schizonts,* which are most commonly attacked today with chloroquine, with or without sulfadoxine–pyrimethamine, depending on whether the parasite is likely to be chloroquine-resistant, and only occasionally with quinine or hydroxychloroquine. The *exoerythrocytic forms* in the liver respond to treatment with primaquine, a drug that also kills the sexual forms (gametocytes) in the person's blood. Pyrimethamine is not gametocidal, but it can sterilize these sexual forms so that they fail to mate. In theory, it is a broad-spectrum an-

Table 10–1. Antimalarial drugs

Generic or official name	Trade name	Oral dosage
Chloroquine phosphate USP	Aralen	Suppressive*: 300 mg chloroquine base (=500 mg chloroquine phosphate) weekly on same day each week beginning 2 wk before exposure and continuing until 6–8 wk after last exposure Therapeutic†: 600 mg chloroquine base (=1 g chloroquine phosphate) followed by 300 mg base (=500 mg phosphate) in 6 hr, and on days 2 and 3
Hydroxychloroquine sulfate USP	Plaquenil Sulfate	Suppressive: 310 mg base (=400 mg hydroxychloroquine sulfate) weekly on same day each week before exposure and continuing until 6–8 wk after last exposure
Primaquine phosphate USP		26.3 mg (=15 mg of the base) daily for 14 days to achieve a radical cure,‡ during or after a course of suppression with chloroquine
Pyrimethamine USP	Daraprim	Suppressive: 25 mg weekly Therapeutic: 25 mg for 2 days
Quinacrine HCl USP	Atabrine	Suppressive: 100 mg/day for 1–3 months Therapeutic: 200 mg given with 1 g of sodium bicarbonate q 6 hr for five doses; then 100 mg tid for 6 days
Quinine sulfate USP	Quinamm; Quine	Therapeutic: 650 mg q 8 hr for 10–14 days
Sulfadoxine 500 mg and pyrimethamine 25 mg	Fansidar	Suppressive: One tablet weekly or two tablets biweekly beginning before departure to malarial area and continuing for 4–6 wk after return. Therapeutic: Two or three tablets as single dose alone or in sequence with quinine or primaquine

* *Suppressive* refers to the use of a single small dose periodically to prevent development of clinical signs and symptoms in a person who may have been bitten and infected with plasmodial parasites (*i.e.*, for *clinical prophylaxis*).
† *Therapeutic* refers to the use of larger or more frequently administered doses to terminate an acute attack (*i.e.*, for *clinical cure*).
‡ *Radical cure* refers to use of drugs of this type to prevent relapses through their effects on the secondary tissue forms of the parasites.

timalarial capable of inhibiting both erythrocytic and exoerythrocytic forms, but in practice it has proved less useful than the administration of a combination of chloroquine and primaquine.

As the above discussion indicates, the currently available antimalarial drugs can act at one or another stage of the plasmodial life cycle. Thus, by the selection of the drug that is most effective against each stage, the following objectives should be achieved:

1. Prevention and treatment of acute attacks
2. Prevention of relapses with a resulting complete cure
3. Disruption of the chain of disease transmission

Actually, the latter objective is not usually practical for the reasons indicated in the discussion of mass prophylaxis.

Mass prophylaxis

Prevention cannot be readily applied to the populations of areas in which malaria is endemic. In theory, these people could routinely receive antimalarial drugs such as *primaquine* or *pyrimethamine* to prevent them from ever getting the disease or transmitting it.

Both these drugs (and *chloroquine*) can destroy the gametocytes of certain *Plasmodium* species in the person's blood or sterilize these sexual forms before they might mate. This could break the human–mosquito–human chain of transmission by which malaria is spread. Similarly, these same drugs are *schizonticides* as well as gametocides. Thus, if taken routinely, they could kill plasmodial parasites in the tissues before they ever got a chance to move back into the bloodstream to invade and destroy red cells.

Unfortunately, these *true causal prophylactic drugs* are considered to be too toxic and expensive for mass administration to uninfected people in endemic areas for the purpose of protecting the population and breaking the chain of transmission. Instead of drugs, public health officials in these areas depend on mosquito control, protective screening, and insect repellents. That is, they try to prevent people from being bitten by the insect vector rather than having them take potentially toxic and expensive drugs in an effort to eradicate the parasites when they enter the blood and tissues.

Suppressive and therapeutic measures

Although it is impractical to use drugs for preventing people from becoming infected, it is possible to prevent them from ever suffering clinical symptoms of the disease, and it is now also practical to eliminate secondary tissue forms of the parasite and thus achieve the complete cure of an infected person.

Suppressive treatment refers to the routine use of small safe doses of certain drugs to prevent a person who has been bitten by the mosquito and infected by plasmodial parasites from suffering an actual clinical attack of malaria. Taken only once weekly, drugs such as *chloroquine* (Aralen), *hydroxychloroquine*, *primaquine*, and *sulfadoxine–pyrimethamine*, alone or in combinations appropriate for the strains of *Plasmodium* endemic to the area, can control the forms of the parasites that enter red blood cells (Table 10-1). This protects the erythrocytes from destruction and thus suppresses the periodic malarial paroxysms of chills, fever, and any other signs and symptoms of an acute attack.

Curative measures

Clinical cure, the relief of an actual attack, can be brought about by the same drugs that are used for suppressive treatment. They act, of course, by stopping the cycles of erythrocytic schizogony through which more and more red blood cells are parasitized by waves of liberated merozoites. By ending the periodic release of toxins responsible for paroxysms of chills and fever, drugs such as *chloroquine* and the other synthetic successors to *quinine* quickly terminate the attacks. With *P. vivax* infections, they do not, however, completely eliminate the parasite from the patient's body. Thus, although the attack is clinically cured, the patient is not truly cured and is subject to relapses of *P. vivax* malaria.

Radical cure of *P. vivax* infection *can,* however, be brought about by chemotherapy. This is accomplished with drugs such as *primaquine,* which wipe out the secondary tissue forms of *P. vivax.* By acting to kill these *exo*erythrocytic schizonts produced by merozoites that have made their way back into liver cells, primaquine prevents the red blood cell parasitizers from ever again emerging. Simultaneous *suppressive therapy* is, of course, needed to keep blood forms from continuing to survive.

In the case of *P. falciparum,* as previously indicated, suppressive treatment alone is adequate, because this organism possesses no persisting secondary exoerythrocytic tissue forms.

Travelers to areas in which malaria is still endemic cannot usually be prevented from being bitten and infected by mosquitoes that are carrying the parasites. However—as was shown with malaria prevention measures employed by the United States Army in Vietnam—people can be protected from developing disease symptoms, and, as was done with soldiers leaving Southeast Asia, any parasites still in their tissues when they leave the malarious country can also be eradicated by drug therapy.

Such suppressive treatment and radical cure can be carried out most conveniently by having the traveler take a single tablet that combines *chloroquine* with *primaquine* in small safe doses once weekly. The first tablet is taken 2 weeks before arriving in the malarious area. This drug combination is then repeated on the same day of the week at weekly intervals during the person's entire stay. Travelers to areas in which chloroquine-resistant strains of *P. falciparum* are known to exist take *chloroquine* and *sulfadoxine–pyrimethamine.*

After leaving the country, the traveler continues to take one tablet weekly for the next 8 weeks. The chloroquine component of such mixtures attacks the primary tissue parasites as they emerge from the tissues and enter the bloodstream. This prevents the traveler from ever suffering any symptoms while in the area. The primaquine portion of the combination tablet eradicates any secondary tissue forms that remain after leaving, as described above in the discussion of radical cure.

Treatment of resistant cases

As described above, reports of patients with malaria resistant to treatment with chloroquine have appeared. Cases caused by infection with resistant strains of *P. falciparum* have been of particular concern because of the seriousness of infections by this plasmodial parasite. The appearance of such cases in American soldiers in Southeast Asia (Vietnam, Cambodia, and Thailand) and in travelers and residents of Central and South America has led to many scientific studies aimed at discovering more effective antimalarial drugs.

Among the drugs now considered most useful for treating a clinical attack of chloroquine-resistant *P. falciparum* malaria or for suppressing its symptoms are some that were discarded when the new synthetic drugs were developed. *Quinine,* for example, is not ordinarily used today because it is less effective and more toxic than the modern synthetic antimalarials. Yet, because strains resistant to quinine have rarely developed, it has proved useful for treating chloroquine-resistant cases. Similarly, as described above, the antibacterial *sulfonamide* drugs (see Chap. 8), which are no longer used in ordinary malaria, have found a place in treating cases caused by chloroquine-resistant strains of *P. falciparum.*

None of these drugs is ordinarily used alone for treating clinical attacks of malaria. Treatment of attacks that occur in geographic areas in which chloroquine-resistant strains predominate is begun with a combination of three drugs. These include quinine, administered orally (or intravenously if the patient is vomiting), together with pyrimethamine and a sulfonamide. A three-drug combination is also employed whenever an attack that was first treated with chloroquine fails to respond promptly.

Other protozoal infections

Protozoal organisms other than plasmodia are a frequent cause of infection. The rest of this chapter will describe mainly the chemotherapy of such protozoan infections as trypanosomiasis and leishmaniasis. The drugs used for treating these disorders are of two main types: organic compounds containing arsenic or antimony, and nonmetallic organic chemicals. All these drugs owe their effectiveness to their *selective toxicity* on certain metabolic processes of the protozoal parasites. However, because such selectivity is only relative, all are also capable of causing toxicity to the patient who is host to the parasites.

Most of these antiprotozoan drugs are not marketed in this country (Table 10-2). They can, however, be quickly obtained when needed by telephoning the Parasitic Disease Drug Service of the Centers for Disease Control (CDC) in Atlanta. Because data on dosage and administration and other information for safe use of these drugs are made available to medical personnel when the drugs are supplied, most of these details will not be described in this text.

Trypanosomiasis

Infection by trypanosomes is spread by insect vectors that are found only in the specific geographic areas in which these diseases are endemic—the tsetse fly in the case of African sleeping sickness and certain bedbuglike species in Chagas' disease, which occurs only in parts of the Americas. Both diseases are severe infections that require treatment with relatively toxic drugs. Thus, prevention by the use of insecticides and other measures for eliminating the transmitter insects from the environment is the best approach to the control of trypanosomiasis. Because the two diseases take different clinical courses and the chemotherapy of each is different, each disorder and its drug treatment will be discussed separately.

African trypanosomiasis

This form, also called sleeping sickness, is a disease that develops in two stages: an early hemolymphatic stage marked by a high fever, and a later meningoencephalitis that is fatal if not treated. Patients treated in the first stage usually make a complete recovery but, once the protozoan parasite has entered the central nervous system, the prognosis for recovery without permanent brain damage is less certain. The hemolymphatic phase usually responds to treatment with nonmetallic trypanocides such as suramin and pentamidine. The presence of trypanosomes in the cerebrospinal fluid indicates the need for

Table 10–2. Drugs for other protozoal infections with insect vectors

Generic or official name	Trade name	Availability in the United States	Indications
Hydroxystilbamidine isethionate USP		Commercially available	Visceral leishmaniasis (kala-azar) and American mucocutaneous leishmaniasis; indicated for North American blastomycosis, but not the drug of choice
Melarsoprol (Mel B)	Arsobal	Available from CDC	Trypanosomiasis (African sleeping sickness)
Nifurtimox	Lampit	Available from CDC	Chagas' disease
Pentamidine isethionate	Lomidine	Available from CDC	Pneumocystosis pneumonia and trypanosomiasis; leishmaniasis
Sodium antimony gluconate or sodium stibogluconate	Pentostam	Available from CDC	Leishmaniasis (kala-azar); American cutaneous leishmaniasis; oriental sore
Suramin	Antrypol; Belganyl; Germanin	Available from CDC	Trypanosomiasis and onchocerciasis (a filarial disease)

treatment with an arsenical, melarsoprol, or *tryparsamide*, which is not available in the United States.

Suramin sodium is the best drug with which to begin treatment of trypanosomiasis while the parasite is still restricted to the blood and lymph and cannot yet be found on examination of the cerebrospinal fluid. Treatment is highly effective, except when the central nervous system has been invaded before treatment of the hemolymphatic phase was started.

Suramin is also employed for treating filariasis (see Chap. 11), and because it stays in the blood for long periods, it has sometimes been used for preventing trypanosomiasis in programs of mass prophylaxis. However, because side-effects are common and sometimes severe, the somewhat safer trypanocide pentamidine (see below) is usually preferred for prophylaxis.

The most common adverse effects of suramin are pruritic skin eruptions, fever, headache, nausea, and vomiting. Rarely, highly sensitive persons may suffer circulatory collapse and coma. Albuminuria is a frequent finding in the urine examinations that are required during courses of suramin treatment. If the urinary protein level rises and casts occur, indicating renal failure, during continued treatment, this drug may have to be withdrawn.

Pentamidine, a drug also employed in the management of other protozoal infections such as leishmaniasis and *Pneumocytis carinii* pneumonia (a disease being seen with increasing frequency as a manifestation of AIDS, acquired immune deficiency syndrome) is effective in the hemolymphatic phase of Gambian trypanosomiasis and for prophylaxis against this infection. It is less useful for treating the Rhodesian form of trypanosomiasis infection that invades the central nervous system much more rapidly. Like suramin, this drug does not pass the blood–brain barrier.

Pentamidine provides a prophylactic effect for 6 months or more after a single intramuscular injection, because it is stored in the liver and other tissues for a prolonged period. When administered by this route, the drug does not cause symptoms of the steep drop in blood pressure that sometimes occur during intravenous administration of therapeutic doses. However, because of the drug's various other side-effects, pentamidine prophylaxis is *not* recommended for most tourists who intend to travel in parts of Africa in which trypanosomiasis is endemic.

Melarsoprol is an organic arsenical compound that has largely replaced other metallic agents, including *tryparsamide*, a less effective trypanocidal agent that was the drug of choice for several decades. It is effective in both phases of trypanosomiasis but, because of its potential toxicity, it is used only when there is evidence of central nervous system invasion. The drug is then administered intravenously in several 3-day courses separated by rest periods of a week or more.

One of this drug's advantages over tryparsamide is that it does not damage the optic nerve or cause blindness. However, encephalopathy often occurs early in the course of treatment of patients sensitive to arsenic or to antigens released from trypanosomes that the drug has killed after passing the blood–brain barrier. Severe arsenic-induced encephalopathy is sometimes responsive to treatment with dimercaprol (see Chap. 5); symptomatic control of sensitization reactions is sometimes achieved by administering corticosteroid or antihistamine drugs.

Melarsoprol has proved effective in infections caused by some trypanosomal strains that have acquired resistance to tryparsamide. However, an occasional infection is resistant to treatment with these drugs and all other arsenicals. In some such cases, the nonmetallic nitrofuran derivative *nifurtimox*, the first truly effective drug for American trypanosomiasis (see below), is also being tried experimentally for treating arsenic-resistant African sleeping sickness infections.

American trypanosomiasis

This form, also called Chagas' disease, is an acute and chronic protozoal infection that afflicts many millions of people in Central and South America. Most survive the acute form of the disease but then develop chronic myocarditis or digestive system disorders as a result of a chronic infection of the heart, colon, or other organs. They may suffer from cardiac arrhythmias, signs and symptoms of heart failure, and severe constipation or other gastrointestinal disturbances.

Until recently there has been no successful chemotherapy for control of this parasitic infection despite the use of various drugs, including the antimalarials primaquine and pyrimethamine, which can clear the parasite from the blood temporarily. However, recent reports of results of treatment with the nitrofuran *nifurtimox* indicate that this drug is more effective than the earlier chemotherapeutic agents. Taken in oral doses for about 2 weeks, it controls the continuous fever and malaise of the acute infection. The chronic condition often responds to a 120-day treatment course, although the drug cannot, of course, counteract chronic damage already done to the myocardium and other organs by the trypanosome. Concurrent administration of antacids helps to relieve symptoms of gastric irritation, the drug's most common side-effect. Phenobarbital controls the effects of drug-induced central nervous system stimulation.

Leishmaniasis

Leishmaniasis is a term used to describe several diseases caused by infection with protozoan parasites of the *Leishmania* genus. These include kala-azar, or visceral leishmaniasis; oriental sore, or cutaneous leishmaniasis; and American mucocutaneous leishmaniasis. Kala-azar is a generalized infection with signs and symptoms involving the liver, spleen, and bone marrow and ranging from vague pains in muscles, bones, and joints to common complications such as bronchitis and pneumonia. The other leishmania infections are limited to the skin, in oriental sore, and to the skin, mouth, nose, and throat in mucocutaneous leishmaniasis.

The current drug of choice for all three types of leishmaniasis is the pentavalent organic antimony compound *sodium stibogluconate.* Most cases of visceral leishmaniasis are cleared up by a single 6-day course of sodium stibogluconate. The small minority of cases resistant to antimony therapy often respond to treatment with intramuscularly administered *pentamidine* (see above) or with intravenous infusions of the chemically related compound, *hydroxystilbamidine isethionate.* American cutaneous and mucocutaneous leishmaniasis sometimes are treated with the antifungal antibiotic amphotericin B (see Chap. 9). The lesions of cutaneous leishmaniasis may be treated adjunctively with various local measures including the application of heat to the lesion for 20 to 32 hours over a 10- to 12-day period.

Pneumocystosis

The protozoan organism *Pneumocystis carinii* is the cause of an acute lung infection, particularly in patients who have been under intensive treatment with immunosuppressive drugs, including high doses of corticosteroids. Death from a rapidly progressive pneumonia can occur in almost all untreated cases. However, when this infection is correctly diagnosed and early treatment is begun with *trimethoprim–sulfamethoxazole* (co-trimoxazole) or *pentamidine* (see above), most patients can make a complete recovery.

The combination of sulfonamides (trisulfapyrimidines) with the antimalarial drug, pyrimethamine, is effective for treating *toxoplasmosis,* an infection caused by the protozoan organism *Toxoplasma gondii* that is also especially serious when it occurs in immunosuppressed patients—for example, during treatment of Hodgkin's disease or other lymphomas with antineoplastic drugs. An alternative drug, not available in the United States, is *spiramycin.*

Other protozoal diseases are discussed in the following chapter, which deals mainly with parasitic diseases that involve infections in the gastrointestinal system.

Additional clinical considerations

The administration of *chloroquine* has been associated with severe and, in some cases, irreversible, retinopathy. Because of this, frequent and regular ophthalmologic examinations should be done if a patient is on chloroquine. Eighth cranial nerve damage has also been seen. This drug has also been reported to be extremely toxic in children, with fatalities reported. If an infant or child is to receive this drug, the dosage should be double-checked at each administration. Anyone taking chloroquine at home should be cautioned to keep this drug securely out of the reach of children to prevent tragedy. *Primaquine* should not be given in combination with any other drug that is hemolytic. The combination could cause severe bone marrow depression. *Pyrimethamine* has been associated with folic acid deficiencies. All these drugs can cause gastrointestinal upset and can be taken with meals, or even with antacids, if this becomes a problem. Pregnancy and lactation are contraindications to the use of all these drugs because of the potential harm to the fetus or infant. The danger is so great with the sulfadoxine and pyrimethamine combination that women should be urged to use contraceptive measures while taking the drug to prevent any possibility of pregnancy.

The patient teaching guide summarizes the teaching points that should be covered. The guide to the nursing process with antimalarial drugs summarizes the application of the nursing process to therapy with antimalarial drugs.

Patient teaching guide: antimalarial drugs

The drug that has been prescribed for you is a drug that suppresses or destroys malaria-causing protozoa that have invaded your bloodstream. These protozoa enter the body through mosquito bites and invade various tissues, including blood cells, and cause such problems as fever and chills. If untreated, these protozoa can cause serious and dangerous tissue damage. Because the drug works at various points in the life cycle of the protozoa, it is necessary to take the drug according to the schedule below. It is *very* important to complete the full course of your prescription.

Instructions:

    1.   The name of your drug is _____ .

    2.   The dosage of your drug is _____ .

(continued)

3. Your drug should be taken _____ . The best schedule for taking your drug is _____ . (A calendar with the days marked for weekly doses is very helpful, especially for travelers who will need to remember once-a-week doses for a long period.)

4. The drug can be taken with meals, with food, or even with antacids to help to decrease the gastrointestinal upset. Be sure to drink plenty of fluids while on the drug.

5. Some side-effects of the drug that you should be aware of include the following:

Nausea, vomiting, anorexia	Taking the drug with food may help; if symptoms are severe, check with your nurse or physician and the dosage can be reduced.
Vision changes, blurring	If this occurs, you should take safety precautions (*e.g.,* do not drive an automobile or operate dangerous equipment).

6. Tell any physician, nurse, or dentist who is taking care of you that you are on this drug.

7. Keep this and all medications out of the reach of children. This drug can cause severe poisoning in children; therefore, it must be stored where children cannot reach it.

8. Take the full course of your prescription. It is very important to take all the medication that has been prescribed for you. Never take this medication to self-treat any other infection or give it to anyone else.

Notify your nurse or physician if any of the following occur:

Severe GI upset
Visual changes
Fever or chills
Rash
Yellowing of skin or eyes
Darkening of urine

Guide to the nursing process: antimalarial drugs

Assessment	Nursing diagnoses	Interventions	Evaluation
Past history—underlying medical conditions (*contraindications*): Renal failure Hepatic failure	Potential alteration in comfort (secondary to GI upset) Potential alteration in bowel elimination	Safe preparation and administration of drug Comfort measures: Hygiene Small frequent meals	Evaluate effectiveness of drug: lack of signs and symptoms Evaluate adverse effects of drug:

(continued)

Assessment	Nursing diagnoses	Interventions	Evaluation

Bone marrow depression
Pregnancy
Lactation
Allergies: *these drugs,* reaction; other allergies
Medication history:
  Current drugs
  (*Cautions:* nephrotoxic drugs, hemolytic drugs, other antimalarials)
	Potential alteration in tissue perfusion (secondary to renal, liver, or bone marrow failure)
	Potential alteration in sensory perception (secondary to visual changes)
	Knowledge deficit regarding drug therapy
		Safety precautions with visual changes
		Patient teaching:
		  Drug
		  Dosage
		  Administration
		  Side-effects
		  Warnings
		  Storage
		Support and encouragement to follow through and comply with drug therapy
			GI upset
			Liver function
			Renal function
			CNS effects
			CBC
			Ophthalmologic tests
			Eighth cranial nerve tests
			Folic acid levels
			Evaluate effectiveness of patient teaching
			Evaluate effectiveness of support and encouragement measures

Physical assessment
Neurologic: orientation, ophthalmologic tests, eighth cranial nerve tests
Cardiovascular: BP, P, baseline rhythm
Respiratory: rate, adventitious sounds
GI: bowel sounds, output, appetite, liver function
Renal: urinalysis, BUN, creatinine
Skin: color, lesions
Tests: CBC

Case Study

Presentation

HH is a student who has earned a fellowship that will allow him to travel to Haiti to work as a student nurse in the public health facilities over the summer. HH will be leaving in 4 weeks and expects to return just before his senior year begins in September. HH must receive malaria prophylaxis because Haiti is one of the islands in the Caribbean in which the disease is endemic. Describe drug treatment and information that HH should be given.

Discussion

The physician or nurse prescribing for HH, or for any traveler to an area in which malaria is endemic, must find out what species of *Plasmodium* causes malaria in the area to be visited and, if *P. falciparum* is a causative agent, whether chloroquine resistance has developed. In Haiti 100% of malaria cases are currently caused by *P. falciparum*, which has not developed resistance to chloroquine. Thus, chloroquine is the drug of choice for HH. Because *P. falciparum* does not have a persistent exoerythrocytic phase, it is unnecessary to add primaquine to the course of suppressive therapy with chloroquine.

The usual protocol would be the following: a single chloroquine tablet (300 mg chloroquine base) given 2 weeks before arriving in the malarial area, and the same dose repeated at weekly intervals thereafter, on the same day of the week, before, during, and for 8 weeks after the visit to the area in which malaria is endemic. Although this is a relatively simple protocol to follow, it is very easy for the patient to omit a dose or completely forget the regimen because it is repeated only once a week. It might be very helpful to prepare a calendar for the patient, plotting out the days the drug should be taken with a box to check as each dose is taken.

HH should be evaluated for renal and liver function and his CBC should be checked. A baseline ophthalmologic exam should be done and recorded, so that a follow-up exam can be done when HH returns. HH will also need teaching about the drug therapy and the importance of compliance to the regimen. HH should be taught to recognize warning signs of drug toxicity, which could be confused with the signs and symptoms of other infections that he might encounter in Haiti. A patient teaching guide should be attached to HH's drug calendar for easy reference. A follow-up visit, on return to this country, and before returning to classes, should be scheduled. At that time, an evaluation of the total patient situation can be performed before this student nurse begins patient care activities again.

Drug digests

Chloroquine phosphate USP (Aralen)*

Actions and indications. This chemical of the 4-aminoquinoline class of synthetic successors to quinine is the drug most widely used for *suppressive treatment* of malaria and for effecting the *clinical cure* of acute attacks. It acts as a schizonticide in the blood against the erythrocytic forms of the asexual stages in the life cycle of *Plasmodium vivax* and *P. falciparum*. In infections caused by susceptible strains of *P. falciparum*, it both terminates the acute attack and brings about a complete cure with no relapses. However, chloroquine does not keep patients with *P. vivax* and similar types of malaria from relapsing later, because it does not act against the secondary tissue (exoerythrocytic) forms of these plasmodia.

Adverse effects, cautions, and contraindications. Side-effects rarely occur with the small amount of chloroquine that is needed for suppressive effects. With the large loading dose given to initiate treatment of an acute attack, epigastric discomfort and headache may occur and, as additional doses are administered for aborting the attack, the patient may also complain of pruritus, blurring of vision as a result of disturbances of accommodation, and diarrhea. These adverse effects pass quickly once the treatment of the malarial attack is completed. Hemolysis may occur in persons with glucose-6-phosphate dehydrogenase (G-6-PD) deficiency. American blacks and persons of Mediterranean ancestry are especially at risk, and their G-6-PD levels should be determined prior to therapy.

Much more serious toxicity may occur during the prolonged employment of chloroquine for treating such chronic diseases as rheumatoid arthritis and discoid lupus erythematosus. These include possible blindness as a result of irreversible retinal damage, blood dyscrasias, and lichenoid skin eruptions. The drug is contraindicated in patients with evidence of visual field or retinal changes. It is used with caution in patients with liver disease. It is discontinued if muscle weakness develops. Overdosage in children and massive ingestion by suicidal patients has resulted in cardiac arrest, circulatory collapse, convulsions, and death. Thus, this drug must be stored where it cannot be reached by children or depressed patients.

Dosage and administration. A single once-weekly oral dose of 500 mg chloroquine phosphate (or 300 mg chloroquine base) is adequate for suppressive therapy. It is administered from 2 weeks before to 8 weeks after the person is in the malarious region. For *clinical cure* of an acute malarial attack, an initial dose of 1 g chloroquine phosphate is followed by 500 mg in 6 hours and by additional doses of 500 mg on the second and third treatment days. These may be given with meals to allay gastric distress.

In *extraintestinal (hepatic) amebiasis* with liver abscess, 1 g is given daily for 2 days and then 250 mg is administered twice a day for at least 2 or 3 weeks.

In *dyscoid lupus erythematosus*, 250 mg is taken orally twice daily for 3 weeks and then followed by maintenance doses of 250 mg daily. *Rheumatoid arthritis* requires prolonged daily oral doses of 250 mg.

Primaquine phosphate USP

Actions and indications. This drug is used for producing radical cure and thus for preventing relapses in malaria. It acts to eradicate the exoerythrocytic (secondary tissue) forms of the plasmodial parasites. However, it does *not* act against an acute attack. It is always administered together with a blood schizonticide, such as chloroquine.

Adverse effects, cautions, and contraindications. Ordinary doses of primaquine cause few side-effects in most people. Complaints are limited to occasional abdominal distress, headache, itching, and blurred vision. Much more serious is the possibility of a hemolytic reaction in a hypersensitive person. Blacks and other darkly pigmented people with a genetic enzyme deficiency are most prone to develop hemolytic anemia. The drug is discontinued if darkening of the urine develops or if the level of hemoglobin, red blood cells, and leukocytes drops. Quinacrine potentiates the toxicity of primaquine, and neither drug should be given with or shortly after the other.

Dosage and administration. A tablet containing 26.3 mg of this phosphate salt—the equivalent of 15 mg of primaquine base—is taken by mouth once daily for 14 days together with chloroquine to produce a radical cure. For prophylaxis, a tablet containing 79 mg—equal to 45 mg of the base—in combination with 300 mg of chloroquine is taken once weekly beginning before entering the area in which malaria is endemic, and continuing for 8 weeks after leaving the area.

---

* Another salt, the hydrochloride (USP), is employed for *parenteral* administration in IM doses not exceeding 800 mg base daily. It should be used only in patients who are vomiting or otherwise unable to take the oral drug.

Pyrimethamine USP (Daraprim)

Actions and indications. This antimalarial drug is effective against several stages of plasmodia species. In practice, however, it is used mainly for suppressive treatment. Its action against blood-borne schizonts is too slow in onset for the drug to be useful in treating acute attacks. It may be administered in combination with other drugs in such cases to control the sexual forms of the parasite responsible for transmission of malaria. Pyrimethamine may also be administered together with sulfonamides for treating chloroquine-resistant cases of *P. falciparum* malaria and for control of *Toxoplasma gondii*, the organism that causes toxoplasmosis.

Adverse effects, cautions, and contraindications. The small doses administered once weekly for malaria suppression produce no side-effects. However, the high doses required in toxoplasmosis may cause signs of folic acid deficiency to develop. Thus, blood counts are carried out, and the drug is discontinued if a drop in white blood cells or platelets is noted. Megaloblastic anemia and pancytopenia may also develop during treatment with large doses.
Anorexia, nausea and vomiting, and inflammation of the tongue (glossitis) may also oc-cur with large doses. Massive overdosage may result in signs of CNS stimulation including convulsions.

Dosage and administration. For malaria prophylaxis, an oral dose of 25 mg is taken once weekly. For transmission control 25 mg to 50 mg is taken for 2 days together with a faster acting agent that controls the blood forms responsible for the acute attack. In toxoplasmosis 50 mg to 75 mg is administered daily for 1 to 3 weeks together with a sulfonamide drug. Treatment may then be continued for several more weeks at about half of this dose.

Quinine sulfate USP and quinine dihydrochloride USP

Actions and indications. These salts of the main alkaloid of cinchona bark are rarely used today for treating ordinary cases of malaria. However, quinine may be lifesaving in some *Plasmodium falciparum* infections caused by strains of this species that are resistant to treatment with chloroquine and the other blood schizonticides that are considered safer and more effective in most cases. It is given with pyrimethamine and sulfadiazine or tetracycline in these cases.
Quinine possesses analgesic–antipyretic properties and has sometimes been used as a substitute for salicylates in the relief of headache, fever, and general malaise. Quinine is often useful for relief of nocturnal skeletal muscle cramps and for relief of mus-cle spasms in the rare condition myotonia congenita.

Adverse effects, cautions, and contraindications. Repeated doses or overdosage is marked by cinchonism, a syndrome similar to that seen when salicylate dosage is pushed to high levels. Ringing in the ears, blurring of vision, nausea, and headache may be followed by further digestive disturbances, impairment of hearing and sight, and confusion and delirium. Death may follow cardiac arrhythmias, collapse, convulsions, and coma when massive amounts are taken in misguided attempts to produce an abortion. Quinine has cardiac effects similar to those of quinidine. Like quinidine, it may increase plasma levels of digoxin and digitoxin. It may potentiate neuromuscular junction blocking drugs (succinylcholine), and may interfere with the synthesis of prothrombin, thereby potentiating oral coumarin-type anticoagulants. It can cause hemolysis in G-6-PD-deficient persons.

Dosage and administration. For treating an acute malarial attack, 1 g is administered daily for 2 days and followed by 600 mg for the following 2 days. Although the oral route is preferred, the dihydrochloride salt may be given by IV drip to patients severely ill with *P. falciparum* malaria affecting the brain. The dihydrochloride is available in the United States only from the Centers for Disease Control in Atlanta.

References

Black RH: The prevention and treatment of malaria. Med J Aust 1:929, 1977

Drugs for parasitic infections. Med Lett Drugs Ther 26:27–34, 1984

Dutz W et al: Therapy and prophylaxis of *Pneumocystis carinii* pneumonia. Natl Cancer Inst Monogr 43:201, 1976

Editorial: Chemoprophylaxis of malaria. Br Med J 2:1215, 1976

Hall AP: The treatment of malaria. Br Med J 1:323, 1976

Lipson A: Treatment of *Pneumocystis carinii* pneumonia in children. Arch Dis Child 52:314, 1977

Lyster A: Nursing care study: Malaria. Nursing Times 72:1796, 1976

Powell RD: Development of new antimalarial drugs. Am J Trop Med Hyg 21:744, 1972

Powell RD, Tiggert WD: Drug resistance of parasites causing human malaria. Ann Rev Med 19:81, 1968

Rollo IM: Drugs used in the chemotherapy of malaria. In Gilman AG, Goodman LS, Gilman A (eds): Goodman & Gilman's The Pharmacological Basis of Therapeutics, 6th ed, pp 1038–1060. New York, Macmillan, 1980

Rollo IM: Miscellaneous drugs used in the treatment of protozoal infections. In Gilman AG, Goodman LS, Gilman A (eds): Goodman & Gilman's The Pharmacological Basis of Therapeutics, 6th ed, p 1070–1079. New York, Macmillan, 1980

Rozman RS: Chemotherapy of malaria. Ann Rev Pharmacol 13:127, 1973

Thompson PE, Werbel LM: Antimalarial Agents: Chemistry and Pharmacology. New York, Academic Press, 1972

Tiggert WD, Clyde DF: Drug resistance in the human malarias. Antibiot Chemother 20:246, 1975

Williamson J: Chemotherapy of African trypanosomiasis. Trop Dis Bull 73:531, 1976

World Health Organization: Chemotherapy of malaria and resistance to antimalarials. WHO Tech Rep No. 529, 1973

The chemotherapy of amebiasis, helminthiasis, and other parasitic infections

11

This chapter, like the previous one, deals with the drug treatment of parasitic diseases. Here, however, the protozoan organisms responsible for infection are transmitted not by insects but mainly by ingestion of contaminated food and water. In addition, unlike the case in malaria, trypanosomiasis, and leishmaniasis, the protozoans that cause *amebiasis* and *giardiasis* exert their ill effects mainly in the intestinal tract. This chapter will also discuss the drug treatment of diseases caused by worms within the human intestinal tract—intestinal *helminthiasis*—and the treatment of diseases in which adult worms or the larvae and eggs of worms make their way to tissues outside the intestine—for example, *filariasis* and *schistosomiasis*.

Protozoan infections

Amebiasis

Amebiasis is an infection with the protozoan organism *Entamoeba histolytica*. More than 10% of the world's people are said to be infected. The disease is endemic mainly in the tropics, where close to half the people in some countries have been found to have this parasite in their stools. However, amebic infection is not limited to the tropics and can occur wherever poor sanitary conditions exist. Between 2% and 5% of Americans are estimated to be infected. Some are people who have picked up the organism while traveling abroad, but the condition is most common in institutions for mentally retarded children and the elderly in which the disease is sometimes spread by direct contact with fecal matter containing the parasite.

Several types of effective drugs are now available for treating amebiasis. The choice of a drug depends mainly on what stage the disease is in when it is detected. This, in turn, depends largely on which of two forms of the parasite is predominant within the patient. Thus, to understand how the various antiamebic drugs are best

employed in the management of amebiasis and the reasons for the usefulness and the limitations of each type of drug, it is necessary to understand the several ways in which amebiasis manifests itself clinically and to understand several significant points about the life cycle of *E. histolytica*.

Amebic disease states

Most of the millions of people who harbor *E. histolytica* in their intestines show no significant clinical symptoms. However, as long as the pathogen exists in the lumen of the large intestine, it can invade the mucosa of the colon at any time. The resulting irritation and ulcerative lesions may lead to mild chronic abdominal complaints or to the sudden onset of severe dysentery. The amebae may also make their way out of the bowel into the bloodstream and then invade other tissues, including the liver, lungs, heart, and brain. They can, for example, cause liver abscesses that lead to death in up to 10% of people who do not get proper treatment.

Asymptomatic carriers of amebae may spread the infection to other people who may not be so resistant to the organisms. In addition, a carrier who has never complained of intestinal symptoms may, in time, develop extraintestinal amebiasis marked by abscesses in the liver, lungs, or brain. Thus, all people who are found to be passing *E. histolytica* in either of its life cycle forms must be treated to eradicate the amebae from the intestine.

Intestinal amebiasis most commonly becomes symptomatic between 1 and 6 months after the person has become infected by ingesting the parasite. If the organisms cause only a few localized lesions in the colonic mucosa, the patient may complain only of flatulence, abdominal cramps or pain, occasional loose stools, or isolated episodes of diarrhea, and may never experience an acute dysenteric attack marked by continued bloody diarrhea, vomiting, fever, and dehydration.

However, even mild amebiasis that becomes chronic can result in widespread ulcerations and scarring of the intestinal mucosa. Amebic colitis of this type causes an irritable bowel syndrome that may sometimes persist and cause periodic acute flare-ups of diarrhea, even after the amebae have been eliminated by late treatment with antiamebic drugs.

Amebic hepatitis and liver abscess is a common complication of invasive intestinal disease. It occurs when amebae make their way into blood vessels in the intestinal wall and are carried to the liver by way of the portal vein. There, they destroy liver cells and produce abscesses made up of liquefied necrotic tissue.

Usually these lesions remain localized, but sometimes they break through the diaphragm in both directions to cause peritonitis or lung abscesses and empyema. Occasionally, amebae are carried from the lungs to the heart, where they can cause a dangerous pericarditis. Amebae that enter the central nervous system can cause fatal brain abscess.

Life cycle of the ameba

Entamoeba histolytica has a two-stage life cycle: (1) a *cystic* stage, in which the organism can live for long periods outside the body, as well as within the human intestine; and (2) a *trophozoite* stage, which occurs only when certain environmental requirements are met in the lower bowel of humans (Fig. 11-1).

The *cystic stage* is the one in which this microorganism is transmitted from one person to another. This form is very resistant to adverse environmental conditions. Passed in the formed feces of infected persons, the cysts can survive outside the body for several weeks, enduring drying, freezing, chemicals, and high heat. Water containing amebic cysts requires prolonged boiling before it is safe for drinking. Contact with the ordinary concentrations of chlorine employed in water purification does not destroy the cysts.

The amebic cysts are transmitted from person to person by ingestion of contaminated food and drink. Flies moving from feces to food are a common source of contamination, as are the fingers of food handlers. These workers, who are themselves often free of intestinal symptoms, can spread the cysts if they do not wash their hands thoroughly after going to the toilet. The swallowed cysts then pass through the stomach unaffected by acid gastric juices.

When the amebic cysts reach the lower level of the small intestine, some of them become activated by digestive juices in the ileum. These amebae break out of their cystic shells and divide to produce tiny daughter cells, called trophozoites. Other cysts never do excyst in this way and pass out of the infected person's intestine unchanged. These, of course, can then continue the transmission chain described above.

The *trophozoite stage* is that in which the amebae feed, multiply, and move about. These motile amebae may stay on the inner surface of the lower intestine without invading it. They may then be carried down toward the terminal end of the bowel where they again become encysted to survive when eliminated from the body during defecation. On the other hand, when they find conditions favorable in the cecal, sigmoid, or rectal portions of the lower intestine, the trophozoites release a substance that digests mucosal cells.

This lets them break through the mucosa to form what are at first only superficial erosions. Later, they may penetrate deep into the muscular wall of the intestine to cause multiple ulcerations. Finally, they may digest their way into mesenteric veins and be carried from these blood vessels to the portal circulation of the liver. Thus, it is the trophozoite form that accounts for both the intestinal and extraintestinal symptoms of amebiasis described above.

Chemotherapy

Treatment of the various clinical stages of amebiasis differs, and dissimilar drug regimens are often preferred in different parts of the world. It is therefore difficult to indicate specific treatment schedules for each stage of amebiasis that all authorities agree to be best (see Fig. 11-1). Nevertheless, certain principles of amebiasis chemotherapy are well established, and these will be emphasized in the following discussion of the management of amebic infections of different types and degrees of severity. Most therapeutic regimens for managing amebiasis use combinations of chemotherapeutic agents to strike at the pathogenic organism in both intestinal and extraintestinal sites (Table 11-1).

Some drugs are poorly absorbed when taken orally. Thus, they reach effective chemotherapeutic concentrations in the large intestine but not in extraintestinal tissues. These drugs are useful only for treating the intestinal forms of the disease. Other drugs are absorbed almost completely from the upper part of the intestine. These reach effective concentrations in extraintestinal tissues but not in the lower parts of the intestinal tract.

Metronidazole[+] (Flagyl), a drug that was introduced originally for treating another protozoal infection, *Trichomonas vaginalis* (see below) has been found to possess properties that make it effective for treating *both* intestinal and extraintestinal amebiasis. Taken by mouth, this drug is rapidly absorbed from the small intestine in amounts that reach amebicidal concentrations in the liver and in all other tissues. Enough of the unabsorbed drug reaches the lower bowel, however, to wipe out the trophozoites responsible for intestinal wall damage and the resulting diarrhea and other intestinal symptoms. The availability of this relatively safe drug has made the management of all the stages of amebic infection discussed below easier than ever before.

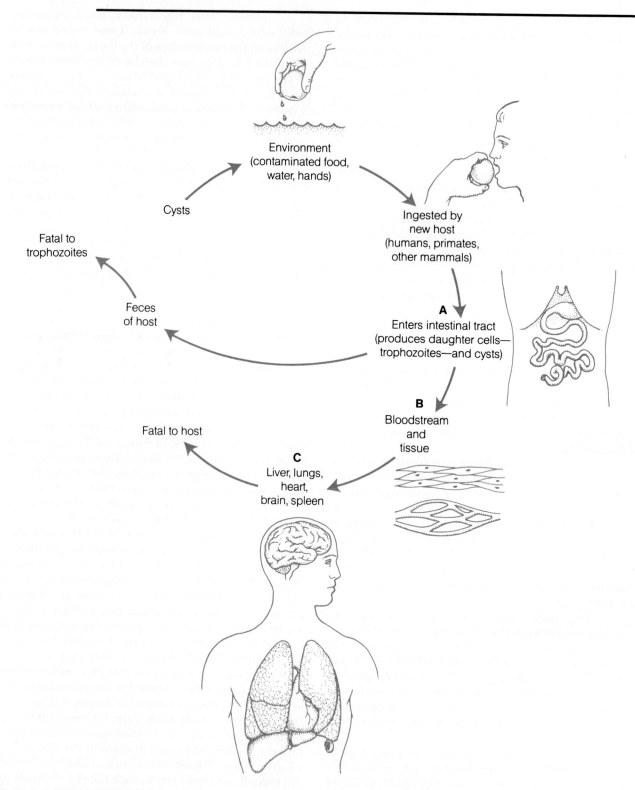

Figure 11-1. Life cycle of *Entamoeba histolytica* and sites of action of some drugs used to treat amebiasis. (*A*) Active site of metronidazole, emetine, and paromomycin. (*B*) Active site of metronidazole, emetine, and chloroquine. (*C*) Active site of metronidazole, emetine, and paromomycin.

Table 11–1. Drugs for treating amebiasis

Generic or official name	Trade name	Adult dosage and administration	Comments
Carbarsone		250 mg orally bid or tid for 10 days	Organic arsenical not now commonly used as an intestinal amebicide (see Drug Digest)
Chloroquine phosphate USP	Aralen Phosphate	250 mg orally qid. for 2 days; then 250 mg bid. for 2 wk*	Antimalarial drug (see Drug Digest, Chap. 10); concentrates in the liver and is effective for prevention and treatment of hepatic amebiasis and liver abscess
Chloroquine HCl	Aralen HCl	200–250 mg by injection every day for 10–12 days*	
Dehydroemetine	Mebadin	1–1.5 mg/kg body weight daily for 5 days, at most, IM	An analogue of emetine sometimes used as an alternative in treating acute amebic dysentery and amebic hepatitis and abscess; available in the United States only from the CDC
Diiodohydroxyquin USP; iodoquinol	Moebiquin; Yodoxin	650 mg tid for a 20-day course in treating intestinal amebiasis	An iodinated hydroxyquinoline for intestinal amebiasis (see Drug Digest)
Diloxanide furoate	Furamide	500 mg orally tid for 10 days	An acetanilid derivative safe enough for routine use in asymptomatic carriers; also often effective in symptomatic intestinal amebiasis; available in the United States only from the CDC
Emetine HCl USP		30–60 mg daily for 10 days as a deep SC or IM injection	Ipecac alkaloid employed for rapid action in severe amebic dysentery and hepatic amebiasis (see Drug Digest)
Furazolidone	Furoxone	100 mg qid orally for 7 days	Nonabsorbable drug used only for GI infections (bacterial and giardial)
Metronidazole USP	Flagyl; Metryl; Protostat; Satric	750 mg orally tid for 5–10 days in intestinal amebiasis and for amebic liver abscess	Very useful for both intestinal and extraintestinal forms of amebiasis; also used for giardiasis and *Trichomonas vaginalis* (see Drug Digest)
Paromomycin sulfate USP	Humatin	25–35 mg/kg body weight/day orally in three divided doses with meals for 1 wk	A direct-acting antibiotic effective for mild or severe, acute or chronic intestinal amebiasis (see Drug Digest)†

* Doses are expressed in terms of the salt, not the base. 1 g chloroquine phosphate = 600 mg base; 250 mg chloroquine HCl = 200 mg base.
† This antibiotic acts directly on amebae as well as on bacteria; other antibiotics employed in intestinal amebiasis, such as the tetracyclines and erythromycin (see Chap. 8), are not directly amebicidal but act instead to alter the composition of the bacterial flora of the intestine and so interfere with the nutrition of the amebae indirectly.

Asymptomatic amebiasis and mild amebic colitis. Asymptomatic carriers and mild chronic cases with only occasional flare-ups of intestinal symptoms are best treated with agents that are relatively free of side-effects. After a person has been found to be an asymptomatic cyst passer, it is often difficult to convince this carrier to receive drug treatment. Obviously, he will be quick to discontinue any drug that causes more discomforting side-effects than the symptomless disorder he is told that he has.

The nurse can play an important role in encouraging carriers to continue with drug therapy. The benefits to the person should be stressed, together with the need to protect family and coworkers. The nurse employed in industry, schools, and other institutions should teach the necessity for thorough handwashing and recommend that all washrooms—especially those used by food handlers—be equipped with plenty of soap and towels.

The drugs traditionally employed in the management of asymptomatic carriers and people with only mild intestinal symptoms are of two main types: (1) the halogenated hydroxyquinoline compound *diiodohydroxyquin*[+] (Diodoquin); and (2) the organic arsenicals, including the phenylarsonic acid derivative *carbarsone*[+], which is now rarely used. Both drug classes cause relatively few discomforting side-effects and, until recently, reports of serious systemic toxicity were rare.

Although these drugs are still used today for treating patients in these stages of amebiasis, the current trend seems to be toward the use of newer antiamebic agents such as *metronidazole, diloxanide furoate,* and the antibiotic *paromomycin*[+] (Humatin). One reason for this is the publication of reports of alarming toxic reactions to the older drugs in occasional cases (see below, and in the Drug Digests).

Another drawback of the older drugs in comparison to metronidazole is the fact that, because they are poorly absorbed, their antiamebic action is limited to trophozoites in the intestinal tract. Thus, to avoid the possible development of amebic hepatitis caused by amebae that may have migrated to the liver, even in people who have shown no symptoms or only occasional mild diarrhea, it is necessary to administer the absorbable amebicide chloroquine (see Chap. 10) when patients are treated with courses of diiodohydroxyquin or carbarsone.

Metronidazole treatment of mild chronic amebiasis does not require such concurrent chloroquine prophylaxis, because it is effective against amebic trophozoites that have reached the liver as well as against those in the intestine. Although some authorities do not think that metronidazole is as reliable as diiodohydroxyquin, diloxanide furoate, or paromomycin for this purpose, others feel that a full course of this drug is as effective as the others. These experts have also suggested that metronidazole should be employed for mass prophylaxis of the population in countries in which amebiasis is endemic, and in mental institutions in this country that have a high incidence of this disease.

In view of the results of studies that have revealed metronidazole's capacity to produce cancerous tumors in experimental animals, its routine use for mass and individual prophylaxis against amebiasis is probably undesirable. An example of the possible risks involved is seen in the recent experience with iodochlorhydroxyquin (Entero-Vioform), a halogenated hydroxyquinoline compound, that was used to treat intestinal amebiasis and was often taken routinely by travelers to treat or prevent "travelers' diarrhea." It was found to cause a disorder called subacute myelo-opticoneuropathy in some people; this drug-induced disease sometimes resulted in blindness. The drug is no longer available in the United States.

The related drug, diiodohydroxyquin, has also caused optic neuritis when used for long periods. It should not be used to treat diarrhea of a nonspecific nature, because the risks of taking the drug routinely outweigh its doubtful benefits. Asymptomatic carriers or patients taking this drug for relief of intestinal amebiasis symptoms should be heeded, and the drug should be withdrawn, if they complain of blurring of vision, because this may be an early sign of optic nerve inflammation and atrophy.

Severe amebic colitis and acute amebic dysentery. Metronidazole is the drug now considered best for control of diarrhea and other colitis symptoms caused by more extensive amebic invasion of the intestinal wall, with resulting deep lesions and ulcerations. As indicated previously, this drug also eradicates any amebae that may have already reached the liver and other extraintestinal sites. In this respect metronidazole is more useful than the nonabsorbable antiamebic drugs that act only in the intestine, such as diiodohydroxyquin, diloxanide furoate, and carbarsone.

Tetracyclines. When patients cannot take metronidazole for any reason, tetracycline or the related antibiotic oxytetracycline (combined with chloroquine for its amebicidal activity at extraintestinal sites) offer an alternative treatment regimen. The tetracyclines do not attack amebae directly, unlike the antibiotic paromomycin, which is a direct-acting amebicide. Instead, these broad-spectrum antibacterial drugs act to affect the amebae indirectly through their ability to alter the bacterial flora of the intestine. (The relationships between bacterial organisms and pathogenic protozoa in the bowel are not well understood, but colonic bacteria seem to play a part in providing the nutrition necessary for survival of the amebae.)

The antibacterial action of the tetracyclines temporarily reduces the numbers of invading amebae, and it is also useful for controlling the secondary bacterial infections that increase the susceptibility of the intestinal wall to amebic invasion. However, the tetracyclines cannot be depended on to eliminate all intestinal amebae permanently, and patients may thus relapse within weeks or months. To prevent this, tetracycline treatment must be followed by a course of treatment with a direct-acting intestinal amebicide such as diiodohydroxyquin.

Emetine therapy. The more rapid-acting amebicides *emetine*[+] and *dehydroemetine* are reserved for patients with severe dysentery who require quicker relief than oral metronidazole or tetracyclines can offer, those whose severe dysentery does not respond to treatment with antibiotics or iodine and arsenical compounds, and those with extraintestinal infections (see below). These drugs, which are injected and carried by the bloodstream to both the intestinal wall and the extraintestinal tissues, are very effective against trophozoites. They give quick relief of such acute symptoms as bloody diarrhea, colicky abdominal pain from intestinal spasm, and tenesmus (involuntary straining and anal sphincter spasm). However, emetine and its derivative are very toxic drugs that can cause severe heart damage and aching pain at the injection sites. (The application of ice to the injection site can help to alleviate this pain. Sites should be rotated to prevent tissue damage.) Thus, patients being treated with emetine are hospitalized, placed on cardiac monitors, and kept at rest in bed.

Close monitoring of cardiovascular function is essential during the course of the emetine therapy. Regular monitoring of vital signs, including cardiac auscultation to detect early signs of congestive heart failure (*e.g.*, development of a third heart sound, S_3), will help to alert the nurse or physician to beginning toxicity. Tachycardia, falling blood pressure, precordial pain, dyspnea, and electrocardiographic changes (inverted T waves, prolonged P–R interval, widening QRS), are all indications that the drug should be discontinued.

Many of the cardiac changes can occur weeks after the emetine has been discontinued. Because of this, the patient needs extensive teaching about the signs and symptoms of cardiac problems. The patient should be urged to try to limit activities. Spacing of activities to avoid any prolonged cardiac stress should be explained. Helping the patient to talk through the usual day while activities are recorded and then spaced appropriately throughout the day may be the most effective way of teaching this idea. Frequent rest periods should be encouraged. The patient should be firmly taught that any activity he is involved in should be stopped if fatigue, shortness of breath, or chest pain is experienced. If any of these occur, the patient should notify the nurse or physician immediately.

Because of the dangerous toxic effects of this drug, it should not be used in patients with known cardiac or renal disease, and should be used with extreme caution in elderly or debilitated patients in whom the risk of toxicity is even greater.

Although emetine is very effective for rapidly eradicating the trophozoites, it does not kill the amebic cysts. Thus, when the symptoms of severe amebic dysentery are controlled and emetine or dehydroemetine is discontinued, the surviving cysts will once more begin to produce invasive trophozoites. To cure the infection completely emetine must be supplemented by a concurrent course of diiodohydroxyquin and tetracycline, or by metronidazole.

Amebic hepatitis and liver abscess. As in the other clinical amebiasis states discussed above, metronidazole alone can control most cases in which amebae have reached the liver and caused hepatitis or abscesses. Administered in safe oral doses, enough of this drug is ab-

sorbed to reach chemotherapeutically effective levels in infected liver tissue. It does not have to be supplemented by amebicides that act only in the intestinal lumen, because enough of the unabsorbed drug reaches the colon to eradicate the amebae in the intestine. Because it is safer than emetine, dehydroemetine, and chloroquine, and does not have to be followed by a course of treatment with an intestinal amebicide, metronidazole is now considered the drug of choice, and emetine alone or combined with chloroquine is used only as an alternative when metronidazole cannot be employed.

Most cases of amebic hepatitis respond to treatment with metronidazole, emetine, or chloroquine. However, patients who do not improve after 5 days of chemotherapy may require other treatment measures. Aspiration of liver abscesses is employed in such cases and when an abscess seems about to rupture. If the abscess tends to keep refilling despite continued chemotherapy and repeated drainage through surface punctures, it may be necessary to perform a laparotomy and surgical drainage. Although amebic lung lesions respond to treatment with amebicidal drugs, surgery is usually required for amebic brain abscesses.

Giardiasis

Another parasitic protozoan, *Giardia lamblia*, has been recognized as the cause of an intestinal infection that frequently disables travelers during a trip abroad or after their return. The feces of a carrier are full of cysts, the form of the organism that transmits the infection by way of contaminated food or water that does not contain enough chlorine to kill them. After ingestion, the pear-shaped flagellated trophozoite excysts and lives in the upper small intestine, where its presence may produce no symptoms at all or set off symptoms about 1 to 3 weeks after infection.

Parasites that invade the duodenal or jejunal mucosa can cause diarrhea that may last for weeks or months. The stool often has a foul, rotten egg odor and may contain mucus but not blood. It may be pale because of unabsorbed fat, and malabsorption of carbohydrate, folic acid, and vitamin B_{12} may also occur, with resulting weight loss and debility. The patient sometimes suffers epigastric distress that may make the physician suspect the presence of peptic ulcer or a gallbladder disorder.

Once the condition is diagnosed by detecting cysts in stool smears or trophozoites in duodenal aspirates, it should be treated by chemotherapy whether or not the patient complains of any symptoms. *Quinacrine*[+] (Atabrine) and *metronidazole* (Flagyl) appear to be equally effective. About 80% of patients respond to treatment with a single course of either drug. Most of the remainder respond to a second course of the same drug or to treatment with the other one. Metronidazole causes fewer side-effects than quinacrine, which has a bitter taste that may cause vomiting. Quinacrine also sometimes discolors the skin and sets off skin reactions. It can also cause central nervous system signs and symptoms including headache, dizziness, and occasionally a toxic psychosis.

Furazolidone (Furoxone), a nonabsorbable drug given orally as tablets or a suspension, is also sometimes used to treat giardial and bacterial diarrhea and enteritis. It has caused orthostatic hypotension, hypoglycemia, and serious allergic reactions. Like metronidazole, it may produce a disulfiram (Antabuse)-like reaction if the patient ingests alcohol (see Chap. 53).

Trichomoniasis

Another flagellated protozoan, *Trichomonas vaginalis*, is a common cause of vaginitis. The infection, which is usually acquired during sexual intercourse, may cause no symptoms. (Most infected men are asymptomatic carriers, and only a few develop trichomonal urethritis.) The organism causes reddening of the inflamed vaginal mucosa with itching or burning and a yellowish green discharge.

Metronidazole (Flagyl) administered orally is effective in most cases when taken in a week-long course or by various other regimens that may be repeated after a month or more if follow-up reveals the presence of the organism in vaginal secretions. Both sexual partners should be treated to prevent reinfection. Metronidazole is no longer available in the form of a vaginal insert, but other types of local therapy may be employed in the small minority of cases that do not respond to treatment with oral doses of this drug. The experimental drugs *carnidazole, flunidazole, ornidazole*, and *trinidazole* are also said to be effective for treating *T. vaginalis*.

Additional clinical considerations

One of the key points in the use of chemotherapy against these protozoa is the goal of complete eradication of the infecting organisms. The patient will need to understand the importance of completing the full course of the prescription. Prophylactic measures should also be taken to prevent reinfection, including sanitation measures, personal hygiene measures—especially hand washing—and avoidance of sexual intercourse (with trichomoniasis infection) until the medication is completed. In some areas, large outbreaks of these infections necessitate a Public Health review to find the source of the protozoa.

Gastrointestinal upsets are common with all these drugs. The patient can take the medication with food to eliminate some of this discomfort. If the GI problems become severe, however, the patient should be reevaluated. There is also a risk of various superinfections with most of these drugs, and the patient should be aware of the possibility. One unpleasant problem has been reported with the use of metronidazole. An oral fungus infection often develops in susceptible people and presents as a furry white growth on the tongue. If this occurs, the patient will need support and reassurances that this will go away when the drug is stopped. None of these drugs has been shown to be safe for use during pregnancy or lactation. They should be avoided during these times, unless the benefit they might bring to the patient outweighs the dangerous risks.

Drug–drug and drug–laboratory test interactions. *Paromomycin* has been associated with ototoxicity and renal damage. Patients on this drug need to be alert for ringing in the ears, vertigo, or difficulty maintaining balance. This drug should not be given concurrently with other *ototoxic* or *nephrotoxic* drugs. *Iodoquinol* interferes with the body's normal use of iodine and may produce false results if *thyroid function tests* are done; this drug may also cause problems with patients on *thyroid replacement therapy*. Patients on *furazolidone* need to avoid *MAO inhibitors, sympathomimetic amines*, and foods containing *tyramine*, because these substances have caused hypertensive crises in these patients. The patient teaching guide and guide to the nursing process summarize the application of the nursing process to this oral drug therapy. *Emetine*, used parenterally, is a very toxic drug that has been previously discussed.

Summary of the adverse effects of drugs used in amebiasis

Carbarsone (see Drug digest)
Nausea, vomiting, epigastric distress, diarrhea

Pruritic skin eruptions (rarely, arsenical exfoliation)

Visual disturbances (contractions of visual field and color changes)

Rare arsenical encephalopathy (mental changes, coma, convulsions)

Rare liver function changes, with possible damage and necrosis

Chloroquine
Loss of appetite, abdominal distress and cramps, nausea and vomiting

Headache, restlessness, sleeplessness

Skin eruptions

Visual disturbances (blurring of vision)

Diiodohydroxyquin (see Drug digest)
Flatulence, abdominal distress, nausea and vomiting

Headache, dizziness

Skin eruptions and pruritus ani

Iodism and interference with tests of thyroid function

Rarely, peripheral neuropathy, including optic neuritis and atrophy; also, spinal cord demyelination

(continued)

Emetine (see Drug digest) and Dehydroemetine
  Cardiotoxicity: chest pains, tachycardia, electro-
      cardiographic changes (T-wave abnormal-
      ities; prolonged Q–T interval)
  Hypotension, dyspnea
  Nausea, vomiting, diarrhea, epigastric distress
  Muscular weakness, aching, and stiffness, espe-
      cially in the region of deep subcutaneous
      injections
  Headache, dizziness, faintness
  Skin eruptions

Metronidazole (see Drug digest)
  Unpleasant metallic taste, loss of appetite, nausea
      and vomiting, epigastric distress, abdominal
      cramps, diarrhea; disulfiramlike interaction
      with alcohol

Paromomycin (see Drug digest)
  Nausea, diarrhea
  Headache and vertigo, skin rash
  Possible superinfections caused by *Candida* and
      Staphylococcus
  Potentially nephrotoxic

Patient teaching guide: oral antiprotozoal drugs

The drug that has been prescribed for you belongs to the class of drugs called anti-
infectives. This drug acts to destroy certain protozoa that have invaded the body.
It acts at specific phases of the protozoan life cycle, and must be taken over a period
of time to be effective. It is very important to take all the drug that has been
prescribed for you. The drug has been prescribed to treat ———————— .

Instructions:

1. The name of your drug is ———————— .

2. The dosage of the drug prescribed for you is ——————— .

3. The drug should be taken ————— times a day. The best time to take
    your drug is ——————— , ——————— , ——————— .

4. This drug frequently causes stomach upset. If it causes you to have nausea,
    heartburn, or vomiting, it is helpful to take the drug with meals or a light
    snack.

5. Some side-effects of the drug that you should be aware of include the
    following:

Nausea, vomiting, loss of appetite	Take drug with meals; have frequent small meals.
Superinfections: mouth, vagina, skin	These will go away when the course of the drug is finished. If they become uncomfortable, notify your nurse or physician for treatment.
Dry mouth; strange metallic taste (metronidazole)	Frequent mouth care and sucking on sugarless candies may help; it will go away when the drug is stopped.
Intolerance to alcohol: nausea vomiting, flushing, headache, stomach pain (metronidazole, furazolidone)	The use of alcoholic beverages or preparations containing alcohol (*e.g.,* cough syrups, elixirs) should be avoided while you are on this drug.

(continued)

6. Tell any physician, nurse, or dentist who is taking care of you that you are on this drug.

7. Keep this and all medications out of the reach of children.

8. Take the full course of your prescription. Never use this medication to self-treat any other infection or give this medication to any other person.

Notify your nurse or physician at once if any of the following occur:

> Sore throat, fever, chills
> Ringing in the ears (paromomycin)
> Blurring vision (iodoquinol)
> Skin rash, redness
> Severe GI upset
> Unusual fatigue, clumsiness,
>   weakness

Guide to the nursing process: oral antiprotozoal drugs

Assessment	Nursing diagnoses	Interventions	Evaluation
Past history—underlying medical conditions (*contraindications*): Renal failure Hepatic failure Pregnancy Lactation *Allergies:* these drugs, reactions; others Medication history: current drugs (*Cautions:* ototoxic drugs; nephrotoxic drugs; MAO inhibitors; tyramine; sympathomimetic amines; alcohol) **Physical assessment** Neurologic: Reflexes; eighth cranial nerve; ophthalmologic screening Respiratory: rate; adventitious sounds	Potential alteration in comfort (GI, superinfections) Potential alteration in nutrition (GI problems) Potential alteration in sensory perception (eye changes, eighth cranial nerve changes) Knowledge deficit regarding drug therapy	Culture area involved Safe and appropriate preparation and administration of drug Comfort measures: Oral hygiene Small frequent meals Drug with food Safety precautions Proper treatment of superinfections Maintain nutrition Patient teaching regarding: Drug Dosage Administration Comfort measures Warnings Hygiene Support and encouragement to comply with therapy	Evaluate effectiveness of drug: resolution of infection Evaluate for adverse effects: Liver function GI problems Neurologic changes Superinfections Evaluate effectiveness of patient teaching Evaluate effectiveness of support measures: compliance Evaluate effectiveness of comfort measures Evaluate for drug–drug interactions. ↑ toxicity of paromymycin with other *ototoxic, nephrotoxic* drugs Severe, ↑ BP with *furazolidone* and MAO inhibitors, *tyramine,*

(continued)

Assessment	Nursing diagnoses	Interventions	Evaluation
GI: liver function tests; bowel sounds; liver palpation Renal: BUN; urinalysis			*sympathomimetic amines* Severe reaction to *alcohol* with *furazolidone*, *metronidazole* Evaluate for drug–laboratory test interactions: Thyroid tests with *iodoquinol*

Case Study

Presentation

JC, a 22-year-old college student, reported to the university health service with complaints of severe diarrhea, abdominal pain and, most recently, blood in the stool. JC was found to have a mild fever and appeared to be dehydrated and very tired. JC denied travel out of the country. He reported eating most of his meals at the local beer spot where he worked in the kitchen each night making pizzas. A stool sample was examined for ova and parasites (O and P), and a diagnosis of amebiasis was made. JC was placed on metronidazole, and a public health referral was made to track down the source of his infection. The public health epidemiologist tracked the source of the infection to the kitchen of the beer–pizza restaurant where JC worked. The restaurant was shut down until all the food, utensils, and environment passed state public health inspection. Although a potential epidemic of amebiasis was averted by this discovery (only three cases were reported), it added a new stress for JC, who was unemployed for several months.

What are the appropriate nursing measures that should have been taken with JC?

Discussion

JC needed reassurance and an explanation of his disease. He was informed that oral hygiene and frequent small meals would help to alleviate some of his discomfort until the drug could control the amebiasis. Specific adverse drug effects to which JC was alerted included the possibility of an adverse response to alcohol (he was advised to avoid alcoholic beverages), a metallic taste in his mouth, GI upset, dizziness or lightheadedness, and superinfections. JC received follow-up evaluation of stools for O and P, and his general state of nutrition was followed. The drug therapy was continued until the amebiasis was eradicated. Because the adverse effects of this drug are somewhat unpleasant and difficult for a student to deal with, along with the other stresses in his life, JC received a great deal of support and encouragement. He was given a telephone number to call to reach a nurse, and a full set of written instructions to serve as a reference.

Drug digests: antiprotozoal drugs

Carbarsone

Actions and indications. This arsenical amebicide is active against both the tropho-zoite and cystic forms of *Entamoeba histolytica.* It is useful when administered in alternation with courses of diiodohydroxyquin in the treatment of mild to moderate diarrhea and other symptoms of acute and chronic intestinal amebiasis. It is *not* effective for *extra*intestinal amebiasis, including hepatic amebiasis.

This antiprotozoal agent is also used topically in treating vaginitis caused by *Trichomonas vaginalis.*

Adverse effects, cautions, and contraindications. This is a relatively safe arsenic compound. However, it may have cumulative toxic effects if taken in successive courses without long enough rest periods to permit its excretion. Toxicity is most common in patients with liver or kidney damage or sensitivity to arsenic, and the use of this drug is contraindicated in patients with such histories.

The most common side-effects include diarrhea, nausea and vomiting, and skin rashes. Patients are observed for signs of pruritic skin eruptions and visual changes, which may call for withdrawal of the drug to avoid possible development of exfoliative dermatitis and arsenical encephalitis.

Dosage and administration. This drug is administered orally, in adult doses of 250 mg bid or tid for 10 days. A rest period of at least 10 days should intervene between such courses of therapy. The total daily dosage for children is 7.5 mg/kg for 10 days.

Diiodohydroxyquin USP (Moebiquin; Yodoxin)

Actions and indications. This organic iodine compound has amebicidal and trichomonacidal properties. It is useful in intestinal amebiasis for the management of mild cases for eradicating cysts in asymptomatic carriers, and for prophylaxis in endemic areas. Although it is effective against trophozoites in the intestinal tract, it is *not* useful for *extra*intestinal infections, including amebic hepatitis and abscess. Topical application is useful for treating vaginal infection caused by *Trichomonas vaginalis.*

Adverse effects, cautions, and contraindications. This drug causes few systemic side-effects, because only relatively small amounts are absorbed from the gastrointestinal tract. Local gastrointestinal effects may cause epigastric distress and diarrhea.

The drug is contraindicated in patients sensitive to iodine and in those with severe liver disease. Symptoms of mild iodism, including pruritic skin rashes, may require discontinuation of therapy. This drug, like other iodides, may affect the accuracy of thyroid function tests.

Dosage and administration. Oral adult dosage for intestinal amebiasis is 650 mg tid for 20 days. This may be repeated after a rest period of 2 or 3 weeks, during which an arsenical compound such as carbarsone may be administered.

Emetine HCl USP

Actions and indications. This ipecac alkaloid kills the trophozoites, or motile forms, of *Entamoeba histolytica* in both the intestinal and extraintestinal tissues. These amebicidal effects make it useful both for treating amebic hepatitis and for controlling severe diarrhea in acute amebic dysentery. However, its routine use in mild cases of amebic dysentery or for treating asymptomatic carriers of amebic cysts is contraindicated because of its high potential cumulative toxicity and low level of effectiveness against the cyst form of the organism.

Adverse effects, cautions, and contraindi- **cations.** The toxic effects of emetine vary from relatively mild and transient—for example, increased diarrhea, nausea, and vomiting—to extremely severe and even fatal reactions. The most serious toxicity is the result of the drug's depressant effects on the myocardium. This may be marked by chest pains, tachycardia, and electrocardiographic (ECG) changes, as well as by hypotension and dyspnea in some cases. The drug is administered to patients with pre-existing heart or kidney disease only when the risk from extraintestinal amebiasis, unresponsive to any other therapy, seems warranted. It is also employed only with extreme caution in children and in elderly and disease-weakened patients.

Dosage and administration. Emetine is administered in doses of 1 mg/kg of body weight, but in a total dose not exceeding 60 mg daily, during a course of 5 to 10 days. Patients taking emetine are kept at rest in bed throughout the entire treatment period and are warned to avoid strenuous activity for some time after completion of the course of therapy. Rest periods of at least 6 weeks are required before further courses of emetine may be safely employed.

Metronidazole USP (Flagyl)

Actions and indications. This antiprotozoal agent is active against *Entamoeba histolytica, Giardia lamblia,* and *Trichomonas vaginalis,* the organisms responsible for amebiasis, giardiasis, and trichomoniasis in humans. It is indicated in both amebic dysentery caused by invasion of the intestinal mucosa and amebic liver abscess resulting from invasion of hepatic tissues by amebae.

When the presence of trichomonads has been confirmed by wet smears and cultures, this drug is indicated for relief of symptoms in men and women with trichomoniasis. It is also indicated for treating women with cervicitis, endocervicitis, or cervical erosion when the organism is found, even though they show no symptoms of trichomoniasis. Because this is a venereal disease, asymptomatic sexual partners should be treated at the same time as the patient to prevent later reinfection of the patient by the sexual partner.

Adverse effects, cautions, and contraindications. The most commonly reported side-effects are gastrointestinal and include anorexia, nausea and occasionally vomiting, gastric distress, abdominal cramps, or diarrhea. Some patients complain of a sharp, unpleasant metallic taste, and others have headaches. Overgrowths of yeastlike *Monilia* organisms in the mouth may cause stomatitis and glossitis with furry tongue. The same fungal organisms may be found in the vagina. Differential leukocyte counts to detect leukopenia are recommended, especially during second courses of treatment. Although no persistent blood abnormalities have been observed, use of this drug is contraindicated in patients with a blood dyscrasia. Similarly, although the drug has not been shown to be teratogenic, its use during the first trimester of pregnancy is not recommended.

Although the risk of carcinogenesis in humans is considered low, results of tests in animals indicating tumorigenic activity make it necessary to consider this drug potentially carcinogenic in humans. Thus, it is recommended that it should be used for treating trichomoniasis during the second and third trimesters of pregnancy only after local treatment measures have failed to control symptoms.

Patients receiving this drug should not drink alcoholic beverages, because they may suffer a disulfiram (Antabuse)-like reaction marked by nausea, vomiting, abdominal cramps, headache, and flushing. The drug, which has occasionally caused dizziness, vertigo, ataxia, and numbness or paresthesia of extremities, is contraindicated in patients with organic disease of the central nervous system.

Dosage and administration. For trichomoniasis in both women and men a single dose of 2 g may be taken, or two doses of 1 g each, taken the same day. Alternatively, the older regimen of one 250-mg tablet taken orally three times daily for 7 days may be used. A second course may be administered after a 4- to 6-week interval if laboratory tests show that the organism is still present. For adults with acute intestinal amebiasis, a dose of 750 mg is administered orally three times daily for 5 to 10 days; for amebic liver abscess, 500 mg to 750 mg is given orally three times daily for 5 to 10 days.

Children with these disorders receive a total 24-hour dosage of 35 to 50 mg/kg, divided into three oral doses, for 10 days.

Paromomycin sulfate USP (Humatin)

Actions and indications. This antibiotic, which has a broad spectrum of antimicrobial activity, is used in the treatment and prevention of gastrointestinal infections caused by pathogenic bacteria and amebae. In amebiasis, it is used mainly in mild to moderately severe chronic cases with subacute or acute exacerbations, rather than for patients critically ill with acute amebic dysentery. It is not effective for treating extraintestinal amebiasis.

Paromomycin is helpful for controlling the secondary infections caused by bacteria that sometimes complicate intestinal amebiasis. Similarly, it is effective for control of gastroenteritis in shigellosis, salmonellosis, and other intestinal infections caused by pathogenic bacteria.

Adverse effects, cautions, and contraindications. The possibility of overgrowths by candidal organisms and resistant staphylococci exists, as does potential nephrotoxicity in the event of systemic absorption. More common is the occurrence of nausea and increased gastrointestinal motility with loose stools or even moderately severe diarrhea. Skin rash, headache, and vertigo may occur. **Dosage and administration.** For amebiasis a minimal daily dose of 25 mg/kg daily is administered in divided doses for at least 5 days. A 2-week rest period is recommended between courses. Hepatic coma patients may require as much as 4 g daily in divided doses for 5 or 6 days.

Helminthiasis

Helminthic infections are among the most common of all diseases. About one billion people are estimated to harbor worms in their gastrointestinal tract or in other tissues. More than 90% of the populations of some tropical countries have helminthiasis. However, these diseases are not limited to the tropics, and cases are often diagnosed in countries with temperate climates, such as the United States, Russia, and Scandinavia. Helminthiasis is still common in the rural South, but it is also not uncommon in major metropolitan areas. Some such infections turn out to have been picked up while the person was traveling in tropical countries, but often the worms were acquired here.

Helminthic infections in humans are caused by worm species that are members of two main groups: the *nematodes*, or roundworms, so called because of their cylindric bodies, and the *platyhelminths*, or flatworms, many species of which are, as their name suggests, flat or ribbonlike.

The nematodes may be subdivided into two groups: (1) those that, as adults, remain mainly in the human intestinal tract (see below and also Table 11-4); and (2) those that, as larvae, invade other body tissues in addition to the intestine (see below). The platyhelminths of medical interest may be subdivided for our purposes into two subgroups: the tapeworms or cestodes, which inhabit the human intestinal tract, and the trematodes or flukes, including particularly four schistosome species, which invade extraintestinal tissues.

The current drug treatment of infestations by the following species of intestinal nematodes will be discussed:

1. *Enterobius vermicularis*, also called oxyurids or, more commonly, pinworms
2. *Ascaris lumbricoides*, the roundworm
3. *Strongyloides stercoralis*, the cause of the infection called *strongyloidiasis*, or threadworm disease
4. *Trichuris trichiura*, the whipworm
5. Two species of hookworm, *Necator americanus* and *Ancylostoma duodenale*

The current treatment of infestations by the following four species of tapeworms will also be presented:

1. *Taenia saginata*, the beef tapeworm
2. *Taenia solium*, the pork tapeworm
3. *Diphyllobothrium latum*, the fish tapeworm
4. *Hymenolepis nana*, the dwarf tapeworm

Finally, drugs used in the management of infections caused by tissue-invading nematode worms, including *Trichinella spiralis*, filariae such as *Wuchereria bancrofti* and others, and by four tissue-invading trematode species—*Schistosoma haematobium, Schistosoma mansoni, Schistosoma japonicum,* and *Schistosoma mekongi*—will be discussed.

Anthelmintics are drugs employed to eliminate worms from the body. Most are taken by mouth to exert their effects locally on intestinal roundworms and tapeworms. Others, usually administered by injection, are carried to extraintestinal tissues to attack flukes, filariae, and other adult worms or larvae that may damage skeletal muscles, skin, and subcutaneous tissues, or even such vital organs as the liver, lungs, heart, and brain.

Diagnosis

Most of these systemically active anthelmintics are toxic drugs that must be employed only after the presence of the invading parasites has been verified by precise diagnostic procedures. A specific accurate diagnosis is also desirable to select the most appropriate anthelmintic for ridding the intestine of parasitic worms.

Thus, to choose the best drug for treating a particular patient, a stool specimen must often first be obtained to send to the laboratory to be examined for ova and parasites. From this or from blood, urine, or other materials obtained from the patient's body, the parasitologist can usually help the physician or nurse to arrive at a correct diagnosis. Once the type of worm has been determined, the anthelmintic that is the safest and most effective for eliminating that specific parasite is selected.

Sometimes, for most efficient use of this medication, other measures must also be employed before or after administration of the anthelmintic. The nurse should be aware of the various specialized procedures and other adjunctive measures that are often part of the total diagnostic and treatment regimen in managing helminthiasis.

Recent advances in therapy

A number of newer intestinal anthelmintics have proved remarkably safe, effective, and convenient to use in comparison with the drugs previously available for treating intestinal helminthiasis. Thus, for example, the traditional drugs oleoresin of aspidium, hexylresorcinol, gentian violet, quinacrine, and tetrachloroethylene, formerly used to treat intestinal worm infections, are presently being replaced by thiabendazole, mebendazole, niclosamide, and pyrantel pamoate.

One reason for the greater safety of the newer anthelmintics is that they are not so readily absorbed into the systemic circulation as are the older drugs. Thus, they are not likely to cause systemic side-effects. Instead, these drugs reach high concentrations in the vicinity of the worms that reside within the intestine. There, these compounds usually exert some effect that proves selectively toxic to a metabolic process of the helminth that is essential for energy production or for the organism's ability to move about and maintain its muscle tone. Because humans do not share the same biochemical processes, their cells are not adversely affected by these drugs.

Another advantage of certain newer anthelmintics, such as mebendazole (Vermox), thiabendazole (Mintezol), and pyrantel pamoate (Antiminth), is that they possess a broad spectrum of activity against several types of intestinal worms. This makes them particularly useful for treating patients with mixed infections—that is, those who harbor several types of helminths simultaneously.

Intestinal and extraintestinal helminths

The most common intestinal infestations are with pinworms, small roundworms, and whipworms. Less frequent are infections with threadworms and tapeworms. Hookworm disease is both common and potentially serious. *Trichinella* adults live in the human intestine, but it is their larvae's entering other body tissues that causes disease symptoms. Other worms that cause systemic disease by invasion of extraintestinal tissues are those responsible for schistosomiasis and filariasis.

The following discussion of all these intestinal and extraintestinal helminthic infections and their management with drug therapy and other measures will be a general one. For detailed information about individual anthelmintic drugs, including their dosage, method of administration, and points on how they are best used for greatest effectiveness and with least toxicity, see the Drug Digest for each and Tables 11-2 and 11-3.

Intestinal worms

Pinworms

Infestation with pinworms is the most common cause of helminthiasis among American schoolchildren (Table 11-4). Fortunately, the infection is not serious and causes little discomfort. The main symptom is itching in the anal area and occasionally in the vulva and vagina. In cases of light pinworm infestations, the only treatment measure needed may be the application of an antipruritic cream or ointment to the perianal and perineal areas. However, several safe, effective, and easy-to-administer anthelmintic drugs are now available for eliminating pinworms.

Treatment. *Pyrantel pamoate*[+] is considered the drug of choice by many authorities. This drug and *pyrvinium pamoate*[+] are usually effective when given in only one dose. A single one-tablet dose of *mebendazole*[+] has also proved capable of eliminating pinworms. *Piperazine*[+], which requires a week-long course of therapy, is also effective. *Thiabendazole*[+] is also effective but may cause a higher incidence of gastrointestinal and central side-effects than the others (see Drug Digests for details of dosage, administration, and other clinically significant aspects of all these agents).

Whipworms

The whip-shaped adult worms of this species attach themselves to the wall of the colon and, when present in large numbers, cause colic and bloody diarrhea. Children with heavy infestations of whipworms can lose enough blood to the worms to develop an iron deficiency anemia. Sometimes a large mass of the whitish worms leads to rectal prolapse.

Treatment. Because no truly effective anthelmintic was available until recently, it was thought best not to try to treat any but the most heavily infested patients. People whose feces contained the eggs but who had only mild diarrhea or no symptoms at all were left untreated. Now, however, with the introduction of two drugs that are effective, safe, and easy to administer, treatment need not be withheld from anyone in whom whipworms or their eggs are detected even when the case of trichuriasis is asymptomatic.

Mebendazole (Vermox), administered orally in a 3-day course, has reportedly cured two out of three whipworm patients. Most of the rest respond to a similar second course administered 3 weeks later. *Thiabendazole* (Mintezol) has proved effective in about a third of cases treated with a 2-day oral course, and additional cures follow repeated treatment 7 days later. Neither of these newer drugs requires complicated adjunctive measures, such as fasting the patient or administering cathartics or enemas.

Threadworms

These parasitic worms burrow beneath the mucosa of the small intestine, and the female lays many eggs that hatch into larvae able to penetrate to all parts of the body, including the lungs, liver, and heart. Lightly infested people may show no symptoms but, in more heavily infested patients, abdominal tenderness and pain resembling peptic ulcer may be reported, and invasion of the lower bowel by larvae may lead to ulcerative lesions and diarrhea resembling ulcerative colitis. Deaths have occurred from bronchopneumonia and lung or liver abscesses caused by the migrating larvae.

Table 11–2. Anthelmintic drugs for treating intestinal helminthic infestations

Generic or official name	Trade name	Adult oral dosage schedule	Comments
Dichlorophen	Antiphen	2–3 g every 8 hr for three doses; or a single 6-g dose on 2 successive days	Taeniacide, chemically related to niclosamide; particularly effective in infestations by the beef tapeworm, *Taenia saginata* (not available in the United States)
Mebendazole	Vermox	200 mg orally once or 100 mg twice daily for 3 days	Broad-spectrum anthelmintic effective for whipworms, as well as for pinworms, large roundworms, and hookworms (see Drug Digest)
Niclosamide	Niclocide	Four 500-mg tablets chewed thoroughly; for children, two or three tablets finely ground and mixed with water; dose is repeated daily for 1 wk for dwarf tapeworm	Cesticide for treating beef, fish, pork, and dwarf tapeworm infestations (see Drug Digest)
Piperazine citrate USP	Antepar; Vermizine	For pinworms, single daily doses of up to 2.5 g daily for 1 wk; for large roundworms, a single daily dose of up to 3.5 g for 2 days	Useful for large roundworm and pinworm infections (see Drug Digest)
Pyrantel pamoate USP	Antiminth	A single oral dose of 11 mg/kg (5 mg/lb) body weight up to a total of 1 g	Effective for pinworm, large roundworm, and hookworm infections (see Drug Digest)
Pyrvinium pamoate USP	Povan	A single oral dose of 5 mg/kg body weight of the base may be followed by the same dose 2 wk later, if necessary, for pinworms	Effective for pinworm and roundworm infestations; this red dye stains stools (see Drug Digest)
Quinacrine HCl USP	Atabrine	800 mg orally in two, four, or eight divided doses at intervals of a few minutes, or all at once by duodenal intubation	Employed for pork tapeworm to avoid release of eggs from worm segments; other taeniacides are now preferred (see Drug Digest)
Thiabendazole USP	Mintezol	25 mg/kg body weight twice daily for 1 day for pinworms and for 2 days in other types of helminthiasis, up to a total of 3 g daily	A broad-spectrum anthelmintic effective against threadworms, trichinosis, and cutaneous larva migrans, as well as for pinworms, whipworms, and mixed infestations with hookworms and large roundworms (see Drug Digest)

Treatment. Because of the potential seriousness of *Strongyloides* infections, all those whose feces are found to contain threadworm larvae should be treated even if they show no symptoms. This is particularly true now that two almost totally effective drugs, *thiabendazole* and pyrvinium pamoate, are available. In the past this infection

Table 11–3. Drugs for treating schistosomiasis, filariasis, and other tissue-invading (systemic) helminthic infections

Generic or official name	Trade name	Chemical category	Adult dosage and administration	Comments
Bithionol	Bithin; Lorothidol	Complex nonmetallic organic compound	30–50 mg/kg body weight orally on alternate days for 10–15 doses	Available in the United States only from CDC for treating infections caused by *Fasciola hepatica* and *Paragonimus westermani**
Diethylcarbamazine citrate USP	Hetrazan	Piperazine derivative	2 mg/kg body weight orally three times daily for 1–3 wk	Effective against the microfilariae and adult worms that cause several types of filariasis
Hycanthone mesylate	Etrenol	A metabolite of the thioxanthone-group compound lucanthone	2.5–3 mg/kg body weight of the base by deep IM injection	Effective in schistosomiasis caused *Schistosoma haematobium* and *S. mansoni*, and less toxic than lucanthone (not available in the United States)
Metrifonate	Bilarcil	Organophosphorus compound	10 mg/kg body weight orally every other week for three doses	Available in the United States only from CDC;* effective against *S. haematobium*
Niridazole	Ambilhar	Nitrothiazole derivative	25 mg/kg body weight orally for 5–10 days	Available in the United States only from CDC;* effective in schistosomiasis caused by *S. japonicum;* also useful in infestations caused by the guinea worm, *Dracunculus medinensis*
Oxamniquine	Mansil; Vansil	Complex nonmetallic organic compound	12–15 mg/kg body weight as a single oral dose	Effective against all stages of *S. mansoni* infection
Praziquantel	Biltricide	Complex nonmetallic organic compound	Three oral doses of 20 mg/kg body weight within a 4 to 6-hr period in 1 day	Effective against all four species of schistosomes causing human schistosomiasis
Stibocaptate; sodium antimony dimercaptosuccinate	Astiban	Trivalent antimony compound	IM as a 10% solution in a dose of 8 mg/kg body weight weekly, up to a total dose of 40 mg/kg body weight	Available in the United States only from CDC;* effective against *S. haematobium* and *S. mansoni*
Suramin sodium	Antrypol; Germanin	Complex nonmetallic organic compound	100–200 mg test dose IV, then 1 g by slow IV at weekly intervals for 5 wk	Effective against the adult filariae of *Onchocerca volvulus* following use of diethyl-carbamazine against the microfilariae (see Drug Digest)

* CDC: Centers for Disease Control, Atlanta.

Table 11–4. Summary of anthelmintic drug therapy in intestinal helminthiasis

Species name	Common name	Name of disorder	Drug(s) preferred
Nematode (roundworm) infections			
Enterobius (Oxyuris) vermicularis	Pinworm; seatworm	Enterobiasis; oxyuriasis	Pyrantel pamoate; mebendazole; piperazine citrate; pyrvinium pamoate
Trichuris trichiura	Whipworm	Trichuriasis; trichocephaliasis	Mebendazole
Strongyloides stercoralis	Threadworm	Strongyloidiasis	Thiabendazole
Ascaris lumbricoides	Large roundworm	Ascariasis	Mebendazole; pyrantel pamoate; piperazine citrate
Necator americanus	Hookworm (New World)	Ancylostomiasis ⎫	Mebendazole; pyrantel pamoate; thiabendazole
Ancylostoma duodenale	Hookworm (Old World)	Ancylostomiasis ⎭	
Tapeworm (cestode) infections			
Diphyllobothrium latum	Fish tapeworm	Diphyllobothriasis ⎫	
Taenia saginata	Beef tapeworm	Taeniasis	Niclosamide; paromomycin
Taenia solium	Pork tapeworm	Taeniasis; cysticercosis ⎭	
Hymenolepis nana	Dwarf tapeworm	Hymenolepiasis	Niclosamide; praziquantel; paromomycin

was difficult to treat. Although the dye *gentian violet* often provided symptomatic relief, it did not eradicate the threadworms. *Dithiazanine*, the first drug effective for eliminating threadworms from the intestine, had to be withdrawn from use in the United States because it resulted in deaths.

Thiabendazole brings about cures in almost all patients who take it orally for only 2 days. It causes no serious toxicity, although some patients complain of epigastric distress, headache, drowsiness, or other gastrointestinal and central nervous system side-effects. Pyrvinium pamoate, which is also effective but requires a longer course of treatment, may be employed for patients who do not tolerate the first-choice anthelmintic or for those with severe liver disease, for whom thiabendazole may be contraindicated.

Roundworms

Ascaris lumbricoides, a large roundworm about the size of an earthworm, is the most common cause of helminth infestations throughout the world. One out of every four people is said to be infected, even though many patients may have no symptoms and are unaware that they harbor these worms until they happen to see one in their stool. Although roundworm infections are most common in the tropics, they can occur wherever sanitation is poor, including parts of the United States.

The first signs and symptoms of roundworm infection may resemble a respiratory infection. This develops a week or two after a person ingests fertilized eggs, when the larvae that hatch in the small intestine make their way to the lungs and produce cough, fever, and other symptoms of pulmonary infiltration. Later, after the larvae migrate back to the stomach and intestine and grow to adult size, the person may have some abdominal pain and distention. Most serious is the danger of intestinal obstruction and other complications caused by masses of tangled worms that have been stimulated into migratory activity.

Treatment. Several very effective drugs for safely eliminating roundworms have replaced earlier less efficient anthelmintics. At present, *mebendazole* or *pyrantel pamoate* are considered the drugs of choice. Mebendazole blocks glucose uptake by the worms, eventually interfering with their reproduction and causing their death. Pyrantel pamoate is believed to act as a neuromuscular junction blocking drug in these worms, thereby paralyzing them. *Piperazine citrate* also paralyzes the roundworms, so that they can no longer lie across the lumen of the intestine feeding on partially digested food. The helpless worms

241

are swept along the intestinal tract by peristaltic activity and passed with the stools.

Mebendazole and pyrantel pamoate are especially useful in mixed infections of *Ascaris* and hookworms. In such cases, they act to remove both types of worms together. (Formerly, it was necessary first to employ an antiroundworm drug such as piperazine before giving an antihookworm drug such as tetrachloroethylene [see below], because the latter drug could stimulate the roundworms into the type of frenzied migration that would lead to intestinal obstruction, peritonitis, and other complications.)

Hookworms

Two types of hookworms infect humans: *Necator americanus,* the cause of the disease in the United States, elsewhere in the New World, and in tropical Africa; and *Ancylostoma duodenale,* the Old World hookworm prevalent in Europe, the Middle East, North Africa, and elsewhere. Both hookworm species attach themselves to the mucosa of the infected person's small intestine and suck blood. Heavy infestations are debilitating because the worms not only damage intestinal mucosa but cause an iron deficiency anemia, with symptoms such as chronic fatigue and apathy. Such patients require treatment with oral or parenteral iron salts or even prompt transfusion of whole blood or packed red cells. Correction of fluid and electrolyte imbalances is desirable before administration of anthelmintic drug therapy.

Treatment. Newer anthelmintics including *pyrantel pamoate, mebendazole,* and *thiabendazole* are now preferred to the previously most frequently employed drug, *tetrachloroethylene.* The main reason is that these broad-spectrum anthelmintics are also effective against the large roundworms with which many hookworm patients are also infected. Thus, their use does not require prior treatment with piperazine to remove the roundworms, and thus prevent their activation by tetrachloroethylene. Another advantage of the newer agents is that, unlike tetrachloroethylene, their use requires no preliminary fasting or posttreatment purging, and they are safer.

Tapeworms (cestodes)

Tapeworms are segmented flatworms, consisting of a scolex, or head, which attaches itself to the intestinal wall, and a variable number of segments that grow from the head, sometimes forming a worm several yards long. However, the presence of lengthy beef or fish tapeworms is not truly serious. The patient may have some mild abdominal symptoms and suffer some weight loss occasionally, but treatment is sought more for psychological than physical reasons. That is, the patient may be frightened by finding worm segments in the stool, even though their passage causes little discomfort.

The pork tapeworm, which is rare in this country, can, however, cause a more serious condition called cysticercosis. In such cases the larval form of the worm makes its way into the bloodstream and may be carried to the muscles, lungs, liver, or brain. Because no specific treatment is available for cysticercosis, it is important to remove the adult worm while it is in the intestinal tract.

Treatment. The once widely used vermifuge, oleoresin of aspidium, and the safer synthetic chemotherapeutic agent, *quinacrine*[+], have both been replaced for this purpose by *niclosamide*[+] and the antibiotic *paramomycin.* These two drugs are used to treat infections caused by the pork tapeworm as well as by the beef, fish, and dwarf tapeworms. The drug *dichlorophen,* which is not available in the United States, is used in other parts of the world to treat tapeworm infestations.

Although all these drugs are highly effective, the main advantage of the newer drugs over quinacrine is that they are less likely to cause nausea and vomiting, and so their use does not require the adjunctive administration of alkaline salts or antiemetic drugs. The newer drugs are also free of the central and skin-type side-effects that sometimes follow administration of large doses of quinacrine (see its Drug Digest). In addition, oral administration of niclosamide or dichlorophen does not need to be preceded by a 24-hour liquid or fat-free diet, as is required with quinacrine.

Niclosamide now seems to be the drug of choice for treating beef tapeworm and fish tapeworm, because a single safe dose cures about 90% of cases. It is also the preferred drug for eliminating adult dwarf tapeworms but, because immature larvae are not affected, this drug must be administered daily for about a week to allow the larvae of this species to develop into the drug-sensitive adult form.

Some authorities also use niclosamide to kill the adult pork tapeworm, but there is one drawback to using it in this species. This drug partially digests the egg-containing worm segments, and the eggs released by the disintegrating segments of the dying worm may lead to development of larvae that can then migrate to the brain, eye, and other organs to cause cysticercosis. For this reason some experts continue to treat this tapeworm infection with quinacrine, which expels the worm segments without digesting them and thus does not allow eggs to be released into the intestine.

Adjunctive measures. Pork tapeworm larvae that invade an infected person's tissues cannot be eliminated by any of the drugs currently available. The newest antischistosomal drug, *praziquantel* (see below) is now being investigated for this purpose. The cysticerci that lodge in the brain can cause convulsive seizures. The occurrence of convulsions may be reduced by management with antiepileptic drugs or by surgical measures to reduce intracranial pressure, and the disorder may occasionally be cured by surgical removal of the larval mass from the brain.

The fish tapeworm, which may grow to a size of about 30 feet in the intestine of an infected person, absorbs large quantities of dietary vitamin B_{12} and folic acid, thus depriving the person of these essential nutrients. This often leads to development of a megaloblastic anemia and, as in pernicious anemia, to neurologic signs and symptoms. Thus, although remission will occur after the parasitic worm is eliminated, the patient's hematologic recovery can be hastened by administration of cyano-cobalamin compounds and folic acid. Remission of neurologic symptoms also occurs if spinal cord tissue has not suffered irreversible degeneration as a result of the parasite-induced nutritional deficiency.

Tissue-invading helminths

The worm infections discussed up to now are largely limited to the intestinal tract and, ideally, the drugs used to treat these disorders should act only on the worms within the intestine without being absorbed systemically. This section will discuss the drug treatment of several helminthic disorders caused by worm forms that invade tissues other than the intestines, including cardiac and skeletal muscles, liver, lungs, urinary tract, and brain (see Table 11-3). These diseases include some that are caused by tissue nematodes, such as *trichinosis* and *filariasis*, and *schistosomiasis*, a type of infection caused by tissue-invading trematodes, or flukes.

Trichinosis

The adult form of the roundworm *Trichinella spiralis* that is responsible for this infection does not enter the tissues after it grows to maturity in the human intestinal tract. However, the larvae that the fertilized female worms deposit in the intestinal mucosa pass into the bloodstream and are carried throughout the body. The larvae penetrate into various skeletal muscles, including those responsible for respiration, and they evoke inflammatory reactions in the myocardium and brain, among other tissues. Severe infections can cause fatal pneumonia, heart failure, and encephalitis, as well as severe muscle pains and other signs and symptoms.

Treatment. *Corticosteroid drugs* help to relieve symptoms that stem from inflammation, including fever, muscle pains, and edema around the eyes and in the brain. The only anthelmintic drug that offers similar symptomatic relief is *thiabenzadole* (Mintezol), which appears to kill some, but not all, of the living larvae encysted in animal and human tissues. *Mebendazole* has the status of an investigational drug for this purpose in the United States. Complications such as congestive heart failure must, of course, also be counteracted if they occur.

Prevention. This requires thorough cooking of pork products to kill the larvae in infected meat. This disease may be eliminated in pigs by heat-sterilizing the garbage that they are fed (or by not feeding them on garbage at all). Keeping cuts of meat frozen at low temperatures for several weeks after butchering of the hogs also helps to kill larvae. The nurse can help by advising people not to eat pork that is still pink.

Filariasis

Filariasis is a term used to describe several helminthic diseases in which the blood and tissues of infected people contain microfilariae, or embryos that are picked up by biting insects and transmitted to previously uninfected people. The adult forms of filarial worms cause various types of damage in the tissues in which they dwell or through which they move.

Wuchereria bancrofti is the worm species that causes the most common form of filariasis. A person becomes infected by being bitten by a mosquito (*Culex* species, especially) that deposits larvae in the skin. Later, the adult females give birth to thin threadlike microfilariae that migrate into the lymphatics and bloodstream. Symptoms are the result of inflammatory reactions to the presence of living and dead worms. Obstruction of the lymphatic system by inflammatory lesions may lead to elephantiasis—gross enlargement of the legs, arms, scrotum, or breast by edema fluid.

Treatment. Until relatively recently no safe drug was available for treatment of filariasis. The relatively toxic arsenical and antimony compounds once employed with only fair success have now been largely displaced by two nonmetallic compounds, diethylcarbamazine, and suramin sodium (see Table 11-3). Dosage varies depending on the response of the particular filarial organism and on the reactions evoked in the tissues of the infected patients.

Diethylcarbamazine, which kills the microfilariae and probably some of the adult worms, is effective for treating bancroftian filariasis and for preventing transmission of this disease. It is best given in small daily doses over periods of several weeks. This minimizes such adverse effects of the drug itself as nausea, vomiting, and headache, and it also reduces the severity of allergic reactions to the proteins of dead filariae. Other medical and surgical measures are also employed in managing lymphedema of the lower extremities, scrotum, and breasts. Preventive measures in addition to prophylactic doses of diethylcarbamazine include spraying of insecticides and destruction of breeding places of mosquitoes.

Onchocerciasis is an infection caused when microfilariae of the worm *Onchocerca volvulus* are deposited in the skin by biting black flies. More serious than the symptoms caused by adult worms in the subcutaneous tissues is possible blindness as a result of migration of microfilariae into the cornea and other tissues of the eye. (The disease is sometimes called river blindness in the areas of Africa and Central or South America in which the insect vector larvae infest river waters.)

Diethylcarbamazine can kill the microfilariae but not the adult worms. It must be administered in much smaller doses than those employed in bancroftian filariasis, because the allergic reaction of the patient's tissues to the proteins of killed filariae of this species can be very severe. Such reactions, particularly when they include acute ocular inflammation, may be minimized by the use of eye drops containing a soluble corticosteroid and by the oral administration of systemic corticosteroid and antihistamine drugs.

After the course of treatment with diethylcarbamazine, *suramin sodium*[+] administration is required to kill the adult worms of this species. Patients who can tolerate a small test dose receive single intravenous injections of 1 g of this drug for 5 or 6 weeks. Adverse reactions much more serious than those with diethylcarbamazine are possible, so patients are observed closely for signs of toxicity. This drug may have to be discontinued, for example, if protein and casts appear in the urine and persist and become worse.

Loiasis, caused by the worm *Loa loa,* is a disease in which microfilariae are transmitted by the bites of deerflies. The adult worms cause repeated painful swellings as they migrate under the skin of the arms, legs, and elsewhere. These parasites can also get into the eyes and affect peripheral and central nerve tissues. Diethylcarbamazine, administered in doses much larger than those used in bancroftian filariasis, destroys both the microfilariae and the adult worms.

The guinea worm or dragon worm, *Dracunculus medinensis,* which is carried in larval form by infected water fleas, can grow up to a yard long under the skin of infected persons. It causes blisters that may be followed by secondary infections of the legs, buttocks, genitalia, and elsewhere. The worm has to be removed surgically or mechanically. Recently, however, two anthelmintic drugs, *niridazole* and *thiabendazole,* have reportedly killed the adult worm and relieved the skin symptoms caused by its toxic secretions. The drug *metronidazole,* used to treat amebiasis and trichomoniasis, is being investigated for use in guinea worm infections.

Schistosomiasis

More than 200 million people in Africa, Asia, and some South American countries and Caribbean islands have this chronic worm infection. Many have only mild symptoms or none at all, but others suffer severe damage to the liver, intestines, urinary tract, and other organs, particularly in the late stages of heavy infestations. This is why early detection and treatment of the disease with modern antischistosomal drugs is so important.

Life cycle. Four different species of flatworms cause the human form of this disease: *Schistosoma haematobium, S. mansoni, S. japonicum,* and *S. mekongi. S. mekongi* is a new species of schistosome that has been found in Laotian refugees. Although they differ in various respects including their responsiveness to drug therapy, all follow essentially the same type of life cycle (Fig. 11-2). Eggs excreted in the urine and feces of infected people hatch in fresh water into a form that infects certain susceptible species of snails. Within the snails, larvae called cercariae develop and are shed back into the freshwater stream, pond, or lake. People become infected while in the water, when the forktailed cercarial larvae of the schistosomes attach themselves to the skin and quickly burrow down into the bloodstream or lymphatics.

These larvae then move to the lungs and later to the liver, where they mature within the portal veins. The mature adult worms mate and move on to areas of the large and small intestines and urinary bladder. Here, the female worms lay large masses of eggs, most of which are eliminated from the body as indicated above.

Signs and symptoms. The eggs that remain, as well as the adult worms acquired by recurrent exposures, are the cause of many varied symptoms as they migrate in the body and set off allergic and inflammatory reactions. A so-called swimmer's itch or pruritic rash, caused by a reaction to larvae that die in the skin, is the first sign of schistosomiasis. About 1 or 2 months later some infected people may suffer fever, chills, headache, and other symptoms that last for several weeks. People heavily infested with some species of shistosomes tend to develop chronic abdominal pain and diarrhea. Infection with *S. haematobium* is often marked by obstruction of the urinary tract, hematuria, and dysuria. Chronic schistosomiasis is also often marked by blockage of blood flow in the veins of the liver, lungs, and central nervous system. These lesions lead to enlargement of the liver and spleen, and to signs and symptoms of heart, lung, and brain involvement.

Chemotherapy. Several types of drugs (see Table 11-3; Fig. 11-2) are available for the treatment of schistosomiasis caused by the various infective species.

Organic antimony compounds. For many years, organic antimony compounds such as *antimony potassium tartrate (tartar emetic), stibophen,* and *stibocaptate (sodium antimony dimercaptosuccinate—Astiban)* were the only drugs available to treat schistosomiasis. The heavy metal in these compounds kills schistosomes by poisoning an enzyme in the metabolic pathway by which the worms convert dietary glucose into energy. Because the same enzyme in human cells is much less sensitive to antimony, these compounds have a degree of selective toxicity. However, because such selective toxicity is quite limited, administration of antimony is marked by many types of adverse effects, which are often more discomforting than the symptoms of schistosomiasis. Thus, it was sometimes difficult to get patients to cooperate and take the many intramuscular or intravenous injections required for completion of a fully effective course of therapy. Now, in the United

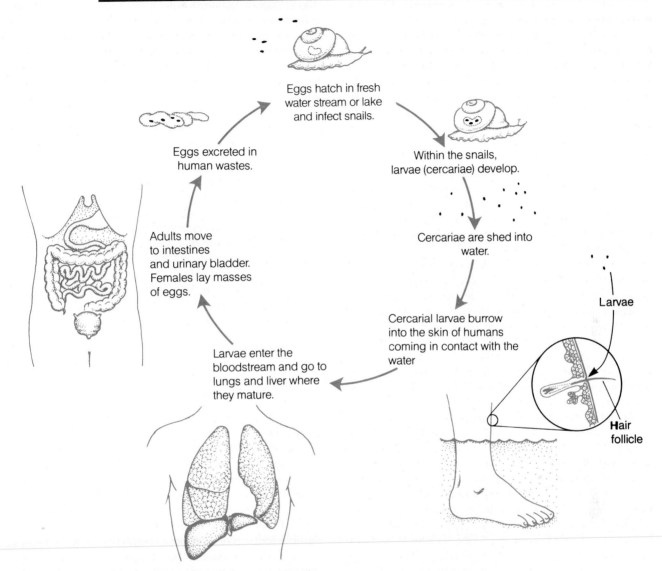

Eggs hatch in fresh
water stream or lake
and infect snails.

Within the snails,
larvae (cercariae) develop.

Eggs excreted in
human wastes.

Cercariae are shed into
water.

Adults move
to intestines
and urinary bladder.
Females lay masses
of eggs.

Cercarial larvae burrow
into the skin of humans
coming in contact with the
water

Larvae

Larvae enter the
bloodstream and go to
lungs and liver where
they mature.

Hair
follicle

Figure 11-2. Life cycle of the schistosome and site of drug action. Molluscicides to kill the snail vector have not proven very effective. The active sites of the drugs are the lungs and liver.

States, the only antimony compound used to treat schistosomiasis is stibocaptate (Astiban). It is not commercially available but may be obtained from the Centers for Disease Control (CDC) in Atlanta. It is effective against *S. hematobium*, *S. mansoni*, and *S. japonicum*. However, if the disease has caused severe liver damage, this drug is contraindicated. It is also contraindicated in cases of renal insufficiency and cardiac disease, and in the presence of bacterial and *herpes simplex* and *herpes zoster* infections. Treatment with any of the antimony compounds can cause bradycardia, arthritis, hepatitis, and many other serious untoward reactions. Use of these drugs has been largely superseded by newer and safer antischistosomal drugs.

Nonantimonials. *Niridazole* (Ambilhar), an orally effective agent that causes less severe side-effects than the antimonials, has proved useful for infections caused by *S. japonicum*, the least susceptible of the schistosome species. This drug is available in the United States only from the CDC. In patients with liver disease, the drug has caused mental symptoms and convulsions. It also reversibly inhibits spermatogenesis. Gastrointestinal upsets and headache are not uncommon.

Hycanthone (Etrenol), also available from the CDC in the United States, is effective in infections caused by *S. haematobium* and *S. mansoni*. It causes a high incidence of gastrointestinal disturbances, and has caused fetal hepatic necrosis. Although some of the drugs described above are still available, it seems likely that they will be replaced by the following three newer and safer drugs.

Metrifonate (Bilarcil) is an organophosphorus

compound that inhibits parasite cholinesterase enzymes. Although plasma cholinesterase levels of the host are also inhibited, it is reported that the drug is well tolerated. It is recommended for use only against *S. hematobium.* Patients receiving this drug, which needs to be taken over a 3-week period, should not be exposed to insecticides containing cholinesterase inhibitors, nor should they receive parasympathomimetic drugs (see Chap. 15) or depolarizing neuromuscular junction blocking drugs (see Chap. 19).

Oxamniquine (Vansil) is clinically effective only against *S. mansoni.* It, too, is generally well tolerated, but a few people have developed convulsions within a few hours after receiving the single oral dose. Patients with a history of seizures need close observation with equipment available to manage convulsions. Dizziness and drowsiness are more common reactions.

The newest antischistosomiasis drug, *praziquantel* (Biltricide), is unlike any of the other relatively nontoxic drugs in this group in that it is clinically effective against all four species of schistosome that cause human systemic infection. It acts by increasing the calcium permeability of the worm's cell membrane. This, in turn, causes the worms to undergo muscle spasms and paralysis. The drug also causes disintegration of the worm's outer covering layer. So far, praziquantel appears to be a very safe drug. No major toxic reactions have been reported. Transient abdominal pain, dizziness, and fever have occurred. This drug is effective orally in a single dose, but dosage is usually divided over 4 to 6 hours to reduce abdominal toxicity. Tablets should be swallowed whole with liquid during meals.

Other measures. Patients with chronic schistosomiasis are often debilitated and anemic. Thus, it is desirable to build up their strength by dietary means and antianemia agents before beginning treatment with antimonial or other toxic drugs. Certain surgical procedures are also sometimes employed as an adjunct to antischistosomal drug therapy.

Measures to prevent this disease are based on avoiding contact with contaminated water, either on an individual basis or by public health procedures for providing clean water for washing and bathing. The latter include measures for destroying the intermediate host—the snails—by means of chemical molluscacides or biologic controls.

Of course, in addition to keeping snails from infecting the waters used by humans, it is desirable to prevent people from infecting the snails in the first place. This can best be accomplished by sanitary disposal of human wastes and by treating large segments of the population with safe oral drugs that reduce the numbers of eggs that people excrete.

Additional clinical considerations

As with many of the other organisms discussed thus far,

prevention of helminth infection should be one of the main goals of patient education efforts by the nurse who practices in endemic areas. None of the available drugs is totally effective without the use of adjunctive measures to eradicate the parasite from the environment, or at least to protect the patient from reinfection with the worm.

Pinworm infestations are good examples of how difficult attainment of these goals can be. Pinworms spread very rapidly among children. Some hygienic measures that can be effective include the following:

1. Keep the child's nails cut short and the hands well scrubbed, because reinfection results from the worm's eggs being carried back to the mouth after becoming lodged under the fingernails during scratching of the pruritic perianal area.
2. Give the child a shower in the morning to wash away any ova deposited in the anal area during the night.
3. Change and launder undergarments, bed linens, and pajamas each day.
4. Disinfect toilet seats daily and the floors of bathrooms and bedroom periodically.
5. Encourage the child to use vigorous handwashing after using the toilet.

Pediatricians, directors of institutions, school officials, and other concerned authorities have the responsibility of deciding how far to go in the direction of instituting special public health measures for coping with pinworm infestations in the family, school, and community. Often, suppression of symptoms in the more heavily infected persons is more sensible and likely to succeed than are attempts to eradicate the worms in all possible contacts or to effect a complete cure in everyone.

After a patient has received the appropriate therapy, the patient or parents may be asked to check for the presence of eggs in the anal area for a period of 5 to 6 weeks. This is done by pressing sticky tape against the anal region before bathing in the morning, and then pressing the tape on a glass slide that has been supplied. The slide is taken to the clinic or laboratory, where it is examined microscopically for the presence of pinworm eggs. This assessment is controversial. Many feel that, because of the relative ease of treating this disease and its relative harmless nature, such a follow-up examination, which can be psychologically traumatic to the patient, is unnecessary.

To prevent trichinosis, certain measures are taken by the farmers who raise the hogs whose meat will be used. In addition to these measures, there is a simple preventive measure that should be taught to all who eat pork or pork products. All pork or pork products should be thoroughly cooked to destroy any trichinellae within the pork muscle. Any pork or pork product that is uncooked or appears pink should probably never be eaten. Although the conditions of hog raising and pork processing have markedly improved in recent years, incidents of trichinosis are still being reported.

Travelers to regions in which schistosomiasis is endemic should be alerted to the possibility of infection with disease if they wade, swim, or bathe in fresh-water streams, ponds, or lakes. Such areas are mainly tropical and include Puerto Rico, a few islands in the West Indies, Africa, parts of South America, the Philippines, China, Japan, and Southeast Asia. Anyone planning a vacation to such areas should be alerted not only to preventive measures but also to signs and symptoms to watch for on return from the visit.

Overall, infestation by worms can be a very frightening and traumatic experience for most people. Seeing the worm can be an especially difficult experience. Patients and their families will need support and encouragement to deal with the infection, as well as with the drug therapy.

Some particular considerations for specific drugs will be discussed briefly. Because *pyrvinium pamoate* will

stain, the patient should be cautioned not to spill the drug. The vomitus and stool will be stained red, and the patient should be alerted to this fact so that he will not be frightened. It is also advisable for the patient to swallow tablets whole to avoid staining the teeth. However, *thiabendazole* tablets should be chewed when they are taken, and not swallowed whole. *Niclosamide* tablets should also be chewed and then swallowed with a small amount of water. *Oxamniquine, praziquantel,* and *thiabendazole* have been associated with drowsiness and dizziness. If these occur, the patient should be cautioned about appropriate safety measures to take (avoid operating an automobile or dangerous equipment; avoid changing position quickly). *Quinacrine* has been associated with aggravation of psoriasis and porphyria, and appropriate measures must be taken to avoid these reactions.

The safety of these drugs during pregnancy and lactation has not been established. They should be avoided during these times, if at all possible.

The patient teaching guide and guide to the nursing process with anthelmintic drugs summarize the clinical considerations of these drugs.

Summary of the adverse effects of anthelmintic drugs

Dichlorophen
Nausea, diarrhea, colic
In *Taenia solium* infestations, cysticercosis (larval invasion as a result of liberation of ova by the disintegrating worms)

Mebendazole
Occasional abdominal pain and diarrhea

Niclosamide (see Drug digest)
Occasional nausea and abdominal pains

Piperazine salts (see Drug digest)
Occasional nausea, vomiting, abdominal cramps, and diarrhea
Rarely, transient dizziness, blurring of vision, vertigo, tremors, and muscle weakness

Skin rash: redness and urticaria, rarely

Pyrantel pamoate (see Drug digest)
Anorexia, nausea, vomiting, abdominal cramps, diarrhea, tenesmus

Pyrvinium pamoate (see Drug digest)
Nausea, vomiting, abdominal cramps, diarrhea; rarely, photosensitization, skin reactions

Quinacrine HCl (see Drug digest)
Nausea and vomiting, dizziness, hallucinations and delusions (toxic psychosis)

Thiabendazole (see Drug digest)
Anorexia, nausea, vomiting, diarrhea
Drowsiness, dizziness, giddiness, headache

Patient teaching guide: Anthelmintic drugs

The drug that has been prescribed for you is of the class of drugs called anthelmintics. This drug destroys specific worms that have invaded the body. Because of the way that this drug works, it must be taken over time to destroy the worm in various phases of its life cycle. You must take the full course of the drug to prevent a recurrence of the infection. Your drug has been prescribed to treat _____ .

Instructions: **1.**   The name of your drug is _____ .

(continued)

2. The dosage of your drug is _____ .

3. Your drug should be taken _____ times a day. The best time to take your drug is _____ , _____ , _____ .

4. Your drug can be taken with meals or with a light snack to help decrease any stomach upset that you may experience. Your tablets should (not) be chewed when taken (to help to increase their effectiveness.)

5. Some side-effects of the drug that you should be aware of include the following:

GI upset	Take drug with food.
Dizziness, drowsiness	If this happens to you, be sure to avoid driving a car or operating dangerous equipment; change position slowly.
Constipation (niclosamide)	Take a mild laxative; drink plenty of water.
Yellow or red color may tint the skin or urine (quinacrine; pyrvinium pamoate)	This will disappear when the drug is stopped.

6. Tell any physician, nurse, or dentist who is taking care of you that you are on this drug.

7. Keep this and all medication out of the reach of children.

8. Take the full course of your prescription. It is very important to take all the medication that has been prescribed for you.

9. As appropriate for intestinal worm infections. Some measures that will help to prevent reinfection with these worms include the following:
    a. Wash hands vigorously after using the toilet.
    b. Shower in the morning to wash away any ova deposited in the anal area during the night.
    c. Change and launder undergarments, bed linens, and pajamas every day.
    d. Disinfect toilet seats daily and the floors of bathrooms and bedrooms periodically.)

Notify your nurse or physician if any of the following occur:

Blurring of vision
Fever, chills
Rash
Headache, weakness, tremors
Swelling or itching of eyes

Guide to the nursing process: anthelmintic drugs

Assessment	Nursing diagnoses	Interventions	Evaluation

History
Past history—underlying medical conditions (*contraindications*)
  Renal failure
  Hepatic failure
  Convulsions
  Pregnancy
  Lactation
Allergies: these drugs, others; reactions
Medications: current medications
 	
Physical assessment
Neurologic: orientation, ophthalmologic exam, reflexes
GI: bowel sounds, output, liver function
Renal: renal function
Skin: color, lesions
	Potential alteration in comfort (GI)
	Potential alteration in self-concept secondary to diagnosis
	Knowledge deficit regarding drug therapy
		Culture for ova and parasites
		Proper administration of drug
		Comfort measures:
		  small frequent meals
		  Hygiene measures
		  Antipruritics for rectal itch
		  Safety precautions
		Support and encouragement to cope with diagnosis, therapy, and preventive measures
		Patient teaching, regarding:
		  Drug
		  Dosage
		  Administration
		  Side-effects
		  Hygiene
		  Warnings
			Evaluate for effectiveness of drug–eradication of helminthiasis
			Evaluate for adverse effects of drugs:
			  GI upset
			  CNS changes
			  Liver changes
			  Hypersensitivity reaction
			Evaluate effectiveness of support measures
			Evaluate effectiveness of patient teaching

Case Study

Presentation

VY is a 33-year-old Vietnamese refugee who came to the United States as part of a church-sponsored resettlement program. VY underwent a complete physical examination in preparation for a training job in custodial work at the local hospital. In the course of the exam it was found that VY had a history of chronic diarrhea, hepatomegaly, pulmonary rales, and splenomegaly. After further tests, it was discovered that VY had chronic schistosomiasis. VY was hospitalized because of his limited use of the English language and so that his disease, which was unfamiliar to the health-care providers, could be monitored. He was given treatment with praziquantel. Outline the nursing care necessary with VY.

Discussion

A language barrier can be a real handicap within the health-care system. Pictures can assist communication in such cases. For example, the need for eating nutritious foods can be conveyed to VY by using appropriate pictures. Frequent reinforcement is very important. The nursing staff should also consult with local authorities about the capability of the local sewer system to deal with the contaminated wastes. (In this case, CDC referral was made, and it was learned that the snail intermediate host does not live in the continental

United States, so the wastes posed no hazard.) Although praziquantel is a relatively nontoxic drug, the patient should be observed for drug fever, abdominal pain, and dizziness. If dizziness occurs, appropriate safety precautions should be taken. The patient should be readied for discharge through careful patient teaching, which in this case may require creative use of pictures, calendars, and clocks to ensure that VY will have the opportunity to comply with the medical therapy.

Drug digests: anthelmintics

Mebendazole (Vermox)

Actions and indications. This broad-spectrum anthelmintic kills a wide variety of worms by preventing them from taking up and using glucose. It is the first drug to prove highly effective for treating whipworm infections (trichuriasis), in which a cure rate of 68% has been reported. The drug is even more effective—cure rates of 95% to 98%—against pinworms (enterobiasis), roundworms (ascariasis), and hookworm infections caused by *Necator americanus*.

Adverse effects, cautions, and contraindi- cations. Abdominal pain and diarrhea sometimes occur but may actually be caused by the movements and expulsion of large numbers of worms in massive infestations. Little of the drug is absorbed systemically, and no toxicity to the liver, kidneys, bone marrow, or other organs has been reported. Use of this drug is not yet recommended in children under 2 years old. Its use is contraindicated in women during pregnancy, because embryotoxicity and teratogenicity have been reported when the drug was fed to pregnant rats in low doses.

Dosage and administration. A single 100-mg tablet is effective for control of enterobiasis. For trichuriasis, ascariasis, and hookworm infection, 100 mg is taken orally twice daily for 3 days in the morning and evening. A second treatment course can be taken in 3 weeks if the first fails to cure the case. No adjunctive measures such as fasting or purging are needed.

Niclosamide (Hydroxychlorbenzamide)

Actions and indications. This cesticide cures a large proportion of infestations caused by the beef, fish, pork, and dwarf tapeworms. Because it causes the partial digestion of worm segments, its use can cause the release of eggs that, in the case of the pork tapeworm, could lead to the formation of larvae that migrate to various tissues to cause cysticercosis. Despite this and the fact that drug-induced digestion of the scolex may make it difficult to determine whether the worms have been completely eliminated, niclosamide is now preferred to quinacrine and is considered the current taeniacide drug of choice.

Adverse effects, cautions, and contraindications. This drug's safety in comparison to quinidine and to oleoresin of aspidium is one of its main advantages. The lack of systemic side-effects presumably stems from the fact that very little of the drug is absorbed. Its presence in the gastrointestinal tract does not cause local irritation, and few patients complain of stomach upset symptoms.

Dosage and administration. A single dose of four 500-mg tablets is taken following an overnight fast. (No special diet is needed to avoid systemic absorption, but the upper GI tract should be empty to ensure maximum contact of the drug with the tapeworm.) Patients are told to chew the tablets thoroughly before swallowing the mass with a watery drink. Children receive one-half (1 g) or one-quarter (0.5 g) of the 2-g adult dose in the form of finely ground tablets mixed with water. Although purging is not necessary, a mild laxative may be taken in an effort to obtain undigested segments and the scolex of the worm for purposes of identification and proof of cure.

Piperazine citrate USP (Antepar)

Actions and indications. This anthelmintic is considered the preferred drug for treating infections caused by roundworms (ascariasis). It is also quite useful against infection caused by pinworms (*Enterobius* or *Oxyuris*). It acts to slow the movements of these worms or to paralyze them, but it does not kill them. This is a desirable feature, because it lessens the likelihood of reactions to absorbed foreign protein from dead worms.

Adverse effects, cautions, and contraindications. Side-effects are uncommon with or- dinary doses, but urticaria may occur in hypersensitive patients, and some patients with epilepsy have reportedly had an increase in seizure activity. Thus, caution is required in such cases.

Overdosage may lead to nausea, vomiting, and diarrhea. Headache, blurring of vision, vertigo, tremors, and muscle weakness may also occur with ingestion of excessive amounts.

Dosage and administration. The official usual dose in pinworm treatment is 50 mg/ kg of body weight daily for 7 days or a dose of up to 3.5 g daily. In practice, half of a flavored tablet or of 1 tsp of syrup, 250 mg, is given to infants weighing up to 15 lb, 1 g to those between 30 lb to 60 lb, and 2 g daily to those over 60 lbs.

The official dose against roundworms is 75 mg/kg for 2 days or 1 g for infants up to 30 lb, 2 g for those weighing from 30 lb to 50 lb, 3 g for those between 50 lb and 100 lb, and 3.5 g for those over 100 lb.

Pyrantel pamoate USP (Antiminth)

Actions and indications. This anthelmintic causes muscular paralysis of worms with which it comes in contact within the intestinal tract. It has proved highly effective for treating enterobiasis (pinworm infection) and ascariasis (roundworm infection). The drug has also cured infections caused by the hookworms *Necator americanus* and *Ancylostoma duodenale*.

Adverse effects, cautions, and contraindications. Signs and symptoms of gastrointestinal upset occasionally reported include an- orexia, nausea and vomiting, abdominal cramps, diarrhea, and tenesmus. Relatively little of the drug is absorbed systemically, but this may account for central nervous system reactions occasionally reported, including headache, dizziness, and drowsiness or insomnia. Because use of the drug has been followed by a minor and transient rise in serum glutamic–oxaloacetic transaminase levels in a few patients, it should be used with caution when patients have a history of a liver disorder. The drug should not be taken repeatedly by patients who develop an allergic skin rash.

Dosage and administration. A single dose of 11 mg/kg of pyrantel base (5 mg/lb) is administered in the form of an oral suspension that contains 50 mg/ml of the base. This may be taken with milk or fruit juices without regard to the ingestion of food or to the time of day. Prior purging with a cathartic is *not* necessary.

Pyrvinium pamoate USP (Povan)

Actions and indications. This salt of a cyanine dye has anthelmintic activity against various worms, but is recommended specifically for the eradication of pinworms. It is so effective against these worms that a single dose very often is enough to cure oxyuriasis. However, the usual hygienic precautions are required to prevent early reinfection. This drug may also be useful for treating threadworm infestation (strongyloidiasis).

Adverse effects, cautions, and contraindications. Side-effects, which are rare with the currently recommended dose of this insoluble salt, take the form of nausea, vomiting, and cramps. Like gentian violet, which it has helped to displace in oxyuriasis treatment, this dye can stain most materials. Thus, patients should be cautioned to protect underclothing and warned that their stools can be colored bright red by this drug.

Dosage and administration. A single oral dose of 5 mg/kg of body weight of pyrvinium base (7.5 mg/kg of this salt) is taken in the form of a suspension containing 10 mg/ml or a tablet containing the equivalent of 50 mg of the base. The tablets should not be chewed but swallowed whole because they may stain the teeth.

Quinacrine HCl USP (Atabrine)

Actions and indications. This antiprotozoal and anthelmintic substance has been used for the suppressive treatment of malaria and in the management of tapeworm infestations. It has been largely replaced by other drugs considered safer and more effective for these purposes, but it is still sometimes preferred for treating pork tapeworm infections. Currently, the drug is most commonly employed for treating giardiasis—intestinal infection caused by the protozoan organism *Giardia lamblia*. However, even here, it may be replaced by metronidazole.

Adverse effects, cautions, and contraindications. The drug is not ordinarily toxic to most patients, but the doses used in treating tapeworms often cause nausea and vomiting. Some patients have had hallucinations or a toxic psychosis following administration of this drug. Thus, its use is contraindicated in persons with a history of psychosis. Caution is also required in patients with psoriasis because this drug may set off severe skin reactions in such cases.

Dosage and administration. The proper use of this drug as a *taeniacide* requires careful pretreatment of the *tapeworm-infested* patient to ensure maximal contact of the drug with the scolex, or head, of the parasite. The patient is placed on a liquid or light fat-free diet for 24 hours before treatment, and the intestine is emptied by the administration of a saline cathartic the night before treatment. The next morning, the fasting patient takes a total of 800 mg of quinacrine in four divided doses over a period of 30 minutes. Each dose is followed by 600 mg of sodium bicarbonate to reduce nausea and vomiting.

Another way in which the drug is given to avoid its bitter taste and possible loss of the drug by vomiting is through a duodenal tube that has previously been inserted and into which the water-dissolved drug is injected. A saline purgative is given about 2 hours following the fourth and final oral dose of quinacrine or after duodenal intubation. The intact worm, its head colored yellow, is often recovered in the patient's stool. Finding the head in this way is an indication of cure, and when pork tapeworm segments are found to be intact, there is no danger that eggs have been released that could form the larvae responsible for cysticercosis.

For giardiasis treatment, 100 mg is given three times daily after meals for 5 to 7 days. For children the dose is 7 mg/kg body weight up to a maximum of 300 mg.

Suramin sodium (Antipyrol; Germanin)

Actions and indications. This complex urea derivative has both filaricidal and trypanocidal properties. In filariasis caused by *Onchocerca*, this drug is given to kill the adult worms after treatment with the less toxic diethylcarbamazine has caused disappearance of the microfilariae.

In the early stages of infection by *Trypanosoma gambiense* and *T. rhodesiense*, suramin may eliminate the protozoal parasite. Similarly, its prolonged presence in the blood after a single dose often offers protection against infection for 2 or 3 months. However, it is not effective in cases in which this pathogen has spread to the central nervous system.

Adverse effects, cautions, and contraindications. The most common of varied early reactions to this drug include acute urticaria and other pruritic dermatoses, nausea, abdominal pain, and fever. Rarely, circulatory collapse and coma may develop shortly after intravenous injection in highly sensitive persons. Later reactions include lacrimation and edematous swelling of periocular tissues, skin rashes, and paresthesia or hyperesthesia.

The drug is contraindicated in patients with renal disorders, and the urine of all patients is examined for the presence of blood, protein, and casts.

Dosage and administration. In trypanosomiasis and onchocerciasis, 1 g is administered by slow IV injection of a 10% solution in warm distilled water. Various course schedules are suggested, but the total dose ranges between no more than 5 g to 10 g.

Thiabendazole USP (Mintezol)

Actions and indications. This broad-spectrum anthelmintic is claimed to be more than 95% effective against enterobiasis (pinworm disease) and strongyloidiasis (threadworm disease). The drug has also been employed in trichuriasis (whipworm disease), ascariasis (large roundworm disease), and in hookworm disease caused by both types of infesting organisms. It is claimed to relieve fever, reduce eosinophilia, and produce other benefits in some patients with trichinosis, and it is said to provide the first successful systemic treatment for cutaneous larva migrans (creeping eruption).

Adverse effects, cautions, and contraindications. Side-effects involving the gastrointestinal tract and the central nervous system may occur with high doses. Anorexia, nausea, and vomiting occur frequently and epigastric distress and diarrhea less often. Drowsiness, giddiness, and headache sometimes develop, and patients should be warned against driving a car or undertaking other potentially dangerous activities requiring alertness. The drug should be used with caution in patients with impaired liver function.

Dosage and administration. This drug is available as a pleasant-tasting suspension that is administered after meals in a dose of 10 mg/lb of body weight twice a day. The length of treatment varies in different infestations. In pinworm disease, for example, the drug is usually given for 1 day and then repeated 7 days later to prevent reinfection. In other intestinal parasitoses, cutaneous larva migrans, and trichinosis, it is given for 2 successive days. In trichinosis treatment may be continued for 4 successive days. The recommended maximal daily dosage is 3 g.

References

Balamuth W, Lasslo A: Comparative amoebicidal activity in some compounds related to emetine. Proc Soc Exp Biol Med 80:705, 1982

Chavarria AP et al: Mebendazole, an effective broad-spectrum anthelmintic. Am J Trop Med Hyg 22:592, 1973

Daha DV et al: Treatment of amebic liver abscess with emetine HCl, niridazole, and metronidazole. Am J Trop Med Hyg 23:586, 1974

Davies A: Clinically available antischistosomal drugs. J Toxicol Environ Health 1:191, 1975

Drugs for parasitic infections. Med Lett Drugs Ther 26:27, 1984

Fierlafjn E: Mebendazole in enterobiasis. JAMA 218:1051, 1971

Fleury FJ et al: Single dose of two grams of metronidazole for *Trichomonas vaginalis* infections. Am J Obstetr 128:320, 1977

Gilles HM: Diseases of the alimentary system: Treatment of intestinal worms. Br Med J 2:1314, 1976

Kean BH: Subacute myelo-optic neuropathy: A probable case in the United States. JAMA 214:519, 1970

Levi G et al: Efficacy of various drugs in the treatment of giardiasis. A comparative study. Am J Trop Med Hyg 26:564, 1977

Mansour TE: Chemotherapy of parasitic worms: New biochemical strategies. Science 205:462, 1979

Miller MJ: Protozoan and helminth parasites—a review of current treatment. Prog Drug Res 20:433, 1976

Miller MJ et al: Mebendazole, an effective anthelmintic for trichuriasis and enterobiasis. JAMA 230:1412, 1977

Most H: Treatment of common parasitic infections of man encountered in the United States. N Engl J Med 287:495; 698, 1972

Powell SJ: Therapy of amebiasis. Bull NY Acad Med 47:469, 1972

Praziquantel: A new antiparasitic drug. Med Lett Drugs Ther 24:108, 1982

Rollo IM: Drugs used in the chemotherapy of amebiasis. In Gilman AG, Goodman LS, Gilman A (eds): Goodman & Gilman's The Pharmacological Basis of Therapeutics, 6th ed, pp 1061–1069. New York, Macmillan, 1980

Rollo IM: Drugs used in the chemotherapy of helminthiasis. In Gilman AG, Goodman LS, Gilman A (eds): Goodman & Gilman's The Pharmacological Basis of Therapeutics, 6th ed, pp 1013–1037. New York, Macmillan, 1980

Rollo IM: Miscellaneous drugs used in the treatment of protozoal infections. In Gilman AG, Goodman LS, Gilman A (eds): Goodman & Gilman's The Pharmacological Basis of Therapeutics, 6th ed, pp 1070–1079. New York, Macmillan, 1980

Seah SK: Mebendazole in the treatment of helminthiasis. Can Med Assoc J 115:777, 1976

Standen OD: Chemotherapy of intestinal helminthiasis. Prog Drug Res 19:158, 1975

Wang CC: Current problems in antiparasitic chemotherapy. Trends Biochem Sci 7:354, 1982

Wolfe MS: Nondysenteric intestinal amebiasis. Treatment with diloxanide furoate. JAMA 18:1601, 1973

Chapter 12

The chemotherapy of cancer

12

Management of malignant neoplastic diseases

Aspects of the nature of neoplastic disease

This chapter deals in detail with the dozens of drugs now available for treating cancer and with their application, alone and in combination, to the chemotherapy of many different types of neoplastic diseases.* Before describing the specific antineoplastic drugs, this chapter will briefly describe the nature of cancer and some of the factors that medical oncologists must consider in planning to control cancer in their patients through the use of antineoplastic chemotherapeutic agents and other types of treatment.

Cancer incidence

Cancer can develop at any age but occurs most commonly among older people. Thus, as the proportion of elderly persons in the population has risen during this century, the number of new cases of cancer occurring in each decade has continued to increase steadily. During the 1980s, an estimated 700,000 Americans are expected to develop cancer annually; one in every four women and one in every five men will develop some form of malignancy during their lifetimes. The disease is expected to claim almost 400,000 lives in this country in each year of this decade—a number second only to the more than a million fatalities from coronary heart disease and other cardiovascular disorders.

Cancer characteristics

All cancers start with a single cell that is genetically different from those of other cells in the tissue in which it

arises. This abnormal cell transfers its fundamentally different properties to daughter cells and to their descendants. The tissues of such tumors, or neoplasms—literally, "new growths"—look and behave differently (in varying degrees) from the normal tissues in which they have their origin. Such cancerous tissues are characterized by *anaplasia:* a loss of cellular differentiation and organization. This, in turn, leads to the loss of their ability to function like the normal cells among which they originate and grow. Another characteristic of cancer cells is *autonomy:* the ability to grow without regard to the restrictions by which bodily homeostatic mechanisms control and limit the growth of normal tissues.

As the neoplastic cells grow aggressively and uncontrolled by such normal "stop" signals, they invade and destroy adjacent tissues. In addition to the damage that the primary tumor does to the local tissues surrounding it, its cells can spread to distant organs by way of the bloodstream or the lymphatic system (metastasize) and, if they find a favorable environment there, the disseminated cancer cells take root and form metastases, or secondary tumors. Thus, for example, malignant tumors that originate at such primary sites as the stomach, pancreas, or colon commonly metastasize to the liver. Breast cancers often travel to the lungs, bones, and brain, where their cells continue to proliferate and form secondary tumor masses.

Types of cancers

Cancers can be divided into solid tumors and into hematologic malignancies, such as the acute and chronic leukemias and the lymphomas, which have their origin in the blood-forming organs. Solid tumors, which can originate in any of the other organs of the body, may be subdivided into *carcinomas* and *sarcomas.* Carcinomas have their start in epithelial cells—for example, the glandular epithelium of the breast serves as the site for primary

---

* Cancer is not a single disease but is a general term employed for the many scores of malignant neoplasms, all of which have certain common characteristics but that also show vast individual differences in their growth patterns.

mammary adenocarcinoma; bronchogenic carcinoma arises in the epithelial cells lining the bronchial tubes; the squamous and basal cell epithelial types are the cause of skin cancers with different growth characteristics.

Sarcomas are malignancies that originate in the mesenchyma and are made up of embryonal connective tissue cells. Thus, osteogenic sarcomas are malignancies made up of the primitive cells from which bone and cartilage form (osteoblasts and chondroblasts), together with other connective tissue elements such as fibroblasts. Sarcomas also develop in soft tissue parts. Rhabdomyosarcomas are malignant tumors of striated muscle, derived from primitive mesenchymal cells of an anaplastic nature. One type is seen mainly in infants and young children.

Malignancies may also be subdivided into pediatric tumors—those that appear primarily in young children and adolescents—and into types of adult tumors differentiated on the basis of their primary site of origin in a particular system or organ—for example, gastrointestinal, genitourinary, head and neck, lung, or skin cancer. Still another type of tumor is trophoblastic in nature—that is, it is derived from cancer cells that have their origin in the fetal membranes of a fertilized ovum. For example, choriocarcinoma is a malignancy made up of abnormal trophoblastic cells—placental epithelial cells, which, instead of forming the fetal part of the placenta and serving to join the mother and child in the uterus, instead metastasize to the lungs and other maternal organs.

History and current status of cancer chemotherapy

History
Modern cancer chemotherapy dates from the discovery during the early 1940s that the chemical warfare agent called nitrogen mustard damaged not only normal cells but also certain types of cancer cells. This led to the synthesis and trial of numerous nitrogen mustard derivatives and other chemicals of several different classes, which were also found to have cytotoxic alkylating activity (see the discussion of alkylating agents, below). Early in the 1950s, introduction of the first *antimetabolites,* drugs that interfered with cancer cell utilization of such essential substances as the B-complex vitamin folic acid, began to change the outlook for children with acute lymphoblastic leukemia. Other antimetabolites in addition to these folic acid antagonists—for example, the purine analogue 6-mercaptopurine—helped to lengthen the life span of patients with this disease from a matter of a few weeks to many months or a year or more. During the 1960s and 1970s, whole new classes of drugs were developed that proved to be active against one or several neoplastic diseases—for example, potent cytotoxic antibiotics and plant alkaloids, as well as new synthetic chemicals.

Cancer chemotherapy was, until recently, used only to treat neoplastic diseases that were too widely disseminated to be responsive to surgical and radiation treatments, for many years the two main types of anti-cancer therapeutic modalities. Cytotoxic drugs were employed first for treating such hematologic malignancies as the leukemias, in which the cancer cells formed in the blood and lymphatic systems are spread throughout the patient's body from the beginning. Later, drug therapy was employed after it had become obvious that cells from primary solid tumors had spread widely even before the localized tumor had been removed by surgery or destroyed by radiation. In such situations, chemotherapy was employed only for palliative purposes—that is, for offering the patient some relief of the symptoms of the advanced metastatic disease.

Current status
During the past dozen or so years, progress in cancer chemotherapy, based on advances in molecular biology and on new knowledge of the nature of cell division, has helped oncologists to make more effective use of anti-cancer drugs. Drugs are now being employed alone and in combination with surgery, radiation and, occasionally, immunotherapy to provide not only palliation, but also more prolonged patient survival and, in some cases, cure—that is, normal life expectancy. The use of drugs with surgery, radiation, or both is referred to as *"combined modality" therapy.* Chemotherapy alone has, for example, produced permanent regression of choriocarcinoma in most drug-treated patients. Drugs are also considered the primary therapy for Burkitt's lymphoma, for which the survival rate is high; for multiple myeloma, in which patient survival time has been prolonged; and the leukemias. Most patients with acute myelocytic leukemia, for example, respond with remissions when treated with combinations of chemotherapeutic agents, and about half of those treated have survived for such prolonged periods that they are considered to be cured.

The types of cancers in which the use of drugs in combination with surgery or radiation has produced prolonged remission and possibly some cures include the pediatric diseases Wilms' tumor, Ewing's sarcoma, retinoblastoma, and embryonal rhabdomyosarcoma. Such lymphomatous disorders as advanced Hodgkin's disease, diffuse histiocytic lymphoma, and mycosis fungoides have also responded well to such a multimodal approach. Some advanced cases of embryonic testicular carcinoma have been halted and perhaps cured when the metastases were attacked with a combination of therapeutic modalities including chemotherapy.

Postoperative adjuvant chemotherapy
The effectiveness of chemotherapy as an adjuvant to surgery and radiation in the treatment of most solid tumors in adults cannot yet be considered to have been established. However, hopes are presently high that the ad-

ministration of chemotherapeutic agents shortly after the surgical removal of a cancerous breast may help to prevent a later recurrence of mammary carcinoma in an advanced metastatic form. The rationale for such adjuvant chemotherapy in patients judged at the time of surgery to have a high risk of developing recurrences of the cancer is that the drugs may be able to destroy the small numbers of cancer cells that may already have spread to distant sites as micrometastases preoperatively. This prevents them from proliferating to form tumor masses too large to be eliminated by later chemotherapy.

Because such adjuvant chemotherapy must be employed in the same large doses as when the drugs are being used for treating clinically apparent metastatic disease, it is possible that patients who may have already been cured by surgery or radiation alone could be exposed unnecessarily to the risks of severe drug toxicity. In addition, such adjuvant drug treatments may suppress the patient's immune system. This not only exposes the patient to the risk of infection but might also interfere with the body's own efforts to eliminate small numbers of remaining cancer cells by means of its own immune mechanisms. Thus, for example, results of some studies suggest that patients treated with drugs following surgical removal of a cancerous lung actually suffer more frequent recurrences of brain and other metastases than those who do not receive such adjuvant chemotherapy postoperatively.

Toxic effects of antineoplastic drugs

One of the main drawbacks of the cytotoxic drugs used in cancer chemotherapy is the fact that they act by mechanisms that cause similar damage to both neoplastic and some normal cells. The healthy cells of the host that are most likely to be injured by cancer chemotherapeutic agents are those with a naturally high rate of proliferation. The cells of such tissues as the bone marrow and the mucosal lining of the gastrointestinal tract are now known to grow and divide even more rapidly than the neoplastic cells of most solid tumors. Cells of hair follicles also divide rapidly.

Types of toxic effects

Bone marrow toxicity. Because of the limited selective toxicity of antineoplastic agents for cancer cells, these drugs often cause a dangerous drop in the formed elements of the circulating blood. Thus, to prevent drug-induced hematopoietic toxicity such as thrombocytopenia, leukopenia, and anemia, it is necessary to monitor closely the levels of leukocytes, platelets, and red cells in the peripheral blood during anticancer chemotherapy.

Drug therapy should be promptly discontinued when granulocyte counts fall to less than about 1000/mm³, because this—together with immunosuppressive effects of many of these drugs—leaves the patient susceptible to severe infection. Similarly, a drug-induced

drop in platelet levels to counts of less than 40,000/mm³ is an indication that the patient may soon suffer from spontaneous bleeding. Because the hematocrit often falls more gradually than the other blood elements, a lack of anemia signs is not a good index of the degree of bone marrow toxicity or of how close the patient is to developing severe hematopoietic toxicity. Interrupted treatment may often be resumed when platelet and leukocyte levels return toward normal as the bone marrow recovers.

Gastrointestinal toxicity. The most common drug-induced side-effects that occur early in treatment are anorexia, nausea and vomiting, and diarrhea. Nausea and vomiting are severe and occur in virtually 100% of patients who are given some of the antineoplastic drugs. Antiemetics such as *prochlorperazine* (Compazine) and *metoclopramide* (Reglan) are often given before and at appropriately timed intervals after antineoplastic therapy. In addition, Δ⁹-*tetrahydrocannabinol* (Δ⁹-THC), the chemical in marihuana that is responsible for most of its pharmacologic effects, is available in states that allow this use of THC from the National Cancer Institute, Bethesda, for use as an antiemetic in cancer patients whose nausea and vomiting caused by chemotherapy are not controlled by commercially available antiemetics. A synthetic congener of tetrahydrocannabinol called *nabilone* (Cesamet) is currently marketed for this purpose in some countries, and is expected to be approved soon for marketing in the United States.

Later manifestations of gastrointestinal toxicity include development of mucosal inflammation and ulcerations in the mouth (stomatitis), esophagus, stomach, intestine, and rectum (proctitis). Patients should receive close clinical checks to detect early signs of such tissue damage, because internal bleeding and even visceral perforations can occur unless cytotoxic drug treatment is promptly discontinued.

Difficulty in swallowing (dysphagia) and persistent nausea and other discomforts often tend to make patients consider stopping their medication. Astute nursing care can often help the patient and family through this difficult time. Support, encouragement, honest and frank patient teaching, and comfort measures (*e.g.*, oral hygiene, environment control, diet modification) are all vital aspects of drug therapy for these patients.

Hyperuricemia. The high turnover of neoplastic cells in some disorders, such as acute lymphoblastic leukemia, often leads to the development of hyperuricemia. In this and other types of cancers, including malignant lymphomas and multiple myeloma, the further increase in the number of cells destroyed by chemotherapy raises the risk of producing plasma uric acid levels so high that crystals of this catabolite of cellular nucleoproteins and purine bases may precipitate in the kidney tubules. To minimize the production of uric acid, it is desirable to administer the antigout drug, allopurinol (Zyloprim) (see

Chap. 38) to all patients whose serum uric acid level is high before treatment is begun or tends to become elevated during chemotherapy. It is also important to maintain a high intake of fluid to help keep uric acid in solution while it is being excreted by the kidneys, and systemic alkalinizers are also sometimes employed to alkalinize the urine and help to prevent uric acid nephropathy, a possible cause of kidney failure in some cases.

Other types of toxicity. Alopecia (loss of hair) occurs with certain classes of chemotherapeutic agents, while some side-effects are seen only with certain individual drugs. Alopecia occurs commonly in patients receiving cyclophosphamide, dactinomycin, doxorubicin, methotrexate, and vincristine—drugs that tend to damage the hair follicle cells of the scalp. The patient should be aware of the possibility of alopecia before the chemotherapy is begun. Many centers suggest that the patient select a wig or hair piece before the hair loss, because it is easier to match style and color beforehand. Patients need to know that their hair will grow back in time, and that the hair might grow in a different color or a different consistency than the original hair. Because of the psychological impact of this hair loss, much nursing research has been done on ways to minimize the loss and to help the patient to cope with this alteration in self-concept. Attempts have been made to ice the scalp during the chemotherapy to cause vasoconstriction and decrease the blood flow, therefore decreasing the dose of the drug reaching the hair follicles; others have used a tourniquet around the head, again to decrease the blood flow to the hair follicles. Neither procedure has proven to be consistently helpful in preventing the alopecia, but further research is being done. Emotional support and encouragement have proven to be very important in helping the patient and family cope with this change in personal image. Alopecia is now considered by the public to be a side-effect of chemotherapy in general. It is very important, therefore, to discuss this adverse effect as a part of patient teaching and to indicate if this side-effect is expected, or if the drugs being used are *not* usually associated with alopecia.

Unusual side-effects that are specific for certain drugs will be discussed later in this chapter and in the summary of adverse effects at the end of the chapter. Examples of these include cyclophosphamide-induced cystitis, the cardiac toxicity that occurs with the administration of doxorubicin after the total dose reaches a critical level, the pulmonary fibrosis that may appear during treatment with bleomycin or busulfan, and the signs of endocrine changes that are also sometimes seen with the latter drug. Peripheral neuropathy can occur with vincristine, and occasionally with vinblastine and procarbazine.

Some drugs, such as mechlorethamine and daunorubicin, can cause local irritation to the lining of the vein into which they are being injected and to surrounding tissues in the event of extravasation. Thus, to avoid thrombophlebitis, these irritating agents are best injected indirectly into a large vein that is receiving a rapidly running saline solution by making the injection into the tubing rather than directly into the venipuncture. If signs such as local itching, redness, and pain appear as a result of leakage, the infusion should be discontinued immediately to avoid a further inflammatory reaction, blistering of the skin and ulceration, and later sloughing. Application of cold compresses helps to lessen local discomfort, and the inflammatory reaction may be reduced by infiltration of hydrocortisone. However, warm compresses and injection of the enzyme hyaluronidase may be better for hastening the drug's absorption and removal from the local site.

Supportive therapy

Patients subject to the toxicity of cytotoxic drugs require many adjunctive therapeutic measures aimed at preventing and minimizing the complications of chemotherapy. As indicated above, the most dangerous drug-induced complications are infection and hemorrhage. Patients whose bone marrow has been infiltrated by tumor tissue are particularly prone to develop overwhelming infections and episodes of severe bleeding during drug therapy.

Patients must be watched carefully for signs of infection such as the sudden spiking of fever. After first taking cultures to identify the infecting organism and its susceptibility to antiinfective drugs, treatment to prevent septicemia and other life-threatening infections is promptly begun with combinations of the antibiotics considered most appropriate for counteracting both the gram-negative pathogens most commonly involved and others, such as protozoa and fungi. In some situations, patients receive transfusions of granulocytes to make up for the granulocytopenia that is both drug- and disease-induced.

Efforts are also made in some centers to minimize contamination of the cancer patient's environment by pathogens brought in from outside sources. These measures include the use of laminar air flow rooms and sometimes so-called Life Islands—enclosed areas that no one may enter. Necessary nursing and medical procedures are performed from outside the island through ports. These methods are said to have increased the number of infection-free days and to have reduced deaths from infection in children with leukemia who were receiving antileukemic chemotherapy.

The incidence of deaths from hemorrhage has also dropped with the introduction of procedures for collecting and transfusing packed platelets. These are transfused not only into patients who are already bleeding but also into those whose platelet counts are seen to fall below 40,000 mm^3, 30,000 mm^3, or 20,000 mm^3. Preventive transfusions of freshly collected platelets are more effective than attempts to treat patients who were hemorrhaging before the bleeding was discovered, and patients managed in this manner now often survive treatment with high doses of anticancer drugs.

Measures to prevent kidney damage secondary to hyperuricemia have been discussed above. In addition, it is important to keep patients well hydrated and in electrolyte balance for other reasons in addition to avoiding renal failure. This is particularly important in patients who become edematous and require diuretic therapy. Other considerations include maintenance of oral hygiene and prevention of constipation, hemorrhoids, and anal fissures. Centrally acting drugs employed for relief of pain, anxiety, and sleeplessness should be used in accordance with the principles that will be discussed elsewhere in this text. Measures to avoid development of skin infections and decubital ulcers are, of course, an important part of the nursing care of bedridden cancer patients, as are fostering activity and ambulation, where possible, and passive exercises and frequent turning to prevent thrombophlebitis, atelectasis, and contractures.

Supportive therapy includes not only physical but also psychological and emotional support and nutritional therapy. This is true for patients in every stage of illness, ranging from people who come to a hospital unit only for periodic diagnostic evaluations and treatment procedures while they are still essentially well, to patients in the terminal stages of their illness who are very close to death.

Oncology nurses are now playing increasingly important roles in teaching and counseling patients about various aspects of their disease and the problems that arise during its treatment. Ambulatory patients who are well enough to continue their normal activities need advice about how to cope with their diagnosis and with the adverse effects of chemotherapy and of other drugs that they may need for pain, nausea, and other symptoms. Nurses who care for terminally ill patients may help them and their families decide whether or not to continue therapy. If they decide to discontinue treatment, these patients and their families will require special support—physical, psychological, and emotional—that will need to be organized and provided by the entire health-care team.

Strategic principles of cancer chemotherapy

The aim of cancer chemotherapy is to destroy cancer cells without doing irreversible damage to too many of the patient's normal cells. However, most of the currently available cytotoxic agents can poison rapidly growing normal tissues almost as readily as they do the neoplastic cells. Thus, medical oncologists have tried to learn how to administer the drugs that seem most active against each type of cancer in doses and dosage schedules that will prove capable of killing the maximum number of cancer cells with minimal toxicity to normal tissues.

Advances in knowledge of cellular biology have helped scientists to understand the mechanisms by which cytotoxic drugs exert their effects. The various types of cancer chemotherapeutic agents act by interfering with the complex biologic processes by which cells grow and divide. Thus, for example, drugs may act to prevent replication of the genetic material deoxyribonucleic acid (DNA) or to interfere with mitosis, the process by which the doubled amount of DNA in a single malignant (or normal) cell is divided between two daughter cells.

Drugs that interfere with the synthesis of DNA or with mitosis are most active against those malignant tumors in which the cancer cells are proliferating rapidly—that is, those with a high proportion of cells undergoing division. Such drugs do not affect the fraction of the cell population that is in a resting stage and is not synthesizing DNA or dividing. Such nonproliferating cells are more drug-resistant and are best attacked with other drugs that can damage cancer cells without regard to whether or not they are actively dividing.

The cell cycle

All cells go through the same general processes of division even though the length of time it takes for the cycles of cells in different types of tissues to reach completion may differ considerably. After the cell has divided, each daughter cell goes into the G_1 phase, during which it synthesizes the substances needed for the formation of DNA. This is followed by the S phase, during which DNA is actively synthesized. When the cell has doubled its total DNA, it passes into the G_2 phase, during which the substances required for construction of the mitotic spindle are synthesized. Finally, in the M, or D, phase, the cell cycle is completed as the cell undergoes mitosis and divides into two more daughter cells.

Rapidly proliferating malignant cells have only a very short G_1 phase following mitosis, before they once again begin to synthesize DNA. On the other hand, in tumors with a slow rate of proliferation, a high proportion of the cells remain in a resting, or G_0, stage for prolonged periods. These cells are not affected by the cytotoxic drugs that injure dividing cells. However, the cells that are capable of surviving can be recruited back into the cell division cycle at some future time. Thus, these survivors can serve as the source of a whole new population of cancer cells that will cause relapses in patients who had seemed free of disease.

Drugs and the cell cycle

Knowledge of the mechanisms by which drugs act and of whether they affect specific phases of the cell cycle or are cytotoxic without regard to the phase of the cycle is of both theoretic and practical importance in planning treatment tactics in different types of cancer. Some chemotherapeutic agents are called *cell cycle-specific* or even *phase-specific*, because they are effective only when cancer cells are actively proliferating. Drugs of the *antimetabolite* type are, for example, most effective against cells that are in the S phase, or DNA-synthesizing phase, of the cell cycle. Similarly, the antineoplastic plant alkaloid *vincristine* is a phase-specific drug that damages cells during the G_2 and M phases of the cell cycle, because it exerts its highest activity while the cells are synthesizing the substances required for mitosis to occur.

Because of their high activity against the so-called *growth fraction* of the cancer cell population, these cell cycle-specific and phase-specific agents are often useful for treating rapidly growing tumors. However, they do not affect that proportion of the cancer cell population that is in the dormant, or G_0, stage. Similarly, these agents are generally not very effective against slowly growing or old tumors, in which a relatively high proportion of the cancer cells are in a resting, or nonproliferating, stage. Such tumors are best attacked initially with those types of chemotherapeutic agents that are active regardless of whether or not the cancer cells are actively dividing.

Such *cell cycle-nonspecific*, or *cell cycle-independent*, drugs include the alkylating agents and certain antineoplastic antibiotics such as *dactinomycin*, which bind to and react with already preformed macromolecules (such as DNA) within cancer cells. These agents are often used for initiating therapy of large, slowly growing tumors to reduce the number of resting cancer cells that make up the bulk of the tumor. This may then lead to more of the remaining cells being recruited into the cell division cycle. As they pass from the G_0 resting stage into such active phases as the S phase, G_2 phase, and M phase, these cells become more vulnerable to the cell cycle-specific or

phase-specific drugs, which can then be added to the regimen. Figure 12-1 illustrates the cell cycle and mechanisms of action of some antineoplastic drugs described in this chapter.

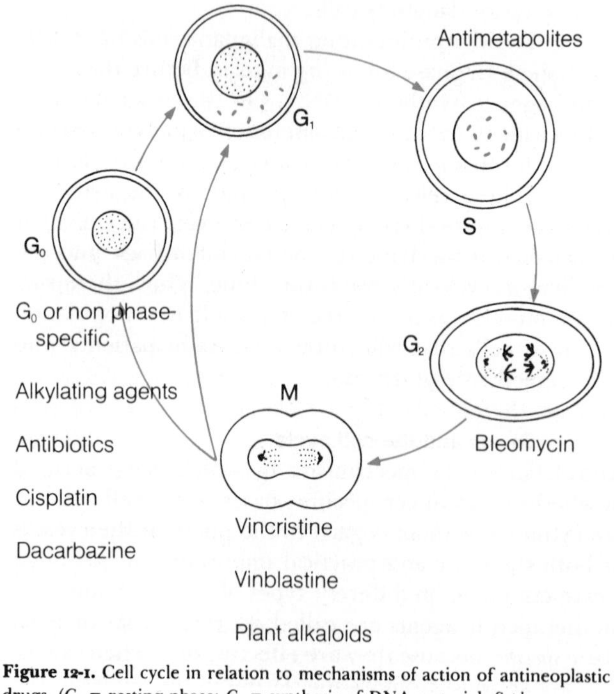

Combination chemotherapy

During the past dozen or so years, it has become clear that many types of cancers respond better to treatment with carefully selected combinations of active drugs than to the administration of a single agent. The main problem with single-drug therapy is that the drug must usually be given in very high, potentially toxic, doses to be effective. An advantage of giving two or more drugs with different types of toxicity to normal cells simultaneously, or in close sequence, is that the degree of effectiveness against the cancer cells is increased while toxicity to normal tissues is reduced. Another advantage of combining drugs with different mechanisms of action or drugs of both the cell cycle-specific and cell cycle-*non*-specific types is that the emergence of resistant clones of cancer cells is delayed or prevented.

Dosage scheduling

Clinical trials of combinations of various types of drugs in accordance with different types of treatment protocols have revealed that the timing and size of doses is often crucial in determining the effectiveness and safety of chemotherapy in different malignancies. The medical oncologist tries to take advantage of the fact that normal bone marrow and mucosal cells possess homeostatic growth-stimulating mechanisms that help them to recover more readily from drug-induced injury than do the cancer cells. Such recovery occurs best when drugs are given intermittently in high doses rather than as small daily doses. Similarly, the patient's immune system recovers more readily when high doses of chemotherapeutic agents are administered at appropriate intervals rather than continuously.

Although the chemotherapist tries to plan dosage scheduling on the basis of the previously discussed theoretic considerations, very little is really known about the optimal times for interactions between the many different types of chemotherapeutic agents and the scores of neoplastic diseases with their differing rates of cell growth. Thus, in practice, no single combination of drugs or type of dosage scheduling is universally accepted as ideal for treating any kind of cancer. Each specialist and each cancer center is constantly engaged in clinical trials of cancer chemotherapy from which new useful information is painfully gained empirically—that is, by actual trial and error experience rather than on the basis of theoretic considerations.

Future prospects

Further advances in cancer chemotherapy depend on new discoveries about the nature of cancer. Thus, for example,

Figure 12-1. Cell cycle in relation to mechanisms of action of antineoplastic drugs. (G_0 = resting phase; G_1 = synthesis of DNA material; *S phase* = active DNA synthesis; G_2 = mitotic spindle synthesis; M = mitosis, cell division)

much remains to be learned about differences in the cycles of malignant and normal cells. Such basic knowledge of cell biology could then be applied in devising dosage schedules that would exert the greatest degree of effectiveness against cancer cells with the least toxicity to vulnerable normal cells. Similarly, because chemotherapy alone is not likely to cure most types of primary or advanced cancers, clinical research must aim to learn how drugs can best be combined with such other therapeutic modalities as surgery and radiation—for example, how best to use adjunctive chemotherapy (see above). New information about how to protect the patient's own immunologic defenses from injury by cytotoxic drugs and how to stimulate production of anticancer antibodies by adjunctive immunotherapeutic measures may also lead to an increase in the number of cancer patients cured by multiple modality therapy. Also, of course, because drugs and other forms of therapy are most effective when the number of cancer cells is relatively small and localized, the development of laboratory tests for detecting the presence of cancer cells before any clinical signs or symptoms of early disease are evident should also prove helpful for increasing the effectiveness of cancer therapy. Finally, as more is learned about the nature of cancer, more will also be learned about preventing the disease. Carcinogens will be identified, as will be measures that can be taken to prevent the growth of neoplasms in people who are at risk. In the distant future, chemotherapy in cancer may become a preventive modality.

Antineoplastic agents

The antineoplastic drugs may be divided into several classes, based on what is believed to be the predominant mechanism by which they produce toxic effects on neoplastic and normal cells (*e.g.*, alkylating agents, antimetabolites), their availability from natural sources (*e.g.*, antineoplastic antibiotics, plant alkaloids, enzymes), and their endocrine activity—that is, their ability to mimic or interfere with the influence of endogenous hormones on hormone-sensitive malignancies. Nonhormonal agents with antineoplastic activity include the radioactive isotopes and certain synthetic chemicals, which at present cannot be readily classified and are listed separately.

Many antineoplastic drugs are classified differently by different authorities. For example, carmustine and lomustine, which are classed as alkylating agents by some and in this text, are classed as "other synthetic

antineoplastic drugs" by others who doubt that their activity as alkylating agents accounts primarily for their antineoplastic activity. Similarly, streptozocin, which is classified as an alkylating agent in this text and elsewhere, is categorized by others as a natural product, which it is, because it is made by molds of the same genus that produces the antibacterial antibiotic streptomycin. Estramustine has both hormonal (estrogenic) and alkylating actions, and may be classified with either group of agents (in this text it is classified as a hormone). Where such controversy exists regarding the classification of a drug, this text will place it in the class that facilitates learning its clinically significant points, especially its toxicity.

In the following discussions of individual drugs in the several classes, emphasis will be placed mainly on those properties of each that account for differences in its indications, adverse effects, and routes of administration from those of other drugs of the same and different classes. Detailed information about dosage and administration of some drugs is found in their drug digests. (Actually, however, so many different treatment protocols are in use at present that it is not possible to offer enough dosage details in a general textbook chapter. Thus, those who require detailed dosage data for drugs employed in a particular center must consult the protocols of that center.)

Table 12-1 lists the antineoplastic drugs currently used, along with their dosage and main clinical indications; a summary at the end of the chapter presents the specific toxic effects of individual antineoplastic agents. Table 12-2 summarizes the current status of the chemotherapy of various types of cancers.

Alkylating agents*

These drugs are of somewhat diverse chemical structure, and are sometimes referred to by a name that denotes the chemical class to which they belong. Thus, mechlorethamine, cyclophosphamide, chlorambucil, melphalan, and uracil mustard are *nitrogen mustards,* and carmustine, lomustine, semustine, and streptozocin are *nitrosoureas.* The other alkylating agents do not fall into any major chemical group.

Mechanism of action. Cytotoxic agents of this type produce their cell-poisoning effects by their ability to react chemically and combine with portions of such cellular macromolecules as DNA, RNA, and proteins. The most significant of several potential cell-damaging actions of these drugs stems from their interaction with the DNA molecules of neoplastic and normal cells. Such cells may then be injured in any phase of the cell cycle, including the resting phase.

These cell cycle *non*phase-specific drugs are often effective against slow-growing tumors in which a high proportion of the cells is in a *non*reproducing state of activity—for example, chronic leukemias, multiple my-

(Text continues p. 270)

---

* The compounds in each of the several chemical subclasses of the alkylating agents have in common the capacity to insert alkyl groups into organic compounds. (Alkyl moieties are monovalent radicals formed by the loss of a single hydrogen atom from an aliphatic hydrocarbon.) The substitution of an alkyl group for an active hydrogen atom of biologically active macromolecules by the alkylating agent interferes with their ability to function normally. This, in turn, prevents the cells that then contain damaged DNA or other altered macromolecules from continuing to carry on processes essential to proliferation and life.

Table 12–1. Antineoplastic agents for cancer chemotherapy

Generic or official name	Trade name or synonym	Usual adult dosage range*	Primary clinical considerations
Alkylating agents			
Busulfan USP	Myleran	4–8 mg orally per day	Chronic myelocytic leukemia
Carmustine	BiCNU; BCNU	200 mg/m² IV every 6 wk	Brain tumors; Hodgkin's disease and non-Hodgkin's lymphomas; multiple myeloma
Chlorambucil USP	Leukeran	4–10 mg orally per day	Chronic lymphocytic leukemia; Hodgkin's disease and other malignant lymphomas
Cyclophosphamide USP	Cytoxan	40–50 mg/kg body weight IV in divided doses over a period of several days, then adjusted to lower maintenance dosage; oral maintenance therapy 1–5 mg/kg body weight daily	Acute and chronic lymphoblastic leukemia and other leukemias; Hodgkin's disease and other malignant lymphomas; mycosis fungoides; neuroblastoma; retinoblastoma; ovarian adenocarcinoma and other solid tumors
Lomustine	CeeNU; CCNU	130 mg/m² orally every 6 wk; or adjust later doses in accordance with response	Brain tumors and Hodgkin's disease as secondary therapy
Mechlorethamine USP	Mustargen; nitrogen mustard	200–600 μg/kg IV in single or divided doses	Hodgkin's disease and other malignant lymphomas
Melphalan USP	Alkeran; L-phenyl-alanine mustard; L-PAM; L-sarco-lysin	6 mg orally for 2 to 3 wk; maintenance, 2 mg daily	Multiple myeloma
Mitobronitol†	DBM; Myelo-bromol; dibro-momannitol	250 mg/m² for 3 days, then 150 mg/m² until remission	Chronic myelocytic leukemia
Pipobroman USP	Vercyte	Initially 1–3 mg/kg body weight orally per day, with very widely variable maintenance doses	Polycythemia vera; chronic myelocytic leukemia
Semustine†	Methyl-CCNU	200 mg/m² orally every 6 wk	Brain tumors; Hodgkin's disease; malignant melanoma; gastric and colorectal adenocarcinoma
Streptozocin	Streptozotocin; Zanosar	1 gm/m² IV weekly for 4 wk	Metastatic pancreatic islet cell carcinoma; malignant carcinoid
Thiotepa USP	Triethylene-thio-phosphoramide; TSPA; TESPA	IV 60 mg initially at 1- to 4-wk intervals usually, or at 5-day intervals in lung cancer; also by intratumor and intracavitary administration	For palliation and control of effusions in breast, ovary, and lung cancer
Uracil mustard USP		1–2 mg orally; or 3–5 mg orally for only 7 days; maintenance, 1 mg daily	Chronic lymphocytic leukemia; lymphomas; polycythemia vera; mycosis fungoides

Table 12–1. Antineoplastic agents for cancer chemotherapy (continued)

Generic or official name	Trade name or synonym	Usual adult dosage range*	Primary clinical considerations
Antimetabolites			
5-Azacitidine†	5-AZC; Ladakamycin	50–400 mg/m² IV	Acute myelocytic leukemia
Cytarabine HCl USP	Cytosar; cytosine arabinoside	2 mg/kg body weight IV for 10 days; raised to 4 mg/kg for maintenance, if necessary	Acute myelocytic leukemia of adults; other leukemias of children and adults
Floxuridine	FUDR	0.1–0.6 mg/kg body weight daily by continuous arterial infusion	Carcinoma of the liver and other organs
Fluorouracil USP	5-FU; Adrucil	12 mg/kg body weight IV for 4 days followed by 6 mg/kg on alternate days through the twelfth day; also by topical application to the skin twice daily for several weeks	Carcinoma of the colon, rectum, breast, stomach, and pancreas; also, topically against solar keratoses
Mercaptopurine USP	Purinethol; 6-MP	2.5 mg/kg body weight daily orally (about 50–100 mg for adults, 50 mg for children)	Acute lymphocytic leukemia; chronic myelocytic leukemia
Methotrexate USP	Amethopterin; MTX; Mexate	2.5–5.0 mg/kg body weight daily orally or parenterally for leukemia; 15–30 mg orally or IM for 5 days in choriocarcinoma	Acute lymphoblastic leukemia; choriocarcinoma; mycosis fungoides; advanced lymphosarcoma; also in severe, disabling psoriasis not responsive to other treatments
Tegafur†	Furanidyl-5-fluorouracil; Ftorafur	2 g/m² IV daily for 5 days every 2 to 4 wk	Colorectal adenocarcinoma
Thioguanine USP	6-TG	2 mg/kg body weight daily orally	Acute myelocytic leukemia
Anticancer agents from natural sources (Antibiotics, alkaloids, enzymes)			
Asparaginase	Elspar; L-asparagine amidohydrolase	1000 IU/kg/day IV for 10 successive days; or 6000 IU/m² IM intermittently in accordance with various dosage schedules in which it is given in combination with other antineoplastic drugs	Acute lymphocytic leukemia
Bleomycin sulfate	Blenoxane; BLM	0.25–0.5 U/kg body weight, or 10–20 units/m² IV, IM, or SC, weekly or twice weekly	Squamous cell carcinoma; lymphosarcoma; reticulum cell sarcoma; testicular sarcoma; Hodgkin's disease
Dactinomycin USP	Actinomycin D; Cosmegen	0.015–0.05 mg/kg body weight IV in divided dosage over 1 wk; repeat for 3 to 5 wk; repeat course after recovery	Wilms' tumor; testicular carcinoma; choriocarcinoma; rhabdomyosarcoma; Ewing's sarcoma; osteogenic and other sarcomas

(continued)

Table 12–1. Antineoplastic agents for cancer chemotherapy (continued)

Generic or official name	Trade name or synonym	Usual adult dosage range*	Primary clinical considerations
Daunorubicin	Daunomycin; Cerubidine; DNR	30–60 mg/m² IV daily for 3 days or weekly	Acute myelocytic and lymphocytic leukemias; neuroblastoma
Doxorubicin HCl	Adriamycin; ADR	60–75 mg/m² IV at intervals of 21 days; or 30 mg/m² on each of 3 successive days repeated every 4 wk	Acute lymphoblastic and myelocytic leukemias; neuroblastoma; soft tissue and bone sarcomas; Hodgkin's and non-Hodgkin's-type lymphomas; carcinomas of breast, ovary, bladder, lung; and other solid tumors
Mitomycin	Mutamycin	20 mg/m² IV as a single dose; or 2 mg/m² IV daily for 5 days, repeated after a drug-free interval of 2 days	Combined with other chemotherapeutic agents for therapy of metastasized adenocarcinoma of the stomach or pancreas
Plicamycin (formerly called mithramycin)	Mithracin	25–30 μg/kg body weight daily by slow IV for 8 to 10 days; also 25 μg/kg for 3 to 4 days	Various types of testicular tumors; also for reversal of hypercalcemia and hypercalciuria
Vinblastine sulfate USP	Velban; VLB	0.1 mg/kg body weight increased weekly by 0.05 mg/kg, up to 0.5 mg/kg	Hodgkin's disease and other lymphomas; choriocarcinoma; reticulum cell sarcoma; breast and testicular carcinoma, and others
Vincristine sulfate USP	Oncovin; VCR	2 mg/m² for children; 1.4 mg/m² for adults	Acute lymphoblastic leukemia; lymphosarcoma; Hodgkin's disease; reticulum cell sarcoma, rhabdomyosarcoma; neuroblastoma, and others

Hormones

Adrenocorticosteroid drugs (Examples)

Prednisolone sodium succinate USP	Meticortelone soluble	10–100 mg orally	Acute and late chronic lymphocytic leukemia; Hodgkin's disease; lymphosarcoma; carcinoma of the lung or breast
Prednisone USP	Deltasone; Meticorten	10–100 mg orally	

Androgenic drugs

Calusterone	Methosarb	200 mg orally	Advanced, inoperable, or metastatic carcinoma of the breast

Table 12–1. Antineoplastic agents for cancer chemotherapy (continued)

Generic or official name	Trade name or synonym	Usual adult dosage range*	Primary clinical considerations
Dromostanolone propionate USP	Drolban	100 mg IM three times weekly for 8 to 12 wk	All used for treating disseminated carcinoma of the breast in premenopausal women, often after ovariectomy and sometimes after adrenalectomy; testolactone, which is claimed to be free of virilizing properties, is also recommended for use in postmenopausal women with advanced or disseminated breast cancer when hormone treatment is indicated
Fluoxymesterone USP	Android-F; Halotestin	20–30 mg orally for maintenance of remissions	
Testolactone	Teslac	100 mg IM three times weekly or 50 mg orally three times daily	
Testosterone cypionate USP	Depo-Testosterone	200–400 mg IM every 2 to 4 wk	
Testosterone enanthate USP	Delatestryl	200–400 mg IV every 2 to 4 wk	
Testosterone propionate USP	—	100 mg IM three times weekly	

Female sex hormones

Estrogens (Examples)

Diethylstilbestrol USP	DES; Stilbestrol	15 mg/day orally	Advanced breast cancer in men and postmenopausal women
		1–3 mg/day orally	Advanced prostatic carcinoma
Diethylstilbestrol diphosphate	Stilphostrol	50–200 mg tid orally; 0.5–1 g/day IV	Advanced prostatic carcinoma
Estramustine phosphate sodium	Emcyt	14 mg/kg/day orally in three or four divided doses	Advanced prostatic carcinoma
Ethinyl estradiol USP	Estinyl	1 mg tid orally	Advanced breast cancer in postmenopausal women
		0.5–2 mg/day orally	Advanced prostatic carcinoma
Polyestradiol phosphate	Estradurin	40–80 mg IM every 2–4 wk	Advanced prostatic carcinoma

Progestins

Hydroxyprogesterone caproate USP	Delalutin	0.5–1.5 g IM twice weekly	Advanced adenocarcinoma of uterus
Medroxyprogesterone acetate USP	Provera; Depo-Provera	400–800 mg IM twice weekly or 200–300 mg orally every day	Recurrent and metastatic endometrial and renal carcinoma
Megestrol acetate	Megace; Pallace	40 mg orally in divided daily doses	Recurrent and metastatic breast and endometrial carcinoma

Adrenal suppressants

Aminoglutethimide	Cytadren	250 mg q 6 hr	Used to suppress adrenal cortex function in postmenopausal breast cancer and in metastatic prostatic cancer

(continued)

Table 12–1. Antineoplastic agents for cancer chemotherapy (continued)

Generic or official name	Trade name or synonym	Usual adult dosage range*	Primary clinical considerations
Mitotane	Lysodren; o,p'-DDD	8–10 g orally per day	Carcinoma of the adrenal cortex
Antiestrogen			
Tamoxifen citrate	Nolvadex	10–20 mg twice daily, morning and evening	Advanced breast cancer in postmenopausal women, especially those with positive estrogen receptor assay
Miscellaneous synthetic chemotherapeutic agents			
Cisplatin	Platinol; cis-di-aminedichloro-platinum; cis-DDP	50–80 mg/m² IV once every 3 wk intravenously; and by other dosage schedules	Ovarian, testicular, and bladder carcinoma
Dacarbazine	DTIC; DIC	2–4.5 mg/kg/day IV for a 10-day course, or 250 mg/m²/day IV for 5 days	Metastatic malignant melanoma
Etoposide	VePesid	50–100 mg/m²/day IV on days 1, 3, and 5 every 3 or 4 wk in combination with other drugs	Approved for use in refractory testicular tumors; also effective in small cell lung cancer
Hydroxyurea USP	Hydrea	20–30 mg/kg body weight orally each day, or 80 mg/kg every third day	Chronic myelocytic leukemia; melanoma
Procarbazine	Matulane	2–4 mg/kg body weight/day orally initially; then maintained at 4–6 mg/kg/day until toxicity or maximum response occurs; maintain at 1–2 mg/kg/day	Hodgkin's disease
Radioactive isotopes			
Chromic phosphate P32	Phosphocol P32	6–20 mc intrapleurally or intraperitoneally	For pleural effusions and ascites caused by cancer
Sodium iodide I131 solution USP	Iodotope	4–10 mc orally for hyperthyroidism; 50–150 mc for thyroid carcinoma	For hyperthyroidism and thyroid carcinoma
Sodium phosphate P32 solution USP	Phosphotope	6–15 mc orally; 1–8 mc IV	For chronic leukemia and polycythemia vera

* These drugs are seldom given alone; they are usually given in a combination protocol. The dosage of each drug used will vary with the combination, the disease being treated, and the particular patient involved. These dosage ranges are some *usual* protocols that may be seen.
† Investigational drug, available in the United States only from the National Cancer Institute.

Table 12–2. Current status of chemotherapy of various types of cancer

Type of neoplastic malignancy	Primarily preferred programs	Secondary drugs active against the disease	Comments
Hematologic malignancies			
Acute lymphocytic leukemia (ALL)	Induction of remission: prednisone and vincristine CNS prophylaxis: methotrexate, intrathecal plus cranial irradiation Maintenance of remission: mercaptopurine (daily); methotrexate and cyclophosphamide intermittently	Daunorubicin Cyclophosphamide Asparaginase Cytarabine Thioguanine	Initial complete remissions can be induced in up to 90% of cases; prolonged survival is possible with proper maintenance therapy; about 50% of patients have survived for 5 years or more, but the median survival rate at present is between 24 and 48 months
Acute myelocytic leukemia (AML)	Induction of remission: cytarabine and daunorubicin with or without thioguanine Maintenance of remission: same as above	5-Azacitidine	Combination chemotherapy produces remissions in over 50% of patients; maintenance with various drug combinations is under experimental investigation
Chronic lymphocytic leukemia (CLL)	Chlorambucil alone, or combined with prednisone	Cyclophosphamide Vincristine	Patients live 7 to 10 years or more when maintained with an alkylating agent and local radiation therapy
Chronic myelocytic leukemia (CML) Stable phase	Busulfan	Mercaptopurine Mitobronitol Hydroxyurea Melphalan Thioguanine 5-Azacitidine	Disease can be controlled for long periods by chemotherapy and splenic irradiation or splenectomy
Acute phase	Daunorubicin and cytarabine and vincristine and prednisone, with or without thioguanine		
Multiple myeloma (plasma cell myeloma)	Melphalan and prednisone, or cyclophosphamide and prednisone	Carmustine Lomustine Vincristine Doxorubicin	Early initiation of chemotherapy often produces remission and lengthens life; supportive therapy for control of complications is important
Polycythemia vera	Radioactive phosphorus (^{32}P)		Chemotherapy is no longer recommended following phlebotomy (venesection)

(continued)

Table 12–2. Current status of chemotherapy of various types of cancer (continued)

Type of neoplastic malignancy	Primarily preferred programs	Secondary drugs active against the disease	Comments
Mycosis fungoides	Combination chemotherapy, as in Hodgkin's disease		Skin signs and symptoms of this type of lymphoma also require drugs for symptomatic relief of pruritis and irradiation of plaques
Burkitt's tumor or lymphoma	Cyclophosphamide with or without vincristine and methotrexate	Methotrexate Carmustine	Can be cured by single-drug therapy if diagnosed in its early localized stages
Hodgkin's disease	The MOPP combination: mechlorethamine, vincristine, procarbazine, prednisone	The ABVD combination: doxorubicin, bleomycin, vinblastine, dacarbazine; other active drugs include carmustine, lomustine, hexamethylmelamine, streptozocin	The MOPP combination has produced complete remissions in advanced (stages III and IV) cases; many of these remissions are prolonged and may be maintained by further treatment; in relapsed cases, treatment with combinations contain-ing chemotherapeutic agents not previously employed often reinduces remission and possible cure
Non-Hodgkin's lymphomas such as malignant lymphomas of the lymphocytic, histiocytic, (*e.g.*, reticulum cell sarcoma), and mixed types	Several complex combinations are used, each of which is made up of four to six of the following drugs: cyclophosphamide, doxorubicin, vincristine, prednisone, bleomycin, methotrexate, cytarabine		Combination chemotherapy has produced prolonged remissions in up to 70% of patients in advanced stages, with possible cure in some cases; results are somewhat better in lymphocytic nodular-type lymphomas than in diffuse histiocytic types

Solid malignant tumors

Pediatric types (in children and adolescents)

Embryonal rhabdomyosarcoma	Combinations of dactinomycin, vincristine, and cyclophosphamide with or without doxorubicin	Methotrexate Thiotepa	Chemotherapy combined with surgery and radiation has helped to lengthen the survival rate

Table 12–2. Current status of chemotherapy of various types of cancer (continued)

Type of neoplastic malignancy	Primarily preferred programs	Secondary drugs active against the disease	Comments
Ewing's sarcoma	Combinations of vincristine, cyclophosphamide, and doxorubicin	Dactinomycin	Chemotherapy combined with radiotherapy has produced lengthened periods of remission
Wilms' tumor	Combinations of dactinomycin and vincristine	Doxorubicin Cyclophosphamide	The rate of cures has increased to 90% as the result of adding chemotherapy to surgery and radiotherapy
Neuroblastoma	Combinations of cyclophosphamide and doxorubicin or vincristine	Daunorubicin Dacarbazine Mechlorethamine, vinblastine, prednisone, and cisplatin	Chemotherapy is being employed as an adjunct to surgery and radiation in advanced cases
Retinoblastoma	Combinations of cyclophosphamide and doxorubicin		Chemotherapy is employed following enucleation in patients with poor prognosis according to current staging classifications
Osteogenic sarcoma	Doxorubicin and high-dose methotrexate followed by leukovorin rescue; bleomycin, cyclophosphamide, and dactinomycin may be added singly or in combination	Melphalan, cisplatin, and mitomycin	Adjunctive chemotherapy following surgery has produced prolonged remissions and possible cures in patients with and without metastases

Types occurring primarily in adults

Breast cancer	*Nonhormonal* chemotherapeutic combinations made up of three to five of the following drugs: cyclophosphamide, methotrexate, fluorouracil, and prednisone; or doxorubicin and cyclophosphamide in combination with or without fluorouracil	Combination of drugs from the preferred group, which were not used previously as primary therapy; other active drugs, including vinblastine, vincristine, mitomycin, and aminoglutethimide	Combination chemotherapy produces palliative responses in 50% to 70% of patients with metastatic breast cancer; single agents are being tested as adjuncts to surgical and radiation therapy of primary breast cancer
	Hormonal therapies, where indicated, include those for (a) *pre*menopausal women—androgens		Hormone and antihormone therapies are likely to be useful mainly in patients whose tumor tissues

(continued)

Table 12–2. Current status of chemotherapy of various types of cancer (continued)

Type of neoplastic malignancy	Primarily preferred programs	Secondary drugs active against the disease	Comments
	(see Table 12–1); and for (b) *post*menopausal women—estrogens with or without progestins (see Table 12–1), but also antiestrogens (tamoxifen) in some cases		contain estrogen receptors
Colorectal carcinoma	Fluorouracil alone or in combination with semustine	Lomustine Mitomycin Semustine Tegafur	Response rate in recurrent or metastatic cases is between 15% and 30%; adjuvant chemotherapy is being employed experimentally following surgery
Gastric adenocarcinoma	Fluorouracil in combination with doxorubicin and mitomycin or semustine		Response rate with new combinations has risen to 40% in some studies as compared with only 15% to 20% previously when fluorouracil alone was employed for palliation of advanced cases
Bronchogenic carcinoma (lung cancer)			
Small or oat cell type	Cyclophosphamide in combination with doxorubicin and vincristine	Cyclophosphamide with lomustine and methotrexate	The combination chemotherapy has moderate activity in this form of lung cancer
Squamous cell and other types	Doxorubicin and cyclophosphamide and cisplatin	Methotrexate Lomustine Fluorouracil Mitomycin	Response rates with combination chemotherapy seem better than with single drugs; however, survival time is not significantly improved
Uterus			
Cervical carcinoma	Cisplatin with or without methotrexate and bleomycin	Cyclophosphamide Mitomycin Vincristine	Combination chemotherapy has moderate activity in both forms of uterine cancer
Endometrial carcinoma	Megestrol acetate; medroxyprogesterone; hydroxyprogesterone caproate	Fluorouracil Tamoxifen	

Table 12–2. Current status of chemotherapy of various types of cancer (continued)

Type of neoplastic malignancy	Primarily preferred programs	Secondary drugs active against the disease	Comments
Choriocarcinoma (and other trophoblastic-type tumors)	Methotrexate alone in low-risk patients, or combined with dactinomycin in high-risk cases	Vinblastine Chlorambucil Bleomycin Cisplatin	Complete prolonged remissions occur in 90% of patients who receive early treatment; results in patients with metastasized disease are also good
Prostatic carcinoma	Diethylstilbestrol; ethinyl estradiol, and other estrogenic hormones such as estramustine	Doxorubicin Cyclophosphamide Fluorouracil Cisplatin	Good responses occur initially in 80% or more of patients treated with hormones; response rates to nonhormonal chemotherapeutic agents range between 20% and 40%
Ovarian carcinoma	Melphalan or cyclophosphamide with or without cisplatin and doxorubicin	Hexamethylmelamine Fluorouracil Chlorambucil Thiotepa Megestrol acetate	Alkylating agents produce initial responses in more than half the patients, fewer relapsing patients respond; however, the survival rate is increased and palliation is good
Testicular cancers	Vinblastine combined with bleomycin and cisplatin	Vinblastine combined with dactinomycin, bleomycin, cyclophosphamide and cisplatin (VAB-6)	Combination chemotherapy produces complete and prolonged remissions and even cures in some cases; however, toxic reactions are common
Bladder cancer	Cisplatin, doxorubicin, or both	Fluorouracil Methotrexate Mitomycin instillation Cyclophosphamide Thiotepa instillation	Response rates of about 35% have been reported in recent studies
Brain tumors	Vincristine and carmustine with or without mechlorethamine and methotrexate	Mechlorethamine and vincristine and procarbazine and prednisone (MOPP)	Primary drugs produce some improvement in a small minority of patients
Malignant melanoma	Dacarbazine or semustine	Dactinomycin	Responses occur in about 20% to 25% of patients; adjunctive immunotherapy is being employed experimentally

(continued)

Table 12–2. Current status of chemotherapy of various types of cancer (continued)

Type of neoplastic malignancy	Primarily preferred programs	Secondary drugs active against the disease	Comments
Head and neck squamous cell carcinomas	Bleomycin and cisplatin with or without methotrexate	Vinblastine Cyclophosphamide Doxorubicin Fluorouracil Mitomycin	Combinations of drugs have moderate activity
Adrenocortical carcinoma	Mitotane	Doxorubicin Aminoglutethimide	Chemotherapy is moderately effective
Sarcomas of soft tissue parts	Doxorubicin with or without dacarbazine plus vincristine plus cyclophosphamide	Methotrexate	Adjuvant chemotherapy (and immunotherapy) are being tried following surgery and radiation therapy

eloma, Hodgkin's disease and other malignant lymphomas.

One problem with these drugs, as with antineoplastic drugs of other classes, is that cancer cells develop resistance to them. Cancer cells develop resistance to alkylating agents by becoming less permeable to them or by producing an increased number of molecules—other than DNA—that react with drug molecules and prevent these drug molecules from interacting with DNA.

Pharmacokinetic factors. Although all the chemicals that possess alkylating activity have a similar general mechanism of action, the individual drugs differ in their suitability for use against specific kinds of cancer, in the manner in which they are best administered, and in various of the adverse effects that they can cause. The main reason for these differences is that the several classes of alkylating chemicals have molecular structures that are quite variable. Thus, their physiocochemical properties differ, as do the ways in which they are handled by the body. As a result, some are readily absorbed from the gastrointestinal tract when administered orally, while others must be given intravenously because they are so irritating (mechlorethamine is a vesicant—it causes blistering) or because they are so rapidly taken up by and metabolized in tissues (carmustine).

Similarly, these drugs vary in lipid solubility. Most are not very lipid-soluble and do not penetrate the blood–brain barrier very well, so they are not useful in treating primary or metastatic brain tumors. The nitrosourea drugs—carmustine, lomustine, and semustine—are an exception; they penetrate the blood–brain barrier well. Streptozocin, another nitrosourea, has a special affinity for cells of pancreatic islet cell tumors, both those that are secreting insulin and those that are nonfunctional.

Although most alkylating agents do not penetrate the central nervous system well, all can and do cause nausea and vomiting (streptozocin does in virtually *all* patients). This effect is very important clinically and has been attributed to effects of the drugs in the central nervous system, perhaps on the chemoreceptor trigger zone and vomiting center, structures that are not protected by the blood–brain barrier.

Toxicity. In addition to nausea and vomiting, these drugs as a group depress the blood cell-forming tissues, cause amenorrhea and depress spermatogenesis, and damage cells of the gastrointestinal tract and hair follicles. In addition, the long-term use of some of these drugs (*e.g.*, the use of chlorambucil to treat polycythemia vera) has been associated with an increased incidence of leukemia and other tumors.

The following discussions of the individual alkylating agents are limited to indicating clinically important differences among these drugs in regard to their toxicity, administration, and usefulness.

Nitrogen mustards

Mechlorethamine[+] (Mustargen) was one of the first chemicals found useful for treating cancer. Its main use is in the treatment of Hodgkin's disease and other lymphomas. It is usually employed in combination with several other classes of antineoplastic agents; for example, it is the first drug in the MOPP regimen (*m*echlorethamine, *O*ncovin— a brand name for vincristine, *p*rocarbazine, and *p*rednisone). It has largely been superseded by other drugs in treating leukemias and solid tumors. It causes a high incidence of nausea and vomiting, and it causes leukopenia and thrombocytopenia, which limit the doses of drug that can be given.

Mechlorethamine must be injected intravenously in the form of a freshly prepared solution, taking care to avoid letting it leak into surrounding tissues, because the chemical can cause severe local reactions. This vesicant agent must not be splashed on the skin or be allowed to come in contact with the eyes. Its local irritating actions in subcutaneous tissues can be counteracted by applying ice-cold compresses to the area, or by infiltrating it with a solution of sodium thiosulfate.

Cyclophosphamide[+] (Cytoxan) differs from mechlorethamine in ways that make it more convenient and safer to use. It does not cause local tissue irritation, vesication, or other damage, and thus may be administered orally as well as by vein. Unlike mechlorethamine, its onset of action is slow and prolonged rather than rapid and short. This occurs because cyclophosphamide must first be metabolized to biologically active alkylating metabolites in the liver and then be broken down further to inactive compounds that are excreted by the kidneys. Obviously, because it is handled by the body in this way, caution is required in patients with impaired liver or kidney function. A possibly significant drug interaction may occur in patients taking cyclophosphamide together with high doses of phenobarbital, which increases induction of liver enzymes. This could unexpectedly speed the formation of active metabolites of cyclophosphamide and later also reduce the amounts that are ordinarily available for producing the prolonged action.

Cyclophosphamide is now probably the most widely used antineoplastic drug. It appears to be able to cure Burkitt's lymphoma when administered alone intermittently in high doses and it is an essential ingredient of many antineoplastic drug combinations, including those used to effect cures of childhood acute lymphocytic leukemia and those used to treat solid tumors.

Like other nitrogen mustards, cyclophosphamide commonly causes nausea and vomiting, whether given orally or IV, and bone marrow depression leading to leukopenia. However, thrombocytopenia and anemia occur less often than with other drugs of this class. Because this drug can suppress immune mechanisms, some patients—particularly those also receiving corticosteroid drugs—may suffer potentially fatal viral infections.

Some types of toxicity are seen more often with cyclophosphamide than with other drugs of this class. Alopecia, for example, is a frequent complication. A more serious complication characteristic of cyclophosphamide is the occurrence of a sterile inflammation of the urinary bladder as a result of irritation by active metabolites. Forcing large quantities of fluid to form a dilute urine and to foster frequent voiding of the bladder helps to prevent hemorrhagic and nonhemorrhagic cystitis.

The drug can also cause the secretion of antidiuretic hormone (ADH; see Chap. 20). Normally, ADH is secreted when the body needs to conserve water; it acts on the collecting ducts of the kidney to facilitate the reabsorption of water into the bloodstream. Cyclophosphamide can cause ADH to be secreted at inappropriate times. Because of this, patients taking cyclophosphamide and forcing fluids to prevent cystitis are especially at risk of water intoxication unless fluid intake and output are monitored and the problem is detected early.

Other nitrogen mustard derivatives that are orally effective and *nonvesicant* include *chlorambucil*[+] (Leukeran), *melphalan* (Alkeran), and *uracil mustard.* These drugs do not cause alopecia, as is often the case with cyclophosphamide; nausea and vomiting are not common; and, with chlorambucil, ordinary therapeutic doses do not damage the bone marrow. Nevertheless, as with other nitrogen mustards, patients being maintained on these drugs must be closely monitored for early signs of neutropenia, lymphopenia, thrombocytopenia, and anemia in order to discontinue therapy before bone marrow damage becomes irreversible.

Although these drugs, like other nitrogen mustards, are active against Hodgkin's disease and other lymphomas, their main indications are for other types of malignancies. Thus, chlorambucil is considered the drug of choice for bringing about remissions in chronic lymphocytic leukemia, and melphalan is the most useful agent available for treatment of multiple myeloma.

Alkyl sulfonates

Busulfan[+] (Myleran), an alkylating agent of another chemical class (alkyl sulfonates), differs from the previously discussed drugs in its lack of lymphoid tissue cytotoxicity and in its degree of specific toxicity on immature malignant bone marrow cells. This accounts for its effectiveness for bringing about remissions in cases of chronic myelocytic leukemia and also for its main toxic effects, which are all the result of dose-related myelosuppression. Patients must have complete blood counts carried out weekly to detect early hematologic changes before hemorrhage and pancytopenia occur. Other complications are rare but can include pulmonary fibrosis with alveolar exudates that interfere with breathing. It frequently causes hyperuricemia, and therefore should be given with allopurinol.

Ethylenimines

Thiotepa[+], an alkylating agent of still another chemical structure, is an ethylenimine compound. It was one of the earliest antineoplastic drugs but currently is not the first-choice drug for treating any neoplasm. It is sometimes used in treating patients with adenocarcinoma of the ovary or breast, and it is sometimes instilled into serous cavities to control effusion of fluid from metastatic malignancies into the pleural space, pericardium, and peritoneum. A chemically related drug, *hexamethylmelamine*, is available from the National Cancer Institute (NCI) for the treatment of ovarian cancer, and *pentamethylmelamine* is a similar drug now under investigation.

Nitrosourea compounds

The two most important drugs of this class with alkylating activity and other cytotoxic actions are *carmustine* (BiCNU) and *lomustine* (CeeNU). The most significant property of these drugs is their ability to cross the blood–brain barrier. Thus, although both these agents have been useful for treating Hodgkin's disease and *non*-Hodgkin's lymphomas, and carmustine is also employed together with prednisone in the management of multiple myeloma, their outstanding clinical use is in the palliative treatment of brain tumors and central nervous system metastases. Among the primary brain tumors in which these agents have produced temporary remissions are glioblastomas and astrocytomas. *Semustine,* the methyl analogue of lomustine, is an investigational drug available from the NCI.

The main type of toxicity with the nitrosoureas is their tendency to cause delayed bone marrow damage. Thus, patients must have their levels of leukocytes, platelets, and red blood cells monitored for at least 6 weeks after a dose, and a second treatment course should not be begun until the formed elements of the blood have returned to safe levels—some time after their low points 4 to 6 weeks after the first dose. Carmustine is administered intravenously every 6 weeks, while patients take the appropriate number of lomustine tablets orally at similar intervals.

Streptozocin (Zanosar), a methylnitrosourea compound that has recently become available commercially in the United States, is useful in treating pancreatic islet cell tumors and malignant carcinoid tumors. In addition to causing nausea, vomiting, and bone marrow depression, this drug causes serious renal and hepatic toxicity. Patients receiving this drug must be monitored closely for signs of toxicity to all three organs.

Other alkylating agents

Pipobroman (Vercyte) has been classified as an alkylating agent, although its mechanism of action is not known precisely. It is used to treat polycythemia vera, a disease characterized by an excess of erythrocytes, and as a substitute for busulfan in the treatment of chronic myelocytic leukemia. Bone marrow depression resulting from this drug is often delayed for weeks or more.

Mitobronitol (*dibromomannitol;* Myelobromol) is also used to treat chronic myelocytic leukemia. It is another alkylating agent that crosses the blood–brain barrier. Like cyclophosphamide, it frequently causes alopecia. In the United States, mitobronitol is available only from the NCI.

Antimetabolites

Cytotoxic drugs of this type possess chemical structures similar to those of various natural metabolites needed for growth and division by both neoplastic and normal cells. These structural analogues are of three main classes: *folic acid analogues* (methotrexate); *purine analogues* (mercaptopurine and thioguanine); and *pyrimidine analogues* (fluorouracil and cytarabine). When these structural analogues of such essential metabolites are taken up by the cells and substituted in biosynthetic steps for the natural metabolites, biosynthetic processes cannot proceed normally. As a result, the cancer cells fail to synthesize essential proteins and nucleic acids. In most cases, the main cause of cell death is a drug-induced block of DNA synthesis—that is, interference with the S phase of the cell cycle. Thus, the antimetabolite-type antineoplastic agents are most effective against rapidly growing tumors and most toxic to rapidly proliferating normal tissues.

A major problem in the use of antimetabolites is the ability of cancer cells to acquire resistance to their adverse effects. The biochemical mechanisms by which cells develop resistance are being investigated in the hope that this will provide a basis for designing drug molecules to which cancer cells will not become resistant.

Folic acid analogues

Methotrexate[+], an analogue of the B-complex vitamin folic acid, is the prototype antimetabolite. This drug was the first chemotherapeutic agent found to be effective against a neoplastic disease. Its use in children with acute leukemia during the late 1940s brought about remissions that extended their life expectancy from fewer than 20 weeks to many months. Later, it was shown to be able to cure choriocarcinoma, a swiftly spreading placental tissue tumor. Today methotrexate is being employed both alone and in combination with other antineoplastic agents in the treatment of many types of cancers, including such solid tumors as breast and lung cancer, as well as acute lymphoblastic leukemia of children.

Methotrexate acts mainly by inhibiting the enzyme *dihydrofolate reductase,* which catalyzes the conversion of dietary folic acid to *tetrahydrofolate,* a coenzyme needed for the formation of an intermediary metabolite that all cells require for synthesis of DNA. Patients who receive high doses of this antifolic agent are prone to develop severe, potentially fatal toxicity that is the result of the death of bone marrow tissues and other rapidly replicating normal cells that are deprived of tetrahydrofolate (see Summary of Adverse Effects). Such toxic reactions cannot be counteracted by administering folic acid, because that vitamin cannot, of course, be converted to the essential active metabolite because the reaction between methotrexate and the enzyme that it has inhibited, is practically irreversible.

Drug-poisoned cells can, however, be salvaged by the administration of an antidote called *leucovorin calcium.* This substance—also called *folinic acid* or the *citrovorum factor*—supplies a tetrahydrofolate derivative that can rescue the bone marrow, intestinal lining, and other normal cells from the lethal effects of methotrexate. Recently, this concept of "leucovorin rescue" has been applied in the treatment of tumors that were previously considered resistant to safe doses of methotrexate. The drug is now often administered in high doses capable of killing previously resistant cells, including those of osteogenic sarcoma and of some lung cancers. Then, several hours after administration of the methotrexate, leucovorin is given to protect the normal cells and thus prevent or reverse toxic reactions. Various dosage schedules are being tried to determine the safest and most effective ways to treat various types of tumors with this combination. Methotrexate does not penetrate the blood–brain barrier, but it is sometimes administered intrathecally to patients whose leukemia has invaded the central nervous system.

Methotrexate causes nausea, vomiting, and toxicity to rapidly proliferating tissues (*e.g.*, gastrointestinal ulceration, diarrhea, alopecia, menstrual irregularities). The bone marrow depression is often manifested by thrombocytopenia, and may require that the patient be given a transfusion of platelets.

Purine analogues

Mercaptopurine[+] (Purinethol), a purine analogue or antipurine, exerts cytotoxic effects by interfering with the synthesis of nucleic acids. This accounts for its effectiveness in maintaining remissions in some children with acute lymphocytic leukemia and in some adults with acute and chronic myelocytic leukemias. Thus, it is often used to maintain patients in remissions that have been induced by the prior administration of combinations of other antileukemic agents considered to be more effective for induction therapy than mercaptopurine.

This drug and the related antipurine agent *thioguanine* are said to cause fewer gastrointestinal-type side-effects than methotrexate and other antineoplastic antimetabolites. However, patients must be carefully observed for early signs of bone marrow depression. A derivative of mercaptopurine, *azathioprine* (Imuran), has a spectrum of activity similar to that of mercaptopurine, but its only approved use in the United States is as an immunosuppressant agent in the treatment of severe rheumatoid arthritis and in the prevention of rejection of renal transplants.

Like other drugs that can destroy large numbers of leukemic cells, mercaptopurine causes an increase in the production of purines. These are then converted to uric acid by the action of the enzyme xanthine oxidase. The resulting hyperuricemia may lead to the precipitation of uric acid crystals in the urine, with resulting kidney injury.

To prevent this potential adverse effect, the antigout drug *allopurinol* (Zyloprim), an inhibitor of xanthine oxidase, may be prescribed. However, blocking the action of this enzyme, which is also responsible for the metabolic degradation of mercaptopurine, can intensify and prolong the cytotoxic effects of that drug on the bone marrow. Thus, when allopurinol is employed as an adjunct to mercaptopurine therapy of the leukemias, it is customary to reduce dosage of the antileukemic drug to only one-third or one-quarter of the normally recommended doses. Patients receiving allopurinol concomitantly with azathioprine need a similar reduction in the dosage of azathioprine.

Pyrimidine analogues

The pyrimidine analogues currently available are poorly and unpredictably absorbed after oral administration, and are therefore given intravenously or intra-arterially.

Fluorouracil[+] (5-FU; Adrucil), an antimetabolite of the pyrimidine subclass, produces its cytotoxic effects by blocking the biosynthesis of thymidylic acid, a substance needed as a precursor of thymine. By preventing this pyrimidine base from being incorporated into DNA, fluorouracil prevents cancer cells from synthesizing that vital substance during the S phase of the cell cycle. Administered intravenously, this drug sometimes causes temporary remissions in patients with carcinoma of the colon, rectum, stomach, and pancreas, and it has been tried in the treatment of breast and bladder cancers.

This drug has only a narrow safety margin, and so normal cells of the gastrointestinal system are commonly damaged. Thus, ulcerations of the mouth, pharynx, and all levels of the gastrointestinal tract may appear, and patients commonly suffer nausea and vomiting following each dose. Gastrointestinal bleeding can be fatal, particularly if drug-induced bone marrow damage has led to severe thrombocytopenia. The patient's formed blood elements are closely monitored, and platelet counts below 100,000/mm^3 are an indication that further administration of this drug should be discontinued. Similarly, to avoid severe infection, the drug is discontinued if the white blood count is found to be falling rapidly to levels under 3,500/mm^3. Patients receiving this drug are often placed on reverse isolation precautions to help to decrease the risk of infection.

The systemic toxicity of this drug, and that of its derivative *floxuridine* (FUDR), may be reduced by injecting them directly into the arteries that carry blood directly to the various involved visceral organs. Floxuridine has proved most effective when infused continuously into the hepatic artery, because much of the drug is metabolized before it enters the systemic circulation after exerting its cytotoxic effect on tumor tissue that may have metastasized to the liver from the stomach, pancreas, or other gastrointestinal organs.

One of the safest and most effective ways in which fluorouracil has been employed is by topical application of the drug in cream form (Efudex; Fluoroplex) to the skin to treat actinic or solar keratosis and some superficial but extensive basal cell carcinomas located at sites not readily accessible to conventional surgical or x-ray treatment. Patients should be advised that the drug-induced inflammatory skin reaction may become unsightly before complete healing occurs several weeks after the 2- to 4-

week treatment course for solar keratosis has been finished. Initial redness and blistering often proceed to an ulcerative stage and to skin necrosis before the drug applications are stopped and new layers of epithelial cells begin to be laid down. Treatment for basal cell carcinomas may take much longer—up to 10 or 12 weeks—before the lesions are obliterated, and these patients should continue to be observed to be sure that their condition is cured.

Cytarabine (Cytosar) is an antimetabolite that produces its cytotoxic effects by interfering with the biosynthesis and function of DNA in leukemic cells and in those of normal bone marrow. This occurs because arabinose, the sugar in this synthetic nucleoside, differs from the natural sugar moieties in the normal nucleosides required in the reactions that produce nucleic acids. This drug has helped bring about remissions in acute leukemias of both the lymphocytic and myelocytic types. However, for best results, it is administered in combination with such other drugs as thioguanine, daunorubicin, and other antineoplastic agents (Table 12-2).

Cytarabine must be administered intravenously in 10-day initial courses. Rapid administration of large divided doses tends to be followed by bouts of nausea and vomiting. This is less likely to occur with continuous infusion of lower doses. However, because bone marrow depression may occur with either dosage regimen, the patient's peripheral blood picture must be monitored every day during the course of treatment with this drug. The drug may also cause hepatic and renal toxicity.

5-Azacitidine (5-AZC; Ladakamycin) is an investigational drug classed as an antimetabolite and available from the NCI for the treatment of acute myelocytic leukemia. *Tegafur* (Ftorafur), another investigational drug, may be obtained from the NCI for treating colorectal cancer.

Natural antineoplastic agents

A number of substances isolated from plants, bacteria, and fungi of the *Streptomyces* genus have been found to possess significant antineoplastic activity against various types of tumors. Although some of these substances act by interfering with the synthesis of cellular proteins and nucleic acids including RNA and DNA, and some act by damaging preformed DNA, they are classified as *alkaloids, antibiotics,* and *enzymes* in terms of their sources rather than in terms of their general mechanisms of action, as is the case with the previously discussed alkylating agents and antimetabolites. The important properties of the main anticancer agents derived from natural sources will be briefly discussed here; their clinical applications and toxic effects are summarized elsewhere.

Asparaginase (Elspar) is an enzyme isolated from the bacterium *Escherichia coli* and made available in purified form for use mainly in the treatment of acute lymphoblastic leukemia. It is not ordinarily used to initiate treatment of that disorder but is, instead, added to the regimen of children who have first been treated with other drugs (see below) to which the disease appears to be becoming resistant. This enzyme acts by depriving leukemic cells of the amino acid L-asparagine, which is broken down before it can be taken up from dietary sources and used in certain essential metabolic processes. Most normal cells synthesize their own supply of L-asparagine, and thus are not as sensitive as neoplastic cells to the action of the enzyme L-asparaginase. Thus, for example, this drug does not depress bone marrow or adversely affect mucosal or hair follicle cells.

Asparaginase is *not,* however, free of adverse effects. The enzyme is, of course, a foreign protein capable of sensitizing patients and causing late hypersensitivity-type reactions ranging from mild skin eruptions to potentially fatal anaphylaxis. Thus, skin tests for sensitivity should be performed before each course of asparaginase treatment, and patients with positive tests should undergo a desensitization procedure. The drugs needed for counteracting allergic reactions must be readily available, because even the intradermal test and desensitization can be dangerous. Another form of this enzyme (*Erwinia* asparaginase; Porton Asparaginase) is available from the NCI for patients sensitive to *E. coli* asparaginase.

Some normal tissues seem subject to direct toxicity induced by this drug. Most patients, for example, show signs of adverse effects on liver function. Drug-induced impairment of liver function may increase the toxicity of other antileukemic medications, including vincristine, particularly if that drug is given after the enzyme treatment instead of well before it. The pancreas also appears prone to suffer toxic reactions to asparaginase, and some deaths from hemorrhagic pancreatitis have been reported. Frequent tests should be made of serum amylase levels during treatment with asparaginase to detect early signs of pancreatic damage. The drug should be discontinued in such situations as well as in those patients who develop hyperglycemia and glycosuria. Such patients may require treatment with insulin and IV fluids to prevent complications similar to those of diabetic hyperosmolar nonketotic hyperglycemia.

Vincristine[+] (Oncovin) and *vinblastine* (Velban) are alkaloids extracted from the periwinkle plant that have shown activity against various types of neoplasms. Both drugs appear to produce their cytotoxic effects by inhibiting the mitotic (M) phase of the cell cycle during which each cell starts to divide its doubled DNA content between the two daughter cells, following the G_2 phase. An advantage of vincristine is that it seems much more likely to kill cancer cells during mitosis than to kill normal bone marrow cells. Thus, it is particularly useful for inducing remissions of acute lymphoblastic leukemia in cases marked by infiltration of the bone marrow by neoplastic cells.

Both vinblastine and vincristine are also useful for treating Hodgkin's disease and other malignant lymphomas, as well as various other types of solid tumors, which—unlike the lymphomas—do not respond to alkylating agents. In the management of the malignancies that are sensitive to treatment with these drugs, they are now commonly administered in combination with other types of antineoplastic drugs for greater effectiveness, reduced toxicity, and lessened development of drug resistance (see the discussion of combination therapy, above). A factor that tends to limit the long-term administration of these drugs for maintenance therapy is their tendency to cause the development of neurologic disorders.

Vincristine tends to cause dysfunction of the motor and sensory components of peripheral nerves. Thus, patients should be questioned concerning the occurrence of numbness and tingling of the fingers and toes. Such paresthesias are a sign that the dosage should be reduced or the drug discontinued entirely to avoid more serious motor disability marked by the loss of deep tendon reflexes. Vincristine may also have adverse effects on autonomic nerves that innervate the gastrointestinal tract. This may account for the constipation that sometimes occurs during its use. Constipation may be kept from advancing to the point of fecal impaction by the adjunctive use of bulk-producing laxatives and fecal softeners. Both vinblastine and vincristine can cause the inappropriate secretion of ADH (as does cyclophosphamide; see above).

A third vinca alkaloid, *vincristine* sulfate (Eldisine), is being investigated. Early results indicate that it is effective in many cancers that have not responded to other drugs, including vincristine and vinblastine.

Bleomycin (Blenoxane) is one of the half-dozen antibiotics with antineoplastic activity that are now available for treating a wide variety of leukemias, lymphomas, and solid tumors of the viscera. This antibiotic has proved particularly useful for treating squamous cell carcinomas of the head and neck, including mouth and throat structures such as the tongue, tonsils, and palate. It is also useful against tumors of the female and male genitourinary organs, such as the cervix, vulva, scrotum, and penis. A high rate of remissions of testicular carcinoma has followed combined treatment with bleomycin and vinblastine. Both drugs are also useful against lymphomas, including advanced stages of Hodgkin's disease.

An advantage of this antibiotic over most antineoplastic drugs is its relative lack of bone marrow toxicity. However, it is unusually toxic to the skin and lungs, possibly because these tissues fail to detoxify the antibiotic as readily as do other body tissues that contain drug-degrading enzymes. Pulmonary toxicity, which develops in up to 10% of patients, is potentially serious, and about 1% of patients treated with bleomycin have died of drug-induced pulmonary fibrosis. Patients, particularly those over 70 years of age and those with pre-existing pulmonary disease, must be very carefully observed during treatment. Chest x-rays are taken every week or two to detect diffuse infiltrates or other signs of pneumonitis that require discontinuation of drug therapy and possible therapy with corticosteroids and antibiotics. Although annoying skin

reactions occur in as many as half the patients, the drug does not ordinarily have to be discontinued for this reason or because of the baldness, nail changes, or mouth ulcers that sometimes develop during its administration.

Dactinomycin (Actinomycin D; Cosmegen) is an antibiotic that binds to cellular DNA and interferes with the synthesis of cellular RNA and proteins. Its cytotoxic effects have been applied in treating pediatric neoplasms such as Wilms' tumor, Ewing's sarcoma, and rhabdomyosarcoma. Combined with chlorambucil and methotrexate, this drug has helped produce regression of metastases of testicular tumor tissue. Women with choriocarcinoma that is resistant to methotrexate have sometimes responded to treatment with dactinomycin. Other adult tumors are not very responsive, but adolescents with osteogenic sarcoma have sometimes had good results when dactinomycin was employed adjunctively following surgery.

Bone marrow depression and gastrointestinal lesions are the most common and dangerous adverse effects that develop during treatment, and patients must be monitored and observed to avoid serious sequelae. The anorexia, nausea, and vomiting that commonly occur within hours of the drug's administration may be lessened by pretreatment with a centrally acting antiemetic of the piperazine group of phenothiazines. Alopecia and erythematous or acneiform skin eruptions occur, and local skin irritation can result from leakage of the drug solution. To avoid this and to minimize phlebitis, the solution is best administered by injection of a free-flowing IV infusion into the tubing. Dosage must be reduced if thrombocytopenia, leukopenia, or anemia appear, or if such late signs of gastrointestinal toxicity develop as glossitis, cheilitis (inflammation of the lips), stomatitis, oral ulceration, abdominal pain, proctitis, and diarrhea. Mouth care is very important for these patients.

Doxorubicin (Adriamycin) and *daunorubicin* (Daunomycin) are chemically related (anthracene) antibiotics, which differ in their degree of effectiveness as antineoplastic agents but share a capacity for causing similar types of toxicity. Daunorubicin is less important than doxorubicin, because its use is limited mainly to cases of acute lymphocytic and myelocytic leukemias. Although doxorubicin has also proved useful in these leukemias, it is in addition often of great value against a much wider spectrum of neoplastic disorders, including carcinomas of the breast, bladder, ovary, testes, prostate, and thyroid; lymphomas of the Hodgkin's and non-Hodgkin's types; sarcomas of bone such as osteogenic sarcoma and Ewing's sarcoma; and pediatric tumors such as Wilms' tumor, rhabdomyosarcoma, and neuroblastoma. Both drugs cause tissue necrosis. They must therefore be injected into a rapidly flowing IV infusion and extra precautions taken to prevent extravasation.

The most common toxic effects of both antibiotics is on the bone marrow and gastrointestinal system, and so patients must be monitored closely in the usual ways to detect early signs that signal that a reduction in dosage is required to avoid bleeding episodes, infections, and ulcerations of the oral and esophageal mucosa. An unusual type of toxicity is the occurrence of cardiomyopathy when continued treatment results in accumulation of the drug in heart muscle tissues. This can lead to sudden, severe, irreversible heart failure. Although monitoring of the ECG is recommended, cardiotoxicity can develop without prior ECG changes. Thus, it is necessary to keep a record of the total dose administered during a course of treatment and to avoid giving a total dose of more than 500 mg/m² of body surface. Patients who are also receiving radiotherapy should get no more than 400 mg/m² of doxorubicin as a total dose, because x-ray treatment and certain other antineoplastic drugs increase the patient's susceptibility to cardiotoxicity. Patients receiving either of these drugs should be warned that their urine may be colored red by the drug for several days after treatment; this does not indicate hematuria.

Plicamycin (Mithracin), formerly called *Mithramycin*, is an extremely toxic antibiotic with only a narrow spectrum of useful antineoplastic activity. However, it has proved of value in the treatment of some patients with metastatic testicular tumors composed of embryonal carcinomatous tissue. Sometimes, signs of tumor regression are seen after 3 or 4 weeks of treatment, and additional courses at monthly intervals occasionally bring about complete regression of the tumor masses for a time. This antibiotic may also be indicated for control of hypercalcemia and hypercalciuria when these complications, which occur in patients with other kinds of cancer, have not been controllable by more conventional measures. These complications usually respond to lower safer doses of plicamycin than are required for tumor treatment.

Patients taking plicamycin must be hospitalized and observed carefully for signs of bleeding, because deaths have occurred from sudden severe hemorrhage. This may be manifested first by nosebleed (epistaxis), but hematemesis may be the first sign of widespread gastrointestinal tract hemorrhage. Laboratory tests are used to check not only for rapid development of thrombocytopenia but also for development of defects in blood coagulation, such as a lengthening of the prothrombin time and bleeding time. Extreme caution is required in patients who show signs of bone marrow depression or of impairment in liver or kidney function.

Mitomycin (Mutamycin), an antibiotic with alkylating activity, is not ordinarily used alone but rather is used in combination with other antineoplastic therapeutic modalities. It has, for example, been employed as an adjuvant to surgery and radiation therapy in the management of advanced adenocarcinoma of the stomach and pancreas and in combination with other chemotherapeutic agents against squamous cell lung cancers and carcinomas of the breast, colon, rectum, and liver. The toxicity of this antibiotic is manifested by signs of bone marrow

suppression, anorexia, nausea, and vomiting, and local irritation of subcutaneous tissues by solution leaking out of the IV infusion.

Hormones and antihormones

Several types of steroid hormones have proved useful for providing symptomatic relief of various types of cancers or for controlling some complications of these neoplastic diseases. The male and female sex hormones are employed in the treatment of metastatic tumors whose growth is influenced by endocrine factors—for example, advanced breast cancer, prostatic carcinoma, and disseminated endometrial malignancies. The adrenocorticosteroids have relatively little direct effect on the growth of breast cancer, but they can be useful against certain complications of this disease, and their direct effect on lymphocytes accounts for the favorable effects that corticosteroids exert on the course of the lymphocytic leukemias and of some malignant lymphomas.

Androgenic hormones sometimes have palliative effects when employed in the management of advanced breast cancer. Favorable responses occur most often in women who developed mammary carcinoma before the menopause, who have had a favorable response to surgical removal of their ovaries, or whose tumors are positive for estrogen receptors. However, women whose breast cancer is detected when they are more than 1 year but less than 5 years past the menopause also sometimes respond to androgenic therapy.

The main drawback of the esters of testosterone that were first used for this purpose is their tendency to produce masculinizing effects on women who are treated with the large doses needed for symptomatic relief. Thus, certain synthetic substances claimed to exert relatively little or no virilizing activity are now preferred. These include calusterone, testolactone, dromostanolone, and fluoxymesterone (Table 12-1).

These androgenic drugs are also less likely than testosterone to lead to edema as a result of fluid retention, and they are claimed to be relatively free of hypercalcemic effects. Nevertheless, all women receiving drugs of this class should have their plasma calcium levels determined routinely. If hypercalcemia is detected, further treatment should be discontinued until the plasma calcium level has been lowered by various measures.

Estrogenic hormones are also used in the management of metastatic mammary carcinoma but are reserved for women who are more than 5 years past the menopause. They are also employed for treating men with metastatic prostatic cancer. Favorable effects are often produced by diethylstilbestrol in such cases, but the drug produces feminizing and other adverse effects on men receiving such hormonal treatment.

Estramustine phosphate, an estrogen linked to a mustard type of molecule, is also used in advanced prostatic cancer. It has been classed with the alkylating agents by some authorities, but its adverse effects are more similar to those caused by estrogens, including gynecomastia and increased risk of vascular accidents; it also causes nausea and vomiting, typical of alkylating agents.

Progestins are employed both in some cases of advanced breast cancer and in metastatic endometrial cancer. Such progestational steroids are thought to antagonize the effects of estrogens on the growth of these two types of hormone-dependent cancers. These female sex hormones have also been claimed to be effective for producing remissions in some patients with renal cell carcinoma.

Antiestrogenic substances such as tamoxifen citrate (Nolvadex), appear to stop cell division in breast cancer by binding to specific estrogen receptors in the target tissues. This prevents circulating estrogens from reacting with these receptors to set in motion the series of biochemical steps that lead to synthesis of DNA in the cancer cells. The main advantage of this drug over androgen therapy of postmenopausal women with advanced breast cancer is its lack of masculinizing effects. The drug causes such minor side-effects as nausea and vomiting, hot flashes, and vaginal discharge, spotting, or bleeding, but these adverse reactions rarely require discontinuation of drug therapy. Similarly, although a reduction in leukocyte and thrombocyte counts sometimes occurs, this drug does not cause bone marrow depression of the type so common with other cancer chemotherapeutic agents.

Adrenocorticosteroid drugs—particularly prednisone—are commonly employed together with vincristine as the initial treatment for inducing remissions in children with acute lymphocytic leukemia. Prednisone is also part of the so-called MOPP combination, which is currently considered to be the most effective treatment for inducing remissions in advanced stages of Hodgkin's disease. In addition to their lympholytic effects against these neoplasms and their occasional beneficial effects in breast cancer, the adrenocorticosteroids are useful for counteracting certain complications of some forms of cancer. They are, for example, useful for reducing fever and other discomforting symptoms and thus help to make patients more comfortable. These steroids also help to counteract cerebral edema secondary to central nervous system metastasis and cranial radiation therapy. Steroid therapy also aids in lowering plasma calcium levels in patients with bone metastases who develop hypercalcemia during treatment with androgens or estrogens.

Mitotane (Lysodren), a drug chemically related to the insecticide DDT, exerts a relatively selective cytotoxic action on malignant and normal cells of the adrenal cortex. It is used only for treating cases of inoperable adrenocortical carcinoma. The drug is best employed after as much as possible of the metastatic masses has been removed surgically.

The most common adverse effects are the result of gastrointestinal disturbances. About four out of five patients suffer anorexia, nausea, and vomiting, or diarrhea. Central nervous system side-effects include drowsiness and dizziness. Impaired neurologic function and brain damage are possible in patients receiving large doses for long periods. As is to be expected, some patients may develop adrenal insufficiency. Thus, in medical or surgical emergencies, this drug must be discontinued, and exogenous corticosteroids should be administered.

Aminoglutethimide (Cytadren) inhibits the synthesis of steroids by the adrenal gland. The administration of this drug has been called a medical adrenalectomy. It is used primarily to treat Cushing's disease, but it is also sometimes effective in breast cancer in postmenopausal women and in metastatic prostatic cancer. Its mechanism of action for producing beneficial effects in these cancers is not completely clear, but may be related to interference with the synthesis of estrogens and androgens by the adrenal cortex. It can cause nausea, skin rashes, and bone marrow depression.

Miscellaneous chemotherapeutic agents

Although for some reason these drugs are not well enough understood to be placed in one of the above categories, they are no less important than those described above. *Hydroxyurea* (Hydrea) is a drug that has shown activity against several types of neoplasms, including some that are particularly resistant to chemotherapy. It is sometimes effective in cases of chronic myelocytic leukemia that have become resistant to busulfan. Some patients with malignant melanoma have shown responses to this drug. Metastatic ovarian carcinoma has also shown some sensitivity. This drug has also been used together with radiation therapy in attempts to control squamous cell carcinomas of the head and neck. (The adverse effects of hydroxyurea and the precautions required to minimize them are reviewed in the summary of adverse effects at the end of this chapter.)

Dacarbazine (DTIC), the triazene-class compound also called imidazole carboxamide, has alkylating activity as well as other cytotoxic actions. It is sometimes classed as an alkylating agent, but also may act as a purine analogue, and it interacts with sulfhydryl groups. It is one of the most effective antineoplastic agents available at present for treating metastatic malignant melanoma. About 20% of patients respond to treatment, most with partial or complete remissions for 6 months or more. Results are even better when it is administered in combination with such other cancer chemotherapeutic agents as carmustine, vincristine, hydroxyurea, and dactinomycin. The first few IV injections of dacarbazine cause nausea and vomiting in over 90% of patients, presumably as a result of central chemoreceptor–trigger zone stimulation. Vomiting is best relieved by treatment with the centrally acting antiemetic prochlorperazine (Compazine) and with phenobarbital. Patients should also not take fluids or food for 4 to 6 hours before treatment.

Vomiting lasts only 1 to 12 hours, but a less frequent type of minor toxicity—an influenzalike syndrome marked by fever, muscle aches, and malaise that occasionally develops a week after treatment—may last up to 3 weeks. The most serious type of toxicity caused by dacarbazine is bone marrow depression, which can lead to fatal thrombocytopenia and leukopenia. For this reason, patients should be hospitalized prior to treatment so that their platelets and white and red blood cells can be carefully monitored and the drug discontinued at the first sign of hematopoietic toxicity.

Etoposide (VePesid) is a semisynthetic derivative of podophyllin, a substance derived from the American mandrake or May apple plant. It has just recently (1984) been approved for use in testicular cancers; preliminary studies indicate that it is also very effective in small cell lung cancers. It is a cell cycle-dependent agent that arrests cell division, acting especially in the S and G_2 phases. It is administered by IV infusion and must be given slowly to avoid hypotension. It causes a high incidence of adverse gastrointestinal effects, alopecia, and bone marrow depression, as well as peripheral neuropathy. A related podophyllin derivative, *teniposide*, is still under investigation.

Procarbazine (Matulane) is a hydrazine compound that was synthesized during a search for monoamine oxidase inhibitor-type antidepressant drugs but discarded because of its hematopoietic toxicity. Later, because of its ability to interfere with the synthesis of lymphoid cell macromolecules and to alkylate and degrade DNA, it was tried as a cytotoxic agent in the treatment of Hodgkin's disease. Today it is one of the components of the most commonly employed type of drug combination employed in treating that malignancy, the MOPP regimen. It is sometimes classed as an alkylating agent, but its mechanism of action is not well defined. Like dacarbazine, it causes nausea, vomiting, and bone marrow depression. Patients receiving this drug should not ingest alcohol because a disulfiramlike reaction may occur (see Chap. 53). Ingestion of foods containing tyramine, the use of sympathomimetic drugs, and other factors may precipitate a hypertensive crisis (see Chap. 46, Drugs Used in the Management of Mental Illness, and the summary of drugs that may interact adversely with MAO inhibitors).

Cisplatin (Platinol) was the first of a new class of platinum-containing cytotoxic agents found to be effective for treating several types of solid tumors. It has proved particularly active against testicular tumors of the nonseminomatous type, when administered alone or simultaneously with combinations of vinblastine and bleomycin. This drug has also produced remissions in cases of bladder cancer and advanced ovarian carcinoma resistant to treatment with alkylating agents. Cisplatin must be administered by IV infusion; contact of the drug with needles or IV sets containing aluminum must be avoided to prevent precipitation and inactivation of the drug.

The most serious type of toxicity seen with this drug is the result of dose-related renal damage. Early signs of nephrotoxicity seen in up to 25% of treated patients include elevations in BUN and serum creatinine levels. Continued administration has led to cumulative toxicity and irreversible kidney damage. However, it has been suggested that this can be prevented by keeping patients well hydrated with intravenous infusions of the osmotic diuretic mannitol with or without furosemide (Lasix).

Other types of toxicity reported for cisplatin include ototoxicity, moderate bone marrow suppression, and severe nausea and vomiting. Auditory monitoring should be performed to detect signs of hearing loss, and patients should be questioned concerning such abnormalities as tinnitus. The patient's blood should be checked periodically for signs of leukopenia, thrombocytopenia, and anemia. Patients with persistent vomiting should receive intravenous fluids to prevent dehydration.

Radioactive isotopes

A few radioactive elements are used to treat certain types of neoplasms (Table 12-1). Ideally, such a substance concentrates in the cancer and selectively damages its cells without affecting normal tissues. In practice, such selective toxicity does not occur with any isotope. Thus, although some do destroy tumor tissues, they also damage normal cells.

Two official radioisotopes in common use in cancer treatment are *sodium phosphate P32$^+$* and *chromic phosphate P32*. A third isotope, *sodium iodide I131*, is employed to destroy thyroid tissue in hyperthyroidism and thyroid carcinoma. In adequate doses, all emit β *particles* or "radiations" in amounts that destroy living tissues in the immediate vicinity. Although β radiations penetrate only a short distance, they can damage enough erythroid or myeloid cells to produce remissions in polycythemia vera and to a lesser extent in chronic myelocytic leukemia.

If overdosage permits too much radioactive phosphate to accumulate in the bone marrow, normal hematopoietic tissues may also be damaged. This can result in leukopenia, thrombocytopenia, and anemia as a result of excessive reduction in all the formed elements of the peripheral blood. Thus, the less toxic alkylating agent busulfan is usually preferred for treating chronic myelocytic leukemia and polycythemia vera.

Additional clinical considerations

The diagnosis of cancer brings with it fear, anxiety, and anger. The patient fears the unknown, the treatment involved, debilitation, loss of income, loss of support, and death. There is anxiety about coping with the problems of daily living as well as dying, about how the family will cope, about what will really happen. There is anger that this has happened. The nursing care of a patient with cancer must incorporate all these fears, anxieties, and anger into a complex approach to help the patient and family deal with the problems of day-to-day existence as well as with the overall impact of this chronic, often fatal, disease. The treatment of cancer is often debilitating, can involve extensive and disfiguring surgery or radiation treatment, and is almost always prolonged. The total care of the patient may involve the physician, the nurse, a social worker, a mental health consultant, rehabilitation experts, and a pharmacologist.

The patient who is to receive antineoplastic drug therapy needs to be totally prepared for what to expect. The adverse effects of the drug therapy can be very uncomfortable, and the patient and family will need support and encouragement to cope with the effects of the drug therapy from the onset of treatment. This encouragement and support are best provided in an atmosphere of honesty, patience, and acceptance. It is important to remember that each patient is experiencing fear and anxiety, and to him the chemotherapy is a unique and important experience. The nurse can often achieve a great deal with a few soothing words, a quiet and relaxed environment, and an accepting and listening attitude.

Comfort measures

The specific side-effects of each drug have been mentioned. Generally, there are four main areas of concern for patients receiving antineoplastic drug therapy; each will be considered in detail.

Anorexia, nausea and vomiting. The exact cause of these symptoms has not been established. They may be a result of direct chemical stimulation of the chemoreceptor trigger zone (CTZ) or a stimulation of the CTZ by chemicals released by the death of cells. Most people who receive chemotherapy suffer some or all of these symptoms, and they are generally thought to be "normal" reactions to chemotherapy. Some studies have shown that people may suffer the nausea and vomiting before they even receive chemotherapy, a reflection of the impact of the anticipation of these side-effects. Helping the patient to deal with this discomfort must begin, therefore, before the chemotherapy is even given. Antiemetic and sedative drugs are often helpful for relaxing the patient and preventing some of the nausea. A quiet relaxed environment with privacy ensured may also be helpful. The patient needs to know that help is readily available if vomiting does occur. Care should be taken to minimize offensive or strong odors, to maintain cleanliness in the patient's environment, and to select the food that is presented to the patient carefully. Small attractive meals, offered frequently, may be the most acceptable to nauseated patients. Many prefer to avoid smoking during therapy. Because it is essential to maintain the nutritional status and fluid intake of these patients to ensure the optimum effect of the chemotherapy, the nurse should work closely with the patient to determine food and beverages that can be tolerated and that will also be nutritious.

Gastrointestinal lesions. These ulcers can be painful, provide an entry source for opportunistic infec-

tions, and further aggravate the problems of anorexia and nausea. Meticulous mouth care performed several times a day can help to alleviate some of the infections and some of the pain. It is helpful to have mouthwash and clean water readily accessible to the patient. If a patient suffers bone marrow depression along with the mouth ulcers, bleeding painful gums may develop. In this case, extreme care must be taken to swab the gums gently, to use soft-bristled toothbrushes, and to avoid hard, spicy, or difficult foods. The patient's underlying nutritional status will be greatly involved with the ultimate healing and recovery of the gastrointestinal ulcers. This is a complex situation, because few patients feel like eating with mouth ulcers. Maintaining such a patient's nutritional status is a real nursing challenge.

Renal toxicity. If the drug being given is nephrotoxic, it is important to preload the patient with fluid before the drug is given. This will dilute the dosage of the drug that reaches the renal tubules. The patient should also be urged to drink 10 to 12 glasses of water daily to maintain hydration and to keep the bladder flushed. The patient's BUN and creatinine levels should be monitored regularly during the chemotherapy and for 6 to 8 weeks after it has been completed.

Bone marrow toxicity. The suppression of the bone marrow presents three major clinical problems. *Anemia*—a decrease in red blood cells—brings with it fatigue and malaise. The patient needs encouragement and support to cope with this frustrating problem. Frequent rest periods and planned activities can be helpful. *Clotting problems—a loss of platelets*—can cause bleeding difficulties. The patient will need to carry out several safety measures to avoid injuries that could cause bleeding or bruising; these must include provision for safety during physical activities as well as during such routine activities as shaving, brushing the teeth, and nail care. *Susceptibility to infection—suppression of leukocytes*—presents a great risk for patients. When the body cannot fight off any infection, many opportunistic infections can ensue. These infections drain the body's resources and often are the cause of death of cancer patients. Prevention is the best method of dealing with these infections. The patient should be taught to avoid crowded public areas and to avoid people with infections. Reverse isolation precautions are often used to protect patients with severely low leukocyte counts until their bone marrow begins to function adequately. No chemotherapeutic agent that suppresses the bone marrow should be given to a patient whose bone marrow is already depressed. It is best to wait until the bone marrow has recovered to administer these agents.

Pregnancy and lactation are contraindications for use of these chemotherapeutic agents. The effect of these drugs on cellular growth can be very detrimental to the fetus or infant. Because of this, patients should use contraceptive measures while receiving these drugs. Nursing mothers should discontinue breast feeding if they are to receive one of these agents.

Technical considerations

The details of drug preparation and administration have been outlined for each drug. An additional point that should be considered is the safety of the nurse who is handling and administering the drugs. Many of these drugs are directly toxic to cells and can destroy the nurse's cells as well as those of the patient. These drugs should be handled with gloves to prevent damage to the nurse's hands. Similar safety precautions should be taken in caring for patients receiving radioisotopes.

The patient teaching guide incorporates the general considerations for teaching patients about antineoplastic agents. The specific points that apply to each drug should be checked and included for each particular drug. The guide to the nursing process with antineoplastic drugs summarizes the general nursing considerations for patients receiving any of these agents.

Summary

This chapter has tried to stress the problems posed by the use of antineoplastic drugs to treat cancer and how these problems may be minimized. No student can be expected to retain all the detailed information that is now available about the individual drugs. Thus, the specific details offered here are useful mainly for reference purposes when required. Because of the rapidly changing nature of cancer chemotherapy, the nurse involved in the management of cancer patients will probably have to supplement the material presented here with the new data that are constantly being published in specialized journals and in books that deal exclusively with cancer and its therapy.

Despite the admitted inability of students (or authors) to master all the details of this area of therapy, it is possible to conclude this long chapter with a summary of some important general principles that are not likely to be changed in the near future:

1. Chemotherapy alone will probably not be successful in eliminating all neoplastic cells, the ultimate aim of cancer treatment. It is best employed together with such other therapeutic modalities as surgery, radiation, and immunotherapy in a regimen prepared specifically for each patient on the basis of the type of cancer from which the patient is suffering and the stage of its advance at the time of diagnosis.
2. Chemotherapy should be begun as soon as possible after a pathologist has made a precise diagnosis of the type of neoplastic disease or after the primary tumor has been surgically removed or treated with local radiation.
3. The drug or, preferably, the combination of drugs selected for initiating therapy, should be chosen on the basis of accumulated evidence of efficacy against the specific type of cancer that requires treatment. Certain pre-existing conditions can limit the choice of an antineoplastic drug. Drugs with toxicity known to aggravate these conditions may need to be avoided.
4. Drugs should be employed in the doses and dosage schedules recommended by the authorities who have had the most experience in using them for treating the types of neoplastic diseases for which they are indicated. This is often reflected in the package inserts of FDA-approved agents but, for experimental drugs, information must be obtained from other sources.
5. At present, it appears that best results are likely to be obtained when combinations of drugs are administered in intermittent, rather than daily, dosage schedules. Even high doses, administered in attempts to obtain the highest possible cancer cell kills, are likely to be less toxic when taken only once weekly or at other intermittent periods that permit normal bone marrow cells and immunologic defenses to recover in the interval between treatment courses.
6. Medical personnel employing cytotoxic drugs should be completely familiar with the types of toxic reactions that they cause, and patients should be closely monitored both clinically and by laboratory tests to detect the earliest signs and symptoms of potential toxicity.
7. Supportive measures should be employed promptly to counteract the expected complications of both the cancer and the chemotherapeutic agents that are being used to treat it. The nurse plays an important role in offering skilled supportive care, as well as in the administration of cancer chemotherapeutic agents and in detection of their adverse effects.
8. Cancer patients need counseling, psychological, and emotional support at every stage of their illness. This includes advice about how a still active, ambulatory patient can best cope with the disease and with the side-effects of chemotherapy and other drugs. The nurse may also be called on to help terminally ill patients make a decision about whether or not to continue therapy.

Summary of adverse effects of antineoplastic agents

Drug class	Types of toxic reactions
Alkylating agents	
Busulfan (Myleran)	Nausea and vomiting; bone marrow suppression; adrenocortical insufficiency syndrome; interstitial pulmonary fibrosis; alopecia; gynecomastia; amenorrhea; sterility
Carmustine (BiCNU)	Frequent nausea and vomiting; local burning at IV injection site; pulmonary fibrosis; delayed bone marrow toxicity; delayed renal damage; liver damage
Chlorambucil (Leukeran)	Bone marrow damage; pulmonary fibrosis; liver damage
Cyclophosphamide (Cytoxan)	Anorexia, nausea, vomiting; hemorrhagic cystitis; anaphylaxis; leukopenia and other possible blood cell deficiencies; alopecia; amenorrhea, temporary azoospermia and sterility; pulmonary fibrosis; ADH secretion
Lomustine (CeeNU)	Nausea, vomiting; delayed bone marrow suppression; stomatitis; abnormal liver function tests; alopecia; neurologic reactions
Mechlorethamine (Mustargen)	Nausea and vomiting; local irritation of subcutaneous tissue, causing sloughing; bone marrow depression with leukopenia and thrombocytopenia; oral ulcers; diarrhea
Melphalan (Alkeran)	Mild nausea and vomiting; bone marrow depression with low leukocyte and platelet counts; pulmonary fibrosis
Mitobronitol (Myelobromol)	Gastrointestinal disturbances; bone marrow depression; alopecia
Pipobroman (Vercyte)	Nausea, vomiting, abdominal cramps, diarrhea; bone marrow depression
Semustine (methyl-CCNU)	Nausea and vomiting; delayed leukopenia and thrombocytopenia; pulmonary fibrosis; renal failure
Streptozocin (Zanosar)	Nausea and vomiting; renal damage; hyperglycemia
Thiotepa (TESPA)	Nausea, vomiting; local pain; bone marrow depression; anorexia
Uracil mustard	Nausea, vomiting, diarrhea; bone marrow depression; amenorrhea; azoospermia; nervousness
Antimetabolites	
5-Azacitidine (5-AZC)	Nausea, vomiting, diarrhea; fever; leukopenia and thrombocytopenia; liver damage; muscle pain and weakness; cardiotoxicity

(continued)

Cytarabine (Cytosar)

Nausea, vomiting, diarrhea; oral ulceration; leukopenia, thrombocytopenia; anaphylaxis; liver dysfunction; renal toxicity

Fluorouracil (5-FU) and Floxuridine (FUDR)

Anorexia, nausea, vomiting, stomatitis, esophagopharyngitis; leukopenia; alopecia and dermatitis; acute and possibly persistent cerebellar syndrome

Mercaptopurine (Purinethol)

Occasional anorexia, nausea, vomiting, diarrhea; bone marrow depression leading to leukopenia and thrombocytopenia; jaundice; possible hyperuricemia

Methotrexate (MTX; amethopterin)

Nausea, abdominal distress, ulcerative stomatitis; bone marrow depression with leukopenia, thrombocytopenia, bleeding, and anemia; possible hepatotoxicity and renal failure; alopecia; menstrual dysfunction

Tegafur (Ftorafur)

Nausea and vomiting; dizziness and lethargy; stomatitis; bone marrow depression; alopecia

Thioguanine (6-TG)

Occasional anorexia, nausea, vomiting; bone marrow depression with leukopenia, thrombocytopenia, and bleeding; stomatitis; possible jaundice and toxic hepatitis

Natural products

Asparaginase (Elspar)

Nausea and vomiting; fever; allergic reactions, including anaphylaxis; hemorrhagic pancreatitis; impairment of liver function; hyperglycemia; CNS depression or stimulation

Bleomycin sulfate (Blenoxane)

Nausea and vomiting; skin reactions marked by redness, vesiculation, and hyperpigmentation; stomatitis; pulmonary fibrosis; idiosyncratic reactions resembling anaphylaxis, marked by hypotension, wheezing, fever, chills, and mental confusion; alopecia

Dactinomycin (Actinomycin D; Cosmegen)

Gastrointestinal effects; anorexia, nausea, and vomiting soon after injection, and later diarrhea, proctitis, and oral lesions; bone marrow depression, rapid and persistent pancytopenia; alopecia; red skin rashes

Daunorubicin (Daunomycin)

Similar to those of doxorubicin (see below)

Doxorubicin (Adriamycin)

Nausea, vomiting, diarrhea, stomatitis, esophagitis; urine dyed red; anaphylaxis; cardiotoxicity leading to heart failure as a result of the cumulative effects of excessive total doses; bone marrow depression leading to leukopenia and thrombocytopenia; alopecia; skin hyperpigmentation; local irritation with cellulitis, blistering, and tissue necrosis

Mitomycin (Mutamycin)

Anorexia, nausea, vomiting, and stomatitis; alopecia; cellulitis and tissue sloughing if extravasated during IV administration; bone marrow depression; pulmonary fibrosis; liver and renal toxicity

(continued)

Plicamycin (Mithracin) (formerly Mithramycin)	Electrolyte imbalances; anorexia, nausea, vomiting, diarrhea, and stomatitis; local irritation and cellulitis at subcutaneous sites of extravasation during IV administration; bone marrow depression and drug-induced coagulation defects; liver damage; hypocalcemia; hypokalemia
Vinblastine (Velban; VLB)	Leukopenia; anorexia, nausea, and vomiting; abdominal pain with constipation or diarrhea; ulcerative stomatitis and pharyngitis; neurologic effects:—peripheral neuritis with signs and symptoms such as numbness, paresthesias, and loss of deep tendon reflexes; mental changes and convulsions; ADH secretion
Vincristine (Oncovin)	Neurologic difficulties first in the form of paresthesias followed by neuritic pain and later neuromuscular signs, such as loss of deep tendon reflexes, footdrop, wristdrop, slapping gait, and muscle wasting; alopecia; abdominal pain and constipation (paralytic ileus); ADH secretion

Hormones

Adrenocorticosteroids	See Chapter 21
Androgenic drugs	See Chapter 24
Estrogens	See Chapter 23
Progestins	See Chapter 23

Adrenal suppressants

Aminoglutethimide (Cytadren)	Skin rash; drowsiness; nausea; fever; bone marrow depression; hypotension
Mitotane (Lysodren)	Nausea and vomiting; diarrhea; CNS depression; adrenal insufficiency; hematuria; hemorrhagic cystitis; brain damage with long use; hypertension; orthostatic hypotension

Antiestrogen

Tamoxifen (Nolvadex)	Hot flashes; nausea and vomiting; occasional vaginal discharge, spotting, bleeding, or menstrual irregularities; occasional increase in bone pain; hypercalcemia; decreased visual acuity; depression

Miscellaneous agents

Cisplatin (Platinol)	Severe nausea and vomiting; kidney damage; ototoxicity; bone marrow suppression; hemolysis; hypomagnesemia; hypocalcemia; hypokalemia
Dacarbazine (DTIC)	Anorexia, nausea, and vomiting; anaphylaxis; influenzalike syndrome; bone marrow depression; alopecia; renal and hepatic toxicity

(continued)

Etoposide (VePesid)	Nausea, vomiting, diarrhea; bone marrow depression; alopecia; peripheral neuropathy
Hydroxyurea (Hydrea)	Anorexia, nausea, vomiting, diarrhea, and constipation; bone marrow depression; occasional impairment of renal function; occasional skin redness and macropapular rash; dysuria; alopecia
Procarbazine (Matulane)	Nausea and vomiting; leukopenia, anemia, and thrombopenia; lethargy, drowsiness, fatigue, and weakness; stomatitis; pneumonitis; antabuselike reaction with alcohol; hypertensive crisis with foods containing tyramine or with sympathomimetic drugs

Patient teaching guide: antineoplastic drugs

The drug that has been prescribed for you is one of a class of drugs called antineoplastic agents. These drugs work to destroy cells at various phases of their life cycle. They are prescribed to destroy cancer cells that are growing in the body. Because these drugs are not active specifically against the cancer cells, they can cause many side-effects, because they also affect normal cells. Your drug has been prescribed to treat ————————————————— .

Instructions:

1. The name of your drug is ————————————————— .

2. The dosage of the drug prescribed for you is ————————————— .

3. The schedule of your drug administration is ————————————— .
   (In many situations it will be helpful to prepare a calendar for the patient indicating "drug" days and "free" days for the proposed course of the therapy.)

4. Some side-effects of the drug that you should be aware of include the following:

Nausea, vomiting	Antiemetic and sedative drugs may help. Someone will be with you to help you if these effects occur.
Loss of appetite	It is very important to keep up your strength. Let your nurse know what you would like to eat, anything that appeals to you, or times that you feel hungry.
Loss of hair	The hair will grow back, but may be a different color and consistency when it does. It may be helpful to purchase a wig early in your treatment. Hats and scarves may also be worn. It is important to cover your head in the sun or in cold weather.

(continued)

Mouth sores	Frequent mouth care is very helpful. Try to avoid spicy or harsh foods.
Fatigue, malaise	Frequent rest periods and careful planning of your day's activities will help.
Bleeding	You may bruise easily and your gums may bleed when you brush your teeth. Special care must be taken when shaving, when brushing the teeth, and in other activities to avoid injury. Avoid any medications containing aspirin.
Susceptibility to infection	You should avoid people with infections or colds, and avoid crowded, public places. In some cases, the people caring for you may wear gowns and masks to protect you from their germs.

5. Tell any physician, nurse, or dentist who is taking care of you that you are on this drug.

6. Try to maintain a balanced diet while you are taking this drug. Drink 10 to 12 glasses of water every day during therapy.

7. Use contraceptive measures while taking this drug.

8. You will have to have periodic blood tests while on this drug.

Notify your nurse or physician if any of the following occur:

Bruising, bleeding
Fever, chills
Sore throat
Difficulty breathing
Flank pain
Swelling of your ankles or fingers

Guide to the nursing process: antineoplastic drugs

Assessment	Nursing diagnoses	Interventions	Evaluation

History
Contraindications:
  Pregnancy
  Lactation
	Potential alteration in self-concept (secondary to side-effects of drug)	Safe preparation and administration of drug
		Comfort measures:
			Evaluate effectiveness of drug
			Evaluate for adverse
			(continued)

Assessment	Nursing diagnoses	Interventions	Evaluation
Bone marrow depression	Potential alteration in comfort	Nutritional support	effects:
Renal failure	Potential ineffective coping	Quiet environment	Monitor CBC
Allergies: reaction	Potential for injury	Clean environment	Monitor renal function
Medication history: drugs being taken	Knowledge deficit regarding drug therapy	Rest periods provided	GI effects
		Safety measures	Nutritional status
		Frequent mouth care	Opportunistic infections
Physical assessment:	Potential alteration in nutrition	Stay with patient	
Complete baseline physical exam is essential	Potential alteration in tissue perfusion	Support and encouragement	Monitor effectiveness of comfort measures
Laboratory tests, including:	Potential for fear	Patient teaching provisions	Monitor effectiveness of patient teaching
CBC		Life support measures, if necessary	Monitor effectiveness of support and encouragement measures
Renal function			
Clotting			Monitor and maintain vital signs, as necessary
Liver function			

Case study

Presentation

BW, a 34-year-old, married, white female school teacher, noted an axillary node on her right side that was slightly painful. About 2½ weeks later, she noted a mass in the upper midline portion of her right breast. She underwent a right radical mastectomy with a biopsy report for grade IV infiltrating ductal carcinoma with 28 of 35 lymph nodes positive for tumor. The patient underwent radiation therapy and was started on a 1-year course of CMF (Cytoxan, methotrexate, 5-FU). Initial patient assessment revealed that the patient had no other underlying medical conditions, no allergies, and took no medications. BW's family history was impressive with respect to the incidence of breast cancer: most women in her family had died of breast cancer in their early thirties. BW's physical examination was unremarkable; all data were recorded for baseline reference.

What initial plans should be made for preparing the patient for this long-term drug therapy?

Discussion

The extent of BW's disease, as evidenced by the biopsy results, does not provide a very hopeful prognosis. The nursing care plan formulated for this patient will have to consider the impact of this disease on the psychological and emotional aspects of BW's life as well as on her physical functioning. The drug therapy prescribed will further complicate the patient's situation, because the adverse effects of the drugs will have further impact on all aspects of BW's life.

BW's immediate needs include comfort measures for her postoperative course and her radiation treatments, preparation for the course of chemotherapy, including all the side-effects, support to deal with the diagnosis, effects of the surgery, radiation, and chemotherapy, and the anticipatory grieving and fear, and encouragement to ventilate her feelings, to cope with the treatment, and to organize her life in the best way possible for her.

Particular drug effects related to the CMF therapy that BW will have to deal with include the following: alopecia—it might be helpful for her to get a wig before the treatment begins, and she should also know that her hair will grow back but may be a different color and texture; nausea and vomiting—antiemetics, sedatives, environmental control, and support will be available; skin and fingernails may become dark and sensitive to sunlight—BW should avoid exposure to sunlight and should be reassured that her skin will return to normal; bone marrow suppression—infection and bleeding are the main concerns here. BW should be taught the warning signs of infection and bleeding, and should be advised to avoid use of aspirin-containing products, to avoid crowded places and people with colds or other infections, and to take special precautions for her own safety. Because the CMF will be long-term therapy, a calendar should be prepared for BW with the projected schedule outlined. Because the methotrexate and fluorouracil are given IV, BW will need to be in a health-care facility for their administration; a long-range calendar can help her to plan for the treatments. She should understand, however, that her response to the drug and the disease may change the schedule over the course of the therapy.

All of BW's treatment should be incorporated and organized into a team approach to help her to deal effectively with all the aspects of her disease and its treatment.

Drug digests

Busulfan USP (Myleran)

Actions and indications. This alkylating agent has a selective action on the myeloid cells of the bone marrow. Thus, it is especially effective for bringing about remissions in many patients with chronic myelocytic leukemia. Patients feel better and eat with more appetite soon after beginning treatment. Later, there is a lessening of immature white cells in the blood, and a reduction in the size of the patient's enlarged spleen. Although this drug does not cure this or the other neoplastic disorders in which it is employed, it often prolongs the patient's life.

Adverse effects, cautions, and contraindications. Complete blood cell counts are made regularly, and the drug is discontinued if there is any sudden drop in leukocyte count or if thrombocytopenia and bleeding develop. Careful hematologic control of this type is necessary to avoid pancytopenia and the danger of irreversible bone marrow depression. Hyperuricemia may be controlled and kidney damage by uric acid crystals avoided by the adjunctive use of allopurinol. Skin pigmentation and other signs resembling those of Addison's disease may

occur in rare cases, as do pulmonary fibrosis, impotence, and sterility. Nausea, vomiting, and diarrhea occur in some cases, as do tongue and lip inflammation (glossitis and cheilitis).

Dosage and administration. The usual daily dosage range is 4 mg to 8 mg orally. Treatment is usually initiated with 4 mg daily and continued until the leukocyte count drops below 10,000/mm³. Therapy is resumed when the WBC count rises above 50,000/mm³. Maintenance therapy at doses between 1 mg and 3 mg daily helps to prevent relapse.

Chlorambucil USP (Leukeran)

Actions and indications. This antineoplastic agent acts primarily on lymphoid tissue. Thus, it is used to bring about remissions in patients with chronic lymphocytic leukemia, Hodgkin's disease, and other malignant lymphomas, including the giant follicular type and lymphosarcoma.

Adverse effects, cautions, and contraindications. This nitrogen mustard derivative is less toxic than other alkylating agents. Therapeutic doses cause relatively few gastrointestinal side-effects or blood cell reductions

other than lymphopenia and neutropenia. However, frequent blood counts are required, and dosage is reduced or the drug discontinued in the event of severe neutropenia. Excessive dosage can cause irreversible bone marrow damage.

Patients with evidence of bone marrow infiltration receive smaller doses. The drug is not administered to patients who have received full radiation therapy or other antineoplastic drugs during the previous 4 weeks. Its use during the first trimester of pregnancy

is also avoided.

Dosage and administration. The usual daily dose is between 4 mg and 10 mg administered at one time—usually an hour before breakfast or 2 hours after the evening meal—for 3 to 6 weeks after treatment is initiated. Dosage is adjusted to lower levels if the WBC count falls abruptly. If maintenance dosage is employed, it is ordinarily between 2 mg and 4 mg daily, depending on the patient's response.

Cyclophosphamide USP (Cytoxan)

Actions and indications. This antineoplastic agent is chemically related to the nitrogen mustards but does not cause local irritation while interfering with the growth of lymphatic and myeloid tissues.

It is employed in the advanced stages of malignant lymphomas, including Hodgkin's disease, lymphosarcoma, reticulum cell sarcoma, Burkitt's lymphoma, and lymphoma of the follicular type. It prolongs remissions of acute lymphoblastic leukemia in children. It may be of some use in advanced mycosis fungoides, multiple myeloma, and such solid tumor neoplasms as neuroblastoma and ret-

inoblastoma.

Adverse effects, cautions, and contraindications. Alopecia is a common complication, about which patients should be warned and also reassured, because the hair will grow back following the course of treatment. Nausea and vomiting are also common, as is leukopenia. Thrombocytopenia also occurs sometimes, and caution is required in patients with these hematopoietic disorders as well as in those with impaired liver or kidney function.

Patients should force fluids and void frequently to prevent possible bladder irritation

that can lead to severe sterile hemorrhagic cystitis. This condition is thought to have led occasionally to secondary malignancies of the urinary bladder.

Dosage and administration. Patients initially receive a total loading dose of 40 to 50 mg/kg body weight IV at a rate of 10 to 20 mg/kg daily for 2 to 5 days. The drug may also be administered orally in doses of 1 to 5 mg/kg daily for maintenance therapy, or it may be given on intermittent-type IV dosage schedules twice weekly, or once every 7 to 10 days.

Fluorouracil USP (5-FU; Adrucil; Efudex)

Actions and indications. This potent antimetabolite of the pyrimidine type is thought to cause a thymine deficiency and thus to interfere with the biosynthesis of DNA and RNA. It may help to produce temporary relief in selected cases of solid tumor cancer that cannot be treated surgically or by x-ray. Among the types of carcinoma that may be benefited by management with this antineoplastic agent are solid tumors of the colon and rectum, stomach, and pancreas, and breast and ovarian cancers. A topical form is used to treat solar keratoses—*non-malignant skin lesions that are the result of* prolonged exposure to sunlight.

Adverse effects, cautions, and contraindications. Patients who are receiving their first treatment course with this agent are hospitalized and carefully supervised, because the drug has a low safety margin. Inflammation and even ulceration of the mouth and esophagus are common, as are vomiting and diarrhea. Skin reactions and alopecia are also frequent. Leukopenia occurs in every case treated with adequate dosage.

Patients are carefully selected to screen out those with certain conditions that make them a poor risk for treatment with this toxic drug.

It is contraindicated in those with bone marrow depression or serious infections, or those in poor nutrition. Extreme caution is required in patients with liver and kidney function impairment.

Dosage and administration. The undiluted drug is injected IV once daily for 4 successive days in a dosage of 12 mg/kg body weight. If no toxicity occurs, treatment is continued at a lower dosage level for a few more days. A cream is applied twice daily for 2 to 4 weeks in treating solar keratoses, and up to 10 or 12 weeks in basal cell carcinomas.

Mechlorethamine HCl USP (Mustargen)

Actions and indications. The first of the nitrogen mustards is still considered to be the most effective of the alkylating agents for bringing about rapid and prolonged remissions in patients in advanced stages of Hodgkin's disease and other lymphomas, such as lymphosarcoma. It is also used in treating some solid tumors, including oat cell carcinoma of the lung, and seminomas.

Adverse effects, cautions, and contraindications. This drug has certain drawbacks in addition to the danger of producing bone marrow depression that limits the usefulness of all antineoplastic agents. It can, for example, cause local tissue damage and must be administered with special care to avoid leakage that can lead to severe pain and even to sloughing of the involved tissues. Anorexia, nausea, and vomiting occur commonly, and headache, drowsiness, and weakness are other complaints.

Dosage and administration. This drug is administered by vein in doses ranging from 200 to 600 µg/kg body weight per course of treatment, which may be spread over several days or given all at once, as a freshly prepared solution. The injection is made directly into the tubing of a fast-flowing IV infusion to dilute the vesicant and thus avoid possible damage to the lining of the vein, which can result in thrombophlebitis. Courses of treatment are not repeated until tests indicate recovery of the bone marrow, usually after an interval of at least 6 weeks.

Mercaptopurine USP (Purinethol)

Actions and indications. This antimetabolite interferes with the biosynthesis of nucleic acids by preventing cells from using certain precursor substances, including purines. It is useful mainly for treating acute lymphocytic leukemia in children, particularly when combined with other antineoplastic drugs for maintenance of remissions. Adults with this acute condition also often respond to treatment, but it is *not* effective for treating the chronic form of lymphatic leukemia. Only a few patients with chronic myelocytic leukemia obtain temporary relief, and the drug is ineffective in Hodgkin's disease or solid tumors.

Adverse effects, cautions, and contraindications. The blood count is carefully observed, and the drug is discontinued at the first sign of a large drop in the number of white cells because bone marrow depression may continue even after the drug is withdrawn. Leukopenia and thrombocytopenia are common toxic hematologic effects, but a change in the number of erythrocytes rarely occurs.

Gastrointestinal upset is uncommon in therapeutic doses, but toxic doses may cause vomiting, diarrhea, and mucosal lesions of the mouth. The drug is withheld from patients with jaundice or other signs of liver damage, and caution is required in those with impaired liver function.

Dosage and administration. The usual first dose is 2.5 mg/kg body weight orally each day. When allopurinol is employed with mercaptopurine to prevent hyperuricemia, this usual dose of about 100 mg to 200 mg daily for adults or about 50 mg for young children is reduced to about one-third or one-fourth, because the antigout drug interferes with the metabolic breakdown of this antineoplastic agent.

Methotrexate USP (Amethopterin; MTX)

Actions and indications. This antimetabolite is employed as an antineoplastic agent and in the chemotherapy of severe cases of psoriasis. Remission in these diseases is the result of this drug's ability to interfere with the reproduction of rapidly growing cells. It does so by preventing these cells from using folic acid, a natural metabolite that takes part in the cellular synthesis of nucleic acids, including DNA. This chemical analogue of folic acid competes with it for the enzyme folic acid reductase and thus inhibits the enzymatic reduction of folic acid to tetrahydrofolic acid, the metabolically active form that the cells require for proliferative activity.

Among the neoplastic disorders most responsive to methotrexate are the following: acute lymphoblastic leukemias and such complications as leukemic meningitis; uterine choriocarcinoma, chorioadenoma destruens, and hydatidiform mole; advanced stages of lymphosarcoma and mycosis fungoides; and carcinomas of the head and neck, cervix, and other areas containing solid tumors.

Adverse effects, cautions, and contraindications. Patients undergoing treatment with this highly toxic drug should be closely observed to detect early signs of toxicity. Blood tests are carried out before and during treatment so that the drug may be discontinued if leukopenia, thrombocytopenia, or anemia develop as a result of bone marrow depression.

Other adverse effects that result from damage to the mucosa of the alimentary tract include ulcerative stomatitis and gingivitis, anorexia, nausea, diarrhea, and bleeding. Skin eruptions of various types and alopecia may occur. Central side-effects include headache and drowsiness.

Particular care is required in patients with impaired renal function, because this drug is excreted by the kidneys. It should not be used to treat psoriasis in patients with severe kidney or liver disorders or during pregnancy, because the drug can cause renal failure, acute hepatic toxicity, and damage to the fetus.

Dosage and administration. Dosage schedules vary depending on the disorder being treated.

Oral dosage for remission of acute leukemia in children is 3.3 mg/m² of body surface administered daily for several weeks; for maintenance of remission, methotrexate may be administered orally or IM in doses of 30 mg/m² twice weekly, or in an IV dose of 2.5 mg/kg body weight every 2 weeks. In meningeal leukemia, a solution of the sodium salt is injected intrathecally in doses of 0.2 to 0.5 mg/kg at intervals of 2 to 5 days.

For choriocarcinoma, doses of 15 mg to 30 mg are administered orally or IM for 5 days and repeated in several more courses, with rest periods of 1 week or more between courses.

In mycosis fungoides, 2.5 mg to 10 mg is taken daily by mouth for weeks or months. Several different dosage schedules (oral, IM, and IV) are employed in the initiation and maintenance of psoriasis treatment.

Sodium phosphate P32 solution USP (Phosphotope)

Actions and indications. Radioactive phosphate concentrates in cells with a high reproductive rate, including the bone marrow, lymph nodes, and spleen, and then gives off β particles that damage the cells that they penetrate. Although the range of penetration is only between 2 mm to 8 mm, it is enough to cause a significant drop in the number of blood cells being produced by the bone marrow.

The ionizing radiations from radiophospho-rus have been used particularly in the treatment of polycythemia vera and to a lesser extent in treating chronic myelocytic leukemia. In these conditions the excessive numbers of cells produced by the erythroid and myeloid bone marrow elements are reduced, and clinical remission follows.

Adverse effects, cautions, and contraindications. The patient's blood is examined between courses of radioactive phosphorus to avoid administering too much too frequently, because this can excessively depress the bone marrow and cause leukopenia, thrombocytopenia, and anemia, and other signs of radiation sickness.

Dosage and administration. An intravenous dose of about 3 mc to 5 mc or an oral dose of 6 mc is administered initially for treating polycythemia vera or chronic myelocytic leukemia. Later doses and the intervals at which they are given are determined by the patient's response.

Thiotepa USP

Actions and indications. Thiotepa is mainly used to control the effusion of fluid into various body cavities containing breast or ovarian cancer metastases. Local instillation often results in relief of symptoms such as cough and dyspnea caused by pressure of fluid effusions from the growth.

The drug is also used as an adjunct to radical mastectomy to reduce the rate of recurrences and to support the palliative effect of the operation. It is also applied topically to treat papillary carcinoma of the bladder.

Adverse effects, cautions, and contraindications. This alkylating agent does not cause tissue irritation, as does nitrogen mustard. It may, however, have toxic hematopoietic effects. Thus, white blood cell counts are employed to check the drug's effect on the bone marrow.

Nausea, vomiting, loss of appetite, and headache may occur, particularly in patients with impaired kidney function. Caution is required in patients receiving other antineoplastic drugs or radiation therapy. The drug is not ordinarily administered during pregnancy.

Dosage and administration. Dosage is individualized using the WBC count as a guide to avoid bone marrow depression. The initial adult dose for local instillation is 45 mg to 60 mg weekly, intraperitoneally, intrapleurally, and elsewhere. Half of these doses is injected intravenously in treating malignant lymphomas. A solution containing 60 mg in 30 ml to 60 ml of water is instilled into the bladder for prolonged retention.

Vincristine sulfate USP (Oncovin)

Actions and indications. This plant alkaloid is used mainly in combination with a corticosteroid drug to treat acute lymphoblastic leukemia in children. It brings about remission in a high proportion of cases but seems ineffective in leukemic meningitis. It is also employed in treating Wilms' tumor, Hodgkin's disease, and other malignant lymphomas, and some solid tumors.

Adverse effects, cautions, and contraindications. Alopecia is the most common adverse effect. More serious are the effects of this drug on neuromuscular function. These include loss of deep tendon reflexes, development of a slapping gait, and wastage of muscles. Impaired sensation and paresthesias followed by neuritic pain may precede the motor impairment and ataxia.

Vomiting, diarrhea, abdominal cramps, and occasionally constipation with fecal impaction in the upper colon are other side effects. Leukopenia may appear early, but the platelets and erythrocytes are not effected.

Dosage and administration. This drug is injected intravenously at weekly intervals, beginning in children with 0.05 mg/kg body weight and raising the dose in increments up to a maximum of 0.15 mg/kg over a period of 5 weeks. The carefully calculated dose is injected either into a running IV infusion or directly into the vein, with care to avoid leakage into surrounding tissues because the drug is quite irritating and can cause pain and possible cellulitis.

References

Breaking down the barriers to cancer nursing. RN 41:55; 56; 59; 63, 1978

Calabresi P, Parks RE Jr: Antiproliferative agents and drugs used for immunosuppression. In Gilman AG, Goodman LS, Gilman A (eds): Goodman & Gilman's the Pharmacological Basis of Therapeutics, 6th ed, pp 1249–1255. New York, Macmillan, 1980

Calabresi P, Parks RE Jr: Chemotherapy of neoplastic diseases. In Gilman AG, Goodman LS, Gilman A (eds): Goodman & Gilman's the Pharmacological Basis of Therapeutics, 6th ed, pp 1256–1313. New York, Macmillan, 1980

Cancer chemotherapy. Med Lett Drugs Ther 25:1, 1983

Carter SK, Bakowski MT, Hellmann K: Chemotherapy of Cancer. New York, John Wiley & Sons, 1977

Chabner BA et al: The clinical pharmacology of antineoplastic agents. N Engl J Med 292:1107; 1159, 1975

Cline MG, Haskell CM: Cancer Chemotherapy, 2nd ed. Philadelphia, W. B. Saunders, 1975

DeVita VT Jr et al: L-Combination versus single chemotherapy: A review of the basis for selection of drug treatment of cancer. Cancer 35:98, 1975

Estramustine for prostate cancer. Med Lett Drugs Ther 24:74, 1982

Etoposide (VP 16-213; VePesid). Med Lett Drugs Ther 26:48, 1984

Fisher B et al: Treatment of primary breast cancer with chemotherapy and tamoxifen. N Engl J Med 305:1, 1981

Jaffe N et al: Adjuvant methotrexate and citrovorum factor treatment of osteogenic sarcoma. N Engl J Med 291:994, 1974

Lawrence W Jr, Terz JS: Cancer Management. New York, Grune & Stratton, 1977

Levitt DZ: Cancer chemotherapy: Those dreaded side-effects and what to do about them. RN 44:56, 1981

Leyland–Jones B: Hormones in cancer. Ration Drug Ther 16:1, 1982

Mattia MA, Blake SL: Hospital hazards: Cancer drugs. Am J Nurs 83:758, 1983

Schabel FM Jr: Rationale for adjuvant therapy. Cancer 39(Suppl 6):2875, 1977

Weiss RB: Streptozocin: A review of its pharmacology, efficacy, and toxicity. Cancer Treat Rep 66:427, 1982

Section 3

Drugs
acting on
the peripheral
nervous
system

3

Drugs that produce their primary therapeutic effects by altering the functioning of the nervous system are described in two sections of this book. Drugs whose primary therapeutic effects are produced in the central nervous system—that is, in the brain and spinal cord—will be described in Section 8; drugs whose primary therapeutic effects are produced in the peripheral nervous system are described in this section. Drugs acting on the peripheral nervous system include local anesthetics (Chap. 14), which produce their therapeutic effects by blocking the conduction of nerve impulses in sensory nerves, drugs that either facilitate (Chap. 15) or block (Chap. 19) transmission at the neuromuscular junction, and the autonomic drugs, which either mimic or block the effects of impulses from the parasympathetic or sympathetic nerves on visceral organs (Chaps. 15 through 18).

To understand how drugs produce therapeutically desirable and adverse effects on the nervous system, there must first be an understanding of the normal functions of the nervous system. Chapter 13 reviews cellular neurophysiology and describes the anatomy and physiology of the autonomic nervous system (ANS), providing the background for understanding how autonomic drugs produce their effects.

Autonomic drugs produce their effects mainly by acting on the smooth muscle, cardiac muscle, and gland cells in which the autonomic nerve fibers end. These autonomically innervated muscle and glandular structures are called *effectors*, or *neuroeffectors*, because they respond to nerve impulses by *doing* something. Thus, the several classes of autonomic drugs produce changes in smooth muscle tone and motility, in the rate and strength of heart muscle contractions, and in the secretions of glandular tissues.

Students often find the study of autonomic drugs difficult. However, this need not be so if time is taken first to understand how this system normally functions and then to learn the "lingo," the special terms for describing the different kinds of drug actions. Thus, the introductory chapter of this section will review not only the anatomy and physiology of the autonomic nervous system, but also the specialized terminology that is employed in discussing *neurotransmitters* and the actions of the drugs that act by affecting chemical neurotransmission of messages to autonomically innervated organs and structures.

The study of autonomic pharmacology can also be confusing because many of the drugs act simultaneously at several different sites, including not only the visceral organs that function involuntarily, or without conscious control, but also voluntary (skeletal) muscles, and even neurons of the central nervous system. However, once certain ground rules are understood, the types of effects that autonomic drugs in each of the different subclasses are likely to have on the functioning of various organs that are innervated by ANS fibers can often be predicted in advance.

Similarly, once the complexities of the synaptic transmission of nerve impulses and the manner in which drugs of different classes alter impulse transmission are understood, the study of autonomic pharmacology offers several rewards. Most immediately important for the nurse, of course, is the fact that these are very potent drugs with a great potential for helping or harming patients. The better the nurse understands what these drugs are actually doing in the patient's body, the more likely it is that the patient can be helped to gain the benefits of autonomic drug therapy while avoiding the adverse effects. In addition, students may find satisfaction from successfully meeting the intellectual challenge posed by the need to apply their reasoning powers to the study of these drugs.

Chapter 13

Introduction to the pharmacology of the peripheral nervous system, including the autonomic nervous system

13

The peripheral nervous system is composed of sensory nerves that carry information into the brain and spinal cord, and of motor nerves that carry information from the brain and spinal cord to effector organs. The peripheral nervous system is much better understood by neuroscientists than is the central nervous system (CNS) because the peripheral nervous system is less complex and more readily accessible to experimentation. To understand the pharmacology of the peripheral nervous system, the properties of nerve cells, the nature of nerve signals, and the nature of communication between nerve cells and between nerve cells and effector organs must first be understood.

Neurons and how they function

The neuron

The structural unit of the nervous system is the neuron, or nerve cell, of which there are about 14 billion in the body—about 10 billion being concentrated in the brain alone. Neurons come in many different sizes and shapes, but all are essentially similar in basic structure (Fig. 13-1).

Each neuron is made up of a cell body, often called the *soma*, containing cytoplasm, a nucleus, and other particles or granules. Thin threads of protoplasm project from the surface of the nerve cell body. Most of the cell's surface is covered by short processes that subdivide and send off branches and smaller twigs to form a treelike crown—the *dendrites*. These receive signals *from* many other interconnecting neurons.

One point on the nerve cell body sends out a more elongated process that does not branch until it comes close to other neurons or to cells of effector organs. This is the *axon*, which transmits messages *to* the dendrites, or directly *to* the cell body or soma of other neurons or *to*

effector cells. Such junctions between the axon of one neuron and the dendrites or soma of another neuron or an effector cell are called *synapses*.

The axons of the nerve cells packed closely together in the brain may extend less than 1 μm (only a few thousandths of an inch) before synapsing with other neurons. However, some axonal fibers run for a meter or more (several feet) before synapsing. The corticospinal nerve tracts—bundles of axons that run between nerve cell bodies in the brain and the spinal cord and make up much of the white matter of the CNS—are one example of the latter. Another example may be seen in the bundles of fibers that pass from the CNS to the skeletal muscles and other peripheral organs.

These axonal cables make up the peripheral nervous system. The nerve fibers that transmit *sensory* signals to the CNS from peripheral receptors are called *afferent* fibers. Those that conduct impulses from the CNS that elicit responses from muscles and glands are called *efferent* fibers, and include *motor* and *secretory* fibers.

The nerve impulse (action potential)

The axons of nerve cells are specialized for conducting electrical signals, called *action potentials. Conduction* of action potentials is the means by which nerve cells send messages to other cells, sometimes over great distances. For example, the axon of a spinal motoneuron that terminates on a flexor muscle in the big toe will carry action potentials for a meter or more. The final step by which this motoneuron communicates with the muscle in the big toe involves another process called *synaptic transmission,* described in the next section.

Nerve cells are specialized for sending out electrical signals. Actually, all living cells possess electrical properties that stem from the nature of their membranes. However, the thin threads of neuronal tissue are capable of conducting electrical signals at a speed much greater

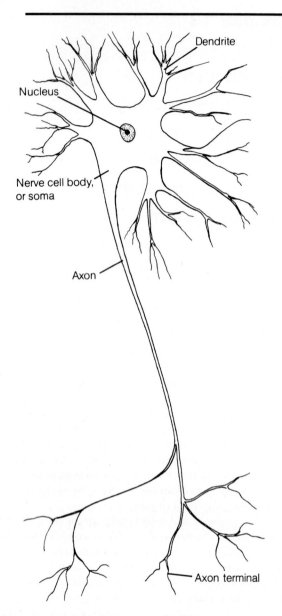

Figure 13-1. A neuron—the structural unit of the nervous system.

stances into the interior of the cells and keep others out. The membranes of neurons that are at rest are impermeable to sodium ions—that is, they keep sodium ions out of the cell. However, they are permeable to potassium ions. Sodium ions thus are in higher concentration in the extracellular fluid than in the intracellular fluid of the neuron, whereas potassium ions are in higher concentration in the intracellular fluid. This differential in the distribution of ions on either side of the cell membrane leads to the buildup of an electrical *potential* between the two sides of the membrane—thus, the interior of the nerve cell becomes negatively charged as compared to the more positively charged exterior of the cell (Fig. 13-2). This is referred to as the neuron's *resting membrane potential* (RMP).

Stimulation of the neuron by an incoming excitatory signal from another neuron *depolarizes* the neuron—that is, the stimulus reduces the membrane potential, making the inside of the cell less negative. In some way, *depolarization* increases the permeability of the cell membrane to sodium ions, and sodium ions rush into the cell, down their concentration gradient, further depolarizing the cell. When depolarization reaches a critical level, called the *threshold membrane potential,* or simply *threshold,* an *action potential* is generated (Fig. 13-3).

The action potential is a sudden, transient change in membrane potential. A single action potential lasts less than 0.001 second (less than 1 msec); the resting membrane potential is then restored. During the depolarizing phase of the action potential, the polarity of the cell membrane actually reverses; the inside of the cell becomes positively charged as a result of the inrush of positively charged sodium ions. The membrane then becomes impermeable to sodium ions but more permeable to potassium ions. Restoration of the resting membrane potential of the cell, or *repolarization,* occurs as potassium ions flow out of the cell, down their concentration gradient.

The action potential thus generated sets up an electrical field in adjacent portions of the cell membrane. This electrical field acts as a stimulus to the adjacent portion of the membrane, which depolarizes, becomes more permeable to sodium ions, reaches threshold, and generates an action potential, which serves as a stimulus to the next adjacent portion of membrane, and so forth. It is in this manner that the action potential is *conducted* along the axon.

Trains of many action potentials may be set up by appropriate stimuli. A neuron cannot respond to a new stimulus, though, until it has been repolarized, as described above. The period of time during which a neuron cannot respond to a stimulus is known as its *refractory period.* This refractory period ordinarily lasts, at most, a few milliseconds. Thus, axons can conduct several hundred action potentials each second. The sodium–potassium pump prevents the buildup of sodium inside the cell and the loss of potassium from the cell that would

than that of other types of tissue. Some drugs act by changing the ability of neurons to conduct and transmit nerve impulses.

Learning how drugs affect neuronal conduction requires an understanding of how action potentials are produced and conducted. This, in turn, requires understanding a few facts about nerve cell membranes, their permeability to various ions, and the resulting distribution of ions inside and outside of the axon.

The membranes of neurons contain a *sodium–potassium pump* (often called simply a *sodium pump*) that pumps sodium ions out of the cell and pumps potassium ions into it. In addition, the membranes of neurons, like those of other cells, contain pores that allow some sub-

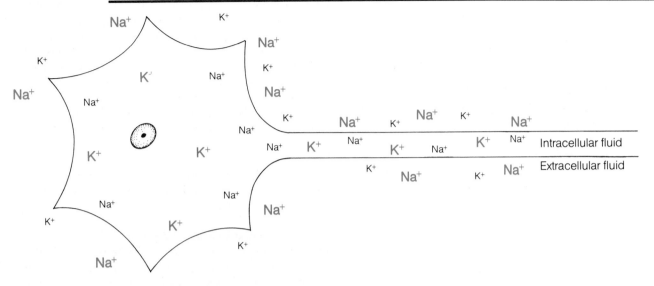

Figure 13-2. Relative concentrations of sodium and potassium ions inside and outside the neuron. In the intracellular fluid, potassium is present in high concentration and sodium in low concentration. In the extracellular fluid, the situation is reversed. The size of the symbol for each ion represents the relative concentration of that ion.

occur during high-frequency firing of action potentials without this pump.

Drugs can affect the conduction of action potentials in various ways. For example, local anesthetics such as lidocaine (Xylocaine) interfere with the conduction of action potentials by blocking the inrush of sodium ions. Thus, local anesthetics block the conduction of pain impulses over peripheral sensory nerves into the central nervous system. Other drugs, such as diuretics, laxatives, and emetics that can alter fluid and electrolyte (sodium and potassium) balance, can also affect the ability of neurons and other excitable cells (cardiac, skeletal, and smooth muscle cells) to generate and conduct action potentials.

Synaptic transmission

When the *nerve action potentials* arrive at the branching ends of the axon, they influence other nearby neurons or effector cells. However, there is a delay of a few thousandths of a second (a few milliseconds) in the spread of the electrical signals to the secondary nerve cells or effectors. One reason for this is that axon terminals do not come into direct contact with the processes of other neurons or with the muscle fibers and secretory cells that they innervate. The electron microscope has shown that there is a microscopic gap, called the *synaptic cleft,* at the synapses between nerve cells and at the junctions between

nerves and muscle or gland cells.* It is now known that, when an action potential reaches the axon terminal, it triggers the release of a chemical substance, called a *neurotransmitter,* from the nerve terminal (Fig. 13-4). That is, the nerve impulse arriving in the axon terminals of the first nerve cell (the *presynaptic neuron*) causes certain granules (the *synaptic vesicles*) concentrated there to release molecules of a neurotransmitter substance. This chemical bridges the gap between the presynaptic nerve endings and the membrane of the *postsynaptic* cell. The molecules of neurotransmitter diffuse across the synaptic cleft, combine with specialized *receptors* on the postsynaptic membrane, and change the membrane's permeability to various ions (sodium, potassium, chloride). The changes in ionic permeability in turn produce small changes in the membrane potential of the postsynaptic cell, and either excite or inhibit it.

The changes in membrane potential produced by neurotransmitters are referred to by various names, depending on the synapse and on the effect produced. Changes in membrane potential produced at the synapse of one neuron with another are called *synaptic potentials;* they are either *excitatory postsynaptic potentials* (*EPSPs*) or *inhibitory postsynaptic potentials* (*IPSPs;* see below). The small changes in membrane potential produced at the synapses of nerves with the cells of visceral effector organs are called *junctional potentials;* they, too, are either excitatory or inhibitory. The changes in membrane potential produced at the synapse of a motoneuron with a skeletal muscle cell are called *end-plate potentials* (*EPPs*).

At some synapses, the change in ionic permeability is produced only after the neurotransmitter stim-

---

* A very few mammalian synapses lack a synaptic cleft. These synapses operate electrically, not chemically, and they operate without a synaptic delay. They will not be discussed further in this book, both because they are seldom encountered and because they are unlikely sites for clinically important drug actions.

A.

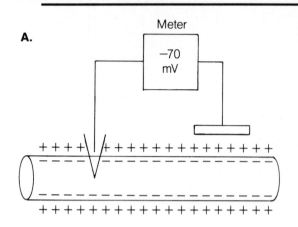

B.

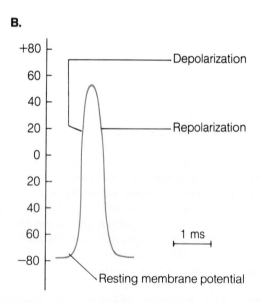

Figure 13-3. Membrane potentials. (*A*) A segment of an axon showing that, at rest, the inside of the membrane is negatively charged and the outside is positively charged. A pair of electrodes placed as shown would record a potential difference of about 70 mV (0.070 V); this is the resting membrane potential. (*B*) An action potential lasting about 1 msec (0.001 sec), such as that shown, would be recorded if the axon shown in *A* were brought to threshold. At the peak of the action potential, the charge on the membrane reverses polarity.

ulates the synthesis of a so-called "second messenger" chemical substance in the postsynaptic cell. Cyclic adenosine monophosphate (*cyclic AMP*, or cAMP) and cyclic guanosine monophosphate (*cyclic GMP*, or cGMP) have been identified as second messengers at some synapses.

The sequence of biochemical events that is initiated by the combination of the neurotransmitter with postsynaptic receptors causes the postsynaptic cell to carry out its characteristic function, or to stop doing so. Nerve cells that are brought to threshold by the summation of

EPSPs will fire an action potential, or they may be prevented from doing so by IPSPs; skeletal muscle cells brought to threshold by EPPs will fire an action potential and contract; exocrine gland cells will secrete more copiously or be prevented from secreting; and intestinal smooth muscle cells will either contract more vigorously or relax their contractions.

Finally, the action of the neurotransmitter is terminated in one or more ways. The molecules of neurotransmitter may diffuse out of the synapse, they may be inactivated by enzymes, or they may be taken up by the nerve terminal that released them or by other cells near the synapse. All these steps in synaptic transmission are shown in Figure 13-4.

Neurotransmitter substances

A chemical must meet certain criteria to be identified as the neurotransmitter at a given synapse. First, it must be synthesized and released by the presynaptic neuron. Then, when the chemical is applied experimentally to the postsynaptic cell, it must produce effects on the postsynaptic cell identical to those of the neurotransmitter, and these effects must be potentiated or antagonized (see Chap. 4) by the drugs that potentiate or antagonize the effects of the neurotransmitter. Finally, a mechanism must exist for terminating the effects of the chemical.

Using these criteria, investigators have identified *acetylcholine (ACh)* as the neurotransmitter at the skeletal neuromuscular junction. Both acetylcholine and *norepinephrine (NE)* have been identified as neurotransmitters at different synapses in the autonomic nervous system. A more detailed description of cholinergic (ACh) and adrenergic (NE) synapses is given below (see Neurotransmission in the Peripheral Nervous System) and in Figures 13-5 and 13-6.

The nature of chemical transmission in the CNS is thought to be essentially similar to that which occurs in the peripheral nervous system. However, because of the difficulty of studying central synapses, it has been hard to prove that a chemical that is present in the brain actually functions as a neurotransmitter at specific synapses. Still, several substances in addition to ACh and NE, the two neurochemicals that control nerve impulse transmission in the autonomic nervous system, have been identified as central neurotransmitters.

Dopamine, a chemical precursor in the biosynthesis of NE, is now known to be a neurotransmitter itself in extrapyramidal motor system pathways. As a result of this knowledge, drugs such as *levodopa* (L-dopa) have been devised to help overcome the deficiency of brain dopamine in patients with Parkinson's disease.

Dopamine and another biogenic amine, the indolamine 5-hydroxytryptamine (5-HT; *serotonin*), also probably play a part in the transmission or modulation of nerve impulses in the limbic system and other brain areas that influence emotional and behavioral responses.

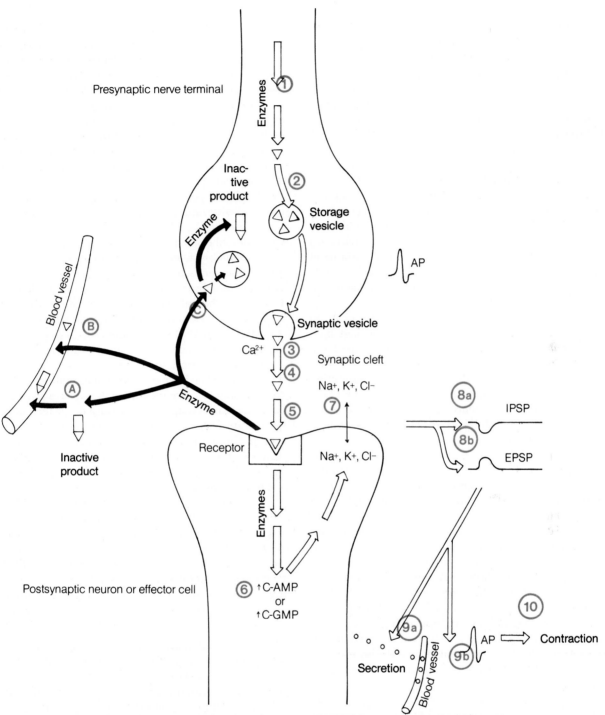

Figure 13-4. Sequence of events in synaptic or junctional transmission (transmission at any one synapse does not involve all these steps). (*1*) Synthesis of neurotransmitter (▽) may require several steps. (*2*) Uptake of neurotransmitter into storage (synaptic) vesicle. (*3*) Release of neurotransmitter by action potential (AP) in presynaptic nerve. (*4*) Diffusion of neurotransmitter across synaptic cleft. (*5*) Combination of neurotransmitter with receptor. (*6*) A series of events leading to synthesis of a "second messenger" (this has been shown only for a few synapses; step 6 is omitted at many synapses). (*7*) Change in permeability of the postsynaptic membrane to one or more ions. (*8*) Small change in membrane potential: (*8a*) inhibitory postsynaptic (IPSP) or junctional potential; (*8b*) excitatory postsynaptic (EPSP) or junctional potential. (*9*) Characteristic response of cell (occurs as result of step *8b*): (*9a*) gland cells secrete; (*9b*) muscle cells fire action potentials. (*10*) contraction of muscle cells.
      The action of the neurotransmitter is terminated by one or more of the following processes: (*A*) inactivation by an enzyme; (*B*) diffusion out of the synaptic cleft; (*C*) reuptake into the presynaptic nerve, followed by storage in synaptic vesicle or by enzymatic inactivation.

Certain psychotropic drugs such as the phenothiazines, haloperidol, and other neuroleptic agents are thought to improve mental function and behavior in schizophrenia and other psychoses by blocking the effects of excess dopamine. The antidepressant drugs that are employed in the management of mental depression are thought to correct a functional deficiency of norepinephrine and 5-hydroxytryptamine and to alter the relationship of these biogenic amines with dopaminergic neural systems.

γ-*Aminobutyric acid* (GABA), an amino acid long known to act as an inhibitory transmitter in lower animals, is now thought to function in similar fashion in the nervous system of mammals, including humans. Certain convulsant poisons such as *picrotoxin* act by blocking the inhibitory effect of GABA on central motor neuron activity. An experimental drug called *muscimol*, which stimulates GABA receptors in the brain, may prove to be therapeutically useful in disorders marked by a deficiency of GABA.

Glycine is another amino acid that acts as an inhibitory neurotransmitter. Its effects are blocked by a different convulsant drug, *strychnine*, and its release from nerve terminals is blocked by *tetanus toxin*. This action of tetanus toxin results in the loss of normal inhibiting mechanisms in the spinal motoneuron circuits in which glycine is an inhibitory neurotransmitter, and it is responsible for the painful and life-threatening muscle spasms that characterize tetanus.

Several other substances, including *histamine*, *prostaglandins*, and a recently isolated class of peptides called *enkephalins*, are claimed to have neurotransmitter or modulator functions centrally. The enkephalins are concentrated in regions of the brain that are involved in the perception of and emotional response to painful stimuli. Although their physiologic function as neurotransmitters is not proved, there is currently considerable interest in research on these compounds. One reason is that the enkephalins, or the larger molecules from which they are probably derived—the *endorphins*—may prove useful for developing potent, nonaddicting analgesic drugs. Also of interest are research observations that suggest a relationship between imbalances in the brain's content of endorphins and the development of mental illnesses such as schizophrenia.

In addition, very recent evidence suggests that substances such as corticotropin (ACTH), vasopressin (ADH), oxytocin, luteinizing hormone-releasing hormone (LH-RH), thyrotropin-releasing hormone (TRH), and somatostatin, which have long been thought to have purely endocrine or neuroendocrine functions, may serve as neurotransmitters or neuromodulators in regions of the brain remote from the endocrine hypothalamus and the pituitary gland.

Synaptic excitation and inhibition

Individual nerve cell fibers fire impulses in an *all-or-none* fashion. That is, weak signals call forth no response at all, while impulses that exceed a certain critical level, or *threshold,* make the axon send along a signal (action potential) of maximum strength. However, the response of *postsynaptic* nerve cell bodies is *not* all or none in nature, but varies instead with the strength of the signals reaching it. The reason for this is that each nerve cell receives excitatory and inhibitory postsynaptic potentials from the endings of not one but *many* other axons. The impulses arriving at the postsynaptic nerve cell can change its membrane potential in either of two opposite directions. The *excitatory* presynaptic fibers release neurochemicals that tend to depolarize the second neuron of the synapse; these depolarizations are the EPSPs described above. At the same time, signals reaching this same nerve cell from still other fibers may tend to reduce its responsiveness. These *inhibitory* fibers release a type of chemical transmitter that tends to stabilize, or *hyperpolarize*, the postsynaptic membrane; these hyperpolarizations are the IPSPs described above. The second cell in the synaptic chain will fire an action potential only when the sum of the EPSPs and IPSPs simultaneously impinging on it in a brief period exceeds the critical threshold level.

In addition to *postsynaptic inhibition* (just described), another form of neuronal inhibition, called *presynaptic inhibition*, occurs in the CNS at sites at which one nerve terminal synapses on a second nerve terminal. The neurotransmitter released by the first nerve terminal decreases the amount of excitatory neurotransmitter released by the second nerve terminal. This decreases the excitation produced in the cell with which the second neuron synapses.

Similarly, some cells of visceral organ effectors receive both excitatory and inhibitory junctional potentials from the autonomic nervous system, with one type of potential coming from sympathetic nerves and the other type from parasympathetic nerves (see below). This dual type of innervation and the modulation resulting from it provide for the moment-to-moment fine tuning of visceral organ responses.

General pharmacology of synaptic transmission

The complex processes involved in chemical transmission at synapses provide many sites at which drugs may act. In studying autonomic and central nervous system drugs, examples will be encountered of drugs that act by each of the following mechanisms:

- Interference with the synthesis of a neurotransmitter
- Facilitation of the synthesis of a neurotransmitter
- Interference with the storage of a neurotransmitter in synaptic vesicles
- Interference with the release of a neurotransmitter

- Stimulation of the release of a neurotransmitter
- Occupation of receptors for a neurotransmitter, leading either to the expected effects of the neurotransmitter or to blocking of these effects
- Inhibition of an enzyme that inactivates a neurotransmitter
- Blocking of the reuptake of a neurotransmitter

A few examples of drugs that interact with specific neurotransmitter processes were given above. As more examples are encountered, it will become apparent that drugs that act this way can produce a wide spectrum of effects.

The autonomic nervous system

General functions

The autonomic nervous system (ANS) regulates the functioning of the viscera, or internal organs, and other structures that function in ways that cannot usually be controlled by an act of will. Although some people can be trained to alter their heart rate or to lower their blood pressure by conditioning and biofeedback techniques, most cannot voluntarily control the functioning of their cardiovascular system or any of the viscera.

The ANS is also called the *visceral* or *involuntary nervous system*. These terms indicate a major functional difference between autonomic nerves and other *nonautonomic*, or somatic, nerves that carry conscious commands from the CNS to skeletal muscles. Although we cannot consciously influence its activity, the ANS *is* influenced by areas of the cerebral cortex and by other CNS nerve centers. Similarly, although we tend to think of the ANS mainly in terms of the nerve fibers that carry motor and secretory messages *from* the CNS, these efferent impulses are actually set off by streams of afferent impulses that travel to the CNS from the viscera and other autonomically innervated structures. The baroreceptor reflex that regulates blood pressure is an example of an autonomic reflex that functions in the way just described.

The main nerve centers for these autonomic reflex arcs are located in the hypothalamus, medulla oblongata, and spinal cord. Nerve impulses that arise in peripheral structures are carried to these centers by afferent fibers. The integrating centers at various levels of the CNS then respond by sending out efferent impulses by way of ANS pathways. These then adjust the functioning of the various visceral organs in ways that keep the body's internal environment constant (homeostasis). The ANS regulates blood pressure, breathing, body temperature, water balance, and urinary bladder and digestive functions, among others. This moment-to-moment con-

trol is exerted by a never ending interplay between two opposing subdivisions of the peripheral part of the ANS: the *sympathetic* and the *parasympathetic systems.*

Divisions

In each of the two divisions of the ANS, nerve impulses are carried from the CNS to outlying organs and structures by way of a two-neuron chain. Nerve cell bodies located at various levels of the cerebrospinal axis send their axons out toward the periphery. However, these axons do *not* pass directly to the organs that they innervate.

Instead, the axons from the first, or central, neuron end in *ganglia*, groups of nerve cell bodies packed together in various locations outside the CNS. These second neurons then receive impulses from the *pre*ganglionic nerve terminals and relay the messages down their postganglionic axons. When these nerve impulses finally reach the terminals of the postganglionic axons, they release chemicals that transmit impulses to the neuroeffector cells located in the innervated smooth and cardiac muscle and exocrine glands. This differs from the way in which messages travel from the CNS to skeletal muscle fibers. That is, messages in the somatic fibers of mixed spinal nerves go directly from the CNS to the skeletal muscle fibers without any intervening nerve cells.

The two-neuron pathways of both subdivisions of the ANS differ from each other in several ways:

1. In the location within the CNS of the first nerve cell body of the two-neuron chain
2. In the location of the ganglia containing the second cells in the link, and
3. In the relative lengths of the preganglionic and postganglionic axons that connect these subdivisions of the ANS with the visceral organs that they innervate (Table 13-1 and Fig. 13-5)

Sympathetic system anatomy

This system is also called the *thoracolumbar* system, because the first nerve cell bodies are located in the part of the spinal cord that runs through the chest, or thorax, down into the lumbar region of the back. These centrally located cells send out relatively short *pre*ganglionic axons that synapse with nerve cells in ganglia located mostly in chains that run like a paired string of beads just outside the spinal cord (Fig. 13-5). Relatively long *post*ganglionic axons then make their way to the autonomically innervated visceral organs.

The adrenal medulla is also part of the sympathetic nervous system. Like sympathetic ganglia, it is innervated by sympathetic preganglionic axons. However, its cells lack axons and, instead of innervating visceral organs, the adrenal medullary cells influence organs by the substances that they secrete into the systemic circulation.

Table 13–1. Comparison of somatic motor, sympathetic, and parasympathetic outflow

Characteristics	Somatic motor system	Autonomic nervous system	
		Sympathetic nervous system	Parasympathetic nervous system
CNS neuron	Motoneuron	Preganglionic neuron	Preganglionic neuron
Location of cell body	Anterior horn of spinal cord	Lateral horn of thoracolumbar spinal cord	Brain: midbrain and medulla; sacral spinal cord
Path of axon	Axons leave spinal cord in ventral roots and go directly to skeletal muscle fibers	Short preganglionic axons leave cord in ventral roots, go through white rami communicantes to vertebral and other ganglia, and to adrenal medulla; terminals synapse with many cells in ganglia	Long preganglionic axons leave CNS in cranial nerves III, VII, IX, and X, and in sacral spinal nerves; go to ganglia in or near organs; terminals synapse with few cells
Neurotransmitter released	ACh	ACh	ACh
Cells innervated	Skeletal muscle fibers	Neurons in sympathetic ganglia; chromaffin cells in adrenal medulla	Neurons in parasympathetic ganglia
Types of receptor	Nicotinic cholinergic	Nicotinic cholinergic	Nicotinic cholinergic
Drugs blocking transmission	Neuromuscular junction blockers: curare, succinylcholine	Ganglionic blockers: trimethaphan	Ganglionic blockers: trimethaphan
Second neuron	None	Neurons in sympathetic ganglia	Neurons in parasympathetic ganglia
Location of cell body		Vertebral and other sympathetic ganglia in abdomen	Parasympathetic ganglia
Path of axon		Long postganglionic axons go to cells of organ innervated	Short postganglionic axons go to cells of organ innervated
Neurotransmitter released		Generally, NE; at sweat glands and some skeletal muscle blood vessels, ACh	ACh
Cells innervated		Visceral organs, vasculature, exocrine glands	Visceral organs, vasculature, exocrine glands
Types of receptor		Generally, α, β_1, or β_2 adrenergic; sweat glands and some blood vessels in skeletal muscle—muscarinic cholinergic	Muscarinic cholinergic

Table 13–1. Comparison of somatic motor, sympathetic, and parasympathetic outflow (continued)

Characteristics	Somatic motor system	Autonomic nervous system	
		Sympathetic nervous system	Parasympathetic nervous system
Drugs blocking transmission		Adrenergic receptor blockers: α receptor blockers—phentolamine; β receptor blockers—propranolol; muscarinic receptors in sweat glands and blood vessels of skeletal muscle: atropine	Atropine

Parasympathetic system anatomy

This system is also called the *craniosacral* system, because its cells of origin lie centrally at the two extreme ends of the cerebrospinal axis. Some nerve cell bodies are located at subcortical levels of the brain (*i.e.,* within the cranium), while others are located in the sacral portion of the spinal cord. Thus, some parasympathetic preganglionic axons run in cranial nerves such as the facial and vagus nerves. Other parasympathetic preganglionic axons, originating at lower levels of the spinal cord, form the pelvic nerves, which send branches to organs such as the urinary bladder and lower large intestine. The ganglia of the parasympathetic nervous system typically lie close to or within the organ that is innervated by the short postganglionic axons.

Comparison of physiologic functions

The sympathetic system, including the adrenal medulla, tends to regulate the expenditure of energy, especially in times of stress. The parasympathetic system, on the other hand, mainly influences functions that help the body to store up and save energy.

Each system is organized anatomically and chemically in ways that serve these differing functions. Thus, the sympathetic system sends out numerous axons that synapse with many different ganglion cells. Its postganglionic axons release sudden spurts of nerve impulse-transmitting chemicals all at once at many different sites. These chemical substances and the related ones released into the systemic circulation by the adrenal medulla are relatively long-lasting in their effects. The parasympathetic system, on the other hand, discharges its impulses to specific organs in a more narrow and localized manner. Its neurochemical transmitter is more rapidly destroyed.

Thus, the sympathetic system helps the organism to react vigorously to emergencies, whereas the parasympathetic system helps to restore the expended energy gradually through a series of separate but interrelated activities of various organs.

The opposing functions of the two divisions of the ANS may be understood by a thoughtful study of Table 13-2. A typical *sympathetic response* is the "fight-or-flight" reaction that occurs when the organism feels threatened and reacts with rage and fear: the heartbeat speeds up, blood pressure rises, and blood leaves the constricted vessels of the skin and viscera and is shunted to the dilated arterioles in the hard-working heart and skeletal muscles; at the same time, the extra amounts of oxygen and glucose that these muscles require are supplied by liver glycogen breakdown and by rapid deep breathing to take in air through widely dilated lung bronchi.

The *parasympathetic system*, on the other hand, slows the heart, constricts the dilated pupils of the eyes to protect the retinas from excessive light, and restarts the temporarily stalled gastrointestinal movements and secretions so that digestion and assimilation of foodstuffs can once more proceed. It helps also to rid the urinary bladder and the rectum of body wastes.

These systems do not function only as emergency mechanisms, however; their work goes on continuously, making possible the delicate adjustments needed to keep up with the ever-changing environment. It is perhaps better to think of the two systems as functioning like the handlebars of a bicycle, which help the rider keep to a straight course when automatically putting pressure on one handle or the other to correct any tendency of the bike to veer too far to the right or the left.

Actually, this picture is somewhat simplified. Both
(Text continues p. 303)

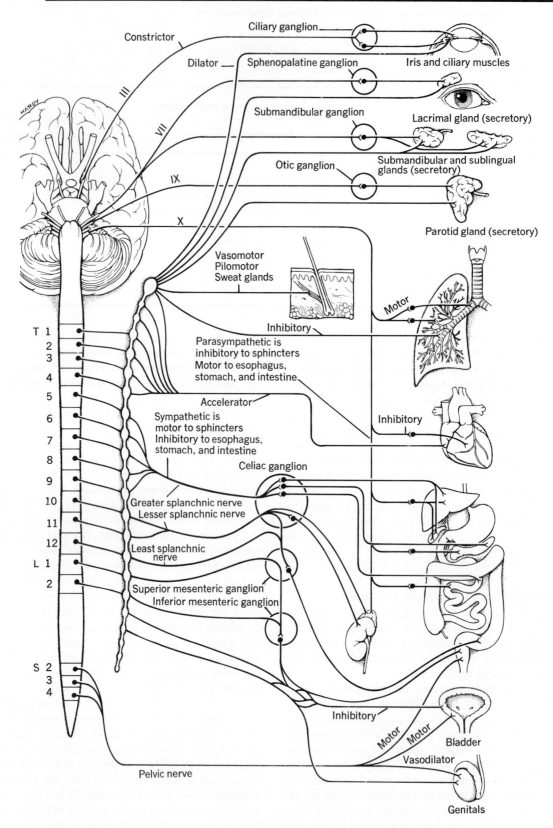

Figure 13-5. The autonomic nervous system. The parasympathetic, or craniosacral, division sends long preganglionic fibers that synapse with a second nerve cell in ganglia located close to or within the organs that are then innervated by short postganglionic fibers. The sympathetic, or thoracolumbar, division sends relatively short preganglionic fibers to the chains of paravertebral ganglia and to certain outlying ganglia. The second cell then sends relatively long postganglionic fibers to the organs that they innervate.

Table 13–2. The most important effects of autonomic nervous stimulation: Comparison of responses to sympathetic and parasympathetic nerve impulses

Organs and structures	Sympathetic nerve impulses	Type of sympathetic receptor	Parasympathetic nerve impulses
Heart	Increase in heart rate and contractility; increase in atrioventricular conduction velocity	β_1	Decrease in heart rate and in atrioventricular conduction velocity
Blood vessels			
Skin and mucous membrane	Constriction	α	—
Skeletal muscle	Dilatation (usually)	Cholinergic,* β_2†	—
Bronchial muscle	Relaxation (lumen dilated)	β_2	Contraction (lumen constricted)
Gastrointestinal system			
Muscle motility and tone	Decrease	β_2	Increase
Sphincters	Contraction (ordinarily)	α	Relaxation (ordinarily)
Exocrine glands	Secretion reduced (?)	(?)	Secretion increased
Gallbladder	Relaxation	(?)	Contraction
Urinary bladder			
Detrusor	Relaxation	β_2	Contraction
Trigone and sphincter	Contraction	α	Relaxation
Ocular structures			
Iris radial muscle	Contraction (pupil dilates)	α	—
Iris sphincter muscle	—	—	Contraction (pupil constricts)
Ciliary muscle	—	—	Contraction (lens accommodated for near vision)
Skin structures			
Sweat glands	Generalized increase in sweating	Cholinergic*	—
Pilomotor muscles	Contracted (gooseflesh)	α	—
Miscellaneous			
Salivary glands	Thick, viscid secretion	α	Copious, watery secretion
Lacrimal and nasopharyngeal glands	—	—	Increased secretion
Liver	Glycogenolysis	β_2	—
Male sex organs	Emission	α	Erection (vascular dilatation)
Uterus	Relaxation	β_2	—

* Cholinergic transmission; nerve cell chain originates in thoracolumbar portion of spinal cord and is, therefore, sympathetic.
† The β_2 receptors in the blood vessels of skeletal muscle may not be innervated; nevertheless, low concentrations of epinephrine, released from the adrenal medulla by sympathetic impulses, may act on these receptors to produce vasodilatation.

divisions of the ANS do not exert equal control over all organs. For example, the parasympathetic system has greater influence on gastrointestinal tract function than does the sympathetic, whereas the latter regulates blood vessel tone and blood pressure to a much greater extent than does the parasympathetic system. Sometimes the term "sympathetic tone" is used to describe the influence of the sympathetic nervous system on the vasculature.

Nonetheless, the general concept of two opposing systems in a state of tonic, or continuous, activity designed to achieve an unstable, shifting functional balance can help the actions of the various autonomic drugs to be understood. By acting at the same synapses and neuroeffectors as do the ANS nerve impulses, these drugs tend to upset the temporary balance in one direction or another. Thus, some drugs may imitate, or *mimic*, the effects either of sympathetic or of parasympathetic stimulation in slowing down or speeding up a particular function. On the other hand, some drugs may prevent nerve impulses from reaching the muscle or gland cells through one or the other division of the ANS. In that case, the still active division tends to exert a disproportionate influence on the functioning of most of the organs, structures, and systems that have had part of their tonic nervous control blocked out.

Neurotransmission in the peripheral nervous system

As stated above, the two neurohormones known to be released by peripheral nerves are *acetylcholine* (ACh) and *norepinephrine* (NE). The complicated processes by which these nerve impulse-transmitting substances are synthesized, stored, released, and inactivated are very vulnerable to interference by foreign chemicals. Autonomic drugs act in various ways: (1) to imitate or mimic the actions of the natural neurohormones; (2) to intensify their activity; or (3) to impair their activity. Thus, to understand how the many complex effects of autonomic drugs are brought about, it is necessary to understand, in some detail, the processes of neurotransmission by ACh and NE.

Cholinergic transmission

Types of cholinergic nerves. Several different types of peripheral nerves transmit nerve impulses by releasing ACh as the chemical transmitter between the neuron and the second cell in the series. *There are three major classes of cholinergic nerves:*

1. *Postganglionic cholinergic nerves.* These include all the parasympathetic postganglionic axons and a few exceptional sympathetic postganglionic axons—those to the sweat glands and to some blood vessels (Tables 13-1 and 13-2).
2. *Preganglionic cholinergic nerves.* These include *all* the preganglionic axons of *both* the sympathetic and parasympathetic

divisions of the ANS. (The cells of the adrenal medulla—a structure similar to autonomic ganglia except that it is made up of gland cells instead of nerve cells—are also innervated by cholinergic preganglionic nerves that originate, along with other sympathetic preganglionic nerves, in the spinal cord.)
3. *Somatic motor nerves.* These nerves, although they are *not* part of the ANS, also release ACh from their endings on skeletal (voluntary) muscle. (Cholinergic transmission is not limited to nerves of the ANS nor even to peripheral nerves alone. ACh is, as previously indicated, also the chemical mediator at certain synapses in nerve pathways that lie entirely within the CNS.)

Acetylcholine synthesis and storage. ACh is an ester of acetic acid and the organic alcohol choline. The last step in its biosynthesis is catalyzed by an enzyme, *choline acetyltransferase,* which is itself synthesized in the nerve cell body and then carried down to the nerve ending, where it performs its function of acetylating choline with acetyl coenzyme A. The ACh molecules are then stored in a bound, or inactive, form, in tiny storage sacs called *synaptic vesicles.* Figure 13-6 summarizes these steps and the overall sequence of steps in cholinergic transmission.

ACh release. The arrival of the action potential (AP) at the nerve ending leads to the release of ACh molecules from such storage vesicles in a reaction that is dependent on the presence of calcium ions. When the nerve cell membrane becomes depolarized by the AP, calcium ions in the extracellular fluid flow into the cytoplasm of the nerve ending. They then promote a process that pushes the ACh-containing vesicles into contact with the nerve cell membrane. Then both the vesicular and the neuronal membranes break down, and a packet of ACh molecules is discharged into the junctional space in a process called *exocytosis.*

Muscarinic and nicotinic cholinergic receptors. The freed ACh molecules that pour out of the nerve terminals cross the junction and make momentary contact with a chemically specialized spot on the postjunctional membrane, called the *cholinergic receptor.* There are two types of cholinergic receptors, referred to as muscarinic and nicotinic. These terms stem from the fact that in early pioneering studies of ANS function, scientists employed muscarine, an alkaloid of the mushroom *Amanita muscaria,* and nicotine, the tobacco plant alkaloid. *Muscarinic receptors* are those cholinergic receptors at which muscarine acts; *nicotinic receptors* are those at which nicotine acts. Neither muscarine nor nicotine is therapeutically useful although they have given their names to receptors at which therapeutically important drugs act.

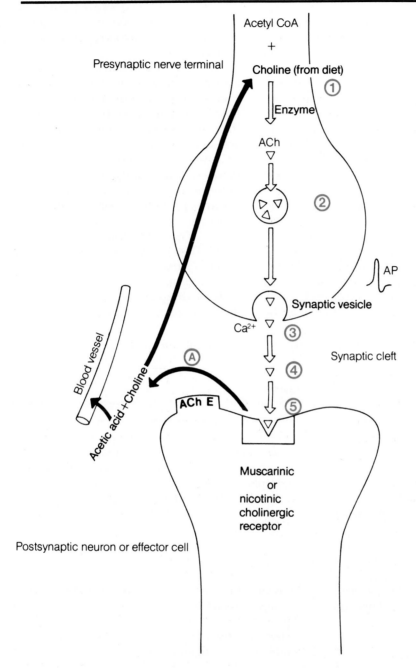

Figure 13-6. Sequence of events at a cholinergic synapse. (*1*) Synthesis of acetylcholine (ACh, ∇) from choline (a substance in the diet) and a cofactor (the enzyme is choline acetyltransferase—no therapeutically important drugs interact with this enzyme). (*2*) Uptake of neurotransmitter into storage (synaptic) vesicle. (*3*) Release of neurotransmitter by action potential (AP) in presynaptic nerve. (*4*) Diffusion of neurotransmitter across synaptic cleft. (*5*) Combination of neurotransmitter with receptor. The events resulting from ACh occupying receptor sites depend on the nature of the postsynaptic cell. ACh excites some cells and inhibits others. (*A*) An enzyme, acetylcholinesterase (AChE) on the postsynaptic cell, inactivates ACh. Some of the products diffuse into the circulation, but most of the choline formed is taken up and reused by the cholinergic neuron. Cholinesterase inhibitors inhibit AChE.

Note that steps 2 through 5 are the same as those shown in Figure 13-4.

Both types of cholinergic receptors are innervated by cholinergic nerves. Muscarinic receptors are innervated by the first class of cholinergic nerves described above, postganglionic cholinergic nerves. Muscarinic receptors are thus located in visceral effector organs that receive parasympathetic innervation and in sweat glands and some vascular smooth muscle.

Nicotinic receptors are innervated by the second

and third classes of cholinergic nerves described above, preganglionic parasympathetic and sympathetic nerves and somatic motor nerves. Nicotinic receptors are thus located in autonomic ganglia, in the adrenal medulla, and at the skeletal neuromuscular junction.

ACh action. The combination of active ACh with this cholinergic *receptor,* or *cholinoceptive site,* changes the permeability of the nerve, muscle, or gland cell membrane. This leads to increased leakage of sodium ions into the cell and—at some sites—to a selective increase in permeability to potassium ions. The resulting depolarization or hyperpolarization of the nerve or muscle cell postjunctional membrane then excites or inhibits cellular activity. There is some evidence to suggest that cGMP may function as a "second messenger" at certain muscarinic receptors.

ACh inactivation. Once the second cell has reacted by sending along the nerve impulse (in the case of neurons), by secreting (in the case of exocrine gland cells), or by contracting or relaxing (in the case of muscle cells), it is essential that any remaining neurotransmitter at the junction be quickly destroyed. An excess of ACh might prevent the membrane from recovering its normal polarity and thus reduce its responsiveness to the next volley of nerve impulses.

The destruction of the excess ACh is carried out almost instantly by an enzyme in the synaptic and neuromuscular junctions. This enzyme, *acetylcholinesterase (AChE),* combines with the ACh molecules and converts them into the neurochemically inactive compounds acetic acid and choline, the same metabolites from which the ACh was made. Once the neurotransmitter is broken down—a matter of thousandths of a second—the membrane of the nerve, muscle, or gland cell repolarizes and becomes ready to respond to the next nerve volley of cholinergic impulses.

Types of drug action at cholinergic synapses. Drugs that affect the functioning of organs and structures that are innervated by the several classes of cholinergic nerves act in several different ways (Table 13-3). Some drugs act by imitating the effects of ACh when their molecules make contact with cholinergic receptors.

Table 13–3. Classification of drugs acting at synapses in the peripheral nervous system

Synapse	Type of receptor	Agonist or mimicking drugs	Antagonist or blocking drugs
Somatic neuromuscular junction Axon of motoneuron → Skeletal muscle fiber	Nicotinic cholinergic	Cholinesterase inhibitors (low doses): neostigmine, edrophonium	Competitive blockers: curare, gallamine; noncompetitive or depolarizing blockers: succinylcholine
Autonomic ganglia Preganglionic axon → Parasympathetic or sympathetic ganglion cell or adrenal medullary cell	Nicotinic cholinergic	No therapeutically useful drug	Ganglionic blockers: trimethaphan
Cholinergic neuroeffector junctions Cholinergic postganglionic axons: parasympathetic and a few sympathetic → Effector cells: smooth and cardiac muscle; glands	Muscarinic cholinergic	Parasympathomimetic drugs: bethanechol, pilocarpine; cholinesterase inhibitor: neostigmine	Parasympathetic blocking drugs: atropine
Adrenergic neuroeffector junctions Adrenergic postganglionic axons: sympathetic → Effector cells: smooth and cardiac muscle; glands	α, β_1, and β_2 adrenergic	Sympathomimetic drugs: α, β_1, β_2— epinephrine; α— phenylephrine; β_1, β_2—isoproterenol	Adrenergic receptor blocking drugs: α blocker—phentolamine, β blocker—propranolol; adrenergic neuron blocking drugs: guanethidine, reserpine

Others, the *anticholinesterase agents,* or *cholinesterase inhibitors,* act by inhibiting the enzyme AChE, which is responsible for the inactivation of ACh. This, of course, causes free ACh molecules to accumulate at all types of junctions between cholinergic nerves and the structures that they innervate, including visceral effector cells, autonomic ganglia, skeletal muscles, and even cells of the CNS, provided, of course, that the anticholinesterase agent can penetrate the blood–brain barrier (see Chap. 4).

Drugs that imitate the effects of acetylcholine—*cholinomimetic drugs*—are sometimes said to produce "muscarinic" or "nicotinic" effects, depending on the type of cholinergic receptor with which they interact to produce the effect. Some cholinomimetic drugs (*bethanechol*—Urecholine) act selectively at muscarinic receptors. One characteristic of cholinergic drug actions at nicotinic sites (ganglia and skeletal muscles) is that small doses stimulate, but large doses that first stimulate are followed by later depression and failure of function.

Cholinergic blocking drugs are agents that prevent cells from responding to the ACh that is released by various types of cholinergic nerves. Most are competitive antagonists of ACh that occupy cholinoceptive sites and thus prevent the molecules of the neurotransmitter from making its normal contact with the cholinergic receptors (see Receptor Theory, Chap. 4). Like some cholinomimetic drugs, cholinergic blocking drugs act with some degree of selectivity, but they are competitive antagonists of ACh. *Atropine,* for example, blocks cholinergic nerve impulses to smooth muscle, cardiac muscle, and exocrine gland cells that receive parasympathetic (and sympathetic) postganglionic cholinergic nerves. Thus, because it acts at muscarinic sites, atropine and other natural and synthetic cholinergic blockers are commonly called *antimuscarinic*-type anticholinergic agents (see Chap. 16).

Curare and related competitive-type neuromuscular blocking agents (Table 13-3 and Chap. 19) block cholinergic transmission selectively at one type of nicotinic site, the neuromuscular junction. Higher doses of these drugs will also prevent ACh from triggering nerve impulses in the other nicotinic-type receptors in autonomic ganglia. However, no clinically practicable dose of curare will cut off cholinergic nervous transmission at the *postganglionic* neuroeffectors in the heart, smooth muscles, and exocrine glands.

Trimethaphan (Arfonad) and most other ganglionic blockers (Table 13-3 and Chap. 18) are specific for blocking the effects of ACh at the other type of nicotinic site—that is, the cholinoceptive site in autonomic ganglia. However, some drugs such as *propantheline* (Pro-Banthine)

are capable of blocking the effects of ACh at both nicotinic ganglionic and muscarinic sites (see Chap. 16).

Adrenergic transmission

Types of adrenergic nerves. Sympathetic postganglionic nerves that synthesize, store, and release NE are referred to as *adrenergic nerves.* Adrenergic nerves also are found in the CNS. In addition, chromaffin cells of the adrenal medulla synthesize, store, and release NE as well as *epinephrine* (adrenaline), which is actually the principal secretory product of these cells.

NE synthesis and storage. NE is a *catecholamine,* which is a chemical term used to refer to molecules that are 3,4-dihydroxyphenylethylamines. Dopamine and epinephrine are other catecholamines that are synthesized and released in the body.

The multiple steps in the biosynthesis of NE are shown in Figure 13-7. The NE that is stored in granules of the peripheral adrenergic nerve endings is formed in each varicosity as the result of a series of chemical steps that are catalyzed by enzymes that are themselves synthesized in the ganglionic nerve cell bodies. These enzymes and the NE storage vesicles are believed to flow from there down the axonal fibers to the terminals at which biosynthesis and storage of the neurotransmitter take place. There, the enzyme tyrosine hydroxylase first converts the amino acid tyrosine to *dopa.* This is then decarboxylated under the influence of the enzyme L-aromatic amino acid decarboxylase, or dopa decarboxylase, to form *dopamine.* A third enzyme, dopamine β-hydroxylase, acts within the many vesicles of each terminal varicosity to convert dopamine to *norepinephrine.**

NE release. When the AP of a stimulated sympathetic nerve arrives at the axonal terminal and depolarizes its outer membrane, the vesicles within each varicosity fuse with the cell membrane. The vesicles are then extruded into the junctional gap by the same sort of calcium-dependent exocytic process previously described for ACh release. The molecules of NE freed in this way then diffuse across the tiny space between the terminal varicosity and the adjacent postjunctional smooth muscle, cardiac muscle, or other effector cells. There the neurotransmitter chemical combines with specialized *adrenoceptive* sites—the α- and β-adrenergic receptors.

Adrenergic receptors. Two main types of adrenergic receptors have been identified, called *α receptors* and *β receptors.* This distinction is necessary because no single drug blocks all the effects of sympathetic nervous system stimulation or all the effects produced by NE or epinephrine. For example, the vasoconstriction produced by an injection of epinephrine is blocked by phentolamine (Regitine), but the increase in heart rate produced by this same injection is not blocked. On the other hand, the increase in heart rate is blocked by propranolol (Inderal), but the vasoconstriction is not. The adrenergic receptors that mediate vasoconstriction (and other effects;

---

* In the chromaffin cells of the adrenal medulla, a fourth enzyme, phenylethanolamine N-methyltransferase, which is *not* present in the adrenergic nerve terminals, catalyzes the conversion of NE to epinephrine.

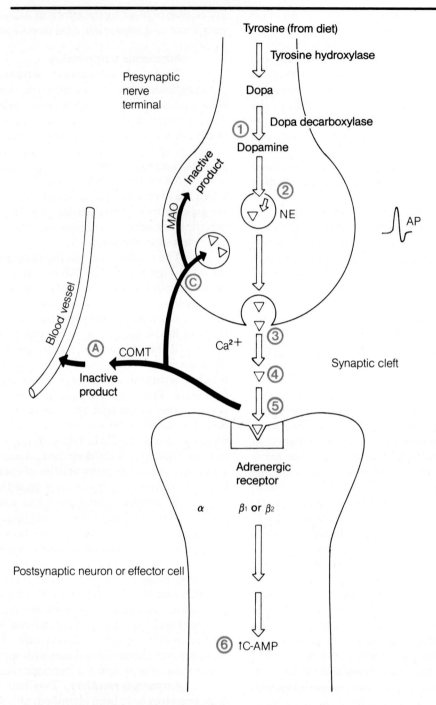

Figure 13-7. Sequence of events at an adrenergic synapse. (*1*) Dopamine, a precursor of norepinephrine (NE), is synthesized from tyrosine in several steps. Metyrosine inhibits tyrosine hydroxylase; a drug given with dopa to parkinsonian patients inhibits dopa decarboxylase. (*2*) Dopamine is taken into the storage vesicle and converted to norepinephrine (NE, ▽). (*3*) Release of neurotransmitter by action potential (AP) in presynaptic nerve. (*4*) Diffusion of neurotransmitter across synaptic cleft. (*5*) Combination of neurotransmitter with receptor. The events resulting from NE occupying receptor sites depend on the nature of the postsynaptic cell. (*6*) Interaction of NE with many β receptors leads to ↑ synthesis of cAMP. (*A*) An enzyme, COMT, inactivates the NE, but the most important way in which the action of NE is terminated is by *C*, reuptake into the presynaptic neuron, where it may be reused or inactivated by another enzyme, MAO. Some antidepressant drugs inhibit this enzyme.

Note that steps 3 through 5 are the same as those shown in Figures 13-4 and 13-6.

see Table 13-2) are designated as α receptors; those that mediate the increase in heart rate (and other effects) are designated as β receptors.

More recently, drugs have been synthesized with yet greater selectivity than NE and epinephrine. This has led to the subdivision of β receptors into two subtypes, called β_1 *receptors* and β_2 *receptors*. β_1 receptors occur only in the heart; they mediate the increase in heart rate and force of contraction produced by an injection of epinephrine and by the sympathetic nervous system in the "fight-or-flight" reaction. β_2 receptors mediate the bronchial relaxation, vasodilatation, glycogenolysis, and uterine relaxation produced by impulses in sympathetic adrenergic nerves (Table 13-2).

Very recently, alpha receptors were also subdivided into two subtypes, α_1 and α_2 receptors. The α_1 receptors occur on postsynaptic and postjunctional membranes and mediate the vasoconstriction and other effects that were for years considered to be mediated simply by α receptors. This book will refer to α_1 receptors simply as α receptors (Table 13-2). Receptors of the other subtype, α_2 receptors, occur presynaptically on adrenergic neurons and have been postulated to mediate a feedback inhibition of NE release. Their significance in explaining drug effects is still largely unknown, and they will be mentioned only a few times more in this text.

NE action at adrenergic receptors. The combination of NE (and other catecholamines) with adrenergic receptors sets into motion a series of intracellular events that results in a change in function of the postjunctional adrenergic neuroeffector cell. The responses mediated by adrenergic receptors have been linked, at least in part, to catecholamine-induced changes at the intracellular level of a cyclic nucleotide system. The neurotransmitter or other catecholamine that occupies a β receptor is believed to activate an enzyme, adenylate cyclase, on the inner surface of the membrane just beneath the β-adrenergic receptor. This enzyme then catalyzes the conversion of the cellular energy carrier adenosine triphosphate (ATP) to adenosine 3',5'-monophosphate, or cyclic AMP (cAMP). This cyclic nucleotide, which acts as a so-called second messenger for many hormones at the intracellular level, then accumulates within the sympathetically innervated cells. In doing so it somehow sets off certain still unknown steps in cellular metabolism that lead to the typical responses of the cardiac, smooth muscle, and other sympathetic neuroeffectors.

Termination of neurotransmission. As in the case of ACh, any excess molecules of the adrenergic neurotransmitter must be promptly disposed of once it has performed its function. That is, after they have transmitted the nerve impulse from the sympathetic postganglionic terminals, the NE molecules must be removed from the vicinity of the responsive α- and β-adrenergic receptors. The main mechanism by which this is accomplished is quite different from the way in which ACh is instantly disposed of by enzymatic action.

Most of the free NE molecules that remain in the junctional gap after activating the adrenergic receptors are taken up again by the same adrenergic nerve terminals that had released them. The molecules that are removed from the extracellular space in this way and recaptured by the nerve endings no longer exert their effects on the postjunctional cells. However, because most of the NE molecules that are taken up by the prejunctional cell membrane are stored in the vesicles of the terminal varicosities, these neurotransmitter molecules are available for release by later volleys of sympathetic nerve impulses.

Although most of the released NE is disposed of by this neuronal reuptake process, enzymes are also available for the biotransformation of the neurotransmitter to inactive metabolites. Free NE that does not get back into the nerve cells diffuses away from the nerve–muscle junction. Molecules of NE that are carried to the liver and to other tissues are destroyed in a series of enzymatically catalyzed steps. The enzymes involved in the destruction of NE and of other endogenous catecholamines, such as the adrenal medulla hormone epinephrine and the CNS neurotransmitter dopamine, are *monoamine oxidase* (MAO) and *catechol-o-methyltransferase* (COMT). The enzyme MAO is also present within adrenergic neurons, where it plays a part in preventing production and storage of excessive amounts of the sympathetic neurotransmitter by inactivating any excess.

Types of drug actions at adrenergic synapses. Drugs that affect one or more of the many steps by which the adrenergic neuronal transmitter is synthesized, stored, released, and recaptured after activating α- or β-adrenoceptive sites can alter normal functioning of the organs and structures that are innervated by postganglionic sympathetic nerves. Some of the various ways in which different types of drugs act to alter the functioning of peripheral—and, in some cases, central—adrenergic nerves are summarized in Table 13-3, and these mechanisms are discussed in more detail at appropriate points in the other chapters of this section and in Sections 5 and 8. Here we shall briefly discuss some of the main mechanisms by which drugs alter adrenergic nerve transmission.

Sympathomimetic (adrenergic) drugs. Some drugs produce effects that imitate, or mimic, those of the sympathetic neurotransmitter that is released by postganglionic adrenergic nerve endings (see Chap. 17). They do so in several ways. Some act by occupying and activating the postjunctional adrenoceptive site. *Isoproterenol*, for example, acts mainly at β-adrenergic receptors (both β_1 and β_2) in this way, while *phenylephrine* activates mainly α receptors when it comes into direct contact with them. *Epinephrine* acts as an agonist at both α- and β-adrenergic receptors.

Still other sympathomimetic drugs act at the adrenergic nerve ending rather than at adrenergic receptors. *Amphetamine* and *tyramine*, an amino acid in certain foods, for example, enter the nerve terminal and displace the stored neurotransmitter from its storage sites. The resulting increase in neurotransmitter concentration in the junctional gap and at the postjunctional adrenoceptive sites produces heightened sympathetic effects in sympathetically innervated organs and structures. Some substances, such as *ephedrine*, are thought to exert *both* this indirect action and effects that result from direct occupancy of adrenergic receptors.

Drugs can also act at adrenergic nerve endings in yet another way. Drugs such as *cocaine* and the tricyclic antidepressant drugs *imipramine* (Tofranil) and *amitriptyline* (Elavil) are thought to act by blocking the reuptake of previously released neurotransmitter at both peripheral adrenergic junctions and central synapses in adrenergic pathways. As a result, the neurotransmitter tends to accumulate in these junctions and to continue exerting its action on the adrenergic receptors, instead of re-entering the nerve terminal with subsequent cessation of its transmitter action, as would normally be the case.

Drugs that inhibit the enzyme MAO within the cytoplasm of the adrenergic peripheral (sympathetic) and central neurons can also sometimes increase the amount of neurotransmitter released by these neurons, thus producing greater effects on the postjunctional cells that they innervate. Thus, for example, the antidepressant drug *tranylcypromine* (Parnate) can cause norepinephrine to accumulate in adrenergic nerves, from which it can then be released in abnormally large amounts by nerve impulses or by indirectly acting neurotransmitter-releasing drugs such as ephedrine (see above).

Adrenergic receptor blocking drugs. These are drugs that can prevent sympathetically innervated cells from responding to the neurotransmitter that is released by nerve impulses and also to circulating natural and synthetic catecholamines such as the adrenal medulla hormone epinephrine or the drug isoproterenol (see Chap. 18). Some of these drugs, such as phentolamine, do so by selectively blocking the α-type adrenergic receptors, while others act by occupying β-adrenergic receptors (Table 13-3). Some of the latter, such as *propranolol* (see Chap. 18, and elsewhere) can block both the β_1 (cardiac) and the β_2 (smooth muscle) types of β receptors. Drugs such as metoprolol (Lopressor) and atenolol (Tenormin) have been synthesized that exert a selective blocking effect on cardiac β receptors without interfering significantly with sympathetic nerve impulse transmission to bronchial and other smooth muscles.

Adrenergic neuron blocking agents. Various drugs interfere with the responses of sympathetically innervated organs and structures by their ability to prevent adrenergic nerves from releasing the neurotransmitter in normal amounts (see Chap. 18). That is, unlike the adrenergic receptor blocking drugs discussed in the previous paragraph, these agents act on sympathetic postganglionic axon terminals rather than on the postjunctional receptors. Thus, they interfere with impulse transmission to both α- and β-adrenergic receptors.

Drugs of this class, several of which are employed clinically in the management of hypertension, can act in any of several different ways to deplete the amount of sympathetic nerve impulse mediator that is synthesized, stored, and released by the adrenergic nerve ending. *Reserpine*, for example, interferes with the cell's ability to store the neurotransmitter in the vesicles of the nerve ending varicosities. As a result, the norepinephrine molecules freed within the nerve cell cytoplasm tend to be destroyed in reactions catalyzed by the enzyme MAO, and the amount of the neurotransmitter that is then available for release by sympathetic nerve impulses is markedly diminished. The diminution in available NE will result in a decrease in sympathetic-stimulated vascular contraction, and the blood pressure will be decreased.

Still other drugs of this class act by altering the amount of neurotransmitter that is synthesized in the cytoplasm and vesicles of the sympathetic nerves. A newly approved drug, metyrosine (Demser), inhibits the first enzyme in the biosynthesis of catecholamines from tyrosine. Thus, the amounts of norepinephrine (as well as dopamine and epinephrine) synthesized are decreased.

Other drugs interfere with sympathetic nerve impulse transmission by several possible mechanisms, not all of which are entirely understood. The potent antihypertensive agent *guanethidine* (Ismelin), for example, acts in various ways to produce prompt and prolonged interference with adrenergic nerve function following its uptake into the nerve endings.

Summary

In this chapter, basic neurophysiology and the anatomy and physiology of the two divisions of the autonomic nervous system have been reviewed. Concepts and terms relevant to chemical neurotransmission have been introduced as background for understanding how autonomic drugs act to alter the functions of organs and structures that are innervated by the autonomic nervous system. At this point, you may be more confused than enlightened by the many and varied mechanisms by which drugs can act to imitate the actions of the natural neurotransmitters or to block their physiologic effects. However, the material presented in this chapter should help you obtain a better understanding of the actions, both therapeutic and adverse, of the various classes of drugs that are taken up in the following chapters of this section and elsewhere in the textbook. Learning about the practical clinical applications of these drugs should, in turn, help to reinforce the general principles that have been set forth in this chapter.

References

Appenzeller O: The Autonomic Nervous System: An Introduction to Basic and Clinical Concepts, 3rd ed. Amsterdam, Elsevier/North Holland, 1982

Bloom FE: Neurohumoral transmission and the central nervous system. In Gilman AG, Goodman LS, Gilman A (eds): Goodman and Gilman's The Pharmacological Basis of Therapeutics, 6th ed, pp 235–257. New York, Macmillan, 1980

Cohen DH, Sherman SM: Peripheral units of the nervous system. In Berne RM, Levy MN (eds): Physiology, pp 77–89. St. Louis, C V Mosby, 1983

Cohen DH, Sherman SM: The autonomic nervous system and its central control. In Berne RM, Levy MN (eds): Physiology, pp 314–335. St. Louis, C V Mosby, 1983

Cohen DH, Sherman SM: The nervous system and its components. In Berne RM, Levy MN (eds): Physiology, pp 69–76. St. Louis, C V Mosby, 1983

Cooper JR, Bloom FE, Roth RH: The Biochemical Basis of Neuropharmacology, 4th ed. New York and London, Oxford University Press, 1982

Johnson RH, Spalding JMK: Disorders of the Autonomic Nervous System. Philadelphia, F. A. Davis, 1974

Kandel ER, Schwartz JH: Principles of Neural Science. Amsterdam, Elsevier/North Holland, 1981

Koizumi K, Brooks CM: The autonomic system and its role in controlling body functions. In Mountcastle VB (ed): Medical Physiology, 14th ed, pp 893–922. St. Louis, C V Mosby, 1980

Krieger DT: Brain peptides: What, where, and why? Science 222:975, 1983

Kutchai HC: Generation and conduction of action potentials. In Berne RM, Levy MN (eds): Physiology, pp 35–49. St. Louis, C V Mosby, 1983

Kutchai HC: Synaptic transmission. In Berne RM, Levy MN (eds): Physiology, pp 50–66. St. Louis, C V Mosby, 1983

Lefkowitz RJ: Direct binding studies of adrenergic receptors: Biochemical, physiological and clinical implications. Ann Intern Med 91:450, 1979

Marshall JM: Vertebrate smooth muscle. In Mountcastle VB (ed): Medical Physiology, 14th ed, pp 120–148. St. Louis, C V Mosby, 1980

Mayer SE: Neurohumoral transmission and the autonomic nervous system. In Gilman AG, Goodman LS, Gilman A (eds): Goodman and Gilman's The Pharmacological Basis of Therapeutics, 6th ed, pp 56–90. New York, Macmillan, 1980

Milnor WR: Autonomic and peripheral control mechanisms. In Mountcastle VB (ed): Medical Physiology, 14th ed, pp 961–985. St. Louis, C V Mosby, 1980

Milnor WR: Properties of cardiac tissues. In Mountcastle VB (ed): Medical Physiology, 14th ed, pp 1047–1060. St. Louis, C V Mosby, 1980

Mountcastle VB, Sastre A: Synaptic transmission. In Mountcastle VB (ed): Medical Physiology, 14th ed, pp 184–223. St. Louis, C V Mosby, 1980

Nastuk WM: Neuromuscular transmission. In Mountcastle VB (ed): Medical Physiology, 14th ed, pp 151–183. St. Louis, C V Mosby, 1980

Shepherd GM: Neurobiology. New York and London, Oxford University Press, 1983

Starke K: Presynaptic receptors. Ann Rev Pharmacol Toxicol 21:7, 1981

Chapter 14

Local
anesthetics

14

General considerations

Local anesthetics are drugs that cause a loss of feeling in limited areas of the body. They are employed mainly to prevent the patient from feeling pain for varying periods after they have been applied to parts of the peripheral nervous system. Depending on which portion of this system's nerve roots and fibers is affected, the loss of sensation may be limited to a small part of the body or may involve quite a large area. However, unlike the general anesthetics, these drugs are *not* used clinically to cause unconsciousness.

The effects of local anesthetics are not limited to the sensory fibers alone. When these drugs are brought into direct contact with mixed spinal nerves, they can also affect the functioning of somatic motor and sympathetic efferent nerve fibers. This can then interfere with the tone of the skeletal and smooth muscles innervated by these nerves.

Manner of action

Local anesthetics cause these effects by temporarily interrupting the production and conduction of nerve impulses.* This reversible block of conduction occurs because local anesthetics, in some way or ways, prevent the increase in permeability of the nerve membrane to sodium ions that normally occurs in response to stimulation. It is this influx of sodium ions that normally depolarizes the nerve to threshold and produces the depolarizing phase of the action potential (see Chap. 13 and Fig. 13-3). Thus, action potentials cannot develop in portions of a nerve that are under the influence of a local anesthetic (Fig.

---

* Prolonged and even permanent interruption of pain impulse conduction can sometimes be produced by injecting so-called *neurolytic* agents such as ethyl alcohol 50% or 95%, or phenol 5% to 10%.

14-1*A*), and action potentials that arise in another part of the neuron "die out" when they reach the segment of an axon that has been blocked by the anesthetic (Fig. 14-1*B*). In actuality, local anesthetics decrease membrane permeability to ions other than sodium (K^+, Ca^{2+}), but it is their effect on permeability to sodium ions that is responsible for their local anesthetic activity.

Pharmacokinetic factors

It is vitally important to understand that the effects of local anesthetics need not be limited to the site of local application. Like other chemicals that are injected, applied, or inhaled, these drugs can be absorbed into the bloodstream and carried to all parts of the body. Rapid systemic absorption may allow high levels of the local anesthetics to reach the heart and brain, for example, with resultant toxic reactions involving the cardiovascular and nervous systems (see the summary of toxic reactions at the end of the chapter).

Such systemic toxicity depends not only on the rate at which the local anesthetics are absorbed into the bloodstream and the amounts that may then rapidly reach the organs susceptible to their toxic effects, but also on the ease or difficulty with which these drugs are destroyed or otherwise eliminated. The various local anesthetics differ in the rates at which they are detoxified by drug-metabolizing enzymes in the blood plasma, liver, and other tissues. The degree to which certain of these drugs are distributed to inactive tissue binding sites and the extent to which some are excreted unchanged by the kidneys also play a part in determining their relative toxicity. How these drugs are handled by the body is related to their chemical structures. Thus, for example, whether a particular local anesthetic is an ester or an amide determines the rate and completeness of its metabolism. Local anesthetics that are esters (*e.g.,* benzocaine, butacaine, chloroprocaine, cocaine, cyclomethycaine, hexylcaine,

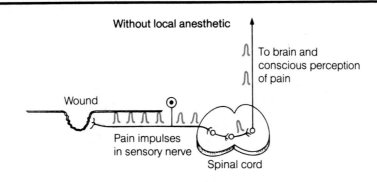

Without local anesthetic

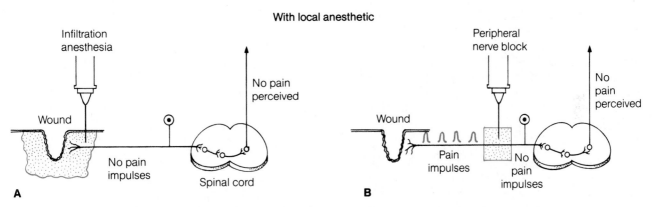

With local anesthetic

A

B

Figure 14-1. Effects of local anesthetics. An injury produces pain impulses (actually, action potentials) that are conducted and transmitted to areas of the brain in which pain is perceived. (*A*) Conduction of the pain impulses has been blocked by infiltration anesthesia at the site of the injury and by (*B*) a nerve block at some distance from the injury.

procaine, proparacaine, tetracaine) are readily hydrolyzed by esterases in the plasma. Local anesthetics that are amides (*e.g.*, bupivacaine, dibucaine, lidocaine, mepivacaine, prilocaine) are metabolized more slowly by liver enzymes; repeated doses of these agents may lead to drug accumulation and systemic toxicity in patients with liver disease.

Techniques of administration

To produce regional anesthesia with local anesthetics, the anesthesiologist employs special techniques of administration. These are intended to

1. Place the local anesthetic solution at some precise local point along the course of the peripheral nerves, and
2. Keep the drug's systemic absorption at a rate so slow that it does not build up to toxic levels.

Several procedures are employed to bring these drugs into direct contact with different parts of peripheral nerves, ranging from their endings in the skin and mucous membranes to the points at which the bundles of nerve fibers, or trunks, enter the spinal cord at the nerve roots (Fig. 14-2).

There are five resulting types of regional anesthesia:

1. *Topical (surface) anesthesia.* This involves applying a cream, ointment, or other vehicle for the local anesthetic to the traumatized skin; or bringing the drug into contact with nerve fiber terminations in mucous membranes of the eye, nose, mouth, and throat, the tracheobronchial tree, or the urethra, anus, and rectum.
2. *Infiltration anesthesia.* Solutions of local anesthetics are injected into tissues that are going to be surgically cut or sutured. This brings the anesthetic into contact with nerve endings in the intracutaneous, subcutaneous, and deeper structures and prevents these sensitive nerve terminals

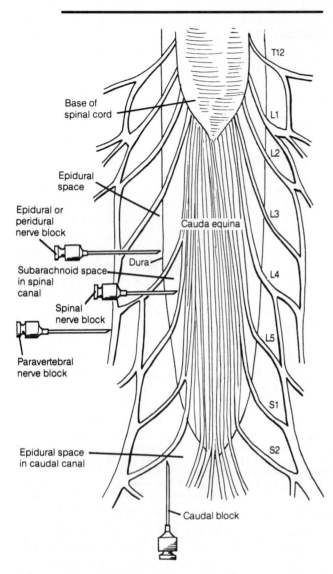

Figure 14-2. Sites of injection for central nerve blocks, showing position of needle for spinal, epidural, caudal, and paravertebral nerve blocks. T12, L1–L5, and S1–S2 indicate the vertebral levels of injection.

from transmitting pain impulses during the subsequent procedure (Fig. 14-1A).

3. *Field (ring) block.* This is a form of infiltration anesthesia in which the local anesthetic is injected all around the area that is to be operated on. The sensory nerve pathways from the operative field are blocked off by a circular ring of

subcutaneously injected solution. It differs from local infiltration (above), in which the injection is made directly into the site that is to be surgically incised or sutured; and it differs from nerve blocks (below), because it is aimed at *all* the nerves arising in the area rather than at any specific nerve.

4. *Nerve block anesthesia.* This is carried out by placing the drug solutions at some point along the course of the nerve or nerves that run to and from the region in which the physician wants to eliminate pain sensation or temporarily relax or paralyze muscles. Nerve blocks of this type are carried out not in the surgical field itself but at a variable distance from it (Fig. 14-1B).

5. *Intravenous regional anesthesia.* This is carried out by injecting the local anesthetic into the vein of the arm or leg after the limb has been exsanguinated (drained of blood). It requires the careful use of a special tourniquet to prevent release of the drug into the systemic circulation before the surgical procedure is complete.

Peripheral nerve blocks affect specific nerves such as the sciatic–femoral, ulnar, or intercostal nerves, or the brachial plexus. Block of both sensory and motor fibers produced by injections at specific sites is often useful for performing not only surgical but also diagnostic and therapeutic procedures that help to determine the cause of acute and chronic pain and to bring about prolonged relief.*

Central nerve blocks affect the roots of nerves near their origin in the spinal cord. *Spinal anesthesia* is not intended to affect the spinal cord itself but blocks the roots of mixed spinal nerves in the subarachnoid space (Fig. 14-2). First the sensory fibers are affected and later the motor fibers. The result of an injection into the spinal fluid in the lumbar portion of the spine is first the loss of all sensation in the area of the body innervated by the blocked nerves and, a little later, the relaxation of the skeletal muscles of this large area. Muscle tone and sensation return in reverse order as the effects of the local anesthetic wear off. *Epidural* (peridural or extradural) anesthesia is achieved by depositing the anesthetic solution in the space in which the nerves emerge from the dural membrane and enter the openings between the vertebrae (the intervertebral foramina). *Caudal* anesthesia is a form of epidural block in which the local anesthetic is deposited in the sacral canal, which is a lower level continuation of the epidural space (Fig. 14-2). All these central nerve blocks can be brought about by single injections of local anes-

---

* Therapeutic nerve blocks with local anesthetics are sometimes useful for relief of very severe pain in many medical disorders, even after the excruciating pain has not proved to be adequately responsive to management with narcotic analgesics.

thetics and maintained by continuous infusions, sometimes through an indwelling cannula.

Properties of individual anesthetics

Hundreds of chemicals can block conduction of nerve impulses. However, only a few dozen, many of which are listed in Table 14-1, have properties that make them effective and safe enough for clinical use. Many drugs are discarded because they tend to cause systemic toxicity or local irritation of nerve and other tissues when they are administered in amounts adequate to produce anesthesia. Chemists continue to synthesize new compounds that they hope will combine greater anesthetic potency with reduced toxicity. Research efforts are also aimed at developing drugs with a duration of anesthetic action long enough to be useful for prolonged surgical procedures and control of chronic pain.

Before discussing the clinical applications of local anesthetics, the properties of some currently important agents that account for their advantages in specific clinical situations or for their disadvantages in certain circumstances will be discussed. (See also the Drug digests for more detailed data on some of these drugs, and the "Comments" section of Table 14-1 for a brief description of agents not taken up here.)

Cocaine[+], an alkaloid extracted from the leaves of the South American coca shrub, was the first important local anesthetic. Cocaine also has sympathomimetic properties; it inhibits the reuptake of norepinephrine by adrenergic neurons, and can cause vasoconstriction by this mechanism. It was first found useful for relief of pain when applied to the conjunctiva prior to eye surgery. However, its high toxicity and abuse properties on injection limited its usefulness. This led to efforts to synthesize local anesthetics that would be safer when injected and would not cause ocular irritation when employed in ophthalmology. Cocaine is still considered quite useful for anesthetizing the throat, larynx, and trachea prior to intubation.

Lidocaine[+] (Xylocaine) is one of the most versatile of the potent long-lasting local anesthetics. It is available in many pharmaceutic forms for use in every type of injection procedure and for topical application to the skin and to the mucous membranes of the eye, nose, throat, and even the gastrointestinal tract. It is also used in the emergency management of ventricular arrhythmias following an acute myocardial infarction and in other cardiac disorders. Lidocaine differs from other local anesthetics in that its most common CNS side-effect is drowsiness.

Procaine[+] (Novocain), one of the first synthetic compounds, is an anesthetic of relatively low toxicity. Unlike cocaine, it is not very effective when applied to the mucosa of the eye. When injected, it is rather rapidly destroyed by enzymes that hydrolyze its ester structure. Thus, compounds of the same chemical series were sought that would have a more prolonged duration of action while retaining the relatively low toxicity of procaine.

Tetracaine[+] (Pontocaine) exerts an anesthetic effect that is more than twice as long as that of procaine. This property once made it the most popular drug for use in spinal anesthesia. However, it is very much more irritating and systemically toxic than the prototype synthetic anesthetic. The availability of several anesthetics of a different chemical class—the amides—that combine prolonged duration of action with relatively high safety has tended to reduce the frequency with which this drug is employed.

Etidocaine (Duranest) produces prompt sensory analgesia and motor blockade that then lasts for several hours. A single epidural injection produces such prolonged effects that continuous administration techniques are not necessary for most surgical procedures. The prolonged duration of action reduces the need for postoperative narcotic analgesics and thus improves pulmonary ventilation in patients in whom opiates might increase the risk of respiratory complications. Of course, its long action makes this drug less desirable for use in short procedures.

Bupivacaine (Marcaine) also produces long-lasting analgesia when used for both peripheral and central nerve blocks. It is claimed to be particularly useful for relief of pain in obstetric patients, because it does so when administered in doses that do not interfere with uterine contractions. Other drugs with a prolonged duration of action are *dibucaine* (Nupercaine), the first amide derivative, introduced almost 50 years ago, and two newer amides, *mepivacaine* (Carbocaine) and *prilocaine* (Citanest), both of which were originally claimed to be more potent and less toxic than procaine and lidocaine. Metabolites of prilocaine have been found to cause methemoglobinemia. This form of toxicity, unique to prilocaine among local anesthetics, has reduced its popularity. However, neither mepivicaine nor prilocaine has been as widely used as procaine and lidocaine, which are still the most popular anesthetics for most procedures.

Proparacaine (Ophthaine) and *benoxinate* (Dorsacaine) are particularly useful for application to the surface of the eye. Unlike cocaine and other topically effective agents, these newer compounds cause relatively little ocular irritation. Their anesthetic effects come on in less than a minute and last long enough both for brief diagnostic procedures such as tonometry and gonioscopy and for more prolonged eye surgery such as extraction of cataracts.

Dimethisoquin (Quotane) is considered too irritating for use in the eye. However, it is safe and effective

Table 14-1. Some drugs used for local anesthesia

Official or generic name	Trade name or synonym	Primary use*	Comments
Benoxinate HCl USP	Dorsacaine	Topical	Used for ophthalmic anesthesia
Benzocaine USP	Ethyl aminobenzoate; Americaine	Topical	Used on broken skin and on mucous membranes
Bupivacaine HCl	Marcaine	Infiltration; central and peripheral nerve blocks	Produces long-lasting nerve blocks in obstetric and surgical procedures
Butacaine sulfate	Butyn sulfate	Topical	Rapid and long action in eye, nose, and throat
Butamben picrate	Butesin picrate	Topical	Used on burns and broken skin
Chloroprocaine HCl USP	Nesacaine	Infiltration and some nerve blocks	More potent and less toxic than procaine
Cocaine USP and cocaine HCl USP		Topical	See Drug digest
Cyclomethycaine sulfate USP	Surfacaine	Topical	Used on urethral, rectal, and vaginal mucosa, as well as on broken skin
Dibucaine HCl USP	Cinchocaine; Nupercaine HCl	Topical, and for central nerve blocks	Most potent, toxic, and long-lasting spinal and surface anesthetic action
Dimethisoquin HCl USP	Quotane HCl	Topical	Used as anogenital antipruritic, and for relief of pain from sunburn and skin lesions
Diperodon monohydrate	Diothane	Topical	Claimed as potent as cocaine and longer lasting for surface anesthesia
Dyclonine HCl USP	Dyclone	Topical	Used to anesthesize mucous membranes prior to endoscopy
Ethyl chloride USP	Monochlorethane; Kelene	Topical	Sprayed on skin prior to making incisions; may cause frostbite
Etidocaine HCl	Duranest HCl	Infiltration; some central and peripheral nerve blocks	Rapid onset and long duration of sensory and motor nerve blocks with relative safety
Hexylcaine HCl USP	Cyclaine	Topical	Used topically prior to intubations; never injected
Lidocaine HCl USP	Lignocaine; Xylocaine HCl	Infiltration; central and peripheral nerve blocks	See Drug digest
Mepivacaine HCl USP	Carbocaine	Infiltration and some nerve blocks	Claimed more rapid and longer acting than lidocaine
Phenacaine HCl USP	Holocaine HCl	Topical	Used mainly in the eye
Pramoxine HCl USP	Tronothane HCl	Topical	Used on broken skin and on anogenital membranes, but not in the eye or nose
Prilocaine HCl USP	Citanest HCl	Infiltration and some nerve blocks	Claimed as effective as lidocaine for nerve block procedures; can cause methemoglobinemia

Table 14-1. Some drugs used for local anesthesia (continued)

Official or generic name	Trade name or synonym	Primary use*	Comments
Procaine HCl USP	Novocain	Infiltration; central and peripheral nerve blocks	See Drug digest
Proparacaine HCl USP	Ophthaine HCl	Topical	Rapid but short-acting ocular anesthesia
Propoxycaine HCl USP	Blockaine HCl	Infiltration and peripheral nerve blocks	More intensive and prolonged action than procaine
Pyrrocaine HCl	Dynacaine HCl	Infiltration and peripheral nerve block	Rapid onset and long duration of action in dental and in other peripheral nerve blocks
Tetracaine HCl USP	Pontocaine HCl	Central nerve blocks	See Drug digest

* Agents for topical use may, in some cases, be applied only to the eye or only to the skin; in other cases, these agents are also administered by injection.

enough when applied to other less sensitive mucosal surfaces or to the skin. *Pramoxine* (Tronothane) is another effective surface anesthetic used in similar clinical situations. *Cyclomethycaine* (Surfacaine) is, like procaine, poorly absorbed when applied to the mucosa of the eye, mouth, or nose, but it can penetrate the rectal and urethral mucosa to reach and anesthetize nerve endings.

Benzocaine (Anesthesin) and *butyl aminobenzoate* (Butesin) exert a relatively long-lasting local anesthetic action when applied to broken skin. This is because they are only slightly soluble and thus are not swept away by the blood and other body fluids.

Ethyl chloride has sometimes been used, literally to freeze the skin prior to superficial surgical procedures. It is now rarely used because it can produce the same local adverse effects as frostbite. Occasionally, it is used before the cosmetic procedure of ear piercing.

Clinical applications

Topical (surface) anesthesia

Dermatologic applications

The skin, when damaged or diseased, permits penetration of topically applied local anesthetics. The drugs' action on nerve endings then deadens pain and itch sensations. Thus, drugs such as *dimethisoquin, pramoxine,* and *benzocaine* (see above) offer effective relief in many dermatologic disorders marked by minor but annoying symptoms.

Among the skin conditions in which topical an-

esthetics of this type are employed are dermatoses marked by pruritus, including poison ivy; burns, including sunburn; fissured nipples in the postpartum period; ulcerations, abrasions, and lacerations from minor injuries; and painful surgical incisions, such as following an episiotomy.

Pain and itching of the anogenital area may also be relieved by application of local anesthetic creams, ointments, jellies, or suppositories. Thus, these products are employed for pruritus ani or vulvae, following hemorrhoidectomy or repair of fissure in ano, or in other proctologic procedures involving the skin and perianal mucosa.

Adverse reactions of the systemic toxicity type are rare with these poorly absorbable agents. However, allergic reactions can occur in patients who have become sensitized to them. Thus, the long-term use of these drugs in chronic dermatoses is not advisable, particularly in patients with atopic dermatitis.

If signs such as redness, swelling, oozing, and pain develop during use of a topical anesthetic, treatment is discontinued. (Sometimes a local anesthetic of a different chemical class can be substituted, but patients whose skin is predisposed to react to chemicals may become sensitized to any of these agents.)

Ocular applications

The ocular mucosa can be anesthetized readily by eye drops containing topical anesthetics. Surface anesthesia produced by *proparacaine* or *benoxinate* (see above) or by *butacaine* or *dibucaine* permits removal of foreign bodies from the cornea. Drops are also applied to the conjunctiva prior to performance of such ophthalmologic diagnostic procedures as conjunctival scraping and tests for the presence of glaucoma.

Simple surgical procedures such as the opening of a small stye or an eyelid tumor (chalazion) can be carried out after topical application of a soluble anesthetic. More complicated ocular surgery such as cataract removal or iridectomy requires retrobulbar injection of local anesthetics. Such injections are made only after the conjunctiva and cornea are first desensitized by surface anesthesia.

Local irritation limits the usefulness of some agents for these purposes. Cocaine, for example, can cause dryness and other damage to the epithelium of the cornea. The newer ophthalmic anesthetics cause little early stinging or burning, and their use is rarely followed by the clouding, pitting, or ulceration of the cornea sometimes seen with cocaine.

Other mucosal applications

The mucosal surfaces of the tracheobronchial, gastrointestinal, and genitourinary tracts are also often anesthetized with local anesthetic solutions that penetrate to the free nerve endings just below the mucosal surface. The resulting reduction in sensation is useful for facilitating passage of instruments and for relief of pain.

The mouth, throat, and upper gastrointestinal tract may be anesthetized by swishing and then swallowing a viscous solution of *lidocaine* or by gargling with a solution of *dyclonine* or other surface anesthetic. This helps to reduce irritation in inflamed oral mucous membranes or to relieve the pain following dental procedures or tonsillectomy. Local anesthesia is also attained by spraying or swabbing the throat prior to passage of a tube down the esophagus for endoscopy.

Endotracheal intubation of patients who require support of respiration is also made easier by reducing the reflex activity that results in gagging and bucking. This is done by spraying the larynx and trachea with a fine aerosol of a local anesthetic solution. This procedure is also used prior to bronchoscopy to prevent laryngeal spasm, coughing, and the dangerous heart-slowing reflexes that are sometimes set off when a tube is introduced into the throat.

Absorption of the local anesthetic from these membrane surfaces or from those of the genitourinary tract (following instillation into the urethra or bladder before cystoscopy) may be dangerously rapid. A sudden rise in the blood levels of certain local anesthetics can cause systemic toxicity similar to that seen with accidental intravenous administration during infiltration and field blocks (see below).

This hazard may be reduced by use of the smallest amount of the lowest concentration of local anesthetic needed to anesthetize mucosal nerve endings. The actual amount of anesthetic (in milligrams) that has been ad-

ministered is generally recorded to ensure that the maximal safe dosage is not exceeded. This applies also when local anesthetics are being administered by the infiltration method.

Nerve block anesthesia

Peripheral nerve blocks

The technically skilled anesthesiologist, other physician, or dentist can effectively prevent or relieve pain in a large variety of clinical situations by procedures that block single cranial or spinal nerves in any part of the body. The specialized techniques employed are, of course, beyond the scope of this text. However, some examples of procedures that are performed following blocks of certain specific nerves will be presented to emphasize some important factors that must be considered.

People are most familiar with nerve blocks employed prior to dental procedures. However, conduction in other cranial nerves in addition to the maxillary nerve is often blocked before more complicated operations are performed on such structures as the scalp, face, and larynx. The success of such anesthesia depends on the ability to locate anatomic landmarks with extreme accuracy to deposit the local anesthetic solution at the precise points required for greatest effectiveness and safety. This is, of course, an equally important consideration when blocks of nerves in the upper and lower extremities, the neck, and elsewhere are being made.

Blocks of the ulnar, radial, and metacarpal nerves are employed prior to surgical procedures on the lower arm, elbow, wrist, and hand. Brachial plexus block affects not only the forearm and hand but also the upper arm, shoulder, and other structures. Blocks of the femoral and sciatic nerves affect the leg, popliteal nerve blocks are employed prior to knee surgery, and anterior tibial and metatarsal nerve blocks provide anesthesia for foot and toe surgery.

An important consideration in all such peripheral nerve block procedures is the proper psychological preparation of the patient. The nurse must gain the patient's confidence and ensure cooperation by explaining what should be expected and by putting the patient in a positive frame of mind. Patients are also often premedicated with barbiturates, narcotic analgesics, or anti-anxiety drugs such as diazepam (Valium) to allay anxiety and ensure tranquility during surgical procedures performed while they are conscious and aware of what is going on.

In other surgical situations, block of peripheral nerves is best supplemented with a general anesthetic that brings the patient down to the upper planes of surgical anesthesia. Intercostal nerve blocks alone, for example, are not likely to be adequate during surgery of the chest and abdomen, including thoracotomy, gastrectomy, and cholecystectomy. However, *postoperative* intercostal blockade with a potent long-acting local anesthetic such as *etidocaine* (Duranest) can be of great value for producing relief of pain following such surgery. Used in this way these drugs reduce the need for narcotic analgesics, with a resulting improvement of pulmonary ventilation. This, of course, helps the postoperative patient to breathe, move, and cough more readily, thus reducing the risk of respiratory complications such as atelectasis.

Central nerve blocks

Regional anesthesia of extensive areas can be obtained by injecting local anesthetic solutions at points close to where the spinal nerves emerge from the cord. Anesthesia of this type includes spinal, saddle, epidural, and caudal blocks—terms that refer mainly to the anatomic sites at which the injections are made.

Spinal anesthesia. Spinal anesthesia is induced by introducing the needle between two lumbar vertebrae, puncturing the dural and subarachnoid membranes, and injecting the local anesthetic solution into the spinal fluid in the subarachnoid space (see Fig. 14-2). The drug then acts on spinal nerve roots, dorsal root ganglia, and to a relatively small extent on spinal cord structures. All three types of axons (sensory, somatic motor, and autonomic) in a mixed spinal nerve are blocked, leading to loss of sensation, muscular relaxation, and a tendency for the blood pressure to fall unless special preventive measures are taken.

This method has some advantages for specially selected patients, but these are often outweighed by its disadvantages for others. Spinal anesthesia is most useful for surgery of the lower extremities and the lower abdomen. It is preferred to inhalation anesthesia for patients with asthma, emphysema, and other pulmonary diseases that might be made worse by the irritating action of some volatile agents. Elderly patients with cardiac or renal disease, and also diabetics, may do better with spinal rather than general anesthesia. For emergency surgery in patients who have eaten recently and have a full stomach, and who thus may aspirate gastric contents into the respiratory tract, spinal anesthesia is indicated. However, nausea and vomiting can occur with spinal anesthesia if blood pressure drops too suddenly or if the patient's position is changed too abruptly.

Spinal anesthesia is not recommended for patients with infections of the central nervous system or of the skin and other tissues through which spinal punctures are to be made. It is not desirable for patients with coronary artery disease or certain other heart diseases that cause cardiac decompensation. Hypotension is another contraindication to spinal anesthesia but, although hypertension is also a relative contraindication, patients with high blood pressure often respond well to spinal anesthesia when precautions are taken to avoid too sudden drops in pressure (see below).

Complications. Spinal anesthesia requires strict adherence to a careful routine to avoid complications during and after the procedure. For example, the patient must be carefully positioned so that the injected local anesthetic solution does not diffuse upward to block the medullary respiratory center or the roots of the phrenic and intercostal nerves, which control the movements of the diaphragm and other respiratory muscles.

In addition to possible respiratory complications, spinal anesthesia is often accompanied by sharp drops in blood pressure. Hypotension is, in part, the result of blockade of sympathetic vasomotor nerve fibers in the thoracolumbar spinal nerves. Reduction in the flow of vasoconstrictor impulses to the arterioles leads to dilatation of these blood vessels and to a steady fall in pressure. Other factors, including skeletal and vascular muscle relaxation and cardiac slowing (see below, Systemic toxic reactions), contribute to this hypotensive reaction to spinal anesthesia. Blood pressure falls may be prevented or counteracted by the administration of vasopressor amines such as ephedrine or mephentermine (Wyamine).

It is usually necessary to give the patient sedative premedication to prevent the natural anxiety that may be felt when fully awake during procedures carried out under regional anesthesia. Patients who are extremely apprehensive are usually given general anesthesia. If the patient is conscious, due consideration must be given to this fact by all operating room personnel.

Postspinal aftereffects. Neurologic complications occur only rarely today, and then mostly in people for whom spinal anesthesia is undesirable because of some pre-existing CNS abnormality. However, patients often fear that they have suffered a spinal injury when they find themselves unable to move their legs after spinal anesthesia. Therefore, it is important to explain in advance that this will occur and will last only a short while. Similarly, patients should also be told to expect feelings of numbness and "pins and needles" as sensation returns, and that these will shortly disappear. Sometimes nerve palsies and paresthesias of longer duration occur, but even these are usually minor and transient.

A more common occurrence is postspinal *headache*, which develops in about 10% of cases, with a somewhat higher incidence in women. Some believe that these are caused by a reduction in cerebrospinal fluid pressure, and suggest the use of needles of narrow diameter for spinal puncture to minimize fluid leakage through the hole made in the dural membrane. It is also advisable to hydrate the patient with saline solution to keep the cerebrospinal fluid pressure up.

A measure commonly employed to reduce the likelihood of headache is to keep the patient flat on his back for 6 to 12 hours after spinal procedures. Patients should be told prior to, as well as after surgery, that they are expected to lie flat for a specific number of hours.

The patient is permitted to turn from side to side, if so desired, without raising his head. The use of side rails is desirable in the care of these patients if they are drowsy because of barbiturates or other adjunctive medications, yet this detail of postoperative care is often overlooked because with spinal anesthesia, the patient has not lost consciousness.

Saddle block. Saddle block is a form of spinal anesthesia in which the local anesthetic solution is brought into contact with the sacral nerves that run to the perineal area. The resulting loss of sensation is limited to the perineum, buttocks, and thighs without affecting feeling or movement in the legs. It is useful for carrying out obstetric procedures during the second stage of labor and delivery, and for gynecologic, urologic, and rectal surgery.

Epidural anesthesia. This method of administration is not followed by headache and the other neurologic complications caused by penetration of the membranes that surround the subarachnoid space, as is the case when spinal anesthesia is performed. Depending on the level at which the anesthetic solution is placed, it is possible to block conduction in thoracic, lumbar, and sacral nerves (see Fig. 14-2). The resulting analgesia may thus involve areas ranging from the neck to the ankles—effects that can be applied clinically in a wide variety of clinical procedures.

Sensory and motor blockade by epidural anesthesia at the lumbar level has, for example, proved useful in such operative procedures as upper and lower abdominal and pelvic surgery. It has been employed prior to total hysterectomies and cesarean section deliveries. Injections at a lower level—that is, into the sacral canal (see caudal anesthesia, above)—is most commonly employed for obstetric anesthesia.

When expertly carried out, using appropriate dilutions of anesthetics with optimal properties, caudal anesthesia can completely relieve labor pains in all three stages. The mother and fetus can be kept totally free of the central depressant effects of systemically acting narcotic analgesics and general anesthetics.

Local anesthetics used in epidural anesthesia, however, are absorbed into the mother's circulation and also cross the placenta, where they can cause neonatal depression. Bupivacaine may be less widely distributed in the circulation. Another possible drawback is that the mother may not be able to cooperate effectively in the delivery because of excessive sensory or motor block. When, for example, etidocaine—a drug that produces profound motor block—is employed during routine vaginal deliveries, its intense relaxing effect on the mother's voluntary muscles may interfere with efforts to expel the fetus. Thus, this drug is best reserved for forceps deliveries or for those that require manual manipulation—procedures that are aided by drug-induced total muscular relaxation. However, if sensory impulses are totally blocked, the mother may not know when to bear down to aid delivery most effectively.

A possible drawback of epidural anesthesia is that it is technically difficult and thus the drug may not be properly deposited. This can lead to failure to produce anesthesia or to unexpected adverse reactions. Even when the epidural space is entered correctly, the anesthetic drug may be absorbed systemically in large amounts, a pharmacokinetic effect that does not occur with spinal anesthesia. The resulting drop in the mother's blood pressure may lead to serious fetal hypoxia. Thus, if hypotensive reactions develop, the patient should receive treatment with a vasopressor drug. However, when a patient in labor has previously received an oxytocic agent (see Chap. 23), a dangerous drug–drug interaction can occur, resulting in conversion of hypotension to severe persistent hypertension and possibly to a stroke.

Infiltration and field blocks

These techniques are especially useful for anesthetizing the abdominal wall. This is accomplished by first making a circle of skin wheals at appropriate points and then piercing these painless areas with longer needles that enter subcutaneous and rectus muscle sites. After the abdomen is surgically entered, the anesthesiologist may perform a splanchnic nerve block that then permits pain-free stomach and gallbladder operations.

A drawback of this and other field block and infiltration procedures is that relatively large amounts of drug must be injected, and the drug may therefore be absorbed into the systemic circulation. If the plasma level rises too rapidly, the anesthetic can adversely affect the functioning of the heart, brain, and other tissues (see Systemic Toxic Reactions, below). Although the rate of absorption can be slowed to some extent by the addition of dilute vasoconstrictor drug solutions such as epinephrine, this can sometimes lead to other complications. Field block of the fingers or penis with such solutions has, for example, reportedly led to tissue-damaging ischemia.

Local infiltration of a highly vascular area such as the scalp or face with a too concentrated solution of a local anesthetic can lead to absorption of toxic doses of the drug. Similarly, during the performance of extensive *field blocks* in preparation for major surgery, large amounts of solution may have to be injected. Thus, care is required to avoid inadvertent intravenous injection or the absorption of high doses from subcutaneous and intramuscular injection sites at a too rapid rate (see Prevention of Systemic Reactions, below).

Systemic toxic reactions

Toxic reactions from abrupt increases in the level of local anesthetics in the systemic circulation are of two types:

1. Central nervous system overstimulation and depression
2. Cardiovascular depression

Central nervous system reactions

Overdoses reaching the brain by way of the bloodstream may make patients nervous, confused, and disoriented; they may begin to tremble and then develop convulsive spasms. Such motor stimulation may be effectively treated by the intravenous injection of diazepam (Valium). The ultrafast-acting barbiturates, such as thiopental[+], have been used for this purpose, but the doses required to arrest convulsions depress respiration and are likely to intensify the CNS depression that often follows initial nervous system stimulation by local anesthetics. Such a double depressant action could result in coma, as well as in respiratory failure. Consequently, an IV line should be established before injecting appreciable quantities of any local anesthetic, and equipment for administering oxygen and supporting respiration should always be available.

Cardiovascular reactions

Cardiac arrhythmias, myocardial depression, and vaso-dilatation of veins as well as arteries may occur as a result of the actions of systemically absorbed local anesthetics on these tissues. All these actions are probably the result of drug-induced decreases in membrane permeability to sodium, potassium, or calcium ions.

Administration of oxygen and manual massage of the heart may revive the rare patient who suffers cardiac arrest from rapid delivery of a large dose of an absorbed anesthetic to the myocardium. In such cases cardiac standstill may occur with dramatic suddenness, and require the immediate use of heroic measures.

Circulatory collapse may occur as a result of drug-induced vasodilatation as well as because of myocardial depression. The resulting fall in blood pressure is slower in onset and easier to correct when the warning signs are noted in time. The patient, in these cases, may turn pale and get drowsy or dizzy; the heart may race, but the beats become progressively fainter until finally the pulse cannot be felt, and the patient becomes comatose. This vascular reaction, the result of direct depression of arteriolar smooth muscle, is best treated in the same way as the hypotensive reactions of spinal anesthesia—that is, by parenteral administration of sympathomimetic vasopressor substances, such as ephedrine or mephentermine.

Prevention of systemic reactions

Precautions employed to prevent rapid systemic absorption from the skin, subcutaneous tissues, fascia, and muscles, or accidental IV injection, include the following:

1. Only the least amount of the most dilute solution effective for producing the desired degree of anesthesia is injected.
2. Aspiration is performed in several injection planes to be sure that the needle has not entered a blood vessel, or the needle and syringe are kept moving back and forth constantly during field block or local infiltration to ensure against the needle's staying in any vein that it may enter accidentally.
3. Injections are not made haphazardly but solutions are instead placed systematically in intradermal, then subcutaneous, and finally intrafascial and intramuscular sites.
4. The maximal safe dosage of the particular local anesthetic is noted (from the package insert or anesthesia texts) before administration. This can vary depending on the site of injection, the concentration of the solution, and whether epinephrine or another vasoconstrictor is added to the solution. The addition of epinephrine allows a higher dose of local anesthetic to be given safely.
5. A record is kept of the total amount of solution injected, and the actual number of milligrams administered is calculated. Thus, the total dose is kept constantly within safe limits for the particular anesthetic that is being employed.
6. Enough time is allowed to elapse for the drug's local action to take effect and for any systemically absorbed drug to be largely eliminated before further injections are made.
7. Observations are made of the patient's behavior, and the pulse, blood pressure, and rate of respiration are carefully monitored.
8. Vasoconstrictor drugs such as epinephrine and phenylephrine are often added in low concentrations to local anesthetic solutions to slow down systemic absorption of the drug so that the body's own detoxifying processes can eliminate it before toxic levels are reached, and keep the anesthetic at the local site and so prolong its blocking effect on conduction in the nerve fibers. This, in turn, decreases the amount of local anesthetic needed.

Solutions that contain epinephrine in the relatively high 1:100,000 concentration are preferred for use in areas rich in blood vessels such as the scalp and face; for less vascular areas such as the skin of the back or the extremities, more dilute solutions (for example, 1:200,000) are adequate and safer. Higher concentrations of epinephrine are no more effective for these purposes and can cause adrenergic side-effects such as a rise in blood pressure, tachycardia, tremors, and nervousness.

Vasoconstrictors are not added to local anesthetic solutions that are to be used for infiltrating areas of relatively restricted circulation such as the fingers, toes, tip of the nose, ears, or penis. Excessive local ischemia and vasospasm in such areas could result in gangrene. Vasoconstrictors need not be added to local anesthetic solutions that are to be sprayed on the mucous membranes of the upper respiratory tract, because their presence does not significantly retard systemic absorption of the inhaled drug particles.

Additional clinical considerations

Patient safety and education

Patient safety measures must include procedures to protect the patient while an area of the body lacks feeling and, in some cases, movement. The anesthetized area must be protected from direct injury and from indirect injuries such as pressure sores. If the patient has received spinal anesthesia and cannot move the lower extremities, it is necessary to turn the patient frequently and to provide skin care until the patient can turn himself and sense pressure-type pain.

The elderly patient is at increased risk for prolonged effects of local anesthetics because of the decrease in vascular perfusion that often accompanies the aging process. Because local anesthetics depend largely on vascular absorption to remove them from the site of deposition and to terminate their effects, a lack of adequate perfusion will result in prolonged anesthesia. Similarly, patients with vascular diseases or poor cardiac output must be observed for prolonged effects of anesthesia. These patients are also at special risk for pressure sores and related injuries, so they must be observed carefully.

Epidural anesthesia can be a problem with elderly or arthritic patients. The narrowed openings of the intervertebral foramina in these patients prevent the drug from being distributed as effectively, and the anesthetic effect is prolonged. These patients will need to be observed and carefully managed until the nurse is assured that all function has returned.

Local anesthetics used in the respiratory tract can produce some particular problems. Loss of sensation in the upper respiratory tract can result in a blocking of the gag reflex, a situation that can lead to aspiration in some patients, and in a feeling of choking and inability to swallow. This sensation is very frightening to patients; they need to be assured, comforted, and constantly observed for any adverse response. The anesthetizing of the trachea and bronchi will paralyze the cilia, whose activity is important for removing secretions and for protecting the lower respiratory tract from foreign material. In patients who have copious secretions, or who are susceptible to respiratory tract infections, the use of these local anesthetics must be accompanied by vigorous respiratory toilet measures and by careful observation for any signs of problems.

Patient teaching regarding the use of local anesthetics is best incorporated into the general teaching protocol about the procedure being performed. The loss of feeling and movement can be very frightening. The patient should know what will be done, what the administration of the anesthetic will feel like (including any discomfort involved), approximately how long the procedure will take, and what the recovery from the anesthesia will involve (including how long the area will remain numb or immobile). The nurse may state that recovery feels like "pins and needles" but will occur with no ill effects to the area.

The patient should also be prepared to anticipate pain in the surgical area when the anesthetic wears off. The patient can help to alleviate the pain in certain areas of the body by gently "pumping" the muscles around the surgical area before feeling returns to that area. This action will stretch the skin around the incision and will help to bring a blood supply to the area to deal with swelling from the trauma. A good example of such an area is in the perineum following an episiotomy. Encouraging the patient to gently "pump" the muscles in the pelvic floor while the area is still anesthesized will greatly decrease her discomfort during her recovery. Facial, dental, and abdominal sutures involve other surgical sites that benefit from this activity.

The patient should also be encouraged to report any discomfort that might occur during the procedure, with the explanation that the effect of the anesthetic can wear off and more may be needed. The patient should be assured that there is no reason to suffer needlessly. The patient also needs to know that things that seem strange or frightening might be seen or heard, and he should be encouraged to ask questions at any time.

Technical considerations

One of the most important nursing functions in caring for the patient receiving a local anesthetic is to serve as a patient advocate: to reassure the patient, to comfort and encourage the patient, and to monitor the environment, reminding all personnel involved, as necessary, that the patient is awake and aware of the surroundings.

Life support equipment should always be at hand to deal with cardiac emergencies—for example, arrhythmias or the hypotension that can occur—and to deal with the potential central nervous system complications (especially seizures) produced by the anesthetic.

Interactions of local anesthetics with other drugs

Patients who are receiving *sulfonamides* can run into problems if they receive procaine or other ester-type local anesthetics that are hydrolyzed to para-aminobenzoic acid (PABA), because these drugs antagonize the antibacterial action of the sulfonamides. These patients may need to be evaluated for treatment with other antibiotics.

If the patient is receiving the local anesthetic as an adjunct to general anesthesia with a *chlorinated agent* (*e.g.,* chloroform, halothane) or with *cycloprane,* epineph-

rine must not be added to the solution of local anesthetic because these general anesthetics predispose the patient to serious cardiac arrhythmias when epinephrine or other catecholamines are given.

The patient teaching guide and the guide to the nursing process with local anesthetics provide a summary of the clinical considerations with these drugs.

Toxic reactions to systemically absorbed local anesthetic drugs

Central nervous system

Stimulation: Excitement marked by nervousness, apprehension, disorientation, confusion, dizziness, vertigo, nausea, vomiting. May progress to tremors and tonic–clonic convulsions

Depression: Convulsions followed by loss of reflexes, coma, respiratory depression and failure

Cardiovascular

Hypotensive reaction: Blood pressure falls gradually or abruptly; pallor, dizziness, fainting; cardiac palpitations occur as reflex response. Drowsiness progressing to coma may occur in shock states

Cardiac: Bradycardia; reduced stroke volume and cardiac output. Cardiac standstill or ventricular fibrillation may develop

Respiratory

Respiratory arrest may occur secondary to cardiovascular depression and inadequate perfusion of the medullary respiratory center in the brain

Miscellaneous reactions

Allergic reactions: Skin rashes, urticaria, bronchospasm, and laryngeal edema may develop in sensitized persons. Local anesthetics that are esters are especially likely to cause allergy

Local tissue damage: Application of cocaine and other topical anesthetics may cause itching, burning, redness, and possible corneal ulcerations

Postspinal sequelae: Headaches and, occasionally, paresthesias (numbness and tingling), palsies, and paraplegia

Cautions and contraindications in the administration of local anesthetics

- Local anesthetics should be used in the lowest concentration and amount of solution that will produce the desired degree of blockade.
- The total amount of the local anesthetic agent (in milligrams) should be recorded each time a solution is injected or applied, and the maximum safe dose for each agent should not be exceeded.
- Local anesthetic solutions should not be injected into areas of infection or applied to traumatized mucous membranes.
- Injections of local anesthetics should always be made slowly and cautiously, and the syringe plunger should be pulled back periodically. If blood is aspirated, the needle should be withdrawn and the injection made in another area.
- Epinephrine or a similar sympathomimetic vasoconstrictor drug should be added to delay systemic absorption of the local anesthetic,

except when patients are known to react adversely to epinephrine-type agents (*e.g.,* severe cardiovascular disease), or in areas with relatively restricted circulation.
- Patients should be placed in proper position for injection of spinal anesthetics to prevent diffusion of the anesthetic in the spinal fluid to levels of the spinal cord at which their effects are not desired.
- Patients should be kept lying flat or with head down (Trendelenburg position) after spinal anesthesia. (This and the use of a narrow-gauge needle may minimize postspinal headache.)
- Oxygen, diazepam, and appropriate vasopressor drugs (*e.g.,* ephedrine, mephentermine), together with apparatus for their proper administration, should be readily available whenever any procedure using local anesthetics is to be carried out.

Patient teaching guide: local anesthetics

Procedure

1. What it will feel like

2. Any discomfort that might occur

3. Feelings to anticipate (numbness, tingling, inability to move, pressure pain, choking)

4. How long the procedure will last

5. Encouragement to report any discomfort and ask any questions as they arise

Recovery

1. How long recovery will take

2. Feelings to anticipate (tingling, numbness, itching, pressure)

3. Pain that will be felt as anesthesia wears off

4. Measures to reduce pain in the area

5. Signs and symptoms to report (pain along a nerve route; palpitations; feeling faint, disoriented)

Guide to the nursing process: local anesthetics

Assessment	Nursing diagnoses	Interventions	Evaluation

Past history:
  Cardiac problems
  CNS problems
  Vascular problems
  Allergies: reactions
Medication history:
  Drugs being taken;
  last dose
  General anesthetic
  given; type
 	
Physical assessment
Neurologic: orientation;
  reflexes, sensation,
  movement
Cardiovascular: BP, P,
  cardiac output, EKG,
  rhythm
	Potential sensory–
	  perceptual alteration
	Potential alteration in
	  mobility
	Potential alteration in
	  comfort: pain
	Potential alteration in
	  cardiac output
	Potential for fear related
	  to the procedure
	Knowledge deficit
	  regarding procedure
	  and recovery
		Monitor dosage and
		  effectiveness of drug
		Support and encourage
		  patient
		Provide comfort
		  measures:
		  explanations,
		  positioning,
		  environment control,
		  pain relief, skin care
		Patient teaching:
		  Preparation
		  Procedure
		  Recovery
		Provision of life support
		  measures, if necessary
			Monitor effect of and
			  response to drug
			Monitor for adverse
			  effects to drug:
			  arrhythmias, BP, CNS
			  response
			Monitor for return of
			  sensation and function
			Evaluate effectiveness of
			  teaching plan
			Evaluate effectiveness of
			  support measures
			Evaluate for drug–drug
			  interaction with
			  sulfonamides

(continued)

Assessment	Nursing diagnoses	Interventions	Evaluation

Respiratory: rate,
  adventitious sounds,
  secretions
GI: bowel sounds
Renal: continence,
  output
Skin: perfusion,
  temperature, wound
  area

Case study

Presentation

AM, a 32-year-old athlete with a prior history of asthma, was admitted to the hospital for an inguinal hernia repair. At the request of the patient, the surgeon elected to use a local anesthetic employing spinal anesthesia. Because the extent of the repair was unknown (the patient had undergone two previous repairs) etidocaine (Duranest), a long-acting anesthetic, was used. The patient remained alert and inquisitive throughout the 1½-hour procedure. BP 120/64, P 62, R 10, remaining stable throughout. Two hours after the procedure the patient appeared agitated—BP 154/68, P 88, R 12. The patient did not complain of discomfort but did state that he still had no feeling and had only limited movement in his legs. What nursing interventions should be done at this point?

Discussion

Etidocaine is a long-acting local anesthetic with effects that might persist for several hours. The patient should be reassured and observed for a period of time to determine if the elevation of vital signs and the agitation are a reaction to the drug or represent a stress response related to fear. An athlete is even more likely than most other people to experience fear and agitation if his legs are numb and if he cannot move them. Life support equipment should be readily available in case the patient is experiencing a drug toxicity response. The most immediate nursing response would be to explain the lack of feeling to the patient and to outline the time frame usually involved in recovery. Other nursing measures would include the following: keeping the patient flat in bed to help to prevent the headache that often follows spinal anesthesia, but encouraging him to turn from side to side; perhaps even offering a back rub to help to alleviate discomfort and prevent pressure sores; and staying with the patient and encouraging him to talk about his reactions. If the elevated vital signs were a reaction to his fear, they should start to return to normal after the patient is reassured. The elevation of systolic pressure with a stable diastolic pressure would tend to support such a sympathetic stress response. Patient teaching and encouragement will often be all that is needed to alleviate this stress.

Drug digests

Cocaine HCl USP and cocaine USP

Actions and indications. This alkaloid obtained from the coca shrub was the first clinically important local anesthetic. It is also a potent psychomotor stimulant and possesses sympathomimetic properties on injection. Cocaine is used mainly for producing topical anesthesia when applied to mucous membranes. It may be sprayed into the throat and tracheobronchial tree prior to passage of an endotracheal tube. Dropped into the eye, it produces prompt surface anesthesia, vasoconstriction, and mydriasis; the latter two effects are caused by its blocking the reuptake of epinephrine.

Adverse effects, cautions, and contraindications. Pupillary dilatation may be a drawback, particularly in patients with narrow-angle glaucoma. Dryness and damage to the cornea (clouding, stippled pitting, and ulcerations) may occur following topical application. The patient's eye should be kept well irrigated with saline solution during the time that the protective wink reflex is inactive.

This drug is not administered by injection, because its systemic absorption can result in a marked rise in blood pressure, tachycardia, tremors, and possible convulsive seizures and respiratory failure. This drug can cause psychological, and possibly phsyical, dependence. Thus, it is handled in accordance with regulations for control of dangerous drugs.

Dosage and administration. For topical application to the nasal and pharyngeal mucosa 5% to 10% solutions are employed. Lower concentrations (1% to 2%) are used for surface anesthesia of the urethra, and solutions as dilute as 0.25% to 0.5% are effective for anesthetizing the cornea, although higher concentrations are often used.

Lidocaine HCl USP (Xylocaine)

Actions and indications. This versatile local anesthetic is administered topically and by injection for producing prompt local anesthetic effects in various clinical situations (see Dosage and Administration, below). It is also employed to control ventricular dysrhythmias.

Adverse effects, cautions, and contraindications. The central nervous system may be stimulated, depressed, or both, if rapid systemic absorption occurs. Drowsiness, dizziness, and unconsciousness may develop; or shivering, tremors, and convulsions may be followed by respiratory and cardiac arrest. Other cardiovascular effects include bradycardia and hypotension. Thus, care is required (slow injection with frequent aspirations) to avoid IV injection. Allergic reactions may occur in hypersensitive patients; thus, the drug is contraindicated in patients known to be hypersensitive to local anesthetics of the amide type.

Dosage and administration. The dosage and strength of solutions for infiltration vary widely, depending on the procedure.

A 1% to 2% solution is usually employed for most peripheral and central (epidural and caudal) nerve blocks in amounts of between 1 ml and 30 ml and total doses of 20 mg to 300 mg when used without epinephrine, or up to 500 mg with epinephrine.

For spinal anesthesia, a 5% hyperbaric solution with glucose is employed in doses of 1 ml to 2 ml (50 mg to 100 mg).

A 4% solution is used for transtracheal or retrobulbar injection and as a spray for the larynx and pharynx prior to endotracheal intubation, laryngoscopy, and bronchoscopy.

Lidocaine is applied topically as an ointment (2%) for relief of minor skin irritations or for control of postoperative anorectal pain and hemorrhoids (5%). The latter ointment is also used for anesthetizing and lubricating oropharyngeal membranes prior to endotracheal intubation. A jelly (20 mg/ml) provides pain relief and lubrication of the urethra in urethritis and prior to instrumentation.

It is also available in suppositories (100 mg) for use prior to proctoscopic and sigmoidoscopic examinations and in anorectal inflammation. A viscous solution (2%) that adheres to the mucous membranes of the mouth and throat is used for relief of oropharyngeal irritation.

Procaine HCl USP (Novocain)

Actions and indications. This prototype local anesthetic is rapidly effective when injected, but it is not effective as a topical anesthetic. Its duration of action is relatively short, but it can be lengthened considerably by the addition of a low concentration of epinephrine. It is used for peripheral and central nerve blocks prior to surgery, and in various diagnostic and therapeutic procedures.

Adverse effects, cautions and contraindications. Procaine possesses relatively low local and systemic toxicity. Injections are not irritating to soft tissues or nerves. The absorbed drug is rapidly destroyed by circulating enzymes before high blood levels are reached.

However, inadvertent intravenous administration, and injection of single doses above 1000 mg, can cause central and cardiovascular toxicity. Central stimulation may be manifested by mental effects such as nervousness, or motor system toxicity, including tremors, muscle twitching, or convulsive spasms. Cardiovascular toxicity includes hypotension, bradycardia, and possible cardiac arrest.

Dosage and administration. Local infiltration and field block is carried out with solutions of 0.5% to 1% in amounts up to 1000 mg, or 300 ml. Solutions of 1% to 2% are employed for central nerve block procedures. The total dose for spinal anesthesia is 50 mg to 200 mg injected intrathecally. For intravenous anesthesia, a 0.1% or 0.2% solution is infused slowly at a rate of 10 to 15 ml/minute for several hours.

Tetracaine HCl USP (Pontocaine)

Actions and indications. This is a potent, long-acting spinal anesthetic that is particularly useful for prolonged (2- to 3-hour) surgical operations. Because analgesia may last as long as 5 or 6 hours, its use reduces the need for potent narcotic analgesics postoperatively. The onset of anesthesia is relatively slow (15 to 45 minutes). This local anesthetic may also be used for infiltration and for peripheral nerve blocks, as well as for epidural, including caudal, anesthesia and as a surface anesthetic in the eye, nose, and throat or on the skin.

Adverse effects, cautions, and contraindications. This anesthetic is about ten times as toxic as procaine but, because it is effective at about one-tenth the dose of procaine, it can be used in solutions of low concentration that are safe when precautions for preventing too rapid systemic absorption are employed. The chief adverse effect in spinal anesthesia is hypotension as a result of depression of conduction in vasomotor fibers. A marked decrease in blood pressure may be manifested by pallor, sweating, restlessness, and vomiting. It should be treated by administration of vasopressor drugs. Oxygen and equipment for artificial respiration should be available for counteracting the effects of respiratory motor nerve or center paralysis from upward diffusion of the anesthetic.

Dosage and administration. Dilute solutions (0.1% to 0.25%) are employed for local infiltration in amounts that should not ordinarily exceed 100 mg. For spinal anesthesia, doses of no more than 15 mg are employed. Topical application of 0.1 ml of a 0.5% solution is sufficient for surface anesthesia. A 2% solution may be applied to the nose and throat in an amount of 1 ml. Ointments of 0.5% to 1% are available for application to the skin.

References

Adriani J, Naraghi M: Pharmacological principles of regional pain relief. Ann Rev Pharmacol Toxicol 17:223, 1977

Adriani J, Zepernick R: Clinical effectiveness of drugs used for topical anesthesia. JAMA 188:711, 1964

Covino BG: Comparative clinical pharmacology of local anesthetics. Anesthesiology 35:158, 1971

Covino BG: Local anesthesia. N Engl J Med 286:975, 1035, 1972

deJong RH: Toxic effects of local anesthetics. JAMA 239:1166, 1978

Fisher AA: Allergic reactions to topical (surface) anesthesia with reference to the safety of Tronothane (pramoxine hydrochloride). Cutis 25:584, 1980

Levy BA: Diagnostic, prognostic, and therapeutic nerve blocks. Arch Surg 112:870, 1977

Ritchie JM, Greene NM: Local anesthetics. In Gilman AG, Goodman LS, Gilman A (eds): Goodman & Gilman's the Pharmacological Basis of Therapeutics, 6th ed, pp 300–320. New York, Macmillan, 1980

Van Dyke C et al: Cocaine: Plasma concentrations after intranasal application in man. Science 191:859, 1976

Chapter 15

Cholinergic drugs: direct-acting parasympathomimetic drugs and cholinesterase inhibitors

General considerations

The cholinergic drugs are chemicals that act at the same sites as the neurotransmitter *acetylcholine.* Their actions on the structures that are innervated by cholinergic nerves are similar to those of stimulation of the same organs by the several types of nerves that transmit impulses by the release of acetylcholine. Thus, these drugs can also be called *cholinomimetic.* Because several different types of cholinergic nerves innervate very many organs and structures, these drugs can cause widespread effects throughout the body.

Cholinergic drugs bring about their cholinomimetic effects in two main ways. Some—the *direct-acting parasympathomimetic agents*—act like the neurotransmitter itself. That is, the chemical structure of their molecules is such that they can approach and directly occupy cholinoceptive sites on the membranes of the effector cells that are innervated by postganglionic cholinergic nerves. They then evoke effects similar to those produced by the acetylcholine (ACh) molecules released by cholinergic nerve impulses. Others—the *cholinesterase inhibitors,* or *anticholinesterase agents*—act mainly by occupying sites not on effector cells but on the surface of the enzyme cholinesterase, which is responsible for the rapid destruction of ACh. Thus, they produce their effects indirectly by bringing about an increase in the amount of ACh in the junctional spaces between cholinergic nerve endings and cholinergic receptor sites on the neuroeffectors.

Direct-acting parasympathomimetic-type cholinergic drugs have effects that are largely limited to the cells that receive postganglionic fibers from the parasympathetic division of the autonomic nervous system (ANS). Cholinergic drugs of this type act directly on postganglionic neuroeffectors of the *muscarinic* type (see Chap. 13). That is, these chemicals combine with the *cholinoceptive sites,* or *cholinergic receptors,* in such structures as smooth muscle, cardiac muscle, and exocrine gland cells. This then produces effects similar to those brought about by stimulation of the parasympathetic nerves that innervate these structures (see Table 13-2).

Anticholinesterase-type cholinergic drugs act *indirectly* to produce ACh-like effects not only at muscarinic but also at "nicotinic" sites. That is, they can affect the functioning of skeletal muscle and ganglion cells as well as of smooth muscle, cardiac muscle, and glandular tissues. (Some even affect transmission at cholinergic nerve pathways in the central nervous system.) As indicated above, these drugs have relatively little direct effect on cholinergic receptors but act, instead, by *inhibiting* the activity of acetylcholinesterase.

As a result of this interference with enzyme function, the ACh that is being constantly freed from cholinergic nerves tends to accumulate at all types of postjunctional cells. At muscarinic sites, the resulting rise in the local levels of free undestroyed ACh leads to intensified parasympathomimetic activity of smooth and cardiac muscle and gland cells. The drug-induced inhibition of the enzyme also leads to the accumulation of undestroyed ACh at nicotinic sites. This, in turn, initially causes stimulation of skeletal muscle and autonomic ganglion cells. Later, however, the excessive accumulation of ACh that occurs indirectly as a result of the enzyme-inactivating action of anticholinesterase-type cholinergic drugs leads to depression of skeletal muscle tone and ganglion nerve cell impulse transmission.

Classes of cholinergic drugs

Direct-acting parasympathomimetic drugs
These are divided into two subgroups (Table 15-1):

1. The *synthetic choline esters*—drugs chemically similar to the neurotransmitter ACh but

Table 15–1. Cholinergic drugs

Official or generic name	Trade name or synonym	Dosage	Comments
Direct-acting parasympathomimetic agents			
Bethanechol chloride USP	Urecholine; Myotonachol	Oral 5–30 mg; SC 2.5–5 mg	See Drug digest
Carbachol USP	Carbacel ophthalmic; Isopto carbachol	Topical ophthalmic	Used mainly in glaucoma
Pilocarpine HCl USP and pilocarpine nitrate USP			See Drug digest in Chapter 42
Anticholinesterase-type agents			
Tertiary amine class			
Physostigmine and its salicylate and sulfate salts USP	Eserine		See Drug digest in Chapter 42
Quaternary ammonium class			
Ambenonium chloride USP	Mytelase	5–25 mg	Antimyasthenic agent
Demecarium bromide USP	Humorsol	Topical ophthalmic	Miotic in glaucoma
Edrophonium chloride USP	Tensilon chloride	5–20 mg	See Drug digest
Neostigmine bromide USP	Prostigmin bromide	10–30 mg, oral	See Drug digest
Neostigmine methylsulfate USP	Prostigmin Methylsulfate	0.25–1 mg IM or SC	See Drug digest
Pyridostigmine bromide USP	Mestinon	180–600 mg daily	See Drug digest
Organophosphorus-type agents			
Echothiophate iodide USP	Phospholine iodide	Topical ophthalmic	See Drug digest in Chapter 42
Malathion	Cythion		Insecticide
Parathion	Etilon		Insecticide
Sarin			Nerve gas
Soman			Nerve gas
Tabun			Nerve gas

with a much longer duration of action; these include *bethanechol* and *carbachol*, esters that resist destruction by cholinesterase-catalyzed hydrolytic reactions.

2. The *cholinomimetic alkaloids*—plant products that differ from ACh chemically but that produce the same types of effects when their molecules occupy cholinergic receptors in postganglionic neuroeffectors. *Muscarine*, the mushroom derivative from which the term "muscarinic" is derived, is one such alkaloid, and *arecoline* is another.

However, *pilocarpine* is the only drug of this subgroup that is still important in clinical therapy.

Muscarine is of only toxicologic significance; people become poisoned by it when they eat certain species of mushrooms. Arecoline is an active substance in betel nuts, which are chewed by many of the inhabitants of Papua New Guinea and of nearby islands in the South Pacific for the pleasurable effects produced. Arecoline is also employed occasionally as an anthelmintic in veterinary medicine. A chemically related synthetic substance, *aceclidine* (Glaucostat), which has potential ophthalmologic usefulness in the treatment of glaucoma (see Chap. 42), has not been introduced into ocular therapy in this country but is available in some other countries.

Anticholinesterase-type agents

These drugs and chemicals have been classified in terms of the duration of their enzyme-inhibitory activity and in accordance with differences in their chemical structures. Thus, for example, those with a relatively short duration of inhibitory effect on the enzyme are often referred to as "*reversible*" inhibitors of acetylcholinesterase. These compounds have the most clinical usefulness. Others with a prolonged inhibitory effect are referred to as "*irreversible*" inhibitors, and are mainly of toxicologic interest.

In chemical terms, most reversible inhibitors can be classed as natural or synthetic *tertiary amino* or *quaternary ammonium* compounds. A point of some clinical significance is that tertiary amines—*physostigmine*, for example—readily pass through biologic membranes, including the blood–brain barrier (see Chap. 4). On the other hand, quaternary ammonium compounds such as *neostigmine* and related carbamates (Table 15-1) are highly charged substances that penetrate cell membranes poorly and pass through them slowly, if at all. Thus, they are not very well absorbed when taken by mouth and are best administered parenterally for full therapeutic effects. They are also relatively free of adverse effects on central nervous system function.

The *organophosphorus*-type anticholinesterase compounds are mostly well-absorbed by any route of administration, including through the skin, and they can penetrate the blood–brain barrier because of their high lipid solubility. Most are irreversible inhibitors of the enzyme cholinesterase and are considered too toxic to be administered systemically for clinical use. One (echothiophate) is administered as eye drops to treat glaucoma. Some of the volatile liquids, the "nerve gases," have been stockpiled in the past for potential employment in chemical warfare. Other organophosphorus compounds are used as insecticides in agriculture. Although less volatile than the nerve gases, substances such as *parathion* have often caused accidental poisoning.

Clinical pharmacology

The cholinergic drugs have actions on the smooth muscles of various visceral organs and other structures and on skeletal muscles that make them potentially useful in several clinical conditions. However, their clinical usefulness is limited by the difficulty of confining their effects to specific target sites. That is, their lack of *specific affinity* (see Chap. 4) makes it almost inevitable that some adverse effects will occur when therapeutic doses of these drugs are administered. To minimize unwanted effects when treating disorders that are responsive to cholinergic drugs, the physician tries to choose the particular agent that is most likely to act primarily at the target organ. Careful adjustment of the drug's dosage is sometimes successful in limiting the drug's actions to these target tissues. It often becomes necessary to turn to adjunctive drugs and measures for relief of discomforting side-effects from the widespread systemic actions of the cholinergic agents.

When such side-effects are expected, the patient should be warned about these ahead of time. Any signs of improvement that may appear as a result of cholinergic drug treatment should also be pointed out. The patient often tends to tolerate annoying drug effects better if what to expect is known in advance and if evidence of the benefits of drug therapy is seen. The patient must be watched closely for early signs of adverse drug effects. It may be possible to reduce the dosage of the cholinergic drug or to administer other medications to relieve some of the almost inevitable side-effects.

In the following discussion, the pharmacologic effects of cholinergic drugs on various visceral organs and on other structures will be described. Then, in each case, the clinical applications of these actions in the treatment of various disorders will be noted. The adverse effects of these drugs on each organ will then be discussed, together with the reasons for the precautions required in their administration.

Gastrointestinal tract

As indicated in the introductory chapter of this section (Chap. 13), the parasympathetic system strongly influences the functioning of the gastrointestinal tract. If the physiologic effects of parasympathetic actions are understood (Table 13-2), the effects of parasympatho*mimetic* drugs on gastrointestinal smooth muscle and on glands should be readily predictable. In general, the effects of cholinergic drugs on smooth muscle cells that are innervated by parasympathetic postganglionic nerves are manifested by an increase in the tone and motility of the musculature. These actions have a certain limited clinical usefulness in some patients with poor gastrointestinal tone and motility that are not responsive to the standard cathartics (see Chap. 41). More commonly, the gastrointestinal actions of the cholinergic drugs are a source of discomforting side-effects when these drugs are given primarily for their effects on structures other than the gastrointestinal tract.

Among the clinical conditions in which the effects of cholinergic drugs on gastrointestinal motility are considered desirable are *postoperative abdominal atony, distention,* and *paralytic ileus*—conditions in which the patient's abdomen becomes bloated and distended with unremoved wastes and gases as a result of bowel wall paralysis. Cholinergic drugs are *contraindicated* when abdominal distention results from bowel obstruction, because increased contractions in the presence of an obstruction can lead to increased intraluminal pressure and to rupture of the intestines. When a cholinergic drug is indicated, *neostigmine*[+] (Prostigmin) is sometimes employed parenterally.

Often, its effects become apparent in only a few minutes. Similarly, the choline ester *bethanechol*[+] (Urecholine; Myotonachol), which has a relatively selective action on the gastrointestinal tract, is often administered to stimulate gastrointestinal motility in such cases. It is given by mouth with meals, or subcutaneously when it cannot be readily absorbed by the oral route. Various physical and mechanical measures may also be tried in these cases; these include enemas, heat applications to the abdomen, and the use of rectal tubes to aid removal of intestinal gases.

Patients with temporary loss of gastric motility following bilateral vagotomy for peptic ulcer are also best treated with bethanechol, which acts directly at the denervated smooth muscle cells of the stomach to overcome gastric atony. The indirect-acting agents such as neostigmine are not effective in this condition because these tissues lack ACh-releasing nerve endings following surgical section of the vagus nerves.

The predictable gastrointestinal side-effects of cholinergic drugs include intestinal cramps and diarrhea. Increased secretion of gastric acid may also cause heartburn and belching. If taken too soon after eating, these drugs may cause nausea and vomiting.

Whenever cholinergic drugs are given systemically, especially by injection, the anticholinergic drug *atropine* (Drug digest, Chap. 16) should be readily available in a syringe to counteract excessive parasympathomimetic effects on the gastrointestinal tract, as well as on the cardiovascular system and respiratory tract (see below). It is also advisable to have a bedpan readily available.

Genitourinary tract

Cholinergic drugs cause the detrusor muscle of the urinary bladder to contract. This action is often useful for treating *bladder atony* and for bringing about micturition (evacuation of urine). Thus, subcutaneous injection of *bethanechol* or of *neostigmine* is sometimes employed for relief of *postoperative* or *postpartum urinary retention* and for patients with neurogenic urinary bladder atony with retention. Before giving these drugs, it is essential to rule out the presence of any obstruction to the flow of urine in the neck of the bladder, because rupture of the bladder could occur if contractions were increased in the presence of an obstruction.

Pharmacologic "catheterization" of this type may help to prevent the urinary tract infections that sometimes follow mechanical catheterization of these patients, or of patients with spinal cord injuries that cause neurogenic atony of the urinary bladder. However, kidney infections may follow the use of these drugs in patients with bacteriuria if the drug's actions cause the detrusor muscle to contract without simultaneously relaxing the trigone and sphincter muscles. This may force the bacteria-containing urine upward into the ureters and the renal pelves.

When any patient is being treated with one of these drugs a bedpan or urinal should be handy, because these drugs sometimes cause a sudden feeling of urgency to void. Atropine should also be available for counteracting any excessive cholinergic side-effects.

Cardiovascular system

Cholinergic drugs tend to slow the heart rate, dilate the blood vessels, and bring about a fall in blood pressure. However, these effects are not entirely predictable, because compensatory reflex responses may counteract the expected circulatory effects in some patients. This and the tendency of these drugs to cause many discomforting side-effects such as abdominal cramps and diarrhea limit the clinical usefulness of cholinergic drugs for treating cardiac and blood vessel disorders.

Paroxysmal atrial tachycardia attacks are sometimes responsive to the vagomimetic actions of parenterally administered cholinergic drugs. *Edrophonium*[+] (Tensilon) has been used for this purpose. However, digitalis glycosides (Chap. 29) and various antiarrhythmic drugs (Chap. 30) are generally preferred to cholinergic drugs for converting the heart to a normal sinus rate and rhythm. Similarly, in the management of *peripheral vascular diseases* (Chap. 33), other vasodilator drugs are considered less toxic than cholinergic drugs and more effective for producing a sustained increase of blood flow to the skin of patients with Raynaud's disease, acrocyanosis, and other disorders marked by ischemia of the skin and skeletal muscles.

Adverse cardiovascular effects are not common when cholinergic drugs are administered in ordinary therapeutic doses. However, overdosage or poisoning may cause not only excessive slowing of the heart (bradycardia) but also such arrhythmias as atrial fibrillation, transient complete heart block, and even cardiac arrest. Patients with hyperthyroidism are particularly prone to develop atrial fibrillation and heart block when cholinergic drugs are employed in attempts to slow a rapid heart rate.

These drugs cause peripheral vasodilatation by actions on muscarinic cholinergic receptors in the vasculature of skeletal muscle and in other vascular beds. This effect, combined with a reduction in cardiac output, lowers blood pressure. However, these drugs are not used clinically in the management of essential hypertension. In fact, hypertensive patients sometimes react with an excessively steep drop in blood pressure when these drugs are employed alone or simultaneously with ganglionic blocking drugs (Chap. 18) or other antihypertensive agents (Chap. 28). Hypotensive reactions of this type are particularly dangerous in patients with coronary artery disease, because the further decrease in coronary perfusion that can result may cause myocardial hypoxia and precipitate an infarction or a fatal arrhythmia.

Ocular effects

Cholinergic drugs have predictable parasympathomimetic effects on smooth muscle structures within the eye. They cause a contraction of the sphincter of the iris that results in constriction of the pupil, or *miosis*. Contraction of the ciliary bodies, structures that control the movements of the lens, causes a spasm of accommodation; that is, the lens will be accommodated for near vision and the patient may be unable to see distant objects clearly. These and other actions tend to cause a reduction in the abnormally high intraocular pressure of glaucoma. (See Chap. 42 for a detailed discussion of the use of cholinergic miotic drugs in the management of open-angle glaucoma and for other ophthalmologic indications.) Patients receiving cholinergic drugs should be warned about these possible visual system effects.

Other muscarinic effects

Cholinergic drugs stimulate increased secretion by various exocrine glands, including those of the skin, mouth, stomach, and respiratory tract. Cholinergic drugs also stimulate sweating, an effect mediated by muscarinic receptors that are innervated by sympathetic cholinergic axons. *Pilocarpine* is particularly likely to cause profuse sweating and salivation when taken by mouth or injected. These effects have few uses in modern treatment, and this parasympathomimetic drug is administered mainly by topical application in the eye in the management of glaucoma (see above).

More serious than excessive salivation, sweating, and flushing are the effects of overdoses of cholinergic drugs on the mucus-secreting glands of the respiratory tract. The outpouring of such secretions, together with drug-induced contractions of the bronchial smooth muscles, causes some patients to cough, choke, or wheeze when these drugs are administered. Such cholinergic side-effects are particularly likely to occur in patients with a history of bronchial asthma. Thus, the use of these drugs is contraindicated in such cases.

Skeletal muscle effects

Certain cholinergic drugs of the anticholinesterase type (Table 15-1, quaternary ammonium class) tend to act more or less selectively at the neuromuscular junctions in skeletal muscles. Small doses of these drugs that indirectly raise the concentration of acetylcholine at the motor endplates of skeletal muscle fibers stimulate transmission of somatic motor nerve impulses and increase the strength of muscular contractions. Thus, cholinergic drugs are sometimes employed postoperatively to counteract the residual muscle paralysis caused by curare and by other neuromuscular blocking agents of the competitive type—that is, those that compete with ACh for the cholinergic receptors of skeletal muscle fiber end-plates (see Chap. 19).

Myasthenia gravis

Myasthenia gravis is a chronic muscular disease caused by a defect in neuromuscular transmission. This leads to rapid development of weakness and fatigue when the person performs simple movements repeatedly. In some

patients the disease is mild and may be marked only by drooping of one eyelid (ptosis). Other untreated patients may be totally incapacitated, and some die of respiratory complications. In some respects the myasthenic patient's muscle weakness resembles that seen in laboratory animals and in human patients who have received an injection of curare.

Very recent evidence indicates that myasthenia gravis is an autoimmune disease. Patients with myasthenia make antibodies to their receptors for ACh, thus reducing the number of cholinergic receptors available to interact with the molecules of ACh released by the somatic motor nerves. Many questions about myasthenia remain unanswered, but this new information about the nature of the disease has provided a basis for understanding the mechanism of action of the drug therapy and other treatment found empirically to be beneficial. Cholinesterase inhibitors, one of the main classes of drugs in this chapter, are a mainstay of therapy. Adrenal corticosteroids (Chap. 21), other immunosuppressive drugs and nondrug manipulations of the immune system (thymectomy and antibody removal by plasma exchange or plasmapheresis) are also used.

It was the resemblance between the signs and symptoms of myasthenia gravis and those of curare poisoning that led doctors to try treating myasthenic patients with *physostigmine* (Eserine), an alkaloidal drug long known to be an antidote to curare. This anticurare agent proved to have a remarkable ability to overcome the muscular fatigue of myasthenia. Shortly after taking the drug the patient's ptosis vanishes, as does the diplopia, or double vision, that stems from weakness of the extraocular muscles. In terms of new information about the nature of myasthenia gravis, cholinesterase inhibitors are beneficial because they prolong the time that ACh molecules have to interact with available ACh receptors.

Unfortunately, this natural anticholinesterase drug causes widespread muscarinic side-effects because its cholinesterase-inhibiting action is not limited to skeletal neuromuscular junctions. This led scientists to search for chemically related drugs that would act selectively on skeletal muscle fibers only. Several synthetic derivatives, including neostigmine, were developed, which do have a somewhat more selective action on the motor end-plates in skeletal muscle. However, these safer antimyasthenic drugs, which have replaced physostigmine, are not free from muscarinic and nicotinic side-effects, including the possibility of causing muscle paralysis if administered in overdoses. (As indicated in Chapter 13, initial cholinergic stimulation at nicotinic sites such as the autonomic ganglia and skeletal muscles is often followed by secondary depression when the drug's dosage is excessive.)

Diagnosis. *Edrophonium* (Tensilon), an anticholinesterase agent with a rapid onset and short duration of action, is used in the differential diagnosis of myasthenia gravis from other disorders in which muscle weakness occurs. Administered by vein in a small dose that has little effect on the muscle weakness of patients who have no defect in neuromuscular junctional transmission, edrophonium brings about a short but dramatic increase in the muscle strength of myasthenic patients.

Treatment. Neostigmine (Prostigmin), a longer acting anticholinesterase drug, is preferred to edrophonium in the long-term management of myasthenic patients. However, it must also be administered fairly frequently and, because myasthenic patients often tend to become resistant to its action, the dose must be raised to high levels to maintain the muscle-strengthening effects. In such cases, the drug's action at autonomic neuroeffectors also increases. This causes various muscarinic side-effects, including abdominal cramps, diarrhea, nausea and vomiting, and increased secretion of sweat, saliva, tears, and bronchial mucus.

Other drugs for treating myasthenia have been introduced, with claims that they have certain advantages over neostigmine. *Pyridostigmine*[+] (Mestinon) has a somewhat longer duration of action, which is further increased by presenting it in a slow-release form. The main advantage is that patients taking the drug at bedtime need not be wakened during the night to take more medication. In addition, patients who used to waken too weak to swallow their morning dose of neostigmine, and who thus had to receive their medication by injection, do not suffer from morning dysphagia when taking the sustained-action oral form of the longer acting drug.

A further advantage claimed for this and another, newer, antimyasthenic drug, *ambenonium* chloride (Mytelase), is that they cause fewer muscarinic side-effects. Pyridostigmine, for example, is said to cause much less gastrointestinal stimulation than neostigmine, a fact that might make it more desirable for myasthenics unable to take effective doses of the latter drug without suffering from severe cramps. Similarly, ambenonium chloride may be better for myasthenics who are being maintained on a respirator, because this agent causes less bronchial secretions than the other anticholinesterase drugs.

Some authorities suggest that a reduction in muscarinic side-effects, such as may be achieved with these newer drugs or by the simultaneous administration of atropine, is not always desirable. They argue that drug-induced gastrointestinal upset and glandular secretions of increasing severity serve as a useful warning against development of the much more dangerous nicotinic effects of overdosage, which may come on insidiously and can result in increasing skeletal muscle weakness and, finally, paralysis.

Dosage adjustment. Because of the tendency of myasthenics to suffer from the effects of underdosage or overdosage of medication, they must be taught the importance of adjusting dosage to their individual needs and then maintaining their muscle strength at optimal levels by regular administration of the drug. Their families should also learn how to help the patient, who may be left helpless either by waiting too long between doses or

by taking too much medication. In either case, the patient may waken in the morning unable to move, swallow, or call for help. Thus, living accommodations must be arranged so that assistance can be obtained from another person when required. Someone in the family, for example, should be able to administer a parenteral form of an antimyasthenic agent if the patient becomes unable to swallow the tablets.

Because the course of the disease is unpredictable, the patient's response to drug treatment must be observed often and with care. Any change in condition must be reported to whoever is superintending the case, who may then order a change in drug dosage. This is true not only for the patient who suffers a flare-up in intensity of the disease, requiring an upward adjustment of dosage, but also for the patient in remission, whose dosage must be reduced to prevent overdosage and an insidious return of muscle weakness that is actually drug-induced. Raising the dosage in such circumstances can cause an acute drug-induced emergency called *cholinergic crisis.*

Detection and treatment of cholinergic crisis. This complication is marked not only by muscarinic side-effects that can be counteracted by atropine but also by skeletal muscle weakness and respiratory difficulties, which do not respond to treatment with this antimuscarinic antidote. This drug-induced muscle weakness stems from the accumulation of excessive amounts of ACh at the motor end-plates, with a resulting reduction in impulse transmission.

It is often difficult to differentiate cholinergic crisis from *myasthenic crisis,* a situation in which, for poorly understood reasons, the patient suffers a sudden flare-up of the underlying disease. This, like cholinergic crisis, is manifested by respiratory muscle weakness. However, whereas cholinergic crisis calls for *withdrawal* of anticholinesterase drug therapy, patients in myasthenic crisis require *more* antimyasthenic medication.

It is, of course, essential to recognize that, regardless of whether the crisis is cholinergic or myasthenic, this is an acute emergency requiring medical intervention. The physician, who then is faced with what has been called "a desperate dilemma" in deciding how to handle the rapidly weakening patient, now has available a useful drug to help determine the myasthenic patient's true status.

Edrophonium (Tensilon) is used to determine whether patients are suffering from cholinergic or myasthenic crisis. A small dose is injected into the vein of a myasthenic patient suffering from severe respiratory difficulties. If the condition *improves* dramatically—even if for only 1 or 2 minutes—the patient is probably suffering from *myasthenic* crisis and requires treatment with larger doses of one of the longer-acting anticholinesterase compounds. If, on the other hand, the edrophonium injection makes the myasthenic patient even *weaker,* this is an indication that all medication except atropine must be withdrawn, and that mechanical and surgical measures, such as endotracheal intubation, suction, tracheotomy, and artificial respiration should be used.

Atropine is useful no matter what the diagnosis. It should always be available in both oral and parenteral form to anyone caring for a myasthenic patient. Small oral doses counteract the common gastrointestinal discomforts; large parenteral doses aid the breathing of patients in cholinergic crisis, although mechanical measures are also often required.

Myasthenic or Eaton–Lambert Syndrome

This syndrome resembles myasthenia gravis in many respects, but can be differentiated from myasthenia gravis by electromyography. It sometimes occurs in patients who have small-cell lung carcinoma. The muscle weakness and fatigability often respond to anticholinesterase drugs, but an alternative is *guanidine HCl* (10 to 15 mg/kg/day in divided doses), a drug that is not indicated in myasthenia gravis. Guanidine is said to act presynaptically to increase the amount of ACh released by nerve action potentials. The effects of guanidine are not typical of cholinergic drugs, although its gastrointestinal side-effects resemble those of cholinergic drugs and are relieved by atropine. Unlike cholinergic drugs, it causes *tachycardia* as well as other serious adverse effects (*e.g.,* bone marrow depression, renal and hepatic toxicity) that cannot be related to the release of ACh.

Central nervous system effects

As indicated earlier, some cholinergic drugs do not cross the blood–brain barrier, and thus exert no effects on the central nervous system. Others, such as the organophosphorus-type compounds, can cause central toxicity (see below and the summary of side-effects at the end of the chapter).

One cholinergic drug, *physostigmine salicylate,* which enters the CNS when administered parenterally, is used as an antidote to the central as well as peripheral toxic effects of anticholinergic drug overdosage. Such poisoning can occur not only with atropine and other belladonna alkaloids (Chap. 16), but also with various other drug classes that exert anticholinergic activity, including the tricyclic-type antidepressant drugs (Chap. 46) and some antiparkinsonism agents (Chap. 49). In such cases, physostigmine can often control such central signs and symptoms of the anticholinergic syndrome as delirium, disorientation, hallucinations, and hyperactivity. However, this antidote must be injected IV at a slow controlled rate, because overdosage can cause convulsions and cholinergic crisis, as well as such typical parasympathomimetic side-effects as bradycardia, bronchoconstriction, and excessive glandular secretions.

Poisoning by irreversible cholinesterase inhibitors (organophosphorus agents)

Systemic absorption of echothiophate eye drops, used to treat glaucoma, can cause a wide spectrum of serious adverse cholinergic effects. The precautions necessary to prevent poisoning by this therapeutic agent are discussed in Chapter 42 in the discussion of eye drugs.

Certain chemicals employed in agriculture as insecticides also exert potent cholinergic activity. *Parathion* and other organophosphorus-type chemicals have been a frequent cause of poisoning in farm workers and in others exposed to them. These poisons that inhibit acetylcholinesterase cause ACh to build up in the body. The accumulation of excess ACh at *all* sites of cholinergic transmission produces very many signs and symptoms of poisoning (see the summary at the end of the chapter).

Those in the field of public health can help to prevent poisoning by parathion and related chemicals by calling attention to the danger of using these insecticides without proper protection. This includes measures to prevent contact of these chemicals with the skin, through which they can be absorbed, and to prevent their vapors from being inhaled. These precautions apply not only to workers who are occupationally exposed to parathion; home gardeners and others using *malathion* and other less toxic pesticides that are cholinesterase inhibitors should also be warned to read the labels of the products they are using and to avoid careless handling. If an accident does occur, the container or a sample of the material should be brought to the hospital emergency room or physician's office.

Treatment. *Atropine,* administered repeatedly in large doses, is a specific antidote against cholinergic poisoning of this type. It often gives dramatic relief of muscarinic-type symptoms and also helps to prevent CNS toxicity, including respiratory center depression and failure. However, atropine does *not* prevent paralysis of the muscles of respiration. Thus, artificial respiration with oxygen inhalation may be required until these muscles resume their function.

Pralidoxime (Protopam; 2-PAM) is an antidote of a different type. Pralidoxime brings about its antidotal effects by breaking the bond between the poisonous chemical and the molecular surface of the inhibited enzyme acetylcholinesterase. Freed of the chemical that had been preventing it from reacting with its natural substrate, the neurotransmitter ACh, the reactivated enzyme becomes capable of carrying out its function once more. The excess of ACh molecules that had accumulated at the neuromuscular junctions of the respiratory muscles is then destroyed by the enzyme, which is made available as a result of the antidotal action of pralidoxime.*

In severe poisoning by parathion and similar pesticide products, pralidoxime is infused by vein in an initial

---

* Pralidoxime does not cross the blood–brain barrier; thus, it does not reactivate cholinesterase in the CNS. Drugs such as diacetyl oxime, not available in the United States but available elsewhere, do cross the blood–brain barrier.

1-g to 2-g dose at the same time that the patient receives 2 mg to 4 mg of atropine IV and mechanical measures for improving ventilation. A second similar dose may be administered if muscle weakness persists about 1 hour after the first infusion. Additional doses may be given IM or subcutaneously later if necessary, along with additional doses of atropine. Occasionally, if gastrointestinal effects of cholinesterase inhibition are not severe, oral doses of pralidoxime may be effective; in the presence of increased gastrointestinal motility, the drug will not be adequately absorbed after oral administration.

This drug is less effective as an antagonist to *carbamate*-type cholinesterase inhibitors such as neostigmine, pyridostigmine, and ambenonium. In fact, some authorities state that pralidoxime is both ineffective *and* contraindicated in poisoning by the carbamate-type reversible cholinesterase inhibitors (*e.g.,* neostigmine), because it is itself a weak cholinesterase inhibitor.

Additional clinical considerations

The cholinergic drugs act to cause predictable autonomic responses. Because these responses may overwhelm the autonomic reflexes that normally prevent excessive parasympathetic effects, they can produce many uncomfortable and often undesirable responses, most of which can be predicted by reviewing the actions of the parasympathetic nervous system. Parasympathetic stimulation will cause bradycardia, bronchoconstriction, increased pulmonary mucus secretion, increased gastrointestinal secretions and motility, increased bladder tone and contractions, and decreased gastrointestinal and urinary tract sphincter tone. Increased parasympathetic activity can cause a reflex sympathetic response, part of the body's attempt to return to a homeostatic state. In patients who experience a sympathetic reflex response, sympathetic activity can be expected: tachycardia; flushing, sweating; increased blood pressure; decreased gastrointestinal activity; decreased bladder tone. In taking care of a patient who is receiving cholinergic drugs, the nurse will need to consider the effects that either excessive parasympathetic activity or rebound sympathetic activity could have on that patient. These two sets of effects provide the bases for the contraindications to the use of cholinergic drugs, as well as the bases for predicting the side-effects. The patient should be informed in advance about these side-effects, and helped to cope with them when they occur.

Patient comfort and education

Patient comfort and safety measures are often as crucial to compliance with therapy as improvement in signs and symptoms. The patient should have ready access to a bedpan or urinal and the opportunity for privacy. A cool, darkened environment can help to make the flushing and eye sensitivity more tolerable. Aspirin or another appropriate analgesic should be offered to help to relieve the headache that frequently develops. Some cholinergics used to treat chronic glaucoma can cause vision changes and night blindness. Patients need to be aware of this possibility, and precautions need to be taken to ensure their safety if these changes should occur.

Patient teaching is very important for patients who are receiving cholinergic drugs. They need to know what effects to expect, how to cope with them, and what warning signs to be aware of and report. The dosage of these drugs often has to be changed as the patient's responses fluctuate. The patient teaching guide presents suggestions for a written protocol to use with these patients. Patients with myasthenia gravis will require very extensive teaching about their drugs and drug dosages as part of their teaching plan.

Technical considerations
Whenever cholinergic drugs are being given, atropine should be readily available for use if drug toxicity occurs. Most institutions stock predrawn syringes of atropine for emergency use. Life support and ventilatory equipment should be on standby if cholinergic drugs are being injected. If a patient with myasthenia gravis should be in crisis, the ventilatory support equipment should be close at hand. If a patient has been poisoned by organophosphorous insecticides, the skin should be washed and all potentially contaminated clothing should be removed, because these drugs are absorbed through the skin, as well as by other routes, such as inhalation or ingestion. All sources of drug exposure should be eliminated. Pralidoxime should be available for these patients.

Ophthalmic preparations containing cholinergic drugs can be absorbed systemically and can cause serious systemic side-effects. This problem can be avoided if careful technique is used when administering the drug. The opening of the nasolacrimal duct must be occluded by applying pressure to the inner canthus of the eye during and for 1 minute after administration of the drug. Blocking the duct will prevent the drug from reaching the nose and throat, being swallowed, and then absorbed into the systemic circulation. The patient should also be instructed in the proper administration of the drug, and the reasons for this technique should be explained. Eye drops should always be clear solutions and should be kept sterile. If there are any doubts about the solution, it should be discarded.

The nursing process table presents a summary of clinical considerations as they apply to the nursing care of a patient receiving cholinergic drugs.

Summary of the pharmacologic actions and therapeutic uses of cholinergic drugs

Pharmacologic actions	Therapeutic uses
Gastrointestinal	
Increased tone and motility of musculature, leading to defecation; increased secretion of gastric and other glands	Relief or prevention of postoperative abdominal distention and of gastric atony following vagotomy; management of megacolon and of constipation induced by ganglionic blocking agents
Genitourinary	
Increased tone of detrusor muscle of bladder and relaxation of trigone and sphincter results in stimulation of micturition	Relief or prevention of postoperative and postpartum urinary retention; management of patients with neurogenic bladder
Cardiac	
Decrease in heart rate (bradycardia); decrease in atrial contractility; decrease in rate of conduction through atrioventricular node	Occasional use in terminating paroxysmal atrial tachycardia, especially when combined with ocular pressure and carotid sinus massage
Vascular	
Vasodilatation resulting in hypotension, rise in skin temperature, and local flushing	Rarely used to relieve local pain, coldness, and cyanosis in selected cases of peripheral vascular disease
Ocular	
Contraction of sphincter muscle of iris causes miosis; contraction of ciliary body causes spasm of accommodation	Reduction of intraocular pressure in chronic simple wide-angle glaucoma; alternated with mydriatics to break up adhesions between the iris and the lens
Respiratory	
Bronchial constriction and increased mucus secretion	Not therapeutically useful
Skeletal muscle	
Only cholinesterase inhibitors act here—direct-acting parasympathomimetics do not affect the skeletal neuromuscular junction; stimulation of muscle fibers improves strength of abnormally weak motor units but causes fasciculation and weakness of normal muscles	Long-term relief of myasthenia gravis; emergency treatment of myasthenic crisis; differential diagnosis of myasthenia gravis and differentiation of myasthenic from cholinergic crisis; curare antidote
Glandular effects	
1. *Diaphoresis*—profuse sweating occurs with some drugs 2. *Sialogogue*—profuse salivary secretion occurs with some drugs	1. Diagnosis of peripheral nerve injuries 2. Used to counteract xerostomia (mouth dryness) in some rare situations
Central nervous system	
Only certain drugs penetrate the blood–brain barrier; low doses stimulate the respiratory center and other central sites; larger doses cause respiratory depression; low doses can counteract central anticholinergic blockade	This is not usually a therapeutically useful action. However, physostigmine salicylate is sometimes useful for antagonizing the central as well as peripheral toxic effects of atropine and other drugs with an anticholinergic component, such as the tricyclic antidepressant agents

Summary of the side-effects of cholinergic drugs

Muscarinic-type effects

Gastrointestinal: Heartburn, belching, epigastric distress, abdominal cramps, tenesmus (painful anal spasms), diarrhea, nausea and vomiting

Genitourinary: Involuntary micturition; increased tone and motility of ureters

Cardiovascular: Bradycardia and hypotension followed by reflex cardioacceleration and hypertension in some persons

Ocular: Blurring of vision and miosis; aching of brow and eyes; other effects such as photophobia, myopia

Respiratory: Bronchoconstriction, increased bronchial mucus secretion, wheezing cough, feelings of tightness and pain in chest

Glandular: Profuse sweating, salivation, lacrimation

Nicotinic-type effects

Initial skeletal muscular fasciculations, twitching and cramps followed by fatigue, weakness, and paralysis of all striated muscles including the diaphragm and intercostals, leading to respiratory distress and failure

Central nervous system effects

The organophosphate (*non*quaternary ammonium) compounds may cause anxiety, confusion, restlessness, disorientation, difficulty in concentrating, slurring of speech, apathy, and drowsiness; also, ataxia, dizziness, headache, weakness, tremor, and convulsions; depression of respiration with Cheyne–Stokes breathing, cyanosis, coma, cardiovascular collapse, arreflexia, respiratory failure, and death

Patient teaching guide: cholinergic drugs

The drug that has been prescribed for you is of the class of drugs that are called cholinergic. The drugs get this name because they act at certain nerve–nerve and nerve–muscle junctions in the body that are called cholinergic sites. This type of drug has been prescribed for you to treat _____ . Because there are many cholinergic sites in the body, the drug may have several effects other than the one you need. It is important for you to understand what to expect and how to deal with it.

Instructions:

1. The name of your drug is _____ .

2. The dose of the drug ordered for you is _____ .

3. Some of these drugs require special storage; note any instructions on your bottle. Eye drops should be clear and should be kept sterile; if you have any doubts about the solution, discard the drug.

4. Your drug should be taken _____ times a day. The best time to take your drug is _____ , _____ , _____ .

(5. If the drug is contained in eye drops, special care should be taken to administer the drug appropriately to avoid side-effects. The head should be tilted backward slightly; the lower eyelid should be pulled down, maintaining pressure over the opening of the tear duct in the corner of the eye; the correct number of drops should be administered; and pressure should be maintained over the tear duct opening for a full minute.)

6. Some common side-effects that you should be aware of are the following:

Nausea, flatulence, diarrhea   It is wise to be near bathroom facilities after taking your drug

(continued)

Flushing, sweating	Staying in a cool environment and wearing lightweight clothing will help
Urgency to void	Again, maintaining access to a bathroom will help
Headache	Aspirin or tylenol (if not contraindicated for other reasons) will help to alleviate this pain

7. Tell any physician, nurse, or dentist who takes care of you that you are taking this drug

8. Keep this and all medications out of the reach of children

Notify your nurse or physician if any of the following occur:

Light-headedness or fainting
Excessive salivation
Abdominal cramping or pain
Weakness, confusion
Blurring of vision

The occurrence of any of these problems could indicate a need to adjust the dose of your medication.

Guide to the nursing process: cholinergic drugs

Assessment	Nursing diagnoses	Interventions	Evaluation
Past history (*contraindications*): Asthma Coronary artery disease Cardiac conduction blocks Peptic ulcer Bowel obstruction–surgery Urinary bladder obstruction–surgery Epilepsy Parkinson's disease Hyperthyroidism Occupation: ask about exposure to organophosphates *Allergies:* reaction	Potential alteration in urinary elimination patterns Potential alteration in bowel elimination: diarrhea Potential alteration in comfort: pain, temperature intolerance Knowledge deficit regarding drug	Preparation and safe administration of drug Provide comfort measures: • Bedpan nearby • Cool environment • Positioning • Pain relief measures Patient teaching: Drug Dose Administration Side-effects Toxic effects Atropine on standby, provision of life support measures if necessary	Monitor response to drug: Bowel sounds Voiding Decrease eye pressure Monitor for adverse effects of drug: excessive cholinergic response Monitor for exacerbation of underlying medical conditions Evaluate effectiveness of comfort measures Evaluate effectiveness of patient teaching plan

(continued)

Assessment	Nursing diagnoses	Interventions	Evaluation
Medication history: last dose; *ganglionic blockers; other cholinergic drugs* **Physical assessment** Cardiovascular: BP, pulses, cardiac output, auscultation, EKG Respiratory: rate, rhythm, secretions, adventitious sounds GI: bowel sounds, output Renal: output, bladder tone, distention Muscular: tone, reflexes, strength			

Case study

Presentation

Mrs. J has been returned to the unit after lengthy abdominal surgery. She has not eaten since the previous evening, but she has no desire for the ice chips that she is offered. Her abdomen appears distended and no bowel sounds are heard on auscultation. The hurried physician who is called decides that she is probably suffering from paralytic ileus and orders an IM injection of neostigmine methylsulfate, which is to be followed by several oral doses of bethanechol chloride. What would the appropriate nursing measures be?

Discussion

The drugs that have been ordered are relatively potent cholinergic drugs. Reviewing the expected effects of these drugs, you would expect to see increased bronchial secretions and bronchoconstriction, increased gastric secretions and increased gastrointestinal tone and motility, increased bladder contractions and tone, and hypotension and bradycardia, followed perhaps by a reflex tachycardia. None of these effects is desirable in a patient who has just been anesthetized for a long period of time and who has just undergone abdominal surgery. The respiratory, bladder, and cardiac effects are undesirable in the postanesthesia period when complications in these systems often occur. The increased gastrointestinal secretions and activity can lead to serious complications after abdominal surgery, such as rupture or obstruction. The most appropriate action in this case would be to question the drug order and to refuse to give the medication until further evaluation determines the exact cause of the problem. In the meantime, baseline assessment should be made of those parameters that are most affected by cholinergic drugs. The patient should be comforted, and appropriate pain relief measures taken. Explain the concerns to the patient and, if an abdominal ultrasound or x-rays are requested, explain the procedures and their rationale to help to allay any further anxieties. If it is determined that the patient does have a paralytic ileus and cholinergic drugs are to be given, extreme care must be taken to observe the patient carefully for the occurrence of any of the adverse effects previously mentioned.

Drug digests

Bethanechol chloride USP (Myotonachol; Urecholine)

Actions and indications. This choline ester exerts parasympathomimetic effects on the smooth muscle of the GI tract, urinary bladder, and other structures innervated by postganglionic cholinergic nerves. Its muscarinic effects on the GI tract are used to increase muscle tone and peristaltic motility in such disorders as postoperative abdominal distention, paralytic or adynamic ileus in patients suffering from severe injury or infections, and gastric atony following bilateral vagotomy or stomach surgery.

The drug's stimulating effect on the urinary bladder is often effective in postoperative and postpartum urinary retention or in similar situations resulting from neurogenic atony or from overdosage of cholinergic blocking drugs, including ganglionic blocking agents. Its use for treating dysphagia in patients with scleroderma has also been suggested.

Adverse effects, cautions, and contraindications. This drug is best administered on an empty stomach to avoid nausea and vomiting. Atropine should be available to counteract cramps, diarrhea, and other undesirable effects that may follow injection. The drug is contraindicated in obstructive GI and genitourinary disorders. Although ordinary doses have few cardiovascular and respiratory effects in most people, this drug is contraindicated in patients with an unstable circulatory system, a history of a recent myocardial infarction, or a history of asthma.

Dosage and administration. Bethanechol may be administered orally in doses of 5 to 30 mg tid or qid before meals. It is also administered subcutaneously—*never* IM or IV—in doses of 2.5 to 5 mg repeated tid or qid. If trial with these doses does not produce the desired response, a single dose of 10 mg may be given subcutaneously.

Edrophonium chloride USP (Tensilon)

Actions and indications. This rapid-acting cholinergic drug of short duration is used mainly in the differential diagnosis of myasthenia gravis and for differentiating myasthenic crisis from cholinergic crisis. However, its muscle-strengthening action is too short to be useful in the maintenance therapy of myasthenia gravis. It is also used occasionally in treating attacks of paroxysmal atrial tachycardia.

Adverse effects, cautions, and contraindications. Overdosage may cause muscarinic side-effects such as abdominal cramps and diarrhea, bronchoconstriction and increased bronchial secretion, and bradycardia and hypotension. These can be corrected by administration of atropine, which should always be available in a syringe for injection. Respiratory failure may also result from possible vagal effects or from skeletal muscle paralysis and respiratory center depression.

Dosage and administration. In the test for differentiating between myasthenia gravis and other disorders marked by muscle weakness, 0.2 ml of a solution containing 10 mg/ml (2 mg) is injected by vein and followed by 0.8 ml (8 mg) more if no cholinergic reactions occur after 45 seconds. The test may also be performed with 1 ml (10 mg) injected IM. These doses increase muscle strength in myasthenic patients but produce no change or slight muscle weakness in others.

In differentiating between myasthenic and cholinergic crisis, 0.1 ml (1 mg) is injected IV, and the patient is observed for improvement of muscle strength (myasthenic crisis) or for further weakness (cholinergic crisis). If no adverse cardiac or respiratory effects occur after a 1-minute interval, an additional 0.1 ml may be injected and observation continued.

If the patient's respiration definitely improves, further treatment with a longer acting anticholinesterase drug administered by vein is indicated. On the other hand, if further respiratory muscle weakness is observed, or if no sign of improved breathing is seen, it is best to discontinue further anticholinesterase drug therapy and to manage the patient with assisted respiration.

Neostigmine bromide and methylsulfate USP (Prostigmin Bromide and Methylsulfate)

Actions and indications. Neostigmine is the prototype cholinergic drug of the anticholinesterase class. By inhibiting the enzyme cholinesterase, it increases the amount of ACh available for transmitting nerve impulses at various junctions, including the neuromuscular junctions of both smooth and skeletal muscles.

It is used to increase the tone and motility of gastrointestinal and genitourinary system smooth muscle in conditions marked by hypotonicity and hypomotility—for example, postoperative distention of the intestine and urinary bladder. The drug is also useful in the management of myasthenia gravis to increase the strength of weakened skeletal muscles. The injectable methylsulfate form is used when patients have difficulty in swallowing the oral tablets and in patients in acute myasthenic crisis.

Adverse effects, cautions, and contraindications. Overdosage causes cholinergic effects of both the muscarinic and nicotinic types. Muscarinic side-effects, including increased salivation, abdominal cramps and diarrhea, bronchoconstriction, and increased bronchial gland secretions, can be counteracted by administration of atropine, which should always be available. The most serious nicotinic effects are muscle cramps, followed by weakness and possible paralysis. This condition, called cholinergic crisis when it occurs in patients being treated for myasthenia gravis, requires immediate discontinuance of neostigmine. This drug is contraindicated in patients with bronchial asthma and in those with obstructions of the GI or genitourinary tracts.

Dosage and administration. For treatment of postoperative abdominal distention and urinary retention, 1 ml (0.5 mg) of the 1:2000 solution of neostigmine methylsulfate is injected SC or IM. Half of this dose (0.25 mg) may be injected postoperatively to prevent these conditions and repeated several times daily for 2 or 3 days.

In myasthenia gravis, oral doses of the bromide salt are administered in highly individualized dosages adjusted to the needs and tolerance of the patient (*e.g.*, 15 to 375 mg daily). The methylsulfate salt solution is injected SC or IM in doses of 1 ml of the 1:2000 solution (0.5 mg) as needed to control severe muscle weakness.

Pyridostigmine bromide USP (Mestinon)

Actions and indications. This cholinergic antimyasthenia drug counteracts the muscle weakness of myasthenia gravis by increasing the duration of action of ACh at the neuromuscular junction. Like neostigmine, it is a cholinesterase inhibitor. It is claimed to cause fewer muscarinic effects on the GI tract than does neostigmine, and its duration of action is said to be longer.

Adverse effects, cautions, and contraindications. Overdosage can cause muscarinic- as well as nicotinic-type side-effects. Muscarinic effects include increased peristaltic activity; the drug is contraindicated in patients with mechanical obstructions of the GI or genitourinary tracts. Increased bronchial secretions and bronchoconstriction can occur. Therefore, the drug is contraindicated in patients with bronchial asthma. It may also cause breathing difficulties that result in weakness or paralysis of the skeletal muscles of respiration when overdosage causes nicotinic interference with transmission. In such cases the drug must be discontinued, atropine administered, and measures taken to control ventilation—for example, by tracheostomy and assisted ventilation. **Dosage and administration.** Daily dosage is adjusted to the needs of each patient individually. Thus, the needs of different patients may vary from 1 tablet to 25 tablets of 60 mg each (average dose 10 tablets). A syrup is now available for easier dosage adjustment when fractions of 60 mg are required. Also available are sustained-action tablets containing 180 mg each, which have a duration of action between two and three times that of ordinary tablets. A dose of one to three of these at intervals of at least 6 hours is usually effective.

References

Barrett DM: Effect of oral bethanechol on voiding in female patients with excessive residual urine: Randomized double blind study. J Urol 126:640, 1981

Drachman DB: The biology of myasthenia gravis. Ann Rev Neurosci 4:195, 1981

Duvoisin RC, Katz R: Reversal of central anticholinergic syndrome in man by physostigmine. JAMA 206:1963, 1968

Gever L: Cholinergics. Nursing 14:41, 1984

Grob D (ed): Myasthenia gravis: Pathophysiology and management. Ann NY Acad Sci 377:1, 1981

Hayes WJ: Parathion poisoning and its treatment. JAMA 192:49, 1965

Hofmann WW: The treatment of myasthenia gravis. Ration Drug Ther 13(2):1979

Lisak RP: Myasthenia gravis: Mechanisms and management. Hosp Pract 19:101, 1983

Namba T et al: Poisoning due to organophosphate insecticides. Am J Med 50:475, 1971

Rowland LP: Diseases of chemical transmission at the nerve–muscle synapse: Myasthenia gravis and related syndromes. In Kandel ER, Schwartz JH (eds): Principles of Neural Science, pp 132–137. New York and Amsterdam, Elsevier/North Holland, 1981

Taylor P: Anticholinesterase agents. In Gilman AG, Goodman LS, Gilman A (eds): Goodman and Gilman's The Pharmacological Basis of Therapeutics, 6th ed, pp 100–119. New York, Macmillan, 1980

Taylor P: Cholinergic agonists. In Gilman AG, Goodman LS, Gilman A (eds): Goodman and Gilman's The Pharmacological Basis of Therapeutics, 6th ed, pp 91–99. New York, Macmillan, 1980

Thanik K et al: Bethanechol or cimetidine in treatment of symptomatic reflux esophagitis. Arch Intern Med 142:1479, 1982

Chapter 16

Parasympathetic blocking drugs

16

General considerations

Drugs that block the effects of parasympathetic nerve impulses on organs and tissues are among the most widely prescribed agents used clinically. When the effects of parasympathetic innervation are blocked, the effects of sympathetic innervation are left unopposed. Thus, many effects of these drugs can be predicted from knowledge of the autonomic nervous system. For example, blockade of the parasympathetic nervous system causes relaxation of the gastrointestinal tract and urinary bladder, a decrease in the secretion of exocrine glands, tachycardia, and mydriasis. These drugs are often employed for their effects on the gastrointestinal tract, but therapeutic use is also made of their effects on the other organs described above, as well as on the CNS. Some clinical uses will be described in more detail in other chapters; reference will be made to these, as appropriate.

These drugs are often called *cholinergic blocking agents* or *anticholinergic drugs* because they block certain effects of acetylcholine (ACh). Specifically, they block the effects of ACh at muscarinic synapses (see Chap. 13). Therefore, these drugs are also called *antimuscarinic*.

Several types of drugs, which are not classed as parasympathetic blocking drugs, have antimuscarinic (anticholinergic) side-effects. For example, the tricyclic antidepressants and the aliphatic phenothiazines (used to treat psychosis) commonly cause side-effects similar to those of *atropine*[+], the prototype agent of this class.

The frequency with which undesired secondary effects occur is a major drawback of these drugs. Drugs of this class are not very selective in the organs that they affect. Thus, for example, when atropine is ordered for its therapeutically desirable effects in reducing motility of the gastrointestinal tract, the patient will often complain of side-effects caused by atropine's concurrent actions on the salivary glands and eyes. Some patients who might profit from a particular action of atropine may not be able to be treated with this drug because they cannot tolerate some of its other actions. Thus, for example, this drug may be contraindicated in some cases because its actions on the urinary bladder or the heart could cause complications more troublesome than its potential beneficial effects. This has led to a not entirely successful search for synthetic drugs with greater specificity for various peripheral sites of action.

The drugs of this class have a particular affinity for the cholinergic receptor sites of visceral effector organs that receive parasympathetic (or sympathetic) postganglionic innervation. However, when the molecules of one of these drugs (atropine, for example) combine with the receptor substance of muscle and gland cells, this reaction does not trigger the series of events that ACh ordinarily sets off. On the contrary, because these blocking molecules prevent the ACh released by nerve endings from making the necessary attachment to the receptors, cellular function fails.

Such *competitive inhibition* or *antagonism* of the natural neurotransmitter (see Chaps. 4 and 13) can sometimes be overcome by raising the local level of ACh at the postganglionic cholinergic receptor sites. Thus, the anticholinesterase agents (*e.g.,* physostigmine; see Chap. 15), which act indirectly to increase the concentration of ACh, can sometimes counteract the actions of atropine; and, of course, atropine is the antidote for overdosage of these cholinesterase-inhibiting chemicals.

Natural and synthetic anticholinergic substances

The earliest (and still the most important) source of chemicals with parasympathetic blocking action was the potato plant family, the Solanaceae. The alkaloids *atropine* (*dl*-hyoscyamine) and *scopolamine* (*l*-hyoscine), called *belladonna alkaloids,* were extracted from plants such as deadly nightshade (*Atropa belladonna*), henbane (*Hyoscyamus niger*), and jimson weed (*Datura stramonium*). They are available both as the purified plant principles and in the form of galenical preparations, including the tincture, extract, and fluidextract of belladonna (Table 16-1).

Because of the many undesired secondary effects of these substances, chemists have long tried to synthesize drugs with an affinity greater than that of the natural alkaloids for specific sites, particularly the gastrointestinal tract. At first, they tried to modify the plant derivatives themselves by treating them chemically. *Homatropine,* which is used mainly for its effects on the eye, is one such semisynthetic derivative. Later, they learned that when the nitrogen atom of the natural alkaloid was quaternized (*i.e.,* altered so that it combines with four, rather than three, other chemical groups), these quaternary ammonium derivatives differed in some of their pharmacologic properties.

For example, atropine *methylnitrate,* scopolamine *methylbromide,* and homatropine *methylbromide* (Table 16-1) have fewer CNS side-effects, because quaternization reduces a drug's ability to cross the blood–brain barrier and enter the CNS. At the same time, these drugs and other synthetic quaternary ammonium compounds, including methantheline bromide, propantheline bromide, and others listed in Table 16-2, are less readily absorbed through the upper intestinal mucosa when they are taken by mouth because of their poor ability to penetrate biologic membranes. Drugs of this synthetic subclass are claimed to be capable also of blocking parasympathetic and sympathetic ganglia—that is, they block *nicotinic,* as well as muscarinic, cholinergic synapses.

A third group of synthetic drugs developed in the search for more selectively acting agents (Table 16-3) is said to relax smooth muscle spasm mainly by a direct action on the muscle fibers rather than by blockade of cholinergic neuroeffectors. Thus, in theory at least, a drug such as *dicyclomine* relieves gastrointestinal spasm and *oxybutynin* relaxes reflex spasm of the urinary bladder while causing few typical anticholinergic side-effects. In practice, these relatively weak spasm-relaxing agents must often be administered in large doses that can produce atropinelike effects on exocrine glands, the eye, and other peripheral sites.

In summary, although some of the parasympathetic-blocking drugs are free of CNS toxicity, all can produce similar peripheral side-effects. In clinical practice, this means that when a drug of this class is administered

Table 16–1. Natural solanaceous alkaloids, preparations, and derivatives

Official or generic name	Trade name or synonym	Usual range of single oral adult doses	Comments
Atropine USP	*dl*-Hyoscyamine	0.4–0.5 mg	Free alkaloid of belladonna, stramonium, and other solanaceous plants
Atropine methylnitrate	Eumydrin	0.5–1.5 mg	Quaternary ammonium derivative of atropine
Atropine sulfate USP		0.3–1.2 mg	See Drug digest
Belladonna extract USP		10–40 mg	Contains about 0.2 mg of atropine
Belladonna (leaf) fluidextract USP		0.06–0.1 ml	Very potent (1 ml contains 3 mg of alkaloids)
Belladonna (leaf) tincture USP		0.3–2.4 ml	Only 1% as potent as the fluidextract
Homatropine methylbromide USP		2.5–7.5 mg	Less potent antimuscarinic activity than atropine
Hyoscyamine sulfate		0.125–0.25 mg	Salts of alkaloid of hyoscyamus
Methscopolamine bromide USP	Scopolamine methylbromide; Pamine	2.5–5 mg	Less potent than atropine orally, but equally potent by IM or SC injection
Methscopolamine nitrate	Scopolamine methylnitrate	2–4 mg	Similar to the above quaternary ammonium derivative of scopolamine
Scopolamine HBr USP	*l*-Hyoscine HBr	0.3–0.8 mg	See Drug digest

Table 16–2. Synthetic quaternary ammonium and other anticholinergic agents

Official or generic name	Trade name	Usual oral adult dose
Anisotropine methylbromide	Valpin	50 mg
Clidinium Br	Quarzan	2.5–5 mg
Glycopyrrolate USP	Robinul	1 mg
Hexocyclium methylsulfate USP	Tral	25 mg
Isopropamide iodide USP	Darbid	5 mg
Mepenzolate bromide	Cantil	25 mg
Methantheline bromide USP	Banthine	50 mg
Oxyphencyclimine HCl USP	Daricon	10 mg
Oxyphenonium bromide	Antrenyl bromide	10 mg
Propantheline bromide USP	Pro-Banthine	15 mg

for a particular purpose, such as relaxing gastrointestinal spasm and reducing excessive gastric secretions, it will almost inevitably cause mouth dryness and blurring of vision. In addition, the development of these ocular effects in the ulcer patient who also happens to have narrow-angle glaucoma is a special danger. On the other hand, such so-called side-effects may, in some situations, be the main action that it is desirable to elicit (*e.g.*, by an ophthalmologist). Thus, atropine is a prime example of a drug with which one man's side-effect is often another's therapeutic action!

Pharmacologic actions and their clinical applications

In the following discussion of the pharmacologic effects of atropinelike drugs, the effects of atropine and its rel-

Table 16–3. Synthetic antispasmodic drugs*

Official or generic name	Trade name	Usual oral adult dose
Dicyclomine HCl USP	Bentyl	10–20 mg
Flavoxate HCl	Urispas	100–200 mg
Oxybutynin chloride	Ditropan	5 mg
Thiphenamil HCl	Trocinate	100–400 mg

* These drugs are claimed to act mainly by a *direct* action on the contractile mechanism of smooth muscle and only slightly by producing blockade of parasympathetic motor impulses. This is the basis for claims that they are likely to cause few atropinelike side-effects. Nevertheless, caution is required in administering these drugs to patients for whom belladonna alkaloids and synthetic anticholinergic drugs would be contraindicated.

atives on the functioning of a particular organ or system will be described, and then the clinically significant aspects of the effects, both beneficial and undesirable, will be described. This will include a description of the various pathologic states that increase a patient's susceptibility to adverse actions which might cause atropinelike drugs to be contraindicated. The pharmacologic actions and therapeutic uses of these drugs will be summarized at the end of the chapter.

Gastrointestinal tract

The actions of parasympathetic blocking drugs on the gastrointestinal tract are the ones most commonly sought clinically. Natural and synthetic atropinelike drugs are used mainly to reduce gastrointestinal spasm and secretions in conditions marked by hypermotility, hypertonicity of smooth muscle, and hypersecretion of gastric acid. Among the disorders in which these drugs are employed are peptic ulcer, gastritis, cardiospasm, pylorospasm, ileitis, diverticulitis, ulcerative colitis, and other functional and organic inflammatory and infectious diseases of the upper and lower gastrointestinal tracts.

Historically, a major use of parasympathetic blocking drugs has been as adjuncts in the management of acid peptic disease, but none of these drugs is entirely satisfactory for this purpose. Although they reduce painful reflex spasms set off by the action of acid gastric secretions on naked nerve endings in the ulcer crater, their ability to inhibit production of the acid itself and to speed healing of the eroded mucosa is limited. The large doses required for adequate antisecretory action almost invariably cause dry mouth, blurred vision, and other side-effects. These drugs have been largely supplanted in the management of peptic ulcer by the histamine H_2 receptor blockers (*e.g.*, cimetidine, ranitidine).

Such adverse reactions also occur with the somewhat more potent synthetic quaternary ammonium antisecretory agents such as *methantheline* (Banthine) and *propantheline*[+] (Pro-Banthine) and their successors (Table 16-2). Drugs of this type are said to produce their antisecretory effects by a double action—blockade of parasympathetic ganglia, as well as of the postganglionic sites; however, the undesired effects of adequate doses often run parallel with increased therapeutic activity.

Although these drugs are seldom used now in the treatment of gastric or duodenal ulcer, most authorities believe that they are probably useful for treating various functional bowel disorders. Thus, for example, the *antiperistaltic–antispasmodic* effect of both the belladonna alkaloids and the several types of synthetic anticholinergic compounds is often effective for treating *irritable bowel syndrome,* a condition marked by spasticity of the colon, and colitis, and in such neurogenic bowel disturbances as the splenic flexure syndrome and neurogenic colitis.

In such conditions, these spasmolytics and inhibitors of intestinal motility sometimes provide symptomatic relief of both diarrhea and constipation. Combined with opiates such as *paregoric,* these drugs often control the patient's cramps and reduce the number of loose bowel movements. On the other hand, when combined with sedatives or tranquilizers and personal reassurances and comfort, the antispasmodics sometimes help patients with constipation of the spastic type by relaxing the hypertonic intestinal segment.

Drugs of this class are not very effective against diarrhea and intestinal spasm caused by chronic inflammatory disorders such as diverticulitis and ulcerative colitis or by acute bacterial, viral, or amebic infections. In such cases, *paregoric* and certain synthetic opium-derived drugs are preferred for control of excessive intestinal motility, corticosteroids are preferred for reducing local inflammation, and antibiotics or sulfonamides are preferred for fighting the pathogenic microorganisms.

Urinary tract

Patients with various urologic disorders including acute urinary tract infections sometimes receive adjunctive treatment with drugs of this class. In such cases, the resulting inflammation causes irritation of the bladder and other structures, which sets off reflex spasms that can cause frequent painful micturition. Such frequency and urgency in cystitis, prostatitis, urethritis, and other infections may be reduced somewhat by administration of adequate doses of belladonna derivatives or of the synthetic anticholinergics. These drugs diminish the number of motor impulses that pass to the fundus of the bladder by way of parasympathetic (sacral) postganglionic axons. This quieting action on the detrusor muscle, together with the drugs' ability to increase the tone of the trigone and vesical sphincter, is useful for increasing the capacity of the bladder—an effect desirable in paraplegics and in others who have become incontinent as a result of reflex, or uninhibited, neurogenic bladder. These actions are also sometimes employed in treating children with a bedwetting problem (nocturnal enuresis).

The loss of bladder tone produced by atropine and even by such synthetic antispasmodics as flavoxate and oxybutynin make micturition difficult in some cases. This is especially true in elderly men with an enlarged prostate gland that already partially obstructs urine flow. Thus, these drugs are contraindicated in patients with prostatic hypertrophy, because their use may result in dysuria and urinary retention. Elderly male patients taking these drugs for gastrointestinal or other problems may be embarrassed to mention difficulty in voiding, or may not associate this difficulty with the drug. To elicit this information, it may be necessary to question these patients specifically about the frequency of urination and whether or not they need to go to the bathroom every few hours during the night.

Other smooth muscles, including those of the ureters and bile ducts, may also be relaxed by the antispasmodic action of these drugs. Atropine is often combined with morphine and meperidine (Demerol) in the treatment of patients with renal or biliary colic to bring about relaxation of the extremely painful reflex spasm set off by the presence of a stone in the ureter or bile duct. Actually, the relaxant action of atropine on these smooth muscles is not very strong. However, the atropine does, at least, help to counteract the spasmogenic effect of morphine. Morphine, which is often very effective for relieving pain by its central analgesic action, actually tends to increase muscle spasm by its peripheral action on smooth muscle.

Cardiovascular system

Low doses of atropine paradoxically slow heart rate; moderate doses tend to speed the rate of the heart by blocking the braking action of vagus nerve impulses on the heart. By reducing the inhibitory influence of the vagus nerves on the sinoatrial (S-A) node pacemaker and on the atrioventricular (A-V) node, atropinelike drugs permit sympathetic cardioaccelerator impulses to predominate.

Atropine-induced tachycardia is not in itself clinically useful. In fact, it is usually considered a side-effect that is especially undesirable for patients with a history of heart disease. Thus, these patients should be monitored for changes in pulse rate after atropine has been administered. Atropine and related drugs must be used cautiously, if at all, in patients with angina pectoris, because they may set off an episode of coronary insufficiency. Too rapid heart action may also cause cardiac decompensation in patients with heart failure by interfering with diastolic filling of the heart's chambers and thus reducing cardiac output.

Atropine is, however, useful for treating cardiac disorders marked by excessive slowing as a result of an increase in vagal tone. Sinus bradycardia and partial heart block commonly occur, for example, following an acute myocardial infarction (AMI). Atropine is often effective for increasing the heart rate, improving A-V conduction, and raising the cardiac output. Because of its possibly adverse effects on cardiac function, atropine is best reserved for AMI patients in whom bradycardia has caused hypotension and in whom the ECG reveals runs of escape beats, indicating an arrhythmia that could be best treated by increasing the heart rate. It should not be administered routinely to all AMI patients with a slow heart rate for prophylaxis against a further fall in the rate and in blood pressure.

The cardiac effects of atropine have proved useful in treating digitalis-induced heart block (see the discussion of digitalis intoxication and its treatment, Chap. 29) and in preventing excessive reflex bradycardia during induction of anesthesia with halothane and other general anesthetics. Given as preanesthetic medication, atropine also protects the heart from the excessive vagal impulses that are set off by certain surgical procedures. Oral doses also help to prevent sudden blackouts in patients with the *carotid sinus syndrome,* a condition in which even slight pressure in the neck sets off a reflex stream of heart-slowing vagus nerve impulses.

Respiratory tract

Historically, one of the main reasons for administering atropine or scopolamine[+] preoperatively was to prevent respiratory complications caused by excessive *respiratory and tracheobronchial secretions.* Ether, for example, can elicit profuse secretions by its irritating effect on the bronchial mucosa, and this can lead to reflex laryngospasm. However, ether is now used infrequently, and the newer fluorinated anesthetics do not cause much irritation or increase secretions. Thus, there is little need today for the routine administration of atropine preoperatively for this reason when these general anesthetics or combinations of nitrous oxide and intravenous barbiturates are employed. (Atropine premedication is, of course, still desirable before administration of an anesthetic known to cause bradycardia, and *scopolamine*[+] may sometimes still be used in obstetrics for its central sedative and amnesic effects.)

Bronchial and nasal gland secretions are dried by these drugs. Drying of nasal secretions by belladonna alkaloids and by antihistaminic drugs that possess an anticholinergic component is the basis for including such agents in products promoted to the public for relief of common cold symptoms (Chap. 39). The reduction of bronchial gland secretions is occasionally useful in the treatment of an allergy-induced cough. More often, though, it is considered undesirable for patients with chronic respiratory difficulties because, when respiratory tract fluids are reduced, they may thicken, harden, and plug up narrow passages. Thus, because asthmatic patients have difficulty in coughing up such secretions, systemically administered anticholinergic drugs are used with caution, if at all, in such cases.

However, the inhalation of the smoke of "asthma cigarettes," made from the leaves of solanaceous plants such as *Datura stramonium,* is an old asthma remedy that is sometimes still employed to relieve bronchospasm, and, very recently, a solution of atropine sulfate (Dey-Dose atropine sulfate), to be given by nebulizer, was approved by the FDA and marketed in the United States for short-term use as a bronchodilator in patients with asthma and other obstructive pulmonary diseases. Another anticholinergic bronchodilator, *ipratropium bromide* (Atrovent), an aerosol drug available in England to treat asthma, is undergoing clinical trials in the United States. The usefulness of these drugs in treating asthma appears to depend heavily on their inhalation route of administration, which limits their systemic toxicity. In addition, ipratropium is said not to inhibit bronchial mucus secretion, an effect that makes systemic anticholinergic drugs dangerous in asthmatics. The role of these inhaled anticholinergic drug preparations in treating bronchial asthma is still unclear. Systemic anticholinergic drugs, once a mainstay of asthma therapy, have been superseded in recent years by adrenergic bronchodilators (Chap. 17), xanthines (Chap. 40), and inhaled corticosteroids (Chap. 21 and 40) and cromolyn sodium (Intal; Chap. 40). All of these drugs have certain drawbacks, at least for some patients, who may find the new anticholinergic drug preparations safe and effective alternatives.

Exocrine glands

The effects of parasympathetic blocking drugs on secretions of exocrine glands other than those of the stomach are not of major therapeutic importance. However, their effect on the patient's salivary glands is a common cause of complaint when these drugs are being employed for other purposes. Anticholinergic drug blockade of bronchial and sweat glands can also cause side-effects and complications in some patients.

Salivary gland secretion is readily reduced by atropine, which blocks transmission of the parasympathetic postganglionic impulses that ordinarily induce secretion of watery saliva. This effect is helpful to anesthesiologists in maintaining a clear airway. Postoperatively, however, the patient who has received atropine or scopolamine as preanesthetic medication is very likely to have an uncomfortably dry mouth that causes difficulty in swallowing and talking. These patients should receive thorough mouth care, including frequent rinsings and ice chips or cold drinks, if permitted. Similar measures may be suggested to patients taking belladonna derivatives for gastrointestinal disorders or other conditions, and the patient should be told that sucking hard candies or chewing a stick of gum may stimulate some salivation when xerostomia (dry mouth) is especially discomforting. Sugarless lozenges are also very helpful, because they do not contribute to tooth decay or to the rebound dryness that can occur after sugar pulls fluid out of the mucosa osmotically.

Sweat gland secretions are reduced by the blocking action of atropinelike drugs on transmission of sympathetic cholinergic postganglionic nerve impulses to these structures. This action is rarely used for relief of excessive sweating (hyperhidrosis) because of side-effects brought about by the doses that reduce perspiration. The sweat-stopping effect of drugs with anticholinergic activity can sometimes cause fever (hyperpyrexia). This is especially likely in warm weather when the body rids itself of excess heat mainly by evaporation of fluid (perspiration) from the skin. By causing cessation of sweating, atropine-type drugs may sometimes precipitate a dangerous hyperpyrexic reaction because the body cannot rid itself of heat. The nurse should be alert to the possibility that a feverish patient with a hot, dry, flushed skin or even a scarlatiniform rash may be suffering from atropine poisoning (see below). Psychiatric patients taking large doses of phenothiazine drugs that possess an anticholinergic component are also subject to similar reactions.

The eye

The actions of atropine and related drugs on the eye are of considerable importance because they bring about effects on the functioning of ocular structures that can be used by the ophthalmologist in diagnosis and treatment, but that can also be harmful to some people. Atropine and similar drugs produce two types of effects in the eye: (1) mydriasis, or dilation of the pupils; and (2) cycloplegia, or paralysis of accommodation, which prevents the patient from making the adjustments of the lens that are needed for near vision. Mydriasis is produced by the blockade of parasympathetic impulses to the sphincter muscle of the iris; cycloplegia results from the blockade of parasympathetic impulses to the ciliary muscles that control the movement of the lens.

Mydriasis and loss of the light reflex, which also often occurs, are useful effects in ophthalmologic examinations. They allow the ophthalmologist to examine the inner structures of the eye, including the retina and optic disk, more easily. Similarly, drug-induced production of cycloplegia permits the examination of the eye for refractive errors without interference by involuntary adjustments of the lens. Relaxation—even paralysis—of these smooth muscles of the eye is desirable in treating various inflammatory ocular disorders. (For a more detailed discussion, see Chap. 42.) Usually, atropinelike drugs (e.g., tropicamide) with shorter durations of action than atropine itself are used as eye drops for diagnostic examinations.

Adverse ocular effects may occur when anticholinergic drugs are administered orally or parenterally for treating gastrointestinal, cardiac, and other disorders. Mydriasis is in itself not usually serious. In fact, Italian women of the Renaissance used to put belladonna drops into their eyes to dilate their pupils for a desired cosmetic effect. (Belladonna means "beautiful lady," and the girl's date may have admired her luminous widely dilated pupils, but the dark-eyed beauty probably saw little of her escort because of the blurring of her own vision brought about by the drug's cycloplegic action.) However, mydriasis can cause discomfort by allowing too much light to reach the retina. Atropinelike drugs are one cause of photophobia. Cycloplegia, even when paralysis of accommodation is incomplete, is a source of annoyance because of the blurring of vision that results, and can endanger the patient who tries to drive a car or operate machinery that requires clear vision. Patients who will receive mydriatic drugs, and those that cause cycloplegia, should be warned beforehand to expect these effects, both to prevent alarm and to allow the patient to plan activities to allow for the expected drug effects. Patients whose eyes will be examined with the aid of atropinelike drugs should always be told to bring sunglasses and to arrange transportation that does not require their driving a car immediately afterward.

More serious than mere discomfort is the danger that these drugs may precipitate an attack of glaucoma. This is not likely to happen to people with normal eyes. However, in those with a congenitally narrow angle in the anterior chamber of the eye, the effect of these drugs on ocular smooth muscle may lead to a sharp rise in intraocular pressure. The relaxing or paralyzing action of atropine on the iris and ciliary bodies may make these structures crowd back into the angle. This may then block the canals through which the aqueous humor ordinarily drains, thus resulting in a buildup of hydrostatic pressure within the chamber. Thus, anticholinergic drugs are usually contraindicated for patients with a history of glaucoma. Their use in patients over 40 years old also requires caution, because in most people ocular smooth muscles tend to undergo changes at about that age, which make them more susceptible to attacks of glaucoma.

Central nervous system

The belladonna alkaloids possess CNS effects of clinical importance. Atropine and scopolamine both penetrate into the CNS, and both presumably block impulse transmission by ACh at certain central synapses. However, the two alkaloids differ somewhat in their effects. Scopolamine produces mainly depressant effects; the actions of atropine on the cerebral centers and medulla are mainly those of a mild stimulant.

Scopolamine acts in relatively small doses to produce drowsiness. This action contributes to the calming and amnesic effects sought when this drug is administered

347

alone or with morphine prior to anesthesia in surgery and obstetrics. However, scopolamine may cause considerable restlessness and even delirium, especially in patients who are in pain. Some doctors now prefer to use diazepam (Valium) or one of the phenothiazines instead of scopolamine for preanesthetic medication and in obstetrics.

Small oral doses of scopolamine, which are not nearly as effective for sedation as the parenterally administered drug, are often combined with centrally depressant drugs of the antihistamine class in nostrums sold directly to the public as "safe sleep" products. Scopolamine and antihistaminic drugs with an anticholinergic component, such as dimenhydrinate (Dramamine), also act centrally to prevent nausea and vomiting in motion sickness and in vestibular disorders such as Meniere's disease (see the section on antiemetic drugs in Chap. 41).

The natural solanaceous alkaloids and certain synthetic anticholinergic drugs, such as those used in the treatment of Parkinson's disease (Chap. 49), cause mental and behavioral changes when taken in overdoses. People suffering from this central anticholinergic syndrome become restless, disoriented, confused, combative, and delirious. Then they may become unresponsive to stimuli and lapse into a coma. Fortunately, fatalities are rare because these drugs are quite rapidly detoxified. Toxicity of this type does not occur with glycopyrrolate, propantheline, and the other quaternary ammonium compounds that do not pass the blood–brain barrier.

Poisoning

Accidental poisonings sometimes occur when children ingest jimson weed seeds or people pick the leaves of a solanaceous plant and use them in preparing a salad. Infants given overdoses of belladonna preparations for colic or who are treated with eye drops that may be absorbed from the ocular and nasal mucosa are sometimes the victims of atropine poisoning. Patients being treated in a coronary care unit after an AMI sometimes become delirious after receiving repeated doses of atropine for treating bradycardia. Elderly patients with organic brain disease who are being treated with antipsychotic drugs combined with anticholinergic medications to counteract drug-induced extrapyramidal symptoms sometimes become behaviorally worse because of the adverse central effects of these drugs (Chap. 46). Reports of atropine–scopolamine-type toxicity in drug abusers deliberately seeking the hallucinogenic effects of these drugs and others with a central anticholinergic component have become increasingly common (Chap. 53).

Poisoning by belladonna alkaloids and by other drugs with an anticholinergic component causes a wide variety of dramatic signs and symptoms. The peripheral and central effects previously described have led to patients poisoned by atropine being described as "Hot as fire, red as a beet, blind as a bat, dry as a bone, and mad as a hatter."

Patients who are poisoned by overdoses of atropinelike drugs or by plant substances containing belladonna alkaloids are effectively treated with repeated parenterally administered doses of 1 mg to 4 mg of *physostigmine,* an anticholinesterase-type cholinergic drug that reverses the central as well as the peripheral effects of anticholinergic drug intoxication.

When administering atropine, scopolamine, and similar drugs, special care should be taken to see that the patient is receiving the right dose. The small doses of these drugs are sometimes ordered in the apothecary system and at other times in the metric system, which could lead to confusion and result in a patient's getting a dangerous overdose. Special caution is necessary when an atropine solution is to be mixed in the same syringe with a narcotic analgesic for preoperative administration. When atropine eye drops are administered, precautions described in Chapter 15 for eye drops containing cholinergic drugs should be taken to prevent the solution from being carried to the throat by way of the nasolacrimal duct and swallowed, because this can lead to systemic absorption and toxicity. Patients should be cautioned to keep anticholinergic eye drops out of the reach of children, because their accidental ingestion can cause poisoning.

Additional clinical considerations

Because of the varied systemic effects of these drugs, many of which are perceived as unpleasant by the patient, compliance to the drug regimen can be a serious problem. The nurse is often in a unique position to help the patient to understand and cope with these unpleasant effects. The patient teaching guide provides an approach to this challenge. Many of the usual procedures for helping the patient to adapt to the side-effects of these drugs have been mentioned in the text. In some cases, additional considerations may be necessary.

The dry mouth can be so severe that the patient has difficulty in swallowing and eating. Artificial saliva can be purchased in the form of crystals that are sprinkled on the food, which are converted to a viscous fluid in the mouth. If the patient is not on fluid restrictions, plenty of fluids will also help the patient during meals.

Constipation is a very common side-effect of these drugs. If a patient has been constipated and develops a watery diarrhea, it could indicate that the patient is developing an obstruction. As the obstruction becomes complete, stool will leak around it. In such a case the drug should be stopped immediately and appropriate measures taken.

The elderly and very young patients are especially susceptible to heat prostration when using these

348

drugs. Those in these two age groups have some difficulty in regulating their body temperatures under normal situations; when parasympathetic blocking drugs are given, the regulation of body temperature may be totally lost. These patients have to be extremely cautious in warm temperatures. They might not be able to accommodate to the heat, and could become hyperpyrexic. These patients also lose the ability to deal with fever, because they have no way of dissipating the heat that their bodies generate. If any of these patients should feel ill or develop a fever, the drug may have to be stopped until the fever subsides. If the drug cannot be stopped, the patient will need to be treated with such measures as antipyretics, cool sponge baths, and a cool environment. The patient will need to be monitored very closely.

These drugs often cause unusual side-effects in the elderly patient. Excitement, agitation, drowsiness, and hallucinations have all been reported. Elderly patients should be monitored carefully, with safety measures provided, the first few times that they take the drug.

Because of the eye changes that can occur with the parasympathetic blocking drugs, any patient over the age of 40 years should be evaluated for glaucoma before the drug is started. Patients also may lose the ability to accommodate to changing levels of light, and need to have that possibility pointed out to them so that appropriate safety measures can be taken.

Although these drugs can be given to patients with cardiac disease, the nurse should be aware of the possibility that the drugs may aggravate the disease by causing tachycardia, thus increasing the workload of the heart. Patients with coronary artery disease may develop angina; patients with congestive heart failure may suffer decompensation and develop the signs and symptoms of congestive failure.

Drug–laboratory test interactions

Because the parasympathetic blocking drugs slow gastrointestinal motility and secretions, they can alter the absorption of other drugs from the gastrointestinal tract. To avoid this situation, parasympathetic blockers should not be taken with other drugs but should be spaced throughout the day.

Any drug that causes effects similar to those of the atropinelike drugs may increase the unpleasant side-effects. Many *over-the-counter (OTC) drugs* contain drugs with these properties, and the patient should be advised to avoid OTC drugs to prevent the development of toxicity.

Isopropamide iodide can interfere with the uptake of *radioactive iodine in thyroid function tests,* yielding results that may be falsely low. If at all possible, the isopropamide should be discontinued about 1 week before the tests are scheduled.

The nursing process guide summarizes the clinical applications of knowledge about the parasympathetic blocking drugs.

Summary of the pharmacologic actions and therapeutic uses of parasympathetic blocking drugs

Pharmacologic actions	Therapeutic uses
Gastrointestinal system	
Smooth muscle: antispasmodic, antiperistaltic *Gastric glands:* decreases acid and digestive enzyme secretion	Decreases motility and secretory activity in the following conditions: peptic ulcer, gastritis, cardiospasm, pylorospasm, regional enteritis, diarrhea (mild dysentery), constipation of the hypertonic or spastic type
Other smooth muscles	
Urinary tract: decreases tone and motility in the ureters and fundus of the bladder, increases tone in the bladder sphincter	Increases bladder capacity in children with enuresis, spastic paraplegics, and in others with urinary incontinence; decreases urinary urgency and frequency in cystitis and in other conditions; used as antispasmodic in renal colic and to counteract spasm caused by morphine
Biliary tract: antispasmodic	Provides relief of biliary colic; counteracts spasmogenic action of narcotics (*e.g.,* morphine)
Bronchial muscle: produces weak relaxation, mild bronchodilatation	Counteracts drug-induced bronchoconstriction; aerosol preparation used in asthma

(continued)

Cardiovascular system

Cardiac: low doses lead to decreased P, high doses lead to increased P
Vascular: local vasodilatation produces "flushing"

Counteracts bradycardia caused by vagal stimulation, surgical procedures, carotid sinus syndrome; used to overcome some heart blocks following myocardial infarction; used to treat hypotension caused by cholinergic drugs

Ocular effects

Pupil dilatation, cycloplegia (paralysis of accommodation)

Ophthalmologic examination of retina, optic disk, refractive errors; relaxes ocular muscles and decreases irritation in iridocyclitis and choroiditis

Glandular secretions

Reduces sweating, salivation, respiratory tract secretions

Used before inhalation anesthesia; used to reduce nasal secretions in rhinitis, colds, hay fever; used to reduce excessive sweating in hyperhidrosis

Central nervous system

Decreases extrapyramidal motor mechanisms
Atropine has excitatory effects: restlessness, disorientation, delirium, or psychosis
Scopolamine has depressant effects: drowsiness, amnesia

Decreases tremor in parkinsonism; helps to prevent motion sickness; scopolamine is in OTC sleep medications

Patient teaching guide: parasympathetic blocking drugs

The drug that has been prescribed for you is called a parasympathetic blocking drug. It "blocks" or stops the actions of a group of nerves that are part of the parasympathetic nervous system. This drug may decrease the activity of your gastrointestinal tract, dilate your pupils, or speed up your heart.

Instructions:

1. The name of your drug is ——————————— .

2. The dose of the drug ordered for you is ——————————— .

3. The drug should be taken ——— time(s) a day.
   The drug should not be taken with any other drugs because it can decrease the amounts of these other drugs that are absorbed. Try to take any other medications you need 1 hour *before* taking this drug or 2 hours *after* taking this drug. If you experience difficulty voiding, take the drug just after you have emptied your bladder. The best times to take your drug are ——— , ——— , ——— .

4. Some common side-effects of this drug that you might experience include the following:

   Dry mouth, difficulty in swallowing

   Frequent mouth care will help to remove dried secretions and keep the mouth fresh; sucking on sour sugarless candies will help keep the
   (continued)

	mouth moist; taking lots of fluids with meals (unless you're on a fluid restriction) will aid in swallowing.
Blurring of vision, sensitivity of eyes to light	If your vision is blurred, avoid driving, operating hazardous machinery, or doing close work that requires attention to details until vision returns to normal; dark glasses will help to protect your eyes from light.
Retention of urine	Taking the drug just after you have emptied your bladder will help; moderate your fluid intake while the drug's effects are high; if possible, take the drug before bed, when this effect will not be a problem.
Constipation	Take fluids and roughage in your diet; follow any bowel regimen you may have; monitor your bowel movements so that appropriate laxatives can be taken, if necessary.
Flushing, intolerance to heat, decreased sweating	This drug blocks sweating, which is your body's way of cooling off; avoid extremes of temperature; dress coolly; on very warm days, avoid exercise as much as possible.

5. Tell any physician, nurse, or dentist who takes care of you that you are taking this drug.

6. Avoid the use of any over-the-counter medication, especially for sleep and for nasal decongestion; avoid antihistamines, diet pills, or cold capsules, because they may contain similar drugs. Consult your nurse or physician if you feel that you need some symptomatic relief.

7. Keep this and all medications out of the reach of children.

Notify your nurse or physician if any of the following occur:

Eye pain
Skin rash
Fever
Rapid heart rate
Chest pain
Difficulty breathing
Agitation, excitement, mood changes
Impotence—a dose adjustment or new drug may alleviate this problem

Guide to the nursing process: parasympathetic blocking drugs

Assessment	Nursing diagnoses	Interventions	Evaluation

History
Past history
(*contraindications*):
  Narrow-angle
    glaucoma
  GI surgery or
    obstruction
  Obstructive bladder
    disease or surgery
  Myasthenia gravis
  Prostatic hypertrophy
  Tachyarrhythmias
  Chronic obstructive
    lung disease
  Pregnancy
  Lactation
  Allergies: reactions
Medication history:
  Other drugs
  OTC drugs
 	
Physical assessment
Neurologic: orientation,
  mental status
Cardiovascular: P,
  auscultation, baseline
  EKG
Respiration: rate,
  adventitious sounds
GI: bowel sounds,
  pattern of functioning
GU: output, bladder
  tone
Skin: temperature, color,
  sweating
	Potential alteration in
	  bowel elimination;
	  constipation
	Potential for injury
	  secondary to vision
	  changes
	Knowledge deficit
	  regarding drug
	  therapy
	Potential alteration in
	  comfort secondary to
	  dry mouth, bladder,
	  and GI changes
	Potential alteration in
	  sexual function
	Potential alteration in
	  urinary elimination
	  patterns
		Prepare and administer
		  drug appropriately:
		  30 min before meals
		  Not in combination
		    with other oral drugs
		  After emptying
		    bladder
		Provide comfort
		  measures:
		  Dark glasses, darkened
		    room
		  Cool temperature,
		    light clothing
		  Bowel maintenance
		    program
		  Sugarless sour candies
		    to suck
		  Fluids and artificial
		    saliva with meals
		Patient teaching
		  program:
		  Drug
		  Dosage
		  Side-effects
		  Warning signs
		Provide encouragement
		  and support
		Provide for patient safety
		Provide physostigmine
		  on standby if toxicity
		  develops
			Monitor response to
			  drug:
			  Pupil dilatation
			  GI inhibition
			  Dry mouth
			Monitor for adverse
			  effects to drug:
			  Severe tachycardia
			  Confusion
			  Hallucinations
			  Chest pain
			  Congestive failure
			  Eye pain
			  Fever
			Evaluate effectiveness of
			  teaching program
			Evaluate effectiveness of
			  comfort and safety
			  measures
			Evaluate for changes in
			  response to other
			  drugs, because their
			  absorption may be
			  altered

Case study

Presentation

EK, a 64-year-old white woman with a long history of valvular rheumatic heart disease, has suffered repeated bouts of cystitis. This time her cystitis is marked by severe pain, urgency, frequency, and even nocturnal enuresis. EK is treated with an antibiotic to which the organism identified in her urine is sensitive, and with hyoscyamine (Anaspaz), 0.125 mg q 4 hours, to relieve the discomfort associated with the cystitis. She is then referred to the nurse for further teaching. What specific points should be considered with this patient?

Discussion

Before any teaching can be undertaken, it is always necessary to assess the total patient situation, diagnose that situation, and develop a teaching plan that is most appropriate to that patient. In assessing EK, it is apparent that, even though her cardiac problems are currently regulated, there is a potential for difficulties in response to the parasympathetic blocking drug. The repeated bouts of cystitis also indicate a serious problem. The patient may require further evaluation as to the cause of the recurrent infection. Because of these factors, the nurse should review for the patient the signs and symptoms of congestive heart failure, the expected side-effects of the drug and ways to deal with them, and the measures used to control bladder infections. These include avoiding citrus juices or other alkaline ash foods, avoiding bubble baths, voiding following sexual intercourse, wiping from front to back after toileting, taking the full course of prescribed antibiotics, and pushing fluids as much as permissible. The patient should be encouraged to take the Anaspaz before bed to help to alleviate the nocturnal enuresis, and to try to empty her bladder as completely as possible before taking each dose of medication. EK's age should alert the nurse to evaluate the situation for other potential problems, such as glaucoma, adverse CNS effects, safety problems with vision changes and slower reflex movements, and interactions with other drugs that she may be taking. The nurse should plan to follow up on the effectiveness of the teaching program and the drug therapy within a few days. Early evaluation of the effects of the drug, the patient's understanding of the therapy, and the problems to watch for can prevent serious complications from developing.

Drug digests

Atropine sulfate USP

Actions and indications. This belladonna alkaloid is the prototype anticholinergic drug. It produces its many peripheral effects by blocking cholinergic nerve impulse transmission to smooth muscle, cardiac muscle, and exocrine glands. It also acts centrally, presumably by blocking central synaptic transmission in cholinergic nerve pathways. Atropine is sometimes used in gastrointestinal disorders marked by smooth muscle hypertonicity and hypermotility and gastric gland hypersecretion. Thus, it is employed as an antispasmodic and antisecretory agent in the management of peptic ulcer, gastritis, and spastic colitis, among other disorders. Atropine is also used to counteract bradycardia and partial heart block that result from excessive vagal influence upon the heart. In conditions of this type, this drug increases the heart rate; it also protects against excessive cardiac slowing caused by halothane and other general anesthetics and by some surgical procedures.

Applied topically to the eye, atropine produces prolonged mydriasis and cycloplegia. These effects make atropine unsuitable for use in routine ophthalmologic examinations, but shorter acting atropinelike drugs are used this way. The central actions of atropine are useful in the management of parkinsonism and in treatment of poisoning by organophosphate-type insecticides and by similar anticholinesterase-type cholinergic drugs.

Adverse effects, cautions, and contraindications. Common side-effects of therapeutic doses include dryness of the mouth and blurring of vision. Other adverse effects are of a type that require cautious use of this drug in patients with various disorders. Thus, atropine-induced tachycardia may be undesirable for patients with coronary insufficiency and other cardiac disorders. It is constipating, and its effect of reduction of GI tract motility makes its use unsafe in patients with organic obstructions, including pyloric stenosis. Atropine is contraindicated in patients with narrow-angle glaucoma and is used only with caution in open-angle glaucoma. It is contraindicated in patients with prostatic hypertrophy, because it can cause dysuria and urinary retention.

Toxic doses can cause CNS stimulation marked by restlessness, confusion, hallucinations, and delirium.

Dosage and administration. Oral doses range from 0.3 mg to 1.2 mg; subcutaneous doses of 0.5 mg may be administered every 4 hours, except in organophosphate poisoning, in which much greater doses (*e.g.,* 2 mg to 6 mg, repeatedly) may be employed. Ophthalmic solutions ranging in strength from 0.5% to 4% are applied topically in drop dosage (*e.g.,* one or two drops bid or tid).

Dicyclomine HCl USP (Bentyl)

Actions and indications. This antispasmodic drug produces its main effects by directly relaxing gastrointestinal smooth muscle. It is used for relief of spasm in organic gastrointestinal disease, including gastritis and peptic ulcer, but it does not reduce gastric acid secretion.

Adverse effects, cautions, and contraindications. This drug does not ordinarily cause atropinelike side-effects. However, in high doses or in susceptible patients, mouth dryness and blurring of vision may occur. Thus, caution is required in patients with narrow-angle glaucoma, as well as in those with a tendency toward urinary retention, or with obstructive gastrointestinal disease such as pyloric stenosis.

Central effects such as drowsiness, euphoria, or feelings of fatigue and headache have sometimes occurred. Nausea, vomiting and, rarely, skin rashes have also been reported.

Dosage and administration. Oral doses of 10 mg to 20 mg may be taken tid or qid in tablet, capsule, or syrup form, alone or combined with phenobarbital. IM injections of 20 mg may be made every 4 to 6 hours.

Propantheline bromide USP (Pro-Banthine)

Actions and indications. This synthetic anticholinergic drug produces peripheral effects similar to those of atropine and scopolamine. It is used mainly as an antispasmodic–antisecretory agent for symptomatic relief in patients with peptic ulcer, pancreatitis, and gastritis. It reduces gastrointestinal hypermotility in functional gastrointestinal disorders, including the irritable bowel syndrome and in diverticulitis, ulcerative colitis, and others. It also relieves spasms of the ureters and urinary bladder.

Adverse effects, cautions, and contraindications. The side-effects are similar to those of atropine—mouth dryness, blurring of vision, tachycardia, and possible urinary hesitation and retention. Thus, it is used with caution in patients with coronary insufficiency and in elderly men with prostatic enlargement, and it is contraindicated in cases of narrow-angle glaucoma. It may cause impotence.

Central toxicity from overdosage is not as likely as with the natural anticholinergic alkaloids. However, the ganglionic blocking effects of this drug can cause episodes of postural hypotension. Massive overdosage may cause a curarelike neuromuscular blockade, leading to muscle weakness and paralysis.

Dosage and administration. Orally, 15 mg is administered with each meal and 30 mg at bedtime. Parenterally, 30 mg is injected IM or diluted with 10 ml of saline solution IV. Up to 60 mg may be injected for prompt action in acute pancreatitis or spasm.

Scopolamine HBr USP (l-Hyoscine HBr)

Actions and indications. This alkaloid of solanaceous plants produces peripheral effects similar to those of atropine. Thus, it is used for its cholinergic blocking effects at several of the same neuroeffector sites. Scopolamine differs from atropine in its effects on the CNS, where it causes depression in therapeutic doses. It is employed as a motion sickness preventive, a sedative–hypnotic, and in parkinsonism treatment. It has also been used for its amnesic effect in obstetrics, and it is given preoperatively to facilitate maintenance of a clear airway and to prevent excessive vagal impulses from reaching the heart.

Adverse effects, cautions, and contraindications. Scopolamine causes peripheral side-effects similar to those of atropine, including mouth dryness, blurring of vision, constipation, and tachycardia. It is used with caution in patients with prostatic hypertrophy, partial gastrointestinal tract obstructions, and angina pectoris, and its use is contraindicated in narrow-angle glaucoma. Overdosage and drug abuse have resulted in signs and symptoms of central toxicity, including excitement, confusion, delirium, and hallucinations.

Dosage and administration. Oral or subcutaneous dosage ranges between 0.3 mg and 0.8 mg (usual dose is 0.6 mg). It is also applied topically to the eyes as a 1% solution (one or two drops).

References

Adami H-O et al: Cimetidine or propantheline combined with antacid therapy for short-term treatment of duodenal ulcer. Digest Dis Sci 27:388, 1982

Effects of systemic drugs with anticholinergic properties on glaucoma. Med Lett Drugs Ther 16:28, 1974

Eger EI: Atropine, scopolamine and related compounds. Anesthesiology 23:365, 1962

Finkbeiner AD, Bissada NK: Drug therapy for lower urinary tract dysfunction. Urol Clin North Am 7:3, 1980

Friend D: Gastrointestinal anticholinergic drugs. Clin Pharmacol Ther 4:559, 1963

Greenblatt DJ, Shader RI: Anticholinergics. N Engl J Med 288:1215, 1973

Heiser JF, Gillin JC: The reversal of anticholinergic drug-induced delirium and coma with physostigmine. Am J Psychol 127:1050, 1971

Inglefinger FJ: The modification of gastrointestinal motility by drugs. N Engl J Med 229:114, 1943

Richman S: Adverse effects of atropine during myocardial infarction. JAMA 228:1414, 1974

Rodman MJ: The anhidrotic action of atropine on human thermoregulatory sweating. J Am Pharmacol Assoc (Sci Ed) 41:484, 1952

Rodman MJ: The effect of Banthine and Prantal on human thermoregulatory sweating. J Am Pharmacol Assoc (Sci Ed) 42:551, 1953

Rotman M et al: Bradyarrhythmias in acute myocardial infarction. Circulation 45:703, 1972

Rumack BH: Anticholinergic poisoning. Treatment with physostigmine. Pediatrics 52:449, 1973

Schwartz B: The glaucomas. N Engl J Med 299:182, 1978

Schweitzer P, Mark H: Effect of atropine on cardiac arrhythmias and conduction. Am Heart J 100:119 and 255, 1980

Sodeman WA Jr et al: Physiology and pharmacology of belladonna alkaloids in acid-peptic disease. Med Clin North Am 53:1379, 1969

Weiner N: Atropine, scopolamine, and related antimuscarinic drugs. In Gilman AG, Goodman LS, Gilman A (eds) Goodman and Gilman's The Pharmacological Basis of Therapeutics, 6th ed, pp 120–137. New York, Macmillan, 1980

Chapter 17

Adrenergic, or sympathomimetic, drugs

17

General considerations

Sympathomimetic drugs, as the name suggests, can mimic the effects of sympathetic nervous stimulation of organs and structures that contain α- and β-type adrenergic receptors (see Tables 13-1 and 13-2). Drugs of this class evoke their effects by occupying these receptor sites on cardiac muscle, smooth muscle, and other cells, where they then act as agonists (see Chap. 4), by acting at the endings of sympathetic postganglionic axons to cause the release of increased amounts of the neurotransmitter norepinephrine, or by a combination of these actions (Table 17-1). Thus, the effects of these drugs may be elicited either by a direct action on the sympathetically innervated organ or indirectly by the action of the neurotransmitter, and in some cases by *both* direct and indirect actions.

In actual practice, the individual adrenergic drugs differ in their ability to imitate the effects of sympathetic nervous system stimulation (Table 17-1). Knowing the types of receptors with which a drug interacts, (Table 17-1), and knowing the effects that these receptors mediate (Table 13-2), many effects of the drug can be predicted. Some drugs—for example, the synthetic catecholamine *isoproterenol*—produce responses that are the result of their affinity for β_1- and β_2-type adrenergic receptors. In this case, it can be predicted that isoproterenol, a *betamimetic* drug, will stimulate the heart and dilate the bronchioles and the blood vessels. Other drugs—for example, *phenylephrine* and *methoxamine*—have an affinity for α-adrenergic receptors and do *not* bind to β receptors. Thus, it can be predicted that these drugs will constrict the blood vessels that respond to sympathetic nerve stimulation by constricting—for example, as indicated in Table 13-2, those of the skin and mucous membranes. These *alphamimetic* drugs will *not* stimulate the heart.

Drugs of this class differ also in the degree to which they produce their effects on various organs. When administered in therapeutic doses, a specifically selected adrenergic drug may produce the desired effects on the functioning of a particular organ or structure without affecting the functioning of other sympathetically innervated organs. Unfortunately, such selectivity is limited with drugs of this class. Thus, side-effects caused by the adrenergic drug's simultaneous actions at various other adrenoceptive sites may be suffered if the patient happens to be *hypersusceptible* to that drug's actions (see Chaps. 4 and 5). In practice, this means that an attempt must be made to choose the adrenergic drug that is best suited for producing a particular effect, taking into account anything in the patient's condition that might make him excessively susceptible to the adverse effects of adrenergic drugs.

The pharmacologic actions of the drugs of this class—both the natural and synthetic catecholamines and the adrenergic drugs that are not catecholamines but that can imitate the effects of the natural transmitters (see Chap. 13 and Table 17-1)—have many important applications in clinical therapeutics. In this chapter, for the most part, the clinical applications of the various pharmacologic actions will be discussed only briefly, and you will be referred to other chapters for more detailed discussions concerning the treatment of specific disorders with adrenergic drugs, among other therapeutic agents. The most important agents of this class are discussed in detail in the Drug digests that appear in this and other chapters.

Pharmacokinetics

The sympathomimetic drugs that are catecholamines have a common fundamental chemical structure (see Chap. 13) that confers on them several properties that they share: (1) they penetrate the blood–brain barrier poorly, al-

Table 17–1. Mechanism of action of some therapeutically important sympathomimetic drugs

Drugs	Receptors activated
Direct-acting sympathomimetic drugs	
Catecholamines	
Epinephrine (adrenaline)*	α, β_1, β_2
Norepinephrine (levarterenol; noradrenaline)*	α, β_1, β_2
Dopamine*	Dopaminergic; $\alpha^\dagger, \beta_1$
Isoproterenol	β_1, β_2
Dobutamine	$\beta_1{}^\ddagger$
Noncatecholamines	
Phenylephrine	α
Methoxamine	α
Albuterol (salbutamol)	$\beta_2 > \beta_1$
Isoetharine	$\beta_2 > \beta_1$
Metaproterenol	$\beta_2 > \beta_1$
Terbutaline	$\beta_2 > \beta_1$
Indirect-acting sympathomimetic drugs§	
Amphetamine	α, β; CNS
Dextroamphetamine	α, β; CNS
Methamphetamine	α, β; CNS
Direct- and indirect-acting sympathomimetic drugs	
Ephedrine	α, β; CNS
Mephentermine	α, β
Metaraminol	α, β

* These are endogenous catecholamines as well as drugs.
† Dopamine activates α receptors only at high doses.
‡ Dobutamine produces mainly a positive inotropic effect; its positive chronotropic effects are much weaker.
§ Drugs that release norepinephrine can theoretically act at all adrenergic receptors that are innervated, including those in the central nervous system, if the drug crosses the blood–brain barrier. In practice, some of these drugs show some specificity and do not affect all receptors equally (see text).

though they cause clinically demonstrable effects (*e.g.,* anxiety, tremors, headache) that are at least partly attributable to actions in the central nervous system; (2) they are rapidly inactivated in the gastrointestinal tract and liver by the enzymes monoamine oxidase (MAO) and catechol-*o*-methyltransferase (COMT), so they are ineffective orally; (3) they have short durations of action as compared to most noncatecholamines; and (4) they are

relatively unstable, especially in solution, and decompose over time to pink, brown, and finally black products that lack the desired pharmacologic activity and should never be administered by any route. Some drugs that are non-catecholamines are also ineffective orally.

The drugs that act indirectly by liberating norepinephrine (NE) from nerve terminals may exhibit *tachyphylaxis,* a rapid form of drug tolerance (see Chap. 4), in which repeated doses of the drug over time lose their effectiveness. Sympathomimetic drugs that act wholly or in part indirectly, such as ephedrine and metaraminol, eventually deplete sympathetic nerve terminals of easily releasable NE so that subsequent doses produce less effect. Ephedrine and metaraminol exhibit tachyphylaxis. It can be demonstrated experimentally that an infusion of NE will restore the body's responsiveness to these two drugs.

Toxicity

The adverse effects of these drugs are referable almost exclusively to unwanted effects mediated by α-, β_1-, or β_2-adrenergic receptors, or by receptors in the central nervous system. The adverse effects of an individual sympathomimetic drug depend on the receptors that it activates (Table 17-1), whether it penetrates the blood–brain barrier, and to some extent on the intended therapeutic effect. Thus, for example, when ephedrine interferes with an asthmatic patient's sleep, it is considered to have produced an adverse effect, but when this same drug prevents a narcoleptic patient from falling asleep at an inappropriate time during the day, it is considered to have produced the desired therapeutic effect.

Epinephrine in many respects is the "complete sympathomimetic" drug, the prototype of the group. It acts on α, β_1, and β_2 receptors, but it has no therapeutically useful CNS effects. It can produce essentially all the effects on organs that are caused by impulses in adrenergic sympathetic postganglionic nerves (see Table 13-2): increased rate and force of contraction of the heart; cardiac arrhythmias; constriction of some blood vessels, or dilatation of others (at low doses); relaxation of the gastrointestinal tract, urinary bladder, and bronchial smooth muscle; contraction of gastrointestinal and urinary bladder sphincters; dilation of the pupil of the eye; increased blood sugar; and relaxation of the pregnant uterus. Some of these are therapeutically useful effects of epinephrine and other sympathomimetics for some patients, and some are unwanted side-effects (see below).

Pharmacology and clinical applications of adrenergic drugs

The catecholamines and other sympathomimetic amines are employed mainly for their effects on the heart, blood vessels, bronchi, and ocular smooth muscles. Some are also employed for their CNS effects, and one is employed for its effect on the pregnant uterus, a relatively new use of sympathomimetic drugs. Table 17-2 indicates the types and locations of receptors that mediate the most important therapeutically useful effects of these drugs. Some of their actions on these organs and structures are excitatory and others are inhibitory. Thus, for example, the primary action of adrenergic drugs on the heart is to stimulate increased activity. On the other hand, the smooth muscle walls of the bronchial tubes are relaxed by adrenergic drugs, and the bronchioles become dilated. The blood vessels in some vascular beds—those in which α-adrenergic receptors predominate, such as those of the skin and mucous membranes—constrict as a result of the increased contractile response of their smooth muscle walls when adrenergic drugs that are α agonists come in contact with them locally or by way of the systemic circulation. On the other hand, other blood vessels, such as those in skeletal muscles, tend to dilate when the natural tone of their smooth muscles is inhibited by adrenergic drugs with β_2-receptor-type activity.

Cardiac effects

Pharmacologic actions

The main actions of such potent catecholamines as *epinephrine*[+] (Adrenalin) and *isoproterenol*[+] (Isuprel) on the heart are similar to those of sympathetic nerve stimulation (see Chap. 13). However, in addition to their *direct* effects, these and other adrenergic drugs can also produce opposing *reflex* effects that are the result of the body's reactions to their direct effects. In addition, overdoses can sometimes set off changes in cardiac rhythm that do not occur physiologically but are the result of a pathologic response of cardiac ectopic pacemaker tissues.

The therapeutic usefulness of adrenergic drugs on the heart stems from the following primary pharmacologic effects of these drugs on cardiac β_1-type adrenergic receptors:

1. An increase in myocardial contractility, a *positive inotropic effect*
2. An increase in the heart rate, a *positive chronotropic effect*

Table 17–2. Receptors mediating clinically useful effects of sympathomimetic drugs*

Effector	Receptor type	Response or effect
Heart		
S-A node	β_1	Increased heart rate
A-V node	β_1	Increased rate of conduction of cardiac impulse; heart block overcome
Ventricular muscle	β_1	Increased force of contraction
Blood vessels		
Skin, mucosa, skeletal muscle, mesenteric and splanchnic beds	α	Vasoconstriction; increased blood pressure; hemostasis
Skeletal muscle	β_2	Vasodilation ⎫ These receptors are
Renal, mesenteric, and splanchnic arteriolar beds	Dopaminergic	Vasodilation ⎬ not innervated but are activated by ⎭ drugs
Bronchiolar smooth muscle	β_2	Relaxation; bronchodilation
Eye		
Radial muscle of iris	α	Contraction; mydriasis
Vasculature	α	Vasoconstriction; decreased production of aqueous humor
Uterus in pregnancy	β_2	Relaxation; prevention of premature labor

* CNS effects are not included in this table.

3. An increase in the velocity with which impulses are conducted from the atria through the A-V node and other specialized conducting tissues, a *positive dromotropic effect*

These combined actions of adrenergic drugs on the heart usually result in an increase in cardiac output, which—together with the vasoconstrictor effect on blood vessels (discussed below)—leads to a rise in arterial blood pressure. Sometimes, if the blood pressure rises rapidly and steeply, it sets off reflex activity, mediated by *baroreceptors* in the carotid sinus and aortic arch, that acts in turn to produce yet another potentially useful cardiac effect—a *slowing* down of the heart rate. Such a *reflex bradycardia*, or negative chronotropic effect, is most likely to occur with those adrenergic drugs that have little or no direct action on cardiac β_1 receptors but that, instead, act as potent agonists when they combine with α-adrenergic receptors in vascular smooth muscle—for example, *phenylephrine* and *methoxamine*, the alphamimetic agents mentioned above.

Ordinarily, the heart muscle itself is the first organ to benefit from the increase in cardiac output brought about by the effects of β_1 agonists. The coronary arterioles, which branch off from the aorta into the myocardium, receive a better flow of oxygenated blood to carry to the myocardium when adrenergic drugs are increasing the speed and strength with which the left ventricle contracts. Sometimes, however, if the myocardium is made to work too hard, the patient's disease-narrowed coronary arteries may not be able to carry enough blood to keep up with the heart muscle's greatly increased demands for oxygen (see Chap. 31). When the heart muscle becomes hypoxic, it is particularly sensitive to yet another cardiac action of catecholamines and other β_1-agonist adrenergic drugs. This is their increased tendency to stimulate spontaneous depolarizations in latent pacemaker tissues. This drug-induced increase in automaticity (Chaps. 26 and 30) at sites other than that of the normal cardiac pacemaker can sometimes cause dangerous cardiac arrhythmias, and can even cause cardiac arrest as a result of ventricular fibrillation.

Clinical uses

The administration of certain adrenergic drugs is indicated mainly for treating those cardiac conditions that are marked by an excessively slow heartbeat or even by sudden stoppage of rhythmic contractions (cardiac arrest). These conditions include the Stokes–Adams syndrome, the carotid sinus syndrome, A-V block and bradycardia in digitalis intoxication or following an acute myocardial infarction (AMI), and in cardiac arrest. Some adrenergic drugs produce reflex bradycardia (see above) and are useful for slowing an excessively rapid ventricular rate.

Stokes–Adams syndrome (Chap. 30) is best managed today by implantation of a permanent electrical pacemaker to keep the cardiac rhythm stable. However, adrenergic drugs are useful adjuncts while the patient is being prepared for insertion of such a pacemaker. *Isoproterenol* (Isuprel) administered intravenously is the most effective adrenergic drug for treating the attacks of asystole that occur periodically in this condition, particularly when a patient with partial heart block goes suddenly into complete A-V block.

Administered during such an attack, isoproterenol acts to overcome the patient's cerebral symptoms (which include syncope–fainting) by stimulating the heart to pump more blood to the brain. It does so by bringing about the three main effects of sympathomimetic amines listed above but, because overdosage can cause a dangerous increase in cardiac irritability, the IV drip of this potent drug must be carefully regulated. To avoid producing a heart rate that is too rapid, the infusion rate is slowed down when the patient's pulse has returned to about 60 beats per minute; if the pulse rises to much higher levels, or if frequent premature ventricular contractions (PVCs; Chap. 30) appear on the electrocardiogram, isoproterenol must be discontinued. Isoproterenol has also been associated with a "cardiac steal" syndrome, in which it actually reduces the oxygen available for use by the injured myocardium. Because of this, isoproterenol is used very cautiously in patients who have suffered a myocardial infarction and who have a precarious blood supply to the heart muscle.

A sublingual dosage form of isoproterenol is available for routine use several times daily for preventing Stokes–Adams attacks. This rapidly disintegrating tablet may also be placed under the tongue for rapid action if the patient complains of feeling faint or light-headed. (The patient is told not to swallow any saliva until the drug is absorbed.) This can help to prevent the falls and physical injuries that can occur when patients with this cardiac condition "black out" as the result of a syncopal attack.

Other adrenergic drugs occasionally ordered for oral administration in this condition include *ephedrine*[+] and *hydroxyamphetamine*. However, these drugs may stimulate the central nervous system and cause nervousness and insomnia, and ephedrine may interfere with micturition in elderly male patients with hyperprostatism. Thus, to avoid such side-effects of daily therapy with adrenergic drugs, the more effective electrical pacemakers are the preferred treatment of this condition.

Supraventricular tachycardias are also best managed by physical measures or by digitalization to protect the ventricles from being driven too rapidly and irregularly by impulses arising in the atria and A-V junctional tissues (Chaps. 29 and 30). However, two adrenergic drugs, *phenylephrine*[+] (Neo-Synephrine) and *methoxamine*[+] (Vasoxyl) are sometimes used for this purpose in paroxysmal atrial tachycardia (PAT). These drugs, as indicated above, act mainly at the α-type adrenergic receptors in blood vessels and have no *direct* effect on the heart itself, which contains mainly β receptors. However, when injected intravenously at a slow rate during an attack, these sympathomimetic agents sometimes rapidly restore normal sinus rhythm. They do so by their ability to constrict blood vessels in the systemic circulation, thus raising the peripheral resistance and blood pressure. This in turn produces a reflex bradycardia, because the rise in blood pressure stimulates the baroreceptors, which in turn signal the brain's cardioinhibitory center to stimulate the vagus nerves, which slow the heart.

Patients who show signs of severe bradycardia or of heart block following an AMI are sometimes treated with *isoproterenol* if atropine fails to increase the heart rate and a temporary transvenous pacemaker has not yet been inserted. This is potentially a very dangerous drug to give an AMI patient, and special precautions are necessary. Cardiac arrest that does not respond to electrical defibrillation or to synchronous electrical shocks is also sometimes managed by parenteral administration of potent catecholamines. The adrenergic drugs most commonly employed in this acute emergency (Chap. 31) are *isoproterenol* (Isuprel) and *epinephrine* (Adrenalin). These drugs are given by intracardiac injection, because in cardiac arrest there is no blood flow to carry the drug from an injection site to the heart. Isoproterenol is preferred for intracardiac administration because it is as useful as epinephrine for restarting a heart that is in standstill (asystole), and even more effective than epinephrine when the heart's failure to pump blood into the arteries is the result of ventricular fibrillation. However, epinephrine sometimes helps to make the fibrillating heart more responsive to electric shock.

Both these sympathomimetic amines are more effective when administered following infusion of sodium bicarbonate solution, a systemic alkalinizer that counteracts the metabolic acidosis caused by the buildup of lactic acid in the heart and in other tissues during periods of hypoxia.

Precautions

As previously indicated, the most dangerous effect of β_1-adrenergic agonist drugs is their tendency to cause rapid cardiac arrhythmias in some circumstances. This is particularly true in patients with coronary heart disease, in whom these drugs can cause myocardial hypoxia by driving the heart beyond the capacity of its coronary arterioles to deliver oxygen. Ventricular premature beats, tachycardia, and fibrillation can also develop when adrenergic drugs are administered to patients under anesthesia with halothane or cyclopropane (Chap. 52).

Sympathomimetic drugs should thus be used with caution, if at all, in patients with angina pectoris. Patients with hyperthyroidism are also hypersusceptible to the cardiac stimulant effects of adrenergic drugs. Patients

with these conditions are particularly likely to complain of cardiac palpitations, pounding heart, and chest pains if they use adrenergic drugs as nasal decongestants (see below), as appetite suppressants (Chap. 47), or for the management of asthma (see below) or other disorders unrelated to their heart ailment.

Vascular effects

Adrenergic drugs that are α-receptor agonists act to constrict arterioles and venules, but other adrenergic drugs act on β_2 receptors in the blood vessels of skeletal muscles to produce local vasodilation (Table 13-2). The vasoconstrictor effects of adrenergic drugs that act on α receptors of blood vessels of the skin and mucous membranes have clinical applications in stopping bleeding and bringing about nasal and ocular decongestion. These and other uses of local vasoconstriction are discussed in this section. The clinical applications of those adrenergic drugs that act on β_2 receptors to dilate the blood vessels of skeletal muscles—for example, nylidrin (Arlidin) and isoxsuprine (Vasodilan)—are discussed in Chapter 33.

Local vasoconstriction

Adrenergic drugs are often applied topically or injected subcutaneously to produce constriction of blood vessels at several local sites. Sometimes, for example, *epinephrine, phenylephrine,* or other sympathomimetic amines are added to solutions of local anesthetics to reduce the rate at which these drugs are absorbed into the systemic circulation. Vasoconstriction serves two purposes here: it prolongs the local pain-preventing effect of the anesthetic; and it prevents the anesthetic from being absorbed too rapidly and causing possible toxic effects on the heart and brain (see Chap. 14).

Epinephrine solution 1:1000 is often applied topically to stop nosebleed or to stem bleeding after a tonsillectomy. The same solution, injected subcutaneously in acute allergic emergencies (Chap. 39), owes some of its effectiveness to its ability to constrict vessels in the skin and mucous membranes. This helps to halt development of urticarial wheals and angioneurotic edema that result from the immune system's reaction to the allergen.

An adrenergic drug that constricts ocular vessels when applied topically is *tetrahydrozoline* (Visine), which is promoted to the public for relief of minor eye irritation. It should *not* be used for treating glaucoma, and patients in whom it does not "get the red out" within 1 or 2 days should be advised to consult an eye-care specialist.

Tetrahydrozoline—under another trade name, Tyzine—is one of a group of adrenergic drugs (Table 17-3) that are employed as nasal decongestants because of their local vasoconstrictor action. These drugs, including phenylephrine, are either applied topically—as nose drops or inhalants, for example—or administered by mouth and absorbed systemically so that they reach the mucous membranes of the nasal passages and sinuses

Table 17–3. Adrenergic nasal decongestant drugs

Generic or official name	Trade name	Dosage form
l-Desoxyephedrine	Vicks Inhaler	Inhaler
Ephedrine USP	Various	Nose drops, nasal jelly
Epinephrine HCl USP	Adrenalin Chloride	Nose drops
Naphazoline HCl USP	Privine HCl	Nose drops, nasal spray
Oxymetazoline HCl USP*	Afrin	Nose drops, nasal spray
Phenylephrine HCl USP	Neo-Synephrine	Nose drops, nasal spray, nasal jelly
Phenylpropanolamine HCl USP	Propadrine HCl	Oral tablets, capsules, elixirs
Propylhexedrine USP	Benzedrex	Inhaler
Pseudoephedrine HCl	Various	Oral tablets, capsules, liquid
Pseudoephedrine sulfate	Afrinol Repetabs	Oral tablets
Tetrahydrozoline HCl USP	Tyzine	Nose drops
Xylometazoline HCl USP	Otrivin	Nose drops, nasal spray

* See Drug digest, Chapter 39.

by way of the bloodstream. In either case, adrenergic drugs such as *oxymetazoline*[+] (Afrin; see Drug digest, Chap. 39) constrict the dilated arterioles and capillaries of the mucous membranes covering the nasal turbinates and paranasal sinuses. This vasoconstriction leads to a shrinking of swollen membranes, tends to open clogged nasal passages, and promotes drainage through the ostia of the sinuses. The common cold sufferer usually gets at least temporary relief from the discomfort of a blocked nose. The use of these decongestant drugs for the symptomatic relief of nasal obstruction in patients with seasonal allergic rhinitis (hay fever) as well as in colds is discussed in Chapter 39.

As indicated in that chapter, the overuse of topically applied nasal decongestants such as naphazoline (Privine) and others can cause an undesirable secondary, or rebound, congestion and a chronic congestive condition called rhinitis medicamentosa. Systemic absorption of drugs such as ephedrine, which is also used as a nasal decongestant, can cause nervousness, heart palpitations, and other side effects of sympathomimetic drugs. To avoid letting the drops trickle down the throat, the patient should be instructed to keep the head tilted back when applying adrenergic vasoconstrictor–decongestant drug nose drops. The orally administered drugs sometimes also cause stimulation of the central nervous system. They can occasionally also cause adverse cardiovascular effects, particularly in patients with heart disease or high blood pressure, and in emotionally depressed patients taking monoamine oxidase (MAO) inhibitor-type antidepressant

drugs (Chap. 46). Many sympathomimetic drugs that are used as nasal and ocular decongestants are available to patients without a prescription as over-the-counter (OTC) drugs. It is important to learn about their use when taking a drug history.

Systemic vascular effects

Adrenergic drugs that are administered parenterally in adequate doses have generalized effects on the blood vessels of vascular beds, including the splanchnic arterioles of the abdominal viscera. Drug-induced changes in the caliber of these vessels play an important part in bringing about changes in systemic arterial blood pressure. Most adrenergic drugs, including the catecholamines *norepinephrine* or *levarterenol*[+] (Levophed) and *epinephrine*, tend to produce vasoconstriction by their effects in blood vessels in which α-adrenergic receptors predominate. *Dopamine* (Intropin) in high doses also constricts these blood vessels by acting on α receptors, but in low doses acts on dopamine receptors in certain blood vessels to cause vasodilatation (see the management of circulatory shock, below).

Norepinephrine, epinephrine, and such other sympathomimetic amines as *ephedrine, phenylephrine,* and *metaraminol*[+] (Aramine) are called *vasopressors* because they raise the blood pressure. The use of these vasoconstrictors and of the potent vasodilator–heart stimulant *isoproterenol,* as well as other adrenergic drugs in the management of acute hypotension and various types of circulatory shock, is discussed in detail in the final section of this chapter.

360

Table 17–4. Adrenergic bronchodilator drugs

Generic or official name	Trade name	Usual adult dosage
Albuterol (salbutamol)	Proventil; Ventolin	2–4 mg orally or two aerosol inhalations
Ephedrine sulfate USP		25–50 mg orally, IM, SC or IV
Epinephrine bitartrate USP	Medihaler-Epi	0.3 mg/inhalation
Epinephrine HCl USP	Adrenalin Chloride	0.2–0.5 mg IM, SC, or by inhalation
Ethylnorepinephrine HCl USP	Bronkephrine	0.6–2.0 mg SC
Isoetharine HCl or mesylate	Bronkosol; Bronkometer	Dosage varies with aerosol form and severity of attack
Isoproterenol HCl or sulfate USP	Isuprel; Norisodrine	10–15 mg sublingually; inhalation dosage varies with aerosol form and severity of attack
Metaproterenol sulfate	Alupent; Metaprel	0.65 mg/inhalation (two to three inhalations), or 20 mg orally
Terbutaline sulfate USP	Brethine; Bricanyl	5 mg orally, or 0.25 mg SC

Bronchial effects

Certain sympathetic amines (Table 17-4) combine with β_2-type receptors in bronchial smooth muscle cells. This sets into motion a series of biochemical events that causes these muscles to relax and results in bronchodilation. This action can be clinically useful for overcoming bronchospasm in patients suffering from bronchial asthma and such other chronic obstructive lung diseases as bronchitis and emphysema.

Mechanism

As indicated in Chapter 13, the interaction of catecholamines such as epinephrine and isoproterenol with β_2 receptors is thought to activate the smooth muscle membrane enzyme adenylate cyclase. The enzyme then acts to increase the intracellular production of the nucleotide cyclic adenosine 3',5'-monophosphate (cAMP), a so-called "second messenger" in chemical transmission at synapses and junctions. A rise in the concentration of this biochemical in bronchial smooth muscle cells leads to a reduction in their tone, or degree of tension. If bronchospasm is present, this action of these catecholamines and other sympathomimetic amines reduces the smooth muscle spasm and leads to dilation, or widening, of the bronchial tubes.

One theory concerning the hypersusceptibility of some persons with asthma to episodes of bronchospasm is that their bronchial cells contain relatively low levels of cAMP compared to the intracellular level of another nucleotide, cyclic guanosine 3',5'-monophosphate (cGMP, Chap. 13). This imbalance is thought to be caused by a partial blockade of the β_2 receptors in bronchial smooth muscle cells, which reduces their capacity to react in ways that maintain normal levels of cAMP. This is said to make them more sensitive to irritants that cause bronchospasm. Administration of adrenergic drugs helps to bring the balance between cAMP and cGMP back to normal, and thus prevents the bronchioles from becoming constricted.*

Selectivity

One drawback of isoproterenol, ephedrine, and other traditional adrenergic bronchodilator drugs is that their effects are not limited to β_2-type receptors in bronchial smooth muscle (Table 17-1). Isoproterenol, for example, also acts as a potent agonist at β_1-type (cardiac) receptors. This can cause cardiac arrhythmias that may be particularly dangerous for patients who are hypoxic, and deaths have in fact occurred from the misuse of pressurized aerosol preparations containing high concentrations of isoproterenol.

Several newer adrenergic drugs have been introduced that have a somewhat greater affinity for β_2-

---

* The intracellular concentration of cGMP in bronchial smooth muscle cells is claimed to be increased by stimulation of the vagus nerves, which release acetylcholine (Chap. 13). Such parasympathetic predominance over sympathetic influences is thought to account for the bronchoconstriction produced by vagal stimulation and by cholinergic drugs (Chap. 15). This bronchospastic effect is blocked by atropine and by other anticholinergic drugs (Chap. 16), which cause contracted bronchial smooth muscle to relax.

type receptors than for β_1-type receptors. Thus, such newer agents as *albuterol, isoetharine, metaproterenol,* and *terbutaline* may be preferred for treating asthmatic patients who also suffer from coronary heart disease, or who have proved prone to develop cardiac arrhythmias when they received the older adrenergic bronchodilator drugs.

Clinical applications

Drugs of this class are available in several different dosage forms for use in the management of bronchial asthma and other obstructive lung disorders. They are administered by aerosol, by mouth, and by subcutaneous injection. The relative efficacy of the various adrenergic bronchodilator drugs and their drawbacks are discussed in detail in Chapter 40, in which the clinical use of the different dosage forms in the long-term management of chronic obstructive lung diseases and in the treatment of acute episodes is taken up. Details concerning the emergency administration of epinephrine for its bronchodilator (and vasoconstrictor) effects in the treatment of anaphylactic reactions are discussed in Chapter 39.

Ocular effects

The main effect of adrenergic drugs on the eye—other than the vasoconstrictive effect on ocular vessels mentioned earlier—is *mydriasis* (dilation of the pupil). This is brought about by topically applied drugs that stimulate α-adrenergic receptors in the radial muscle of the iris. This causes that muscle to contract in a direction that makes the pupillary aperture widen.

The mydriatic action of sympathomimetic drug solutions is useful for diagnostic purposes when the ophthalmologist wants to examine internal structures within the patient's eyes. Application of a strong (10%) solution of phenylephrine, for example, widens the pupil in a way that allows the physician to see the internal structures of the eye more readily and thus facilitates ophthalmoscopic examination of the eyegrounds. Unlike atropine and other anticholinergic drugs (Chap. 16), the adrenergic drugs do *not* ordinarily cause cycloplegia (paralysis of accommodation). Thus, they are *not* used alone to prepare the eye for refraction, although they are occasionally combined with cycloplegic drugs of the anticholinergic class such as atropine and homatropine for this diagnostic purpose. On the other hand, the lack of a cycloplegic effect can be desirable because blurring of the patient's vision does not occur. Thus, when only mydriasis is desired, such adrenergic drugs as *hydroxyamphetamine, phenylephrine,* and *ephedrine* are preferred to the anticholinergic mydriatic–cycloplegics for topical ocular application. (See Chapter 42 for a further discussion of the diagnostic and therapeutic uses of adrenergic drugs in ophthalmology.)

Epinephrine, phenylephrine, and some other sympathomimetic drugs that are α-receptor agonists are sometimes used in the management of cases of open-angle glaucoma. These drugs cause mydriasis, as indicated above, so this use may seem paradoxical. Parasympathetic blocking drugs such as atropine, that also cause mydriasis, are contraindicated for patients with glaucoma (Chap. 16). Epinephrine and the other sympathomimetic drugs used to treat open-angle glaucoma probably act to reduce intraocular pressure by interfering with the secretion of aqueous humor. However, these drugs are contraindicated in narrow (closed)-angle glaucoma because the mydriatic effect of adrenergic drugs may make the iris muscle crowd back into the angle, thus blocking fluid outflow. The resulting rise in intraocular pressure could set off an attack of acute glaucoma in such patients.

Effects on other organs

Various adrenergic drugs exert sympathomimetic effects on the smooth muscles of the gastrointestinal and genitourinary tracts that, in theory, have potential clinical usefulness. In practice, the doses required to influence the functioning of such organs as the stomach, uterus, and bladder tend to cause cardiovascular and central nervous system side-effects. Thus, the desired therapeutic effects can ordinarily be obtained more effectively and with less risk by employing drugs of other classes.

Ephedrine and other orally administered adrenergic drugs are sometimes employed to contract the trigone and sphincter of the *urinary bladder* (α-receptor effects) while reducing the tone of the detrusor muscle of that organ (β_2-receptor effect; see Table 13-2). As is the case with atropine and other belladonna alkaloids (Chap. 16), which produce the same effects by their blocking actions at cholinergic receptors rather than by stimulating adrenergic receptors, such drug-induced effects may have some clinical usefulness in the treatment of nocturnal enuresis and incontinence. However, the central stimulating effect of ephedrine can disturb the sleep of enuretic children when the drug is used to increase the capacity of the bladder and to prevent or delay micturition. At present, *imipramine* (Chap. 46) is preferred to ephedrine and other autonomic drugs for this purpose.

Uterine muscle responses to adrenergic drugs vary considerably. Small doses of epinephrine injected subcutaneously are said to relax spasms of the uterus during labor. However, the drug is rarely used clinically for this purpose in obstetrics, although its presence in solutions of local anesthetic drugs employed to relieve labor pains sometimes interferes with uterine contractions. Recently, the β_2-adrenergic agonist *ritodrine* (Yutopar) has been approved for use as a uterine relaxant in patients in premature labor. Ritodrine has some selectivity for β_2 receptors, but it also can interact with cardiac β_1 receptors. It has produced changes in cardiac function in both the mother and fetus. Furthermore, when it has been given with corticosteroids, pregnant mothers have developed pulmonary edema.

Gastrointestinal smooth muscle in spasm is occasionally relaxed by epinephrine and ephedrine, as would be predicted from the effects of sympathetic nervous system stimulation on the gastrointestinal tract (Chap. 13). However, the slight inhibitory action on the gastrointestinal tract elicited by safe doses of these adrenergic drugs is of little clinical usefulness as compared to the gastrointestinal antispasmodic action of drugs that act directly or by blocking parasympathetic motor activity (*e.g.,* atropine, propantheline, dicyclomine; Chaps. 16 and 41).

Central nervous system effects

Ephedrine, amphetamine, and some other sympathomimetic drugs cross the blood–brain barrier and produce therapeutically useful effects in the central nervous system (Table 17-1). As indicated above, ephedrine can interfere with sleep, an unwanted side-effect when this drug is used to treat enuresis and asthma. However, this is a therapeutically useful effect of ephedrine for patients suffering from narcolepsy, who fall asleep inappropriately in the middle of daytime activities. Amphetamine can be used to offset the sedation produced by some antiepileptic drugs. Other therapeutic uses of the central nervous system effects of dextroamphetamine and some related drugs include the following: the treatment of children with hyperkinetic syndromes (an apparently paradoxical use of drugs that are CNS stimulants); the suppression of appetite in obese patients; and the treatment of patients with Parkinson's disease who cannot tolerate newer and more effective drugs. (See Section 8, Drugs Acting on the Central Nervous System, for a more detailed description of the therapeutic uses of sympathomimetic drugs with CNS effects.)

Additional clinical considerations

The adrenergic drugs produce a wide range of systemic effects that are normally seen with stimulation of the sympathetic nervous system. Ordinarily, these effects are balanced with reflex controls involving the parasympathetic nervous system. When adrenergic drugs are given, they may overwhelm these reflex controls. Thus, patients receiving adrenergic drugs may experience many side-effects that can be predicted by reviewing the organ system effects of stimulation of the sympathetic system (see Table 13-2). To benefit from one particular desired effect—for example, bronchodilation—the patient may have to cope with a series of undesired effects (*e.g.,* tachycardia, urinary retention, flushing, sweating). Patient teaching is thus a vital part of this drug therapy, because the patient needs to know what to anticipate and how to deal with it. Patient assessment is also very important, because many underlying medical conditions can be adversely affected by uncontrolled sympathetic stimulation. Cardiac disease, diabetes mellitus, hypertension, seizure disorders, and narrow-angle glaucoma are examples of such conditions. As with many other drugs, the use of these drugs in pregnancy and lactation is not recommended.

Technical considerations

As mentioned previously, these drugs are unstable over time. Before any adrenergic drug is administered the solution should be checked to make sure that it is clear and not pink, brown, or black. It is important to remember this when checking drugs on emergency carts.

When given IV, adrenergic drugs must be administered very carefully. The IV site needs to be evaluated regularly for any evidence of infiltration, and an emergency bottle of phentolamine (see Chap. 18) should be readily available. Extra caution also needs to be taken to secure the site when moving the patient.

Sublingual administration needs to be done with precise instruction to the patient not to swallow until the tablet has totally dissolved or else the patient will not receive the prescribed dose. If the drug is to be administered through an inhaler, the manufacturer's directions should be followed because proper use of each type of inhaler is slightly different. To prevent alarm, patients using isoproterenol through an inhaler should be cautioned that their saliva will turn pink.

Patient comfort and safety

Patients who receive these drugs in acute situations require constant monitoring to evaluate not only the therapeutic effectiveness of the drug but also the occurrence of any undesired effects. IVs often need to be titrated very specifically to obtain the desired results. Because these drugs are very powerful, only a few milliliters of fluid can mean the difference between the desired effect and a toxic reaction. Patients receiving these drugs are often very sick, and it is important to remember that they and their families are still entitled to know about the drug therapy the patient is receiving. They will also need constant support and encouragement throughout the acute period. As with all acute situations, emergency life support equipment should be readily available.

Patients who are receiving adrenergic drugs need assurance that the effects that they are experiencing are a result of the drug's activity. Ambulatory patients who experience restlessness, "nervousness," insomnia or "jitters" as a result of taking these drugs should be advised to avoid operating dangerous machinery, driving cars, or attempting to perform delicate tasks. They can also be advised to avoid caffeine, nicotine, or other stimulants that can further increase these effects. Men with prostatic hypertrophy should be advised to void before taking a dose of the medication so that the bladder will be empty when the drug's effects are maximum, and to report any problems with urinary retention. It may be necessary to monitor the urinary output of these patients if the urinary retention becomes a problem. Some patients will experience a photophobia (eye discomfort in bright light), which can be helped by sunglasses and by avoiding extremes of light. Patients who experience flushing and sweating should be advised to avoid warm temperatures and heavy clothing. If any of the undesired effects becomes intolerable, the dosage should be evaluated and reduced, if possible.

Drug–drug interactions with adrenergic drugs

Several drugs are known to cause potentially dangerous drug–drug interactions with the adrenergic drugs. *MAO inhibitors* and *tricyclic antidepressants* will increase the pressor effect of adrenergic drugs, leading to a greater increase in blood pressure than expected. If a patient is on one of these drugs and an adrenergic drug is needed, the dosage of the adrenergic drug should be small. *Oxytocic drugs* used in obstetrics should not be given concurrently with adrenergic drugs because severe persistent hypertension and even cerebrovascular accidents (CVAs) have been reported. *Cyclopropane* and *halogenated hydrocarbon anesthetics* can increase myocardial irritability and serious cardiac arrhythmias may result if sympathomimetics are given. *Insulin* requirements often increase with diabetic patients receiving dobutamine, secondary to the glycolytic effect of dobutamine. *Diuretics* may produce an increased diuresis if used in combination with dopamine, which dilates the renal arteries and causes an increase in renal blood flow. *Phenytoin* and dopamine in combination have caused seizures; this effect is more likely to be seen in patients with a history of seizures. *Guanethidine's* effects (Chap. 18) are decreased by epinephrine, and the patient will not experience the desired antihypertensive effect. An increase in guanethidine dose may be required. *Propranolol's* blood pressure-lowering effect (Chap. 18) is often lost if the drug is given concurrently with epinephrine; hypertension can result. The effects of epinephrine are enhanced by several drugs, including various antihistamines and sodium L-thyroxine.

The concurrent use of two or more sympathomimetic drugs increases the incidence of serious adverse effects. The intentional combination of two such drugs should be done only with careful patient monitoring. Many patients who use OTC preparations unknowingly take several similar adrenergic drugs. Adrenergic drugs are ingredients in countless OTC preparations—for example, diet pills, cold pills, antihistamine combinations, and nasal sprays. Patients should be warned to avoid the use of any OTC drug until they have consulted their nurse or physician. This is particularly important in patients who have an underlying medical condition that could be exacerbated by this sympathetic stimulation.

The patient teaching guide for adrenergic drugs presents a summary of important points to include in patient teaching. The guide to the nursing process summarizes important clinical points for application of the nursing process to adrenergic drug therapy. A discussion of the use of adrenergic drugs in shock states will follow as an example of the clinical use of these complex drugs.

Patient teaching guide: adrenergic drugs

The drug that has been prescribed for you is called an adrenergic drug. The drug acts by mimicking the effects of the sympathetic nervous system. Because this drug causes many effects in the body, you may experience some undesired side-effects. It is very important to discuss the effects of the drug with your nurse or physician and to try to make them as tolerable as possible. This drug has been ordered for

_____ .

Instructions:

1. The name of your drug is _____ .

2. The dosage of your drug is _____ .

3. Your drug should be taken _____ times a day. The best time to take your drug is _____ , _____ , _____ .

4. If your drug is in solution, you should check the solution before use. If the solution is pink, brown or black it should be discarded.
    * Men with prostate problems should void before taking the medication.

(continued)

- If the drug is to be taken sublingually, you must be careful to avoid swallowing the tablet; do not swallow until the tablet has completely dissolved.
- If the drug is to be taken with an inhaler, check the instructions that come with the inhaler before use. Each inhaler is slightly different and you should read the instructions for its use to ensure that the proper amount of drug is delivered.

5. Some side-effects of the drug that you should be aware of include the following:

Restlessness, shaking, sleeplessness	If these occur, you should be very careful when performing delicate tasks, driving, or operating heavy machinery.
Flushing, sweating	If these occur, avoid warm temperatures and heavy clothing; frequent washing with cool water may also help.
Heart palpitations	If you feel that your heart is beating too fast or skipping beats, sit down and rest for a while; if it becomes too uncomfortable, check with your nurse or physician.
Sensitivity of eyes to light	Avoid glaring light; use sunglasses; be careful if moving between extremes of light.
Saliva turns pink	This is the effect of inhaled Isuprel and is not blood. Do not be concerned.

6. Notify any physician, nurse, or dentist who is taking care of you that you are taking this drug.

7. Keep this and all medications out of the reach of children.

8. Do not use any over-the-counter medications—for example cold capsules or diet pills—while you are taking this medication. If you feel that you need some of these medications, call your nurse or physician.

Notify your nurse or physician if any of the following occur:

Difficulty voiding
Chest pain
Difficulty breathing
Dizziness
Headache
Changes in vision

Guide to the nursing process: adrenergic drugs

Assessment	Nursing diagnoses	Interventions	Evaluation
Past history—underlying clinical condition (*contraindications*): • Cardiac arrhythmias • Coronary artery disease • Idiopathic hypertrophic subaortic stenosis (IHSS) • Pheochromocytoma • Hypertension • Narrow-angle glaucoma • Urinary retention–prostatic hypertrophy • Seizures • Pregnancy • Lactation *Allergies:* these drugs, others; reaction Medication history (*cautions*): MAO inhibitors Tricyclic antidepressants Oxytocic drugs Propranolol Guanethidine Phenytoin Cycloprane Halogenated hydrocarbon anesthetics OTC drugs **Physical assessment** Neurologic: mental status, orientation, reflexes, muscular strength Cardiovascular: BP, P. baseline EKG, auscultation, perfusion Respiratory: rate, adventitious sounds Excretory: bladder tone, output GI: tone, output Skin: perfusion	Potential alteration in cardiac output Potential sensory-perceptual alteration Potential alteration in tissue perfusion Potential alteration in urinary elimination patterns Knowledge deficit regarding drug therapy	Safe and appropriate preparation and administration of drug Provision of comfort measures Provision of safety measures: • IV site • Seizure precautions • Orientation Support and encouragement to deal with effects of drug and to comply with therapy Patient teaching measures Life support measures, as appropriate	Evaluate for effectiveness of desired drug effect Evaluate for side-effects of drug: Cardiovascular CNS Respiratory GI Renal Evaluate effectiveness of safety measures Evaluate effectiveness of support and encouragement measures Evaluate patient teaching measures Evaluate effectiveness of life support measures, as appropriate Evaluate for drug–drug interactions: ↑ BP with: *MAO inhibitors, oxytocic drugs, propranolol, trycyclic antidepressants, antihistamines* ↑ Cardiac irritability with: *cycloprane* or *halogenated hydrocarbon anesthetics.* Seizures with *phenytoin*

Case Study

Presentation

JD, a 26-year-old man, recently moved to the northeastern United States from New Mexico. He has been suffering from sinusitis, runny nose, and coldlike symptoms for 2 weeks. He appears at an outpatient clinic with complaints of headache, "jitters," inability to sleep, loss of appetite, and a feeling of impending disaster. He states that he feels "on edge" and has not been productive in his job as a watch repairman and jewelrymaker. According to the history, JD had been treated by several drugs for nocturnal enuresis, a persisting childhood problem; only ephedrine, which he has been taking for 2 years, has been successful. He has no other significant health problems. He denies any side-effects of ephedrine. JD does admit to self-medicating his nagging cold with OTC cold preparations: a nasal spray used four times a day and a combination decongestant–pain reliever. A physical exam reveals a pulse of 104, BP of 154/86, R of 16. The patient appears flushed and slightly diaphoretic.

While JD is being evaluated, cultures are done, and he is started on a 5-day course of tetracycline to treat his sinusitis. What appropriate actions should be taken with JD?

Discussion

The first step in the care of JD is the establishment of a trust relationship with him to help to alleviate some of the anxiety that he is exhibiting. The complete patient history is necessary to determine the presence of any underlying medical conditions: the chronology of his presenting signs and symptoms; the history and details of his nocturnal enuresis and its treatment, including any side-effects he has experienced from the drug; a history of any known allergies; and the use of any other medications, including OTC drugs. In this case, a careful review of the OTC preparations JD has been taking indicates that JD is receiving a toxic dose of ephedrine, leading to his presenting signs and symptoms.

JD needs extensive patient teaching about his drug, its effects and side-effects, and what type of OTC drugs he should avoid. JD should be reassured that his signs and symptoms are most likely drug-related, and will pass when the drug levels fall. He should be advised to avoid any OTC drug containing ephedrine, and to avoid such other stimulants as caffeine or nicotine while his "jitters" remain.

Written patient teaching information can be given to JD; he should be asked to call the next day to check on his cultures and to see if the appropriate drug therapy is being used, and he should be asked to return in 1 week for follow-up evaluation of his presenting problems.

Adrenergic drugs in management of shock

Adrenergic drugs are commonly employed as adjuncts to fluid administration and to the other general measures used to treat acute hypotension and circulatory collapse. These drugs help to attain the main goal in the therapy of shock: producing an increased flow of blood to underperfused body organs. This is the result of the effects of adrenergic drugs on the heart and blood vessels.

However, the various adrenergic drugs differ in their cardiac and vascular effects. Some are more effective than others for strengthening myocardial contractions; some cause blood vessels to constrict, while others exert vasodilator effects. No single drug is ideal in all the different kinds of shock syndromes, so drugs have to be selected for each case on an individual basis after diagnosis of the hemodynamic defect responsible for the circulatory collapse. This section of the chapter will briefly describe the nature of shock, and will then discuss the properties of several adrenergic drugs most often used for treating shock syndromes.

Circulatory shock

The main characteristic of this condition is a reduction in the flow of blood to the tissues, particularly those of such vital organs as the brain, heart, kidneys, liver, and lungs. Such *hypoperfusion* prevents the tissues from getting enough of the oxygen and nutrients they need for energy production. The lack of bloodborne oxygen leads to damage to intracellular structures, including the mitochondria and lysosomes. This, in turn, results in further metabolic derangements and the release from the cells of toxic metabolites and other substances that accumulate and cause further derangements. If hypoxic cellular destruction is not promptly reversed by restoring normal blood flow to the vital tissues, the state of shock may become irreversible and refractory to all treatment.

Shock occurs as a complication of many disorders, including trauma and hemorrhage, myocardial damage, and severe infection. The primary hemodynamic defect responsible for the reduction in blood flow differs, depending on the cause of the shock state. These are the main types of mechanisms that trigger the sequence of events that end in circulatory collapse:

Hypovolemia—a reduction in blood volume
Cardiac failure—a reduction in the ability of the heart to pump enough blood to meet the needs of the tissues
Microcirculatory malfunction—a reduction in blood flow through the capillary beds and the very small precapillary arterioles and postcapillary venules

Treatment

The most direct way to treat shock is to determine the specific cause and to remove it by medical or surgical procedures. In shock caused by massive bleeding, an essential first step in management is to find and repair the torn vessels. Unless this is done, transfusions of whole blood or the infusion of plasma substitutes or other fluid and electrolyte solutions (Chap. 54) will not be successful in returning the blood volume to normal. Similarly, in shock caused by bloodborne infection, antibiotic treatment capable of eradicating the pathogenic gram-negative bacilli in the bloodstream is necessary for control of the septic shock state. To prevent cardiogenic shock, a complication in about 5% of patients hospitalized following an AMI, drugs or cardiac pacing are used to keep the injured heart beating at an efficient rate and rhythm and to decrease its workload. (See discussion of management of AMI complications, including cardiogenic shock, in Chapter 31.)

Often, however, the specific etiologic factor cannot be readily corrected. In such situations it is desirable to detect and counteract the primary source of the patient's circulatory disturbance. In hypovolemic shock, for example, it is essential to replace the fluid that has been lost from within the vascular system (see Chap. 54). In cardiogenic shock the myocardial pump must be stimulated to increase its output enough to maintain blood flow through the coronary vessels. In septic shock, which is characterized by poor microcirculatory function, treatment is aimed at reversing this defect and promoting flow of the peripherally pooled blood back to the heart.

Drugs for shock

Among the adrenergic drugs most commonly employed in managing shock are those that act at both α and β receptors, particularly *levarterenol* (Levophed), and a more recently introduced agent, *dopamine* (Intropin) (Table 17-5). The two drugs are similar in one important respect: by their action on β_1-type receptors, these drugs increase the strength of cardiac contractions. They do so without at the same time speeding up the heart rate or excessively raising the oxygen demands of the myocardium. One reason for this is that these drugs, by their stimulating effects on α receptors in the blood vessels, raise peripheral arterial resistance and raise systemic blood pressure. This in turn sets off reflex activity (baroreceptor reflexes) that tends to reduce the heart rate. These effects make the $\alpha-\beta$ agonists preferable to isoproterenol (Isuprel) in cardiogenic shock. Isoproterenol, a pure β agonist, also increases cardiac contractile strength. However, its use can be harmful to a patient with a damaged heart muscle, because isoproterenol tends to raise the heart rate and cause an increase in oxygen consumption greater than the patient's occluded coronary arteries can deliver, leading to further myocardial damage. The same drawback applies to epinephrine, which is sometimes also used in shock. Both isoproterenol and epinephrine are likely to cause cardiac arrhythmias.

Levarterenol and another drug, *metaraminol* (Aramine), also have vasopressor effects that may be useful for cardiogenic and other kinds of shock. That is, through their stimulation of vascular α receptors, these drugs cause a generalized vasoconstriction that results in a rise in arterial pressure. The increase in pressure within the aorta leads in turn to an increase in coronary and cerebral arterial perfusion pressure—that is, in a better flow of blood to the heart muscle and the brain. In addition, drug-induced venoconstriction helps to return blood to the heart, and this increase in venous return adds to the therapeutically desirable increase in cardiac output that these drugs bring about in shock patients.

Dopamine (Intropin) differs from the other $\alpha-\beta$ agonists in one important respect: when administered in moderate doses, this drug does not cause the sometimes too intense vasoconstriction seen with the other vasopressors. In fact, by acting on dopamine receptors, it exerts a dilating effect on the renal arterioles. This leads to a rise in renal blood flow, glomerular filtration, and urine production, even in shock patients with oliguria that had not improved significantly as a result of an increase in cardiac output after treatment with the other vasopressors. Patients with failing cardiac and renal function who have not responded to treatment with the potent diuretic drugs furosemide and ethacrynic acid alone sometimes have a marked increase in urine volume when cautious dopamine infusion is added to their regimen.

When dopamine is administered in high doses, it loses its advantages over the other adrenergic drugs

Table 17–5. Main adrenergic drugs used in shock and acute hypotension

Official or generic name	Trade name	Sites and mechanism of action	Usual adult dosage and administration	Comments
Catecholamines				
Dobutamine	Dobutrex	Relatively cardioselective action on β_1-adrenergic receptors increases cardiac contractility and output with few vascular or cardioacceleratory effects	Rate of infusion ranges usually from 2.5 to 10 $\mu g/kg/min$, but rates up to 40 $\mu g/kg/min$ have occasionally been required to raise the cardiac output	Increases cardiac output in patients with decompensation because of depressed myocardial contractility resulting from organic heart disease or cardiac surgical procedures
Dopamine HCl	Intropin	1. Direct action on cardiac β_1-adrenergic receptors increases cardiac contractility and heart rate. 2. Acts on dopaminergic receptors in renal and mesenteric vessels to cause vasodilation at doses <10–12 $\mu g/kg/min$ 3. Releases norepinephrine from sympathetic nerves in blood vessels, thus indirectly stimulating α-adrenergic receptors to cause vasoconstriction in skeletal muscles	Initiate IV infusion at a rate of 2–5 $\mu g/kg/min$ and increase in accordance with the patient's response to rates of 20–50 $\mu g/kg/min$ or more (see Drug digest for further details)	Effective for increasing cardiac output, blood pressure, and urine flow in patients with septic, hypovolemic, and cardiogenic shock, and for treating acute heart failure following cardiac surgery
Epinephrine HCl USP	Adrenalin Chloride	1. Direct action on cardiac β-adrenergic receptors increases cardiac contractility and heart rate 2. Acts directly on vascular α receptors to constrict splanchnic and other vessels 3. Very low doses act on vascular β_2 receptors to cause vasodilation	0.5–1.0 mg IV	Increases cardiac output and systemic blood pressure, but is less used than some other agents because it can cause myocardial ischemia and cardiac arrhythmias
Isoproterenol HCl USP	Isuprel	1. Direct action on cardiac β_1-adrenergic receptors increases myocardial	Dilute a 1:5,000 solution to 1:500,000 and infuse at rates adjusted to the	Useful in some cases of septic and hypovolemic shock; can be dangerous in cardio-

(continued)

Table 17–5. Main adrenergic drugs used in shock and acute hypotension (continued)

Official or generic name	Trade name	Sites and mechanism of action	Usual adult dosage and administration	Comments
		contractility and heart rate 2. Direct action on β_2-adrenergic receptors in blood vessels causes vasodilation in skeletal muscle and splanchnic vascular beds	shock patient's response (see Drug digest for further details)	genic shock because excessive stimulation of heart can cause myocardial ischemia and cardiac dysrhythmias
Levarterenol bitartrate USP	Levophed	1. Acts directly at cardiac β_1-adrenergic receptors to increase cardiac contractility 2. Acts directly at vascular α-adrenergic receptors to constrict splanchnic vessels and those of other vascular beds 3. Heart rate tends to be slowed by reflex action as blood pressure rises	IV infusion of a dilution containing 4 μg/ml is begun at a rate of 2–3 ml/min and adjusted to reach and maintain blood pressure between 80 mm and 100 mm Hg systolic (see Drug digest for further details)	Useful for cases of cardiogenic shock, because it raises blood pressure and increases coronary blood flow without excessively increasing myocardial oxygen consumption

Sympathomimetic amines (*Noncatecholamines*)

Ephedrine sulfate USP		1. Acts directly and indirectly (by release of neurotransmitter) to stimulate cardiac β_1 receptors 2. Acts similarly at α-adrenergic receptors in blood vessels to cause constriction	20 mg IV or 15–50 mg IM or SC (see Drug digest for further details)	Raises blood pressure by increasing cardiac output and by systemic vasoconstriction in treating and preventing acute hypotension in various clinical situations
Mephentermine sulfate USP	Wyamine Sulfate	1. Acts directly and indirectly (by release of neurotransmitter) to stimulate cardiac β_1 receptors 2. Acts similarly at α-adrenergic receptors in blood vessels to cause constriction	IV infusion of a solution of 1 mg/ml is preferable, with rate adjusted depending on patient's response; may also be given IM, 10–30 mg	Raises blood pressure by increasing cardiac output and by systemic vasoconstriction in treating and preventing acute hypotension in various clinical situations Not recommended in hypovolemic shock, but may be used to maintain blood pressure until whole blood is obtained

Table 17-5. Main adrenergic drugs used in shock and acute hypotension (continued)

Official or generic name	Trade name	Sites and mechanism of action	Usual adult dosage and administration	Comments
Metaraminol bitartrate USP	Aramine	1. Acts directly and indirectly (by release of neurotransmitter) to stimulate cardiac β_1 receptors 2. Acts similarly at α-adrenergic receptors to cause constriction	2–10 mg IM or SC; 0.5–5 mg IV bolus, followed by an infusion of 15–100 mg in the form of a dilute solution administered at a flow rate adjusted as required to maintain the desired pressure (see Drug digest for further details)	Raises blood pressure by increasing cardiac output and by systemic vasoconstriction in treating and preventing acute hypotension associated with spinal anesthesia, hemorrhage, and other conditions including cardiogenic and bacteremic shock
Methoxamine HCl USP	Vasoxyl	1. Acts only at vascular α-adrenergic receptors with little or no effect at β_1 or β_2 receptors 2. The heart rate is not increased but, instead, tends to slow as a result of carotid sinus reflex bradycardia	3–5 mg IV slowly, supplemented if needed by 10–15 mg IM to provide a more prolonged effect (see Drug digest for further details)	Raises blood pressure primarily by peripheral vasoconstriction during spinal and general anesthesia; it is safer than most sympathomimetic amines for use with cyclopropane and other anesthetics
Phenylephrine HCl USP	Neo-Synephrine	1. Acts only at vascular α-adrenergic receptors with little or no effect at β_1 or β_2 receptors 2. The heart rate is not increased but, instead, is slowed as a result of stimulation of carotid sinus pressoreceptors, with resulting reflex bradycardia	2–5 mg IM or SC; 0.1–0.5 mg IV; a 1:50,000 dilution of the 1% solution may be infused continuously at rates that raise blood pressure rapidly and then maintain it at the desired level (see Drug digest for further details)	Raises and maintains blood pressure by peripheral vasoconstriction and by increased cardiac output; it does not disturb cardiac rhythm in ordinary doses, and so is used with inhalation anesthetics as well as during spinal anesthesia

used for treating shock. In large doses dopamine can cause cardiac dysrhythmias similar to those sometimes set off by isoproterenol, epinephrine, or levarterenol. It may also cause excessive generalized vasoconstriction, as is the case with overdoses of other adrenergic vasopressor drugs.

Dobutamine (Dobutrex), the most recently introduced synthetic catecholamine, possesses properties that make it preferable to previously available adrenergic drugs. It increases cardiac output by strengthening weak-

ened myocardial contractions and thus increasing left ventricular stroke volume. In this respect it differs from isoproterenol, which can also increase cardiac output but does so mainly by increasing the heart rate, an action that, as indicated above, leads to increased myocardial oxygen demand.

Because dobutamine acts mainly on cardiac β_1-type receptors rather than on the α and β_2 receptors of blood vessels, it has relatively few vascular effects. That is, it neither dilates the vessels as isoproterenol does, nor constricts them as norepinephrine and large doses of dopamine may do. Thus, unlike the latter two drugs, which can cause severe local ischemia leading to gangrene if they leak from the vein into surrounding tissues (see below), such accidental infiltration by dobutamine would not cut off the local blood supply.

Like low doses of dopamine, dobutamine does not ordinarily cause systemic vasoconstriction and an excessive rise in mean aortic pressure, which would add to the work of a failing left ventricle. However, patients must be closely monitored, and the IV infusion rate of this drug should be reduced promptly in the minority of patients who develop a marked rise in systolic blood pressure or in heart rate. Fortunately, this drug is rapidly metabolized, and blood pressure then quickly stabilizes at a lower level.

Dobutamine is presently employed mainly for the short-term treatment of patients with severe heart failure following a weakening of cardiac contractility as a result of organic heart damage or cardiac surgery that has required the cardiopulmonary bypass procedure. Although its safety for patients who have suffered a massive AMI has not yet been established, some cardiologists have stated that the use of dobutamine in such cases may be beneficial for selected patients with cardiogenic shock.

Vasodilator therapy. Excessive vasoconstriction is often a drawback in treating shock. Frequently the patient's blood vessels have responded to the condition of shock itself by maximal vasoconstriction, and the addition of a vasoconstrictor drug either is ineffective in raising perfusion pressure, or it further compromises already compromised blood flow to vital organs and tissues. When prolonged, vasoconstriction leads to a loss of fluid from within the vessels and makes it difficult to maintain blood volume. It can also cause a sudden rise in peripheral arterial resistance and blood pressure. Drug-induced hypertension is especially dangerous for older patients with atherosclerotic cerebral arterioles, because a sudden rise in pressure can cause a cerebral vascular accident. Too high a rise in intra-aortic pressure is also undesirable in cardiogenic shock patients, because the left ventricle is then required to work too hard to eject its load of blood (the afterload) into the arterial circulation.

In shock states marked by excessive reflex vasoconstriction, many authorities now recommend the use of vasodilating drugs. Sometimes, excessive vasoconstriction caused by the α-adrenergic agonist effect of levarterenol or of high doses of dopamine may be counteracted by adding an α-adrenergic blocking agent (Chap. 18) to the infusion. For example, *phentolamine* (Regitine) and *phenoxybenzamine* (Dibenzyline) help to antagonize the action of the α–β agonists on the α receptors of the blood vessels. They do so without interfering with the action of these adrenergic agonists on cardiac β_1 receptors, and thus the desired increase in cardiac contractile strength and cardiac output continues.

Isoproterenol (Isuprel), the most potent β-adrenergic agonist, and low doses of dopamine are also often advocated for use in similar situations—that is, when the patient shows signs of excessive reflex vasoconstriction, or when the shock state fails to respond to treatment with α–β agonist-type vasopressors. Septic shock is the type of shock in which this is most likely to occur, and isoproterenol or dopamine may therefore be used in such cases. These drugs are also effective in some cases of hypovolemic shock that have not responded to fluid replenishment alone or to fluids and vasoconstrictor drugs.

In such situations, isoproterenol may be beneficial not only by its stimulating action on cardiac β_1 receptors, but also by its action on vascular β_2 receptors. This often leads to the dilation of constricted microcirculatory vessels in visceral vascular beds. As a result, blood that may have been trapped in the capillary beds is released and may then be returned to the right side of the heart from these peripheral pools. This increase in venous return, together with the drug-induced strengthening of cardiac contractions and output, is thought to account for the occasional benefits of isoproterenol in some cases of septic shock.

Direct vasodilators, such as *sodium nitroprusside* (Nipride; Chap. 31), are also sometimes used to overcome excessive vasoconstriction and to restore blood flow to the kidneys and other vital organs.

Acute hypotension. Drugs that act only at α-type adrenergic receptors such as phenylephrine (Neo-Synephrine) and methoxamine (Vasoxyl) are not now considered desirable for treating the shock syndromes. They cannot, of course, stimulate cardiac β receptors, and thus do not increase cardiac contractile strength or output. In fact, excessive doses of these drugs may reduce cardiac output by raising the peripheral arterial resistance against which the left ventricle must work. However, these and other vasoconstrictors, including the *non*adrenergic vasopressor angiotensin (Hypertensin), may sometimes help to *prevent* shock from developing in some patients suffering an acute hypotensive episode.

During spinal anesthesia, for example, the regional anesthetic that has been injected close to the roots of mixed spinal nerves tends to block the flow of tonic vasoconstrictor impulses to the blood vessels by way of sympathetic nerve fibers (see Chap. 14). The resulting reduction in vasomotor tone leads to dilation of the arterioles, pooling of blood in the venous capacitance vessels, and a steady drop in the patient's blood pressure. Overdoses of the adrenergic neuron blocking drugs that are used in treating high blood pressure—for example, guanethidine and reserpine (Chap. 18)—or of drugs with an α-adrenergic blocking or ganglionic blocking action (Chap. 18), including chlorpromazine (Chap. 46), can also cause a similar loss of sympathetic vasomotor tone.

The prophylactic intramuscular administration of one of the two pure α-adrenergic agonists (or of ephedrine, or *mephentermine, α–β* agonists), at about the same time that a local anesthetic is being injected to produce spinal anesthesia, helps to prevent hypotension from developing during the surgical procedure. These drugs also often help to raise the steeply falling arterial pressure of patients in whom overdoses of autonomic blocking drugs have cut off the flow of sympathetic vasoconstrictor impulses to peripheral vessels (Ephedrine and, to a lesser extent, mephentermine, also act to raise the cardiac output by increasing the contractile force of the myocardium.) However, to maintain tissue perfusion of the brain and heart when acute hypotension has progressed to actual shock, the intravenous infusion of levarterenol is preferred for its more rapid and dependable effects.

Monitoring the shock patient

Before treatment of shock is begun, preparations are made to monitor the patient's response to the administration of fluids and drugs. To determine the patient's need for fluid replenishment and the ability of the heart to handle the load during fluid infusion, central venous pressure (CVP) is sometimes measured continuously. Pulmonary artery wedge pressure measurement serves as an even more accurate guide to fluid administration in cardiogenic shock cases (Chap. 31). The response of the patient's blood pressure to vasopressor drugs is now often recorded directly following insertion of a catheter into a peripheral artery. Such brachial or femoral artery pressure measurements are more accurate than the traditional cuff method, which may be misleading when a vasoconstrictor such as levarterenol is being infused. When isoproterenol is employed, the patient's heart rate and rhythm are closely monitored, preferably with an electrocardiographic monitor, to avoid a too rapid and irregular response. Careful and continuous monitoring of urine output, respiratory function, and general perfusion are also important aspects of patient care.

Drug administration

During IV infusion of a vasopressor such as levarterenol, methoxamine, or metaraminol, the patient should not be left unattended. Blood pressure is checked every 2 minutes at first and, even after the patient's pressure has stabilized, it should be taken at frequent intervals so that the infusion rate can be promptly adjusted downward if pressure rises

too high. The systolic pressure should not be raised to normal with vasopressors but only to about 90 mm to 100 mm Hg. (In general, the patient's pressure is kept at a level about 30 mm below the mean arterial pressure.)

If the patient is conscious, it is also important to be aware of any complaints of headache, because this symptom may indicate an excessive buildup of cerebrovascular pressure. Projectile vomiting is a dangerous sign of a drug-induced pressure rise in the vascular bed of the brain. Excessive cardiac slowing may result from a reflex vagal response to arterial hypertension induced by vasopressor overdosage, and a too rapid rate—110 beats per minute or more during isoproterenol infusion—indicates that the rate of flow should be slowed or discontinued entirely.

The injection site should also be checked to see that the solution is flowing freely. Leakage of levarterenol or any potent vasopressor drug into the tissues can cause local vasoconstriction that, if allowed to continue, can result in ischemia, necrosis, and sloughing. The needle is best inserted into a large vein—the antecubital or femoral vein is preferred. The needle is advanced well into the vein and is then securely taped to the skin rather than tied in, because a tie may block blood flow and the resulting stasis tends to concentrate the levarterenol locally. Extra care is taken to avoid dislodging the needle when turning the patient.

If the skin above the site becomes blanched, cold, and hard, the infusion is stopped immediately, and the patient's physician is notified. A change of infusion site, local application of hot packs, and immediate infiltration of the ischemic area with phentolamine (Regitine) may be required. Phentolamine, an α-adrenergic blocking agent, may help to dilate the constricted arterioles and to increase local blood flow. (It will not help to reverse intense vasoconstriction produced by angiotensin.) Sometimes phentolamine is added to the levarterenol infusion at the start in small amounts intended to antagonize local vasoconstriction without reducing the desired systemic vasopressor effects.

In general, patients in shock should not receive drugs by intramuscular or subcutaneous injection because poor circulation to the injection site can delay the absorption of the drug, and thus also delay the production of its desired effects. Furthermore, when the patient's circulation is restored, excessive amounts of previously unabsorbed drug may enter the circulation from an IM or SC reservoir. If the drug is a vasopressor (*e.g.,* metaraminol is sometimes given by these routes), a sudden and dangerous rise in blood pressure may result. Similarly, toxic blood levels of other drugs may be reached under these circumstances.

Summary of chief pharmacologic actions and clinical uses of adrenergic drugs

Cardiac actions and uses

1. Increase in rate and strength of heartbeat useful in treating cardiac slowing and heart block in Stokes–Adams disease and the carotid sinus syndrome; may help to resuscitate heart in cardiac standstill, or asystole; in ventricular fibrillation, epinephrine may make the heart more responsive to electrical defibrillation.
2. Decrease in heart rate as a result of reflex vagal stimulation may be useful for terminating paroxysmal atrial (supraventricular) tachycardia.
3. Strengthening of heart contractions, slowing of heart rate, and coronary vasodilation: these actions may be desirable in adrenergic drugs used in cardiogenic shock and in other states of circulatory collapse marked by low cardiac output.

Vascular actions and uses

Local vasoconstriction is useful in many circumstances:

1. Nasal decongestant in acute and chronic inflammatory and allergic disorders, including the common cold, hay fever, and vasomotor rhinitis.
2. Ocular decongestant in conjunctivitis.
3. Intraocular pressure reduction in some forms of glaucoma.
4. Hemostatic in epistaxis (nosebleed) and after tonsillectomy and other throat surgery.
5. Additive to local anesthetic solutions for reducing systemic absorption of these drugs.
6. Antiallergic action in urticaria, angioneurotic edema, and anaphylactoid reaction.

Local vasodilation by some adrenergic drugs may be useful for treating certain peripheral vascular diseases.

Systemic vasoconstriction to raise blood pressure in the following conditions:

1. Acute hypotension caused by drug-induced reduction of sympathetic vasomotor tone (*e.g.*, spinal and inhalation anesthetics, ganglionic and adrenergic blocking agents).
2. Shock of cardiac origin (cardiogenic shock) following an AMI or severe dysrhythmias.
3. Septic (endotoxic, or gram-negative bacteremic) shock.
4. Circulatory collapse from other causes, including that resulting from severe hemorrhage (here, replacement of blood or restoration of blood volume with plasma or other fluids is the most important measure, and the use of adrenergic vasopressors is only adjunctive).

Bronchial muscle actions and uses

Stimulation of β_2-type receptors in smooth muscle of bronchi relaxes spasm and dilation of bronchial tubes in the following conditions:

1. Acute and chronic asthmatic states
2. Pulmonary emphysema and fibrosis
3. Chronic bronchitis and bronchiectasis

Miscellaneous actions and uses

1. Stimulation of α-type receptors in radial muscle of the iris results in mydriasis, which facilitates ophthalmologic examinations.
2. Uterine musculature may be relaxed to delay premature labor.
3. Skeletal muscle is sometimes strengthened by ephedrine in myasthenia gravis.
4. Increased tone of trigone and sphincter of urinary bladder brought about by ephedrine may be helpful in nocturnal enuresis (bed wetting).
5. Central stimulation by amphetamines and ephedrine may be useful in narcolepsy and in other clinical situations.

Summary of side-effects of adrenergic drugs: receptor type or site generally associated with effect

Cardiovascular system effects

Tachycardia (β_1 receptors)
Palpitations (β_1 receptors)
Arrhythmias (β_1 receptors)

Angina → AMI (β_1 receptors)
Hypertension (α receptors)
Flushing (β_2 receptors)

Central nervous system effects

Nervousness, tremors, and restlessness (CNS receptors; effect may also be secondary to cardiovascular and metabolic effects)

Anorexia (CNS receptors)

Convulsions (CNS receptors)

Insomnia (CNS receptors)

Psychoses (CNS receptors)

Urinary bladder effects

Urinary retention (α and β_2 receptors)

Ocular effect

Pupil dilatation $\rightarrow$ photophobia (α receptors)

Other effects

Increased blood sugar, glycosuria (β_2 receptors)

Sweating (Mechanism unclear—possibly secondary to anxiety and CNS effects)

Drug digests

Dopamine HCl (Intropin)

Actions and indications. This naturally occurring catecholamine has hemodynamic effects that make it safer and more effective for treating the shock syndrome than the related sympathomimetic amines norepinephrine and isoproterenol. Like these other adrenergic drugs, dopamine increases the strength of myocardial contractions and the cardiac output. However, optimal doses cause less of an increase in heart muscle oxygen consumption than isoproterenol and less peripheral vasoconstriction than norepinephrine. This amine is unique in its ability to dilate mesenteric and renal blood vessels. Renal blood flow, glomerular filtration rate, and urine output are increased, even in oliguric patients.

Administered after blood volume has been restored with plasma expanders or whole blood, this drug helps to correct hemodynamic imbalances in cardiogenic shock following open heart surgery with cardiopulmonary bypass. Used with other measures, including circulatory assist devices, this drug may help to increase the survival rate of patients in cardiogenic shock following AMI. Administered with potent diuretics such as furosemide or ethacrynic acid, it may help to overcome the effects of acute myocardial depression from general anesthetics and chronic cardiac decompensation in congestive heart failure. It has also been used in treating traumatic shock and endotoxic, or septicemic, shock.

Adverse effects, cautions, and contraindications. Overdosage may cause ectopic heartbeats, tachycardia, and anginal chest pains or dyspnea. These signs and symptoms and others caused by generalized vasoconstriction and by a rise in diastolic blood pressure may be corrected by reducing the infusion rate. This drug should not be administered until tachyarrhythmias and hypovolemia have been corrected. Its use in patients with pheochromocytoma is contraindicated. Nausea, vomiting, and headache are other possible side-effects.

Monitor patients with a history of vascular disease for darkening of skin color or a drop in skin temperature, because this may indicate a drug-induced decrease in circulation to the extremities. Decrease the flow rate or discontinue entirely to avoid the risk of possible necrosis. If extravasation occurs, infiltrate the area with phentolamine as soon as possible to prevent possible sloughing and necrosis in ischemic areas.

Dosage and administration. A 5-ml ampule containing 200 mg of drug is diluted with 250 ml or 500 ml of 5% dextrose injection or other sterile IV solution and administered at a controlled flow rate by needle or IV catheter. Initially, doses of 2 to 5 μg/kg/min are usually administered. This may be increased gradually to 20 to 50 μg/kg/min or more. The patient's urine flow, cardiac output, and blood pressure must be constantly monitored during administration, and the rate of drop flow in an IV drip chamber or other metering device should be adjusted in accordance with the patient's response.

Ephedrine and its HCl and sulfate salts USP

Actions and indications. This adrenergic drug produces sympathomimetic effects on bronchial and vascular and other smooth muscles and on the heart. It is most useful when administered orally as a bronchodilator in the management of asthma. Taken alone or combined with a theophylline compound and a sedative, it is effective for preventing and treating mild asthmatic attacks. Applied topically to the nasal mucosa, the drug has a decongestant effect in acute and chronic rhinitis. Topical application to the eye produces mydriasis.

Administered parenterally, ephedrine produces prolonged vasopressor effects by increasing cardiac output and causing generalized vasoconstriction. It is used to prevent blood pressure from dropping during spinal and general anesthesia. This adrenergic drug has central effects similar to those of the amphetamines and, like the latter drugs, it has been employed in the management of narcolepsy. It is occasionally used as an adjunct to cholinergic drugs in treating myasthenia gravis. It may also be given alternately with atropinelike drugs in nocturnal enuresis (bed-wetting).

Adverse effects, cautions, and contraindications. Like other adrenergic drugs, ephedrine requires caution in patients with hyperthyroidism, diabetes, coronary insufficiency, and hypertension. It should not be taken by patients receiving antidepressant drugs of the MAO inhibitor or tricyclic types, because it may precipitate a hypertensive crisis in such patients. Caution is also required in men with enlarged prostate glands, because the drug's effect on the bladder may lead to urinary retention. Central stimulation may cause insomnia, restlessness, and nervousness.

Dosage and administration. Ephedrine salts are administered orally to adults in doses of 25 mg to 50 mg; dosage for children usually ranges between 12.5 mg and 25 mg. It is applied topically in nose drops and nasal sprays, usually in a concentration of 0.5% to 1%. For ophthalmic use a 3% solution is applied in drop dosage. Injectable solutions containing 20 and 50 mg/ml are available for subcutaneous, intramuscular, and slow intravenous administration in doses of 25 to 50 mg for adults or 3 mg/kg body weight daily for children divided into four to six doses.

Epinephrine (Adrenalin) and its bitartrate and HCl salts USP

Actions and indications. This potent sympathomimetic amine has many actions on the heart, blood vessels, bronchi, and other smooth muscles. It is most useful for treating acute asthmatic attacks and anaphylactic shock. In these conditions its rapid bronchodilator and vasoconstrictor effects can be lifesaving. However, too frequent use results in reduced effectiveness in asthma. It is also sometimes useful for speeding and strengthening cardiac contractions in cases of cardiac arrest and complete heart block.

Applied topically it is useful for producing a hemostatic effect in epistaxis (nosebleed) and for stemming local oozing of blood from other mucous membranes (e.g., following tonsillectomy) and the skin. It is commonly added to local anesthetic solutions in low concentration to delay their systemic absorption, thus prolonging the local effect and reducing toxic anesthetic reactions. It is occasionally used as a nasal and, more commonly, as an ocular decongestant. Applied to the eye in wide-angle glaucoma (usually together with a miotic), it helps to bring about a rapid and prolonged fall in intraocular pressure.

Adverse effects, cautions, and contraindications. Overdosage, particularly as the result of accidental intravenous injection of a dose intended for subcutaneous administration, can cause a rapid rise in blood pressure that may lead to severe hypertensive headache and, possibly, intracranial hemorrhage. High doses, particularly in patients with coronary insufficiency, can set off severe rapid arrhythmias, including fatal ventricular fibrillation. More common side-effects of smaller doses include pallor, heart palpitations, chest pain, feelings of anxiety, fear, dizziness, restlessness, and tremulousness. Care is required in diabetic patients because of this drug's effect on glycogen metabolism, and caution is, of course, needed in patients with angina pectoris, hypertension, and hyperthyroidism.

Dosage and administration. A 1:1000 solution is available for injection subcutaneously or IM in doses of 0.2 ml to 0.5 ml for asthma attacks, or, diluted in 10 ml of dextrose or saline solution, intravenously or by intracardiac injection in cardiac arrest and other extreme emergencies. A 1:500 suspension in peanut oil produces longer lasting bronchodilator effects when injected IM, and a 1:400 aqueous suspension is employed in the same way. Solutions for inhalation (0.1% to 1%) are inhaled as a mist; some supply a measured dose of 0.3 mg. A 1% aqueous solution is used intranasally, and one drop of a 0.5%, 1%, or 2% solution may be instilled into the conjunctival sac for topical ocular vasoconstrictor action.

Isoproterenol HCl USP (Isuprel)

Actions and indications. This potent synthetic catecholamine produces the following important pharmacologic effects: cardiac stimulation, peripheral vasodilation, and bronchial spasm relaxation. These make it useful for treating certain cardiac arrhythmias, shock states, and chronic bronchopulmonary disorders. The arrhythmias that respond to treatment with this drug include cardiac standstill and excessively slow rhythms such as those seen in Stokes–Adams disease, A-V heart block caused by digitalis intoxication, and the carotid sinus syndrome. Shock states treated with this agent include bacteremic, cardiogenic, and hypovolemic shock marked by poor cardiac output. Bronchopulmonary disorders, in which this drug often offers symptomatic relief, include bronchial asthma, bronchitis, bronchiectasis, bronchospasm during anesthesia, pulmonary fibrosis, and pulmonary emphysema.

Adverse effects, cautions, and contraindications. Although this drug causes few side-effects when inhaled as a mist, adverse reactions typical of adrenergic drugs are common when it is administered by other routes. These include tachycardia with heart palpitations felt as a pounding in the chest. Thus, the drug is contraindicated in patients with tachystolic arrhythmias, including those with digitalis intoxication manifested by a rapid, irregular rhythm. This drug should not be given together with epinephrine, because their combined cardiac stimulation can lead to serious arrhythmias. When this drug is administered by IV infusion for shock the rate of flow should be slowed or discontinued if the patient's heart rate goes above 110 beats per minute. Caution is required in patients with coronary insufficiency such as angina pectoris and in those with hyperthyroidism and diabetes to avoid producing chest pains. Headache, flushing, sweating, tremors, and nervousness are other side-effects.

Dosage and administration. This drug is available as solutions of 1:100, 1:200, and 1:400 strengths for nebulization and oral inhalation in dosage adjusted to the patient's needs for control of acute asthma attacks. It is also administered sublingually in doses of 10 mg or 15 mg four times daily. (Doses by this route should not exceed 60 mg daily for adults or 30 mg for children.) Five ml of a 1:5000 solution may be diluted with 500 ml of 5% dextrose and infused IV at carefully adjusted flow rates for treating shock. One ml may be administered undiluted by the IM and SC routes, or even directly into the heart in extreme emergencies such as cardiac standstill.

Levarterenol bitartrate USP (Levophed)

Actions and indications. When used as a drug, norepinephrine is called levarterenol. This potent vasopressor is used in the management of acute hypotension and shock from all causes, including coronary occlusion and septicemia, as well as that following injury, burns, bleeding, and spinal or general anesthesia. It may be used to treat hypotension developing during and after surgery, particularly following sympathectomy and pheochromocytomectomy. It acts mainly by constricting arterioles and venules; the resulting increase in venous return of blood to the heart, coupled with the drug's ability to strengthen cardiac contractility, produces a desirable increase in cardiac output, aortic pressure, and coronary artery perfusion. This may make the drug particularly useful in cardiogenic shock, provided that precautions are taken to avoid development of drug-induced ventricular arrhythmias.

Adverse effects, cautions, and contraindications. Too rapid administration of excessive doses can cause hypertension and reflex bradycardia or other arrhythmias, including ventricular tachycardia and fibrillation. The risk of arrhythmias is greatest in patients anesthetized with halothane, cyclopropane, and other agents that sensitize the heart to catecholamines. Thus, the drug is contraindicated during anesthesia with these drugs. Local leakage can cause intense vasoconstriction in the injection area, which may be followed by death of the tissue, with sloughing or gangrene. Thus, the infusion site is checked often to ensure that the solution is flowing freely. Particular care is required in patients with obstructive peripheral vascular disorders such as Buerger's disease; in such patients and in the elderly, infusions should not be made into leg veins or into those on the back of the hand. The drug should not be administered when blood clots have formed in mesenteric arterioles.

Dosage and administration. Levarterenol is infused IV in individually adjusted dosage following dilution of 4 ml of a 0.2% solution in 1000 ml of 5% dextrose solution. Patients are observed constantly for complaints of headache and signs of hypertension, or for excessive bradycardia. The rate of infusion flow is checked frequently by use of a drip bulb for observing the number of drops entering the plastic IV catheter each minute through the thin-walled needle and tubing. Blood pressure is taken every 2 minutes at first, then every 5 minutes once pressure has been stabilized at the desired low normal level.

Metaraminol bitartrate USP (Aramine)

Actions and indications. This sympathomimetic amine is used mainly as an adjunct to other measures such as blood volume replacement in the management of acute hypotensive states and shock. It acts primarily by constricting the arterioles to raise the reduced peripheral resistance. However, the drug also increases the strength of cardiac contractions without causing tachycardia or arrhythmias. This results in increased cardiac output and in a better flow of blood to the brain and coronary blood vessels. These effects may make it useful for treating cardiogenic shock following an AMI. It has also been employed to prevent and counteract acute hypotensive reactions to spinal anesthesia and other medications and for shock caused by infections (*e.g.*, endotoxic shock in gram-negative septicemia).

Adverse effects, cautions, and contraindications. Although cardiac arrhythmias are less likely than with other adrenergic vasopressor drugs, its use should be avoided in hypotensive surgical patients inhaling halothane or cyclopropane for anesthesia. Care should be taken to keep blood pressure from rising too high and too rapidly, because hypertensive reactions can also cause cardiac arrhythmias. Caution is required in patients with a history of hyperthyroidism, diabetes, hypertension, and heart disease.

Dosage and administration. Injection of 2 mg to 10 mg IM produces a prompt and relatively prolonged pressor response (in about 10 minutes compared to up to 20 minutes when administered by the subcutaneous route). Given by direct IV injection (only in extreme emergencies), doses of 0.5 mg to 5 mg produce peak effects in only 1 or 2 min-

utes. IV infusion of a solution containing 15 mg to 100 mg in 500 ml of 5% dextrose or isotonic salt solution is safer, because it permits more careful dosage adjustment. The preferred injection sites are the larger veins of the antecubital area and the thighs to avoid tissue infiltration or thrombosis.

Methoxamine HCl USP (Vasoxyl)

Actions and indications. This sympathetic vasopressor amine raises blood pressure by stimulating α-type adrenergic receptors in the arterioles. Because it does not act on cardiac β-type receptors, the drug does not stimulate or overwork the heart. It is particularly useful for overcoming hypotension during surgery conducted under cyclopropane or halothane anesthesia, because this drug—unlike most other adrenergic drugs—does not tend to set off cardiac arrhythmias in hearts sensitized by these general anesthetics. Methoxamine is also useful for preventing falls in blood pressure during spinal anesthesia or for bringing pressure back to normal in such cases. It is used also to restore normal cardiac rhythm in patients with paroxysmal supraventricular tachycardia through its ability to slow the heart by setting off vagal reflex activity.

Adverse effects, cautions, and contraindications. Doses that cause blood pressure to rise to too high levels may lead to severe headache, projectile vomiting, and excessive cardiac slowing. Patients with severe hypertension or with hyperthyroidism require particular care in dosage adjustment and overdosage detection if this drug is used at all in such cases. Obstetric patients who have received ergot alkaloid oxytocic drugs may be particularly subject to dangerous rises in blood pressure if methoxamine is adminis-

tered.

Dosage and administration. The usual IM dose for preventing or correcting hypotension in adults is 10 mg to 15 mg; in children, it is 0.25 mg/kg body weight. Slow IV injection of 3 mg to 5 mg is useful in emergencies. In cases of prolonged shock and in treating hypotension following an acute coronary attack, a solution containing 35 mg to 40 mg diluted in 250 ml of 5% dextrose in water is infused at a rate that keeps blood pressure slightly below normal. An IV dose of 10 mg is slowly injected for restoring normal rhythm in cases of paroxysmal supraventricular tachycardia.

Phenylephrine HCl USP (Neo-Synephrine)

Actions and indications. This synthetic adrenergic drug produces prolonged vasoconstriction on topical application and systemic administration. It is useful as a decongestant for symptomatic relief of rhinitis and sinusitis in treating the common cold and hay fever. Drops applied to the eye constrict intraocular vessels. This helps to reduce pressure in wide-angle glaucoma and reduces congestion in uveitis. Higher concentrations have a mydriatic action that is useful in ophthalmology for diagnostic and therapeutic procedures that require pupillary dilation without paralysis of accommodation.

Administered by injection, this drug produces a rise in blood pressure and reflex bradycardia, thus often terminating attacks of supraventricular tachycardia. Systemic vasoconstriction also prevents hypotension during spinal anesthesia and counteracts shock resulting from overdosage of other drugs, including chlorpromazine and various antihypertensive agents.

Adverse effects, cautions, and contraindications. Overdosage may cause an excessive rise in blood pressure and hypertensive headache. Thus, this drug should not be administered to patients who are also receiving MAO inhibitor drugs for treating mental depression or essential hypertension, or oxytocic drugs in obstetrics. Caution is also suggested in patients with heart disease, diabetes, and hyperthyroidism. Parenteral overdosage may precipitate various types of cardiac arrhythmias, including both bradycardia and tachycardia.

Solutions of low concentration cause little nasal or ocular irritation. However, higher concentrations can cause stinging and lacrimation. This is prevented by prior application of a drop of a local anesthetic solution. Ophthalmic solutions are contraindicated in narrow-angle glaucoma because of the mydriatic effect.

Dosage and administration. For intranasal application, concentrations of 0.125%, 0.25%, 0.5%, and 1% are available for instillation as drops, as a spray, and in jelly form. Solutions of 2.5% and 10% for ophthalmic use are applied topically. An elixir is available for oral use as a nasal and bronchial decongestant in a dose of 10 mg tid.

For treating moderate hypotension, doses of 2 mg to 5 mg may be injected intramuscularly or subcutaneously as a 0.2% solution. In severe hypotension and shock, 1 ml of a 1% solution is diluted in 500 ml of dextrose or saline solution and infused continuously—first at a rapid rate and later more slowly. For halting attacks of tachycardia, 0.5 mg is rapidly injected by vein.

References

Ahlquist RP: A study of adrenotropic receptors. Am J Physiol 153:586, 1948

Finkelstein BW: Ritodrine. Drug Intell Clin Pharm 15:425, 1981

Lefkowitz RJ: Direct binding studies of adrenergic receptors: biochemical, physiological and clinical implications. Ann Intern Med 91:450, 1979

Moyer JH et al: Vasopressor agents in shock. Am J Nurs 75:1168, 1975

Rodman MJ: Drugs for treating shock. RN 39:77, 1976

Rodman MJ: Adrenergic drugs and adrenergic blockers. RN 37:55, 1974

Rosenblum R: Physiologic basis for the therapeutic use of catecholamines. Am Heart J 87:527, 1974

Shubin H, Weil MH: Bacterial shock. JAMA 235:421, 1976

Sutherland EW: On the biological role of cyclic AMP. JAMA 214:1281, 1970

Webb–Johnson DC, Anderson JL Jr: Bronchodilator therapy. N Engl J Med 297:476, 758, 1977

Weiner N: Norepinephrine, epinephrine, and the sympathomimetic amines. In Gilman AG, Goodman LS, Gilman A (eds): Goodman and Gilman's The Pharmacological Basis of Therapeutics, 6th ed, pp 138–175. New York, Macmillan, 1980

Drugs that block adrenergic receptors and autonomic ganglia

18

This chapter is concerned with some drugs that are used therapeutically for their ability to interfere with the functioning of the sympathetic nervous system (SNS). These drugs are sometimes called *sympatholytic drugs.* The desired therapeutic effects of these drugs all depend on their interfering, directly or indirectly, with the function of sympathetic *adrenergic* nerves, although the ganglionic blocking drugs also interfere with the function of sympathetic *cholinergic* nerves (see Chap. 13, Tables 13-1 and 13-2). These drugs are used primarily for their effects on the cardiovascular system. For example, they are useful in treating hypertension, angina, and cardiac arrhythmias.

The drugs that interfere with SNS function do so by four different mechanisms of action, and may be classified according to these mechanisms:

1. *Adrenergic receptor blocking drugs,* either α blockers, such as phentolamine, or β *blockers,* such as propranolol
2. *Adrenergic neuron blocking drugs,* such as guanethidine, that interfere with the synthesis, storage, or release of the neurotransmitter norepinephrine by adrenergic nerves
3. *Ganglionic blocking drugs,* such as trimethaphan
4. *Centrally acting sympatholytic drugs,* such as methyldopa, that depress SNS outflow from the CNS

Only two classes of these drugs will be discussed in this chapter, the adrenergic receptor blocking drugs and the ganglionic blocking drugs. The other two groups of drugs are used almost exclusively for reducing the blood pressure of hypertensive patients, and are described, along with other drugs, in Chapter 28, Drugs Used in Treating Hypertension.

Adrenergic receptor blocking drugs

General considerations

Nerve impulses are transmitted from the sympathetic nervous system to muscle and gland cells when the neurotransmitter *norepinephrine* is released from nerve endings and interacts with specialized receptor sites on these effector cells. These sympathetically innervated neuroeffectors contain adrenergic receptors of two general types, α and β *receptors* (see Chap. 13).

This section will discuss drugs that interfere with the transmission of nerve impulses to adrenergic neuroeffectors by their ability to occupy adrenergic receptors without activating them. These drugs are pharmacologic antagonists; most are competitive antagonists (see Chap. 4). By these actions, these drugs prevent the neurotransmitter norepinephrine from producing the effects typical of SNS stimulation. In addition, they prevent other catecholamines, such as epinephrine (released from the adrenal medulla), and sympathomimetic drugs (see Chap. 17) from producing their characteristic effects.

Adrenergic receptor blocking drugs show different degrees of specificity. Most act *either* on α receptors (*e.g.,* phentolamine) *or* on β receptors (*e.g.,* propranolol) (Table 18-1). Recently, several drugs with yet greater specificity have been marketed in the United States: prazosin blocks α_1 receptors to a much greater extent than α_2 receptors; atenolol and metoprolol block β_1 receptors to a much greater extent than β_2 receptors (see Chap. 13, and below). A new drug, *labetalol* (Trandate; Normodyne) is unusual in that it blocks *both* α and β receptors competitively; it is available in Europe and may soon be available in the United States for the treatment of hypertension.

Table 18-1 lists the adrenergic receptor blocking drugs currently available in the United States, along with their uses and dosage.

Table 18–1. β-Adrenergic receptor blockers

Official or generic name	Trade name	Clinical indications	Usual adult dosage
Atenolol	Tenormin	Selective β_1 blocker used for hypertension	50 mg PO once a day (less in renal failure)
Metoprolol tartrate	Lopressor	Selective β_1 blocker used for hypertension; investigational in acute myocardial infarction	Initially, 100 mg/day PO; may gradually increase to 450 mg/day for maintenance
Nadolol	Corgard	Hypertension; angina	Initially, 40 mg PO once a day; may gradually increase to 240 mg (angina) or 320 mg (hypertension) for maintenance (reduce dose in renal failure)
Pindolol	Visken	Hypertension	Initially, 10 mg PO bid; may gradually increase to 60 mg/day for maintenance
Propranolol HCl USP	Inderal	Cardiac arrhythmias; pheochromocytoma; hypertension; angina; hypertrophic cardiomyopathy; migraine; thyrotoxicosis; anxiety; prevention of reinfarction after AMI	10–30 mg tid or qid, PO (varies with indication for use); may also be given by slow IV injection in life-threatening cardiac arrhythmias
Timolol maleate	Blocadren; Timoptic	Hypertension; prevention of reinfarction after myocardial infarction; wide-angle glaucoma	10 mg PO bid in hypertension, may gradually increase dose to 60 mg/day; one drop of 0.25% ophthalmic solution in each eye, bid

β-Adrenergic blocking drugs

Although drugs that block α-adrenergic receptors have been known and used much longer than the β blocking drugs, β blockers will be discussed first. The reason for this is that although most of the α blockers have relatively limited clinical usefulness, the prototype β-blocking agent, *propranolol*[+] (Inderal) has proved very useful in a number of important types of disorders, including cardiac arrhythmias, coronary heart disease, and hypertension.

Mechanism of action

Propranolol and other drugs of this class act mainly as competitive antagonists. That is, they bring about their pharmacologic effects by competing with agonists for receptor sites and by combining reversibly with these receptor sites. Thus, they prevent the receptors from responding to sympathetic nerve impulses or to circulating catecholamines and adrenergic drugs. Propranolol blocks both β_1 (cardiac) and β_2 receptors. Therefore, propranolol produces therapeutic effects on the heart in certain disease conditions, but can also precipitate or aggravate asthma and other bronchoconstrictive diseases by blocking SNS influences on the β_2 receptors of bronchial smooth muscle.

Newer drugs of this class, such as *metoprolol* (Lopressor) and *atenolol* (Tenormin) act more selectively at the β_1-type receptors; that is, they are *cardioselective*.

The newest drug of this group, *pindolol*, is actually a *partial agonist* (see Chap. 4). That is, in addition to blocking β receptors, it has some *intrinsic sympathomimetic activity* (ISA). The clinical significance of this property is a controversial subject. Some authorities claim that pindolol is less likely than other nonselective β blockers to precipitate asthma and heart failure (see below), but others believe this property only reduces the therapeutic effectiveness of the drug.

Pharmacologic effects

Cardiac actions. The most important actions of propranolol and related drugs are those that result from their ability to reduce sympathetic tonic influences on the functioning of the patient's heart. Administered in adequate doses, these drugs have the following effects on cardiac function:

1. A reduction in the heart rate (negative chronotropic)

379

2. A reduction in cardiac contractility (negative inotropic)

3. A slowing of atrioventricular (A-V) conduction (negative dromotropic)

4. A decrease in the automaticity of ectopic pacemakers*

These cardiac effects account for the therapeutic usefulness of propranolol in the management of such heart disorders as supraventricular and ventricular arrhythmias (Chap. 30) and angina pectoris (Chap. 31). However, the drug-induced reduction in sympathetic tone can also have serious adverse effects in patients for whom the stimulating effects of sympathetic nerve impulses to the heart are necessary. The reduction in myocardial contractile force that follows β-adrenergic blockade can, for example, cause congestive heart failure in a patient whose badly damaged heart requires reflex sympathetic stimulation to maintain adequate cardiac output (see Chap. 29). Similarly, patients with sinus bradycardia or partial heart block may suffer complete heart block and cardiac arrest when deprived of the effects of sympathetic stimulation on the heart rate and cardiac impulse conduction. Thus, to gain the benefits of β-adrenergic blockade without risking its dangers, the patients who can profit from treatment must be carefully selected, and the drug's dosage is then adjusted to individual needs.

Vascular effects. Circulating epinephrine and sympathomimetic drugs with β_2 agonist activity (see Table 17-1) can act on β_2 receptors in arterioles of skeletal muscles and elsewhere to cause vasodilatation. β_2 receptor blockers might be expected to lessen local blood flow by interfering with this action of epinephrine. In actual practice this is seldom a clinically significant effect, but patients with peripheral vascular disorders, such as Raynaud's disease, sometimes complain of coldness of the extremities when given propranolol.

Similarly, when propranolol is employed to lessen the cardiac symptoms of pheochromocytoma (see below), it should always be administered only after α-adrenergic blocking drugs have first been administered. If this is not done, the drug-induced blockade of β_2-type adrenergic receptors in the patient's blood vessels will cause the vasoconstrictor effect of circulating epinephrine (from the tumor tissue) on vascular α receptors to remain unopposed by any vasodilating action. This can then lead to a marked increase in peripheral resistance and to a dangerous rise in blood pressure.

In view of the above discussion, it should be surprising to learn that one of the most important therapeutic uses of propranolol and other β blockers is to *lower* the blood pressure of hypertensive patients. Unlike most of the therapeutic and adverse effects of autonomic drugs, this effect would not be predicted from an understanding of the effects of the sympathetic nervous system and the receptors that mediate these effects. The cardiac effects of β_1 receptor blockade account in part for the ability of these drugs to lower blood pressure, but other sites of action (the renin–angiotensin system, the CNS) are also probably involved (see Chap. 28). All the β blockers listed in Table 18-1 are used to treat hypertension, often in combination with a direct vasodilator drug. A new drug under investigation, *prizidolol*, combines the properties of a β_1 receptor blocker and a direct vasodilator in one molecule, and may provide some hypertensive patients effective therapy with only one drug.

Bronchial effects. Drug-induced blockade of β_2-type receptors in bronchial smooth muscle can cause bronchoconstriction. Bronchospasm does not develop in most patients, but it can occur in those with asthma and other chronic obstructive lung disorders. Thus, propranolol must not be administered to patients with bronchial asthma, because it may cause a dangerous increase in airway resistance. Its use in patients with chronic bronchitis and emphysema requires caution, because competitive β_2 blockade can, of course, interfere with the therapeutic action of aerosols of isoproterenol and other adrenergic bronchodilator drugs that are often employed daily in the long-term management of patients with chronic pulmonary obstruction. The cardioselective β-adrenergic blocking drugs are much less likely to cause bronchospasm than propranolol and other drugs that act at both types of β receptors, as the blocking action of the new drugs is limited largely to β_1 receptors.

Metabolic effects. Epinephrine plays a part in the conversion of glycogen to glucose by an action on β-adrenergic receptors in skeletal muscles and the liver. When these receptors are blocked by propranolol or by other β blockers, glucose cannot be as readily mobilized when required. Most people taking propranolol do not show any significant fall in blood glucose levels. However, the degree of hypoglycemia induced by insulin injections in patients with labile diabetes mellitus may be markedly increased. This is particularly dangerous because the diabetic patient may not be aware that acute hypoglycemia is developing; the β blocking agent tends to prevent the tachycardia, flushing, diaphoresis, and feeling of anxiety that are the main warning signs. Thus, diabetics who are put on propranolol therapy should be observed for hypoglycemic reactions and warned that these are possible following insulin administration. In addition, because β receptors mediate the release of insulin in response to hyperglycemia, patients on β blockers may show prolonged hyperglycemia. Atenolol is safer than the other β blockers for diabetics because it is less likely to influence carbohydrate metabolism.

Central nervous system effects. Propranolol passes the blood–brain barrier and enters the CNS. This may

---

* Some of these drugs, including propranolol, also have a direct action on cardiac cell membranes similar to that of local anesthetics (Chap. 14) and antiarrhythmic drugs such as quinidine (Chap. 30). However, this membrane-stabilizing, or quinidinelike, effect is not considered significant compared to β-adrenergic blockade, when these drugs are employed clinically in the doses ordinarily administered to treat patients with cardiac arrhythmias.

account for its effectiveness in preventing migraine headache, and it is thought to account for the feelings of fatigue and tiredness that are a common complaint early in propranolol therapy. It may also be responsible for the occasional development of such psychic changes as depression, insomnia, vivid dreams, and hallucinations. Metoprolol, the only other β blocker that crosses the blood–brain barrier that is available in the United States, also causes feelings of fatigue, dizziness, and mental depression.

On the other hand, the central effects of propranolol may be responsible for favorable responses that have been reported when it has been employed experimentally in psychiatric treatment. β blockers are presently being studied in the management of anxiety states and phobias, alcoholism, opiate addiction, and psychoses, as well as in patients with parkinsonism.

Ocular effects. Timolol is available as an ophthalmic preparation (Timoptic) for use in treating wide-angle glaucoma. Its mechanism of action in lowering intraocular pressure is unclear. To allay the anxiety of the astute student, it would perhaps be helpful to point out here that several classes of drugs with apparently opposing effects on important parameters of ocular function (pupil size, accommodation of the lens) *are* used to treat glaucoma. These include parasympathomimetics, sympathomimetics (*e.g.*, epinephrine) with α- and β-receptor agonist activity, and a β blocker (timolol; see also Chap. 42).

Therapeutic uses and dosage considerations

The established clinical indications for propranolol appear in the Drug digest and are also summarized in Table 18-1. The current therapeutic applications of this drug are also discussed in detail in the following chapters of the text and elsewhere: Chapter 28 (hypertension); Chapter 30 (cardiac arrhythmias); Chapter 31 (angina pectoris); Chapter 22 (thyrotoxicosis). Thus, this section will describe only general topics related to the management of such disorders that are not discussed elsewhere.

Patients often vary very widely in the amounts of orally administered propranolol that they require for optimal control of the cardiovascular disorders for which it is prescribed. The main reason for this is that patients differ considerably in *sympathetic tone*. In some patients, even such small initial doses as 10 mg to 20 mg can precipitate heart failure and acute hypotension, because—as indicated above—the drug's β-blocking action deprives these patients of the sympathetic nervous system support required for maintaining cardiac compensation. Others may require (and be able to tolerate) relatively enormous doses—2 g daily, for example—that must finally be administered to attain the full benefit of β-blockade therapy.

Pharmacokinetic factors also play a part in determining optimal dosage of propranolol in different patients. Although oral doses are readily absorbed from the upper gastrointestinal tracts of all patients, the plasma

propranolol levels reached in different patients who have been receiving the same dosage regimen are sometimes very variable. Some patients, for example, are found to have plasma concentrations only 5% or 10% of the level attained in others. This is believed to occur because a large proportion of any administered dose is *destroyed in the liver* of such patients as it passes through the portal circulation (first-pass effect; see Chap. 4). Thus, the drug never reaches the systemic plasma concentrations required to produce adequate β-adrenergic blockade.

A final factor that determines the wide difference in dosage range is *the nature of the disorder* being treated. In patients with *supraventricular arrhythmias*, for example, relatively small doses of propranolol are often sufficient for protecting the ventricles and reducing the rapid rate at which they are being driven—particularly when the patient is also digitalized. Patients with *angina pectoris* usually require much larger doses to counteract the oxygen-consuming response of the myocardium to the increased sympathetic stimulation set off by physical and emotional stress.

Some *hypertensive patients* require unusually large doses of propranolol to attain maximal lowering of their high blood pressure. Some authorities suggest that this depends primarily on their plasma renin status when treatment is started. Thus, for example, patients with high renin or normal renin pretreatment levels respond to treatment with moderate doses of propranolol, while those with low renin levels do not. Raising their dosage to much larger amounts does help to reduce the blood pressure of these patients, possibly because high doses of the drug act by another mechanism that is independent of the patient's plasma renin concentrations (see Chap. 28 for further discussion of treatment of essential hypertension with propranolol alone and with combinations of propranolol with diuretics.)

Establishing optimal dosage levels for each patient is important, because the main adverse effects of propranolol are extensions of the same pharmacologic actions that are responsible for its therapeutic effects. Thus, if dosage is not carefully titrated, the desired cardiac effects may be followed by an excessive degree of bradycardia, heart block, or myocardial weakness. Actually, the incidence of side-effects with propranolol is relatively low, provided that the drug is not ordered for patients with heart failure, heart block, or bronchial asthma, and that those for whom it is prescribed are started on small doses that are then raised gradually at recommended intervals.

Patients with angina pectoris have reportedly suffered a worsening of coronary heart disease symptoms when they suddenly stopped taking their daily propranolol dosage. Thus, patients with coronary heart disease should be warned not to interrupt this treatment without the knowledge and approval of their nurse or physician. If it becomes necessary to discontinue propranolol therapy for any reason, including elective surgery, the drug should be withdrawn only gradually to avoid development of severe chest pains, dysrhythmias, and even fatal myocardial infarction. Although this advice applies primarily to patients with angina pectoris, propranolol should probably also not be abruptly withdrawn from hypertensive and elderly patients, because they may have hidden, previously undetected coronary atherosclerosis.

In summary, propranolol is a drug with a wide, and still enlarging, spectrum of clinical applications. Properly employed in patients for whom it is not contraindicated and in doses that are raised from initially low levels to often much larger amounts, it is relatively free of adverse effects. However, those caring for patients taking propranolol should be aware of its potential toxicity in some patients, and should employ the precautions required to ensure its safe use. The cardioselective β blockers are safer than the nonselective β blockers for patients with pulmonary problems, but their cardioselectivity is only relative, not absolute, and it should be noted that these drugs, too, could produce the entire spectrum of adverse effects caused by β-receptor blockade. Metoprolol, more than atenolol, blocks β_2 receptors as the dose is raised.

Additional clinical considerations

Contraindications in the presence of certain clinical conditions. β-Adrenergic receptor blocking drugs should be avoided in patients with clinical conditions that require SNS activity to maintain their stability. Such conditions include the following:

1. *Chronic obstructive pulmonary disease* and *asthma* (at times when the disease is likely to be activated readily; for example, pollen season). These conditions need the bronchodilation mediated by the β_2 receptors; if these receptors are blocked, bronchoconstriction and exacerbation of the diseases may occur.
2. *Congestive heart failure* (CHF). The decrease in cardiac output and loss of reflex sympathetic activity can precipitate CHF in predisposed patients, and worsen the condition in patients who are already in failure.
3. *Hypotension, shock.* The decrease in blood pressure and cardiac output, together with the loss of sympathetic reflexes, will worsen these states.
4. *Bradycardia, heart block.* The decrease in heart rate and conduction velocity can exacerbate these conditions.
5. *Diabetes mellitus.* β blockers may increase insulin-induced hypoglycemia, and they also block the normal warning signs of hypoglycemia (flushing, sweating, tachycardia). Thus, diabetic patients may not be aware of an acute hypoglycemic episode. If a β blocker must be used,

atenolol is the drug of choice, because it is less likely to cause these effects.
6. *Surgery.* Patients who are to undergo surgery should be withdrawn from β-adrenergic blockers 1 to 2 weeks before surgery. The loss of sympathetic reflexes caused by β blockers could otherwise result in prolonged hypotension and reduced cardiac output following the surgery and anesthesia. If emergency surgery is required, a β-adrenergic agonist (see Chap. 17) should be administered.
7. *Pregnancy and lactation.* As with many other drugs, the β-adrenergic blockers should not be used in either of these conditions unless the benefit clearly outweighs the risks involved.

In addition to these adverse effects and others summarized at the end of this section, these drugs frequently cause impotence. The patient should be aware of the possibility of this problem and should have every opportunity to discuss it. Such patients will, of course, need constant support and encouragement.

The β-adrenergic blocking drugs should not be withdrawn abruptly. Acute myocardial infarction, angina, and ventricular arrhythmias have occurred with acute withdrawal of these drugs. It is thought that a hypersensitivity to catecholamines occurs, and that the sudden withdrawal of these drugs results in intense β-adrenergic stimulation. If a patient is to be discontinued from β-adrenergic blocking drugs, it should be done slowly over a 1- to 2-week period. During this time the patient should be alert for any signs of angina or cardiac problems. Patient teaching needs to emphasize that these drugs should not be stopped abruptly.

Propranolol is being successfully used for prophylaxis of migraine headaches. Its mechanism of action in migraine has not been established, but it may be due to blockade of cerebral vasodilation or to inhibition of arteriolar spasms in blood vessels in the pia mater (a membrane covering the brain) that overlies the cerebral cortex. Propranolol may interact with β receptors in the smooth muscle of these blood vessels. Propranolol is also currently being investigated for use in acute myocardial infarction, gastrointestinal bleeding in cirrhotic patients, schizophrenia, and even stage fright.

Drug–drug and drug–laboratory interactions. Concurrent use of β blockers and *monoamine oxidase (MAO) inhibitors* is contraindicated. Use of *digitalis* while on β blockers may result in increased depression of A-V conduction resulting in A-V heart block, and the β blocker's negative inotropic effect may reduce the positive inotropic effect expected from digitalis. *Catecholamine-depleting drugs* may have an additive effect when taken with β-blocking drugs. Patients who are taking both these drugs must be monitored very carefully for signs of severe side-effects.

Concomitant use of *aminophylline* and β blockers may produce antagonistic effects, resulting in no therapeutic effect for the patient. The hypoglycemic effects of *insulin* are prolonged by β-blocking drugs. Diabetic patients are at high risk with this combination, and must be monitored very carefully. The plasma levels of propranolol are increased by concurrent use of *chlorpromazine, cimetidine, furosemide,* and *hydralazine*. Propranolol used with any of these drugs should be started with a lower than expected dose to compensate for the higher plasma levels. *Phenytoin* and *phenobarbital*, on the other hand, induce increased activity of liver enzymes that metabolize propranolol, and lower than anticipated serum levels result. *Cigarette smoking* also reduces the blood levels of propranolol by increasing its clearance, resulting in lessened therapeutic effects of propranolol. If patients are smokers, the propranolol dosage will need to be increased to achieve the desired therapeutic effect.

Propranolol may increase *blood urea* levels in certain physical states. *Timolol* may cause an increase in *BUN* and in *potassium* and *uric acid* levels. Pindolol has been associated with increased *SGOT* and *SGPT* levels. Any of these agents can interfere with *glucose tolerance test* results.

The patient teaching guide for patients on β-adrenergic blockers presents points to include in patient teaching. The guide to the nursing process with adrenergic blockers (at the end of the chapter) summarizes the clinical application of this drug therapy in nursing practice.

Summary of pharmacologic actions of and clinical indications for β-adrenergic blocking drugs

Pharmacologic actions*

Cardiac: decreases heart rate and cardiac output

Vascular: decrease systemic blood pressure

Bronchial: increase tone of bronchial smooth muscle

Metabolic: increases hypoglycemic response to insulin

Plasma renin activity (PRA): decreases PRA, especially in patients with high predrug levels (PRA)

CNS: fatigue, lethargy, weakness

Clinical indications

Cardiac arrhythmias: supraventricular arrhythmias—sinus tachycardia associated with thyrotoxicosis, and paroxysmal atrial tachycardia caused by excess catecholamines, digitalis toxicity, or Wolff–Parkinson–White syndrome; ventricular arrhythmias—ventricular tachycardia caused by excess catecholamines or digitalis toxicity, or unresponsive to other drugs, or developing during anesthesia as a result of catecholamine actions on the anesthetic-sensitized myocardium

Pheochromocytoma (only after prior treatment with α-adrenergic blockers)

Hypertrophic subaortic stenosis

Angina pectoris

Postmyocardial infarction

Hypertension

Migraine headaches

* The actions of greatest clinic usefulness are those on the heart. Reduction of plasma renin activity probably plays a part in the antihypertensive effect of these drugs. The central actions may have some clinical usefulness in certain psychiatric and neurologic disorders. However, the CNS and other listed actions are mainly a cause of adverse effects in patients suffering from secondary disorders that make them excessively susceptible (see the summary of adverse effects, below).

Summary of adverse effects of β-adrenergic blocking drugs

Cardiovascular system

Bradycardia, atrioventricular block, congestive heart failure, peripheral arterial insufficiency, hypotension

Respiratory system

Bronchospasm*

Central nervous system

Weakness, fatigue, lethargy; mental depression progressing to suicide in susceptible patients; memory loss; disorientation, hallucinations, psychoses; visual disturbances

Gastrointestinal system

Nausea, vomiting, epigastric distress, abdominal cramping, diarrhea, constipation

Miscellaneous effects

Loss of vigorous sympathetic response may mask many of the early signs and symptoms of hypoglycemia, angina pectoris, myocardial infarction, or hyperthyroidism.

Abrupt withdrawal of the drug may precipitate such conditions as hypertensive crisis or myocardial infarction.

* The newer *cardioselective* β-blocking drugs are less likely to cause bronchospasm. However, caution is required in patients with allergic bronchial asthma and in patients prone to develop nonallergic bronchospasm—for example, those with chronic bronchitis or emphysema.

Patient teaching guide: β-adrenergic blockers

The drug that has been prescribed for you is called a β blocker. This type of drug works to prevent certain stimulating activities that normally occur in your body in response to such factors as stress, injury, or excitement. In your case the drug has been prescribed to treat _____ .

Instructions:

1. The name of your drug is _____ .

2. The dosage that has been prescribed for you is _____ .

3. The best time to take your drug is _____ , _____ , _____ .
   Propranolol and metoprolol should be taken with food to help to increase their absorption.

4. *Never* discontinue this medication suddenly. If you find that your prescription is running out, notify your nurse or physician at once.

5. Some side-effects of the drug that you should be aware of include the following:

   Fatigue, weakness — These are often discouraging effects. Space your activities throughout the day and allow rest periods.

   Dizziness, drowsiness — If these occur, you should take care to avoid driving, operating dangerous machinery, or doing delicate tasks. Change position slowly to avoid dizzy episodes.

   Change in sexual function — This can also be a discouraging effect. Be assured that it is a drug effect, and discuss it with your nurse or physician.

   Nausea, diarrhea — The gastrointestinal discomforts often pass over time; if they become too uncomfortable or persistent, notify your nurse or physician.

   Dreams, confusion — Again, these are drug effects. If they become too uncomfortable, notify your nurse or physician.

6. Avoid the use of OTC (over-the-counter) medications unless you have discussed it with your nurse or physician. Many of these preparations can block the desired effects of this drug.

7. If you have angina you must be careful while on this drug, because it may block the normal chest pain and warning signs that indicate that your heart needs more oxygen. If you are diabetic, you may not experience the usual signs and symptoms of an acute hypoglycemic attack. You will have to learn other ways of monitoring your blood glucose levels.

(continued)

8. You should learn to take your own pulse and monitor it on a daily basis. Your current pulse rate is —————— .

9. Tell any physician, nurse, or dentist who is taking care of you that you are on this drug.

10. Keep this and all medications out of the reach of children.

Notify your nurse or physician at once if any of the following occur:

Unusually slow pulse
Need to sleep on more pillows at
    night
Difficulty breathing
Swelling in ankles or fingers
Sudden weight gain
Mental confusion or personality
    change
Rash, fever

Case study

Presentation

Mr. R, a 59-year-old white man, suffered a diaphragmatic myocardial infarction (DMI) in August. He recovered very well and returned to work as a salesman within 8 weeks. He began to experience vague, pressure-type chest pains and was maintained on propranolol (Inderal), 10 mg qid, with no further problems. The following July Mr. R developed acute respiratory distress while picnicking with his family. On the way to an emergency room, he suffered an apparent respiratory arrest. He was admitted to the hospital and placed in the respiratory ICU. It was found that Mr. R had a history of hay fever and allergic rhinitis during the pollen season, but had never experienced such severe problems. Why did Mr. R have such a severe reaction? What appropriate measures should be taken after Mr. R recovers?

Discussion

Propranolol is a nonspecific β-adrenergic blocker. It was originally prescribed for Mr. R, postmyocardial infarction, for its β_1 sympathetic blocking effects, which decrease myocardial oxygen consumption. The blocking of the β_2-adrenergic receptors also prevents the bronchodilatation that normally occurs in response to sympathetic stimulation. In Mr. R's case, the inability of his sympathetic nervous system to respond with bronchodilatation during an attack of hay fever led to severe bronchoconstriction and respiratory arrest. Mr. R had probably never experienced a severe reaction to his hay fever in the past because his sympathetic nervous system produced adequate reflex bronchodilatation to compensate for the bronchoconstriction caused by the allergies. Mr. R was slowly tapered from his Inderal. It was very important to withdraw the β blocker slowly, in spite of Mr. R's respiratory problems, because of the danger that rapid withdrawal of the Inderal could pose to his heart.

After complete respiratory recovery and weaning from the Inderal, Mr. R was begun on a cardioselective β-adrenergic blocker, metoprolol. A very thorough patient history was taken to ensure that any other contraindications to drug therapy were not missed. Teaching measures were then reinforced for Mr. R regarding his coronary disease, his medications, and all the signs and symptoms of drug toxicity to which he should be alert.

α-Adrenergic blocking drugs

Mechanism of action

Drugs of this class act by occupying α-adrenergic receptors in smooth muscle and glands that are innervated by sympathetic postganglionic nerve fibers. By their ability to block access of the neurotransmitter and of circulating catecholamines or sympathomimetic drugs to these adrenoceptive sites, these agents reduce the responsiveness of the innervated cells and prevent the inhibited structures from functioning normally.

Pharmacologic action

Clinically, the most important action of α blockers occurs at the α receptors of *vascular smooth muscle* cells. By occupying these receptors, molecules of these drugs prevent the excitatory response to sympathetic stimulation (and to adrenergic drugs) that, it will be recalled, results typically in tonic constriction of the blood vessels. Other excitatory effects of sympathetic stimulation (*e.g.*, contraction of the radial muscle of the iris) may also be blocked, but pharmacologic effects of the α-adrenergic blockers that affect the patient's blood vessels are by far the most clinically significant.

As you should be able to predict (see Chap. 13), blockade of tonic sympathetic nerve impulses to a patient's arterioles results in relaxation of the smooth muscle walls. The resulting dilatation of the vessel should then lead to two effects: (1) an increased local flow of blood into the skin and other organs; and (2) a tendency for the arterial blood pressure to fall as a result of reduced peripheral resistance. Thus, one should expect these drugs to be tried in clinical conditions marked by poor local circulation or by excessively high diastolic blood pressure. These conditions (*e.g.*, peripheral vascular disease and hypertension) have, indeed, been the ones for which the α-adrenergic blockers have been employed. The older drugs have not been very successful clinically in these conditions, but a new α blocker, *prazosin*, differs significantly and is effective in controlling the blood pressure of patients with mild to moderately severe hypertension (Table 18-2).

Clinical uses

Hypertension. The older drugs of this class, *phenoxybenzamine*, *phentolamine*, and *tolazoline*, are no longer used in the treatment of primary hypertension, and have been replaced by newer and more effective drugs. A primary reason for the disappointing

Table 18–2. α-Adrenergic receptor blockers

Official or generic name	Trade name	Clinical indications	Usual adult dosage
Phenoxybenzamine HCl USP	Dibenzyline	Control of blood pressure in pheochromocytoma; vasospastic peripheral vascular disease	Initially, 10 mg/day PO; dose may be increased gradually up to 60 mg/day
Phentolamine HCl and mesylate USP	Regitine HCl; Regitine mesylate	Control of blood pressure in pheochromocytoma; diagnosis of pheochromocytoma; prevention and treatment of dermal necrosis caused by extravasation of α agonists	Hydrochloride: PO, 50 mg, 4–6 times/day, to control BP in pheochromocytoma; mesylate: parenterally, 2.5–5 mg IV, for diagnosis of pheochromocytoma; 10 mg is added to 1 liter of vasopressor IV solution to prevent necrosis or excessive vasoconstriction; 5–10 mg in 10 ml solution are infiltrated in area in which extravasation of an α agonist has occurred
Prazosin	Minipress	Hypertension	Initially, 1 mg bid or tid; first dose may cause syncope—observe patient up to 1½ hr; dose may be increased slowly up to 20 mg/day, in divided doses
Tolazoline HCl USP	Priscoline	Vasospastic peripheral vascular disease	10–50 mg qid SC, IM, or IV

performance of these older drugs in most cases of high blood pressure is the fact that they often cause adverse cardiac effects. Thus, their blockade of α-adrenergic receptors in the patient's blood vessels brings about a drop in pressure (especially when in the standing position), and this fall in systemic blood pressure activates baroreceptor reflexes that increase impulse activity in the sympathetic cardioaccelerator nerves (and in other sympathetic nerves to the heart). This causes reflex tachycardia. Such an increase in the speed and work of the hypertensive patient's heart can cause coronary insufficiency and set off anginal attacks, or it may even put the patient into heart failure. This is, of course, particularly likely in patients with a history of hypertensive heart disease.

The newest drug of this group, *prazosin* (Minipress), has proved to be clinically useful in hypertension because it is much less likely than the older α blockers to cause reflex tachycardia. The explanation of this difference between prazosin and the other, older α blockers is somewhat complex and requires reference to the α_2 receptors that were described in Chap. 13.

The α_2 receptors occur on the terminals of adrenergic nerves and mediate a feedback inhibition of norepinephrine release. That is, when norepinephrine is released by an adrenergic nerve terminal, some of the molecules act on postsynaptic adrenergic receptors (α or β) but some also act on the presynaptic α_2 receptors to inhibit the continued release of norepinephrine. The older α blockers are nonselective and block both the postsynaptic α receptors (sometimes now called α_1 receptors) and the presynaptic α_2 receptors. By contrast, prazosin blocks only the postsynaptic (α_1) receptors, and does not interfere with the negative feedback of norepinephrine release. This means that, when prazosin causes a decrease in blood pressure, the resulting reflex activation of cardiac sympathetic nerves releases less norepinephrine than when the older drugs cause a decrease in blood pressure; less reflex tachycardia results.

Pheochromocytoma. Some drugs of this class have also proved useful for both treatment and diagnosis of a type of *secondary* hypertension that develops in patients with *pheochromocytomata*. These are chromaffin cell tumors of the adrenal glands and elsewhere that secrete excessive amounts of epinephrine and norepinephrine into the patient's bloodstream. The abnormally high levels of these sympathomimetic substances cause chronically sustained high blood pressure in some patients and sudden attacks of paroxysmal hypertension in others.

Diagnosis. Although pheochromocytoma is a relatively rare disorder, some feel that all patients with a significant degree of hypertension should be tested to determine whether their abnormally high blood pressure is caused by a catecholamine-secreting tumor. This is because the condition, once discovered, is usually curable by surgery. Today, pheochromocytoma is usually best

diagnosed by biochemical screening tests to determine the amounts of catecholamines (and their metabolites) in the patient's urine and plasma. However, a pharmacologic test in which phentolamine mesylate (Regitine) is employed may also be used to confirm the biochemical diagnosis.

The fact that phentolamine is a relatively weak blocker of sympathetic nerve impulses is a factor in its efficacy when used for the differential diagnosis of pheochromocytoma. This screening test is based on the fact that a dose of phentolamine, too small to lower blood pressure by blocking sympathetic vasoconstrictor nerve impulses, can prevent the adrenergic receptors from responding to circulating catecholamines, thus causing a sharp drop in blood pressure that had been elevated by abnormally high levels of these sympathomimetic substances.

A *positive* test is one in which the patient's blood pressure quickly falls more than 35 mm Hg systolic and 25 mm Hg diastolic. Such a response to the phentolamine screening test in a patient with sustained hypertension alerts the physician to the possibility that the patient's high blood pressure may be the result of tumor-produced catecholamines.

Patients whose high blood pressure is stable or changes very little following a diagnostic injection of phentolamine are considered to have hypertension of other etiology. Because false negative and false positive test results sometimes occur in patients taking other drugs, patients should be told to take no medication for at least a day or two before being tested with phentolamine.

Treatment. The definitive treatment of pheochromocytoma requires the location and surgical removal of the tumor masses. However, orally administered phentolamine HCl and *phenoxybenzamine*[+] (Dibenzyline), a much longer acting α-adrenergic blocking agent, are useful for preparing the patient for surgery and for use during the surgical procedure. By blocking vascular α receptors, these drugs prevent the pressor response to circulating catecholamines. This lowers the patient's blood pressure and increases blood volume. The tachycardia and ventricular arrhythmias that occur in patients with epinephrine-secreting tumors are best prevented by adding the β-adrenergic blocker *propranolol* to the patient's regimen.

Phentolamine mesylate is administered by vein just before the patient is anesthetized to prevent sharp rises in blood pressure during intubation. Additional bolus doses are injected during the operation as the surgeon explores the patient's abdomen for tumors, because handling such tissue tends to force jets of epinephrine into the patient's bloodstream. This α-adrenergic blocker helps to prevent hypertension attacks and reflex supraventricular arrhythmias. Intravenously administered small doses of propranolol or of lidocaine, another antiarrhythmic drug, are employed to control ventricular arrhythmias.

In the period immediately following removal of

the pheochromocytoma, the patient's blood pressure often tends to fall. Often, restoring blood volume by infusing a plasma expander will return the pressure to a normal level. Sometimes, however, it may be necessary to employ an adrenergic vasopressor such as *levarterenol* (see Chap. 17). An advantage of having employed the relatively short-acting agent phentolamine during the operation, rather than the long-acting phenoxybenzamine, is that it has little residual blocking effect. Thus, the competitive vasopressor agonist can occupy the vascular α receptors to bring about vasoconstriction and a rise in peripheral resistance and blood pressure.

On the other hand, phenoxybenzamine is the best drug to use in patients with inoperable chromaffin tumors or in those too ill to tolerate surgery. Its long-lasting blockade of vascular α-adrenergic receptors usually keeps the patient's blood pressure at safe levels during long-term maintenance therapy. Some pheochromocytoma patients who have failed to respond to phenoxybenzamine have been treated with *metyrosine* (α-methyl-*p*-tyrosine; Demser). This drug is neither an α- nor a β-adrenergic blocker. It acts, instead, by inhibiting the enzyme tyrosine hydroxylase, which catalyzes the first step in the series of reactions by which the catecholamines dopamine, norepinephrine, and epinephrine are biosynthesized (see Chap. 13). Adverse effects of this drug are mainly referable to the CNS and include sedation, anxiety, psychic disturbances, and extrapyramidal signs sometimes accompanied by parkinsonism. These may be caused by the drug's interfering with the synthesis of dopamine and norepinephrine in the brain.

Other clinical uses. The α-adrenergic blocking drugs have their greatest clinical usefulness in the management of certain peripheral vascular diseases, particularly those in which a strong vasospastic component is responsible for the patient's poor local blood flow, such as Raynaud's disease, acrocyanosis, and the sequelae of frostbite. The use and status of such α-adrenergic blocking agents as phenoxybenzamine and tolazoline (Priscoline) for this purpose are discussed in Chapter 33.

Circulatory shock treatment is also sometimes facilitated by the use of phentolamine or phenoxybenzamine. Patients suffering from severe infection by gram-negative invaders of the bloodstream are said to benefit from treatment with α-adrenergic blockers, because shock caused by bacteremia (*endotoxin shock*) is marked by excessive reflex vasoconstriction. In such cases, intravenous injection of *phentolamine* or *phenoxybenzamine,* after the blood volume has first been restored by the administration of appropriate fluids, is said to result in improved blood flow.

Phentolamine mesylate (Regitine) is also sometimes employed as an adjunct to the potent vasopressor levarterenol, which is employed in treating other forms of shock. The addition of small doses of this drug to solutions of levarterenol helps to prevent necrosis and sloughing of the skin in case of leakage of levarterenol from the vein into the surrounding tissues. As indicated in Chapter 17, this α-adrenergic blocker may also be injected directly into the area of levarterenol extravasation to help dilate the extremely constricted local blood vessels. Phentolamine infiltration of the ischemic area is also now recommended within 12 hours of similar accidents with the vasopressor drug *dopamine* (Intropin). Occasionally, phentolamine or phenoxybenzamine may be administered by vein in conjunction with levarterenol or dopamine. Their use tends to counteract any excessive α-agonist vasoconstriction caused by these vasopressors without interfering with their desirable cardiac effects.

Additional clinical considerations

Prazosin often produces what is called a "first-dose effect." In many patients, the first dose of prazosin produces dizziness, syncope, and loss of consciousness within 30 to 90 minutes. The exact mechanism of this reaction is unclear. There is often a severe drop in blood pressure, associated with a reflex tachycardia. Because of this first-dose effect, the patient is started on a low dose of prazosin, which is slowly increased. If starting the drug at home, the patient should probably be advised to take the drug at bedtime to avoid any falls or serious injury if fainting does occur. The α-adrenergic blocking drugs should not be used during pregnancy or lactation because of the potential risk to the fetus and infant.

Some special problems involved with the use of prazosin include reddened sclera, blurred vision, tinnitus, and nasal congestion. The patient needs to be aware of the possibility of these effects. The nasal congestion, or feeling of "stuffiness," can sometimes be relieved by use of a saline nasal solution. The patient must be cautioned, however, about the use of OTC allergy medications, cold preparations, or nasal sprays that contain sympathomimetic drugs (*e.g.,* ephedrine). If absorbed systemically, these OTC drugs can antagonize the desired effects of the prazosin.

As with the β blockers, this drug should not be discontinued suddenly. The patient will need to receive teaching about the dangers involved.

Prazosin is a highly protein-bound drug, and could interact with other highly protein-bound drugs. This is an important consideration to keep in mind if unexpected drug effects should occur in a patient on this combination of drugs. No specific clinically significant drug–drug interactions have been reported.

The patient teaching guide for prazosin summarizes the points that should be incorporated into the patient education plan. The guide to the nursing process with adrenergic blocking drugs summarizes the application of the nursing process to this drug therapy.

Patient teaching guide: prazosin

The drug that has been prescribed for you is called an α-adrenergic blocking drug. It acts to block the stimulation of blood vessel muscles, and thus causes blood vessels to dilate. This relaxation of the blood vessels lowers the blood pressure. Your current blood pressure is _____ .

Instructions:

1. The name of your drug is Minipress.

2. The dosage of your drug is _____ .

3. Your drug should be taken _____ times a day. The best time to take your drug is _____ , _____ , _____ . The first dose of this drug may cause dizziness or fainting. Because of this, it would be advisable to take the first dose of the drug, or the first dose of any increased dosage of drug, at bedtime.

4. Some side-effects of this drug that you should be aware of include the following:

Nasal "stuffiness," red eyes	Saline nasal solution might help, but do *not* use over-the-counter cold or allergy medications.
Dizziness	Avoid sudden changes in position; take safety precautions to avoid falls.
Drowsiness	Avoid driving a car or operating dangerous machinery if this occurs.
Change in sexual function	This can be very upsetting; be assured that it is a drug effect; discuss it with your nurse or physician.
Headache	This will usually pass after a few days on the drug.

5. Never discontinue this drug suddenly. If you find that your prescription is running out, notify your nurse or physician.

6. Avoid the use of over-the-counter medications; if you feel that you need some of these preparations, discuss this with your nurse or physician.

7. Tell any physician, nurse, or dentist who is taking care of you that you are on this drug.

8. Keep this and all medications out of the reach of children.

Notify your nurse or physician if any of the following occur:

> Difficulty in breathing
> Swelling in fingers or ankles
> Sudden weight gain
> Rash, fever

Assessment	Nursing diagnoses	Interventions	Evaluation
Past history—underlying medical conditions (*contraindications*): Chronic obstructive pulmonary disease Asthma Congestive heart failure Hypotension–shock Bradycardia–heart block Diabetes mellitus Pregnancy Lactation *Allergies: these drugs;* others; reactions Medication history (*cautions*): MAO inhibitors Catecholamine-depleting drugs Aminophylline OTC drugs Propranolol and: chlorpromazine, insulin, furosemide, cimetidine, hydralazine, phenytoin, phenobarbital, cigarette smoking, OTC drugs	Potential alteration in cardiac output Potential alteration in tissue perfusion Potential sexual dysfunction Potential alteration in sensory–perceptual status Potential for impaired gas exchange Knowledge deficit regarding drug therapy	Safe and proper drug administration Provision of comfort measures: Safety measures with dizziness, drowsiness Spacing of activities and provision of rest periods Warm clothing on extremities in cold weather Support and encouragement to cope with sexual dysfunction, fatigue, drowsiness, other drug effects Patient teaching: Drug Dosage Side-effects Cautions Warnings Taking pulse	Evaluate effectiveness of drug: desired therapeutic effect Evaluate side-effects of drug: CHF Heart block Respiratory failure Hypoglycemia Sexual dysfunction CNS effects Peripheral vasoconstriction Evaluate for drug–drug interactions: No effect of therapy with *MAO inhibitors, aminophylline* Hypoglycemia with *insulin* (β blockers) ↑ Propranolol toxicity with *chlorpromazine, cimetidine, furosemide, hydralazine* ↓ Propranolol effects with *phenytoin, phenobarbital, cigarette smoking* Evaluate for drug–laboratory test interaction: ↑ *BUN* levels with propranolol, timolol ↑ K, *uric acid* levels with timolol ↑ *SGOT*, ↑ *SGPT* levels with pindolol Altered *glucose tolerance tests*

Physical assessment
Neurologic: mental status, orientation, affect
Cardiovascular: BP (supine, standing, sitting), P, apical pulse (extra sounds, rate, rhythm), EKG (baseline reading), peripheral perfusion
Respiratory: rate, rhythm, adventitious sounds
Skin: color, temperature, vascular filling
Tests: blood sugar, BUN

* Some contraindications and nursing diagnoses do not apply equally to β- and α-blockers. Please refer to text for specific details of the drug you are using.

Table 18–3. Ganglionic blocking drugs

Official or generic name	Trade name	Clinical indications	Usual adult dosage
Mecamylamine HCl USP	Inversine	Severe hypertension	Initially, 2.5 mg bid PO; dose may be increased gradually to 25 mg/day in divided doses
Pentolinium tartrate	Ansolysen	Severe hypertension	20–60 mg/day, PO (no longer available in United States)
Trimethaphan camsylate USP	Arfonad	To produce controlled hypotension during surgery; hypertensive crises	Initially, 3–4 mg/min by IV infusion of 1 mg/ml solution in 5% dextrose; adjust dosage according to response

Ganglionic stimulation and blockade

Acetylcholine (ACh) is the neurotransmitter responsible for transmission of nerve impulses from preganglionic to postganglionic nerves in both divisions of the autonomic nervous system. When the neurotransmitter is released by preganglionic nerve impulses from storage sites in the nerve endings of the first neurons in the chain, it acts to depolarize the nerve cell bodies of the second neurons, located in the ganglia. This results in the propagation of nerve impulses that pass down the postganglionic parasympathetic and sympathetic fibers to the smooth muscle and gland cells that they innervate (see Chap. 13).

This stimulating action of ACh on the ganglia is called *nicotinic,* because early investigators noted that the tobacco alkaloid nicotine produced the same sort of stimulating effects as ACh at autonomic ganglia and on skeletal muscles. An excess of nicotine, however, can block ganglionic and skeletal muscle transmission by making the cells insensitive to ACh. Thus, the initial stimulating effects of nicotine may be followed by depression and paralysis of the ganglia if the amount administered is large enough.

Neither nicotine nor any other substance that acts to *stimulate* the ganglia is employed clinically. However, the ganglion-stimulating effects of nicotine play a significant part in the effects it has when inhaled during tobacco smoking.* Neither these effects nor the other deleterious effects of cigarette smoking will be discussed here, even though these subjects are of infinitely more importance to the public health than the drugs taken up in the following section.

The drugs that are employed clinically for their effects on autonomic ganglia are agents that block transmission at this site *without* first stimulating the ganglia (like nicotine). That is, the ganglionic blocking drugs—like the α- and β-adrenergic blocking drugs discussed above—act as competitive antagonists when their molecules occupy receptor sites on the membranes of postganglionic nerve cell bodies in both sympathetic and parasympathetic ganglia. These drugs also block receptors of the adrenal medullary cells that secrete epinephrine and norepinephrine into the circulation. Thus, they also block the transmission of sympathetic impulses to these cells. Drugs of this type have been used mainly for their blocking effects on sympathetic ganglia and on the adrenal medulla in the treatment of hypertension.

Today, however, the ganglionic blocking agents have been largely replaced by newer more selective and less toxic drugs (Table 18-3). The newer drugs (see Chap. 28) are not only more reliable for lowering blood pressure but also have the advantage of not interfering with transmission in parasympathetic ganglia. Thus, the drugs that act only on sympathetic nerves are free of the adverse effects on gastrointestinal tract and urinary system function of the ganglionic blocking agents—for example, constipation, paralytic ileus, and urinary bladder paralysis with urine retention. Only two ganglionic blockers are still available in the United States, *trimethaphan* (Arfonad) and *mecamylamine* (Inversine). *Pentolinium, chlorisondamine, pempidine,* and *tetraethylammonium* are still used in other countries.

The use of the ganglionic blocking agent trimethaphan (Arfonad) in the emergency management of acute hypertensive crisis is discussed in Chapter 28, and the status of this class of drugs in the treatment of peripheral vascular diseases is taken up in Chapter 33. Refer to these chapters for clinical considerations and the application of the nursing process in the use of these drugs.

---

* Stimulation of sympathetic ganglia and of the adrenal medulla by the small amounts of nicotine inhaled with tobacco smoke causes constriction of blood vessels and an increase in heart rate and blood pressure. These effects can be harmful to people with various cardiovascular disorders, and probably play a part in the higher death rate from coronary and cerebrovascular disease among cigarette smokers. Stimulation of parasympathetic ganglia can stimulate gastric acid secretion and gastrointestinal motility. These effects can be harmful to patients with peptic ulcer disease and other gatrointestinal disorders. However, other substances in tobacco smoke are actually much more significant than nicotine in causing fatal illnesses among the several hundred thousand people who die prematurely each year as a result of habitual smoking of tobacco.

Drug digests

Phenoxybenzamine HCl USP (Dibenzyline)

Actions and indications. This α-adrenergic blocking agent produces dilation of blood vessels in the skin. The better flow of blood to the skin of patients with certain peripheral vascular disorders may provide some symptomatic relief. Among vasospastic conditions benefited are frostbite, Raynaud's disease, acrocyanosis, and causalgia. It is *not* useful for treating thromboangiitis obliterans (Buerger's disease) or other disorders in which vessel walls are damaged.

Although this drug is also not very useful for reducing blood pressure in essential hypertension, it can help to prevent pressure rises in patients with pheochromocytoma when administered before and during surgery. The drug is being used experimentally to improve circulation in shock cases resistant to other treatment measures.

Adverse effects, cautions, and contraindications. Minor side-effects of blockade of sympathetic nerve impulses include nasal congestion, bronchoconstriction, and miosis. More serious effects of overdosage are postural hypotension and reflex tachycardia, because these effects can lead to a heart attack, congestive heart failure, stroke, or kidney failure in patients with coronary or cerebral atherosclerosis or renal damage.

Dosage and administration. Treatment is started at a dosage level of 10 mg daily. This is increased gradually to levels high enough to offer symptomatic relief without causing discomforting or dangerous side effects. The usual individually adjusted optimum daily dosage is between 20 mg and 60 mg.

Phentolamine mesylate USP (Regitine)

Actions and indications. This α-adrenergic blocking agent is used mainly for the diagnosis of pheochromocytoma. A positive test for this tumor is suggested by a prompt and persistent fall in blood pressure by more than 35 mm Hg systolic and 25 mm Hg diastolic. This drug is also injected intravenously during surgery for pheochromocytoma, if manipulation of the tumor leads to sudden release of large amounts of epinephrine with a resulting rapid rise in blood pressure to dangerous levels (hypertensive crisis).

Adverse effects, cautions, and contraindications. The drug-induced fall in blood pressure may set off reflex tachycardia. Thus, this drug is contraindicated in patients with coronary artery disease, including angina pectoris. Overdosage may also cause a severe sustained fall in blood pressure. This is best treated by infusion of fluids to fill the dilated vascular tree, followed by administration of levarterenol to counteract adrenergic blockade of the blood vessels.

Dosage and administration. For diagnosis, a single dose of 2.5 mg or 5 mg is injected intravenously or intramuscularly under standard conditions. For treatment of hypertensive crisis, this dose may be administered repeatedly or the drug solution may be infused continuously.

To prevent sloughing from leakage of levarterenol infusion solutions, infiltration of the affected area with 10 ml to 15 ml of phentolamine solution (5 mg to 10 mg) is recommended.

An oral dosage form, phentolamine HCl USP, is available for use in doses of 50 mg four to six times daily in the period prior to surgery.

Propranolol HCl USP (Inderal)

Actions and indications. This prototype β-adrenergic blocking agent is employed mainly in the management of cardiac arrhythmias, angina pectoris, and essential hypertension. It is also used in treating such relatively rare conditions as hypertrophic subaortic stenosis, an obstructive cardiomyopathy, and pheochromocytoma, a type of chromaffin cell tumor that releases catecholamines into the systemic circulation.

The drug's effectiveness for control of several supraventricular arrhythmias and some ventricular arrhythmias stems from its ability to block cardiac, or β_1-type, adrenergic receptors by reversible competitive inhibition. This decreases the responsiveness of cardiac tissues to sympathetic nerve stimulation and to circulating catecholamines.

The drug's beneficial effects in angina pectoris are the result of its ability to reduce the demands of the ischemic myocardium for oxygen. This is also a result of reduced responsiveness of the heart to sympathetic stimulation, which leads to a slowing of the heart and a lessening of its contractile force and of the cardiac output. Improvement is manifested by an increase in exercise tolerance as indicated by delayed development of electrocardiographic changes and chest pains.

Reduction in blood pressure is probably brought about by several actions that include not only a decrease in cardiac output, but also a reduction in the release of renin by the kidneys, and an effect on the vasomotor center.

Adverse effects, cautions, and contraindications. Adverse cardiac effects include excessive slowing of the heart rate, block of A-V conduction, and decreased myocardial contractility. Thus, the drug is contraindicated in sinus bradycardia and second- or third-degree heart block and in most patients with congestive heart failure.

Because its use can cause bronchoconstriction, it is contraindicated in bronchial asthma and used only with caution in such other chronic obstructive lung diseases as emphysema and chronic bronchitis. Its use during the pollen season is contraindicated for allergic rhinitis patients. Caution is required in labile diabetics who are being treated with insulin or oral hypoglycemic agents, because this drug may mask signs and symptoms of diabetes drug overdosage.

Central side-effects include fatigue and lightheadedness. Occasionally, psychiatric disturbances develop, including mental depression, disorientation, and hallucinations. Gastrointestinal side-effects such as nausea, vomiting, abdominal cramps and distress, and diarrhea are occasionally reported.

Dosage and administration. Dosage must be adjusted for each patient, because the dosage range varies widely in different patients and for different indications. In general, treatment is initiated with small doses that are gradually raised until an optimal response is achieved.

In angina pectoris, the patient is started on 10 to 20 mg tid or qid and then increased at intervals of 3 to 7 days. The average optimal dose is 160 mg, but some patients may require up to 320 mg or more. The drug should not be abruptly discontinued, because this may lead to a worsening of anginal symptoms and to more severe degrees of coronary heart disease. Thus, dosage should be gradually reduced.

Hypertensive patients are started on daily doses of 80 mg, which are then raised to as high as 640 mg or more. The usual dosage range required for optimal blood pressure control is between 160 and 480 mg a day. For treating arrhythmias, oral doses ranging from 10 to 30 mg tid or qid are administered before meals and at bedtime. For life-threatening arrhythmias, including those which occur during anesthesia, this drug may be administered intravenously in doses of 1 mg to 3 mg at a rate of not more than 1 mg/min with careful electrocardiographic and clinical monitoring.

References

Aellig WH: Clinical pharmacology of pindolol. Am Heart J 104:346, 1982

Alderman EL et al: Coronary artery syndromes after sudden propranolol withdrawal. Ann Intern Med 81:625, 1974

Aviado DM: Hemodynamic effects of ganglionic blocking drugs. Circulation Res 8:304, 1960

Buhler FR et al: Antihypertensive action of propranolol. Am J Cardiol 32:511, 1973

Epstein SE, Braunwald E: Beta adrenergic receptor blocking drugs. Mechanisms of action and clinical applications. N Engl J Med 275:1106, 1966

Frishman WH: β-adrenoceptor antagonists: New drugs and new indications. N Engl J Med 305:500, 1981

Gibson DG: Pharmacodynamic properties of beta adrenergic blocking drugs in man. Drugs 7:8, 1974

Harris A: Long-term treatment of paroxysmal cardiac arrhythmias with propranolol. Am J Cardiol 18:431, 1966

Hjalmarson A et al: Effect on mortality of metoprolol in acute myocardial infarction. Lancet 2:823, 1981

Johnson GP, Johnson BC: Beta blockers. Am J Nursing 83:1034, 1983

Koch–Weser J: Metoprolol. N Engl J Med 301:698, 1979

Kvale WF et al: Present-day diagnosis and treatment of pheochromocytoma. JAMA 164:854, 1957

Manger WM, Gifford RW, Jr: Pheochromocytoma: Diagnosis and management. NY State J Med 80:216, 1980

Nies AS, Shand DG: Clinical pharmacology of propranolol. Circulation 52:6, 1975

Rangno RE: Stopping beta blockers in patients with angina. Ration Drug Ther 15:1, 1981

Salem MR: Therapeutic uses of ganglionic blocking drugs. Int Anesthesiol Clin 16:171, 1978

Scriabine A: β-adrenoceptor blocking drugs in hypertension. Annu Rev Pharmacol Toxicol 19:269, 1979

Shand DG: Propranolol. N Engl J Med 293:280, 1975

Sharpe CJ: Propranolol in the treatment of migraine. Br Med J 3:522, 1974

Soffer A: Phentolamine (Regitine) and piperoxan (Benodaine) in the diagnosis of pheochromocytoma. Med Clin North Am 33:375, 1954

Spergel G et al: A modified phentolamine test for the diagnosis of pheochromocytoma. JAMA 211:266, 1970

Taylor P: Ganglionic stimulating and blocking agents. In Gilman AG, Goodman LS, Gilman A (eds): Goodman & Gilman's The Pharmacological Basis of Therapeutics, 6th ed, pp 211–219. New York, Macmillan, 1980

Weiner N: Drugs that inhibit adrenergic nerves and block adrenergic receptors. In Gilman AG, Goodman LS, Gilman A (eds): Goodman & Gilman's The Pharmacological Basis of Therapeutics, 6th ed, pp 176–210. New York, Macmillan, 1980

Widerbe TE, Vigander T: Propranolol in the treatment of migraine. Br Med J 2:699, 1974

Chapter 19

Neuromuscular junction blocking drugs

19

General considerations

This chapter will discuss the actions and clinical applications of drugs that produce profound relaxation and even paralysis of skeletal muscles. These drugs should *not* be confused with *centrally acting skeletal muscle relaxants* (Chap. 48), which act in the brain or spinal cord and produce relatively mild effects on spastic skeletal muscles, nor should they be confused with parasympathetic blocking drugs (Chap. 16), which can relax spasms of gastrointestinal and urinary tract smooth muscle and are sometimes called *antispasmodics*. The very potent skeletal muscle paralyzing drugs described in this chapter bring about their effects by acting at peripheral sites. Specifically, these drugs interfere with the transmission of nerve impulses from motor nerve terminals to the skeletal muscle fibers that they innervate. These drugs are sometimes referred to as skeletal muscle relaxants, or just as muscle relaxants. To avoid confusion this text will refer to them by the more cumbersome term, neuromuscular junction blocking drugs.

As discussed in Chapter 13, transmission of impulses at the neuromuscular junctions is mediated by the neurotransmitter *acetylcholine* (ACh), which is released from the nerve terminals in which it is stored in presynaptic vesicles. The molecules of this chemical transmitter then diffuse across the synaptic cleft and combine with cholinergic receptors on the postjunctional muscle membranes (Fig. 19-1; see also Fig. 13-6). This, in turn, makes the membranes more permeable to sodium and potassium ions with resulting local depolarization and development of an action potential, which excites the muscle fibers of the motor units and causes them to contract.

Mechanism of action

Drugs and toxins can interfere in various ways with this sequence of events. Those therapeutic agents

that are used clinically as neuromuscular junction (NMJ) blockers act on cholinergic receptors on the postjunctional membranes. They bring about flaccid paralysis in two different ways and are classified on this basis as *competitive nondepolarizing* and as *depolarizing* neuromuscular blocking agents.

Drugs such as *tubocurarine*[+] (Tubarine) and the others listed in Table 19-1 as *non*depolarizing NMJ blockers compete with molecules of ACh for cholinergic receptor sites and prevent the muscle membranes from being depolarized and from producing the action potential that causes muscles to contract. Unlike the neurotransmitter ACh, the bulky molecules of these curariform drugs occupy the cholinergic receptors without activating the train of metabolic events that ordinarily occurs when ACh molecules released by nerve endings reach these receptors. The continued presence of the blocking drug prevents ACh from binding to and depolarizing the membrane and from triggering contractions of the muscle fibers of the motor unit. However, the loss of muscle tone caused by this type of competitive blockade can be counteracted by increasing the number of ACh molecules that accumulate at the NMJ. This can sometimes be accomplished clinically by administering repeated small doses of drugs that inhibit *acetylcholinesterase*, the enzyme responsible for the metabolic breakdown of the neurotransmitter ACh (see Chap. 13 and discussions of neostigmine and physostigmine in Chap. 15).

Drugs such as *succinylcholine*[+] (Anectine; Quelicin; Sucostrin) that are classified as *depolarizing*-type muscle relaxants (Table 19-1) act somewhat differently. These drugs also occupy cholinergic receptors on the postjunctional muscle membrane. However, unlike the *non*depolarizing blockers discussed above, these drugs act initially like ACh. That is, they also depolarize the motor end-plate membranes and, by doing so, they at first set off a series of transient muscle fiber contractions seen

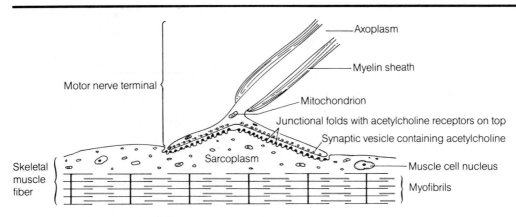

Figure 19-1. The mammalian neuromuscular junction. The motor nerve loses its myelin sheath as it contacts the specialized area of skeletal muscle membrane on which acetylcholine receptors are found.

clinically as fasciculations, or twitchings, of isolated muscle groups.

A major difference between these depolarizing drugs and the natural neurotransmitter ACh, which is instantly destroyed by the enzyme acetylcholinesterase, is that the drug molecules resist such destruction and remain attached to the cholinergic receptors for a relatively long period. This leads to a *persistent depolarization* of the membrane that prevents its *re*polarization, and thus reduces its responsiveness to further volleys of nerve

Table 19–1. NMJ blocking drugs

Official or generic name	Trade name	Usual adult dosage range
Competitive, *non*depolarizing blockers		
Atracurium besylate	Tracrium	0.4–0.5 mg/kg as IV bolus
Gallamine triethiodide USP	Flaxedil	1.0 mg/kg body weight with a total dose of 40–80 mg, at one time
Hexafluorenium bromide USP	Mylaxen	0.4 mg/kg
Metocurine iodide USP	Metubine iodide	0.2–0.4 mg/kg body weight, depending on the anesthetic to be employed
Pancuronium bromide	Pavulon	0.04–0.1 mg/kg body weight initially, with later increments starting at 0.01 mg/kg
Tubocurarine chloride USP	Tubarine	0.1–0.3 mg/kg body weight initially
Depolarizing blockers		
Decamethonium bromide USP	Syncurine	0.5–3.0 mg initially
Succinylcholine chloride USP	Anectine; Quelicin; Sucostrin	2.5–4 mg/kg body weight after an initial test dose of 10 mg

Table 19–2. Interactions of NMJ blocking drugs with other drugs

Drugs	Effect(s)
Competitive nondepolarizing blocking drugs with:	
Volatile general anesthetics such as diethyl ether, enflurane, halothane, methoxyflurane, isoflurane	Depth and duration of NMJ blockade are intensified; dosage of the blocking agent should be reduced by at least one-third initially
Quinine and quinidine	May increase NMJ blockade and cause recurarization and respiratory paralysis if administered during postoperative recovery period
Magnesium sulfate; calcium salts; propranolol; trimethaphan	May increase NMJ blockade
Aminoglycoside antibiotics; bacitracin; polymyxin-B; tetracyclines	Increase the degree of NMJ blockade
Neostigmine and physostigmine (anticholinesterase drugs)	Antagonize NMJ block
Depolarizing blocking drugs with:	
Neostigmine and physostigmine (anticholinesterase drugs)	Prolong and intensify NMJ blockade
Procaine-type local anesthetics	Tend to prolong the NMJ blockade
All antibiotics except penicillin; oxytocin, chloroquine; furosemide	May increase the intensity of NMJ block
Hexafluorenium	Prevents early contractions by SCC and may prolong duration of action of SCC

impulses. After the initial drug-induced increase in muscle fiber contractions, therefore, a flaccid paralysis soon sets in that appears similar clinically to that produced by the *non*depolarizing NMJ blocking drugs. The patient's muscles remain relaxed or paralyzed until the molecules of the depolarizing drugs finally leave the receptors and diffuse away into the bloodstream, where they are destroyed in chemical reactions catalyzed by *plasma* enzymes called *pseudocholinesterases.**

One difference between these two types of NMJ blockers is that the block caused by drugs such as succinylcholine (SCC), which produce persistent depolarization, *cannot* ordinarily be counteracted by administering acetylcholinesterase inhibitor drugs. In fact, as indicated in Table 19-2, drugs such as the anticholinesterase agents neostigmine and physostigmine may actually intensify and prolong the NMJ blockade that results from SCC-induced

persistent depolarization of the skeletal muscle fiber motor end-plates.

Competitive nondepolarizing NMJ blockers

History
Curare is a term employed traditionally to describe various substances that South American Indians have used for centuries to paralyze and kill the small game that they hunted for food. These primitive people learned to prepare crude extracts of certain tropical plants from various *Chondodendron* and *Strychnos* species, which they then applied to the tips of their arrows, darts, and spears. Animals wounded even superficially by these poisoned points were unable to run far before collapsing as a result of skeletal muscle paralysis. The flesh of small game immobilized or killed in this manner could be safely eaten, because the poison is not absorbed from the gastrointestinal tract.

Although crude curare was first studied scientifically more than a century ago, its composition and

---

* This term is used to distinguish this enzyme from the above-mentioned acetylcholinesterase found at NMJs, which is sometimes referred to as "true" cholinesterase.

strength were, until rather recently, too variable and its action too uncertain to permit its safe use in clinical medicine. It was only after the purified alkaloid *d*-tubocurarine was isolated from the plant *Chondodendron tomentosum* in 1935 that these peripherally acting muscular relaxants could be put to use in clinical practice.

Once the chemical structure of the natural alkaloid was known, chemists were able to synthesize substances of similar but simpler structure that also proved potent as neuromuscular blocking agents. Most natural and synthetic curarelike substances contain positively charged quaternary ammonium groups, as does ACh. Some are several times as potent as *d*-tubocurarine in their ability to compete with ACh and to stabilize the muscle cell membrane against the depolarizing action of the neurotransmitter.

Pharmacologic effects

By far the most important effect of the curariform drugs, when administered in the doses employed clinically, is the skeletal muscle relaxation and paralysis produced by their *non*depolarizing competitive action described above. Occasionally, however, some of these drugs also act at the other type of nicotinic site—the autonomic ganglia (see Chaps. 13 and 18)—and, in some cases, at such muscarinic sites of cholinergic transmission as the vagal postganglionic cholinergic receptors in the heart. In addition, as discussed below, some of these drugs release histamine from mast cells and other tissues (Chap. 39).

Muscle paralysis

The paralysis produced by these drugs progressively affects various muscle groups in a specific sequence that can be observed when small doses are administered intermittently. Although patients usually receive a general anesthetic that makes them unconscious before NMJ blockers are given, these drugs are sometimes given to conscious patients suffering from tetanus. In such cases the sequence of paralysis can be observed. The first muscles to show signs of weakness are those innervated by motor fibers of cranial nerves. Thus, the patient may first find it difficult to keep the eyelids up or vision focused, and this is quickly followed by difficulty in swallowing and in talking. It is of interest that these small muscles are also often the first to show weakness when a patient develops myasthenia gravis (see Chap. 15); patients with this neuromuscular disorder are extremely sensitive to small doses of curariform drugs.

The next muscles to lose their tone and relax during a slow infusion of an NMJ blocking agent are those of the limbs and abdomen. Finally, the muscles responsible for respiratory movements become paralyzed—that is, the *intercostal* muscles that control rib cage movements, and the *diaphragm,* the sheet of skeletal muscle fibers which separates the thoracic and abdominal cavities. Clinically, these drugs are most often employed to produce relaxation (paralysis) of the muscles of the abdomen and the extremities. However, the dosage that will bring about these desired effects is so close to the dosage that will paralyze the muscles of respiration that breathing difficulties are a common occurrence. This narrow safety margin, which makes some degree of respiratory embarrassment and even apnea almost unavoidable, makes it imperative to have readily available the necessary equipment for maintaining the patient's respiration artificially until the effects of the NMJ blocking agents wear off.

Other actions

The actions at other sites and by other mechanisms mentioned above account for certain adverse cardiovascular and respiratory effects sometimes seen with tubocurarine, particularly when it is injected too rapidly by the intravenous route. Some of the synthetic nondepolarizing agents, such as *pancuronium bromide* (Pavulon) and *atracurium besylate* (Tracrium), for example, are claimed relatively free of such side-effects. Thus, these drugs and *gallamine* (Flaxedil), an NMJ blocking drug that also exerts an atropinelike vagal blocking action, are said to be superior to tubocurarine for some patients and when certain anesthetics are to be employed.

Although tubocurarine primarily blocks the skeletal NMJ, it may also sometimes block autonomic ganglia. That is, the molecules of this drug may occasionally prevent ACh from transmitting nerve impulses at some of the synapses between preganglionic fibers and ganglionic neurons, as well as at the NMJs in skeletal muscles. Such a partial blockade of the sympathetic ganglia, which relay tonic vasoconstrictor nerve impulses to the smooth muscle walls of the blood vessels, may lead to a loss of their tone. The resulting vasodilation is one cause of the circulatory collapse that sometimes occurs from overdosage with tubocurarine.

Pancuronium, *metocurine*, and *alcuronium* (Alloferin; not available in the United States), unlike tubocurarine, do *not* cause ganglionic blockade or hypotension, but pancuronium and gallamine *can* block vagal influences on the heart and cause a slight rise in the heart rate and blood pressure. Thus, these two drugs may be preferred when the general anesthetic *halothane,* which tends to cause bradycardia and hypotension, is to be inhaled. On the other hand, gallamine may cause cardiac arrhythmias.

Another disadvantage of tubocurarine, compared to pancuronium and the other competitive blockers, is that this curare alkaloid sometimes causes some tissues to release *histamine*. The vasodilating effects of free histamine on the arterioles and capillaries (Chap. 39) may add to the danger of circulatory depression from tubocurarine. Histamine freed by the curare alkaloid may also cause bronchial constriction, thus adding to the breathing difficulties the patient may be suffering. Because such reactions are especially undesirable in patients with bronchial asthma, pancuronium and SCC (see below), which rarely cause histamine release, are the preferred muscle relaxants for these and other patients with chronic obstructive respiratory diseases. *Hexafluorenium,* listed in Table 19-1 as a competitive blocker, is used only as an adjunct to SCC (see below).

Pharmacokinetic factors

When these drugs are administered by vein, they are quickly carried to their principal site of action and are rapidly taken up by cholinergic receptors at the NMJ. Their molecules are unaffected by the presence of the enzyme acetylcholinesterase at that site, and termination of the relatively long blockade produced by these drugs begins only as their molecules diffuse away to other sites in the body. Little biotransformation to inactive metabolites occurs with tubocurarine or other drugs of this group as a result either of the action of plasma pseudocholinesterase-type enzymes (see below) or of degradation by hepatic drug-metabolizing enzymes.

Drugs of this group are, instead, eliminated almost entirely by the kidneys, except for atracurium, which is rapidly inactivated in the plasma by a nonenzymatic reaction, and pancuronium and *fazadinium* (another competitive blocker not available in the United States), which are also partially inactivated by the liver. Clinically, this means that the duration of tubocurarine's action may be prolonged in patients with severe renal disease, and caution is required when pancuronium or fazadinium is employed in patients with liver disorders, as well as in those with kidney disease.

These quaternary ammonium compounds do not pass the blood–brain barrier (Chap. 4). Thus, they have no effect on a patient's consciousness or ability to perceive pain. Because of this, it is important to remember that, unless they are under general anesthesia, patients paralyzed by these drugs have normal hearing, vision, and pain perception, but are unable to ask questions or to communicate the fact that they are feeling severe pain, if that is the case.

Drug–drug interactions

The prior administration of thiopental or nitrous oxide to produce unconsciousness or of potent narcotic analgesics or droperidol to prevent awareness of or reaction to painful stimuli does *not* prolong the duration of the NMJ blockade produced by these drugs. However, *ether* and *halothane* or such other fluorinated inhalation anesthetics as *methoxyflurane* and *enflurane* can intensify the block and lengthen the period of paralysis. Thus, when these anesthetics are used, the blocking agents must be administered, at first, in smaller doses than usual. The patient's response to infusion of the smaller dose should be observed and noted as a guide to determining the size of any supplemental doses that may be necessary.

Other drugs that may potentiate the action of curariform muscle relaxants include such aminoglycoside-class antibiotics as *gentamicin, kanamycin, neomycin,* and *streptomycin. Quinidine* may also cause deeper curarization. On the other hand, the administration of *potassium salts* may interfere with the effectiveness of the NMJ blockade produced by these drugs. As indicated previously, blockade of the skeletal NMJ can be antagonized by *neostigmine, edrophonium,* and other anticholinesterase-type cholinergic drugs.

Depolarizing NMJ blockers

Succinylcholine (SCC) is by far the most important neuromuscular blocking agent of this subclass, and decamethonium is now rarely used in this country (Table 19-1). SCC has a very rapid onset and brief duration of action. These properties make it particularly suited for use in short procedures. *Decamethonium* is long-acting and, when a long-acting agent is needed, one of the competitive blockers, whose actions can be reversed by a cholinesterase inhibitor, is usually preferred.

Pharmacologic actions

Muscular effects

As previously indicated, SCC and similarly acting NMJ blocking drugs produce a flaccid paralysis that looks no different from that which follows administration of a nondepolarizing blocking agent.

Initial stimulation. The major difference in the muscular effects of SCC as compared to those of tubocurarine is that the depolarizing-type blocker first causes groups of muscle fibers to fibrillate before they are paralyzed. This is particularly true when the intravenous injection is administered rapidly as a bolus dose and after repeated administration of many small doses. This preliminary fasciculation-producing effect has potentially harmful consequences in the patient in whom SCC is employed clinically.

Pain. A high proportion of patients complain of postoperative muscle pain, particularly in the abdomen, trunk, and shoulders. This is thought to be caused by local damage to the muscles resulting when some muscle groups contract while others are unaffected—a circumstance that leads to a muscle shearing or tearing effect. Patients do not ordinarily feel such pain during injection of SCC, because they have first been given a general anesthetic.

Another way in which postoperative muscle pain may be reduced is by first administering a small dose of the *nondepolarizing* blocker *hexafluorenium* (Mylaxen). This double-drug procedure is also sometimes used in patients with fractures, in whom the initial muscle contractions produced by SCC alone would be especially injurious. Hexafluorenium has the additional property of inhibiting pseudocholinesterase, and it is sometimes given with SCC to delay the metabolism of SCC and to prolong its duration of action.

The initial muscle contraction trauma caused by SCC also has secondary effects with possibly serious significance for some patients. Injury to the muscle cells is often followed by release of potassium ions, certain enzymes, and myoglobin into the systemic circulation. The drug-induced hyperkalemia can cause cardiac arrhythmias and possibly even cardiac arrest in certain categories of patients, including those under treatment with digitalis or quinidine (Chaps. 29 and 30). Other patients who might become seriously hyperkalemic following use of SCC are those with muscular dystrophies, paraplegics with spinal cord injuries, and people who have suffered severe burns, crushed limbs, or other muscle-damaging injuries. Thus, SCC may not be a good choice for patients with preexisting hyperkalemia secondary to injury or disease, and for cardiac patients who are on digitalis or quinidine.

Other effects

SCC does not ordinarily have any direct effects on the heart. However, in some circumstances, this drug may stimulate sympathetic and parasympathetic ganglia to bring about changes in cardiac rate and rhythm or in blood pressure. Children, for example, sometimes develop a slowed heart and a drop in blood pressure after repeated SCC injections, particularly during passage of an endotracheal tube and when halothane is the inhaled anesthetic. However, such bradycardia and hypotension tend to be transient and can be readily counteracted with atropine. More common during prolonged procedures in which SCC is infused continuously is a tendency of the heart rate to increase with an accompanying rise in blood pressure—effects that are attributed to its stimulating effect on sympathetic ganglia.

Pharmacokinetic factors

When administered by vein in an adequate dose, SCC reaches an effective concentration at the NMJ to bring about muscle paralysis within 1 minute. If no further doses are administered, recovery occurs promptly as the drug diffuses away from its primary site of action. Ordinarily, the peak paralytic effect lasts about 2 minutes, after which muscle tone returns to normal within the next few minutes. Thus, if more prolonged paralysis is required, additional fractions of the first dose must be injected intermittently or, as in the more common practice, the drug is administered by continuous IV drip.

Plasma levels of the enzyme pseudocholinesterase are the most important factors in determining the fate of SCC and the duration of its action. Less than 10% of administered SCC is excreted unchanged by the kidneys. The duration of SCC-induced muscle paralysis may be prolonged and intensified by the presence of pathologic and pharmacogenetic factors that reduce the amount of

available active plasma pseudocholinesterase molecules. Thus, for example, because this detoxifying enzyme is synthesized in the liver and then sent out into the bloodstream with other plasma proteins, patients with a history of liver disease, malnutrition, or anemia are considered poor candidates for SCC administration.

Others in whom the use of this agent is undesirable are those with a genetic defect that results in a lack of the enzyme required for eliminating this drug. As indicated in Chapter 4, pharmacogenetic factors can affect people's responses to drugs. Some persons are born with atypical esterase enzymes in their blood. As a result of failure to destroy the circulating drug, an abnormally large proportion of any intravenously administered dose of SCC reaches the NMJ and remains at this site of action in high concentrations for long periods. Thus, a dose that would ordinarily be entirely eliminated within 8 to 10 minutes may continue to exert a profound and prolonged paralyzing effect in such people. Instead of the ordinarily brief period of respiratory paralysis that is followed by spontaneous breathing within a few seconds, or at most, minutes, those with this enzymatic defect tend to suffer from prolonged apnea that requires long-continued controlled respiration with oxygen.

Drug–drug interactions. Drugs that can inhibit cholinesterases also tend to prolong the muscle-paralyzing effects of SCC and other depolarizing-type neuromuscular blocking agents. In addition to the *anticholinesterase-type drugs* previously discussed, the local anesthetic procaine can act in this way. *Procaine, lidocaine* and *other local anesthetics* are rapidly hydrolyzed by plasma cholinesterase—a factor that accounts for their relative safety (Chap. 14). However, their presence in the bloodstream together with SCC can potentiate its muscle-paralyzing effect, because these drugs compete with SCC for the circulating enzyme and reduce the number of enzyme molecules available for destroying SCC.

Clinical uses

Neuromuscular junction blocking drugs are employed mainly as adjuncts to general anesthesia (Chap. 52) and for preparing emotionally depressed patients for electroconvulsive therapy (ECT). In addition, they are sometimes used to facilitate certain diagnostic and orthopedic procedures, and in rare instances to prevent convulsions caused by drugs or by tetanus toxin.

Adjuncts to anesthesia

These peripherally acting drugs are *not* themselves anesthetics. They are administered as *supplements* to central depressant drugs to facilitate endotracheal intubation, when this is desirable, and to reduce the amount of inhalation anesthetic required to bring about the relaxation of abdominal and other skeletal muscles that may be necessary, for example, in intra-abdominal procedures or in alignment of fractures. Ordinarily, large amounts of even the most potent general anesthetics are required to depress the spinal reflex centers that control muscle tone. The continued administration of high concentrations of such anesthetics to produce and maintain muscular relaxation may lead to various adverse reactions, ranging from postoperative vomiting to depression of the respiratory and cardiovascular systems. By bringing about relaxation of skeletal muscles through their *peripheral* blocking effects, drugs such as tubocurarine and SCC permit a marked reduction in the amount of general anesthetic required, and this lessens the likelihood of anesthetic complications.

Precautions
Of course, the NMJ blockers are themselves often a cause of dangerous complications, and must be employed with great caution if these are to be avoided. It is essential, for example, that these drugs not be employed in patients with underlying disorders that make them excessively sensitive to the cardiovascular and respiratory complications that can occur even in the best of circumstances (see the summary of adverse effects at the end of this chapter). Even in properly selected patients, it is important to employ only the smallest amount of blocking agent needed for attaining and maintaining the desired degree of muscular relaxation. Patients must be kept under constant observation, and the state of their respiratory muscle function must be closely monitored. These drugs must, of course, be employed only by personnel experienced in the use of the apparatus that may be required for administering oxygen under positive pressure during periods of respiratory muscle paralysis and apnea.

Adjuncts to electroconvulsive therapy
SCC is commonly used today as part of the premedication of psychiatric patients prior to electroshock therapy. Its use helps to prevent the convulsions set off by passage of the current through the brain. This lessens the likelihood of the massive muscular contractions that might otherwise occur and the consequent vertebral fractures or dislocations. Because the use of this drug together with thiopental increases the likelihood of postseizure apnea, the patient is well oxygenated prior to the procedure and oxygen is kept readily available for administration through an endotracheal tube. Patients also receive a small dose of atropine or of scopolamine before administration of thiopental, SCC, and the electric shock.

Other uses
NMJ blocking drugs are sometimes employed for other intubations in addition to insertion of an endotracheal tube. These include laryngoscopy, bronchoscopy, esophagoscopy, and sigmoidoscopy. Among orthopedic pro-

cedures facilitated by prior curarization are reductions of fractures and dislocations of the jaw, the knee, and the shoulder. In ophthalmologic surgery, the relaxant effect of relatively small doses of curariform drugs on the muscles of the eye has been used to ease procedures such as the removal of cataracts. The use of SCC and similar depolarizing-type blocking agents is undesirable in the latter two clinical situations, because of the initial muscular contractions that drugs of this class can cause.

Muscle spasm and convulsive seizures
In the past, attempts were made to employ tubocurarine in the management of chronic disorders marked by muscle spasm and rigidity. Although this and related curariform drugs often produced muscle relaxation and relief of pain, their effects were of short duration and difficult to control, and excessive muscle weakness often also resulted. Thus, the use of curare-type drugs for treating patients with cerebral palsy, hemiplegia, and chronic states of dystonia and athetosis has declined since the introduction of diazepam and centrally acting skeletal muscle relaxants (Chap. 48).

NMJ blocking agents are sometimes employed in the management of patients severely ill with tetanus in some special treatment centers. The patient is kept completely paralyzed with repeated doses of tubocurarine for several weeks until the tetanus toxin is eliminated from his poisoned nerve cells. During this prolonged period of artificial respiration, meticulous nursing care is required, because the patient cannot breathe, eat, or even communicate in any way.

This patient requires total nursing care. All the care provisions necessary for the immobilized patient must be observed, as well as respiratory hygiene measures, while the patient is on a respirator; these provisions include nutritional support and, in this case, particular concern for the patient's psychological and emotional well-being because the patient can be completely alert but unable to make any voluntary responses.

Management of adverse reactions

As indicated previously, the main danger in the use of blocking agents of both types is that paralysis of the diaphragm and chest muscles may cause respiratory difficulty and even apnea. For this reason, these drugs are never used when facilities for controlled respiration are unavailable, nor are they ever to be administered by those not completely skilled in their use. The occurrence of apnea following administration of these drugs is no great problem to the experienced anesthesiologist, who merely ventilates the patient artificially until the effects of the drug wear off—usually in a matter of minutes. Indeed, apnea is sometimes deliberately induced in chest and heart surgery without harm, as long as the patient continues to get oxygen by mechanical means.

Prolonged apnea produced by overdosage of tubocurarine, pancuronium, or other *non*depolarizing blocking agents may sometimes be reversed by the intravenous administration of such antagonists as neostigmine and edrophonium. These anticholinesterase drugs may help to overcome the curare block mainly by indirectly increasing the amount of endogenous ACh at the NMJs. That is, they prevent the enzymatic destruction of the nerve-released neurotransmitter by acetylcholinesterase. This helps the ACh molecules to accumulate to levels at which they can compete successfully with the curariform compounds for the cholinergic receptors. Atropine administration is also often desirable to counteract salivation, bronchial mucus secretion, and other muscarinic side-effects of curare-drug antidotes such as neostigmine.

Administration of anticholinesterase drugs does not ordinarily counteract the effects of overdosage with the *depolarizing*-type blocking agents. On the contrary, because neostigmine and edrophonium are themselves direct and indirect depolarizing agents, they make an SCC- or decamethonium-induced block even worse by their additive actions.

It is often also important to maintain the patient's blood pressure at adequate levels. In cases of hypotension resulting from curare-induced histamine release and ganglionic blockade, the administration of ephedrine or of other adrenergic vasopressor drugs may prevent circulatory collapse. Similar sudden drops in blood pressure are not likely with SCC, which only rarely causes release of histamine and which stimulates sympathetic ganglia. However, because SCC may trigger malignant hyperthermia (see Chap. 5), the patient's body temperature should be monitored.

Additional clinical considerations

The list of cautions that need to be observed before using any of these drugs is quite lengthy. The drug effects can aggravate many underlying medical conditions, including such problems as *chronic obstructive lung disease*—the increase in histamine release and the resultant bronchoconstriction can cause severe problems for these patients; *cardiovascular disease*—the bradycardia, reflex tachycardia, blood pressure changes, and arrhythmias that often occur in response to these drugs can cause cardiac arrest, congestive heart failure, or myocardial infarction in susceptible patients; *pregnancy*—as with many other drugs, the safety of NMJ blocking drug use has not been established.

A condition called malignant hyperthermic crisis has been reported with the use of the depolarizing blocking drugs during anesthesia with some agents. A situation of hypermetabolism of skeletal muscle develops with rising temperature, metabolic acidosis, and a generalized rigidity. In these situations, anesthesia must be stopped immediately and supportive measures begun to reverse the condition. (See also the discussion of this problem in Chap. 52.)

The drugs should never be used without full life support and ventilatory equipment available. When the competitive blockers are used, the antidotal drugs (*e.g.,* neostigmine, edrophonium) should be on standby in case of an emergency. As mentioned above, some people lack the genetic ability to metabolize certain of these drugs (SCC) and may experience prolonged muscular paralysis. Unless such people know that they have this predisposition, it is not readily possible to identify who may be at risk. For this reason, all patients receiving NMJ blocking drugs should be constantly monitored until it is certain that full function has returned.

If a patient is to receive one of these drugs without general anesthesia, it is very important to remember that the drug blocks the patient's ability to speak and to respond in any way, but the drug does *not* alter pain sensation or consciousness. The patient will require emotional support throughout the procedure, and will need to be alerted to any potentially painful moment. The nurse will need to serve as a patient advocate and will need to anticipate pain and take appropriate measures to alleviate it; the nurse will also need to monitor the environment and remind others that the patient is alert and can feel pain.

The teaching points that should be considered for a patient receiving NMJ blocking drugs are outlined in the patient teaching guide. The drug information should be incorporated into the total patient teaching protocol involving pre- and postoperative information.

The *drug–drug interactions* involved with these drugs are numerous. Ideally, some drugs should be withdrawn several days before an NMJ blocking drug is used. These include the following: *propranolol*, which can increase the neuromuscular block; the *thiazide diuretics*, which can cause hypokalemia and increase the blocking effect; and *digitalis preparations*, which in the presence of SCC are more likely to cause serious ventricular arrhythmias. The mechanism of this interaction is not understood.

It is often impossible to change all the drugs that a patient is taking before use of an NMJ blocking drug. It is wise to note all the drugs that a patient is taking on the front of the chart, or on the anesthesia flow sheet, to alert the anesthesiologist to any possible drug–drug problems. As a technical point, curare, gallamine and metocurine should not be mixed with *alkaline solutions* (*e.g.,* barbiturates) because an insoluble precipitate may form.

The guide to the nursing process summarizes the clinical aspects to consider in the nursing care of a patient on an NMJ blocking drug.

Summary of adverse effects of NMJ blocking drugs and precautions required in their use

Respiratory depression and prolonged apnea

1. Dosage must be individualized on the basis of a careful assessment of each patient's sensitivity.
   a. Patients with pulmonary, hepatic, and renal diseases are particularly sensitive to *non*depolarizing blockers, as are those with myasthenia gravis, carcinomatosis, extreme debilitation, dehydration, and electrolyte or acid–base imbalances.
   b. Patients with low levels of plasma cholinesterase or with hereditary abnormalities of this enzyme are especially sensitive to the *depolarizing* blocker succinylcholine.
2. These drugs must be administered only by personnel skilled in artificial respiration and only when facilities and apparatus for endotracheal intubation and for providing assisted or controlled ventilation with oxygen under positive pressure are available.
3. The degree of NMJ blockade and the adequacy of the patient's respiratory function must be continuously observed. A peripheral nerve stimulator may be employed to monitor skeletal muscle tone.

Circulatory complications

1. *Hypotension* may occur with high doses of these drugs, especially of tubocurarine, as a result of histamine release and sympathetic ganglionic blockade.

2. Initial *bradycardia* and later *tachycardia* may occur with succinylcholine. Increased pulse rates occur with gallamine and pancuronium.
3. *Cardiac arrhythmias or cardiac arrest* may occur with succinylcholine in patients who have been recently digitalized or are receiving quinidine. Hyperkalemia caused by this drug may endanger patients with pre-existing high plasma potassium levels, including patients with severe burns or crushing injuries, paraplegics, and others with spinal injury or neuromuscular dystrophic or degenerative diseases.

Other adverse effects

1. Succinylcholine and decamethonium can cause muscle injury and pain as a result of early muscular contractions with fasciculations. Caution is required in patients with fractures.
2. Succinylcholine-induced contractions of extraocular muscles and elevation of intraocular pressure make its use undesirable for patients undergoing ophthalmic surgery.
3. Succinylcholine may precipitate malignant hyperthermia in genetically predisposed patients, particularly when it is employed with inhalation anesthetics such as halothane, methoxyflurane, cyclopropane, and diethyl ether.

Patient teaching guide: NMJ blocking drugs

Preparatory measures

For example, diet, respiratory toilet

Drug effects

- Paralysis
- Inability to speak or respond
- *No* effect on consciousness (if used alone)
- *No* effect on pain

Recovery

- Back, neck, pharynx pain, secondary to intense muscular contractions (depolarizing agents)
- Recovery time anticipated

Guide to the nursing process: NMJ blocking drugs

Assessment	Nursing diagnoses	Interventions	Evaluation
Past history—underlying medical conditions (*contraindications*): Cardiovascular disease Hepatic failure Renal failure Chronic obstructive pulmonary disease Myasthenia gravis Electrolyte imbalances Pregnancy Fractures (depolarizing blockers) *Allergies: these drugs; iodine sensitivity* (gallamine, metocurine); others; reactions Medication history: *all drugs being taken;* last dose	Potential alteration in respiratory function Potential alteration in cardiac output Potential fear related to procedure and anesthesia Impaired physical mobility Knowledge deficit regarding drug Potential sensory–perceptual alteration Potential alteration in comfort, pain from procedure, intense contractions	Safe and appropriate preparation and administration of drug Comfort measures: Reduce pain Positioning Environmental control Support and encouragement before, during, and after procedure Provision of life support measures, as needed Patient teaching regarding procedure: Signs and symptoms to anticipate What it will feel like Recovery time	Evaluate effectiveness of drug: paralysis Monitor for adverse effects of the drug: Tachycardia Respiratory distress Slow recovery of vital functions ↑ Respiratory secretions Evaluate effectiveness of patient teaching measures Evaluate effectiveness of support and encouragement offered Evaluate effectiveness of comfort measures Constant monitoring of vital functions and return to normal muscular function
Physical assessment Neurologic: orientation, reflexes, sensation Cardiovascular: BP, P, heart sounds, baseline EKG Respiratory: R, adventitious sounds GI: bowel sounds, liver function tests Renal: output, urinalysis, BUN, electrolyte status General: T, perfusion			

Case study

Presentation

Mrs. N, an 82-year-old white woman in very good health, has been admitted to the hospital for an exploratory laparotomy to evaluate what seems to be a palpable abdominal mass. The admission interview revealed that Mrs. N had a history of mild hypertension that has been regulated by diuretic therapy. Her baseline physical status was noted and preoperative instruction was begun. On the morning of surgery, it was noted that, along with a general anesthetic,

Mrs. N would be receiving succinylcholine chloride to ensure muscle paralysis. Describe the measures that should be taken with Mrs. N.

Discussion

Before Mrs. N goes to surgery, the preoperative teaching program should be reviewed with her again. Because of the succinylcholine, Mrs. N should be advised that her back, neck, and pharnyx may be painfully sore after surgery. She should know that this is anticipated and is a result of medication received during the operation. Her chart should indicate the prolonged use of diuretics, and her current serum potassium level should be checked and noted prominently on her chart.

Following surgery, Mrs. N should be constantly monitored until it is certain that the effects of muscle paralysis have totally worn off. This will include careful monitoring of BP, P, cardiac rhythm, respiratory function, and urinary output. Because of Mrs. N's age and increased susceptibility to circulatory disorders, Mrs. N should receive meticulous skin care, turning, and careful positioning during the recovery period. Analgesics may be necessary if muscular pain or postsurgical pain are severe. Mrs. N will need further teaching regarding the diagnosis, potential treatment, and prognosis. At this time she may also need support and encouragement to deal with her situation.

Drug digests

Succinylcholine chloride injection USP (Anectine; Quelicin; Sucostrin)

Actions and indications. This is the prototype NMJ blocking agent of the *depolarizing* type. It causes skeletal muscle paralysis by occupying cholinergic receptors at the NMJ. Depolarization at first causes muscle contractions (fasciculations), but this is soon followed by flaccid paralysis as the depolarization persists and blocks neural transmission of impulses to the muscle fibers.

This drug is employed mainly as an adjunct to anesthesia with inhalation anesthetics such as nitrous oxide, which do not produce adequate skeletal muscle relaxation, or to lessen the amount of more potent general anesthetics required to maintain prolonged muscle paralysis.

It is also used prior to electroconvulsive therapy to lessen the severity of electrically induced convulsions. Its use facilitates endotracheal and other intubation procedures.

Adverse effects, cautions, and contraindications. Profound and prolonged respiratory depression to the point of apnea can occur.

Thus, this drug should be used only when personnel and facilities are available for intubating the patient and administering oxygen by artificial respiration.

Respiratory difficulties are most likely to occur in patients with low levels of plasma pseudocholinesterase, the drug-detoxifying enzyme. Such patients include, in addition to those with a pharmacogenetic defect, those with severe liver disease, anemia, or malnutrition. If this abnormality is suspected, patients should first be checked by determining their response to a small test dose of the drug.

Cardiovascular complications including bradycardia and serious cardiac arrhythmias leading to cardiac arrest can occur in some circumstances. Caution is required in patients who are receiving quinidine or who have recently been digitalized, and in those with hyperkalemia or other electrolyte imbalances.

Caution is required during ocular surgery and in patients with glaucoma because of a possible transient drug-induced rise in intraocular pressure. Use of this drug with certain general anesthetics may set off an episode of malignant hyperthermia in genetically predisposed people.

Dosage and administration. Dosage is individualized in accordance with the response of the patient and the length of the procedure. After the patient has been anesthetized with a hypnotic dose of thiopental or a similar basal anesthetic, a test dose of 10 mg IV may be administered to determine sensitivity. For procedures of short duration, muscle relaxation may be achieved with average doses of 2.5 to 4 mg/kg. For more prolonged procedures, the first effective dose may be repeated intermittently, or the patient may receive a continuous IV infusion at an average rate of 2.5 mg/min. The rate of infusion can be varied to provide different degrees of muscle relaxation as required.

Tubocurarine chloride injection USP (Tubarine)

Actions and indications. This drug is the prototype of the competitive *non*depolarizing class of NMJ blocking agents. It causes skeletal muscle relaxation and paralysis by competing with the neurotransmitter ACh for cholinergic receptors at the NMJ. By occupying these sites, molecules of this drug prevent ACh from depolarizing the muscle cell membrane and from transmitting nerve impulses required for muscular contraction. The drug is used mainly as an adjunct to anesthesia to bring about muscular relaxation when general anesthetics are employed that

do not provide adequate relaxation when administered alone in safe concentrations (*e.g.*, nitrous oxide), or to lessen the large amounts of more potent inhalation anesthetics that might otherwise be required to maintain adequate muscular relaxation during prolonged surgical procedures.

It is also used prior to electroconvulsive therapy to reduce the intensity of the electrically induced muscle contractions. The drug is sometimes employed to facilitate the management of patients who require prolonged mechanical ventilation—for example,

to prevent acute ventilatory failure in patients with status asthmaticus or those suffering from tetanus.

Adverse effects, cautions, and contraindications. Because this drug can cause respiratory depression and apnea, it must be administered by personnel experienced in the use of facilities for intubation and administration of oxygen by assisted or controlled respiration.

This drug is contraindicated in persons known to be hypersensitive to it or excessively reactive to the histamine which it may release from body tissues. Hypotension can occur as a result of histamine-induced vasodilation or of blockade of sympathetic ganglia by large doses. Caution is required in patients with depressed respiration or renal function. Muscular paralysis may be potentiated in patients with low plasma potassium levels (hypokalemia).

Dosage and administration. Dosage is individualized in accordance with a prior evaluation of each person and after consideration of other clinical circumstances. Average initial IV doses range from 0.1 to 0.3 mg/kg body weight. However, when ether or other inhalation anesthetics with a potentiating effect on NMJ blockade are to be employed,

the dose may be reduced by about one-third. The calculated dose should be administered in fractions of the full dose when the patient is thought to be especially sensitive and, if additional doses are required, only one-third to one-quarter of the first full dose should be administered at any one time.

References

Argov Z, Mastaglia FL: Disorders of neuromuscular transmission caused by drugs. N Engl J Med 301:409, 1979

Atracurium. Med Lett Drugs Ther 26:53, 1984

Christensen NA: Treatment of the patient with severe tetanus. Surg Clin North Am 49:1183, 1969

Cronnelly R, Morris RB: Antagonism of neuromuscular blockade. Br J Anesth 54:183, 1982

Fisher DM et al: Pharmacokinetics and pharmacodynamics of d-tubocurarine in infants, children, and adults. Anesthesiol 57:203, 1982

Foldes FF: The pharmacology of neuromuscular blocking agents in man. Clin Pharmacol Ther 1:345, 1960

Hubbard JI, Quastel DMJ: Micropharmacology of vertebrate neuromuscular transmission. Ann Rev Pharmacol 13:199, 1973

Kalow W: Genetic factors in relation to drugs. Ann Rev Pharmacol 5:9, 1965

Katz RL: Clinical neuromuscular pharmacology of pancuronium. Anesthesiology 34:550, 1971

Lee C, Katz RL: Neuromuscular pharmacology: Clinical update and commentary. Br J Anesth 52:173, 1980

Riker WF, Ohamoto M: Pharmacology of motor nerve terminals. Ann Rev Pharmacol 9:173, 1969

Rodman MJ: Drugs for treating tetanus. RN 34:43, 1971

Speight TM, Avery GS: Pancuronium bromide: A review of its pharmacological properties and clinical application. Drugs 4:163, 1972

Taylor P: Neuromuscular blocking agents. In Gilman AG, Goodman LS, and Gilman A (eds): Goodman and Gilman's The Pharmacological Basis of Therapeutics, 6th ed, pp 220–234. New York, Macmillan, 1980

Thesleff S, Quastel DMJ: Neuromuscular pharmacology. Ann Rev Pharmacol 5:263, 1965

Young RR, Delwaide PJ: Spasticity. N Engl J Med 304:96, 1981

Section 4

Endocrine
drugs

4

This section deals with drugs that affect the endocrine system or, more accurately, the neuroendocrine system, which includes not only the glands of internal secretion but also the sites within the central nervous system with which the glandular system interacts.* It is now well known, for example, that the activities of both the anterior and posterior portions of the pituitary gland are controlled by nerve cells in the hypothalamus at the base of the brain—specialized neurons that can secrete hormones from their endings.†

The coordinated activity of these two major systems is responsible for maintaining the stability of the body's internal environment, and their integrated functioning also influences the body's behavioral responses to the external environment. Thus, the administration of hormones and other drugs that influence the neuroendocrine system can cause a wide range of effects, not only on the metabolic, or biochemical, processes of all of any person's cells and tissues, but also on the ways in which he thinks and acts.

The natural hormones and their synthetic analogues, which often have even more powerful and prolonged effects, combine with specialized receptors on the surface of target cells, activating cAMP to alter cellular activity, or at sites within the cells. The interaction of the hormone with its specific receptor site sets off a series

---

* The term "endocrine" (from the Greek *endo,* within, and *krino,* separate) refers to the system of glands and other tissues or structures that synthesize substances (hormones) that are secreted into the circulatory system. In contrast to these glands of internal secretion, the *exocrine* glands secrete substances such as sweat, or saliva and other digestive juices, directly onto body surfaces such as skin and mucous membranes.

---

† *Hormones* are chemical substances produced endogenously by endocrine glands, certain nerve cells, and other tissues or structures. They are carried throughout the body but influence the activity only of specific target tissues, the cells of which contain specialized receptors that can bind hormones.

of biochemical events within the cells that finally causes the different types of cells to respond in a characteristic manner. The effects of hormones, which are brought about by their ability to stimulate or to inhibit intracellular biochemical processes, are manifested in many ways.

Various hormones interact in complex ways to influence the intermediary metabolism of body cells. Thus, for example, two hormones produced and released by the pancreas—insulin and glucagon—help to regulate carbohydrate metabolism by their effects on the processes by which glucose is stored, released, and used. However, carbohydrate metabolism and the metabolism of fat and proteins also involve a subtle interplay between these pancreatic hormones and those of the thyroid, pituitary, and adrenal glands.

The adrenal cortex synthesizes and releases hormones that not only affect the metabolism of carbohydrates, proteins, and fats, but also help to maintain mineral and water balance. Its hormones also aid in mobilizing the body's defenses to meet stressful situations such as infection and trauma, and some of its hormones even influence the growth and development of the reproductive organs. Most important in that regard, however, are the hormones produced by the gonads—the ovaries and testes—that are essential for turning immature girls and boys into women and men capable of reproduction.

The various chapters of this section are concerned mainly with the clinical applications of the hormones, their synthetic analogues, and certain other synthetic drugs that are used to antagonize endocrine gland overactivity—the antithyroid drugs, for example. Hormones are often administered in small doses intended to replace the amounts that would ordinarily be produced physiologically by a normally functioning gland when that gland is failing to secrete adequate amounts of its hormones. However, in addition to their use for such replacement or substitution therapy, hormones are also often employed in larger doses for their pharmacologic effects. Thus, for example, although the natural adrenocortical hormones and their synthetic analogues are sometimes administered in small daily doses that substitute for the missing hormones of patients with acute or chronic adrenal insufficiency, their use as adrenocorticosteroid drugs that are administered in pharmacologic, or *supra*physiologic, doses is of infinitely greater clinical significance in the management of scores of *non*endocrine disorders.

Despite this emphasis on the therapeutic applications of hormone action, some aspects of the natural physiologic functions of each group of hormones as regulators of metabolism, growth, reproduction, and responses to stress will be discussed. Similarly, the regulation of the functioning of various glands will be reviewed. The reason for this is that such knowledge of normal endocrine gland function and the regulation of secretory activity is necessary to understand both the beneficial effects of hormone therapy in treating endocrine disorders and many of the adverse effects that can develop when hormones and related drugs are administered in pharmacologic doses for treating the many medical conditions that do *not* stem from endocrine dysfunction. In addition, it is becoming apparent that many nonendocrine drugs can affect the secretion of hypothalamic and pituitary hormones; they may produce both therapeutically useful and adverse effects by this mechanism.

Advances in analytic chemistry—particularly the application of radioimmune assay techniques—have made possible the detection of the tiny amounts of hormones that circulate in the blood. This, in turn, has added to the understanding of how endocrine functions are regulated and to the knowledge of what specifically goes wrong in the pathogenesis of various endocrine disorders. Such advances have now made it possible to diagnose and to treat various endocrinopathies more precisely and appropriately than was once the case. However, because the details of diagnosis and treatment of all but the most common endocrine disorders are beyond the scope of this textbook, those who specialize in endocrinology will want to consult more specialized books and other literature.

Hypothalamic and pituitary gland hormones and drugs

20

Anatomic aspects

Pituitary gland

The *pituitary gland* is a tiny organ, hardly larger than a fingertip. It is located deep in the head, nestled in a protective depression in the skull called the *sella turcica*. It lies just below the brain—more specifically, just below the hypothalamus—to which it is connected by a stalk containing nerve fibers and blood vessels. Its true importance went unrecognized until this century and, in fact, the name *pituitary*, derived from the Latin word for mucus, indicates the fact that for a long time its function was thought to be merely to supply moisture for the mucous membranes of the nose. (Another name for this body is *hypophysis*, which comes from the Greek for "undergrowth" and this, at least, describes its anatomic relation to the brain accurately.)

The pituitary gland consists of two separate parts, called the anterior and posterior lobes. They have their origins in different parts of the embryo and then move toward each other to meet midway. The anterior lobe, or *adenohypophysis* (from the Greek *adenos*, gland), which starts out in the embryo as part of the mouth, is made up of true glandular secretory tissue. This tissue contains several types of cells, each of which can biosynthesize and secrete a particular type of anterior pituitary hormone.

The posterior portion develops from the floor of the brain, to which it remains connected, and is made up largely of nerve fibers. Thus, this so-called *neural lobe*, or *neurohypophysis*, does not make its own secretions at all but only stores and releases hormones, which are made in the hypothalamic portion of the brain and transported to the posterior pituitary. These hormones are nevertheless called posterior pituitary hormones. The target tissues for its hormones are not other glands but rather such structures as the uterus, breast, and certain kidney tubule cells.

Hypothalamus

The *hypothalamus* is an area of the brain that integrates information about stresses and imbalances in the body, and allows appropriate behavioral, autonomic, and endocrine responses to be made to restore and maintain equilibrium, or *homeostasis*. The hypothalamus is involved in hunger and satiety, thirst, water loss and water retention, regulation of body temperature and blood pressure, reproduction, sleep and waking, and emotional reactions. It exerts important control over the endocrine system, and is itself an endocrine organ. Many functions of the hypothalamus (*e.g.*, water loss and retention, reproduction) are mediated in large part by the endocrine system and by the hypothalamus functioning as an endocrine organ.

Anatomically, the hypothalamus is at the base of the forebrain. It receives input, directly or indirectly, from virtually all other areas of the brain, including the limbic system and the cerebral cortex. In addition, the hypothalamus is one of the brain areas that is least protected by the blood–brain barrier. Thus, hormones and many other substances in the blood that never reach neurons in most other brain areas can influence hypothalamic neurons. The output from the hypothalamic neurons, in turn, influences neurons in many other parts of the CNS, including neurons of the autonomic nervous system. The hypothalamus thus influences the function of almost every organ system through the autonomic nervous and endocrine systems.

Two different aspects of hypothalamic function justify its inclusion in the endocrine system. First, neurons in several hypothalamic areas synthesize hormones that either release or inhibit the release of specific hormones from the anterior pituitary. The axons of these neurons terminate in the median eminence (near the pituitary stalk) on the capillaries of the *hypothalamoadenohypophyseal portal system*, which is part of the circulatory supply to the anterior pituitary gland (Fig. 20-1). The hypothalamic releasing and release-inhibiting hormones enter this portal system and are carried by it directly to the cells of the anterior pituitary.

Second, the hypothalamus itself secretes two hormones that influence target organs directly. Specialized neurosecretory neurons in the paraventricular and supraoptic nuclei synthesize oxytocin and antidiuretic

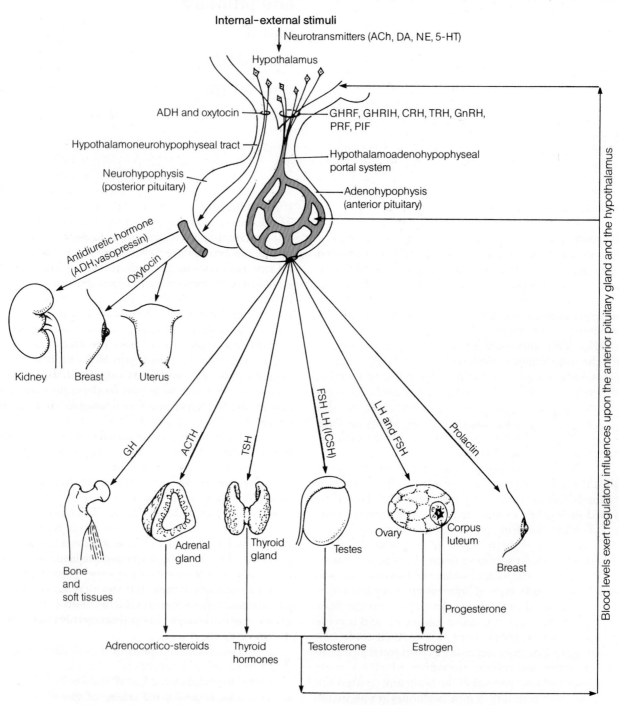

Figure 20-1. The pituitary gland and its interrelationships with the brain and peripheral target tissues and glands. Some hypothalamic hormones influence anterior pituitary gland function. Anterior gland tropic hormones affect the production and secretion of various responsive glands. The secretions of these glands influence metabolism of various peripheral tissues and also exert feedback effects on the adenohypophysis and the hypothalamus. The neurohypophysis stores and releases other hypothalamic hormones, which also affect the functioning of peripheral target tissues.

hormone (ADH; also called vasopressin). These hormones are transported by the axons of the neurons that synthesize them to the posterior pituitary gland, where they are stored (Fig. 20-1). The axons that transport these two hormones make up the *hypothalamoneurohypophyseal tract.* Action potentials in these axons release the hormones into the systemic circulation, which carries them to their target organs. (The hypothalamic hormones that influence the anterior pituitary are described below in Regulation of secretion in the discussion of the anterior pituitary hormones; oxytocin and ADH are described below in Posterior pituitary hormones and synthetic substitutes.)

The anterior and posterior pituitary and hypothalamic hormones have a profound influence over many metabolic functions. Through its connections with the hypothalamus by blood vessels and nerve fibers, the pituitary works together with the nervous system to maintain a stable internal environment and to regulate behavioral responses to the external environment. Thus, even though pituitary and hypothalamic hormones have relatively few uses in treatment or diagnosis, the physiologic effects of these hormones need to be understood to understand the functioning of the other endocrine glands discussed in the following chapters of this section— the adrenal cortex, the ovaries and testes, the thyroid gland, and the pancreas—and to understand the beneficial and adverse effects of drugs that act on the endocrine system.

Anterior pituitary gland and its hormones

Before the discovery of the hypothalamic releasing factors and their activity, the anterior pituitary gland (adenohypophysis) was called the "master gland" of the entire endocrine system. Six hormones of physiologic significance to humans have been obtained from this portion of the pituitary gland (see Fig. 20-1). These are often referred to as *tropic* (or *trophic*) *hormones*. The first five of these hormones, described below, directly control cells of target glands; the sixth, growth hormone, influences metabolic processes in many types of body tissues.

Adenohypophyseal hormones and other substances

The adenohypophyseal hormones, all of which are glycoproteins or polypeptides, include the following:

1. *Corticotropin* or *adrenocorticotropic hormone (ACTH),* which stimulates the adrenal cortex to synthesize steroid hormones
2. *Thyroid-stimulating hormone (TSH)* or *thyrotropin,* which stimulates the thyroid gland to synthesize and secrete thyroid hormones

3. *Follicle-stimulating hormone (FSH),* a *gonadotropic hormone,* which in men stimulates spermatogenesis and in women stimulates follicle development in the ovaries, leading to estrogen production
4. *Luteinizing hormone (LH),* also called *interstitial cell-stimulating hormone (ICSH),* another gonadotropic hormone, which in women causes ovulation and the secretion of estrogen and progesterone by the corpus luteum, and in men stimulates interstitial or Leydig cells of the testes to produce testosterone
5. *Prolactin,* which stimulates milk production in breast tissue
6. *Growth hormone (GH),* also called *somatotropin (STH),* which stimulates the growth of long bones, skin, and connective tissue, and has complex effects on protein, carbohydrate, and lipid metabolism

In addition to these six hormones, a number of other substances with biologic activity have been isolated from the anterior pituitary, but the physiologic role, if any, of these pituitary substances is unclear. These substances include the following:

1. *Melanocyte-stimulating hormone (MSH),* which is responsible for skin pigment changes in amphibia and, like ACTH, can darken the skin of humans when injected repeatedly over a period of time
2. *Endorphins* and *enkephalins,* which bind to opiate receptors in the CNS (and in the gastrointestinal tract); these substances are found in nerve terminals in other areas of the CNS in which they may have a physiologic role in modulating pain impulses
3. *Lipotropins,* which stimulate fat mobilization

Actually, all three of these biologically active pituitary substances that have unknown physiologic roles are found in one large molecule that appears to be the parent compound of ACTH. Thus, their presence in the mammalian pituitary may only reflect the use by mammalian cells of an evolutionarily old biochemical pathway for synthesizing ACTH.

Regulation of secretion
The secretion of the tropic hormones of the anterior pituitary gland is controlled in two ways—by the hypothalamus and by feedback inhibition exerted by hormones from the endocrine target glands that are regulated by a particular tropic hormone. Other feedback controls are described below. All these control mechanisms allow the body to keep the levels of these crucial endocrine hor-

mones within a small range of physiologic concentrations. Knowledge of these control systems is important for understanding the various ways that drugs can produce beneficial and adverse effects on the endocrine system.

Hypothalamic control

The hypothalamus integrates the influences from the limbic system, the cerebral cortex, and other areas of the CNS, as well as information about blood levels of hormones and other substances. It uses this information to regulate the anterior pituitary gland.

As described above, cells in various areas of the hypothalamus synthesize releasing factors, also called *hypophysiotropic factors,* and release-inhibiting factors that are carried from the median eminence by the portal system to the anterior pituitary, where they regulate the synthesis and secretion of the anterior pituitary tropic hormones. There are seven factors that regulate the pituitary tropic hormones listed above; four of these have been identified chemically and are more properly referred to as "hormones," not as "factors." These hypothalamic factors and hormones, all of which are peptides (except possibly PIF), include the following (see Fig. 20-1):

1. *Corticotropin-releasing hormone (CRH; formerly corticotropin-releasing factor, CRF)*—a peptide hormone recently identified chemically, that causes the release of ACTH
2. *Thyroid-stimulating hormone-releasing hormone or thyrotropin-releasing hormone (TRH)*—a tripeptide that causes the release of TSH (and prolactin)
3. *Gonadotropin-releasing hormone (GnRH)*—a peptide hormone that causes the release of both LH and FSH; it is sometimes called *LHRH or LRH,* but increasing evidence indicates that the hormone initially found to release LH also releases FSH
4. *Prolactin-releasing factor (PRF)*—although TRH can cause the release of prolactin, there is evidence for a separate prolactin-releasing factor
5. *Prolactin release-inhibiting factor (PIF)*—a substance, possibly dopamine, that inhibits the release of prolactin
6. *Growth hormone releasing factor (GHRF)*—an unidentified substance that releases growth hormone (GH)
7. *Growth hormone release-inhibiting hormone (GHRIH; also called somatostatin)*—an identified peptide that inhibits the secretion of GH (and of ACTH, TSH, insulin, glucagon, and many hormones of the gastrointestinal tract)

In addition, substances that have melanocyte-stimulating hormone-releasing and release-inhibiting activity have been isolated from the amphibian and mammalian hypothalamus. Because the function of MSH in mammals is unclear, these substances will not be considered further.

Some hypothalamic hormones, or substances very similar to them chemically and biologically, are found in high concentration in tissues other than the hypothalamus and pituitary. For example, CRH, TRH, LHRH, and somatostatin are found in nerve terminals outside the hypothalamus, where they may function as neurotransmitters or as neuromodulators. Somatostatin is found in delta cells of the pancreas and in the gastrointestinal tract. Elucidation of the functional significance of these high concentrations of hypothalamic hormones in other parts of the body represents an area of important current research interest and activity.

Another important area of current research involves discovering which neurotransmitters influence the hypothalamic neuroendocrine cells, both those that secrete the releasing or release-inhibiting factors and those that secrete ADH and oxytocin. Drugs that influence these neurotransmitters, as well as drugs that act on the pituitary, the peripheral endocrine organs (*e.g.,* thyroid gland, adrenal cortex, ovary), and endocrine target organs, can alter the endocrine responses of the body.

Feedback controls

The hormone-producing and hormone-secreting activity of the anterior pituitary gland hormones is also influenced by the hormones of their target glands. That is, the functioning of the pituitary gland is influenced by a feedback from the very same glands that it influences. Thus, for example, when the plasma levels of hormones of the adrenal, thyroid, or sex glands become high, the rising plasma levels signal the appropriate anterior pituitary gland cells to slow down their production and secretion of the tropic hormones corticotropin, thyrotropin, or gonadotropin (Fig. 20-2).

Such so-called *negative feedback* mechanisms are of particular clinical significance, because they may be brought into play purposefully—for example, to prevent ovulation through the administration of ovarian sex hormones—or they may be the cause of undesired adverse effects, as when the administration of adrenocorticosteroid drugs in supraphysiologic doses depresses the production of endogenous hormones by the adrenal cortex, with resulting adrenal insufficiency and failure.

The possible mechanisms by which endocrine target hormones inhibit the secretion of their pituitary tropic hormones are rather complex, and involve the hypothalamic releasing factors described above. Some evidence suggests that high levels of an endocrine target hormone cause a decrease in the secretion of the hypothalamic releasing hormone, or a decrease in the sensitivity

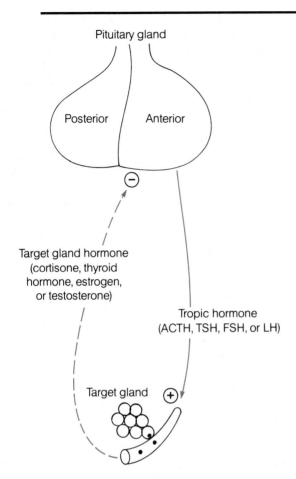

Figure 20-2. Feedback inhibition exerted by hormones of endocrine target glands on secretion of anterior pituitary tropic hormones. Stimulation of secretion is shown by solid arrows and +; inhibition of secretion is shown by dashed arrows and −.

of the anterior pituitary cells to the hypothalamic releasing hormone (Fig. 20-3A). Thus, for example, high circulating levels of adrenal corticosteroids decrease the secretion of CRH and may decrease the responsiveness of the pituitary ACTH-secreting cells to CRH. These effects would in turn decrease the secretion of ACTH resulting in a decreased secretion of corticosteroids.

Two anterior pituitary hormones, growth hormone and prolactin, lack endocrine target organs; therefore, the secretion of these two pituitary hormones cannot be regulated by any form of feedback inhibition exerted by a hormone of an endocrine target gland. It is interesting that these are the two anterior pituitary hormones for which hypothalamic release-inhibiting factors (somatostatin, or GHRIH, and PIF) have been demonstrated. (Factors that inhibit the release of other anterior pituitary hormones may, of course, be described in the future.) High circulating levels of GH do decrease the secretion of GH; high circulating levels of prolactin decrease the secretion of prolactin. Both these effects may be mediated by the appropriate hypothalamic release-inhibiting hor-

mones, somatostatin or PIF. There is evidence that this is true for GH, but little is known about the control of prolactin secretion.

Elucidation of the mechanisms controlling the anterior pituitary hormones and the hypothalamic releasing and release-inhibiting factors is another area of great current research interest. The mechanisms are much more complicated than once thought. Figure 20-3 indicates that, in addition to the control mechanisms described above, pituitary tropic hormones may exert feedback inhibition on the release of hypothalamic releasing factors, and hypothalamic releasing and release-inhibiting factors may exert feedback inhibition on their own secretion.

Posterior pituitary gland and its hormones

The posterior lobe of the pituitary body (*neurohypophysis*), stores secretions that are made by nerve cells of the paraventricular and supraoptic nuclei of the hypothalamus. The same hypothalamic nerve fibers that transport these neurosecretions to the pituitary storage sites also send down the signals that release these hormones into the bloodstream. The two main types of posterior pituitary hormones that then affect the functioning of peripheral target tissues are the oxytocic hormone, *oxytocin*, and the antidiuretic hormone (ADH), *vasopressin*.

Oxytocin

Oxytocin is thought to play a part in parturition, or childbirth, and in releasing the flow of milk from the mother's breast. This hormone may be responsible for the initiation of labor when it is released from the pituitary lobe as the result of a reflex set off by distention of the uterus and dilatation of the cervix.

Similarly, the suckling infant causes afferent nerve impulses to pass from the breast to the hypothalamus. Certain nerve cells in this portion of the brain then both secrete oxytocin and send down the nerve impulses that release the previously synthesized hormone from its storage sites in the posterior pituitary neural lobe. The hormone then drains into the bloodstream, which carries it to target tissues in the breast. This results in the ejection of milk from the alveoli of the mammary gland into the large ducts and sinuses that direct it into the baby's mouth.

Antidiuretic hormone

ADH is also called vasopressin because it is a potent vasoconstrictor substance that can elevate blood pressure. These vascular effects are not produced by concentrations of the hormone normally found in the circulation, but may be produced when the drug is injected. ADH has a physiologic regulatory function that is even more important than that of oxytocin, because it operates continuously rather than only occasionally. It acts constantly

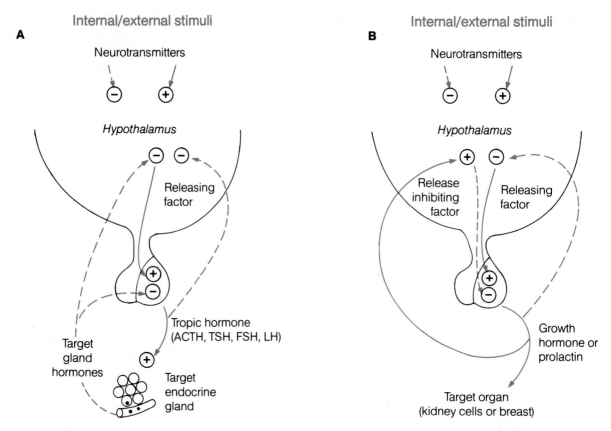

Figure 20-3. Regulation of the synthesis and release of anterior pituitary hormones by hypothalamic releasing factors by (*A*) feedback inhibition exerted by target gland hormones, and by (*B*) hypothalamic release-inhibiting factors. In addition to the sites of feedback shown, the releasing and release-inhibiting factors may regulate their own release. None of the anterior pituitary hormones has been shown to be regulated by all the processes shown.

to prevent the body from becoming excessively dehydrated by acting on the kidneys in a manner that helps to conserve water that might otherwise be lost in the urine. Released from the posterior pituitary as required, ADH is carried by the blood to its primary target tissues—certain portions of the renal tubular epithelium. Here, the hormone's action helps to increase the permeability of this tissue to the filtered water still contained in the tubules. Thus, this water re-enters the bloodstream, instead of remaining in the tubules and collecting ducts of the kidneys to be carried out of the body in the urine.

Clinical uses

Hypothalamic hormones and synthetic substitutes

None of the naturally occurring hypothalamic hypophysiotropic hormones is used clinically, but synthetic analogues of two of these hormones are now available for clinical use in diagnostic tests (see Chap. 56, Drugs Used for Diagnosis).

Protirelin (Thypinone; Relefact TRH), a synthetic tripeptide that is believed to be identical to TRH, is used in diagnosing thyroid, pituitary, and hypothalamic dysfunction; *gonadorelin HCl* (Factrel), a synthetic gonadotropin-releasing hormone, is used to evaluate suspected hypothalamic and anterior pituitary gonadotropin deficiency. Gonadorelin is being investigated as a therapeutic agent to induce or inhibit ovulation and to treat precocious puberty. *Arginine HCl* (R-Gene 10), levodopa, and insulin act like GHRF (their use in diagnosing anterior pituitary dysfunction is described in Chapter 56).

The usefulness of the hypothalamic hormones in treating chronic endocrine deficiency states is limited by their chemical nature; except possibly for PIF, they are all peptides and therefore must be administered by injection.

Anterior pituitary hormones and synthetic substitutes

Disease of the anterior pituitary gland leads to the partial failure of the endocrine target glands that depend on the pituitary hormones for tropic stimulation. Although patients suffering from pituitary gland failure could be treated by replacement therapy with pituitary tropic hormones, their use is not generally considered clinically practicable at present.

Patients who show deficiencies of the target endocrine glands are treated with the hormones of those glands (Table 20-1). Thus, thyroid hormones, sex steroids, and adrenocorticosteroids from an outside source are administered because the pituitary hormones that might be given to make the person's own glands produce these secretions are more expensive, less reliable, and more difficult to administer than the target organ's hormones. Because the pituitary hormones are proteins or polypeptides that would be digested if taken by mouth, they must be given by injection; also, as foreign proteins, they stimulate production of antibodies that may lead to allergic reactions as well as eventually to a lessening of their effectiveness.

Nevertheless, there are some circumstances in which certain of the anterior pituitary hormones are employed. Their use may well increase in the future as purified human pituitary hormones or their synthetic or semisynthetic modifications become more readily available. Thus, it seems desirable to discuss the current clinical status of several anterior pituitary hormones in the treatment and diagnosis of various disorders.

Adrenocorticotropic hormone

Actions and regulation of secretion. The adrenocorticotropic hormone (corticotropin[+]; ACTH) is produced by certain cells of the anterior pituitary gland and is released into the systemic circulation when that gland receives stimuli from the brain. The hypothalamus secretes a neurohormone, the corticotropin-releasing hormone (CRH), which signals the pituitary cells to secrete the previously synthesized hormone. Carried by the bloodstream to the adrenal glands, corticotropin then stimulates the outer coat, or cortex, to increase production of hormones—the several types of adrenocortical steroids (glucocorticoids, mineralocorticoids, and sex hormones) that are discussed in Chapter 21.*

These adrenal steroids in the bloodstream tend in turn to regulate the further secretion of corticotropin by the pituitary gland. When high levels of the circulating steroids reach the brain, they suppress the secretion of CRH. Deprived of this hypothalamic stimulus, the

pituitary cells stop secreting stored corticotropin. This negative feedback mechanism from the adrenal glands, in turn, shuts off adrenocortical hormone production.

In times of physical and emotional stress, the hypothalamic–pituitary secretion mechanism is *not* turned off by the usual amounts of adrenal hormones reaching the brain by way of the bloodstream. The continued outpouring of pituitary and adrenal hormones that results from this failure of negative feedback then helps the body to meet and to overcome the stressful situation. However, patients who have been treated for various diseases with high doses of adrenocortical steroid drugs may suffer suppression of pituitary production of corticotropin. This then can result in atrophy of the adrenal glands and thus subject the steroid-treated patient to the danger of adrenal insufficiency and failure (Chap. 21).

Status of corticotropin. The adrenocorticotropic pituitary hormone was formerly employed for treating most of the same disorders that are relieved by corticosteroid therapy (Chap. 21). This is understandable, because injections of this hormone stimulate normal adrenal glands to secrete increased amounts of all three types of endogenous adrenocorticosteroid hormones. However, the treatment of choice is exogenously administered corticosteroid drugs rather than this adrenal cortex-stimulating hormone for most of the clinical conditions that are responsive to both types of hormones.

One reason for the superiority of steroids in most conditions is that the foreign protein in the ACTH preparation may cause allergic reactions in sensitive patients. Skin tests are sometimes done before beginning treatment, and patients should be observed for a few minutes following injections to detect and to counteract anaphylaxis. In addition, oral doses of corticosteroid drugs are more convenient to administer and less expensive than corticotropin injections. The synthetic steroids produce a more predictable anti-inflammatory effect, and they are free of the usually undesirable mineralocorticoid and sex hormone effects that corticotropin produces by its actions on the patient's own adrenal glands.

Some physicians, however, still prefer ACTH to the synthetic adrenal steroid hormones for some patients, because ACTH stimulates the adrenal cortex to release *all* the natural steroid hormones, including the male sex hormone, which has *anabolic,* or protein-building, effects (Chap. 24). These are thought to be beneficial for patients with neuromuscular conditions that might be made worse by the muscle-wasting effects of therapy with synthetic glucosteroids alone. (See the index for further discussions of disorders in which corticotropin is employed.)

Treatment and diagnosis of adrenal insufficiency with corticotropin. Patients with failing adrenal function that is the result of hypopituitarism may respond to continued injections of ACTH. However, the preferred treatment for such cases of adrenal insufficiency secondary to pituitary failure is replacement therapy with adrenal

---

* The mechanism of action of corticotropin (and of other polypeptide hormones) is similar in many respects to that of the catecholamines (Chap. 13). That is, it first binds to specific receptors on the membranes of adrenal cortex target cells. The hormone–receptor complex then activates the membrane enzyme, adenylate cyclase. This, in turn, raises the rate at which the intracellular cyclic nucleotide, cyclic adenosine $3',5'$-monophosphate (cAMP), is formed. The increased intracellular quantity of this second messenger—corticotropin is the first chemical messenger here—then stimulates the rate of the enzymatic reactions that catalyze key steps in the biosynthesis of both adrenal cell protein and the adrenocortical steroid hormones.

Table 20–1. Pituitary gland hormones and synthetic substitutes

Official or generic name	Trade name or synonym	Usual adult dosage and administration	Comments
Anterior pituitary hormone activity			
Chorionic gonadotropin for injection USP	Human chorionic gonadotropin; HCG (many trade names)	1,000–10,000 U, depending on the indication for its use	Has LH (ICSH) activity
Corticotropin injection USP	Acthar; ACTH	25–40 U IM, or SC tid; 10–25 U IV infusion in 500 ml of 5% glucose	See Drug digest
Corticotropin injection, repository USP	H.P. Acthar Gel	25–40 U IM, or SC every 24–72 h	Long-acting form
Corticotropin zinc hydroxide sterile suspension, USP	Cortrophin-Zinc	20–60 units IM every 24–72 hr	Long-acting form
Cosyntropin	Cortrosyn	0.25–0.75 mg IM, or IV	Synthetic subunit of corticotropin employed as a diagnostic screening test in patients with presumed adrenocortical insufficiency
Growth hormone, human	Asellacrin; Crescormon; HGH; somatotropin; STH	2–5 mg SC three times a week	Used for treatment of pituitary dwarfism
Menotropins	Pergonal; HMG; human menopausal urinary gonadotropin	75 U of FSH and 75 U of LH daily for 9–12 days	Follicle-stimulating hormone from the human pituitary; used in treatment of female sterility as an ovulatory agent (Chap. 23)
Thyrotropin USP	Thytropar	10 U IM, or SC daily for 1 to 8 days, depending on the indication for its use	Thyrotropic activity; used to stimulate the thyroid gland in diagnostic and therapeutic procedures
Posterior pituitary hormone activity			
Desmopressin	DDAVP	5 μg twice daily by nasal insufflation	Synthetic 8-arginine vasopressin
Lypressin	Diapid nasal spray	One or two sprays to one or both nostrils qid	Synthetic 8-lysine vasopressin
Oxytocin injection USP	Pitocin; Syntocinon; Uteracon	2–10 U IM, IV, or by IV infusion, depending on the specific indication	Used for its oxytocic effect in the induction and management of labor and postpartum hemorrhage

(continued)

Table 20–1. Pituitary gland hormones and synthetic substitutes (continued)

Official or generic name	Trade name or synonym	Usual adult dosage and administration	Comments
Oxytocin, synthetic	Syntocinon nasal spray	One spray into one nostril	Used for its galacto-kinetic effect to make breast milk more readily available
Posterior pituitary injection USP	Pituitrin injection	5–10 U IM	Contains the activity of the antidiuretic hormone (ADH)
Posterior pituitary USP	Pituitrin powder	Variable	Same as above
Vasopressin injection USP	Pitressin	5–10 U IM, or SC or by intranasal application, tid or qid	Purified antidiuretic hormone (ADH) for treating diabetes insipidus
Vasopressin tannate injection USP	Pitressin Tannate	1.25–5 U IM every 1 to 3 days, or at other required intervals	Long-acting form of ADH for treating diabetes insipidus

steroids (Chap. 21). Similarly, the hypopituitary patient's lack of endogenous thyroid and sex gland hormones is best treated by administering these hormones directly rather than by trying to stimulate the glands with the thyroid-stimulating and gonadotropic hormones of the pituitary glands.

Corticotropin is not, of course, useful for treating adrenal insufficiency in patients who have had their adrenal glands removed. It is also ineffective in patients with Addison's disease or other disorders in which the damaged adrenal glands do not respond to the patient's own pituitary adrenocorticotropic hormone. Although corticotropin has, in the past, been advocated for stimulating the partially atrophied adrenal glands of patients who have been on long-term steroid therapy, it is rarely recommended today for reactivating adrenal function. (Some authorities suggest that, once spontaneous recovery of adrenal secretion begins, corticotropin injections may help to shorten the lengthy recovery period.)

Corticotropin is, however, used in laboratory tests of adrenal function. *Cosyntropin* (Cortrosyn), a synthetic polypeptide made up of a chain of 24 of the 39 amino acids of corticotropin, is often preferred for diagnostic purposes (its only use) because it is as effective as ACTH for stimulating the adrenal glands but is less likely than ACTH to cause allergic reactions. (The use of corticotropin, cosyntropin, and *metyrapone ditartrate* (Metopirone), an inhibitor of corticosteroid synthesis, in diagnostic tests of the hypothalamopituitary–adrenal axis is described in Chapter 56, Drugs Used for Diagnosis.)

Thyrotropin

The anterior pituitary gland secretes thyrotropin (thyroid-stimulating hormone; TSH), a tropic hormone that stimulates the thyroid gland to increase its secretion of thyroid hormones. TSH is itself secreted by the pituitary in response to stimulation by the hypothalamus, which produces a thyrotropin-releasing hormone (TRH). The hormones of the thyroid gland exert a negative feedback effect that controls the secretion of TRH by the hypothalamus and of TSH by the anterior pituitary gland (see Chap. 22 for a further discussion of thyroid–pituitary regulatory relationships).

Thyrotropin (Thytropar) is a purified extract of TSH obtained from bovine anterior pituitary glands. It is used mainly as a diagnostic agent to differentiate between primary hypothyroidism and that which occurs secondary to pituitary failure (see Chap. 56, Drugs Used for Diagnosis).

Gonadotropic hormones

The anterior pituitary gland produces two hormones that affect the functioning of the male and female sex glands, or gonads. These are the follicle-stimulating hormone (FSH), and the luteinizing or interstitial cell-stimulating hormone (LH or ICSH). These hormones and gonad-stimulating substances obtained from *non*-pituitary sources (see below), as well as drugs that promote or inhibit the release of gonadotropins, have important clinical application in the treatment of infertility, endometriosis, and other reproductive organ dysfunctions. In addition, it is necessary to understand the functions of the gonadotropins to understand the actions and clinical uses of the natural and synthetic gonadal hormones (estrogens, progestins, and androgens) discussed in Chapters 23 and 24.

Follicle-stimulating hormone. FSH is first secreted at puberty, when a preset "biologic clock" within the brain makes the hypothalamus increase its secretion of GnRH, which stimulates pituitary cells to produce this gonadotropic hormone.

Actions on the ovary. After puberty, FSH continues to affect ovarian function cyclically all through the reproductive years of a woman's life. Early in each cycle, FSH released by the pituitary stimulates several primordial follicles in the ovary to grow. As they enlarge and develop under the influence of FSH (together, probably, with small amounts of LH), these follicles secrete *estrogens.* These ovarian sex hormones then act on the reproductive system, including the inner lining of the uterus or *endometrium*, which gradually grows in thickness during this so-called *proliferative phase* of the ovulatory cycle (see Fig. 23-2).

Actions on the testis. In men, FSH has only one function. It does *not* stimulate secretion of androgens, or male sex hormones, but it does have an effect on sperm production analogous to its role in helping to produce ova in women. Specifically, FSH produces this gametogenic effect in men by stimulating the development of the seminiferous tubules of the testes. Such stimulation of testicular germinal epithelium influences *spermatogenesis,* the complex series of steps by which spermatozoa are produced and brought to maturity.

Luteinizing hormone. LH, or ICSH, the second gonadotropin produced by the anterior pituitary gland of both men and women, serves to stimulate hormone production by the gonads of both sexes.

Actions on the ovary. LH plays an important role in the final ripening of the ovarian follicles that leads to *ovulation*, the release of an ovum by the ovary. The small amounts of LH produced by the pituitary gland during the first half of the menstrual cycle aid FSH stimulation of follicular growth. Then, at midcycle, a sudden steep rise in serum levels of LH is seen. This burst of LH activity, together with a brief resurgence of FSH to peak plasma levels, causes the wall of one ripened follicle to become thinner and finally to rupture. The mature ovum is then flushed out of the ruptured follicle by the pressure of follicular fluid. It floats away from the ovary and is picked up by the ends of an oviduct (fallopian tube), within which it may be fertilized by arriving sperm. Anything that interferes with the precisely timed release of hypothalamic GnRH and the pituitary gonadotropins may prevent the release of the ovum and thus affect fertility (see discussion of oral contraceptives in Chapter 23).

After the ovarian follicle breaks, LH continues to act on the cells of the collapsed sac. Under the influence of this gonadotropic hormone, the follicle capsule is converted into a thick bright orange body called the *corpus luteum* (see Figs. 23-1 and 23-2). The continuing secretion of LH stimulates the cells of the corpus luteum to secrete a second ovarian hormone, *progesterone*, during the latter 2 weeks of the menstrual cycle.

The rising level of progesterone in the bloodstream exerts a negative feedback effect on the hypothalamus and on pituitary production of gonadotropins. Suppression of pituitary secretion of LH, in turn, causes the corpus luteum to shrivel and die. This then deprives the lining of the uterus, or *endometrium*, of its support by the ovarian sex steroids. The deteriorated endometrium and the unfertilized ovum leave the body during the process of *menstruation* that then begins.

However, if the ovum has been fertilized while in the oviduct, or fallopian tube, and has become attached to the uterine wall, menstruation does not occur. This is because the corpus luteum continues to produce progesterone under stimulation by a *luteotropic* gonadotropin. This gonadotropic hormone is produced *not* by the anterior pituitary gland but by the early pregnancy tissues, or trophoblast, that eventually form the placenta, or *chorion.*

This *non*pituitary hormone is *human chorionic gonadotropin* (HCG), which begins to appear in a woman's urine within a week or so after conception—a fact that forms the basis for several pregnancy tests. HCG obtained from the urine of pregnant women has been the gonadotropin chiefly employed clinically in the treatment of both men and women deficient in the pituitary luteinizing hormone, LH (see below, Therapeutic uses).

Actions on the testis. In men, LH is known as the interstitial cell-stimulating hormone (ICSH), because it stimulates the Leydig cells located in the interstices, or spaces, between the seminiferous tubules. These cells then secrete *androgens* (male sex hormones)—mainly testosterone, the growth hormone of the male accessory sex organs (Chap. 24). Thus, in theory at least, this gonadotropin might be expected to stimulate sluggish male gonads to secrete more testosterone when administered from an outside source.

Therapeutic uses. Purified gonadotropic hormones obtained from human pituitary glands postmortem have proved effective for favorably altering sex gland functions in clinical experimental studies. However, because of the limited supply available from this source, the human gonadotropins employed clinically are extracted from the urine of pregnant and postmenopausal women. Pregnancy urine is a rich source of HCG, which—as previously indicated—has high luteinizing (LH) activity. Postmenopausal urine has high levels of both types of pituitary gonadotropins, because the low level of estrogen resulting from menopausal ovarian failure releases the pituitary gland from negative feedback inhibition.

Female infertility. *Menotropins,* a purified preparation of human menopausal gonadotropin (HMG; Pergonal), is employed together with chorionic gonadotropin in a treatment regimen that has helped some infertile women to conceive and bear children. It is useful only in women who have failed to ovulate because of a lack of the pituitary gonadotropins needed to bring about maturation of ovarian follicles. The treatment is not effective in primary ovarian failure, or when infertility is caused by disease of the fallopian tubes or the uterus. Thus, patients must undergo extensive tests to rule out organic disease and primary ovarian failure before this treatment is undertaken.

Patients with secondary ovarian failure are first treated with daily intramuscular injections of menotropins for 9 to 12 days. Although this preparation has both FSH and LH activity, the doses of menotropins alone that can be safely employed do not usually produce ovulation. Thus, after this treatment has brought about ovarian follicular maturation (as indicated by tests for increased estrogenic activity), it is followed by an injection of human chorionic gonadotropin 1 day after the last dose of menotropins. The ovulation that then occurs in about three out of four patients can be confirmed by various tests that show the presence of progesterone, which has been produced by the corpus luteum following HCG stimulation. To ensure insemination of any ovum that is produced, women desiring pregnancy are encouraged to have daily intercourse from the last day of menotropins administration until well after the tests for progesterone are all positive.

Pregnancy occurs in about 25% of the treated women, with multiple births—mostly twins—in about 20% of cases. The patient should be made aware of the possibility of multiple pregnancies, including occasional triplets and, more rarely, quadruplets and quintuplets. The patient should also be advised of other possible adverse effects of ovarian overstimulation. Most commonly this is manifested by abdominal distention and pain. Further administration of menotropins should be stopped in such cases, and the patient should be hospitalized because of the hazard of ovarian cyst rupture.

Clomiphene citrate (Clomid; Serophene), an orally effective drug, is also used to induce ovulation in women with ovulatory failure. It is thought to act by competing for estrogen receptors in cells of the hypothalamus or pituitary and releasing these cells from feedback inhibition by endogenous estrogen. Thus, it brings about an increased output of gonadotropins by the patient's own pituitary gland. The pituitary FSH and LH then stimulate maturation of the ovarian follicle, followed by ovulation and the later development of a functioning corpus luteum. This drug is therefore indicated for treating anovulatory women who are shown to have a functioning pituitary gland and ovaries. It is not effective in patients with either primary pituitary or primary ovarian failure, which must be ruled out by a battery of preliminary tests.

This *non*gonadotropic drug has helped to produce pregnancies in about the same proportion of patients as the menotropins–HCG injection series described above. It has the advantage of being relatively simple to use, because most patients who respond do so after a single 5-day course of daily oral doses (50 mg/day). Some side-effects of the two types of infertility treatments, such as abdominal discomfort and ovarian enlargement, are sim-

ilar, and multiple births occur more often than normally with both treatments.

Additional adverse reactions to clomiphene include occasional vasomotor symptoms such as hot flashes and visual symptoms, including blurring and the appearance of spots or flashes in the visual field. Neither of these side-effects is severe, and both disappear promptly after treatment is discontinued. Clomiphene and HCG are also used diagnostically in male patients when hypogonadism is suspected (see Chap. 24).

Male infertility. Menotropins and HCG are given concomitantly for 3 months to stimulate spermatogenesis in men with pituitary hypofunction. These men have usually been pretreated with HCG alone until secondary sexual characteristics develop and testosterone levels are normal.

Cryptorchidism. HCG is the preferred treatment for cryptorchidism, or undescended testicle. This is a condition in which the testes of young boys fail to descend from their fetal position in the abdomen. If uncorrected, this can lead to sterility as a result of damage to the germinal epithelium, with subsequent failure of sperm production. In such cases, provided that there is no mechanical obstruction requiring surgery, a course of HCG injections can often bring the testes down into the scrotal sac.

Apparently, the interstitial cell-stimulating (ICSH) activity of this extract leads to production of the male hormone, the action of which brings about descent of the testis. Failure of HCG to accomplish this or to elicit any other androgenic responses means that the patient's testes are either absent or atrophied and that he will require treatment with testosterone itself, preferably at puberty, to develop his accessory sex organs and secondary sex characteristics (see Chap. 24). On the other hand, youngsters being treated with HCG must be watched for signs of sexual precocity—the result of stimulation of excessive testosterone secretion at too early an age. The occurrence of frequent penile erections in such children serves as a warning that HCG dosage should be reduced or that the hormone should be administered less frequently.

Antigonadotropic drugs

The female sex hormones estrogen and progesterone, and synthetic substances with similar activity, can suppress production of FSH and LH by the anterior pituitary gland. This, in turn, interferes with ovarian function, an effect that accounts for the use of these drugs as oral contraceptives and in the treatment of such disorders as dysfunctional uterine bleeding, dysmenorrhea, and endometriosis (Chap. 23). However, because of the adverse effects of sex steroids, scientists have been seeking other safer drugs with antigonadotropic activity.

Danazol (Danocrine), a synthetic drug that is a weak androgen, can depress the release of both FSH and

LH (ICSH) from male and female pituitary glands. It is used for treating *endometriosis*, a disorder that sometimes leads to infertility in women, and has recently been approved for treating fibrocystic breast disease when breast pain is severe and does not respond to analgesics. It is also being employed experimentally as a male oral contraceptive. The recommended dose is 800 mg/day for endometriosis and 100–400 mg/day for fibrocystic breast disease. Doses are usually divided, and the drug is administered twice daily.

As indicated in the more detailed discussion of endometriosis in Chapter 23, drugs that suppress pituitary function and thus prevent ovulation and menstruation from occurring are useful for symptomatic relief of this disorder. Such drugs, including danazol, help to prevent pathologic bleeding from bits of endometrial tissue that have been carried back from the uterus and become implanted on pelvic organs including the ovaries and fallopian tubes. When the drug is withdrawn after many months of treatment, the displaced uterine lining tissue may remain atrophied, even though normal ovulation and menstruation resume. Thus, this drug has helped some women who were infertile because of endometriosis to conceive and bear children.

Danazol is not any more effective than the progestins that are used for this purpose (Chap. 23), and it can cause masculinizing and other side-effects. It is presently reserved for treating women with endometriosis that has not been helped by progestin treatment or by other medical measures. It should not be used for treating cases of endometriosis that require surgical removal of the intra-abdominal masses or panhysterectomy.

Prolactin

The anterior pituitary gland also secretes a hormone called *prolactin* that plays a part in milk production by nursing mothers. This hormone is not ordinarily produced by nonpregnant women, because the hypothalamus secretes a prolactin release-inhibiting factor (PIF) that inhibits the pituitary gland. During pregnancy, however, there seems to be a reduction in such hypothalamic inhibition of prolactin production and secretion, which reaches peak plasma levels at the time of delivery. The infant's suckling of the mother's breast stimulates further secretion of prolactin (and of the posterior pituitary hormone, oxytocin; see below), with a resulting increase in milk secretion by the breast.

Certain antipsychotic drugs including chlorpromazine (Thorazine) and haloperidol (Haldol), which block dopamine receptors (see Chap. 46), sometimes cause milk secretion (galactorrhea) in women who have not been pregnant. There is much evidence for a dopaminergic inhibitory synapse in the neural pathway controlling prolactin release. PIF (prolactin release-inhibiting factor) may itself be dopamine. The antipsychotic drugs may cause galactorrhea by blocking the effects of PIF and by allowing greater amounts of prolactin to be secreted.

Dopaminergic agonists inhibit the release of prolactin. One of these, an ergot alkaloid derivative, *bromocriptine mesylate* (Parlodel) has recently been approved for use in syndromes marked by both galactorrhea and amenorrhea. This drug is believed to prevent inappropriate lactation in women with hyperprolactinemia by its ability to inhibit excessive prolactin secretion. Bromocriptine is also used to suppress unwanted lactation after delivery, and also restores menses in women whose amenorrhea is associated with failure to ovulate because of certain complex effects of high plasma levels of prolactin on gonadotropic and ovarian function. Thus, this drug is also useful for treating infertility in women whose failure to ovulate is a result of hyperprolactinemia. However, if pregnancy occurs, the drug should be stopped immediately because there is not yet enough evidence to prove that bromocriptine does not produce birth defects in babies whose mothers have taken the drug during pregnancy. The dose of bromocriptine is 2.5 mg, bid or tid, with meals.

Human growth hormone (somatotropin)

Certain cells of the anterior pituitary gland secrete a hormone that stimulates the growth of all body tissues. The secretion of this growth hormone (GH; somatotropin) is, in turn, influenced by two types of hypothalamic-releasing hormones: GHRF (growth hormone-releasing factor), and GHRIH (growth hormone release-inhibiting hormone), or somatostatin.

Hypopituitary dwarfism. Some children do not grow because the pituitary gland cells responsible for secreting growth hormone fail to do so. If their growth failure is found to be caused by a deficiency of this growth hormone, they can now be treated successfully by replacement therapy with a growth hormone obtained from human pituitary glands. This substance, which is available as *Asellacrin*, is a purified dried extract that is reconstituted with bacteriostatic water and injected intramuscularly.

Children whose dwarfism has been shown to result from a lack of growth hormone are started on a course of three IM injections per week. If growth definitely accelerates over the next 8 to 12 months, the somatotropin treatment is continued for several years until the patient reaches a satisfactory height. If growth slows to 1 inch or less in 6 months, the dose is doubled during the next 6 months.

This treatment is not effective for children whose dwarfism results from other factors, nor does it work once the epiphyses—the growing ends of the long bones—have closed. Almost 50% of patients treated with this protein antigen develop antibodies to it, but this seldom causes allergic reactions or interferes with the growth-stimulating effect of the drug.

Patients must be monitored in various ways to ensure maximal effectiveness with minimal adverse effects. Those who are close to puberty or who are also receiving thyroid replacement therapy must have their bone age determined before continuing with the treatment course, which would be ineffective after the rapid epiphyseal closure that tends to occur under those circumstances. Patients whose lack of growth hormone has been caused by an intracranial lesion must be examined frequently. If the underlying disease process continues to progress, somatotropin treatment must be stopped.

Somatotropin has many metabolic effects. The one most important in producing growth is its stimulation of amino acid transport into body cells. It also interferes with the intracellular metabolism of glucose, an effect that is called *diabetogenic*, because it can lead to hyperglycemia and ketosis. This is why caution is required when somatotropin is administered to dwarfed children with a personal or family history of diabetes mellitus.

Scientists have been trying to separate the diabetes-producing component of somatotropin. If they succeed in so doing, and then synthesize the pure growth-promoting factor, the synthetic growth hormone would *not* cause hyperglycemia. More important, if it could be made cheaply in unlimited amounts, growth hormone would no longer have to be obtained from human pituitary glands, a source that supplies only a small fraction of the amount required.

Somatotropin has also been used experimentally to raise the blood sugar levels of *hypo*glycemic patients. On the other hand, *somatostatin*—the growth hormone release-inhibiting hormone of the hypothalamus (see above)—is being used in the experimental treatment of *hyper*glycemia in diabetes, because it can cause hypoglycemia (see Chap. 25). Its effects on blood sugar levels and the fact that it must be administered by injection limit its usefulness for treating disorders marked by excessive growth.

Acromegaly and gigantism. These and other forms of hyperpituitarism, in which growth hormone is secreted in excessive amounts, are treated mainly by irradiation or by surgical excision of the pituitary gland tumors that are the usual cause. However, these treatments do not always succeed in destroying or removing all the hyperactive secretory cells. In these cases, bromocriptine, the dopaminergic drug described above that inhibits prolactin secretion, is now sometimes used as an adjunct. Bromocriptine, administered orally, has proved effective for lowering plasma levels of growth hormone

in most patients in whom it has been employed. It causes no side-effects other than nausea at the start of treatment, and it does not affect the secretion of other pituitary hormones except prolactin (see above). It should be noted that the ability of bromocriptine to lower plasma levels of growth hormone in patients with acromegaly is paradoxical. Levodopa and other dopaminergic agonists facilitate the release of GH in people with normal pituitary function.

Posterior pituitary hormones and synthetic substitutes

Oxytocin

The clinical use of oxytocin and drugs with oxytocic activity in initiating and managing labor and postpartum is described in chapter 23 (Table 20-1).

Antidiuretic hormone

The main clinical use of drugs with the activity of ADH is as replacement therapy in patients with diabetes insipidus.

Diabetes insipidus. This condition, marked by the excretion of copious quantities of sugar-free urine, is caused mainly by a deficiency of ADH. The lack of this secretion is, in turn, usually the result of a brain tumor or of trauma affecting the hypothalamic neurosecretory cells and their nerve fiber tracts running in the pituitary stalk. Such so-called central diabetes insipidus is now also sometimes seen postoperatively in patients who have undergone a hypophysectomy (surgical removal of the pituitary gland) for treatment of breast cancer, diabetic retinopathy, or other serious and life-threatening illnesses.*

Extracts of the posterior pituitary glands of animals have been employed to prevent patients with diabetes insipidus from becoming dehydrated. Patients with a relatively mild form of this disease may keep it under control by inhaling a powdered form of the extract through the nose for systemic absorption from the nasal mucous membranes. The more potent *posterior pituitary injection* (Pituitrin) is needed for more severe cases. However, when injections are necessary, most specialists now prefer to use the purer form of the hormone, *vasopressin injection* (Pitressin), or a longer-lasting preparation *vasopressin tannate injection* (Pitressin Tannate; see Table 20-1).

Administered in proper dosage at optimal intervals, all these forms of ADH are effective for reducing the large volume of urine voided daily (*polyuria*). However, overdosage can lead to *fluid retention* and to excessive loss of sodium (*hyponatremia*). Patients are watched for such signs of water intoxication as drowsiness and mental confusion. If this occurs, the hormone is withheld until

---

* Occasionally, diabetes insipidus proves to be nephrogenic, rather than central. That is, the patient's kidneys are not responsive to the antidiuretic hormone. Such cases cannot be treated with the drugs discussed here. Instead, they sometimes respond—paradoxically—to treatment with thiazide-type diuretics (see Chap. 27).

the patient's production of urine rises again to abnormal levels. Treatment is resumed at reduced dosage and less frequent intervals.

Other adverse effects of posterior pituitary extracts, including vasopressin, may occur as the result of contraction of the smooth muscles of the intestine (cramps and diarrhea), uterus, and blood vessels. Constriction of arterial smooth muscle may cause a mild rise in blood pressure. More serious is constriction of the coronary arteries of patients with angina pectoris, because it may set off chest pains or even cause an acute coronary attack. Thus, these preparations are administered cautiously in the smallest dose effective for control of diabetes insipidus when the patient also suffers from disease of the coronary arteries. Patients also occasionally become allergic to the foreign protein in even the purified extracts of animal glands. This can be avoided by the use of certain synthetic substitutes with antidiuretic activity.

Lypressin (Diapid) is a synthetic form of the antidiuretic hormone that has several advantages over the natural posterior pituitary gland hormone. Because it is completely free of any oxytocin impurity or foreign proteins, it produces the desired renal reabsorption of water in diabetes insipidus patients with fewer allergic reactions or other side-effects than are caused by the animal-derived hormone, vasopressin.

This drug is available as a liquid nasal spray that is less irritating than the dry posterior pituitary gland powdered extract and more convenient to take than the conventional injections of the natural hormone. Patients learn to titrate their own dosage, taking one or two sprays in each nostril as needed to control polyuria and thirst, usually for up to 6 hours.

Lypressin has relatively little vasoconstrictor and vasopressor activity compared to vasopressin. However, it has to be used cautiously by diabetes insipidus patients with coronary heart disease or hypertension. It can also occasionally cause abdominal cramps and increased bowel movements.

Nasal membrane irritation and ulceration are rare, but the drug's effectiveness may be reduced in patients with nasal congestion caused by a cold or allergic rhinitis. In such cases, patients may require pretreatment with a nasal decongestant followed some time later by a larger than usual dose of the lypressin nasal spray.

Desmopressin (DDAVP) is another synthetic substitute for natural vasopressin that is also administered intranasally. Its main advantage over lypressin lies in its longer lasting renal action—6 to 20 hours. This makes it effective for most patients when taken only twice daily, in the morning and at bedtime. Like lypressin, desmopressin possesses a therapeutic ratio superior to that of vasopressin. That is, the very small (5 μg) doses often effective for reducing the patient's daily urinary output to normal do not ordinarily cause such systemic side-effects as a rise in blood pressure or abdominal cramps.

Headache is the only systemic side-effect thus far reported with any frequency, and this has occurred mainly in patients who occasionally become resistant to desmopressin's antidiuretic effect and require doses several times higher than those that had proved initially effective. Drug interactions with the antilipemic agent clofibrate (Atromid-S) and the oral hypoglycemic agent chlorpropamide (Diabinese) have occasionally been reported. However, such interactions—which involve a potentiation and prolongation of the antidiuretic effect of desmopressin—may actually prove useful in the management of some patients with diabetes insipidus. Each is sometimes used alone in treating diabetes insipidus in patients with some ability to produce ADH. Clofibrate may act by stimulating the secretion of ADH; chlorpropamide may act by increasing the kidney's sensitivity to ADH.

Other uses. Some other actions of vasopressin mentioned previously as a cause of adverse effects in patients with diabetes insipidus are sometimes sought in the treatment of other disorders. The vasoconstrictor effect of vasopressin is, for example, employed to control bleeding from swollen vessels in the esophagus of patients with cirrhosis of the liver that has led to a rise in pressure within the portal circulation. This use of vasopressin as a hemostatic in the management of bleeding esophageal varices is discussed in the section on liver disease treatment in Chapter 41.

Vasopressin has also been employed to increase the propulsive motility of the intestinal smooth muscle of patients with postoperative abdominal distention. However, drugs such as the cholinergic agents neostigmine and bethanechol (see Chap. 15) are preferred for this purpose, as are various mechanical measures for aiding the elimination of gas. Similarly, although vasopressin has been used prior to x-ray of the gallbladder, a drug called *sincalide* (Kinevac) seems safer as a means of evacuating this organ in preparation for radiography (see Chap. 56). Vasopressin is also no longer employed in the management of shock, because the adrenergic vasopressor drugs (Chap. 17) are now considered more reliable in such cases.

Additional clinical considerations

Many hypothalamic and pituitary drugs are used for diagnostic purposes; clinical considerations relating to these drugs are discussed in the chapter on diagnostic agents. The ovulatory stimulants menotropins and clomiphene should be administered only after a thorough evaluation of the probable causes of the infertility, and after an evaluation of the woman's overall physical condition. The woman has to be carefully evaluated to rule out fibrocystic breast disease, ovarian enlargement, uterine disorders, and pregnancy, all of which are contraindications to the use of these drugs. Side-effects that the patient, male or female, may experience include the signs and symptoms of elevated sex hormone levels—nausea, vomiting, flushing, and breast tenderness and enlargement. Blurring of vision is a frequent problem of which the patient should be aware, so that driving an automobile or working with dangerous machinery can be avoided, should blurring of vision occur. Women need to be counseled about the possibility of multiple births if they succeed in conceiving; the multiple births are a result of the actions of the drug on the developing ovarian follicles.

Danazol, which acts to block the release of FSH and LH, causes adverse effects as the body responds to lower than normal levels of estrogen—for example, vaginitis, hot flashes, vaginal atrophy, and skin changes. The drug also can cause some masculinizing effects, such as lower voice, skin changes, and breast changes. The patient needs to know about these possibilities, and she should be encouraged to discuss her feelings about them as she learns to cope with them.

Technical factors

ADH should never be given IV because of its vasoconstricting properties. When given IM or SC, the area should be rubbed vigorously after administration to facilitate drug absorption. In general, ADH is contraindicated in people with cardiovascular diseases, because the vasoconstriction it causes can seriously aggravate such conditions as hypertension, angina, and peripheral vascular disease. When a patient is taking ADH as a nasal spray, it is important that it be administered with the head upright—not tilted back, as is the normal procedure for nose drops. The patient should be upright, and the bottle should also be held upright. This position will ensure that the drug is absorbed properly and rapidly. Problems can occur if the patient has a "cold" or allergic rhinitis. In these conditions, the mucous membranes are edematous and cannot absorb the drug adequately. When these conditions result in an exacerbation of the patient's diabetes insipidus, it may be necessary to administer the drug by a different route until the nasal congestion has cleared. ADH is also contraindicated in pregnancy, because it may have harmful effects on the pregnant uterus and the fetus.

Drug–drug and drug–laboratory test interactions. The systemic effects of these hormones can influence the effects of a number of other drugs that the patient might be taking concomitantly. *Danazol* decreases the synthesis of clotting factors in the liver, which in turn tends to delay clotting. Because of this, if a patient is on *warfarin*, the prothrombin time will be greater than expected, and the patient will require a smaller dose of warfarin for safe anticoagulation. *Danazol* also increases blood glucose levels, increasing the body's *insulin* requirements. A patient stabilized on insulin may need to be reregulated at higher doses when danazol is started. The *menotropins* have been reported to cause an increase in *serum thyroxine* levels, an effect often associated with increases in estrogen levels.

The patient teaching guide and guide to the nursing process for most of these drugs are included in the chapter on drugs used for diagnosis (Chap. 56) and in the chapters on hormones and drugs affecting the female and male reproductive systems (Chaps. 23 and 24). ADH is the only drug that is not discussed in any of these other chapters. The patient teaching guide and guide to the nursing process that follow will address the patient on ADH therapy.

Patient teaching guide: antidiuretic hormone

The drug that has been prescribed for you is called antidiuretic hormone, ADH. This drug acts in the kidneys to limit the loss of water in the urine.

Instructions:

1. The name of your drug is _____ .

2. The dose of the drug ordered for you is _____ .

3. The drug should be taken _____ times a day. The best time to take your drug is _____ . It is important to take a dose before you go to bed to cover you through the night. You might be asked to monitor your fluid intake while you are taking this drug.

4. (If the drug is to be injected, the patient and a significant other will need instruction in preparation and administration, including rotating sites.)
   If the drug is to be given intranasally, it should be administered with the head held upright and the bottle held upright.

(continued)

5. Some side-effects of the drug that you might experience include the following:

Nasal irritation or congestion	The nasal passages may adjust to the effects of the drug after a time.
Heartburn	This often is caused by excess drug dripping down the pharnyx; more careful administration may alleviate the problem.
Abdominal cramps	If mild, they are a side-effect that must be tolerated.

6. Tell any physician, nurse, or dentist who takes care of you that you are taking this drug.

7. Keep this and all medications out of the reach of children.

Notify your nurse or physician if any of the following occur:

Drowsiness, listlessness, headache
Chest pain, shortness of breath,
    severe abdominal cramps
Prolonged nasal congestion
Return of signs of diabetes
    insipidus—passing large volumes
    of urine and experiencing excessive
    thirst

Guide to the nursing process: antidiuretic hormone

Assessment	Nursing diagnoses	Intervention	Evaluation
Past history (contraindications) include:	Alteration in urinary elimination patterns	Prepare and safely administer drug: IM, SC, intranasally	Monitor response to drug: Decreased urinary output
Coronary artery disease	Knowledge deficit regarding drug therapy	Patient teaching regarding:	Monitor for adverse effects:
Angina	Potential excess in fluid volume	Drug Administration	Water intoxication
Hypertension		Side-effects	Nasal congestion
Peripheral vascular disease		Warning signs	Heartburn
Chronic nephritis		Monitor and limit fluid intake, especially in the elderly	GI problems
Pregnancy			Evaluate effectiveness of teaching program
Current history: Medications: allergies, reactions			

Assessment	Nursing diagnoses	Intervention	Evaluation
Physical assessment Neurologic: orientation Cardiovascular: BP, perfusion, pulses, apical pulse, baseline EKG Respiratory: rate, adventitious sounds GI: bowel sounds, pattern Renal: output, complete urinalysis Urine: specific gravity			

Case study

Presentation

BT, a 56-year-old teacher, developed diabetes insipidus and was eventually regulated on lypressin (Diapid) nasal spray, one or two sprays per nostril qid. BT seemed very much interested in her disease and therapy and learned to control her own dosage by symptom control. BT managed for several years, in good control of her symptoms. At her last clinical visit, it was noted that she had developed postnasal ulcerations and nasal rhinitis. She complained of several GI symptoms, including "upset stomach," severe abdominal cramps, and diarrhea. What nursing measures should be taken?

Discussion

An essential aspect of the ongoing nursing process is the continual evaluation of the effectiveness of drug therapy. In BT's case, an evaluation of the situation shows that the postnasal mucosa is ulcerated, possibly as a result of overexposure to the vasoconstrictive properties of the drug, and the GI tract seems to show evidence of increased ADH effects. All these points seem to indicate that perhaps the drug is not being administered properly—excessive exposure of the postnasal mucosa to the drug, increased absorption, and increased levels reaching the systemic circulation and renal systems. In such situations, the nurse should ask the patient to give herself a dose of the drug and to discuss the signs and symptoms for which she is supposed to be alert. (In this case, although BT remembered most of the details of her drug teaching, when she administered the drug she tilted her head back and, tipping the bottle up, squirted the drug into each nostril. When the nurse questioned BT about her technique, it was discovered that she had seen an advertisement about nasal sprays and realized that she had been "doing it wrong" all this time. The nurse explained the misunderstanding and reviewed the entire teaching protocol with BT. The drug was discontinued, and BT was placed on SC ADH until the nasal ulcerations healed.)

As a patient becomes comfortable with a drug therapy, the details about the drug often become lost or forgotten. It is very important to remember that patient teaching needs regular updating and evaluation. This point is often forgotten with patients who have been on a drug for years, but re-membering to assess the patient's knowledge about the drug can prevent problems such as BT's from developing.

Drug digest

Corticotropin injection USP (ACTH; Acthar)

Actions and indications. This purified pituitary gland preparation stimulates the patient's adrenal glands to produce and secrete glucocorticoid, mineralocorticoid, and sex steroid hormones. It has been used to treat the many types of disorders that respond to treatment with adrenocorticosteroid hormones, including gout and other rheumatic disorders. However, the latter drugs are now preferred for most purposes because of their greater convenience and safety compared to corticotropin.

Corticotropin is sometimes claimed to have special advantages for some types of patients, including those with multiple sclerosis and ulcerative colitis. It is also said to be less likely than the corticosteroids to suppress growth in children. However, these advantages have not been clearly established. Special experimental uses of corticotropin are in the treatment of infantile convulsive spasms and in the management of severe cases of myasthenia gravis. It is also used in the diagnosis of adrenal insufficiency.

Adverse effects, cautions, and contraindications. Corticotropin is capable of causing all the types of toxicity seen in corticosteroid therapy, including sodium and water retention and potassium loss, a type of toxicity that is minimal with most of the synthetic steroids. It can cause signs both of Cushing's syndrome and of adrenocortical insufficiency, which are the result of metabolic and endocrine toxicity. It may also bring about changes in behavior and in mental function, including psychotic changes. In addition, the foreign protein in this preparation may produce allergic reactions in sensitive patients. Thus, patients should be observed for signs of anaphylaxis.

Dosage and administration. Dosage is individualized, depending on the response of each patient's adrenal glands. In general, an attempt is made to obtain and maintain the desired therapeutic effect with the smallest dose that will do so.

Most commonly, treatment is initiated with daily doses of 40 U administered intramuscularly or subcutaneously. Doses of 10 U to 25 U may be dissolved in 500 ml of a 5% solution of dextrose in water and infused intravenously over a period of 8 hours. Doses up to 80 to 120 U daily may be required in some cases.

Repository forms with a more prolonged duration of action may be administered once daily in doses of 40 to 80 U intramuscularly or subcutaneously. In diagnostic procedures, 10 U to 25 U are usually administered intravenously or intramuscularly.

References

General reviews of hypothalamic and anterior pituitary gland hormones

Brooks CM, Koizumi K: The hypothalamus and control of integrative processes. In Mountcastle VB (ed): Medical Physiology, Vol I, 14th ed, pp 923–947. St. Louis, C.V. Mosby, 1980

Goodman HM: The pituitary gland. In Mountcastle VB (ed): Medical Physiology, Vol II, 14th ed, pp 1468–1494. St. Louis, C.V. Mosby, 1980

Guillemin R: The hormones of the hypothalamus. Am J Med 57:591, 1974

Hall R, Gomez–Pan A: The hypothalamic regulatory hormones and their clinical application. Adv Clin Chem 18:173, 1976

Iversen LL: Nonopioid neuropeptides in mammalian CNS. Ann Rev Pharmacol Toxicol 23:1, 1983

McCann SM: Physiology and pharmacology of LHRH and somatostatin. Ann Rev Pharmacol Toxicol 22:491, 1982

Murad F, Haynes RC Jr: Adenohypophyseal hormones and related substances. In Gilman AG, Goodman LS, Gilman A (eds): Goodman and Gilman's The Pharmacological Basis of Therapeutics, 6th ed, pp 1369–1396. New York, Macmillan, 1980

Reichlin S: Anterior pituitary—six glands in one. N Engl J Med 287:1351, 1972

Reichlin S: Hypothalamic hormones. Ann Rev Physiol 38:389, 1976

Root AW et al: Current status and clinical application of the hypothalamic hormones. Adv Pediatr 23:151, 1976

Schally AV et al: Hypothalamic hormones: The link between brain and body. Am Scient 65:712, 1977

Schally AV et al: Hypothalamic regulatory hormones. Science 179:141, 1973

Vale W et al: Regulatory peptides of the hypothalamus. Ann Rev Physiol 39:473, 1977

Wade N, Guillemin R, Schally AV: The years in the wilderness. Science 200:279, 1978

Yallow RS: Radioimmunoassay: A probe for the fine structure of biologic systems. Science 200:1236, 1978

Corticotropin (ACTH) and related drugs

Collip JB et al: The adrenocorticotropic hormone of the anterior pituitary lobe. Lancet 2:347, 1933

Ganong WF et al: ACTH and the regulation of adrenocortical secretion. N Engl J Med 290:1006, 1974

Hench PS: Cortisone and ACTH in clinical medicine. Proc Mayo Clin 25:474, 1950

Thyrotropin, prolactin, and related drugs

Boyd AE et al: Galactorrhea–amenorrhea syndrome: Diagnosis and therapy. Ann Intern Med 87:165, 1977

Carlson HE, Hershman JM: The hypothalamic–pituitary–thyroid axis. Med Clin N Am 59:1045, 1975

Del Pozo E et al: Clinical and hormonal response to bromocriptine (CB-154) in the galactorrhea syndromes. J Clin Endocrinol Metab 39:18, 1974

Duchesne C, Leke R: Bromocriptine mesylate for prevention of postpartum lactation. Obstet Gynecol 57:464, 1981

Greenblatt RB: Amenorrhea–galactorrhea syndromes. Prog Clin Biol Res 112 Pt A:245, 1982

Kolata GB: Infertility: Promising new treatments. Science 202:200, 1978

Ramey JN: Clinical uses of thyrotropin-releasing hormone. Am Fam Physician 12:93, 1975

Thorner MO et al: Long-term treatment of galactorrhea and hypogonadism with bromocriptine. Br Med J 2:419, 1975

Turkington RW: Prolactin secretion in patients treated with various drugs. Arch Intern Med 130:349, 1972

Gonadotropic and antigonadotropic drugs and hormones

Dmowski WP et al: Treatment of endometriosis with an antigonadotropin, danazol. Obstet Gynecol 46:147, 1975

Gemzell CA: Induction of ovulation with human pituitary gonadotropins. Fertil Steril 13:153, 1962

Gonadorelin: Synthetic LH-RH. Med Lett Drugs Ther 25:106, 1983

Rust LA et al: Individualized graduated therapeutic regimen for clomiphene citrate. Am J Obstet Gynecol 120:785, 1974

Vaitukaitis JL, Ross GT: Recent advances in evaluation of gonadotropic hormones. Ann Rev Med 24:295, 1973

Yen SS: Clinical applications of gonadotropin-releasing hormone and gonadotropin-releasing hormone analogs. Fertil Steril 39:257, 1983

Human growth hormone (somatotropin), somatostatin, and related substances

Braunstein GD et al: Response of growth-retarded patients with Hand–Schüller–Christian disease to growth hormone therapy. N Engl J Med 292:332, 1975

Cassar J et al: Bromocriptine treatment of acromegaly. Metabolism 26:539, 1977

Gerich JE: Somatostatin: Diabetes and acromegaly. Adv Intern Med 22:251, 1977

Phillips LS, Vassilopoulou–Sellin R: Somatomedins. N Engl J Med 302:371, 1980

Root AW et al: Diagnosis and management of growth retardation with special reference to the problem of hypopituitarism. J Pediatr 78:737, 1971

Rosenbloom AL: Growth hormone replacement therapy. JAMA 198:364, 1966

Sachdev Y et al: Bromocriptine therapy in acromegaly. Lancet 2:1164, 1975

Tanner JM: Human growth hormone. Nature 237:433, 1972

Vasopressin and related drugs with ADH activity

Cannon JF: Diabetes insipidus. Arch Intern Med 96:215, 1955

Cobb WE: Neurogenic diabetes insipidus: Management with DAVP. Ann Intern Med 88:183, 1978

Du Vigneaud V: Hormones of the posterior pituitary gland: Oxytocin and vasopressin. Harvey Lect 50:1, 1954–55.

Hays RM: Agents affecting the renal conservation of water. In Gilman AG, Goodman LS, Gilman A (eds): Goodman and Gilman's The Pharmacological Basis of Therapeutics, 6th ed, pp 916–928. New York, Macmillan, 1980

Lee WP: Vasopressin analog DDAVP in the treatment of diabetes insipidus. Am J Dis Child 130:166, 1976

Mimica N et al: Lypressin nasal spray. JAMA 203:802, 1968

Rallison ML, Tyler FH: Treatment of diabetes insipidus in children with lysine-8-vasopressin. J Pediatr 70:122, 1967

Randall RV: Treatment of diabetes insipidus. Mod Treat 3:180, 1966

Robinson AG: DDAVP in the treatment of central diabetes insipidus. N Engl J Med 294:507, 1976

Swanson LW, Sawchenko PE: Hypothalamic integration: Organization of the paraventricular and supraoptic nuclei. Ann Rev Neurosci 6:269, 1983

Chapter 21

Adrenocorticosteroid drugs

The adrenocorticosteroid drugs are among the most widely employed of all therapeutic agents. These substances sometimes exert dramatic effects that help to tide patients over the critical stages of acute illnesses. They also control the symptoms of many chronic disorders and thus help patients to avoid disability and to continue their normal activities.

However, these drugs do not actually cure any of the many diseases for which they are so often ordered. When taken to suppress the signs and symptoms of chronic disorders, these drugs do not prevent the progress of the underlying disease process. In addition, prolonged administration of corticosteroid drugs in such chronic cases leads inevitably to the development of adverse effects. Often, serious complications occur in patients with conditions that make them particularly susceptible to steroid toxicity.

To make the most effective use of corticosteroid drugs, certain therapeutic principles must be applied. To understand these principles, it is necessary to understand the control of the synthesis and secretion of the natural adrenal hormones, the physiologic and pharmacologic effects of the natural and synthetic corticosteroids, and the toxic effects and complications that can arise during the use of these drugs. Thus, this chapter will discuss these topics before finally summarizing the principles that must be employed during the use of these drugs in clinical therapeutics.

Physiology of adrenal cortex hormones

The two adrenal glands are flattened bodies that fit like a cap over the top of each kidney. Each gland is made up of an inner core, the medulla, and an outer shell or bark, the cortex. The adrenal medulla is part of the sympathetic nervous system. It is composed of dark brown chromaffin cells which secrete the catecholamines *epinephrine* and *norepinephrine*. The physiologic functions of these catecholamines were discussed in Chapters 13 and 17, which deal with the actions of the autonomic nervous system and of sympathetic nervous system neurotransmitter substances.

The adrenal cortex, which surrounds the adrenal medulla, consists of three layers of cells, each of which biosynthesizes chemically different types of steroid hormones that exert different physiologic effects. There are three types of natural steroid hormones produced and secreted by the adrenal cortex:

1. The *glucocorticoids*—substances such as *cortisol* (hydrocortisone) and *cortisone*, which mainly affect carbohydrate metabolism but also affect protein and fat metabolism
2. The *mineralocorticoids, aldosterone* and *desoxycorticosterone*, which influence salt and water metabolism and promote the retention of sodium in exchange for potassium ions in the renal tubules
3. Certain *male* and *female sex hormones*, which are of only minor importance in normal metabolism compared to similar substances secreted by the testes and the ovaries; however, their presence in excess sometimes causes pathologic symptoms

The glucocorticoids and mineralocorticoids, on the other hand, play an important part in *homeostasis*—that is, in helping the body adjust to changes in the external environment. Through their metabolic effects on body tissues, these hormones influence the functioning of the organs and systems in ways that help to keep the human internal environment constant. When these hormones are lacking and are not replaced from an outside source, survival is not possible, particularly when the person is subjected to severe environmental stress.

Metabolic effects of mineralocorticoids

Among the hormones most important for survival are those with high *mineralocorticoid* activity. When *aldosterone,* for example, is deficient, the kidney tubules lose their ability to return some of the sodium that was filtered through the glomeruli to the blood. As a result of the steady drain of sodium that then develops, the volume of the blood and extracellular fluid declines steadily. If this condition is unchecked, blood pressure falls to shock levels and the patient dies of circulatory collapse.

Metabolic effects of glucocorticoids

These hormones (and synthetic drugs with similar effects) exert complex effects, not only on carbohydrate metabolism, but also on protein and fat metabolism.* One of their functions may be part of a homeostatic mechanism for maintaining reserves of carbohydrate for emergency use. Thus, glucocorticoids tend to increase the production of glucose and to decrease the rate at which the body's tissues burn up this sugar. Under the influence of these hormones, greater amounts of glucose are stored as glycogen in the liver, skeletal muscles, and other tissues.

One source of such *gluconeogenesis,* or new glucose formation, is the breakdown of protein to amino acids. These are then shunted to the liver, where they are converted by enzymatically catalyzed reactions to glucose and stored there as glycogen. Glucocorticoid hormones affect protein metabolism in two main ways: they increase the rate of protein breakdown to amino acids (*catabolic* effect), and they decrease the rate at which dietary and other amino acids are built up into new protein molecules (*antianabolic* effect).

Glucocorticoids also play a part in *lipid* metabolism through complex interactions with the hormones produced by the adrenal medulla, the pancreas, and the anterior pituitary gland. These adrenocortical hormones act directly to break down the triglycerides in the body's fat depots to fatty acids (lipolysis). However, they may also indirectly increase the formation of fat and its storage in adipose tissue reservoirs. Such *lipogenesis* occurs through the action of insulin, which is released from the pancreas

as a result of the rise in blood sugar levels induced by the effects of glucocorticoids on carbohydrate metabolism.

The glucocorticoid hormones secreted by the adrenal cortex also possess some *mineralocorticoid* activity. Their effect on electrolyte and water metabolism is seen clinically when hydrocortisone and cortisone are administered in doses greater than the amounts produced daily by the patient's own adrenal glands. These patients then tend to retain sodium and water and to lose potassium and hydrogen ions, with resulting side-effects and complications. The complexly interrelated effects of glucocorticoids on carbohydrate, protein, and fat metabolism also account for many of the other adverse effects and complications of corticosteroid drug therapy (see below).

Regulation of hormone secretion

The biosynthesis and secretion of glucocorticoid hormones are regulated by the anterior pituitary gland, or *adenohypophysis* (see Chap. 20), which releases a hormone that is carried by the bloodstream to the adrenal glands (Fig. 21-1). When this adrenocorticotropic hormone, *corticotropin* or *ACTH,* reaches the tissues of the adrenal cortex, it stimulates an increase in their production of cortisol and cortisone. The ACTH-secreting cells of the anterior pituitary are in turn regulated by corticotropin-releasing hormone (CRH) from the hypothalamus (see Figs. 20-1, 20-2, and 20-3). The secretion of the adrenal and pituitary hormones does not occur at a steady rate but varies at different times of day.

Diurnal rhythm

The anterior pituitary gland of a person in an ordinary cycle of sleep and wakefulness begins to produce greater amounts of corticotropin in the hours after midnight. At that time, neurosecretory cells in the hypothalamus stimulate the ACTH-secreting cells of the pituitary through CRH. The corticotropin that is biosynthesized and released by the pituitary gland during the night reaches a peak in the blood plasma at about 6 AM. This, in turn, causes the *adrenal cortices* to secrete large amounts of glucocorticoids between the hours of 6 and 9 AM.

The high level of circulating corticosteroids in the morning hours acts to cut off further production of corticotropin. This inhibitory or negative feedback effect is believed to be exerted at the level of the hypothalamus, as well as the pituitary. That is, the glucocorticoids in the blood that reaches the brain are thought to suppress the production of the CRH of the hypothalamus, and this in turn prevents the anterior pituitary from producing ACTH. High levels of circulating glucocorticoids probably also act on the ACTH-secreting cells of the pituitary, perhaps by decreasing their sensitivity to CRH. As a result of these negative feedback mechanisms, the adrenal glands are no longer stimulated to synthesize and release more glucocorticoids.

---

* The mechanism by which glucocorticoids affect the metabolic processes of their target cells is uncertain. However, as is the case with other steroid hormones (Chaps. 23 and 24), these adrenal steroids stimulate increased synthesis of important cellular enzymes. After passing through the cell membrane, the steroids bind to specific receptor proteins in the cell's cytoplasm. This hormone–receptor complex is then carried to the cell's nucleus, where its presence leads to changes in the regulatory functions for protein synthesis. For example, by promoting the transcription of messenger RNA, the steroids induce the production of enzyme proteins that then catalyze intermediary metabolic reactions.

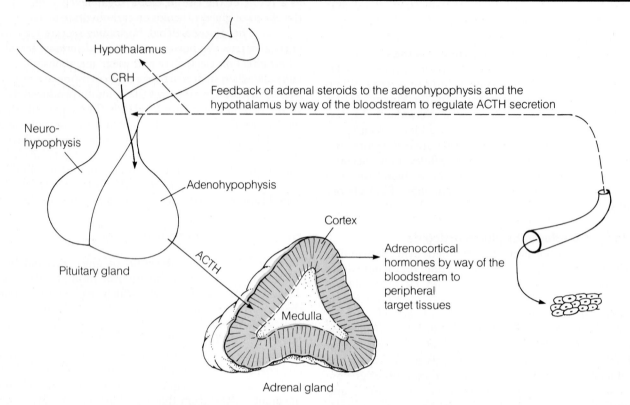

Figure 21-1. Interrelationships between corticotropin secretion and adrenocortical function. The secretion of corticotropin (ACTH) by the pituitary stimulates the synthesis and release into the bloodstream of adrenal glucocorticoid hormones such as cortisol. Their level in the blood in turn regulates the pituitary's production of ACTH. Low levels of cortisol stimulate ACTH production, while high levels exert a negative feedback action (*dashed arrows*) on the adenohypophysis and on the hypothalamus, which results in a reduction of ACTH production.

In addition, corticotropin and corticosteroid production are regulated by nervous system influences. These come into play regularly as a result of a diurnal rhythm and periodically in response to stress. Nerve impulses result in the release by the hypothalamus of the corticotropin-releasing hormone, which then stimulates the adenohypophysis to increase its output of ACTH (see text in this chapter and in Chapter 20).

During the day, the glucocorticoids that were secreted in the morning are gradually used up as they exert their metabolic effects on the body's tissues, and are themselves metabolized. As a result, the steroid levels in the blood drop during the day and reach their lowest level late in the evening. This leads to the *release* of the hypothalamic–hypophyseal mechanism from the negative feedback effect of the glucocorticoids. The anterior pituitary gland then again begins to produce corticotropin in the hours after midnight, and the diurnal cycle of corticosteroid hormone production proceeds as described above.

Effects of stress

This diurnal rhythm may be disrupted when a person is subjected to physical or emotional stress. Under stressful conditions, excitatory stimuli within the central nervous system tend to counteract the negative feedback effect of circulating steroids on the hypothalamus. The anterior pituitary gland is then released from inhibition and can continue producing and releasing corticotropin at any time during the day. This stimulates the adrenal glands to produce and pour out large quantities of corticosteroid hormones. Thus, the glands of a person who is under severe stress may secrete ten times more cortisol than their normal daily output of about 25 mg.

This increased secretory response of the adrenal glands to stress can be lifesaving following accidental or surgical trauma, during severe infections, and in other stressful situations. The abnormally high levels of glucocorticoids in the blood and tissues seem to strengthen the body's ability to cope with stress. On the other hand, a person who is subjected to severe stress may die if the adrenal glands cannot increase their production and secretion of corticosteroids.

Adrenal insufficiency and its treatment

Chronic adrenal insufficiency

People whose adrenal glands fail to synthesize adequate amounts of corticosteroids sooner or later develop symptoms of adrenal deficiency. Such symptoms may be mild or severe, depending on the extent of the patient's hormonal lack. In some cases, the patient may get along well enough ordinarily and show symptoms only when subjected to unusual stress. Other patients may have such a complete lack of cortical hormones that they are in continuous danger of going into acute adrenal crisis unless they receive substitution therapy with exogenous adrenal hormones.

Adrenal insufficiency can occur as a result of failure of the adrenal glands to respond to pituitary ACTH, or because the anterior pituitary gland fails to produce enough of that adrenal-stimulating hormone. In *Addison's disease,* the adrenal glands may be damaged or destroyed by tuberculosis or become atrophied from the effects of other pathogenic factors. *Hypopituitarism* also often leads to secondary adrenal atrophy, among other endocrine gland disorders (see Chap. 20).

Modern surgical and medical treatment is another cause of adrenal insufficiency. Adrenalectomy and hypophysectomy—surgical procedures that are sometimes employed in the management of some forms of cancer—obviously completely deprive these patients of adrenal hormones. However, the most common cause of *partial* loss of adrenal function is the prolonged administration of corticosteroid drugs. This occurs because the continued presence of high levels of steroid drugs suppresses the hypothalamic–hypophyseal–adrenal axis. Instead of recovering its capacity to produce corticotropin in the hours after midnight, as it does during ordinary diurnal cycle regulation (see above), the anterior pituitary gland fails to function properly because of drug-induced inhibition. The resulting lack of corticotropin prevents the adrenal glands from being stimulated to produce corticosteroid hormones. In time, the adrenal glands become partially atrophied. Although the glands may recover their ability to function some time after withdrawal of corticosteroid drug therapy, the patient may not be able to cope with stress for many months after these drugs are discontinued (see below, Endocrine Toxicity and Steroid Withdrawal).

Adrenal crisis

People with chronic adrenal insufficiency often get along well enough under ordinary conditions, despite their subnormal production of adrenocortical hormones. However, they may become critically ill if they develop an infection or are subjected to anesthesia and surgery or to some other form of stress. This occurs, as indicated above, because of the failure of the adrenals to respond to stress with an outpouring of extra hormones.

Patients who show sudden signs of acute adrenal insufficiency require prompt treatment with massive doses of steroids. The soluble salts and esters of *hydrocortisone*[+] are commonly infused by vein along with a large volume of fluid in the form of isotonic sodium chloride and glucose solutions. These patients, who are often in an intensive care unit, must have their central venous pressure

closely monitored to avoid fluid overload while the effect of this treatment on arterial blood pressure is checked. The underlying stressful cause of adrenal cortex insufficiency—severe injury, overwhelming infection, or heavy bleeding, for example—must also be treated at the same time, while the steroids are helping to tide the patient over the life-threatening crisis.

Replacement therapy

Patients who have been supported through an acute adrenal crisis may often be maintained on only small physiologic doses of hydrocortisone taken together with ample amounts of sodium chloride. Many patients with chronic adrenal insufficiency following adrenalectomy or from addisonian atrophic lesions require only 15 mg to 30 mg of hydrocortisone daily to replace the amount of the natural hormone that would ordinarily be secreted. Patients whose adrenal insufficiency stems from a lack of corticotropin following hypophysectomy or from disease of the anterior pituitary gland need even less hydrocortisone—usually only about 5 mg after each meal.

However, hydrocortisone alone may not have enough mineralocorticoid activity to keep most patients adequately hydrated and in electrolyte balance. Thus, to prevent possible dehydration and hypotension, it is desirable to add small doses of a drug with strong mineralocorticoid activity to the patient's regimen. *Fludrocortisone acetate* (Florinef), a synthetic corticosteroid with potent effects on fluid and electrolyte metabolism, has the advantage of being effective when taken orally. Doses of only 0.1 mg to 0.2 mg daily are often enough to maintain most patients. Others are treated with daily injections of the natural mineralocorticoid hormone *desoxycorticosterone*[+] in the form of the acetate (Doca Acetate; Percorten). Although aldosterone is a much more potent hormone, it is not commonly employed for this purpose and is not commercially available.

Pharmacologic effects of corticosteroids

The use of corticosteroids in small physiologic doses for replacement therapy in patients with adrenocortical insufficiency is an important indication for steroid therapy, but one that applies to only a few patients. Most clinical conditions for which natural and synthetic steroids are employed require their administration in much larger amounts. Such *supra*physiologic, or pharmacologic, doses produce the changes in function of cells, tissues, organs, and body systems that account for their effectiveness in the treatment of so many clinical disorders.

Among the important therapeutic effects of corticosteroid drug action are the following: *anti-inflammatory, antiallergic,* and *antistress.* Most of these interrelated effects of supraphysiologic doses of steroids probably stem from their actions on protein, carbohydrate, and fat metabolism, and on the hypothalamic–pituitary–adrenal system discussed above. This also accounts for the fact that the sustained use of these drugs also leads to toxic effects that are the result of excessive disruption of normal metabolic processes and of hypothalamic–hypophyseal–adrenal axis.

Anti-inflammatory activity

The corticosteroids have a remarkable ability to inhibit the inflammatory responses of body tissues to all the types of stimuli that evoke such reactions. That is, these drugs suppress the expected signs and symptoms that follow exposure to such insults to tissue integrity as mechanical trauma; invasion by infecting microorganisms; irritating chemical substances; damaging radiation; and injurious antigen–antibody reactions. Both the early and late phases of the inflammatory process are inhibited by administration of these drugs.

Despite considerable research that has led to many speculative hypotheses, there is at present no single complete explanation of how the corticosteroids exert their anti-inflammatory effect or their probably interrelated effects on allergic and immune responses and on fever. One important effect appears to be the ability of steroids to strengthen, or stabilize, biologic membranes. These include, in particular, the endothelial membrane of the capillaries and the lining of the other tiny blood vessels that make up the microvasculature. The steroids also seem to stabilize the membranes of blood cell elements, such as the leukocytes, and of intracellular particles of all cells such as the lysosomes. (See Chapter 36 for a discussion of the roles that such cells and intracellular organelles play in inflammatory processes.)

These membrane-stabilizing effects of the steroids may help to explain how corticosteroid drugs suppress such signs of the early defensive phase of inflammation as heat, redness, and swelling. Thus, for example, by preventing the synthesis or release of such vasodilator substances as bradykinin, prostaglandins, and histamine from tissue cells, the corticosteroids could prevent the injured area from becoming red and hot secondary to the resulting increased blood flow to the area and, by preventing the expected increase in capillary permeability, the corticosteroids could prevent fluid from leaking out of the blood vessels into the extravascular spaces to cause swelling and pain.

Corticosteroid effects on capillary permeability also seem to interfere with the movement of polymorphonuclear leukocytes from the blood to the site of injury or irritation. This lessens the amount of tissue-damaging lysosomal enzymes that can be released locally during phagocytosis. Finally, the effect of steroids on fibroblast formation and on other elements that take part in the late healing phase of the inflammatory process tends to prevent scar tissue from forming and damaging delicate structures such as those of the eye.

Antiallergic activity

The therapeutically desirable effect of corticosteroids in various types of allergic disorders is probably the result of actions similar to those that account for their anti-inflammatory activity. They may, for example, suppress immediate hypersensitivity reactions by interfering with steps in the processes by which histamine is released to act on capillary membranes and other sites, such as the smooth muscle of the microvasculature. Delayed hypersensitivity reactions may be suppressed by the effects of steroids on the activity of such cellular mediators of immune reactions as macrophages, monocytes, T cells, and B cells. These actions could then help to suppress the signs and symptoms of allergic reactions in the skin, mucous membranes, and other tissues.

Antistress activity

Just how corticosteroids help the body to mobilize its defenses in stressful situations is also still uncertain. One way that they may do so is by bringing about an improvement in cardiovascular function. This results not only from the salt- and water-retaining effect of natural hormones such as hydrocortisone, which can prevent hypovolemia in patients with adrenocortical insufficiency. It may also stem from the ability of corticosteroids to increase the responsiveness of the heart, blood vessels, and other tissues to circulating catecholamines such as epinephrine, released by the adrenal medulla, and norepinephrine, released from adrenergic nerve endings.

This synergistic effect of natural and synthetic corticosteroids with adrenergic stimuli brings about better cardiac functioning and a rise in peripheral resistance and blood pressure. The resulting increase in cardiac output and local perfusion pressure may then help to keep blood flowing to the brain and other vital organs. This could account for the reported effectiveness of these drugs in preventing or counteracting circulatory collapse, not only in acute adrenal crisis but also in other clinical conditions in which shock tends to develop, such as septicemia.

Synthetic corticosteroids

Organic chemists have tried to alter the naturally occurring steroid molecules in ways that would intensify their desirable anti-inflammatory action while eliminating the other pharmacologic effects, which are considered clinically undesirable. Although they have succeeded in developing new synthetic steroid molecules of much greater potency than those built by the body, the molecule-manipulating chemists have been only partially successful in separating the therapeutically useful actions of these synthetic steroids from the adverse effects that limit their usefulness.

The first synthetic corticosteroids to be devel-

Table 21–1. Adrenocorticosteroid drugs*

Generic or official name	Trade name or synonym	Usual adult doses and dosage ranges†
Mineralocorticoids		
Desoxycorticosterone acetate USP	DOCA; Doca Acetate; Percorten Acetate (pellets)	2–5 mg/day, IM; pellets are implanted surgically after optimum daily DOCA dose has been determined
Desoxycorticosterone pivalate USP	Percorten Pivalate (repository injection)	25–100 mg, IM, once every 4 wk; dose is calculated after optimum daily dose has been determined
Fludrocortisone acetate USP	Florinef Acetate	0.1–0.2 mg/day, orally
Glucocorticoids		
Betamethasone USP	Celestone	600 µg–7.2 mg/day, orally
Betamethasone sodium phosphate USP	Celestone Phosphate	Up to 9 mg/day systemically (including IV) and locally
Cortisone acetate USP	Cortone Acetate	20–300 mg/day, orally or IM
Dexamethasone acetate USP	Decadron-LA	8–16 mg, IM, repeated in 1–3 wk, if necessary; 0.8–1.6 mg, intralesional; 4–16 mg, intra-articular, repeated in 1–3 wk
Dexamethasone, oral USP	Decadron; Hexadrol	Initially, 0.75–9 mg/day
Dexamethasone sodium phosphate USP	Decadron Phosphate	0.5–9 mg/day, IV, IM, intra-articular
Fluprednisolone	Alphadrol	2.5–30 mg/day, orally
Hydrocortisone USP	Cortisol; Cortef; Hydrocortone	Initially, 20–240 mg/day, orally; 6–120 mg, IM, q 12 hr
Hydrocortisone acetate USP	Cortef Acetate	10–50 mg intra-articular
Hydrocortisone cypionate USP	Cortef Fluid	Initially, 20–240 mg/day orally
Hydrocortisone sodium phosphate USP	Hydrocortone Phosphate	15–240 mg/day, IM, IV, SC
Hydrocortisone sodium succinate USP	A-hydroCort; Solu-Cortef	Initially, 100–500 mg IV, IM
Methylprednisolone USP	Medrol	Initially, 4–48 mg/day, orally; dose is often tapered

(continued)

Table 21–1. Adrenocorticosteroid drugs* (continued)

Generic or official name	Trade name or synonym	Usual adult doses and dosage ranges†
Methylprednisolone acetate USP	Depo-Medrol	40–120 mg, IM, at various intervals, depending on use
Methylprednisolone sodium succinate USP	Solu-Medrol	Initially, 10–40 mg, IV; subsequent doses may be IV or IM
Paramethasone acetate USP	Haldrone	2–24 mg/day, orally
Prednisolone USP	Cortalone; Delta-Cortef; Sterane	Initially, 5–60 mg/day, orally
Prednisolone acetate USP	Meticortelone Acetate	5–100 mg, intra-articular; 4–60 mg/day, IM
Prednisolone sodium phosphate USP	Hydeltrasol	Initially, 4–60 mg/day, IM or IV
Prednisolone tebutate USP	Hydeltra-T.B.A.	4–30 mg, intra-articular or intralesional
Prednisone USP	Deltasone; Meticorten	Initially, 5–60 mg/day, orally
Triamcinolone, oral USP	Aristocort; Kenacort	Initially, 4–48 mg/day, orally
Triamcinolone acetonide USP	Kenalog	Initially, 2.5–60 mg/day, IM; 2.5–40 mg, intra-articular
Triamcinolone diacetate USP	Aristocort Forte	40 mg/week, IM; 5–40 mg, intra-articular; 5–48 mg intra- or sublesional
Triamcinolone hexacetonide USP	Aristospan	2–20 mg, intra-articular; up to 0.5 mg/inch^2 of affected area, intra- or sublesional

* The preparations and uses of adrenocorticotropin (ACTH) are described in Chapter 20. Topical and ophthalmic preparations are described in Chapters 43 and 42; preparations dispensed from an inhaler by patients with chronic obstructive pulmonary disease are described in Chapter 40; intranasal steroids are described in Chapter 39.
† Doses vary widely, depending on the nature and severity of the condition being treated.

oped were *prednisone*[+] and *prednisolone*, which proved not only to be four to five times more potent than hydrocortisone and cortisone, but also to have much less sodium-retaining activity (Tables 21-1 and 21-2). This property has made them safer for use in patients with heart disease and hypertension—disorders that are adversely affected by drug-induced accumulation of salty fluids in the tissues.

Further research has resulted in the discovery of other new families of steroid compounds, in which the anti-inflammatory action is selectively increased and the electrolyte–water-retaining effect is entirely eliminated. In practice, this means not only that less than 1 mg of potent synthetic steroids such as *dexamethasone*[+] and *betamethasone* will do the work of 25 mg of cortisone (Table 21-2), but that they will do so without causing the tissues to become edematous, as equivalent anti-inflammatory doses of cortisone and hydrocortisone do.

These potent steroids also have a relatively long duration of anti-inflammatory activity and can cause prolonged suppression of the hypothalamic-pituitary-adrenal axis. Although this makes them ideally suited for treating certain disorders that require prolonged inhibition of pituitary function, other clinical situations are best controlled with corticosteroids of intermediate duration of action. For example, in alternate day treatment schedules (see below), prednisone and prednisolone are preferred to betamethasone and dexamethasone, which are not considered suitable for use in such dosage regimens.

Table 21–2. Comparison of common corticosteroid drugs

Name of Glucocorticoid	Relative Anti-Inflammatory Potency*	Relative Mineralocorticoid Activity†	Relative Duration of Activity (hr)‡
Hydrocortisone	1 (20 mg)	Strong (2+)	Short (8–12)
Cortisone	0.8 (25 mg)	Strong (2+)	Short (8–12)
Prednisone	3.5 (5 mg)	Moderate (1+)	Intermediate (18–36)
Prednisolone	4 (5 mg)	Moderate (1+)	Intermediate (18–36)
Methylprednisolone	5 (4 mg)	Little (0+)	Intermediate (18–36)
Triamcinolone	5 (4 mg)	Little (0+)	Intermediate (18–36)
Paramethasone	10 (2 mg)	Little (0+)	Long (36–54)
Fluprednisolone	10 (1.5 mg)	Little (0+)	Long (36–54)
Dexamethasone	30 (0.75 mg)	Little (0+)	Long (36–54)
Betamethasone	25 (0.60 mg)	Little (0+)	Long (36–54)

* Compared to hydrocortisone, which here has the arbitrary value of 1 and the actual dosage of 20 mg. (The weaker compound cortisone, only 0.8 times as potent as hydrocortisone, requires a higher dose [25 mg]. The synthetic steroids are arranged in accordance with their increasing potency and consequently lower dosage for equivalent anti-inflammatory activity.)
† Compared to the purely mineralocorticoid compound fludrocortisone with an activity of 5+. (Only hydrocortisone and cortisone cause enough sodium retention to make them useful for treating some cases of acute and chronic adrenal insufficiency.)
‡ Compared in terms of duration of the biologic half-life of the compounds.

Adverse effects of corticosteroid drugs

Despite their increased potency and their relative freedom from mineralocorticoid activity, the synthetic corticosteroids can cause all the other types of chronic toxicity that occur with the natural glucocorticoid hormones. Because scientists have never succeeded in separating the therapeutically desired effects of the synthetic steroids from the undesirable effects that cause toxicity to develop with the natural hormones, the prolonged use of *any* of these drugs—natural or synthetic—eventually leads to characteristic complications. Some of their many side-effects can be grouped together as *metabolic,* while others are called *endocrine.* These classes of adverse reactions will be discussed here in detail, along with those that are the result of corticosteroid effects on the brain and the eyes.

Metabolic toxicity

Many adverse effects of corticosteroid therapy are more or less obviously the result of their effects on carbohydrate, protein, and fat metabolism. How long it takes for signs and symptoms to develop depends mainly on the dose level being administered. Patients who require large daily doses of steroids to suppress signs and symptoms of a potentially disabling disease can develop signs of dangerous metabolic toxicity in only 2 or 3 weeks of treatment. On the other hand, if a patient can be maintained on the minimal dose that is effective for symptomatic relief, the appearance of adverse effects may be postponed for many months, and such effects may never become intolerably severe.

Cushingoid features. Some signs of steroid overdosage are the result of a peculiar redistribution of the body's adipose tissue. Because the patient's appearance resembles that of people with Cushing's syndrome, a disorder caused by certain hypersecreting tumors of the adrenal or pituitary gland, these signs and symptoms of *hypercorticism* are often called "cushingoid." The patient's face often becomes full or rounded as a result of fat being deposited in the cheeks ("moon face"). The skin of the face may be flushed, and sometimes an acnelike eruption and growth of excess hair are also seen.

Fat deposits often develop in the area of the shoulder girdle. Rolls of fat at the back of the neck and between the shoulder blades have been called "buffalo hump" and, at the front of this area, fat piles up over the collarbones (supraclavicular fat pads). The patient's abdomen becomes distended with fat, and the stretched skin is often marked by red lines, or striae, that run vertically over its surface.

Despite the obese appearance, the steroid-treated patient's arms and legs are often very thin. This is the result of a wasting away of skeletal muscle tissue in the extremities. It is thought to occur because of the catabolic and antianabolic effects of these drugs on protein metabolism. Myopathy is mainly the result of negative nitrogen balance, which develops despite the fact that these drugs increase the patient's food intake. One synthetic steroid, *triamcinolone*[+], which—unlike other steroids—is said *not* to stimulate appetite and lead to a gain in weight, seems more likely than other drugs to cause this type of muscle wasting.

Patients taking steroids often develop increased blood levels of glucose (hyperglycemia), and some of this spills over into the urine (glycosuria). This is the result of gluconeogenesis that is related to the conversion of some of the amino acid residue of protein catabolism to glucose and glycogen. Patients with a family history of diabetes should have their blood and urine tested periodically for sugar. However, the appearance of hyperglycemia and glycosuria does not necessarily mean that corticosteroid therapy must be discontinued.

Counteracting complications. Patients with steroid-raised blood sugar levels, and even those with actual diabetes, can often continue to take these drugs. Adjustments may be made in their diet, and oral hypoglycemic agents may be added to their regimen to restore more normal carbohydrate metabolism. Diabetic patients may require increased insulin dosage during corticosteroid therapy, but the use of these drugs need not be contraindicated.

Osteoporosis. Patients who are prone to develop other complications may also be continued on corticosteroid therapy, provided that they are closely observed and preventive measures are promptly employed when required. Thus, for example, when patients who are immobilized by rheumatoid arthritis, or elderly patients, receive steroids, they should be examined frequently for signs of *osteoporosis*. This condition, which can lead to compression fractures of the vertebrae, ribs, and femur, may develop as a result of steroid-induced negative nitrogen balance and negative calcium balance.

In addition, x-rays of the patient's spine should be taken periodically during steroid therapy. If signs of bone demineralization and thinning appear, it may be necessary to withdraw this treatment to avoid development of osteoporotic fractures. This complication may possibly be prevented by having the patient eat a protein-rich diet and take such dietary supplements as calcium lactate, sodium fluoride, and vitamin D.

The administration of anabolic agents (Chap. 24) has also been recommended to counteract the steroid-induced negative nitrogen balance that can lead both to osteoporosis and myopathy.

Potassium salt supplements may be employed when muscle weakness is caused by potassium loss as a result of the mineralocorticoid activity of a natural steroid hormone such as hydrocortisone or cortisone. In such cases, the patient can also be switched to one of the synthetic steroids that do not affect electrolyte metabolism. However, this would not, of course, prevent the development of muscle wasting from the effects of steroids on protein metabolism.

Peptic ulcer. This is another possible complication of corticosteroid therapy, particularly in patients with rheumatoid arthritis. These patients should not ordinarily continue to receive other potentially ulcerogenic anti-inflammatory drugs. That is, drugs such as indomethacin and phenylbutazone are best withdrawn when steroid treatment is begun.

Despite the risk of reactivating a healed peptic ulcer, steroid therapy may be warranted in some selected cases because of the benefit that the patient may derive from their use.* If so, considerable caution is required, because steroids may mask such a symptom of gastrointestinal ulceration as abdominal pain. Thus, to avoid development of a peptic ulcer that is recognized only when signs of such complications as internal bleeding, perforation, and penetration appear, it is desirable that gastroduodenal x-rays be made at the start of steroid treatment and periodically during the use of these drugs.

Patients with a history suggesting susceptibility to peptic ulceration should also be warned against taking aspirin or concentrated alcoholic drinks during steroid drug treatment. Even coffee may be contraindicated because of its caffeine content, which may stimulate stomach acid secretion. Patients may also receive antiulcer medications such as antacids, histamine-2 receptor blockers (cimetidine; ranitidine), or anticholinergic–antisecretory drugs prophylactically while taking corticosteroids. Because the ulcerogenic effects of steroid drugs may stem from their interference with mechanisms for protecting the gastrointestinal mucosa from injury, the antiulcer agent, carbenoxolone (not available in the United States), which appears to stimulate production of substances that protect the mucosa, may also prove to be a useful adjunctive medication. This drug has mineralocorticoid activity, however, and thus can alter fluid and electrolyte balances.

Infections. The presence of an active infection or even of the healed lesions of a former infection such as pulmonary tuberculosis can lead to yet another complication of steroid therapy: the sudden spread of the infection from its localized site. This can occur because corticosteroids tend to interfere with the inflammatory and immune responses by which the body defends itself against further invasion of its tissues by pathogenic microorganisms. The danger is compounded by the fact that steroid drugs tend to mask such local and systemic signs and symptoms of an advancing infection as redness, heat, swelling, pain, fever, and leukocytosis.

Despite this danger, the use of corticosteroids is not necessarily contraindicated in the presence of infection. The main criterion for determining whether to continue corticosteroid therapy is whether antimicrobial che-

---

* Some internists have even recently questioned the entire concept of steroid-induced ulcers (see References). However, most authorities still believe that caution is required when these drugs are employed in particularly susceptible persons.

motherapeutic drugs are available that can control the pathogenic microorganism. Thus, even though steroids are often said to be contraindicated in patients with pulmonary tuberculosis, these drugs are sometimes employed, provided that tests prove that the patient's tubercle bacilli are sensitive to treatment with standard antituberculosis drugs. The patient's response to combined steroid and anti-infective drug treatment is followed by periodic chest x-rays and sputum studies.

Corticosteroid therapy is usually contraindicated in the presence of viral and fungal infections for which no effective anti-infective therapy is yet available. Thus, topical and systemic steroid therapy, which is often helpful in *bacterial* infections of the eye when combined with appropriate antibacterial agents (*e.g.*, neomycin), is considered contraindicated in *fungal* infections of various eye structures and in *herpes simplex virus* invasions of the cornea. The viruses of chickenpox and of other exanthematous diseases may be disseminated during administration of steroid medication. This is one reason why some physicians avoid long-term administration of steroids to children, who are especially susceptible to such virus infections (another reason is the fact that long-term treatment with corticosteroids tends to suppress the growth of children).

Although corticosteroids are usually contraindicated in viral infections, they *are* sometimes employed to control certain complications of these and other serious infections. For example, in men with orchitis caused by mumps virus infection, corticosteroids may be used to reduce the painful swelling of the testes and, in severe infectious mononucleosis, the beneficial effects of steroid therapy for reducing discomforting symptoms may outweigh the risks of further spread of the still-unknown virus.

Steroids may also be employed for control of brain inflammation in cases of measles complicated by encephalitis. Here, and in cases of bacterial meningitis, corticosteroids help to prevent cerebral edema and brain swelling. These drugs also tend to interfere with formation of fibrotic tissue that could block the flow of cerebrospinal fluid and cause a dangerous rise in pressure on nervous tissues. Specific antibacterial therapy must also be employed against the pathogen responsible for the meningitis.

Another reason for continuing corticosteroids when an infection develops in a patient who has been taking these drugs for a long period is the possibility that steroid-induced adrenal insufficiency may have developed (see below, Endocrine Toxicity). Instead, it may be necessary to *raise* corticosteroid drug dosage in such cases to make up for the inability of the patient's own partially atrophied adrenal glands to respond to the stress of the infection. In patients with septicemia caused by gram-negative bacilli, it is now customary to administer massive doses of soluble corticosteroid drugs by vein to manage the patient during the critical period and to help prevent

or counteract endotoxic shock. Again, specific antibacterial drugs must also be administered to control the infecting pathogens, and other antishock measures, including vasopressor or vasodilator drugs, are also employed.

Endocrine toxicity

As stated in the discussion of chronic adrenal insufficiency (see above), long-term treatment with steroid drugs suppresses the hypothalamic–hypophyseal mechanism responsible for production and secretion of the ACTH of the anterior pituitary gland. This, in turn, leads to a reduction in the size of the adrenal glands. The partially atrophied adrenal cortices then produce and secrete abnormally low amounts of the natural endogenous glucocorticoid hormones. More important is the fact that the adrenal glands cannot respond by stepping up their production of these hormones when the patient is subjected to stress (see above, Effects of Stress).

Thus, patients who have been taking corticosteroids may be unable to cope with sudden stressful situations, such as a severe injury or an infection. It is also important to be aware that a patient who is on steroid therapy requires additional steroid dosage when undergoing general anesthesia for elective or emergency surgery.

Because steroid drug-induced adrenal insufficiency may last for many months after treatment has finally been discontinued it is important that the drug history elicit information about any chronic illnesses that may recently have required steroid therapy for control of acute flare-ups. Information acquired in this way during the assessment of the patient should be transmitted to the surgical team, which will then prepare the patient by preoperative administration of steroid drugs, if further tests indicate that adrenal function is, indeed, deficient.

Patients whose adrenal glands may be in a partial state of atrophy because of long-term corticosteroid therapy are also often advised to carry a card to indicate that they are taking these drugs. This could serve to alert medical personnel to the need for intravenous infusion of a soluble steroid drug, such as hydrocortisone sodium succinate, during the emergency management of the patient following an accident. Such support of the patient's circulation with exogenous steroids may help survival by making up for the lack of endogenous hormone production from the atrophied adrenals.

Failure of growth in children who are required to take steroids for long periods may be caused, in part, by steroid suppression of the growth hormone of the anterior pituitary gland (see Chap. 20). However, other factors, such as the antianabolic action of these drugs, may also play a part in the child's lack of linear growth. In any case, it is desirable that steroid therapy be gradually discontinued periodically, if possible, to permit resumption of the child's growth. Intermittent schedules of steroid administration (see below) have also been devised for children in attempts to prevent this type of adverse endocrine or metabolic toxicity.

Behavioral effects

Corticosteroid therapy often affects the patient's mental state. Most commonly, the patient becomes happy and talkative. This sometimes happens so soon after treatment with steroids is started that it was thought to be the patient's natural response to the drug-induced relief of pain or other discomforting physical symptoms. Actually, this euphoric effect is now known to result from an action of corticosteroids on the CNS. Some patients so enjoy this feeling of well-being that they become, in effect, psychologically dependent on steroids. This is one reason why they resist attempts to reduce dosage or to withdraw these drugs.

The continued use of corticosteroids sometimes leads to excessive excitement, restlessness, and sleeplessness. The patient's mood may become manic and then swing back to a stage of agitated depression. Such mood swings and behavioral changes should be looked for, because they may necessitate a reduction in corticosteroid dosage to avoid possible psychotic complications, including suicide attempts. Such mood swings require nursing intervention—for example, reducing stimuli, thus helping the manic patient to become calmer, or supporting the patient who is depressed, thus helping him to combat this distressing symptom.

Serious reactions of this type are relatively rare. More often, the main difficulty caused by drug-induced mental changes is a decrease in the patient's ability to cope with the chronic illness constructively. The patient must be helped to meet problems realistically and to maintain relationships with other people, despite the adverse effects of steroid medication on mood and emotional state.

The cause of manic–depressive, schizophrenic, and other psychotic reactions to corticosteroids is uncertain. Unlike other types of steroid toxicity, the adverse central effects are not closely related to the length of time patients have been taking high supraphysiologic (pharmacologic) doses. A more important factor in determining which patients will react abnormally is the patient's personality before treatment is begun. People with a history of emotional and psychological difficulties develop these types of complications more often than other patients. Thus, steroid use should, if possible, be avoided in such cases, particularly in patients who are already psychotic.

Ocular toxicity

Two types of ocular complications may occur during corticosteroid therapy: a rise in intraocular pressure resembling that seen in patients with open-angle glaucoma, and the development of clouding of the lens of the eye, or cataract. These adverse effects may develop both in patients who apply topical corticosteroid solutions to the eye for treating ocular inflammatory disorders and in those who are receiving oral steroids in the management of *non*ocular chronic conditions, such as rheumatoid arthritis.

Glaucoma. The steroid-induced rise in intraocular pressure appears to occur most commonly in patients with a family history of open-angle glaucoma. Thus, patients should be questioned about this before prolonged steroid drug treatment is begun. Those who appear to be genetically prone to develop this disorder should have their intraocular pressure measured by tonometry periodically during treatment.

Steroid-induced glaucoma can cause the same type of irreversible loss of vision as that which occurs in primary open-angle glaucoma. Thus, if elevation of intraocular pressure occurs, drug treatment should be discontinued to permit the pressure to return to normal, as it almost always does within a few weeks. Some authorities suggest that patients who require prolonged steroid therapy despite their tendency to develop this adverse ocular effect should be treated adjunctively with antiglaucoma medications (Chap. 42). This, of course, applies particularly to patients who already have primary glaucoma.

Cataracts. The tendency to develop posterior subcapsular cataracts seems most common in patients with rheumatoid arthritis who require chronic corticosteroid drug treatment. The reason for this is as uncertain as is the increased susceptibility of these patients to development of peptic ulcers. In any case, they and others who must take these drugs for long periods should have an ophthalmologic examination every few months. If such a check reveals early signs of cataract formation, it may be necessary to discontinue corticosteroid therapy.

Therapeutic uses in clinical disorders

The adrenocorticosteroid drugs have been tried in the treatment of diseases of almost every type by practitioners of nearly every medical specialty. Before discussing how these useful but potentially dangerous drugs are best used to obtain their maximal benefits with minimal adverse effects, some of the main types of disorders for which corticosteroids are commonly ordered will be outlined with references to other chapters in the text in which these uses are discussed in more detail.

Adrenocortical insufficiency. As described above, corticosteroid drugs can both *cause* hypocortism and yet be lifesaving in patients with that condition who develop an acute adrenal crisis. Injections of soluble hydrocortisone salts are preferred for this latter purpose, because they possess both glucocorticoid and mineralocorticoid activity. When a soluble synthetic steroid is used, it may have to be supplemented with a drug that has mineralocorticoid activity.

Other endocrine disorders in which corticosteroids may prove effective are *thyroiditis* and *congenital ad-*

renal hyperplasia, a condition in which the adrenal glands of patients who cannot biosynthesize glucocorticoids become enlarged as a result of a compensatory increase in pituitary corticotropin secretion. Treatment is aimed at replacing the missing hormones with physiologic doses of steroid drugs. In thyroiditis, on the other hand, the steroids are administered in supraphysiologic doses to suppress the thyroid gland inflammation.

Rheumatic disorders. The use of these drugs in rheumatoid arthritis and in related inflammatory diseases of the joints is discussed in Chapter 38 and below as part of the summary of general principles for the proper administration of corticosteroids in the management of chronic nonfatal disorders.

Other collagen diseases. These are conditions in which certain characteristic changes occur in the connective tissue of various organs (*collagen* is a connective tissue protein found in the deeper layers of the skin, in the joints, and elsewhere). Although the diseases of this tissue are grouped together, they probably do not have a common cause and they vary considerably in their end results. All are serious—some are disabling rather than deadly, and others are invariably fatal. They have in common a responsiveness to treatment with corticosteroids, which often afford temporary relief. In addition to rheumatoid arthritis, they include the acute stages of such potentially fatal disorders as disseminated lupus erythematosus, acute rheumatic carditis, periarteritis nodosa, and pemphigus.

Allergic disorders. The use of these drugs in the management of such chronic disorders as pollinosis and perennial rhinitis is taken up in Chapter 39, together with a discussion of their role in the emergency management of anaphylactic shock reactions. Steroid therapy in the management of bronchial asthma and other chronic obstructive respiratory diseases is discussed in Chapter 40. Steroid treatment of urticarial reactions and atopic and contact dermatitis is taken up in Chapter 43, as is steroid therapy of certain *non*allergic skin conditions.

Dermatologic disorders. In addition to their use in the allergic skin conditions mentioned above, steroids are also effective for treating psoriasis, seborrheic dermatitis, and severe disorders as dangerous as the previously mentioned pemphigus. These include erythema multiforme, the cause of the Stevens–Johnson syndrome and bullous dermatitis herpetiformis (Chap. 8).

Ophthalmic diseases. The use of corticosteroids for control of ocular inflammation caused by infections or allergic processes is taken up in Chapter 42, together with a discussion of the potentially adverse effects of these drugs on the eye when they are applied topically or taken internally.

Respiratory diseases. In addition to their use in the upper and lower respiratory tract disorders mentioned above and discussed elsewhere, the corticosteroids are employed for such serious lung disorders as aspiration penumonitis caused by ingestion of petroleum distillates such as kerosene or gasoline and in certain stages of pulmonary tuberculosis, a condition for which these drugs were previously considered to be contraindicated. As mentioned previously, appropriate antituberculosis chemotherapy must be administered simultaneously.

Other infectious diseases. Massive doses of steroids are sometimes employed in overwhelming infections for their antistress effects, despite their admitted tendency to spread infection. For example, patients in shock from severe blood poisoning or meningitis who have not been responding adequately to vasopressor drugs and antibiotics have sometimes been aided remarkably and helped to survive by such steroid medication. Among patients reportedly saved by the timely addition of steroids to their regimen have been some with severe bacteremias and endotoxic shock.

Corticosteroids are sometimes used to control the complications of serious infections such as tuberculous meningitis and even of viral infections for which there is still no effective anti-infective chemotherapy—mumps orchitis, for example, or measles encephalitis. Although topical treatment of eye infections is probably best discontinued if keratitis caused by herpes simplex virus develops, systemically administered steroids are now sometimes employed in treating this ocular infection. The use of corticosteroids is contraindicated in patients suffering from systemic infections caused by disseminated fungal organisms.

Hematologic disorders. Blood dyscrasias, including acquired, or autoimmune, hemolytic anemia, are treated with corticosteroids, as are idiopathic thrombocytopenia (Chap. 34) and that which may develop secondary to drug therapy. Infants with erythroblastosis and congenital hypoplastic anemia sometimes require corticosteroid treatment.

Neoplastic diseases. Corticosteroids are employed as part of the multiple drug therapy regimens for acute lymphocytic leukemia in children and for the palliative treatment of chronic lymphocytic leukemia in adults. These uses are discussed in Chapter 12.

Gastrointestinal diseases. Steroid therapy is employed in severe flare-ups of ulcerative colitis and regional enteritis, as well as in sprue that has proved intractable to other treatments. It is also used in chronic active hepatitis, a common cause of cirrhosis of the liver. Although the effectiveness of corticosteroids for controlling liver inflammation in other forms of hepatitis is more controversial, these drugs are also sometimes employed for inducing diuresis when administered to patients with cirrhosis of the liver and ascites that had proved refractory to diuretic therapy alone (Chap. 27).

Miscellaneous. The corticosteroids are used in conditions so varied in etiology and so numerous that any attempt to classify the steroid-responsive diseases finally breaks down. Among renal, respiratory, dermatologic, neuromuscular, cardiac, and other disorders not mentioned above, but in which corticosteroids are sometimes employed, are the following: the idiopathic type of nephrotic syndrome in children; sarcoidosis, berylliosis, Löffler's syndrome; dermatomyositis; myasthenia gravis; multiple sclerosis; and diuretic–refractory congestive heart failure. (See the summary at the end of the chapter for a further partial listing of the endocrine and *nonen-docrine* disorders in which corticosteroids are employed.)

Clinical considerations in corticosteroid therapy

Corticosteroid drugs have been called a two-edged sword, because they can do both great good and great harm. When they were first introduced in the years after the 1948 discovery of the potent anti-inflammatory activity of cortisone, attention focused on their dramatic effectiveness for relief of the disabling symptoms of many severe illnesses. However, as these drugs began to be used more widely and indiscriminately, their many drawbacks and dangers became known.

Fortunately, it was gradually learned how to use these drugs in the ways that were most likely to benefit properly selected patients and yet keep adverse effects to a minimum. This section will discuss some general principles of corticosteroid drug dosage and administration that have evolved during almost forty years of experience with their use in various clinical situations (see also the summary of principles at the end of this chapter).

Chronic nonfatal disorders

In chronic diseases such as *rheumatoid arthritis* and *bronchial asthma,* corticosteroids are never used until these conditions can no longer be controlled by safer, more conservative measures. Thus, corticosteroids should be introduced for the management of arthritic symptoms only when the patient's condition is worsening despite vigorous use of other antirheumatic medications and physical therapy. Similarly, in bronchial asthma, oral steroids are introduced only after safer, standard measures have failed to halt the progress of disabling symptoms that threaten the patient's ability to function.

Once the decision is made to employ steroid drugs, it is important to try to determine the smallest daily dose that will keep the individual patient comfortable. The aim is not to eliminate all the patient's rheumatic or asthmatic symptoms and, in fact, the dosage should be gradually reduced whenever these disorders seem to be going into remission. If patients require relatively high doses that cause hypercorticism, or when complications tend to develop, progressive toxicity may be minimized in some cases by switching the patient to a schedule of intermittent steroid therapy (see below). Similarly, signs of systemic steroid toxicity may be lessened by the use of drugs that are administered locally at the desired sites of action. Examples include the use of the corticosteroid *inhalation* preparation beclomethasone diproprionate in

asthma, *intra-articular* injections of poorly absorbable steroids such as triamcinolone diacetate in rheumatoid arthritis and osteoarthritis, and the *intralesional* injection of the latter and related steroids in psoriasis and other chronic skin disorders. Relatively small amounts of corticosteroids given in these ways are absorbed into the systemic circulation.

Acute stages of chronic diseases

Patients who are seen during an acute flare-up of arthritis or asthma are started on large doses of steroids rather than on small doses added to their regular regimen, as is done in less severe cases. This is particularly true in life-threatening complications such as status asthmaticus (Chap. 40) or in cases of rheumatic fever with signs of myocarditis (Chap. 38). The high dosage level is gradually lowered as the acute episode is brought under control.

Patients with chronic diseases such as systemic lupus erythematosus and pemphigus—conditions marked by periodic acute exacerbations that are potentially fatal—also receive very large daily doses of steroids during these acute stages. However, in these diseases, it may also be necessary to keep the patient on lower but still relatively large doses for long periods after the severe flare-up has subsided. Although signs of metabolic toxicity develop during steroid maintenance therapy, and endocrine toxicity is also certain to occur, such high steroid dosage may be necessary to prevent life-threatening complications from developing. Yet, patients must also be watched closely for signs of severe and possibly fatal complications of high steroid dosage, such as hemorrhage from a perforated peptic ulcer.

Acute crises

The administration of even massive doses of corticosteroids for only brief periods to manage a patient during an acute crisis is a relatively safe procedure. Such situations include not only adrenal crisis but also anaphylactic shock (Chap. 39) and—as previously stated—endotoxic shock, in which corticosteroids are often administered as adjuncts to therapy with more specific drugs such as epinephrine, antibiotics, and vasopressors. When steroids are used in this way for only a few days, metabolic and endocrine toxicity are unlikely to develop. However, patients should be observed for signs of behavioral disturbances, because central nervous system toxicity sometimes occurs even during short courses of steroids.

Acute episodes of self-limiting disorders

Patients with annoying symptoms of conditions that take some time to run their course when untreated can often get quick relief from oral or topical corticosteroid therapy. In pollinosis (Chap. 39) or poison ivy (Chap. 43), for example, symptoms are often quickly controlled by taking a large oral dose at once and then reducing the dose each day over a period of a week or two, until therapy is finally discontinued entirely. When administered by such a "step-down" dosage regimen, steroids rarely cause any adverse effects. Topical application of steroid preparations in acute contact dermatitis (Chap. 43) and in ocular allergic or other inflammatory disorders (Chap. 42) is also effective and relatively free of typical corticosteroid toxicity.

Intermittent dosage schedules

Some patients who require long-term corticosteroid therapy for symptomatic control of chronic disorders are now being maintained on dosage schedules that differ from the traditional way of administering these drugs. Instead of taking several small doses at different times during the day, patients take the total daily steroid dosage at about 8 AM, or they may even take the entire dosage for a 2-day period every other morning at that hour. Such intermittent dosage schedules are said to minimize the signs and symptoms of metabolic toxicity and to delay the development of endocrine toxicity, including both chronic adrenal insufficiency and retarded growth of children.

Alternate day therapy (ADT) is a dosage regimen that is never used to start patients off on steroid therapy. Instead, after patients have been brought under symptomatic control in the usual way, they may sometimes be switched gradually to this safer way of taking steroid drugs. The reason for the relative safety of this method of administration is that it reduces the time during the day in which the patient's tissues are kept exposed to high concentrations of corticosteroid drugs.

High levels of steroids circulating continuously in the blood interfere with cellular intermediary metabolism and soon lead to cushingoid signs and symptoms. In addition, when doses of steroids are taken in the late afternoon and evening, the normal diurnal rhythm of hypothalamic–pituitary–adrenal function is disrupted. That is, the artifically high levels of steroids that reach the brain late at night tend to keep the hypothalamic-hypophyseal mechanism from becoming active, as it ordinarily does when circulating adrenal hormones fall to low levels late in the evening (see above, Regulation of Hormone Secretion).

Morning administration of the total daily steroid dosage imitates the normal cycle of natural adrenal hormone secretion, which reaches its height between 6 and 9 AM. Similarly, when corticosteroid drugs with a short or intermediate duration of action are administered, their concentration in the blood drops gradually during the day in a manner that mimics the decline in the level of natural hormones in the circulation as the day progresses (Table 21-2). As a result, there is less chance that metabolic toxicity or suppression of hypothalamic–pituitary–adrenal gland function will develop. (As indicated previously, the long-acting steroids are not suited to alternate day therapy. If they were to be employed at all for intermittent

therapy, they would have to be administered every 3 or 4 days.)

Unfortunately, some patients cannot profit from ADT because their discomforting or disabling symptoms tend to return too severely on the second, or no-steroid, day. To make the conversion from divided daily doses of steroids to ADT easier for such patients to bear, various programs have been devised for accomplishing the transition. These individually tailored programs include, for example, first consolidating the several daily divided doses into a single daily dose on the morning of each day before attempting to employ double doses every other morning.

To profit from ADT and other intermittent dosage schedules, many patients require emotional support. The patient must be taught the reasons for continuing to take steroid drugs in this way, and should understand that, even though this method does not give complete relief of all symptoms, it helps to prevent toxicity that might otherwise make it necessary to discontinue corticosteroids completely. In any case, the patient who receives personal assurance of concern for his health and well-being is more likely to profit from long-term treatment of the chronic disorder.

Steroid withdrawal

One reason for avoiding steroid therapy in patients whose symptoms can be controlled by other measures is that it is usually difficult to discontinue these drugs. Sometimes the withdrawal of steroids sets off an acute flare-up of the underlying disorder. In rheumatoid arthritis, for example, the patient's joint symptoms return with increased severity when an attempt is made to reduce dosage too rapidly. Bronchial asthma patients often develop breathing difficulties if steroids are discontinued too abruptly.

Patients resist attempts to wean them from steroids for another reason, also. These drugs can produce both psychological and physiologic dependence (see Chapter 53, Alcoholism and Drug Abuse, for definitions of these terms). Thus, some patients want to continue taking these drugs for the euphoria that they feel as a result of their central effects. Others resist giving up steroid medication because they feel worse physically without it. That is, they seem to develop a steroid withdrawal syndrome characterized by feelings of fatigue, muscle weakness and aching, lethargy, loss of appetite, and even fever.

Although such symptoms are not caused by chronic adrenal insufficiency, patients who have been taking large doses of steroid drugs are actually in such a deficiency state during treatment and for up to a year after these drugs are discontinued. It has been suggested that the rate of recovery of the drug-suppressed adrenal glands may be increased by reducing the patient's daily dosage very gradually. This may be done by first consolidating the several divided doses into a single daily morning dose (see above). After a while, all dosage may be gradually withdrawn on alternate days and, finally, further administration may be eliminated entirely.

Patients from whom steroids are being withdrawn should receive all possible medical and emotional support. Thus, for example, such other medications as salicylates may be substituted for some of the steroid dosage withdrawn from rheumatic patients, and cromolyn sodium (Chap. 40) may be employed in asthma patients to ease the difficulties of withdrawal of steroids.

Some authorities have suggested that also administering injections of the adrenal-stimulating pituitary hormone corticotropin increases the rate at which the adrenal glands recover their function. Others deny that such administration helps to hasten a return to normal pituitary–adrenal function, and even claim that corticotropin dosage may actually delay the process. All agree, though, that patients who become seriously ill during the year after they have been withdrawn from prolonged steroid therapy should be put back on supplemental doses of these drugs during the course of the acute illness.

It is essential that the patient receive a careful explanation of the reasons for discontinuing the medicine that may have been giving gratifying relief. If the drugs are withdrawn without adequate discussion of why this is necessary, the patient who is left with little to sustain him may make the rounds of physicians' offices, trying to find someone who will prescribe the continued use of steroids. The patient is likely to do better physically if both personal reassurance and continued treatment with other medications are provided, than if both the drugs and his feeling of the physician's concern for his well-being are withdrawn.

Additional clinical considerations

The mineralocorticoids, or combinations of mineralocorticoids and glucocorticoids, are used as replacement therapy for patients with specific deficits; the glucocorticoids are used alone mainly for their anti-inflammatory effects. The patient receiving glucocorticoids often "feels good," experiences the return of appetite and the reduction of pain to a tolerable level, and is free of many of the uncomfortable signs and symptoms of the inflammatory response for which the drug has been ordered. Because of these effects of the glucocorticoids, the clinical management of the patient receiving corticosteroids can be a complex problem.

The anti-inflammatory immunosuppressive effects of the glucocorticoids are therapeutically very useful, and even lifesaving. However, along with the desired anti-inflammatory or immunosuppressive effects comes the generalized decrease in body defenses in addition to the absence of the usual signs and symptoms of infection. Patients receiving these drugs are therefore very susceptible to infection and, if they do develop an infection, can have a very difficult time recovering from it. The patient should be taught to avoid high-risk situations— for example, to avoid crowded public places, people with "colds," visiting friends in the hospital—and should be evaluated regularly for any possible infectious process. It needs to be kept in mind that if a patient on steroids is found to have an infection, the usual signs and symptoms used to evaluate the severity of the problem are "masked" by the steroid's anti-inflammatory and immunosuppressive effects. The patient should be treated vigorously with high doses of the appropriate anti-infective drug. Patients who may have latent infections that are normally controlled by their own immune systems should probably receive prophylactic antibiotics when the corticosteroids are started—for example, tubercular patients. No vaccinations with live virus should ever be given to a patient on glucocorticoids because of the body's inability to deal with the virus.

The patient on corticosteroids is also less able to respond to stress, whether it is emotional, physiologic, or traumatic. Because of this, if an emergency situation arises, the patient will require careful monitoring and, in many cases, an increase in steroid dosage and prophylactic, protective measures. The patient should be advised to wear a medical identification tag at all times to alert any medical personnel to these particular needs. Hospital inpatients should have their charts clearly noted in red to alert all personnel about their steroid therapy. The patient on corticosteroids needs to be taught about the risks of stressful events so as to be alert to special needs during such elective stresses as dental work or elective surgery.

Certain susceptible patients need to be closely monitored for adverse effects of the drugs. Patients with diabetes mellitus will need careful monitoring if they receive glucosteroids because these drugs raise blood glucose levels. Insulin requirements will need to be evaluated daily to cover the patient's needs adequately. Patients with a known history of peptic ulcer have had their ulcers perforate; the exact mechanism involved is not understood. These patients should be monitored very closely, with stool guaiac tests being done regularly and periodic gastrointestinal x-rays taken if the patient is on prolonged therapy. Children maintained on corticosteroids may experience growth retardation; if the therapy must be continued for several years the epiphyseal plates may close, and their growth may be permanently retarded. Attempts are usually made to avoid this occurrence by tapering steroids as much as possible in children. Patients on prolonged therapy may develop hypernatremia from the sodium retention that occurs as a result of the corticosteroid activity. Patients on prolonged therapy should be advised to restrict their salt intake—by avoiding foods with high salt content and by not adding salt at the table—to help alleviate this problem. Patients on prolonged therapy should also be advised to have a liberal amount of protein in their diets to help counteract the protein catabolism brought about by the corticosteroids.

The psychological dependence that can develop as a result of the "good" feeling brought about by the corticosteroids is another complicating factor of drug therapy. The corticosteroids are not curative, but palliative. The patient needs to know the following: that the disease will be a chronic problem; that the steroids just help to cope with the signs and symptoms; and that, because therapy presents many problems for the body, they cannot be used indefinitely. Patients who are being tapered from the drug will need a great deal of support and encouragement. They may also need a calendar clearly marked with dates and dosages. All patients need to be encouraged to seek regular medical consultation to evaluate the effects of therapy and the disease process.

Drug–drug interactions. Patients on these drugs need to be evaluated carefully if they are taking any other *hormones*—for example, birth control pills, other sex hormones, thyroid hormone replacement, insulin—because the normal body regulatory mechanisms are not maintained, and the anticipated effects may not be seen. When *aspirin* is given with glucocorticoids, the steroids may decrease serum aspirin levels and the desired aspirin effect may not be achieved; this often leads to the patient's overuse of aspirin compounds. Several drugs increase the metabolism of the corticosteroids and decrease the levels of the steroid; these include *phenytoin, rifampin,* and *ephedrine.* Patients on these drugs require increased doses of steroids. *Over-the-counter* drugs, many of which contain such ingredients as ephedrine or aspirin, should be avoided while the patient is on corticosteroids, and the patient should be taught to consult with the physician or nurse if such a medication is needed.

The patient teaching guide presents some key points for teaching a patient on corticosteroids; the guide to the nursing process summarizes the clinical application of this drug therapy in nursing.

Summary of some clinical conditions responsive to corticosteroid therapy

Collagen diseases and nonarticular musculoskeletal disorders

Rheumatoid arthritis (and related disorders, such as rheumatoid spondylitis, Still's disease, psoriatic arthritis, acute and chronic gout, and gouty arthritis)

Acute rheumatic fever and carditis

Bursitis, fibrositis, synovitis, myositis, tendinitis

Disseminated lupus erythematosus

Pemphigus

Scleroderma

Periarteritis nodosa

Dermatomyositis

Allergic, infectious, and other inflammatory disorders of the skin and ocular and respiratory mucous membranes

Bronchial asthma, including status asthmaticus

Pulmonary fibrosis and emphysema

Pollinosis (hay fever)

Rhinitis (perennial vasomotor; allergic)

Skin disorders such as atopic dermatitis (eczema), contact dermatitis, poison ivy dermatitis, neurodermatitis, exfoliative dermatitis, angioneurotic edema, urticaria, seborrheic dermatitis, pruritus vulvi or ani, dermatitis herpetiformis

Eye disorders such as allergic conjunctivitis, iritis, iridocyclitis, choroiditis, chorioretinitis, keratitis, uveitis, corneal ulcers, secondary glaucoma

Severe allergic reactions including anaphylactic shock, transfusion reactions, Stevens–Johnson syndrome

Hematologic and neoplastic conditions

Acute leukemia; chronic lymphocytic leukemia

Autoimmune hemolytic anemia

Acquired hemolytic anemia

Idiopathic thrombocytic purpura

Blood dyscrasias such as agranulocytosis and aplastic anemia

Breast cancer (advanced metastatic mammary carcinoma)

Hodgkin's disease and other lymphomatous neoplasms

Pulmonary granulomatosis

Miscellaneous

Nephrotic syndrome

Adrenogenital syndrome

Ulcerative colitis and regional enteritis

Thyroiditis (subacute nonsuppurative)

Sarcoidosis

Chronic active hepatitis and cirrhosis of the liver

Parotitis (mumps)

Neuritis

Bell's palsy

Myocarditis and other cardiac conditions, including heart block and congestive heart failure

Shock—hemorrhagic, endotoxic, bacteremic, postoperative, etc.

Adrenocortical insufficiency

Infectious mononucleosis

Adrenal hyperplasia (congenital)

Hypercalcemia (varied etiology)

Berylliosis

Löffler's syndrome

Dermatomyositis

Myasthenia gravis

Summary of principles of corticosteroid dosage and administration

Chronic nonfatal disorders (*e.g.*, rheumatoid arthritis; asthma)

Steroids are reserved for use in cases not controlled by safer, more conservative measures.

Steroids are added to the patient's regular regimen in small doses that are then raised slowly.

Administration is continued at the lowest daily dose levels needed for symptomatic relief and for the shortest possible time.

Acute exacerbations of these chronic conditions can be treated with large doses for short periods with relatively little danger, but dosage must be slowly reduced once the acute stage is brought under control.

During periods of disease remission, drug dosage is gradually reduced and, if possible, an attempt is made to discontinue steroid therapy.

If possible, steroids are administered locally rather than systemically (*e.g.*, intra-articular injections; topical application).

If the patient's condition can be kept under control by intermittent rather than daily drug administration, such a method of administration should be tried (such as alternate day therapy).

Acute stages of chronic, possibly fatal, diseases (*e.g.*, lupus erythematosus; pemphigus)

Massive doses of steroids are administered during the life-threatening episodes and then reduced to some-

what lower levels. (To avoid the dangerous complications of these chronic conditions, the development of hypercorticism from large daily doses is considered acceptable.)

Acute crises caused by severe infection or other forms of stress (*e.g.*, gram-negative bacterial endotoxic shock; surgical shock; anaphylactic shock)

Massive doses of a soluble steroid are administered by vein several times daily during the critical period, whether or not there is acute adrenal insufficiency. (Steroids are adjuncts to other drugs such as vasopressors, vasodilators, antibiotics, and replacement fluids and electrolytes.)

Acute, self-limiting episodes of allergic and other disorders (*e.g.*, in conditions not of a dangerous nature, such as hay fever or poison ivy)

Large oral doses are administered at once, and dosage is then "stepped down" every day or two until discontinued entirely after 7 to 10 days.

Topical corticosteroid therapy is employed promptly whenever the symptoms can be controlled with this alone.

Summary of side-effects and toxicity of adrenocorticosteroid drugs

Neurologic effects

Headache, vertigo, psychic disturbances, insomnia, fatigue, increased intracranial pressure, convulsions

Ophthalmic effects

Increased intraocular pressure, posterior subcapsular cataracts

Cardiovascular effects

Hypertension, thrombophlebitis, thromboembolism, petechiae, purpura, necrotizing angiitis

Gastrointestinal effects

Peptic ulcer, gastrointestinal hemorrhage, ulcerative esophagitis, acute pancreatitis

Metabolic changes

Protein depletion, osteoporosis, myopathies, aseptic necrosis of hip or humerus, suppression of growth in children, diabetes mellitus, amenorrhea

Immune–inflammatory effects

Infection, absence of signs and symptoms of infection

Cushingoid signs

"Moon" face, flushing, sweating, hirsutism, thinning scalp hair, supraclavicular fat pads, buffalo hump, abdominal distention, striae, weight gain

Patient teaching guide: corticosteroid drugs

The drug that has been prescribed for you is called a corticosteroid. Similar steroids are produced naturally in the body and affect a number of bodily functions. Your drug has been prescribed to treat ————————— .

Instructions:

1. The name of your drug is ————————— .

2. The dosage of your drug is ————————— .

3. Your drug should be taken ——————— . The drug may cause stomach upset, so it often helps to take the drug with food. If your drug should be taken once a day, it should be taken by 9 AM. If your drug is taken on intermittent days, you should mark a calendar for each drug day and cross off the date as you take the medication.

4. You should never stop taking this drug suddenly. If your prescription is low or you are unable to take the medication for *any* reason, notify your nurse or physician.

5. Some side-effects of the drug that you should be aware of include the following:

Increase in appetite	This may be a welcome change but, if you notice a continual weight gain, you may want to watch your calories.
Restlessness, trouble sleeping	Some patients feel elation and new energy; frequent rest periods should be taken.
Increased susceptibility to infection	Your body's normal defenses are decreased; you should avoid crowded places and people with known infections; if you notice any signs of illness or infection, notify your nurse or physician at once.

6. If you are on this drug for a prolonged period of time you should decrease your intake of salt and salted products, and should supplement your diet with a liberal amount of proteins (*e.g.*, meat, fish, eggs).

7. Tell any dentist, nurse, or physician who is taking care of you that you are on this drug.

8. Because this drug affects your body's natural defenses, you will require special care during any stressful situations. You should wear an identification tag stating that you are maintained on corticosteroids to alert any medical personnel to your particular needs.

(continued)

9. Avoid the use of any over-the-counter medications while you are on this drug. If you feel a need for any of these preparations, consult your nurse or physician.

Notify your nurse or physician if any of the following occur:

Sudden weight gain
Fever, sore throat
Black, tarry stools
Swelling of hands or feet
Any signs of infection
Easy bruising

If you are being tapered from the drug, notify your nurse or physician if any of the following occur:

Fatigue
Nausea, vomiting
Diarrhea
Weight loss
Weakness
Dizziness

Guide to the nursing process: corticosteroid drugs

Assessment	Nursing diagnoses	Intervention	Evaluation
Past history—underlying medical conditions (*contraindications*): Cardiovascular disease, CHF Hypertension Renal insufficiency Active infection— especially fungal; tuberculosis; herpes; chronic active hepatitis Metastatic carcinoma Osteoporosis Myasthenia gravis Peptic ulcer Diverticulitis Diabetes mellitus Hyperthyroidism Psychiatric disorders	Potential alteration in cardiac output Potential fluid volume excess Knowledge deficit regarding drug therapy Potential sensory– perceptual alteration Potential alteration in tissue perfusion Potential ineffective coping with drug changes	Safe and proper administration of drug Provision of comfort measures: Dietary Protection from infection Positioning Patient teaching regarding: Drug Dosage Warnings Diet Side-effects Support and encouragement to cope with: Physical changes Dependency	Monitor for desired effects of drug Monitor for side-effects of drug: Weight gain Edema ↑ or ↓ BP Serum K$^+$ levels Serum glucose levels GI changes Infections Renal function Monitor for drug–drug interactions: Aspirin Insulin Birth control pills Phenytoin Rifampin Ephedrine

(continued)

446

Assessment	Nursing diagnoses	Intervention	Evaluation

Pregnancy
Lactation
Vaccination with a live
  virus
Allergies:
  These drugs
  Tartrazine (certain
    preparations)
  Others
Medication history:
  current drugs
 	
Physical assessment
Neurologic: mental
  status, affect, reflexes
Cardiovascular: BP, P,
  heart auscultation,
  peripheral perfusion,
  edema
Respiratory: R,
  adventitious sounds,
  chest x-ray
GI: stool check, bowel
  sounds, appetite
Renal: BUN, urinalysis
General: lesions,
  temperature
		Withdrawal
		Life support as needed
		  during stress
			Monitor for laboratory
			  test changes:
			  ↑ urine glucose levels
			  ↑ serum cholesterol
			    levels
			Evaluate effectiveness of
			  patient teaching
			Evaluate effectiveness of
			  support and
			  encouragement
			  offered
			Monitor patient during
			  stress situations

Case study

Presentation

MW, a 48-year-old white woman, was diagnosed with severe rheumatoid arthritis 7 years ago. She has been retired, on disability, from her job as an art teacher in the local high school. Her pain was no longer controlled by aspirin, and her physician ordered 5 mg of prednisone tid. Over the next 4 weeks, MW's symptoms were markedly relieved, she was able to start painting again, and she became much more mobile. She also noted that for the first time in years she felt "really good." Her appetite had increased, she wasn't as fatigued as she had been, and her outlook on life was markedly improved. At her follow-up visit, MW was noted to have a weight gain of 9 pounds, slight edema in both ankles, and BP 150/92. An inflamed oozing lesion was found on her right hand, which she stated became infected a couple of weeks ago after she cut her hand while peeling potatoes. Her range of motion and joints were markedly improved. The physician decided that MW should be tapered to 5 mg qd of prednisone over a 4-week period. Describe the appropriate nursing interventions for MW at this visit.

Discussion

The most urgent problem for MW at this time is the infected lesion on her hand. Because steroids interfere with the normal inflammatory and immune responses to this infection, the lesion could progress to a serious problem. The lesion should be cultured, cleansed, and dressed. MW can be instructed in how to care for her hand and how to protect it from water or further injury. An antibiotic will probably be prescribed, and then evaluated for its appropriateness when the culture report comes in. The real nursing challenge with MW will be helping her to cope with and understand the need to taper her prednisone. The drug teaching measures for prednisone should be thoroughly reviewed with MW, pointing out the side-effects of drug therapy that she is already experiencing and explaining, again, the effects that prednisone has on the body. A calendar should be prepared for MW to help her schedule the tapering; usually it progresses from 5 mg bid for 2 weeks to 5 mg qd. MW will need a great deal of encouragement and support to cope with the decrease in therapeutic benefit caused by the need to reduce the prednisone dosage. She has felt so good and done so much better on the drug that she may have a real dread of losing those benefits. She should be encouraged to discuss her feelings, and to call in for support if she needs it. MW should be given an appointment for a return visit in 2 weeks to evaluate the lesion on her hand and to check her progress in the tapering of the drug. She should be urged to call if the lesion looks any worse to her or if she has any difficulties with her drug therapy.

MW's case is a common example of the clinical problems that are encountered when a patient with a chronic inflammatory condition is started on steroid therapy. These patients require strong nursing support and continual teaching.

Drug digests

Desoxycorticosterone acetate USP (Doca Acetate; Percorten)

Actions and indications. This steroid possesses almost pure mineralocorticoid activity and produces prompt retention of sodium and water. Administered as replacement therapy to patients with primary and secondary adrenal insufficiency including Addison's disease, Simmonds' disease, or the Waterhouse–Friderichsen syndrome, this hormone helps to overcome the characteristic hypotension, salt loss, and potassium retention (hyperkalemia) of these disorders. A glucocorticoid must be administered as well as this mineralocorticoid for total replacement therapy.

Adverse effects, cautions, and contraindications. Overdosage of this drug together with an excessive salt intake may lead to the development of edema, high blood pressure, and cardiac enlargement, particularly in patients with essential hypertension or heart disease. Treatment is stopped if a significant gain in weight or rise in blood pressure is detected. Local irritation and symptoms of hypersensitivity may develop occasionally.

Dosage and administration. An oily suspension is administered in initial doses of 2 mg daily by intramuscular injection into the upper outer quadrant of the buttocks. Dosage for maintenance is then adjusted between 1 and 5 mg daily. Initial dosage for the first few days of treatment of patients with the salt-losing adrenogenital syndrome may be somewhat higher but should never exceed 10 mg.

Pellets for implantation in subcutaneous sites have long-lasting effects. The amount implanted for a 6- to 8-month period is based more or less on the daily maintenance dose of the oily suspension.

Dexamethasone USP (Decadron)

Actions and indications. This is one of the most potent and long-acting of the synthetic corticosteroids. It has little or no mineralocorticoid activity, and so is not used for replacement therapy in adrenal insufficiency. Small oral doses are used for anti-inflammatory effects in rheumatic disorders and in chronic collagen and dermatologic diseases. Its antiallergic action is useful for symptomatic relief of respiratory ailments such as seasonal rhinitis (hay fever) and bronchial asthma and skin conditions, such as contact dermatitis.

The sodium phosphate salt of dexamethasone, which is highly soluble and rapidly absorbable, is useful as an adjunct to other specific measures in the management of severe allergic reactions, including status asthmaticus, shock—particularly if adrenal insufficiency is also present—cerebral edema, and the acute life-threatening stages of chronic diseases such as systemic lupus erythematosus.

Adverse effects, cautions, and contraindications. Treatment for periods of over 10 to 14 days with moderate doses may produce signs and symptoms resembling Cushing's syndrome. Psychological disturbances may develop. Long-term use may suppress growth in children and lead to suppression of pituitary–adrenal function. Increased gastric acidity may occur with possible peptic ulcer formation. Diabetes mellitus may be precipitated in patients in whom the condition has been latent, and diabetic patients may require higher dosage of insulin.

This drug is not ordinarily administered to patients with a history of healed or active tuberculosis, but it may be used in some situations together with antituberculosis drugs. It is also contraindicated in patients with herpes simplex virus eye infections and in overtly psychotic patients.

Dosage and administration. Dosage is individualized and varies usually from 0.5 to 3 mg (oral) daily in mild cases to 10 mg in more severe disorders. The sodium phosphate salt is sometimes employed in even more massive doses—20 mg IV or IM, for example, repeated several times if necessary in severe shock and in other acute life-threatening emergencies. It is also injected into joints for local effects in doses of about 2 to 4 mg, depending on the size of the joint, and it may be administered by inhalation to exert effects on respiratory tract membranes, or applied topically to the skin and eyes.

Hydrocortisone USP and its esters and salts* (Cortisol; Cortef; Cortril)

Actions and indications. This is the main natural glucocorticoid secreted by the adrenal cortex; it also has some mineralocorticoid activity. These actions account for its effectiveness as maintenance replacement therapy in many cases of chronic adrenal insufficiency. In acute cases and in various stressful situations resulting from severe trauma and infection, the highly soluble sodium succinate ester and sodium phosphate salt are the preferred forms because of the relative rapidity of their actions.

Hydrocortisone is an effective anti-inflammatory agent when administered by both systemic and local routes. The poorly soluble acetate ester exerts a prolonged antirheumatic effect when injected directly into inflamed joints. It may be applied topically to the skin and to the eyes and other inflamed membranes. The parenterally administered forms are most effective for emergency use in acute allergic emergencies such as status asthmaticus and anaphylaxis, and also as an adjunct in the management of shock from other causes.

Adverse effects, cautions, and contraindications. The relatively high mineralocorticoid activity of this steroid tends to cause sodium and fluid retention leading to weight gain and edema; loss of potassium leading to muscle weakness and possibly to cardiac irregularities may also occur as a result of this secondary effect. Thus, the synthetic steroids are preferred for patients with cardiovascular disorders, including hypertension and a tendency toward cardiac decompensation.

Prolonged use may also lead to the typical metabolic effects of glucocorticoid therapy, including cushingoid signs and symptoms. Mental changes ranging from euphoria to depression may also develop. Following withdrawal, the patient's own adrenals may be unable to secrete cortisol in the amounts required for meeting stressful emergencies. This occurs secondary to the drug-induced depression of hypothalamic–pituitary function.

Dosage and administration. Dosage must be adjusted for each patient in accordance with the nature of the condition and the response to therapy. For replacement therapy, doses of 15 to 30 mg daily are usually adequate, while 40 to 80 mg a day are needed for control of inflammation. In emergencies, 100 mg to 250 mg of the soluble preparations may be administered by vein or intramuscularly and repeated if needed. Intrasynovial injections of the acetate range from 10 mg for small joints to 50 mg for larger ones.

Prednisone USP (Deltasone; Meticorten)

Actions and indications. This synthetic derivative of cortisone has greater glucocorticoid activity and much less mineralocorticoid activity than the natural steroid. It is used for its anti-inflammatory and antiallergic effects in the treatment of rheumatic and collagen diseases, and in dermatologic and ophthalmic disorders marked by acute or chronic inflammatory and allergic processes. It is also used in hematologic disorders and in neoplastic diseases and numerous other conditions in which it offers symptomatic relief.

Adverse effects, cautions, and contraindications. It is not as likely to cause sodium retention as the natural hormones, but is more likely to do so at higher dosage levels than the newer steroids that have relatively greater anti-inflammatory activity. It causes the typical metabolic, endocrine, central, and other adverse effects of all corticosteroids. Susceptible patients may develop peptic ulcer with perforation and bleeding, hypertension and congestive heart failure, signs of diabetes mellitus, muscle weakness and wastage, and osteoporosis.

Dosage and administration. Dosage varies depending on the severity of the disease and on the patient's response. Thus, depending on the disease, treatment may be begun with doses ranging from 5 to 60 mg daily. Later, the first dosage is gradually adjusted downward to the least amount required for maintaining adequate symptomatic relief with minimal toxicity. When treatment is to be discontinued, the drug is withdrawn very gradually.

Triamcinolone USP and its derivatives† (Aristocort; Kenacort)

Actions and indications. This synthetic corticosteroid is used for its potent anti-inflammatory effect when administered locally or systemically. Some forms, such as the *diacetate* and *hexacetonide* suspensions, are injected directly into inflamed joints, where they exert a prolonged local effect useful for symptomatic relief in rheumatoid arthritis and osteoarthritis. The diacetate is also injected directly into the skin lesions of psoriasis and various dermatoses.

The *acetonide* is applied topically for relief of itching, burning, oozing, and other discomforting symptoms of contact dermatitis, atopic and seborrheic dermatitis, eczema, neurodermatitis, exfoliative dermatitis, anogenital pruritus, and—under occlusive dressings—in psoriasis. Other forms are administered orally or parenterally for the systemic effects of corticosteroids in a wide variety of clinical disorders.

Adverse effects, cautions, and contraindications. Taken internally, this synthetic steroid can produce most of the adverse metabolic, endocrine, central, and other adverse effects of other corticosteroids. It has relatively little mineralocorticoid activity and is thus less likely than hydrocortisone and prednisolone to cause sodium and water retention or potassium loss. It does not stimulate appetite, and its use is thus not as likely to lead to weight gain as when other steroids are employed. However, it may cause more muscle wastage and weakness of the muscles of the thighs, lower back, and pelvis than other corticosteroids.

Injection directly into joints may cause an early increase in inflammatory symptoms, including swelling and pain. Later relief of pain may result in the patient's becoming excessively active, thus leading to acceleration of degenerative processes in the joint. Joint injections should not be made when there is evidence of infection. Aseptic technique is required for both the intra-articular and intralesional administration of these products. Topical use is contraindicated in the presence of fungal and viral skin diseases or tuberculosis of the skin.

Dosage and administration. Dosage varies widely, depending on the nature and severity of the disorder that is being treated, but it usually ranges between 4 and 16 mg daily. The amounts administered by intralesional injection vary from 5 mg to 50 mg, depending on the size of the lesion and other factors. The dosage injected into joints may range between 2 mg and 20 mg, depending on the size of the joint.

---

* Hydrocortisone acetate; cypionate; sodium phosphate; sodium succinate.

† Triamcinolone acetonide, diacetate, and hexacetonide.

References

Axelrod L: Glucocorticoid therapy. Medicine 35:39, 1976

Baxter JD, Forsham PH: Tissue effects of glucocorticoids. Am J Med 53:573, 1972

Conn HO, Blitzer BL: Nonassociation of adrenocorticosteroids and peptic ulcer. N Eng J Med, 294:473, 1976

Fanci AS, et al: Glucocorticosteroid therapy: Mechanism of actions and clinical considerations. Ann Intern Med 84:304, 1976

Fenster LF: The ulcerogenic potential of glucocorticoids and possible prophylactic measures. Med Clin N Am 57:1289, 1973

Genuth SM: The adrenal glands. In Berne RM, Levy MN (eds): Physiology, pp 1033–1068. St. Louis, C.V. Mosby, 1983.

Gotch PM: Teaching patients about adrenal corticosteroids. Am J Nurs 81:78, 1981

Harter JG et al: Studies on intermittent corticosteroid dosage regimen. N Eng J Med 269:591, 1963

Haynes RC Jr, Murad F: Adrenocorticotropic hormone; adrenocortical steroids and their synthetic analogues; inhibitors of adrenocortical steroid biosynthesis. In Gilman AG, Goodman LS, Gilman A (eds): Goodman and Gilman's The Pharmacological Basis of Therapeutics, 6th ed, pp 1466–1496. New York, Macmillan, 1980

Melby JC: Clinical pharmacology of systemic steroids. Annu Rev Pharmacol Toxicol 17:511, 1977

Melby JC: Systemic corticosteroid therapy, pharmacology, and endocrinologic considerations. Ann Intern Med 81:505, 1975

Rodman MJ: The corticosteroids. RN 32:69, 1969

Streeten DHP: Corticosteroid therapy. 1. Pharmacologic properties and principles of corticosteroid use. JAMA 232:944, 1975

Thompson EB, Lippman MF: Mechanism of action of glucocorticoids. Metabolism 23:159, 1974

Zurier RB, Weissmann G: Anti-immunologic and anti-inflammatory effects of steroid therapy. Med Clin North Am 57:1295, 1973

Chapter 22

The thyroid hormones and antithyroid drugs

22

The thyroid gland

General considerations

Anatomy. The thyroid (from the Greek *thyreos*, shield, and *eidos*, form) gland is located in the neck, where it surrounds the trachea and seems to protect the windpipe like a shield. It is composed of cells arranged in circular follicles. The lumen of each follicle contains colloid, in which the thyroid hormone is stored (Fig. 22-1).

History. The prominence of the thyroid gland in the neck, and the ease with which it can be palpated, made it possible for endocrinologists in the last century to associate the signs and symptoms of thyroid hyperfunction with enlargement of the gland, and to associate the signs and symptoms of hypofunction with thyroid atrophy. These pioneering endocrinologists also noted what happened when they removed this gland from the necks of experimental animals; they then prepared and injected thyroid extracts that could overcome most of the signs and symptoms produced by the prior surgical ablation of the gland. Later, physicians found that they could counteract the low metabolic rate of hypothyroid patients simply by giving them powdered thyroid gland by mouth.

Actions. It is now known that the thyroid gland regulates the rate of metabolism in almost all body cells. That is, the thyroid gland secretes hormones that control the speed of the combustion processes by which body tissues burn food to derive the energy needed for normal function and for growth and development. Despite findings that thyroid hormones act on cell membrane enzymes and bind to a protein in the cell nucleus, the precise mechanism by which they act to control the rate of cellular metabolic processes is still unknown. However, it is clinically obvious what happens to a person whose thyroid gland fails to function properly. This chapter will discuss the drugs used to treat clinical conditions caused by the underfunctioning and the overactivity of the thyroid gland.

Disorders. Thyroid gland disorders may be divided into two general categories:

1. *Hypothyroidism*—conditions marked by a decrease in the production and secretion of thyroid hormones
2. *Hyperthyroidism*—conditions in which the thyroid gland produces and secretes excessive amounts of its hormones into the systemic circulation

In hypothyroid conditions, body metabolism slows down to subnormal levels, rates of growth and development are reduced, and the effects of sluggish metabolism are apparent in many body systems, including the central nervous system. In hyperthyroidism, on the other hand, the metabolic rate is abnormally elevated, with far-reaching effects on many systems, particularly the cardiovascular system. (The signs and symptoms accompanying full-blown hypo- and hyperthyroidism are summarized in Table 22-1.)

Simple nontoxic goiter is a thyroid disorder of another type. The thyroid gland is enlarged but the secretion of its hormones may be more or less normal. This so-called *euthyroid* or essentially normal state occurs because the gland has grown enough to compensate for conditions that would otherwise result in deficient secretion. The most common cause of simple goiter is a lack of dietary iodine, which tends to reduce thyroid hormone production. However, this causes an elevation in thyroid-stimulating hormone, or thyrotropin (TSH; see Chap. 20), and this in turn leads to an increase in the size of the thyroid gland and an increase in the gland's ability to extract iodine from the circulation. As a result, enough thyroid hormones are usually produced to maintain nor-

451

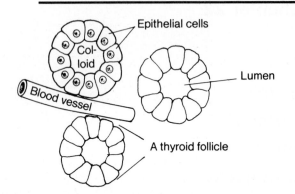

Figure 22-1. Histology of the thyroid gland. Synthesis of the thyroid hormone from its constituents, including iodide, which are brought to the thyroid gland by the blood, begins in the epithelial cells, which are arranged in follicles. A precursor form of the hormone is then secreted into the colloid in the lumen of the follicles, where further synthetic steps produce a storage form of the hormone. Secretion of the final hormone product requires the reuptake of the storage form into the cell, and further processing. The hormone is then released into the bloodstream.

mal metabolism. Nonetheless, such thyroid enlargement indicates an abnormal functional state that requires correction.

Biosynthesis and regulation of thyroid hormone release

Before discussing the treatment of hypothyroidism, hyperthyroidism, and simple goiter, it is desirable to review the way in which the production and secretion of thyroid hormones are controlled and carried out. The reason for this is that nearly every type of thyroid function disorder stems fundamentally from some defect that alters the normal state of thyroid hormone synthesis and release.

Biosynthesis
The thyroid gland produces two slightly different hormones:

1. *Tetraiodothyronine* (T_4) or *thyroxine,* which contains four atoms of iodine
2. *Triiodothyronine* (T_3), which contains three atoms of iodine, and which is called *liothyronine* when used as a drug

These hormones are made in the following biosynthetic steps (Fig. 22-2):

1. Iodide trapping
2. *Iodination:* attachment of one or two iodine atoms to the amino acid tyrosine, which is contained in molecules of a mucoprotein called *thyroglobulin*

3. Coupling of two types of iodotyrosine molecules (*mono-* and *diiodotyrosine*) to form triiodothyronine and thyroxine

Iodide trapping. The thyroid gland removes iodide from the blood that passes through it and concentrates the ion within the gland in much higher amounts than are present in the plasma. The trapping or pumping of iodide into the thyroid cell is an active energy-requiring process that is stimulated by TSH and by low concentrations of iodide, but is inhibited by some drugs (see below) and by high concentrations of iodide ions.

A dietary deficiency of iodine, resulting in reduced synthesis of thyroid hormones and in simple goiter, was once common in some parts of the world, including the midwestern United States.* Now, however, people who cannot get this element from seafood, drinking water, or leafy vegetables grown in soil that contains it can avoid iodine deficiency diseases by using table salt to which iodine salt supplements (iodides) have been added.

Iodination. The thyroid cells that take up iodide from the blood contain enzymes that oxidize it to active iodine atoms that are then attached to the amino acid tyrosine, which is contained in thyroglobulin molecules synthesized in the thyroid cells. The iodination step occurs in or near the lumen of the follicle. Some tyrosine residues receive one iodine atom (monoiodotyrosine, MIT); others receive two (diiodotyrosine, DIT). Some drugs that are used in treating *hyper*thyroidism (Table 22-2) act by inhibiting the enzymes responsible for this oxidative reaction. Thus, even though the overactive gland continues to trap large amounts of iodide, hormone production is reduced, as are the signs and symptoms of *thyrotoxicosis* (see hyperthyroidism, Table 22-1).

Coupling. In the final biosynthetic step, oxidative enzymes cause two molecules of diiodotyrosine to couple and to form *tetra*iodothyronine, or one molecule of *di*iodotyrosine may couple with one molecule of *mono*-iodotyrosine to form *tri*iodothyronine. Both of these iodinated molecules are still attached to the thyroglobulin molecule, and this complex constitutes a storage form of the hormones in the colloid. Before these hormones can be secreted into the bloodstream, the storage complex must be taken back up into the thyroid cell; this uptake process is called *endocytosis.* The complex is then acted on by proteolytic enzymes that release the T_3 and T_4 hormones, which are then secreted into the bloodstream. Depending on conditions, the thyroid gland normally produces about four times more T_4 than T_3. However, T_3 is about four times as active as T_4, and it is believed that most of the T_4 released from the thyroid is converted to the more active T_3 form in peripheral tissues.

Regulation of secretion
As indicated in Chapter 20, the secretion of stored thyroid hormones into the bloodstream is stimulated by the anterior pituitary gland hormone *thyrotropin* (TSH), which

---

* The average daily dietary intake is 150 µg. About 70 µg is taken up by the thyroid gland and the rest is excreted by the kidneys.

Table 22–1. Signs and symptoms of thyroid dysfunction

	Hypothyroidism	Hyperthyroidism
Central nervous system	*Functions depressed:* hypoactive reflexes (hyporeflexia), lethargy, emotional dullness, sleepiness, slow speech, stupid appearance	*Functions stimulated:* hyperactive reflexes, anxiety, nervousness, restlessness, insomnia, tremors
Cardiovascular–renal	*Functions depressed:* bradycardia, hypotension, increased circulation time, oliguria, anemia, decreased sensitivity to catecholamines and to adrenergic drugs	*Functions stimulated:* tachycardia, palpitations, decreased circulation time, increased pulse pressure, systolic hypertension, and increased sensitivity to catecholamines and to adrenergic drugs
Skin and other epithelial structures	Skin pale, coarse, dry, thickened, especially on hands and face, which is puffy about the eyelids, cheeks, and elsewhere; hair coarse and thinned on scalp and in eyebrows; nails thick and hard	Skin flushed, thin, warm, moist because of vasodilation and sweating; hair fine and soft; nails soft and thin
Metabolic rate	*Decreased,* with body temperature reduced, intolerance of cold, decreased appetite, with more of food intake converted to fat, including cholesterol (*i.e.*, tendency toward weight gain and definite hypercholesterolemia)	*Increased,* with body temperature raised (low-grade fever), intolerance of heat, increased appetite, but with tendency toward weight loss, which may be severe sometimes and accompanied by muscle wasting and weakness (thyrotoxic myopathy)
Generalized myxedema	Including accumulation of mucopolysaccharides in heart (cardiomegaly), tongue and vocal cords (hoarseness and thickened speech), periorbital areas	Localized, with accumulations of mucopolysaccharides in the orbits, eyeballs, and ocular muscles; periorbital edema, puffiness of eyelids, lid lag, and exophthalmos; occasional pretibial edema
Ovarian function	*Decreased,* with tendency toward menorrhagia, possible habitual abortion, or sterility	Altered, with tendency toward oligomenorrhea or amenorrhea
Goiter	Relatively rare and of simple nontoxic type	Diffuse, highly vascular, and murmurous (bruit); very frequent

also stimulates the steps of iodination, coupling, endocytosis, and proteolysis. Under the influence of this pituitary tropic hormone, the thyroid gland grows in size and increases in vascularity.

The secretion of TSH is itself stimulated by a tripeptide, *thyrotropin releasing hormone* (TRH), which is synthesized in the hypothalamus and carried to the anterior pituitary by the hypothalamoadenohypophyseal portal system. A very delicate balance exists between the hypothalamic, pituitary, and thyroid gland hormones. Ordinarily, if the level of thyroid hormones in the blood rises even slightly above normal, this suppresses the secretion of TSH by the pituitary gland. (Negative feedback may also occur at the level of the hypothalamus.) This negative feedback leads in turn to a reduction in thyroid

hormone production. The reverse is also true; if the blood level of thyroid hormones is reduced, the pituitary gland increases its secretion of TSH. This then causes the thyroid to synthesize and to secrete more of its hormones. The failure of these reciprocal mechanisms to regulate function in normal fashion often results in thyroid gland disorders such as hypo- and hyperthyroidism and in the development of simple nontoxic and toxic goiters.

Hypothyroidism

Technical advances have made it simple not only to detect a deficiency of circulating thyroid hormones but also to determine the type of hypothyroidism. On the basis of

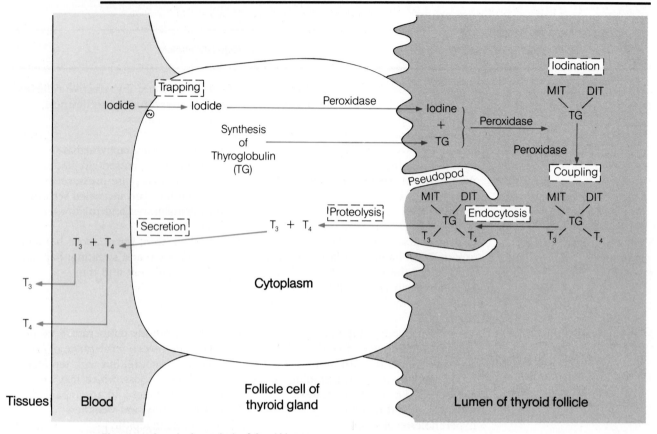

Figure 22-2. Steps in the synthesis of thyroid hormones.

certain sensitive diagnostic tests (see the summary at the end of the chapter), this disorder can be subclassified:

1. *Primary*—the result of thyroid gland disease or absence of functioning thyroid tissue
2. *Secondary*—caused by pituitary gland disease and a lack of TSH
3. *Tertiary*—stemming from a tumor or other lesion in the hypothalamus that impairs the production or secretion of TRH

Disorders

Primary hypothyroidism may occur congenitally, or it may develop in adulthood. Such failure may be functional and of uncertain origin, or it may result from acute or subacute (viral) thyroid inflammation or from chronic (Hashimoto's) thyroiditis, which is an autoimmune disorder. It also commonly occurs as a result of overtreatment of *hyper*thyroidism with antithyroid drugs, radiation therapy, or surgery (see below). A lack of thyroid hormone leads to two clear-cut deficiency syndromes:

1. *Cretinism*, which is the result of glandular failure in infancy

2. *Myxedema*, a condition that sometimes develops in adults and in older children (juvenile myxedema)

In addition to these obvious deficiency states, some patients apparently suffer from a partial or *borderline* type of hypothyroidism. These patients, who often seem to have more or less normal thyroid activity, complain of various vague symptoms that are often dramatically improved by the administration of thyroid.

Cretinism

Cretinism, or congenital hypothyroidism, may result from an inborn enzymatic defect that interferes with iodine uptake and use. More commonly, the child is born without a thyroid gland (athyreosis) or with one that has failed to develop properly. Although the routine use of iodized salt has largely eliminated endemic goiter in this country, a lack of iodine in the mother's diet may still account for cases of cretinism in certain isolated mountainous regions elsewhere in the world.

Growth and development of the nervous and skeletal systems are retarded in congenitally hypothyroid infants. If the condition is recognized early and treated with adequate doses of thyroid hormones, the child may

Table 22–2. Drugs used in treatment and diagnosis of thyroid disorders

Official, generic, or USAN name	Trade name or synonym	Route of administration	Usual adult daily dosage
Drugs used in hypothyroidism			
Levothyroxine sodium USP	Levothroid; Noroxine; Synthroid; T_4	Oral	Initially 25–100 μg daily; maintenance 150–300 μg daily
Liothyronine sodium USP	Cytomel; triiodothyronine; T_3	Oral	Initially 5–25 μg daily; maintenance 50–100 μg daily
Liotrix	Euthroid; Thyrolar	Oral	Initially one tablet daily containing 25–30 μg of levothyroxine and 6.25–7.5 μg liothyronine; later, maintenance with mixtures of levothyroxine 50–180 μg and liothyronine 6.25–45 μg daily
Thyroglobulin USP	Proloid	Oral	Initially 32–60 mg daily; maintenance 32–200 mg
Thyroid USP	Desiccated thyroid	Oral	Initially 16–65 mg daily; maintenance 65–195 mg
Drugs used in hyperthyroidism			
Thioamides (antithyroid drugs)			
Methimazole USP	Tapazole	Oral	Initially, 15 mg/day in three divided doses; maintenance, 5–15 mg/day in three divided doses
Propylthiouracil USP	Propacil	Oral	Initially, 300 mg/day in three divided doses; maintenance, 100–150 mg/day in divided doses
Iodides			
Iodine solution, strong USP	Lugol's solution	Oral	2–6 drops bid for 10 days before surgery
Potassium iodide solution USP	SSKI	Oral	0.3–0.6 ml (300–600 mg) tid or qid
Sodium iodide USP		IV	2 g/day

(continued)

Table 22–2. Drugs used in treatment and diagnosis of thyroid disorders (continued)

Official, generic, or USAN name	Trade name or synonym	Route of administration	Usual adult daily dosage
Radiation therapy			
Sodium iodide ^{131}I USP	Iodotope Therapeutic; Sodium iodide ^{131}I therapeutic	Oral	Hyperthyroidism: 4–10 mc; thyroid carcinoma: 50 mc initially, 100–150 mc subsequently
Supplementary sympatholytic (adrenergic receptor or neuron blocking) drugs			
Guanethidine USP	Ismelin		See Drug digest, Chapter 28
Propranolol USP	Inderal		See Drug digest, Chapter 18
Reserpine USP	Serpasil		See Drug digest, Chapter 28
Drugs used in diagnosis			
Anterior pituitary hormone			
Thyrotropin	Thyroid-stimulating hormone (TSH); Thytropar	IM, SC	10 international U
Hypothalamic hormone			
Protirelin	Thypinone; Relefact TRH; synthetic thyrotropin-releasing hormone (TRH)	IV bolus	200–500 μg

develop normally. However, in those who are hypothyroid during fetal development and in infants whose condition goes unrecognized and untreated for more than a few months, the likelihood of permanent mental retardation is very high.

Treatment. Once the cretinous condition is recognized, thyroid replacement therapy is promptly instituted. Physicians may differ in regard to the particular thyroid product that they prefer, but all agree that it is desirable to administer full doses of any preparation from the start. Infants apparently require relatively large doses and are able to tolerate them. After thyroid treatment has been initiated, the maintenance dose is determined through frequent checks of the levels of thyroxine by radioimmunoassay of T_4 (see Summary of Tests of Thyroid Function at the end of the chapter) and by periodic x-rays to follow the baby's bone development.

Myxedema

Myxedema, the adult form of thyroid hormone deficiency, is marked by characteristic signs and symptoms (see Table 22-1). The condition most often develops slowly as the thyroid gland gradually atrophies and functioning cells are replaced by fibrous connective tissue. Occasionally, myxedema follows acute viral thyroiditis or chronic inflammatory destruction of the gland—as in Hashimoto's (autoimmune) thyroiditis, for example. Overtreatment of hyperthyroidism with antithyroid drugs, excessive radiation therapy, or excessive tissue removal by surgery may also cause this severe form of hypothyroidism.

Some cases of myxedema are secondary to pituitary gland failure following childbirth complications or tumor development. Patients with pituitary myxedema have a thyroid gland that can function but that does not because of a lack of TSH. Primary and secondary myxedema can be differentiated by administering the tropic pituitary hormone, *thyrotropin*. A normal thyroid gland then markedly increases its uptake of radioactive iodine despite the pituitary gland disorder. Patients with primary myxedema continue to show low iodine uptake despite administration of thyrotropin. It is now also possible to distinguish between myxedema of pituitary and hypothalamic (tertiary) dysfunction by the use of protirelin (Thypinone), a synthetic form of TRH.

Treatment. The administration of adequate doses of thyroid hormones has a remarkable effect on the mental and physical condition of the myxedematous patient. Even small amounts of thyroid quickly make a great difference in the patient's appearance and behavior. Puffiness disappears as most of the retained fluids are removed from the tissues by way of the kidneys. The dull expressionless look is replaced by an alert interested appearance, and physical sluggishness gives way to normal activity. Once the patient achieves normal hormonal balance, such functional equilibrium can be kept indefinitely by maintenance thyroid therapy.

The aim of treatment in primary myxedema is to bring about the greatest possible improvement with the lowest dosage of thyroid. That is, the patient is returned to as close to normal a state as possible without being pushed into a *hyper*thyroid state. Ordinarily this is done by administering relatively small doses, which are gradually raised to exert a cumulative effect over a period of several weeks. Special care is taken to avoid overdosage in elderly patients and in those with a history of cardiac complications. The organ systems of patients who have been in a hypothyroid state are often extremely sensitive to small increments in levels of circulating thyroid hormone.

In myxedema that arises secondary to pituitary gland damage—as in hemorrhagic postpartum necrosis—thyroid treatment is helpful. Here, however, and in the case of hypophysectomized patients, it may also be necessary to give sex hormones and adrenal corticosteroids to make up for the lack of these secretions following the loss of the gonadotropic and adrenocorticotropic hormones of the pituitary. Replacement of corticosteroids is especially important when thyroid hormones are being administered, because the increased tissue metabolism brought about by the latter may send the patient into a state of adrenal insufficiency.

Myxedema coma is a severe complication with a high mortality rate. Treatment of this emergency requires not only the immediate intravenous administration of relatively large doses of one of the synthetic thyroid hormones, such as sodium liothyronine, but also various adjunctive drugs. Digoxin in small doses may, for example,

be required to control congestive heart failure. Intravenous glucose may be necessary to counteract hypoglycemia, and IV hydrocortisone is employed to overcome adrenal insufficiency. Antibiotics may be required for treating any concurrent infection. Other medications may also be administered as needed, but sedatives, narcotics, and other central nervous system depressants should be avoided.

Borderline hypothyroidism. *Hypometabolism* is a term sometimes used to describe the state of a group of patients who do *not* show the multiple symptoms of fullblown myxedema but who nonetheless complain of various vague symptoms, traceable to a thyroid gland that is functioning at only a low normal level. When symptoms such as muscle weakness and pain, fatigue, lethargy, headaches, and emotional upsets are recognized through diagnostic testing to be the result of a mild, or borderline, hypothyroidism and thyroid therapy is administered, the patient may respond with a remarkable improvement.

Misuses of thyroid medications

Thyroid medication has long been advocated for treating many conditions marked by the presence of one or more signs and symptoms found in hypothyroidism. Obviously, because inadequate thyroid secretion can affect the functioning of nearly every body tissue, there are a great number of signs and symptoms that might in theory respond to thyroid replacement therapy. There is no reason to believe, however, that thyroid treatment will be effective for these conditions in the absence of hypothyroidism. Nonetheless, the fact that patients with seemingly normal thyroid gland activity sometimes respond well to thyroid administration has encouraged the *misuse* of thyroid drugs as a panacea.

Obesity. Thyroid medication has often played a part in weight reduction regimens. Its use for this purpose is unjustified and potentially dangerous.* Although thyroid replacement therapy often reduces the flabbiness and puffiness of a myxedematous patient, it will speed neither fat metabolism nor removal of fluids from the tissues of a patient whose thyroid function is normal.

High doses of thyroid products may accelerate the patient's metabolism enough to cause some loss of weight. However, overdosage not only is dangerous (see below), but also may stimulate the patient's appetite. This, of course, makes it difficult for the most effective weight-reducing measure to be carried out—to lower the caloric intake. Patients need to be taught that thyroid medication is not a quick answer to weight problems, but is a potentially dangerous medication that should be used only for patients whose blood tests reveal that they lack the hormone.

Obstetric-gynecologic disorders. The reproductive system tissues are adversely affected by a lack of thyroid secretion. Frequently, hypothyroid women may

---

* Deaths have occurred following the administration of thyroid hormones combined with diuretics and digitalis in so-called "rainbow capsules."

suffer, for example, from a secondary deficiency of ovarian hormones. This lack of estrogens or progesterone often leads to menstrual irregularities, including menorrhagia. The fact that the administration of thyroid hormones sometimes helps to regulate the menstrual cycle of such *hypothyroid* patients does *not* mean that thyroid drug administration will be useful for treating abnormal menses in *euthyroid* women, yet thyroid has been administered routinely in *unselected* cases of amenorrhea, dysmenorrhea, premenstrual tension, and other gynecologic disorders, including sterility and habitual abortion.

Other misuses. The use of thyroid seems much less justified—even in theory—in dermatologic, musculoskeletal, and other conditions marked by signs and symptoms similar to some found in hypothyroidism. Thus, although the myxedematous patient's skin may be dry and scaly, thyroid is no panacea for such symptoms when they occur in *euthyroid* patients. Similarly, thyroid often relieves muscular cramps and joint pains in overt hypothyroidism, but it is no cure-all in arthritis and myositis, nor does the reversal of anemia by thyroid treatment of hypothyroidism mean that thyroid is ever a substitute for the adequate diagnosis and specific treatment of anemia with iron salts or other hematinics.

Other indications

Suppression of thyrotropin by the administration of a thyroid product has several applications in treatment and diagnosis. In *simple goiter,* for example, giving thyroid often helps to reduce the size of the gland that has grown in size in response to stimulation by the pituitary hormone TSH. Similarly, in hyperthyroid patients whose glands have undergone compensatory enlargement as a result of prolonged treatment with antithyroid drugs (or *goitrogens*), the addition of thyroid medication in doses that suppress the thyroid-stimulating pituitary hormone sometimes stops further growth of the gland. The growth of thyrotropin-dependent thyroid cancer may also be slowed by administering thyroid. (The use of thyroid products in the diagnosis of hyperthyroidism and for evaluating the patient's response to antithyroid drugs is discussed below.)

Adverse effects

Overdosage with thyroid products results in the appearance of adverse cardiac effects and in other signs and symptoms similar to those of hyperthyroidism or thyrotoxicosis (see the summary at the end of this chapter and Table 22-1). The heart muscle is forced to work harder to meet the demands of the rapidly metabolizing peripheral tissues for blood. As a result, the rapidly beating heart may tend to outrun the capacity of its own coronary vessels to supply the myocardium with oxygenated blood. Anginal chest pains then occur as a result of such myocardial ischemia.

Older patients with some prior degree of coronary insufficiency may be precipitated into congestive heart failure if they receive too high a dose of a thyroid preparation. Patients taking thyroid should not be treated with catecholamines or with other adrenergic drugs because of the possible adverse cardiac effects of the combination. Both these patients and poorly controlled hyperthyroid patients are unusually sensitive to catecholamines. Experimental evidence suggests that these patients may have a greater number of adrenergic receptors, especially cardiac β_1 receptors, than normal.

Thyroid products

Several types of thyroid products are available for correcting hypothyroidism (see Table 22-2). Opinions differ as to which preparation is preferable, and each type has its advocates. Actually, all exert the same type of metabolic effects and differ mainly in potency and in the time they take to act and to stop acting. *Thyroid*[+] and *thyroglobulin* (Proloid) are dried defatted powders prepared from the thyroid glands of animals. They are, of course, less potent than the pure hormones that they contain. Thus, for example, 60 mg of these substances is equivalent to 100 μg of thyroxine or 25 μg of liothyronine, and the latter hormone is the most rapid in onset and shortest in duration of action.

Today most patients are started on one of the potent pure hormones of synthetic origin rather than on one of the natural preparations, which have been known to vary in their composition and potency. However, when given in adequate dosage, these products can produce all the desired effects of the purified or synthetically prepared hormones. The official thyroid powder is relatively cheap and serves as entirely satisfactory replacement therapy in most cases of hypothyroidism. Thus, there is little reason to switch a patient who has been maintained for many years on dessicated thyroid tablets to one of the synthetic thyroid hormones.

Levothyroxine sodium[+] (Synthroid) is usually preferred, even though its absorption is variable and incomplete on oral administration. Because of this and its greater degree of binding to plasma proteins, it produces its effects more slowly than liothyronine, but its effects, once fully attained, are longer lasting—a desirable property in a product that is to be taken indefinitely. Thus, for example, some patients may be maintained with once-weekly doses of T_4 and, in any case, rapid effects can be attained in emergencies such as myxedema coma by administering doses high enough to saturate the protein binding sites.

Liothyronine sodium[+] (Cytomel; triiodothyronine) is the faster acting of the two natural hormones. This may make it most useful for emergency treatment of myxedema coma. However, the relatively short duration of its action may be a drawback during long-term maintenance therapy of hypothyroidism. An additional disadvantage may be the tendency toward adverse cardiac effects following rapid attainment of high concentrations of T_3 in the heart and other tissues.

Liotrix (Euthroid; Thyrolar) is a mixture containing four parts of levothyroxine to one part of liothyronine. This 4:1 ratio of the two hormones is claimed to imitate closely the effects of the natural thyroid gland secretion. Actually, however, because thyroxine is now known to be partially converted in the body to liothyronine, the same effect—that is, attainment of natural ratios of T_4 and T_3—can be attained less expensively by the use of thyroxine sodium alone. Another possible advantage claimed for administering this mixture, instead of either hormone individually, is that its use permits better interpretation of the laboratory tests employed to determine the patient's response to treatment (see Summary of tests of thyroid function at the end of the chapter).

Average dosage levels of all thyroid products are now much lower than they once were. It is now known that patients with primary hypothyroidism should be maintained on a dosage that is just large enough to lower the level of circulating TSH to normal by its negative feedback effect on secretion of that pituitary hormone. With the development of a very sensitive radioimmune assay for TSH, it was learned that this therapeutic goal could be achieved by administering about half the amount of thyroid that was previously employed.

Of course, the clinical response of the patient to thyroid therapy is still the best guide to regulating dosage. The patient's general condition on initiation of treatment is also an important factor in determining starting dosage. Thus, because patients with severe myxedema are often very sensitive to thyroid therapy, they are usually started on very small doses that are then raised only gradually. A similar regimen is also recommended for hypothyroid patients with angina pectoris or other forms of heart disease and for elderly myxedematous patients.

Once a hypothyroid patient's condition has responded to treatment with appropriate doses of a thyroid preparation, he must continue to take the daily dosage to which he has been titrated indefinitely to maintain the gratifying improvement. Unfortunately, many people think that they can stop taking their medication once they feel well again. Such failure to take thyroid replacement therapy regularly or at all then leads to the gradual redevelopment of myxedema.

The mental effects of myxedema may keep such relapsing patients from realizing what is happening to them, even when signs and symptoms become apparent to others. To avoid development of increasingly severe deficiency symptoms or even of myxedema coma, the patient and a responsible member of the family should be made aware of the importance of continuing to take daily replacement doses of the prescribed thyroid product and the need to keep all appointments for periodic checkups.

Hyperthyroidism (thyrotoxicosis)

Etiology and diagnosis

Several different disorders can lead to the secretion of excessive quantities of thyroid hormones and to the characteristic signs and symptoms that are summarized in Table 22-1. Actually, however, the most common cause of hyperthyroidism—Graves' disease—is not primarily a thyroid disorder but is a generalized, or constitutional, condition stemming from a still poorly understood autoimmune mechanism. Several circulating immunoglobulins are suspected as being responsible for stimulating the thyroid gland to secrete abnormally.

One such substance, called the long-acting thyroid stimulator, or LATS, continues to act on the thyroid gland for many years. Unlike the thyroid-stimulating hormone of the pituitary gland (TSH), production of LATS is *not* shut off by an abnormally high plasma level of thyroid hormones, as demonstrated in the so-called thyroid-suppression test.

In this test, *liothyronine sodium* is administered daily for a week. This reduces radioactive iodine uptake of *euthyroid* patients to less than 20% of normal by suppressing pituitary production of thyrotropin. In the *hyperthyroid* patient, on the other hand, such suppression of pituitary TSH by the thyroid hormone does not prevent the thyroid gland from continuing to take up the radioactive iodine. This indicates that the thyroid gland is functioning autonomously and is not responsive to the normal negative feedback regulatory mechanism described above. (The diagnosis of Graves' disease can now be confirmed by a test in which the intravenous injection of a synthetic TRH, protirelin [Thypinone], fails to stimulate increased production of TSH, which has been suppressed by the high circulating levels of thyroid hormones.)

Treatment

Control of hyperthyroidism symptoms or complete cure of thyrotoxicosis can be brought about by three types of therapy that are employed alone or in sequential combination:

1. *Subtotal thyroidectomy,* the surgical excision of most of the thyroid gland
2. *Radiation therapy,* in which the radioactive isotope ^{131}I is administered to destroy some of the thyroid tissue that is producing excessive amounts of hormones
3. *Antithyroid drugs,* which act specifically on the thyroid gland to interfere in different

ways with the steps by which thyroid hormones are biosynthesized, or that prevent hormones already synthesized and stored within the gland from being released into the bloodstream for transport to peripheral target tissues. (Various other drugs that do not affect thyroid gland function—for example, the β-adrenergic blocking agent propranolol—are also often employed to interfere with the peripheral effects of the thyroid hormones on the heart and other tissues or to support the patient suffering from the effects of thyrotoxicosis.)

Each type of treatment has its advantages and disadvantages (see Summary of adverse effects of antithyroid drugs at the end of this chapter). The use of surgery or of radiation is, for example, followed by the fewest number of recurrences and by the most frequent occurrence of permanent remissions. However, *hypo*thyroidism as a result of excessive loss of thyroid tissue is a common complication of these types of definitive therapy. Thus, although relapses are more common following treatment with antithyroid drugs, these agents are now preferred for initiating treatment of patients with Graves' disease, because drug therapy does not damage the thyroid gland beyond repair and so is less likely to cause permanent hypothyroidism. Patients who fail to respond fully to drug treatment can still receive radiation therapy or be treated surgically, if necessary.

Drug therapy: mechanisms of action

The drugs that interfere specifically with thyroid gland function do so in three main ways (Table 22-3):

1. The *thioamides* (Table 22-2) block biosynthesis of thyroid hormones, probably by inhibiting the oxidative enzymes that catalyze the iodination and coupling processes in the formation of thyroxine (T_4) and liothyronine (T_3) discussed above. Propylthiouracil also inhibits the conversion of T_4 to the more active T_3 form in peripheral tissues.
2. The *iodides*, substances that are needed for formation of thyroid hormones, can, paradoxically, also interfere with iodine metabolism in several ways when present in excessively high concentrations compared to those required for physiologic function. Most significant is the fact that the

---

* The term "antithyroid drugs" is commonly employed to refer *only* to the thioamides, even though the other categories of agents that depress thyroid function directly are also antithyroid drugs.

Table 22–3. Sites of action of antithyroid drugs

Step in hormone synthesis	Inhibitor
Iodide trapping	High iodide concentration
	Ion inhibitors*: thiocyanate, perchlorate
Iodination and coupling	Thioamides*: propylthiouracil, methimazole
	High iodide concentration
	Ion inhibitors: thiocyanate
Endocytosis	High iodide concentration
Proteolysis	High iodide concentration
Secretion	High iodide concentration*
Tissue conversion of T_4 to T_3	Propylthiouracil

* Probable chief site of therapeutic action of this agent or class of drugs.

---

presence of high concentrations of iodides inhibits the secretion of hormones by the thyroid gland.

3. The *monovalent ions,* such as potassium perchlorate and potassium thiocyanate, also interfere with hormone synthesis. Like high concentrations of iodides, they inhibit the extraction of iodide from the blood by the thyroid gland. Thus, these *ionic inhibitors* of the gland's ability to trap and concentrate circulating iodide prevent the thyroid from accumulating the iodine needed to form the hormone precursors mono- and diiodotyrosine. However, because of their toxicity, these agents are no longer used therapeutically. *Potassium perchlorate* (Perchloracap), which caused sometimes fatal aplastic anemia when used chronically to treat hyperthyroidism, is sometimes given in a single dose prior to diagnostic tests in which radioactive pertechnetate (TcO_4) ion is used to aid imaging of the brain or placenta. Used this way the perchlorate is relatively safe and prevents excessive uptake of the radioactive pertechnetate into the thyroid and salivary glands and choroid plexus.

Thioamides. Drugs of this class, including *methimazole*[+] (Tapazole) and *propylthiouracil*, are by far the most commonly employed of the antithyroid drugs.* This is because they are much safer than the ionic inhibitor-type agents and are more predictably and permanently effective than iodides. Improvement in the condition of Graves' disease patients is usually seen within 1 or 2 weeks after treatment is initiated, and many patients attain a euthyroid state in about 6 to 8 weeks. The slow onset of therapeutic benefit is a result of the fact that these drugs act primarily to inhibit early steps in the biosynthetic pathway of thyroid hormones. Thus, preformed, stored hormone must be "used up" before circulating levels of the hormones are reduced. Maintenance therapy may then be continued with reduced doses for from 6 to 18 months in patients whose response to therapy offers promise of a permanent remission.

The prognosis is most favorable for those patients whose toxic goiter is not very large to begin with and in whom the thyroid gland grows somewhat smaller during the first weeks of thioamide treatment. More than half of the hyperthyroid patients who take these antithyroid drugs faithfully for a year or more may never again suffer a recurrence of thyrotoxicosis. A second course of drug therapy administered following relapse a few months after the first frequently succeeds in controlling the condition for a longer period or even in producing permanent remission in additional patients.

It is important to encourage patients to take the drug regularly and exactly as directed because, if they neglect to continue taking the drug daily for many months and at the proper times of day until control is established, the condition may recur. They should also be urged to report any symptoms of illness immediately; sore throat, fever, rash, or jaundice may be signs of drug reactions calling for prompt withdrawal of these drugs. Only a small minority of patients develop adverse reactions. However, these may include hepatitis and such serious blood disorders as agranulocytosis (see the summary at the end of the chapter).

*Hypo*thyroidism is not a common adverse effect, but it can occur if dosage is not reduced during prolonged maintenance therapy. Thus, after the patient has become euthyroid, only the lowest daily doses needed to prevent thyrotoxicosis symptoms from returning should be administered. Patients should be observed not only for signs of myxedema, but also for any enlargement of the thyroid gland. To counteract this goitrogenic effect, which is caused by increased secretion of TSH by the pituitary gland when it is released from negative inhibition by circulating hormones, patients should receive a thyroid preparation together with the antithyroid drug. Such hormone supplements are particularly important during pregnancy to prevent hypothyroidism from developing in the fetus—a condition that could lead to cretinism in the newborn infant.

The addition of the thyroid hormone, liothyronine sodium, to the patient's regimen may also have prognostic value. Thus, it is often possible to determine

during the course of treatment with antithyroid drugs whether or not further treatment is likely to result in a cure. The patient is given a thyroid suppression test after 6 months of drug treatment. If the test dose of liothyronine now suppresses the uptake of radioactive iodine, the chance of a permanent remission is good; if uptake is not suppressed, remission is unlikely, and surgery or radioactive isotope therapy will probably be required.

In such cases and in those patients whose thyrotoxicosis is too severe from the outset to be cured by these antithyroid drugs alone, treatment with these agents prior to thyroid surgery or radiation is desirable. The use of antithyroid drugs for several weeks preoperatively reduces the risks of subtotal thyroidectomy by stabilizing the patient's metabolism and thus reducing the heart rate and other cardiovascular abnormalities of the hyperthyroid state. These drugs may also be supplemented by propranolol and by the administration of daily doses of an iodide solution for 7 to 10 days before the surgical procedure is to be performed.

Iodides. Inorganic salts of iodine were once the only drug treatment available for control of hyperthyroidism. However, although their beneficial effects come on rapidly, the iodides do not offer prolonged and permanent control of thyrotoxicosis symptoms. In fact, if patients on long-term therapy failed to take full doses at frequent intervals or stopped taking these drugs entirely, the disease would often return in more severe form. Thus, the iodides are used mainly for their rapid ability to reduce the size and vascularity of the thyroid gland, and so prevent excessive bleeding during thyroidectomy.

In addition to their preoperative use for reducing the size and fragility of the enlarged thyroid gland, iodine salts are sometimes effective in other clinical situations. For example when administered following methimazole[+], iodides are sometimes helpful for treating *thyroid crisis* (see below) because of the rapidity with which they inhibit the release of hormones by the thyroid gland. Iodides are also sometimes administered following radioactive iodine therapy (see below) to control symptoms of thyrotoxicosis during the several weeks before the delayed response to the radioisotope develops. In all such situations the small amounts of Lugol's solution or of saturated solution of potassium iodide that are ordered for this purpose must be accurately measured, and the drops should be added to fruit juice or milk to disguise the unpleasant taste.

Radiation therapy: radioactive iodine
The iodine isotope ^{131}I is trapped by the thyroid gland in the same manner as ordinary iodides. Reaching very high concentrations there, it gives off β and γ radiations in amounts that are useful for both the diagnosis of thyroid disorders and the treatment of some cases of hyperthyroidism. Tiny tracer doses are administered to determine the thyroid gland's capacity to store iodine; much larger

amounts are administered deliberately to destroy thyroid tissue—for example, in patients for whom surgery does not seem safe and whose hyperthyroidism has not responded to drugs.

The *diagnostic use* of sodium radioiodide solution is based on the measurable differences in retention and excretion of iodine. In myxedema, only a small proportion of any administered dose is taken up by the thyroid gland, and the rest is excreted in the urine. In the hyperthyroid patient, on the other hand, the thyroid retains a high percentage of the amount administered, and relatively little radioactivity is detected in the urine. The small doses of radioiodide give off enough γ rays so that such determinations may readily be made; the β rays are so few that there is little danger of damage to the thyroid or other tissues.

The *therapeutic use* of sodium iodide $^{131}I^+$ involves the administration of perhaps a thousand times as high a dose of the radioisotope. The drug is given either as a single large dose or in a series of smaller cumulative doses. In either case, the iodine isotope accumulates in the thyroid in amounts as much as 10,000 times as high as those in other body tissues. The very short-range β rays that are then given off thus destroy thyroid tissue without harming other cells. As a result of the gradual reduction in hormone secretion, the symptoms of hyperthyroidism are gradually reduced, and the patient's metabolic rate may become normal in about 12 weeks.

The main difficulty with radioactive iodine is that the β rays may destroy too much thyroid tissue. Therefore, the patient is examined periodically for signs of *hypothyroidism* and, if any tendency toward myxedema is noted, thyroid therapy is instituted. Just as in hypothyroidism caused by surgical removal of too much thyroid tissue, the patient who is made myxedematous by too great a destructive action of radioactive iodine may require life-long replacement thyroid therapy.

Dosage in radioactive iodine therapy is much smaller than was once employed to minimize the chances of hypothyroidism developing long after the treatment. If a second dose of ^{131}I is necessary to produce a euthyroid effect—as it may well be in about half the patients treated with the present smaller initial doses—it is administered between 6 to 12 months after the first dose, instead of after only about 3 months as was once done when it became apparent that further treatment would be needed.

During the long interlude between the administration of radioactive iodine and development of its full effects, patients are customarily treated with daily doses of ordinary iodides and other antithyroid drugs such as methimazole or propylthiouracil to suppress the symptoms of thyrotoxicosis. When these drugs are being administered in the intervening periods before a second or third small dose of radioactive iodine, their use is interrupted for several days before and after the isotope treatment to prevent them from interfering with uptake of the radioactive iodide by the thyroid gland.

The personnel involved in caring for a patient who is to receive radioactive iodide must follow the appropriate precautions necessary for their own safety. The patient, as well as visitors, will also need to know what precautions are taken and why they are necessary.

Supplementary therapy

Because the effects of the antithyroid drugs and of radioactive iodine develop relatively slowly, it is sometimes desirable to use other drugs to bring the discomforting and potentially dangerous signs and symptoms of thyrotoxicosis under quicker control.

Propranolol (Inderal) is commonly employed today to bring about rapid improvement by relieving such signs of excessive sympathetic activity in hyperthyroidism as tachycardia, sweating, and heat intolerance, as well as anxiety, restlessness, and tremor. There are a few clinical situations in which drug-induced β-adrenergic blockade (see Chap. 18) is desirable: (1) in the period of several weeks or more before the definitive antithyroid drugs gradually bring about a euthyroid state; (2) in the preparation of patients for surgery to reduce the heart rate and lessen the risk of arrhythmias developing during anesthesia and surgery; and (3) in the management of thyroid crisis, or thyroid storm.

Thyroid storm, or *thyroid crisis*, is a syndrome that occasionally develops in patients whose hyperthyroidism has not been recognized and treated or in those who have received inadequate treatment. This very severe form of thyrotoxicosis, which has a high mortality rate unless promptly and vigorously treated, is usually precipitated by an acute infection, trauma or surgery, diabetes mellitus with ketoacidosis, toxemia of pregnancy and childbirth, and other stresses that cause metabolic abnormalities in hyperthyroid persons.

Although the most effective specific treatment of thyroid storm involves the use of iodine solutions and such antithyroid drugs as propylthiouracil, propranolol is particularly useful for rapid control of tachycardia to prevent possible congestive heart failure or fatal cardiac arrhythmias as a result of myocardial ischemia and hypoxia. Lithium salts have also sometimes been used to control excessive secretion of thyroid hormone more quickly than is possible with the thioamides. These salts, which are *approved* for use only in managing manic–depressive mental illness, block the proteolytic step in the formation of the thyroid hormones and thus interfere with their secretion. Lithium has caused thyroid toxicity in patients receiving it for mental illness.

Other adjunctive drugs may also be employed to treat the illness responsible for setting off thyroid storm or to provide the patient with general support. Thus, for example, antibiotic therapy may be used against acute infections, antipyretic drugs (and physical hypothermic measures) for reducing fever, IV corticosteroids for their antistress effects, and IV glucose and vitamin solutions for nutrition and for counteracting dehydration.

Additional clinical considerations

Whenever a patient is being treated with drugs that alter thyroid function, the patient should be scheduled for regular evaluation of thyroid function (blood tests) and physical functioning. The best method for most accurately determining the dose of drug for an individual patient is a precise assessment of the patient's physical response to drug therapy. Overdosage with thyroid hormone or undertreatment with antithyroid drugs will result in the signs of hyperthyroidism—for example, tachycardia, arrhythmias, fever, flushing, increased gastrointestinal activity—while overdosage with antithyroid drugs or undertreatment with thyroid hormone will result in the signs of hypothyroidism—for example, hyporeflexia, bradycardia, hypotension, edema, weight gain. During the course of therapy, many patients learn to regulate their own medication by how they feel. They should be encouraged to discuss this with their nurse or physician, however, so that the reasons for a changed response to the drug can be determined and dealt with accordingly.

Thyroid replacement therapy is usually a lifelong therapy. The patient needs to understand this, and will need to be taught about the drug and the need to continue taking it daily. It is helpful for the patient to wear a medical identification tag stating the need for daily medication in the event of an emergency situation. Special support measures may need to be taken if the patient is in an acute stress situation and the thyroid gland cannot respond normally.

Patients receiving thyroid hormones should take the drug at the same time each day. The best time is first thing in the morning, before breakfast. This timing will allow the drug therapy to fit into the patient's normal hormonal rhythm. The patient should know the signs and symptoms of hyperthyroidism.

Patients who are receiving antithyroid drugs will be taking the medication for a prolonged period of time, although usually not for life. These patients need to be cautioned about the importance of taking their medication exactly as it is prescribed. The drugs should be taken around the clock to ensure the best therapeutic results. It is important to determine an appropriate schedule with the patient. The patient will need to know the signs and symptoms of hypothyroidism, and should be cautioned to return for regular evaluations.

Drug–drug interactions

Both thyroid and antithyroid drugs are known to increase the effectiveness of *oral anticoagulants;* this can lead to bleeding in patients receiving the drugs concurrently. Patients receiving thyroid drugs and oral anticoagulants should receive reduced doses of the anticoagulant, and their prothrombin time should be monitored closely. Patients with diabetes mellitus need to be monitored very closely if they are started on thyroid hormone replacement therapy because the thyroid hormone may cause an increase in the required dosage of *insulin.* A reduction in thyroid hormone dose may also necessitate a reduction in the required insulin dose. *Cholestyramine* binds T_3 and T_4, preventing absorption. Patients who must receive both drugs should wait 4 to 5 hours between taking the cholestyramine and the thyroid drug. Patients receiving *cardiotonic glycosides* (digoxin) are especially vulnerable to the toxic cardiac effects of the glycosides if they are also receiving thyroid hormone; these patients need to be monitored carefully.

The patient teaching guide presents a summary of points to include when teaching the patient who is receiving thyroid hormone. A similar teaching guide can be developed for the patient receiving antithyroid drugs, incorporating the teaching points that have been discussed in the text. The guide to the nursing process summarizes the clinical aspects of the drug therapy for patients receiving thyroid and antithyroid drugs.

Summary of tests of thyroid function*

Direct methods for determining hormone levels

Protein-bound iodine (PBI). Normal range is 4 to 8 $\mu g/100$ ml of serum. It is lower (2.5 to 4 $\mu g/100$ ml) in patients with hypothyroidism and higher in those with hyperthyroidism. A difficulty with this test is that patients receiving *thyroxine* (T_4) show PBI values in the hyperthyroid range—for example, 10 $\mu g/100$ ml—when they are actually euthyroid; on the other hand, patients taking *liothyronine* (T_3) have abnormally low PBI levels, even after full replacement therapy has made them euthyroid. The use of *natural thyroid* or of *liotrix* permits this test to be interpreted in terms that are more consistent with the patient's true response to replacement therapy.

Butanol extractable iodine (BEI). This test is not interfered with by the presence of iodides from outside sources. That is, it measures only the thyroxine content of the plasma and *not* other circulating iodine-containing compounds that may also be present in addition to the hormone. However, because—like the PBI test—it is influenced by the degree to which protein binding may be altered in various clinical circumstances, the BEI has been superseded by certain tests which measure the free, or unbound, fraction of the circulating thyroid hormones.

Thyroxine by column (T_4C). This test, like the two above, is a laboratory procedure that depends on iodometry, the measurement of the iodine content of the

(continued)

serum, as a means of estimating thyroid hormone content. Like the other two, it has also been largely superseded by more specific techniques for measuring the actual hormones.

Competitive protein-binding displacement assay. Responses in this test, which measures the amount of labeled tracer thyroxine (T_4) displaced from binding protein, are measurements of the actual T_4 molecule rather than of its iodine content. (Normal range is 4 to 11 μg T_4/100 ml.)

Radioimmunoassays for serum thyroxine (T_4) and liothyronine (T_3). These are especially useful for determining the concentration of T_3, which is quite low compared to T_4 (about 100 ng/100 ml in euthyroid adults and only 20 to 80 ng/100 ml in hypothyroid patients). Serum T_3 radioimmune assay is also the most specific test for the diagnosis of hyperthyroidism.

Free thyroxine and T_3 resin uptake tests. These tests directly reflect the available free, or unbound, fraction of the thyroid hormones, and they thus offer the best indication of the patient's true status. These tests also offer an evaluation of the amount of circulating thyroxine-binding globulin (TBG) indirectly. This makes it possible to estimate the free hormones accurately even in patients with an excess of TBG—for example, in pregnancy—or with a TBG deficiency, as in hypoproteinemic states.

Radioactive iodine uptake ($RA^{131}I$). This test is intended to measure the thyroid gland's capacity for trapping and concentrating radioiodide. The gland of hypothyroid patients takes up only a small fraction of the orally administered tracer dose of the isotope, whereas hyperthyroid patients show accumulation of a large percentage of the amount of ^{131}I that was taken 24 hours before. The iodine uptake of a normal gland is suppressed by prior administration of the hormone liothyronine sodium; in Graves' disease, the patient's hyperplastic gland continues to concentrate radioactive iodide even after thyroid suppression of pituitary TSH production. $RA^{131}I$ has also been used for thyroid scanning, but sodium pertechnetate T is now preferred for thyroid scans.

Indirect tests of thyroid hormone function

T_3 suppression test. This test helps to differentiate the euthyroid state from hyperthyroidism in patients whose ^{131}I uptake is in the borderline high range. The administration of sodium liothyronine for 1 week will not affect uptake of $RA^{131}I$ significantly in the *hyper*thyroid patient whose gland continues to function autonomously. Thyroid $RA^{131}I$ uptake falls to less than 20% in euthyroid patients because of suppression of pituitary thyrotropin (TSH) by liothyronine.

Thyroid-releasing hormone (TRH) testing. This offers an alternative to radioactive iodine uptake as a means of monitoring suppression of thyrotropin by thyroid hormones. In addition, it aids in differentiating between primary, secondary, and tertiary *hypo*thyroidism. Intravenous administration of synthetic TRH (protirelin; Thypinone) causes increases in serum TSH levels as measured by radioimmune assay in euthyroid patients and in those with primary hypothyroidism (in whom TSH levels are elevated in any case).

In patients with pituitary disease (secondary hypothyroidism), the basal serum TSH level is low and rises very little after TRH stimulation. In patients with hypothalamic disease (tertiary hypothyroidism), the low TSH level tends to rise somewhat and with a delayed peak response. This alone is not, however, diagnostic of this disorder and must be supplemented by other laboratory tests, physical examination, and a careful history.

Basal metabolic rate (BMR). This test is intended to measure the extent to which the patient's tissues are using up oxygen in carrying out combustion processes when the patient is in the resting state. When properly performed, it not only helps to differentiate euthyroid from hyperthyroid and hypothyroid patients, but also aids in following the patient's response to circulating thyroid hormones administered as replacement therapy, or in determining the drop in tissue response to such hormones under the influence of antithyroid drugs. (This test is used much less often today than it once was because of the availability of the less cumbersome and more accurate methods discussed above.)

Neuromuscular function evaluation. Achilles tendon reflex time measurements are lengthened in hypothyroid patients and shortened in those with hyperthyroidism. The difficulty with these tests is that there is considerable overlap with the normal range of euthyroid patients. The tests are most useful for detecting delayed muscle contraction and relaxation times in hypothyroid patients when specialized instrumentation procedures are employed.

Lipid abnormality evaluation. The concentration of serum cholesterol tends to be raised above normal in patients with hypothyroidism. Patients with hyperthyroidism often show a decrease in serum cholesterol levels. However, the range of cholesterol readings is rather broad, even in euthyroid patients. Thus, such evidence is only suggestive or partially confirmatory.

Serum enzyme abnormality evaluation. In severe hypothyroidism, the concentrations of circulating creatine phosphatase, LDH, and SGOT are elevated. In hyperthyroidism, the serum alkaline phosphatase level is often elevated to some extent. Because these enzyme levels are also elevated in several other conditions, these tests are not definitively diagnostic.

---

* All these laboratory diagnostic tests are often useful when evaluated simultaneously. However, all are subject to error and serve best when the results are used to supplement clinical judgment based on the patient's history and physical examination.

Summary of the clinical uses of thyroid preparations

Hypothyroidism (replacement therapy)

Myxedema (adult and juvenile)

Cretinism (after very early diagnosis)

Gynecologic disorders (*e.g.,* amenorrhea, dysmenorrhea, habitual abortion, *when* these are the result of thyroid hormone deficiency)

Male infertility (as a result of oligospermia stemming from reduced thyroid function)

Hypometabolism as a result of borderline hypothyroid deficiency, with signs and symptoms such as dry skin and hair, loss of scalp hair, brittle nails, intolerance to cold, feelings of fatigue and sluggishness, and obesity

Other uses (suppression of thyrotropin)

Simple nontoxic goiter in the following:

1. Euthyroid patients (normally functioning thyroid gland)
2. Hypothyroid patients (*e.g.,* chronic thyroiditis)
3. Hyperthyroid patients treated with antithyroid drugs

Treatment of thyrotropin-dependent thyroid gland malignancies

Thyroid suppression test (using liothyronine sodium):

1. Differential diagnosis of response of hyperthyroid and euthyroid patients to radioactive iodine uptake test
2. Evaluation of response of hyperthyroid patients to treatment with antithyroid drugs

Summary of adverse effects, cautions, and contraindications with thyroid products

Signs and symptoms of overdosage

Tachycardia, cardiac arrhythmias, elevated pulse pressure, anginal-type chest pains, dyspnea, possible precipitation of congestive failure; excessive sweating, intolerance to heat, fever, flushing, nervousness, irritability, insomnia, headache; increased gastrointestinal motility, abdominal cramps, diarrhea, nausea, increased appetite

Cautions and contraindications

Caution in patients with a history of angina pectoris, recent myocardial infarction or congestive heart failure, and hypertension

Contraindicated in adrenal insufficiency, or in hypopituitarism, unless adrenal deficiency is first corrected by administration of adequate doses of cortisone or hydrocortisone

Summary of adverse effects of antithyroid drugs

Thiocarbamides (*e.g.,* Methimazole; propylthiouracil)

Skin rashes: mild hives, papules, purpura

Gastrointestinal upset: nausea, epigastric distress

Arthralgia: pain, stiffness in joints of wrists and hands

Nervous system: headache, dizziness, drowsiness

Blood dyscrasias: mild leukopenia and rarely agranulocytosis, signaled by severe sore throat and fever

Hepatitis: jaundice requires discontinuation

Iodine (potassium iodide; sodium iodide; strong iodine solution)

Mouth: brassy taste; burning sensation; gum soreness, salivary gland swelling, excessive salivation

Respiratory tract: irritation resembling common cold; sinusitis with frontal headache; conjunctivitis

Skin: acnelike lesions; rarely, bulbous lesions

Gastric: irritation with nausea and vomiting

Radioactive iodine (sodium iodide ^{131}I)

Thyroid gland: early soreness or tenderness and swelling, with rare asphyxial reactions; late hypothyroidism

Late development of acute leukemia or thyroid carcinoma is possible but considered unlikely

Contraindicated in pregnant women and nursing mothers

Potassium perchlorate

Gastric irritation, nausea, vomiting

Hypersensitivity reactions: skin rashes, fever

Lymphadenopathy; nephrotic syndrome

Agranulocytosis and, rarely, aplastic anemia

Patient teaching guide: thyroid hormones

The drug that has been prescribed for you is called a hormone and is designed to replace the thyroid hormone that your body is not able to produce. The thyroid hormone is responsible for regulating your body's metabolism, or the speed with which the body's cells burn energy. Because of this action of the thyroid hormone, it affects many body systems. It is very important that you take this medication only as prescribed.

Instructions:

1. The name of your thyroid replacement is ——————— .

2. The dosage prescribed for you is ——————— .

3. Your drug should be taken at the same time each day, preferably in the morning, before breakfast. The best time for you to take your drug is ————— .

4. Never stop taking this drug without consulting with your nurse or physician. The drug is used to replace a very important hormone, and will probably have to be taken for life. Stopping the medication can lead to serious problems.

5. This drug usually causes no adverse effects. You should notice, over a period of time, that the symptoms of your thyroid deficiency—for example, puffiness, fatigue, weight gain—will disappear and, when your thyroid hormone levels return to normal, you will also feel "back to normal."

6. Tell any physician, nurse, or dentist who is taking care of you that you are taking this drug.

7. It might be useful to wear a medical alert tag stating that you are on this medication. This will alert any medical people who are responsible for emergency care to the fact that you are on this drug.

8. Avoid the use of any over-the-counter (OTC) preparations. Many OTC drugs contain medicines that can interfere with the action of thyroid hormones. If you feel that you need such a medication, consult with your nurse or physician.

9. You will need to have periodic blood tests and physical examinations to evaluate the effectiveness of the drug therapy. It is important to keep your scheduled appointments.

10. Keep this and all medications out of the reach of children. Do not give this medication to anyone else, or take any similar medication that is not prescribed for you.

Notify your nurse or physician if any of the following occur:

Chest pain
Difficulty breathing
Sore throat, fever, chills
Weight loss

(continued)

Sleeplessness
Nervousness, irritability
Unusual sweating, intolerance to
heat

Guide to the nursing process: thyroid and antithyroid drugs*

Assessment	Nursing diagnoses	Intervention	Evaluation
Past history—underlying medical conditions (*contraindications*): Angina Myocardial infarction Hypertension Congestive heart failure Addison's disease Lactation† Pregnancy† (iodine: radioactive iodine) *Allergies: these drugs†; tartrazine* (certain preparations); others Medication history (*cautions*): Oral anticoagulants† Insulin Cholestyramine Cardiotonic glycosides **Physical assessment** Neurologic: orientation, affect, reflexes Cardiovascular: pulse, auscultation, baseline ECG, BP Respiratory: R, adventitious sounds GI: appetite General: skin—texture, lesions, perfusion; T; CBC†, prothrombin time†	Potential alteration in cardiac output Knowledge deficit regarding drug and drug therapy Potential alteration in nutrition Potential alteration in tissue perfusion secondary to hypo- or hyperthyroidism	Proper and safe administration of the drug Patient teaching regarding: Drug Dosage Warnings Identification Symptoms to watch Support and encouragement to deal with long-term therapy, drug effects, evaluation Life support and appropriate interventions in emergency situations	Evaluate patient for therapeutic effects of drug Monitor for adverse effects of drug: • T_3, T_4 levels • CBC† • Prothrombin time† • Cardiac status • Neurologic changes (reflexes, affect) • Rash • Weight loss or gain • Fever Monitor for potential drug–drug interactions: Bleeding with oral anticoagulants† ↑ hypoglycemia with insulin ↓ absorption of thyroid hormone with cholestyramine ↑ cardiotoxicity with cardiotonic glycosides Evaluate effectiveness of patient teaching program Evaluate effectiveness of support and encouragement measures Monitor vital functioning and response in emergency and high-stress situations

* The basic principles to be considered are very similar for the thyroid and antithyroid drugs.
† These points are of special importance with the *antithyroid* preparations.

Case study

Presentation

HR, a 38-year-old, white woman was seen in the clinic with complaints of "exhaustion, lethargy, and sleepiness." HR's past history was very sketchy; her speech seemed slurred and her attention span was very limited. HR's husband reported a feeling of frustration with HR, stating that she had become increasingly lethargic, disorganized, and uninvolved at home, and that she had continually gained weight and lost interest in her appearance. A physical exam revealed the following remarkable findings: heart rate 52; BP 90/62; Hct 32%; T 96.8°F (oral); skin—pale, dry, thick; periorbital edema; tongue—thick, asymmetric; weight 165 lb; height 5'3". The immediate impression was that of an advanced case of hypothyroidism. Laboratory tests confirmed this; TSH levels were elevated, with very low T_3 and T_4 levels. The patient was begun on Synthroid, 0.2 mg, qd, orally. What teaching plans should be developed for this patient?

Discussion

HR developed myxedema over a period of time. One problem with this disorder is that with it comes fatigue, lethargy, and lack of emotional affect that results in the patient losing interest in appearance, activities, and self-care. HR's husband, not knowing the reason for the changes in his wife, admits to a sense of frustration. The teaching plan should involve HR's husband as well as HR, and should be written down for easy reference and so that HR can read it as the drug begins to work and her affect and interest begin to return. It is often helpful with these patients to have them bring in a photograph, from about a year before, and to review with them the changes that have occurred as a result of the lack of thyroid hormone. Because these changes occur so gradually, many patients, surprisingly, are not aware of the changes that have occurred in their appearance. The patient will need to know about the thyroid gland and about the drug and its dosage, as well as the points outlined in the patient teaching guide. HR and her husband will need to understand the importance of regular follow-up visits. A return visit in 2 weeks would be advisable to evaluate the effectiveness of the drug therapy, to reinforce the teaching program, and to help the patient and her husband to cope with the changes in her behavior and appearance. The replacement therapy works rapidly and, as HR begins to regain some of her normal functioning, she may experience some of the same frustration that her husband has felt as she becomes aware of the changes in her appearance and behavior but still lacks the energy to return to "normal" rapidly. Both people will need support and encouragement. As the situation stabilizes, further teaching will be needed to help the patient cope with this lifelong therapy.

Drug digest

Levothyroxine sodium USP (Letter; Synthroid)

Actions and indications. This synthetic salt of the natural thyroid hormone L-tetraiodothyronine produces a gradual but long-sustained stimulation of tissue metabolism, growth, and development. This makes it effective for long-term replacement therapy of patients with hypothyroidism. It is useful as substitution therapy in cretinism and in other pediatric cases, in myxedema, and in hypothyroidism without myxedema in other adults, including pregnant women and elderly patients. It also reduces the size of the enlarged thyroid gland in simple nontoxic goiter.

Adverse effects, cautions, and contraindications. Patients are watched closely for the gradual development of signs of hypermetabolism and thyrotoxicosis. These include loss of weight, abdominal cramps, diarrhea and vomiting, nervousness, tremors, sweating, and heart palpitations. Caution is required in patients with cardiovascular diseases, including angina pectoris and hypertension. The drug is contraindicated in patients with uncorrected adrenal insufficiency. Dosage of anticoagulant drugs is reduced by one-third because of possible potentiation of their hypoprothrombinemic effects by the action of this drug. The dosage of insulin or oral hypoglycemic agents may have to be increased when this thyroid hormone is added to the regimen of a patient with diabetes mellitus.

Dosage and administration. Dosage at the start of therapy and the rate at which increments are added depend on the patient's age, physical condition, and response to therapy as determined primarily by the patient's appearance and only to a lesser extent by laboratory tests of thyroxine levels. Thus, most adults in good physical condition can receive full replacement doses of 0.10 mg to 0.2 mg (100 μg to 200 μg) immediately. On the other hand, elderly patients with evidence of cardiovascular disease may receive starting doses less than 0.10 mg daily with increments of that dose added at intervals of 3 to 4 weeks if warranted by the need for a further response to attain full replacement therapy. Infants and children require much higher doses than adults for maintaining full growth and development. Thus, they may need 0.3 to 0.4 mg daily (300 to 400 μg per day). Most patients with myxedema coma receive 200 μg to 500 μg by vein immediately and an additional 100 μg to 300 μg on the following day. Smaller IV doses are continued daily until the patient can take a daily oral dose.

Liothyronine sodium USP (Cytomel)

Actions and indications. This synthetic salt of the natural thyroid hormone L-triiodothyronine has a rapid onset and short duration of action. These properties may make it more useful in emergency situations than other thyroid preparations but less useful than forms with a longer action for long-term maintenance therapy of hypothyroidism.

It may be most useful for patients in coma from myxedema and for patients made suddenly hypothyroid as a result of overtreatment of hyperthyroidism. This hormone is also useful in the differential diagnosis of borderline hyperthyroidism from euthyroidism. In this situation and in the treatment of simple (nontoxic) goiter, it acts by suppressing the production of thyrotropin by the anterior pituitary gland.

Adverse effects, cautions, and contraindications. Overdosage produces signs and symptoms of hyperthyroidism, including nervous irritability, sweating, headache, diarrhea, menstrual irregularities, and tachycardia. These adverse effects can be quickly controlled and the dosage readjusted because of this drug's short action. Caution is required in patients with cardiovascular diseases such as angina pectoris and in patients with hypopituitarism and others with adrenal insufficiency. It should not be administered until supplemental adrenal steroids have corrected any tendency toward adrenal insufficiency.

Dosage and administration. Initiating and maintenance dosage is determined by the patient's condition at the start of therapy, clinical response, and such confirmatory laboratory tests as radioactive iodine T_3 resin uptake, thyroid-binding index (TBI), basal metabolic rate (BMR), and the Achilles tendon reflex test. In myxedematous patients, treatment is begun with only 5 μg daily because of their high sensitivity to thyroid hormones. Then the dose may be increased every 1 or 2 weeks by 5 to 10 μg daily until a dose of 25 μg is attained. If further treatment to a total daily dose of 50 to 100 μg daily is required, the dose is raised in increments of 12.5 or 25 μg every 1 or 2 weeks. Patients with only mild hypothyroidism may be begun on 25 μg daily, which may then be maintained indefinitely in some cases; others may require as much as 75 to 100 μg daily—a total dose that is attained with increments of 12.5 or 25 μg every 1 or 2 weeks. The recommended starting dose for infants with cretinism is 5 μg daily, with increments of that amount every 3 or 4 *days* until a satisfactory response is seen. Maintenance dosage is increased from about 20 μg daily in infants a few months old to full adult doses in children 3 years of age and older.

Methimazole USP (Tapazole)

Actions and indications. This antithyroid drug is used in the treatment of hyperthyroidism to reduce the rate of biosynthesis of thyroid hormones. Continued treatment for up to a year or more often brings about remission of thyrotoxicosis. Patients who require thyroid surgery or radioisotope treatment often benefit from pretreatment with methimazole. It is also used as part of the management of thyroid crisis, or storm.

Adverse effects, cautions, and contraindications. Minor side-effects that occur in a small proportion of patients include skin rash, gastrointestinal upset, headache, and joint pain. The potentially most serious adverse effect is the development of blood dyscrasias such as agranulocytosis and thrombocytopenia. Although this is not common, all patients are cautioned to report such signs as severe sore throat and fever so that differential blood counts can be made and the drug discontinued if necessary. Further treatment is contraindicated in patients who have shown signs of hypersensitivity.

Care is also required in administering this drug during pregnancy, because it can cross the placenta and induce goiter and cretinism in the fetus. To avoid this in treating hyperthyroidism, dosage of this drug is kept at minimal effective levels and supplemented with a thyroid preparation to prevent hypothyroidism from developing in the mother and the fetus, and the newborn infant should not be nursed when treatment is continued in the postpartum period.

Dosage and administration. This drug is taken by mouth in three daily doses at intervals of 8 hours. Mild cases in adults can often be controlled with a daily dose of 15 mg. More serious cases may require a rise in dosage to 30 or 40 mg daily, and 60 mg may be required for the most serious cases. Dosage can later be reduced to maintenance levels of 5 to 15 mg daily. The latter is also the dose used for initiating treatment of children aged 6 to 10 years.

Sodium iodide ¹³¹I USP (Iodotope; Radiocaps)

Actions and indications. This radioactive isotope of iodine is taken up by the thyroid gland and concentrated there. With small doses, the amount taken up serves as an index of thyroid function because the γ radiation that is given off is low in hypothyroidism and abnormally high in hyperthyroidism.

High doses are used to destroy glandular tissue in hyperthyroidism. This (and the resulting reduction in secretory activity) is brought about by the β rays that are given off by the iodide that has accumulated in the gland.

Adverse effects, cautions, and contraindications. Use of this isotope is contraindicated during pregnancy and in nursing mothers. It is given only with caution in children and young adults, because the question of whether this compound can cause thyroid cancer, leukemia, or chromosome damage has not yet been resolved.

Pain in swallowing and soreness in the neck often follow treatment, but severe swelling and thyroiditis are relatively rare. Hypothyroidism may develop as a late result of treatment. Large doses may cause bone marrow depression or set off thyroid storm.

Dosage and administration. The solution may be administered orally or by vein in doses that depend on the intended use and on the size of the gland. Doses for treatment of hyperthyroidism are very much higher than those used for diagnosis. Currently recommended doses are about 4 mc to 10 mc. For treating thyroid carcinoma, doses of 50 mc to 150 mc are sometimes used.

Thyroid USP

Actions and indications. This preparation, a dried powder made from animal thyroid glands, contains the natural hormones. Thus, it exerts the same therapeutic effects as the pure compounds when administered in adequate dosage as replacement therapy in hypothyroidism, myxedema, cretinism, and nontoxic goiter. In such cases the full effects of thyroid administration come on slowly but are then relatively prolonged.

Adverse effects, cautions, and contraindications. Overdosage causes cardiac palpitations and rapid rhythmic irregularities, sweating, nervousness, headache, tremors, and insomnia. Thyroid is used only with caution in patients with a history of hypertension or angina pectoris, and it is contraindicated in patients with an acute myocardial infarction. In patients who also suffer from Addison's disease, hypothyroidism should be treated only after hypoadrenalism is first corrected with corticosteroid drug therapy. The same is true in cases of hypothyroidism that occur secondary to hypopituitarism. Patients taking anticoagulant drugs of the coumarin type may require a reduction in dosage of about one-third when thyroid is added to their regimen.

Dosage and administration. Dosage of thyroid varies widely, depending on the degree of hypothyroidism that requires correction. Treatment may be begun with 16 to 65 mg daily, depending on pretreatment PBI values. Dosage is then gradually increased until the desired effect is attained. The usual maintenance dose is between 65 and 195 mg daily, but may range from 30 to 600 mg daily depending on the individual patient's response.

References

Blum M: Myxedema coma. Am J Med Sci 264:433, 1972

Editorial: Treatment of Graves' disease. N Engl J Med 298:681, 1978

Feck CM et al: Combination of potassium iodide and propranolol in preparation of patients with Graves' disease for thyroid surgery. N Engl J Med 302:883, 1981

Genuth SM: The thyroid gland. In Berne RM, Levy MN (eds): Physiology, pp 1013–1032. St. Louis, C V Mosby, 1983

Goodman HM, Van Middlesworth L: The thyroid gland. In Mountcastle VB (ed): Medical Physiology, 14th ed, pp 1495–1518. St. Louis, C V Mosby, 1980

Haibach H: Hyperthyroidism in Graves' disease. Arch Intern Med 136:725, 1976

Haynes RC Jr, Murad F: Thyroid and antithyroid drugs. In Gilman AG, Goodman LS, Gilman A (eds): Goodman and Gilman's The Pharmacological Basis of Therapeutics, 6th ed, pp 1397–1419. New York, Macmillan, 1980

Larsen PR: Tests of thyroid function. Med Clin North Am 59:1063, 1975

Larsen PR: Thyroid–pituitary interaction: Feedback regulation of thyrotropin secretion by thyroid hormones. N Engl J Med 306:23, 1982

Levey GS: The heart and hyperthyroidism. Use of beta adrenergic blocking drugs. Med Clin North Am 59:1193, 1975

Mackin JF et al: Thyroid storm and its management. N Engl J Med 291:1396, 1974

McKenzie JM et al: Graves' disease. Med Clin North Am 59:1177, 1975

Oppenheimer JH: Initiation of thyroid hormone action. N Engl J Med 292:1063, 1975

Potency of oral thyroxine preparations. Med Lett Drugs Ther 26:41, 1984

Refetoff S: Thyroid hormone therapy. Med Clin North Am 59:1147, 1975

Ridgway EC et al: Rational therapy in hypothyroidism. Ration Drug Ther 10:1, 1976

Senior RM et al: The recognition and management of myxedema coma. JAMA 217:16, 1971

Sterling K: Radioactive iodine therapy. Med Clin North Am 59:1217, 1975

Sterling K: Thyroid hormone action at the cell level. N Engl J Med 300:117, 1979

Stock JM et al: Replacement dosage of L-thyroxine in hypothyroidism. N Engl J Med 290:529, 1974

Chapter 23

Hormones and drugs affecting the female reproductive system

23

There are a number of hormones that affect the female reproductive system:

1. The anterior pituitary hormones: prolactin and the gonadotropins—FSH (follicle-stimulating hormone) and LH (luteinizing hormone)
2. The posterior pituitary hormone, oxytocin
3. The female sex hormones: estrogens and progesterone

The hypothalamic-releasing and release-inhibiting hormones and factors (GnRH, PRF, and PIF) influence the female reproductive system indirectly through their effects on circulating levels of FSH, LH, and prolactin. These hypothalamic hormones, the gonadotropins, and prolactin have been discussed in Chap. 20, and will not be discussed in detail here. The drugs to be described in this chapter are the estrogens, the progestins (including progesterone), and oxytocin and other drugs that affect the uterus.

Physiology of the female reproductive system

The female sex hormones: Estrogens and progesterone

The female hormones—the estrogens and progesterone—are produced by the ovaries, by the placenta during pregnancy, and by the adrenal glands, which also produce small amounts of androgens, including testosterone. In the nonpregnant female, plasma levels of these hormones follow a cyclical pattern that, although subject to the influence of physical, emotional, and other stimuli that act through the hypothalamus (see Chap. 20), is established

at puberty and normally continues, except during pregnancy, until the menopause.

The primary action of the female sex hormones is to prepare the body, primarily the reproductive system, for pregnancy, and to maintain pregnancy until delivery is appropriate. However, these hormones also have effects on other organ systems. These effects can influence the response of the body to stressors, including disease and drugs. Before attempting to understand the therapeutic effects of the estrogens, progestins, and drugs that act like these hormones, or that intervene in normal hormone function, it is necessary to understand the cyclical nature of female hormone secretion, the controls of this secretion, and the influence of female hormones on body systems.

The menstrual cycle

The periodic cycling of the female sex hormones is called the menstrual cycle because its effects are most obviously seen in the regular sloughing of the endometrium, the uterine lining, in the menses or menstrual flow. The cycle depends on the interaction of the pituitary hormones FSH and LH with the ovarian hormones estrogen and progesterone (Fig. 23-1). The first day of menstruation is commonly considered as day 1 of the menstrual cycle (Fig. 23-2).

The hypothalamus, which is itself influenced by higher levels of the central nervous system, releases gonadotropin-releasing hormone (GnRH) into the portal circulation that perfuses the anterior pituitary. This hormone stimulates the pituitary to release FSH and LH into the systemic circulation. The pituitary hormones stimulate follicles in the ovaries to develop. This phase of the menstrual cycle is sometimes called the *follicular phase* because of the ovarian changes taking place. The developing follicles produce estrogens, which stimulate the endometrial lining of the uterus to proliferate and

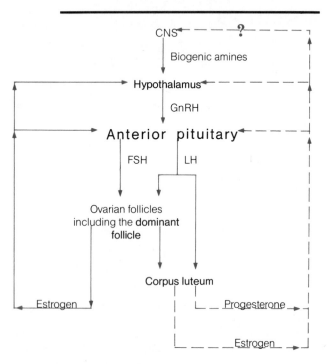

Figure 23-1. The interaction of hypothalamic, pituitary, and ovarian hormones that underlies the menstrual cycle. (*Solid arrows:* stimulatory effects and positive feedback; *dashed arrows:* inhibitory effects and negative feedback)

to increase in vascularity in preparation for supporting a fertilized ovum. This phase of the menstrual cycle is also called the proliferative phase because of the type of changes that are occurring in the uterine lining (Fig. 23-2).

The rising plasma concentration of estrogen reaches a level that causes the pituitary to release a large amount of LH in what is called the "LH surge." FSH is also released, but the "FSH surge" is not as dramatic (see Fig. 23-2). This is an example of a *positive feedback* mechanism; that is, ovarian estrogen secretion, which has itself been stimulated by FSH and LH, in turn stimulates greater secretion of FSH and LH.

The high level of LH causes one developed follicle, the dominant follicle, to rupture, and the remaining follicles then involute. The rupture of the dominant follicle releases a mature ovum and the fluid surrounding it in the process called *ovulation*. This usually occurs around the fourteenth day of the menstrual cycle, but the timing is quite variable. The remaining cells of the ruptured follicle then form a new endocrine organ, the corpus luteum, which secretes progesterone and estrogen and heralds the beginning of the *luteal phase* of the menstrual cycle.

Rising levels of estrogen and progesterone, produced by the corpus luteum, stimulate the uterine lining to accumulate glycogen and to undergo secretory changes that prepare it to support a developing embryo. This

phase of the menstrual cycle is thus sometimes called the *secretory phase* because of the type of endometrial changes that are occurring.

Rising levels of estrogen and progesterone also "turn off" the production of FSH and LH by the pituitary and "turn off" the production of GnRH by the hypothalamus; these are examples of *negative feedback*. Negative feedback is more typical of hypothalamic–pituitary–endocrine target organ systems than positive feedback (see Chap. 20). It is intriguing but not well understood how, during the follicular or proliferative phase of the cycle, high levels of circulating estrogens exert *positive* feedback on the pituitary to cause the LH surge but, during the luteal or secretory phase, high concentrations of estrogen exert *negative* feedback on the pituitary. This difference is believed to be related, at least in part, to the high levels of progesterone that accompany the elevated estrogen levels during the *post*ovulatory luteal phase but not during the *pre*ovulatory follicular phase.

The corpus luteum, however, will regress and cease to produce hormones unless a pregnancy occurs and its growth is stimulated by placental hormones (human chorionic gonadotropin, HCG). The corpus luteum ceases to function completely after about 14 days. At this point, the hypothalamus and pituitary are released from negative feedback, GnRH is again released from the hypothalamus and FSH and LH released from the pituitary, and the process begins again—thus forming a cycle. The uterine lining, no longer stimulated by estrogen and progesterone, sloughs off and sheds the innermost endometrial cells as the menses.

It is theorized that, before puberty, the hypothalamus is very sensitive to the small amounts of circulating estrogen. These levels of estrogen prevent the hypothalamus from releasing GnRH. As the hypothalamus matures, it loses its sensitivity to these estrogens, and puberty occurs when GnRH reaches a level high enough to stimulate the pituitary secretion of FSH and LH. Menopause usually occurs when the ovarian follicles have been "used up" and none are left to develop and cause the cycling levels of the hormones.

Understanding the cycling of the various sex hormones will lead to an understanding of the periodic effects that these hormones have on the female body. First, the actions of the estrogens on the body and then those of progestins will be reviewed briefly.

Estrogens

Physiologic effects on reproductive tissues. The estrogens—principally *estradiol* and its metabolites *estrone* and *estriol*—are first produced at puberty. The estrogens released at that time stimulate the growth and development of all the tissues involved in the reproductive process, including the uterus, oviducts, vagina, and breasts.

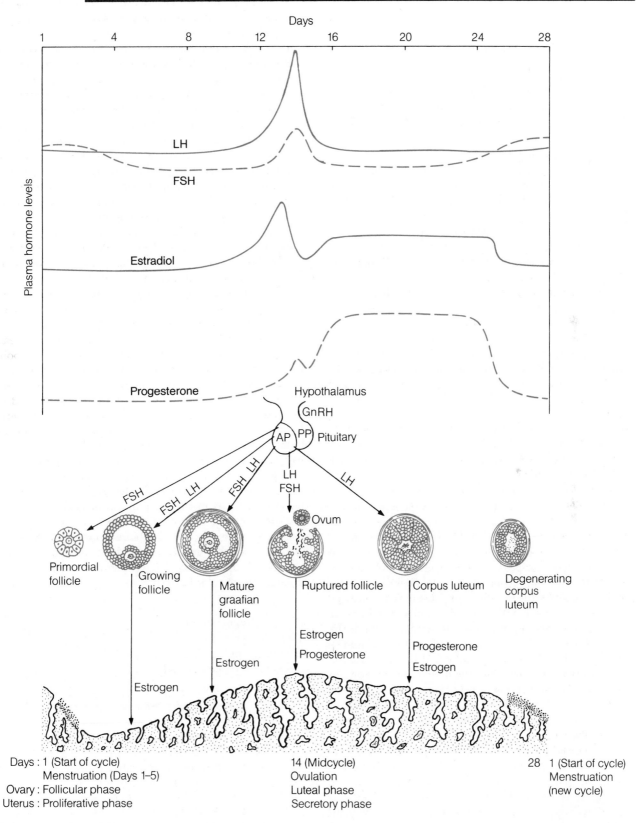

Figure 23-2. Relation of pituitary and ovarian hormone levels to the menstrual cycle and to ovarian and endometrial function.

Effects of estrogens on the body
  Growth of genitalia
  Growth of breasts
  Characteristic female hair distribution pat-
    tern
  Protein anabolism
  ↓ blood cholesterol level
  Sodium and water retention
  Inhibition of calcium resorption from bone
  Alteration of pelvic bone structure
  Epiphyseal closure
  ↑ thyroid hormone-binding globulin
  ↑ elastic tissue in skin
  ↑ vascularity of skin
  ↑ uterine motility
  Thin, clear cervical mucus
  Proliferative endometrium
  Anti-insulin effect → ↑ blood glucose level

Estrogenic hormones are thought to exert their effects on growth by stimulating cellular protein synthesis. The steroid hormones cross the cell membrane, bind to specific receptor proteins in the cytoplasm, and are carried, in the form of a hormone–receptor complex, into the cell nucleus, where they stimulate synthesis of messenger RNA. The messenger RNA then directs the synthesis of new proteins in the cytoplasm. These proteins are responsible for the hormonal effects. Because these processes are slow, it takes time for estrogens to exert their effects; thus, if estrogens are given as drug therapy, the patient will need to be evaluated over time for evidence of therapeutic benefit.

Uterus. Estrogens influence the growth and development of both the muscular and mucosal elements of the uterus and the oviducts, or fallopian tubes. Estrogens stimulate uterine and tubal muscular activity. When coitus occurs at about the time of ovulation, these contractions help to propel the man's sperm toward the recently released ovum. As previously mentioned, estrogens are responsible for the proliferative phase of the menstrual cycle, causing growth of the endometrium and an increase in its blood supply in preparation for implantation if the ovum is fertilized. The cervical glands are stimulated to produce a thin clear cervical mucus that facilitates the penetration of the sperm into the uterus and encourages pregnancy. Women trying to become pregnant can learn to evaluate their cervical discharge and, on the basis of this evaluation, can encourage intercourse at appropriate times in their cycle.

Vaginal tract mucosa. This is kept thick by the action of ovarian estrogens on its epithelium, and a reduction in the glandular secretion of these hormones at the menopause is accompanied by a thinning of these epithelial layers and an increased susceptibility to vaginal infections.

Breast tissues. These are affected by estrogens both at puberty and during pregnancy, as well as in each ovulatory cycle. Through the complicated interactions between these and other hormones, the mammary gland ducts and alveoli (the secreting sacs) grow and develop to full functional maturity. (The actual milk production that occurs after pregnancy is regulated by prolactin, a pituitary hormone described in Chap. 20.)

Other effects of estrogens. Estrogens are also responsible for many of the changes that occur in the female body at puberty (see above). The growth spurt and the closing of the epiphyses of the long bones that results in an end to growth in height are both stimulated by estrogens. Estrogens are also responsible for the growth and characteristic female distribution of body hair, the deposition of fat over the hips, and the smooth thin skin characteristic of women. By its effects on the skin and on the vasculature, it allows the skin to stretch in pregnancy and provides a large vascular bed for dissipation of the heat generated by the developing fetus.

The estrogens have effects on many other body tissues that are not as apparent. Estrogens promote protein anabolism or growth (a factor that is needed during pregnancy); decrease the blood cholesterol level; have an anti-insulin effect that results in an increase in the blood glucose level (another factor needed for fetal growth); increase sodium and water retention (another factor needed for fetal growth but one that is also responsible for the fluid weight gain and edema associated with the latter part of the menstrual cycle); inhibit the resorption of calcium from the bones (a factor that is apparent when estrogen levels fall at menopause and many women develop osteoporosis as the calcium leaves the bone); increase hepatic synthesis of the globulin proteins that carry the thyroid hormone cortisol and the sex steroids in the circulatory system; and alter the bone structure of the pelvic girdle. This last effect is responsible for the characteristic female gait and for the enlargement of the pelvic inlet to allow delivery of the fetus.

Progesterone

The other primary female hormone is progesterone. Like estrogen, this hormone is produced by the ovaries, the placenta, and the adrenal glands.

Effects of progesterone on the body
  Growth of breasts
  ↓ uterine motility
  Thick cervical mucus
  Secretory endometrium
  ↑ body temperature
  ↑ blood glucose level
  ↑ appetite
  ↓ T-cell function

Physiologic effects on reproductive tissue

Uterus. Progesterone acts on both the thick muscle mass of the uterus and on its inner mucous lining in ways that are significant for the survival of the fertilized ovum and the embryo.

The endometrial actions of progesterone prepare the uterine mucosa for reception and implantation of the egg, and the relaxing effect of this luteal secretion on the myometrium prevents the embryo and later the placenta and developing fetus from being dislodged by muscular contractions of the uterus. A fall in progesterone production late in pregnancy is thought to be one stimulus that initiates labor because, in the absence of progesterone, the uterus is sensitive to the contractile effects of estrogen, oxytocin, and the prostaglandins.

The *endometrium*, which has been previously primed by the proliferative effects of the estrogens, undergoes so-called *secretory* changes under the influence of progesterone. Its glands multiply rapidly and secrete large amounts of glycogen, a carbohydrate that will serve as the first source of energy for the rapidly dividing fertilized ovum. The accumulating secretions fill the glands and make them swell and twist into corkscrew shapes that give the pregravid endometrium a characteristic lacelike appearance in microscopic cross section (Fig. 23-2).

During pregnancy, however, under the continued influence of progesterone, the dilated glands become narrow and their spirals straighten out as a result of secretory exhaustion (Fig. 23-2). These atrophic changes in the glands and in their underlying framework, or stroma are also seen during long-term treatment with progesterone or synthetic progestins. This pregnancy-type endometrium offers an *unfavorable* environment to the ovum that might be released from the ovary and fertilized. The glands in the inner lining of the cervix—the endocervical glands—produce a secretion under the influence of progesterone that is quite different from that induced by estrogens. This pregnancy-type secretion is thick and viscid. It tends to form a cervical plug that acts as a barrier to sperm cells and invading bacteria during pregnancy and progestin administration.

Other effects. Progesterone also has effects on other body tissues (see above). Breast tissue growth is stimulated by progesterone, but lactation following pregnancy does not occur until levels of both estrogen and progesterone have fallen. Progesterone stimulates an increase in appetite during pregnancy, and this can occur with administration of exogenous progestins. Many women can recognize an increase in their progesterone levels by their cravings for food and by their ravenous appetites.

A unique characteristic of progesterone is its action on the thermoregulatory area of the hypothalamus to reset the body temperature at a higher level. This aspect of progesterone activity is used in the "rhythm method" of family planning. Daily temperature recordings will show an abrupt increase of about 0.5°C (1°F) shortly after ovulation, when progesterone levels increase. This persists for about 14 days, until menstruation occurs, and then the temperature drops back to preovulatory levels. The increase in temperature can be used as a guide to the timing of coitus by a woman desiring to become pregnant or, conversely, it can be used by women desiring to avoid pregnancy as a guide to times to avoid coitus. Clinically, a woman presenting with a low-grade fever should be questioned about the phase of her menstrual cycle.

Like estrogens, progesterone can produce some effects that are adaptive during pregnancy but that are maladaptive to the nonpregnant woman who is taking exogenous progesterone. As an example, progesterone decreases T-cell activity. This constitutes a useful adaptation to protect the foreign cells of the fetus from the mother's immune system but constitutes the loss of a potentially necessary protective mechanism for a nonpregnant woman.

Premenstrual syndrome (PMS)

The combined physiologic effects of estrogen and progesterone produce a group of signs and symptoms called premenstrual syndrome (PMS). The individual response to the cyclical changes brought about by these hormones varies from a mild awareness to severe discomfort and incapacitation. Reviewing the effects of the hormones, and the times during the menstrual cycle when the level of each is high, indicates the possible reactions: water retention; weight gain; swollen or tender breasts; increased appetite; aches and pains in muscles and joints; irritability, restlessness, and tension (thought to be a result of the change in body fluid); headaches; and depression. Cramping and abdominal pain often occur with the onset of the menses, and are thought to be caused by the release of prostaglandins within the uterus. Teaching women about the physiology of their bodies and helping them to cope with these changes are important aspects of total patient care.

Menopause

This syndrome results from a physiologic process that occurs most often during a woman's middle to late forties. It is set in motion by a gradual reduction in ovarian function. The resulting deficiency in estrogen secretion is accompanied by menstrual irregularities and by various other more or less discomforting physical complaints. As menopause begins, the decrease in ovarian function will also lead to an increase in FSH and LH, because neither estrogen nor progesterone is available to "turn off" these hormones. This can result in many signs and symptoms: irregular and atypical menses; vasomotor instability (flushing); increased sweating ("hot flashes" or "hot flushes''); and temperature irregularities. Emotional instability sometimes accompanies such physical instability; this may be characterized by depression, mood swings, and irritability. Once the menses have ceased entirely, and ovarian function has virtually stopped, the body adapts to the new levels of hormones. In the absence of most estrogen and progesterone, however, there is a slow atrophy of these tissues that were dependent on these hormones for stimulation. Breast tissue atrophies; the vaginal mucosa becomes dry and atrophies, making it more susceptible to infection; the uterus becomes smaller and less contractile; bone loses calcium, causing osteoporosis and fractures in many women; and the skin and joints lose much of their elasticity. The syndrome is a normal process of aging, and patients can be helped to cope with the physiologic and emotional changes they will be experiencing through educational programs, understanding, and support.

Pregnancy, labor, and delivery

If a fertilized ovum is implanted in the uterus, the placenta takes on endocrine functions, secreting by about the ninth day of pregnancy *human chorionic gonadotropin*, HCG, that maintains the corpus luteum (corpus luteum of pregnancy) and, like LH, stimulates the ovarian secretion of progesterone and estrogens. This prevents menstruation. Later, the placenta itself begins to secrete these hormones. Structurally, HCG resembles TSH (thyroid-stimulating hormone; see Chaps. 20 and 22) as well as LH and FSH. It has significant TSH activity that can stimulate thyroid function during pregnancy and can even cause hyperthyroidism. The increased thyroid activity is also caused, in part, by another placental hormone called *human chorionic thyrotropin.*

The placenta also secretes other hormones, including *human chorionic somatomammotropin* (HCS; also called *human placental lactogen*, HPL). This hormone resembles both human growth hormone (HGH or somatotropic hormone, STH) and prolactin (see Chap. 20). HCS stimulates the breakdown of fats and raises the plasma glucose level by an anti-insulin effect. Both these metabolic effects help to ensure an adequate supply of nutrients for the fetus.

The corpus luteum of pregnancy also secretes a substance called *relaxin*, which relaxes the pelvis, softens the cervix, and inhibits uterine contractions, thus preparing the pelvis for delivery and tending to prevent abortion.

Structure and function of the uterus

The uterus is a hollow organ in which the fertilized ovum develops into the embryo and fetus. Its rounded upper part, the *fundus*, is joined at its two sides by the fallopian tubes, through which ova pass from the ovary to the main body of the uterus. The lower part—the neck, or *cervix*—tapers to the *external os*, or mouth, which opens into the

vaginal tract. The uterus of a nonpregnant nulliparous woman is only about 3 inches long, but it grows enormously during pregnancy. This organ is made up mainly of two types of tissue: the *endometrium*, a layer of mucous membrane that lines its inner surface, and the *myometrium*, a thick wall of muscle that constitutes the bulk of the uterus.

Uterine tissue of both kinds responds to circulating chemical substances. The glandular epithelium of the endometrium undergoes continual changes during the menstrual cycle and in pregnancy in response to steroid hormones secreted by the ovaries, as previously discussed.

The *myometrium* is made up of interlacing bands of muscle fibers that circle the uterus on the inside and run lengthwise and obliquely in its outer layers. Blood vessels pass between the intertwining fibers, bringing a rich flow of nutrient fluids to the placenta, the organ formed from fetal and maternal tissues in the pregnant uterus. The fetal surface of the placenta sends fingerlike projections into openings, or *sinuses,* in the wall of the uterus. The blood in the sinuses bathes the placental extensions and thus transfers oxygen and nutrients to the fetal circulation. The mother's vessels and those of the developing fetus are not directly connected. Materials contained in the blood supply of the fetus, including carbon dioxide and other wastes, pass through the umbilical cord and diffuse across the vascular membranes of the placenta into the maternal circulation. Substances in the mother's blood supply (*e.g.*, nutrients, O_2) pass in the opposite direction.

The size and weight of the uterus increase greatly during pregnancy. It grows from only 1 or 2 ounces to 2 pounds or more, exclusive of its contents. The fiber bundles of the myometrium stretch to accommodate the rapidly growing fetus. Their contractions, which are weak in early pregnancy, become stronger and occur more often as pregnancy advances. Finally, at term, myometrial irritability is markedly increased, possibly because of sudden changes in the levels of various circulating hormones, and the contractions of labor begin.

Parturition (labor) and delivery

The exact nature of the complex chemical and physical factors that initiate labor is still uncertain. Catecholamines may play a role; α receptors mediate uterine stimulation by these agents, while β receptors mediate relaxation. Another theory is that the secretion of certain steroids by the adrenal glands of the fetus controls the timing mechanism. These steroid hormones may stimulate the release of arachidonic acid, a precursor of the *prostaglandins*. These local hormones then stimulate contractions of the uterus. Stretching of the cervix and vagina as a result of these contractions then sets off a reflex that results in the release of the posterior pituitary gland hormone *oxytocin*. The continued outpouring of this hormone then causes the uterus to contract strongly, with a steadily increasing rhythm.

Labor, or parturition (the process by which the baby is delivered), is divided into three stages. The first stage begins with the onset of strong contractions of the fundus, the rounded upper portion of the uterus, and continues until the opening of the cervix is fully dilated. In the second stage, mounting contractions, becoming stronger and occurring more frequently, propel the fetus's head through the open cervical mouth, or os, into the vaginal tract and continue to push the fetus along the birth canal until delivery is completed. The third stage is marked by separation of the placenta from the wall of the uterus and its expulsion from the body. This stage is followed by the *puerperium,* the period during which the uterus gradually returns to its pregravid state.

Immediately after the delivery of the baby and the placenta, the uterus becomes completely relaxed. During this period of uterine atony, the mother may lose a good deal of blood through the sinuses in the uterine wall where the placenta separated. A pint or more of blood may be lost before the flaccid myometrium begins to contract spontaneously and becomes firm once again. Once such contractions start, the muscle fibers clamp down on the blood vessels like ligatures. This shuts off the flow of blood from the uterus, thus halting any further significant hemorrhaging. During the next few days of the puerperium, the uterus regains much of its tone and, in the next 6 to 8 weeks, *involution*—a reduction in size—gradually takes place. These natural processes can often be speeded by the administration of certain oxytocic drugs.

Hormones and drugs with therapeutic effects on the female reproductive system

The estrogens

Therapeutic uses

Estrogens are employed in many clinical conditions. Most often these hormones are used in small doses for *replacement* purposes in girls or women who have menstrual cycle disturbances arising from partial or complete lack of natural ovarian steroid secretions. On the other hand, natural and synthetic estrogens are sometimes administered in pharmacologic, rather than physiologic, doses to inhibit pituitary gonadotropic activity and to produce various other effects, not only on female genital tissues but also elsewhere in the body. Indeed, doses of these female hormones are sometimes administered to men as well as to women.

The menopause. This has been described above. Estrogens are sometimes given to treat the discomforting signs and symptoms that accompany this change in endocrine status. There is no evidence that estrogens are effective treatment for the depression or nervous symptoms that sometimes accompany the menopause, and they should not be used for these purposes, but they are effective treatment for the hot flashes and other vasomotor symptoms and for atrophic vaginitis. Topical preparations are preferable to systemic estrogens for the latter use. Cyclic therapy with progestational steroids (discussed below) can also control the menstrual irregularities of the menopause.

Because of reports suggesting that the risks of prolonged estrogen therapy may be greater than was previously believed, the present practice is to administer these steroids for only short periods and to employ the smallest effective doses. The current conservative view is that women should take replacement estrogens for only the few months—or at most a year or two—when the physical discomforts of the menopause are at their peak. Even then, estrogens are not taken continuously but on a cyclic schedule of 3 weeks on and 1 week off. This tends to prevent overstimulation of the breast tissues and the endometrium.

Menstrual bleeding tends to occur during the 1-week rest period, when the endometrium is deprived of estrogen stimulation. If menstruation fails to occur, progestin administration and withdrawal may be employed as described below. However, if spotting or breakthrough bleeding develops during the several weeks of estrogen therapy, it is best counteracted by doubling the dosage of the estrogen for a while.

Atrophic vaginitis. This can occur in young girls as well as in menopausal and postmenopausal women. Estrogens are used in immature girls (along with antibiotics) to convert the vaginal mucosa to a more mature, infection-resistant state.

Postmenopausal uses. Some physicians advise women to continue taking estrogens indefinitely following the menopause. They claim that these hormones exert *non*sexual metabolic effects that play an important part in protecting the well-being of practically every tissue, organ, and system in the body, not only helping to keep breasts firm and skin supple but also helping to avoid serious disorders such as osteoporosis and coronary atherosclerosis.

Osteoporosis. This skeletal disorder, which sometimes thins the bones of elderly men as well as women, is sometimes treated with conjugated estrogens (see below). It is believed that the anabolic effects of these hormones are helpful for providing the protein framework into which calcium is laid down by bone cells. Patients are also often put on a diet high in protein and milk, with supplementary calcium salts and perhaps vitamin D and fluorides.

Estrogens seem to relieve back pain caused by weakened vertebrae, even though there seems to be no clear-cut x-ray evidence that these bones are thickened or that compression fractures are less likely to occur.

Nevertheless, the continued use of these hormones for preventive purposes during the postmenopausal period has been recommended as a means of keeping the bones strong and hard and less liable to fracture. Prophylactic therapy with estrogens or other anabolic steroids is considered especially desirable during treatment of menopausal or postmenopausal patients with corticosteroid drugs (see Chap. 21).

Coronary atherosclerosis. The prophylactic use of estrogens for preventing heart attacks in both men and women was advocated until recently. The theoretic basis for this therapy is the fact that *pre*menopausal women are relatively free of coronary artery disease, whereas women who have had their ovaries removed show a sharp rise in atherosclerosis. Similarly, postmenopausal women have about the same rate of myocardial infarctions as men in the same age range.

Actually, there is little evidence that the administration of estrogenic drugs delays the development of artherosclerosis in coronary vessels. In fact, it has been suggested that some dose levels of estrogen may actually cause a rise in plasma triglyceride levels and an increase in atheromatous blood vessel lesions and complications, with a resulting reduction in the survival time of some patients with a previous history of heart attacks.*

The lack of objective proof of the efficacy of estrogens for these purposes, coupled with recent reports of toxic effects during prolonged estrogen therapy (see below), has led the Food and Drug Administration to try to discourage the long-term postmenopausal use of these drugs. However, many physicians continue to prescribe estrogens for indefinite periods following the menopause because they feel that the benefits of such therapy outweigh the risks for most patients. Women in this situation should be offered factual information that will help them to decide, in consultation with their physician, whether or not they want to keep taking these hormones.

Other uses

Female hypogonadism. Estrogens have dramatic effects when administered to girls of adolescent age who have failed to develop sexually because of *primary ovarian failure.* This condition may be caused by inadequate hypothalamic or pituitary function, or it may result from failure of the ovaries to respond to stimulation by pituitary gonadotropic hormones at the time for the normal onset of puberty. Of course, congenital absence of the ovaries or their removal by surgery or destruction by irradiation in treatment of childhood cancer can have the same result.

Patients who suffer from such *sexual infantilism* respond to estrogen therapy with development of the breasts and other accessory sex organs. This, and development of adult female sex characteristics, exert desirable emotional and psychological effects. Although these girls cannot bear children because of their lack of ovaries, they can marry and have normal sexual relationships. They can even have menstrual periods despite the absence of a normal ovulatory cycle.

Primary amenorrhea. In a normal menstrual cycle, female sex hormones of both types must be secreted in adequate amounts and exert their sequential proliferative and secretory effects on the endometrium. Then, when ovarian secretion drops off late in the menstrual cycle, the mucous membrane breaks down and menstruation occurs. Thus, in the hypogonadal girl, menarche (*i.e.,* the beginning of menstrual function) never does occur (*primary* amenorrhea) because she lacks ovarian estrogens. Successful treatment of the hypoovarianism by exogenous gonadotropic stimulation (Chap. 20) or by estrogen replacement therapy helps to produce the proliferative endometrium on which progestational compounds can then act. Withdrawal of these hormones then leads to breakdown of the secretory endometrium and menstrual bleeding. (In girls and women without functioning ovaries, this is, of course, *pseudo*menstruation. See below for further discussion of the use of estrogen–progestin combinations in the management of menstrual disorders.)

Abnormal uterine bleeding. Estrogens are sometimes useful for treating episodes of uterine bleeding that have been diagnosed as being caused by a lack of adequate estrogen production by the ovaries. In such cases, the administration of large doses for a few days may bring profuse bleeding to a halt. Treatment may then be continued at lower dose levels together with the cyclic use of a progestational steroid (see below). Often, after several such treatment cycles have been completed, the patient's own ovaries may recover the ability to produce balanced amounts of estrogens and progesterone. Then, bleeding will occur only during the normal menstrual period, and the amount of blood lost will no longer be excessive.

Estrogens are also sometimes used in other disorders that require pharmacologic doses rather than the physiologic amounts employed in replacement therapy. This, of course, tends to increase the risk of toxicity. Thus, it is particularly important that the patient be given an opportunity to take part in deciding whether she wants to be treated with these drugs for these purposes.

Suppression of lactation. Synthetic estrogens, such as *diethylstilbestrol*+ (DES), for example, have been commonly used to overcome painful postpartum engorgement of the breasts with milk. Once the woman's breasts have been first freed of milk by pumping or by the use of oxytocin, high doses of estrogens are administered for several days to suppress production of prolactin by the pituitary gland and thus inhibit further lactation. This

---

* Conjugated estrogen administration to patients participating in the Coronary Drug Project (Chap. 32) was discontinued after early results indicated that the larger dose seemed to increase the incidence of cardiovascular complications in the patient population, and that lower doses were no more effective than a placebo while possibly being responsible for some observed illnesses that developed during the course of long-term treatment.

practice risks thromboembolic disorders, and the use of analgesics is preferable for treating painful postpartum breast engorgement.

Control of height. One effect of the increased flow of estrogens at puberty is to bring growth in height to a halt after a final spurt of increased growth. This happens because the sex hormones cause the cartilage at the ends of the long bones (the epiphyses) to be invaded by bone cells. Closure of the epiphyses stops further growth, and the girl's final adult stature is attained. However, a *lack* of female hormones as a result of ovarian failure may allow her to keep on growing. Thus, high doses of estrogens are sometimes administered well before puberty to stop expected excessive growth in girls whose personal or family history suggests this possibility.

Children who require estrogen therapy prior to puberty run the risk of having their adult height shortened. Thus, when estrogen therapy seems indicated—in treating *juvenile vaginitis*, for example—girls are treated with locally acting estrogens rather than with the systemically administered hormones. This converts the vaginal mucosa into the thicker infection-resistant adult type without setting off precocious pubertal changes or interfering with the girl's further growth in height.

Cancer treatment. Estrogens are sometimes employed in the treatment of cancer in men and in women with mammary carcinoma who are more than 5 years past the menopause (Chap 12). In such cases of breast cancer that continues to progress as inoperable metastases that no longer respond to x-ray treatment, high doses of estrogens are sometimes administered. In such cases, the drugs may give symptomatic relief for many months even though their action does not affect the final outcome.

Men with advanced prostatic carcinoma are also treated with estrogens. Although the doses required in such cases are relatively low, they cause feminizing effects such as growth of the male breasts (gynecomastia) and lead to a lack of libido. They also increase the likelihood of thromboembolism. These patients will need a great deal of support to cope with the change in body image.

Acne treatment. Another use of estrogens to counteract the effects of the male hormone is in the management of acne. The growth of sebaceous glands in this skin disorder is stimulated by androgens and can thus be reduced by the antiandrogenic action of estrogen therapy. As indicated in Chapter 43, this treatment may be helpful for young women with acne or hirsutism whose ovaries or adrenal glands produce excessive androgens. The feminizing effects of estrogen therapy may not be acceptable in the case of young men with acne. Other ther-

apy, such as topical or systemic antibiotics, should be tried before estrogens are used.

Postcoital contraception. DES is effective as a postcoital contraceptive when given in doses of 25 mg twice a day for 5 days. This is an emergency use only—for example, for rape victims. Other estrogens (*e.g.*, ethinyl estradiol, 5 mg/day, for 5 days; conjugated estrogens, 30 mg/day, for 5 days) have also been shown to be effective. Therapy is most effective when begun within 24 hours after coitus. At present the use of these drugs as emergency postcoital contraceptives has investigational status in the United States.

Adverse effects

Low-dose estrogen replacement therapy is generally considered safe, especially when limited to the few months or at most a year or two when menopausal symptoms are at their height. In most such cases, the only side-effects reported are occasional gastrointestinal upset, breakthrough bleeding, and breast tenderness. However, when estrogens are employed in larger doses or for long periods, the risk of toxicity tends to rise in some patients whose personal or family history may make them particularly susceptible to the adverse effects of these hormones.*

The results of studies in special groups of women suggest that estrogens can sometimes cause types of toxicity that were once not associated with their use for replacement therapy in the menopause. Some of these adverse effects—such as an increased incidence of blood clotting episodes, for example—were first observed in women taking daily doses of oral contraceptives containing an estrogen component. More recently, epidemiologic evidence has been presented that indicates an apparent relationship between the prolonged use of estrogens by postmenopausal women and an increased incidence of cancer of the endometrium.

These findings suggest that caution is required even in prescribing low-dose replacement therapy for menopausal patients. All women must be carefully examined to rule out estrogen therapy for those whose physical condition or medical history indicates a possible increased risk. All patients should also be observed periodically during treatment to detect early signs of toxicity. Some current concepts concerning certain types of possible toxicity resulting from estrogen therapy will now be discussed.

Cancer. Three studies have documented an increase in the incidence of endometrial cancer in postmenopausal women taking estrogens for long periods of time. The risk was 5 to 14 times greater in estrogen users than in nonusers, and appeared to be related both to the duration of use and to the dose. Thus, both dose and duration should be kept to a minimum, and women taking estrogens should be examined frequently.

In addition, women exposed *in utero* to DES, a synthetic estrogen, have an increased risk of developing

---

* Patients can get information in the form of a patient package insert (PPI) when they receive a prescribed estrogen-containing product. However, What You Should Know About Estrogens may raise more questions than it answers. Thus, nurses, as well as pharmacists and physicians, should prepare themselves to offer the patient fuller explanations of any topic that is taken up in the PPI.

vaginal or cervical cancer. Male offspring similarly exposed to DES have shown congenital malformations of the urogenital tract and abnormal semen. Whether or not cancer will develop or fertility will be affected is still unknown. Other congenital malformations (*e.g.*, of the heart or limbs) have also been associated with maternal use of sex hormones during pregnancy. For these reasons, and because there is no evidence that estrogens or progestins are beneficial in preventing abortion (the rationale for giving them in pregnancy), these hormones should be avoided during pregnancy.

Results of animal studies have shown that chronic administration of estrogens increases the incidence of cancer of the breast, cervix, vagina, liver, and kidney. Although there is no evidence that estrogens increase the incidence of these malignancies in women, they should be used with caution in women with a family history of breast cancer or in women with benign breast disease. Women on oral contraceptives (OCs) containing estrogens (see below) have developed benign hepatic adenomas that appear to be related to OC use. These may rupture and cause death from intra-abdominal hemorrhage. Some women on OCs have also developed hepatocellular carcinoma, and there are very recent reports of a greater risk of breast and cervical cancer with OCs.

Thromboembolic disorders. Reports of an increased risk of intravascular blood clot formation in healthy women taking oral contraceptives have also led authorities to limit the use of estrogens in some women with clinical disorders for which these drugs are indicated. At this time, estrogens have not been shown to cause blood clotting in menopausal or postmenopausal women. However, estrogens should not be used for such patients if they have a history of having suffered a thrombotic episode while taking estrogens in oral contraceptives or for other medical reasons. Cigarette smoking greatly increases the risk of thromboembolic episodes in patients using these drugs. Patients should be advised of this, and should be cautioned to decrease their use of cigarettes while taking estrogen preparations.

These drugs should be used with caution in patients who have a history of coronary heart disease or cerebrovascular disease. Patients who require high doses of estrogens for conditions in which they are clearly needed—men with prostatic cancer, for example—should be observed closely and warned to report what may be early manifestations of drug-induced thrombotic disorders. Complaints of pain in the calves, for example, may indicate development of thrombophlebitis, and sudden shortness of breath may be a sign of a pulmonary embolism. Estrogen therapy should be discontinued immediately in such situations and also when patients report visual changes (possible retinal thrombosis), or if they have sudden headaches, dizziness, and symptoms of sensory or motor function loss that suggest a possible stroke.

Another condition that requires high doses of estrogens is postpartum breast engorgement. Because some women are already prone to develop blood clots in pelvic area veins following labor and delivery, the risk of thromboembolism may be increased if estrogens are administered to suppress lactation. Thus, the physician must determine whether the benefits of using estrogens for this purpose may not be outweighed by the risk of puerperal thromboembolism in a particularly susceptible woman. The patient should be informed and consulted about this decision. It may be desirable to avoid estrogen therapy if the discomfort is not severe, or if it can be controlled by analgesics, restriction of fluid intake, ice packs, or binding of the breasts.

Other problems. Women taking only replacement doses of estrogens should also be watched for other side-effects that were first reported following the widespread use of oral contraceptives. *Gallbladder disease*, for example, seems to have doubled in incidence among such women, as has *hypertension*. Thus, it is now suggested that all women taking estrogens for any purpose should be carefully observed for signs of these disorders during the course of therapy. (See the section on oral contraceptives for a further discussion of possible added risks from sex steroid therapy; also see the summary of adverse reactions to estrogens at the end of this chapter.)

Common side-effects

Gastrointestinal. The most common complaint of women taking large doses of estrogens (especially the synthetic type, such as DES), is a tendency toward loss of appetite, nausea, and even vomiting and diarrhea. Such symptoms are similar to those of early pregnancy and, like the latter, they tend to disappear as the patient becomes tolerant to the gastrointestinal side-effects of the female hormones. These symptoms or the headaches and dizziness of which a few patients sometimes complain rarely require permanent withdrawal of estrogen therapy.

Breakthrough bleeding. Also called spotting, this sometimes occurs in women taking relatively low doses of estrogens. This can often be prevented by raising the dose. However, high doses of estrogens administered for long intervals can also cause irregular uterine bleeding. This is best avoided by withdrawing estrogenic medication for 1 or 2 weeks after several weeks of treatment. Often, a normal menstrual period occurs during such a rest period. (Predictable *cyclic bleeding* of this kind can be ensured by taking a progestational steroid together with the estrogen for the last few days before both sex hormones are withdrawn, as described below.)

Postmenopausal women who are placed on cyclic estrogen therapy should understand that they will have a menstrual period when the hormones are withdrawn every few weeks. It should be explained that this is actually *pseudo*menstruation, and that they are neither fertile nor likely to become pregnant. They should, of course, be cautioned to report any bleeding that occurs while the drug is being administered, so that the physician can make a pelvic examination and rule out the possibility of bleeding from an organic lesion.

Types of estrogens

Substances with estrogenic activity can be broadly classified: (1) *the natural steroids* (and their esters and semisynthetic derivatives); and (2) certain *non*steroidal synthetic chemicals that can elicit essentially similar effects (Table 23-1). Compounds of both types are available in oral and parenteral preparations. The products that can be given by mouth are preferred for most purposes because of their convenience and the fact that their effects are more predictable and more readily controlled.

In addition to two of the natural hormones (*estradiol* and *estrone*), a commonly employed mixture of natural estrogens is *conjugated estrogens*[+] (Premarin), which is claimed to have certain special properties. These sub-

Table 23–1. Natural and synthetic estrogens

Official or generic name	Trade name or synonym	Usual adult dosage and administration	Comments
Natural steroid hormone estrogens and derivatives			
Estrogens, conjugated USP	Premarin Intravenous; Premarin	25 mg IM or IV 0.3–10 mg PO at various intervals	See Drug digest
Estrogens, esterified USP	Evex; Menest	0.625–3.75 mg daily PO at various intervals	Mixture of water-soluble estrogens, mainly sodium estrone sulfate
Estradiol USP	Estrace	1–2 mg daily PO	Most potent natural ovarian hormone
Estradiol cypionate USP	Depo-Estradiol	1–5 mg IM every 3–4 wk	Long-acting ester
Estradiol valerate USP	Delestrogen	10–40 mg IM at various intervals	See Drug Digest
Estrone	In various parenteral preparations	0.1–4 mg IM at various intervals	Metabolite of estradiol
Ethinyl estradiol USP	Estinyl; Feminone	0.02–0.05 mg daily PO, cyclically	Highly potent synthetic steroid (see also Table 23-3)
Piperazine estrone sulfate USP	Ogen	0.625–7.5 mg daily PO, cyclically	Sulfate ester of estrone
Quinestrol	Estrovis	100 μg daily for 7 days, then 100 μg PO once weekly	Stored in body fat, with slow release and metabolism to ethinyl estradiol
Nonsteroidal synthetic estrogens			
Chlorotrianisene USP	Tace	12–25 mg PO in menopause; 72 mg twice daily for 2 days for preventing postpartum breast engorgement	Long-acting synthetic estrogenic substance
Dienestrol USP	AVC/Dienestrol suppositories; DV Cream	Topical application in various dosage schedules	For symptomatic relief of senile vulvovaginitis, atrophic vaginitis, pruritis vulvae
Diethylstilbestrol USP	Stilbestrol; DES	0.2–0.5 mg daily PO, cyclically	See Drug digest

stances are effective when administered orally, as is *ethinyl estradiol,* a semisynthetic derivative that is especially potent, in part because its chemical side chain structures protect the natural estrogenic nucleus from rapid inactivation in the liver and other tissues. The injectable esters of estradiol (*e.g.,* the *cipionate* and *valerate*+) are also long-acting, primarily because they are absorbed very slowly from intramuscular injection sites. These esters may exert effects for as long as a month or more after a single injection. They are used ordinarily only in certain special situations, because the orally administered products bring about menstruation in a more natural manner when discontinued.

The prototype of the *non*steroidal estrogenic substances is *DES,* which is inexpensive in comparison to the natural hormones and can produce all their physiologic effects. The two other synthetic estrogens listed in Table 23-1 are similar in their actions but may be less likely to cause nausea and vomiting than is DES. This may be only because they are less rapidly and completely absorbed from the intestinal tract than the latter (when DES is made available in more slowly absorbed forms, gastrointestinal upset is minimized).

Progesterone and progestins

Therapeutic uses

When progesterone first became available, gynecologists tried to employ it in the treatment of menstrual and reproductive difficulties that stemmed from a lack of the natural hormone. They reasoned that many women failed to menstruate, or bled excessively, because a deficiency of endogenous progesterone led to endometrial abnormalities. Similarly, many women with no organic defects of the reproductive tract remained childless as a result of deficient production of this hormone.

In practice, progesterone proved disappointing. Although the natural hormone seemed helpful in some menstrual disorders and in certain selected cases of endocrine infertility and habitual or threatened abortion, the need to administer either massive oral doses or frequent painful injections put severe practical limitations on its use. Fortunately, the development of synthetic substances that produce many effects of the natural hormone when taken by mouth in small doses has greatly simplified the treatment of some gynecologic disorders. These drugs have also proved convenient to use for other purposes, including contraception.

However, few of these drugs have purely progestational properties. Some, such as *medroxyprogesterone* (Table 23-2), exert some mild androgenic (masculinizing)

---

* It is important to distinguish between two types of uterine hemorrhage: (1) *menorrhagia,* which is marked by excessive blood loss during a normal menstrual period; and (2) *metrorrhagia,* a term that refers to bleeding at irregular intervals at times other than menstrual periods.

activity. Others either have some inherent estrogenic activity or are, like *norethindrone,* metabolized by the body to biologically active estrogen.

Thus, some progestins are preferred to others for treating particular patients and conditions and some should not, in fact, be employed at all in certain of the conditions discussed below and summarized at the end of the chapter. However, progesterone or one or another of the synthetic progestogens can be selected for effective use when a drug seems indicated in most of the various clinical situations discussed below. (In some situations—for example, in patients known or suspected to be pregnant—progestational therapy is not now recommended because of its possible hazards to the embryo or fetus.)

Menstrual disorders. As described earlier in this chapter, the menstrual cycle requires the sequential production of estrogens and progesterone by the ovary under the influence of the pituitary gonadotropins FSH and LH. The two sex steroids, in turn, affect the endometrium in ways that prepare it for pregnancy or result in menstruation. If any link in the timed production and release of the gondotropins or of the ovarian hormones fails, various types of menstrual disturbances may result, including the following: (1) *hypermenorrhea* (excessive uterine bleeding);* (2) *amenorrhea* (the absence of menstruation); and (3) *dysmenorrhea* (painful menstruation).

In all these conditions, and in others such as *endometriosis* and *PMS,* the introduction of convenient, orally effective synthetic progestins has led to better control. Combined with estrogens, or administered alternately with them in accordance with the principles of menstrual cycle physiology, the progestins seem to help correct many of the hormonal imbalances responsible for menstrual abnormalities.

Uterine bleeding. Hemorrhage from the uterus may be the result of an organic lesion. An examination is always done to rule out this possibility before employing estrogens or progestins. These medications are used only for controlling bleeding that is the result of glandular disturbances. *Dysfunctional bleeding* of this type occurs most commonly at puberty and at the menopause, when the ovaries are most likely to secrete sex hormones irregularly and in less than normal amounts. Such bleeding episodes are the end result of either too little estrogen production or too long continued estrogen secretion in the absence of a source of progesterone.

The latter situation may occur as the result of ovulatory failure. In such an anovulatory cycle, no corpus luteum is formed; as a result, a progesterone deficiency occurs and the proliferative endometrium is not converted to the secretory type. Because it is then being stimulated solely by estrogens, it continues to proliferate and grows quite thick. Finally, however, this proliferative endometrium outgrows its blood supply and begins to break down at various weak spots. This leads to bleeding that is irregular and often prolonged and excessive, because

Table 23–2. Progestational steroids (progestins or progestogens)

Official or generic name	Trade name	Usual adult dosage and administration	Therapeutic indications
Hydroxyprogesterone caproate USP	Delalutin	250–1000 mg IM	See Drug digest
Medroxyprogesterone acetate USP	Amen; Provera; Depo-Provera	2.5–10 mg PO, or 100–400 mg IM	See Drug digest
Megestrol acetate	Megace	40–320 mg daily	Endometrial carcinoma (see Chap. 12)
Norethindrone USP	Norlutin; in several combinations with estrogens (see Table 23–3)	0.35–20 mg PO	See Drug digest
Norethindrone acetate USP	Norlutate	2.5–15 mg PO	Amenorrhea and abnormal uterine bleeding; endometriosis; contraception
Norethynodrel USP	In Enovid and Enovid-E (see Table 23-3)	5–30 mg PO	Oral contraceptive; endometriosis; hypermenorrhea
Norgestrel	In Ovral; Lo-Ovral (see Table 23–3)	0.3–0.5 mg	Oral contraceptive
Progesterone USP	Progesterone in oil; Progesterone aqueous	5–10 mg IM	Functional uterine bleeding; amenorrhea

the hyperplastic endometrial tissue does not slough off completely and all at one time.

Acute bleeding can often be controlled by estrogens or androgens, but hemostasis is best accomplished today by administering an oral progestogen such as norethindrone+ (Norlutin), which may be given by mouth several times a day for a week or two to repair the necrotic endometrial areas. The withdrawal of the progestational steroids at the end of that time is then followed by shedding of the endometrium, with what appears to be essentially normal bleeding. Such a hormone-induced removal of the uterine mucous membrane frequently does away with the need for dilatation and curettage (D & C), a procedure considered undesirable in young unmarried women. Often after several such intermittent "medical curettage" treatments with oral progestins, combined estrogens and progestins, or injections of a long-acting progestin such as hydroxyprogesterone caproate+ (Delalutin) or progesterone itself, the woman's normal cycles are re-established and excessive bleeding episodes no longer occur.

To prevent recurrences, it is desirable to use the sex steroids in ways that imitate their release by the ovary in a normal ovulatory cycle. Often, bleeding is the result of the ovary's failure to produce enough progesterone in proportion to estrogen secretion. This may occur when there is no ovulation and consequently no formation of a corpus luteum (Fig. 23-2). In such an anovulatory cycle,

the proliferative endometrium is not converted to the secretory form. This leads to irregular and, often, prolonged and excessive bleeding from an endometrium that fails to slough off. Regular menstrual bleeding can be brought about by the administration and withdrawal of a progestin in such cases.

Amenorrhea. This may have many causes. Failure to menstruate can be entirely physiologic—in pregnancy, for example, or following the menopause; absence of menstruation may, on the other hand, be secondary to many systemic diseases and endocrine malfunctions. Once the cause has been determined by various diagnostic tests, treatment to establish normal menstrual bleeding can be undertaken. The potent synthetic progestins such as medroxyprogesterone+ (Amen; Provera), hydroxyprogesterone caproate, and others are often useful for both the diagnosis and treatment of amenorrhea.

In a normal menstrual cycle, female sex hormones of both types must be secreted in adequate amounts and exert their sequential proliferative and secretory effects on the endometrium. Then, when ovarian secretion drops off late in the menstrual month, the mucous membrane breaks down and menstruation occurs.

In both primary amenorrhea—the type seen in a hypogonadal patient who has never menstruated—and in secondary amenorrhea—which occurs in women who have previously menstruated—the two types of female hormones may be administered cyclically to bring about menstruation. In girls and women who do not have functioning ovaries, combination therapy of this type must be continued indefinitely. In *secondary amenorrhea* the administration of estrogen–progestin combinations in a way that imitates normal cyclic production can, of course, also be used to bring about menstruation on periodic withdrawal. Therapy of this type often results, after several such artificial cycles, in spontaneous menstruation—presumably because this treatment stimulates pituitary hormone production, and the gonadotropins in turn stimulate natural ovarian hormone secretion in proper amounts and timing.

Diagnostic tests

Endogenous estrogen production. To determine whether the ovaries of a patient with amenorrhea can produce estrogens, a progestational steroid may be administered (see Table 23-2). Because this produces a secretory endometrium and withdrawal bleeding only when the endometrium has first been primed by estrogens, failure to menstruate indicates that the patient's ovaries are not producing enough natural estrogen. Bleeding a week or so after withdrawal shows that her ovaries *can* secrete enough estrogen to produce a proliferative endometrium.

Endogenous progesterone production (pregnancy test). If a patient is producing estrogen, the administration and withdrawal of a progestin will produce menstrual bleeding. Failure to menstruate means that the corpus luteum is still producing progesterone. This occurs because the corpus luteum is still being stimulated by a gonadotropic hormone, the *chorionic* gonadotropin that is released by the trophoblastic tissues. This was formerly the basis for a pregnancy test. That is, when a woman who received a combination of estrogen and a progestin failed to menstruate a few days after withdrawal of the hormones, she was considered most probably to be pregnant. This type of pregnancy test is now contraindicated because of evidence that intrauterine exposure to female sex hormones for even a few days is associated with congenital heart and limb defects. Also, there are immunoassays available that can detect minute amounts of chorionic gonadotropin within a few days after fertilization, so tests employing progestins—particularly those with an estrogenic component—are not justified.

Dysmenorrhea. Many women with no evidence of organic pelvic disease suffer disabling uterine cramps during their menstrual periods. Progesterone injections just prior to the menstrual period were first employed as replacement therapy on the assumption that the uterine contractions in this condition are the result of a lack of this myometrium-quieting hormone. Although this *premenstrual* treatment did not help many patients, the oral administration of either synthetic progestins or estrogens, or a combination of the two steroids, *early in the menstrual month* has been reported to be followed by painless menstruation after withdrawal.

Such treatment, which suppresses pituitary gonadotropin secretion, prevents ovulation from occurring. It is now thought that inhibition of ovulation is somehow responsible for the resulting relative freedom from menstrual cramps. Thus, the same steroid combinations employed as oral contraceptives are used to treat women with dysmenorrhea. When the combined oral estrogens and progestins are withdrawn at the end of each cycle, painless menstrual bleeding usually occurs. If such cyclic steroid therapy is continued indefinitely it will, of course, interfere with fertility.

More recently, reports have indicated that many women who suffer from primary dysmenorrhea produce excessive amounts of prostaglandins that cause uterine hyperactivity. Three relatively new nonsteroidal anti-inflammatory agents (ibuprofen—Motrin, Rufen; mefenamic acid—Ponstel; and naproxen—Anaprox; Naprosyn), that inhibit the synthesis of prostaglandins have been found effective in relieving dysmenorrhea and have been approved for this use. Progesterone may be effective in dysmenorrhea by interfering in a different way with the production of prostaglandins.

Premenstrual edema and tension. Many women tend to retain fluid as their menstrual periods approach. As described earlier, weight gain, painful breast fullness, backache, and headache are part of this syndrome. In addition, some women suffer from emotional upsets of varying intensity. Although its cause is uncertain, it has been suggested that PMS results from inadequate production of progesterone by the corpus luteum and a resulting relative excess of fluid-retaining estrogens.

The oral progestins have been administered as replacement therapy, alone or combined with oral diuretics and sedatives, during the latter half of the menstrual cycle. This regimen is claimed to provide effective relief of some of these signs and symptoms.

Progestin–estrogen combinations administered early in the menstrual cycle have also proved effective for counteracting premenstrual emotional distress. As in the dysmenorrhea treatment mentioned above, the benefits may stem from suppression of ovulation.

Endometriosis. In this condition, according to one theory, pieces of endometrial tissue, which have been carried (by retrograde menstrual flow) from the uterus through the oviducts up into the abdominal cavity, become implanted on pelvic organs. These vagrant bits of uterine mucosa form masses on organs such as the ovaries, fallopian tubes, ureters, urinary bladder, and colon. These transplanted tissues are under the same hormonal influences as other uterine tissue. Periodic bleeding then causes surface swellings that may be painful and may interfere with the proper functioning of these organs. By blocking the tubes, for example, such masses may cause infertility, and the rupture of blood-filled ovarian cysts may result in sterility.

Until recently, severe endometriosis was treated

mainly by surgical removal of the ovaries and uterus. Such hysterectomy and castration, of course, halted the disease but also ended the woman's childbearing years and brought about a premature menopause. This serious condition is now successfully treated by the continuous administration of progestins, alone or combined with estrogens, for many months. Such a regimen not only prevents the painful menstruation of this condition but also often leads to regression of the growths within the abdomen.

The *pseudo*pregnancy brought about by such progestin therapy is effective for several reasons. By suppressing pituitary function, ovulation, and menstruation, such steroid treatment prevents the pathologic extra-uterine bleeding that otherwise occurs in this condition at the time of each menstrual period. Even more important than the drug-induced amenorrhea is the fact that the bits of displaced endometrial tissue often become fibrotic and reduced in size during prolonged progestin therapy. When the drug is withdrawn after 6 to 9 months, normal ovulation and menstruation soon resume but, in most cases, the ectopic endometrial implants do not become reactivated. As a result, many women with endometriosis-induced infertility become able to conceive and bear children.

Other uses of uninterrupted progestational therapy

Threatened abortion. Spontaneous abortion occurs in about 20% of all pregnancies and thus accounts for the termination of very many desired pregnancies. Some women abort repeatedly, and those who have had three or more consecutive miscarriages are termed "habitual" or "recurrent" aborters. Drugs cannot, of course, prevent spontaneous abortions that are caused by defects in the embryo. Many miscarriages are inevitable because of some fundamental defect in the germ plasm. In some cases, the embryo has died even before signs such as vaginal staining and colicky pains in the lower abdomen appear.

Progesterone has been employed for many years on the assumption that at least some abortions result from a failure of the placenta to secrete enough of the hormone to keep the uterus quiet. Administered in large and frequent doses all through pregnancy, progesterone is claimed to counteract the contractile effects of estrogens on the myometrium and thus to prevent premature expulsion of the embryo or fetus from the uterus. There may be a role for this treatment in women who can be proven to have a progesterone deficiency. However, because of reports that women who receive sex hormones during pregnancy have a higher risk of bearing children with birth defects involving the heart, nervous system, limbs, and gastrointestinal tract, prescribing synthetic progestogens for this purpose does not seem desirable and is not now recommended. This is particularly true for those progestins that possess a masculinizing component in their spectrum of actions. These include the

testosterone derivatives *norethindrone* and *medroxyprogesterone acetate*, which possess a slight androgenic action. This has occasionally led to clitoral enlargement and to other masculinizing effects on the external genitalia of female fetuses. Such virilizing effects have, in rare instances, occurred after treatment with progesterone itself as well as after use of norethynodrel—a progestin that, if anything, has slight estrogenic rather than androgenic activity. (See the discussion of the carcinogenic effects on the female fetus of the synthetic estrogen DES, above.)

Infertility. Infertility, of course, may have many causes including, not infrequently, the man's inability to produce adequate numbers of lively motile sperm or obstruction of the woman's fallopian tubes. The usefulness of progestins is limited, even in theory, to those cases in which their use may help to correct some hormonal abnormality—only about 15% of all cases. They are best reserved for cases in which ovulation occurs but the endometrium appears to be inadequately prepared for implantation of a fertilized egg.

The new synthetic steroids seem to have proved most effective in those women whose infertility can be traced to a poorly functioning corpus luteum that fails to produce enough progesterone to maintain an adequate secretory endometrium. The administration of small daily oral doses of synthetic progestins (combined with estrogens) during the *post*ovulatory phase of the menstrual cycle is claimed to have helped some women with luteal phase defects to conceive and bear children.

In such cases of infertility, the progestins serve as substitutional therapy. That is, when administered daily from the time when a rise in the woman's body temperature indicates that ovulation has occurred, these synthetic hormones supplement the patient's own inadequate progesterone production. Under their influence, the proliferative endometrium is converted into the secretory type that can receive and nourish a fertilized egg. Repetition of such steroid replacement therapy during several menstrual cycles eventually permits pregnancy, provided that the woman with luteal phase deficiency can produce an ovum, and that viable sperm reach it during its descent through the oviduct.

Anovulation. Progestins have also been used to treat women whose infertility stems from failure to ovulate. This may seem strange, because the ovarian sex steroids themselves *suppress* ovulation (see discussion of oral contraceptives, below). The manner in which the progestins stimulate ovulation in such cases is still uncertain. Unlike treatment with gonadotropins or clomiphene, the preferred agents for infertility (Chap. 20), progestins do not stimulate either the ovaries or the pituitary gland directly. However, it has been suggested that, after withdrawal of progestin therapy, there may be increased hypothalamic activity leading to secretion of GnRH and production of the pituitary gonadotropins FSH and LH that stimulate the ovaries to produce ova.

Reportedly, when progestin–estrogen therapy was stopped after several such cycles, the ovaries of some women whose infertility stemmed from failure to ovulate were indirectly stimulated to produce ova, and the women soon became pregnant. This so-called rebound effect, which may result from the rest afforded a sluggish pituitary gland, is said to account for the seeming *increase* in fertility of women who stop taking oral steroid contraceptives when they wish to become pregnant.

Cancer. The use of such progestins as megestrol acetate (Megace) and medroxyprogesterone acetate (Depo-Provera) in the treatment of endometrial and other carcinomas has been discussed in Chapter 12, together with the use of other sex steroids in treating hormone-dependent neoplastic diseases.

Oral contraceptives

The most common indication for progestins and estrogens is the prevention of conception. Taken orally in tablet form, combinations of synthetic sex steroids have proved highly effective for this purpose. However, doubts have arisen about whether it is safe for women to continue taking these potent drugs for prolonged periods.

Many methods of birth control are now available. Women have the right to know the benefits and risks involved of the particular method(s) they are considering. If oral contraceptives are to be used, the nurse taking care of the patient must be fully aware of the beneficial and adverse actions of these drugs to advise and teach the patient about the drug appropriately.

This section of the chapter will briefly review the ways in which oral contraceptives act. Then, after indicating the types of products that are available and how they must be used to ensure maximum effectiveness, their potential toxicity and measures to avoid adverse reactions will be discussed.

Mechanism of action. The main way in which steroid combination contraceptives are believed to act is through suppression of ovulation. This effect is thought to be brought about by their ability to inhibit the release of the ovulation-regulating gonadotropins of the pituitary gland. However, this is probably not the only way in which these drugs prevent conception. Evidence indicates that they also exert direct actions on such reproductive system organs as the ovaries, oviducts, and uterus.

Actions of this type not only prevent the ovaries from releasing ova but also prevent any ova that might be freed from being fertilized, or—if fertilized—from taking root in the lining of the uterus. For example, one effect of progestational steroids is to make the cervical glands produce a thick mucous secretion. This makes it difficult for sperm cells to pass into the uterus and to fertilize an ovum in the fallopian tubes. Other steroid actions interfere with fallopian tube function so that, even if an egg were to be fertilized there, its movement down the oviduct to the uterus would be impeded. Finally, any fertilized egg that managed to reach the uterus would find it impossible to become implanted in the lining of the uterus because of steroid-induced atrophic changes in the endometrium.

Contraceptive products. Several types of steroid products are currently available (Table 23-3). Most common are combinations of estrogens and progestins for oral use. However, a few products contain only a progestin. The emergency use of 5-day estrogen therapy for postcoital contraception in rape victims has been described above. Other contraceptive methods involve the intramuscular administration of a long-acting synthetic progestational steroid, or the addition of progesterone to an intrauterine device (IUD) from which it is released locally in the uterus at a very slow controlled rate.

Steroid combinations. Most oral contraceptives are combinations of the following: (1) a potent estrogen, either *ethinyl estradiol* or its methyl ether derivative, *mestranol;* and (2) any one of several progestins such as *norethindrone* and its acetate ester; *norgestrel; norethynodrel;* and *ethynodiol diacetate.* The main difference between these products and the first steroid combinations introduced for this purpose is that they contain relatively low doses of the two types of steroids. Estrogen dosage has been reduced to particularly low levels—as little as 20 μg or 30 μg of ethinyl estradiol and 50 μg or 75 μg of mestranol. This reflects the fact that such small doses of estrogen have been found to be adequately effective and less likely to cause side-effects than larger doses.

These products are almost 100% effective when properly employed. That is, the rate of pregnancies is far less than 1/100 woman years of use with any of the available combinations. However, for full effectiveness, the tablets must be taken exactly as directed. One tablet is taken each day from day 5 through day 25 of the woman's menstrual cycle. (The first day of menstrual flow is day 1.) Then, following 20 or 21 consecutive days of medication, no tablets are taken for 7 days, or a tablet containing inert material or an iron salt is taken from day 22 through day 28.

Menstrual bleeding begins within a few days after withdrawal of the steroid combination. A new course of tablet taking should be begun following the 1 week off medication, whether the menstrual flow has stopped or not. If a woman forgets to take a tablet at the usual time—often, bedtime each night is most convenient— she should take the missed tablet as soon as she remembers and then take the next tablet at the usual time. If two tablets are missed on consecutive days, dosage should be doubled on the next 2 days. Even after the regular regimen is resumed, an additional method of contraception is recommended for the rest of the cycle, because ovulation may have occurred because of failure to take the tablets on more than 1 day.

Progestin-only products. Several available antifertility preparations contain no synthetic estrogen but only a progestin in dosage as low as 75 μg (Table 23-3). Such so-called minipills may be less likely to cause adverse effects

Table 23–3. Oral contraceptive products

Trade name	Progestational content	Estrogen content
Brevicon	Norethindrone 0.5 mg	Ethinyl estradiol (EE) 0.035 mg
Demulen	Ethynodiol diacetate 1 mg	EE 0.035 mg and 0.05 mg
Enovid	Norethynodrel 5 mg	Mestranol (ME) 0.075 mg
Enovid-E	Norethynodrel 2.5 mg	ME 0.10 mg
Loestrin	Norethindrone acetate 1 mg and 1.5 mg	EE 0.02 mg and 0.03 mg
Lo-Ovral	Norgestrel 0.3 mg	EE 0.03 mg
Micronor	Norethindrone 0.35 mg	
Modicon	Norethindrone 0.5 mg	EE 0.035 mg
Nordette	Levonorgestrel 0.15 mg	EE 0.030 mg
Norinyl	Norethindrone 1 mg and 2 mg	ME 0.035 mg, 0.05 mg, 0.08 mg, and 0.10 mg
Norlestrin	Norethindrone acetate 1 mg and 2.5 mg	EE 0.05 mg
Nor-Q.D.	Norethindrone 0.35 mg	
Ortho-Novum	Norethindrone 0.5 mg, 1 mg, and 2 mg	ME 0.05 mg, 0.08 mg, and 0.10 mg
Ovcon	Norethindrone 0.4 mg and 1 mg	EE 0.035 mg and 0.050 mg
Ovral	Norgestrel 0.5 mg	EE 0.05 mg
Ovrette	Norgestrel 0.075 mg	
Ovulen	Ethynodiol diacetate 1 mg	ME 0.10 mg

of the types associated with estrogens. However, this is uncertain at present, and the labeling of these products bears warnings similar to those of the combination-type contraceptives.

These products are somewhat less reliable than the combinations that also contain estrogens. The rate of pregnancies is about 3/100 woman years compared to less than one pregnancy per year in 100 women taking combination products. Another drawback is that, because the minipill must be taken every day of the year without interruption, no withdrawal bleeding occurs. Instead, the user's menstrual pattern may become quite irregular and the flow very variable. Thus, these products have proved less acceptable to many women, and the dropout rate has been much higher than in patient populations maintained on combination contraceptives.

Long-lasting pregnancy protection. Two types of contraceptive products that eliminate the need for taking daily oral doses of steroids seem to have proved effective in extended clinical trials. However, their final status is uncertain. One of these products, medroxyprogesterone acetate (Depo-Provera) is injected intramuscularly to provide protection for 3 months or more when given at intervals of 90 days. It is used in this way abroad, but its use in the United States is presently, however, restricted to experimental use in patients who must be fully informed

of the possible risks of this method. These include, in addition to the usual adverse effects of sex steroids, the possibility of prolonged or even permanent infertility after the drug is discontinued.

Progesterone contraceptive system (Progestasert). The hormone progesterone has been made available in an IUD that delivers a small daily dose for 12 months. The mechanism of action is unknown, but adverse effects on sperm, and prevention of implantation of a fertilized ovum, have been hypothesized as mechanisms. The hormone acts locally within the womb and does not enter the general circulation. Thus, it prevents pregnancy without interfering with ovulation or causing any of the adverse systemic effects associated with oral contraceptives (see below). The pregnancy rate is about 2/100 woman years of use.

The drawbacks of this product are those of IUDs in general. Although this contraceptive method has many advantages, it sometimes causes uterine cramps, backache, and bleeding between menstrual periods. The device sometimes has to be removed because of heavy bleeding or, much more rarely, because of such complications as pelvic infections or perforation of the uterus.

The physician or nurse inserts the Progestasert IUD contraceptive system only after a complete pelvic examination has ruled out the presence of pregnancy, malignancy, and infection. Patients who become pregnant despite the presence of devices of this kind may suffer spontaneous—and sometimes septic—abortion. The incidence of ectopic pregnancies is about ten times higher in women using IUD devices than in those who become pregnant while employing other mechanical contraceptive measures such as a diaphragm.

Adverse effects. In addition to its relative reliability compared to mechanical methods of contraception, oral steroid administration has various other advantages that make it more acceptable to most women, yet some who start out on oral contraceptives switch to other birth control devices. Sometimes this is because of minor side-effects (See also the summary at the end of this chapter). Increasingly, however, women have been deciding against taking sex steroids for this purpose because of their anxiety about possible long-term toxicity, including blood clot-induced disabilities and cancer, and concern that they may later be unable to become pregnant and bear a normal child.

Minor side-effects. The most common undesirable effects resemble those of early pregnancy and, like the latter, they tend to diminish or disappear after several monthly cycles. These include nausea and vomiting, headache and dizziness, weight gain, breast fullness and discomfort and, occasionally, acne and chloasma (an increase in skin pigmentation). Another reaction that some women find frightening and confusing is the occurrence of breakthrough bleeding, or spotting, during their cycle or, on the other hand, failure to menstruate on withdrawal of the drugs at the end of the cycle.

Despite these distressing symptoms, many women continue taking oral contraceptives through the first few cycles, after which—as in pregnancy—nausea and other discomforts lessen. Most side-effects are, in any case, controllable. Nausea, for example, can be reduced by taking the tablet at bedtime with a glass of milk. Breakthrough bleeding can be overcome by *increasing* the steroid dosage to prevent premature endometrial breakdown.

Long-term toxicity. It now seems quite clear that some women have been harmed by taking oral contraceptives, and that a small number of deaths have occurred. However, although the risks seem greater statistically in users than nonusers, the actual number of cases is small, and the danger to any individual patient appears to be low. Nevertheless, the nurse should know the types of complications that can occur and be able to answer questions about them in ways that will help each woman make her own decision about whether or not to use this method.*

Circulatory side-effects. As indicated in the discussion

of estrogens and thromboembolic disorders (above), some women are prone to suffer blood-clotting episodes while taking oral contraceptives containing sex steroids. The risk is close to six times as high in users as in comparable women who have not taken this medication, but this reaction is so rare in both groups that the actual risk of death from thrombophlebitis complications such as pulmonary embolism is quite low—about 15 per every million women under 35 years old taking these drugs. (In comparison, the risk of death from this and other complications of pregnancy is more than ten times as great.)

Although such statistics are encouraging, the risk for any particular woman may be greater depending on her age, whether or not she smokes cigarettes, and possibly on factors still unrecognized. Thus, no woman should take oral contraceptives if she already has a medical history of a thromboembolic disorder, or if a physical examination reveals the presence of an active clotting disease process. The risk of myocardial infarction rises steeply in women over 35 years of age, and stroke is also somewhat more likely.

Cerebral complications of this type are more likely in patients with high blood pressure. Hypertension has been found more frequently in users of oral contraceptives, just as it develops in some women during pregnancy. Thus, a check of blood pressure should be made each time a patient on the pill comes to the clinic, just as is done during pregnancy. When oral contraceptives are discontinued—as they should be in any woman with persistent hypertension—blood pressure usually drops to normal levels.

Cancer risk. The question of whether oral contraceptives can cause breast or genital cancer still cannot be answered at this time. The findings concerning an increased risk of *endometrial cancer* in postmenopausal women taking estrogens (see above) does not necessarily indicate that the same risk applies to young women taking low doses of estrogens and progestins. This type of uterine cancer *has* been reported in users of oral contraceptives, but these steroids have not been proved to be the cause. (Endometrial cancer may have been present and gone undetected before treatment was begun.) However, results of one recent study indicate a 75% greater risk of *cervical cancer* in patients on OCs than in patients using an IUD. Previous studies showed only a slightly increased risk. Because many factors are associated with cervical cancer, it is difficult to explain the discrepancies in the results of these studies.

The relationship of oral contraceptives to *breast cancer* is also still uncertain. Some studies have suggested that sex steroids tend to protect against benign fibrocystic breast disease, a condition that may make women more susceptible to later development of mammary carcinoma. Other reports suggest that breast cancer is more likely to develop in women with nonmalignant breast disease when they take oral contraceptives for several years. A recent study has reported that women under 25 years of

---

* Women now receive a patient package insert (PPI) when they obtain their prescribed oral contraceptive products. However, the teaching effectiveness of such PPIs is currently a subject of controversy. Thus, consumers will still have questions for physicians, pharmacists, and nurses about the safety and effectiveness of these products.

age who had taken OCs for at least 5 years were four times more likely to develop breast cancer. These women had taken the high hormone preparations available in the early 1970s. Whether the newer, lower dose formulations also carry this risk is uncertain. However, these products should probably not be prescribed for women with a family history of this disease or be taken by those who already have even benign breast nodules or who show other abnormalities in mammograms.

In summary, whenever a patient is to be put on OCs, she should be examined before the drugs are prescribed and periodically during the years of their use. Perhaps women who return regularly for physical, including pelvic, exams and Pap tests are better protected against serious malignancies than women who take no drugs but who do not receive such regular examinations.

Fertility. Fears that taking oral contraceptives for several years might affect a woman's future fertility seem to be unfounded. Occasionally, a woman may not menstruate or ovulate for up to 3 months after she stops taking these drugs. However, in most cases, the pretreatment menstrual cycle returns promptly and with it comes the ability to conceive.* Rarely, a woman who had been childless before taking oral contraceptives (and who may have been sterile without being aware of it) fails to ovulate after discontinuing the drugs. Such cases may respond to infertility treatment with gonadotropins or clomiphene (Chap. 20).

Babies born to women who have employed this contraceptive method seem to have no more birth abnormalities than infants of women who had used other contraceptive methods. However, because of the possible adverse effects of estrogens on the embryo, it is probably best for a woman who wishes to become pregnant to employ another contraceptive method for a couple of months after discontinuing these drugs. Similarly, because the long-term effects of excess sex steroids on the development of newborn infants is not known, nursing mothers may be well advised to use another contraceptive method for a time.

Risk-to-benefit ratio. No one can answer the question of sex steroid safety with total assurance at this time. No drug can ever be considered completely safe for everyone, and so it is customary to weigh the benefits of drug therapy against the risk of toxicity. This is difficult to do in the case of oral contraceptives, because the degree of risk—of some cancers, for example—is still uncertain. However, most authorities continue to claim that these drugs can still be considered safe—for healthy women under 35 years old, anyway—because the benefit-to-risk ratio is high enough. Of course, in some women with various underlying medical disorders, the balance may

shift in favor of the risk factors, and the use of oral contraceptives would, of course, be unwarranted in such cases.

Additional clinical considerations

Patients who are treated with estrogens, progestins, or combinations should be screened carefully to ensure that they are free of any underlying medical condition that might be aggravated by the systemic effects of these drugs. Such conditions include thrombophlebitis or a history of thrombophlebitis; cancer of the breast or any genital tissue (a family history of breast cancer is also a contraindication); abnormal vaginal bleeding with no known cause; liver failure; metabolic bone diseases (hypercalcemia can result); pregnancy or lactation; cardiac or renal disease that can be aggravated by fluid retention; gallbladder disease; diabetes (a glucose intolerance can occur).

Patients also need to be fully informed about some of the usual side-effects of this particular drug therapy. Fluid retention is common. Patients with a predisposition to such problems may experience migraine headaches, asthma attacks, or seizures as a result. Corneal curvature is often altered, which can cause problems for patients who wear contact lenses. Bleeding usually occurs when estrogens are withdrawn, and patients need to understand that this is a natural response, and does not indicate a return to menstruation and fertility for postmenopausal women. However, bleeding at any time other than withdrawal should be a cause of concern and should be reported. Young girls who are treated with these drugs should be fully informed about the changes in secondary sex characteristics that should occur. They, and their parents, will need to be able to discuss and ask questions about these changes and how to cope with them. Mental depression has been reported frequently with the use of these drugs. It is more likely to be a serious problem in patients with a past history of mental depression, but patients should be aware of the possibility and helped to cope with it if it does occur.

Proper administration of the medication can be a problem for patients. Patients who are using local estrogenic medications should be instructed in the proper use of vaginal suppositories and creams. The following recommendations should be made: refrigerate suppositories before use; have the patient wash her hands before and after insertion of the suppository; peel off the foil of the suppository before use; and do *not* use the suppository orally but always insert it into the vagina. The patient should be advised to lie down for about 30 minutes after insertion and to use a perineal pad to prevent soiling of clothes. If external creams are being used, it is again advisable to suggest that the patient use a perineal pad to protect her clothing. Sex hormones that are taken orally in a cyclical pattern usually come in a prepacked dispenser to help increase the patient's compliance. The patient needs to know the specific information about making up missed doses: because each preparation is somewhat different, the specifics for each drug should

---

* Prolonged infertility has been a more frequent problem in women who have received injections of medroxyprogesterone. This is one reason for the FDA's having withdrawn its once limited approval of the use of this injectable contraceptive in some categories of patients.

be written down for the patient. If gastrointestinal upset occurs, these drugs can be taken with meals.

Drug–drug interactions. Use of an oral contraceptive (OC) has been associated with several drug–drug interactions. Reduced effectiveness of the OC and an increase in breakthrough bleeding have been associated with concurrent use of *rifampin, barbiturates, phenylbutazone, phenytoin, primidone, carbamazepine, isoniazid, neomycin, penicillin V, chloramphenicol, sulfonamides, nitrofurantoin, analgesics, tranquilizers,* and *broad-spectrum antibiotics (e.g.,* tetracycline). Any patient taking OCs who is started on any of these drugs may experience an unwanted pregnancy or breakthrough bleeding, and should be cautioned to use another means of contraception and to report any side-effects. OC preparations may decrease the effects of *oral anticoagulants, antiepileptic drugs, tricyclic antidepressants, oral hypoglycemic agents, vitamins,* and various *antihypertensive agents.* Patients maintained on any of these drugs should be carefully monitored and may require an increased dosage if OCs are taken concurrently.

Drug–laboratory test interactions. The OCs are also associated with numerous alterations in laboratory test results, including the following: increased *prothrombin time* and other coagulation factors; increased *renin activity;* increased *triglyceride levels;* increased *high-density lipoprotein* (HDL) *levels;* increased *protein-bound iodine* (PBI) and T_4 levels as a result of increased thyroxine-binding globulin; increased *aldosterone levels,* secondary to the increase in renin–angiotensin activity; increased *amylase levels;* and slightly decreased *glucose tolerance.* If any patient on OCs shows an abnormal result in any of these tests, the drug effect should be carefully considered in the total clinical picture.

The patient who is to receive estrogens or progestins will need a great deal of teaching and counseling to deal with the effects of the drug, as well as the condition for which they are receiving it. The patient teaching guide summarizes the key points to include in teaching a patient who is receiving oral contraceptives. The guide to the nursing process presents the clinical points to consider in the nursing care of a patient receiving estrogen, progesterone, or combined therapy.

Patient teaching guide: oral contraceptives

The method of contraception that you have elected to use involves taking an oral contraceptive (OC) preparation, commonly called a birth control pill. These tablets contain specific amounts of female sex hormones that work to make the body unreceptive to pregnancy and to prevent ovulation (combination OCs)—the release of an egg from the ovary. The hormones affect many systems in your body and it is important to have regular physical check-ups while you are on this drug.

Instructions:

1. The drug that has been prescribed for you is _____ .

2. The dosage that has been prescribed for you is _____ .

3. Your pill should be taken at the same time each day. If your stomach becomes upset with this medication, it can be taken with meals. The pattern of your drug cycle is _____ . If you skip a pill, you can "catch up" pills for _____ days. It would be advisable to use another method of birth control during the cycle in which the pills were missed.

4. Avoid the use of other drugs, including over-the-counter medications, without checking with your nurse or physician. Many drugs affect the way that these drugs work; to be safe, you should discuss the use of any other drug with your nurse or physician.

5. Some side-effects of the drug that you should be aware of include the following:

Headache, nervousness   Check with your nurse or physician for analgesia if the headache is severe. These effects usually pass after a few months on the drug.

(continued)

490

Nausea, loss of appetite	These usually pass with time; consult with your nurse or physician if they persist.
Swelling, weight gain	Water retention is a normal effect of these hormones, and limiting salt intake may help. Usually, this also adjusts over time.

6. Cigarette smoking can aggravate a serious adverse effect of these drugs—the formation of blood clots. If you are taking these drugs, it is advisable to cut down, or preferably to stop, cigarette smoking.

7. Tell any physician, nurse, or dentist who is taking care of you that you are taking this drug.

8. Keep this and all medications out of the reach of children.

9. Bleeding, a false menstrual period, should occur during the time that the drug is withdrawn (combination OCs). Bleeding at *any* other time should be reported to your nurse or physician.

10. It is very important to have a regular physical exam, including a Pap smear, while you are taking this drug. If you decide to stop the drug to become pregnant, consult with your nurse or physician.

11. A patient package insert is available with this drug. Read this information and feel free to ask any questions.

Notify your nurse or physician if any of the following occur:

Pain in the calves or groin
Chest pain, difficulty in breathing
Lumps in the breast
Severe headache, dizziness, visual changes
Severe abdominal pain
Yellowing of skin
Suspected pregnancy

Guide to the nursing process: estrogens and progestins

Assessment	Nursing diagnoses	Intervention	Evaluation
Past history (*contraindications*): • Family history–breast cancer • Breast cancer	Potential alteration in comfort Potential alteration in fluid volume Knowledge deficit	Proper and safe administration of the drug Provision of comfort measures:	Evaluate therapeutic effects of drug Monitor for adverse effects of drug: • GI upset

(continued)

Assessment	Nursing diagnoses	Intervention	Evaluation
• Genital cancer • Coronary disease • Hepatic failure • Thromboembolic disorders • Idiopathic vaginal bleeding • Metabolic bone diseases • Pregnancy • Lactation • Renal disease • Diabetes *Allergies:* these drugs; tartrazine (specific preparation) Medication history: other drugs being taken **Physical assessment** Neurologic: mental status, affect, reflexes Eyes: ophthalmologic exam (special concern with contact lenses) Cardiovascular: BP, P, perfusion, edema, cardiac auscultation, baseline ECG (if appropriate) Respiratory: rate, adventitious sounds GI: liver, abdominal exam Genitourinary: urinalysis, pelvic exam, Pap smear Other: lesions, breast exam, skin	regarding drug therapy Potential alteration in tissue perfusion Potential alteration in thought processes	• Use of perineal pad as needed • Drug with meals for GI upset • Analgesics for headache, mylagias Patient teaching regarding: Drug Precautions Side-effects Warnings	• Liver changes • Changes in secondary sex characteristics • Edema • Headaches • Thromboembolic episodes • Breakthrough bleeding Evaluate effectiveness of patient teaching plan Evaluate effectiveness of comfort measures offered Evaluate effectiveness of support and encouragement offered Monitor for drug–drug interactions (several) Monitor for drug–laboratory test interactions: ↑ prothrombin time and other clotting factors ↑ renin levels ↑ aldosterone levels ↑ triglyceride levels ↑ HDL levels ↑ PBI, T_4 (by certain tests) ↑ amylase levels Slightly ↓ glucose tolerance Monitor patient's total physical condition with regular and complete examinations

Drugs acting on the uterus

The uterus is responsive to the actions of many types of drugs when studied under laboratory conditions. However, only a few types of drugs are effective enough for clinical use in obstetrics and gynecology. One reason for this is that few drugs exert their *primary* effects on the muscles of the uterus, and those that have only *secondary* effects on the uterus would cause too many side-effects if given in doses large enough to influence uterine function. The rest of this chapter will consider the actions of three groups of drugs: (1) oxytocics, including the posterior pituitary hormone, oxytocin, and ergot alkaloids; (2) abortifacients; and (3) uterine relaxants.

Oxytocics

Oxytocics are drugs that act on the smooth muscle of the uterus to increase its tone and motility (Table 23-4). They act most strongly late in pregnancy, particularly during labor and in the period immediately following it. The response of the myometrium to oxytocic agents is also dose-related. Very small amounts may set off contractions followed by relaxation, as in normal labor. Larger doses

Table 23-4. Oxytocic agents

Official or generic name	Trade name	Usual adult dosage and administration
Ergonovine maleate USP	Ergotrate	See Drug digest
Methylergonovine maleate USP	Methergine	0.2 mg (200 μg) orally tid or qid, or by IM injection (IV injection only with extreme caution)
Oxytocin injection USP	Pitocin; Syntocinon	See Drug digest
Oxytocin, synthetic, nasal	Syntocinon	One spray into one or both nostrils 2–3 min before nursing

cause more powerful and longer lasting contractions that come at a more rapid rate and with shorter rest periods. Excessively high doses produce sustained tetanic contractions of the uterus that can often by relaxed only by having the patient inhale a general anesthetic

Indications for oxytocic drugs (see summary at the end of this chapter). The most important use of the oxytocic drugs is the prevention of postpartum bleeding by contracting the muscle fibers of the uterus around the blood vessels that course through its tissues. Their administration late in labor also aids in the removal of the placenta from the uterus. Some of the available oxytocics are used cautiously to induce labor in selected patients or to restart stalled labor in selected cases of uterine inertia. Other oxytocic substances are too dangerous to be used to stimulate contractions of the uterus while it still contains the head of the fetus.

Oxytocin (Pitocin; Syntocinon). As indicated above, this posterior pituitary gland hormone (Chap. 20) plays an important physiologic role in labor and delivery. It is released in increasing quantities as a result of a reflex that is set off when the uterine cervix and the vagina are first forcibly dilated and their muscles stretched at the onset of labor. The continued action of the hormone, which is carried from the pituitary to the uterus by the bloodstream, accounts for the crescendo of contractions that culminates in delivery of the baby and expulsion of the placenta.

Oxytocin of exogenous origin is used clinically to contract the uterus before, during, and after labor. Extracts of the natural gland are no longer the source of the solutions that are injected for various purposes, because these contain a contaminating impurity—the other posterior pituitary gland hormone, the antidiuretic component (ADH; vasopressin; see Chap. 20). Instead, a highly purified synthetic form of oxytocin is employed clinically.

Induction of labor. Oxytocin is now commonly used to set off labor when it is decided that early delivery is desirable for the safety of the mother and fetus in several clinical situations (see the summary of clinical indications at the end of this chapter). This procedure is employed in selected patients, after the presence of factors that could lead to drug-induced complications has been ruled out. The patient is kept under close observation to detect and deal with any difficulties that may arise during the drug-induced labor.

Patient selection and precautions. Labor is induced with oxytocin only when the fetus is mature and its head is in proper proportion to the mother's pelvis. The fetus should also be in a position that favors normal delivery without any need for turning it from a transverse or other unusual presentation. The mother should have no past history of traumatic delivery or of uterine sepsis. She should not have had a previous cesarean section or major cervical or uterine surgery. In every case, including elective induction or obstetric emergencies, the potential benefits of oxytocin-induced induction are weighed against the risks of setting off too strong uterine muscle spasm.

Oxytocin must be administered in doses that set off contractions similar to those that occur in normal labor. Care is required not to overstimulate the uterus, because hypertonic contractions can harm both the mother and the fetus. Strong contractions that force the fetus against a hard, unyielding and only partially dilated cervix can tear the cervical tissues or even rupture the muscles of the fundus itself. The infant's head or other parts may be damaged when shoved against the unripe cervix in this way. Sustained uterine spasms may also choke off the child's only source of oxygen—the blood that flows from the mother's arteries into the placenta during periods of relaxation. Thus, tetanic contractions of the uterus can cause serious birth defects, fetal death, or fatal trauma to the mother.

Dosage and administration. For induction of labor, oxytocin is administered in only a small fraction of the dose that is injected after delivery to control postpartum bleeding (see below). The amount employed is determined by the response of the uterus in each patient individually. For induction or stimulation of labor, only the IV route is used. A dilute solution is infused at the rate of 1 to 2 mU/min, initially; this may be increased gradually (see Drug digest) to establish a pattern of contractions similar to that of normal labor. Careful monitoring of the mother and fetus is necessary. Too strong spasms must be avoided in case they interfere with blood flow to the fetus. When caring for any patient who is receiving oxytocin for induction, the frequency, strength, and duration of uterine contractions are carefully observed and the fetal heart sounds are listened to or, preferably, fetal monitoring is used to evaluate the condition of the fetus continually.

Other indications

Uterine inertia Oxytocin is not ordinarily injected during the first and second stages of labor. However, it has been used to stimulate labor that has stopped or that is proceeding so slowly that the mother is close to exhaustion. Infused intravenously in carefully regulated amounts, very dilute solutions of oxytocin sometimes succeed in restoring rhythmic contractions in selected cases of arrested labor. The criteria for selection of cases are the same as those employed in deciding whether oxytocin should be used for inducing labor. Such a patient should receive a careful explanation of why the drug dosage cannot be increased too rapidly to hasten delivery.

Incomplete abortion. Oxytocin is occasionally used to rid the uterus of a fetus that has died. Because the uterus is not very responsive to stimulation in the earlier months of pregnancy, the drug must be administered in much larger doses than are employed at term. Excessive amounts of oxytocin have sometimes caused water intoxication because of an antidiuretic action similar to that of the related posterior pituitary hormone, vasopressin (ADH), discussed in Chapter 20. In the first trimester, curettage (not oxytocin) is considered as primary therapy.

Postpartum hemorrhage. Oxytocin is sometimes employed to stop uterine bleeding following delivery. Much larger doses are administered than during induction of labor—for example, as many as 40 U may be added to 1 liter of dextrose solution for IV infusion; or 3 U to 10 U may be given as a single IM injection. Some personnel inject the desired dose immediately after the infant's right shoulder is delivered, while others wait until after the placenta has been delivered before injecting the dose of oxytocin required for contracting the uterine muscle fibers about the open bleeding sinuses. Often, today, ergot alkaloids are preferred for this purpose because they cause longer lasting postpartum contractions (see below).

Oxytocin and the breast. Oxytocin released by the posterior pituitary gland in response to a baby's suckling plays a part in the ejection of milk from the breast. This hormone is not responsible for the process by which the mammary glands make milk, but it does make it easy for the baby to obtain the mother's milk. Synthetic oxytocin is now available in the form of a nasal spray for use when the natural reflex fails. When the mother sprays the solution into her nostrils, oxytocin is absorbed and carried to the smooth muscle cells surrounding the alveoli of the breasts. This causes them to contract and to force the milk into the larger ducts, from which the baby can draw it more readily.

Ergot alkaloids. Ergot is a parasitic fungus that grows on rye and other cereal grains. It contains many potent chemical substances, including the alkaloids ergotamine and ergonovine, which are widely used in modern medicine for their dependable actions in certain chemical conditions. (The use of ergotamine in the management of migraine headache is discussed in Chap. 38.) *Ergonovine* and a semisynthetic derivative, *methylergonovine,* are used in obstetrics because of their relatively selective action on the uterus at term.

Effects on the uterus. Small doses of these drugs, administered parenterally toward the end of the second stage or during the third stage of labor, are used in the management of *postpartum hemorrhage* and *uterine atony.* The ergot alkaloids act directly on the smooth muscle fibers of the flaccid uterus. The resulting contraction makes the fibers clamp down on the open arterioles. This keeps postpartum bleeding from the now firm uterus to a minimum.

Administration. Ergonovine and methylergonovine are usually administered intramuscularly in a dose of 0.2 mg during the third stage of labor. The drug reaches the uterus 2 to 5 minutes later, at about the time when the placenta is being expelled. This causes the uterus to become hard instead of staying relaxed, thus preventing excessive blood loss in the period of atony that ordinarily follows delivery of the afterbirth.

Some prefer to give the ergot alkaloids earlier—following delivery of the infant's anterior shoulder but before expulsion of the placenta. The drug's action on the uterus then aids in completing the second stage and shortening the third stage of labor. A possible difficulty with this method is that—if the placenta does not separate spontaneously—the drug's action on the uterus may trap the placenta in the uterus, from which it may then have to be removed manually.

Involution of the uterus. Ergot alkaloids are sometimes given during the puerperium to help hasten return of the normal tone of the uterus. This is thought to lessen the likelihood of infection by closing the gaping sinuses through which bacteria might enter. For this purpose, tablets for oral administration are given three or four times a day during the first week when the process of involution is normally most rapid. Longer use is undesirable because of possible chronic toxicity, or ergotism (see below).

Partial abortion. Like oxytocin, ergot is sometimes

ordered after a spontaneous partial abortion. Whereas oxytocin is often considered superior for initiation of contractions, ergonovine may be more effective for reducing the bleeding that follows expulsion of the dead fetus and the membranes. Persistent hemorrhage may require a dilatation and curettage of the uterus. Surgical repair is necessary for control of hemorrhage from cervical tears or lacerations of the birth canal, because ergot alone does not stop bleeding from trauma to such sites.

Side-effects and toxicity. Ergonovine is a remarkably safe drug when given in proper dosage, because its effects are largely limited to myometrial smooth muscle. Occasionally, however, it may have effects on blood vessels. Sometimes, for example, when given intravenously for immediate action in an emergency, methylergonovine may cause a sudden rapid rise in blood pressure that can lead to a hypertensive crisis or cerebral hemorrhage. Thus, even when IV injection is considered to be a necessary lifesaving measure, the methylergonovine infusion is made slowly and with constant monitoring of the patient's blood pressure.

Even though ergonovine and methylergonovine have very little vasoconstrictor activity as compared to other ergot alkaloids, including ergotamine, their use is best avoided in patients with the obliterative type of peripheral vascular diseases. The main danger of overdosage with ergot products is that the patient's peripheral circulation may be severely impaired. Narrowing of the vessels and damage to the inner lining of the arterioles may lead to the formation of blood clots and finally to gangrene of the toes, fingers, and other parts.

Signs and symptoms of accidental ergotism. These are sometimes seen in women who take a prescribed ergot alkaloid for too long a time during the puerperium. Early side-effects to watch for include nausea, vomiting, and complaints of abdominal cramps. Sometimes the patient may have a headache and show signs of confusion. Most serious are signs of circulatory stasis, including itching, tingling, numbness, and cold in the fingers and toes.

Ergot poisoning. This is relatively rare today but may still occur as the result of attempts to produce an abortion with drugs of this type. During the early months of pregnancy the uterus does not react as strongly to ergot alkaloids as do the blood vessels. Thus, the danger of gangrene from overdosage is great when an abortion is rashly attempted by taking large doses of preparations such as the fluidextract, which contains vasoconstrictive alkaloids. Such efforts are misguided at best and are especially dangerous because, in the early months of pregnancy, a woman's blood vessels are much more reactive to these drugs than is her uterus.

There is at present no safe and effective method for inducing pharmacologic contraction of the uterus during the first weeks of pregnancy. Suction curettage is most commonly employed for evacuation of the uterine contents during the first trimester. In the early weeks of the second trimester, saline induction is the method most often used. Now, however, an oxytocic drug of the prostaglandin group is available for intra-amniotic use, and another is employed in the form of a vaginal suppository for abortion and certain related indications.

Abortifacients

Prostaglandins. Drugs of the prostaglandin family have found their first clinical applications in the field of obstetrics and gynecology. Two types of prostaglandins, dinoprost ($PGF_{2\alpha}$) and carboprost, a methylated derivative, and dinoprostone (PGE_2), have been employed experimentally for various purposes and are now approved and available for early termination of pregnancy (Table 23-5).

Dinoprost. This drug is available as *dinoprost tromethamine* and is marketed under the trade name Prostin F_2 alpha), for a single indication—termination of pregnancy in the second trimester, between the 16th and 20th weeks—by a single route of administration—transabdominal intra-amniotic injection.

Therapeutic or elective abortion. The procedure, involving the slow instillation of a dinoprost solution into the amniotic sac by needle or catheter, is at present restricted to specially trained physicians in university medical centers with intensive care and acute surgical services. Actually, however, the need for such services has not proved necessary, except in a few cases in which oxytocin was administered intravenously together with intraamniotic instillation of dinoprost. Because this resulted in perforation of the cervix or rupture of the uterus in some primiparous patients, this combination should be administered with caution (if at all) when the cervix is not yet adequately dilated.

Dinoprost, administered alone, has proved relatively safe and effective as an abortifacient. In about four out of five cases the uterine contents were completely expelled within 24 hours and the remainder aborted within 48 hours, sometimes with the assistance of suction curettage or with hypertonic saline solution administration. Side-effects were mainly gastrointestinal—nausea, vomiting, abdominal cramps, or diarrhea—the result of absorption of dinoprost into the maternal circulation. Caution is required in patients with asthma because of occasional bronchospasm after administration of dinoprost. A history of epilepsy, hypertension, or glaucoma should also suggest the need for caution in employing this procedure.

Dinoprostone. Dinoprostone is currently available as vaginal suppositories under the trade name Prostin E_2. The suppositories have been approved for evacuating the uterine contents in several gynecologic situations, including the production of abortion in the second trimester of pregnancy and the management of missed abortion. In all such cases, the oxytocic action of this prostaglandin product is brought about by inserting the suppositories

Table 23–5. Abortifacients

Official or generic name	Trade name	Usual dosage and administration
Carboprost tromethamine	Prostin/15 M	0.250 mg (250 μg) IM at 1½–3-hr intervals (maximum dose = 12 mg for 2 days)
Dinoprost tromethamine (prostaglandin F₂ alpha)	Prostin F₂ alpha	40 mg (8 ml) by very slow injection into the amniotic sac; later, an additional 10–40 mg (2–8 ml) may be administered if necessary
Dinoprostone (prostaglandin E₂)	Prostin E₂ vaginal suppositories	Insert suppositories high into the vagina; repeat every 3–5 hr until contractions occur
Sodium chloride 20%		250 ml by transabdominal intra-amniotic injection

high in the vaginal vault to stimulate contractions similar to those of normal labor. The process may be repeated every 3 to 5 hours until effective contractions occur.

Therapeutic or elective abortion. This agent is employed to produce abortion from the 12th week of pregnancy through the second trimester. It is successful in terminating pregnancy in about 90% of cases within 30 hours. The abortion induced by the drug is complete in about two-thirds of the patients. In the remaining third the uterine evacuation must be completed by other means. Thus, the suppositories are employed for this purpose only by hospital personnel trained to provide intensive medical and surgical care when required.

Other uses. Intravaginal administration of dinoprostone also achieves complete evacuation of the dead fetus and other products of conception in nearly 90% of cases when it is employed in the management of missed abortion. It is approved for this use up to the 28th week of gestation. In the remaining cases, placental fragments can be removed by suction or gentle curettage without anesthesia.

Dinoprostone suppositories are also employed to set off uterine contractions in patients with benign hydatidiform mole, a nonmetastatic disorder involving the trophoblastic tissues of pregnancy. In these hydatidiform mole cases, even when drug-induced evacuation of the uterus appears to be complete, curettage is performed in all patients to obtain tissue samples for the histopathologic examination required to rule out possible malignancy.

This product cannot be used in the presence of pelvic inflammatory disease or in patients known to be allergic to the prostaglandin. Almost two-thirds of patients vomit at some point during the drug's absorption and about 40% suffer diarrhea, possibly because the systemically absorbed portion of the drug stimulates contractions of gastrointestinal smooth muscle.

Temperature elevations of 2°F or more develop in about half of the patients. Fever develops early and soon disappears. However, it must be differentiated from fever caused by endometritis or infection of the uterus in women carrying a dead fetus. An advantage of the suppository in such cases is that it obviates the need to invade the uterus with instruments, thus reducing the risk of introducing pathogens that might grow in the necrotic tissue.

Carboprost. This methylated prostaglandin (PG) F₂α derivative is the latest PG derivative approved for use as an abortifacient. It has two main advantages over the two drugs described above: it is given intramuscularly, a route that is safer and less difficult than the intraamniotic route required for use of dinoprost; and it can be given in the presence of profuse vaginal bleeding that would expel dinoprostone vaginal suppositories. It is used for terminating pregnancies in the 13th to 20th weeks. Nausea and diarrhea are common, but can be allayed by prophylactic administration of antiemetic and antidiarrheal drugs, which are recommended. Adverse effects, cautions, and contraindications are similar to those for the first two PGs described above. Like dinoprostone, carboprost sometimes causes fever (1.1°C or 2°F elevation in temperature) that must be differentiated from fever of other causes.

Hypertonic saline solution. A 20% solution of sodium chloride (a 0.9% solution is isotonic with body fluids) is sometimes instilled intra-amniotically to induce abortion in the 16th to 22nd weeks of pregnancy. This procedure usually causes fewer adverse effects than the use of prostaglandins, but there is generally a longer interval until induction is complete.

Uterine relaxants

Researchers have long been seeking drugs that would be as dependable for depressing uterine hypermotility as the oxytocic drugs are for stimulating contractile activity. Drugs that could reduce uterine hypertonicity would be useful for preventing premature labor, a common cause of perinatal death, and for relaxing tetanic uterine contractions during abnormal labor. An effective myometrial relaxant might also be helpful for relief of the cramplike pains of dysmenorrhea.

Unfortunately, no drugs are available that selectively depress the uterine musculature. The many drugs that have been tried experimentally are only moderately effective, and the large doses that are required can cause severe side-effects by their actions on other organs and systems. Thus, in practice, the most common means of coping with a threatened miscarriage and for preventing premature labor at term is to order bed rest and central nervous system depressant drugs. The new β_2- adrenergic agonist, ritodrine, can stop premature labor, but it can cause many serious adverse effects (see below).

Although heavy sedation with barbiturates, diazepam, and opiates may lessen uterine motility or even occasionally relax contraction rings in abnormal labor, the main reason for administering sedatives, antianxiety agents, and narcotic analgesics is not to relax the uterus directly but to keep the patient calm.

Ethyl alcohol. This is sometimes administered intravenously for its sedative and analgesic effects, and has also been found to reduce uterine contractions when administered in this way during premature labor. Although alcohol inhibits the secretion of *oxytocin* from the posterior pituitary gland by depressing the hypothalamic nerve cells that control the release of this hormone into the systemic circulation (see Chap. 20), this is probably not its mechanism of action, because oxytocin does not play an important role in the early stages of labor. More likely, it is the direct uterine relaxant effect of alcohol that is responsible for its therapeutic benefit. In addition to causing inebriation, a major disadvantage of alcohol is that it stimulates gastric acid secretion. If general anesthesia is needed for delivery, aspiration of stomach contents is more likely. There is also a great deal of research being done on the effects of alcohol on the fetus. It appears that alcohol ingested at any time during pregnancy can be detrimental to the fetus (perhaps resulting in the fetal alcohol syndrome), and alcohol should be thus avoided during pregnancy.

β-adrenergic receptor stimulants. The uterus contains both α- and β-adrenergic receptors. Stimulation of the β receptors by sympathetic nerve impulses or by sympathomimetic drugs tends to relax the uterine musculature. However, the doses of such adrenergic drugs as *epinephrine* that are required to relax the myometrium produce prohibitive side-effects by their actions on the cardiovascular and central nervous systems. Adrenergic drugs have been introduced for treating bronchial asthma that act more specifically on the β_2-type receptors in smooth muscle than on the β_1 receptors in cardiac muscle. This has led to attempts to use these same drugs and their derivatives for control of the activity of uterine smooth muscle.

One β_2 selective agonist, *ritodrine* (Yutopar), has been approved for use in the United States, and is used abroad, for inhibiting uterine activity in advanced labor and thus preventing premature expulsion of the fetus. Administered by slow intravenous infusion, this drug helps to delay delivery. However, its use requires close patient monitoring: it often causes a moderate to marked increase in the maternal and fetal heart rates and either an increase or a decrease in maternal blood pressure. Central side-effects include jitteriness, apprehension, and tremors. Metabolic effects (decreased serum potassium level, increased glucose level) have also occurred. When given with corticosteroids (to prevent fetal respiratory distress syndrome), ritodrine has caused pulmonary edema and maternal death.

Prostaglandin antagonists. One current theory concerning the mechanism that triggers labor suggests that an increased production of prostaglandin by the muscle cells of the uterus is the cause. Thus, a rational approach to the control of excessive contractions may be the administration of drugs known to inhibit the biosynthesis of prostaglandins. Among such substances are aspirin and certain other anti-inflammatory agents, such as indomethacin and fenoprofen (see Chap. 37).

Aspirin has not been used clinically for reducing the rate of uterine contractions during premature labor. However, it has been noted to do so in patients who had received the prostaglandin dinoprost for terminating a pregnancy (see above). Thus, aspirin should not be used for pain relief during labor. Also contributing to contraindications to its use during pregnancy are aspirin's antiplatelet effects (see Chap. 34), which can cause excessive loss of blood during delivery, and its ability to inhibit the binding of bilirubin, which can cause jaundice or even kernicterus in the infant.

Additional clinical considerations

The availability of legal medical abortions to end pregnancy has decreased the use of oxytocic and ergot drugs to induce abortions. Patients should be urged to seek assistance if abortion is the only acceptable solution for them. If a patient has used an abortifacient, she will need support and understanding to cope with her situation, as well as careful monitoring to evaluate the adverse effects of the drug. If the attempted abortion is unsuccessful the patient will need continued support to deal with the pregnancy, as well as careful counseling to discuss the effects the drug may have had on the fetus and the alternatives available to her.

Several situations constitute contraindications to the use of oxytocics during labor because of the possible risk to the mother or fetus. These situations include the following: cephalopelvic disproportion, abnormal fetal position, abnormal fetal presentation, or fetal distress— all of which could result in fetal injury or even death; premature cervix, primiparous patients over the age of 35 years, multiparous patients, previous cesarean section, history of traumatic delivery, and hypertonic labor—all of which could result in uterine rupture if oxytocic drugs are given. Severe toxemia and *abruptio placentae* are other contraindications. If any of these conditions pertains, or if continual monitoring is not available to evaluate both mother and fetus during drug administration, the oxytocic drugs should not be used during labor and surgical intervention should be considered. The woman who receives an oxytocic drug during labor will need constant support and encouragement. She may become exhausted and frustrated, and will need comfort measures and reassurance. She will also need frequent monitoring, and the fetal and maternal monitoring should be explained to her. Patients who receive oxytocic drugs over a prolonged period are at risk for developing water intoxication. The patient's fluid intake should be monitored and the patient should be monitored for any signs of water intoxication—for example CNS changes, increased blood pressure, nausea.

The delivery room nurse will need to be responsible for the proper timing of administration of the oxytocic drugs following delivery. Before the actual delivery it is advisable to check with the physician or midwife who is attending the delivery so that appropriate preparations can be made.

The ergot derivatives often affect the systemic vasculature, and patients receiving the drugs should be monitored for blood pressure changes as well as for peripheral vasoconstriction and changes in tissue perfusion. Because of their vascular effects, these drugs should not be used in patients with peripheral vascular disease, kidney disease, or hypertension.

Patients undergoing abortions, elective or nonelective, require emotional support and understanding. They should have the opportunity to ventilate their feelings and should be monitored for adverse effects to the drugs used, as well as for common adverse reactions associated with delivery.

Drug–drug interactions. The oxytocic drugs should not be given concurrently with *sympathomimetic pressor amines,* because the pressor effect is potentiated and severe hypertension with serious consequences can occur.

Teaching points to consider with the use of oxytocic drugs are summarized in the patient teaching guide. Patients who receive these drugs are in a clinical situation that requires a great deal of teaching and support; therefore, these points can be incorporated into the overall teaching plan. The guide to the nursing process summarizes clinical considerations in the care of patients receiving oxytocic drugs.

Patient teaching guide: oxytocic drugs

Administration:	Route and rate: IV, IM, or PO
Reason for use:	Induce labor Improve labor Prevent postpartum bleeding
Reactions to expect:	Nature of contractions Continued contractions postdelivery Peripheral "tingling" or "cold"
Monitoring to anticipate and the frequency of monitoring:	Maternal: BP, P, uterine contractions, uterine tone, bleeding Fetal: heart rate, activity

Guide to the nursing process: oxytocic drugs

Assessment	Nursing diagnoses	Intervention	Evaluation
Past history (*contraindications*) • Cephalopelvic disproportion • Abnormal fetal position • Abnormal fetal presentation • Fetal distress • Premature cervix • Primipara over 35 years old • Multipara • Previous cesarean section • Previous traumatic delivery • Hypertonic labor • Renal disease • Toxemia • *Abruptio placentae* • Peripheral vascular disease • Hypertension *Allergies:* these drugs; others Medications: *cautions*—sympathomimetic amines **Physical assessment** Neurologic: affect, orientation Cardiovascular: BP, P, ECG (if appropriate), perfusion Respiratory: R, adventitious sounds GI: nausea Genitourinary: uterine contractions—tone, timing; bladder tone	Potential alteration in comfort: pain Potential alteration in tissue perfusion Potential fluid volume excess Potential ineffective coping Knowledge deficit regarding drug and monitoring	Proper and accurate administration of drug Provision of comfort measures Provision of support, encouragement, and reassurance Patient teaching regarding drug and monitoring Provision of emergency support and surgical preparation, if needed	Monitor effects of drug: • Uterine contractions • Uterine tone • Fetal status Monitor for adverse effects: • BP • GI status • Fetal changes • Water intoxication Evaluate comfort measures being used Evaluate support, encouragement, and reassurance being given Evaluate patient teaching protocol Evaluate effectiveness of emergency support, if needed

Summary of clinical indications for estrogens and progestins

Estrogens

Menopause: relief of *vasomotor symptoms* of moderate to severe degree

Postmenopausal osteoporosis, atrophic vaginitis, and kraurosis vulvae

Abnormal uterine bleeding caused by estrogen deficiency

Female hypogonadism, or hypogenitalism, to bring about maturation of secondary sex organs and other bodily changes

Amenorrhea, primary and secondary

Postpartum breast engorgement: to suppress lactation and reduce discomfort

Mammary carcinoma: in women more than 5 years postmenopausal with progressing disease not treatable by surgery or x-ray

Prostatic carcinoma: when castration has failed or is not feasible

Contraception, including postcoital pregnancy prevention

Prevention of excessive growth in height

Control of acne and hirsutism in females with excessive androgen secretion

Progesterone and progestins*

Contraception

Abnormal uterine bleeding

Amenorrhea, primary and secondary

Dysmenorrhea

Endometriosis

Premenstrual tension

Habitual and threatened abortion

Premature labor

Diagnostic test for evaluating ovarian capacity to produce endogenous estrogen

Infertility with luteal phase efficiency

Endometrial carcinoma, advanced metastatic adenocarcinoma

* Some of the indications listed do not have FDA approval at the present time—for example, use in treating threatened abortion.

Summary of clinical indications for the use of oxytocic and abortifacient drugs

Oxytocin

Induction of labor at term in selected cases—for example:

1. Maternal problems: diabetes, preeclampsia; premature rupture of membranes; postterm pregnancy
2. Fetal problems: Rh incompatibility

Uterine inertia in selected cases of arrested labor

Postpartum hemorrhage and uterine atony

Incomplete abortion management to control postabortal bleeding after spontaneous or therapeutic abortion

Expulsion of the placenta in management and control of the third stage of labor

Facilitation of *breastfeeding* (by its galactokinetic action)

Ergonovine and methylergonovine

Prevention of postpartum hemorrhage and uterine atony after delivery of the placenta

Control of postabortal bleeding

To hasten involution of the uterus in cases of puerperal subinvolution

Dinoprost

Termination of pregnancy in the second trimester

Dinoprostone

Evacuation of the uterine contents in the management of abortion, missed abortion, and benign hydatidiform mole

Summary of adverse reactions to estrogens, progestins, and oral contraceptives*

Relatively common side-effects

Nausea, vomiting, abdominal cramps

Breakthrough bleeding or spotting

Breast enlargement and tenderness

Increase in size of uterine fibroid tumors

Headache, including migraine, and dizziness

Mental depression, nervousness, and fatigue

Chloasma (irregular brown spots on skin)

Fluid retention leading to edema and weight gain

(continued)

Relatively rare increased risks

Cervical cancer

Breast cancer

Endometrial carcinoma (in postmenopausal women)

Vaginal adenocarcinoma (in offspring of women treated during pregnancy)

Thromboembolic disorders: thrombophlebitis, pulmonary embolism; cerebral thrombosis or hemorrhage; myocardial infarction; and possibly retinal thrombosis and optic neuritis

Hypertension

Gallbladder disease, and possibly liver tumors with intra-abdominal bleeding

Glucose tolerance impairment

Hypercalcemia (in patients with breast cancer and bone metastases)

Jaundice (especially in patients with a prior history of its occurrence during pregnancy)

Premature bone closure and precocious puberty in children

* Most of the listed adverse effects apply mainly to estrogens. However, the labeling of FDA-approved products containing only progestational steroids lists essentially similar side-effects.

Summary of adverse effects of the oxytocic and abortifacient drugs

All oxytocics: administered under unfavorable obstetric conditions

Tetanic contractions of the uterus can interfere with placental blood flow to the fetus, resulting in fetal distress, hypoxic cardiac irregularities, or asphyxia

Laceration of the cervical tissues and perineum of the mother and trauma to the fetus

Rupture of the fundus of the uterus

Too rapid labor and precipitous delivery may damage the infant's head and cause intracranial hemorrhage

Oxytocin

Severe water intoxication with convulsions and coma following prolonged IV infusion

Premature ventricular contractions (PVCs)

Possible increased blood loss following hypofibrinogenemia or afibrinogenemia

Nausea and vomiting

Ergonovine and methylergonovine

Elevation of blood pressure: usually transient, but possibly extreme and resulting in hypertensive crisis and cerebral hemorrhage in case of injection into a vein

Headache, dizziness, drowsiness, ringing in the ears, sweating

Nausea, vomiting, abdominal cramps, diarrhea

Cardiac palpitations, chest pains, dyspnea

Circulatory changes: itching, tingling, numbness and cold in the fingers and toes, possible thrombophlebitis with necrosis of tissue and gangrene

Dinoprost

Nausea, vomiting, abdominal cramps, diarrhea, bronchospasm, hypertension, tachycardia

Dinoprostone and carboprost

Fever, in addition to effects listed for dinoprost

Case study

Presentation

NN is a 21-year-old nursing student, in excellent health, who is getting married in a few weeks. She has been seen in the gynecologic clinic for a routine exam and to discuss birth control methods available to her. After much thought, NN has decided that the use of oral contraceptives is the best method for her. Ovral-28 has been prescribed for the patient, and she has been referred for patient teaching regarding her drug therapy. What specific points should be covered with this patient?

Discussion

The age and health of the patient probably minimize many potential risks of OC drugs. The patient should be questioned about any family history of breast or genital cancer, and the risks associated with the use of the drug should be explained. The risks of thromboembolic episodes should also be included in the discussion and, if NN smokes cigarettes, it should be recommended that she stop. Because NN is a nursing student, she might find the package insert understandable and useful. She should be encouraged to read it and to ask any questions that she might have about potential risks and effects.

The nurse should discuss the basic action of the drug, not assuming that the patient knows all of this because the patient is a nursing student. The Ovral-28 comes in a dispenser with 21 tablets containing hormones and 7 inert tablets for the withdrawal period. This helps to increase patient compliance, because a tablet is taken every day and the patient doesn't need to keep a schedule. She should be advised to use an additional means of birth control during the first month of therapy. She should take the tablet at the same time each day. If one day is missed, two tablets can be taken the next day. If 2 days are missed, two tablets can be taken daily over the next 2 days. If three tablets are missed, the drug should be stopped and started again as a new cycle in 7 days. It is advisable to use another method of birth control during a cycle with missed doses.

NN should be told that some spotting might occur during the first month of therapy, but after that bleeding should only occur during the withdrawal days. The side-effects and warnings, including drug–drug interactions, should be discussed, and NN should be encouraged to have regular physical examinations to assess the effects of the drug therapy. If NN decides to become pregnant, she should first consult her nurse or physician.

It is best to give NN written instructions to refer to in the future. It should never be assumed that, because she is a nursing student, she doesn't require this information. The level of patient teaching may be different than with other patients, but this patient also has a right and a need to know about the drug and its effects on her body.

Drug digests

Conjugated estrogens USP (Premarin)

Actions and indications. This mixture of esterified natural estrogenic substances offers effective replacement therapy in various disorders marked by a deficiency of natural ovarian estrogens. Its administration during the menopause helps to control various discomforting symptoms, including hot flashes and sweating, heart palpitations, headache, and irritability. It has been recommended for prolonged *post*menopausal maintenance therapy to help protect against various degenerative changes in the aging woman, including senile osteoporosis and atrophic vaginitis.

This preparation may be employed in female hypogonadism to bring about development of the secondary sex characteristics and to promote menstruation in primary amenorrhea. It is also effective in cases of secondary or functional amenorrhea and in the management of dysfunctional uterine bleeding. Conjugated estrogens are employed for symptomatic relief in men with prostatic carcinoma, and in women with mammary carcinoma who are more than 5 years past the menopause.

Adverse effects, cautions, and contraindications (see text and appropriate summaries for fuller statements). Overdosage in women may cause nausea, fullness and tenderness of the breasts, vaginal discharge, and irritability, malaise, or mental depression. Withdrawal bleeding may occasionally be excessive but, more commonly, *under*dosage causes spotting, or breakthrough bleeding, which is overcome by raising the dose. If bleeding continues, curettage may be required. Estrogens are employed to treat uterine bleeding only after ruling out the possibility that the bleeding may have organic causes.

The prolonged administration of estrogens to postmenopausal women is now thought to increase the risk of endometrial cancer, and their use during the menopause may also increase the risk of later development of breast cancer. This drug must not be administered to women with known or suspected genital or breast cancer, and caution is required when there is a family history of mammary carcinoma or in the presence of breast nodules, fibrocystic disease, or abnormal mammograms.

Dosage and administration. Dosage varies with the type of disorder being treated and with the patient's response. In the menopausal syndrome treatment is begun with 1.25 mg. This dose may be adjusted upward if necessary, but it is best to employ the lowest dose that will control symptoms and to discontinue the medication as soon as possible. Control of abnormal bleeding requires 3.5 to 7.5 mg daily, followed by maintenance dosage of 3.5 mg daily for 20 days of each cycle and 1 week without medication. Doses as high as 10 mg three times daily for at least 3 months may be required for relief of symptoms in properly selected postmenopausal women and men with breast cancer, and men with progressing prostatic cancer receive 1.25 to 2.5 mg three times daily.

Diethylstilbestrol USP (DES; Stilbestrol)

Actions and indications. This nonsteroidal synthetic substance produces all the effects of the natural estrogens. It offers effective replacement therapy when women lack ovarian estrogens—for example in the menopause and afterwards, or in senile vaginitis and kraurosis vulvae resulting from estrogen deficiency. It is administered alone or combined with an androgen–anabolic agent to stimulate osteoblastic activity in the bones of women with postmenopausal osteoporosis.

It is also used in the management of mammary cancer in women who are more than 5 years past the menopause, and in men with prostatic carcinoma. DES is employed to suppress lactation and for relief of painfully engorged breasts in postpartum women. Suppositories containing this substance are inserted for relief of itching and other symptoms of senile vaginitis. It has also been administered in large doses as a postcoital contraceptive, but its routine use is not recommended.

Adverse effects, cautions, and contraindications (see text and appropriate summaries for fuller statements). High doses may cause nausea and vomiting, particularly in menopausal women at the start of treatment. Less common gastrointestinal side-effects include abdominal distress and diarrhea. Fluid retention may cause breast tenderness and possibly such symptoms as headache and ir-

ritability. Patients with epilepsy and migraine must be watched for signs of any increase in seizures induced by fluid and electrolyte imbalance. Caution is required in patients with cardiac, kidney, or liver disorders.

Use of this drug is contraindicated in women with known or suspected breast cancer or other estrogen-dependent malignancies, and caution is recommended in those with a strong family history of mammary carcinoma.

This drug must not be administered during pregnancy, because it use in attempts to prevent threatened abortion has led to development of vaginal adenocarcinoma in female offspring who were exposed to it while *in utero*. Like other estrogens, it can be expected to increase the risk of endometrial carcinoma in postmenopausal women and the possibility of breast cancer years after its use during the menopause. Physical examination with

special reference to the breasts and pelvic organs should be performed prior to initiating therapy and periodically thereafter.

Dosage and administration. In the menopause daily oral doses of 0.1 to 1 mg are administered depending on the patient's response, and for other disorders doses of 5 mg may be administered several times daily. Postmenopausal breast cancer patients receive 15 mg daily, while men with prostatic carcinoma can be managed with doses of as little as 1 to 3 mg daily. (Longer acting esters and salts such as the diproprionate and phosphate are available for oral, intramuscular, or intravenous use in large doses for intensive cancer therapy.)

For use as a postcoital contraceptive, the currently recommended dose of DES is 25 mg twice a day for 5 continuous days beginning within 24 hours after exposure and, in any case, not later than 72 hours.

Ergonovine maleate USP (Ergotrate)

Actions and indications. This ergot alkaloid produces prompt and prolonged contraction of the smooth muscle of the uterus. It is administered *only after* delivery of the infant and the placenta and *not* to induce labor *nor during* labor. It is, however, an oxytocic drug of choice for preventing postpartum uterine atony and hemorrhage, and it may also be used to stop postabortal bleeding. Oral doses of this drug are sometimes also used to speed return of the uterus to normal size (that is, to hasten involution) and to reduce possible bleeding and infection during this period.

Adverse effects, cautions, and contraindi-

cations. This drug is not ordinarily administered before the placenta is delivered because the "afterbirth" may become trapped in the persistently contracted uterus, and its use during pregnancy or in the first two stages of labor is always contraindicated. It is not administered to patients with a history of allergic hypersensitivity or idiosyncrasy to ergot derivatives.

This alkaloid causes relatively little constriction of blood vessel smooth muscle as compared to ergotamine. However, its prolonged use is undesirable because of the possibility that particularly sensitive patients may suffer

excessive vasoconstriction and other chronic toxic effects (ergotism). Its use is contraindicated in patients with severe peripheral vascular disease, and caution is required in patients with cardiac disease or hypertension. (The drug occasionally causes elevation of central venous pressure or of arterial blood pressure.)

Dosage and administration. Intramuscular or intravenous injection of 0.2 mg usually controls postpartum bleeding. An additional dose of 0.2 mg to 0.4 mg may be given every 6 to 12 hours for the first 2 days postpartum (or longer) if uterine atony persists.

Estradiol valerate USP (Delestrogen)

Actions and indications. This ester of estradiol produces prolonged estrogenic effects. The fact that injections are required only every 2 or 3 weeks makes this form of the hormone useful for treating cancers such as prostatic carcinoma in men and advanced mammary carcinoma in women who are more than 5 years past the menopause. It is also employed for suppression of lactation and for relief of postpartum engorgement of the breasts. It is recommended for cyclic use with a long-acting progestational preparation in the management of various menstrual cycle disorders and ovarian deficiency syndromes.

Adverse effects, cautions, and contraindications. Patients with prostatic or mammary carcinoma are observed for hypercalcemia, which requires discontinuation of the medication. They are also watched for signs of thromboembolic disorders such as thrombophlebitis and for irregular uterine bleeding. Caution is required in patients with heart, kidney, and liver disease, and in those with epilepsy, migraine, diabetes, or a history of cerebrovascular disease. Men may develop gynecomastia and suffer a loss of libido.

Dosage and administration. This prepration

is injected deep into the upper outer quadrant of the gluteal muscle in doses of 10 mg to 40 mg depending on the condition being treated. A single injection of 10 mg to 25 mg is used for suppressing lactation, while the treatment of prostatic carcinoma requires 30 mg every week or two. For menstrual and ovarian deficiency syndromes, 20 mg is administered alone on the first day of the cycle, and 5 mg is administered 2 weeks later in combination with a long-acting progestational steroid.

Hydroxyprogesterone caproate USP (Delalutin)

Actions and indications. This long-acting ester derivative of a natural progestational substance changes an estrogen-primed proliferative endometrium into the secretory phase. It also inhibits gonadotropic hormone production by the pituitary gland.

These actions account for its main clinical uses: (1) as a test to determine whether or not the patient's own ovaries are producing estrogen; (2) to remove a proliferative endometrium from which abnormal uterine bleeding is occurring ("medical D & C"); (3) to bring about menstruation in primary and

secondary amenorrhea when its action on the endometrium wears off (desquamation of the secretory endometrium); (4) to treat advanced (stage III or IV) uterine adenocarcinoma.

Adverse effects, cautions, and contraindications. Patients with abnormal uterine bleeding must be examined to rule out organic causes such as genital malignancy before beginning treatment. The drug is contraindicated in mammary carcinoma and in patients with liver function impairment. It is also contraindicated in patients who have

or develop signs and symptoms of blood-clotting disorders, including thrombophlebitis, pulmonary embolism, and retinal thrombosis. Although further injections are not made in such cases, the drug may continue to exert for long periods any adverse reaction with which it is associated.

Caution is required in patients in whom progesterone and its derivatives are known to set off migraine headaches, asthmatic attacks, or epileptic seizures, or in whom fluid retention may lead to congestive heart failure.

Dosage and administration. For treating

amenorrhea and abnormal uterine bleeding, 375 mg is injected intramuscularly and repeated cyclically in doses of 250 mg every 4 weeks in alternation with a long-acting estrogen product.

As a test of whether or not endogenous estrogen is being produced by the patient's ovaries, 250 mg is administered IM. If the patient is not pregnant, bleeding that occurs between 1 and 2 weeks after injection indicates that this hormone has converted an estrogen-primed endometrium to a secretory one that is then in the process of being shed.

For uterine adenocarcinoma, 1000 mg is repeated one or more times each week—that is, up to seven times a week. This may be continued for up to 12 weeks in attempts to produce improvement. If relapse occurs after initial improvement, treatment is stopped.

Medroxyprogesterone acetate USP (Amen; Provera)

Actions and indications. This synthetic derivative of progesterone can produce the various effects of the natural hormone and also some androgenic and anabolic effects. It can convert a proliferative endometrium to the secretory state, an action that accounts for its usefulness in control of dysfunctional uterine bleeding and in secondary amenorrhea.

Only the oral dosage form is recommended for treating menstrual disorders. The injectable suspension (Depo-Provera), which produces the same effects on the uterine lining, is recommended for use only in the treatment of endometrial carcinoma that has metastasized and is inoperable. Unlike the usually recommended oral doses, usual doses of the parenteral product interfere with follicular maturation and ovulation. Because of this, it has been employed experimentally to prevent pregnancy for prolonged periods after a single IM injection. However, it does not have FDA approval for this purpose at present.

Adverse effects, cautions, and contraindications. Because of its slight androgenic component, this progestin has occasionally caused acne and hirsutism. This virilizing effect has led to clitoral hypertrophy in infant girls born to mothers treated with medroxyprogesterone during pregnancy. As with all other progestational steroids, its use during the first 4 months of pregnancy is not recommended because of the possibility of other types of congenital damage to the fetus, including cardiac and limb reduction defects. This drug has occasionally caused development of malignant mammary nodules in beagle dogs, but this has not been shown to occur in humans. Nonetheless, its use in women with known or suspected breast (or genital) malignancies is contraindicated. It should also not be used in patients with thromboembolic disorders or cerebral apoplexy (stroke syndrome), and it should be immediately discontinued at the first signs of such disorders. As with other drugs of this class, breakthrough bleeding, edema, mental depression, cholestatic jaundice, and cervical erosion can occur and should be watched for.

Dosage and administration. Oral doses of 5 to 10 mg daily are administered for from 5 to 10 days, beginning at any time in cases of secondary amenorrhea or, in abnormal uterine bleeding, beginning preferably on the calculated 16th day of the menstrual cycle. For treating endometrial carcinoma, doses of 400 mg to 1000 mg are injected initially at weekly intervals. Later, it may be possible to maintain any observed improvement with monthly doses of 400 mg.

Norethindrone USP* (Norlutin)

Actions and indications. This is a potent oral progestin with some estrogenic, androgenic, and anabolic activity. It is combined with either of the two potent estrogens, ethinyl estradiol or mestranol, in many oral contraceptive products. It is also used alone in treating amenorrhea and abnormal uterine bleeding of a functional nature. In these disorders it acts to convert a proliferative endometrium to the secretory phase, and its action is followed on withdrawal by desquamation and menstrual bleeding. Larger doses are employed in the management of endometriosis.

Adverse effects, cautions, and contraindications. Breakthrough bleeding and other menstrual flow changes are common and may require diagnostic tests to rule out organic causes. Patients should also be watched for signs of cervical erosion, fluid retention, thrombosis, and mental depression. Gallbladder disease, benign liver tumors, and hypertension have been reported during use of drugs of this class.

Discontinue if there is sudden loss of vision, severe headache, or signs of serious psychic depression. Do not use in patients with active or past thromboembolic disorders, known or suspected breast cancer, or impaired liver function. Cholestatic jaundice may occur.

Dosage and administration. For amenorrhea or abnormal uterine bleeding, doses of 5 to 20 mg are taken daily from the 5th through the 25th day of the menstrual cycle. In endometriosis, treatment is begun with 10 mg daily and raised gradually to 30 mg. Doses for contraception are 0.35 mg alone, or 0.5 to 2 mg in combination with low doses of estrogens.

Norethindrone acetate and ethinyl estradiol tablets USP (Norlestrin)

Actions and indications. The acetate ester of the progestational steroid norethindrone is used alone in conditions marked by a deficiency of progesterone, including abnormal uterine bleeding, amenorrhea, and endometriosis. Ethinyl estradiol is a potent estrogen employed in management of the menopause and in other conditions for which estrogen therapy is indicated. However, a combination of this type is used mainly as an oral *contraceptive* for prevention of pregnancy. Employed properly in accordance with the recommended course schedule, the progestin–estrogen mixture is close to 100% effective for this purpose.

Adverse effects, cautions, and contraindications. The most common side-effects resemble the discomforts of early pregnancy, such as nausea, vomiting, loss of appetite, and abdominal bloating. These and such other side-effects as headache, dizziness, breast tenderness, and weight gain tend to lessen after the first one or two cyclic courses. Brownish skin blemishes appear occasionally, and some susceptible patients may have a small rise in blood pressure.

Products of this type are contraindicated in patients with thromboembolic disorders, undiagnosed vaginal bleeding, suspected breast or genital cancer, or severely impaired liver function. Patients with a history of heart or kidney disease, diabetes, mental depression, migraine, epilepsy, or asthma are watched closely for any worsening of these disorders during treatment.

Dosage and administration. The combination is taken daily for three weeks (21 days) from day 5 to day 24 of the menstrual cycle. During the final 7 days of the menstrual cycle, the patient takes no pill, or—in some forms—an inert tablet, or one containing therapeutically inactive amounts of an iron salt. Tablets should be taken at a regular time—at bedtime or with a meal.

---

* The acetic acid ester derivative, norethindrone acetate USP, differs only in being twice as potent as norethindrone. Thus, the dosage of the derivative is only half that of the parent compound for all indications.

Oxytocin injection USP (Pitocin; Syntocinon)

Actions and indications. This drug's ability to raise the muscle tone of the uterus and to start contractions or increase their frequency makes it useful in several obstetric situations. These include the following: (1) induction of labor in carefully selected cases; (2) stimulation of slow or arrested labor in cases of true uterine inertia; (3) management of cases of incomplete abortion; and (4) management of the third (placental) stage of labor and of postpartum uterine atony and hemorrhage.

Adverse effects, cautions, and contraindications. Oxytocin should be administered only by trained professional personnel in closely controlled dosage and to carefully selected patients. Too strong stimulation of the uterus may be dangerous to both mother and fetus. Excessive contractions that cause severe spasms may cut off the circulation to the fetus, with resulting hypoxia that causes cardiac irregularities. Rupture of the uterus can occur, especially in patients predisposed to this danger. Thus, the drug is not administered to women with a history of uterine surgery, including cesarean section, or when the uterus is already overdistended. Unlike the natural hormone, synthetic oxytocin does not increase the tone of blood vessel smooth muscle. It may, however, occasionally cause water intoxication because of some small antidiuretic activity.

Dosage and administration. This varies with the particular indication. For control of postpartum hemorrhage, oxytocin is usually administered intramuscularly in a dose of 3 U to 10 U. For induction of labor, 1 ml (10 U) is added to 1 liter of a 5% solution of dextrose and dripped into a vein at a controlled rate—usually 10 to 14 drops/minute initially.

References

Barden TP et al: Ritodrine hydrochloride: A beta-mimetic agent for use in preterm labor. Obstet Gynecol 56:1, 7, 1980

Baum JK et al: Possible association between benign hepatomas and oral contraceptives. Lancet 2:926, 1973

Baxi LV et al: Induction of labor with low-dose prostaglandin F$_{2\alpha}$ and oxytocin. Am J Obstet Gynecol 136:28, 1980

Berczeller PH et al: The therapeutic use of progestational steroids. Clin Pharmacol Ther 5:216, 1964

Boston Collaborative Drug Surveillance Program: Surgically confirmed gallbladder disease, venous thromboembolism and breast tumors in relation to postmenopausal estrogen therapy. N Engl J Med 290:15, 1974

Brengman S, Burns M: Ritodrine hydrochloride and preterm labor. Am J Nurs 83:537, 1983

Chan L, O'Malley BW: The mechanism of action of sex steroid hormones. N Engl J Med 294:1322, 1976

Collaborative Group for the Study of Stroke in Young Women: Oral contraceptives and stroke in young women: Associated risk factors. JAMA 231:718, 1975

Dickerson J: The pill: A closer look. Am J Nurs, 83:1392, 1983

Drill VA: Oral contraceptives: Relation to mammary cancer, benign breast lesions, and cervical cancer. Ann Rev Pharmacol 15:367, 1975

Edmonson HA et al: Liver cell adenomas associated with use of oral contraceptives. N Engl J Med 294:470, 1976

Gambrell RD, Jr: Menopause: benefits and risks of estrogen–progestogen replacement therapy. Fertil Steril 37:457, 1982

Genuth SM: The reproductive glands. In Berne RM, Levy MN (eds): Physiology, pp 1069–1115. St. Louis, CV Mosby, 1983

Goodman HM: Reproduction. In Mountcastle VB (ed): Medical Physiology, 14th ed, pp 1602–1637. St. Louis, CV Mosby, 1980

Greenwald P, et al: Vaginal cancer after maternal treatment with synthetic estrogens. N Engl J Med, 285:390, 1971

Grimes DA et al: Midtrimester abortion by intraamniotic prostaglandin F$_{2\alpha}$: Safer than saline? Obstet Gynecol 49:612, 1977

Herbst AD et al: Adenocarcinoma of the vagina. Association of maternal stilbestrol therapy with tumor appearance in young women. N Engl J Med 284:878, 1971

Herbst AD et al: Prenatal exposure to stilbestrol. A prospective comparison of exposed female offspring with unexposed controls. N Engl J Med 292:334, 1975

Hulka BS et al: Predominance of early endometrial cancers after long-term estrogen use. JAMA 244:2419, 1980

Hulka BS et al: Protection against endometrial carcinoma by combination-product oral contraceptives. JAMA 247:475, 1982

Inman WHW et al: Thromboembolic disease and the steroidal content of oral contraceptives. Br Med J 2:241, 1970

Kaplan NM: Clinical complications of oral contraceptives. Adv Int Med 20:197, 1975

Knab DR: Estrogen and endometrial cancer. Obstet Gynecol Surv 32:267, 1977

Lauersen NH: Inhibition of premature labor: Multicenter comparison of ritodrine and ethanol. Am J Obstet Gynecol, 127:837, 1977

Lauersen NH et al: Management of intrauterine fetal death with prostaglandin F$_{2\alpha}$ vaginal suppositories. Am J Obstet Gynecol 137:753, 1980

Lindsay R et al: Long-term prevention of osteoporosis by estrogen. Lancet 1:1038, 1976

Mack TM et al: Estrogens and endometrial cancer in a retirement community. N Engl J Med 294:1262, 1976

Mann JI, Inman WHW: Oral contraceptives and death from myocardial infarction. Br Med J 2:245, 1975

Marx JL: Estrogen drugs: Do they increase the risk of cancer? Science 191:838, 1976

Mays EI et al: Hepatic changes in young women ingesting contraceptive steroids. JAMA 235:730, 1976

Moir JC: The present day use of ergot. Can Med Assoc J 72:727, 1955

Murad F, Haynes RC Jr: Estrogens and progestins. In Gilman AG, Goodman LS, Gilman A (eds): Goodman

& Gilman's The Pharmacological Basis of Therapeutics, 6th ed, pp. 1420–1447. New York, Macmillan, 1980

Oral contraceptives and the risk of cardiovascular disease. Med Lett Drugs Ther 25:69, 1983

Rall TW, Schleifer LS: Oxytocin, prostaglandins, ergot alkaloids, and other agents. In Gilman AG, Goodman LS, Gilman A (eds): Goodman & Gilman's The Pharmacological Basis of Therapeutics, 6th ed, pp 935–950. New York, Macmillan, 1980

Rice–Wray E et al: Return of ovulation after discontinuance of oral contraceptive. Fertil Steril 18:212, 1976

Rodman MJ: What we now know about oral contraceptives. RN 42:133 (Sept), 1979

Rosenberg L et al: Myocardial infarction and estrogen therapy in postmenopausal women. N Engl J Med 294:1256, 1976

Smith DC et al: Association of exogenous estrogen and endometrial cancer. N Engl J Med 293:1164, 1975

Smith ED: Women's Health Care: A Guide for Patient Education. New York, Appleton–Century–Crofts, 1981

Utian WH: Current status of menopause and postmenopausal estrogen therapy. Obstet Gynecol Surv 32:193, 1977

Visscher RD et al: Guidelines for elective induction of labor with oral prostaglandin E_2. Obstet Gynecol 49:15, 1977

Weiss NS, Sayvetz TA: Incidence of endometrial cancer in relation to oral contraceptives. N Engl J Med 302:551, 1980

Wentz AC: Assessment of estrogen and progestin therapy in gynecology and obstetrics. Clin Obstet Gynecol 20:461, 1977

Ziel HK, Finkle WD: Increased risk of endometrial carcinoma among users of conjugated estrogens. N Engl J Med 293:1167, 1975

Chapter 24

Hormones and drugs affecting the male reproductive system

24

The male sex hormone

The male sex glands, or testes, secrete a hormone called *testosterone;* it is also secreted to a lesser extent by the adrenal glands. This substance is responsible for the development and maintenance of the male sex organs and secondary sex characteristics. Even primitive peoples were well aware that castration (removal of the testes) at an early age was accompanied by the loss of male physical features. It is now felt that, once a male has passed puberty, the adrenal androgens are sufficient to maintain the secondary sex characteristics associated with "maleness," although castration will cause a loss of fertility and libido. The extraction and purification of the testicular hormone and the preparation of more potent, longer acting derivatives for use in therapy did not occur until earlier in this century.

Now available for use in treating men and boys who lack the natural hormone are several esters, including *testosterone cypionate*[+], that have a much more prolonged action when injected than testosterone itself. Also available are *fluoxymesterone*[+] and other synthetic substances that are effective when taken by mouth—unlike the natural hormone, which is largely destroyed in the liver after oral ingestion. However, all the available substances with male sexual (*androgenic*) activity and with tissue-building (*anabolic*) effects on metabolism are essentially similar to the testicular hormone in their physiologic effects. Thus, the physiology of the male hormone will be reviewed before discussing its use in therapeutics.

Physiology

Regulation of androgen secretion

The production of testosterone is not cyclical like the production of the female sex hormones. The production of testosterone is regulated by a negative feedback system involving the pituitary gonadotropic hormones, the hypothalamic gonadotropin-releasing hormone (GnRH), and the testicular hormones testosterone and estrogen (Fig. 24-1).

The hypothalamus, under the influence of other areas of the central nervous system, releases GnRH into the hypothalamoadenohypophyseal portal system. GnRH stimulates the pituitary to release follicle-stimulating hormone (FSH) and luteinizing hormone (LH). In the male LH is often referred to as ICSH, or interstitial cell-stimulating hormone. These hormones are carried by the systemic circulation to their target organs, the testes.

In the testes, FSH stimulates spermatogonia in the seminiferous tubules to become spermatozoa (sperm) in a process called *spermatogenesis.* FSH also stimulates the *Sertoli cells* in the seminiferous tubules to secrete estrogens that feed back negatively onto the pituitary and hypothalamus, causing a decrease in the release of GnRH, FSH, and LH. This decreases spermatogenesis and estrogen production, which then allows an increase in FSH and LH again. The Sertoli cells produce another substance, *inhibin,* which also acts on the pituitary to decrease FSH production and thus decrease spermatogenesis. Through the production and interaction of the substances described above, the body maintains a relatively constant production of sperm.

LH, on the other hand, acts not on cells of the seminiferous tubules but on the *Leydig* or *interstitial cells* of the testes (Fig. 24-1). It stimulates these cells to produce testosterone, which, like the estrogens from the Sertoli cells, negatively feeds back onto the hypothalamus and pituitary. High levels of testosterone decrease the release of LH (and FSH), which eventually leads to decreased testosterone secretion. This allows an increase in FSH and LH levels, spermatogenesis, and production of testosterone and estrogens.

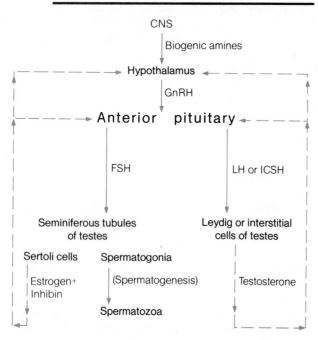

CNS

Biogenic amines

Hypothalamus

GnRH

Anterior pituitary

FSH

LH or ICSH

Seminiferous tubules
of testes

Leydig or interstitial
cells of testes

Sertoli cells

Spermatogonia

Estrogen+
Inhibin

(Spermatogenesis)

Testosterone

Spermatozoa

Figure 24-1. The interaction of hypothalamic, pituitary, and testicular hormones in the male. (*Solid arrows:* stimulatory effects; *dashed arrows:* inhibitory effects and negative feedback)

As in the female, puberty in the male is thought to occur when the hypothalamus matures enough to lose its sensitivity to low levels of circulating testosterone and estrogens. It ceases to be inhibited by these low hormonal levels and releases enough GnRH to stimulate the anterior pituitary to produce FSH and LH, which stimulate the testes to function as described above and as shown in Figure 24-1.

Males do not experience the extensive cyclical variations in reproductive hormone levels that females experience. After puberty, the circulating levels of male sex hormones remain relatively constant. However, recent research has found some convincing evidence that levels of male sex hormones may undergo slight seasonal fluctuations. These fluctuations may be mediated by the pineal gland, which in turn is influenced through the visual system by changing levels and durations of light and darkness. Further research may eventually lead to changes in the concepts of regulation of the male sex hormone and of male sexual function.

Physiologic functions of testosterone

The functions of testosterone may be broadly classified as *sexual* and *metabolic.* These actions become dramatically evident at puberty when previously suppressed gonadotropic hormones are released in large amounts on a signal from the hypothalamus. The outpouring of testosterone that follows such gonadotropic stimulation of the boy's testes produces effects of the two types (sexual and metabolic) on all the tissues of the body. That is, the testicular secretions act as a growth hormone not only to the sex organs but also to such structures as the skeletal muscles and the bones. The skin and hair are also affected, and protein metabolism in general is stimulated, so that dietary nitrogen is retained in the tissues in larger amounts (an *anabolic* action).

Sexual function. The accessory sex organs—the penis, prostate gland, seminal vesicles, and vas deferens—grow in size and functional capacity under the influence of pubertal testosterone. The testosterone that is secreted into the circulation and transported to these target tissues enters their cells and is bound by protein receptors in the cytoplasm. It is then reduced by an enzyme-catalyzed reaction to dihydrotestosterone (DHT), which is the active form of the hormone. The protein-bound DHT is then moved to the cell nucleus where it activates enzymes that increase the synthesis of RNA and, as a result, of cellular protein. These steps that precede the actions of testosterone take time. Thus, a therapeutic response to exogenous testosterone will also take time. A patient who is receiving testosterone for therapeutic reasons will have to be assessed over time for the effectiveness of the drug.

The testes themselves grow in size, as does the scrotal sac in which they are contained. The seminiferous tubules of the testes share in this growth, and, under the combined influence of testosterone and FSH, spermatogenesis begins. Sperm production is maintained throughout the man's reproductive life by the balanced effects of these testicular and pituitary hormones. Oddly, oligospermia, or low sperm counts, can result from either too little or too much testosterone. In the latter case, too much testosterone shuts off pituitary secretion of the FSH needed to maintain seminiferous tubule function.

The *secondary sex characteristics* of the male also make their appearance at puberty under the influence of testosterone. At this time, the boy's high-pitched voice deepens as his vocal cords thicken under the influence of this hormone. Hair begins to grow, not only in the axillary and pubic areas, but also on the arms, legs, and trunk. Interestingly, some young people predisposed to baldness by heredity begin to show the first signs of future loss of hair at this time. Apparently, testosterone plays a part in producing so-called male pattern baldness. Facial hair makes its first appearance at this time, and the beard continues to come in gradually over the next few years. Testosterone also stimulates the skin's sebaceous glands to grow in size and secretory capacity. This plays a part in the pathogenesis of acne, a condition very common in adolescence.

Metabolic function. The greater growth of the male's skeletal structures is also attributable to testosterone. This hormone somehow stimulates tissue-building processes by aiding retention of the dietary protein nitrogen needed for formation of the amino acids from which new muscle is built. At the same time, less nitrogen is lost from the pool of chemical fragments formed in the constant breakdown of body tissues. This hormone-regulated combination of increased anabolism and decreased catabolism of protein helps to produce the larger, more powerful muscles of the male.

The boy's bones also begin to grow in thickness and in length. However, after stimulating a sudden spurt of growth at puberty, this action of testosterone finally puts an end to any further growth in height. This happens because the hormone converts the cartilaginous tissues at the ends of the long bones (the *epiphyses*) into bone. The shafts of the limb bones can then no longer lengthen.

Testosterone is also responsible for the thick, rough skin of the male, and for the prominent veins. It may also account for firmer, tighter cartilage that gives the characteristic male gait. Much research has been done in an attempt to correlate testosterone levels with aggressive or hostile behavior, felt to be "male" characteristics. No conclusive results have been documented.

The male climacteric. This condition is caused by testicular (Leydig cell) failure and is analogous to the menopause in women, which is the result of ovarian failure. Some symptoms—hot flashes, heart palpitations, and other vasomotor effects, nervous irritability, or fretting over minor matters, failure of concentration and memory, and insomnia—are also somewhat similar. However, these are often so vague and subjective that some authorities feel that the condition is psychogenic rather than the result of an endocrine imbalance stemming from testicular failure. Reviewing the physiologic activities of testosterone demonstrates the range of problems that can occur when testosterone levels fall: a loss of muscle mass, a weakening of joints and ligaments, a thinning of the skin, a loss of body and facial hair, and possible CNS effects, such as irritability. These signs and symptoms may all be seen in aging male patients. These patients can be helped to cope with this phase in their lives through education, support, and understanding.

Testosterone preparations and derivatives

Testosterone itself is rapidly metabolized when injected intramuscularly as an aqueous or oily solution. Because various esters of testosterone are absorbed more slowly from tissue depots, and thus have a more prolonged duration of action, they are usually preferred for the long-term replacement therapy that ordinarily is necessary.

The propionic acid ester, testosterone propionate, is administered in an oily solution that is absorbed at a moderately slow, steady rate that produces hormonal effects for a period of 2 or 3 days. Testosterone cypionate and testosterone enanthate (Table 24-1) are much longer lasting in their hormonal activity, and the oily solutions of these esters need be given only once every 1 to 6 weeks for replacement therapy and other purposes.

Testosterone's action can be still further extended by implanting pellets subcutaneously. This can be done quickly and conveniently by the use of a special injector, or a small incision may be made in the skin and a pocket prepared in the underlying tissues, into which the pellet is placed. In either procedure the skin is cleansed with iodine and alcohol, and aseptic precautions are employed. Depending on the number of pellets employed, the procedure need not be repeated for from 2 to 6 months. The number of pellets that are needed is established first by oral or parenteral administration.

Although testosterone is absorbed when taken by mouth, the hormone is largely destroyed in the liver after absorption from the upper gastrointestinal tract. Thus, it and its derivative *methyltestosterone* are best given by the buccal route for greater effectiveness. Patients are advised not to chew or swallow the tablets, which are intended to be absorbed through the oral mucous membranes between the gum and the cheek. They are also told not to eat, drink, or smoke while the tablets are in place. The synthetic androgen *fluoxymesterone* (Halotestin) is, however, fully effective when swallowed in tablet form.

Therapeutic uses of the androgens

Androgen therapy in men

Testosterone and its derivatives are used in medicine mainly as replacement therapy in males who lack the hormone. Such hypogonadism may become apparent at puberty when the boy fails to develop normally, or it may occur in men at some time after the masculinizing changes of adolescence have taken place. **Eunuchism,** as a result of castration before puberty, and *eunuchoidism,* from either prepubertal or postpubertal testicular failure, are forms of hypogonadism that can be successfully treated with testosterone replacement therapy.

Disorders

Eunuchoidism. Male hypogonadism may result from a primary defect of the testes, or it may occur secondary to a defect in the hypothalamus or in the anterior pituitary gland. At present, the best way to treat both the primary and secondary types of eunuchoidism is by replacement therapy with androgenic hormones. However, the more precise diagnosis of those hypogonadism cases that stem from a lack of pituitary gonadotropins can now be made, and experimental treatments for such cases of secondary, or hypogonadotropic, hypogonadism are available for use in certain selected patients (see below).

Delayed puberty. Puberty in boys begins at about the age of 11 years, and pubertal changes become readily apparent by the age of 13 years. Sometimes, however, the onset of such changes fails to occur because of diseases

Table 24–1. Androgenic and anabolic agents*

Official or generic name	Trade name	Usual adult dosage and administration
Preparations used mainly for their androgenic effects		
Calusterone	Methosarb	50 mg qid oral for advanced breast carcinoma in selected female patients
Fluoxymesterone USP	Halotestin; Ora-Testryl	Oral, 2–10 mg
Methyltestosterone USP	Metandren; Oreton Methyl	Buccal, 5–40 mg; oral, 10–80 mg
Testolactone USP	Teslac	250 mg qid oral or 100 mg three times/wk IM for advanced breast carcinoma in selected female patients
Testosterone (in aqueous suspension)	Andro 100; Android-T; Histerone; Testaqua; Testoject	IM, 10–50 mg daily or three times/wk
Testosterone pellets	Oreton	Two to six pellets (each 75 mg) SC q 3–4 months after dosage is established by oral or parenteral administration
Testosterone cypionate in oil USP	Depo-Testosterone	IM, 100–400 mg every 1–6 wk
Testosterone enanthate in oil USP	Delatestryl	IM, 100–400 mg every 1–6 wk
Testosterone phenylacetate USP	Perandren Phenylacetate	IM, 50 mg
Testosterone propionate in oil USP	Testex	IM, 10–50 mg daily or three times/wk
Preparations used mainly for their anabolic effects		
Dromostanolone propionate USP	Drolban	100 mg three times/wk for advanced breast carcinoma in selected female patients
Ethylestrenol	Maxibolin	4–8 mg/day oral
Methandriol	Anabol; Andriol; Durabolic	IM, 10–40 mg/day (aqueous) or 50–100 mg once or twice a week (oil preparation)
Nandrolone decanoate USP	Deca-Durabolin	IM, 50–100 mg every 3 or 4 wk
Nandrolone phenpropionate USP	Durabolin	IM, 25–50 mg once weekly

(continued)

Table 24–1. Androgenic and anabolic agents* (continued)

Official or generic name	Trade name	Usual adult dosage and administration
Oxandrolone USP	Anavar	5–20 mg/day oral in two to four divided doses
Oxymetholone USP	Anadrol	1–5 mg/kg/body weight/day oral
Stanozolol USP	Winstrol	2 mg oral tid

* See also Table 12–1.

of the testes that make them unresponsive to the gonadotropins that are being secreted by the anterior pituitary gland, or because the brain's "biologic clock" that ordinarily triggers such pituitary secretions (Chap. 20) has failed to function properly.

When the defect is primarily in failure of the testes to respond, diagnostic tests will show that the level of testosterone in the plasma is very low despite high blood levels of the gonadotropic hormone LH. On the other hand, when hypogonadism occurs secondary to a failure of the hypothalamic–hypophyseal trigger mechanism, or possibly because of the presence of a hypothalamic or pituitary gland tumor, plasma testosterone and LH levels are *both* very low. At present, such *hypogonadotropic* hypogonadism in young men 20 years of age or older is treated in the same way as are cases of eunuchoidism that are caused by testicular dysfunction.

The effects of male hormone replacement therapy on the young patient's physical and psychic development are often truly dramatic. Administered in doses and intervals intended to imitate the natural rate of testicular hormone secretion, these preparations almost literally make a man of the boy. Some of these changes—in height, depth of voice, size of sex organs, and pattern of hair distribution, for example—are permanent. However, hypogonadal patients must continue to receive hormone replacement therapy indefinitely to maintain muscular strength, physical vigor, and libido or sex drive. In addition, the administration of testosterone alone does not produce spermatogenesis in patients with disease-damaged testicular germinal tissues.

In theory, the sexual maturation of boys in whom the onset of puberty is delayed because of some defect in hypothalamic function rather than by failure of diseased testes to respond can be brought about by treatment with a hypothalamic hormone or by substances with gonadotropic activity. Thus, for example, cases of hypogonadotropic eunuchoidism have been treated experimentally with the GnRH (Chap. 20) of the hypothalamus. A larger

number have been treated with *human chorionic gonadotropin* (HCG; Chap. 20), which has LH, or ICSH, activity on the cells of Leydig that leads to production of endogenous testosterone. Occasionally, to provide FSH-type activity, *menotropins* (HMG; Pergonal) is added to the HCG regimen, as described below in the discussion of the management of male infertility. However, because of the expense and inconvenience of maintaining sexual maturation with these gonadotropic hormones, teen-aged patients are all eventually switched to a regimen of androgen replacement therapy.

Postpubertal hypogonadism. Men who have experienced a natural puberty resulting in normal sexual development sometimes later have signs or symptoms of hypogonadism because of diseases that lead to pituitary or testicular failure. The resulting androgen deficiency does not cause regression to the prepubertal stage. However, certain secondary sex characteristics may be altered and there is often a loss of libido and of sexual potency.

Androgen replacement therapy is the preferred treatment of postpubertal hypogonadal patients, particularly because treatment need not be as intensive as it is with young eunuchs or eunuchoid boys. These patients, whose primary and secondary sex characteristics had been previously established during a natural pubertal period, can often be maintained on relatively low oral doses of androgens rather than by repeated parenteral administration of testosterone esters. The use of gonadotropic therapy is reserved for those hypogonadotropic hypogonadal males in whom it is thought desirable to attempt restoration of fertility, at least temporarily (see below).

Impotence. Treatment with testosterone as described above is of value in only a small minority of men who complain of failure to achieve and maintain an erection. In over 90% of cases the cause is functional rather than organic. However, hormone replacement therapy for hypothyroidism, diabetes mellitus, and other endocrine causes of impotence may sometimes prove helpful, as can specific treatment for genitourinary, vascular, and nervous system diseases that can lead to impotence. In addition, a complete drug history may be helpful. Many autonomic, antihypertensive, and CNS drugs can cause sexual dysfunction. One recent study found medication to be the most common cause of impotence. However, when no underlying physical condition or medication-related cause can be found, psychotherapy, rather than treatment with testosterone or other drugs, is the preferred method of management. Patients may also be referred to a clinic that deals exclusively with problems of sexual maladjustment, now recognized as among the most common causes of impotence.

Male infertility. In more than half of all couples who want a child but fail to conceive, the cause is a defect in the man's reproductive system. Failure to form large numbers of motile sperm is not usually the result of an endocrine imbalance. *Azoospermia,* a lack of live sperm in the semen, stems mainly from blockage in the vas deferens or in other parts of the ductal system. Such obstructions and the presence of varicoceles are treated surgically, if possible, rather than with hormones. Occasionally, however, *oligospermia,* a deficiency of viable, motile sperm in the semen, may respond to treatment with testosterone or with gonadotropins. (This condition may also be caused by drugs—for example, the sulfonamide, sulfasalazine.)

Testosterone alone has been employed to treat oligospermia with occasional success in properly selected patients. Actually, testosterone tends to suppress spermatogenesis by inhibiting the secretion of the pituitary gonadotropin FSH. However, when testosterone is withdrawn at the end of a course of treatment, there is sometimes a *rebound* rise in the sperm counts. This is thought to occur because the testosterone-induced suppression of spermatogenesis has given the germinal tissues time to rest and become more responsive to stimulation by the pituitary gonadotropin when the hypothalamus was released from the temporary feedback inhibition by testosterone.

Testosterone therapy of male infertility is not effective when abnormal spermatogenesis results from fibrosis following damage to the germinal and peritubular tissues. Even when the germinal epithelium is normal, testosterone alone cannot ordinarily stimulate the production of complete spermatogenesis in men with hypogonadotropic hypogonadism. In some such cases, combinations of the same gonadotropins that have been employed successfully in *female* infertility (Chap. 20) have also been tried in men. The patients are first treated with a course of HCG for several months. Then menotropins is added to the regimen for its FSH effects. Although fertility has been reported to follow this experimental regimen, the treatment is expensive and time-consuming and the results have varied widely and unpredictably in different patients.

Cryptorchidism. As indicated in Chapter 20, undescended testicle is a condition caused by either an obstruction of the inguinal canal or a lack of testosterone. In the latter case, it is customary to treat the boy with a course of HCG injections. Even if this LH-like containing substance fails to stimulate enough secretion of endogenous testosterone by the Leydig cells to let the testes descend from the abdomen into the scrotum, it helps to facilitate the surgery that may be required later. If, instead, testosterone from an outside source is used, the dosage must be regulated very carefully to avoid precipitating premature puberty in the youngster. As when HCG is used in such patients, the sex hormone may cause too early development of accessory sex structures and secondary sex characteristics.

Male contraception. Various substances are now known that can inhibit spermatogenesis and thus interfere with male fertility. The practical employment of such compounds seemed limited by their potential toxicity or by the fact that they often interfered with the desirable physiologic effects of testosterone. At present, several approaches that attempt to overcome these drawbacks appear promising, and research efforts are being pursued that some authorities think will result in effective male contraceptive products within the next decade.

One type of approach involves the combined administration of testosterone or one of its derivatives with small amounts of a progestin or an estrogen in the form of a rubber–silicone capsule implant, from which the natural hormones are slowly released. The female sex hormones are intended to suppress secretion of the gonadotropin FSH without exerting effects on other tissues of the man, while the male hormone helps to support his accessory sex organ tissues.

A substance called inhibin, isolated from Sertoli cells (see above), is claimed to be able to block sperm production by inhibiting FSH without interfering with pituitary production of the other gonadotropin LH, which is responsible for stimulating testicular secretion of testosterone. It may be possible to synthesize this substance and make it available for routine use as a contraceptive. Certain derivatives of testosterone have also been synthesized that are claimed to be able to suppress sperm production without inducing other potential adverse effects of the prolonged use of testosterone itself.

Adverse effects and precautions

In addition to the possibility of producing precocious puberty in prepubertal boys and masculinizing effects in females (see below), androgen administration can have potentially harmful effects in adult men (see summary at the end of this chapter). Before treating patients for prolonged periods with testosterone or with other androgenic compounds, it is important to rule out the presence of prostate gland growths, which are not uncommon in men of late middle age. By hormone treatment, the already hypertrophied gland might be stimulated to grow more rapidly and thus interfere with voiding of the urinary bladder. Similarly, such men are examined frequently during treatment to detect any signs of possible prostatic carcinoma, because such a hormone-dependent neoplasm might grow rapidly and metastasize.

There are other adverse effects of excessive amounts of testosterone that must be guarded against:

1. A steroid-induced retention of salty fluids, which may tend to raise the patient's blood pressure or send a person with previous cardiovascular difficulties into congestive heart failure
2. Psychological and physical changes, including a tremendous increase in libido. Both these reactions, including increased sex drive, are unlikely with carefully regulated replacement therapy

Androgen therapy in women

Gynecologic disorders. Women are sometimes treated with the male hormone for two reasons: it antagonizes the effects of excessive amounts of estrogens; and it suppresses the secretion of pituitary gonadotropic hormones. These effects sometimes help to control uterine bleeding and relieve dysmenorrhea, premenstrual tension, and postpartum breast engorgement. However, it is now preferable to use oral estrogen–progestogen combinations for treating these gynecologic conditions (Chap. 23).

Metastatic mammary carcinoma (see also Chap. 12). Cancer of the breast that has spread beyond the reach of surgery or radiation therapy is a condition in which large doses of androgens are sometimes administered to women. The symptomatic relief sometimes obtained in such cases is occasionally accompanied by masculinizing effects. Thus, these patients are watched for early signs, such as growth of facial hair and development of acne. Withdrawal of hormone treatment results in clearing of these skin symptoms and prevents permanent signs of virilization, such as deepening of the voice and clitoral enlargement. The patient is often willing to endure such virilizing effects to obtain the feeling of well-being and the relief of pain that hormone treatment often offers.

Hypercalcemia. Cancer patients being treated with the male hormone are also watched for signs and symptoms of hypercalcemia. This condition requires prompt withdrawal of androgen therapy and the forcing of fluids to avoid formation of kidney stones. Because the action of the long-acting esters still in the intramuscular depots cannot be turned off, these forms of the hormone can cause hypercalcemia that continues even after their further administration is stopped. Thus, the short-acting ester, *testosterone propionate,* is often preferred for treating cancer patients. *Fluoxymesterone* and certain other synthetic derivatives are also claimed to be less likely to cause hypercalcemia in cancer patients or to

produce masculinizing effects in women (see the summary at the end of this chapter).

Anemia. Androgens and the less masculinizing anabolic agents discussed below are now sometimes employed to treat certain severe anemias in women (as well as in men and children). Among patients treated with these nonspecific stimulants of erythropoiesis are patients with acquired or congenital hemolytic and aplastic anemias, cancer patients under treatment with antineoplastic drugs that suppress bone marrow function, and patients with chronic renal failure who are undergoing frequent maintenance hemodialysis treatments.

These androgenic and anabolic hormones are believed to act by stimulating the kidneys to produce erythropoietin. However, because even bilaterally nephrectomized patients respond to some extent, it is thought that these substances may also have a direct stimulating effect on the bone marrow or that they may act on extrarenal sites of erythropoietin production that respond to androgenic anabolic therapy. In any case, patients who continue to be treated for 3 months or more often show a rise in the hematocrit level—a significant rise in red cell mass over the pretreatment levels.

Although the use of these hormones lessens the need for frequent blood transfusions and the risk of hepatitis, the drugs can themselves sometimes cause liver damage and other adverse effects. Patients must be watched for signs of cholestatic jaundice, which would require withdrawal of those androgens with a chemical structure that could cause this form of hepatitis. To avoid virilizing effects in women and children, dosage should be individualized at the lowest level needed to bring about a bone marrow response. Anabolic agents such as nandrolone are now preferred to testosterone for this purpose.

Actions and therapeutic uses of anabolic agents

It is often desirable to stimulate the flagging appetites of debilitated patients and to reverse the processes responsible for protein wastage and subsequent weight loss. When it was found that testosterone possessed anabolic activity that could produce positive nitrogen balance in patients who were in negative nitrogen balance, physicians tried administering the hormone to them. Although it often brought a return of appetite and a feeling of well-being, the hormone's sexual effects limited its usefulness for women and children and caused mental and physical changes undesirable even in men.

Chemists have tried to modify the testosterone molecule in attempts to devise compounds free of sexual effects, yet able to stimulate muscle growth and strength in the manner of the hormone. Several synthetic anabolic steroids are available (Table 24-1) that can increase protein anabolism when administered in doses that are less likely to cause undesired masculinizing activity than are doses of testosterone that cause comparable anabolic activity. However, a complete separation of the sexual effects from the anabolic effects has not yet been achieved. Thus, patients taking any of these drugs must be watched for possible development of virilizing and other toxic effects of testosterone. Hepatic carcinoma, and impotence and azoospermia that outlast drug therapy, are among these adverse effects.

Clinical uses

The clinical uses of these anabolic steroids with reduced androgenic activity are potentially quite varied. These substances might prove useful in any of many conditions marked by inadequate protein biosynthesis or by excessive protein breakdown. However, it has been hard to prove that patients actually do better on these drugs, which tend to stimulate the appetite, than they would by simply eating a diet adequate in proteins and other food factors. This difficulty, as well as the possibility of causing undesired side-effects, particularly in women and children, has limited the acceptance of these agents.

Patients being treated with *corticosteroid drugs* sometimes receive adjunctive anabolic steroids. The catabolic, or protein breakdown, effects of the corticosteroids are especially dangerous for patients with arthritis who are confined to bed or inactive. These patients are subject to osteoporosis resulting from disease of their limbs. Like elderly patients with senile osteoporosis, they may suffer bone fractures as a result of calcium loss from the protein matrix of osseous structures. Administration of anabolic steroids in such cases is said to help prevent osteoporosis.

Convalescent patients sometimes receive a course of treatment with an anabolic agent. Patients who have suffered the stress of surgery or other trauma are often in negative nitrogen balance. Administration of anabolic agents in such cases or in patients who have suffered fractures, deep extensive burns, or weakening virus infections such as influenza sometimes helps to retain nitrogenous compounds that would otherwise be lost to the body, and to convert them into the amino acids from which new tissues are built. Here too, however, it has been hard to prove that patients actually recover more rapidly than they would with good nursing care and an adequate diet only.

Some patients with wasting diseases such as tuberculosis and cancer are claimed to benefit from the protein-building action of these drugs. They cannot, of course, be used in patients with prostatic carcinoma, because the retained androgenic component, although less potent than that of testosterone, may be sufficient to stimulate the growth and spread of the hormone-dependent cancer.

Children whose growth is retarded or who eat poorly and are weak and anemic may sometimes respond to small doses of these drugs. However, most physicians do not lightly undertake such therapy, because children may be especially sensitive to the androgenic component in all these drugs. This could, of course, have adverse effects on the child's ability to achieve full height. That is, an initial increase in weight and a spurt in growth might be bought at the expense of early closure of the epiphyses.

To avoid this, the physician may consult an authority on growth and development before beginning treatment with anabolic drugs. Then, in the intervals between courses, the ends of the long bones are examined by x-ray to detect any early changes that might indicate the start of premature ossification that could keep the child from further growth. The child is also watched for signs of premature puberty, which would require withdrawal of the anabolic agents.

As indicated above, these substances may stimulate production of erythrocytes by the bone marrow when administered in doses that are less likely than testosterone to produce undesirable masculinizing effects. Thus, some patients with *refractory anemias*—renal failure and cancer patients or those with aplastic anemia and other blood disorders that do not respond readily to treatment with iron alone, or B-complex vitamins such as folic acid and vitamin B_{12}—sometimes recover when maintained on anabolic steroids for from 3 to 5 months.

Perhaps further research in this field will succeed in entirely separating the sexual from the metabolic effects of these compounds. Such drugs could then be used with greater safety in children, women with senile or disuse-type osteoporosis, and men debilitated by metastatic prostate cancer.

Additional clinical considerations

The androgens and anabolic agents must be used with caution because of their varied and potentially dangerous systemic effects. The prostatic growth that they can cause poses a potentially serious problem for patients with prostatic cancer or with known prostatic hypertrophy. This is a particular concern with geriatric patients, who have an increased risk of both these prostatic conditions. These drugs need to be used with caution in diabetic patients because the androgens and anabolic agents alter the patient's glucose tolerance. A diabetic patient who is given one of these drugs will need to be monitored closely to adjust insulin dosage or the dosage of oral hypoglycemic agents appropriately. Because liver dysfunction and liver cancer have been reported with these drugs, they should be used very cautiously in patients with any hepatic dysfunction or abnormal liver function test results. Patients on long-term therapy should have their liver function monitored on a regular basis. The male hormones cause an increase in serum cholesterol levels, and thus should be used with caution in any patient with a known history of coronary artery disease. The edema and changes in serum electrolyte levels that occur with these drugs can precipitate congestive heart failure in compromised patients with heart or kidney disease. The use of these drugs is contraindicated in pregnancy because of their proven teratogenic effects. Because no data are available on the safety of the use of male hormones during lactation, they should be avoided during lactation.

Many adverse effects of these drugs can be predicted by reviewing the effects described earlier in this chapter. Patients need to know what to anticipate with these drugs. Women or prepubertal boys who receive these hormones may experience dramatic side-effects. They will need extensive teaching, support, and encouragement to cope with the change in body image. The patient teaching guide summarizes the key points to include in a teaching program for these patients. The guide to the nursing process summarizes the clinical aspects of the nursing care of a patient on anabolic steroids or androgens.

Drug–drug interactions

The concomitant use of the male hormones and *adrenal steroids* or *adrenocorticotropic hormone* (ACTH) can cause edema and the complications that it will precipitate. The *oral anticoagulants* will need to be given at lower than normal doses if given with the male hormones. *Insulin* and *oral hypoglycemic agents* may need to be given in lower dosage to a patient on these drugs because of the body's changing glucose tolerance.

Drug–laboratory test interactions

Patients receiving anabolic steroids or androgens may show changes in the following laboratory tests: *glucose tolerance, blood coagulation,* and *thyroid and liver function* tests.

Patient teaching guide: androgens and anabolic agents

The drug that has been prescribed for you belongs to a class of drugs called androgens or male hormones. The properties of this drug are similar to those of the male sex hormones. Because the drug has widespread effects, there are often many side-effects associated with its use. Your drug has been prescribed to treat _____ .

Instructions:

1. The name of your drug is _____ .

2. The dosage of your drug is _____ .

3. Your drug should be taken _____ times a day. The best time to take your drug is _____ . If your stomach is upset after taking the drug, you can take it with a snack or with meals.

4. Some side-effects of the drug that you should be aware of include the following:

GI upset, nausea, vomiting	Taking the drug with meals usually helps; if this persists discuss it with your nurse or physician.
Acne	This is an effect of the hormone; meticulous face washing and avoidance of oily foods may help.
Increase in facial hair; decrease in head hair	Again, these are hormonal effects; if these occur and cause great concern, discuss the effects with your nurse or physician.
Menstrual irregularities (women)	Report any problems to your nurse or physician; irregular and abnormal periods can be expected;

(continued)

	if you suspect that you are pregnant, however, notify your nurse or physician at once.
Weight gain, increased muscle development	Again, these are common effects of the drug.
Changes in sex drive	This can be distressing or difficult to adjust to; discussing your feelings about this drug effect can be helpful.

5. Tell any physician, nurse, or dentist who is taking care of you that you are on this drug.

6. Keep this and all medications out of the reach of children.

7. Take this medication only as directed. Do not lend this medication to others, or take similar medication from anyone else.

Notify your nurse or physician if any of the following occur:

> Swelling in legs, fingers
> Continual erection
> Uncontrollable sex drive
> Yellowing skin
> Fever, chills, rash
> Chest pain or difficulty in breathing
> Hoarseness, baldness, facial hair
> (women)

Guide to the nursing process: androgens and anabolic agents

Assessment	Nursing diagnoses	Intervention	Evaluation
Past history (*contraindications*): Prostatic hypertrophy Prostatic cancer Male breast cancer Coronary artery disease Diabetes Hepatic dysfunction Renal disease Pregnancy Lactation *Allergies:* these drugs; tartrazine—certain	Potential alteration in cardiac output Potential ineffective coping Potential excess fluid volume Knowledge deficit regarding drug therapy Potential alteration in self-concept Potential sexual dysfunction	Safe preparation and administration of drug Patient teaching regarding: Drug Side-effects Cautions Warning Support and encouragement to cope with side-effects of drug	Monitor effectiveness of drug therapy Monitor side-effects of drug: • ↑ male sex characteristics • Liver function tests • Electrolyte level changes • Edema • Glucose tolerance changes • Serum Ca^{2+} levels (women)

(continued)

Assessment	Nursing diagnoses	Intervention	Evaluation
preparations; others; reactions Medication history (*cautions*): Insulin Oral hypoglycemics Oral anticoagulants ACTH Adrenal steroids **Physical assessment** Neurologic: affect, reflexes, muscle tone Cardiovascular: BP, P, auscultation, ECG—if appropriate, perfusion Respiratory: adventitious sounds GI: liver function tests Genitourinary: prostatic exam, genital evaluation Skin: texture, hair distribution Laboratory tests (for long-term therapy): CBC Serum electrolyte levels Coagulation factors Ca^{2+} in women with breast cancer			• Sexual changes • Prostatic changes Monitor for drug–drug interactions: ↑ effect of insulin ↑ effect of oral hypoglycemics ↑ effect of oral anticoagulants ↑ edema with ACTH, adrenal steroids Monitor for drug-induced alterations in laboratory tests of: Thyroid function Blood clotting Glucose tolerance Evaluate effectiveness of patient teaching program Evaluate effectiveness of support and encouragement

Summary of clinical indications for the use of androgens and anabolic agents

Male patients

Male hypogonadism (eunuchism and eunuchoidism). Eunuchism: complete functional failure of the testes (prepubertal, or in surgically castrated adult men)

Eunuchoidism: partial *primary* testicular failure caused by diseases affecting the testes directly (*e.g.*, following severe mumps, orchitis, or trauma); also *secondary* to a deficiency of gonadotropin as a result of pituitary or hypothalamic disease (*e.g.*, pituitary tumor or insufficiency, following head injuries)

Oligospermia. Discontinuing male hormone administration may result in rebound recovery of spermatozoa production

Cryptorchism. Undescended testicle may move from the abdomen under the influence of testosterone administered from an outside source or produced endogenously by the patient's testes following stimulation with human chorionic gonadotropin (HCG)

Anemias. Caused by defective production of erythrocytes by the bone marrow of patients with renal failure who are undergoing regular hemodialysis treatment; also in the treatment of aplastic and hemolytic anemias and for patients with bone marrow suppression caused by antineoplastic drugs

Osteoporosis. Of the senile type or occurring during long-term treatment of inactive rheumatoid arthritis patients with corticosteroid drugs

(continued)

Female patients

Metastatic mammary carcinoma. Relief of pain and discomfort of advanced inoperative breast cancer between 1 and 5 years postmenopausal

Gynecologic disorders. Menorrhagia, metrorrhagia, dysmenorrhea, premenstrual tension; also for suppression of postpartum breast engorgement

Negative nitrogen balance

In convalescence following surgical operations, severe injuries, burns, or infections

During chronic illnesses marked by tissue wastage (*e.g.,* tuberculosis, carcinosis)

In children with dwarfism or other forms of retarded growth, weakness, or anemia

Summary of adverse effects of androgens and anabolic agents

Virilizing (masculinizing) effects
Adult men

Chronic priapism (persistent erections)
Increased libido (excessive sex drive)
Oligospermia
Prostate growth

Prepubertal boys

Precocious puberty
Premature closure of the epiphyses

Adult women

Hirsutism (growth of facial hair)
Acne: secondary to increased sebaceous gland growth and secretion
Baldness: male pattern—hair recedes at temples, thins at crown

Clitoral enlargement
Hoarseness (deepening of voice)
Menstrual irregularities, amenorrhea
Increased libido

Cardiovascular–renal effects

Edema: secondary to steroid-induced sodium and water retention

Other effects

Hypercalcemia: in advanced breast cancer
Cholestatic hepatitis*
Jaundice*
Liver function test abnormalities*

* This does *not* occur with testosterone and its esters but may develop during treatment with *methyl*testosterone and certain synthetic androgens with a particular chemical structure.

Case study

Presentation

KS is a senior nursing student who has recently become engaged to a college senior. He is training as a javelin thrower and hopes to be in the Olympics. KS has noticed that her fiancé has been suffering from chronic gastrointestinal upset for about 3 weeks and more recently has developed tremors and muscle cramps. KS at first suspected that her fiancé was suffering from a viral infection but, as his symptoms continued, she became concerned. When KS tried to persuade her fiancé to see a physician in the university health service, he admitted to her that he had begun taking anabolic steroids to help develop his muscles and increase his athletic prowess. He told KS that his friend, who gave him the drugs, told him to expect stomach upset. He now refuses to seek medical advice because he knows that the use of such drugs is not permitted in athletic competition, yet he feels that using these drugs for a period of time will help him to reach his goal. KS accepts her fiancé's decision, but is still upset about his symptoms and has come to the university health service to discuss the effects of these drugs with the nurse. What does KS need to know about the use of anabolic steroids and the effects of these drugs?

Discussion

KS is obviously concerned about her fiancé's welfare, but doesn't feel secure in her knowledge or her position to discuss this with him. It is important to assure KS of the confidentiality of the discussion and to allow her the opportunity to discuss her feelings and the approaches she might take in discussing her concerns with her fiancé. KS should be taught about the effects and potential dangers of the anabolic steroids. First, it is important for her to know that there is no evidence that these drugs improve athletic ability. The drugs do cause an increase in muscle development, to an extent, as a result of their anabolic activity. Body builders, weight lifters, and other athletes in competition have reportedly used these drugs to increase muscle mass more rapidly in attempts to increase their athletic ability. At the Olympic Games, athletes are routinely screened to ensure that they are not using these drugs. Use of anabolic steroids is illegal in most competitive amateur sports. The use of these drugs can also be quite dangerous, especially if used in dosages that are not within the established safe range. Potential adverse effects include GI problems—nausea, vomiting, and abdominal pain; hepatotoxicity and liver cancer; insomnia; chills; muscle tremors; acne; oligospermia, impotence; baldness; gynecomastia; bladder irritability; electrolyte imbalances involving sodium, potassium, chloride, calcium, and phosphate ions, and the resulting acid–base and neuromuscular disturbances. These can be distressing and potentially serious problems for anyone, and many of them can interfere with athletic ability and concentration.

Ideally, KS should discuss the risks and problems of these drugs with her fiancé. Because he is receiving the drugs from a friend and not from a medical professional, he is at greater risk of developing toxic effects from improper dosage. Knowing how important this man's goals for the Olympics are, and understanding the relatively insecure position of a new fiancé, the nurse should be aware that KS will need a great deal of support and encouragement to deal with this situation. KS may be able to point out to her fiancé that he is already experiencing some adverse effects of the drug, and she may be able to use this fact to explain the further complications that could develop, and how they could adversely affect his athletic ability. KS should be encouraged to discuss her feelings and the approaches to use with her fiancé, and to seek out further support as needed.

Drug digests

Fluoxymesterone USP (Halotestin; Ora-Testryl)

Actions and indications. This synthetic derivative of testosterone exerts the androgenic and anabolic effects of the male hormone when taken by mouth. Although less potent than the longer acting testosterone esters, it is effective as replacement therapy in various disorders marked by a deficiency or complete absence of natural male hormone. In primary eunuchism and eunuchoidism, for example, its actions bring about maturation of the accessory sex organs in prepubertal boys and prevent atrophic changes in castrated men. It is also effective for counteracting symptoms of hypogonadism that are secondary to pituitary gland disorders and those symptoms of the male climacteric that stem from a deficiency of the male hormone.

In women, its main use is in the management of metastatic breast cancer of a type that has been proved to be hormone-dependent by the patient's previous beneficial response to removal or destruction of her ovaries. In such cases, it is administered only to women who are at least 1 year past the menopause and still less than 5 years postmenopausal.

Adverse effects, cautions, and contraindications. Virilizing changes in men, boys, women, and the fetus are the main undesired effects. Men may develop persistent erections (chronic priapism) but at the same time show reduced sperm production (oligospermia). Boys may show signs of premature pubertal changes in their sex organs and secondary sex characteristics. They must be watched for signs of skeletal system maturation, because this requires discontinuation of the drug to prevent premature stopping of their growth in height. Women may develop a deep voice, growth of hair on the face, and menstrual irregularities. The sex organs of the female fetus may show signs of masculinization.

This drug is contraindicated in men with carcinoma of the prostate and even in those with benign prostatic enlargement. It is also contraindicated in patients with severe nephrosis or nephritis and severe heart and liver disease. Patients with milder forms of these disorders must be treated cautiously to avoid edema and jaundice development.

Dosage and administration. For eunuchoid male patients, a daily oral dosage of 2 mg to 5 mg is employed and occasionally raised cautiously to as high as 10 mg. Prepubertal boys are begun on doses of 2 mg daily, which may be increased gradually if necessary and if studies of skeletal development during rest periods show no excessive bone maturation. Women with advanced breast cancer may receive as much as 20 to 30 mg daily in several divided doses.

Testosterone cypionate USP (Depo-Testosterone Cypionate)

Actions and indications. This ester of testosterone produces prolonged androgenic–anabolic effects. Single intramuscular doses administered to eunuchoid males and to others deficient in the male hormone have masculinizing effects for from 2 to 4 weeks. It is one of the preferred forms of testosterone for initiating and maintaining development of the accessory sex organs and secondary sexual characteristics in hypogonadal males. It is also used for symptomatic relief of the male climacteric, when such symptoms are the result of androgen deficiency.

Although testosterone tends to suppress sperm production, this ester has been tried in the treatment of oligospermia in subfertile men on the assumption that rebound spermatogenesis may occur when it is discontinued and its effects wear off. It may be useful in the management of senile osteoporosis in both men and women when administered for its adjunctive anabolic effects to patients who are receiving an adequate diet.

Adverse effects, cautions, and contraindications. Adult men may develop chronic priapism as a result of excessive dosage, together with suppression of sperm production and other testicular functions. Caution is required in prepubertal boys to avoid precocious development of the accessory sex organs and characteristics, and to avoid premature closure of the epiphyses with re-

sulting reduction in adult height. Women may show such signs of masculinization as deepening of the voice (which is irreversible), growth of facial hair, male pattern baldness, amenorrhea or other menstrual irregularities, and other physical and mental signs of virilization, which tend to disappear when the drug is discontinued.

Elderly patients with cardiac or renal disorders should be watched for signs of fluid retention. Bedridden patients and women with metastatic breast cancer should be monitored for signs of hypercalcemia, which requires the treatment to be discontinued. (Shorter acting forms of compounds with male hormone activity are preferred because

of the persisting effects of this long-acting compound even after its withdrawal.)

This compound is contraindicated in pregnancy because of its possible masculinizing effects on the female fetus. It is also contraindicated in patients with carcinoma of the prostate and in those with cancer of the male breast.

Dosage and administration. The most common dosage regimen is the intramuscular administration of 100 to 400 mg every 3 or 4 weeks. For oligospermia, 200 mg may be administered weekly for 6 to 10 weeks and further injections stopped to permit rebound of the suppressed spermatogenic function of the testes.

References

Alexander MR: Use of androgens in chronic renal failure patients on maintenance hemodialysis. Am J Hosp Pharm 33:242, 1976

Drugs that cause sexual dysfunction. Med Lett Drugs Ther 22:108, 1980; 25:73, 1983

Genuth SM: The reproductive glands. In Berne RM, Levy MN (eds): Physiology, pp 1069–1115. St. Louis, CV Mosby, 1983

Goodman HM: Reproduction. In Mountcastle VB (ed): Medical Physiology, 14th ed, pp 1602–1631. St. Louis, CV Mosby, 1980

Lipsett MB: Physiology and pathology of the Leydig cell. N Engl J Med 303:682, 1980

Murad F, Haynes RC Jr: Androgens and anabolic steroids. In Gilman AG, Goodman LS, Gilman A (eds): Goodman and Gilman's The Pharmacological Basis of Therapeutics, 6th edition, pp 1448–1465. New York, Macmillan, 1980

Rodman MJ: The male sex hormone and anabolic steroids. RN 30:41, 1967

Segal S: Male fertility control studies: An editorial comment. Contraception 8:173, 1978

Shahadi NT: Anabolic androgenic hormones. Am J Med 62:546, 1977

Von Hartitzich B et al: Androgens in the anemia of chronic renal failure. Nephron 18:13, 1977

Wilson JD, Griffin JE: Use and misuse of androgens. Metabolism 29:1278, 1980

Chapter 25

Drugs
used
in diabetes

Diabetes mellitus

Diabetes is the most common of all the metabolic diseases. About three million Americans are known diabetics, and an estimated two million more have not yet come to medical attention. The number of diabetics is expected to double as more people live to middle and old age, during which four out of five cases are first recognized.

Diabetes is characterized by complex disturbances in intermediary metabolism. The most prominent sign of such metabolic abnormalities is *hyperglycemia* (fasting sugar levels of over 110 mg/100 ml of venous blood) and *glycosuria* (the presence of any sugar in the urine). However, despite this focusing of attention on sugar (the Latin *mellitus* means honeyed), diabetes mellitus is a disease not only of carbohydrate metabolism but also of protein and fat metabolism. In fact, even though screening tests and diagnostic techniques for detecting diabetes are based on finding evidence of defects in carbohydrate metabolism, the most dangerous of both the acute and chronic complications of diabetes are the result of abnormalities in fat and protein chemistry that follow from the diabetic's altered carbohydrate metabolism.

Most authorities believe that the altered intermediary metabolism of diabetics accounts for the complications that commonly occur late in the course of the disease. These long-term effects of the disease, which are related to changes in both large and small blood vessels, are responsible for the higher than normal rates of disability and death. Thus, for example, diabetic retinopathy is one of the major causes of blindness, and renal vascular disease—diabetic nephropathy—is a frequent cause of fatal kidney failure. The accelerated development of atherosclerosis that occurs in diabetics accounts for the high incidence of peripheral, cerebral, and coronary vascular disease. Ischemic heart disease—like kidney vessel disease—is more common than in nondiabetics, and myocardial infarction is now the leading cause of death in diabetics.

Insulin and diabetes

The metabolic abnormalities of diabetes stem from a lack of effective insulin activity. Insulin is a hormone secreted into the bloodstream by one of the endocrine portions of the pancreas. These are the so-called β (beta) cells located in tiny islets of tissue scattered through the rest of the pancreas, an organ that also produces exocrine digestive juices (the Latin *insula* means island).

The relationship between the pancreas and carbohydrate metabolism was first recognized late in the last century, when dogs whose pancreases had been surgically removed developed diabeteslike signs. In 1922, the Canadian scientists Banting and Best gave an extract of pancreatic islet tissue to a boy dying of diabetes. His dramatic recovery demonstrated the ability of insulin to correct the metabolic abnormality responsible for this severe illness.

Later, insulin was prepared in pure crystalline form from extracts of the pancreatic tissues of animals. This led to its use as replacement therapy in patients with diabetes mellitus whose pancreatic β cells failed to secrete enough active insulin. Before discussing the use of insulin in diabetes, the physiologic functions of this hormone will be discussed, as well as the metabolic abnormalities that develop when its actions are lacking.

The role of insulin in regulating metabolism

Body cells burn fragments of digested foodstuffs to produce energy. The products of the digestion of carbohydrates, fats, and proteins must first be absorbed into the blood from the intestine. They are then transported to the tissues and released into the extracellular fluids and, finally, they make their way through the membranes of all the various tissue cells. Only after it gets inside the cell can a molecule of a substance such as glucose enter the metabolic mill—the series of enzymatically catalyzed intracellular oxidation–reduction reactions—and be converted into sources of energy.

The insulin released by the β cells of the pancreas during the digestion of a meal and during the absorption of the products of digestion plays an important role in intermediary metabolism. That is, this hormone participates at several points in the series of complex intracellular biochemical reactions that convert glucose, lipids, and amino acids into glycogen, fat, and protein. The storage forms of carbohydrates and other metabolic fuels can be quickly reconverted to glucose and fatty acids when the cells require more energy.

The main stimulus for the secretion of insulin is a rise in the level of glucose as it enters the blood. The release of insulin is brought about by glucose molecules binding to glucoreceptors on the membranes of pancreatic β cells. Similarly, insulin itself binds to specific receptors on the membranes of muscle and other target cells. This activates transport mechanisms for carrying glucose and other products of digestion into the cells. Insulin then also seems to activate a so-called second messenger, which is somehow involved in the cellular synthesis of glycogen and fat from glucose and of proteins from amino acids.

Metabolic abnormalities in insulin deficiency

An absolute or a relative lack of insulin activity is the main reason for the development of the metabolic abnormalities of diabetes. The use of radioimmune assays able to detect extremely minute amounts of circulating hormones has helped to explain differences in the development and course of the disease among diabetics. A minority (10%–15%) of patients—mostly those with *juvenile-onset* diabetes, now more accurately called type I or insulin-dependent diabetes mellitus (IDDM), the type that leads to development of signs and symptoms during childhood or youth—fails to show any rise in plasma insulin levels after eating a carbohydrate-containing meal. Most diabetics—mainly those with *maturity-onset* diabetes, now more accurately called type II, or noninsulin-dependent diabetes (NIDDM), which usually is manifested after the age of 40 years—still can produce and release insulin. However, in these people, the secretion of insulin in response to rising blood glucose levels is abnormally delayed.

The course and severity of the disease varies in these two types of diabetics. In those with juvenile-onset diabetes, the disease develops suddenly and sometimes explosively. They are quick to develop such acute complications as diabetic ketoacidosis (see below), and the incidence of complications that occur after 15 or 20 years is very high: over 90% develop nephropathy, retinopathy, and nervous or circulatory system, skin, and other dis-

orders. These insulin-dependent patients always require insulin from an outside source to replace that which their pancreatic β cells cannot biosynthesize.

In the 85% to 90% of patients whose disease develops in later life, insulin is not routinely required for control of diabetes symptoms. Episodes of ketosis rarely occur. Most such patients are overweight or even obese, and their diabetes can usually be kept under control when they lose weight and then adhere to an individually prescribed diet. The rest often respond when drugs that can stimulate their still functioning β cells to secrete insulin more rapidly are added to their dietary regimen.

Despite these differences in onset and severity of symptoms, prognosis, and treatment, both types of diabetics can develop similar metabolic abnormalities as a result of an insufficiency of insulin and the influence of other hormones that exert diabetogenic effects when insulin is lacking. Hyperglycemia, the most prominent sign of deranged metabolism, occurs because glucose is not taken up from the extracellular fluids and stored in the cells as glycogen. In fact, there is not only an underuse of glucose but an increase in its production from glycogen in muscle and liver cells that then release it into the circulation.

Decreased insulin activity can also lead to lipolysis, the mobilization of free fatty acids (FFA) from fat stored in adipocytes. Hyperlipemia, increased levels of circulating FFA, probably plays a role in development of vascular damage over a prolonged period. The more immediate effect in many patients is development of ketosis because of cellular oxidation of fatty acids instead of glucose in the absence of insulin.

The burning of FFA in various body tissues produces large amounts of energy rapidly, but the waste products of fat metabolism in the liver are not removed as readily as those produced when glucose alone is being metabolized to carbon dioxide and water by way of the Krebs tricarboxylic acid cycle. Instead, as a result of oxidation of fatty acids, the ketoacid acetoacetic acid and its by-product β-hydroxybutyric acid and acetone, are formed. Some of these ketone bodies are metabolized in the muscle tissue, but the accumulation of excess ketones in the blood that occurs when insulin is lacking leads also to development of ketosis and acidosis.

The lack of insulin also results in the breakdown of muscle proteins and an inability of the released amino acids to pass into liver cells for protein synthesis. Some of these amino acids are converted to glucose—a further cause of hyperglycemia. In addition, there is a rise in production of the nitrogenous waste products urea and ammonia. Their excretion in the urine leads to azoturia in some patients with inadequately controlled diabetes.

In the absence of adequate insulin activity, other hormones that play roles opposing that of insulin in regulating intermediary metabolism tend to exert unopposed actions that are diabetogenic. Thus, for example, *glucagon*, a hormone produced by the α (alpha) cells of the pancreas, causes hyperglycemia by actions that increase glucose production from liver glycogen and other sources. The *growth hormone* of the pituitary gland also increases glucose production while decreasing the cellular uptake and use of glucose by its anti-insulin action. Adrenal gland *glucocorticoids* and *catecholamines* also tend to increase blood glucose levels.

Signs and symptoms of diabetes

The onset of acute diabetes in a person who had previously shown no overt signs may be slow and insidious, or it may occur with dramatic suddenness. At one extreme, the patient may complain only of being chronically tired; at the other, the first sign may be a swift slide into diabetic coma. People with only mild diabetes may have no specific signs and symptoms of this disorder. Their condition is often diagnosed during a clinical workup, which includes a detailed history and laboratory studies of blood and urine in addition to the physical examination. Most often the diagnosis is made on the basis of the laboratory findings. These include a possible elevation of the fasting blood glucose level and of the sugar level in the urine, or an abnormality of the person's responses to glucose tolerance tests. Most type II or maturity onset diabetics who are obese show a delayed but adequate rise in plasma levels of insulin in response to a glucose challenge when insulin is measured by radioimmune assay.

In general, however, acute diabetes of moderate severity is marked by a classic clinical picture. It is essential that those providing primary care be alert to early symptoms of diabetes. Older people, especially, require vigilance, particularly if their family history shows the disease. Prompt referral for diagnosis and therapy is necessary.

In addition to feelings of fatigue and complaints of pruritus (itching of the skin and genital area), the patient may become aware of being excessively thirsty (polydipsia) and hungry. These symptoms persist even when the patient drinks large amounts of fluid and eats heavily (polyphagia). Weight loss is common in young patients; obesity frequently occurs in older ones. The patient produces large amounts of urine (polyuria), which tests reveal to be loaded with sugar (glycosuria) and, often, with acetone or other ketones (ketonuria). Blood tests also reveal high glucose and ketone levels.

All these features of this phase of diabetes can be explained in terms of the underlying metabolic defect. The hyperglycemia, as indicated, stems from the lack of effective insulin for shunting blood glucose into muscle cells, adipose tissues, and liver glycogen. The polyuria and glycosuria develop when the amount of sugar filtered by the glomeruli of the kidneys is greater than the renal tubules can reabsorb. Because the sugar dissolved in the tubular fluid drags water along with it by osmotic action as it drains out into the ureters, the diabetic patient tends to become dehydrated and to develop a hyperosmolar state. The polydipsia is a response to the loss of water, and the polyphagia is a response to the cellular starvation, because cells are not getting the glucose they require for metabolism.

Diabetic ketoacidosis and coma

This acute complication resulting from a lack of insulin is most dangerous. It occurs most frequently in youngsters with juvenile-onset or type I diabetes—that is, diabetes diagnosed between birth and about the age of 20 years. However, older people, in whom so-called maturity-onset or type II diabetes usually manifests itself after the age of 40 years in a relatively mild form, sometimes go suddenly from an asymptomatic state into a comatose one, which may be the first sign of their disturbed diabetic-type intermediary metabolism. In such cases, this severe syndrome may be set off by an extremely stressful situation, such as surgery, physical injury, or infection. (More commonly, elderly patients become comatose as a result of entering a hyperosmolar state without ever developing ketoacidosis—that is, they develop *nonketotic* coma.)

The derangements of intermediate metabolism that contribute to the development of ketoacidosis in patients with poorly controlled diabetes have been described above. The complex metabolic processes are initiated when the patient's insulin lack and consequent failure to use glucose leads to the breakdown of tissue proteins and fats for use as fuel. The fatty acids formed in this way flood the liver with metabolic fragments that are converted to ketones. When these pile up to levels higher than the tissues can handle by burning for energy, they accumulate in the blood and are carried to the kidneys for excretion in the urine. Some are also carried to the lungs for elimination, and account for the fruity odor on the patient's breath. Other ketoacids are excreted by the kidneys combined with bicarbonate, sodium, and potassium ions. This reduces the body's alkaline reserves and leads to a loss of fluids and electrolytes that may send the dehydrated patient into shock. The patient's respiratory center is at first stimulated (Kussmaul-type hyperpnea) and then depressed. Finally, the higher brain centers are depressed and coma and death ensue unless adequate insulin is administered and other supportive measures are taken.

Insulin in the treatment of diabetes

Indications

The injection of insulin is the most important measure in the management of diabetes. All patients whose condition cannot be adequately controlled by diet and weight reduction must receive properly adjusted doses of insulin, unless various complications make its use impractical. In some such cases, oral hypoglycemic agents can be substituted for insulin.

Specific clinical situations in which the use of insulin is required include the following:

1. All cases of juvenile-onset or type I (IDDM) diabetes and those underweight maturity-onset or type II diabetic patients who fail to secrete adequate insulin in response to a carbohydrate challenge
2. Patients who are hyperglycemic and are thought likely to become ketotic when subjected to surgery or during such other stressful situations as severe infections, or following injury
3. Pregnant hyperglycemic patients
4. Patients with maturity-onset or type II diabetes who fail to respond to a regimen of diet supplemented by oral hypoglycemics
5. All patients who present with such acute diabetic complications as ketoacidosis, lactic acidosis, or the hyperosmolar state—both during coma and before or after that clinical condition has developed

Preparations

Various forms of insulin are available for use in different clinical situations (Table 25-1). Some, such as *regular insulin*[+], are rapid in onset and relatively short in duration of action. Others exert very long-lasting effects following a single subcutaneous injection. A third group of preparations produces effects intermediate between these two extremes. Increasing use is apparently being made of the latter preparations—for example, *isophane insulin suspension* (NPH insulin) and *insulin zinc suspension*[+] (lente insulin)—while the use of the longest lasting preparations such as *protamine zinc insulin suspension*[+] appears to be declining.

Insulin has traditionally been prepared from animal pancreatic tissue. Insulin from the porcine pancreas is generally considered to resemble human insulin more closely than bovine insulin, and porcine insulin is less likely to be antigenic. Insulin is now available in preparations that are relatively free of certain antigenic foreign proteins. The elimination of such impurities has helped to reduce the tendency of administered insulin to stimulate the production of antibodies responsible for some patients' becoming allergic to the hormone and for some cases of insulin resistance. As a result, patients employing the purer preparations are now much less likely to become sensitized and to develop local skin reactions at the injection site. However, because only a minority of cases of insulin resistance are the result of an immune response, the availability of the purified preparations has not entirely

Table 25–1. Insulin preparations used in the treatment of diabetes

Generic or official name	Trade name or synonym	Onset of action (hr)	Peak effect (hr)	Duration of action (hr)
Rapid-acting preparations				
Insulin injection USP	Actrapid Human; Humulin R; Regular insulin; Regular Iletin I	½–1	2–5	6–8
Prompt insulin zinc suspension USP	Monotard Human; Semilente Insulin; Semilente Iletin I; Semitard	½–1½	5–10	5–10
Intermediate-acting preparations				
Isophane insulin suspension USP	NPH insulin; NPH Iletin; Humulin N	1–1½	8–12	24
Insulin zinc suspension USP	Lente Insulin; Lente Iletin I; Lentard; Monotard	1–2½	7–15	24
Long-acting preparations				
Extended insulin zinc suspension USP	Ultralente Insulin; Ultralente Iletin; Ultratard	4–8	10–30	>36
Protamine zinc insulin suspension USP	Protamine, Zinc & Iletin	4–8	14–20	36

solved the problem of acute and chronic resistance some-times seen clinically in patients being treated with insulin.

Human insulin (Humulin S; Actrapid Human; Monotard Human) is now available. This form of insulin is synthesized by *Escherichia coli* using recombinant DNA techniques. Early results indicate that human insulin is less antigenic than insulin from animal sources and is less likely to cause lipodystrophy (see below). Its use is considered especially advantageous in patients who are newly diagnosed, to lessen the chance of their developing insulin allergy, and in those patients who need insulin only intermittently and who may thus be most likely to develop insulin allergy.

As indicated below, a concentrated preparation containing 500 U/ml is available for treating insulin-resistant patients. Another advance—one that simplified the measurement of insulin and reduced dosage errors—was the use of a single uniform dosage form, the U-100 concentration. The American Diabetes Association advocates the elimination of U-40, U-80, and other concentrations of insulin so that patients need to use only a single syringe calibrated to measure U-100 insulin. None of the new insulin preparations need to be refrigerated, but extremes of temperature and exposure to direct sunlight should be avoided.

The type of insulin preparation or combination of preparations that is employed to initiate treatment of a newly diagnosed patient and for use during long-term maintenance management depends on various considerations. However, no matter which preparations are selected or what dosages of insulin are required, the main aims of hormone replacement therapy are the same: control of the signs and symptoms of diabetes and prevention of its complications. That is, insulin dosage and the duration of its action should be sufficient to keep blood sugar at normal levels both before and after meals and for most of the rest of the day. This should be accomplished without causing any significant episodes of hypoglycemia (see below, and the summary at the end of the chapter).

Administration of insulin in individualized dosage and at appropriate intervals will prevent hyperglycemia and the symptoms that stem from excessive blood glucose, including, in addition to those listed above, such common complications as frequent urinary tract infections in women, impotence in men, and growth failure in children. Evidence is also accumulating that using insulin in doses that maintain close control of the blood sugar level may also help to prevent the late kidney, ocular, and other vascular complications of the disease. Some specific examples of how insulin is employed in different clinical situations will be described in the section on the management of diabetic patients with hormone replacement and with such other measures as diet and oral hypoglycemic drugs (below).

Oral hypoglycemic drugs

The need to administer insulin by injection has various disadvantages. Scientists have not yet succeeded in preparing a practical oral insulin. However, two classes of synthetic chemicals have been developed that are effective for reducing high blood sugar when taken by mouth. These chemicals—the sulfonylureas and the biguanides (Table 25-2)—offer some patients the convenience of symptomatic control of diabetes without the need for repeated daily injections.

Current status

The orally effective hypoglycemic agents have been employed almost entirely for patients whose diabetes has developed during adult life—the maturity-onset or type II (NIDDM) diabetes. The drugs are never used alone in cases that were first diagnosed during childhood—the juvenile-onset or type I (IDDM) diabetes—nor are they employed in patients likely to develop ketoacidosis or other complications of this disease. The main reason for this is that the sulfonylurea-type drugs act mainly by stimulating the secretion of endogenous insulin by pancreatic β cells. Obviously, they cannot be effective for treating patients in whom the pancreas has lost its ability to produce insulin.

The present clinical indications for use of these drugs in the management of diabetes are more limited than ever before. This is mainly because of the publication of reports that have questioned both their safety and efficacy. The first such reports came from a cooperative study carried out in a dozen American clinics. According to the results reported by the University Group Diabetes Program (UGDP), diabetic patients who received drugs from each class—the sulfonylurea compound *tolbutamide* or the biguanide *phenformin*—had a death rate from cardiovascular disease that was much higher than the mortality rate of patients being treated with diet alone, insulin, or placebos.

The manner in which the UGDP study was performed has been severely criticized, and controversy concerning the validity of the reported results continues. The Food and Drug Administration has *not*, however, seen fit to withdraw tolbutamide on the basis of its reputed cardiovascular toxicity. Thus, this and the other available sulfonylurea compounds are still being employed by those who feel that these are essentially safe drugs for use in certain categories of patients who are responsive to their action.

At present, it appears that these drugs are *not* indicated in any case that can be controlled by diet and a weight-reducing regimen alone, or by these measures together with insulin. They are, however, claimed to be useful for control of mild to moderately severe but non-ketotic cases of the maturity-onset type when insulin can-

Table 25–2. Oral hypoglycemic agents

Generic or official name	Trade name	Usual adult daily dosage range	Doses/day	Duration of action (hr)
Sulfonylurea compounds				
First generation				
Acetohexamide USP	Dymelor	250 mg–1.5 g	1–2	12–24
Chlorpropamide USP	Diabinese	100–250 mg	1	Up to 60
Tolazamide USP	Tolinase	100 mg–1.0 g	1–2	10–16
Tolbutamide USP	Orinase	250 mg–2.0 g	2–3	6–12
Second generation				
Glipizide	Glucotrol	5–15 mg	1–2	10–24
Glyburide; glibenclamide	DiaBeta; Micronase	1.25–20 mg	1–2	24
Biguanide compound				
Phenformin HCl USP*				

* Formerly marketed as DBI or Meltrol; removed from the market in the United States in 1977, but now available from the FDA to physicians who file an IND application (for use in selected patients).

not be employed for any reason. Among the cases of type II diabetes in which the sulfonylurea-type agents may sometimes be substituted for insulin are the following:

1. Patients allergic to insulin
2. Patients unwilling to take insulin because they find the frequent injections painful or a cause of disfiguring skin lesions
3. Patients who fail to follow directions for correct use of insulin
4. Patients with physical disabilities such as blindness or other visual difficulties, or with arthritis and other neuromuscular disorders that make self-administration of the hormone difficult

On the other hand, phenformin was withdrawn from the American market late in 1977 on the basis of reports indicating that its use was sometimes a factor in the development of another type of serious toxicity: *lactic acidosis.* This frequently fatal metabolic disorder has long been known to develop occasionally in some diabetic patients as a complication of kidney disease, shock and hypoxemia, or alcoholic intoxication. After the use of phenformin was found to be a factor sometimes involved in the production of this disorder, the Secretary of Health, Education, and Welfare (now Health and Human Services)

ordered that it be taken out of general use. The drug is currently available to diabetologists, who must file an Investigational New Drug (IND) application with the FDA, for use *only* in patients who meet *all* requirements on a long list of criteria. This unusual circumstance results from the recognition that a select group of patients may benefit uniquely from this potentially dangerous drug.

Individual drugs

The currently available sulfonylurea drugs differ mainly in the ways in which they are handled by the body. Most of these compounds are metabolized in the liver to active metabolites that are then excreted by the kidneys at varying rates that determine the duration of their action. Thus, to avoid prolongation of their action and an excessive drop in blood sugar level, these drugs should not be used in patients with severe liver or kidney disease. However, the individual drugs differ in the degree to which they depend on hepatic metabolism and on renal excretion for their elimination.

Tolbutamide[+] (Orinase) is more rapidly and completely metabolized than the other sulfonylurea compounds. Thus, its duration of hypoglycemic action is shorter than that of the other drugs and it must usually be taken in several doses daily. This can be a drawback in patients who tend to omit doses of drugs that require multiple daily administration. On the other hand, its relatively short duration of action is a safety factor in any patients who may develop hypoglycemia and, because most of its renally excreted metabolites are inactive, tolbutamide is probably safer than other sulfonylureas for elderly patients and for others with reduced kidney function.

Chlorpropamide+ (Diabinese) differs from tolbutamide and the other sulfonylureas in not being subjected to metabolic degradation by hepatic enzyme systems. It is, instead, excreted by the kidneys in unchanged form over a prolonged period. Thus, patients need to take only a single dose of this drug before breakfast to maintain its therapeutic effects for 24 hours. This drug is also the safest for diabetic patients with liver disease. On the other hand, because of its dependence on renal excretion for elimination, chlorpropamide is more likely to cause hypoglycemia in elderly patients and in others with reduced renal function. Hypoglycemic reactions sometimes require treatment for several days because of the relatively prolonged duration of its action (see below).

Tolazamide (Tolinase) and acetohexamide (Dymelor) are most commonly reserved for use in patients who have not responded adequately to treatment with tolbutamide or chlorpropamide. Tolazamide, for example, is claimed effective in about one-third of such cases of failure with the leading drugs of this class. Both these drugs have a duration of action about midway between that of tolbutamide and chlorpropamide, tolazamide because of its slower absorption and acetohexamide because it is converted in the liver to an active metabolite that is slowly excreted by the kidneys. Both drugs can often be given on a once-daily dosage schedule, and both require caution in patients with renal insufficiency because of possible accumulation that could lead to hypoglycemic reactions.

Other adverse effects

The incidence of hypoglycemia is relatively low when these drugs are administered to properly selected patients in initially low doses that are raised only gradually. Similarly, despite the UGDP study findings discussed above, it has been difficult to prove that most patients suffer cardiac arrhythmias or other signs of increased cardiovascular toxicity. However, patients prone to develop congestive heart failure may do so sometimes when treated with chlorpropamide, a drug that can cause retention of water and dilutional hyponatremia. This is thought to occur because chlorpropamide tends to potentiate the activity of the antidiuretic hormone of the posterior pituitary gland. (See Chap. 20 for a brief discussion of the adjunctive role of chlorpropamide in treating diabetes insipidus.)

These drugs have only rarely had to be discontinued because of toxicity, mainly hypersensitivity-type reactions affecting the skin, liver, or bone marrow (see summary at the end of the chapter). Adverse interactions

have also been reported in patients taking certain other drugs together with the sulfonylureas. Thus, for example, caution is required in patients taking the coumarin-type anticoagulant dicumarol or anti-inflammatory agents such as phenylbutazone, because both these types of drugs tend to interfere with the metabolism of the sulfonylureas and to increase their hypoglycemic effects. The sulfonylureas may increase the anticoagulant effect of the coumarin-type drugs by displacing them from binding sites on plasma proteins. On the other hand, patients taking thiazide-type diuretics may show reduced responsiveness to the usual therapeutic doses of sulfonylurea drugs because of the tendency of the thiazides to suppress insulin secretion and to cause hyperglycemia. Drinking alcohol is undesirable while taking these drugs, not only because it adds to the hypoglycemic effects, but also because some patients have suffered a disulfiramlike reaction (see Chap. 53).

Patient management in major types of diabetes

The methods employed in the treatment of diabetic patients differ in their details. The approach to the patient depends primarily on the severity of the symptoms. Thus, the initial treatment of a middle-aged patient, who is relatively asymptomatic and whose condition has been diagnosed from a history and a battery of laboratory tests, will be very different from that required when a diabetic child is seen for the first time in a hospital emergency room to which he has been brought in a state of severe ketosis or even in coma. Discussions of the details of management in all the many and varied clinical circumstances are beyond the scope of this chapter and are best sought in specialized texts of diabetology. However, this section will present the use of the several major therapeutic modalities for managing diabetes in some common clinical situations that require the use of insulin or oral hypoglycemic drugs as well as dietary therapy.

Maturity-onset, type II, noninsulin-dependent diabetes

Diet

Most adults who develop mild symptoms of diabetes after the age of 40 years can keep their condition under control by bringing down their body weight and adhering to an individually prescribed diet. Maintaining body weight at levels ideal for each person's height, frame, and age is necessary in all types of diabetes. It is particularly important in these patients, most of whom are obese. Some scientists suggest that the body cells of overweight diabetics contain fewer receptors for insulin than those of thin people, and that this is why they are hyperglycemic despite also having relatively high levels of insulin in their blood. These authorities claim that when obese patients diet and attain their ideal weight, their body cells regain normal concentrations of insulin receptors, which then help the cells to take in and utilize the excess circulating glucose.

In any case, the hyperglycemia and impaired carbohydrate tolerance of many overweight adult diabetics can often be corrected by dietary therapy that leads to weight loss. They may then maintain this new normoglycemic state with a long-term program based on a carefully calculated daily diet divided into several small meals and snacks and controlled physical activity. Often, patients with type II diabetes then remain asymptomatic without any need for insulin or oral hypoglycemic drug therapy. (See other sources for the standard exchangeable dietary lists recommended by the American Diabetes Association.)

Oral hypoglycemic drugs

The addition of a sulfonylurea compound to the dietary regimen of patients whose symptoms are not completely controlled by diet alone sometimes succeeds in keeping their blood sugar at normal levels. These drugs appear to make the pancreatic β cells of adult diabetics more sensitive to plasma glucose levels. Thus these cells, which in older diabetics ordinarily respond sluggishly to rising plasma glucose levels following food intake, then release their insulin reserves more rapidly. As indicated above, patients with type I diabetes should not be treated with these drugs, because they possess no reserves of insulin that could be released by this sensitizing action of the sulfonylurea compounds.

Even among type II patients, as many as 40% may not respond adequately to sulfonylurea drug therapy. In addition to such so-called primary failures, a substantial number of patients who respond to drug therapy at first fail to do so after a while (secondary failure). Some critics of oral drug therapy claim that fewer than 15% of patients who are started on hypoglycemic drugs continue to take them successfully after a few years.

Despite such criticism of their efficacy and the evidence suggesting possible long-term toxicity (see above), most physicians continue to employ these drugs in the management of many adult diabetic patients whose condition has not responded adequately after several months of dietary therapy. Some claim that all available sulfonylurea compounds are equally effective for treating those patients who respond at all. However, tolbutamide and chlorpropamide are the most commonly employed drugs, while tolazamide and acetohexamide are most often reserved for use in patients who have failed to respond to a trial with the first two drugs.

Tolbutamide, the prototype agent, is still often preferred for initiating treatment, particularly in patients with impaired kidney function who might have difficulty in excreting chlorpropamide. However, the latter drug is more desirable for patients with liver disease who might not be able to metabolize tolbutamide to inactive metabolites. Whichever drug is employed, treatment should be initiated with small doses, especially in elderly patients who are often sensitive to the hypoglycemic effects of the sulfonylurea drugs. Dosage is then adjusted upward (or occasionally downward) on the basis of the patient's reports of urinary glucose tests carried out daily at home and blood glucose tests performed once weekly by the nurse or physician, or daily by home glucose monitoring.

It was formerly preferred to initiate treatment with phenformin because (except for gastrointestinal side-effects) it caused fewer adverse effects than the sulfonylureas. This drug was also sometimes combined with a sulfonylurea compound because it acts by a different mechanism and thus tends to potentiate the hypoglycemic activity of the sulfonylureas in patients who respond inadequately to full doses of drugs of that class alone.* Unfortunately, that option is no longer open to most patients because of the severe restrictions that have been placed on the availability of phenformin as a result of its use having been linked to fatal lactic acidosis in patients prone to develop that disorder (see above).

Insulin dosage scheduling

Because of the cautious attitude toward oral hypoglycemic drug therapy that has been provoked by the UGDP study and by the withdrawal of phenformin from general use, many more maturity-onset, type II diabetics whose condition cannot be controlled by dietary therapy alone are being treated with insulin. Treatment may be initiated in a hospital setting, because this offers better opportunities to teach the patient how best to use insulin and because laboratory facilities allow more rapid adjustment of insulin dosage levels. However, adult patients who have few, if any, symptoms may be managed with insulin on an ambulatory basis, provided that the patient receives instruction concerning how to adjust its dosage on the basis of blood glucose home monitoring or urine sugar tests and how best to administer the hormone. (See the section on patient education, below.)

Treatment of the nonketotic, nearly asymptomatic adult outpatient is now most commonly begun with an intermediate-acting preparation such as *insulin zinc suspension* (lente insulin) or isophane insulin suspension (NPH insulin). Usual treatment begins with the injection of 10 to 20 U about 30 minutes before breakfast. Adjustments in dosage are made on the basis of the patient's reports of the results of self-performed tests for glucose in urine samples taken three or four times daily before meals and at bedtime, or preferably on the basis of results of self-monitoring of blood glucose levels done two or three times daily until the insulin dose is regulated. Dosage is ordinarily increased in increments of 2 to 4 U daily,

---

* Three actions have been described to account for the therapeutic efficacy of phenformin: (1) increased glucose utilization; (2) decreased intestinal absorption of glucose; and (3) decreased gluconeogenesis. Phenformin does *not* act by stimulating the release of insulin.

or every other day until blood glucose or urine glucose levels are within acceptable limits.

Regular insulin is occasionally employed in the nonketotic adult (as it always is in the younger and other patients with ketosis). An initial dose of about 10 U is injected before breakfast and followed with similar or different doses before other meals and at bedtime, depending on the results of blood and urine tests. After an adjusted total daily dose of regular insulin is determined on the basis of blood and urine test results for glucose, the patient may be switched to a single daily dose of one of the intermediate-acting preparations to avoid the need for frequent injections of the short-acting preparation.

The total dose of the suspension—usually somewhat less than the daily total of regular insulin units—is administered as a single dose before breakfast. Usually this is enough to maintain control of most mild cases of maturity-onset, type II diabetes. Occasionally, a small amount of regular insulin may be added to the morning injection of intermediate insulin to provide coverage in the hours before lunch when the latter has not yet reached its peak effect. Based on current research results, it is now recommended that, in adult patients, it may also be most advisable to supplement the morning injection of the suspension with a late afternoon injection of regular insulin or even to split the total dose of the intermediate-acting insulin into two injections, with most being administered before breakfast and the rest (about one-third) before the evening meal. This protocol more closely approximates the insulin release pattern in "normal" adults. (See insulin dosage adjustment in type I diabetes, below.)

The objective of all these varied insulin regimens for adult diabetics (and also of the modifications employed for control of juvenile-onset, type I cases) is to keep the patient's blood glucose as close to normal for as long periods as possible without precipitating episodes of hypoglycemia.

Juvenile-onset, type I, insulin-dependent, diabetes: insulin dosage adjustment

Many children may present for the first time in a state of acute diabetic ketoacidosis or even diabetic coma. The management of such acute cases is discussed below. Once the condition of these patients has been stabilized by frequent regular insulin injections—as indicated by their requirements for each succeeding 5- or 6-hour period remaining essentially the same—they are transferred to one of various maintenance regimens based on the use of one or another of the several intermediate-acting preparations.

A first step in accomplishing this is to add up the total amount of regular insulin that had been required in each 24-hour period. The total of these divided doses may then be given as a single prebreakfast dose of an intermediate-acting insulin. (Actually, because of the greater efficiency of these longer acting preparations, the patient may receive only 75% to 80% of the number of units of regular insulin than was previously required.) Often, a mixture containing about one-quarter regular and three-quarters intermediate insulin is prepared and administered.

As indicated above, the inclusion of the regular insulin component is intended to keep blood sugar levels down during the morning, and the intermediate-acting insulin is intended to prevent hyperglycemia and glycosuria from developing between noon and the next morning. Occasionally, a supplementary dose of regular insulin may be needed late in the evening to prevent nocturnal glycosuria. (The longest acting preparations such as protamine zinc insulin suspension and extended insulin zinc suspension [Ultralente Insulin] were also formerly employed for persistent glycosuria often, however, with hypoglycemic episodes.)

Sometimes the administration of a single morning injection of an insulin mixture may not be enough to provide 24-hour control. Attempting to do so by increasing the number of insulin units in the single injection can lead to late afternoon hypoglycemic reactions. To avoid this, some authorities advocate a split dosage regimen. This involves the administration in the morning of about two-thirds of the daily total of the mixture of intermediate-acting and regular insulin. The remaining third of the mixture is given about 15 minutes before the evening meal to prevent hyperglycemia and glycosuria during the night by stimulating body cells to utilize the late glucose intake. The closer control of diabetes achieved in this way is claimed to help prevent retinopathy and other late complications of diabetes.

After the patient's daily insulin needs have been determined by blood glucose tests before breakfast, lunch and at bedtime, and the condition has been stabilized during the hospital stay, further adjustments may be necessary after the patient goes home. Often, for example, the now ambulatory patient requires less insulin because physical activity has increased. To avoid episodes of afternoon hypoglycemia, the number of insulin units injected in the morning is adjusted downward, and the patient is advised to take a snack at times of peak insulin action. On the other hand, some young patients may become careless in sticking to their diet when not under hospital supervision, which may lead to an increase in their insulin requirements. Of course, in any case, as young diabetics grow, their insulin needs become greater. Thus, these type I diabetics must have their insulin requirements reviewed about every 3 to 6 months. Most of these patients learn to regulate their own insulin, based on how they feel, and actually cover their needs very effectively.

Diabetic ketoacidosis treatment

Before the discovery of insulin, ketoacidosis and related metabolic derangements were the most common cause of death in diabetes. The death rate from this cause has dropped from almost 50% to about 2% because of advances in the emergency medical care of patients in coma resulting from developments of diabetic ketoacidosis or from the hyperosmolar nonketotic state, syndromes that, as described above, tend to develop in uncontrolled juvenile-onset, type I cases or in elderly diabetic patients, respectively.

Various types of stressful conditions may increase a diabetic patient's need for insulin. Most commonly, the occurrence of an acute infection and fever raises the patient's insulin requirements. However, if nausea and vomiting prevent eating, the patient may think that insulin is not needed. Patients are instructed not to neglect taking their insulin in such circumstances. They should, in fact, administer an additional dose of rapid-acting regular insulin if their tests of urine specimens reveal a rising glucose level or persistent ketonuria. It is desirable that a member of the family be instructed to call the nurse or physician and perform the testing of the patient's urine or blood and make the necessary adjustments in insulin dosage, because the acutely ill patient may become too drowsy or confused to do so.

The patient with definitely diagnosed ketoacidosis or diabetic coma requires prompt and vigorous treatment. Injections of relatively large doses of rapid-acting insulin are given together with fluids and electrolytes and, occasionally, with a vasopressor drug to raise blood pressure.

The first step in treatment is to replace the patient's fluid deficit and reverse the hypovolemia by infusing 1 or 2 liters of a solution of isotonic saline solution (0.9%) or, if necessary, even more of a less concentrated (0.45%) salt solution. After infusion of the first 2 or 3 liters and production of a brisk flow of urine, some authorities recommend that IV administration of potassium chloride be begun under electrocardiographic monitoring to restore that lost electrolyte or to prevent hypokalemia. Others think that it is safer to wait until the patient can take the prophylactic dose of the potassium salt by mouth. Infusion of sodium bicarbonate is also sometimes recommended to counteract exhausting Kussmaul respirations.

Immediately after the rehydrating fluid infusion is begun, regular insulin injections are made, preferably by the intravenous route. In comatose patients, some prefer to administer several successive bolus doses of 100 to 200 U of insulin every hour until the blood glucose and plasma ketones fall to lower levels. Then, each following dose of insulin is reduced to half of the previous dose, as long as frequent monitoring shows continued improvement in the patient's condition and a steady drop in the blood glucose concentration to below 300 mg/dl. Others advocate the continuous infusion of low doses of insulin, a procedure that is said to bring about a slow steady drop in blood glucose levels with much smaller total amounts of insulin than when it is administered

intermittently. The rate of infusion can be raised if the response to insulin seems too slow.

When facilities and personnel for close monitoring are not readily available, regular insulin may be administered intramuscularly, or even subcutaneously, provided that the patient is not in shock. Ordinarily, doses of 25 to 50 U repeated every 1 or 2 hours will bring about a significant drop in blood glucose and ketone levels. Rarely, a patient may prove resistant to even large doses of insulin, possibly because of the development of antibodies to the foreign protein or as a result of infection, trauma, or other forms of stress. Such patients may have to receive enormous amounts of insulin before their blood sugar begins to come down. A concentrated solution containing 500 U/ml of regular insulin, prepared from porcine sources, is available for IM or SC use in patients markedly resistant to beef insulin. However, special care is required to avoid late developing hypoglycemic reactions.

Hypoglycemia

Causes

Reactions as a result of drops in blood sugar to abnormally low levels—40 mg/dl and below, usually—can occur clinically in a large number of disorders, including liver and kidney disease, various types of pancreatic and extrapancreatic cancers, diseases of the anterior pituitary gland with corticotropin or growth hormone deficiencies, and adrenocortical insufficiency (Chap. 21). In diabetic patients, insulin and the sulfonylurea compounds are, of course, the most common causes of hypoglycemic reactions. These occur most commonly, not only as a result of errors in dosage and timing of administration of these drugs, but also because of the patient's failure to take in adequate amounts of food or because of performing excessive physical activity.

Insulin reactions

Signs and symptoms

These are mainly the result of changes in functioning of the autonomic and central nervous systems. The clinical manifestations vary considerably from patient to patient (see the summary at the end of this chapter) and—because the severity of hypoglycemic reactions depends on how rapidly as well as on how far the blood sugar level falls—the type of preparation employed also affects the nature of the patient's response to insulin overdosage. Thus, some of the early signs of autonomic nervous system stimulation, which are observed with regular insulin when it reaches its peak of action (only a couple of hours after injection), are largely absent with the more slowly absorbed insulins that lower blood sugar levels gradually as

530

successive increments slowly enter the blood from the depot site.

The earliest autonomic signs and symptoms are partially parasympathetic in origin. Parasympathetic hyperactivity often causes gastrointestinal contractions that feel like hunger pangs and increased peptic acid secretions that cause epigastric distress and nausea. Slowing of the heart and mild hypotension may occur and also make the patient feel weak or faint. However, tachycardia and a rise in blood pressure are more common cardiovascular manifestations of a hypoglycemic reaction. These and such other signs and symptoms as profuse sweating, anxiety, and tremulousness are the result of increased sympathoadrenal activity and a rise in plasma epinephrine levels. The discharge of epinephrine serves to break down liver and muscle glycogen to glucose; it also releases FFA for use as fuel in place of sugar.

Such symptoms serve as early warnings to which the patient should respond by ingesting a carbohydrate-containing substance such as candy, a cola drink (*not* a "diet" soft drink), orange juice, sugar, or honey. Unfortunately, some patients may miss the signs of an autonomic reaction to hypoglycemia, possibly because of diabetic neuropathy. The β-adrenergic blocking agents such as propranolol (Chap. 18) may also mask those premonitory signs and symptoms of hypoglycemic reactions that are the result of release of epinephrine and of its actions on cardiac and other β receptors. Because α receptors in blood vessels are *not* blocked, the hypoglycemic reaction may be marked by a steep rise in blood pressure and, because propranolol prevents compensatory glycogenolysis by the liver, patients with labile diabetes who are taking this drug may be subjected to hypoglycemic reactions of severe intensity.

Early signs and symptoms of abnormal central nervous system function, particularly when blood sugar is dropping slowly, include headache, drowsiness, double vision, and mental confusion or irritability. The patient and family should be taught to recognize these effects of falling blood sugar on the brain, which largely burns sugar alone as a source of energy. Further reduction in the fuel required for cerebral oxidative metabolism may lead to hypoglycemic coma and convulsions.

Such severe reactions, which must be differentiated from those of diabetic coma (see signs and symptoms of hypo- and hyperglycemia at the end of this chapter), are most likely to occur in patients who fail to recognize hypoglycemic symptoms or who do nothing to counteract them. This sometimes happens with long-acting insulin preparations, not only because the changes in the patient's personality and mental efficiency may come on more slowly and subtly, but also because these products often reach their peak action during the night while the patient is asleep. As a result, the patient may feel no muscular weakness and fatigue before the sudden onset of motor symptoms such as twitching, athetoid (twisting) movements, clonic spasms and, finally, full-blown tonic seizures. Repeated episodes of continuing convulsions and respiratory insufficiency, followed, as they often are, by coma, may result in permanent cerebral cortical damage (the organic brain syndrome).

Treatment

Treatment of even severe hypoglycemic reactions is simple enough, once the condition is recognized (Table 25-3). Sublingual or buccal sugar is rapidly absorbed and frequently very effective. Treatment usually involves giving glucose by vein if the patient cannot swallow. Often, simply the injection of 1 or 2 oz of a concentrated (50%) solution of glucose will produce dramatic recovery. Occasionally, when it is difficult to find a good vein or the patient is thrashing about in delirium, drugs such as epinephrine, hydrocortisone, or glucagon may be administered subcutaneously.

Glucagon, a purified polypeptide extracted from pancreatic α cells, acts to speed conversion of the liver's glycogen stores to glucose. It may be useful when no one capable of injecting glucose intravenously is available. Members of the family can readily be taught to give a dose of 1 mg of glucagon SC or IM while awaiting the arrival of a physician or transport to an emergency care facility; ordinarily, the patient responds in 5 to 20 minutes, provided that the liver glycogen has not been previously depleted. If the patient does not respond and remains in deep coma, additional 1-mg doses may be administered, preferably by the intravenous route. If the patient con-

Table 25–3. Glucose-elevating agents

Generic or official name	Trade name or synonym	Usual adult dosage and administration
Diazoxide, oral	Proglycem	3–8 mg/kg body weight/day, divided into two or three equal doses
Glucagon		0.5–1 mg SC, IM, or IV
Glucose	Glutose; Insta-Glucose	10 g dextrose orally

tinues to stay in a comatose state, intravenous glucose must then be administered.

Once the patient recovers consciousness, more carbohydrate should be given by mouth to avoid lapsing into unconsciousness as the effects of the glucagon injections wear off. If the patient's hypoglycemia was caused by a long-acting agent that continues to enter the blood, sources of rapidly available sugar, such as the contents of a tube of glucose paste, corn syrup, or Coca-Cola syrup, should be supplemented by a more slowly digestible form of carbohydrate, such as bread and honey. The physician should always be informed of any hypoglycemic reaction so that the patient may be questioned and examined and measures taken to prevent future episodes of the same type.

Prevention

Avoiding episodes of hypoglycemia is better than having to treat them after their occurrence. This is particularly true in diabetic patients with coronary artery disease, in whom the compensatory sympathoadrenal discharge might cause an acute myocardial infarction to occur during a hypoglycemic reaction. Some authorities suggest that the blood glucose level be allowed to remain well above normal in such cases rather than risk hypoglycemia and a possible heart attack.

Other diabetologists, who advocate close rather than loose control of all patients, deny that loose blood sugar control is ever desirable. They claim that occasional episodes of mild hypoglycemia are less serious than continued hyperglycemia, which they believe can lead not only to acute infections and ketotic or hyperosmolar reactions, but also to the late vascular renal and visual complications of diabetes. Presumably, a compromise can be reached between these two extreme positions, and it should be possible for insulin to be administered in doses adequate for control of hyperglycemia but not high enough to lower blood glucose levels excessively.

Prevention of hypoglycemic reactions requires careful adjustment of insulin dosage. Management of the insulin-dependent patient requires working out a schedule of injections suited to individual needs. This is sometimes difficult to accomplish in patients whose condition has become unstable. For example, patients with juvenile-onset, type I diabetes who have grown older may suddenly become "brittle" in their response to insulin. They may suffer sudden episodes of severe hypoglycemia that seem to come on with little warning. This calls not only for reevaluation of their therapeutic program but also for reminders to be constantly on the alert for any unusual feelings that may signal the onset of a reaction that requires quick carbohydrate ingestion.

In some cases, patients may have repeated episodes of hypoglycemia that go undetected because they occur while the patient is asleep. When the patient awakens in the morning, the blood sugar level may actually be abnormally high, and glucose may be spilling into the urine. Such periods of rebound hyperglycemia and glycosuria—the so-called Somogyi effect—occur as a result of the release of epinephrine in the compensatory reaction to the patient's nighttime or early morning hypoglycemia. Often, such patients are subjected to increasingly high doses of insulin, which are intended to control their rising blood glucose levels but instead cause recurrent episodes of hypoglycemia followed by further rebound phenomena. The way to stop this vicious cycle is to reduce the patient's insulin dosage by about one-quarter to one-third. (Other aspects of the prevention of insulin reactions are discussed below in the section dealing with patient education.)

Hypoglycemic reactions to sulfonylurea drugs

Severe reactions to oral hypoglycemic agents have been relatively rare. However, to prevent their occurrence, it is essential to start patients on small doses and to monitor blood sugar responses carefully during the period when the dosage is being individually adjusted to optimal levels. Although most reactions are the result of overdosage in especially sensitive patients during the first few days of treatment, an occasional patient may suffer a severe prolonged hypoglycemic episode after months of successful maintenance therapy.

Older patients with impaired renal function are most susceptible to hypoglycemia, and chlorpropamide is the drug most commonly involved. Reactions in such cases may require extended treatment because of the slow rate at which chlorpropamide is eliminated by the kidneys. Patients must often be closely supervised for several days after such drug-induced hypoglycemia is diagnosed. They should receive frequent feedings or continuous IV infusion during this time.

These drugs should be kept out of reach of children, because severe hypoglycemia has sometimes occurred as a result of accidental ingestion. As indicated previously, efforts should be made to avoid adverse interactions with drugs such as dicumarol and phenylbutazone, which can potentiate the hypoglycemic action of the sulfonylurea agents. Patients should be advised against drinking alcohol, which itself can cause hypoglycemic reactions.

Other types of hypoglycemia

People without a history of having taken insulin or sulfonylureas are sometimes found to have very low levels of blood sugar. Before their hypoglycemia is treated symptomatically with glucose infusion or drugs, it is necessary to determine the cause. If, for example, the patient is found to have pancreatic islet cell tumors, surgical removal of such insulinomas or adenomas can often eliminate the cause and cure their condition. In cases of pituitary malfunction, repository injections of corticotropin (Chap. 20) can often raise the patient's blood sugar level, and administration of glucocorticoids may correct hypoglycemia caused by chronic adrenal insufficiency.

Diazoxide (Proglycem), an oral form of the same *non*diuretic thiazide drug that is administered parenterally for treating hypertensive emergencies (see Hyperstat, Chap. 28), has recently been introduced for raising blood sugar levels in children and in others suffering from certain rare organic disorders that cause persistent hypoglycemia. (It should not be used to treat the forms of functional hypoglycemia discussed above.) This drug is thought to reverse hypoglycemia and to produce hyperglycemia by blocking the release of insulin from pancreatic β cells and from extrapancreatic cells that secrete insulinlike substances. Thus, it has been employed prior to surgical procedures in infants and children for removal of islet cell adenomas and extrapancreatic cancers. It is also used postoperatively when hypoglycemia persists, and it may be administered to counteract hyperinsulinism in adults with inoperable insulin-secreting tumors.

Oral doses of this drug do not ordinarily cause a drop in blood pressure, despite the potent hypotensive effect of the parenteral preparation. Transient hypotension may occur, however, when this drug is given together with a thiazide diuretic as is sometimes necessary in patients who retain sodium and fluids as a result of the *anti*diuretic effect of diazoxide. This combination may also cause increased retention of uric acid (hyperuricemia). Blood glucose levels must be closely monitored to avoid development of hyperglycemia, ketoacidosis, and hyperosmolar nonketotic coma. However, this reaction responds to prompt insulin administration.

Additional clinical considerations

Diabetes mellitus is a chronic disease whose management requires that the patient understand the disease and therapy, and that the nurse and patient work together to detect any changes in the disease process or in the response to the therapy being used.

The oral hypoglycemic agents, as indicated earlier, are used with caution and only in particular patients with type II diabetes who can benefit from the pancreatic stimulation. These drugs should not be used in patients who have an immediate need for insulin, such as those with diabetic ketoacidosis, coma, fever, infections, or impending surgery. The drugs should also be avoided in patients with hepatic, thyroid, or renal disease. The safe use of these drugs in pregnancy has not been established and, because pregnancy is a high-stress situation, pregnant diabetics must be closely monitored and treated with insulin therapy. Any patient who is started on oral hypoglycemic agents should be closely monitored for response to therapy and compliance to diet and weight control measures. The patient should be advised to wear a medical identification tag to ensure proper treatment in emergency situations.

The effective use of insulin therapy requires a careful balance between diet, exercise, and appropriate insulins. The patient needs an extensive and thorough education program about the disease, the insulin, and the signs and symptoms of adverse reactions. The insulin is usually administered subcutaneously and a graph of rotation sites should be used to remind the patient, in the home setting, and the nursing staff in the hospital setting, where the injections have been given. It is important to rotate the injection sites to ensure adequate absorption of each dose and to prevent lipodystrophy, a destruction of the subcutaneous tissue with resultant scarring and fibrotic changes. Insulin is best given at room temperature; the vial should be rotated gently to disperse the crystals adequately. It is important, of course, to check the expiration dates carefully before use. The conversion to U-100 insulin has made the measurement of insulin much safer and more convenient. Some patients, who have been using insulin for a long period of time, may still use U-40 insulin, which is still available. In such cases, a notice should be clearly posted on the hospital unit to ensure that all nursing personnel are aware of the situation and that appropriate equipment is used.

Once insulin has been given, it is important to make sure that the patient eats. This can be a crucial factor in preventing hypoglycemic reactions. It can also be a difficult task in the hospital; for example, the patient's tray may be late arriving, or the patient may be taken off to tests or may be NPO (nothing by mouth). The nursing staff of a unit in which there are diabetic patients must be prepared with standby supplies of orange juice, sugar, and IV dextrose in severe cases.

It has been found that insulin adheres to plastic IV tubing and that much of the dose is lost if insulin is given this way. It is very important, therefore, to monitor the patient's response to such therapy closely and not to rely on measured dosage to provide adequate treatment.

It is also important to remember that the body's response to stress, as part of the sympathetic nervous system's activity, includes an increase in blood glucose levels. For this reason, whenever a patient undergoes a stressful event—for example, infection or surgery—the need for insulin may increase. Such patients require very careful monitoring and regulating of their insulin dose.

Drug–drug interactions

Oral hypoglycemic agents may increase the metabolism of *digitoxin*, so that patients receiving both drugs concurrently may require an increased digitoxin dosage. Several drugs increase or prolong the activity of the oral hypoglycemic agents, with a resultant increased risk of hypoglycemia: *sulfonamides, oxyphenbutazone, phenylbutazone, salicylates, nonsteroidal anti-inflammatory drugs, probenecid, MAO inhibitors, clofibrate, dicumarol*. Some drugs increase the metabolism of the oral hypoglycemic agents, leading to a decrease in their effectiveness: *thyroid hormones, oral contraceptives, estrogens, corticosteroids, rifampin*.

The patient's insulin requirements are increased by *oral contraceptives, corticosteroids, epinephrine, thyroid hor-*

mone, *dobutamine, cigarette smoking,* and *thiazide diuretics.* The hypoglycemic effects of insulin are increased by *MAO inhibitors, phenylbutazone, sulfinpyrazone, tetracycline, alcohol,* and *anabolic steroids.* The *β-adrenergic blockers* may mask the signs and symptoms of hypoglycemia by blocking the effects of sympathetic nervous system outflow. Patients receiving insulin should probably not be given these drugs.

The guide to the nursing process presents a summary of clinical considerations as they apply to the nursing care of a patient receiving insulin therapy, and the section following presents a discussion of some points to consider in patient education. As discussed above, patient education is the most important component of a successful patient care regimen for the diabetic patient.

Guide to the nursing process: insulin

Assessment	Nursing diagnoses	Intervention	Evaluation
Past history—underlying medical conditions (*contraindications*): Allergies: *pork products; beef products; other*	Potential alteration in bowel elimination— secondary to diabetes	Proper preparation and administration of drug	Evaluate effectiveness of drug therapy: Blood sugar level Subjective reports
Medication history: current drugs	Potential alteration in breathing patterns	Provision of comfort measures:	Evaluate patient for progression or
Cautions:	Potential alteration in cardiac output	• Skin care	complications of
Oral contraceptives	Potential ineffective coping secondary to diagnosis and therapy	• Diet	diabetes
Corticosteroids		• Safety measures	Evaluate effectiveness of
Epinephrine	Potential for injury, secondary to disease and therapy	Patient teaching regarding:	patient teaching measures
Thyroid hormone		• Disease	Evaluate effectiveness of
Dobutamine		• Drug	comfort measures
Cigarette smoking	Knowledge deficit regarding disease and therapy	• Administration	Evaluate effectiveness of
Thiazide diuretics		• Adverse effects	support and
MAO inhibitors		• Cautions	encouragement
Phenylbutazone	Potential alteration in nutrition	• Warnings	offered
Sulfinpyrazone		Provision of support and maintenance in cases of:	Monitor and maintain
Tetracycline	Potential sensory– perceptual alteration		patient if adverse
Alcohol		Hypoglycemia	effects occur:
Anabolic steroids	Potential alteration in tissue perfusion secondary to diabetes	Hyperglycemia	Hypoglycemia
β-adrenergic blockers		Provision of encourage- ment, support to cope with diagnosis, therapy, prognosis	Hyperglycemia
Physical assessment	Potential impairment of skin integrity secondary to disease, insulin injections		Monitor possible drug– drug interactions
Neurologic: orientation, reflexes, affect, peripheral sensation			
Ocular: vision, retinas			
Cardiovascular: BP, P, baseline EKG, auscultation, peripheral pulses, perfusion, edema			
Respiratory: rate, adventitious sounds			
GI: bowel sounds, elimination function			
Renal: output, bladder tone, urinalysis			

(continued)

Assessment	Nursing diagnoses	Intervention	Evaluation

Sexual: normal libido;
women—menstruation
history
Laboratory tests:
pH
Serum K$^+$ level
Fasting glucose level
GTT (glucose
tolerance test)

Patient education

The success of diabetes treatment depends on the patient's understanding the nature of the disease and on the patient's ability to carry out a self-care program. This is, of course, true of other chronic illnesses, including cardiac disease, hypertension, and obstructive lung disorders. However, no other chronic condition requires the patient to acquire and apply as much general and specifically detailed knowledge as does diabetes.

The patient should be given a realistic perspective about how a diagnosis of diabetes is likely to affect life style and future prospects, and should be advised that diabetes is a serious disease that will require daily compliance with instructions for carrying out detailed technical self-care procedures. On the other hand, the patient can be reassured that the disease does not have to rule out leading a life that will be nearly normal in all respects. A diagnosis of diabetes does not have to prevent a young person from preparing for almost any career. Most diabetics can participate in athletics, marry, and have children. It is necessary, though, that they learn to regulate their own lives in ways that will keep them in optimal health, avoid minor and major acute complications, and delay the late disease sequelae.

Among the specific points that must be emphasized in instructing diabetic patients are the following:

1. *How to take insulin and care for it and the syringes, needles, and other supplies that will be needed*

Thus, for example, although insulin no longer needs to be refrigerated, it should still not be subjected to extremes of temperature. Syringes appropriate for the prescribed concentration of insulin should be purchased. Thus, with U-100 insulin, U-100 syringes calibrated to measure preparations of that strength precisely should be obtained. The patient should be taught how to draw up the precise amounts of evenly distributed insulin suspensions and how to mix insulins in the same syringe.

Special syringes are available for patients with limited vision and these should be used, if appropriate.

Patients should be shown the preferred sites for making injections—for example, the deltoid muscle area at the back of the arms, the front of the thigh, the skin of the front and sides of the abdominal wall, and the buttocks—and should be advised to alternate between these injection sites. This helps to lessen the likelihood of developing insulin lipodystrophy and hypertrophy—changes in subcutaneous fat content that occur when injections are made repeatedly at the same sites over a prolonged period, and that can have adverse cosmetic effects or interfere with normal absorption of the hormone. The patient should be instructed not to change syringe or insulin types without consulting with the nurse or physician. The proper disposal of needles and syringes should also be discussed.

The patient should not only be taught what to do but should also be observed to see how the instructions are actually carried out. (One nurse explained that insulin must be injected rather than swallowed. She then proceeded to demonstrate the technique of giving oneself an injection by making an injection through the skin of an orange. Later that day, when she asked the patient to show her how he would go about taking his insulin, he injected the insulin into an orange, which he then began to eat!)

2. *How to check on whether the treatment measures that the patient is employing are effective for controlling the condition*

Most important both in initiating treatment and during long-term maintenance management are the urine or blood tests that the patient makes routinely. Thus, the patient learns to remember to void the bladder before each meal and at bedtime to obtain samples and how to use such aids as Clinitest reagent tablets or various types of reagent strips that indicate the urine glucose content, which reflects blood glucose levels, Acetest reagent tablets for determining urinary ketone levels, and Keto-Diastix for indicating the presence and levels of both ketones and glucose. Blood glucose monitoring in the home is done using various equipment to facilitate the finger prick to obtain the blood, and reagent strips that indicate the blood glucose level. The patient needs to practice this technique and to use it before injecting the insulin.

Patients should know how to make adjustments in insulin dosage on the basis of such tests and how to make mixtures of regular and intermediate-acting insulins when the administration of combinations of such preparations appears indicated for achieving closer control at particular times of day. Most important, patients must learn to recognize early clinical signs and symptoms of acute complications such as ketosis and hypoglycemic reactions (see the summary at the end of this chapter), so that they and their family can take immediate action, including notifying the physician. Patients should be urged to wear a tag or ID bracelet to help others recognize the nature of their disease in emergencies.

3. *How to keep insulin and drug dosage in balance with food intake and exercise*

Thus, the patient should know what to eat, when to eat, and the type and amount of physical activity in which to indulge to help determine the response to the insulin that is injected. The nurse can help the patient remember the need for adjusting the times of the main meals to the peak activity of the type of insulin preparation that is being taken. The patient is told to replace any meals not eaten with amounts of food containing the missing carbohydrates, fats, and proteins. Snacks between meals and at bedtime may also be suggested as a means of neutralizing the amounts of insulin being absorbed at certain hours. (In difficult or unusual cases, the nurse consults closely with the dietitian or nutritionist who has helped to set up the patient's dietary program.)

The nurse can also help the patient become aware of the effect of exercise on the insulin requirements. It can be pointed out that sudden strenuous exercise of an unusual nature is undesirable for diabetics taking insulin (regular moderate exercise is, of course, considered de-

sirable). The importance of compensating for the carbohydrate that is burned up in unaccustomed physical activity must be made clear to the patient, who is told that this can be done by taking extra sugary snacks up to a point, and that it may also be necessary to reduce the next insulin dose after unusually prolonged exercise.

Children with diabetes—and their parents—require special instruction. When youngsters are told to carry candy or some other source of quick carbohydrates, they may consume these sweets and then not have them when needed for combating a hypoglycemic reaction. They should be warned against this practice and be taught the importance of not missing meals and of not changing their exercise patterns suddenly from day to day, so that sudden drops of blood sugar levels are avoided.

4. *How to prevent infections of the skin of the feet, upper and lower respiratory tracts and urinary tract, which could lead to serious complications for diabetics*

Thus, for example, poor circulation in the feet can lead to dry gangrene in some patients. Therefore, the nurse must teach patients the principles of proper foot care. Hyperglycemia and glycosuria can set the stage for frequent urinary infections. In addition, of course, the nurse can recognize the development of visual problems, hypertension, and the other common complications of diabetes.

In summary, diabetes is a disease that requires the patient's close personal cooperation for its proper control. The patient must be taught all that can be understood to be as able and willing as possible to comply with instructions for self-care. The nurse who participates in the group or individual instruction and counseling of diabetic patients must be knowledgeable about all aspects of this complex condition, which is one of the most challenging of all the diseases about which nurses are required to develop special skills and competence.

The patient teaching guide presents points for teaching the patient the specifics about insulin therapy.

Patient teaching guide: insulin

The drug that has been prescribed for you is called insulin. Insulin is a hormone that is normally produced by your pancreas and helps your body to regulate your energy balance by affecting the way it uses sugars and fats. The lack of insulin produces a disease called diabetes mellitus. By injecting insulin each day, you can help your body use the sugars and fats in your food effectively.

Instructions: 1. The type(s) of insulin that has been ordered for you is called _____ . There are several types of insulin available. It is important to only use that type of insulin that has been prescribed for you.

(continued)

2. The dosage of insulin prescribed for you is _____ . The insulin should be taken _____ and _____ . It is important to eat after taking your insulin. If you know that a meal will be delayed, you should also delay your insulin. Monitor your blood or urine glucose levels. You may adjust your insulin as follows: _____ .

3. Check the expiration date before using the insulin. Store the insulin at room temperature, and avoid extremes of heat and light. Gently rotate the vial between your palms before use to disperse any crystals. *Do not shake it; such vigorous treatment will inactivate the drug.*

4. Keep your syringes sealed up and sterile until use. Dispose of your syringes and needles appropriately. Rotate your injection sites regularly to prevent tissue damage and to ensure that the proper amount of insulin is absorbed.

5. Tell any physician, nurse, or dentist who is taking care of you that you are on insulin therapy. Wear a medical identification tag to alert any medical personnel of your need for insulin in an emergency situation.

6. Keep your medication and syringes out of the reach of children.

7. You should be aware of the signs and symptoms of hypoglycemia (too much insulin). If any of these occur, eat or drink something high in sugar—for example, candy, orange juice, honey, or sugar. The signs and symptoms to watch for include the following: nervousness; anxiety; sweating; pale, cool skin; headache; nausea; hunger; shakiness. These may happen if you skip a meal, exercise too much, or experience extreme stress. If it happens very often, notify your nurse or physician.

8. Avoid the use of over-the-counter drugs. If you feel a need for one of these preparations, consult with your nurse or physician. Avoid the use of alcohol, because this will increase the chances of hypoglycemic episodes.

9. Maintain regular visits with your nurse or physician to monitor your blood glucose level and to evaluate you for any of the adverse responses to diabetes.

Notify your nurse or physician if any of the following occur:

Loss of appetite
Blurred vision
Fruity odor to your breath
Increased urination
Increased thirst
Nausea
Vomiting

Recent research developments

Despite research advances in understanding the underlying causes of diabetes and the manner in which its pathologic changes and complications are produced, diabetologists still cannot apply the new information to development of a cure. However, some recent discoveries seem to offer leads that indicate new directions for further research efforts. These may, in the future, have results that could be applied successfully for more effective therapy and, possibly, for the prevention of diabetes.

Somatostatin

This is a hormone produced in the hypothalamus, the pancreas, and possibly the gastrointestinal tract, which was first found to inhibit the release of the growth hormone (somatotropin) by the anterior pituitary gland (see Chap. 20). Thus, it was first referred to as GHRIH—the growth hormone release-inhibiting hormone—but it is now more commonly called somatostatin. Somatostatin has also been found to act directly on the pancreas to suppress the release of *glucagon* by the α cells (and to suppress the release of insulin by the β cells). (As indicated above, glucagon is a hormone that can restore the blood glucose level to normal in hypoglycemic states mainly because of its ability to release glucose that had been stored in the liver. It is also thought to play a significant part in producing hyperglycemia in diabetes.) Somatostatin is secreted by δ (delta) cells of the pancreatic islets, and has recently been postulated to have a physiologic role in controlling glucagon (and insulin) secretion.

Somatostatin has been employed experimentally in diabetic animals and humans to counteract hyperglycemia, prevent ketoacidosis, and alleviate other signs and symptoms of diabetes. Unfortunately it cannot be given by mouth and its action, when infused by vein, lasts only a few minutes because it is very rapidly destroyed by blood and liver enzymes. Thus, the same scientists who first succeeded in isolating the peptide and in making it available in synthetic form are now trying to prolong the duration of its action or to prepare related compounds more resistant to enzymatic degradation.

The synthetic hypothalamic hormone has been physically bound to zinc and protamine in a pharmaceutical form from which it is gradually released to produce a long-acting depot preparation with effects that last up to 6 hours following IM injection. Administered together with insulin, this has protected patients with juvenile-onset, type I diabetes from ketoacidotic coma. However, the routine long-term use of somatostatin in diabetic children could interfere with their growth.

Thus, although its suppressive effect on the release of growth hormone might be minimized by injecting somatostatin in the morning or during the day to avoid its antagonizing somatotropin (which is released during sleep), efforts are also being directed toward the development and synthesis of somatostatin analogues without any growth hormone release inhibitory action. If such an analogue, which would suppress only glucagon and not growth hormone, could be prepared in a long-acting form, it could be used along with intermediate-acting insulin in the maintenance management of juvenile-onset, type I diabetics and other insulinopenic, or insulin-dependent, diabetics.

New oral hypoglycemic agents

Two new sulfonylurea derivatives, *glyburide*, also called *glibenclamide* (DiaBeta; Micronase) and *glipizide* (Glucotrol) have recently become available in this country. These drugs, called "second-generation sulfonylureas," have several advantages over the first-generation drugs. They are excreted by both the biliary and renal routes, making them safer in patients with renal impairment; they are less likely to be displaced from plasma protein binding sites by other drugs because they bind by a different mechanism; and they have a longer duration of action than some first-generation drugs and are therefore effectively administered only once or twice a day, a feature that should increase patient compliance, but that also could increase the duration of hypoglycemic episodes and other adverse effects, should these occur. Their efficacy, and their adverse effects, resemble those of the first-generation drugs. As is always the case with new drugs, evaluation of the role of these drugs in therapy requires their use in clinical practice for a longer period of time.

Diabetes vaccine

Research results suggest that at least some cases of juvenile-onset, type I diabetes are the result of virus infections. Certain viruses have been shown able to destroy pancreatic β cells directly, or indirectly through initiation of an autoimmune process. Thus, some scientists are optimistic about the possibility of developing a vaccine that could prevent diabetes. However, other less sanguine scientists say that it could be several decades, if ever, before such a vaccine could be produced, particularly if—as is the case with the common cold—a dozen or more different viruses are involved.

Insulin pumps

A portable external infusion pump has been developed, which delivers a constant infusion of insulin through a needle implanted in subcutaneous tissue, usually in the abdomen. The pump, which consists of a syringe connected to the needle by a catheter, is worn on a belt. A battery-powered plunger in the syringe delivers continuous, low-dose insulin throughout the day. At high-stress times—for example, meals or exercise—the patient can press a button on the pump to deliver an increased amount of insulin. The needle needs to be moved every 2 or 3 days, the syringe needs to be filled daily, and the patient must be highly motivated to monitor his own activities and to wear and maintain the apparatus. Despite these potential drawbacks, patients who have used the pump have done very well with it and seem pleased with the therapeutic results.

The goal of the insulin pump is to achieve as normal a release of insulin as possible, avoiding the peaks of hypo- and hyperglycemia that inevitably occur as a result of other insulin therapy. Much research is being done on an implantable insulin pump, an "artificial pancreas," that would sense blood glucose levels and release insulin appropriately, similar to what happens with the normal pancreas. There is also research being done on the possibility of pancreatic tissue or pancreatic cell transplants. New developments in immunosuppressive drugs may make this possible in the future.

Summary of adverse reactions to oral hypoglycemic agents of the sulfonylurea class

Hypoglycemic reactions
Relatively rare; can be severe in cases of overdosage, or unexpectedly high sensitivity during the period of conversion from insulin

Allergic dermatologic reactions
Itching, redness, wheals, measleslike maculopapular eruptions

Blood dyscrasias
Leukopenia, agranulocytosis, thrombocytopenia, pancytopenia

Liver disorders
Hepatocellular and cholestatic jaundice types of liver disorders (tests of liver function are made on initiation of therapy and periodically during treatment)

Gastrointestinal upset
Anorexia, nausea, vomiting, epigastric distress, diarrhea

Nervous system side-effects
Headache, tinnitus, paresthesias (tingling), weakness, alcohollike intoxication

Summary of signs and symptoms of hypo- and hyperglycemia

Type of parameter involved	Hypoglycemia (insulin reaction)	Hyperglycemia (diabetic ketoacidosis)
Central nervous system	Headache; blurred vision, diplopia; drowsiness → coma; ataxia; hyperactive reflexes	Decreased level of consciousness; sluggishness → coma; hypoactive reflexes
Neuromuscular effects	Paresthesias; weakness; muscle spasms; twitching → seizures	Weakness; lethargy
Cardiovascular effects	Tachycardia; palpitations; normal to increased BP	Tachycardia; low BP
Respiratory effects	Rapid, shallow R	Rapid, deep respirations (Kussmaul's), acetonelike or fruity odor to breath
Gastrointestinal effects	Hunger Nausea	Nausea; vomiting; thirst
Other effects	Diaphoresis (sweating); cool, clammy, pale skin; normal eyeballs	Dry, warm, flushed skin; soft eyeballs
Laboratory tests	Presence of urine glucose—negative; blood glucose level—low	Presence of urine glucose—strongly positive; urine ketone levels—positive; blood glucose level—high
Presentation	Sudden onset; patient appears anxious, "drunk"; associated with overdose of insulin, missing a meal, increased stress	Gradual onset; patient is slow, sluggish; associated with lack of insulin, increased stress

Case study

Presentation MJ, a 22-year-old woman, has newly diagnosed type I diabetes mellitus. She was stabilized on 20 U of NPH insulin daily while hospitalized for diagnosis and management. One week after discharge from the hospital, MJ experienced anorexia and nausea. She was unable to eat but she took her insulin as usual in the morning. That afternoon she experienced profuse sweating and was tremulous and apprehensive, and she went to the hospital emergency room. The initial diagnosis was insulin reaction, brought about when MJ omitted her usual food intake because of her gastrointestinal upset. MJ was treated at the emergency room with intravenous glucose to relieve hypoglycemia, and with chlorpromazine to relieve nausea. After she had rested for an hour, she was ready to return home. What instructions should be given to MJ before she leaves the hospital?

Discussion

MJ, as a young, newly diagnosed type I diabetic, has several life changes to cope with all at once. She was stabilized on NPH insulin while hospitalized for her initial diagnosis and management. She was then discharged to home after a thorough diabetic teaching program, including the techniques of self-injection and home blood glucose monitoring, adverse insulin effects to be expected, and information about the course of diabetes. Patients who are hospitalized for insulin stabilization often develop problems at discharge because of changes in the levels of stress and resulting changes in sympathoadrenal discharge. As reviewed earlier, the sympathetic nervous system's response to stress includes an elevation of blood glucose levels. Some hospitalized patients perceive the hospital situation as stressful. If the blood sugar level is monitored and regulated while the patient is under this stress, problems can occur at discharge when the stress is removed. The sympathetic response can then decrease and the blood sugar level can fall. If the patient takes the same amount of insulin as that taken during hospitalization, there is a chance for a hypoglycemic episode. Other patients may do well in the hospital and experience stress at discharge, increasing their need for insulin. Because of these problems, it is no longer considered most beneficial to admit a patient to the hospital for regulation of insulin dosage. Patients are, instead, closely followed as outpatients, using blood glucose monitoring, and regulated in their usual environment. Patients who are regulated in the hospital are encouraged to wear street clothes and to be as active and "normal" as possible. MJ's reaction was a classic hypoglycemic response, which was probably precipitated by taking insulin and not eating. MJ should be thoroughly evaluated to make sure that this is the only reason for the reaction. The teaching program should be reviewed, with special emphasis on the need to eat after insulin administration and what should be done if eating is not possible. MJ should be asked to draw up an insulin dose and to demonstrate administration technique. She should be encouraged to verbalize her feelings and any anxieties she may be experiencing. Before she leaves the hospital, MJ should be given a follow-up visit in 2 or 3 days and a telephone number to call if any questions arise. The management of type I diabetes is challenging and often frustrating to the nurse. Developing trust and support can help the patient to cope with and adapt to this chronic disease.

Drug digests

Chlorpropamide USP (Diabinese)

Actions and indications. This sulfonylurea-type oral hypoglycemic compound is similar to tolbutamide and other drugs of the same chemical class. That is, it stimulates pancreatic β cells to synthesize and release endogenous insulin. As a result, its use may be indicated in selected cases of maturity-onset, type II diabetes that do not respond to a regimen of diet and weight reduction alone or to the use of these measures together with insulin. Its use may be necessary in mild to moderately severe cases, in which insulin cannot be employed for various reasons.

Adverse effects, cautions, and contraindications. Like other oral hypoglycemic agents, this one is contraindicated in type I diabetes (IDDM), in severe unstable or "brittle" cases, and in those complicated by ketoacidosis or coma, severe infection or injury, and conditions that require major surgery.

Hypoglycemic reactions may be prolonged and require close observation of the patient for several days because of this drug's long duration of action. The drug is slowly excreted unchanged by the kidneys, and its use is consequently contraindicated in patients with chronic kidney disease. The drug is discontinued if jaundice develops as a result of hepatic tissue hypersensitivity, allergic dermatologic reactions, or blood dyscrasias. Gastrointestinal and neurologic side-effects are usually reversible when dosage is reduced.

Dosage and administration. A single daily dose of 250 mg is usually adequate for control of symptoms. Elderly patients are started on smaller doses, such as 100 mg. Patients who do not respond to high doses of this drug alone (up to 500 mg) can sometimes have their condition controlled by combining it with up to 150 mg of phenformin in the timed-release form. However, the latter drug is now no longer generally available.

Insulin injection USP (Iletin; Regular Insulin)

Actions and indications. This form of insulin is the most prompt-acting of the available insulin preparations that act to aid diabetic patients to use dietary carbohydrate and fat in a manner that controls hyperglycemia, glycosuria, and ketosis.

It is often used alone for stabilizing newly diagnosed cases and later as a supplement to various of the longer acting modified insulin products. (It may, for example, be employed in the morning when use of an intermediate-acting product does not prevent prelunch glycosuria.) It is particularly useful in unstable cases of diabetes in which glucose tolerance fluctuates widely, and for patients with severe infection, injuries, or surgical trauma and shock who are likely to develop ketoacidosis or coma.

Adverse effects, cautions, and contraindications. Overdosage can cause the rapid onset of hypoglycemic reactions. Thus, frequent blood sugar level determinations are desirable, and patients should be watched for such early signs as sweating and anxiety reactions. Failure to detect and to treat these and other early manifestations of insulin shock may result in more severe reactions that include coma and convulsions, and even death.

Dosage and administration. Dosage varies very widely. Treatment is usually initiated with 10 to 20 U administered subcutaneously about 30 minutes before breakfast. The intravenous route is used in patients in diabetic coma and with circulatory collapse.

Insulin zinc suspension USP (Lente Insulin; Lente Iletin)

Actions and indications. This mixture has a duration of action midway between that of the prompt-acting zinc insulin suspension and protamine zinc insulin, preparations of rapid and prolonged duration. Like isophane insulin suspension, with which it can be used interchangeably, this preparation has its onset of action in over 2 hours, exerts its peak effects between 8 and 12 hours after administration, and lasts over 24 hours. It is not suited for intravenous administration in emergencies.

Adverse effects, cautions, and contraindi- cations. Hypoglycemic reactions may not have a dramatic onset but tend to be prolonged and recurrent, because any overdose continues to be absorbed from the injection site. To ensure withdrawal of a uniform suspension of particles and thus avoid dosage irregularities, the vial is inverted several times from end to end. It should not, however, be shaken vigorously, nor be exposed to freezing or warm temperatures. Local sensitivity reactions do not occur with this preparation, which contains no protamine or other modifying protein.

Dosage and administration. This preparation is administered subcutaneously in initial doses of 10 U, but final dosage may range up to 80 U in some cases. It is best given before breakfast to counteract the expected rise in blood sugar levels after that meal. During the later hours of the morning it may have to be supplemented by injection of a more rapid-acting insulin and, during the night, the addition of a long-acting insulin may be necessary.

Protamine zinc insulin suspension USP (Protamine, Zinc & Iletin)

Actions and indications. This preparation possesses a prolonged duration of action. Its effects come on only after 4 to 6 hours but may last 36 hours or longer. It is most useful for treating cases in which the patient's condition is stable and timing is not of primary importance. Its use is desirable in patients whose blood sugar level begins to rise at night and stays high during sleep. This form is never used in diabetic emergencies, nor is it ever substituted for other ordered insulin preparations except when such a change is directed.

Adverse effects, cautions, and contraindications. Dosage adjustment is necessary to avoid long-lasting and recurrent episodes of hypoglycemia. If such reactions occur they are counteracted by administering a combination of a soluble, rapidly utilized source of carbohydrate, such as orange juice, together with a more slowly digestible food substance. It is desirable for patients to take snacks between meals and essential that they eat something before going to sleep. Presence of the protein protamine may lead to development of local sensitivity reactions.

Dosage and administration. Subcutaneous injections are made once daily about 30 to 60 minutes before breakfast. It is never given by vein.

Tolbutamide USP (Orinase)

Actions and indications. This oral hypoglycemic agent lowers blood sugar levels by stimulating the synthesis and release of insulin by β cells of the pancreas. Its use is now limited largely to cases of adult or maturity-onset, type II diabetes mellitus that are not adequately controlled by diet and weight reduction alone, or by these measures plus insulin. Its use is also justified in mild to moderate cases of maturity-onset diabetes in which insulin cannot be used for any of various reasons.

Adverse effects, cautions, and contraindications. This drug is contraindicated in juvenile- or growth-onset, type I diabetes, or in cases complicated by ketosis, acidosis, or the presence of infection, fever, severe injury, or major surgery. Hypoglycemic reactions may occur with overdosage or in patients with severe liver disease that interferes with metabolic degradation of the drug. Caution is necessary when other drugs such as the coumarin-type anticoagulants, salicylates, or phenylbutazone are also employed to prevent potentiation of the hypoglycemic effect. Other adverse effects include gastrointestinal disturbances and allergic skin reactions.

Dosage and administration. Dosage is individualized in accordance with the patient's response. Treatment is usually begun with 1 to 2 g daily administered in divided dosage. This is adjusted downward to as little as 0.5 g or upward to as much as 3 g daily. The usual maintenance dose is 2 g daily administered in several divided amounts.

References

Cahill GF Jr et al: "Control" and diabetes. N Engl J Med 294:1004, 1976

Cavalier JP: Crucial decisions in diabetic emergencies. RN 43:32 (Nov) 1980

Chalmers TC: Settling the UGDP controversy. JAMA 231:624, 1975

Davidson JK: Controlling diabetes mellitus with drug therapy. Postgrad Med 59:114, 1976

Dupre J: Insulin therapy: Progress and prospects. Hosp Pract 18:171, 1983

Fletcher HP: The oral antidiabetic drugs: Pro and con. Am J Nurs 76:596, 1976

Genuth SM: Whole body metabolism and the hormones of the pancreatic islets. In Berne, RM, Levy MN (eds): Physiology, pp 915–948. St. Louis, CV Mosby, 1983

Gerich JE: Somatostatin: Diabetes and acromegaly. Adv Intern Med 22:251, 1977

Gerich JE et al: Prevention of human ketoacidosis by somatostatin. Evidence for an essential role of glucagon. N Engl J Med 292:285, 1975

Hansen AP et al: Somatostatin: A review of its effects, especially in human beings. Diabetes Metab 2:203, 1977

Hayter J: Fine points in diabetic care. Am J Nurs 76:594, 1976

Human insulin: Med Lett Drugs Ther 25:63, 1983

Larner J: Insulin and oral hypoglycemic drugs: Glucagon. In Gilman AG, Goodman LS, Gilman A (eds): Goodman and Gilman's The Pharmacological Basis of Therapeutics, 6th ed, pp 1497–1523. New York, Macmillan, 1980

Larner J, Haynes RC Jr: Insulin and oral hypoglycemic drugs; Glucagon. In Goodman LS, Gilman A (eds): The Pharmacological Basis of Therapeutics, 5th ed, pp 1507–1533. New York, Macmillan, 1975

Mecklenburg R et al: Clinical use of the insulin infusion pump in 100 patients with Type I diabetes. N Engl J Med 307:513, 1982

Meyers SA: Diabetes management by the patient and a nurse practitioner. Nurs Clin North Am 12:415, 1977

Murray P: When hyperglycemia goes critical: Distinguishing between hyperosmolar and ketoacidotic coma. RN 46:56 (March) 1983

National Diabetes Data Group. Classification and diagnosis of diabetes mellitus and other categories of glucose intolerance. Diabetes 28:1039, 1979

Nemchick R: Diabetes Today (Part 2): A very different diet; a new generation of oral drugs. RN 45:41 (Nov) 1982

Nemchick R: Diabetes Today (Part 3): The news about insulin. RN 45:49 (Dec) 1982

Nemchick R: Diabetes Today (Part 6): The new insulin pumps: Tight control at a price. RN 46:52 (May) 1983

Page M: Treatment of diabetic ketoacidosis. N Engl J Med 294:1183, 1976

Salans LB: Diabetes mellitus: A disease that is coming into focus. JAMA 247:590, 1982

Self-monitoring methods for blood glucose. Med Lett Drugs Ther 25:42, 1983

Shagan BP: Diabetes in the elderly patient. Med Clin North Am 60:1191, 1976

Shen SW, Bressler R: Clinical pharmacology of oral antidiabetic agents. N Engl J Med 296:493, 787, 1977

Unger RH, Orci L: Glucagon and the A cell. N Engl J Med 304:1518, 1981

Yue DK et al: New forms of insulin and their use in the treatment of diabetes. Diabetes 26:341, 1977

Section 5

Drugs acting on the cardiovascular system

5 This section will discuss the actions and uses of drugs employed in the management of cardiovascular diseases. Although many cardiac and vascular diseases are now treated surgically or with electronic devices, most patients are still maintained by medical means. Thus, the nurse must be thoroughly familiar with the many potent drugs employed in treating these disorders, and must also be prepared to help patients and their families deal realistically with the emotional aspects of heart disease.

Cardiovascular disease is the leading cause of disability and death in this country. Most people are, of course, aware of the high mortality rate of heart disease and only need to watch TV or read a newspaper to be freshly reminded of the suddenness with which cardiac death can strike. Thus, a diagnosis of heart disease usually has a tremendous emotional impact on the patient and family.

Because heart disease is often associated with sudden death, people who hear that they have a heart rhythm disorder, a coronary condition, or a failing heart may be overwhelmed by fear and hopelessness. Their families often share this despair and are, in addition, alarmed by the thought that, if an emergency should arise, the responsibility of obtaining help or even giving the patient emergency care might be theirs alone. Family members may worry about how helpless they would feel in such a situation, and their uneasiness in the presence of the patient may add to the patient's anxiety and tension.

The nurse who is called on to care for a heart patient may often be troubled by the responsibilities involved in a life-or-death situation. A thorough understanding of the mechanisms of action of the various cardiovascular drugs will prepare the nurse to deal effectively with the responsibilities of patient teaching, daily patient care, and the acute cardiovascular emergency.

A meaningful discussion of the various classes of pharmacologic agents that affect heart and blood vessel function requires first a brief review of certain significant properties of the organs and structures that comprise the circulatory system.

Chapter 26

Review
of cardiovascular
function

26

This chapter will review some aspects of the anatomy, physiology, and pathophysiology of the cardiovascular system. Some highlights of the subject will be emphasized to provide the foundation for the study of the various drugs used in treating cardiovascular disorders that will be discussed in the following chapters of this section. An understanding of the terms and concepts presented here should be helpful in studying the drug actions that alter circulatory system function.

The heart

The heart is a hollow muscular organ with four chambers (Fig. 26-1). Actually, there are two joined hearts—a right and a left—and each is divided into two parts, an upper *atrium* and a lower *ventricle*. The right half of the heart, which is separated from the left heart by a partition, or septum, directs the deoxygenated blood brought to it from the body tissues by the veins (a vein is any vessel carrying blood toward the heart) into the lungs. The left heart receives the blood after it has been reoxygenated in the lungs and pumps it out into the aorta, from which it flows through the rest of the systemic circulation by way of the arteries (an artery is a muscular vessel carrying blood away from the heart).

Before following the flowing blood to the tissues that it nourishes, the properties of this muscular pump that propels blood through the 60,000 miles of tubes comprising the rest of the circulatory system will be examined.

The cardiac cycle

The heart, which in its healthy state beats thousands of millions of times in a lifetime, possesses structural and functional properties different from those of other muscles. The fibers of the myocardium form two intertwining

networks, or *syncytia*—an atrial syncytium and a ventricular syncytium. This interlacing structure enables first both atria and then both ventricles to contract synchronously when excited by the same rapidly traveling stimulus. Completely simultaneous contraction is a necessary property of a muscle that acts as a pump. A hollow pumping mechanism must also pause long enough in its pumping cycle to allow its chambers to fill with fluid. Heart muscle does relax long enough to ensure adequate filling and, the more fully it fills, the stronger is the contraction that follows as the muscle fibers, stretched by the volume of blood that has been returned, spring back like elastic bands (a property defined in the Frank–Starling law of contraction).

As indicated below, during diastole—the period of cardiac muscle relaxation—blood that returns to the heart from the systemic and pulmonary veins flows into the atria. When the pressure generated by the blood volume in the atria becomes greater than intraventricular pressure, the blood flows through the open atrioventricular valves directly into the ventricles. Atrial contractions complete the process of ventricular filling, pumping approximately 1 tbsp (15 ml) of blood into each ventricle just before the ventricles are stimulated to contract (systole). The much more powerful ventricular contractions then pump the blood into the large arteries that carry it to the lungs and to the systemic circulation (Fig. 26-1).

Each period of systole followed by diastole is referred to as a *cardiac cycle*. The heart is equipped with four one-way valves to keep the blood flowing in the right direction. The tricuspid valve, between the right atrium and right ventricle, allows blood to flow from the atrium into the ventricle but closes tightly when the ventricle contracts to prevent any backward flow of blood. The mitral valve serves the same function on the left side of the heart. The pulmonic valve, at the base of the pulmonary artery, allows blood to flow from the right ven-

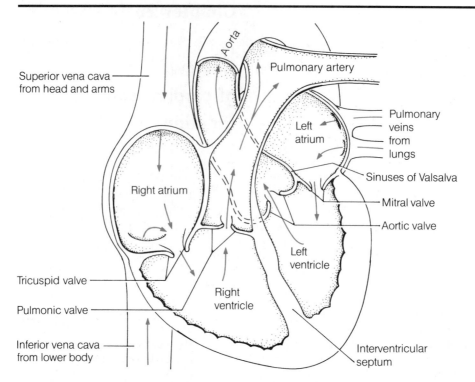

Figure 26-1. Blood flow into and out of the heart. Deoxygenated blood enters the right atrium from the superior and inferior venae cavae and falls through the tricuspid valve into the right ventricle, which contracts and sends the blood through the pulmonic valve into the pulmonary artery and to the lungs. Oxygenated blood from the lungs enters the left atrium through the pulmonary veins and passes through the mitral valve into the left ventricle, which contracts and ejects the blood through the aortic valve into the aorta and out to the systemic circulation.

tricle into the pulmonary artery during ventricular systole. It closes tightly during diastole to prevent blood from flowing backward into the right ventricle. The aortic valve, between the aorta and the left ventricle, serves the same function on the left side of the heart. The proper functioning of the cardiac valves is important in maintaining the direction of blood flow and adequate perfusion of vital organs with oxygenated blood.

Normal cardiac rhythm

Each cycle of cardiac diastole and systole is controlled by impulses that arise spontaneously in certain *pacemaker cells* of the sinoatrial node of the heart. These impulses are conducted from the pacemaker cells by a specialized conducting system that activates all parts of the myocardium almost simultaneously (Fig. 26-2). The continual rhythmic contraction of the mammalian heart is controlled within the heart itself. This allows the heart to continue to beat as long as it has enough nutrients and oxygen, regardless of the functional status of other systems of the body. This property protects the vital cardiovascular function in many disease states; it is this same property that allows the heart to go on functioning normally in a patient who is "brain-dead."

The special system for initiating and conducting the impulses that control cardiac rhythm is comprised of the following structures: (1) the *sinoatrial (S-A) node*, the usual pacemaker of the heart, which sends impulses over (2) the *atrial bundles* to (3) the *atrioventricular*, or *A-V, node*, from which the impulses are passed on to (4) the *bundle of His*, a large fiber bundle that carries the impulses into the ventricle and then divides into (5) three *bundle branches* (the left anterior, left posterior, and right bundle branches), which break up into (6) a network of fine conducting fibers, the *Purkinje fibers*.

Automaticity. The cells of this impulse-forming and conducting system are very primitive uncomplicated cells called pale or P cells. Because of their simple cell membranes, these cells possess a special property that differentiates them from other cardiac muscle cells: they can generate impulses without being excited to do so by external stimuli. This property is called *automaticity*. These cells undergo *spontaneous depolarizations*, called *diastolic depolarizations*, because they occur during diastole, and also called *pacemaker potentials* because it is these potentials in cells of the S-A node that normally set the pace of the heart contractions. These pacemaker potentials are due mainly to a decreasing flow of potassium ions out of the

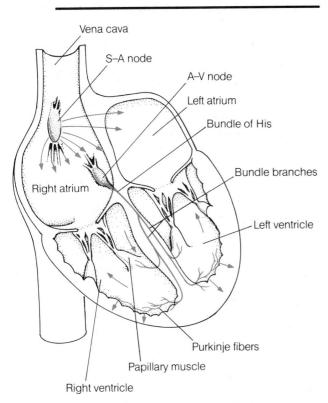

Vena cava

S–A node

A–V node

Left atrium

Bundle of His

Bundle branches

Right atrium

Left ventricle

Purkinje fibers

Papillary muscle

Right ventricle

Figure 26-2. The conducting system of the heart. Impulses originating in the S-A node are transmitted through the atrial bundles to the A-V node and down the bundle of His and the bundle branches by way of the Purkinje fibers through the ventricles.

cell, although for many years they were believed to be due to a leak of sodium ions into the cell. Leakiness to sodium may also contribute to the depolarizations.

These pacemaker potentials actively move the electrical potential across the membrane, or the *resting membrane potential*, toward a trigger point—the *threshold potential*. When this point is reached, sodium ions rush into the interior of the cell at a very rapid rate and cause further depolarization of the cardiac cell membrane and the development of an *action potential.*

The classic action potential of a cardiac muscle cell consists of five phases, phase 0 through phase 4 (Fig. 26-3). Phase 0 occurs when the cell reaches the threshold potential and sodium gates open along the cell membrane, allowing sodium ions to rush into the cell. This causes a change in transmembrane electrical potential, and is an all-or-none phenomenon. Phase 1 is a short period during which the sodium concentrations equalize on either side of the cell membrane. Phase 2 is often called the plateau stage, because the transmembrane potential is relatively constant during this time. The cell membrane becomes less permeable to sodium, calcium slowly begins to enter the cell (through what is called the "slow channel"), potassium begins to leave the cell, and the cell begins to

return to its electrical resting state. Phase 3 is a period of rapid repolarization when sodium and potassium leave the cell and the slow channel becomes inactive. During phase 4, repolarization is completed as the sodium pump actively pumps sodium out and pumps potassium in, until the transmembrane potential reaches its normal resting state of about −80 mV. During phase 4, cells in the specialized impulse-forming and conducting tissue undergo the spontaneous depolarizations described above. (The membrane potential of ventricular muscle cells remains constant during phase 4.) The proper operation of this impulse-forming and conducting system depends on appropriate concentrations of sodium, potassium, and calcium ions, as well as on energy in the form of ATP to operate the sodium pump.

The actual appearance of the action potential differs in different areas of the heart. The action potentials of the specialized tissue have less well-defined phases 1 and 2 (Fig. 26-3A), while the action potentials of ventricular

A

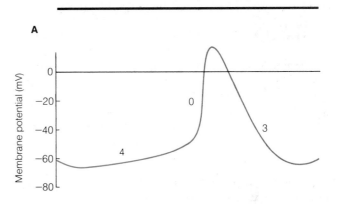

B

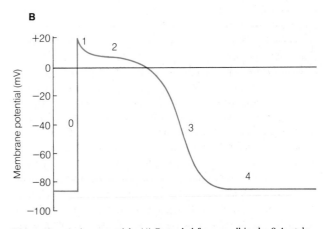

Figure 26-3. Action potentials. (A) Recorded from a cell in the S-A node, showing diastolic depolarization in phase 4; (B) recorded from a ventricular muscle cell. (*Phase 0*) The cell is stimulated, sodium rushes into the cell, and the cell is depolarized; (*phase 1*) sodium levels equalize; (*phase 2*) the plateau phase, in which calcium enters the cell (the slow current), and potassium and sodium leave; (*phase 3*) the slow current stops, and sodium and potassium leave the cell; (*phase 4*) the resting membrane potential returns and the pacemaker potential begins in the S-A node cell.

muscle cells have all phases well defined, including a relatively long plateau phase (Fig. 26-3B). Because of these differences, the *rhythmicity* of each area of the heart is different—that is, the rate at which spontaneous action potentials are fired differs. The S-A node will simultaneously generate action potentials at the rate of 70 to 80/minute, the A-V node at 40 to 50/minute, and the ventricular muscle cells at only 10 to 20/minute.

Conductivity. Thus, under normal conditions, the cells of the S-A node depolarize at a more rapid rate than any cells of the other specialized cardiac tissue. Although these other cells of the impulse-generating and conducting system all can also generate impulses actively, they do so at a slower rate than the S-A node. Thus, the S-A node is the *pacemaker* that triggers the passive firing of the rest of the conducting system cells by means of its excitatory action potentials.

The speed at which the propagated impulses set by the sinus rhythm pass through the specialized conducting tissues and the atrial and ventricular musculature differs from tissue to tissue within the heart. The *conduction velocity* is slowest in the A-V node and fastest in the Purkinje system fibers. The delay in impulse conduction from the atria to the ventricles accounts for the fact that the atria contract a fraction of a second before the ventricles, as described above. This allows the ventricles to fill completely just before contracting. The almost instantaneous spread of the impulse to the terminations of the Purkinje fibers in the ventricular muscle walls permits their simultaneous stimulation and accounts for their powerful, efficient pumping action.

The rate at which an action potential is conducted depends partly on the height and rate of increase of the action potential—that is, on the amount of potential change during phase 0 and on how rapidly this change occurs (Fig. 26-3). A "tall," steeply rising action potential will bring the next adjacent patch of membrane to its threshold faster than a "sickly," gradually rising action potential (see also Chap. 13, The Action Potential), indicating that conduction velocity will be faster. Conduction velocity also depends on the threshold potential.

After a patch of cell membrane has conducted an action potential, it may not be at all responsive to a succeeding impulse for a time. This *absolute refractory period* is followed by a period of partial and then full recovery of the ability of the membrane to be stimulated. The absolute refractory period corresponds to the time from the beginning of the action potential (phase 0) until repolarization (phase 3) is one-half to two-thirds complete. Sometimes one sees the term, *functional* or *effective* refractory period, or *ERP*. This is the minimal time that must elapse between two stimuli applied at one site on the heart for each of them to elicit an action potential at another site. This parameter is a measure not only of refractoriness but also of conduction velocity. Cardiac drugs can lengthen or shorten the refractory periods of the various heart tissues. This reduces or raises the responsiveness of these cardiac tissues to stimuli that reach them at a normal or an abnormal rate.

Autonomic influences. The rate at which cardiac impulses are rhythmically generated and conducted depends primarily on the intrinsic electrophysiologic properties of the heart cell membranes, as described above. However, the heart's rate, rhythm, and contractile strength are also influenced by nerve impulses from both branches of the autonomic nervous system (Chap. 13). These extrinsic impulses affect the rate of S-A nodal firing, the speed with which action potentials pass through the A-V node and the specialized conducting tissues, and the strength of ventricular contraction.

The extrinsic nerves that carry the impulses that alter the heart's inherent sinus rhythm are of two types. The vagus nerves, which are part of the parasympathetic nervous system (Chaps. 13 and 15) innervate the S-A and A-V nodes. Vagal impulses slow the heart rate and decrease the rate of conduction of the cardiac impulse through the A-V node. Their activity tends to allow the heart to rest and conserve its strength. The other nerves that exert an outside influence on the heart are part of the sympathetic nervous system (Chaps. 13 and 17). These nerves innervate the S-A and A-V nodes and ventricular muscle. Sympathetic impulses speed the heart rate, increase the rate of conduction of the cardiac impulse through the AV node, and strengthen the force of contraction of ventricular muscle.

The sympathetic nervous system sends more impulses to the heart during exercise, when the tissues raise their demands for oxygen and the heart responds by beating more rapidly and powerfully to send added blood surging through the arterial circulation. Heart disease may also set off the same kind of compensatory reflexes for counteracting a lack of adequate tissue oxygenation.

Tissue hypoxia is one cause of the accelerated heart rate often seen in patients with heart failure. When drugs of the digitalis group (see Chap. 29) help the failing heart to beat more effectively, the activity of the cardioacceleratory nerves is reduced in response to the increased cardiac output, and that of the vagus nerves is reflexly increased. As a result, the rate of the heart's beating slows as an indirect response to the cardiotonic action of these drugs. (There are also direct effects of digitalis on the heart to cause it to slow.)

In addition, drugs can slow or speed the heart directly by imitating the actions of autonomic nerve impulses or by blocking such extrinsic impulses. Thus, sympathomimetic drugs accelerate the heart, as do vagus blocking drugs such as atropine; on the other hand, parasympathomimetic drugs slow the heart rate, as do β-adrenergic blocking agents.

Mechanical activity

The end result of the electrical activity in the heart is stimulation of the two cardiac syncytia, leading to a unified contraction of first the atria and then the ventricles. These unified contractions move the blood through the vascular system.

The basic unit of the cardiac muscle is called a sarcomere. The sarcomere is composed of two contractile proteins: *actin*, a thin filament, and *myosin*, a thicker filament with projections on it. The two proteins have a great affinity for each other but are normally prevented from interacting by the presence of the protein *troponin*. During phase 2 of an action potential calcium enters the cell and inactivates the troponin, and the actin and myosin proteins then interact. The myosin projections form "bridges" of *actomyosin*, with active sites on the actin filament. The bridge breaks quickly and the myosin moves to the next active site, sliding the fibers along and shortening the sarcomere. This process requires energy. The group of sarcomeres shortening at the same time produces a contraction of the muscle. In the case of the cardiac ventricle, the contraction forces the volume of blood out of the ventricles, producing what is known as the *stroke volume* or volume ejected per beat or contraction (Fig. 26-4).

Muscle contraction occurs as a result of *excitation–contraction coupling*. The electrical activity causes the release of calcium into the cell, and contraction occurs. If more calcium is available, more actomyosin bridges will form, resulting in a stronger contraction that uses more energy. If less calcium is available, fewer bridges are formed, the contraction is weaker, and less energy is used.

Frank–Starling's law of the heart (see above) states that, the more a cardiac muscle is stretched, the more it will contract, up to a certain point. This is an important concept of cardiac function. The further the actin and myosin are stretched apart, the more bridges can be formed and, thus, the stronger the contraction. However, if the proteins are stretched too far apart, they will not be able to interact, no bridges will be formed, and the contraction will not occur. This can occur in several pathologic conditions involving the heart.

Cardiac arrhythmias

Various factors in addition to drugs can alter cardiac rate and rhythm. Cardiac arrhythmias result most often from an inadequate flow of oxygenated blood to the heart's tissues. The resulting hypoxia and acidosis, the rise in carbon dioxide content of the blood perfusing the heart, and changes in the content of electrolytes such as potassium may all lead to irregular rhythms. Any irregularity in the cardiac rhythm will influence the work of the heart and can result in serious alterations in cardiac output. Changes in cardiac output will influence every organ of the body, and are very serious clinical problems.

Cardiac arrhythmias can arise as a result of abnormalities in either or both of the fundamental electrophysiologic properties discussed above: *automaticity* and *conductivity*. Impulses may be generated at an excessively rapid or slow rate from the S-A node and other pacemaker cells. Similarly, impulses may be conducted too slowly,

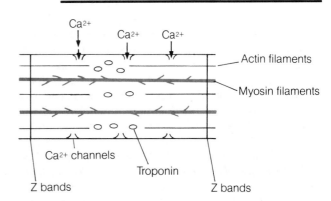

Figure 26-4. A sarcomere, the functional unit of cardiac muscle.

they may be blocked, or they may follow abnormal pathways that can then cause the heart to beat rapidly and irregularly.

Some arrhythmias are marked by a shift in the pacemaker from the S-A node to some other site of automatic impulse production called an *ectopic* focus. This occurs most commonly as a result of pathophysiologic factors that cause the usually latent pacemakers to begin firing. Such firing from ectopic foci causes *premature contractions*, or *extrasystoles*. Premature beats of this type may not be serious, but in certain clinical situations—after a heart attack, for example, or during overdosage with digitalis—their presence may be the prelude to more serious arrhythmias such as ventricular tachycardia or fatal ventricular fibrillation.

A decrease in the ability of impulses to pass through the A-V node or the bundle of His leads to varying degrees of *heart block*. In first-degree block, all the impulses that originate at the S-A node pass through to the ventricles, but they are delayed at the A-V node for an abnormally long time. Second-degree block is marked by failure of some atrial impulses to reach the ventricles. No impulses from the atria reach the ventricles in complete heart block, and the ventricles then beat at a slow rate that is set by automatic cells in Purkinje fibers—so-called *idioventricular* pacemakers.

Other changes in the rate of impulse conduction along a cardiac cell fiber can lead to *circus reentry rhythms*. These result from disturbances in conduction that progressively slow the action potential in one area (*decremental conduction*) or that bring it to a complete halt in one area (*unidirectional block*). Impulses that move very slowly or take an abnormally long pathway may then get back to their original starting point at a time when the tissue has recovered from the first passage of the impulses. This no longer refractory tissue then responds once more to the returning impulses. Reentry of these impulses sets up a self-sustaining circular movement of action potentials. (Reentry can also occur when the refractory period of the heart muscle tissue is shortened.)

Some serious arrhythmias result from a combination of both the rapid firing of impulses from ectopic foci and a reduction in the speed with which the impulses are conducted through some, but not all, areas of heart muscle tissue. Impulses that travel at irregular rates through many abnormally lengthened pathways with different refractory periods activate smaller and smaller areas of heart muscle. Such fractionation of depolarizing currents results in fibrillatory activity. This is a condition marked by chaotic incoordinated twitching of atrial or ventricular muscle, in which blood cannot be pumped out of the heart's chambers. People can live quite normally with atrial fibrillation but death occurs quickly in ventricular fibrillation, unless the heart is rapidly defibrillated and a regular rhythm is restored.

The electrocardiogram

Electrocardiography is a very important diagnostic tool for detecting cardiac arrhythmias. The electrocardiograph records patterns of electrical activity that are generated in the heart and spread to the surface of the patient's body, where they are picked up by recording electrodes. These patterns of cardiac electrical activity are made visible on the electrocardiogram (ECG), a record traced on a strip of moving calibrated paper. It is important to remember that the ECG is simply a measure of electrical activity and provides no information about the mechanical activity of the heart. The patient, himself, needs to be assessed to determine the adequacy of cardiac output.

Nurses in intensive coronary care units (ICCUs) are expert in reading and rapidly interpreting ECG recordings. When the presence of potentially dangerous abnormalities in cardiac rhythm is detected, prompt action is taken to terminate the arrhythmia with drugs or other measures. The nature of the normal ECG and some abnormal patterns that appear during various arrhythmias, whose treatment with drugs is discussed in several of the chapters in this section, will be reviewed briefly.

Normal sinus rhythm

The normal ECG is made up of five main waves: a P wave, a QRS complex that is composed of three separate smaller waves, and a T wave (Fig. 26-5). The P wave is formed as impulses originating in the sinus node pass through and depolarize atrial tissues. The QRS complex indicates passage of impulses down the bundle of His (Q) and through the ventricles (RS). The P wave immediately precedes the contraction of the atria; the QRS complex immediately precedes the contraction of the ventricles. The T wave appears during the repolarization and relaxation of the ventricles. The repolarization of the atria (T_a wave) is normally hidden in the larger QRS complex; it is seen only in certain pathologic conditions.

The critical intervals of the ECG are the P–R interval, reflecting the normal delay of conduction at the AV node; the Q–T interval, reflecting the critical timing of repolarization in the ventricles; and the S–T segment, which provides important information about the repolarization of the ventricles (Fig. 26-5). Abnormalities in the configuration and timing of each part of the tracing reveal the presence of functional or organic cardiac disorders.

The ECG in the diagnosis of cardiac arrhythmias

Sinus arrhythmias. The S-A node normally fires in response to the changing demands of the body's tissues for blood. This is reflected in changes in the number of complexes that appear on the ECG per unit of time. Arrhythmias that stem from changes in S-A nodal depolarization rates follow similar patterns of normally shaped complexes that appear at abnormal rates. *Sinus tachycardia,* for example, is marked by complexes that are measured at 100 or more per minute. In *sinus bradycardia,* the rate of complex formation falls below 60 per minute. In one type of sinus arrhythmia seen commonly in children, the complexes are also normal but their rate is irregular, increasing with each inhalation of a breath and decreasing with each expiration.

Supraventricular arrhythmias. These cardiac irregularities originate above the ventricles in atrial tissue outside the S-A node. Abnormally shaped P waves indicate that the source of the often rapid ventricular rate is not in the ventricles but in the atria. Impulses that arise at ectopic atrial sites more rapidly than those from the S-A node now set the pace for the rest of the heart. Arrhythmias of this type include premature atrial contractions (PACs), paroxysmal atrial tachycardia (PAT), atrial flutter, and atrial fibrillation.

In these conditions, the QRS complexes have normal configurations because there is no defect in ventricular condition. When every rapidly generated atrial impulse passes through the A-V node—as in PAT, for example—each abnormal P wave is followed by a normal QRS complex. However, in atrial flutter and atrial fibrillation, many of the abnormal P waves fail to pass through the A-V node. Thus, the QRS complexes—although normal in shape—do *not* appear in a 1:1 ratio to the ectopic atrial waves.

The P waves in atrial flutter form a regular sawtooth pattern, because they arise in a single rapidly firing ectopic focus. If one of every two atrial impulses is blocked at the A-V node, there will be only one QRS complex for each abnormally shaped P wave. Atrial fibrillation is characterized by very irregularly shaped P waves, often appearing as a wavy line, because they originate from various atrial ectopic sites and each takes a different pathway to the A-V node. Because these impulses do not pass to the ventricles in any regular ratio, the QRS complexes

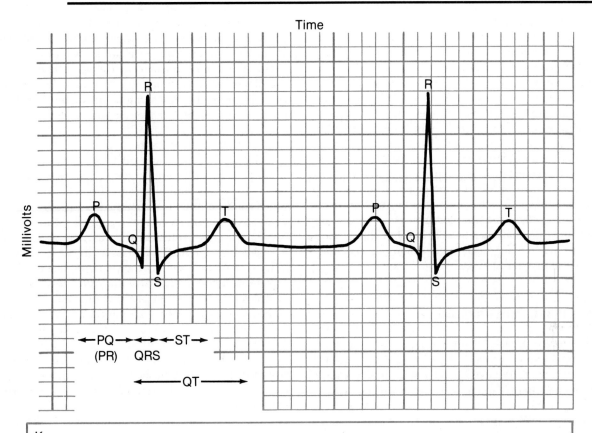

Figure 26-5. The normal ECG pattern.

occur in a completely irregular rhythm. Most of the several hundred atrial impulses are blocked at the A-V node, but enough get through to drive the ventricles to beat in a rapid, irregular, inefficient manner.

Atrioventricular (A-V) block. First-degree heart block is characterized by a prolongation of the P–R interval, which is lengthened to well beyond the normal 0.16 to 0.20 second. Each P wave is followed by a QRS complex, because—as indicated earlier—each atrial impulse activates a ventricular beat. In second-degree heart block, conduction ratios of 2:1, 3:1, 4:1, or other combinations, reflect the fact that only a single QRS complex follows every two, three, four, or more P waves. Third-degree, or complete, heart block is marked by a total

dissociation of P waves from QRS complexes and T waves. Because the P waves can come at any time, the P–R intervals are not constant. The QRS complexes appear at the slow rates that are set by the idioventricular pacemakers.

Ventricular arrhythmias. Impulses that originate in pacemaker cells below the A-V node and that set off extrasystoles produce wide, or prolonged, QRS complexes and inverted T waves in the ECG, reflecting the conduction of the action potential across tissue that is not using the rapid conduction system. Such premature ventricular complexes (PVCs) on the ECG record may arise from a single ectopic focus or from multifocal sources. PVCs that appear in groups, each of which has a different shape, are considered particularly ominous, because they reflect several different irritated foci within the muscle. Runs of several wide PVCs that come at a rapid rate are characterized as ventricular tachycardia. In ventricular fibrillation, the impulses arising at numerous sites and moving in many directions produce a bizarre pattern of irregular, distorted waves on the ECG. This arrhythmia is fatal if untreated, because no ventricular contraction occurs and no blood is delivered to the body or the brain.

Other ECG abnormalities. The presence of myocardial ischemia and hypoxia is marked by elevation of the S–T segment of the complexes recorded on the ECG. After a myocardial infarction, this is followed by an inversion of the T wave and often by an abnormally large Q wave. After the infarct has healed, the T wave returns to its normal upright position, but the Q wave of a once-damaged heart can remain enlarged, reflecting a loss of healthy conducting tissue.

The cardiovascular system

The purpose of the heart's unceasing pumping action is to keep blood flowing to and from all the body's tissues. Blood brings the cells the oxygen and nutrients they need for producing energy, and it carries away carbon dioxide and other metabolic waste products. This steady circulation of blood is essential for proper functioning of all the body's organs, including the heart itself. Certain aspects of blood flow through the heart and the pulmonary and systemic circuits will be reviewed. The various clinical conditions that develop when such circulation is interfered with, as well as the actions of the drugs used to treat these disorders, will be better understood by learning about the basic physiology of the system.

Circulation

Heart–lung circulation

The blood that returns to the right heart by way of the venous portion of the systemic circulation first enters the right atrium (Fig. 26-6). Most of the blood that enters the right atrium will fall, with pressure changes, into the right ventricle. Following electrical activation of the atria, a contraction of the thin muscular wall of this chamber sends the remaining oxygen-deficient blood into the right ventricle, which squeezes it, in turn, into the pulmonary artery. This vessel enters the lungs and divides into smaller and smaller vessels through which the blood flows until it spreads out in a thin sheet in the pulmonary capillaries. These thin-walled vessels are in direct contact with another wispy membrane lining the alveoli, the terminal cells for air inhaled with each breath. Here, oxygen diffuses across these thin walls and is picked up by the blood pigment hemoglobin in the red blood cells.

The oxygenated blood now flows into vessels that grow from capillary size into venules and, finally, into the pulmonary veins, which carry it into the left atrium. From here the oxygenated blood spills into the left ventricle. The thick muscular wall of this chamber drives the blood out into the aorta, the body's largest artery. Branches of the aorta carry blood to the heart, head, lungs, liver, kidneys, and other vital organs.

Systemic circulation

The aorta and other large arteries have thick muscular walls. The entire arterial system contains muscles in its walls all the way to the terminal branches or arterioles, which consist of fragments of muscle and endothelial cells. These offer resistance to the surging blood that is forced through the arterial tree by the pumping pressure at the left ventricle. These so-called *resistance vessels* can be constricted or dilated to meet the changing needs of various organs for blood. Thus, some arterioles can be closed off completely to help shunt blood to other dilated vascular beds that have a greater need for blood at a particular time. This ability makes the arterioles one of the major regulators of blood pressure.

Blood from tiny terminal arterioles of the microvasculature flows into the thin-walled capillaries, which are merely connected endothelial cells. Fluid containing oxygen and nutrients diffuses through the arterial end of these vessels into the interstitial spaces between tissue cells. Fluid containing waste products of tissue metabolism is drawn back into the vascular system at the venous end of the capillaries. This shift of fluid is carefully balanced by hydrostatic (fluid pressure) forces and by oncotic pressures (the pulling pressure of vascular proteins). Understanding this regulation of fluid is important in understanding the development of edema and other signs of cardiovascular disease (Fig. 26-7). These capillaries then merge with venules, the smallest veins, and larger vessels of the venous system then carry blood back to the right side of the heart.

The venous system is not only a conduit for the venous return of deoxygenated blood to the right atrium. These vessels can also hold large quantities of blood in reserve because of the distensibility of their relatively thin, flexible walls. This function of these so-called *capacitance vessels* plays a part in regulating the pressure within the heart's right atrium—the *central venous pressure* (CVP).

The volume (load) of blood that is brought back to the heart by the large veins (the superior and inferior vena cavae) and by the coronary veins that drain into the right atrium is referred to as the *preload,* and the resistance offered to the left ventricle by blood pumped into the aorta and the rest of the peripheral systemic arterial tree is called the *afterload.* These terms and concepts concerning the hemodynamics of the systemic circulation are significant for understanding the response of the heart

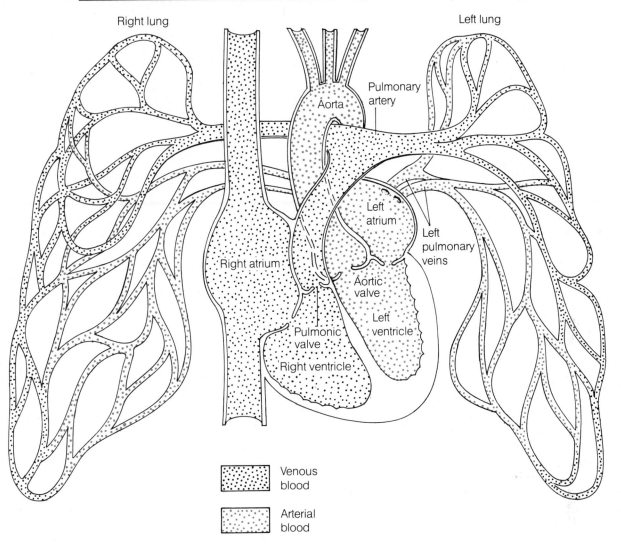

Figure 26-6. The pulmonary circulation.

and the coronary circulation to the drugs that are used in treating patients with coronary heart disease.

Coronary circulation

The heart muscle itself requires a constant supply of oxygenated blood to keep contracting. The myocardium receives its own nourishment through two main coronary arteries. These vessels are called "coronary" because they branch off from the base of the aorta just as it leaves the left ventricle (an area called the *sinuses of Valsalva*) and then encircle the upper part of the heart in a pattern resembling a coronet, or crown. The coronary arteries fill during diastole, when the heart muscle is at rest and relaxed, and they can thus receive the flow of blood. When the ventricle contracts, the aortic valve covers the openings of the coronary arteries as the blood is ejected into the aorta. When the ventricle suddenly relaxes, the blood is dropped back against the aortic valve, snapping it shut and filling the coronary arteries at the same pressure. This force, the dropping of a column of blood from systolic ejection pressure to resting diastolic pressure, is reflected clinically in the pulse pressure (systolic blood pressure reading − diastolic blood pressure reading). The pulse pressure is monitored to evaluate adequate filling pressure of the coronary arteries and therefore perfusion of the cardiac muscle. The oxygenated blood that is thus immediately fed back into the heart by the coronary circulation reaches every cardiac fiber, because these main vessels branch, divide, and subdivide throughout the myocardium. The heart has a pattern of circulation referred to as end-artery circulation. The arteries go into the heart muscle and end, without the back-up collateral circulation provided to most of the rest of the body's tissues.

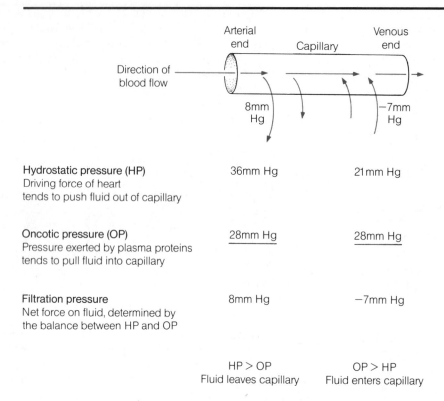

Figure 26-7. The net shift of fluid out of and into the capillary is determined by the balance between the hydrostatic pressure (*HP*) and the oncotic pressure (*OP*). HP tends to push fluid out of the capillary, and OP tends to pull it back into the capillary. At the arterial end of the capillary bed, blood pressure (HP) is higher than at the venous end. At the arterial end, HP exceeds OP, and fluid filters out. At the venous end, HP has fallen and HP is less than OP; fluid is pulled back into the capillary from the surrounding tissue. The lymphatic system also returns fluids and substances from the tissues to the circulation.

Normally, when the heart's own output of blood is adequate, enough of the flow from the aorta is forced through the coronary vessels to meet the demands of the myocardium for oxygen and nutrients. However, in heart failure (with low cardiac output) and in circulatory collapse (when the arterial blood pressure drops to shock levels) the coronary flow may be reduced and the myocardium may become hypoxic, thus further reducing its capacity to contract efficiently.

Another cause of inadequate heart muscle circulation may be disease of the coronary arterioles themselves. These vessels are often so narrowed by atherosclerosis that they carry a markedly reduced quantity of blood to the myocardium. If the vessels do not widen when physical exertion or emotional stress make the heart beat more vigorously, the failure to deliver as much oxygen as the myocardium demands may lead to painful attacks of angina pectoris.

If a major branch of a coronary vessel is blocked off completely, the prolonged coronary occlusion can result in death of the heart tissue that is deprived of its blood supply because the heart lacks the collateral backup that other body tissue has. Such a myocardial infarction can then prevent the heart from pumping with enough contractile force to keep the blood circulating adequately throughout the body.

Systemic arterial pressure

The contraction of the left ventricle, which sends blood surging out into the aorta, creates a pressure that continues to force the blood into all the branches of the aorta. This pressure against the arterial walls is greatest during systole (the contractile phase of the cardiac cycle), and it falls to its lowest level during diastole. Thus, in determining a patient's blood pressure, both the systolic and diastolic pressures are measured.

Hypotension and shock

The pressure in the arteries must remain high enough to ensure a sufficient flow of blood to all the body tissues, because all body tissues require the oxygen carried by the blood to survive. If the pressure falls too steeply for any reason—for example, through a reduction in cardiac output—tissue function soon fails. A sharp drop of pressure in the carotid arteries is followed by a marked reduction of blood flow to the brain. This leads to loss of consciousness in just a few seconds. Reduced renal arterial pressure interferes with kidney function. Change in pressures plays an important part in producing edema in congestive heart failure and in keeping patients with other illnesses edematous. A very severe fall in pressure following sudden circulatory collapse can kill very quickly by bringing about a state of irreversible shock that leads to the death of blood-deprived vital organs.

Hypertension

On the other hand, too high a level of arterial blood pressure is also undesirable. Such hypertensive pressure may damage the arterioles and even lead eventually to rupture of a major blood vessel in the brain or other vital organs. Hypertension puts an added burden on the heart, which must use up more energy in driving blood out into a relatively resistant circulatory tree.

The cause of most cases of hypertension remains unknown (so-called *essential hypertension*), despite numerous hypotheses. These theories are all based on the presence of some abnormality in one or another of the complex nervous, hormonal, and kidney mechanisms known to play a part in regulating the level of a person's arterial pressure. Although high blood pressure is not necessarily caused by excessive vasoconstrictor nerve impulses, many of the drugs employed in treating hypertension produce their pressure-reducing effects by lessening the flow of such impulses to the blood vessels; thus, a brief review of the ways in which arterial pressure responds to variations in nervous regulation will be discussed.

Vasomotor tone

The smooth muscle walls of the blood vessels receive nerve fibers from the sympathetic nervous system. Impulses passing continuously over these fibers to the vascular walls keep the vessels in a constant, or tonic, state of moderate constriction. Any increase in the output of vasoconstrictor impulses by the vasomotor center in the brain stem tends to raise the tone of the vascular musculature and to increase the pressure of the blood passing through the narrowed arterioles. A reduction in the number of tonic nerve impulses reaching the smooth muscle walls allows them to relax. This dilates the arterioles and results in a lessening of the pressure of the blood on the walls of the vessels.

Although impulses carried by certain nerves may also relax vascular smooth muscle directly, such vasodilator nerves do not play an important role in the control of systemic arterial pressure. Instead, when the blood pressure tends to rise too high, the vasomotor center lessens its output of vasoconstrictor signals. This is accomplished by so-called buffer reflexes, which are intensified by pressure rises in the carotid arteries carrying blood to the brain. Many drugs act to lower (or raise) arterial pressure by their effects on these vasomotor reflex mechanisms (see Chap. 28 and elsewhere).

Renin–angiotensin system

Blood pressure is now known to be regulated in part by a mechanism located in the kidneys. This system is activated when any of many physiologic factors cause the release of an enzyme called *renin* from certain specialized cells in the smooth muscle walls of renal arterioles. The liberation of renin sets in motion a series of complex chemical and physiologic reactions, which tend to raise the peripheral resistance and systemic arterial pressure (Fig. 26-8).

There is now reason to believe that when this system fails to be adequately controlled by the negative feedback factors that normally shut it off, hypertension tends to develop. This occurs in such cases because high plasma renin activity (PRA) leads to production of an excessive amount of a potent vasopressor substance called *angiotensin* II and of an adrenal cortex hormone, *aldosterone*. Several antihypertensive drugs are now thought to bring about their blood pressure-reducing effects—at least, in part—by lowering the level of renin or by antagonizing the production and effects of angiotensin II and of aldosterone.

Venous pressure

Pressure in the veins may also sometimes rise above normal. This may happen, for example, when the heart cannot adequately cope with all the blood being returned to it by the venous circulation. One sign of the heart's failure to handle this load of blood is a rise in pressure in the right atrium. This, in turn, leads to increased pressure in the veins that empty into this chamber as the venous blood that is attempting to flow into the atrium meets with resistance and begins to "back up" in the system.

Heat failure and edema

Blood that becomes dammed in the veins behind a weakened heart causes a rise in the venous pressure of many organs, including the lungs, liver, spleen, and kidneys. The hydrostatic pressure in the capillaries rises, leading to leakage of fluid into the tissue spaces (Fig. 26-7). This accounts for the pulmonary edema that makes breathing difficult in acute left ventricular failure. It is also a factor in the congestive signs and symptoms of right heart failure—the enlarged liver, fluid-filled abdomen, and pitting edema of the extremities.

However, other mechanisms in addition to raised venous pressure operate in the production of congestive heart failure. For example, as a result of the reduction in renal arterial pressure already mentioned and the lessened blood flow that follows, another mechanism contributes to the kidneys' reduced ability to remove sodium and to the resulting retention of salty fluids in the tissues: the kidneys increase their rate of renin secretion, which leads, in turn, to production of angiotensin, and a vicious cycle develops.

In addition to its vasopressor action, discussed above, angiotensin II acts to stimulate the secretion of the mineralocorticoid hormone aldosterone by the adrenal glands. This hormone then causes the kidney tubule

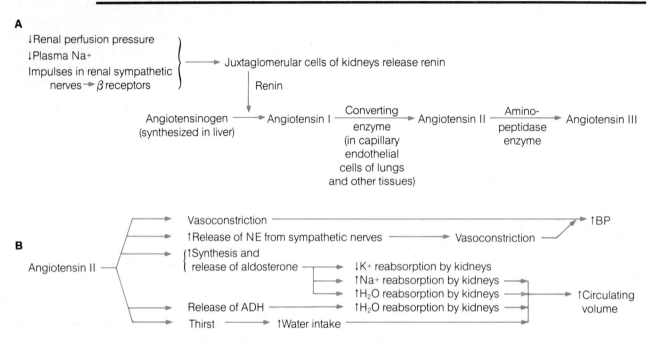

Figure 26-8. The renin–angiotensin system. (*A*) The synthesis of angiotensin II; (*B*) some effects of angiotensin II (angiotensin III also causes some of these effects).

cells to transport more sodium back from the glomerular filtrate into the blood and the fluids bathing the body tissues. This sodium takes with it water, which increases the circulatory volume and pressure and results in edema. Angiotensin II has other effects that tend to increase blood pressure and circulating volume. It increases norepinephrine release from sympathetic postganglionic nerve terminals and it stimulates a sense of thirst that results in increased fluid intake. It also increases the release of antidiuretic hormone (Chap. 20) from the posterior pituitary, which then acts on the kidney tubules to cause the reabsorption of water.

Hypoproteinemia (a reduced amount of plasma proteins) may be a cause of reduced blood volume. This is because these colloid molecules exert an osmotic force (oncotic pressure), which ordinarily helps to retain fluids within the circulatory tree. When the synthesis of plasma proteins is reduced (in liver disease, for example), or when albumin is lost through a leaky glomerular membrane (in nephrosis), fluid tends to move out of the plasma and into the extravascular spaces to form pools of edema.

In summary, some aspects of the functioning of the circulatory system have been briefly reviewed. Some things that sometimes go wrong with cardiovascular function have been emphasized. An understanding of the importance of the circulation and of the necessity to keep this system working as close to normal as possible will lead to a better appreciation of the value of the drugs administered to patients with disorders of the heart and blood vessels. Drugs acting on the cardiovascular system

in various ways will be discussed in the following chapters of this section.

References

Berne RM, Levy MN: The cardiovascular system. In Berne RM, Levy MN (eds): Physiology, pp 439–636. St. Louis, CV Mosby, 1983

Karch AM: Cardiac Care: A Guide for Patient Education. New York, Appleton–Century–Crofts, 1981

Milnor WR: Cardiovascular system. In Mountcastle VB (ed): Medical Physiology, 14th ed, pp 951–960. St. Louis, CV Mosby, 1980

Milnor WR: Principles of hemodynamics. In Mountcastle VB (ed): Medical Physiology, 14th ed, pp 1017–1032. St. Louis, CV Mosby, 1980

Milnor WR: The heart as a pump. In Mountcastle VB (ed), Medical Physiology, 14th ed, pp 986–1006. St. Louis, CV Mosby, 1980

Milnor WR: Normal circulatory function. In Mountcastle VB (ed): Medical Physiology, 14th ed, pp 1033–1046. St. Louis, CV Mosby, 1980

Milnor WR: Autonomic and peripheral control mechanisms. In Mountcastle VB (ed): Medical Physiology, 14th ed, pp 1047–1060. St. Louis, CV Mosby, 1980

Milnor WR: The cardiovascular control system. In Mountcastle VB (ed): Medical Physiology, 14th ed, pp 1061–1084. St. Louis, CV Mosby, 1980

Reder RF, Rosen MR: Mechanisms of cardiac arrhythmias. Cardiovasc Rev Rep 2:1007, 1981

Chapter 27

Diuretic drugs

27

Normal kidney function

All the body's cells need a constant internal environment in which to function efficiently. The kidneys play a very important part in adjusting the amount of fluid and essential chemicals inside body cells and in the extracellular fluids that surround these cells. In carrying out their function of keeping *the volume and composition of the body fluids within normal limits,* the kidneys work in various ways to retain substances vital to the body and to discard chemicals that are present in excess.

As a result of renal functioning, the body is cleared of the nitrogenous waste products of protein metabolism; is maintained in acid–base balance; and maintains such substances as sodium, potassium chloride, and bicarbonate ions in homeostasis within the body's several separate fluid compartments.

The importance of the kidneys in the control of the volume and composition of the body fluids is evidenced by the fact that, although the kidneys make up less than 0.5% of body weight, they receive almost 25% of the blood pumped out of the heart. About 1700 quarts (1600 liters) of blood pass through the kidneys for cleansing each day. From this huge volume of liquid, the kidneys filter out the waste products, foreign materials, and excesses of electrolytes. Most of the filtered fluid is sent back to the blood, along with other essential substances. The filtered wastes, together with some undesirable substances secreted by the kidneys themselves, are dissolved in a relatively small amount of water and passed out of the body as urine.

Body water compartments

Water makes up more than half of the body's weight. This fluid is distributed between two major compartments: *intracellular* and *extracellular*. The fluid outside the cells, the extracellular compartment, is subdivided into an *intravascular* portion—the blood plasma—and a portion that is *extravascular* (as well as extracellular), called the *interstitial fluid* because it fills the interstices, or small spaces, between the cells.

Ordinarily, about 75% of the extracellular fluid is found in the interstitial spaces and 25% remains within the blood vessels. The distribution of fluid in these two segments of the extracellular compartment normally remains in a steady state, despite the constant interchange, or turnover, of water and sodium and other solutes between the two subcompartments. Many mechanisms are involved in maintaining this dynamic balance, including hydrostatic and oncotic pressures (Chap. 26).

Sometimes, the processes regulating the relationship between the intravascular and interstitial compartments may become temporarily disturbed. However, the kidneys help to keep the volume and ionic composition of extracellular fluid in a steady state by adjusting the rate of renal excretion in response to various signals from within the circulatory system. The pathologic changes that occur when the kidneys fail to do so produce the signs and symptoms of renal failure.

Review of renal function

Basic processes

The kidneys employ three processes in performing their vital functions: glomerular filtration, tubular secretion, and tubular reabsorption. All three types of processes are performed by each of the two million functional units called nephrons (Fig. 27-1). Each nephron consists of a *glomerulus,* which is a microscopic ball of blood vessels enclosed in a membranous capsule, called Bowman's capsule, and a hair-thin *tubule* made up of several segments, which runs a twisted course before it empties into a collecting duct. The collecting ducts empty into the ureters, which lead to the urinary bladder. Each tubule spans a

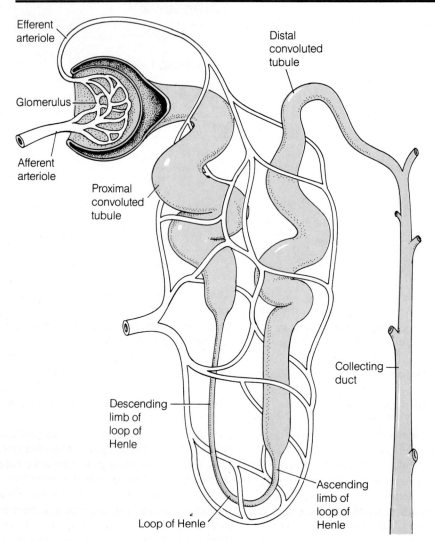

Figure 27-1. The nephron, the functional unit of the kidney. Secretion and reabsorption of water, electrolytes, and other solutes in the various segments of the renal tubule, the loop of Henle, and the collecting duct can be influenced by diuretics, other drugs, and endogenous substances, including certain hormones.

distance of less than 2 inches, but so serpentine are its windings that the total length of all the renal tubules is estimated to be between 60 and 75 miles!

Glomerular filtration. The *glomerulus* functions as an ultrafine filter. Normally, its semipermeable membranes keep blood cells, plasma proteins, and lipids inside the capillary vessels, while hydrostatic forces push plasma constituents of smaller molecular size, along with the water in which they are dissolved, through the tiny membranous pores. About 125 ml of fluid are filtered each minute, or a total of around 180 liters/day. Most of this filtered fluid (about 99 ml of every 100 ml) is returned to the blood as the filtrate makes its way through the tubules. Thus, the total volume of fluid that is lost as urine averages less than 2 liters daily.

Tubular secretion. The epithelial cells that line the kidney tubules can secrete substances *from* the blood *into* the tubular fluid by an active, energy-using process. Secretion of hydrogen ions helps to keep body fluids from becoming acidic. Excess potassium ions may also be secreted into the tubular fluid to be passed out of the body in the urine. Uric acid is another natural substance that is removed from the blood by tubular secretion as well as by glomerular filtration. Drugs such as penicillin that are organic acids are also both secreted by the tubules and filtered by the glomeruli.

Tubular reabsorption. About 99% of the glomerular filtrate is, as indicated above, returned to the blood during its passage down the tubules. The cells that line the tubules can reabsorb substances from the filtrate that the body needs, including glucose, vitamins, and dissolved electrolytes, such as sodium chloride and sodium bicarbonate. A small amount of sodium (about 1%) normally is not reabsorbed and ends up in the urine along with other filtered waste materials and the water in which they are dissolved. This reabsorptive process is very important for maintaining the extracellular fluids at just the right volume and composition for serving the needs of the surrounding tissue cells.

Tubular transport systems. The sodium and other ions in the glomerular filtrate are returned to the blood by several separate tubular transport systems. The different classes of drugs that alter renal function interfere with one or more of these processes in ways that determine both the ionic content and the acidity or alkalinity of the urine and the electrolyte pattern of the interstitial fluids. Thus, to understand how these several types of drugs, called diuretics, are best administered to obtain their beneficial effects in edematous patients and to avoid drug-induced electrolyte and acid–base imbalances, the mechanisms by which reabsorption of sodium is normally accomplished in the several segments of the renal tubules must be reviewed.

Regulation of fluids and electrolytes by the kidneys

Sodium and water regulation. The *proximal segment* of the convoluted tubule reabsorbs most of the glomerular filtrate that enters it from Bowman's capsule (Fig. 27-2). At this first site, sodium is removed from the filtrate by an *active* (energy-consuming) process that passes this cation into the network of plasma-containing capillaries that surround the tubules. The sodium is accompanied by the chloride anion and by large amounts of water—effects that are brought about by passive diffusion because of the need to maintain electrochemical and osmotic balances on both sides of the tubular epithelial membrane.

A second sodium transport system also operates here and along the entire length of the tubule, all the way down to where it meets the collecting tubule or duct (Fig. 27-2). Sodium ions contained in the tubular lumen filtrate are reabsorbed into the peritubular blood in exchange for *hydrogen* ions. The source of these hydrogen ions is the epithelial cells that line the proximal and other parts of the tubule. These hydrogen ions are produced by a reaction that combines cellular carbon dioxide with water to form carbonic acid (H_2CO_3). This reaction is catalyzed by the enzyme *carbonic anhydrase*. The carbonic acid that is formed dissociates immediately into bicarbonate (HCO_3^-), which is retained in the peritubular blood along with the reabsorbed sodium, and hydrogen ions (H^+), which are secreted into the tubular filtrate that is then carried downstream to other tubular segments and finally out of the body in the urine. This is one of the processes by which the body normally retains its so-called alkaline reserve, or stores of base, while producing an acidic urine.

The *loop of Henle* continues these reabsorptive processes. In its descending limb water is drawn out of the tubule and into the surrounding saline fluid within the renal tissues. However, after the tubular fluid moves around the bend at the base of the loop and enters the thick ascending limb of the loop of Henle, water is no longer reabsorbed (Fig. 27-2). This is because the tubular epithelial membrane at this site and in the segment of the distal tubule just beyond it is impermeable to water.

Sodium ions, however, readily penetrate the tubular membrane at these sites and leave the luminal fluid for the peritubular blood. In fact, up to 25% of all the sodium filtered by the glomeruli—a large fraction of the total—is actively reabsorbed in the loop of Henle. Chloride is actively pumped out of the ascending limb and the sodium passively flows out with it to maintain electrical neutrality. The loss of sodium and chloride, combined with the impermeability of the tubule to water, results in a tubular fluid that is hypotonic compared to the plasma in the surrounding peritubular capillaries. The osmotic gradient that results is an important part of the medullary countercurrent mechanism (see below).

The *distal convoluted tubule* reabsorbs much of the sodium that has not been returned to the blood. The main mechanism by which this reabsorption is accomplished is the exchange of sodium ions in the tubular fluid for potassium ions that are secreted by the tubular epithelial cells. Part of this cation exchange mechanism is controlled by *aldosterone*, an adrenal mineralocorticoid hormone, which stimulates a sodium–potassium ion exchange pump and leads to the loss of potassium and the retention of sodium. The brain also releases a *natriuretic hormone* that causes a decrease in sodium reabsorption in the tubules and leads to a dilute urine of increased volume. In addition, the exchange of sodium for hydrogen ion that was discussed above also operates at this distal site. The transport system that will predominate depends on several factors, including the acid–base and potassium balances of the body and on the amount of sodium that has been delivered to the distal convoluted tubule.

The urine flows from the distal tubule into the *collecting duct*, where the final concentration of the urine is adjusted. As the tubular fluid flows down the collecting duct it passes through the medullary region of the kidney, which has been made hypertonic by the reabsorption of sodium without water from the fluid in the ascending limb of the loop of Henle. The urine is either concentrated or diluted by a process called the *countercurrent mechanism* in response to the body's need either to conserve water or to rid itself of excess water. The actual tonicity of the urine that is excreted depends on the circulating levels of antidiuretic hormone (ADH; Chap. 20), a hormone

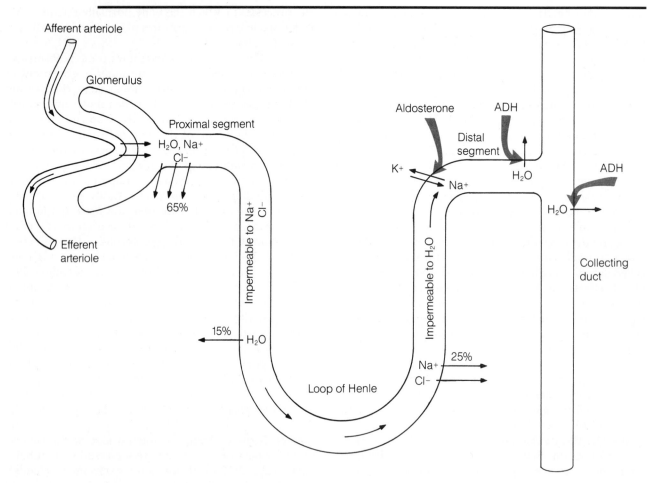

Figure 27-2. Renal regulation of sodium chloride and water. (*Arrows* (→): Direction of net flow of substances with respect to the renal tubule; *Arrows* (➔): sites of hormone action; %: refers to portion of filtered load that is reabsorbed at the labeled site)

that increases the permeability of the distal convoluted tubule and collecting duct to water. In the presence of ADH, these areas of the kidney tubule become permeable to water; water flows out of the tubule into the hypertonic interstitium of the medulla and is reabsorbed into the peritubular capillaries. Thus, water is retained in the body and a concentrated urine results. In the absence of ADH, these areas of the kidney tubule remain impermeable to water and the water stays in the tubule and is passed through the collecting duct into the ureters. A dilute urine is excreted.

Potassium regulation. Potassium, another cation that, like sodium, is essential for the proper functioning of excitable tissues (*e.g.*, neurons, the heart, skeletal muscle) throughout the body, is also regulated by the renal tubules. Most of the potassium filtered through the glomerulus (65%) is reabsorbed at Bowman's capsule and at the proximal convoluted tubule (Fig. 27-3). Another 25% to 30% of the potassium is reabsorbed from the ascending limb of the loop of Henle. The fine tuning of potassium

regulation occurs in the distal convoluted tubule where aldosterone activates a sodium–potassium ion exchange mechanism that retains sodium and secretes potassium into the urine to maintain electronegativity. If body potassium levels become too high, the release of aldosterone is directly stimulated and more potassium is excreted in the urine. It must be remembered that in these situations more sodium and, therefore, more water are retained; edema can result from the increased extracellular fluid volume. In addition, the cells of the distal tubule contain a potassium secretory mechanism that is not influenced by aldosterone. This secretory mechanism is normally stimulated by a transtubular electrical potential.

Calcium regulation. The kidneys play an important role in the regulation of calcium levels in the body. Calcium, like other electrolytes, is reabsorbed from the proximal tubule and the ascending limb of the loop of Henle. The fine tuning of calcium regulation occurs at the distal convoluted tubule, where the parathyroid hormone (PTH) stimulates the reabsorption of calcium

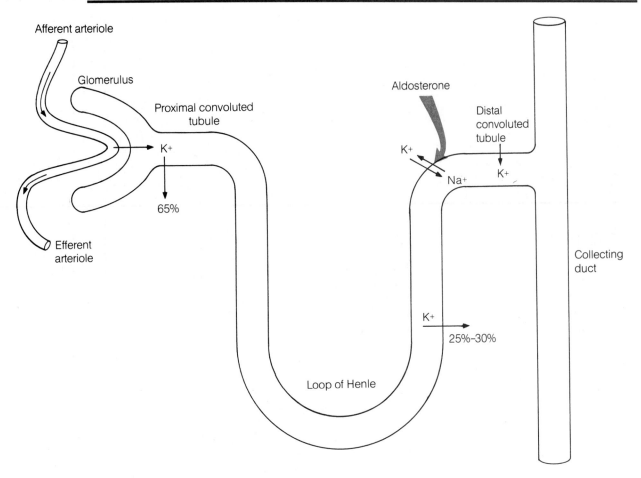

Figure 27-3. Renal regulation of potassium. (*Arrows* (→): direction of net flow of substances with respect to the renal tubule; *arrows* (➤): sites of hormone action; %: refers to portion of filtered load that is reabsorbed at the labeled site)

to increase serum calcium levels (Fig. 27-4). The kidneys are also responsible for the final activation of vitamin D, which is necessary for the absorption of calcium from the intestinal tract.

Renin–angiotensin system

The many regulatory systems of the kidneys work together to maintain body homeostasis and to guarantee an adequate blood flow to the fragile nephrons. The renin–angiotensin system is an example of this activity (see Fig. 26-8). This complex system, which plays an important part in the regulation of salt and water metabolism and in the control of blood pressure, depends on the presence of renin, an enzyme found mainly in the outer portion, or cortex, of the kidney. Renin is synthesized and stored in groups of cells located close to each glomerulus within the afferent arteriole and in the macula densa, an area between the afferent and efferent arterioles (Fig. 27-1). Renin is released from this complex of so-called juxtaglomerular (next to the glomerulus) apparatus

cells in response to various physiologic stimuli, and in pathologic states including hemorrhage, dehydration, ascites, congestive heart failure, and other conditions that produce a reduced cardiac output and subsequent fall in renal blood flow.

Renin is secreted into the renal afferent arteriole and is then carried into the systemic and pulmonary circulations. Here renin acts on a plasma protein substrate called *angiotensinogen* (that is synthesized in the liver) to form a decapeptide, *angiotensin I,* which is then acted on by another so-called converting enzyme, in the lungs and elsewhere, to generate *angiotensin II,* an octapeptide. This is a powerful constrictor of vascular smooth muscle and a very potent vasopressor substance that is believed to play an important part in the regulation of blood pressure. In addition, angiotensin acts on the cortices of the adrenal glands, possibly after its conversion to angiotensin III, to stimulate the synthesis of aldosterone.

As indicated above, this adrenal hormone helps to conserve sodium and thus to maintain blood volume

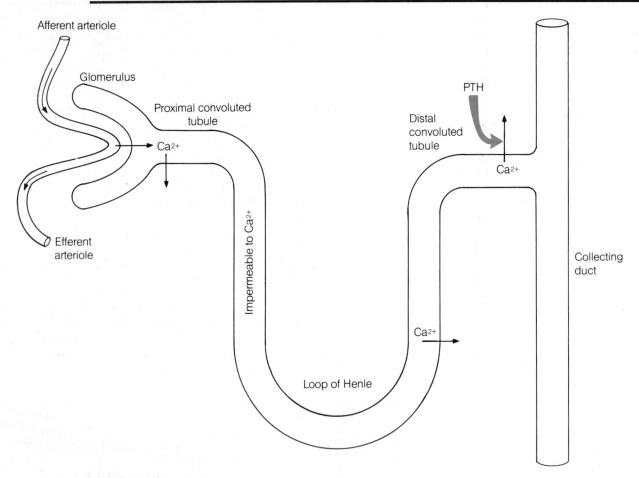

Figure 27-4. Renal regulation of calcium. (*Arrows* (→): direction of net flow of substances with respect to the renal tubule; *arrows* (➡): sites of hormone action; %: refers to portion of filtered load that is reabsorbed at the labeled site)

by stimulating the exchange of sodium and potassium ions. However, when present in excess, because of inappropriate oversecretion by the adrenal gland or because of inadequate metabolic breakdown by the liver, aldosterone can play an important role in sodium and fluid retention and thus, can be active in edema formation and in development of hypertension.

The retention of sodium that is stimulated by aldosterone causes a rise in plasma osmotic pressure that stimulates the posterior pituitary gland to secrete increased quantities of ADH. Thus, production of aldosterone can lead to a greater release of ADH, which then adds water retention to sodium retention. The net result is an increase in blood volume, which increases renal blood flow, causing the decrease of one of the stimuli that results in renin release. Clinically, it is important to remember that the renin–angiotensin system is part of a complex set of interrelated reflexes, and manipulating one aspect of this system will cause an imbalance in the rest of the system, with resultant clinical manifestations.

Diuretics

Diuretics are commonly defined as drugs that increase the amount of urine produced by the kidneys. Actually, of greater clinical significance than their effect on the volume of urinary output is the ability of most diuretics to increase the excretion of *sodium* and other ions along with water. The drug-induced elimination of sodium accounts for the main clinical indications for the diuretic drugs: the management of edema; and the treatment of hypertension (see Chap. 28).

Sodium retention and edema

In many diseases of differing etiology, the kidney tubules reabsorb sodium and water in amounts that are disproportionately large. That is, in patients with heart failure and cirrhosis of the liver, for instance, the amount of salt that is returned to the blood from the glomerular filtrate is abnormally high. The retained salt and water result first in an expansion of the total volume of blood within the circulatory system. Then, as pressure rises within the venous capillaries, salty fluids leak out into the extravascular compartment to expand the volume of interstitial fluid, as described in Chapter 26.

In *congestive heart failure,* the kidneys receive signals from various sources that set off renal compensatory mechanisms intended to maintain circulatory homeostasis. That is, the decreased ability of the failing heart to maintain an adequate cardiac output causes the kidneys to retain more salt and water as a means of raising the volume of intravascular fluid and thus increase the amount of blood that is being returned to the heart by the veins. Unfortunately, the disease-weakened heart cannot increase its output or handle the increased venous return adequately. As a result, pressure rises within the pulmonary and systemic veins and fluid transudes out into interstitial and serous spaces.

The resulting edema is both discomforting and, in some situations, life-threatening. Fluid that accumulates within the abdomen (ascites) or in the subcutaneous tissues of the legs and ankles and elsewhere (anasarca) makes movement difficult. Fluid accumulating in the lungs interferes with breathing and, if lung edema develops suddenly, the patient can quickly die unless emergency treatment is provided, along with diuretics and other drugs designed to decrease the vascular volume and to increase the contractility of the failing heart.

The sources of all the signals that stimulate such an overcompensatory response by the renal tubules in congestive heart failure have not yet been determined. However, the kidneys themselves contain receptors that respond to an *actual* loss of blood volume—such as that caused by severe bleeding, loss of fluid from burns, or severe diarrhea, for example—by setting into motion a series of events that is intended to counteract hypovolemia. When, for instance, the amount of blood received by the kidneys is reduced as a result of plasma volume depletion, blood flow within the kidneys is shifted to intrarenal areas that contain the most efficient tubular reabsorptive transport mechanisms.

As a result of this intrarenal hemodynamic redistribution, these tubules reabsorb a greater than normal amount of salt and water from the glomerular filtrate. Unfortunately for the patient in congestive heart failure—whose blood volume is *not* actually diminished, but who suffers from a decline in cardiac output secondary to the failing of the heart muscle—this renal hemodynamic response is inappropriate and results in hypervolemia and edema. Similar false signals set off a complex *hormonal* response that also stimulates an increase in sodium and water retention that is unwarranted.

In *hepatic ascites,* a common complication of cirrhosis of the liver, several factors contribute to the formation of fluid in the abdominal cavity. One cause is a rise in pressure within hepatic and splanchnic capillaries

because of obstruction of normal blood flow within the portal system. Another factor in addition to the increased intravascular pressure that tends to force fluid out of the capillaries is a reduction in the plasma colloidal osmotic pressure that normally helps to retain fluid within the vessels. This occurs because the patient's damaged liver cannot synthesize adequate amounts of plasma proteins. In addition, the damaged liver has a relatively low detoxifying capacity. Thus, it does not readily inactivate the aldosterone that is commonly secreted in abnormally large amounts in this liver disorder. The resulting secondary hyperaldosteronism stimulates the sodium–potassium exchange mechanism that leads to sodium reabsorption, increased vascular volume, and perpetuation of the patient's persistent ascitic state.

The *nephrotic syndrome* is a condition in which damage to the glomerular membranes causes plasma proteins that would ordinarily not be part of the ultrafiltrate to leak out into the tubules. This loss of protein from the plasma and the resulting reduction in intravascular colloidal osmotic pressure also leads to edema and eventually to ascites. The low plasma volume (hypovolemia), which stimulates secretion of renin and of aldosterone (secondary hyperaldosteronism), is also a factor in the edema formation of nephrosis.

Other types of edema occur in various clinical situations. Those glucocorticoid drugs that possess a mineralocorticoid component—hydrocortisone, for example—can cause retention of sodium and water. Such steroid drugs can be therapeutically useful, though, when combined with diuretic therapy for patients with the nephrotic syndrome, and for congestive heart failure (CHF) patients. For reasons that are uncertain, CHF patients who are pretreated with corticosteroids for several days sometimes show an increased response to diuretic therapy. The edema of pregnancy and premenstrual edema are the result of female hormone imbalances. Diuretic drugs can reduce this edema, but these agents have not been proven safe for use in pregnancy and do not prevent the toxemia of pregnancy or the emotional tension sometimes present in the premenstrual period (premenstrual syndrome).

Classes of diuretic drugs

Although diuretic drugs are dissimilar in their chemical structures and differ also in the exact mechanisms by which they produce diuresis, all classes of diuretics that are most useful for treating edema perform one main function: *they interfere with the tubular reabsorption of sodium.* That is, these drugs prevent the cells that line the tubules from reabsorbing an excessive proportion of the sodium ions from the glomerular filtrate. As a result, sodium and other ions such as chloride enter the urine along with the water in which they are dissolved, instead of being returned to the blood where they would cause an increase in intravascular volume, and therefore an increase in hydrostatic pressure, which could cause a leaking of fluid into interstitial spaces and body cavities.

The several different types of diuretics act in different ways to prevent sodium from being carried back into the blood plasma. Depending on which of the several different renal tubular transport systems they affect, these drugs also remove other ions, such as potassium, hydrogen, chloride, and bicarbonate. Excessive diuretic actions can cause complications that are the result of the ensuing electrolyte and acid–base imbalances, which can lead to the development of many discomforting and dangerous signs and symptoms.

Knowledge of where and how the various diuretics act on the renal tubules helps in the selection of the most appropriate drug for treating a particular patient's edematous disorder. Differences in the sites and mechanisms of action also help to explain why some diuretics often cause one type of electrolyte imbalance while others cause excessive loss of different ions.

Sulfonamides

Diuretics of this class are related chemically to the antibacterial sulfonamides but possess no anti-infective activity (Table 27-1). Most sulfonamide diuretics, including the prototypes *chlorothiazide* (Diuril) and *hydrochlorothiazide*[+] (Esidrix; HydroDiuril; Oretic) are derived from benzothiadiazine and are known as thiazide diuretics. Other sulfonamide diuretics, such as *chlorthalidone* (Hygroton), *quinethazone* (Hydromox), and *metolazone* (Diulo), differ somewhat in their chemical structure, but these *nonthiazides* are essentially similar in site and manner of action, as is the new indoline diuretic *indapamide* (Lozol).

Site of action. The thiazides and related sulfonamide diuretics act mainly at a point in the distal convoluted tubule just beyond the ascending limb of the loop of Henle. Their action at this first part of the distal tubule is to block the chloride pump, which then prevents the reabsorption of both chloride and sodium. Because this segment of the tubule is impermeable to water there is little change in the actual volume of tubular fluid but rather a *saluretic,* or salt-removing, effect. The urine produced is more concentrated than usual. Some of these diuretics also inhibit the enzyme carbonic anhydrase, preventing the reabsorption of sodium and bicarbonate in the proximal convoluted tubule.

Adverse effects. Many adverse effects of these drugs are caused by interference with the normal regulatory mechanisms of the nephron. Hypokalemia is the most frequent problem encountered. The thiazides increase the secretion of potassium by the cells of the distal tubule and thus promote the urinary excretion of potassium. This loss of potassium from the body can lead to hypokalemia. As a result, the patient may exhibit adverse effects on excitable tissues of the body. These are manifested by weakness, muscle cramps, and cardiac irregularities. Hypokalemia also predisposes patients on digitalis to ventricular arrhythmias. The sulfonamide di-

uretics can also decrease calcium excretion, an effect that can lead to parathyroid problems, because this gland attempts to compensate for the resulting elevated serum calcium levels.

The sulfonamide diuretics decrease the excretion of uric acid by interfering with the renal tubular secretory mechanism for uric acid. This can lead to elevated serum uric acid levels and, in severe cases, it may precipitate an attack of gout. Patients who would benefit from the use of a sulfonamide diuretic, but who are experiencing a gouty reaction, are often treated with an antigout drug to counteract this effect.

For unidentified reasons, the thiazides sometimes cause an elevation of blood glucose levels. If this occurs, latent diabetes mellitus may be activated, or control of their disease may be lost by frankly diabetic patients. These patients need to be followed closely to restore stable management of their condition.

These drugs also can lower blood pressure, a therapeutically useful effect (see Chap. 28), but one that is potentially dangerous in the presence of alcohol and barbiturates that may potentiate it.

Specific clinical considerations. These drugs are not as effective against severe edema as many of the other diuretics that are available, but they have several important advantages. The orally effective thiazides are, for example, convenient to administer and relatively safe as compared to some other classes of diuretics. The thiazides are less likely to cause excessive diuresis and severe electrolyte imbalances than are the more potent but often less readily controllable loop diuretics (see below). For these reasons, treatment of most edematous patients is often begun with a moderately potent diuretic such as hydrochlorothiazide.

The relative safety of the thiazide diuretics also makes their use preferable to more potent but potentially more dangerous diuretics in patients with minor degrees of edema, such as that which develops in some women premenstrually or during treatment with some corticosteroid drugs. The thiazides are also employed clinically in conditions not marked by edema, particularly in the treatment of hypertension. Paradoxically, these diuretics have proved useful for controlling the excessive production of dilute urine in some patients with diabetes insipidus who cannot tolerate vasopressin (ADH) or who are not helped by treatment with that posterior pituitary hormone.

The sulfonamide diuretics are more efficiently absorbed when taken with food. Because of this, patients can be instructed to take them with meals. Care must be taken to correlate drug administration times with times of convenient access to bathroom facilities. Taking the drug at bedtime, for instance, can interrupt sleep and pose a safety hazard for the patient who has to get up frequently to void.

The action of the sulfonamide diuretics is terminated mostly by renal excretion of the unchanged mol-

Table 27–1. Diuretic drugs

Generic or official name	Trade name	Usual adult daily dosage range and administration	Comments
Oral sulfonamide-type diuretics			
Bendroflumethiazide USP	Naturetin	2.5–20 mg PO	Potent, long-acting
Benzthiazide USP	Aquatag; Exna	50–200 mg PO	Moderate duration and potency
Chlorthalidone USP	Hygroton	50–200 mg PO 3 times weekly	Long-acting nonthiazide
Chlorothiazide USP	Diuril	500–1000 mg PO	Prototype thiazide
Cyclothiazide USP	Anhydron	1–2 mg PO	High potency; long duration
Hydrochlorothiazide USP	Esidrix; HydroDiuril; Oretic	25–200 mg PO	See Drug digest
Hydroflumethiazide USP	Diucardin; Saluron	25–200 mg PO	Moderate duration and potency
Indapamide	Lozol	2.5 mg PO	New antihypertensive–diuretic of a new chemical class (indoline)
Metolazone	Diulo; Zaroxolyn	5–20 mg PO	Long-acting nonthiazide
Methyclothiazide USP	Enduron	2.5–10 mg PO	Long-acting; high potency
Polythiazide USP	Renese	1–4 mg PO	High potency; long duration
Quinethazone USP	Hydromox	50–200 mg PO	Nonthiazide of moderate potency and duration
Trichlormethiazide USP	Metahydrin; Naqua	1–4 mg PO	High potency; long duration
High-ceiling or loop diuretics			
Bumetanide	Bumex	0.5–10 mg IV or IM; 0.5–2 mg PO	Very potent—40 times as potent as furosemide
Ethacrynate sodium USP	Edecrin sodium	0.5–1 mg/kg body weight IV	See Drug digest
Ethacrynic acid USP	Edecrin	25–200 mg PO	See Drug digest
Furosemide USP	Lasix	40–80 mg PO	See Drug digest
Carbonic anhydrase inhibitors			
Acetazolamide USP	Diamox	250–375 mg PO	See Drug digest
Acetazolamide sodium USP	Diamox Parenteral	250–500 mg IV	See Drug digest
Dichlorphenamide USP	Daranide; Oratrol	25–200 mg PO tid	Used to reduce intraocular tension in glaucoma
Methazolamide USP	Neptazane	50–100 bid or tid PO	Lowers intraocular pressure in glaucoma
Osmotic diuretics			
Isosorbide	Ismotic	1–3 g/kg body weight PO bid to qid	Used to decrease intraocular pressure
Mannitol USP	Osmitrol	50–200 g IV in 15–20% solution	Infused slowly in oliguria or in certain types of edema
Urea, sterile USP	Ureaphil	40–120 g IV in 4% or 30% solution	See Drug digest

(continued)

Table 27–1. Diuretic drugs (continued)

Generic or official name	Trade name	Usual adult daily dosage range and administration	Comments
Potassium-sparing diuretics			
Amiloride	Midamor	5–10 mg PO	Used in combination therapy
Spironolactone USP	Aldactone	25 mg PO, bid to qid	See Drug digest
Triamterene USP	Dyrenium	100–200 mg PO	Used with thiazides to counteract potassium loss
Acid-forming salt			
Ammonium chloride USP		1 g qid PO	Used as adjunct with more potent diuretics

ecule. Thus, renal failure or decreased renal function can cause these drugs to accumulate in the body and lead to toxicity. The new nonthiazide diuretic indapamide is metabolized and excreted by the gastrointestinal tract as well as by the kidneys; it is claimed, therefore, to be less likely to accumulate. Patients with electrolyte disturbances are also at risk from these diuretics.

Certain potential drug–drug interactions should be evaluated when a patient is receiving a sulfonamide diuretic. The effects of the diuretic can be increased if it is taken with any drugs that have similar effects—for example, increased hypotension if given with other antihypertensives, increased hypokalemia if given with steroids, and problems with antidiabetic dosages.

The cardiac drug *quinidine* is not excreted as efficiently when urine is alkaline. Because these diuretics block the reabsorption of bicarbonate, they tend to alkalinize the urine. Patients on concomitant thiazide and quinidine therapy may have increased serum levels of quinidine. A lower dose of quinidine will thus need to be ordered to avoid its toxic effects.

High-ceiling or loop diuretics

Three diuretics—*furosemide*[+] (Lasix), *ethacrynic acid*[+] (Edecrin) and *bumetanide* (Bumex)—are more efficacious than any other diuretics currently available (Table 27-1). They are known as high-ceiling diuretics because they can cause a greater degree of diuresis than other drugs, and are also known as loop diuretics because their primary action is in the loop of Henle. Their diuretic action often comes on promptly, even in patients with impaired renal function and in others who do not respond well to treatment with thiazides or other diuretics. They have, in fact, replaced the older mercurial diuretics, because—unlike the latter, which must generally be injected and are very

toxic—these drugs are effective when administered by the more convenient oral route.

Site of action. The primary site of action of these diuretics is in the ascending limb of the loop of Henle, where up to 30% of all the filtered sodium is normally reabsorbed. These drugs block the chloride pump, which decreases the reabsorption of both sodium and chloride. This and their similar actions in the proximal and perhaps the distal tubules accounts for their prompt and often dramatic production of a copious flow of urine high in sodium chloride. Unlike most other diuretics, these drugs continue to be effective even in the presence of drug-induced electrolyte or acid–base imbalance, nitrogen retention, and renal failure; large losses of fluid, up to 20 lb/day, can be produced.

Adverse effects. Although the continuing action of these drugs even in the presence of diuretic-induced electrolyte imbalances adds to their effectiveness for removing fluid, it also makes more likely the possible development of serious fluid–electrolyte disturbances, such as hypokalemia. Because of these drugs' potent effects in inhibiting sodium reabsorption at more proximal tubular sites, an extraordinarily large load of sodium reaches the most distal portion of the tubule. The efforts of transport systems in this portion of the renal tubule to retain some of this heavy sodium load by exchanging potassium ions for sodium can lead to severe depletion of the latter important cation and often also of hydrogen ions. There is consequently a very great probability of inducing hypokalemia and, in some cases, alkalosis.

The patient can experience all the signs and symptoms of hypokalemia and alkalosis, any of which can be dangerous in particular patients. When given parenterally, these high-ceiling diuretics can cause severe and rapid volume depletion. In certain compromised patients this rapid diuresis can lead to hypotension, shock, cardiac arrhythmias, and vascular problems. The clinical management of patients on loop diuretics should include careful adjustment of dose to regulate fluid loss to a steady, relatively slow (1 lb to 2 lb/day) rate.

Ototoxicity, including ringing in the ears and deafness, has been associated with the use of these drugs. Although deafness is usually reversible, prolonged use of the drug can lead to permanent hearing loss in susceptible patients. Glucose metabolism is altered in some patients, leading to increased blood glucose levels and glycosuria. Patients having known problems with glucose metabolism need to be followed closely.

Unlike the thiazide diuretics, these drugs have the potential for lowering calcium levels and causing tetany. However, like the thiazides, they can increase uric acid levels.

Specific clinical considerations. The loop diuretics are the drugs of choice for reducing the edema associated with CHF, hepatic cirrhosis, and renal disease, including nephrotic syndrome. They are used in emergency situations when a rapid intense diuresis is necessary. Because of their high ceiling, these drugs always have the potential for causing electrolyte imbalances and dehydration, with the resultant clinical problems. Close clinical management to avoid these problems should include accurate recording of weight loss, observation of urinary output, and adjustment of dose to the minimum level that produces the desired fluid loss. For example, this may involve giving doses only on alternate days. Care should be taken when administering bumetanide to check the dosage carefully. This drug is approximately 40 times more potent than furosemide, and is administered in appropriately smaller doses.

Some clinically important drug–drug interactions have been documented with these drugs. *Ethacrynic acid* and *furosemide* interact with *aminoglycoside antibiotics* to cause increased ototoxicity; this combination of drugs should be avoided. *Furosemide* has been shown to antagonize the effects of *tubocurarine* but may potentiate *succinylcholine,* leading to prolonged paralysis; for this reason, furosemide should be discontinued a few days before surgery. *Furosemide* can block the renal excretion of *salicylates,* causing salicylate toxicity if the two drugs are taken together; if a patient must receive both drugs, a low dose of salicylates should be used and the patient should be carefully watched for signs of toxicity. *Ethacrynic acid* can displace *warfarin* from plasma protein-binding sites, leading to elevated levels of warfarin and greater anticoagulant effects than expected; the dosage of warfarin will need to be decreased, accordingly, in patients receiving ethacrynic acid.

Organic mercurial diuretics

Sites of action. These drugs block the chloride pump at several sites, including the loop of Henle as well as portions of the proximal and distal tubules. This leads mainly to the loss of large amounts of sodium and chloride and a tendency to retain bicarbonate as the chief anion. Their diuretic action depends on the release of mercuric ion, which combines with sulfhydryl groups on enzymes involved in sodium and chloride transport. Mercuric ion is released more readily in an acidic medium. Thus, acid-forming salts (*e.g., ammonium chloride;* Table 27-1) are sometimes given with the mercurial to increase its efficacy.

Status. Historically, these are the oldest high-ceiling diuretics. They are, however, rarely used clinically because newer diuretics are less toxic and patients are less likely to become refractory to their beneficial effects with continued administration. Other drawbacks of the mercurials include the need for administration by injection for full effectiveness and the tendency of mercury to cause direct tissue toxicity. The mercury ion can cause many systemic toxic effects, including bone marrow depression, renal necrosis, gastrointestinal problems, and severe electrolyte imbalances.

Carbonic anhydrase inhibitor-type diuretics

Site and mechanism of action. The enzyme carbonic anhydrase (CA) plays an important role in certain cellular chemical reactions throughout the body. In the kidney tubule cells, its action helps to produce free hydrogen ions. These are then secreted into the tubular fluid in exchange for sodium ions. This sodium–hydrogen ion exchange takes place—as indicated earlier—along the entire length of the renal tubule, and is one of the ways in which the kidney forms an acid urine while conserving its stores of base by reabsorbing filtered bicarbonate anions along with the sodium that is returned to the blood and interstitial fluids.

Drugs such as *acetazolamide*[+] (Diamox) that inhibit CA interfere with this ability of the renal tubular cells to produce and secrete hydrogen ions (Table 27-1). As a result there are fewer hydrogen ions available for exchange with filtered sodium, and the sodium is then eliminated along with bicarbonate ions and the water in which these ions are dissolved, producing a diuresis of alkaline urine. By preventing the production of a normally acid urine, these drugs lead to a buildup of acidity in the interstitial fluid that can result in the acid–base imbalance called *metabolic acidosis.*

The inhibition of CA will also decrease the secretion of aqueous humor in the eye, resulting in a decrease in intraocular pressure. Because of this action, these drugs can be effectively used in the treatment of glaucoma.

CA inhibitors are also sometimes administered together with antiepileptic drugs for the control of seizures of the *petit mal* type. Their usefulness in this condition may be due in part to their ability to dehydrate the patient and to acidify tissues. Their use together with a systemic alkalinizer such as sodium bicarbonate has also been recommended for increasing the rate of excretion of aspirin in children suffering from salicylate intoxication.

Adverse effects. Potassium excretion is increased

by these diuretics, and hypokalemia is one of the most common side-effects. Metabolic acidosis is also a frequent and often dangerous effect of these diuretics. The patient's acid–base balance and electrolyte status need to be evaluated regularly to prevent complications. Fortunately, the action of the drugs is somewhat self-limiting because, with a decrease in serum bicarbonate levels, the mechanism responsible for diuresis no longer operates.

Specific clinical considerations. The CA inhibitors were among the first orally effective modern diuretics. Their action is relatively weak compared to that of the thiazides, and the CA inhibitors are rarely employed today as primary diuretics. Instead, these drugs are sometimes used alternately with other diuretics, or in combination with them, in patients whose edema has become relatively refractory to treatment with thiazide diuretics and even with the loop diuretics. Combination therapy with thiazides is said to be not merely additive but actually synergistic, and the effects of even the potent loop diuretics are claimed to be potentiated.

In evaluating the drug therapy, it should be noted that one of the frequent complaints of patients starting on the drug is a paresthesia (tingling) of the extremities or at mucocutaneous junctions (around the lips and anus). Other adverse effects include confusion and drowsiness. Patient teaching and safety measures need to incorporate this information. Some patients also develop photosensitivity while on these drugs; they need to be reassured and cautioned to avoid ultraviolet light, to use appropriate sunscreens, and to protect their skin and eyes from the sun.

The cardiac drug *quinidine* needs an acidic urine to ensure its excretion. When the urine is alkalinized by these diuretics, the quinidine is not excreted and can build up to toxic levels in the blood. Patients who would benefit from both drugs should receive a smaller than normal dose of quinidine and should be evaluated carefully for any signs of toxicity.

If gastrointestinal upset occurs, these drugs can be taken with food without loss of efficacy.

Potassium-sparing (antikaliuretic) diuretics

Spironolactone[+] (Aldactone), *triamterene* (Dyrenium), and *amiloride* (Midamor) can remove sodium-containing edema fluid without causing a loss of potassium (Table 27-1). Spironolactone acts as a competitive antagonist of aldosterone. By preventing the action of aldosterone in the distal tubule, this drug blocks the sodium–potassium exchange mechanism and causes the loss of sodium along with water, while potassium is retained (Fig. 27-2). Spironolactone thus acts only when aldosterone is present. Amiloride and triamterene also inhibit the distal tubule reabsorption of sodium, sparing potassium and hydrogen. These drugs, however, are *not* aldosterone antagonists and do not depend on the presence of aldosterone to cause a diuretic effect. They act on the other potassium secretory site in the distal tubule (Fig. 27-3).

Adverse effects. As with the other diuretics, most adverse effects of the potassium-sparing diuretics are caused by the imbalances in the system brought about by the changes in the normal regulatory mechanisms. In certain people—for example, those with renal failure or diabetes—hyperkalemia can occur as potassium is retained. This can cause muscle cramps, central nervous system toxicity (lethargy, confusion, ataxia), and cardiac arrhythmias. Patients can sometimes experience the signs and symptoms of dehydration, but this is a relatively infrequent occurrence with these weak diuretics.

Specific clinical considerations. These potassium-sparing diuretics are employed mainly in combination with the thiazides and other diuretics that act at more proximal sites. Such combined therapy of spironolactone, triamterene, or amiloride with the thiazides and other diuretics not only leads to an increased excretion of sodium, but also counteracts the tendency of the other diuretics to cause hypokalemic alkalosis. However, if patients have been taking a potassium salt supplement together with the other diuretic, the potassium is discontinued when one of these drugs is added to the patient's treatment regimen. This is because the potassium-retaining effects of these diuretics could lead to *hyper*kalemia, particularly in patients with renal insufficiency.

Spironolactone is most effective in disorders marked by secondary hyperaldosteronism—conditions in which the adrenal cortex secretes high levels of *aldosterone.* The level of this hormone is often high in patients with cirrhosis of the liver and the nephrotic syndrome.

Patients should be evaluated for signs of increased serum potassium levels, and potassium levels should be determined periodically, especially in elderly or diabetic patients. Patients should not be receiving any other drugs that might increase serum potassium levels. The patient should also be advised to avoid excessive intake of potassium-rich foods. Apparently, because of its steroid structure, spironolactone has caused gynecomastia, impotence, and menstrual abnormalities. The patient should be aware of these possibilities.

Osmotic diuretics
Mechanism of action. Certain substances that, unlike sodium, are *non*electrolytes are sometimes administered intravenously to increase the volume of urine that the kidneys produce. When molecules of such substances appear in the glomerular filtrate in large amounts, the fraction that is not reabsorbed by the tubules acts osmotically to prevent water from leaving the tubule. The diuresis seen in diabetes mellitus is the result of the glomerular filtration of more glucose molecules than the renal tubules can reabsorb. The large glucose molecules exert an osmotic pull to bring extra water into the tubules.

Glucose solutions are not commonly used to produce clinical diuresis. However, another sugar, *mannitol,* very little of which is reabsorbed by the tubules following filtration, is often employed for this purpose

(Table 27-1). *Urea*, another nonelectrolyte, only about half of which is reabsorbed, is also used to trap water within the tubule in several clinical situations other than the management of edema. (Although large doses of urea and mannitol may interfere with the reabsorption of filtered sodium and lead to the increased excretion of this electrolyte, these osmotic diuretics are not ordinarily used to counteract sodium retention.) *Isosorbide* (Ismotic) is an oral osmotic diuretic that is used to decrease intraocular pressure (see below).

Adverse effects. The most frequent adverse effects seen with these drugs are a sudden drop in blood volume followed by hypotension and cardiovascular imbalance. The drugs are given in acute situations, and the patient must be carefully monitored to detect and deal with the acute changes that could occur.

Specific clinical considerations. Careful monitoring of fluid and electrolyte balance and renal function is a very important aspect of caring for patients receiving osmotic diuretics. *Urea$^+$* (Ureaphil) and *mannitol* (Osmitrol) are used mainly to keep the kidneys producing urine in circumstances that might cause renal shutdown. Thus, in clinical situations in which blood flow through the kidneys and the rate of glomerular filtration are severely reduced, these diuretics help to prevent renal failure. In certain severely injured and burned patients, and in others following extensive surgery, a marked reduction in urine production occurs that can in itself lead to kidney damage. These osmotic substances can, by their ability to hold water within the renal tubules, maintain urine production and in this way overcome oliguria and prevent renal tubular necrosis.

The effects of these drugs are not limited to the kidneys. The osmotic action of molecules of these substances circulating *in the bloodstream* tends to draw fluid from the extravascular spaces into the plasma. This action is useful for reducing abnormally elevated intracranial and intraocular pressures. The reduction of cerebral edema and of pressure on the brain is often useful during neurosurgery and in patients who have suffered head injuries. Reduction of pressure within the eye with these drugs is sometimes employed prior to surgery for acute closed-angle glaucoma or for a detached retina. Use of these drugs is undesirable in patients with severely impaired kidney, liver, or cardiac function; if however, it is necessary to use these drugs in such a patient, extreme caution must be exercised to monitor the patient's vital signs.

The signs and symptoms of acute fluid loss—nausea, vomiting, light headedness, confusion, headache—can occur. Measures should be taken to provide for the patient's safety and comfort if any of these occur. Before administering mannitol, the solution should be carefully warmed and then allowed to return to room temperature. Patients often complain about the bitter taste of isosorbide—pouring the drug solution over cracked ice may make it more palatable.

Use of diuretics in specific clinical situations

Congestive heart failure

Not all patients with heart failure need diuretic therapy. In fact, it is best to avoid using these drugs and risking the complications that they can cause by first directing treatment at the failing heart itself. Thus, the use of digitalis in doses adequate for increasing the cardiac output and normalizing renal blood flow can often produce sufficient diuresis to counteract edema. Restricting the patient's daily dietary sodium intake is also often helpful, as is moderating physical activity. Reduced physical activity lessens the workload of the failing heart, and the rate of glomerular filtration often increases if the patient's feet are elevated for a while. However, if the patient continues to show signs of pulmonary congestion, ascites, or dependent edema, a diuretic should be added to the regimen.

Selection of a diuretic. The choice of a diuretic depends first on the severity of the patient's edema and on the urgency of the situation. For example, in a medical emergency such as acute pulmonary edema, intravenous injection of the high-ceiling diuretics—furosemide, sodium ethacrynate, or bumetanide—may be required for rapid mobilization of fluid from the lungs. On the other hand, in a patient who has been relieved of edema but who still requires diuretic therapy to prevent fluid from reaccumulating, it may be better to employ a less potent diuretic. This is administered orally in the smallest doses and at the longest intervals that will achieve the therapeutic goal, without causing electrolyte or acid–base imbalances or other complications.

Hydrochlorothiazide or one of the other thiazide or nonthiazide sulfonamide diuretics is most commonly employed for maintaining congestive heart failure patients at their "dry weight." A relatively low dose of the drug is ordered and the patient's response to it is evaluated. If no significant increase in urine volume is produced, or if the patient begins to show some gain in weight after a day or two, the dose is increased. When an effective dose is found, the intervals at which it is best administered should also be determined. Some patients may require daily doses of their diuretics, while others may get along well enough when taking the drug every other day, or only two or three times a week. Such intermittent therapy also has the advantage of allowing the patient's kidneys to help adjust homeostasis and thus avoid excessive losses of potassium along with sodium and chloride ions. However, it does cause some problems with patient compliance. It is more difficult for patients to remember which days are "drug days" than to remember to take a dose of drug *every* day. Patients should be encouraged to use a calendar to plan their drug doses, and to mark off the doses as they take them.

Potassium-sparing diuretics are sometimes added to thiazide therapy to avoid the need to raise the dose of the potassium-losing drugs in patients who appear to require more vigorous diuretic drug therapy. Such combinations are likely to produce increased natriuresis, without any added kaliuresis. In fact, less potassium may be lost than with thiazide therapy alone, while the loss of sodium chloride and water is even greater than before. The dose of the added spironolactone or triamterene should be adjusted to an optimal level in relation to the thiazide diuretic. If the effective dosage ratio of both types of diuretics turns out to be similar to that of one of the commercially available fixed-dosage combination products, the patient may then be switched to one of these for the convenience and better compliance that can be obtained by taking the two diuretics in a single capsule or tablet.

Patients who continue to accumulate fluid and to show signs of persistent pulmonary congestion may require treatment with one of the more potent diuretics. Such *refractory edema* has many possible causes, including increased severity of the patient's underlying cardiac disease or deterioration of his kidney function. One advantage of the loop diuretics over other diuretics is that these high-ceiling drugs remain active even in patients with renal impairment. Another advantage in such patients is that, unlike the older mercurial diuretics, these high-ceiling (loop) drugs do not do further damage to the failing kidneys, even when quite large daily doses are required to obtain the desired diuretic response. However, daily weight loss should be limited to only 1 lb or 2 lb, because more massive diuresis could lead to loss of circulating blood volume, reduced renal blood flow, and kidney-damaging oliguria or anuria.

Initial adjustment of the loop diuretic dosage is best carried out in the hospital, where laboratory facilities are available for following the effects of these diuretics on kidney function—for example, by checks of blood urea nitrogen (BUN) levels—and for early detection of any tendency toward development of hypokalemia, hyponatremia, or alkalosis. Ordinarily, it is possible to attain a dose level that is both safe and effective by starting the patient on small doses of potent diuretics and increasing the amount administered in several incremental steps. Sometimes, however, it is safer to stop such treatment with a single potent diuretic even when the saluretic response is less than optimal, because attempts to push dosage to higher levels can lead to toxicity.

Combination therapy is sometimes effective in such cases of refractory cardiac edema. As indicated previously, the addition of an antikaliuretic drug such as spironolactone or triamterene to a thiazide or a loop diuretic may both increase the desired loss of sodium and decrease the risk of potassium depletion. Similarly, adding acetazolamide to furosemide or ethacrynic acid occasionally brings about a much greater diuretic response than would have been expected from the usually weak action of the CA inhibitor-type diuretic.

In summary, a diuretic can be a useful adjunct to digitalis, dietary salt and fluid restrictions, and other measures for control of edema in patients with congestive heart failure. Properly employed, these drugs can help to improve the patient's myocardial function by reducing the load of blood that must be pumped by the failing heart. On the other hand, a diuretic-induced loss of excessive amounts of fluid can lead to a further reduction in cardiac output and to an even greater degree of cardiac decompensation. In addition, these drugs can cause electrolyte imbalances that may further endanger these patients—for example, diuretic-induced hypokalemia can intensify digitalis toxicity, and the dilutional hyponatremia that some diuretics induce, by favoring a greater loss of sodium in relation to water, can cause a worsening of this complication of severe heart failure.

Cirrhosis of the liver

Ascites is a common complication of hepatic cirrhosis and portal hypertension. The amount of fluid that accumulates in the abdominal cavity may be small, and its removal may require no specific treatment other than measures to improve liver function. On the other hand, when a patient's abdomen is severely distended, the ascitic fluid should be removed to relieve respiratory distress and to avoid development of further complications. However, the overuse of diuretics in an attempt to drain fluid from the peritoneal cavity can precipitate hepatic coma. Thus, other measures, such as restriction of the patient's daily dietary sodium and water intake, are often tried first.

Initiating diuretic therapy. If this and other conservative measures fail, *spironolactone* therapy may be initiated. This aldosterone-antagonizing diuretic is favored, not only because of the frequency with which cirrhotic ascites is accompanied by secondary hyperaldosteronism, but also because it does not cause hypokalemic alkalosis. This complication of treatment with thiazide and loop diuretics is especially dangerous for liver-damaged patients, because it aids the movement of ammonia from the gastrointestinal tract into the arterial blood and thence into the brain, leading to hepatic coma.

Unfortunately, only a minority of cirrhotic patients respond to the ordinarily recommended doses of spironolactone. Thus, some authorities suggest that treatment should begin with double the usual dose. Sometimes, after several days, a satisfactory diuresis may occur. If not, the dose of spironolactone is doubled for a few more days and then, if necessary, redoubled. It is, of course, essential that the patient's kidneys be functioning properly to avoid drug-induced retention of potassium. Ordinarily, despite such high doses, hyperkalemia does not occur, because patients with liver disease have relatively low plasma levels of potassium, and treatment with a potassium-sparing diuretic tends, if anything, to replenish their depleted potassium stores. Of course, the patient's serum potassium level must still be monitored during treatment with all diuretics.

Further treatment. If spironolactone alone fails to remove much ascitic fluid, a *thiazide diuretic* can be added to the patient's regimen. The two drugs may then exert the additive diuretic effect that was previously described. In addition, the presence of the potassium-sparing spironolactone helps to prevent the hypokalemic alkalosis that could occur if thiazide diuretics alone were being administered.

Refractory edema. Patients whose ascites remains refractory to treatment with these diuretics together with dietary sodium and fluid restrictions may require therapy with one of the more potent diuretics. They should, however, be hospitalized before beginning more vigorous treatment so that their serum electrolyte concentrations and BUN levels may be more carefully monitored. *Furosemide* and *ethacrynic acid* are considered safe and effective for treating resistant ascites in severe cirrhosis. However, quite large doses of these potent drugs may have to be injected intravenously to produce diuresis. These should be administered at well-spaced intervals—at least 6 hours apart—and for only 2 or 3 days at a time. During the intervals patients sometimes receive spironolactone or triamterene and, during such intermittent diuretic treatment, the patient's fluid and electrolyte loss is carefully measured and attempts are made to replace the lost potassium, chloride, and other ions and to prevent dehydration. In severe cases, when the ascites is not relieved by drug therapy, a peritoneal tap, called a paracentesis, is often done to drain off the fluid directly and to relieve the patient's symptoms. Once the accumulation of fluid has been removed, diuretic therapy may be effective enough to prevent a reaccumulation. Some patients remain refractory to even the most aggressive diuretic therapy, possibly because of severe protein depletion. One approach in such cases is to infuse salt-poor *serum albumin* to raise the patient's low plasma protein levels. Sometimes this may succeed in increasing the low colloidal osmotic pressure of the plasma, thus helping to pull fluid back into the bloodstream.

Renal disease

Diuretics were, at one time, considered ineffective or even contraindicated in patients with primary kidney diseases. However, with the availability of the safer and more potent thiazide and high-ceiling diuretics, the edema of both acute and chronic kidney disorders can now be better managed. Because patients with renal disease are less responsive to diuretic therapy, quite large doses are sometimes required, and patients must be closely observed for signs of drug-induced electrolyte imbalances.

The *nephrotic syndrome* is best treated with the glucocorticoid drug *prednisone,* which can both produce diuresis and favorably affect the underlying disease process. However, corticosteroids can also cause sodium and water retention under some circumstances. Thus, the *thiazide* diuretics and *furosemide* are sometimes employed before and during prednisone therapy. In addition, *spironolactone* may be useful for patients who develop secondary hyperaldosteronism, and the intravenous infusion of *serum albumin* is sometimes effective in this protein-losing syndrome. The use of albumin in edematous and ascitic patients with hypovolemia helps to reduce the risk of further reduction in plasma volume as a result of treatment with potent diuretics.

Acute glomerular nephritis following streptococcal infections results in hypervolemia and edema that may now sometimes be treated successfully with furosemide. In the past the almost equally potent organic mercurial diuretics could not be employed, because ordinary doses were ineffective, and because high doses could cause further damage to the inflamed glomerular membranes.

Acute renal failure may sometimes be prevented by employing an osmotic-type diuretic to keep adequate amounts of fluid in the nephrons and thus avoid further damage.

Other types of edema are also responsive to treatment with thiazides and with similar safe, modern diuretics. Mild diuretics are sometimes used to relieve the edema associated with premenstrual syndrome. However, in the much more serious clinical situation, toxemia of pregnancy—preeclampsia or eclampsia—edema-reducing diuretics have not been shown to affect hypertension favorably or to prevent eclamptic convulsions and other possible complications of this condition. In fact, the use of any diuretic during pregnancy must be carefully weighed against the possible harm to the fetus, as well as to the mother.

Additional clinical considerations

Safe use of diuretics can best be ensured by establishing a slow and consistent weight loss and avoiding rapid changes in fluid and electrolytes. A 1- to 2-lb/day weight loss is usually sufficient. Ideally, the effectiveness of diuretic therapy should be evaluated by weighing the patient early in the morning. The patient should be weighed, wearing the same amount of clothing, before eating and at the same time each day. An outpatient being maintained on diuretics should be taught to weigh himself in a similar manner and to record the weight on a calendar for easy reference. The weight fluctuation is the best indication of body water changes. Intake and output measurements, another useful monitor of fluid loss, are difficult to perform accurately. The actual output of fluid is complicated by water loss from the lungs, the skin, and the stools, and should not be the only parameter assessed.

With most of the diuretics, the patient needs to be constantly evaluated for the occurrence of hypokalemia (Table 27-2). It should be remembered that a natural loss of potassium occurs during stress or other times when aldosterone levels are high. Patients who have been regulated on a diuretic for a long period of time can still

Table 27–2. Signs and symptoms of hypokalemia

Signs	Symptoms
Decreased reflexes	Weakness
Orthostatic	
hypotension	Lethargy
Cardiac arrhythmias	Confusion
Weak pulses	Muscle cramps, pain
U waves on ECG	Anorexia
Prolonged P–R interval	
on ECG	Palpitations
Vomiting	
Trembling	

suffer from hypokalemia during times of stress, when their dietary potassium intake falls, or when increased amounts of potassium are lost, as with diarrhea. Many signs and symptoms are apparent before a significant change in serum potassium levels occurs. The patient should receive appropriate dietary potassium, or a potassium supplement, if any of these occur, and potassium levels should be carefully monitored.

Commercial potassium supplements may be necessary if diet alone proves inadequate for any reason, and if the potassium level of the patient's serum is seen to drop to 3.0 mEq/liter or below during prolonged daily diuretic therapy. Enteric-coated or other tablets should not be employed in such cases, because patients have sometimes suffered severe damage to the small intestine when they were given products containing potassium chloride combined in this manner. The tablets can become stuck at certain points in the bowel, and the salt reaches a high local concentration in the delicate tissues of the jejunum and ileum. This can lead to bleeding and ulceration, with perforation in some patients and scarring and contraction at the site of the gut lesion in others. Stenosis, or narrowing, of a portion of the intestine has caused serious obstruction. Such complications can also occur even with the slow-release or controlled-release potassium chloride tablets that are claimed to be safer than earlier oral dosage forms. Thus, if these products are employed, they should be promptly discontinued if abdominal pain, distention, nausea and vomiting, or gastrointestinal bleeding develops.

Liquid preparations containing the *chloride* salt of potassium are preferred because presence of the chloride anion helps to correct the *hypochloremic alkalosis* that often occurs together with hypokalemia. In such cases, replacing the lost potassium by the administration of such other salts as potassium bicarbonate (and acetate, citrate, or gluconate anions, which are converted to bicarbonate in

the body) will not overcome the alkalosis. To prevent the acid–base imbalance from persisting in patients who have lost too much chloride through excessive chloriuresis (with a resulting retention of excessive bicarbonate anion), potassium chloride is required.

Patients sometimes complain of the unpalatable saltiness of potassium chloride solution, which is not always adequately masked with fruit or other flavorings. However, the unpleasant taste may be minimized by diluting the prescribed dose of the potassium salt solution with water or fruit juice, or drinking it ice cold or over ice chips. A dose of 5 ml of a 20% solution or 10 ml of a 10% solution of potassium chloride is usually diluted in a glass of water or orange juice and taken one or more times daily—depending on the results of frequent checks of the patient's serum potassium level—to prevent depletion during daily diuretic therapy. (Dosage adjustment is necessary to prevent possible *hyper*kalemia and potassium toxicity.)

Specific clinical situations such as renal failure, hepatic failure, gout, and diabetes mellitus can be aggravated by these drugs. If a patient is known to have any of these conditions and a diuretic is used, very careful clinical monitoring of the patient will be necessary.

Pregnancy and lactation are contraindications for the use of diuretics. The research is not complete, but the diuretics have been associated with fetal malformations and death, as well as with maternal complications. Most of the diuretics pass into breast milk and can cause rapid fluid and electrolyte imbalances in a neonate. If a pregnant patient must receive a diuretic, careful consideration must be given to the risks and benefits of each type of drug, and the patient must be very carefully monitored.

Drug–drug interactions

The various effects of diuretics may be potentiated when they are given with other drugs that cause similar effects. For example, *adrenal steroids* cause a loss of potassium. When adrenal steroids are given with diuretics such as the thiazides or loop diuretics, hypokalemia is more likely to occur. *Alcohol* inhibits the release of ADH from the posterior pituitary, leading to a water diuresis. A patient on diuretics who takes alcohol could suffer a rapid fluid loss that would result in the signs and symptoms of dehydration—for example, nausea, confusion, headache, weakness. *Lithium*, an ion used to treat manic–depressive mental illness, should not be given with diuretics if it can be avoided. The diuretics prevent the renal clearance of lithium and serum blood levels of lithium increase, causing toxicity. For other specific drug interactions, review each type of diuretic discussed.

Patient teaching

This is a very important aspect of the nursing care of patients receiving diuretics. The patient needs to understand the drug and its actions, and will be expected to make some significant changes in daily activities, because availability to a bathroom is essential while the drug is at its effective levels. The patient will need help and encouragement in adjusting to the drug, and should be assured that, once regulated on the drug, he will know exactly how long the diuresis lasts and will be better able to plan activities around it. The daily weighing and recording of body weight that is necessary and the restricted dietary intake of fluid and salt also must be incorporated into the patient's life style. These take time and patience, and the patient will need frequent encouragement and reassurance. A summary of the various points that should be incorporated into the teaching plan for patients on diuretics is found in the patient teaching guide.

Technical considerations

For the most part, increasing the dosage of any of the diuretics does not increase urine output considerably, but does increase the risk of electrolyte imbalances. In acute situations, large doses of loop diuretics are sometimes given in a zealous attempt to increase urinary output. The nurse is often in a position to add a gentle reminder that giving large intravenous doses of these drugs can increase the vascular volume with which the heart has to deal, without producing appreciable therapeutic benefit.

The nursing process table presents a summary of considerations that should be made for the patient who is receiving diuretic therapy.

Patient teaching guide: diuretics

The drug that has been prescribed for you is called a *diuretic,* or a "water pill." This medication helps to reduce the amount of fluid that is in your body by causing the kidneys to pass large quantities of water and salt from the bloodstream into the urine. By removing this fluid from the bloodstream, the diuretic helps to decrease the work of the heart and to get rid of edema or swelling in your tissues.

Instructions:

1. The name of your drug is _____ .

2. The dose of the drug ordered for you is _____ (tablets).

3. The drug should be taken _____ time(s) a day. The best time to take your drug is in the morning, or at a time when you will have ready access to a bathroom for several hours. Try not to take your diuretic any later than 6 PM; taking the drug later than that will cause you to be disturbed during the night when you get up to go to the bathroom.

4. The drug can be taken with meals, and this may alleviate any stomach upset. While you are taking a diuretic, you should be careful about fluid intake and you should not add salt to your food. (The diuretic causes potassium loss so it is also necessary to try to eat foods high in potassium—for example, orange juice, raisins, other fruits—or to take a potassium supplement, because this important chemical is often lost in the urine.)

5. Some common effects of the drug that you should be aware of include the following:

Increased volume and frequency of urination	Have ready access to a bathroom; once you are used to the drug and its actions, you will be able to plan how long this effect will persist.
Dizziness, feeling faint on arising, drowsiness	The loss of fluid often lowers blood pressure and causes these feelings. They can be lessened if you avoid rapid position changes. If you tend to become drowsy, it is important to avoid dangerous activities, such

(continued)

		as driving a car. These feelings can be increased if alcohol is consumed, and safety precautions should be taken if you use alcohol.
	Increased sensitivity to sunlight	Avoid sunlight, use sunglasses, and wear protective clothing.
	Decrease in sexual functioning	This can occur with the change in body fluid and electrolyte levels; if severe, report the occurrence; it may be possible to try a new drug.
	Increased thirst	The loss of fluid may cause an increase in thirst; try to avoid increased fluid intake. Sucking on lozenges or frequent mouth care (brushing your teeth, or using a mouthwash) can help to overcome the thirst.

7. Avoid the use of any over-the-counter medications without first checking with your nurse or physician. Several of these medications can interfere with the effectiveness of the diuretic.

8. Report the use of this diuretic to any physician, nurse, or dentist who takes care of you.

9. Keep this and all medications out of the reach of children.

10. Weigh yourself each morning on arising, and record your weight on a calendar.

Notify your nurse or physician if any of the following occur:

Muscle cramps or pain
Loss or gain of more than 3 lb in 1
   day
Swelling in your fingers or ankles
Nausea or vomiting for no
   apparent reason
Unusual bleeding or bruising
Drowsiness, fatigue, or trembling
   or weakness

Guide to the nursing process: diuretics

Assessment	Nursing diagnoses	Intervention	Evaluation
Past history (*contraindications*)	Potential deficit in fluid volume	Daily weighing, monitor intake and output	Monitor response to drug:

(continued)

Assessment	Nursing diagnoses	Intervention	Evaluation
include: Pregnancy Lactation Renal failure Hepatic failure Known electrolyte imbalances Gout *Allergies:* reactions Medication history: drugs being taken (*cautions*); lithium; adreno- orticosteroids **Physical assessment** Neurologic: reflexes, orientation, muscle strength, hearing Cardiovascular: pulses, baseline ECG, BP, orthostatic BP, edema, cardiac output Respiratory: rate, pattern adventitious sounds Renal: output, pattern, electrolyte levels Skin: perfusion, edema, lesions	Knowledge deficit regarding drug therapy Potential alteration in nutrition Potential sexual dysfunction Potential alteration in urinary elimination	Provide comfort and safety measures: Easy access to bathroom Side rails, if necessary Encourage slow position changes Patient teaching regarding: Drug actions Dose Timing Side-effects Toxic effects Encourage increased potassium intake; limiting of dietary fluids and salt (unless diuretic spares potassium) Provide encouragement and reassurance for: Sexual dysfunction Changes in diet Recording of weight Compliance to drug therapy Provide for preparation and administration of drug: timing is im- portant—outpatients on alternate-day drugs (or on other patterns) need measures to help them to remember to take their drug	Output levels Weight changes Loss of edema Monitor for adverse effects: Hypoglycemia Hypokalemia Increased uric acid levels (gout) Increased blood sugar levels Orthostatic hypotension Evaluate for drug–drug interactions: Lithium Steroids Alcohol (Other specific drugs) Evaluate for environmental changes leading to adverse effects: Stress Diet changes Diarrhea Evaluate effectiveness of teaching plan and reassurance Evaluate effectiveness of comfort measures

Summary of diuretic-induced abnormalities in electrolyte and acid–base balances

Type of imbalance	Diuretic involved	Prevention and treatment
Acidosis, metabolic Results from accumulation of chloride ions in relative excess compared to bicarbonate, which is excreted in the urine; retention of hydrogen ions occurs along with this decrease in alkali reserve.	Carbonic anhydrase inhibitor-type diuretics; ammonium chloride and other acidifying salts; potassium-sparing type diuretics	Discontinue diuretic therapy to allow readjustment by homeostatic mechanisms including increased renal excretion of chloride and secretion of hydrogen ions; if severe administer bicarbonate

(continued)

Alkalosis

Results from a relatively excessive loss of chloride ions with retention of bicarbonate; also caused by excessive excretion of hydrogen ions

High-ceiling, or loop, diuretics; sulfonamides (*e.g.*, thiazides)

Provide chloride ions, preferably as potassium chloride, but also as sodium or ammonium chloride, lysine monohydrochloride, or arginine monohydrochloride; or use other acidifiers such as a carbonic anhydrase inhibitor diuretic intermittently to correct alkalosis

Hyperchloremia

Results from excessive accumulation of chloride ions in the extra-cellular fluid (see Acidosis, above)

See Acidosis, above

See Acidosis, above

Hyperkalemia

Results from excessive accumulation of potassium ions in plasma and extracellular fluid as a result of reduced distal tubular secretion of potassium

Potassium-sparing diuretics; possible also with any diuretic-induced hypovolemia leading to oliguria, renal failure, and anuria

Avoid by discontinuing previously administered potassium supplements and by not using these diuretics in patients with renal failure; correct by discontinuing these drugs

Hypochloremia

Results from low levels of chloride ions in plasma and other extracellular fluids caused by excessive urinary excretion of chloride in relation to sodium

See Alkalosis, above

See Alkalosis, above

Hypokalemia

Results from low levels of potassium in plasma and other extracellular fluid, caused by excessive urinary excretion of the ion

High-ceiling, or loop, diuretics; sulfonamides (*e.g.*, thiazides); carbonic-anhydrase-inhibitor-type diuretics

Administer more dietary potassium, potassium supplements, preferably, potassium chloride, combine these potassium-losing diuretics with a potassium-sparing diuretic such as spironolactone

Hyponatremia, dilutional

Results from a decrease in the proportion of sodium in the extracellular fluid relative to its water content; this may be related to the patient's disease state and may occur spontaneously, or it may be caused by diuretics that interfere with the kidneys' ability to excrete an adequately dilute urine

Sulfonamide (*e.g.*, thiazide) diuretics; high-ceiling, or loop, diuretics

Discontinue diuretic therapy; restrict patient's daily water intake; salt is *not* ordinarily administered; an osmotic diuretic may be employed in severe cases

(continued)

Hyponatremia, true

Results from low levels of sodium in the plasma and other extracellular fluid caused by an actual depletion of the body's salt reserve by excessive activity of saliuretic diuretics	Loop diuretics, when employed in excessive doses and too frequently, particularly during hot weather, when sodium is lost in perspiration	Avoid excessive salt loss by employing small doses of diuretics and not restricting sodium intake too severely; treat by increasing oral salt intake, or by IV infusion of 5% sodium chloride solution in severe cases

Summary of side-effects, toxicity, cautions, and contraindications of certain diuretic drug classes

High-ceiling or loop diuretics (furosemide, bumetanide, ethacrynic acid)

Fluid and electrolyte imbalances. Vigorous diuresis may lead to excessive loss of water and electrolytes, including sodium, chloride, and potassium ions. Reduction in blood volume can cause acute hypotension, circulatory collapse, and, particularly in elderly patients, thromboembolism, secondary to hemoconcentration.

Other adverse effects. Mild diarrhea may occur; the occasional profuse watery diarrhea caused by *ethacrynic acid* requires discontinuation of drug treatment. Readministration of this diuretic in such cases is contraindicated.

Hearing loss, usually reversible, has been reported, especially in patients with impaired kidney function and in those receiving other ototoxic drugs. These drugs may increase possible kidney damage when administered with aminoglycoside and other antibiotics that are potentially nephrotoxic.

Cautions and contraindications. These drugs are contraindicated in the presence of anuria and should be withdrawn if increasing oliguria or azotemia is noted during treatment. Particular caution is required in the following situations:

1. Advanced liver cirrhosis: diuretic drug-induced electrolyte imbalances may lead to encephalopathy, hepatic coma, and death
2. Patients receiving digitalis for cardiac decompensation: diuretic drug-induced hypokalemia can cause fatal arrhythmias
3. Patients taking antihypertensive drugs, who are subject to episodes of postural hypotension
4. Diabetic patients, in whom hyperglycemia may develop
5. Gout patients, in whom an acute gout attack may be precipitated by a rise in plasma levels of uric acid (hyperuricemia)
6. Patients who have previously exhibited sensitivity to these drugs resulting in leukopenia or thrombocytopenia
7. Patients taking lithium should not receive these or other diuretics, because their use may decrease its renal excretion and lead to lithium intoxication

Sulfonamide (*e.g., benzothiadiazide*) diuretics

Fluid and electrolyte imbalances. Evidenced by: mouth dryness, thirst, nausea and vomiting, muscle weakness or cramps, drowsiness, lethargy, and possible hypotension and oliguria.

Hypersensitivity reactions. Skin eruptions of maculopapular type, photosensitivity, leukopenia, agranulocytosis, thrombocytic purpura.

Cautions and contraindications. Patients with anuria should not receive these drugs. Those with less severely impaired kidney function may retain blood urea nitrogen (BUN), nonprotein nitrogen (NPN), and creatinine; gout patients may get acute attacks from higher uric acid levels; diabetes patients may need more insulin; heart irregularities may occur in digitalized heart patients.

Potassium-sparing diuretics (spironolactone; triamterene; amiloride)

Fluid and electrolyte imbalances. Increased retention of potassium can lead to fatal cardiac arrhythmias and to other adverse effects of hyperkalemia. These drugs should not be taken by patients who have high plasma potassium levels, and patients—particularly those with impaired kidney function, the elderly, and diabetics—should be checked for rises in serum potassium levels during treatment. Potassium supplements should be discontinued if patients were previously taking them with a potassium-losing diuretic. Two drugs of this type should not ordinarily be taken together because of the increased possibility of causing potassium retention.

Excessive loss of sodium may occur and be reflected by mouth dryness, thirst, lethargy, and drowsiness. Mild metabolic acidosis may sometimes develop.

Other adverse effects. Spironolactone is a steroid that can cause gynecomastia and such other signs of endocrine effects as deepening of the voice, hirsutism, irregular menses or amenorrhea, and impotence. It has

(continued)

caused tumors to develop in animals during chronic toxicity studies, but no cause-and-effect relationship relative to potential mammary carcinogenicity has been established in humans.

Carbonic anhydrase inhibitors

Fluid and electrolyte imbalances. Potassium depletion and sodium bicarbonate loss cause hypokalemia and mild metabolic acidosis.

Other adverse effects. Paresthesias, drowsiness, tremor, anorexia.

Hypersensitivity reactions. Skin rashes, fever, bone marrow depression, crystalluria, and renal calculi.

Cautions and contraindications: Patients with renal failure; Addison's disease and adrenocortical insufficiency; respiratory disorders with reduced pulmonary ventilation can lead to hyperchloremic acidosis.

Ammonium chloride and other acidifying salts

Acid–base imbalance. These drugs produce metabolic acidosis through loss of bicarbonate. Ordinarily, the kidneys compensate for this by excreting excess chloride and secreting hydrogen ions. However, uncompensated acidosis can occur in patients with chronic kidney disease that has led to impaired renal function. These drugs should be avoided in such patients, and their prolonged use alone is contraindicated.

Other adverse effects. Local gastrointestinal irritation may lead to nausea and vomiting, enteric-coated tablets should be employed.

Case study

Presentation

HL, a 68-year-old retired bank executive, has been taking Lasix, 40 mg qd, along with several other medications to control his congestive heart failure. HL has been regulated on these drugs for 2 years and has been doing very well. Today, HL appeared in the emergency department complaining of shortness of breath, dizziness, weakness, and lethargy. While waiting to be seen, HL's weakness evolved into lower limb paralysis and he was then in acute respiratory distress. The patient was placed on a cardiac monitor and oxygen was started through nasal prongs. Clinical laboratory reports revealed severe hypokalemia. The patient's potassium level was returned to normal limits after IV infusion of KCl, and he was stabilized.

When questioned, HL reported that he began having muscle cramps in his legs about a week ago. They were not intolerable, and he was playing golf daily for exercise and enjoyment. He denied any increase in stress, diarrhea, or decrease in dietary potassium. The only real change he could identify in his diet was a rather sudden licorice binge. He reports that he got "hooked" on black licorice bits and thought he was eating two or three bags every couple of days.

The patient is very concerned about what happened, and about the possibility of another episode. What nursing measures should be taken at this point?

Discussion

Because the patient has been regulated on Lasix for an extensive period of time, and because he has been regularly evaluated, the most reasonable approach to his teaching was to determine what change occurred in his environment that could have precipitated the hypokalemia. The culprit in HL's case was his love for licorice. Licorice contains glycyrrhizic acid, a compound that acts in the renal tubules like aldosterone: it causes a loss of potassium in exchange for sodium ions. Inveterate consumption of licorice causes a pseudoaldosteronism. The combined loss of potassium from the diuretic and the licorice pushed HL into a progressive but severe hypokalemia. HL needs to be reassured about the cause of this episode. He will need reinforcement of his basic teaching—encouraging him to be alert for, and to report, any of the signs and symptoms of hypokalemia. He will also need to be taught that excesses of any substance, especially one that may contain chemicals or "drugs," should be avoided. Moderation should be the key. The patient will need to be reassured and encouraged to ask questions and voice his concerns to ensure compliance to drug therapy. This case will also provide a good teaching base for staff and other patients regarding the unknowing abuse of a potentially harmful substance.

Drug digests

Acetazolamide USP (Diamox)

Actions and indications. This is the prototype of the carbonic anhydrase inhibitor class of diuretics. It is not potent enough for use in mobilizing already accumulated fluid in congestive heart failure. However, once "dry weight" is attained by use of other more potent diuretics, this drug is sometimes effective for keeping the patient free of edema. It is most useful when administered on alternate days with a diuretic of another class, such as a thiazide being given on the day when this drug is skipped. Other types of edema that may respond to oral doses include that induced by corticosteroid drugs and premenstrual edema. This drug is also used as an adjunct to anticonvulsant therapy in the management of various forms of epilepsy and of glaucoma.

Adverse effects, cautions, and contraindications. This drug does not ordinarily cause serious side-effects, but hypersensitivity-type reactions including fever, rash, and blood dyscrasias are possible. The most common side-effects are drowsiness and paresthesias, including feelings of tingling and numbness. The drug causes a metabolic acidosis as a result of the excretion of sodium bicarbonate in the urine and retention of chloride ions in the tissues. This is usually self-limiting, however, and acid–base balance may be restored by a day or two of rest from the drug. Administration of a thiazide diuretic that tends to cause a metabolic alkalosis also corrects acidosis, as does the administration of bicarbonate.

This drug is contraindicated in patients with low levels of plasma potassium, particularly if they suffer from severe liver or kidney disease. It is also contraindicated in cases of chronic narrow-angle glaucoma, although it is useful in the acute congestive phase.

Dosage and administration. For treating edema in congestive heart failure, a single daily dose of 250 to 375 mg is administered in the morning for 1 or 2 days alternating with a rest day. Raising the dose or administering the drug too frequently may actually cause a reduced diuretic response.

In glaucoma, doses range from 250 mg to 1 g daily in chronic open-angle cases; in acute closed-angle glaucoma, 250 mg is administered orally or IV every 4 hours preoperatively. In epilepsy, daily doses range between 375 mg and 1 g daily.

Ethacrynic acid USP and sodium ethacrynate USP (Edecrin; Edecrin Sodium)

Actions and indications. This is one of the most potent diuretics for management of edema in patients with advanced cardiac, kidney, and liver disease, including those who are no longer responsive to thiazides and other diuretics. The rapid onset of action of this diuretic—within 30 minutes of oral administration and 15 minutes after intravenous injection—is particularly useful for patients with acute pulmonary edema for whom the drug has sometimes proved lifesaving.

The drug is also useful in patients with ascites from hepatic cirrhosis. It is effective in patients with significant degrees of chronic renal insufficiency, including children and others with the nephrotic syndrome.

Adverse effects, cautions, and contraindications. Care is required to avoid too strong a diuretic effect, because this may lead to dehydration and to depletion of essential electrolytes. Patients are weighed before and during treatment as a check against too great a loss of weight in water, because the resulting reduction in plasma volume might cause an acute hypotensive or a thromboembolic episode, particularly in elderly patients. Patients are closely observed for signs and symptoms of electrolyte imbalance, and laboratory determinations are made of serum levels of potassium, chloride, and other ions to detect and avoid hypokalemia, hypochloremia, and alkalosis. These conditions may be manifested by a loss of appetite, nausea and vomiting, muscle cramps and weakness, and feelings of fatigue and drowsiness. Dangerous direct actions of this drug that may make it necessary to discontinue its use are the development of deafness or of a profuse watery diarrhea.

Dosage and administration. Treatment is initiated with a single small oral dose (50 to 100 mg) taken after a meal. Dosage is then gradually raised by increments of 25 or 50 mg as needed to keep the daily weight loss at only 1 or 2 lb. Once dry weight is reached, patients may be maintained on lower daily doses, or even receive the drug only on alternate days or intermittently—that is, with intervening rest periods of several days. In emergencies or when oral administration is not feasible, a single dose of 50 to 100 mg of the sodium salt may be injected IV.

Furosemide USP (Lasix)

Actions and indications. This sulfonamide diuretic is more potent than the thiazide diuretics. This may be because it interferes with the reabsorption of filtered sodium in the ascending limb of the loop of Henle as well as in the proximal and distal portions of the renal tubules. Thus, it is often useful for treating edematous patients who have proved resistant to therapy with thiazides and other diuretic drugs.

Treatment of patients with impaired kidney function, including those with acute and chronic kidney failure, has sometimes been effective in producing diuresis. It has also been useful in treating the nephrotic syndrome, hepatic cirrhosis, and congestive heart failure. Because of its rapid onset of action when administered parenterally (5 minutes to 10 minutes), it is used in the emergency treatment of acute pulmonary edema and in hypertensive crisis.

Adverse effects, cautions, and contraindications. This potent drug can cause an excessively strong diuretic effect that can result in dehydration, depletion of electrolytes, and a drop in blood volume. Elderly patients may develop blood clots and emboli or circulatory collapse as a result of hemoconcentration. Drug-induced potassium loss can be particularly dangerous for patients taking digitalis, because ventricular arrhythmias may result. Loss of potassium in excess causes leg cramps. Alkalosis leads to such symptoms as anorexia and vomiting, feelings of weakness and lethargy, dizziness, and mental confusion.

Other metabolic imbalances include a rise in blood sugar and in serum uric acid levels— conditions that occasionally precipitate diabetes and gout attacks. High doses have caused tinnitus and deafness, particularly in patients with severely impaired kidney func-

tion. The drug should be discontinued in such patients, if it fails to produce diuresis and blood urea nitrogen (BUN) levels rise. Patients with hepatic cirrhosis should be started on this drug in the hospital where fluid and electrolyte balance can be carefully observed to avoid precipitating hepatic coma.

Dosage and administration. For rapid action, a single IV or IM dose of 20 to 80 mg is usually administered. If it fails to produce the desired effect, a dose 20 to 40 mg higher is injected after at least 2 hours. Oral doses of 40 to 80 mg are given in the morning; if the response is unsatisfactory, the dosage may be raised by 40 mg no sooner than 6 to 8 hours later. Daily dosage is usually maintained at 20 to 40 mg, qd or bid. If doses greater than 80 mg/day are given, clinical laboratory tests are essential. In acute emergencies, up to 600 mg/day can be given.

Hydrochlorothiazide USP (Esidrix; HydroDiuril; Oretic)

Actions and indications. This close relative of the prototype thiazide diuretic chlorothiazide is commonly used in the management of chronic essential hypertension as well as in many disorders in which edema develops. It is often effective for reducing mild to moderately elevated blood pressure when administered alone. In more severe degrees of hypertension, this drug is commonly administered in combination with such other antihypertensive drugs as hydralazine, methyldopa, pargyline, and guanethidine. In congestive heart failure it is frequently used as an adjunct to digitalis treatment. Other edematous states in which it is employed include cirrhosis of the liver, nephrosis, premenstrual edema, and drug-induced (e.g., steroid) edema, and as an adjunct in the management of obesity.

Adverse effects, cautions, and contraindications. This drug rarely causes side-effects secondary to direct tissue toxicity. Hypersensitivity-type reactions are also rare but include skin rashes and blood dyscrasias such as agranulocytosis and aplastic anemia. Ill effects are much more commonly the result of an excessive loss of fluids and electrolytes including sodium, chloride, bicarbonate, and potassium. Warning signs include mouth dryness and thirst, feelings of weakness, restlessness, and drowsiness, muscle fatigue, cramps, and pain, and nausea, vomiting, and diarrhea. Special care is required in patients with severe kidney and liver disease, because this drug may precipitate hepatic coma or azotemia in such cases. The drug is absolutely contraindicated in patients with renal shutdown and relatively contraindicated in rapidly progressive liver disease.

Dosage and administration. In initiating treatment of edema, oral doses of 25 mg to 200 mg or more may have to be administered daily for several days. Once dry weight is attained, patients may be maintained on 25 mg to 100 mg administered daily or intermittently on alternate days.

For reducing high blood pressure a single morning dose of 25 mg to 100 mg or two daily doses of 50 mg may be adequate. Dosage during maintenance may range from 25 mg to 100 mg. If this drug is administered as part of a program of combined therapy, the dosage of the more potent sympatholytic drugs should be reduced to about half of the usual doses for these agents to avoid too great a drop in blood pressure.

Spironolactone USP (Aldactone)

Actions and indications. This is a potassium-sparing diuretic, a drug that relieves edema and ascites by removing sodium-containing fluids without causing depletion of potassium ions. It is indicated for treating edema in disorders marked by development of secondary hyperaldosteronism, including congestive heart failure, hepatic cirrhosis, and the nephrotic syndrome. The drug, a steroid, blocks the sodium-retaining and potassium-losing effects of the adrenal mineralocorticoid hormone aldosterone on the most distal portion of the renal convoluted tubule. This drug is commonly administered in combination with a thiazide diuretic, both in treating edematous disorders and for reducing high blood pressure in patients with essential hypertension.

Adverse effects, cautions, and contraindications. Adverse reactions of a direct tissue toxicity type are relatively rare. However, this steroid drug has occasionally caused effects of an androgenic (male hormone) type, including hirsutism and deepening of the voice; female hormone effects in men, manifested by gynecomastia (painful breast swelling) has occasionally been reported.

A more common concern is the possibility that this drug may cause potassium retention resulting in hyperkalemia. To avoid this, the drug is administered with caution to patients with impaired kidney function, and its use is contraindicated in patients whose kidney function is rapidly progressing toward acute renal insufficiency and anuria, because hyperkalemia may lead to cardiac arrest in such cases. Mild metabolic acidosis and hyponatremia (marked by thirst and drowsiness) sometimes occur as a result of reduced excretion of hydrogen ions and depletion of sodium ions.

Dosage and administration. Treatment of edema is begun with daily doses of 100 mg, divided into four doses of 25 mg each. This dose is continued if the diuretic response after 5 days is adequate; if not, this drug may be administered in larger doses and in combination with a thiazide diuretic. For treating essential hypertension, daily doses of 50 mg to 100 mg may be adequate, particularly when the drug is administered with a thiazide or other antihypertensive agent.

Urea, sterile, USP (Ureaphil; Urevert)

Actions and indications. This osmotic diuretic is used clinically for various purposes other than control of edema because of its ability to keep water within the renal tubules and thus bring about an increase in the amount of urine produced. This helps to prevent oliguria and possible kidney damage in patients with severe injuries or burns, or following surgery. In addition, the osmotic activity of the intravenously injected solution tends to draw fluid from the extracellular spaces into the blood. This is useful for reducing excessively high cerebrospinal pressure during neurosurgical operations and cerebral edema following head injuries. Intraocular pressure may also be reduced. The drug is used to promote an increased flow of urine in patients who have undergone prostate surgery, but it is not very effective for relief of resistant cirrhotic or nephrotic edema.

Adverse effects, cautions, and contraindications. Care is required in administering this drug to patients with kidney disease, and its use is contraindicated in those with severely impaired renal function. Care is also needed to avoid leakage of the hypertonic solution into the tissues around the injected vein, because local irritation may lead to possible tissue necrosis. The infusion should not be made into veins of the lower extremities in elderly patients because of possible development of thrombophlebitis and thrombosis. The drug should not be administered to severely dehydrated patients or to those with active intracranial bleeding. Disorientation, confusion and headache, and nausea and vomiting have occasionally been reported.

Dosage and administration. Solutions are prepared by mixing the powder with diluent fluids in amounts needed to make 4% and 30% solutions. To make a 4% solution, 40 g of sterile urea are mixed with 1 liter of dextrose injection or other diluent; the 30% solution is made by mixing 40 g of sterile urea with 105 ml of diluent to make 135 ml of solution.

The 30% solution, which is used for reducing intracranial pressure, is infused slowly by vein at a rate of 3 or 4 ml/minute in amounts of 1 to 1.5 g/kg of body weight in adults and usually in lesser dosage for children. The 4% solution employed against oliguria is administered at the same slow intravenous infusion rate in amounts of 1500 to 3000 ml daily, which is equal to a maximum of 120 g of urea daily.

References

Arroyo V: A rational approach to the treatment of ascites. Postgrad Med 51:558, 1975

Aspinall MJ: A simplified guide to managing patients with hyponatremia. Nursing '78 8:32, 1978

Beyer KH: Chlorothiazide. Br J Clin Pharmacol 13:15, 1982

Bumetanide (Bumex)—a new "loop" diuretic. Med Lett Drugs Ther 25:61, 1983

Carriere S et al: Bumetanide, a new loop diuretic. Clin Pharmacol Ther 20:424, 1976.

Duling BR: The kidney. In Berne RM, Levy MN (eds), Physiology, pp 823–892. St. Louis, CV Mosby, 1983

Fenster LF: Therapy of cirrhosis of the liver. Ration Drug Ther 10:1, 1976

Frakes JT: Physiologic considerations in medical management of ascites. Arch Intern Med 140:620, 1980

Freis ED: Salt in hypertension and the effects of diuretics. Ann Rev Pharmacol Toxicol 18:13, 1979

Gifford RW Jr: A guide to the practical use of diuretics. JAMA 235:1890, 1976

Gottschalk CW, Lassiter WE: Mechanisms of urine formation. In Mountcastle VB (ed): Medical Physiology, 14th ed, pp 1165–1205. St. Louis, CV Mosby, 1980

Kemp G, Kemp D: Diuretics. Am J Nurs 78:1006, 1978

Kósman ME: Management of potassium problems during long-term diuretic therapy. JAMA 230:743, 1974

Lassiter WE, Gottschalk CW: Urine formation in the diseased kidney. In Mountcastle VB (ed): Medical Physiology, 14th ed, pp 1206–1217. St. Louis, CV Mosby, 1980

Lassiter WE, Gottschalk CW: Volume and composition of the body fluids. In Mountcastle VB (ed): Medical Physiology, 14th ed, pp 1149–1164. St. Louis, CV Mosby, 1980

Mudge GH: Diuretics and other agents employed in the mobilization of edema fluid. In Gilman AG, Goodman LS, Gilman A, (eds): Goodman and Gilman's The Pharmacological Basis of Therapeutics, 6th ed, pp 892–915. New York, Macmillan, 1980

Mudge GH: Introduction: Drugs affecting renal function and electrolyte metabolism. In Gilman AG, Goodman LS, Gilman A (eds): Goodman and Gilman's The Pharmacological Basis of Therapeutics, 6th ed, pp 885–892. New York, Macmillan, 1980

Newma KS, Diuhy RG: Hyperkalemia and hypokalemia. JAMA 231:631, 1975

Perez-Stable EC, Materson BJ: Diuretic drug therapy of edema. Med Clin North Am 55:359, 1971

Rovner DR: Use of pharmacologic agents in the treatment of hypokalemia and hyperkalemia. Ration Drug Ther 6:1, 1972

Teyel IH (ed): Perspectives on Bumetanide (Symposium). J Clin Pharmacol 21:531, 1981

Vidt DG: Diuretics, use and misuse. Postgrad Med 59:143, 1976

Chapter 28

Drugs used in treating hypertension

28

The nature of hypertension

More than 25 million Americans have hypertension—excessively high blood pressure. The upper limit of normal blood pressure is now often set as 140 mm Hg systolic and 90 mm Hg diastolic. Blood pressure can, of course, rise briefly far above this arbitrary borderline, without the person being considered hypertensive. Physical exercise or emotional stress may, for example, cause a person's blood pressure to become elevated for a while, and the blood pressure may drop below this level when resting or sleeping.

Diagnosis

The blood pressure should be measured after the patient has been at rest for a few minutes. Even then, a single high reading does not necessarily indicate hypertension. The person's pressure should be taken on several different occasions, and while the patient is sitting, standing, and lying down. Only when several separate examinations of this type have shown that the blood pressure stays persistently at an abnormally high level can the patient be classified as being hypertensive.

The diagnosis of hypertension is made, of course, on the basis of additional tests. These may include the following: examination of the patient's eyegrounds with an ophthalmoscope to see if the arterioles in the fundus of the eye are excessively constricted or whether the optic disk is edematous (papilledema); chest x-rays and an electrocardiogram to see whether the heart is enlarged or shows signs of strain from overloading; and urinalyses and tests of blood urea nitrogen (BUN) and serum creatinine levels to determine the state of the patient's kidney function.

Complications

The studies of ocular blood vessels and cardiac and kidney functions are done to determine whether the patient's high blood pressure has led to damage in the vascular walls of the brain and other vital organs. Pressure that stays steadily at levels only slightly above normal tends to cause an accelerated rate of atherosclerotic and other degenerative changes in cerebral, renal, and coronary vessels. This increases the risk of strokes, kidney failure, and congestive heart failure or coronary heart disease. Thus, the death rate from cardiovascular–renal disease is several times higher in people with untreated hypertensive disease than in normotensive persons.

Etiology

The cause of chronic hypertension is unknown in about 90% of cases. *Primary, or essential, hypertension* of this type has been attributed to abnormal functioning of the sympathetic nervous system (neurogenic), the kidneys (nephrogenic), and the adrenal glands (hormonal). However, although research findings suggest that scientists may be at the threshold of discovering specific causes for essential hypertension, there is at present still no single factor that can account for this disorder, nor is there any specific cure for it.

Secondary hypertension, on the other hand, has been found to occur as a result of any one of several specific organic causes. These include stenosis, or narrowing, of one or more of the major arteries in the kidneys—*renovascular hypertension*. Much less frequently a patient's high blood pressure may be traced to the presence of small tumors in the adrenal glands. These are pheochromocytoma, a catecholamine-secreting chromaffin cell tumor of the adrenal medulla (Chap. 18), and growths of cells in a zone of the adrenal cortex that secretes the mineralocorticoid hormone aldosterone (Chap. 21).

Hypertension caused by pheochromocytoma or by primary hyperaldosteronism can often be cured by surgical procedures. Another curable type of hypertension is that which develops in some women while they are taking an oral contraceptive. When these women stop taking such sex steroid products and switch to another form of contraception, their blood pressure often returns to normal.

Drug treatment

Despite the lack of a cure for most cases of hypertension, many drugs are now available that can bring elevated blood pressure down toward normal and keep it there. Drugs developed during the past 35 years have proved capable of preventing the cerebral, renal, and coronary vascular complications caused by sustained hypertension. These antihypertensive agents have helped to reduce the rate of illness and death from stroke, hypertensive heart disease, and uremia.

The goal of drug treatment of chronic hypertension is not only to maintain the patient's blood pressure at a safe level, but also to do so with a minimum of discomforting or disabling adverse effects. To keep each patient's blood pressure under control while avoiding such side-effects, the drug or combination of drugs that seems best suited to the clinical situation must be selected. Before discussing the basis for drug selection decisions, it is necessary to understand the pharmacologic properties of the various drugs now available. Thus, this chapter will discuss the following topics: (1) where and how each type of drug is thought to act; (2) what effects these actions have on the hemodynamic function of the hypertensive patient's circulation; and (3) how these and other effects of these drugs can cause undesirable results, as well as therapeutically beneficial changes.

General considerations regarding antihypertensive drugs

As indicated in Chapter 26, several complex, interacting homeostatic mechanisms play a part in regulating arterial pressure and in adjusting blood flow to the body's organs and tissues. Despite the never-ending need to shunt blood from one area to another to meet the constantly changing demands of different organs, a person's mean blood pressure—except for brief periods—ordinarily continues to stay within normal limits. This stability stems from the body's ability to make continual finely tuned adjustments in cardiac output and in peripheral resistance. It is not known exactly what goes wrong with the pressure control mechanisms of patients with essential hypertension. However, when a patient's blood pressure remains persistently at elevated levels, the normal relationship between the volume of fluid that fills the arterial side of the vascular system and the resistance that this fluid meets as it moves through these vessels has been altered. Thus, in chronic hypertension, the volume of blood in the arterial tree may be excessive, *or* the arterioles may be excessively constricted.

Effects of drugs on hemodynamics

All currently available drugs for treating hypertension affect the circulation in two main ways: (1) by *reducing peripheral resistance;* or (2) by *decreasing the volume of circulating blood that the heart must pump.* Some drugs do both. That is, they lower the elevated pressure within the patient's circulatory system both by dilating the arterioles so that the vessels offer less resistance to blood flowing through them, and by making the heart pump less blood out into this increased circulatory space. Clinically, the most significant of these two types of drug-induced effects are those that are the result of actions that affect the caliber of the blood vessels directly or indirectly.

Sites and mechanisms of drug actions

The drugs used to treat hypertension act at many different sites in the blood pressure-regulating system. For some drugs the precise site and mechanism of action is unknown; for other drugs several sites and mechanisms of action are known or have been postulated. The following drugs and groups of drugs are used to reduce high blood pressure: diuretics; α- and β-adrenergic receptor blockers; a drug that acts in the renin–angiotensin system to inhibit synthesis of angiotensin II; adrenergic neuron blocking drugs; drugs that act in the central nervous system to reduce sympathetic outflow; direct vasodilators; ganglionic blocking drugs; and a drug that is a monoamine oxidase (MAO) inhibitor but whose mechanism of action as an antihypertensive drug is unknown. Figure 28-1 illustrates these sites of drug action.

The direct vasodilators act directly on vascular smooth muscle to cause it to relax, thus lowering peripheral resistance and reducing blood pressure. Captopril, the drug that blocks synthesis of angiotensin II, is effective in some forms of hypertension by reducing the plasma concentration of angiotensin II, a potent vasoconstrictor and the most potent pressor substance known. All the other drugs act, at least in part, to inhibit sympathetic vasoconstrictor tone; that is, they interfere with the flow of sympathetic nerve impulses to vascular smooth muscle. The main adverse effect of many (but not all) of these drugs is the result of an extension of the therapeutic effects—they can cause blood pressure to fall too far. This is most likely to occur when a patient who has been lying down stands up too suddenly (*postural* or *orthostatic hypotension*). The brain is then deprived of blood, because these drugs tend to block the reflex responses that ordinarily compensate for the fall in pressure that occurs on standing.

Individual antihypertensive drugs

Diuretics

Mechanism of action. As discussed in detail in Chapter 27, thiazides and other diuretics remove sodium

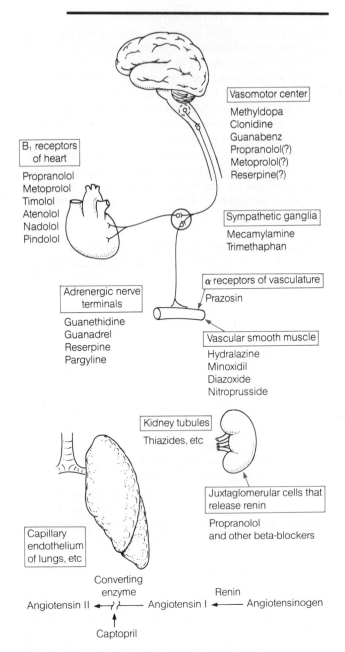

Figure 28-1. Sites of action of antihypertensive drugs.

a result of diuretic-induced salt and water loss leads to a reduction in cardiac output. The drug-induced reduction in blood volume and cardiac output may, indeed, account for the fact that hypertensive patients with low plasma renin activity (PRA) and high plasma volume respond better to diuretic therapy than do those with high or normal PRA and low plasma volume.

However, as patients continue to take diuretics, their blood volume gradually returns to almost normal as a result of certain homeostatic mechanisms. This readjustment of the volume of blood in the vascular tree, however, is *not* accompanied by a reversal of the early decrease in blood pressure. That is, even after the plasma volume and cardiac output return to pretreatment levels, the total peripheral resistance of patients who continue to take diuretics shows a persistent reduction, as does their blood pressure. One explanation of this is that the diuretics reduce the responsiveness of the blood vessel walls to the vasoconstrictive influence of sympathetic (adrenergic) nerve impulses and of circulating catecholamines. They are thought to do so because a drug-induced reduction of the sodium content of the vascular tissues lessens the sensitivity of the vessels to sympathoadrenal influences. However, there is little direct evidence to support this concept of a sodium-depleting vasodilator effect of the diuretics as an explanation for the persistent reduction in peripheral resistance and arterial pressure that continues during chronic therapy with these drugs.

Current status. The thiazide-type diuretics such as *hydrochlorothiazide* (Esidrix; HydroDiuril) are the drugs most commonly employed in treating hypertension (Table 28-1). The more potent diuretics, such as furosemide (Lasix), are no more effective for reducing blood pressure, and they are more likely to cause excessive loss of potassium along with sodium ions. Although the use of furosemide or other so-called loop, or high-ceiling, agents may be preferable for treating hypertensive patients who also have advanced kidney disease, most patients respond adequately to low doses of the thiazide diuretics, which produce blood pressure reduction in about two out of three patients with a *mild* degree of hypertension. They do so without ordinarily causing the electrolyte and water imbalances or other types of side-effects that occur more commonly when larger doses of diuretics are employed in treating patients with edema.

Other diuretics that are used in treating hypertension include the potassium-sparing diuretics *spironolactone* (Aldactone) and *amiloride* (Midamor), which are used in combination with thiazide diuretics to prevent hypokalemia, and the new diuretic *indapamide* (Lozol), which is given alone or with other antihypertensive drugs.

Diuretics can also increase the effectiveness of other antihypertensive drugs when administered in *combination*. Patients with moderately severe hypertension get a much greater decrease in blood pressure, for example, when *methyldopa* (Aldomet; see below) is admin-

from the body by their renal action. This sodium-depleting effect is also thought to account for the hypotensive effect of these diuretic drugs. However, despite considerable study and speculation, the precise way in which natriuresis—the elimination of sodium in the urine—helps to lower elevated blood pressure and to keep it at the lower level during long-term therapy is still uncertain.

Hemodynamic effects. Of course, one way in which diuretics may reduce blood pressure is by their ability to cause a contraction of plasma and extracellular fluid volume. This lessening of intravascular volume as

Table 28–1. Antihypertensive drugs

Generic or official name	Trade name	Usual adult oral dosage range
Diuretics		
Amiloride HCl	Midamor	5–10 mg/day
Furosemide USP	Lasix	20–80 mg, once or twice a day
Hydrochlorothiazide USP	HydroDiuril	25–100 mg, as a single or divided dose
Indapamide	Lozol	2.5 mg, once a day
Spironolactone USP	Aldactone	50–100 mg, once a day
α-Adrenergic receptor blocker		
Prazosin HCl	Minipress	Initially, 1 mg bid or tid; may gradually increase dose to 20 mg/day in divided doses
β-Adrenergic receptor blockers		
Atenolol	Tenormin	Initially, 50 mg/day; may increase to 100 mg/day
Metoprolol tartrate	Lopressor	Initially, 100 mg/day, in single or divided doses; may increase to 450 mg/day
Nadolol	Corgard	Initially, 40 mg/day; may increase to 80–320 mg/day
Pindolol	Visken	Initially, 10 mg, bid; may increase gradually to 60 mg/day
Propranolol HCl USP	Inderal	Initially, 40 mg bid; dose may be gradually increased to 160–480 mg/day, in divided doses
Timolol maleate	Blocadren	Initially, 10 mg bid; may increase gradually to 60 mg/day
Renin–angiotensin system inhibitor		
Captopril	Capoten	Initially, 25 mg tid, 1 hr before meals; dose may be raised to 50 mg tid if needed after 1–2 wk
Adrenergic neuron blocking drugs		
Guanadrel sulfate	Hylorel	Initially, 5 mg bid; may increase to 20–75 mg/day in divided doses
Guanethidine sulfate USP	Ismelin	Initially, 10 mg/day; may increase gradually to 25–50 mg/day
Reserpine USP	Sandril; Serpasil	Initially, 0.5 mg/day; maintenance, 0.1–0.25 mg/day
Centrally acting antihypertensive drugs		
Clonidine HCl	Catapres	Initially, 0.1 mg bid; may increase gradually to 0.8 mg/day in divided doses
Guanabenz monoacetate	Wytensin	Initially, 4 mg bid; may increase gradually (maximum dose studied is 32 mg bid)
Methyldopa USP	Aldomet	Initially, 250 mg bid or tid, may increase or decrease gradually (usual maintenance dose is 0.5–2.0 g/day in two to four divided doses)

(continued)

Table 28–1. Antihypertensive drugs (continued)

Generic or official name	Trade name	Usual adult oral dosage range
Direct-acting vasodilators		
Hydralazine HCl USP	Apresoline	Initially, 10 mg qid; may increase gradually to 50 mg qid
Minoxidil	Loniten	Initially, 5 mg/day as single dose; may increase gradually to 40 mg/day in single or divided doses (maximum dose: 100 mg/day)
Ganglionic blocking drug		
Mecamylamine HCl USP	Inversine	Initially, 2.5 mg bid; may increase dose gradually (average daily dose is 25 mg in three divided doses)
Antihypertensive–MAO inhibitor		
Pargyline HCl	Eutonyl	25 mg, once a day; may increase dose gradually (maximum dose; 200 mg/day)

istered together with a diuretic than when it is given alone. *Guanethidine* (Ismelin) is also more effective for treating severe degrees of hypertension when combined with a diuretic.

One reason for this is that the presence of a diuretic in the patient's regimen helps to prevent the compensatory increase in plasma volume that is set off when the other antihypertensive drugs reduce peripheral resistance and arterial pressure.* Thus, by their ability to prevent such a rise in plasma volume and, subsequently, a rise in peripheral vascular resistance and blood pressure, diuretics make it possible to maintain the continued effectiveness of the other antihypertensive agents, even when they are administered in lower doses than would otherwise be necessary. The reduction in the dosage of antihypertensive drugs when they are combined with diuretics, results, of course, in fewer noncirculatory side-effects. (Combination therapy is discussed further in the final section below, which deals with the drug therapy of various grades of hypertension.)

Adverse effects. Adverse effects of the diuretics—other than the hypokalemia and other electrolyte imbalances mentioned above—are summarized at the end of Chapter 27.

α-Adrenergic receptor blocking drugs
These drugs lower blood pressure by blocking the α receptors in the vasculature that mediate sympathetic va-soconstrictor tone. As described in Chapter 18, the older drugs of this class were among the first drugs to be tried in treating hypertension. These older drugs—that is, phentolamine, phenoxybenzamine, and tolazoline—are almost never used now in treating essential hypertension, although they are sometimes used to control blood pressure in patients with pheochromocytoma. The main problem with the older drugs is that they cause reflex tachycardia. However, a new α blocker, prazosin, *is* used to treat hypertension.

Prazosin
Mechanism of action. This new drug blocks α_1 receptors selectively; the older drugs also block the presynaptic α_2 receptors (see Chap. 13). This difference accounts for the fact that prazosin HCl (Minipress) is much less likely than phentolamine and the other older α blockers to cause reflex tachycardia and coronary insufficiency (see Chap. 18). Unlike the adrenergic neuron blockers (*e.g.,* guanethidine) and the ganglionic blockers (see below), prazosin does not reduce cardiac output or renal blood flow. It is useful in mild to moderately severe hypertension; it is often given with a diuretic, as explained above.

Adverse reactions. Despite these advantages, this drug *can* cause postural hypotension, particularly if its dosage is raised too rapidly. With the 1-mg oral dose recommended for initiating therapy, dizziness is the most common side-effect. However, raising the dose to 2 mg has led to syncope (a sudden loss of consciousness) in some patients, presumably because a postural hypotensive reaction has briefly deprived the brain of part of its blood supply. Patients being started on prazosin should be ob-

---

* The kidneys respond to a drop in renal arterial pressure by releasing increased quantities of *renin* into the patient's circulation. The resulting rise in circulating *angiotensin II* and *aldosterone* levels (Chap. 27) promotes compensatory sodium and water retention, increased body fluid volume, and increased peripheral resistance.

served for up to 1½ hours and should be advised to sit or lie down if they get dizzy and light-headed to avoid being injured in a fall caused by a sudden syncopal attack. If a diuretic is added to the antihypertensive regimen of a patient on prazosin, the dose of prazosin should be reduced. Other side-effects include headache, drowsiness, feelings of fatigue and weakness, and nausea.

β-Adrenergic receptor blocking drugs

The oldest drug of this group, *propranolol*[+] (Inderal), was accepted as an antihypertensive drug considerably after its introduction as an antiarrhythmic drug, and after its acceptance for use in treating angina. Now one of its major uses is in the management of hypertension. Five other β blockers are also marketed in the United States and are officially approved for use in hypertension (see Tables 18-1 and 26-1).

Propranolol

Mechanism of action. The manner in which this prototype β-adrenergic receptor blocking drug lowers high blood pressure is still disputed, although there is no question of the drug's efficacy. Actually, as discussed in Chapter 18, if an attempt were made to predict the effect of propranolol on the arterioles, it might be assumed that it could cause generalized vasoconstriction and, consequently, a *rise* in peripheral resistance and arterial pressure. That is, blockade of β (vasodilator) receptors in the blood vessels could, in theory, cause unopposed stimulation of α (vasoconstrictor) receptors in the arterioles.

In clinical practice, however, this does not happen and—particularly with the administration of much higher doses than those employed in the treatment of angina pectoris and cardiac arrhythmias—a hypotensive effect of varying degree is produced in most patients. Large doses are, at present, thought in some way to reduce the outflow of sympathetic nerve impulses from the medullary vasomotor center. This may also be part of the mechanism of action of metoprolol, the other β blocker that crosses the blood–brain barrier, but it is unlikely to be a mechanism of action of the other β blockers, which do not cross the blood–brain barrier to a significant extent. Much smaller doses are effective for reducing the cardiac output in some patients. Another patient population subgroup—those with high levels of PRA—respond to propranolol therapy as a result of this drug's ability to reduce the release of renin from juxtaglomerular cells of the kidney by blocking their β-adrenergic receptor sites, thus interfering with their stimulation by sympathetic nerve impulses (see summary of effects of antihypertensive drugs at the end of this chapter).

Hemodynamic effects. Propranolol causes a reduction in cardiac output, peripheral resistance, and blood pressure. The time required for a full hypotensive response ranges from a few days to several weeks. When propranolol is employed alone, it is desirable for patients to reduce their dietary sodium intake to help avoid an expansion of plasma volume, which might counteract some of the drug's desired hypotensive effect. The addition of a thiazide diuretic to the patient's propranolol regimen also helps to avoid such an increase in plasma volume. Combined therapy of this type also reduces blood pressure still further, particularly in the large patient subgroup in whom PRA is normal. The role of renin and the renin–angiotensin–aldosterone system in the regulation of salt and water metabolism and in the control of blood pressure is discussed in Chapters 26 and 27. The manner in which propranolol blocks sympathetic nerve impulses is discussed in Chapter 18. Propranolol is sometimes given in combination with a direct vasodilator such as hydralazine (see below).

Adverse effects. The potentially harmful effects of propranolol and the precautions required in its use are summarized at the end of Chapter 18. Patients with hypertension require and can usually tolerate much larger doses of propranolol than are usually employed in treating the various other cardiovascular disorders for which this drug is recommended. Because some hypertensive patients may also have undiagnosed coronary heart disease—a condition that may be made much worse by abrupt withdrawal of propranolol—the high-dose schedules (640 mg or more in some cases) on which some patients have been stabilized should be only gradually reduced, if it becomes necessary to discontinue β-blocker therapy. In patients who suffer an exaggerated hypotensive response to propranolol that requires treatment with vasopressors, epinephrine may be preferred to levarterenol. Propranolol may also precipitate heart failure and A-V nodal block in predisposed patients.

Nadolol, Pindolol, and Timolol

These three newer β blockers are, like propranolol, nonselective (*i.e.*, β_1 and β_2 blockers), and are therefore quite similar to propranolol in their pharmacologic effects (see Chap. 18 for differences). Nadolol is excreted unchanged by the kidneys and should be given in reduced dosage to patients with compromised renal function. The other drugs, like propranolol, are metabolized in the liver.

Metoprolol and Atenolol

Metroprolol tartrate (Lopressor) and *atenolol* (Tenormin) differ from propranolol in having a more selective blocking effect on β_1-type adrenergic receptors. As indicated in Chapter 18, such relative cardioselectivity reduces the likelihood of adverse effects from blockade of β_2-type receptors in the bronchioles and elsewhere. Thus, these drugs are, in theory, safer than propranolol for treating patients who have both hypertension and bronchial asthma.

In practice, however, hypertensive patients with obstructive lung disease who require high doses of these drugs could suffer from a drug-induced episode of bronchospasm. Thus, use of these β-blocking agents is at present recommended in such cases only when the patient's high blood pressure has not been brought down by treatment with other antihypertensive agents such as diuretics or vasodilators, or when other medications for hypertension are poorly tolerated.

The dosage of these drugs should be individualized. Determining the smallest amount of medication required for a therapeutic effect in each patient makes it more likely that these drugs will block β_1 receptors without blocking bronchial and other β_2 receptors.

The precautions described for propranolol to avoid cardiac toxicity apply to these drugs. They should, for example, be employed with caution, if at all, in patients who are prone to heart failure or who have advanced degrees of heart block. In addition, neither of these drugs should be discontinued abruptly, because such sudden withdrawal might precipitate chest pains in hypertensive patients with previously undiagnosed heart disease.

Drugs that interfere with the renin–angiotensin system

Captopril

Recent research has aimed at developing drugs that would be particularly effective for treating patients with high PRA. Such patients seem to be most subject to the life-threatening complications of severe hypertensive disease. The vascular damage seen in such patients is not caused directly by renin itself but is thought to be caused, at least in part, by the presence of certain peptides—especially angiotensin II—that are produced in high quantities when the PRA is abnormally high, as for example in malignant hypertension and renovascular hypertension (see Chap. 26 and Fig. 26-8).

Captopril (Capoten) acts by blocking the conversion of angiotensin I to angiotensin II. It inhibits the enzyme, called converting enzyme, in vascular endothelial cells that catalyzes this reaction. Angiotensin II is the most potent pressor substance known. It is believed that the reduction of angiotensin II is the mechanism by which captopril lowers blood pressure, but no consistent correlation has been found between therapeutic response to the drug and circulating levels of renin. Because of the risk of serious toxicity (*e.g.*, renal and glomerular damage, neutropenia, agranulocytosis, angioedema), the drug is approved for use only in those patients whose hypertension has not responded to other safer drugs, although physicians are prescribing it less discriminately and the manufacturer has requested broader FDA approval. An experimental long-acting converting enzyme inhibitor, *enalapril,* is currently being investigated.

Captopril should usually be given with a thiazide diuretic. Because captopril decreases aldosterone production, potassium-sparing diuretics or potassium supplements should be given only when hypokalemia is demonstrated (see Fig. 26-8). The sympathetic nervous system (SNS) may be especially important in supporting the blood pressure of patients on captopril, so drugs that interfere with SNS function need to be given cautiously.

Another drug group, the angiotensin II antagonists, acts by competing with the natural vasoconstrictor for its receptors at various sites. One drug of this subclass, called *saralasin* (Sarenin), prevents angiotensin II-induced rises in blood pressure by occupying its receptors and thus blocking its pressor action. (The use of this drug in diagnosing angiotensin II-dependent hypertension is described in Chap. 56, Drugs Used for Diagnosis.) Saralasin is not used therapeutically.

Adrenergic neuron blocking drugs

These drugs act in various ways to interfere with the synthesis, storage, release, and reuptake of norepinephrine by sympathetic nerves. *Reserpine,* which is used less often now than formerly, also acts on adrenergic (and serotoninergic) nerve terminals in the *central* nervous system. *Metyrosine* (Demser), a drug that blocks synthesis of catecholamines, belongs in this class of drugs, but it is not used to treat hypertension except when the hypertension is caused by pheochromocytoma (see Chap. 18). *Bretylium tosylate* (Bretylol), a drug that blocks norepinephrine release, also belongs in this class of drugs, but it is used only to treat cardiac arrhythmias (Chap. 30). These drugs not only block sympathetic vasoconstrictor tone but also interfere with sympathetic impulse activity to the heart and to other organs (*e.g.*, the gastrointestinal tract and the reproductive organs).

Guanethidine

Mechanism of action. Guanethidine sulfate[+] (Ismelin) produces its pressure-reducing effects by preventing sympathetic nerve impulses from releasing the neurotransmitter norepinephrine from postganglionic adrenergic nerve endings located in the heart and blood vessels. Part of its impulse-inhibiting effect appears to result from a slow depletion of the catecholamine content of the nerve endings during prolonged oral administration of the drug.

Drug interactions. To bring about its hypotensive effect, this drug must be taken up into the adrenergic nerve endings from which it displaces norepinephrine. Thus, the desired therapeutic effect can be prevented in patients who simultaneously take other drugs that interfere with the uptake of guanethidine. Among chemicals capable of doing so are drugs used in the management of mental illness, such as the tricyclic-type antidepressant agents and the phenothiazine-type antipsychotic agents.

The hypotensive action of guanethidine may also be prevented by amphetamine or ephedrine administration, because these and other sympathomimetic amines, which act in part by releasing the natural neurotransmitter from nerve endings (Chap. 17), can also cause the release of guanethidine from these same sites and thus reduce its activity. Patients who have been taking the MAO-type antidepressant drugs should not receive guanethidine simultaneously, because it might then rapidly release the large amounts of norepinephrine stored in the adrenergic nerve endings—an effect that could lead to a sharp *rise* in blood pressure. For the same reason, this drug is contraindicated in patients whose elevated pressure results from the presence of pheochromocytomata (Chap. 18). That is, guanethidine could cause the sudden release of pressure-raising chemicals from such catecholamine-containing chromaffin cell tumors. Sympathomimetic drugs (levarterenol and other vasopressors) may produce exaggerated cardiovascular effects in the presence of guanethidine.

Hemodynamic effects. The adrenergic nerve blocking effect of this drug very dependably produces the typical effects of potent sympatholytic drugs on arterial, venous, and cardiac function. That is, it reduces the tone of smooth muscle in the walls of arterioles and venules, and causes dilation of these vessels. Arterial vasodilation results in reduced peripheral resistance and reduced blood pressure. Dilation of the veins leads to pooling of blood and to a reduction in the amount of blood that is returned to the heart. This reduction in preload and direct drug effects on cardiac sympathetic nerves reduce cardiac output. The drug-induced pooling of blood in the venous capacitance vessels, and the blockade of reflex compensatory responses to the resulting reduction in cardiac output, also account for the frequency with which patients suffer from postural hypotension.

Adverse effects. Other reactions, which are the result of excessive sympathetic blockade at sites other than the circulatory system, include diarrhea and interference with normal ejaculation in sexually active men. This drug must be used with caution when patients have a history of peptic ulcer or spastic colitis, because these conditions may be aggravated by the unopposed parasympathetic stimulation of the intestinal tract that often follows administration of this potent sympatholytic agent. Similarly, the vagal slowing of the heart brought about by sympathetic blockade can prove undesirable for patients with certain types of cardiac difficulties. The reduction in cardiac output and, consequently, in glomerular filtration may lead to edema and congestive heart failure. Patients should be watched for signs of weight gain from fluid. This can be prevented by the simultaneous administration of a thiazide-type diuretic. Combining guanethidine with a diuretic also permits reduction in the dosage of the potent sympathetic blocker. This then helps to reduce such other dose-related side-effects as diarrhea, as well as those that stem from postural hypotension, such as feelings of faintness, dizziness, and weakness.

Such side-effects are, of course, best avoided by careful dosage adjustment to prevent postural hypotension. Patients and their significant others should be taught how to take a blood pressure reading. Many health insurance policies now cover the purchasing of a sphygmomanometer. If self-monitoring of blood pressure is not possible, patients should be urged to come to a clinic for frequent checks or to use various blood pressure monitoring services available in their community. Many patients learn to monitor their own antihypertensive drug therapy by the drug-induced symptoms that they are experiencing. An antihypertensive agent should not be administered in the hospital until the patient's current blood pressure is determined and recorded.

Guanadrel

Guanadrel sulfate (Hylorel), a close chemical and pharmacologic relative of guanethidine, was recently approved for use in treating hypertension. It produces the same hemodynamic effects by the same mechanism of action. It differs from guanethidine in that maximum reduction of blood pressure occurs in 4 to 6 hours, whereas with guanethidine this may not occur for 1 week. Its duration of action is also shorter. Its adverse effects are similar to those of guanethidine; in addition, it causes water retention and should always be given with a diuretic. It is contraindicated in patients with congestive heart failure. It is also contraindicated, or needs to be used with great care, in patients with coronary artery disease or cerebrovascular insufficiency.

Rauwolfia alkaloids

Reserpine[+] (Serpasil) is the most widely used of the various available natural and semisynthetic derivatives of the *Rauwolfia*, or snakeroot, plant, which has been used for centuries in India for treating many ailments. Because it acts in the brain as well as peripherally on the circulation, this adrenergic nerve blocker was once widely used in this country as a tranquilizer, but it has now been largely replaced by the phenothiazines and other more effective antipsychotic agents. However, it still has a role in the management of hypertension.

Mechanism of action. Drugs of this type interfere with transmission of impulses from sympathetic postganglionic and central adrenergic nerve endings by gradually depleting their content of the neurotransmitter norepinephrine. They do so by preventing norepinephrine from remaining within the synaptic vesicles in which it is normally stored. The molecules of free norepinephrine that are then released within the nerve cell, as well as those molecules of the neurotransmitter that are taken back up into the nerve terminal after transmitting sympathetic nerve impulses, are metabolized intraneuronally to inactive products as a result of chemical reactions that are catalyzed by the mitochondrial enzyme MAO.

Hemodynamic effects. The depleting effect of reserpine and its relatives on the catecholamine content of sympathetic nerves results in a gradual reduction in peripheral resistance and in arterial blood pressure. This drug also slows the heart and reduces cardiac output. Because it has a long duration of action, a single daily dose is often enough to maintain the blood pressure at normal levels in mild cases that respond to its gradual pressure-reducing effect. Reserpine and the other rauwolfia alkaloids are commonly administered with one or another of the thiazide-type diuretics, which increase their pressure-reducing effectiveness while helping to reduce side-effects (see below).

Adverse effects. Reserpine and the other rauwolfia alkaloids cause many minor side-effects, but these are not usually severe enough to require that the drugs be discontinued. Some of these adverse effects are the result of reduced sympathetic nervous system transmission and a relative increase in parasympathetic predominance. Thus, local vasodilation in the nasal sinus mucosa often leads to nasal congestion and obstruction and occasionally to nosebleed. The increased gastrointestinal secretion and motility that often occur with these drugs can cause cramps and diarrhea or even make a healed peptic ulcer become active again.

In addition to these and other effects of autonomic imbalance, the rauwolfia alkaloids cause various central effects. Least serious is the drowsiness that often develops during the early days of treatment. Most dangerous is emotional depression, at times so serious that the patient may try to commit suicide. Thus, all patients, especially those with a history of depression, should be monitored for signs of personality change while they are taking rauwolfia alkaloids for hypertension. Psychiatric patients who have been taking these drugs may suffer severe convulsions and prolonged apnea if subjected to electroshock therapy. Reports of an increased incidence of breast carcinoma in women who had taken reserpine as an antihypertensive for long periods have led some to avoid the use of this group of drugs in women; other studies have failed to corroborate this finding.

Centrally acting antihypertensive drugs

The antihypertensive effects of propranolol and metoprolol, as well as reserpine, may be explained in part by actions in the central nervous system (CNS). However, these drugs have peripheral actions that are primarily responsible for their antihypertensive effects. In contrast, methyldopa, clonidine, and guanabenz lower blood pressure *primarily* by actions in the CNS.

Methyldopa and methyldopate HCl

Mechanism of action. Like reserpine, *methyldopa*[+] (Aldomet) may act at both central and peripheral sites to reduce transmission of impulses by adrenergic nerves. It is used by the catecholamine-synthesizing enzymes in place of the normal substrate levodopa (see Fig. 13-6), and a so-called false neurotransmitter, α-methylnorepinephrine, is synthesized instead of norepinephrine. For several years it was believed that this false neurotransmitter was less effective than norepinephrine as a vasoconstrictor. The antihypertensive effect of methyldopa was explained by postulating that this false neurotransmitter replaced norepinephrine in synaptic vesicles and was released by sympathetic nerve

impulses. This sequence of events occurs in nerve terminals, but α-methyl-norepinephrine has been found to be almost as effective as norepinephrine as a vasoconstrictor. It is now believed that the primary site of action of methyldopa is in the CNS. α-Methylnorepinephrine is thought to act on adrenergic receptors in or near the vasomotor center that mediate a reduction in sympathetic outflow from the brain (see mechanism of action of clonidine, below).

Methyldopate HCl is the ethyl ester of methyldopa. It is used parenterally and has the same pharmacologic spectrum as methyldopa.

Hemodynamic effects. Methyldopa reduces peripheral resistance and, in some patients, decreases heart rate. It also reduces plasma renin levels. Methyldopa, unlike such other sympatholytic agents as the ganglionic and α-adrenergic receptor blockers and guanethidine, is effective for reducing blood pressure while the hypertensive patient is lying down as well as while standing upright. As is the case with reserpine and clonidine (see below), oral doses of this drug cause only a small degree of postural hypotension, and such orthostatic effects occur relatively infrequently. Because cardiac output and kidney perfusion are not reduced, this drug is considered to be desirable for patients with poor kidney function that might be worsened by pressure-reducing drugs that reduce renal blood flow excessively.

Adverse effects. The most common complaint of patients—particularly in the early stages of treatment—is drowsiness and a feeling of weakness. Less frequent central side-effects include emotional depression, nightmares, dizziness and light-headedness, and occasional signs of extrapyramidal motor system disorders such as parkinsonism and choreoathetotic movements resembling those described in Chapters 46 and 49. Adverse effects attributable to loss of sympathetic nerve impulses include nasal congestion, diarrhea, and other signs of predominant parasympathetic influence on the gastrointestinal tract, and impotence and failure to ejaculate.

Occasional hypersensitivity reactions involving the liver and the formed elements of the blood require discontinuation of further therapy with methyldopa. Liver function tests are performed during the first weeks of therapy to detect any drug-induced abnormalities before such clinical signs as fever and jaundice appear. Much later in the course of methyldopa therapy, a significant proportion of patients shows a positive Coombs' test (the presence of protein—usually a gamma globulin—on red cell surfaces). This only rarely indicates that a drug-induced hemolytic anemia has developed, which would make the immediate withdrawal of the drug mandatory. If, as is very likely in most cases, blood counts reveal no dyscrasia, drug treatment may be continued. Because this test abnormality may make cross matching of blood confusing, a hematologist should be consulted if the patient should ever need a blood transfusion during therapy with this drug.

Clonidine

Mechanism of action. *Clonidine* (Catapres) acts like methyldopa or, more precisely, like α-methyl-norepinephrine. That is, it acts centrally to reduce the outflow of sympathetic nerve impulses by stimulating certain nerve nuclei that exert inhibitory control over the vasomotor and cardioacceleratory centers located in the medulla oblongata. Clonidine does this by acting as an agonist at central α-adrenergic receptor sites. A similar stimulating action at *peripheral* α-adrenergic receptors in vascular smooth muscle is thought to account for a paradoxical *rise* in blood pressure that occurs in some circumstances.

Hemodynamic effects. This drug, when administered orally in appropriately adjusted dosage, produces a rapid and prolonged drop in blood pressure. This occurs with the patient in the supine as well as in the erect position, as is the case with methyldopa (see above). The effects of this drug also resemble those of methyldopa in other respects. It does not, for example, reduce renal blood flow or cause more than mild orthostatic hypotension in most patients, and it reduces plasma renin. This drug produces an early reduction in the heart rate and cardiac output. However, during long-term therapy, the drug's ability to maintain blood pressure at lower levels appears to depend on reduced peripheral resistance rather than on decreased cardiac output, as output gradually returns to pretreatment levels.

Adverse effects. The most common patient complaints early in therapy with clonidine are drowsiness and dry mouth. Occasionally, as with reserpine and methyldopa, this centrally acting drug can cause mental depression. Patients should be told not to stop taking this drug without consulting with their nurse or physician, because this can lead to nervousness, agitation, and nightmares. A potentially more serious manifestation of the abrupt withdrawal of clonidine can be the development of a rapid rise in blood pressure to levels high enough to cause brain damage. Such a sudden blood pressure elevation is presumably the result of an unmasking of the drug's sympathomimetic action at peripheral adrenergic sites, because it can be controlled by the intravenous injection of an α-adrenergic blocking agent such as phentolamine (Regitine; see Chap. 18).

Guanabenz

Guanabenz monoacetate (Wytensin) is the newest drug of the group of centrally acting sympatholytic drugs. It is very similar pharmacologically to clonidine, although its name suggests a relationship to the peripherally acting adrenergic neuron blockers, guanethidine and guanadrel. Guanabenz, like clonidine, acts on CNS α receptors to depress sympathetic tone on the vasculature. Like clonidine, it seems to spare cardiovascular reflexes—that is, it causes relatively little orthostatic hypotension. It also resembles clonidine in that it frequently causes drowsiness and dry mouth, and it can cause a serious rebound of hypertension if therapy is stopped abruptly. Unlike most antihypertensive drugs, it does *not* appear to cause salt and water retention.

Direct-acting vasodilators

These drugs act directly on smooth muscle in the walls of blood vessels to cause it to relax. Two of these drugs, *diazoxide* (Hyperstat) and *sodium nitroprusside* (Nipride) are used in hypertension only as intravenous preparations and only in emergencies, or to produce controlled hypotension during surgery (see the final section of this chapter, Hypertensive Emergencies). *Hydralazine HCl* (Apresoline) is also given IV in hypertensive emergencies but, in addition, it is used orally in controlling essential hypertension. This is the only use of the newest drug of this group, *minoxidil* (Loniten).

Hydralazine

Mechanism of action. This drug acts mainly by its ability to relax arterioles by a direct action on their smooth muscle walls rather than by blockade of sympathetic nerve impulses. Advantages of the resulting vasodilation and reduction in peripheral resistance are that they are usually not accompanied by postural hypotension, and that renal blood flow is increased rather than reduced. These advantages over adrenergic nerve blocking agents, such as guanethidine and ganglionic blocking agents are, however, counterbalanced by the drug's tendency to cause reflex tachycardia—the result of activation of baroreceptor reflexes by the drug-induced reduction in peripheral resistance. The cardiac efferent pathway of these reflexes is not blocked at any point, as it would be with the sympatholytic drugs or the ganglionic blockers.

Adverse effects. This drug is rarely used alone in treating essential hypertension because of its tendency to cause cardiac stimulation. Such drug-induced tachycardia can lead to anginal chest pains or even to a myocardial infarction in patients with coronary artery disease. Thus, its use in patients with a history of myocardial ischemia or with rheumatic heart disease and mitral valve insufficiency is contraindicated. However, hydralazine is often given in combination with the β-adrenergic blocking agent propranolol (Inderal), which is very effective in preventing hydralazine-induced reflex tachycardia.

Patients taking this drug sometimes develop a syndrome that resembles systemic lupus erythematosus (SLE). Signs and symptoms include fever and joint pains. Complete blood counts, examinations for LE cells, and antinuclear antibody titers should be done at the start of hydralazine therapy and periodically during prolonged therapy, even if the patient develops no unusual symptoms.

Minoxidil

The exact mechanism of action of minoxidil (Loniten) in relaxing vascular smooth muscle is not known. It may act by blocking calcium uptake.

Like hydralazine, this direct vasodilator lowers blood pressure and causes reflex tachycardia. It should usually be given with a β blocker, as well as with a diuretic; it causes marked sodium and water retention that are sometimes difficult to control with even high doses of furosemide. It also causes hirsutism in about 80% of patients. In fact, a topical preparation of this drug is currently being investigated as a potential treatment for baldness. Because of its serious toxicity, it should be used only in severe organ-damaging hypertension that has not responded to other antihypertensive regimens.

Ganglionic blocking drugs

As described in Chapter 18, only two ganglionic blockers, *trimethaphan camsylate* (Arfonad) and *mecamylamine HCl* (Inversine), are still available in the United States. Trimethaphan is given only parenterally in hypertensive emergencies (see below) or to produce controlled hypotension to reduce bleeding during surgery. Mecamylamine is given orally, but only infrequently, to treat essential hypertension. These drugs lower blood pressure by blocking sympathetic ganglia, and by preventing impulses in sympathetic preganglionic nerves from releasing epinephrine and norepinephrine from the adrenal medulla. Thus, they decrease peripheral resistance and prevent sympathetic influences on the heart. However, they also block parasympathetic ganglia. Because of their lack of selectivity they cause many adverse effects, including orthostatic hypotension, dry mouth, blurred vision, constipation, urinary retention, and impotence. Thus, whenever possible, newer and more selective drugs are used to control essential hypertension.

Antihypertensive—MAO inhibitor

Pargyline

Pargyline HCl (Eutonyl) is one of the class of drugs called MAO inhibitors that are used mainly as antidepressants in the management of emotionally depressed patients (see Chap. 46). By inhibiting MAO, the enzyme that normally inactivates norepinephrine in adrenergic nerve terminals, these drugs allow norepinephrine to accumulate. Nerve impulses would be expected to release more norepinephrine, and therefore an *increase* in blood pressure would be expected, but this does *not* happen with pargyline. Despite its ability to increase the stores of norepinephrine in adrenergic nerve endings, it tends to interfere with impulse transmission from sympathetic nerves to the cardiovascular system. The mechanism is unclear. One suggestion is that in the presence of pargyline a false neurotransmitter, perhaps octopamine, is formed, and that this false neurotransmitter is a weaker vasoconstrictor than norepinephrine. This leads to a drop in peripheral resistance and in blood pressure. This effect, which is

considered an adverse reaction when it occurs in patients who are being treated for emotional depression with other drugs of this class, is considered desirable in the treatment of some hypertensive patients.

Pargyline can cause all the varied adverse effects and drug interactions that have limited the usefulness of this drug class in patients with affective disorders. The most serious of these interactions occurs with sympathomimetic drugs, and with certain foods that contain tyramine (*e.g.,* cheese, wine, fava beans), and can result in hypertensive crisis. For the same reasons, the use of this drug as an antihypertensive agent is reserved for the relatively few patients with moderately severe hypertension who have not responded to treatment with such other antihypertensive agents as propranolol (Inderal), reserpine, methyldopa, and guanethidine. It is not used in treating either mild or malignant hypertension or in patients whose pressure is elevated because of the presence of pheochromocytoma. As is true with depressed patients taking drugs of this type, the patient on pargyline must be warned about self-treatment with nonprescription cold remedies and about eating certain cheeses and other foods that could cause dangerous drug or food interactions with this agent.

Experimental antihypertensive agents

Two drugs now under investigation for use in treating hypertension are of interest because they do not follow the usual pharmacologic principle that new drugs have greater specificity in their sites of action. *Labetalol HCl* (Trandate; Normodyne) is a combined α-, β_1-, and β_2-adrenergic receptor blocker (it is more potent as a β blocker than as an α blocker), as well as a direct vasodilator.* It decreases peripheral resistance and cardiac output and, so far, appears to have a low incidence of side-effects. *Prizidolol* is a β-adrenergic receptor blocker and a direct vasodilator, thus combining the properties of two classes of drugs that are often given together to treat hypertension (see below). It therefore has the potential for simplifying drug regimens for those hypertensive patients who would otherwise need to remember to take two different drugs. Other classes of drugs being studied as potential antihypertensives include calcium channel blockers (now used in cardiac arrhythmias and angina; Chaps. 30 and 31) and certain derivatives of prostaglandins (PGE_2).

Additional clinical considerations

Hypertension is a widespread disorder that is uniquely difficult to treat. Patients may have hypertension for years with no symptoms. The drug therapy that is effective in treating this "silent" disease is often very uncomfortable and difficult to live with because it causes many side-effects, including sexual dysfunction, nasal congestion, drowsiness, dizziness, and restlessness. Because the treatment seems to be worse than the disease, noncompliance

---

* Labetalol is now available in the United States.

with medical regimen is one of the biggest clinical problems confronting those who treat hypertensive patients.

Numerous studies have been conducted to determine the best way to increase patient compliance. The key element seems to be a thorough and continuous patient education program and a consistent support system to encourage patient compliance and to help the patient adapt to the drug therapy. Specific guidelines about drug therapy that should be incorporated into a total hypertensive teaching program are presented below in the patient teaching guide.

One of the most frequently encountered problems with the antihypertensive agents is orthostatic hypotension. The loss of normal blood pressure control reflexes results in a slow cardiovascular adaptation to changes in position. The patient's blood pressure should be assessed in the supine, sitting, and standing positions, which will give an indication of the patient's orthostatic changes and allow appropriate safety measures to be taken to prevent falls or fainting spells. The patient experiencing orthostatic hypotension should be taught the following: change position very slowly; avoid squatting down to lift or to garden, for example; and take extra care when the weather is warm and when peripheral vasodilation, which occurs in hot weather, may reduce blood pressure further and aggravate the problem.

Various forms of sexual dysfunction are associated with many of the antihypertensive drugs. Male impotence and failure to ejaculate and female amenorrhea and inability to conceive are common problems associated with the use of various drugs. The patient needs to be aware of this problem, have the opportunity to ventilate feelings, understand that the problem is drug-related, and have the opportunity to change medication if the problem becomes severe and is one that the patient cannot accept. A problem called Peyronie's disease, a fibrotic process involving the corpus cavernosum of the penis, has recently been associated with long-term use of propranolol and metoprolol. Male patients who are maintained on either of these drugs should be carefully evaluated for this problem, and the drug(s) should be discontinued if this occurs.

The use of methyldopa and of hydralazine have been associated with a lupuslike syndrome. Both drugs should be discontinued if a rash, joint pains, blood changes, or liver changes are noted. Clonidine use has been associated with degenerative retinal changes. Patients maintained on this drug should receive regular ophthalmologic examinations. Both guanethidine and guanadrel should be withdrawn 2 weeks before elective surgery to prevent severe cardiovascular collapse. If emergency surgery is needed for a patient on one of these drugs, the last dose should be prominently noted on the front of the patient's chart, and complete life-support and emergency equipment should be immediately available.

The antihypertensive agents should not be stopped suddenly. A rebound hypertensive crisis has been associated with sudden cessation of many of these drugs. The patient needs to understand this and should be cautioned to notify the nurse or physician if for any reason the medication cannot be taken. Inhospital personnel also need to be constantly aware of the potential danger of sudden stoppage of these drugs if patients are NPO for tests and inadvertently miss several doses of drug.

As mentioned above, patients receiving the MAO inhibitor *pargyline* (Eutonyl) to treat their hypertension should be cautioned to avoid foods and beverages that are high in tyramine. Tyramine is an amino acid found in many "aged" food products that have been acted on by molds or bacteria. Thus, it is found in cheddar, camembert, and other cheeses, beer, and wine (especially Chianti). Tyramine and other pressor amines are also found in high concentrations in yogurt, sour cream, fermented sausages, pickled herring, ripened bananas, avocados, papayas (and the meat tenderizer *papain* made from them), figs, raisins, chocolate, yeast extract, fava beans, and chicken livers. Tyramine is an indirectly acting sympathomimetic (Chap. 17) that releases norepinephrine (NE) from adrenergic nerve terminals. It is normally inactivated by MAO enzymes in its first passage through the liver after it is absorbed into the circulation from the gastrointestinal tract, which prevents it from reaching high enough levels to produce appreciable effects on NE-containing nerve terminals. However, when the MAO enzymes in the liver and in adrenergic nerve terminals are inhibited, tyramine levels are increased *and* the amount of releasable NE in nerve terminals is also increased. Thus, the ingestion of tyramine-rich foods can lead to release of large amounts of NE that in turn can cause hypertensive crises.

Patients who are traveling to warmer climates should have their drug dosage adjusted before they go to prevent a severe hypotensive response when vasodilation occurs in response to the warm climate and lowers blood pressure further. Patients who live in environments with wide seasonal temperature variations may require a seasonal dosage adjustment.

Drug–drug interactions

Most of the important drug–drug interactions have been described previously in the discussion of each individual drug. Patients taking *MAO inhibitors* to treat emotional depression, or who are on the MAO inhibitor pargyline for hypertension, should be withdrawn from the MAO inhibitor 2 weeks before therapy is begun with any of the antihypertensive drugs that release NE from nerve terminals. These drugs include *reserpine* and other *rauwolfia alkaloids, guanethidine,* and *guanadrel.* These NE-releasing drugs could cause an initial serious hypertensive episode by releasing the increased stores of NE from adrenergic nerve terminals in patients on a MAO inhibitor.

Over-the-counter (OTC) drugs are often involved in drug–drug interactions with antihypertensive drugs. Many OTC compounds—diet pills, cold capsules, decongestants, cough mixtures, sinus medications—contain sympathomimetic substances that can be dangerous for hypertensive patients, or at least can decrease the desired effectiveness of any antihypertensive drug. Patients on guanethidine and guanadrel especially may show an exaggerated response to *sympathomimetics*. In general, all patients on antihypertensive therapy should be advised to avoid the use of any OTC drugs unless they have first discussed the specific drug with their nurse.

The guide to the nursing process with antihypertensive drugs summarizes the clinical application of this drug therapy in nursing care. The final section of this chapter presents examples of commonly used hypertension treatment protocols.

Patient teaching guide: oral antihypertensives

The drug(s) that has (have) been prescribed for you is (are) known as an antihypertensive drug. It is used to treat high blood pressure. High blood pressure is a disorder that may have no symptoms but that can cause serious problems—for example, heart attack, stroke, kidney problems—if it goes untreated. It is very important to take your medicine every day, as prescribed. You may feel perfectly well, or you may feel bad as a result of the side-effects of the drug, but it is very important that you continue to take the drug. If side-effects become too uncomfortable, or if you have problems with your drug therapy, consult your nurse or physician.

Instructions:

1. The name of your drug is _____ .

2. The dosage of your drug is _____ .

3. Your drug should be taken _____ times a day. The best time to take your drug is _____ , _____ , _____ . Your drug can(not) be taken with food.

4. *Never* stop taking this drug suddenly. If your prescription becomes low or you are unable to take your medicine for any reason, notify your nurse or physician.

5. If your drug is pargyline, you should avoid the use of foods that are high in natural pressor, or blood pressure-raising, substances. These foods include the following:

Aged cheeses	Chicken livers	Yeast
Wine (especially Chianti)	Bananas	Meat tenderizers
Beer	Pickled herring	
Yogurt	Avocado	
Sour cream	Chocolate	

6. Some side-effects of the drug that you should be aware of include the following:

Dizziness, drowsiness	Avoid driving automobiles, operating dangerous machinery, or performing delicate tasks when you are so affected.
Fainting, dizziness with position change	Change position slowly; when rising from a supine position, sit first for a few minutes and then stand slowly; avoid prolonged squatting;

(continued)

take extra care in hot weather when these problems are often worse.

Changes in sexual function, fertility	Impotence, failure to ejaculate, amenorrhea, and inability to conceive are all common problems; discuss these problems with your nurse or physician—they can be frustrating.
Nasal congestion	This "stuffy" feeling can be uncomfortable, but do *not* self-medicate with over-the-counter preparations; consult with your nurse or physician for the most appropriate medication for this problem.
Swelling in ankles, fingers	This is a frequent problem—rings may become tight and shoes may become uncomfortable; elevate your legs when resting; limit salt intake; consult your nurse or physician if this swelling becomes severe or too uncomfortable.
Nausea, loss of appetite, diarrhea	These effects often subside after a time on the drug; if they persist, consult your nurse or physician.

7. Avoid the use of over-the-counter medications while you are on this drug. If you need such a medication for a particular problem, consult with your nurse or physician.

8. You may find that you are very sensitive to the effects of alcoholic beverages while you are on this drug. Try to avoid the use of alcoholic beverages; if that is not possible, be very careful and limit your consumption.

9. Tell any physician, nurse, or dentist who is taking care of you that you are taking this drug.

10. Keep this and all medications out of the reach of children.

11. Consult with your nurse or physician if you are planning on traveling to a different climate. Dosage alterations may be necessary.

Notify your nurse or physician if any of the following occur:

Chest pain
Difficulty in breathing
Fever, skin rash
Numbness, tingling, or pain in hands or feet
Severe diarrhea

Guide to the nursing process: oral antihypertensives

Assessment	Nursing diagnoses	Intervention	Evaluation

Past history—underlying medical conditions (*contraindications*):
  Coronary artery disease
  Renal failure
  Liver failure
  Peptic ulcer
  Pregnancy
  Lactation
Allergies: *these drugs; tartrazine* (certain preparations); other allergies; reactions
Medication history: current drugs
	Potential alteration in cardiac output
	Knowledge deficit regarding disease and drug therapy
	Potential noncompliance secondary to side-effects of drug
	Potential sexual dysfunction
	Potential alteration in tissue perfusion
	Potential for injury secondary to side-effects of drug
		Appropriate and safe administration of drug
		Patient teaching program regarding:
		  Disease
		  Drug
		  Diet
		  Dosage
		  Side-effects
		  Warning signs
		Provision of comfort measures:
		  Slow position change
		  Safety precautions
		  Positioning and dietary changes
		  Medication for side-effect problems
		Support and encouragement to cope with drug therapy, side-effects, sexual dysfunction
			Monitor desired effects of drug: BP control
			Monitor adverse effects of drug:
			  Congestive heart failure
			  Liver problems
			  Reynaud's disease
			  Peyronie's disease
			  Postural BP changes
			  CNS changes
			  Lupuslike reaction
			  Sexual dysfunction
			Monitor for drug–diet, drug–drug, drug–environment interactions
			Monitor effectiveness of patient teaching program
			Monitor effectiveness of encouragement and support offered:
			  • Patient appointments kept
			  • Patient verbalizes fears and problems
			  • Patient stabilizes in BP control

Physical assessment Neurologic: orientation, state of mind, reflexes, sensations, pupillary response Cardiovascular: BP—sitting, standing, lying; P—peripheral pulses; cardiac auscultation—baseline ECG; edema check Respiratory: R, adventitious sounds GI: liver function, bowel sounds Renal: output, urinalysis, electrolyte levels			

Hypertension treatment programs

The goal of treatment in primary hypertension is to bring the patient's blood pressure down to a normal or nearly normal level and to keep it there without causing discomforting or dangerous side effects. To achieve this goal, treatment of essential hypertension is begun—after ruling out surgically curable causes of (secondary) hypertension—by trying to arrive at the drug or drug combination that is best suited to the needs of each patient. Treatment programs are advocated that differ in their details. In general, however, treatment is tailored to each patient's requirements on the basis of the level of the diastolic pressure and the presence or absence of signs and symptoms of complications caused by sustained blood pressure elevation. Whether or not to treat a particular patient also requires consideration of such factors as age, sex, race, and family history.

Types of hypertension

Mild hypertension

Many patients with diastolic pressure above 90 mm Hg but less than about 100 mm to 105 mm Hg may need no drug treatment at all, particularly when a physical examination reveals no signs of organic damage. In such cases, the presence of other factors that can increase the risk of cardiovascular complications is sought and elimination of these factors is attempted. Often, for example, an overweight woman in her middle forties will be able to keep her pressure from rising further if she follows her physician's recommendation that she reduce her dietary intake of calories and salt. A somewhat younger woman who smokes cigarettes and takes oral contraceptives may also not require antihypertensive drug therapy if she is willing to stop smoking and switches to some other means of birth control. A young man who shows signs of nervousness and emotional tension may be able to keep his pressure from rising to higher levels if he can manage to maintain a less hectic life style and get more rest and regular exercise.

If such risk factors as overweight, high salt intake, sedentary life style, and stress cannot be eliminated, and the patient's diastolic pressure stays persistently in the 90 mm to 105 mm Hg range, antihypertensive drug therapy is indicated. This is particularly true for young black men because of the higher incidence of illness and death resulting from hypertensive complications in this population. People with a family history of strokes, heart failure, or other complications of hypertension may also be candidates for antihypertensive drug treatment even though their own blood pressure is only in the borderline range between normal and high.

In all such cases, and in the large group of people with diastolic pressure that stays persistently above 105 mm Hg but rarely rises above about 115 mm Hg, treatment is usually begun with small doses of a diuretic drug. The patient may, for example, be started on a 50-mg dose of *hydrochlorothiazide* (Esidrix; HydroDiuril) once a day, and this dose may later be taken twice daily if needed to bring blood pressure down still further. *Spironolactone* (Aldactone) may also be employed, either alone or together with one of the thiazide-type diuretics. An advantage of such diuretic combinations is that taking spironolactone—or another potassium-sparing diuretic such as *triamterene* (Dyrenium)—prevents excessive loss of potassium ions from thiazide drug therapy, while the presence of a thiazide-type diuretic counteracts any tendency toward excessive retention of potassium as a result of spironolactone or triamterene therapy.

Most patients with mild hypertension respond to diuretic therapy with an adequate drop in pressure, and few suffer any significant side-effects. However, if the patient's blood pressure stays above normal after a trial of diuretics in maximal doses, a second drug is then usually added to the regimen in the first of what may be a series of steps aimed at complete control. Until recently, *reserpine* was the drug most commonly given together with a diuretic. The appearance of several reports suggesting a possible increased risk of breast cancer in women who took reserpine for long periods seems to have set off a trend away from this drug. Although the reported carcinogenic effect of reserpine has not been confirmed, many who had prescribed *methyldopa* at that time have continued to employ that drug for those of their patients who require a second drug. Clonidine, guanabenz, prazosin, or propranolol or another β blocker are all "second-step" drugs.*

Numerous combinations of thiazide diuretics with reserpine, methyldopa, clonidine, prazosin, propranolol, and timolol are available commercially. Patients should *not* be started out on such fixed dosage combinations. Instead, the preferred practice is for the dosage ratio of the two drugs that is most effective and best tolerated for each individual patient to be found. Then, if the individually adjusted double dosage can be matched in a commercial product containing similar fixed doses of each drug in a single tablet, the patient may be switched to such a product because compliance is likely to be better when fewer drugs and doses need to be taken.

Moderate hypertension

Combinations of the type described above are also employed in the stepped care approach to the management of patients with diastolic pressures above 115 mm Hg but below about 125 mm to 129 mm Hg. If such a patient does not respond fully to such two-drug treatments, it has been customary to add *hydralazine* to the regimen. The cautious addition of this direct-acting vasodilator to the diuretic agent and one of the sympathetic blocking drugs that act centrally or peripherally to reduce the outflow of sympathetic vasomotor impulses helps to bring moderately high blood pressure down to close to normotensive levels in about three out of four cases. Such three-drug combinations not only have additive hypotensive effects but also produce the advantage of a reduction in the potential adverse effects of the individual drugs. Thus, for example, the undesirable reflex tachycardia caused by hydralazine is counteracted when it is taken together with propranolol or with another β blocker. Similarly, the lupuslike syndrome sometimes seen during long-term therapy with large doses of hydralazine is unlikely to occur when its combination with other hypotensive drugs permits a reduction in its daily dosage.

Severe hypertension

Patients with diastolic pressures above 129 mm Hg require rapid control of their elevated blood pressure. Those whose condition is not complicated by cardiac, kidney, or cerebrovascular disease can often be treated successfully with one of the triple combinations described above. Here, however, treatment is begun with a full dose of diuretic followed promptly by a fairly large starting dose

---

* Some authorities now favor propranolol or another β blocker as the *first* drug with which to begin treatment of a previously untreated patient. A diuretic is added to the patient's regimen if he fails to respond fully or at all to the β blocker.

of propranolol, to which hydralazine is then added. Dosage increments of both the latter drugs are raised at a more rapid rate than in patients with less dangerously high blood pressure levels. The purpose of such an approach is to stop promptly the possible progress of this stage toward the accelerated or malignant phase of hypertension, which can rapidly damage the vessels of such vital organs as the brain, heart, and kidneys.

In some such cases, guanethidine is the first drug added to the diuretic with which therapy was initiated. In others, guanethidine is withheld until a trial of the three-drug combinations discussed above has not proved able to control the patient's accelerated hypertension. Guanethidine's potent hypotensive effect is considered necessary if such symptoms as headache, nosebleed, and dyspnea appear. However, although aggressive therapy with guanethidine may be required, its addition as a supplement to other antihypertensive agents should always be carried out cautiously. This is particularly true in the case of patients whose hypertension has already been complicated by damage to vital organs, as indicated by the presence of such signs and symptoms as pulmonary edema, chest pains, or azotemia. Too abrupt a drop in the pressure of such patients can further reduce the flow of blood through their vital organs and actually *cause* a

stroke, acute myocardial infarction, or renal failure. The newer drugs, minoxidil and captopril, may be added to the antihypertensive drug regimen of patients with severe hypertension who have not responded to safer drugs in combination.

Hypertensive emergencies

Patients are sometimes seen who have extremely elevated blood pressure—for example, 250/150 mm Hg. This is considered an emergency, or *hypertensive crisis,* which requires prompt parenteral therapy with antihypertensive agents to bring the diastolic pressure down to a level closer to 100 mm Hg or less (Table 28-2). This is thought necessary because the very high blood pressure is believed to be accompanied by spasm of the arterioles, which can damage the vessels and lead to irreversible injury to the brain, kidneys, and heart.

The most common cause of such a crisis and of the *hypertensive encephalopathy* that is its most dangerous complication is failure to control the accelerated or malignant phase of essential hypertension by use of the measures described above. However, other causes of critical emergencies include hypertensive heart disease with left ventricular failure and pulmonary edema, renovascular hypertension, and acute severe rises in pressure secondary

Table 28–2. Drugs used in hypertensive emergencies

Generic or official name	Trade name	Usual adult dosage range and administration
Rapidly acting drugs		
Diazoxide, parenteral USP	Hyperstat IV	1–3 mg/kg body weight by IV push in 30 sec or less (150 mg maximum dose) at intervals of 5–15 min, as needed
Sodium nitroprusside USP	Nipride; Nitropress	3 μg/kg body weight/min by precisely metered IV infusion
Trimethaphan camsylate USP	Arfonad	Infuse 1 mg/ml solution IV; initial rate: 3–4 mg/min; adjust as necessary (usual range is 0.3–6 mg/min)
Slower acting drugs		
Hydralazine HCl USP	Apresoline	20–40 mg IM or IV
Methyldopa HCl USP	Aldomet Ester Hydrochloride	250–500 mg q 6 hr by IV infusion over ½–1 hr
Reserpine USP	Sandril; Serpasil	0.5–1.0 mg IM followed by doses of 2 mg and 4 mg at 3-hr intervals

to such other kidney diseases as acute and chronic glomerulonephritis and chronic pyelonephritis. Severe hypertension may also develop during pregnancy as part of such pathologic states as preeclampsia and eclampsia. Hypertensive crisis in pheochromocytoma has been discussed in Chapter 18, and the occurrence of this condition as a complication of certain drug–drug and drug–food interactions will be discussed in Chapter 46.

General principles

The choice of drugs for dealing with hypertensive emergencies depends, in part, on how rapidly the patient's arterial pressure must be reduced and partly on the nature of the underlying disorder that has led to the very high pressure. Thus, when the high blood pressure is not yet accompanied by acute severe signs and symptoms, or when too rapid a drop in pressure may endanger the patient, it may be preferable to employ a parenteral preparation of *reserpine* or *methyldopa*—drugs with a slow onset of hypotensive action. In patients who have signs and symptoms of hypertensive encephalopathy, the most desirable drugs are those with an almost immediate hypotensive effect, such as *diazoxide, sodium nitroprusside,* and *trimethaphan.* In emergencies secondary to hypertensive heart disease, direct-acting vasodilator drugs such as diazoxide or hydralazine, which tend to cause reflex stimulation of the heart, should be avoided, while drugs which decrease the work of the heart, such as sodium nitroprusside or trimethaphan, are preferred.

Hypertensive encephalopathy

This complication of a very rapid rise in pressure to high levels is often heralded by development of a severe occipital headache, nausea and vomiting, and mental confusion. If the patient's pressure is not brought down very promptly, there may be convulsive seizures, intracranial bleeding, coma, and death. The ability to manage this life-threatening disorder has been greatly improved by the addition of diazoxide (Hyperstat) and sodium nitroprusside (Nipride) to the drug armamentarium.

Diazoxide solution is injected undiluted in an IV bolus dose of 1 to 3 mg/kg body weight, which must be completed within 30 seconds to be effective. This is often followed by a steep fall in pressure within 5 minutes or less. If the drop in diastolic pressure is not fully adequate, this dose may be repeated in 30 minutes. Once a satisfactory pressure level has been attained, it may be maintained by repeated injections of diazoxide at appropriate intervals.

Although diazoxide is chemically related to the thiazide diuretics, it does *not* have a diuretic effect. On the contrary, it tends to cause retention of sodium and water. For this reason, *furosemide*[+] (Lasix) is often also administered by vein to maintain the urinary output, particularly in patients in whom diazoxide induced edema might cause congestive heart failure. However, this com-

bination can cause an excessive fall in blood pressure. Thus, the patient's pressure should be monitored at frequent intervals, and vasopressor drugs should be available for treating hypotensive reactions.

Sodium nitroprusside solution acts within seconds after the start of an intravenous infusion. Its prompt and powerful pressure-reducing effect produces the most rapid relief of hypertensive encephalopathy signs and symptoms. However, its use requires very close monitoring of the patient's blood pressure and frequent adjustment of the infusion rate to avoid too precipitous a fall in pressure and to maintain the diastolic pressure at the desired level.

Sodium nitroprusside is preferred to diazoxide for those patients with hypertensive heart disease in whom a sudden rise in pressure may have precipitated left ventricular failure and pulmonary edema. This drug helps to improve myocardial performance in such patients by its dilating action on both the arterioles and the venules. That is, it does not stimulate the heart directly as does digitalis, nor indirectly as does diazoxide. Instead, it lessens the load on the left ventricle by reducing both the venous return of blood to the heart and the peripheral arterial resistance—the preload and afterload (Chap. 26).

Trimethaphan (Arfonad) is one of the few ganglionic blocking agents (Chap. 18) still employed for reducing high blood pressure. Like sodium nitroprusside, it acts promptly to lower very high blood pressure when administered by carefully controlled IV drip. Although its site and mechanism of action differ from that of sodium nitroprusside, it has a similar hemodynamic effect. That is, this drug also reduces the venous return of blood to the heart. The resulting decrease in cardiac output helps to lessen leakage of blood in hypertensive patients who have an aortic aneurysm. This drug's lack of a cardiac-stimulating effect makes it safer for patients with heart disease than diazoxide or hydralazine.

Hydralazine is not as rapid-acting as the three drugs discussed above. However, when injected intravenously, it can reduce blood pressure in less than 30 minutes. It is considered by some to be especially useful for patients with poor kidney function, including women with preeclampsia, because of its ability to maintain renal blood flow. It should not, however, be used in hypertensive patients with coronary heart disease unless its tendency to increase cardiac work can be counteracted by concomitant administration of reserpine or propranolol.

Reserpine injections and the parenteral form of methyldopa are not considered desirable drugs for treating cases of hypertensive crisis complicated by encephalopathy. In part, this is because these drugs have too slow an onset of action for use in that emergency, because they take several hours to achieve their full effects. In addition, the central depressant action of these drugs may make it difficult to evaluate the mental status of patients with hypertensive brain symptoms.

However, in still asymptomatic cases of malignant

hypertension, and in other situations in which immediate action is unnecessary, or when a gradual reduction in blood pressure is desirable, methyldopa (Aldomet Ester) and reserpine, administered intramuscularly, can be quite useful for lowering dangerously elevated blood pressure. Among patients for whom these drugs may be the best choice are elderly patients with cerebral or coronary atherosclerosis, in whom too sudden and deep a drop in pressure should be avoided. Others for whom methyldopa may be preferred are patients with severe renal impairment caused by acute or chronic glomerulonephritis. In such cases and in women with preeclampsia and eclampsia, the use of methyldopa may help to maintain renal perfusion and to prevent oliguria and possible renal failure.

Preeclampsia and eclampsia

Patients with preeclampsia may often be managed without resorting to specific antihypertensive agents. Sometimes bed rest and sedation with diazepam (Valium) may be helpful for control of this condition. If the preeclamptic state progresses to eclampsia, larger doses of diazepam or carefully controlled injections of magnesium sulfate may be required to prevent or treat convulsions and to reduce the patient's high blood pressure.

Summary of effects of antihypertensive drugs on the renin–angiotensin system and on plasma renin activity (PRA)

1. *Propranolol* and other β blockers decrease renin secretion and decrease PRA, in part, by blocking β-adrenergic receptors on juxtaglomerular cells of the kidney. This *antirenin* action reduces production of angiotensin II, and, in turn, of aldosterone. As a result, *both* the excessive vasoconstrictor and the increased blood volume components of some forms of hypertension are reduced.

2. The converting enzyme inhibitor *captopril* prevents biologically inactive angiotensin I from being converted to the very potent vasopressor angiotensin II.

3. The angiotensin II antagonist *saralasin* prevents that vasopressor polypeptide from activating its receptors at peripheral (vascular and adrenal cortical) and central sites. This drug is actually a partial agonist. It is used only in diagnosis, not in therapy.

4. The centrally acting antihypertensives *reserpine, methyldopa, clonidine* and *guanabenz* may reduce renin release and PRA by their actions at central sites. (This is responsible for only part of their pressure-reducing effects.)

5. The vasodilator drugs *hydralazine, minoxidil, diazoxide,* and *sodium nitroprusside* tend to *increase* PRA. They do so because they cause a reflex increase in sympathetic stimulation of kidney cell β-adrenergic receptors, as well as reflex tachycardia.

6. *Diuretic drugs* counteract vasodilator drug-induced sodium and fluid retention. However, the diuretic-induced depletion of blood volume—despite its antihypertensive effect—sets off increased renin secretion and PRA. (This can be counteracted by combining diuretics with propranolol or with another β blocker.)

Summary of some adverse effects, cautions, and contraindications of antihypertensive drugs*

Captopril (Capoten)

Adverse effects. Renal glomerular toxicity; neutropenia–agranulocytosis; dysgeusia (taste impairment); hypotension; rash and fever.

Cautions. Discontinue nitrates and other vasodilators; use caution in patients on diuretics and other antihypertensives.

Clonidine (Catapres)

Adverse effects. Mouth dryness, drowsiness, dizziness, headache.

Cautions. Discontinue gradually to avoid possible rapid rise in blood pressure.

Diazoxide (Hyperstat)

Adverse effects. Sodium and water retention; hyperglycemia, tachycardia.

Cautions. Employ in conjunction with a diuretic to avoid edema in patients prone to develop congestive heart failure. Monitor blood sugar levels of patients with diabetes mellitus. Monitor ECG of patients with coronary artery disease for signs of arrhythmias caused by myocardial ischemia.

(continued)

Contraindications. Patients with compensatory hypertension associated with aortic coarctation or arteriovenous shunt; patients with a history of hypersensitivity to benzothiadiazine and other sulfonamide derivatives.

Diuretics

See summaries in Chapter 27.

Guanabenz monoacetate (Wytensin)

See adverse effects and cautions for clonidine (above).

Guanadrel Sulfate (Hylorel)

See adverse effects and cautions for guanethidine (below).

Guanethidine Sulfate (Ismelin)

Adverse effects. Postural or exertional hypotension causes dizziness, weakness, possible syncope, diarrhea, nausea, vomiting; interference with male sexual function (ejaculation).

Cautions. Employ a diuretic to avoid edema; watch for weight gain and bradycardia. Caution in patients with a history of peptic ulcer or bronchial asthma.

Contraindications: Patients with pheochromocytoma or those being treated with MAO inhibitors; also not for patients with congestive heart failure.

Hydralazine HCl (Apresoline)

Adverse effects. Headache, heart palpitations, tachycardia, anginal chest pain; anorexia, nausea, vomiting, diarrhea.

Cautions. Patients with suspected coronary or cerebral artery disease. Discontinue in patients who develop a syndrome resembling systemic lupus erythematosus.

Contraindications. Patients with coronary artery disease and mitral valvular rheumatic heart disease.

Methyldopa (Aldomet)

Adverse effects. Early drowsiness, headache, weakness; mouth dryness, nausea, vomiting.

Cautions. Patients with a history of liver disorders. Periodic blood counts should be performed to detect hemolytic anemia. Coombs' tests should be performed before beginning therapy and periodically during treatment.

Contraindications. Patients with active hepatitis, cirrhosis, or other liver disease.

Minoxidil (Loniten)

Adverse effects. Edema; pericardial effusion and tamponade; hirsutism; hematologic depression; nausea and vomiting.

Cautions. Give with a β blocker and a diuretic.
Contraindications. Pheochromocytoma.

Pargyline (Eutonyl)

See summary, Chapter 46, concerning MAO inhibitor drugs.

Prazosin (Minipress)

Adverse effects. Dizziness, drowsiness, weakness, headache, palpitations.

Cautions. First dose has caused syncope; patient should not drive or operate machinery for 4 hours after first dose.

Propranolol (Inderal) and other β blockers (e.g., Atenolol, Metoprolol Tartrate, Nadolol, Pindolol, Timolol)

See summary, Chapter 18, concerning β-adrenergic blocking agents. In addition, chronic use of metoprolol and propranolol has caused Peyronie's disease in some men.

Reserpine (Serpasil) and other rauwolfia alkaloids

Adverse effects. Gastrointestinal: anorexia, nausea, vomiting, hypersecretion, diarrhea; *CNS:* drowsiness, nervousness, nightmares, anxiety, mental depression; *Other:* weight gain, nasal congestion, impotence and decreased libido.

Cautions. Watch for signs of mental depression and discontinue promptly.

Contraindications. Emotionally depressed patients and those receiving electroconvulsive therapy; patients with active peptic ulcer or ulcerative colitis.

Sodium nitroprusside (Nipride)

Adverse effects. Too rapid infusion can cause nausea, retching, and abdominal pain; also sweating, restlessness, headache, and heart palpitations.

Cautions. Blood pressure must be very closely monitored, and the infusion rate carefully regulated with devices for measuring the flow of fluid precisely.

Contraindications. Not for use in patients with compensatory hypertension caused by coarctation of the aorta or arteriovenous shunt.

Trimethaphan (Arfonad) and other parenterally administered ganglionic blocking agents

Adverse effects. Excessive hypotension can occur with overdosage and when other drugs that cause a fall in blood pressure are also being employed.

Cautions. Patient's circulation must be very closely monitored and supplies, equipment, and trained personnel should be available for rapidly reversing excessive hypotension.

Contraindications: Patients with hypovolemia, anemia, respiratory difficulties, or asphyxia.

---

* All potent antihypertensive drugs should be used with caution in patients with severe coronary or cerebrovascular disease or in those with chronically impaired kidney function. Symptoms of postural hypotension occur in varying degrees with all sympathetic blocking drugs.

Case study

Presentation

BR, a 46-year-old black male business executive, was seen in the outpatient department for a routine physical examination associated with his company's insurance plan. His exam was negative except that BR was estimated to be 20 lb overweight and his BP was 164/102. Urinalysis was negative. Standard blood work was also within normal limits. He was started on a 1200-calorie, no salt-added diet and asked to return to the department several times over the next 3 weeks to have his BP checked by the nurse. Three weeks after first being seen, BR had lost 7 pounds and his average BP reading was 140/96. Because of the many factors that put him at high risk (see below), he was started on captopril, a drug usually reserved for patients who have failed to respond to other antihypertensive medication. The dose was 25 mg tid. He was evaluated after 2 weeks and found to have lost a total of 11 lb and to have a BP of 132/84. The decision was made to maintain BR on captopril therapy. Explain what nursing measures should be taken with this patient.

Discussion

Because of his high-risk factors—age, sex, race, occupation—for complications of hypertension, BR will need a thorough and continuous teaching program regarding his disease and drug therapy. The end results of hypertension should be discussed as a motivation for helping the patient to cope with the diet and drug therapy throughout his life. A diet history should be taken to help the patient adapt his own life style to the diet restrictions and to assess the incidence of natural pressor foods in his diet. The patient and his significant other can help to select the foods most appropriate and acceptable to the diet limitations. The patient should receive positive reinforcement regarding his weight control at every opportunity. The usual drug teaching protocol should be followed with the following specific adaptations. The patient should be told to take captopril 1 hour before meals and to report any skin rash, mouth sores, or sore throat. He should be warned that loss of taste perception or an unusual taste can occur. He should receive all this information in writing for easy reference. He should also be scheduled for routine follow-up exams that include time for teaching evaluation and support measures. Essential hypertension is a chronic, usually lifelong, problem, which will require continual medical follow-up. Therefore, the development of a positive, trusting relationship with the patient is one of the most important initial tasks of the nurses taking care of BR.

Drug digests

Guanethidine sulfate USP (Ismelin)

Actions and indications. This potent, long-acting, and dependable antihypertensive agent is used mainly in the management of moderate to severe degrees of essential hypertension and to reduce blood pressure that is high as a result of renal disease. It interferes with the transmission of sympathetic nerve impulses to the cardiovascular system by depleting sympathetic postganglionic nerves of norepinephrine. This ability to block transmission in adrenergic nerves without affecting functioning of the parasympathetic system as do the ganglionic blocking agents accounts for its freedom from the atropine-like side-effects often seen with the latter class of drugs. This, together with its better absorption and reliability, has resulted in its largely having replaced that class of drugs in treatment of chronic cases of moderately severe and malignant hypertension.

Adverse effects, cautions, and contraindications. This drug's ability to block vasomotor reflexes often results in orthostatic (postural) hypertension, particularly on arising in the morning and during periods of suddenly increased activity. To avoid weakness, dizziness, and fainting, patients should be taught to change position slowly.

Caution is required in patients with coronary, cerebral, or renal vascular disease, because too sudden and steep a fall in blood pressure can dangerously reduce blood flow in the brain, heart, and kidneys. The drug is contraindicated in patients with congestive heart failure; to avoid a tendency toward cardiac decompensation in susceptible patients, it is best administered together with a diuretic and sometimes also with digitalis.

Patients with high blood pressure secondary to pheochromocytoma should not receive this drug. Its use is also undesirable in patients with peptic ulcer or colitis, because it may cause increased gastrointestinal motility (diarrhea) and secretion.

Dosage and administration. Treatment is

ordinarily begun with a single daily dose of 10 mg orally. The dose is then raised gradually until the best response is obtained, usually with single daily doses of 25 mg to 75 mg. Doses are raised in increments of about 10 mg after 5 or more days of treatment with the lower dose, and daily dosage is later regulated in accordance with the patient's day-to-day response. In severe hypertension, this drug may be employed in larger doses or in lower doses combined with diuretics, hydralazine, or methyldopa.

Methyldopa and methyldopate HCl USP (Aldomet; Aldomet Ester)

Actions and indications. This is the preferred antihypertensive agent for patients with renal insufficiency, because it does not tend to reduce blood flow through the kidneys when it produces falls in blood pressure. It may be used alone in patients with moderate hypertension but it is more effective when combined with diuretics or other pressure-reducing drugs in hypertension of more severe degree, including that seen in women with eclampsia. The drug's effects come on promptly, when it is administered orally, but intravenous administration is preferred for patients in hypertensive crisis. The drug produces its effects by actions in the central nervous system that reduce sympathetic outflow.

Adverse effects, cautions, and contraindications. This drug causes less orthostatic hypotension than do other adrenergic neuron blocking drugs. However, weakness, dizziness, and light-headedness are likely to occur in older patients who are sensitive to its hypotensive action and thus require reduced dosage. Lower doses are also desirable in patients with renal insufficiency whose kidneys may not excrete the drug adequately, with resulting systemic cumulation. Drowsiness is the most common side-effect of early treatment or of periodic increases in dosage. Headache and gastrointestinal upset, including diarrhea, also occur. Potentially more serious are various hypersensitivity reactions involving the liver, blood and skin. Drug-induced hepatitis may be manifested by loss of appetite, malaise, fever, and other signs and symptoms in addition to jaundice. Caution is required in patients with a history of liver disease, and the drug is contraindicated during active hepatic disease. It is also administered with caution to mentally depressed patients, because the drug itself sometimes causes psychic depression. Routine liver function and blood tests, including the Coombs' test (for possible hemolytic anemia) are recommended.

Dosage and administration. Oral doses of this drug may be added to the regimen of patients previously unresponsive to diuretic therapy alone. Initial doses of 250 mg three times daily may gradually be raised to between 1 and 2 g daily if necessary, or reduced if desirable. Intravenous administration of 250 to 500 mg may be used in starting treatment of acute crises, but repeated higher doses may be necessary, or lower doses may be employed in patients with poor kidney function.

Reserpine USP (Serpasil)

Actions and indications. This rauwolfia alkaloid produces gradual drops in blood pressure by partially blocking transmission of tonic vasomotor and cardioacceleratory impulses from sympathetic (adrenergic) nerves. Its effects are thought to result from the release and depletion of the neurotransmitter norepinephrine in adrenergic nerve endings.

Small oral doses are commonly combined with a diuretic in treating chronic essential hypertension of mild to moderate degree of severity. For treating resistant cases, hydralazine is sometimes added to the reserpine–diuretic combinations. The parenteral form is employed in the management of hypertensive crisis. However, because of the slow onset of its action (about 3 or 4 hours for maximal effects) a more rapid-acting hypotensive agent such as trimethaphan is often first administered.

Adverse effects, cautions, and contraindications. Postural hypotension is *not* common with the orally administered drug but does occur following parenteral administration. Nasal congestion and stuffiness is a more common result of vasodilation occurring locally in the mucosa of the nose. Also common is drowsiness with feelings of weakness and fatigue. More serious is the mental depression that develops in some patients, particularly those with a prior history of suicidal tendencies, in whom this drug is contraindicated. Caution is also required in patients with a history of epilepsy.

An increase in gastrointestinal motility and secretion that can cause epigastric distress, cramps, and diarrhea calls for caution in patients with a history of past peptic ulcer or ulcerative colitis; it is contraindicated in active cases. This drug is discontinued 2 weeks before electroshock therapy or surgical anesthesia because of possible severe convulsions, bradycardia, and hypotension.

Dosage and administration. Oral administration of 0.1 to 1 mg (usual dose is 0.5 mg) daily may be used for initiating therapy; later patients may be maintained on 0.25 mg daily or less. Parenteral doses of 0.5 mg to 1.0 mg may be administered IM to initiate treatment in hypertensive emergencies. These may be followed by doses of 2 mg and 4 mg at intervals of 3 hours.

Sodium nitroprusside USP (Nipride)

Actions and indications. This intravenously administered antihypertensive agent is used in hypertensive emergencies for rapid reduction of high blood pressure. The drug has a direct relaxing action on the smooth muscle walls of blood vessels. The resulting arteriolar vasodilation leads to a reduction in peripheral resistance. Pooling of blood peripherally tends to decrease the return of blood to the heart and results in some decrease in the cardiac output.

These drug-induced hemodynamic effects make the drug most suitable for hypertensive crisis complicated by acute left ventricular failure and pulmonary edema, intracranial bleeding, and aortic aneurysms of the acute dissecting or leaking abdominal types. However, it has also been used in cases of hypertensive encephalopathy, and in acute or chronic glomerulonephritis, because a significant decrease in blood flow to the brain and kidneys does *not* occur.

Adverse effects, cautions, and contraindications. Too rapid reduction in blood pressure may cause cardiac palpitations and chest pain, nausea, retching, and abdominal pain, headache, dizziness, restlessness, anxiety, and sweating. These symptoms can be avoided by close monitoring of the patient's blood pressure, and they disappear rapidly when the rate of infusion is slowed, or the flow is briefly discontinued.

Elderly patients, who tend to be sensitive to the hypotensive effect of this drug, should be started on low doses. Caution is also required in patients with hypothyroidism or with poor renal function.

The drug is converted to cyanmethemoglobin and free cyanide, which is converted in the liver to thiocyanate. If the drug accumulates or if sulfur (to form thiocyanate) is depleted from the body, cyanide toxicity may occur. Metabolic acidosis is an early sign of this problem. Sodium nitroprusside should be stopped at once, and the cyanide poisoning should be treated with IV sodium nitrate followed by IV sodium thiosulfate (see Table 5-1).

This drug is contraindicated when hypertension is compensatory, as in aortic coarctation (compression) or arteriovenous shunt.

Dosage and administration. A stock solution is prepared by dissolving 50 mg in 2 ml to 3 ml of dextrose in water. This is *never* injected directly but is, instead, diluted in 500 ml to 1000 ml of 5% dextrose in water. The container is then wrapped in aluminum foil or some other lightproof material to delay deterioration of this light-sensitive drug. The dosage range is 0.5 to 8 μg/kg body weight/min (average 3 μg/kg/min), infused under close monitoring with the use of an infusion pump, microdrip regulator, or other similar device for measuring the flow rate precisely.

References

Blaschke TF, Melmon KL: Antihypertensive agents and the drug therapy of hypertension. In Gilman AG, Goodman LS, Gilman A (eds): Goodman and Gilman's The Pharmacological Basis of Therapeutics, 6th ed, pp 793–818. New York, Macmillan, 1980

Blythe WB: Captopril and renal autoregulation. N Eng J Med 308:390, 1983

Clark, AB et al: A nurse's clinician's role in the management of hypertension. Arch Intern Med, 136:903, 1976

Dollery CT: Hypertension and new antihypertensive drugs: Clinical perspectives. Fed Proc 42:207, 1983

Finnerty FA: The nurse and care of the hypertensive patient. Ann Intern Med 84:746, 1976

Freis ED: Changing attitudes to hypertension. Ann Intern Med 78:141, 1973

Freis ED: Prazosin: Clinical symposium proceedings. Postgrad Med (Spec Rep) 1975

Freis ED: Salt in hypertension and the effects of diuretics. Ann Rev Pharmacol Toxicol 18:13, 1979

Guanadrel (Hylorel)—a new antihypertensive drug. Med Lett Drug Ther 25:95, 1983

Hansson L, Werko L: Beta adrenergic blockade in hypertension. Am Heart J 93:394, 1977

Heel RC et al: Captopril: A preliminary review of its pharmacological properties and therapeutic efficacy. Drugs 201:409, 1980

Hollifield JW et al: Proposed mechanisms of propranolol's antihypertensive effect in essential hypertension. N Engl J Med 294:68, 1976

Indapamide (Lozol)—a new antihypertensive agent and diuretic. Med Lett 26:17, 1984

Jones LN: Hypertension: Medical and nursing implications. Nurs Clin North Am 11:283, 1976

Kaplan HR et al: Survey of new antihypertensive drugs: 1982. Fed Proc 42:154, 1983

Koch–Weser J: Hypertensive emergencies. N Engl J Med 290:21, 1974

Koch–Weser J: Metoprolol. N Engl J Med 301:698, 1979

Laragh JH et al: Modern system for treating high blood pressure based on renin profiling and vasoconstriction volume analysis. Am J Med 61:797, 1976

Long ML et al: Hypertension: What nurses need to know. Am J Nurs 76:765, 1976

Moser M: Report of the joint national committee on detection, evaluation, and treatment of high blood pressure: A cooperative study. JAMA 237:255, 1977

Nies AS: Clinical pharmacology of antihypertensive drugs. Med Clin North Am 61:675, 1977

Palmer RF, Lassiter KC: Sodium nitroprusside. N Engl J Med 292:294, 1975

Pettinger WA: Recent advances in the treatment of hypertension. Arch Intern Med 137:679, 1977

Robinson AM: The RN's goal: Under 90 mm Hg diastolic. RN 37:43, 1974

Rodman MJ: How to cope with those new antihypertensive drugs. RN 42:109 (Oct) 1979

Rodman MJ: Managing those tricky emergency antihypertensives. RN 44:85 (Sept) 1981

Scriabine A: β-adrenoceptor blocking drugs in hypertension. Ann Rev Pharmacol Toxicol 19:269, 1979

Weber MA: Saralasin testing for renin-dependent hypertension. Arch Intern Med 139:93, 1979

Chapter 29

Digitalis
and
related
heart
drugs

29

The foxglove plant and digitalis

The foxglove plant has been employed for hundreds of years in the treatment of congestive heart failure. The British physician William Withering brought this old vegetable drug into modern medicine. In 1775 he singled out the foxglove plant as the active ingredient of an old wives' secret recipe for treating "dropsy," as edema was then called. After studying the effects of the leaf and its aqueous extracts for 10 years, he published his findings in An Account of the Foxglove—a classic paper that still makes fascinating reading. Withering, although he thought of the drug as a diuretic rather than a heart stimulant, had obviously learned both the value of digitalis and its dangers.

Today, the active principles of foxglove plants—the glycosides—are still among the most commonly prescribed of all medications. In this country two species of foxglove, *Digitalis lanata* and *D. purpurea*, are the sources of the most commonly employed plant principles *digoxin*[+] and *digitoxin*[+] (Table 29-1). Another glycoside of *D. lanata*, *deslanoside*[+], is still available, but the manufacture of many preparations has been discontinued. A mixture of amorphous (*non*crystalline) glycosides of *D. purpurea*, called gitalin, is also available, as is the powdered dried leaf of this plant.

This chapter will discuss mainly the two most important digitalis glycosides. However, principles ob-

tained from other families of plants also have the same type of *cardiotonic*, or heart-strengthening, activity. For example, ouabain, a rapidly acting drug available until recently, comes from the plant *Strophanthus gratus*. Plants of other families that contain principles with digitalislike cardiac actions include the lily of the valley (*Convallaria majalis*), the sea onion (squill; *Urginea maritima*), the oleander shrub (*Nerium oleander*), and the Christmas rose (*Helleborus niger*). These plants and their principles are rarely used for medicinal purposes in this country, but cases of accidental poisoning from eating parts of ornamental shrubs or flowers may occasionally be of clinical concern.*

Pharmacologic actions
and pharmacokinetics

The cardiac glycosides of digitalis continue to be the most valuable drugs for the long-term treatment of chronic congestive heart failure. These drugs are also useful adjuncts to antiarrhythmic agents and other measures in the management of certain cardiac arrhythmias (see Chap. 30). However, digitalis is also the cause of one of the most common and most dangerous of all drug poisonings: a potentially fatal intoxication marked by many types of cardiac irregularities.

To use digitalis effectively and safely, it is necessary to understand the drug's pharmacologic actions and the manner in which the various glycosides are handled by the body after they are administered orally or parenterally. Much has been learned about the actions and pharmacokinetics of the digitalis glycosides. This knowledge can be applied in adjusting dosage of digoxin, digitoxin, and other glycosides to the needs and tolerance of individual patients to ensure maximum efficacy and to minimize the development of digitalis toxicity. Thus,

---

* Not of similar clinical significance but nevertheless of some interest is the fact that substances with the same pharmacologic and toxic effects have been found in the skin secretions of toads and in the bodies of certain beetles and other insects, including monarch butterflies (*Danaus plexippus*). The larvae of the latter feed on certain species of milkweed plants (*Asclepias*) that contain cardiac glycosides. The presence of these poisons in the wings and other body parts of the adult butterflies has some survival value. Birds that eat these butterflies quickly become ill, retch, and vomit. Thus, they learn the lesson that this is a species of butterfly that they should shun in the future as a source of food.

Table 29-1. Cardiotonic drugs and dosage schedules*

Generic or official name	Trade name	Range of total (full) digitalizing dosages†	Usual adult daily oral maintenance dosage‡
Deslanoside injection USP	Cedilanid-D; desacetyllanatoside C	1.6 mg IV or 0.8 mg at each of two IM sites	
Digitalis, powdered (dried leaf) USP	Digifortis	1.2 g oral, in divided doses, q 6 hr	100–200 mg
Digitalis glycosides mixture USP	Digiglusin	Oral: 6 USP U then 4 USP U 4–6 hr later and 2 USP U q 4–6 hr until full therapeutic effect is achieved	0.5–3 USP U/day
Digitoxin USP and digitoxin injection USP	Crystodigin; Purodigin	IV or oral: 0.6 mg, then 0.4 mg 4–6 hr later and 0.2 mg every 4–6 hr until full therapeutic effect is achieved (8–12 hr)	0.05–0.3 mg
Digoxin USP and digoxin injection USP	Lanoxin	IV: 0.6–1.0 mg; oral: 0.75–1.25 mg	0.125–0.25 mg
	Lanoxicaps have greater bioavailability than the other oral preparations. The 0.2-mg Lanoxicap is equivalent to the 0.25-mg tablets, the 0.1-mg Lanoxicap is equivalent to the 0.125-mg tablet, and so forth.		
Gitalin (amorphous)	Gitaligin	Oral: 2.5 mg, then 0.75 mg q 6 hrs	0.25–1.25 mg

* Dosage must be adjusted to the needs and tolerance of each patient. Thus, these doses are offered only as a guide for initiating therapy.
† Rapid digitalization is usually achieved by administering a large fraction of the calculated total, the loading dose, which is then followed by one to three smaller fractions at intervals of several hours. Occasionally, the entire digitalizing dose of *digitoxin* is administered at once.
‡ Digitalization with *digoxin* may be achieved within 5 to 7 days by administering daily small fractions of the calculated total, which are then continued as the maintenance dose.

before taking up the clinical applications of these drugs in the treatment of the cardiac disorders for which they are employed, their basic cardiovascular actions will be summarized and some aspects of the metabolism of the two most commonly prescribed glycosides, digoxin and digitoxin, will be discussed.

Cardiac and circulatory effects
Digitalis has two main types of actions on the heart:

1. It increases the strength of the heartbeat (positive inotropic action).
2. It alters the electrophysiologic properties of the heart and thus affects its rate and rhythm.

Positive inotropic action
The ability of digitalis to make the myocardium contract more forcefully when this muscular pump is weakened

by disease is the main action that accounts for the drug's usefulness in treating congestive heart failure. Administered to patients with hypodynamic heart action, digitalis glycosides help the heart muscle to drive more blood out of its chambers with each beat. This increase in stroke volume and cardiac output improves the patient's pulmonary and systemic circulations and leads to relief of the signs and symptoms caused by fluid that has accumulated in the tissues as edema.

Other drugs such as the sympathomimetic catecholamines norepinephrine, epinephrine, isoproterenol, and dobutamine (Chap. 17) also strengthen the heartbeat. These adrenergic drugs are contraindicated for most chronic cardiac patients, however, because they can force the heart to work too hard, causing tachycardia and a demand for more oxygen than its coronary vessels can deliver. Digitalis, on the other hand, tends to slow the heart as it strengthens it, and this slowing of the heart rate together with a drug-induced decrease in the size of the dilated ventricular chambers results in a reduction in the amount of oxygen that the failing heart muscle consumes during its contractions.

The *mechanism* by which digitalis produces its positive inotropic action is still not fully understood. However, it is thought that the drug does so by an indirect action that makes more free calcium ions available within the cardiac muscle cell. The increased influx of calcium through the cell membrane favorably affects the process by which electrical excitation of the cell membrane is linked to the mechanical contraction of the muscle fibers—the so-called excitation–contraction coupling process. This increases the efficiency with which energy produced by the heart muscle cells is converted into contractile force.

The digitalis-induced movement of calcium from the cell membrane to the inner protein (troponin) with which it combines to activate contraction of cardiac muscle seems to be an indirect result of the drug-induced inhibition of a membrane enzyme called sodium–potassium-activated adenosine triphosphatase (Na, K-ATPase). This enzyme runs the so-called sodium pump, the mechanism by which cells pump sodium ions out of their interior in exchange for potassium ions. Thus, the drug's depressant effect on the activity of this enzyme reduces the cell's ability to move sodium out of the cell. The resulting increase of intracellular sodium (as well as of calcium), together with the loss of potassium ions, is also thought to account for the electrophysiologic effects of digitalis that are both therapeutically beneficial and the cause of cardiac toxicity (see below).

Other cardiac actions

In addition to its primary positive inotropic effect, digitalis slows heart rate (a negative chronotropic effect) and slows the conduction of the cardiac impulse through the atrioventricular (A-V) node. The slowing of heart rate can be therapeutically beneficial to the heart in failure by providing more time for the ventricles to fill. The slowing of heart rate is a result of a decrease in the rate of firing of the sinoatrial (S-A) node pacemaker that, in turn, is caused largely by an increase in firing in the parasympathetic vagal nerve but in part by a decrease in firing in the cardiac sympathetic nerves. Digitalis acts at many sites, including the central nervous system, to produce these effects. The improvement in cardiac contractility, and thus in arterial blood pressure, is sensed by baroreceptors; thus, baroreceptor reflexes may also be active in the increased parasympathetic and decreased sympathetic outflow and in the reduction of sinus rhythm. Atropine (Chap. 16) blocks most of the digitalis-induced cardiac slowing.

The reduction in A-V nodal conduction rate is progressive with increasing doses of digitalis. This is the second major therapeutic effect of digitalis. (It can also be an unwanted, adverse effect, under certain circum-

stances.) At high doses, A-V nodal conduction block may be complete (complete heart block). The increased vagal activity and decreased sympathetic nerve activity described above are partly responsible for this effect of digitalis on the A-V node, but direct effects of digitalis on the A-V node are probably more important. Digitalis decreases the height and rate of rise of the action potential in A-V node cells, thus making the action potential a less effective stimulus to adjacent tissue, and slowing conduction velocity.

At the same time that digitalis is producing these effects on cardiac contractility and on the S-A and A-V nodes, it can produce clearly adverse and dangerous effects on other areas of the heart. Some of these effects result from the drug's direct action on cardiac cell membranes and on ion flow across these membranes. Electrophysiologic properties of these cells are thus altered, predisposing them to become ectopic (*i.e.,* abnormal) pacemaker sites and leading to dangerous cardiac arrhythmias. The clinical significance of these complex effects on the rate and rhythm of the heart in terms of the drug's therapeutic effectiveness and potential toxicity is discussed below and in the next chapter.

Vascular effects

In people with *normal* cardiac function, digitalis acts directly on the smooth muscle walls of the blood vessels and causes them to contract. It might seem that this vasoconstrictor effect would tend to prevent any increase in cardiac output from the drug's positive inotropic, or contraction-strengthening, action on the heart. However, in *heart failure patients,* oral or slow intravenous doses of digitalis rarely cause enough peripheral vasoconstriction to prevent an increase in cardiac output. Instead, the drug acts to reduce the high sympathetic impulse outflow in these patients, with a resulting slowing of the heart (described above), dilation of blood vessels, and improved peripheral blood flow.

Pharmacokinetic properties of digoxin and digitoxin

Digoxin, digitoxin, and all the other available cardiotonic glycosides exert essentially similar actions on the heart. These drugs differ mainly in their pharmacokinetic properties—that is, in the manner in which they are absorbed and then move about the body to their sites of action and to the organs that metabolically degrade or eliminate them (Chap. 4). It is important for those who administer digitalis products and observe their effects on patients to understand the clinical applications of each drug's pharmacokinetics and its final fate. Such knowledge is necessary to obtain the therapeutically beneficial effects of these potent drugs for the patient while preventing digitalis overdosage and intoxication.

How the body handles each digitalis preparation after it is swallowed and enters the gastrointestinal tract or is deposited in an intramuscular site or injected directly into the bloodstream determines the level that the drug attains and maintains in the plasma. Such plasma, or serum, concentrations are, in turn, correlated with the amounts of these drugs that reach the heart and other reactive tissues at any time after their administration, and determine for how short or long a time the therapeutically desirable or the toxic effects of these drugs continue. As indicated below in the discussion of digitalis toxicity, it is now possible to measure the presence of less than one billionth of a gram (0.000000001 g) of digoxin in the blood and to correlate such serum concentrations with the patient's clinical responses to the drug.

Absorption and bioavailability

Digitoxin and digoxin are both rapidly absorbed when taken by mouth. Thus, except in emergency situations, these drugs do not have to be injected. Another glycoside, deslanoside, a close chemical relative of digoxin that differs from it only in the presence of a single residual glucose substructure in its molecule, is so poorly and unreliably absorbed that it is ineffective if taken orally, and so must be injected.

Unlike digitoxin, which is almost totally absorbed from the gastrointestinal tract, digoxin is incompletely absorbed. Only about 60% to 80% of any tablet that is taken orally is absorbed. More of the available digoxin elixir, 70% to 85%, reaches the bloodstream, and 70% to 85% of liquid digoxin contained in Lanoxicap capsules also enters the blood from the duodenum (Table 29-1). Thus, dosage should be adjusted, depending on the preparation used. In any case, enough digoxin is absorbed by the oral route to begin producing its therapeutic effects within 1 or 2 hours. However, its incomplete and often variable absorption has led to problems when patients who were stabilized with one tablet brand were switched to another in which the digoxin content was more or less bioavailable than in the first.

As indicated previously (Chap. 4), differences in the bioavailability of different brands of digoxin or even in different batches of the same brand have led to either overdosage or underdosage in patients who continued to take the same maintenance dose but who then actually absorbed greater or smaller amounts of the drug. Thus, generally speaking, many physicians try to avoid such difficulties by selecting and staying with a digoxin product manufactured by a pharmaceutical company that has an established reputation for reliability.

A result of efforts to develop products with a higher degree of bioavailability has been a need to reduce digoxin dosage to about half of what had previously been recommended. One reason for this is that overdosage might occur when patients who had been stabilized on products of low bioavailability started taking the same dose of a product with a higher bioavailability. Another reason for using lower doses of digoxin has been a change in the traditional idea that every patient should receive the highest dose of digitalis that can be tolerated. (See below for a further discussion of the current status of the "full digitalization" concept.)

Other factors in addition to differences in the formulation of digoxin tablets may also affect the amount absorbed and consequently the serum level attained. Patients who take laxatives may absorb less digoxin, while those taking antispasmodic or other constipating drugs may absorb more. A patient who routinely takes digoxin on an empty stomach will have an altered serum level if he starts to take the drug with meals, which change gastrointestinal activity and acidity. The absorption of both digoxin and digitoxin can be prevented by resins such as the hyperlipidemic drugs cholestyramine and colestipol (Chap. 32), which should never be taken at the same time as these glycosides. Patients suffering from abnormalities in the mucosal lining of the gastrointestinal tract that lead to a malabsorption syndrome may not be able to take these drugs by mouth.

Fate following absorption

Although digoxin and digitoxin are both adequately absorbed when taken by mouth, they differ somewhat in the time required for their effects to become evident and to rise to a peak. Differences in the biologic half-life (Chap. 4) of the two glycosides and in the duration of their cardiac actions are even greater. These differences in onset and duration depend on such factors as the following:

1. The extent to which each drug is bound to plasma proteins after absorption, or is available in a free form that more readily diffuses from the blood
2. The extent to which each drug is excreted into the gut and then once more reabsorbed from that site (enterohepatic circulation)
3. The degree to which each drug undergoes metabolic degradation in the liver
4. The speed with which the drug and any still active metabolites are excreted by the kidneys

Plasma binding. Most *digitoxin* molecules that enter the blood become tightly bound to serum albumin, from which they are then released at a relatively slow rate. This slow diffusibility of digitoxin accounts for the slowness with which its effects come on and rise to a peak—4 to 12 hours—even when it is injected directly into a vein. The fact that over 90% of digitoxin circulating in the bloodstream is bound to albumin also means that its actions might be intensified as the result of unexpected drug interactions (Chap. 4). For example, simultaneously taken doses of warfarin (Coumadin) and other drugs with a high affinity for albumin might displace digitoxin from its plasma protein-binding sites. More of the daily doses of this drug might then diffuse to the heart and cause toxic effects by accumulating in the myocardium to a greater extent than expected.

Digoxin, on the other hand, circulates in a form that is mostly free to diffuse out of the bloodstream. Thus, digoxin accumulates more rapidly in the myocardium and begins to exert its cardiotonic effect more quickly—in 30 minutes or less when injected intravenously. Digoxin also diffuses readily from the blood, passing through the glomeruli of the kidneys for excretion from the body. This accounts, in part, for the moderately rapid renal excretion of digoxin and for its relatively short half-life of about 36 hours, or 1½ days, in patients with normal kidney function.

Metabolism and enterohepatic circulation. Both these orally administered digitalis glycosides pass through the liver, which then tends to convert *digitoxin* to other inactive and active substances but does not alter *digoxin* to any extent.

Digitoxin is enzymatically degraded to metabolites that are mainly inactive but include a small amount of active digoxin, among other active breakdown products. The process of enzymatically catalyzed inactivation of digitoxin can be accelerated if a patient is simultaneously taking phenobarbital, phenytoin, oral hypoglycemic agents, phenylbutazone, rifampin, or some other enzyme-inducing drugs (Chap. 4). This type of drug interaction could cut the serum concentration of digitoxin to half of the steady state level at which the patient had originally been stabilized. To avoid the resulting loss of therapeutic effectiveness in a patient who requires both drugs, it would be necessary to raise the dose of digitoxin. (Actually, it would be preferable to discontinue phenobarbital, if possible, and to substitute a benzodiazepine or other antianxiety drug [see Chap. 45] or anticonvulsant drug that was *not* an enzyme inducer.)

A portion of the digitalis glycosides that have passed through the liver is excreted in the bile that enters the duodenum. Some of this stays in the body by being reabsorbed and recirculated through the liver, instead of being eliminated in the stool. This accounts, in part, for the prolonged biologic half-life of *digitoxin* (about 1 week), which undergoes such enterohepatic circulation to a much greater extent than does digoxin.

The bile-binding resins cholestyramine and colestipol (Chap. 32) can interfere with this recycling process by removing bile-dissolved digitoxin before it can be reabsorbed. This drug interaction decreases the half-life of digitoxin and could reduce its effectiveness in patients who are taking both types of drugs together. On the other hand, digitoxin-poisoned patients treated with colestipol are claimed to have been helped to recover because of the drug's ability to increase the rate of removal of digitoxin from the body (see treatment of intoxication, below).

Renal excretion. Both of the important digitalis glycosides are filtered from the blood by the glomeruli of the kidneys. Most of the filtered *digitoxin* is reabsorbed into the blood, and only a small proportion appears in the urine. *Digoxin*, on the other hand, is not reabsorbed by the renal tubules. Thus, renal excretion is the main route by which the largely unmetabolized, still active, digoxin molecules are eliminated from the body. The proportion of digoxin that is removed by renal excretion each day is between 35% and 40% of the total amount that has accumulated during daily dosing.

Although this *fraction* is a constant one, the *amount* of digoxin eliminated between doses increases as the total amount of drug stored in the body becomes greater. Finally, a point is reached at which patients with adequate kidney function can eliminate all of the last, previously administered dose before the following dose is due to be administered. Then, the residue of digoxin remaining in the body and exerting its desired therapeutic effects can be kept at the same effective steady state concentration by continuing to administer the same dose at the intervals that were previously established (see maintenance of digitalization, below).

Patients with impaired renal function and many elderly people do not adequately eliminate digoxin (Chap. 4). If the drug were to be administered in the same dose and at the same intervals as in younger patients with normal kidney function, it would soon accumulate to toxic levels. Fortunately, the ability of any patient's kidneys to filter digoxin is correlated with their ability to filter and remove creatinine. Thus, by checking the results of creatinine clearance tests, the degree to which the patient's glomerular filtration of digoxin is also impaired can be determined. This then permits calculation of the lower doses and the longer intervals between doses that are required to attain and maintain safe and effective stores of digoxin.

Therapeutic applications of digitalis glycosides

As indicated earlier, the actions of digitalis are applied clinically in the management of heart failure and certain cardiac arrhythmias. This chapter will focus on describing the nature of congestive failure and the manner in which the digitalis glycosides can best be employed to reverse the pathophysiology of this disorder and to safely relieve its signs and symptoms. The clinical use of digitalis for treating supraventricular arrhythmias will only briefly be discussed in this chapter and will then be reviewed more fully in the following chapter, which describes these and other arrhythmias and their management with antiarrhythmic drugs more completely. To appreciate the benefits brought about by digitalis in heart failure, it is first necessary to discuss the syndrome itself and how it develops.

The nature of congestive heart failure

The term *congestive heart failure* refers to a pathophysiologic state in which the heart *fails* to fulfill its function—pumping enough blood to the body's organs and tissues to meet their needs for oxygen and nutrients. Failure of the ventricles to force out into the arteries an adequate amount of the blood that is brought back to the heart by the veins leads in turn to venous engorgement as the blood backs up into the venous system waiting to get into the ventricles. This swelling of the veins within various organs, together with leakage of fluid from the venous capillaries into the tissue spaces and cavities, is what is meant by the term *congestive*. The accumulation of fluid in the lungs and elsewhere as a result of primary pump failure accounts for the discomforting and often dangerous signs and symptoms of congestive heart failure.

Etiology

Heart failure (formerly called cardiac decompensation) is not a specific cardiac disease but rather an acute or chronic syndrome that develops as a result of any of many other disorders that tend to overstress the normal functioning of the heart. The primary cardiac and extracardiac conditions that cause the heart to fail may do so in any of several ways, or sometimes by a combination of mechanisms. Three types of primary cardiovascular disorders account for about 95% of all heart failure cases. These are coronary artery disease (Chap. 31), hypertension (Chap. 28), and valvular heart disease.

In coronary heart disease, the myocardium fails gradually or suddenly because its ability to contract is impaired by the damage done to the heart muscle that is deprived of an adequate supply of the oxygen and nutrients needed for normal function. In hypertension, the heart is forced to work too hard to pump blood out into the arterial tree against the elevated peripheral resistance in the systemic circulation. Increased cardiac workload is also a factor that leads to failure in patients in whom mitral, aortic, or other heart valves have been scarred, narrowed, or made incompetent by primary valvular diseases. In other clinical situations, particularly those in which obstructions interfere with the free flow of blood into and out of the heart, the myocardium may fail as a result of *both* myocardial damage and mechanical factors.

Compensatory mechanisms

Many people with coronary, hypertensive, or valvular heart disease can carry on normal active lives for many years before they begin to show any signs of chronic congestive heart failure. This is because the cardiovascular system can put several efficient compensatory mechanisms

into play (Fig. 29-1). These help to maintain an adequate flow of blood to the vital organs, despite the presence of underlying diseases that adversely affect cardiac function. Heart failure develops only when these mechanisms can no longer compensate for the stresses put on the heart by the various primary disease states.

Some short-term adjustments to disease-induced stresses are similar to those by which the heart normally increases its output to meet a temporary increase in the demands of the tissues for more oxygenated blood. For example, as indicated in Chapter 26, increased sympathetic nerve impulses help the heart to pump more blood out into the arterial circulation. The activation of the renin–angiotensin system and the increased release of aldosterone increase blood volume and blood pressure and aid in maintaining perfusion of the kidneys and other tissues. Similarly, the myocardial fibers lengthen under an increased load of blood, filling the ventricles during diastole, and this, in accordance with the Frank–Starling mechanism, then leads to a more powerful pumping action

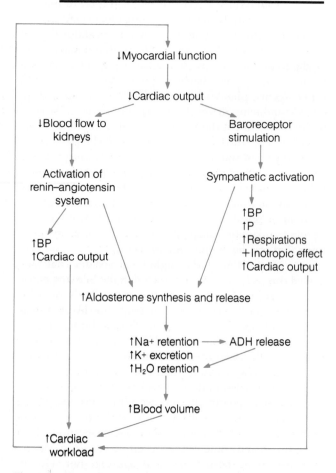

Figure 29-1. Compensatory mechanisms in congestive heart failure. The body's reflexes respond to the decrease in cardiac output through activities that increase blood pressure, blood volume, and cardiac output. Prolonged activity of the compensatory mechanisms, however, also increases cardiac workload, leading to further heart failure.

and increased stroke volume during the following systolic contraction.

Long-term compensatory mechanisms for maintaining normal cardiac output in the face of handicaps that force the heart to work harder lead to a gradual enlargement of the heart. Cardiac *hypertrophy*, an increase in thickness of the ventricular wall and in the weight of the heart, is one way in which the heart responds to a constant increase in the workload with which it must cope. Thus, for example, the left ventricle of patients with chronic arterial hypertension or with aortic valve narrowing grows in size when stimulated by the need to continue pumping blood into the systemic circulation against the increased resistance that occurs in these disorders—the so-called postload or afterload (Chap. 26).

The chambers of the heart also enlarge to accommodate a greater load of blood carried back to them by the pulmonary and systemic circulations—the venous return, or preload. The resulting increase in end diastolic volume and pressure leads to a more powerful systolic contraction. Thus, up to a point, the dilated heart can maintain an adequate stroke volume and cardiac output for a time, at least while the patient is at rest.

Unfortunately, the capacity of the cardiovascular system to compensate is limited and, if the primary underlying disorder cannot be corrected surgically or controlled by antihypertensive, antiarrhythmic, or other drugs, the patient eventually uses up the cardiac reserve and becomes decompensated. The failing compensatory mechanisms may, in fact, prove counterproductive. Thus, for example, the retention of sodium and water causes a fluid overload for the failing heart and leads to increased edema, putting even more demands on the myocardium. When the heart's chambers dilate excessively, the ventricular walls waste too much energy and oxygen while building up the tension required for contractions. Similarly, if reflex tachycardia becomes too rapid, the time needed for ventricular filling during diastole is excessively reduced, and the amount of blood that can be pumped with each contraction is actually decreased, as is the total cardiac output. Here, too, the amount of energy and oxygen consumed by the myocardium in performing its pumping function is increased, and the weakened heart beats inefficiently and with decreasing effectiveness.

Defects in failing heart cells

A greater understanding of how cardiac muscle cells produce their energy and use it in the contraction process has provided some insight into the decreased ability of the failing heart to convert the energy that it produces into productive pumping. It is thought that a defect in the ability of the failing heart's cells to shift calcium ions from the cells' outer and inner membranes to its contractile proteins is responsible. Reversal of this defect in calcium ion movement may also account for the ability of digitalis to increase the cells' conversion of biochemical energy into mechanical energy, and thus increase the

strength of the failing heart's contractions. (See also the above discussion of how digitalis strengthens the hypodynamic heart.)

Clinical signs and symptoms

As indicated in Table 29-2 and Figure 29-2, the appearance of the decompensated patient tends to reflect the mechanisms by which the body has attempted to adjust to the stresses put on the heart. The patient's signs and symptoms vary, of course, with the degree of decompensation and with whether failure developed suddenly—during a myocardial infarction, for example—or, as in most cases, as the end result of a prolonged process that had finally led to a loss of cardiac reserve. In addition, the presenting signs and symptoms vary in accordance with which heart chamber is primarily involved. That is, patients with left ventricular failure differ in appearance from those in whom the right side of the heart has failed first. (Actually, because the most common cause of right ventricular failure is prior failure of the left ventricle, patients in the later stages show signs of both left and right congestive heart failure.)

In either case, or both, the signs and symptoms involve changes in the size, rate, and rhythm of the heart, and congestion and edema in various organs and body cavities as a result of retention of excessive amounts of sodium and water. Diagnosis is not difficult on the basis of these cardiac and peripheral effects of heart failure, after other causes—primarily pulmonary diseases—have been ruled out.

Cardiac signs and symptoms of decompensation may be detected by physical examination and through use of x-rays and electrocardiograms (ECGs). *Cardiomegaly*, or cardiac enlargement is, for example, often present in patients who have been compensating for the effects of an increased workload or of myocardial disease by the mechanisms discussed earlier—cardiac dilation and left or right ventricular hypertrophy. It can be detected clinically by percussion or by palpation—that is, feeling for movements of the apex of the heart to determine the degree of its displacement. More precise measurements of heart size are made by chest x-ray or fluoroscopy.

Sinus tachycardia, often accompanied by palpitations or gallop rhythm, is also common. An ECG helps to determine whether the patient's rapid heart rate is caused by atrial fibrillation or by one of the other supraventricular arrhythmias that sometimes accompany heart failure (see below and Chap. 30). The presence of varying degrees of heart block (Chap. 26) that may be either a cause or a complication of congestive heart failure may also be detected electrocardiographically. In patients with heart muscle damage and left-sided failure, *pulsus alternans*, a condition in which strong beats are regularly followed by weak ones, can be detected by auscultating the peripheral pulses, or while taking the patient's blood pressure with a sphygmomanometer. *Heart murmurs* may be heard in patients in failure from the effects of damage

Table 29–2. Congestive heart failure and response to digitalis glycosides

Signs and symptoms*	Response	
	During congestive heart failure	After full digitalization†
Heart rate, rhythm, and size	Heart hypertrophied, dilated; rate rapid, irregular; "palpitations"; auscultation—S_3, S_4, pulsus alternans	Dilatation decreased, hypertrophy remains; rate, 70–80, may be regular; auscultation—S_4 may remain, no S_3, no pulsus alternans
Lungs	Dyspnea on exertion; orthopnea; tachypnea; paroxysmal nocturnal dyspnea; wheezing, rales, cough, hemoptysis (pulmonary edema)	↓ rate of respiration; wheezes, rales gone; diuretics, morphine, aminophylline may be needed to clear pulmonary edema
Peripheral congestion	Pitting edema of dependent parts; hepatomegaly; ↑ JVP; cyanosis; oliguria; nocturia	↑ cardiac output and renal blood flow leads to ↑ urine flow, ↓ edema, ↓ signs and symptoms of poor perfusion
Other	Weakness, fatigue, anorexia, insomnia, nausea, vomiting, abdominal pain	↑ appetite; ↑ strength, energy

* Because the clinical picture in heart failure varies with the stage and degree of severity, the signs and symptoms may vary considerably in different patients.

† Digitalis will not overcome similar symptoms when they are caused by conditions other than heart failure. Overdosage may actually cause symptoms similar to those of heart failure (*e.g.*, anorexia, nausea, and vomiting, cardiac arrhythmias, peripheral congestion).

to the various cardiac valves, most commonly mitral or aortic.

Peripheral effects of heart failure may be observed in the various organs and tissues in which the veins are distended or fluid is passing out of permeable venous capillaries. The signs and symptoms caused by congestion and edema reflect the heart's inability to transfer the blood brought back by the veins—the venous return or preload—into the arterial circulation. That is, the decrease in cardiac output of the decompensated heart causes the venous capillaries to become engorged with blood. This alters the balance between the physical forces that control the exchange of fluids between the bloodstream and the tissue spaces. The increased intravascular hydrostatic pressure within the swollen venous capillaries tends to force fluid out of the vessels and into the tissues. This accumulation of extravascular fluid, or edema, is

the main cause of the discomforting and dangerous signs and symptoms of congestive heart failure.

Left ventricular failure. This is marked mainly by engorgement of the pulmonary veins that leads to difficulty in breathing. *Tachypnea* (rapid shallow breathing) can be detected in patients with advanced heart failure even when they are at rest, and even those with milder degrees of failure often develop this sign during slight physical exertion. Such patients also often complain of *dyspnea*, a discomforting feeling of breathlessness that becomes more alarming during effort. Often, however, the patient's respiratory distress worsens when lying down (called *orthopnea*) because the pattern of blood flow changes in the supine position, increasing the pulmonary pressure and making the pulmonary congestion more severe. The distress is relieved when the patient sits up with the legs hanging down. This decreases the blood

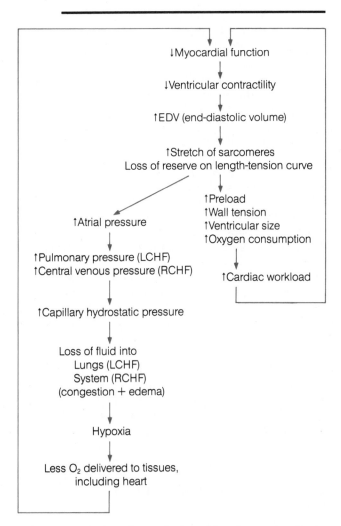

↓Myocardial function

↓Ventricular contractility

↑EDV (end-diastolic volume)

↑Stretch of sarcomeres
Loss of reserve on length-tension curve

↑Atrial pressure

↑Preload
↑Wall tension
↑Ventricular size
↑Oxygen consumption

↑Pulmonary pressure (LCHF)
↑Central venous pressure (RCHF)

↑Cardiac workload

↑Capillary hydrostatic pressure

Loss of fluid into
Lungs (LCHF)
System (RCHF)
(congestion + edema)

Hypoxia

Less O₂ delivered to tissues,
including heart

Figure 29-2. Mechanisms of congestive heart failure. Increased workload of a heart with decreased contractility leads to venous congestion and further increased workload.

return to the heart and relieves the workload on the heart, which in turn relieves the pulmonary congestion.

Sometimes patients with left-sided failure suffer sudden attacks of dyspnea during the night. Such *paroxysmal nocturnal dyspnea* wakens the patient from sleep in a state of anxiety. The attack usually subsides after the patient sits on the edge of the bed for a few minutes. Occasionally, however, the attack is a prelude to acute pulmonary edema, a condition in which fluid forms at first in the interstitial lung tissues and later in the alveoli or air sacs. (The emergency management of this life-threatening complication following a massive myocardial infarction is discussed in detail in Chapter 31.)

Presence of fluid in the air spaces causes a cough that produces varying amounts of frothy sputum that may be tinged pink by traces of blood (hemoptysis). The rales (abnormal lung sounds) that develop are somewhat similar to those of bronchial asthma, but this condition

does not respond well to treatment with the adrenergic bronchodilators that often relieve the obstructive lung disorder's symptoms. Aminophylline is more effective and less dangerous than the adrenergic bronchodilators when administered cautiously to these cardiac patients. (See Chapter 40 for details of IV infusion therapy of bronchial asthma, and Chapter 31 for treatment of pulmonary edema.)

Right ventricular failure. This occurs in patients with acute exacerbation of emphysema and other chronic pulmonary diseases (cor pulmonale) as a result of pulmonary hypertension that is also marked by such symptoms as dyspnea and cyanosis. However, most other signs and symptoms of right ventricular failure are the result of a rise in systemic (rather than pulmonary) venous pressure. The elevated pressure is readily detectable in the patient's elevated JVP (jugular venous pressure), which may make the neck appear to be swollen and throbbing.

Hepatomegaly or liver enlargement is another indication of an increase in systemic circulation pressure in right-sided heart failure. Continued liver congestion can cause pain and tenderness, jaundice, and cirrhotic damage. In patients with advanced failure, the long-continued high hydrostatic pressure in the venous capillaries of the liver, spleen, and other viscera forces fluid out into the peritoneal cavity—a form of edema called *ascites* that causes a discomforting feeling of abdominal fullness and loss of appetite.

Fluid may also collect in such other serous spaces as the pleural cavity (hydrothorax) and even within the pericardium, another cause of cardiac enlargement. Edema may develop in subcutaneous tissues throughout the body in right ventricular failure, a condition called *anasarca*. A *pitting edema* on pressure is usually seen first in the feet and ankles of ambulatory patients but tends to disappear during the night when the patient's feet are elevated. This positioning will also help to increase the venous return to the heart. The return of fluid to the systemic circulation will increase the blood being pumped to the kidneys, and this increases nocturnal urine formation. It is important to remember that patients who tend to retain fluid during the day with an accompanying decrease in urination (*oliguria*) may need to void a large volume of urine shortly after going to bed or early in the morning (*nocturia*).

Management of heart failure

Clinical indications for digitalis

Digitalis glycosides are remarkably effective drugs for relief of congestive heart failure signs and symptoms that develop as a result of chronic malfunction of the myocardium. In such cases, the administration of adequate doses produces a prompt improvement in cardiac function and in the patient's signs and symptoms. Relief of peripheral congestion soon follows. However, all patients with congestive heart failure do not respond equally well, and some may even be made worse by attempts to treat their condition with digitalis.

Digitalis is most effective for patients in whom the primary defect is a gradual reduction in myocardial contractility. It is particularly useful when the resulting reduction in cardiac output and coronary artery perfusion sets off atrial fibrillation, a disorder that speeds up the rate of ventricular contractions (see below; also see Chap. 30). However, when failure is the result of mechanical defects that interfere with the flow of blood out of the heart—for example, in constrictive pericarditis or hypertrophic subaortic stenosis (Chap. 30)—digitalis is less likely to give a good result. Similarly, digitalis is not very useful for cases of high output failure—for example, in hyperthyroidism—in which the heart finally fails to meet the abnormally elevated demands of the peripheral tissues for oxygen, and in other disorders marked by excessively high metabolic requirements. Use of digitalis may be dangerous in patients with acute myocarditis of rheumatic or other origins and in other disorders (see the discussion of digitalis toxicity, below).

Cardiac function improvement

The positive inotropic action of digitalis (see above) helps the failing heart to function more efficiently. Its chambers do not need to fill as fully nor do the muscular walls of the ventricles have to build up as much filling pressure. The drug-induced increase in contractile force and velocity that leads to a rise in the volume of blood pumped during each systolic contraction also results in a decrease in intraventricular end diastolic pressure and in intraventricular volume. This, in turn, results in a reduction in the size of the dilated cardiac chambers.

The decrease in the size of the dilated heart also adds to myocardial efficiency, because a smaller heart uses up less oxygen and energy in developing increased pumping power. Thus, as the digitalis-induced increase in stroke volume reduces the amount of residual blood within the ventricles, excessive stretching of heart muscle fibers is reversed. Chest x-rays reveal that the size of the heart's chambers has become smaller during digitalization—another indication that the ventricles are beating more efficiently.

Digitalis also exerts desirable direct and indirect effects on the rate and rhythm of the failing heart. The early benefits are brought about by the drug's positive inotropic action. Later changes that help to slow a rapid irregular heartbeat are the result of the direct and reflex effects of digitalis on the specialized pacemaker and conducting tissues. The initial positive inotropic effect and the resulting increase in stroke volume and cardiac output that improve the peripheral circulation help to reverse the compensatory increase in sympathetic impulses that sometimes occurs in heart failure. As the tissues begin

to receive adequate quantities of blood, the stimuli that had set off the cardioacceleratory compensatory reflexes are removed. The heart rate of patients whose hearts had speeded up (sinus tachycardia) in an effort to meet the needs of the tissues for blood commonly drops by about 30% after adequate digitalization has helped to improve the circulation. Other digitalis actions described earlier help to slow the heart's rapid rate when this is caused by an arrhythmia that has developed in patients with poor coronary perfusion.

In *atrial fibrillation*, for example, impulses arise in atrial tissues other than the S-A nodal pacemaker. These ectopic pacemakers may fire at rates between 400 and 600 beats/minute. Although the A-V node and other conducting tissues are refractory to most of these atrial impulses, enough get through to drive the ventricles at rates of between 100 and 200 beats/minute. In such cases, digitalis acts to prolong the refractory period of the A-V conducting tissues and to reduce A-V junctional conduction velocity. It does so by a combination of vagal and extravagal effects—by increasing the sensitivity of the A-V nodal tissues to the braking action of the vagus, and by directly depressing the conducting tissues.

These cardiac actions of digitalis help to protect the ventricles against bombardment by rapid atrial impulses. As a result, the ventricular rate of patients with this atrial arrhythmia is controlled and may fall to between 70 and 80 beats/minute. Following full digitalization, any pulse deficit that may previously have been detectable in the heart failure patient with rapid, irregular cardiac rhythm is no longer present. That is, the apical pulse is now promptly followed by a pulse that *can* be felt brachially.

Digitalis is sometimes used to treat another cardiac irregularity, *atrial flutter*. In part it is used here, again, to protect the ventricles by producing a partial block of A-V conduction. In addition, the drug may sometimes help to convert the flutter to a normal sinus rhythm. Oddly, this often happens only after digitalis has first sent the fluttering atria into fibrillation. If the drug is then discontinued, the atria often stop fibrillating spontaneously and begin beating normally. If they fail to do so, atrial fibrillation can usually be overcome by careful administration of the antiarrhythmic drugs quinidine and procainamide or by such measures as cardioversion (Chap. 30).

Paroxysmal atrial tachycardia (PAT) is another cardiac arrhythmia that responds very well to digitalis. In this disorder, which often develops in patients with rheumatic, arteriosclerotic, and hypertensive heart disease, digitalis not only prevents the rapidly generated atrial impulses from reaching the ventricles but also often brings about a normal sinus rhythm. This is best accomplished by intravenous injection of a relatively rapid-acting glycoside such as digoxin or deslanoside. (See Chapter 30 for a more detailed discussion of the use of digitalis and antiarrhythmic drugs and other measures in the management of this supraventricular arrhythmia.)

Circulatory improvement

Because the ventricles empty more completely, they can cope more readily with the load of blood being brought back to the heart by the veins. This circulatory improvement, which is a hemodynamic consequence of the primary positive inotropic action of digitalis, permits edema fluid to be reabsorbed from the tissues. As this fluid is transferred into the arterial portion of the circulation, the pressure in the previously engorged veins falls. This reduction in venous hydrostatic pressure leads, in turn, to relief of lung congestion and of the peripheral congestion and signs of edema in the skin, limbs, abdomen, and elsewhere.

As fluid leaves the lungs of a patient with pulmonary edema, the dyspnea is usually relieved. With easier breathing, the patient's anxiety and restlessness are reduced, skin color is restored, and cyanosis lessens. In patients with right heart failure, abdominal distention lessens, and pitting no longer occurs when the skin of an extremity is pressed. Better kidney function is manifested by a marked increase in urine production, which may rise from as little as half a pint (250 ml) or less (oliguria) to as much as several quarts (2 or 3 liters) each day.

Diuresis

Patients often show a marked weight decrease, because the train of circulatory events set in motion by the inotropic action of digitalis helps to drain edema fluid from the tissue spaces and carries it to the kidneys for excretion. The diuresis may also be produced by a digitalis-induced reduction in sympathetic outflow to the kidneys, which improves renal perfusion. The patient's urinary output and extent of the weight loss should be carefully recorded, because these signs are a useful index of the drug's desirable action. If improvement of edema is incomplete, a diuretic (Chap. 27) may be added to the treatment regimen to bring the patient down to a "dry weight."

Digitalis is not a true diuretic, because it has little direct effect on the kidneys. However, the drug improves renal circulation in ways that help to reverse the complex renal compensatory processes that had led to sodium and water retention in the heart failure patient. As indicated in Chapter 27, a decrease in cardiac output sets off a cycle of hemodynamic and hormonal events that causes the kidneys to retain more sodium and water.

These compensatory mechanisms help to maintain cardiac output by increasing the blood volume and the amount of blood that is brought back to the right side of the heart. However, because the patient's damaged heart may not be able to cope with this increased venous return, or preload, the resulting hypervolemia can actually become counterproductive, as is the case with the cardiac compensatory mechanisms. Thus, renal retention of sodium and water accounts for the venous congestion and resulting edema that lead to the signs and symptoms of heart failure.

Digitalis-induced diuresis is another beneficial result of the drug's primary positive inotropic effect. The increased cardiac output brings a better blood supply to the kidneys, and the improvement in renal hemodynamics restores the normal pattern of perfusion through these organs. This redistribution of the intrarenal blood flow somehow reduces the abnormally high proportion of filtered sodium that the renal tubules reabsorb in heart failure.

In addition, improved renal perfusion reverses the hormonal mechanism that also plays a part in sodium and water retention—that is, the renin–angiotensin-aldosterone-producing reaction (Chap. 27) by which the kidneys compensate for loss of blood volume. This mechanism, which helps to prevent the body from losing further fluid when hypovolemia is actually present—in hemorrhage, for example—operates inappropriately in heart failure and leads to congestion and edema. Digitalis reverses this sodium-retaining process by counteracting heart failure. This puts a stop to the persistent stimuli that, in heart failure, lead to continued release of renin and excessive adrenal secretion of the mineralocorticoid hormone aldosterone (Chap. 21). Presumably, the cardiac action of digitalis leads to a rise in blood flow through the renal afferent arterioles, and the greater filling of these vessels and increased stretching of their walls cut off the signals that had been stimulating excess renin secretion.

Digitalis toxicity

Digitalis is remarkably effective for reversing the signs and symptoms of congestive heart failure and for slowing the rapid ventricular rate of supraventricular arrhythmias, but this very useful drug can also *cause* dangerous cardiotoxicity. About 10% of patients taking digitalis are said to show signs of such toxicity, and two or three times as many of those taking this drug together with a diuretic have been found to be suffering from digitalis intoxication. According to one survey, about one of every three digitalis-toxic patients dies.

Recognizing toxicity

The nurse should suspect possible overdosage in any patient who becomes more ill while taking digitalis. The nurse may be the first to detect early signs and symptoms while checking the rate and rhythm of the patient's heart. Complaints of gastrointestinal upset and of disturbances in vision should also alert the astute nurse to the onset of digitalis toxicity. The drug's effects on nervous system function can also cause behavioral changes and neuro-muscular signs and symptoms that indicate overdosage.

The nurse should be able to recognize the characteristic cardiac and *non*cardiac changes induced by digitalis overdosage. If a patient exhibits any of the signs and symptoms of digitalis toxicity, the drug should be discontinued until a blood sample for serum digitalis determination has been drawn. Appropriate adjustment in dosage can then be made, if necessary.

Digitalis-induced arrhythmias

Digitalis overdosage can lead to almost every type of cardiac arrhythmia. Thus, no abnormality that may be detected on an ECG is specifically characteristic of digitalis-induced toxicity. Certain ECG patterns occur so often with digitalis overdosage, however, that their appearance raises the possibility of toxicity. Some clinical signs should also suggest digitalis overdosage—for example, a drop in the patient's apical pulse rate to below 60 beats/minute, and "coupling," the occurrence of a regular beat followed almost immediately by a weak one. Thus, cardiac slowing, coupled beats, and also the presence of pulse deficit— the lack of a pulse at the wrist when an apical pulse is heard—may be indications of the presence of drug-related extrasystoles.

Digitalis-induced arrhythmias may be broadly categorized as those caused by disturbances in *automaticity,* and those caused by impaired impulse *conduction*. Sometimes arrhythmias develop that are the result of both these processes occurring together. Thus, digitalis overdosage may manifest itself by an *increased* heart rate as well as by *bradycardia,* and the patient's cardiac rhythm may be *regular* as well as *irregular*. The following discussion offers examples of digitalis-induced cardiac disturbances that stem from all three types of electrophysiologic abnormalities.

Effects of digitalis-induced automaticity. The most common digitalis-induced arrhythmia is the development of extrasystoles—particularly premature ventricular contractions (PVCs). This shows up easily on the ECG, but it may also be detected clinically as coupling and pulse deficit (see above) when a weak beat is heard through the stethoscope placed above the apex of the patient's heart while no corresponding pulsation is felt at the patient's wrist. As indicated in Chapter 26, such impulses arising at multiple ectopic foci can be precursors of dangerously rapid ventricular tachyarrhythmias that can lead to fatal ventricular fibrillation. Thus, such rhythm

---

* Premature ventricular contractions are also common in patients with coronary artery disease (Chap. 31) and can, of course, occur in such patients when they are developing heart failure. Thus, to determine whether these and other extrasystoles are caused by overdosage or underdosage, other diagnostic methods in addition to the ECG may have to be employed, such as measurement of the patient's serum concentration of digitalis glycosides.

irregularities as bigeminy and trigeminy may indicate the need for reduction in digitalis dosage when they appear in a patient who had shown no previous sign of an ectopic arrhythmia.*

Digitalis intoxication can also cause supraventricular tachyarrhythmias that develop as a result of the complex effects of the drug on the electrical properties of cardiac tissues. Premature atrial contractions, atrial tachycardia, and supraventricular tachycardia can develop when digitalis increases the rate at which impulses arise spontaneously from ectopic automatic cells in the atrial and A-V nodal tissues. However, similar rapid arrhythmias may occur when digitalis depresses the S-A pacemaker. That is, when digitalis increases vagal action on the pacemaker while increasing automaticity in other atrial and nodal tissues and reducing their refractory period, latent pacemakers at these sites may take control of the cardiac rhythm.

Effects of digitalis on conduction. Digitalis can cause varying degrees of A-V block and dissociation of atrial and ventricular rhythms (Chap. 26). Digitalis-induced first-degree block—marked only by some prolongation of the P–R interval on the ECG—is usually considered to be a desirable effect when digitalis is being employed clinically in the management of supraventricular arrhythmias (see above and Chap. 30). That is, this effect plays a part in the therapeutically useful slowing of the ventricular rate in patients with atrial fibrillation and similar atrial beat disorders. However, too great a lengthening of the P–R interval may be an early sign of digitalis overdose that precedes more serious second-degree blocks and complete heart block.

In both the latter disorders, and in digitalis-induced S-A nodal block and sinus bradycardia, the heart may beat at an abnormally slow rate. A drop in the heart rate to levels below 60 beats/minute usually signals an excessive effect of the drug. Too slow a heartbeat is bad in itself, because it may reduce blood flow to the brain or through the coronary vessels that supply the myocardium. In addition, excessive slowing can set the stage for escape rhythms that may terminate in ventricular fibrillation. Ordinarily, for example, when the A-V node is blocked, ectopic automatic cells set up a slow *idioventricular* rhythm. However, if digitalis then increases the rate at which such escape pacemakers fire, while the drug at the same time reduces the refractory period of ventricular tissues, dangerous re-entry type rhythms (Chap. 26) may result.

Combined effects of digitalis. A more common cause of a combined digitalis-induced increase in automaticity together with a decrease in conduction is seen in the frequent development of PAT together with A-V block of varying degrees. This common toxic effect of digitalis—called PAT with block—tends to be marked by very irregular rhythms, because some of the impulses that arise in the atria at a rapid rate reach the ventricles while others fail to penetrate the A-V node. On the other hand, digitalis toxicity can be marked by a quite regular rhythm and either a rapid or an almost normal ventricular rate. This can occur through a drug-induced combination of A-V block together with development of an A-V junctional rhythm caused by automatic nodal cells at the junction firing regularly at a moderate or a rapid rate.

Hemodynamic consequences of cardiotoxicity

Digitalis toxicity, by causing the heart to beat too slowly or too rapidly, can lead to a reduction in cardiac output. This effect—the opposite of that produced by the drug's positive inotropic action—can cause signs of congestive heart failure to reappear. Thus, the patient may appear to be underdigitalized but, if digitalis dosage is increased, this will only worsen the cardiotoxicity of the already overdosed patient. To help avoid such potential catastrophes, other noncardiac, or extracardiac, side-effects that often accompany digitalis overdosage should be evaluated and recorded.

Extracardiac signs and symptoms. Although the first and occasionally the only sign of digitalis toxicity is the development of an abnormal cardiac rate and rhythm, most patients first show signs and symptoms of gastrointestinal upset and central nervous system stimulation. Most commonly, the patient complains of headache and nausea, and may also display a marked aversion to food. Such anorexia should be promptly reported to the physician, because it is often a sign that the patient is fully digitalized and is entering an early toxic state.

Anorexia and nausea are often followed by salivation, vomiting, abdominal pain, and diarrhea. Late vomiting is significant, because it means that digitalis has accumulated in the brain in amounts sufficient to stimulate the central vomiting mechanism. This vomiting is *not* the result of gastrointestinal tract irritation; it can even occur when digitalis glycosides are given by vein rather than orally. Of course, if a patient vomits shortly after receiving the very first dose of digitalis, it is probably *not* caused by overdosage. Some products, such as powdered digitalis, tend to cause early gastrointestinal tract irritation. Also, patients with congestive heart failure are often nauseated to begin with. In such cases giving the digitalis preparation with meals may reduce the local irritation that causes vomiting.

Other direct effects of digitalis on the central nervous system include drowsiness, feelings of fatigue, dizziness and, rarely, convulsions. Sometimes, elderly patients with cerebral arteriosclerosis develop disorientation, confusion, delirium, and even hallucinations and delusions. Some patients may suffer severe facial neuralgia or other neuralgic aches and pains that they do not recognize as toxic effects of digitalis.

Such complaints should alert the nurse to the possibility that the patient may be suffering from overdosage, even though cardiotoxic effects are not yet ap-

parent. The patient should also be questioned about eyesight; such common signs of drug-induced ocular toxicity as flickering flashes of yellow-green lights, the presence of white dots or "snowflakes," and blurring or double vision may then be mentioned. All these visual and neurologic effects are an indication that digitalis should be discontinued before cardiotoxicity develops.

Treatment

The simplest measure, and sometimes the only one that is required, is to discontinue digitalis immediately when toxicity is suspected. When the drug's next scheduled doses are withheld while the patient continues to be closely observed, signs and symptoms of overdosage may soon disappear. This is particularly true with glycosides such as digoxin that are eliminated relatively rapidly, especially when the drug's adverse effects are of the *noncardiac* type. With digitoxin, and particularly when signs of cardiotoxicity have already appeared, specific treatment may be required for a week or more.

Tachyarrhythmia treatment

Oral or intravenous administration of potassium salts is often the first specific treatment to be tried in patients whose ECG reveals PVCs or supraventricular tachycardias such as PAT. This usually corrects the digitalis-induced loss of potassium from within myocardial cells and thus reduces the rise of impulses from ectopic automatic cells that account for the extrasystoles and other rapid rhythms (see above). Potassium chloride is considered to be the best salt for correcting hypokalemia and hypochloremia (Chap. 27) if these electrolyte imbalances are seen—as they often are—in patients who have been receiving too high doses of diuretics together with digitalis.

Patients who receive potassium salt treatment—particularly by intravenous drip—should be constantly monitored electrocardiographically. If signs of conduction abnormalities appear the drip is discontinued, because potassium overdosage can lead to heart block and cardiac arrest. Potassium therapy is probably best avoided in most patients whose ECGs already show a digitalis-induced decrease in A-V conduction (see below).

Antiarrhythmic drugs of all types are also sometimes employed to suppress ventricular ectopic beats and more serious rapid arrhythmias such as ventricular tachycardia that have been induced by digitalis. Procainamide[+] and quinidine[+] (see Drug digests, Chap. 30) are effective for this purpose, but today the antiarrhythmic agents phenytoin[+] (see Drug digests, Chap. 50) and lidocaine[+] (see Chaps. 14 and 30, and Drug digests of Chap. 14) are preferred. The main reason for this is that, unlike the two older drugs, these newer agents are not likely to depress the A-V conducting tissues or to affect ventricular conduction velocity adversely when infused intravenously. Propranolol[+] (see Chaps. 18 and 30, and Drug digests of Chap. 18) is also sometimes employed, particularly when the digitalis-toxic patient's rapid heart rate appears to originate at a supraventricular site and when there is no sign of A-V block. However, its effects—like that of all these potent drugs—should be carefully monitored by ECG to detect early signs of a drug-induced slowing of conduction or depression of myocardial contractility.

Treatment of bradycardia and heart block

Patients with very slow heart rates or with advanced degrees of digitalis-induced heart block are best managed today by transvenous insertion of a temporary electronic pacemaker into the right ventricle. However, certain drugs including *atropine*+ (see Chap. 16 and its Drug digests), which counteracts the vagal effects of digitalis on the S-A and A-V nodes, may sometimes prove effective for increasing the heart rate and reducing the degree of block. *Isoproterenol*+ (see Chap. 17 and its Drug digests) is a more dangerous drug for increasing the heart rate, because this catecholamine may add to the digitalis-induced increase in ventricular automatic cell activity that causes extrasystoles. Such ectopic activity is especially hazardous in patients with complete heart block. *Phenytoin*, which—as mentioned above—suppresses automaticity without decreasing conductivity, sometimes actually reduces digitalis-induced A-V block.

Other measures

Because calcium tends to increase digitalis cardiotoxicity of both the heart block and heart-stimulating types, chelating agents (Chap. 5) that bind calcium ions have been employed in treatment. *Disodium edetate* (Endrate), has sometimes proved successful, for example, in treating the digitalis-induced type of toxicity that is marked by a combination of PAT with A-V block. However, this drug is today reserved mainly for digitalis-toxic patients who also have hypercalcemia, rather than for routine treatment of those with normal serum calcium levels.

Several new types of treatments are still in experimental stages. One of these involves the oral administration of the bile-binding agents cholestyramine and colestipol (Chap. 32) to speed the removal of digitoxin from the body when it is excreted into the upper intestine with liver bile. By removing this digitalis glycoside in the stool along with the bound bile, these substances prevent it from re-entering the enterohepatic cycle (see above). This helps to lower its serum concentration and shortens its half-life and the duration of its toxic effects.

A new experimental immunologic approach to treatment involves the preparation of antibodies called *Fab fragments* (antigen-binding globulin fragments), which interact specifically with digitalis glycosides. When administered to digitalis-poisoned animals, such antibodies have combined with the glycosides, corrected the drug-induced cardiac arrhythmias, and prevented the expected death of the animals. In human trials, this preparation has also rapidly and completely reversed the signs and symptoms of overdosage, and led to complete recovery in more than 80% of cases.

Prevention

Research findings have led to a better understanding of the factors that contribute to the high incidence of digitalis intoxication. Application of this knowledge has helped to reduce the frequency of this dangerous type of toxicity in hospitals that have provided educational programs for their staffs.

General considerations

Digitalis glycosides all have a relatively narrow safety margin between the doses needed for therapeutic effectiveness and those that can cause cardiotoxicity. In addition, individual patients vary widely in the dosage of digitalis that they require and can tolerate. Thus, it is very important to recognize those patients who are most sensitive to digitalis and to adjust the average drug dosage downward to avoid overdosage.

Caution is also necessary, even with heart failure patients who do not seem especially predisposed to develop toxic reactions. In contrast to the traditional view that dosage of digitalis for these patients should be pushed to the point of early toxicity, there is a current trend toward the use of moderate doses rather than the largest dose that the patient can tolerate. It is now also felt that, except in emergencies, patients should be digitalized slowly with frequent observation of how they are responding. Finally, as indicated below in more detail, new knowledge of the pharmacokinetics of digoxin has led to a reduction in the average digitalizing and maintenance doses of that drug considerably below those previously recommended.

Specific factors

The single most significant factor associated with digitalis toxicity is the concurrent use of diuretic drugs in excessive dosage. Loss of potassium from the extracellular fluids increases the sensitivity of the myocardium to digitalis-induced tachyarrhythmias. Thus, to avoid *hypokalemia* and the resulting increase in digitalis-induced automaticity in ectopic pacemakers, diuretics should be employed cautiously in accordance with the principles discussed in Chapter 27 for preventing potassium depletion.

Other electrolyte imbalances may also predispose patients to digitalis toxicity, even when they are taking ordinary doses of the glycosides and their serum concentrations do not rise to excessive levels. Excessively high serum levels of potassium are—as indicated above—associated with digitalis-induced bradycardia and heart block. *Hyperkalemia* may develop in a digitalized patient who takes excessive amounts of a potassium salt supplement or who continues to take such a supplement after the regimen has been changed from a potassium-losing diuretic to one of the potassium-sparing diuretics, such as *spironolactone* (Chap. 27).

Hypomagnesemia also tends to increase sensitivity to digitalis. This electrolyte deficit occurs most commonly in alcoholics. When magnesium levels are checked and hypomagnesemia is detected, it can be corrected by administering soluble, absorbable magnesium salts. As indicated earlier, *hypercalcemia* also favors development of digitalis toxicity. Calcium levels should be checked in heart failure patients with hyperparathyroidism or with certain types of cancer that cause calcium to move from bones to the blood. It is not caused by taking oral calcium supplements.

Predisposing diseases

As indicated earlier, some heart failure patients do not respond well to digitalis because of the nature of their primary cardiac defect and some, in fact, are harmed by this drug. Ironically, among those most prone to develop toxicity are those with the most severe degrees of heart disease. Patients with advanced heart disease are so sensitive to digitalis that drug-induced arrhythmias may occur with only a fraction of the dose needed for digitalization of most patients and toxicity can, in fact, occur before any beneficial effects are seen. Sometimes, patients who had been maintained on the same dose of digitalis for many years slide into a state of toxicity as their myocardium deteriorates with advancing age.

Caution is also required in administering digitalis following an acute myocardial infarction (AMI). Some physicians feel that its use is dangerous, because the drug may set off arrhythmias in the ischemic hypoxic myocardium of AMI patients. Others claim that its use is both safe and beneficial for patients with pump failure (Chap. 31) when small doses are administered at intervals with ECG monitoring. Prophylactic use of digitalis in uncomplicated AMI cases is usually considered inappropriate. The vasoconstricting effect of intravenously injected glycosides may raise peripheral resistance and thus increase the work of the damaged myocardium.

Patients with cor pulmonale—right-sided heart failure secondary to chronic lung diseases—may also be excessively sensitive to the arrhythmia-producing effects of digitalis. This may be because the hypoxia and acid–base imbalances in such patients tend to lead to arrhythmias. Thus, these physiologic abnormalities should be corrected, if possible, before digitalis is employed in patients with emphysema and other obstructive lung disorders.

Thyroid disease also influences the response of patients to digitalis. *Hypothyroid* patients, for example, may suffer severe bradycardia after only relatively small doses. *Hyperthyroid* patients are relatively resistant to digitalis when attempts are made to increase the cardiac output in heart failure. However, it is not desirable to push digitalis dosage in such patients, because the drug may set off arrhythmias before it favorably affects heart failure symptoms or reduces the rapid ventricular rate.

Kidney disease, as indicated earlier, usually requires a reduction of digoxin dosage, because renal excretion is the main route of elimination of this glycoside. Patients with renal impairment require much smaller than average doses for digitalization, and maintenance doses may be administered at longer than usual intervals to avoid the accumulation of digoxin in the body. Digitoxin also depends on the kidneys for elimination of its metabolites, which include digoxin. However, because most of any dose of digitoxin is excreted as conjugated inactive metabolites, the presence of kidney disease is less serious in patients taking this glycoside. On the other hand, severe *liver disease* may interfere with the metabolism of digitoxin and may raise its potential toxicity unless the dosage is adjusted downward when signs of accumulation appear.

Radioimmune assay

Toxicity can today often be prevented through use of this analytic technique, which can be done by most hospital laboratories. The test, which is an important tool for determining whether the doses that patients have been taking are safe and effective, can determine minute amounts of digoxin, digitoxin, and other glycosides. The glycosidal serum levels correlate well—within limits—with the patient's clinical responses.

Thus, for example, most heart failure patients found to have digoxin serum levels of between 0.8 and 1.6 ng/ml of serum show evidence of clinical improvement without significant signs of toxicity.* When serum concentrations of the drug rise well above 2.0 ng/ml, many patients have symptoms of excessive drug effects, and almost all with digoxin levels above 3.0 ng/ml show signs and symptoms of toxicity.

Patients, of course, vary somewhat in their sensitivity to the same serum concentration, as previously indicated. However, evaluation of the radioimmune assay report, in conjunction with the patient's clinical condition and ECG, can usually clarify whether the drug's dosage is safe or has to be reduced to avoid more serious toxicity. The test can also be performed with patients who are taking digitoxin. The ratio between therapeutic and toxic concentrations is about the same as with digoxin, but the serum concentrations of this glycoside are about ten times as high—with about 10 ng/ml of serum digitoxin indicating therapeutic activity, and 30 ng/ml indicating toxicity, for instance.

Dosage and administration of digitalis preparations

The most commonly used products today are the pure crystalline glycosides *digoxin* and *digitoxin*. *Deslanoside* injections are sometimes employed in emergencies because of their rapid onset of action and the speed with which peak effects are reached. However, most physicians prefer to inject the only slightly slower glycoside digoxin in such urgent situations; oral digoxin can then be employed for

---

* A nanogram (ng) is one billionth (0.000000001) of a gram.

maintenance, as it is in the management of routine cases. This is because digoxin's relatively rapid onset and intermediate duration of action offer flexibility both in establishing relatively quick therapeutic activity and in maintaining long-term control with relative stability and safety. Some physicians continue to employ digitoxin because its long elimination half-life allows a stable level to be maintained even when patients miss a few doses occasionally.

Digitalization

It has long been customary to begin digitalis therapy by administering a relatively large *loading dose* (Chap. 4) over a period of about 12 to 24 hours. After the drug level in the body has reached a concentration that can produce the therapeutically desired effects on myocardial function, treatment is continued with a much lower daily *maintenance dose*. This is an amount of the drug that is just enough to replace the amount that had been eliminated by the body in the interval since the previous dose was administered. Thus, the therapeutic level that was attained in the initial, relatively rapid loading dosage process can be maintained for very long periods, provided that there is no change in the underlying heart disease.

Rapid digitalization. This is a relatively dangerous procedure that is best reserved for patients whose condition requires quick control—for example, those who show signs of serious heart failure such as acute pulmonary edema (Chap. 31), or patients with a very rapid ventricular rate caused by atrial fibrillation or other supraventricular tachyarrhythmias (Chap. 30). It does not appear appropriate to administer large loading doses to patients with mild heart failure or with only sinus tachycardia or no increase at all in their ventricular rate.

Slow digitalization. There seems to be a trend toward the administration of relatively small daily doses of *digoxin* over a period of about 1 week to attain digitalization more slowly and safely. After 5 to 7 days of treatment with the same properly chosen fixed dose of digoxin, a plateau drug level, or steady state (Chap. 4) is attained. The same dose may then be administered daily to maintain the total body stores of this drug at the same level indefinitely.

It is also thought that, even when the use of a loading dose seems desirable because of an urgent need for rapid digitalization, that dose of digoxin should be much lower than was previously employed. The initial loading dose does not need to be any larger than the total amount of this drug that is stored in the body after about 1 week of treatment with the small daily doses that are administered in the slow digitalization procedure. In addition, the recommended intervals at which fractions of the full, rapidly administered digitalizing dose are given have been lengthened. (See the Dosage and administration section of the Drug digests for digoxin, in which the loading doses for oral and intravenous use are 50% of those previously recommended, and the additional frac-

tional doses are timed to follow the initial doses at longer intervals than had been customary.)

Digitoxin is not administered gradually for slow digitalization, as is done with digoxin. This is because this drug's long half-life—5 to 7 days—and the small fraction of the total body stores eliminated daily—only 10% of what had previously accumulated—makes such a procedure impractical. That is, unlike digoxin, which has a half-life of only about $1\frac{1}{2}$ days and a daily elimination rate of about 35% of the total body stores, digitoxin would require about 1 month to attain a steady state plateau concentration if it were administered slowly in small, safe therapeutic doses. Thus, a loading dose is always employed to digitalize patients with digitoxin rapidly. However, the full digitalizing dose is not given all at once; rather, the total dose is divided into two or more smaller doses administered several hours apart (see the Drug digests).

Maintenance management

To sustain the therapeutic effect that is achieved by either slow or rapid digitalization, it is necessary to keep the total accumulated body stores of the drug at the initial level. As indicated above, the amount of drug that is eliminated in a certain period must be replaced by administering the proper maintenance dose at appropriate intervals. Although the doses that are administered for maintenance are low as compared to the amounts that were initially accumulated over a relatively short period, the risk of toxicity caused by overdosage remains, as does the possible development of an underdigitalized state.

Digitalis toxicity or edema and other signs of failure often develop gradually during long-term maintenance therapy. The main reason for this is that many patients fail to comply with the directions that they were first given for taking their medication. Diet, other drugs, and sometimes the patient's condition may change with increasing age and as progressive deterioration of cardiac or renal function occurs. Taking the same maintenance dose may then lead to overdosage and cardiotoxicity.

It is agreed that patients should be seen often and observed carefully to be sure that the maintenance dosage of digitalis originally ordered is still keeping their cardiac activity at an optimal functional level.

Thus, *in summary,* digitalis is considered to be the most effective drug for managing heart failure. However, the potential toxicity of these glycosides and their relatively slow rise to peak effects make their use dangerous in some clinical situations and not optimally effective in other cases. Thus, for example, in pump failure following an AMI, some now prefer to try other positive inotropic agents or even various arterial vasodilator drugs that can also improve the performance of the patient's failing heart. (See Chapter 31 for discussions of the use of *adrenergic* inotropic drugs for treating cardiogenic shock and of vasodilators such as nitroglycerin and sodium nitroprusside in the management of AMI-induced left ventricular failure and acute pulmonary edema.)

Because of the problems and limitations in the use of digitalis, as well as in the use of the adrenergic agents and the vasodilators, researchers have sought new drugs as alternative treatment for managing heart failure. Two chemically related drugs, *amrinone* (Inocor)* and *milrinone,* that both increase myocardial contractility, appear promising in the results of preliminary studies. Amrinone is being investigated for intravenous use, and milrinone for oral use. Neither drug appears to cause significant adverse effects by the proposed route of administration. The mechanism of their therapeutic effects is not known; however, they do not act through cardiac β_1-adrenergic receptors and thus do not increase heart rate.

Additional clinical considerations

Because of the varied effects of digitalis, there are several conditions in which the drug either should not be used or should be used with extreme caution. These conditions include the following: sick sinus syndrome, ventricular fibrillation, ventricular tachycardia, heart block, and bradycardia, all of which could be exacerbated; electrolyte imbalances that could alter the effects of the digitalis on the cell, including increased K^+, and Ca^{2+} and decreased Mg^{2+} levels; and thyroid diseases. Hypothyroid patients respond to a lower dose of digitalis and hyperthyroid patients need a higher dose. In addition, patients with renal disease may not excrete the drug as readily and may therefore experience drug toxicity if the dosage is not reduced. Elderly patients, who may have decreased body mass and decreased renal perfusion, are also at high risk for the development of toxicity. The safety of the use of these drugs during pregnancy and lactation has not been established.

A complicating factor of digitalis therapy is that the signs and symptoms of toxicity are also the signs and symptoms that the digitalis is often used to treat. Determining the patient's clinical status requires astute evaluation of the total situation. Measuring serum digitalis levels is very helpful in determining the state of the patient's digitalization. The blood sample should be drawn just before a dose of the drug is due to be given or, if that is impractical, 6 to 8 hours after the last dose has been given. It must be remembered that each patient has an individual response to the drug, and the serum drug level should be considered along with the total clinical picture. Because the margin of safety with the digitalis glycosides is so small, extreme care must be taken when administering these drugs. The name of the preparation and the dosage prescribed should be carefully checked several times. The names of preparations are very similar,

but the appropriate dosage for each preparation can be quite different. Small children and the elderly are at particular risk for toxicity because of their small body mass and inefficient renal and liver functions. Before administering a digitalis preparation to any patient at these extremes of age, the dose prepared should be double-checked by another nurse. Many institutions require that two nurses sign for administering digitalis preparations to infants to ensure that the dose has been checked very carefully.

Before each dose of a digitalis preparation is administered, the patient should also be carefully evaluated for the effects of the drug: an apical pulse should be taken for a full minute, noting rate, rhythm, and presence of S_3 (a cardinal sign of congestive heart failure); the degree, if any, of peripheral edema should be checked; and the patient should be asked about appetite, gastrointestinal disturbances, headache, or visual changes. If the heart rate is slow or irregularly irregular, the dose should be withheld and the serum digitalis level should be determined. When the results are known and the patient has been evaluated clinically, a new dosage regimen can be determined.

Patients started on a digitalis drug usually notice a remarkable improvement in their condition: a decrease in edema; loss of weight; relief of dyspnea, orthopnea, and cyanosis; increase in urinary ouput; and relief of the anxiety and restlessness associated with congestive heart failure. The patient who has been stabilized on digitalis therapy will have to know the importance of monitoring the continued effectiveness of the drug. The patient should be taught to weigh himself daily or every other day and to record the weight for easy reference. Such regular weight checks should alert the patient to steady or rapid weight gain that could indicate fluid retention and tissue congestion. The patient should also be advised to monitor himself for the signs and symptoms of congestive heart failure and to report the occurrence of any of these to the nurse or physician.

Patient teaching is an essential aspect of the drug therapy with digitalis preparations. Maintaining the appropriate serum concentration of the drug requires a careful balance of dose, timing, and use of other drugs. The patient needs to understand the disease; the action of the drug; the need to monitor the pulse (for rate and regularity), weight, and physical activity; the cautions needed with the drug; and the signs and symptoms to report. All this information should be written down for reference. It is often helpful, especially with older patients or patients who are easily confused, to prepare a calendar for the patient to record the pulse and weight and to check off each day as the medication is taken. The patient also needs to understand the importance of regular medical follow-up to evaluate the response to the drug. The patient teaching guide summarizes points to incorporate into a teaching program for the patient on digitalis. Effective and continued patient teaching can increase the

---

* Available in IV preparation in the United States short-term management of CHF patients.

benefits of the digitalis therapy and prevent serious problems from developing.

Drug–drug interactions

Drugs that induce the microsomal liver enzymes that metabolize digitoxin can decrease the effectiveness of the digitoxin. These drugs include *barbiturates, hydantoins, rifampin, oral hypoglycemic agents,* and *phenylbutazone.* Patients receiving these drugs concurrently with digitoxin will require increased doses of the digitoxin and will be at risk for developing digitalis toxicity if the second drug is stopped. The gastrointestinal absorption of digitalis preparations is decreased if they are given concurrently with *cholestyramine* or *colestipol.* If a patient needs to receive these drugs concomitantly, they should be given several hours apart. Because of the increased potential for digitalis-induced arrhythmias in the presence of hypokalemia,

caution should be used if giving digitalis with *potassium-losing diuretics,* or with *mineralocorticoids.* The *potassium-sparing diuretics* also alter the effects of digitalis, and a patient receiving these drugs concurrently must be monitored very carefully. *Quinidine* blocks the renal excretion of digoxin and, if these two drugs are given concurrently, the patient should receive very small doses of digoxin to prevent accumulation of digoxin and digoxin toxicity. Synergistic effects occur if digitalis preparations are given with various *adrenergic drugs.* Because many of these drugs are contained in over-the-counter (OTC) preparations, the patient needs to know that it is important to avoid the use of OTC preparations unless he has consulted with the physician or nurse.

The guide to the nursing process with digitalis preparations summarizes the clinical points applicable to the care of the patient receiving these drugs.

Patient teaching guide: digitalis preparations

The drug that has been prescribed for you is called a digitalis preparation. Digitalis has several helpful effects on the heart to help it beat more slowly and efficiently. These effects lead to better circulation and should help to reduce swelling in your ankles or legs and to increase the amount of urine you produce each day. Digitalis is a powerful drug and must be taken *exactly* as prescribed; never skip doses and never "catch up" on any missed doses. It is important to have regular medical checkups to make sure that the dosage of the drug is correct for you and to be sure that it is having the desired effect on your heart.

Instructions:

1. The name of your digitalis preparation is _____ .

2. The dosage that has been prescribed for you is _____ . Take your drug in the morning. Try to take it at the same time each day.

3. Do not stop taking the drug without consulting with your nurse or physician. If you miss a dose, do not "catch up" or take more than has been prescribed.

4. You should learn to take your pulse. You should take your pulse each morning before engaging in any activity. Your normal pulse rate is _____ .

5. You should monitor your weight fairly closely. Weigh yourself every other day, at the same time of day, and wearing the same amount of clothing. Record the weight on a calendar for easy reference.

6. Keep this and all medications out of the reach of children.

7. Tell any physician, nurse, or dentist who is taking care of you that you are on this drug.

8. Do not take any other medicine unless it has been prescribed for you. Do not take over-the-counter preparations while you are taking this drug. Many of these drugs contain ingredients that can interfere with the action

(continued)

of digitalis. If you feel that you need one of these preparations, consult with your nurse or physician.

9. It might be helpful to wear or carry a medical alert tag to alert any medical personnel who may take care of you in an emergency that you are taking this drug.

10. Regular medical follow-up is important to evaluate the actions of the drug and to adjust the dosage, if necessary.

Notify your nurse or physician if any of the following occur:

> Unusually slow or irregular pulse
> Rapid weight gain
> Loss of appetite, nausea, vomiting
> "Yellow vision" or blurred vision
> Unusual tiredness, weakness,
>   drowsiness
> Skin rash or hives
> Swelling of the ankles, legs, fingers
> Difficulty in breathing

Guide to the nursing process: digitalis preparations

Assessment	Nursing diagnoses	Intervention	Evaluation
Past history (*contraindications*): Ventricular tachycardia Ventricular fibrillation Heart block Sick sinus syndrome IHSS (idiopathic hypertrophic subaortic stenosis) Renal insufficiency Pregnancy Lactation $\downarrow K^+$, $\downarrow Mg^{2+}$, $\uparrow Ca^{2+}$ levels Allergies: *these drugs; tartrazine* (certain preparations) Medication history (*cautions*): Thyroid drugs Adrenergic drugs	Potential alteration in cardiac output Potential alteration in fluid volume Potential impaired gas exchange Knowledge deficit regarding drug therapy Potential alteration in tissue perfusion Potential alteration in patterns of urinary elimination	Safe and proper administration of the drug Provision of comfort measures for patient: • Positioning • Environmental control • Bathroom facilities provided • Rest periods Patient teaching regarding: • Disease • Drug • Cautions • Warnings • Weight • Pulse check Provision of support and encouragement to cope with drug and chronic therapy	Monitor for therapeutic effects of drug: ↑ peripheral perfusion ↓ heart rate ↓ signs of failure • Serum digitalis levels Monitor for toxic effects of drug: • Arrhythmias • CNS changes • Visual disturbances • GI upset, anorexia • Electrolyte levels Monitor for lack of drug effect: • Weight gain • Edema ↓ perfusion • Return of congestive heart failure Monitor for drug–drug interactions (many possible) *(continued)*

Assessment	Nursing diagnoses	Intervention	Evaluation
Quinidine (with digoxin) Barbiturates Hydantoins Rifampin Oral hypoglycemic agents Phenylbutazone } (with digitoxin) Cholestyramine Colestipol Diuretics Mineralocorticoids Spironolactone		Provision of appropriate life support measures in toxicity situations	Monitor for effectiveness of comfort measures Evaluate effectiveness of patient teaching program Evaluate effectiveness of support and encouragement offered Monitor support measures used and response in toxic situations

Physical assessment
Neurologic: orientation affect, reflexes, vision
Cardiovascular: P, BP, baseline ECG, cardiac auscultation, peripheral pulses, peripheral perfusion, edema
Respiratory: R, adventitious sounds
GI: abdominal percussion, bowel sounds, liver evaluation
Genitourinary: urinary output
Laboratory tests: electrolyte levels, liver and renal function tests
General: weight

Summary of clinical indications for digitalis therapy

Congestive heart failure

Both right- and left-sided failure, especially in hypertensive heart disease or failure secondary to valvular and coronary heart disease.

Supraventricular arrhythmias

Paroxysmal tachycardia. Both atrial (PAT) and A-V nodal types may be converted to a normal sinus rhythm.

Atrial fibrillation. Digitalis does not ordinarily convert this arrhythmia to a normal sinus rhythm but it protects the ventricles from overstimulation, thus reducing their rapid rate and restoring myocardial efficiency.

Atrial flutter. Digitalis acts indirectly to restore sinus rhythm in some cases but, even if the flutter is not converted, the ventricles are prevented from being driven at an excessively rapid rate.

Summary of pharmacologic and toxicologic effects of digitalis glycosides

Cardiac effects (therapeutically desirable)

Increased contractility (positive inotropic). Strengthening of the beats of the hypodynamic heart increases the stroke volume and cardiac output. This sets in motion a series of circulatory changes that relieve congestion.

Slowing of the heart (negative chronotropic)

1. Heart slows as circulation improves, and the stimuli that had caused reflex cardioacceleration are removed, thus increasing vagal tone
2. Heart slows as a result of sensitization of the vagal mechanism, which leads to increased vagal (braking) control over the heart
3. Heart rate may slow because of direct (as well as vagal) depression of the A-V node and subsequent development of partial heart block

Cardiac effects (toxic)

Partial or complete heart block. Slowing of the ventricular rate (apical pulse) well below 60 beats/minute may lead to poor cerebral and coronary circulation, manifested by dizziness, weakness, fainting spells, and even signs and symptoms of congestive heart failure.

Increased automaticity. Leads to patterns of premature beats, including bigeminy or coupling, trigeminy, pulse deficit, and ventricular tachycardia; together with depressed ventricular conduction, this action can result in fatal ventricular fibrillation.

Extracardiac effects (signs and symptoms of toxicity)

Gastrointestinal. Anorexia, nausea and vomiting—caused by CNS actions—are early signs of over-digitalization; epigastric pain and diarrhea occur less frequently.

Nervous System. Drowsiness, fatigue, and headache are common; facial pain as a result of neuralgia is relatively rare as are convulsions.

Elderly patients may show such mental symptoms as confusion, disorientation, and even delirium.

Visual effects. Vision may be blurred and diplopia (double vision) may also develop; flashes and flickering lights, halos, white or colored dots may be seen; yellow or green vision is common, brown, blue, and red less frequent.

Miscellaneous. Gynecomastia (painful breast swellings) occurs sometimes in male patients treated with these glycosides, which are chemically related to sex hormones such as the estrogens; dermatologic reactions include urticarial eruptions (hives) and scarlatiniform rashes.

Case study

Presentation

GJ is an 82-year-old white woman, with a 50-year history of rheumatic mitral valve disease. GJ has been stabilized on digoxin for 10 years in a compensated state of congestive heart failure. GJ has recently moved into a nursing home, having had difficulty caring for herself alone. GJ was examined by the nursing home physician when she arrived and he found her to be stable, noting only an irregularly irregular pulse of 76, with ECG documentation of atrial fibrillation (a chronic state). Three weeks after arrival at the nursing home, GJ began to develop progressive weakness, dyspnea on exertion, two-pillow orthopnea and peripheral, 2^+ pitting edema. These signs and symptoms became worse and, 5 days after the initial complaint of shortness of breath, GJ was admitted to the hospital in severe congestive heart failure. The physical examination revealed a heart rate of 96, atrial fibrillation, S_3, rales, wheezes, 2^+ pitting edema bilaterally up to the knees, elevated JVP, cardiomegaly, weak pulses, and poor peripheral perfusion. GJ's serum digoxin level was 0.12 ng/ml (therapeutic range of 0.5–2.0 ng/ml). A diuretic was ordered to dry out GJ's edematous tissues. GJ was digitalized in the hospital and, with careful monitoring of her serum digoxin levels and clinical status, she was stabilized on 0.25 mg Lanoxin qd.

Once GJ was out of immediate danger and comfortable, a careful history was taken to determine why GJ's digoxin level was so low. GJ was sure that she had been given her digoxin as usual, with the only change being the timing. She said that at the nursing home she was taking the drug in the afternoon, with a dish of ice cream, instead of in the morning. The nursing home confirmed that GJ had been given the drug daily in the afternoon and that it was GJ's usual brand of digoxin, allaying some concerns of a change in bioavailability. They also stated that none of GJ's drugs had been changed, no OTC preparations had been given, and her diet was being closely regulated. What nursing actions should be taken?

Discussion

GJ's immediate needs were to alleviate the alteration in her cardiac output and decrease in tissue perfusion. Positioning—preferably a semi-Fowler's position—can help her respiratory distress and decrease the workload for her failing heart.

In this case, the low serum digoxin level, below the therapeutic range, was not adequate to keep GJ stabilized and out of congestive heart failure. As GJ was prepared for discharge back to the nursing home, the question of the fall in serum digoxin levels at the nursing home remained a concern. Extensive patient teaching was done, reviewing the signs and symptoms of congestive heart failure, the actions of digoxin, and precautions needed. The clinical pharmacologist was consulted and it was determined that the ice cream—which is cold and decreases gastrointestinal activity, and contains milk products (calcium) that stimulate gastric acid secretion—could decrease the amount of digoxin available for absorption by allowing the drug to remain too long in the acid environment of the stomach. This could destroy some of the drug. It was determined that the decrease in available digoxin was significant enough to lead to the low digoxin level and thus to cause the patient to return to congestive heart failure over the 3-week period. The nursing home nurse was consulted, and the problem was discussed. It was decided that GJ should continue taking her digoxin in the morning, on an empty stomach, as she had in the hospital. Blood for serum digoxin levels was to be drawn in 1 week to determine if GJ's serum level was being maintained.

The factors that keep the serum digoxin levels within a therapeutic range are varied. Diet, brand of drug, environmental stresses, disease state, and interactions with other drugs are often involved in a change in response to digitalis. Helping the patient and the staff in the nursing home to understand and regulate these factors can help to prevent similar problems from occurring in the future.

Drug digests

Deslanoside USP (Cedilanid-D)

Actions and indications. This is a more soluble and stable derivative of the orally administered *Digitalis lanata* glycoside, lanatoside C. It is available as an injection for use in clinical situations that require rapid digitalization. These urgent clinical situations include acute left-sided heart failure with pulmonary edema, paroxysmal supraventricular tachycardia (for attempting conversion to sinus rhythm), and atrial fibrillation and flutter (for protecting the ventricles against excessive impulses originating in ectopic atrial and junctional tissues). The drug's effects begin in from 10 to 30 minutes and are fully developed in 1 or 2 hours. The fully digitalized patient may be maintained with

oral doses of a glycoside of intermediate duration (*e.g.*, digoxin) or of long duration (*e.g.*, digitoxin).

Adverse effects, cautions, and contraindications. The solution of this glycoside is said to be less irritating than other digitalis preparations and may be administered intramuscularly as well as by vein, but some pain may be expected. The cardiac toxicity characteristic of all digitalis glycosides is likely to occur at about the same time, or even before, the extracardiac side-effects. Thus, electrocardiographic monitoring is desirable to detect evidence of advancing heart block or of premature ventricular extrasystoles.

These may appear concurrently with such extracardiac warning signs as anorexia, nausea, and vomiting or headache, listlessness, and confusion, and with such visual disturbances as blurring, flickering colored dots, and flashes.

The relatively rapid elimination of this glycoside is a safety factor in cases of overdosage. However, as with other digitalis preparations, caution is required in patients with depletion of plasma potassium (hypokalemia), or with high blood calcium levels (hypercalcemia). Patients should not be given calcium salt injections, because this may sensitize the heart to digitalis toxicity.

Dosage and administration. This glycoside may be administered as a single intramuscular or intravenous injection of 1.6 mg (8 ml) or divided into two doses of 0.8 mg (4 ml) at half-hour intervals. (The IM dose is administered at two different sites.) Patients who have already been receiving digitalis should receive reduced doses, as should elderly or debilitated patients.

Digitoxin USP (Crystodigin; Purodigin)

Actions and indications. This crystalline cardiotonic glycoside of *Digitalis purpurea* has the same actions as digoxin, but these reach peak effects much more slowly—4 to 12 hours, for example—even when it is administered IV, and the duration of its action is more prolonged. The long-lasting effects of this glycoside and its complete absorption when taken orally help to produce dependably smooth and stable digitalization during maintenance therapy.

Digitoxin has the same pharmacologic effects on the heart as other glycosides, and it is indicated in the same disorders. Its ability to strengthen the heartbeat and to lessen sympathetic nervous system stimulation of the sinoatrial node and to increase vagal control accounts for its effectiveness in heart failure patients with compensatory sinus tachycardia. The drug's depressant effect on atrioventricular conduction helps to control rapid ventricular rates that are the result of supraventricular arrhythmias.

Adverse effects, cautions, and contraindications. Digitoxin, like other digitalis glycosides, can cause almost any type of cardiac arrhythmia, including some that are similar to the supraventricular arrhythmias for which it is employed, such as paroxysmal atrial tachycardia. It should not be used to treat ventricular tachycardia, because it may itself cause this dysrythmia that can lead to fatal ventricular fibrillation. The appearance of premature ventricular contractions often precedes these dangerous arrhythmias and may require discontinuing the drug. However, because of the relatively slow rate of elimination of digitoxin, cardiotoxicity may continue to develop even after it is withdrawn, and prolonged treatment may be required before the drug's toxic effects gradually disappear.

Atrioventricular conduction block can occur with or without supraventricular and ventricular tachyarrhythmias. The patient's pulse should be checked for signs of excessive slowing, and the electrocardiogram should be employed to detect increasing degrees of drug-induced heart block. The drug should not be administered to most patients with incomplete heart block or to those prone to suffer Stokes–Adams attacks. Caution is also required in patients with acute myocarditis, acute myocardial infarction, and advanced heart failure; in severe lung, liver, and kidney disease; and in myxedema (hypothyroidism).

Dosage and administration. Patients may be digitalized slowly by oral administration of 0.2 mg of digitoxin twice daily for 4 days, and they may then be maintained with about 0.15 mg daily. (Maintenance dosage may, however, vary from 0.05 to 0.3 mg daily depending on the sensitivity or tolerance of the patient to digitoxin.)

More rapid oral digitalization may be accomplished by administering an initial loading dose of 0.6 mg followed at intervals of 4 to 6 hours by additional doses of 0.4 mg and 0.2 mg.

Rapid parenteral digitalization is employed only when patients cannot take digitoxin by mouth. IV injections should be made slowly, starting with an initial loading dose of 0.6 mg, which is followed at intervals of 4 to 6 hours by doses of 0.4 mg and 0.2 mg until the effects of full digitalization are apparent. The average digitalizing dose is 1.2 mg to 1.6 mg, but patients vary considerably in their requirements.

Digoxin USP (Lanoxin)

Actions and indications. This crystalline glycoside extracted from the leaves of *Digitalis lanata* has the same pharmacologic actions as other cardioactive plant principles, but its special pharmacokinetic properties make it useful in a wider variety of clinical situations than most other glycosides.

Like other glycosides, digoxin increases the contractile strength of the failing myocardium and is indicated in the management of congestive heart failure. It can reduce the too rapid ventricular rate of such supraventricular arrhythmias as atrial fibrillation, atrial flutter, and paroxysmal atrial tachycardia by its ability to lengthen the refractory period of the atrioventricular (A-V) node.

Digoxin's effects develop relatively rapidly compared to those of digitoxin. Maximum myocardial effects are reached in between 1 and 2 hours following injection or 6 to 8 hours after oral administration. Its elimination from the body is also relatively rapid, but the duration of its action is long enough to allow long-term maintenance therapy with daily doses.

Adverse effects, cautions, and contraindications. Because digoxin depends on the kidneys for excretion caution is required, and it is often necessary to adjust dosage downward in patients with impaired renal function and in the elderly to avoid accumulation of the drug to toxic levels. Cardiotoxicity is also most likely to occur in older people with advanced heart disease. Caution is also required in patients with obstructive cardiomyopathies and others with disorders that increase sensitivity to the cardiotoxic effects of digoxin.

Among the many types of cardiac arrhythmias induced by overdosage are premature ventricular contractions, atrioventricular block, and paroxysmal atrial tachycardia and block. Electrocardiographic signs of these drug-induced dysrhythmias sometimes appear before noncardiac adverse effects. More commonly, however, the first indication of overdosage is development of anorexia, followed by nausea and vomiting. Other early warning signs are complaints of colored (yellow, green, or white) vision and headache. Confusion and other signs of mental disturbances are other extracardiac side-effects.

Dosage and administration. The average oral digitalizing dose for adults and children over 10 years old is 0.75 mg to 1.25 mg; and the average parenteral (IV or IM) digitalizing dose is 0.6 mg to 1.0 mg. However, average doses should be considered to be only guidelines for initiating therapy, and dosage should be adjusted in accordance with the individual response.

Dosage may be accomplished rapidly or slowly, but the rapid IV route is best reserved for emergencies. Rapid parenteral administration is usually begun with an initial loading dose of 0.25 mg to 0.50 mg, which may be followed, if necessary, by additional doses of 0.25 mg every 4 to 6 hours as needed for full digitalization. Accumulation of the total required amount may also be accomplished rapidly by the oral route with an initial loading dose of 0.5 to 0.75 mg followed by additional doses of 0.25 to 0.50 mg every 6 to 8 hours.

Slow oral digitalization can be carried out by administering maintenance doses (without any loading dose) daily for about 7 days. The average maintenance dose is between 0.125 mg and 0.25 mg, but this may be much lower for patients with poor renal function and the elderly, or as high as 0.5 mg daily in those resistant to digoxin. Lanoxicaps have a greater bioavailability than standard tablets: 0.2-mg Lanoxicaps are equivalent to 0.25 mg, 0.1 mg is equivalent to 0.125 mg, and the 0.5-mg capsule is equivalent to 0.625 mg of the standard tablets. Care should be taken to carefully check the dose of Lanoxicaps being used.

References

Aronson JK: Clinical pharmacokinetics of digoxin, 1980. Clin Pharmacokinet 5:137, 1980

Baim D et al: Evaluation of a new bipyridine inotropic agent—milrinone—in patients with severe CHF. N Engl J Med 309:748, 1983

Bigger JT, Leahey EB: Quinidine and digoxin—an important interaction. Drugs 24:229, 1982

Cannon PJ: The kidney in heart failure. N Engl J Med 296:26, 1977

Cavanaugh AL, Manconi RE: Drug interactions and digitalis toxicity. Am J Nurs 80:2170, 1980

Cohn J: Physiologic basis of vasodilator therapy for heart failure. Am J Med 71:135, 1981

Farah AE et al: Positive inotropic agents. Ann Rev Pharmacol Toxicol 24:275, 1984

Foster SB: Pump failure. Am J Nurs 74:1830, 1974

Greenblatt DJ: Bioavailability of drugs: The digoxin dilemma. Clin Pharmacokinet 1:36, 1976

Hoffman BF, Bigger TJ Jr: Digitalis and allied cardiac glycosides. In Gilman AG, Goodman LS, Gilman A (eds): Goodman and Gilman's The Pharmacological Basis of Therapeutics, 6th ed, pp 729–760. New York, Macmillan, 1980

Huffman DH, Azarnoff D: The use of digitalis. Ration Drug Ther 8:1, 1974

Karch AM: Cardiac Care: A Guide for Patient Education. New York, Appleton–Century–Crofts, 1981

Lindenmayer GE: Mechanism of action of digitalis at the subcellular level. Pharmacol Ther 2:813, 1976

Mathers DH Jr et al: Current management of digitalis intoxication. South Med J 69:1079, 1976

McCauley K, Burke K: Your detailed guide to drugs for CHF. Nursing 14:47, 1984

Moss AF et al: Digitalis-associated cardiac mortality after myocardial infarction. Circulation 64:1150, 1981

Rodman MJ: Latest thinking on drug therapy post MI: Congestive heart failure—acute pulmonary edema. RN 44:74 (Jan) 1981

Schick D, Scheuer J: Current concepts of digitalis. Parts I and II. Am Heart J 87:253, 391, 1974

Smith TW: Digitalis glycosides. N Engl J Med 288:719, 942, 1973

Weber KT: New hope for the failing heart. Am J Med 72:665, 1982

Weintraub M: Interpretation of serum digoxin concentrations. Clin Pharmacokinet 2:205, 1977

Winslow EH: Digitalis. Am J Nurs 74:1062, 1974

Chapter 30

Antiarrhythmic drugs

Cardiac arrhythmias

This chapter will describe the drugs most commonly employed clinically in the management of cardiac disorders characterized by development of premature atrial or ventricular contractions and tachycardias.* Cardiac arrhythmias of this type occur because of disease-induced changes in certain fundamental electrophysiologic properties of cardiac muscle cells and of the cells of the heart's specialized conducting system. Thus, before beginning to study this chapter—or while doing so—it would be desirable to review the discussion of the nature of normal and abnormal cardiac rhythms in Chapter 26.

Causes

As indicated in that chapter, there are several reasons for disturbances in cardiac rhythm:

1. Abnormalities in *automaticity*, the special properties of certain cardiac cells that allow them to depolarize spontaneously and to generate pacemaker impulses
2. Abnormalities in the *conduction* of impulses, which cause them to be slowed or blocked or to take abnormal pathways
3. Abnormalities in *both* the rate and site of impulse production and in the manner of their conduction through the specialized conducting tissues and the atrial or ventricular musculature.

---

* Other drugs that can also affect cardiac rate and rhythm are discussed elsewhere—for example, edrophonium and other cholinergic drugs (Chap. 15); atropine and other anticholinergic drugs (Chap. 16), isoproterenol and other adrenergic drugs (Chap. 17), and the digitalis glycosides (Chap. 29).

Drug actions

The antiarrhythmic drugs, which are employed clinically to convert cardiac irregularities to a normal sinus rhythm or, at least, to control the rapid ventricular rate, act mainly by exerting favorable effects on the electrophysiologic properties of cardiac cell membranes. They may do so by depressing automaticity in ectopic foci—that is, in latent or subsidiary pacemakers that can come to dominate the cardiac rhythm by generating impulses at a rate more rapid than that of the sinoatrial (S-A) node. Drugs may also abolish arrhythmias by altering conduction velocity or cardiac cell membrane responsiveness to stimuli and by lengthening or shortening the refractory period—effects that help to terminate circus re-entry rhythms.

Hemodynamics

The ability of the heart to pump blood with power depends on the coordinated contraction of the atria and ventricles. The muscular walls of these cardiac chambers are activated to contract by impulses that arise regularly at the S-A pacemaker. These impulses, spreading swiftly through the atria, the atrioventricular (A-V) node, and the His–Purkinje system, the specialized conducting tissues in the ventricles, trigger the powerful beats that propel blood into the pulmonary and systemic circulations.

When this orderly initiation and conduction of impulses is interfered with, the resulting rapid, often poorly coordinated contractions of the ventricles may be unable to supply an adequate flow of oxygenated blood to the brain and to other vital organs, including the myocardium itself. These adverse hemodynamic consequences of cardiac arrhythmias can lead to serious and sometimes fatal complications. Rapid irregularities that reduce cardiac output and lessen the flow of blood to the brain can, for example, cause syncopal blackouts and possibly precipitate strokes. Reduction in blood flow from the left ventricle and aorta into the coronary vessels can lead to anginal chest pains or even to ventricular fibrillation, a frequently fatal complication.

Antiarrhythmic drugs

General considerations

Remarkable advances have been made in scientific understanding of the electrophysiology of myocardial cells and of how their fundamental properties are affected by the actions of drugs and by changes in serum levels of such electrolytes as potassium and calcium. Employing sophisticated techniques for inserting microelectrodes into single cardiac cells and then recording their transmembrane action potentials, scientists are continuously obtaining more information about the electrical and ionic bases for the spontaneous firing of impulses and the conduction of the action potentials that are then propagated through the fibers of the cardiac conduction pathway.

Despite this explosion of detailed data, much of what is known cannot be applied by the practicing cardiologist in the treatment of a cardiac arrhythmia in any particular patient. This is because it is still rarely possible to know which one of several possible pathophysiologic alterations of cardiac cell electrophysiology is responsible for setting off a particular patient's specific arrhythmia. Thus, the physician cannot yet select the antiarrhythmic drug that would act most specifically to reverse the underlying abnormality responsible for the patient's cardiac irregularity.

Nevertheless, even though the physician's choice of drugs must still be made on an empiric—that is, a trial-and-error—basis rather than by more rational methods such as an exact understanding of the patient's underlying arrhythmia mechanism, knowledge of the electrophysiologic actions and pharmacokinetic properties of the available drugs is very important in obtaining their therapeutic benefits and avoiding their potential toxicity. Thus, after the arrhythmia has been identified by electrocardiographic and clinical diagnostic measures, a drug is chosen that has been shown clinically to be most effective for controlling that type of cardiac irregularity. It is then administered in doses that will promptly attain plasma concentrations known to correlate well with therapeutic effectiveness. The patient's responses to drug therapy are closely monitored to determine whether the drug is producing the desired effect or causing signs of toxicity. On this basis the drug's dosage may be raised or reduced,

* These discussions emphasize functional factors of current clinical significance, rather than some of the newer concepts concerning drug actions at the ionic and electrical level, which are not yet of practical significance for drug selection and monitoring.

or it may be discontinued entirely, and an alternative antiarrhythmic drug may be tried.

The following discussion of individual antiarrhythmic drugs will describe first those electrophysiologic actions that are thought to account for the agent's effects in therapeutic and toxic doses.* It will also describe the pharmacokinetic factors that help to determine the dosage schedules for each drug that are most likely to bring about beneficial results while minimizing the likelihood of cardiotoxicity and adverse drug reactions. The main clinical indications for each different drug will be mentioned, but fuller discussions of the applications of some of these drugs and of other measures in the management of specific supraventricular arrhythmias will be reserved for the last section of this chapter. The applications of these and other antiarrhythmic drugs in the treatment of cardiac rhythm disorders resulting from such causes as acute myocardial infarction (Chap. 31) or digitalis intoxication (Chap. 29) are discussed in detail in those chapters.

Individual antiarrhythmic drugs

The currently available antiarrhythmic drugs are similar in some of their effects on the electrophysiologic properties of cardiac cell fibers but differ from one another in other of their actions. All, for example, can counteract arrhythmias by their ability to suppress excessive automaticity in one or another of the subsidiary or latent types of hyperactive ectopic pacemaker tissues. Paradoxically, all can, in addition, *cause* cardiac arrhythmias and even cardiac arrest. Some, however, differ from others in their effects on such properties as conduction velocity, excitability, and membrane responsiveness to stimuli (see Chap. 26).

Quinidine, procainamide, and disopyramide, for example, reduce conduction velocity and decrease the excitability and membrane responsiveness of cardiac cells (Table 30-1). Lidocaine and phenytoin, on the other hand, have little effect on cardiac excitability, and in low therapeutic doses may actually increase conduction velocity and cardiac cell membrane responsiveness. Propranolol is similar to quinidine and procainamide in most respects, but differs in some properties because it possesses a β-adrenergic blocking action not shared by any of the other antiarrhythmic drugs.

As indicated in the following discussions, some of these drugs are superior to others for treating various specific types of arrhythmias. The differences in their electrophysiologic effects account in large part for the greater effectiveness of one or another drug or drug group in the management of the different types of atrial and ventricular tachyarrhythmias.

Table 30–1. Antiarrhythmic drugs*

Generic or official name	Trade name or synonym	Usual daily adult dosage and administration	Clinical applications
Bretylium tosylate	Bretylol	IV or IM 5–10 mg/kg of body weight	Treatment of immediately life-threatening ventricular arrhythmias, such as ventricular fibrillation and ventricular tachycardia
Disopyramide phosphate	Norpace	400–800 mg daily, divided into four oral doses following an initial loading dose of 300 mg	Suppression and prevention of premature ventricular contractions (PVCs) and episodes of ventricular tachycardia
Lidocaine HCl USP	Xylocaine	Single IV bolus dose of 50–100 mg followed by a continuous IV infusion at a rate of 1–4 mg/min; also by IM injection of about 3 ml of a 10% solution (300 mg/150 lb body weight, or 2 mg/lb)	Suppression and prevention of PVCs and episodes of ventricular tachycardia, particularly in patients who have suffered an acute myocardial infarction and in cases of digitalis intoxication (see also Drug digests)
Phenytoin sodium USP	Dilantin	100 mg q 5 min by slow IV injection, repeated until arrhythmia is terminated; also 100–200 mg orally	Suppression and prevention of atrial and ventricular tachyarrhythmias, especially in digitalis intoxication (see also Drug digests, Chap. 50)
Procainamide HCl USP	Pronestyl	Initial oral doses of 1–1.25 g are followed by doses of 250 mg, 750 mg, or 1000 mg, depending on the disorder; IM, 0.5–1 g; IV, 0.2–1 g	Suppression and prevention of PVCs and ventricular tachycardia; also in atrial fibrillation and paroxysmal atrial tachycardia (see also Drug digests)
Propranolol HCl USP	Inderal	Orally 10–30 mg tid or qid; IV, 1–3 mg at a rate of no more than 1 mg/min with careful monitoring	Various supraventricular and ventricular arrhythmias, particularly those induced by catecholamines—for example, in pheochromocytoma, thyrotoxicosis, and during general anesthesia; also in digitalis intoxication and in the Wolff–Parkinson–White syndrome (see also Drug digests, Chap. 18)
Verapamil HCl	Calan; Isoptin	0.075–0.15 mg/kg IV followed in 30 min by 0.15 mg/kg, if needed	Control of supraventricular tachycardia; control of ventricular rate in atrial flutter and fibrillation
		80–160 mg bid oral†	Paroxysmal supraventricular tachycardia†

(continued)

Table 30–1. Antiarrhythmic drugs* (continued)

Generic or official name	Trade name or synonym	Usual daily adult dosage and administration	Clinical applications
Quinidine salts			
Quinidine sulfate USP	Quinora	Orally 200–300 mg tid or qid	Suppression and prevention of premature atrial contractions (PACs) and premature ventricular contractions (PVCs); paroxysmal atrial tachycardia (PAT), and A-V junctional tachycardia; atrial fibrillation and flutter; paroxysmal ventricular tachycardia without complete heart block (see also Drug digests)
Quinidine gluconate USP	Quinaglute	Orally, 200–300 mg; IM, 600 mg followed by 400 mg repeated as often as every 2 hr; IV 300–750 mg at a rate of 1 ml/min of a dilute solution	
Quinidine polygalacturonate	Cardioquin	Orally 275–825 mg for conversion, repeated in 3 or 4 hours if necessary; for maintenance, 275 mg AM and PM	

* Other drugs employed in the management of cardiac arrhythmias include edrophonium and other cholinergic drugs (Chap. 15), atropine and other anticholinergic drugs (Chap. 16), isoproterenol, phenylephrine, and other adrenergic drugs (Chap. 17), and digitalis glycosides (Chap. 29).
† Investigational use only.

Quinidine salts

Pharmacologic effects. The effects of quinidine sulfate[+] (Quinidex; Quinora) and other salts of this *Cinchona* alkaloid are mainly the result of their direct actions on cardiac cell membranes, which alter such electrophysiologic properties as automaticity, excitability, conduction velocity, and effective refractory period (Chap. 26). In addition, quinidine has an indirect action—an atropinelike ability to block vagal impulses—which may sometimes also influence its pharmacologic effects on cardiac function when the drug is administered in therapeutic doses.

Quinidine, like all the other antiarrhythmic drugs listed in Table 30-1, depresses automaticity in cardiac pacemaker cells. Fortunately, when ordinary doses are administered, such suppression of spontaneous depolarizations occurs much more readily in subsidiary, or latent, pacemakers than at the S-A node. Thus, this action is useful for treating arrhythmias caused by impulses arising at a rapid rate at ectopic foci in the atria, A-V junction, bundle of His, and Purkinje fibers.

Quinidine also reduces myocardial excitability and conduction velocity while it lengthens the effective refractory period in relation to the duration of the action potential passing through the Purkinje fibers and the muscle fibers of the ventricle. These actions are thought to account for its effectiveness in treating arrhythmias that are the result of re-entry phenomena—self-sustaining circular movements of impulses that cause rapid irregular rhythms (Chap. 26). In such cases, quinidine can abolish the re-entry-type arrhythmias by converting a unidirectional block to a bidirectional block. That is, this drug—by slowing impulse conduction through healthy cardiac tissue or by increasing the refractoriness of responsive cardiac cell membranes to stimuli—causes the circling impulses to arrive when the tissue is unresponsive, thus breaking up the cycle responsible for the continuous circus re-entry rhythm (see Chap. 26 for a discussion of decremental conduction as a cause of arrhythmogenesis).

Although all the above actions tend to terminate rapid atrial and ventricular rhythms and to cause conversion to a slower more regular sinus rhythm, quinidine can sometimes cause an already rapid ventricular rate to become even more rapid. This paradoxical response even to therapeutic doses can occur if the drug's *indirect* anticholinergic action predominates over its direct depressant action at the A-V junction. That is, by blocking the influence of the vagus nerve that helps to slow A-V conduction, this atropinelike action of quinidine increases the rate of impulse transmission from the atria to the ventricles. This action can complicate the use of quinidine in the treatment of disorders marked by rapid atrial impulse formation at ectopic sites (see the discussion of atrial flutter and fibrillation treatment, below).

Pharmacokinetics. Orally administered quinidine is readily absorbed into the bloodstream, in which about 80% is bound to plasma protein. The therapeutically beneficial effects of this drug occur when the plasma level is between about 3 and 6 mg/liter (3 to 6 μg/ml). Patients vary widely in the doses required to attain therapeutic concentrations. Some people with atrial arrhythmias may fail to respond to ordinary doses of quinidine because these do not attain minimal therapeutic levels. In others the same doses may produce plasma concentrations that cause cardiotoxic effects—for example, 8 mg/liter or more. Toxic effects are most likely to occur in patients with liver or kidney disease. Hepatic cirrhosis, for example, is marked by low levels of serum albumin, a condition that favors movement of free unbound quinidine molecules from the blood to the myocardium. Reduced renal clearance of quinidine in patients with kidney disease can also lead to cardiac toxicity. Quinidine may be given parenterally (IV or IM) to patients who cannot take the drug orally. Parenteral quinidine therapy has been largely replaced by IV lidocaine therapy.

Cardiotoxic effects. The most common toxic effect of quinidine is the development of various degrees of A-V block caused by slowing of conduction through the junctional tissues. This may be detected by observing an increase in the P–R interval on the electrocardiogram. A widening of the QRS complex on the ECG indicates that conduction velocity of impulses through the ventricles is also being slowed. If excessive intraventricular slowing of conduction develops, sudden cardiac asystole may occur. On the other hand, re-entry phenomena may also develop during intraventricular conduction depression. This can lead to premature ventricular contractions (PVCs), ventricular tachycardia, and ventricular fibrillation followed by cardiac arrest.

Quinidine overdosage may also lead to a weakening of myocardial contractions that can cause congestive heart failure. Early detection of the signs and symptoms of congestive heart failure can prevent serious problems from developing.

When quinidine is administered by the IV route, the drug-induced depression of cardiac contractility combined with its tendency to produce generalized vasodilation can lead to a sudden drop in blood pressure. The patient's blood pressure must be constantly monitored, and the IV drip of quinidine gluconate or of a similar soluble salt should be discontinued if hypotension develops.

Extracardiac toxicity. Quinidine can cause adverse reactions of many types other than those involving cardiovascular function. Some reactions occur immediately in patients with an idiosyncrasy to the drug. Thus,

it is desirable to administer a single-tablet test dose of quinidine sulfate orally to rule out such possible hypersensitivity. Other adverse effects that tend to develop during long-term therapy often force patients to discontinue further use of quinidine.

The most frequently observed side-effects involve the gastrointestinal tract. Oral doses may cause gastrointestinal irritation that leads to nausea, vomiting, cramps, and diarrhea. The polygalacturonate salt of quinidine (Cardioquin) is claimed to cause less gastrointestinal distress than the sulfate or the hydrochloride. However, all quinidine salts can cause certain other central and peripheral signs of overdosage (cinchonism) and various types of hematologic and hypersensitivity-type reactions.

Cinchonism, a syndrome also sometimes seen in malaria patients being treated with quinine, is manifested by tinnitus (ringing in the ears), visual disturbances (blurred or double vision), dizziness, headache, confusion, and delirium. Hypersensitivity reactions may be of the histamine-release type—for example, urticaria, angioneurotic edema, and asthma. Another type of idiosyncrasy occasionally results in destruction of blood platelets by an antigen–antibody reaction. This may lead to bleeding into the mucous membranes of the mouth and to petechial hemorrhages in the skin. Thus, quinidine is contraindicated in some patients, especially elderly women with a history of thrombocytic purpura. Bleeding can also occur in patients previously stabilized on coumarin-type anticoagulants, because quinidine may also depress the biosynthesis of blood-clotting factors by the liver. Another drug–drug interaction that must be remembered involves quinidine and digoxin, and probably also digitoxin. By one or more mechanisms quinidine may increase digoxin levels, which could lead to digoxin toxicity. Thus, when quinidine therapy is initiated in a patient on digoxin, the digoxin dose should be halved. The dose of digitoxin should also be reduced, although this interaction is less well documented.

Clinical indications. Quinidine salts are employed primarily in the management of atrial and other supraventricular arrhythmias (see below). Although it can also control ventricular arrhythmias, other newer antiarrhythmic agents such as lidocaine are considered safer than parenteral quinidine administration for treating episodes of ventricular tachycardia in emergency situations. In the long-term therapy of patients with PVCs, the antiarrhythmic drug disopyramide may now be preferred to oral quinidine medication because it is less likely to cause development of the discomforting or dangerous side-effects that often require quinidine treatment to be stopped.

Procainamide

Pharmacologic effects. The effects of this synthetic relative of the local anesthetic procaine (Chap.

14) are essentially similar to those already described for the natural *Cinchona* alkaloid quinidine. Like the latter drug, procainamide HCl[+] (Pronestyl) depresses automaticity, reduces the rate of cardiac impulse conduction, and lengthens the refractory period of both the specialized conducting tissues and the cardiac muscle fibers. In addition to these direct effects on electrophysiologic function, procainamide possesses an indirect or vagus-blocking effect, which can cause a paradoxical increase in the heart rate in some circumstances.

Pharmacokinetics. As is the case with quinidine, procainamide is promptly absorbed from the gastrointestinal tract. Taken orally, this drug reaches therapeutic plasma levels—4 to 8 mg/liter (4 to 8 µg/ml) within 1 hour. Similar concentrations are attained in about 15 minutes by the intramuscular route and almost immediately when the drug is administered by vein. However, to avoid reaching toxic levels (16 mg/liter and above), intravenous doses are best administered intermittently in small amounts—for example, 100 mg every 5 minutes until the drug accumulates to an effective concentration.

The main advantage of procainamide over procaine, which can also terminate cardiac arrhythmias when injected intravenously, is its longer duration of action. The presence of the amide grouping in the chemical structure of this drug prevents it from being destroyed by the plasma esterase enzymes that rapidly hydrolyze procaine. Nevertheless, procainamide has a relatively short half-life (2 to 3 hours), and its plasma concentrations drop below effective arrhythmia control levels before long. Thus, to maintain its effectiveness in ventricular arrhythmias, this drug must be readministered at least every 3 hours, which can cause a real problem for patients who must take the drug around the clock. Continued control of atrial arrhythmias may be maintained with larger doses administered at somewhat longer intervals. (Because this drug is eliminated mainly by renal excretion, patients with poor kidney function receive smaller doses at longer intervals.)

Cardiovascular toxicity. Procainamide overdosage causes cardiotoxicity similar to that seen with quinidine. Its ability to depress A-V conduction means that it must be administered with caution to patients who already have A-V block or such other conduction defects as bundle–branch block. On the other hand, in patients with atrial flutter or fibrillation this drug's atropinelike, or vagolytic, action may set off a sudden increase in the ventricular rate even while the atrial rate is slowing. Procainamide can also cause an excessive decrease in conduction velocity in the ventricles, as indicated on the ECG by a progressive widening of the QRS complex. This effect must never be allowed to go to more than 50% above normal, because such slowing of intraventricular conduction can lead either to cardiac asystole or to ventricular fibrillation types of cardiac arrest. (The physician should be informed of QRS widening of 25% or more.)

Procainamide overdosage can also cause acute hypertension, which is mainly the result of the drug's peripheral vasodilator effect when it is administered by vein. This can be especially dangerous when drug-induced depression of myocardial contractility, leading to a reduction in cardiac output, occurs simultaneously. To prevent any sudden steep drop in blood pressure during IV administration, procainamide is infused very slowly with continuous electrocardiographic monitoring. Patients are kept lying flat during the infusion, and blood pressure readings are taken continuously.

Extracardiac reactions. The most common side-effects of large oral doses of procainamide are anorexia, nausea, vomiting, and diarrhea. In addition to gastrointestinal upsets and allergic reactions, procainamide has reportedly produced two much rarer but more dangerous toxic reactions. These are a syndrome resembling the collagen disease lupus erythematosus, and the blood dyscrasia agranulocytosis. Therefore, for early detection of the latter, patients should be instructed to report symptoms such as sore throat or upper respiratory infections that develop during long-term procainamide maintenance therapy. They should also have measurements made regularly during prolonged therapy to detect any rise in the level of antinuclear antibody (ANA). If a positive ANA titer develops, or if clinical signs of the lupuslike syndrome develop, such as fever, arthritis, or pleuritic pain, it may be necessary to discontinue therapy and to employ another antiarrhythmic agent.

Clinical indications. Procainamide is employed for control of both atrial and ventricular arrhythmias. It is used more commonly than quinidine for the emergency management of ventricular tachycardia, because the parenteral administration of procainamide is considered somewhat safer than quinidine. However, in such cases—and particularly when ventricular arrhythmias develop following an acute myocardial infarction—procainamide is usually reserved for patients who have failed to respond adequately to intravenously administered lidocaine (see below).

Following control of acute atrial or ventricular arrhythmias by lidocaine, electrical conversion, or any other means, procainamide may then be taken orally to prevent their recurrence. Quinidine is more commonly employed for such prophylactic purposes, because its long-term adverse effects seem less serious than the blood dyscrasia or systemic lupus syndrome that occasionally develops during procainamide therapy. Some physicians have preferred procainamide to quinidine for prophylaxis against recurrences of *ventricular* arrhythmias. However, with the introduction of the safer drug disopyramide for prevention of PVCs and of ventricular tachycardia, the use of procainamide for this purpose may decline. (Further discussion of the use of procainamide in *supraventricular* arrhythmias appears in the final section of this chapter.)

Disopyramide

Pharmacologic effects. This drug, which differs in its chemical structure from quinidine, procainamide, and other previously available antiarrhythmic agents, resembles them all in some of its electrophysiologic effects while differing in others. Like the others, disopyramide phosphate (Norpace) decreases the rate of spontaneous depolarizations in ectopic cardiac pacemaker cells that are discharging impulses automatically at an excessively rapid rate. Like quinidine and procainamide, it slows the rate of conduction velocity and increases the effective refractory period in atrial and ventricular muscle cells. However, disopyramide differs from the prototype drugs in its effects on A-V and His–Purkinje system refractory periods and conduction times, which are *not* significantly altered. In theory, these properties should make this drug safer for suppressing rapid arrhythmias in patients who also have conduction defects. In practice, however, this drug is used cautiously, if at all, in patients with abnormalities in conduction, and its use in patients with higher degrees of heart block is contraindicated.

Pharmacokinetics. Disopyramide is rapidly absorbed when administered orally. It reaches therapeutic plasma levels—about 2 to 6 mg/liter (2 to 6 µg/ml)—somewhat more slowly than procainamide, unless a large loading dose is administered in initiating treatment. However, it has a relatively long half-life, a fact that permits dosage scheduling at intervals of 6 hours, or only four times daily.

Most of this drug is eliminated unchanged in the urine, and the rest is excreted as metabolites produced by hepatic enzyme degradation. Thus, patients with impaired renal or hepatic function can quickly attain toxic levels of this drug—thought to be above 9 mg/liter (9 µg/ml)—unless precautions are taken to avoid its accumulation. Depending on the degree to which the patient's creatinine clearance capacity is depressed, the dosing interval may be lengthened from the usual 6 hours to as long as 10, 20, or 30 hours. The drug's dosage should also be reduced in the presence of hepatic impairment, and the ECG should be monitored for signs of prolongation of the P–R interval or widening of the QRS complex.

Cardiovascular toxicity. This drug is claimed less likely to have adverse cardiac and hemodynamic effects than quinidine and procainamide. However, its use requires the same precautions as when other antiarrhythmic drugs are employed. Thus, while this drug is said to cause an *increase* in peripheral arteriole resistance rather than the decrease and resulting vasodilation that occurs with the other antiarrhythmic drugs, some patients may develop a fall in blood pressure sufficiently severe to require

discontinuation of the drug. Similarly, although the drug is claimed not to decrease cardiac contractility significantly, its use in patients with poorly compensated heart failure requires caution to prevent drug-induced decompensation. As indicated previously, despite its relative lack of effect on A-V conduction, use of this drug in patients with greater than first-degree block is considered undesirable because of the possible drug-induced development of second-degree, or even complete (third-degree), heart block.

Extracardiac adverse effects. The main advantage claimed for this drug is its relative freedom from serious toxicity and side-effects compared to quinidine and procainamide. Most patients appear to tolerate its prolonged use much better than they do the older drugs and, according to some studies, only a small fraction of patients have been forced to discontinue this drug compared to the sizable proportion who must stop taking quinidine or procainamide because of discomforting side-effects or serious chronic toxicity reactions. However, this drug has significant anticholinergic activity, and this is responsible for the fairly frequent occurrence of atropinelike side-effects, including mouth dryness and blurring of vision. A smaller percentage of patients, including particularly men with prostatic hypertrophy, may suffer urinary retention. The drug's use may also be unsafe for patients with glaucoma.

Clinical indications. At the present time, the Food and Drug Administration has approved only an oral form of disopyramide for use in suppressing PVCs and episodes of ventricular tachycardia and in preventing their recurrence. An intravenously administered form is being employed experimentally for treating these ventricular arrhythmias when they occur as complications following an acute myocardial infarction or as a result of digitalis intoxication.

The effectiveness of the oral drug for treating patients with purely atrial arrhythmias is also being tested clinically. Because the electrophysiologic effects of disopyramide resemble those of quinidine and procainamide, it is expected to prove useful for control of premature atrial contractions (PACs) and paroxysmal atrial tachycardia (PAT). However, the drug's anticholinergic, or vagolytic, effect could be dangerous in atrial flutter patients, and its safety and efficacy for atrial arrhythmias has not yet been demonstrated in a sufficiently large patient population to permit its approval for use in these disorders.

Lidocaine*

Pharmacologic effects. This drug differs from quinidine and procainamide, the older, "classic" antiarrhythmic drugs, in its effects on some electrophysiologic properties of cardiac cells. These differences are thought to account for its greater safety and effectiveness in the treatment of the ventricular

---

* The local anesthetic properties of this drug and their applications for producing various kinds of regional anesthesia are discussed in Chapter 14 and summarized in *another* drug digest that appears in that chapter.

arrhythmias that often follow an acute myocardial infarction (Chap. 31). Unlike the classic, or prototype, antiarrhythmic agents, lidocaine[+] (Xylocaine) has little effect on the atria, and it does not depress conduction velocity or increase the effective refractory period in A-V and His–Purkinje system tissues when administered in doses that attain therapeutic levels (see the following section on pharmacokinetic aspects). In practice, this means that lidocaine is less likely to cause heart block, cardiac asystole, or ventricular ectopic rhythms. In addition, ordinary therapeutic doses of lidocaine do not depress myocardial contractility, an effect of quinidine and procainamide that can cause cardiac decompensation and failure.

The efficacy of lidocaine in terminating ventricular arrhythmias stems from its actions on the electrophysiologic properties of the cardiac conducting tissues and the muscle cells of the ventricles. Like quinidine, procainamide, and disopyramide, it depresses automaticity, particularly in ectopic sites such as Purkinje fiber pacemakers. Thus, this drug helps to stop PVCs (or extrasystoles) by suppressing spontaneous depolarizations that readily arise at an excessive rate from such subsidiary, or latent, pacemakers in the presence of heart cell ischemia and hypoxia following an acute myocardial infarction (Chap. 31). The drug is believed to be effective in abolishing those ventricular arrhythmias that are the result of re-entry phenomena because of its ability either to overcome a unidirectional block or to convert it to a bidirectional block. That is, this drug helps to counteract the conditions in depressed cardiac cells, which, as explained in Chapter 26, are thought to be responsible for the development of potentially fatal fibrillatory activity in hearts that have been damaged by coronary artery disease or adversely affected by the cardiotoxic effects of overdosage with such drugs as quinidine and digitalis.

Pharmacokinetics. Lidocaine does not reach therapeutically effective levels—1.5 to 5 mg/liter (1.5 to 5 μg/ml)—when it is taken by mouth. The drug must be administered by rapid intravenous injection to be effective for terminating ventricular arrhythmias. To prevent the return of cardiac irregularities, this drug must then often be infused into a vein for a relatively prolonged period. All these facts, which were first learned through clinical experience, can now be explained on the basis of how this drug is handled by the body.

Lidocaine is ineffective when taken orally because much of any administered dose is metabolized by hepatic enzymes during the drug's passage through the liver after its absorption from the duodenum into the portal circulation (first-pass effect). When injected intravenously in a large loading, or bolus, dose, this drug is quickly distributed to the myocardium and other organs with a rich blood supply, and its antiarrhythmic effects develop very rapidly—usually within 1 or 2 minutes after completion of the injection. However, the drug is soon re-distributed by the blood to other body tissues and, although this is a factor that accounts for its relative safety, it also causes the plasma and cardiac concentrations of lidocaine to fall quickly below the level required to maintain therapeutic activity.

Because the plasma level of lidocaine falls to a subtherapeutic point in only 10 to 20 minutes after a single IV bolus dose, additional doses are often required to raise the drug's concentration to levels needed to maintain antiarrhythmic activity. Once the blood level has been built up by repeated bolus doses, it is best maintained by a continuous infusion of a more dilute lidocaine solution. The flow of this infusion can usually be gradually tapered off after 24 hours. During the slow decline in the blood level of lidocaine from the steady state attained by infusion—a result of the drug's metabolism by liver enzymes—the patient is carefully observed to determine whether an increase in the infusion rate is required to counteract any recurring arrhythmias.

Cardiotoxic effects. Adverse effects on cardiac function rarely occur when lidocaine is injected even in large loading doses, because the drug is so rapidly redistributed and diluted in the total mass of body tissues. However, cardiotoxicity can occur during prolonged infusion, particularly in patients with severe liver or kidney disease in whom the plasma level of lidocaine accumulates more readily to the toxic range above 7 mg/liter. Caution is also required in patients with severe congestive heart failure, hypovolemia, or shock, because ordinary safety factors such as rapid redistribution and steady hepatic metabolic degradation do not operate properly in these patients as a result of their circulatory impairment.

The toxic effects of high plasma levels and accumulation of lidocaine in cardiac tissues are similar to those of the antiarrhythmic drugs previously discussed. To avoid depression of A-V and His–Purkinje system conductivity or of myocardial contractility, the patient's ECG is monitored for such signs as lengthening of the P–R interval and widening of the QRS complex. The drug should not be administered to counteract rapid ventricular arrhythmias in patients who also have a high degree of heart block, unless a temporary cardiac pacemaker has previously been inserted to counteract possible drug-induced complete heart block.

Extracardiac effects. Lidocaine, like other local anesthetics, tends to cause central nervous system toxicity when administered in overdoses. The most common symptom is drowsiness, but signs of psychomotor stimulation may also develop. If the infusion is not discontinued, convulsive seizures can occur. Actually, earlier signs of CNS stimulation such as muscle twitching, slurring of speech, mental confusion, or disorientation, which usually develop before signs of cardiotoxicity occur, should serve to warn observant ICCU personnel that plasma concentrations of lidocaine are rising to levels toxic to the heart.

Clinical indications. Lidocaine is the current drug of choice for abolishing premature ventricular beats and preventing ventricular tachycardia in patients who develop cardiac irregularities as a complication of an acute myocardial infarction (Chap. 31). It is safer than quinidine and procainamide for most patients with digitalis-induced cardiotoxicity and is sometimes more effective than phenytoin in such cases. This drug is also used to manage any ventricular arrhythmias that may develop during cardiac catheterization or open heart surgery. It is not as effective as quinidine and procainamide for treating supraventricular arrhythmias.

Phenytoin

Cardiac effects. This antiepileptic drug also has a combination of actions on cardiac cell membranes that make it especially useful for treating some types of ventricular tachyarrhythmias, although it is not approved for this use by the FDA. These actions cause electrophysiologic changes that differ in most respects from those produced by quinidine and procainamide and, instead, resemble those of lidocaine. Specifically, phenytoin[+] (Dilantin; see Drug digests, Chap. 50) causes either no change in conduction velocity or an actual *increase* in the rate at which impulses are conducted through the A-V tissues and Purkinje fibers. It is similar to all the other antiarrhythmic drugs in its ability to suppress automaticity at ectopic pacemakers when administered in doses that do not depress the patient's S-A pacemaker cells.

Clinical indications. The combination of electrophysiologic effects noted above makes phenytoin safer than the traditional antiarrhythmic drugs in clinical disorders marked by *both* premature atrial and ventricular beats and by partial atrioventricular block. This is a common occurrence in digitalis intoxication. As indicated in detail in Chapter 29, overdoses of digitalis can cause many types of arrhythmias, including PAT with block. In such situations, the administration of quinidine or procainamide to terminate atrial and ventricular extrasystoles could lead to complete heart block and ventricular asystole. In contrast, phenytoin—like lidocaine—can abolish premature atrial and ventricular beats without decreasing conduction velocity or increasing the degree of conduction block in the drug-depressed cardiac tissues. In fact, phenytoin can often counteract a partial A-V block while terminating the rapid irregular cardiac rhythms of digitalis intoxication and of other disorders marked by ventricular tachyarrhythmias (see the summary of clinical indications at the end of this chapter).

Cardiotoxicity. Phenytoin should *not*, however, be employed in patients with advanced degrees of heart block, because its use could lead to complete heart block and to simultaneous suppression of the subsidiary ventricular pacemakers that would then be responsible for driving the heart to beat by producing an idioventricular

rhythm. Cardiac arrest of this type has occurred occasionally when phenytoin has been injected intravenously at too rapid a rate in the treatment of status epilepticus (Chap. 50). Thus, to avoid cardiotoxicity during the use of phenytoin for treating ventricular arrhythmias, it must be injected at a rate of no more than 50 mg/minute or in IV doses of 100 mg administered at 5-minute intervals up to a total dose of 1 g.

Other aspects of phenytoin dosage and administration, dosage adjustment to maintain therapeutic plasma levels while avoiding toxic cardiac and central nervous system concentrations, and precautions required to avoid adverse drug interactions are discussed in Chapter 50.

Propranolol

As discussed in detail in Chapter 18, this prototype β-adrenergic blocking agent possesses cardiac actions that are mainly the result of its ability to block some of the tonic sympathetic influences on the functioning of the heart. In this respect, propranolol[+] (Inderal; see Drug digests, Chap. 18) differs from all the previously discussed antiarrhythmic drugs. This drug *does* also affect electrophysiologic properties of cardiac cell membranes by what is sometimes called "quinidinelike" activity. However, ordinary therapeutic doses do not cause such direct depression of cardiac activity, except possibly when this drug is used in treating some cases of digitalis intoxication.

Arrhythmia treatment. Propranolol is particularly effective in the treatment of those cardiac irregularities that are caused entirely or partially by excessive stimulation of the heart by sympathetic nerve impulses or by circulating catecholamines. It is, for example, effective for controlling sinus tachycardia in cases of pheochromocytoma when administered in combination with an α-adrenergic blocking agent such as phentolamine (Regitine; see Chap. 18 for a full discussion of the management of patients with this catecholamine-secreting tumor).

This drug's adjunctive use against similar arrhythmias that arise in other disorders is discussed in several other chapters of the text. It is, for example, employed for slowing the heart in hyperthyroidism (Chap. 22). As indicated in more detail in that chapter, propranolol—when administered by vein—can even counteract the extreme tachycardia of the life-threatening complication of thyrotoxicosis called thyroid storm. Its use for slowing the heart and reducing myocardial oxygen consumption in patients with angina pectoris during periods of emotional stress and physical exertion is discussed in detail in Chapter 31. Intravenously administered propranolol may also counteract arrhythmias that develop during anesthesia as a result of the effects of excessive circulating catecholamines on the myocardium (Chap. 52).

Propranolol is particularly effective for the treatment of atrial and ventricular arrhythmias caused by digitalis intoxication (Chap. 29). Its use can abolish premature ventricular beats produced by digitalis overdosage, and it can sometimes restore sinus rhythm in digitalis-induced PAT. However, if the patient's PAT is accompanied by a high degree of A-V block, propranolol may cause complete heart block by further depression of A-V conduction. For this reason, and because propranolol may also depress myocardial contractility, the safer drug phenytoin is preferred for treating digitalis intoxication, as is discussed above and in Chapter 29.

The role of propranolol alone or together with digitalis for controlling the ventricular rate of patients with such supraventricular arrhythmias as atrial flutter and atrial fibrillation is discussed in the final section of this chapter.

Bretylium

Pharmacologic effects. This more recently introduced drug differs from all the previously discussed antiarrhythmic agents in its mechanism of action and electrophysiologic properties. A unique feature of its cardiac action is a lack of depressant effects on conductivity or on myocardial contractility. Because bretylium tosylate (Bretylol) acts initially to release norepinephrine from adrenergic nerve endings, it can actually increase conduction velocity and strengthen the heartbeat.

Despite this potential advantage, bretylium is not considered a desirable drug with which to begin treatment of severe ventricular arrhythmias, and it is at present recommended for use only after such first-line antiarrhythmic agents as lidocaine, procainamide, or phenytoin have failed to restore a stable cardiac rhythm. One of this drug's main drawbacks is its tendency to cause a decrease in blood pressure, particularly when infused continuously during maintenance therapy. Such hypotension occurs because, after the initial release of norepinephrine, this drug blocks further release of that neurotransmitter from sympathetic nerve endings. Bretylium is actually a member of the class of drugs called adrenergic neuron blockers (Chaps. 18 and 28).

Clinical indications. Bretylium is employed only in the treatment of life-threatening ventricular arrhythmias. It is, for example, used as an adjunct to electrical cardioversion and other standard measures for management of ventricular fibrillation. Patients who develop recurrent episodes of ventricular tachycardia that do not respond to treatment with other antiarrhythmic drugs and measures have sometimes had a sinus rhythm restored by parenterally administered bretylium. For treating ventricular fibrillation, the undiluted drug solution is injected rapidly into a vein. Recurrences of rapid, irregular ventricular arrhythmias are best prevented or treated by injecting bretylium intramuscularly or by the constant IV infusion of a dilute solution of the drug.

Verapamil

Mechanism of action and cardiovascular effects. Verapamil HCl (Calan; Isoptin) is the newest of the antiarrhythmic drugs. It is a member of yet a different class of drugs called *calcium channel blockers* or *slow channel blockers* (Chap. 26). It blocks rather selectively the influx of calcium ions across the cell membranes of the specialized tissue and muscle of the heart and of the smooth muscle of blood vessels. It thus depresses the rate at which pacemaker cells in the specialized tissue, including the S-A node, fire; it slows conduction velocity through the A-V node; and it decreases the contractility of vascular smooth muscle. These drug effects are supportive evidence for the fairly new concept that action potentials in the cells of these tissues are calcium-dependent rather than sodium-dependent, a difference from action potentials in neurons and skeletal muscle cells. The result of these effects is that verapamil can slow the heart, suppress ectopic pacemakers in the specialized tissue, protect the ventricles from an excessive rate of firing of atrial pacemakers, and cause vasodilatation in the coronary and in the peripheral arteries.

Clinical indications. The effects of this drug on the heart make it useful as an antiarrhythmic agent in treating supraventricular tachyarrhythmias. Its negative chronotropic and vascular effects make verapamil useful in treating angina pectoris (Chap. 31). However, the drug can further reduce blood pressure in hypotensive patients, and can cause exacerbations of sinus bradycardia and heart block. By depressing calcium influx to the contractile mechanism of ventricular muscle, it can interfere with excitation–contraction coupling (Chap. 26) and weaken the contractions of cardiac muscle, thus exacerbating congestive heart failure. The drug is therefore contraindicated in patients with such problems. In addition, patients with impaired liver function need a reduction in dosage, and special caution must be used when giving the drug to patients with impaired kidney function. The drug is extensively metabolized in the liver and its metabolites are excreted in the urine.

Verapamil is approved only for IV use in cardiac arrhythmias; however, the oral preparation that is used in angina is under investigation for use in paroxysmal supraventricular tachycardia.

Two other calcium channel blockers, *nifedipine* (Procardia) and *diltiazem* (Cardizem), that are approved for oral use in angina pectoris (Chap. 31), are being investigated for IV use in supraventricular tachyarrhythmias.

The management of tachyarrhythmias*

Rapid arrhythmias originate either in the ventricles or in the cardiac tissues above the ventricles—the *supraventricular cells of the atria and of the atrioventricular junc-

---

* *Bradyarrhythmia* treatment with drugs such as atropine and isoproterenol is discussed in Chapters 16, 17, and 31 and elsewhere in the text.

tion. Some aspects of the treatment of ventricular arrhythmias have been taken up in the earlier discussions of individual drugs such as lidocaine, phenytoin, and propranolol, and more detailed discussions of the use of these and other agents in treating such arrhythmias as PVCs, ventricular tachycardia, and ventricular fibrillation appear in Chapters 29 and 31.

Thus, this section will deal only with the clinical applications of antiarrhythmic drugs in the management of supraventricular tachyarrhythmias. The most common of these are atrial extrasystoles, or PACs, atrial flutter, atrial fibrillation, and tachycardias that originate in the atria and in the A-V junctional tissues.

General considerations

Supraventricular arrhythmias can have serious hemodynamic consequences of the type discussed at the beginning of this chapter. The reason for this is that many impulses that arise in the atrial and junctional tissues are transmitted to the His–Purkinje system of the ventricles. The impulses that pass down from above then depolarize ventricular muscle fibers at a rapid, and most often an irregular, rate. Ventricular contractions that occur as a result of supraventricular arrhythmias can be just as hazardous as those that are the result of ventricular arrhythmias.

This is particularly true in the case of older patients with pre-existing organic heart disease. Thus, while a young person may develop PACs or even PAT without suffering serious consequences, an elderly patient with advanced rheumatic, coronary, or hypertensive heart disease may develop a potentially fatal reduction in cardiac output when the ventricles are being driven at a rapid regular or irregular rate. Such situations constitute medical emergencies requiring prompt treatment.

The main goal of drug treatment is to protect the ventricles from being driven at too rapid a rate. A secondary aim is to terminate the atrial arrhythmias. Although drugs can be effective for abolishing abnormal atrial and junctional rhythms, they are not often the treatment of choice in extreme emergencies. In such cases, most cardiologists prefer to employ direct current electric shock to convert atrial flutter or fibrillation to a normal sinus rhythm. Drugs may then be employed for a third therapeutic objective: to prevent further recurrences of the original supraventricular arrhythmia.

Treatment of specific arrhythmias

Premature atrial contractions

Atrial extrasystoles are isolated beats set off by impulses generated at ectopic sites—that is, in atrial tissues outside of the S-A node. These and the ventricular beats that the abnormal atrial impulses may elicit when they make their way through the junctional tissues into the His–Purkinje system do not in themselves have any serious

hemodynamic consequences. In fact, when PACs occur in people with a normal heart (as they sometimes do) no treatment is ordinarily necessary.

On the other hand, PACs can set off more serious arrhythmias when they occur in patients with organic heart disease such as congestive heart failure or following an acute myocardial infarction (AMI). To prevent possible atrial fibrillation or even ventricular fibrillation, drug treatment is desirable in such cases. Control of congestive heart failure by digitalis, diuretics, and other measures described in the previous chapter will ordinarily prevent PACs. If they persist in this and other situations, such antiarrhythmic drugs as quinidine or procainamide may be employed to suppress automaticity in the ectopic atrial foci. PACs that appear on the ECG of AMI patients being monitored in the ICCU are best treated by IV infusion of lidocaine, just as are PVCs (Chap. 31), because both types of extrasystoles can set off more serious arrhythmias in a damaged, ischemic myocardium.

Atrial fibrillation and flutter

These arrhythmias tend to develop in patients with advanced degrees of such disorders as coronary heart disease, valvular damage as a result of rheumatic heart disease, and congestive heart failure. Atrial flutter occurs less commonly than atrial fibrillation, causes fewer complications, and is somewhat easier to control (Fig. 30-1). Both conditions are marked by impulses generated in the atria at a rapid rate either from ectopic foci or as a result of reentry (circus) movements.

In atrial fibrillation, impulses arise in the atria at rates of 400 to 600/minute; in atrial flutter the rate of fluttering beats is between 260 and 340/minute. Fortunately, only a fraction of these atrial impulses trigger ventricular responses. Thus, for example, because most of the impulses from the atria fail to pass through the A-V junction, the ventricular rate of patients with atrial fibrillation is usually between 120 and 160 beats/minute, and is highly irregular. In atrial flutter, the ventricular rate is somewhat lower and may be more regular, because of the development of a high degree of physiologic A-V block. Only one of every two atrial impulses elicits a ventricular contraction in most cases—a 2:1 conduction ratio. Patients with higher—3:1 or 4:1—conduction ratios may have very little increase in their ventricular rate and may even be unaware of any signs and symptoms of atrial flutter.

Treatment. The main method employed today to convert these atrial arrhythmias to a normal sinus rhythm in emergency situations is direct current (DC) shock cardioversion rather than drug therapy. However, to protect the ventricles from being driven too rapidly in less urgent situations, rapid digitalization is the method of choice. Patients with atrial arrhythmias of relatively recent onset usually respond with a drop in their ventricular rate to between 70 and 80 beats/minute when

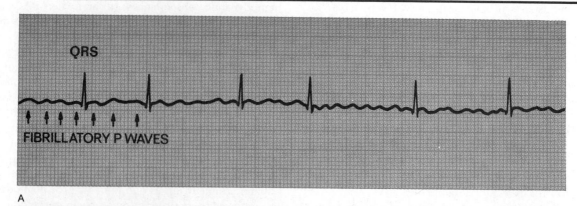

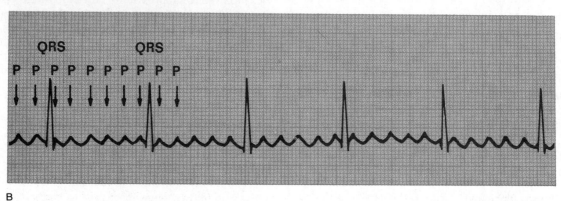

Figure 30-1. (*A*) ECG for atrial fibrillation; (*B*) ECG for atrial flutter. (Blowers MG, Smith RJ: How to Read an ECG (rev ed). Oradell, NJ, Medical Economics, 1977)

they are digitalized within 24 hours with several divided doses of digoxin (Chap. 29).

Digitalis acts in these disorders by interfering with passage of atrial impulses to the ventricles through its ability to increase the degree of the natural A-V block mentioned above. This drug does not depress automaticity at the atrial ectopic sites in which the aberrant impulses responsible for these arrhythmias originate. Thus, its use alone does *not* ordinarily convert the atrial arrhythmia to a sinus rhythm. Occasionally, however, patients with atrial fibrillation attain a normal sinus rhythm, possibly because of better myocardial circulation following digitalization. Many more patients with atrial flutter respond favorably to digoxin therapy, particularly when this arrhythmia developed suddenly and treatment was started promptly. Actually, the flutter is often first converted to fibrillation, which then converts to a sinus rhythm when digitalis dosage is reduced or withdrawn.

Quinidine and procainamide, which—unlike digitalis—depress automaticity, can restore a sinus rhythm and prevent recurrences of the atrial arrhythmias. Thus, after patients are first digitalized, they then often receive quinidine or the synthetic antiarrhythmic drug with similar actions. Prior digitalization is essential because the

administration of these drugs may actually *increase* the ventricular rate instead of slowing it, particularly in patients with atrial flutter. As indicated above, quinidine can do this by an atropinelike action, which removes vagus nerve influence over the A-V node—a so-called *vagolytic* effect. This possible drug-induced change of a 2:1 conduction ratio to a 1:1 ratio with a resulting doubling of the ventricular rate is avoided by digitalis pretreatment, which increases vagal control over the A-V node by its *vagomimetic* or *vagotonic* action (Chap. 29).

Although quinidine and procainamide can produce a sinus rhythm in previously digitalized patients, they are rarely used for this purpose today when immediate emergency conversion of atrial fibrillation or flutter is required. This is because the intravenous administration of these drugs is less dependable than DC cardioversion, and because adequate doses commonly cause cardiotoxicity. In patients who are to receive cardioversion, digitalis must be discontinued (if it was previously employed), because DC shock can set off ventricular arrhythmias in the digitalized myocardium. In such cases quinidine is substituted for digitalis during the preconversion period. After conversion to a sinus rhythm, digitalis treatment is resumed—sometimes together with quinidine—to prevent recurrences of atrial flutter and fibrillation and to maintain normal sinus rhythm. (The dosage precautions that must be considered when these drugs are used concurrently have been discussed above.)

Many patients whose chronic atrial fibrillation is a result of mitral stenosis or of other residual effects of rheumatic heart disease are prone to develop blood clots because of blood flow stasis in the auricle, an appendage of the atrium. Thus, these patients are often placed on anticoagulant therapy to prevent mural thrombi and possible arterial emboli (Chap. 34), particularly following conversion with DC electroshock or with quinidine. It is important to check such patients carefully for signs of bleeding whey they are receiving both quinidine and warfarin (Coumadin), because these drugs can interact in ways that increase the likelihood of hemorrhage.

Propranolol (Inderal) is sometimes employed with patients in atrial fibrillation, because it causes fewer side-effects than quinidine or procainamide. Although it is less effective than the traditional drugs for producing a normal sinus rhythm, propranolol is quite effective for preventing the ventricles from being driven at a too rapid rate. It is particularly useful in patients with atrial fibrillation that stems from thyrotoxicosis, because these patients often do not respond adequately to digitalis alone. The addition of propranolol to the digitalis regimen increases the degree of A-V block and helps bring the ventricular rate down to the desired 70 to 80 beats/minute.

Tachycardias of supraventricular origin

Three types of tachycardia have their origin in impulses arising at an abnormally rapid rate in the tissues above the ventricles. In one of these—*sinus tachycardia*—the automaticity of the normal pacemaker, the S-A node, is increased. In the other arrhythmias, the source of the rapid ventricular rhythm that invariably develops lies in tissues outside the S-A node. Such *atrial* or *junctional tachycardia* may develop suddenly and end just as abruptly—for example, in episodes of PAT, bouts of

which sometimes occur even in a patient with a healthy heart (Fig. 30-2). However, supraventricular tachycardias can also be continuous, or *non*paroxysmal, particularly in patients with underlying heart damage. In such cases these tachycardias can be quite dangerous to patients with severe organic heart disease, because the impulses that arise in ectopic supraventricular sites at rates of 140 to 220/minute are conducted to the ventricles at a 1:1 conduction ratio.

Treatment. *Sinus tachycardia* with a heart rate of 100 beats/minute or more does not ordinarily require or respond to specific treatment with antiarrhythmic drugs. Instead, it is best to determine the underlying cause of the rapid sinus rhythm and correct it. Thus, when sinus tachycardia occurs in patients with congestive heart failure, the sinus rate slows when treatment with digitalis (Chap. 29) succeeds in counteracting the cardiac decompensation. Similarly, in hyperthyroidism (Chap. 22), sinus tachycardia reverts to a more normal sinus rhythm when the thyroid disorder is brought under control with specific surgical and medical measures.

In *atrial and A-V junctional tachycardias,* treatment depends in part on whether the patient's heart is diseased or essentially healthy and on whether or not the rapid heart rate leads to development of hazardous hemodynamic disturbances such as congestive heart failure. Thus, a young patient with PAT but no other symptoms may respond to rest and reassurance.

Vagal stimulation by physical or pharmacologic measures is employed in patients who do not respond to rest and sedation or who require more rapid conversion to a sinus rhythm. The physician may first try carotid sinus massage or have the patient perform the Valsalva maneuver. If these attempts to induce reflex vagal stimulation of the atrial or A-V junctional tissues fail to terminate the tachycardia, the physician may resort to intravenous administration of certain autonomic drugs or digitalis glycosides to increase vagal tonic influences upon the heart.

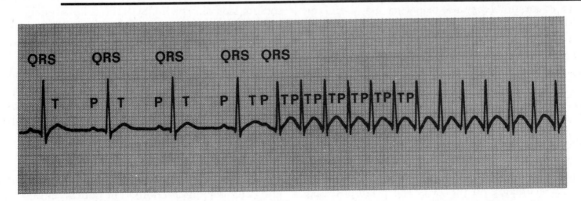

Figure 30-2. ECG for paroxysmal atrial tachycardia (PAT). (Blowers MG, Smith RJ: How to Read an ECG (rev ed). Oradell, NJ, Medical Economics, 1977)

Parasympathomimetic drugs such as edrophonium (Tensilon), which has a rapid action of short duration, or neostigmine (Prostigmin) may be employed together with carotid sinus pressure to increase vagotonia (Chap. 15).

This can also sometimes be accomplished with a single injection of one of the adrenergic drugs that act mainly at α receptors in the blood vessels. As indicated in Chapter 17, phenylephrine (Neo-Synephrine) and methoxamine (Vasoxyl) can slow the rapid heart rate, even though these "alphamimetic-type" sympathomimetic agents do not act directly on the heart. Phenylephrine, injected as a single IV bolus or by slow IV infusion, acts, instead, by constricting the patient's blood vessels and raising the systolic pressure. This, in turn, stimulates baroreceptors in the carotid sinus and elsewhere and sets off reflex activity that slows the heart by increasing vagal tone.

Digitalization (Chap. 29), which as indicated above is a procedure that also increases vagal control over the A-V node, is next used in the event that the more immediately effective cholinergic or adrenergic drugs fail. A relatively rapid-acting glycoside such as digoxin (Lanoxin) or deslanoside (Cedilanid-D) is injected IV in several divided doses with application of carotid sinus massage periodically to aid in converting the tachycardia to a sinus rhythm. Oral digoxin may then be ordered as maintenance therapy for patients who tend to suffer frequent recurrences of PAT.

Antiarrhythmic drugs such as quinidine, procainamide, propranolol, or verapamil are also occasionally used for conversion in some circumstances, as are direct current countershock and atrial pacing. More commonly, these drugs are added to the regimen of patients who tend to suffer recurrent episodes of PAT despite digitalization. Propranolol and verapamil are claimed to be particularly effective for control of supraventricular tachycardias in patients with the Wolff–Parkinson–White syndrome, a disorder in which the patient's rapid ventricular rate is thought to result from excessively frequent conduction of impulses from the atria through abnormal pathways. Propranolol may also be particularly useful for control of PAT induced by digitalis overdosage. However, as previously indicated, when digitalis toxicity causes PAT with a high degree of A-V block, phenytoin is often preferred.

Additional clinical considerations

The effects of these drugs on various body systems contraindicate their use in certain conditions. A very slow heart rate, presence of A-V nodal heart block, or a prolonged QRS complex on the ECG will predispose the patient to serious cardiac problems if an antiarrhythmic is given. Congestive heart failure and hypotension can be exacerbated by the cardiovascular depression produced

by these drugs. Precautions also have to be taken with patients who have hepatic or renal dysfunction, because the drugs can accumulate to toxic levels if they are not metabolized and excreted efficiently. As with many other drugs, the safety of the use of these drugs during pregnancy and lactation has not been established. The drugs should be avoided during pregnancy and, if they are indicated in a lactating woman, another method of feeding the baby should be used.

Quinidine toxicity is characterized by a syndrome called cinchonism. The signs and symptoms of this toxic reaction include ringing in the ears, headache, nausea, dizziness, vertigo, and fever, which are similar to the signs and symptoms of aspirin overdose. This can occur in predisposed persons after only one dose of quinidine. If possible, it is recommended that a test dose of quinidine be given to establish its safety in a particular patient. Patients receiving quinidine should be taught the signs and symptoms of cinchonism so that they can be alert to the development of a toxic response.

Procainamide use has been associated with the development of a lupuslike syndrome. If a patient is maintained on chronic procainamide therapy, he should receive periodic blood tests to monitor for antinuclear antibody (ANA) development. If ANAs are found, the drug should be stopped; in most cases, the lupus syndrome will then resolve.

Disopyramide has been associated with many anticholinergic side-effects, such as urinary retention and dry mouth. It should be used very cautiously in patients who can be adversely affected by these effects—for example, patients with prostatic hypertrophy or glaucoma. This drug has been frequently associated with the development of congestive heart failure (CHF), and patients who are receiving this drug should be alerted to the early signs of CHF to prevent serious problems from developing.

Any patient whose cardiac status is unstable enough to require the use of an antiarrhythmic should be carefully monitored and emergency equipment should be on standby. Quinidine toxicity can be treated with sodium lactate, which blocks the cellular effects of quinidine. Dopamine and norepinephrine can be used to reverse the hypotension associated with toxicity from procainamide, disopyramide, or verapamil. Infusion of calcium may also be useful in reversing the toxicity of verapamil. Life support equipment, emergency cart drugs, and electronic cardiac pacemakers may be needed in extreme situations, and should be readily accessible if a patient is on these drugs.

Drug–drug and drug–diet interactions

Quinidine has been associated with several drug–drug and drug–diet interactions. The concurrent use of quinidine with *oral anticoagulants* has been associated with bleeding and even with frank hemmorhage. If a patient on oral anticoagulants is to receive quinidine, the dosage of the oral anticoagulant should be markedly reduced. Quinidine also increases the effectiveness of *neuromuscular blocking* and *anticholinergic drugs. Rifampin, phenytoin,* and *phenobarbital* induce liver enzymes that decrease the effective levels of quinidine. Patients taking these drugs will require increased dosage of quinidine to achieve a therapeutic effect. Quinidine blocks the excretion of *digoxin,* and patients who receive these drugs concurrently will require a reduced dosage of digoxin to prevent the development of digoxin toxicity. Quinidine requires an acidic urine for excretion. Foods that have an *alkaline ash*—citrus juice, vegetables, milk products—as well as excessive use of *antacids* can cause the urine to become alkaline and lead to elevated serum quinidine levels. Patients need to be taught to avoid excess ingestion of these foods, and should be taught the signs and symptoms of quinidine toxicity so that they can promptly detect any problems.

The hypotension produced by verapamil may add to that produced by *oral antihypertensives;* antihypertensive drugs should be used at a lower dosage if verapamil is started. Verapamil can also increase the serum levels of *digitalis preparations.* Calcium-containing drugs and excess dietary calcium can interfere with the effectiveness of verapamil. *Phenytoin* induces enzymes that metabolize *disopyramide,* thus decreasing its therapeutic effect. *Phenytoin* and *lidocaine* used concurrently can lead to serious cardiac depression. The concurrent use of two antiarrhythmic drugs can produce additive–adverse effects on the heart and lead to potentially serious cardiac problems.

The patient teaching guide summarizes the points that should be incorporated into a teaching program for patients who are receiving antiarrhythmics. The guide to the nursing process summarizes the clinical considerations necessary in the nursing care of the patient receiving antiarrhythmics.

Patient teaching guide: antiarrhythmics

The drug that has been prescribed for you is called an antiarrhythmic. This drug acts to stop irregular rhythm in the heart, helping it to beat more regularly and therefore more efficiently. The drug may work by making the heart less irritable and by slowing it down to a more effective rate.

Instructions:

1. The name of your drug is ——————— .

2. The dosage that has been prescribed for you is ——————— .

3. Your drug should be taken ———— times a day. The best time to take your drug is ——————— .
   (*Procainamide* must be taken around the clock. You will need to have an alarm clock at night to awaken you to take your medication. Procainamide should be taken on an empty stomach. The best times for you to take your drug are ————— , ————— , ————— .)
   (*Quinidine* and *disopyramide* may be taken with food if gastrointestinal upset occurs.)
   (*Verapamil* should be taken on an empty stomach, 1 hour before or 2 hours after meals.)

4. If your drug is quinidine, you should limit your intake of foods, and avoid over-the-counter drugs that make your urine alkaline—for example, citrus juices, milk, vegetables, and antacids. If your urine becomes alkaline you may develop signs of an overdose of quinidine.

5. It is helpful to take your pulse on a regular basis. You should count the number of beats in 1 minute and determine if the pulse is regular or irregular. Your usual resting heart rate is ——————— . Record your pulse on your calendar for quick reference.

(continued)

6. Some side-effects of the drug that you should be aware of include the following:

Nausea, vomiting, loss of appetite	These problems may pass over time; taking the drug with meals, if appropriate may help; small, frequent meals may help.
Diarrhea or constipation	These problems are very common; if either occurs and becomes too uncomfortable, consult with your nurse or physician.
Tiredness, weakness	Spacing your activities throughout the day and taking periodic rests will help to conserve your energy and will also help your heart.
Sensitivity to light (*disopyramide*)	Avoid prolonged exposure to ultraviolet light and sunlight.

7. Tell any physician, nurse, or dentist who is taking care of you that you are on this drug.

8. Avoid the use of over-the-counter drugs while you are taking this drug. If you feel that you need one of these drugs, consult with your nurse or physician.

9. Keep this and all medications out of the reach of children.

10. It is important to see your nurse or physician regularly to have your heart and your response to this drug evaluated.

11. Do not stop taking this medication. If you have to stop the medication for any reason, contact your nurse or physician.

Notify your nurse or physician if any of the following occur:

Chest pain
Difficulty in breathing
Ringing in your ears
Fever, sore throat, skin rash
Swelling in your ankles, legs or
    hands
Unusually slow pulse (less than 55
    beats/minute)
Unusually fast pulse (more than 15
    beats/minute above your
    normal rate)
Suddenly irregular pulse

Guide to the nursing process: antiarrhythmics

Assessment	Nursing diagnoses	Interventions	Evaluation
Past history—underlying medical conditions (*contraindications*): Myasthenia gravis A-V heart block Congestive heart failure Renal disease Hepatic failure Hypotension Electrolyte imbalance Pregnancy Lactation *Allergies:* these or related drugs; tartrazine (in some preparations) Medication history (*cautions*) Oral anticoagulants Anticholinergics Neuromuscular blockers Rifampin Phenytoin Phenobarbital Digitalis preparations Other antiarrhythmics Oral antihypertensives **Physical assessment** Neurologic: orientation, affect, reflexes Cardiovascular: P, BP, ECG, auscultation, peripheral perfusion Respiratory: rate, adventitious sounds GI: normal habits, bowel sounds, liver function tests Renal: urine output, renal function tests Laboratory tests: ANA, blood glucose level	Potential alteration in bowel elimination Potential alteration in cardiac output Potential alteration in fluid volume Knowledge deficit regarding drug therapy Potential alteration in tissue perfusion	Safe and appropriate drug administration Provision of comfort measures: • Small frequent meals • Accessible bathroom facilities • Rest periods • Avoidance of exposure to light • Positioning • Diet precautions Patient teaching regarding: • Drug • Cautions • Warning signs Support and encouragement to cope with diagnosis, therapy and side-effects Provision of monitoring, life support, and emergency equipment, as needed	Monitor the therapeutic effects of the drug: cardiac rhythm Monitor for side-effects of drug: • Arrhythmias • Renal function • Hepatic function • ANA levels • Signs of CHF • Rash, fever • Chest pain • Cinchonism Evaluate effectiveness of patient teaching program Evaluate effectiveness of support and encouragement offered Monitor for drug–diet interactions: • Alkaline foods → ↓ effect of quinidine Monitor for drug–drug interactions (several possible) Monitor for cardiovascular instability: ↑ QRS ↑ P–R interval ↓ BP Severe CHF Monitor effectiveness of supportive measures, as needed

Summary of clinical indications and objectives of antiarrhythmic drug treatment

Clinical indications	Objectives
Atrial tachyarrhythmias Atrial premature beats Atrial flutter Atrial fibrillation Atrial tachycardia (paroxysmal and *non*paroxysmal)	Used mainly to protect the ventricles from excessive supraventricular impulses May also prevent recurrences of atrial arrhythmias when administered as maintenance therapy, following electrical cardioversion to restore normal sinus rhythm
Ventricular tachyarrhythmias Premature ventricular contractions (ventricular extrasystoles; PVCs) Ventricular tachycardia Ventricular fibrillation	Used to restore normal rhythm by abolishing PVCs and thus preventing their extension to more serious arrhythmias in various clinical situations*

* Among the clinical situations of varied etiology in which various antiarrhythmic drugs are employed are the following: (1) patients who have suffered an acute myocardial infarction (AMI); (2) patients who have received overdoses of digitalis; (3) patients with arrhythmias set off by anesthetics such as cyclopropane and halothane; (4) patients undergoing cardiac (open heart) surgery and other types of thoracic surgery; and (5) patients with conditions marked by excessive sympathetic nervous system stimulation or excessive circulating catecholamines (pheochromocytoma).

Summary of toxic effects of antiarrhythmic agents

Cardiovascular toxicity

Various degrees of atrioventricular (A-V) dissociation, or heart block, as indicated by lengthening of the P–R interval on the electrocardiogram

Depression of ventricular conduction, as indicated by a widening of the QRS complex on the electrocardiogram

Cardiac arrest: either asystole or ventricular fibrillation, possibly preceded by premature ventricular contractions and tachycardia

Acute hypotension as a result of depression of myocardial contractility combined with peripheral vasodilation (quinidine and procainamide)

Paradoxical tachycardia in patients with atrial flutter, or fibrillation, as a result of drug-induced reduction in the degree of A-V block to a 1:1 ratio (because of the vagolytic effect of quinidine, procainamide, and disopyramide, such patients should first be digitalized)

Arterial embolism as a result of conversion to a sinus rhythm in patients with atrial mural thrombi

Extracardiac toxicity

Disopyramide. Dry mouth, blurred vision, urinary hesitancy or retention, constipation

Lidocaine. Drowsiness, dizziness, nervousness, confusion; paresthesias (generalized numbness and tingling); muscular tremors, twitching, convulsions

Procainamide. Nausea, vomiting, bitter taste, loss of appetite; macropapular skin rash, urticaria, angioneurotic edema, fever; dizziness, weakness, mental depression; rare idiosyncrasies include agranulocytosis and collagen disease syndrome resembling lupus erythematosus

Phenytoin. Dizziness, weakness, fatigue, muscular incoordination, and ataxia, nystagmus; nausea and vomiting; skin rash, itching (see also Chap. 50)

Propranolol. Nausea, vomiting, light-headedness; weakness, fatigue, possible mental depression; rarely, respiratory distress, wheezing, laryngospasm (contraindicated in patients with bronchial asthma and allergic rhinitis); rarely, a red rash and paresthesias (see summary, Chap. 18)

Quinidine. Cinchonism: tinnitus, visual disturbances, dizziness, headache, confusion; gastrointestinal: nausea, vomiting, abdominal cramps, and diarrhea; hypersensitivity: fever, skin rashes, angioneurotic edema, asthma, respiratory depression, cyanosis, thrombocytic purpura

Verapamil. Nausea, constipation, headache, dizziness

Case study

Presentation

RA, a 56-year-old post-MI patient with a documented duodenal ulcer, has felt very "stressed" lately. He called the clinic nurse with complaints of dizziness, occasional confusion, headaches, nausea, vomiting, and a very slow pulse. The nurse requested that RA come right into the clinic. On examination BP was 82/60 and P 52, with ECG tracing showing second-degree heart block with escape beats. It was discovered that RA was being maintained on quinidine to regulate post-MI arrhythmias. On questioning, he said that his vomiting was minimal, but that he had been medicating himself with Mylanta tablets (about 12 a day) for his ulcer pain, and drinking "lots of orange juice" (1 to 2 quarts a day) to treat a "cold."

What happened to RA, and what nursing actions should be taken with him?

Discussion

RA has many of the signs and symptoms of quinidine toxicity. The initial therapy for his present condition will include withholding all medication, drawing a blood sample for serum quinidine level determination, and carefully monitoring RA's condition, with emergency equipment on standby in case his cardiovascular status deteriorates further. (This emergency equipment should include sodium lactate, which blocks the effects of the drug on the myocardium, and adrenergic stimulants, which can increase heart rate, BP, and cardiac output.) RA was rapidly stabilized, and patient teaching was begun on the drug therapy that the patient had been using. The effects of foods and drugs on urine pH and on quinidine excretion were stressed with RA. Foods that have an alkaline ash—milk, citrus juices, vegetables—cause an alkaline urine, which prevents the excretion of the quinidine, leading to toxic levels in the bloodstream. Antacids, such as Mylanta, especially when taken in large quantities, also increase the alkalinity of the urine. This combination of drug and diet factors probably made RA's urine quite alkaline, leading to increased serum levels of quinidine and a toxic response to the drug. The signs and symptoms of quinidine toxicity should be reviewed with RA, as well as precautionary measures that he should take. RA should be told that he did the correct thing in calling and should be encouraged to do so again should he have problems. The teaching program should be directed at preventing future problems.

While RA is within the health-care system, it is important to offer him support and encouragement. His ulcer can be evaluated at this time, as well as his feelings of "stress." The patient may need to ventilate his feelings and explore new ways of coping with stressful situations or of avoiding them. The effects of such stress on the heart can be reviewed with RA in attempts to help him realize the importance of minimizing it. It would also be helpful to review the problems of self-medication for various complaints while on a prescription drug. When the teaching session is complete, RA should receive all this information in writing for future reference. This time, his quinidine toxicity was discovered before serious complications developed; with effective teaching, such problems should be minimized or avoided in the future.

Drug digests

Lidocaine HCl USP (Xylocaine)

Actions and indications. This very versatile local anesthetic is used not only for relief of pain during and after surgery, obstetrics, and other clinical situations, but also for treatment of cardiac arrhythmias. It is particularly useful for rapid control of premature ventricular contractions in patients with an acute myocardial infarction; this prevents development of dangerous ventricular tachycardia. The drug also suppresses digitalis-induced ventricular tachyarrhythmias and abolishes the various arrhythmias that may arise during or following cardiac manipulation, surgery, or catheterization. It has also been employed in neurology for controlling the seizures of status epilepticus.

Adverse effects, cautions, and contraindications. To avoid cardiovascular toxicity (manifested mainly by bradycardia and hypotension) this drug must be administered with constant monitoring of the patient's electrocardiogram and frequent blood pressure checks. The IV infusion flow is discontinued if the P–R interval becomes prolonged, if the QRS complex widens, or if actual arrhythmias appear or get worse. The drug is not administered to patients with severe degrees of heart block or Stokes–Adams syndrome; patients with sinus bradycardia

should first receive isoproterenol or rapid electric pacing before this drug is administered to control premature ventricular contractions.

The first central effect of overdosage is drowsiness rather than the restlessness usually seen with other systemically absorbed local anesthetics. However, higher doses can also cause excitation of central motor systems leading to muscular twitching, tremors, and convulsions, which may require control by administration of an ultrashort barbiturate.

Dosage and administration. For relief of pain this local anesthetic is available in various concentrations for infiltration and regional anesthesia, and for topical application as solutions, jelly, or ointment. (See the Drug digests in Chapter 14 and other sources for details of administration.)

The 2% intravenous solution is employed for cardiac arrhythmias in two ways: (1) *a single injection* of 50 to 100 mg is administered (using the 5-ml ampule containing 20 mg/ml) at a rate of 25 to 50 mg/min; this dose may be repeated, but only up to a total of no more than 200 to 300 mg in 1 hour; (2) *continuous infusion* of 1 to 4 mg/min of a solution containing 1 or 2 mg/ml may be administered until the patient's rhythm has stabilized. (Such solutions are prepared by adding one or two 50-ml vials of the 2% solution to 1 liter of 5% glucose and water solution.)

An intramuscular injection of about 3 ml of a solution containing 100 mg/ml may be made in certain exceptional circumstances. It may be repeated, if necessary, after 1 to 1½ hours.

Procainamide HCl USP (Pronestyl)

Actions and indications. This drug, a derivative of the local anesthetic procaine, is used for its effects on cardiac function in the treatment of arrhythmias. It acts by suppressing automaticity in ectopic tissues and by slowing conduction in atrial and ventricular musculature and in the specialized transmission system.

Procainamide is particularly effective for control of ventricular extrasystoles and tachycardia, and it is employed for that purpose in treating arrhythmias arising as a complication of an acute myocardial infarction, digitalis intoxication, cyclopropane anesthesia, and surgery within the chest. It is also sometimes effective for terminating supraventricular tachycardia resulting from atrial fibrillation.

Adverse effects, cautions, and contraindications. Patients must be carefully observed during intravenous administration of this

drug to detect tendencies toward hypotension and electrocardiographic changes indicative of progressive conduction defect. The drug is discontinued if signs of heart block appear. Caution is required in patients with digitalis poisoning and others with A-V conduction disturbances. Complete heart block constitutes a contraindication to the use of procainamide. Patients with atrial flutter or fibrillation should be digitalized before conversion to a normal sinus rhythm is attempted to avoid sudden speedup of the ventricular rate as a result of a reduction in A-V block by this drug's anticholinergic activity. Overdosage or too rapid IV administration can cause cardiac arrest.

High oral dosage can cause loss of appetite, nausea, and vomiting. Prolonged oral administration often causes the appearance of lupus erythematosus cells and occasionally clinical signs and symptoms of that syndrome.

The drug should be discontinued if a test for the presence of increasing antinuclear antibodies (ANA) becomes positive. It is also withdrawn if blood tests reveal a markedly reduced white blood cell count, because cases of fatal agranulocytosis have been reported.

Dosage and administration. The drug is injected intravenously in emergencies at rates between 25 and 50 mg/min with electrocardiographic and blood pressure monitoring. Dosage should not exceed 1 g.

Intramuscular administration of between 250 mg and 750 mg is employed when patients cannot take procainamide by mouth; larger doses—1 g to 2 g—may be administered IM prior to intrathoracic surgical procedures. Oral doses of 1 g are given initially for ventricular tachycardia and 1.25 g for atrial tachycardia. These may be followed by doses of 500 mg, 750 mg, or 1000 mg every 3 to 6 hours.

Quinidine sulfate USP (Quinora)

Actions and indications. This *Cinchona* alkaloid is used to prevent and treat atrial and ventricular arrhythmias. It acts mainly by suppressing automaticity in ectopic pacemaker tissues and by increasing the effective refractory period of cardiac muscle and conducting tissues. Although still sometimes employed to terminate attacks of atrial tachycardia, fibrillation, and flutter, quinidine is now used mainly to prevent recurrences of these disorders following their conversion to a normal rhythm by direct current electric shock or by other drugs. It is used occasionally to abolish atrial extrasystoles but, for reverting ventricular premature beats and tachycardia, other drugs or electric techniques are now preferred. Quinidine may then be used for maintaining a normal sinus rhythm.

Adverse effects, cautions, and contraindi-

cations. Cardiotoxic effects tend to develop as a result of overdosage, particularly during emergency intravenous administration. In such situations, the electrocardiogram is monitored for signs of impaired conduction or for the development of ventricular extrasystoles. Quinidine is contraindicated in patients with heart block. Ordinarily, drug-induced cardiac arrhythmias occur mainly when plasma levels of quinidine exceed 8 mg/liter, but cardiotoxicity can occur at much lower blood levels in sensitive patients who are taking relatively small oral doses.

Other signs of idiosyncrasy or drug allergy include development of skin rashes, fever, and thrombocytic purpura. A syndrome called *cinchonism* is marked by gastrointestinal disturbances (nausea, vomiting, abdominal cramps, and diarrhea), tinnitus (ringing in the ears), blurring of vision, light-headed-

ness, dizziness, and tremors. Some authorities suggest administering a test dose to detect hypersensitivity before beginning treatment. Patients unable to tolerate quinidine can usually be maintained on procainamide.

Dosage and administration. Patients are usually first treated with oral doses of 0.2 to 0.6 g every 2 to 4 hours (or five doses daily) for several days. Once therapeutic blood levels of about 3 to 6 mg/liter have been attained, the patient may usually be maintained on daily doses of about 0.2 g administered by mouth up to six times a day. An extended-action tablet containing 300 mg of quinidine sulfate is claimed to maintain more sustained blood levels and antiarrhythmic action during sleep as well as during the day. It is administered for maintenance in doses of two tablets (600 mg) every 8 to 12 hours.

References

Bassett AL, Witt AL: Recent advances in electrophysiology of antiarrhythmic drugs. Prog Drug Res 17:35, 1973

Bigger JT Jr: Arrhythmias and antiarrhythmic drugs. Adv Intern Med 18:251, 1972

Bigger JT Jr et al: Quinidine and digoxin: An important drug interaction. Drugs 24:229, 1982

Bigger JT Jr, Hoffman BF: Antiarrhythmic drugs. In Gilman AG, Goodman LS, Gilman A (eds): Goodman and Gilman's The Pharmacological Basis of Therapeutics, 6th ed, pp 761–792. New York, Macmillan, 1980

Gettes LS: The electrophysiologic effects of antiarrhythmic drugs. Am J Cardiol 28:526, 1971 (also reprinted in abridged form in RN 36:1 (ICU ed,), 1973 and 36:1 (ICU ed), 1973

Gettes LS: Physiology and pharmacology of antiarrhythmic drugs. Hosp Pract 16:89, 1981

Hayes AH: The actions and clinical uses of the newer antiarrhythmic drugs. Ration Drug Ther 6:1, 1972

Karch AM: Cardiac Care: A Guide for Patient Education. New York, Appleton–Century–Crofts, 1981

Koch–Weser J: Bretylium. N Engl J Med 300:473, 1979

Koch–Weser J, Klein SE: Procainamide dosage schedules, plasma concentrations and clinical effects. JAMA 215:1454, 1971

Lown B et al: Ventricular tachyarrhythmias. Circulation 47:1364, 1973

Nademanee K et al: Advances in antiarrhythmic therapy: The role of newer antiarrhythmic drugs. JAMA 247:217, 1982

Reder RF, Rosen MR: Mechanisms of cardiac arrhythmias. Cardiovasc Rev Rep 2:1007, 1981

Rosen MR, Hoffman BF: Mechanisms of action of antiarrhythmic drugs. Circ Res 32:1, 1973

Rusy BF: Pharmacology of antiarrhythmic drugs. Med Clin North Am 58:987, 1974

Scheinman MM: The treatment of paroxysmal supraventricular tachycardia. Ration Drug Ther 10:1, 1976

Treatment of cardiac arrhythmias. Med Lett Drugs Ther 25:21, 1983

Warner HW: Therapy of common arrhythmias. Med Clin North Am 58:995, 1974

Zipes DP: Editorial: New approaches to antiarrhythmic therapy. N Engl J Med 304:475, 1981

Chapter 31

Drugs used in coronary artery disease

31

The nature of coronary artery disease

Coronary artery disease (CAD) is the most common cause of death in the United States and other Western countries, and accounts for one out of every three deaths in people between the ages of 34 and 65 years. This epidemic of premature deaths is a public health problem that nurses can help to combat through their teaching role as well as by patient care.

General considerations
As discussed in Chapter 26, the myocardium must receive a constant supply of oxygen and nutrients to perform its pumping function. The blood that carries these sources of energy to the heart muscle reaches the tissues by way of the coronary arteries. These blood vessels branch off from the aorta in the sinuses of Valsalva, just above the aortic valve, and spread down through the myocardium. The subdividing vessels form arterioles and capillaries through which oxygenated blood reaches every fiber of the heart muscle mass.

The myocardium ordinarily receives enough oxygenated blood to meet its needs, as long as the left ventricle pumps forcefully enough to maintain the perfusion pressure of the aorta and coronary arteries, as reflected in the pulse pressure. However, in patients with CAD, the coronary arterial channels become too narrow to carry the quantities of blood needed to meet the needs of the myocardium for oxygen under all circumstances. The underlying cause of this narrowing of the coronary arteries is most often *atherosclerosis* (Chap. 32).

In this disorder lipid deposits are laid down within the intima, the inner lining of the coronary arteries. The formation of such fatty masses (atheromas) in the walls of the vessels narrows their channels and interferes with the blood flow to the mycoardial tissues. In addition, the disease-hardened arteries lose their natural elasticity and become unable to dilate adequately in response to the demands of the myocardium for more oxygenated blood during increased physical activity.

The main clinical manifestation of the myocardial *ischemia* and *hypoxia* that occurs in patients with coronary atherosclerosis is chest pain. This pain, which is thought to be set off by a lack of oxygenated blood in local areas of heart muscle tissue, varies in the degree of its severity and in its duration. Depending on various factors, including how long and how completely the local blood supply is cut off, the heart muscle tissue may suffer no permanent damage or it may die and degenerate.

Syndromes
On the basis of the patient's pain pattern, the degree of residual damage, and the threat posed to the patient's life, CAD attacks may be divided into several symptom complexes, or syndromes:

1. *Angina pectoris,* which is classified as *stable; unstable* (also sometimes referred to as *angina decubitus,* preinfarction syndrome, or acute coronary insufficiency); or *variant angina (Prinzmetal's angina);* and
2. *Acute myocardial infarction*

Stable angina pectoris
The episodes of chest pain that occur in this condition are transient, lasting less than 3 minutes in most attacks. The temporary ischemia and hypoxia do not lead to detectable myocardial damage. Thus, although the pain is often frightening, it usually stops spontaneously when the patient ceases all activity, and sits down or lies down to rest. Anginal attacks are usually set off by physical exertion or emotional stress, situations that increase the myocardial oxygen demand.

In either case, there is an increased discharge of nerve impulses to the heart by way of the sympathetic nervous system. The resulting increase in heart rate and contractile force makes the heart muscle work harder and thus increases its consumption of oxygen. When the narrowed inflexible atherosclerotic coronary arteries cannot meet the demands of the myocardium for more oxygenated blood, pain impulses pass from the ischemic tissue to the brain by way of sympathetic afferent nerve fibers.

The anginal pain pattern varies in different patients but remains fairly stable in the same person. Pain often begins substernally and spreads from under the breastbone up into the throat. Often, it causes a feeling of suffocation or strangling. (The Latin *angina pectoris* means literally "a choking of the chest.") Pain may also be referred to the jaw, the back of the neck, and both the left and right arms and shoulders. Occasionally referred pain may predominate, with little or no chest pain. (Pain in the teeth or the mandible and maxilla has led some angina patients to the dentist rather than to the internist following their first attacks.)

Unstable angina

In this form of CAD, chest pain may develop even with the patient at rest. The pain is more severe and lasts longer than that of stable angina. The attack does not ordinarily lead to permanent heart damage. However, for a while following an attack, the patient's electrocardiogram (ECG) may show persistent abnormalities. Patients with this intermediate CAD syndrome (preinfarction angina) are considered to be likely candidates for the most serious type of coronary attack, an acute myocardial infarction (AMI).

Variant (Prinzmetal's) angina

In this form of CAD, chest pain also develops while the patient is at rest. Attacks often occur at the same time each day. Coronary arteriograms of patients made during an attack have shown that actual spasms of the large coronary arteries occur. This is an unusual form of angina; most angina is caused by the atherosclerotic narrowing of coronary arteries, rather than by spasms of the vessels.

Acute myocardial infarction

Here, an area of heart muscle tissue is so completely cut off from its blood supply that it is destroyed. The chest pain, which is usually persistent and often excruciating, is not relieved by rest. The area of dead tissue, or infarct, is gradually replaced, over an 8- to 10-week period, by a fibrous connective tissue scar, provided the patient survives the complications of the heart attack.

The precipitating cause of an AMI is usually the complete obstruction (occlusion) of a coronary artery, sometimes by a blood clot—in coronary thrombosis, for example—or by a piece of atherosclerotic plaque that breaks off from the inner lining of an artery and is carried down to a narrower part of the same arterial channel. The ischemic hypoxic myocardium becomes electrically unstable and subject to sudden cardiac dysrhythmias, including cardiac arrest. If the infarct area is relatively large, the heart may be unable to pump enough blood to meet the needs of the body's tissues. Such pump failure may lead to congestive heart failure and cardiogenic shock.

This chapter will discuss the use of drugs in the management of the several coronary heart disease syndromes, taking up first the antianginal drugs employed to relieve or prevent acute attacks of angina pectoris, unstable angina, and variant angina. This will be followed by a discussion of the use of drugs of several different types in the management of uncomplicated myocardial infarctions and in AMIs complicated by the development of cardiac arrhythmias, congestive heart failure and acute pulmonary edema, cardiogenic shock, and thromboembolic episodes.

Antianginal agents

The chest pains of angina pectoris are precipitated by situations that create an imbalance between the heart muscle's need for oxygenated blood and the amount of blood that can be delivered by the diseased coronary arteries. Such anginal attacks can be relieved by restoring the normal balance between the oxygen demands of the myocardium and the amounts of oxygen that can be supplied by coronary artery blood flow. As indicated, rest alone relieves most anginal attacks by reducing the work of the heart and by lowering its consumption of oxygen to a level that can be met even by the lessened amount of blood flowing through the patient's narrowed, inelastic coronary vessels.

Drugs useful for treating and preventing anginal attacks also act to correct the temporary imbalance between myocardial oxygen consumption and the less than adequate amount of oxygen that the narrowed coronary arteries can carry to heart muscle tissues during periods of excessive physical activity or emotional stress. Effective drugs act to relieve or prevent chest pains in one or both of the following ways:

1. By improving the flow of oxygenated blood through the coronary vascular system and thus relieving the myocardial ischemia and hypoxia
2. By reducing the work of the heart and thus decreasing its demand for oxygen

At present, the three main types of antianginal drugs that are thought to act in one or both of these ways include:

1. *Vasodilators* of coronary arteries and other vessels—for example, the organic nitrates such as nitroglycerin
2. *β-adrenergic blocking agents—propranolol* (Inderal) is the prototype of its class
3. *Calcium channel blockers,* such as nifedipine, verapamil, and diltiazem

Nitrate-type vasodilators

Pharmacologic actions. Chemicals of this class can relax all types of smooth muscle by a direct depressant action on muscle tone. That is, the nitrate ion acts directly on muscle fibers rather than by blocking autonomic nerve impulses that cause these muscles to contract. In the past, some nitrates (and nitrites) were employed clinically as

Table 31–1. Drugs used for treating angina pectoris

Official or generic name	Trade name or synonym	Usual adult dosage and route of administration
Nitrates and nitrites		
Amyl nitrite	Aspirols; Vaporoles	Vapor of 0.18–0.3 ml, inhaled as needed to relieve pain
Erythrityl tetranitrate USP	Cardilate	Sublingual, 5–15 mg prior to anticipated stress; oral, 10–30 mg tid
Isosorbide dinitrate USP	Isordil; Sorbitrate	Sublingual, 2.5–10 mg as needed to relieve pain, or q 4–6 hr; oral, 5–30 mg as needed or qid; 40 mg of sustained-release oral preparation q 6–12 hr
Nitroglycerin USP	Glyceryl trinitrate; Nitrostat	Sublingual, 0.15–0.6 mg q 5 min as needed to relieve pain; transmucosal, 1 mg tid; topical, 1–2 inches (15–30 mg) q 8 hr; transdermal system, 1 pad/day (pads release 2.5–15 mg, depending on preparation used); oral, 1.3–9 mg sustained-release tablet or capsule q 8–12 hr; IV, dilute solution infused at the rate of 5 μg/min
Pentaerythritol tetranitrate USP	P.E.T.N.; Peritrate	Oral, 10–20 mg tid or qid—may increase gradually to 40 mg qid; 30–80 mg sustained-release capsule q 12 hr
β-Adrenergic receptor blockers		
Nadolol	Corgard	Oral—initially 40 mg once a day; may increase gradually to 80–240 mg once a day
Propranolol	Inderal	Oral—initially, 10–20 mg tid or qid; may increase gradually to 160–320 mg/day in divided doses
Calcium channel blockers		
Diltiazem HCl	Cardizem	Oral—initially, 30 mg qid; may increase gradually to 240 mg/day in divided doses
Nifedipine	Procardia	Oral—initially, 10 mg tid; may increase gradually to 120–180 mg/day in divided doses
Verapamil	Calan; Isoptin	Oral—initially, 80 mg tid or qid; may increase gradually to 240–480 mg/day in divided doses

antispasmodics to relieve visceral pain. They have now been largely replaced for this purpose by antispasmodic drugs that act more selectively on the smooth muscles of the gastrointestinal tract, the bile ducts and ureters, and the bronchioles. The use of nitrates is now largely limited to situations in which it is desirable to relax *vascular* smooth muscle.

Nitrate-induced relaxation of all types of blood vessels—arterioles, venules, and capillaries—leads to vasodilation. The enlargement of the lumen of the arterioles leads, in turn, to a local increase in the flow of blood to the tissues served by these vessels. In addition, generalized vasodilation can lead to a drop in systemic arterial blood pressure and to complex changes in cardiovascular hemodynamics.

Local vasodilation of coronary arteries is thought to play a minor part in the relief of most types of angina pectoris pain by nitrates. These drugs do not have much effect on the diseased coronary arteries, because atherosclerotic arterial walls cannot relax and the vessels cannot dilate. However, the nitrates are thought to dilate healthy coronary vessels. As a result, the blood in the collateral coronary circulation is believed to be redistributed to ischemic areas of the myocardium. This shunting of oxygenated blood to the hypoxic portions of heart muscle may help to relieve anginal pain. In Prinzmetal's angina, these drugs are thought to be able to overcome the spasms of the coronary arteries.

In most cases of angina, however, the nitrates are thought to produce their beneficial effects mainly by acting indirectly to reduce myocardial oxygen requirements. These indirect effects on cardiac function are brought about by the relaxant action of nitrates on two types of peripheral blood vessels: the systemic venules and the arterioles. Dilation of these vessels acts in two main ways to lessen the heart muscle's need for oxygen:

1. When the venules (or *capacitance vessels*) widen, blood tends to pool in the veins of the legs and elsewhere. This reduces the return of blood to the right side of the heart (the *venous return*), which in turn lessens the load of blood (the *preload*) that the heart has to pump.
2. When the systemic arterioles (or *resistance vessels*) dilate, peripheral resistance falls. This makes it easier for the left ventricle to eject its load of blood (the *afterload*) into the aorta.

Because of these actions of the nitrates on the peripheral circulation, the heart has a decreased load of blood to pump into a less constricted arterial tree. The resulting reduction in volume and pressure within the ventricles reduces the work that the heart has to perform and the amount of oxygen that it requires. Thus, in sum-

mary, the nitrates are now thought to exert their antianginal effects in both of the ways that drugs may act to relieve or prevent angina pectoris attacks: by increasing the flow of oxygen-rich blood to ischemic hypoxic heart muscle areas and, more importantly, by reducing the work that the heart has to do, thus decreasing the myocardial oxygen demand.

Clinical uses. The nitrates are used in three ways in the management of angina pectoris: to abort an acute attack; to prevent an expected attack just before physical activity is undertaken (*immediate prophylaxis*); and to reduce the total number of daily attacks over a long period of time and to lessen their severity (*sustained prophylaxis*).

Acute attacks. Aborting an acute attack is best accomplished by use of nitrates that have a relatively rapid onset of action. *Nitroglycerin*[+], administered sublingually, is the drug most commonly employed for this purpose (see below). A volatile compound, *amyl nitrite*, acts even faster than nitroglycerin when inhaled. Its effects come on within seconds as compared to the minute or two or more required with sublingual nitroglycerin. However, this drug is rarely prescribed today because it is inconvenient to use. Amyl nitrite is a liquid that comes in a fabric-covered glass ampule. The patient has to wrap it in a handkerchief, break it, and inhale the vapors. Its unpleasant odor permeates the room and draws attention to the often embarrassed patient. In addition, amyl nitrite is sometimes abused by people seeking the sensation of light-headedness that results from its hypotensive vasodilator effect. An angina patient may, mistakenly, be accused of this form of drug abuse.

Nitroglycerin, on the other hand, can be quietly slipped under the tongue in the form of a tiny soluble tablet whenever the patient feels an attack coming on that cannot be relieved by rest alone. Usually, this provides rapid relief of pain in patients with stable angina. The full effect is reached in 2 or 3 minutes, and relief then lasts even after the drug's effects have worn off.

The patient who is hospitalized with angina for the first time often has to be instructed in how to store and use this drug to get the dramatic relief it offers while avoiding most of its adverse effects. The patient should, for example, be informed that nitroglycerin is volatile and likely to evaporate if exposed to air. The tablets should be kept in the dark glass bottle in which they are dispensed and a day's supply should not be transferred to a plastic container. The bottle should be closed tightly each time after a tablet is removed; the bottle should not be kept too close to the body but in a relatively cool place. A potent tablet usually causes a brief stinging or burning sensation under the tongue; lack of this effect may indicate that the tablet has deteriorated.

Ordinarily, after the nitroglycerin tablet is put under the tongue, the patient should sit down or lie down. If standing, the blood pressure may fall excessively, and the patient may then feel faint, weak or dizzy. Although this peripheral pooling of blood in the extremities tends at first to reduce the work of the heart, too steep a drop in blood pressure while standing (postural hypotension) may precipitate reflex tachycardia and thus cause an increase in myocardial oxygen consumption.

The patient should learn to take the smallest dose needed to relieve the anginal chest pains, because larger doses tend to cause side-effects such as the characteristic throbbing headaches. Once the drug has relieved the patient's pain, any portion of the tablet still undissolved under the tongue can be spit out to prevent this vascular headache from developing. The patient should also be warned not to take an alcoholic drink while the drug's vasodilator effect lasts. The interaction between this drug and alcohol can intensify the fall in blood pressure and cause a severe shocklike syndrome called nitrite syncope. This occasionally occurs in patients hypersusceptible to the action of nitrates, even when they have not been drinking. In either case, the patient may become pale, perspire profusely, feel nauseated, and vomit, and may also faint and even go into a state of cardiovascular collapse.

The patient should also be taught what to do if the ordinary dose of sublingual nitroglycerin fails to relieve the chest pain. A second and even a third tablet can be taken sublingually at 5-minute intervals. However, if the pain has not been relieved by three tablets taken over a 15-minute period, probably no more should be taken, and the physician should be notified.

Ordinarily, when a patient who has not developed tolerance to nitroglycerin takes tablets that have not deteriorated, relief of pain occurs promptly. Thus, if several sublingual tablets fail to provide relief, the CAD may have become more serious. The patient may be suffering from one of the more severe CAD syndromes—unstable angina (or acute coronary insufficiency) or even an acute myocardial infarction. Taking nitroglycerin during an AMI may, in some circumstances, set off fatal cardiac arrhythmias (see below). The patient should be instructed to report any change in the response to nitroglycerin for proper evaluation.

Hospitalized patients who need nitroglycerin for quick use when an attack strikes are often allowed to keep a supply at the bedside, because they will need the drug immediately if an attack occurs.

The patient should be asked to report the use of any of the tablets to the nurse, who is still responsible for signing for the drugs on the hospital records. The patient's vital signs and response to the drug should be recorded. This is a good time to evaluate the cause of chest pain with the patient. Numerous teaching opportunities arise with the use of the nitroglycerin. The patient can be helped to identify stressful situations and activities and to determine other methods of coping with these effectively.

Immediate prophylaxis. Patients do not have to wait for an anginal attack before taking nitroglycerin. This drug and other nitrates that act rapidly when taken sublingually can also be used to prevent attacks from occurring. Especially useful for this purpose are *isosorbide dinitrate*[+] (Isordil; Sorbitrate) and *erythrityl tetranitrate*[+] (Cardilate), which have a somewhat slower onset of action than nitroglycerin but exert a much longer lasting effect. Once their vasodilator effects begin (in about 5 minutes or more) and reach a peak (30 to 45 minutes), the protective antianginal action may last for 2 hours or longer.

The patient puts a tablet of one of these drugs under the tongue a few minutes before engaging in activity that is known from experience can cause chest pains. Such situations include walking outdoors in cold, windy weather, eating a heavy meal, or having sexual intercourse. The patient's ability to tolerate physical activity or excitement is increased for a while after taking one of these nitrates sublingually. Too much activity should not, however, be attempted.

Thus, excessive stress should also be avoided. The patient should, for example, stay indoors in cold and windy weather, or, if it is necessary to go outdoors, warm clothing should be worn and the mouth and nose kept covered. Instead of eating a heavy lunch or dinner, patients whose anginal attacks often occur after meals should eat several small meals daily instead of one or two large ones. Those who suffer anginal attacks when they become emotionally upset should try to avoid situations that make them anxious or angry.

It is not always possible for the patient to control or anticipate all attack-precipitating environmental factors. In any case, trying to stick to an excessively restrictive regimen may be a source of stress in itself. The patient should be encouraged to walk and to perform other light exercises that are within his physical capacity. In such situations, the prophylactic use of nitrates taken alone sublingually or taken together with oral sedatives, antianxiety agents, or propranolol (see below) often helps to reduce the number of attacks the patient might otherwise suffer during periods of activity. Most patients learn to regulate their own activities by monitoring their limitations and scheduling activities accordingly.

Sustained prophylaxis. Oral forms of the above nitrates and others (Table 31-1), including *pentaerythritol tetranitrate*[+] (Peritrate), are also available. These products are too slow in onset to be useful for aborting an acute attack or for immediate prophylaxis in most situations. They are employed, instead, in the long-term management of angina. In theory, when taken daily, orally administered nitrates are supposed to help stimulate the development of the collateral coronary circulation. Their use is commonly claimed to reduce the number, duration, and intensity of the patient's anginal attacks. These benefits of oral therapy are said to be measurable in terms of a reduction in the number of sublingual nitrate tablets that the patient has to take daily.

The use of these oral preparations has been controversial. As a result, oral products containing pentaerythritol tetranitrate, isosorbide dinitrate, and nitroglycerin have a DESI rating (a rating of safety and efficacy in the Drug Efficacy Study Implementation that is being carried out by the National Academy of Sciences—National Research Council; see Chap. 1) of only "possibly effective," which means that they may be withdrawn from the market if further convincing clinical evidence of their efficacy is not presented in the future.

There have been three main concerns about the use of oral nitrates:

1. Can they produce adequate blood levels for therapeutic benefit?
2. Does sustained prophylaxis prevent the development of collateral coronary circulation?
3. Does sustained prophylaxis with oral nitrates favor the development of tolerance to the therapeutic effects of all nitrates?

One view is that the orally administered nitrates are taken up from the upper intestine by the portal vein, and the drug is then destroyed in the liver by drug-metabolizing enzymes before it can get into the systemic circulation. Others claim that, when taken orally in adequately large doses, enough nitrate escapes enzymatic destruction to exert its therapeutically desirable vasodilator effects. Evidence seems to be accumulating that sufficiently large oral doses *are* effective.

Those who argue against the use of nitrates for sustained prophylaxis suggest that, even if some of the oral nitrate is absorbed systemically, it will not stimulate development of the collateral coronary circulation. The best stimulus for producing local vasodilation is the lack of oxygen (hypoxia) in ischemic myocardial tissue. Thus, they say, if the nitrates actually did produce some vasodilation, the drugs would tend to reduce the natural hypoxic stimulus to the collateral circulation. There is little evidence to support this contention. The third concern is that the continuous presence of the drug might favor the development of cross tolerance to all nitrates and that, if a patient were to take sublingual nitroglycerin to treat an acute attack, it might fail to produce the expected rapid relief. Evidence has accumulated to suggest that this does not happen. Tolerance develops to the headache and to certain other effects of the nitrates, but results of several studies have shown that long-term therapy with oral isosorbide does not produce tolerance to its antianginal effect or cross tolerance to the antianginal effect of sublingual nitroglycerin.

An ointment containing nitroglycerin is claimed to be more effective than oral products for sustained prophylaxis. Applied to the skin in a thin uniform layer without rubbing or massage, the ointment permits absorption of enough nitroglycerin to produce beneficial circulatory effects for several hours. This is manifested by a persistent increase in the patient's capacity to tolerate exercise and by favorable electrocardiographic findings. The greatest benefits have been reported in patients with nocturnal angina, who often sleep through the night without being awakened by an attack after applying the ointment at bedtime.

The cutaneous absorption of nitroglycerin is variable, and the drug's onset of action is too slow for use in an acute attack. However, it is usually possible to obtain beneficial responses by gradually raising the dosage of the ointment. The usual effective dose is 1 or 2 inches of the amount applied with a special applicator, but some patients may require as much as 4 or 5 inches for a full effect.

There may be psychological benefits in having the patient apply the nitroglycerin ointment to the left side of the chest. Actually, however, it may be applied to the skin of the abdomen or the front of the thighs with similar effects and without interfering with the stethoscoping and palpation of the left chest. A piece of polyethylene plastic can be used to cover the area, a procedure that also helps to increase absorption of nitroglycerin and prevent it from volatilizing.

Several new transdermal dosage forms of nitroglycerin (Nitro-Dur, Nitrodisc, Transderm-Nitro) are available that liberate a predetermined amount of the drug for percutaneous absorption over a 24-hour period. Pads containing different doses are available. Although these pads or patches are convenient for the patient, several recent clinical studies suggest that tolerance may develop rapidly to nitroglycerine delivered this way.

Nonnitrate vasodilators

Most other types of chemicals traditionally employed for treating angina pectoris have not been proved useful, and they are rarely used today for this purpose. Although these nonnitrate vasodilators are occasionally prescribed for angina patients who have become tolerant to nitrates, they are now more commonly employed in treating other disorders. *Theophylline* and its derivatives, including *aminophylline* and *oxtriphylline*, are, for example, used mainly for their bronchodilator effects rather than as coronary vasodilators. *Papaverine* and its synthetic analogues *ethaverine* and *dioxyline* are used mainly in the management of cerebrovascular disorders, and their efficacy in any clinical situation is questionable.

Dipyridamole (Persantine) is being employed experimentally to prevent arterial blood clots from forming by interfering with platelet function. Despite animal experiments that are said to demonstrate drug-induced coronary vasodilation and a large increase in intercoronary perfusion through the collateral circulation, results of double-blind experiments have failed to establish that dipyridamole decreases the incidence or severity of anginal attacks.

β-adrenergic blocking drugs

Propranolol[+] (Inderal; see Drug digests, Chap. 18), the prototype of this class, has been approved fairly recently for use in treating angina. *Nadolol* (Corgard), a newer β blocker, is also approved for this use. Like propranolol, nadolol is a nonselective β_1 and β_2 blocker (Chaps. 13 and 18), but it has a longer duration of action that allows once-daily dosage.

Indications. Propranolol has proved particularly useful for patients whose stable angina suddenly becomes unstable—that is, attacks begin to occur even when the patient is resting in bed, and the attacks last half an hour or longer despite sublingual nitroglycerin treatment. Some cardiologists have used surgical treatment in such cases of acute coronary insufficiency. Others consider such surgical procedures as the coronary bypass operation to be too risky for routine use. Controversy has surrounded this type of surgery. Many cardiologists believe it is clearly indicated in selected patients when the left main coronary artery is narrowed or when angina pain is crippling and not controlled by drugs. The results of a recent study indicate that, for patients with mild to moderate pain, bypass surgery decreases the number of angina attacks and improves exercise tolerance, but does not increase survival rates when compared to drug therapy. One factor that must be considered in deciding between surgical and medical (drug) treatment of angina is that the underlying atherosclerotic process usually continues after surgery and that the grafted vessels, too, may become clogged. A second bypass operation may then be needed, but this is both more difficult and more dangerous. Thus, many cardiologists would advise delaying surgery and using drugs as long as possible. These patients should then be maintained on a medical regimen of propranolol alone or in combination with a sublingual nitrate, or on one of the calcium channel blockers (see below).

Dosage. Propranolol dosage (see Drug digests, Chap. 18) must be adjusted carefully for each patient. The reason for close control of dosage is that propranolol has properties that can both improve angina pectoris and make it worse. The drug's benefits stem from its ability to reduce blood pressure (Chap. 28) and to block the sympathetic nervous system impulses that stimulate the heart during physical exertion and emotional upsets. The resulting slowing of the heart reduces the work and oxygen requirements of the myocardium.

In overdoses, however, propranolol can actually *increase* the oxygen demands of the heart. This occurs when drug-induced impairment of myocardial contractility causes a buildup of left ventricular end diastolic pressure. As the ventricles become dilated with blood,

their muscular walls must build up more tension and use up more oxygen to move the blood into the pulmonary and systemic circulation. In such cases, angina pectoris would be aggravated rather than improved.

Precautions. Particular care is required in coronary heart disease patients who have a history of congestive heart failure episodes and only limited cardiac reserve. In such cases, sympathetic stimulation is needed to keep the myocardium in a compensated state, and adrenergic blockade can cause decompensation and heart failure. The drug should also be used cautiously in patients with sinus bradycardia or with more than first-degree heart block, because it can further depress atrioventricular (A-V) conduction and so cause excessive cardiac slowing or even arrest.

As indicated in Chapter 18, dosage is initiated with quite small amounts of propranolol to avoid precipitating heart failure in the few elderly and other patients with angina pectoris who are dependent on sympathetic nervous system stimulation of the heart to maintain cardiac compensation. If the patient suffers no weakening of cardiac contractions or excessive slowing of the heart rate, the drug's dosage is gradually raised and adjusted to the needs and tolerance of the patient. If it becomes necessary to discontinue treatment, propranolol dosage should be reduced gradually over 7 to 10 days to avoid the increased severity of coronary heart disease symptoms sometimes reported following abrupt withdrawal of this drug.

Synergism. Despite these potential dangers, some cardiologists recommend a regimen of propranolol and sublingual isosorbide dinitrate as the best available long-term treatment for severe angina. Properly employed, these two drugs exert synergistic, or supra-additive, effects that benefit patients in two ways:

1. Both drugs act in different ways to reduce the work of the heart and its demands for oxygen.
2. Each drug helps to antagonize the potentially undesirable cardiac effects of the other.

This ability to counteract each other's adverse effects on the heart occurs in this way:

1. When nitrates cause excessive dilation of peripheral blood vessels, the blood pressure may drop rapidly, thus setting off reflex tachycardia. This potentially dangerous increase in heart rate is prevented by propranolol, which blocks the sympathetic cardioacceleratory impulses at the β receptors in heart muscle cells.
2. As indicated above, propranolol tends to depress cardiac contractility and thus to

increase intraventricular volume, end diastolic pressure, and oxygen consumption. This can be counteracted by the ability of sublingual nitrates to reduce the venous return of blood to the right side of the heart (the preload) and to reduce the resistance of the peripheral arterial system to blood pumped by the left ventricle (the afterload). These effects of the nitrates tend to decrease the size of the heart and to lessen the intraventricular volume and pressure.

Administration. The nitrates and propranolol are not actually taken together. To achieve their maximal synergistic effects, the two types of drugs are administered separately in ways that result in each reaching its peak effects at the same time. The patient is directed to take his propranolol dose by mouth about 1½ hours before taking the nitrate sublingually. Thus, for example, if a patient suffers chest pains after eating, the medications may be taken in this way:

1. About half an hour before eating, the patient takes a propranolol tablet, then lies down, and rests until lunch or dinner.
2. After slowly eating the meal, the patient rests again for half an hour.
3. About 5 minutes before resuming physical activity, the patient puts a tablet of isosorbide dinitrate or other sublingual nitrate under the tongue.

Then when the patient gets up, the propranolol, a drug of slow onset, and the relatively rapid-acting nitrate produce their peak effects together. The sublingual nitrate may be repeated in about 2 hours, when it has worn off and the longer acting β blocker is still working.

As indicated above, nadolol has also been approved for use in angina. Other new β-adrenergic blocking agents have been employed experimentally as antianginal drugs (Table 18-1). All have been found as effective as propranolol for increasing the patient's ability to tolerate exercise. The cardioselective β_1 blockers, atenolol and metoprolol, may be preferable to propranolol for angina patients who also suffer from a chronic obstructive pulmonary disease. Propranolol may be contraindicated in patients with bronchial asthma, for example, because it may cause bronchoconstriction by its blockade of β_2-type receptors in the bronchioles.

---

* The indications described here relate only to CAD treatment. Verapamil is also used as an antiarrhythmic drug (Chap. 30). The calcium channel blockers described here, and others, are being investigated for use in managing essential hypertension and migraine headache.

Calcium channel blockers

This class of drugs, the newest class of drugs to be approved for use in treating angina pectoris, has been briefly discussed in Chapter 30.

Mechanism of action. As described previously, these drugs block rather selectively the calcium channels in the specialized tissue and muscle cells of the heart and in smooth muscle cells in the walls of blood vessels. These effects can slow the heart rate, decrease the rate of A-V node conduction (an unwanted effect in treating angina), decrease myocardial contractility, and decrease peripheral vascular resistance. The negative chronotropic and negative inotropic effects reduce cardiac work, and thus reduce cardiac oxygen consumption. The decrease in resistance of peripheral arterioles also decreases cardiac work by decreasing afterload. In addition, these drugs dilate coronary arteries and inhibit coronary artery spasm.

Indications. These drugs are approved for use in Prinzmetal's angina and in chronic stable angina.* Verapamil is approved for use in unstable angina. Their effect on coronary artery spasm makes them especially useful in Prinzmetal's angina. It is unclear whether they have significant actions on the coronary arteries of patients with other forms of angina, but their effects on the heart and peripheral vasculature (described above and explained earlier in the chapter) are potentially beneficial in all forms of angina. Patients taking these drugs still need a sublingual nitrate, and some will benefit from concomitant therapy with a beta blocker.

Individual Drugs. Three calcium channel blockers have been approved for use in angina in the United States: *diltiazem* (Cardizem), *nifedipine* (Procardia) and *verapamil* (Calan; Isoptin). The three drugs differ somewhat in their cardiovascular effects. Nifedipine has the greatest effect on the peripheral vasculature; it is also less likely than verapamil to depress myocardial contractility, and it may actually increase cardiac output in some patients with angina and heart failure. The increase in cardiac output in these patients is effected in two ways: by the decrease in afterload, and by a reflex increase in heart rate, both of which result from arteriolar dilation. Diltiazem is intermediate between nifedipine and verapamil in its cardiovascular effects. As the above discussion should suggest, the effects produced in a given patient will depend, to some extent, on the patient's baseline cardiovascular status and on other drugs that are given concomitantly. For example, a patient receiving a β blocker along with nifedipine would be unlikely to show reflex tachycardia.

Adverse effects. The most serious adverse effects are hypotension and bradycardia, extensions of the therapeutic effects. Light-headedness, dizziness, weakness, nausea, and headache have been reported. Nifedipine has been reported to cause edema, primarily in the lower extremities, in 10% of patients; this is usually related to arteriolar dilation rather than to drug-induced ventricular failure but, if edema occurs, its cause should be established in the individual patient. Oral verapamil has caused constipation in more than 6% of patients.

All three drugs are metabolized in the liver, and their metabolites are excreted in the urine. Dosage should therefore be reduced in patients with hepatic failure, and the drugs should be used with caution in patients with compromised renal function.

Additional clinical considerations

Most patients with angina pectoris are probably best managed initially with sublingual nitrates for the rapid prevention and control of symptoms. These may be combined with an oral drug—an oral nitrate preparation, a β blocker, or one of the new calcium channel blockers. Selected patients may benefit from coronary artery bypass surgery or from angioplasty, the opening of a blocked coronary artery by mechanical means after a catheter is threaded into it.

The patient should be taught to look for and then to try to eliminate types of emotional and physical factors that tend to set off the anginal attacks. A great deal of support and encouragement may be needed for this. Having the patient recount the activities before angina attacks is usually helpful; often the patient cannot recognize the stressful factors until they are concisely pointed out to him.

The patient will also have to learn to reduce the workload on the heart to minimize angina attacks. It should be suggested, as appropriate, that the patient lose weight, avoid stimulants, avoid engaging simultaneously in more than one energy-requiring activity, and learn to pace himself through the day. The patient may need to change life style, and this will require a great deal of adjustment on the part of the patient. Patient teaching and support are key elements in the care of these patients. The patient needs to develop a trust in the nurses and physicians, and to feel free to ventilate concerns, anger, and frustrations. Angina is a chronic disease that will be part of the patient's life, and the patient will require strong support to adjust to it.

As with many drugs, the antianginal agents are contraindicated for use during pregnancy and lactation. The specific considerations for the β-adrenergic blockers have been described in Chapter 18, and those for the calcium channel blockers in Chapter 30. The nitrates should be avoided in patients with head trauma or cerebral hemmorhage because these drugs can increase intracranial pressure, which can be especially detrimental in these patients. The drugs must also be used with extreme care in patients with postural hypotension who may suffer serious hypotension and syncope as a result of the vasodilation that these drugs can cause.

Technical considerations

Special technical points apply to the nitrates regarding storage and administration. The transdermal patches should be applied to an area that is free of body hair. One patch should be applied daily, and the site changed slightly each day to prevent local irritation and skin breakdown. Patients should be evaluated for local reactions to the preparations. The sublingual nitrates are very unstable and need to be stored in dark glass bottles. The patient needs to know how to tell if the drug is active and how to store the drug properly. The patient will also need instruction in how to take the drug sublingually. Patients taking long-acting oral nitrates will require extra coverage with another form of nitrates if they are experiencing any gastrointestinal hyperactivity, because they will not be absorbing the drug adequately. When a patient is first given a nitroglycerin tablet to relieve acute chest pain, the response to the drug should be evaluated and recorded. The total number of tablets that need to be taken to relieve the pain should be noted on the medical record. Failure of the patient to obtain pain relief later in the course of therapy after taking that number of tablets could indicate a myocardial infarction, and the patient should receive medical attention as soon as possible.

Tolerance and cross tolerance to the antianginal nitrates have been reported after prolonged use of these drugs. These problems can be minimized by using the smallest effective dose and by changing nitrate preparations periodically. Patients on long-term maintenance with the long-acting nitrates should be cautioned not to stop the drug suddenly. The drug should be withdrawn slowly, because rapid withdrawal has been known to precipitate angina attacks.

The nitrates can cause some uncomfortable side-effects—headache, flushing, postural hypotension, dizziness—that are all related to the vasodilation and fall in blood pressure that they produce. Patients can be advised to sit or lie down after taking the drug, to remain in a cool environment, and to use analgesics for headache, if indicated. The patient teaching guide summarizes points that should be included in a patient teaching program for patients on antianginal nitrates.

Drug–drug interactions

Patients receiving nitrates should not use *alcohol*. Severe hypotension and even cardiovascular collapse have occurred.

The guide to the nursing process with antianginal nitrates presents a summary of the clinical considerations that should be incorporated into the nursing care of a patient receiving these drugs.

(*Text continues p. 663*)

Patient teaching guide: antianginal nitrates

These drugs are given to patients with angina or chest pain that occurs because the heart muscle is not receiving enough oxygen. The nitrates act by decreasing the work that the heart must do, and this decreases the heart's need for oxygen, which it uses for energy, and the pain is relieved.

In addition to taking the drugs as prescribed, you can do other things to help your heart by decreasing the work that it must do. These include the following:

1. Reduce your weight, if necessary.

2. Decrease or avoid the use of coffee, cigarettes, and alcoholic beverages.

3. Avoid going outside in cold weather; if this can't be avoided, dress warmly and avoid exertion while outside.

4. Avoid stressful activities in combination—for example, if you eat a big meal, don't drink coffee or alcoholic beverages, and if you have just eaten a big meal, don't climb the stairs but rest for a while, and so forth.

5. Determine what social interactions cause you to feel stressed or anxious; find ways to limit or avoid these situations.

6. Determine ways to ventilate your feelings—throwing things, screaming, diversions, expressing your feelings—are very helpful for decreasing the work of your heart.

7. Learn to space your activities throughout the day, slow down, rest periodically, and schedule your activities so as to allow your heart to pace its use of energy throughout the day and to help you to maintain your activity without pain.

Instructions:

1. The drug that has been prescribed for you is _____ .

2. The dosage of your drug is _____ .

3. If your drug is a long-acting nitrate, it should be taken _____ times a day. The best time to take your drug is _____ .
    Nitroglycerin tablets are taken sublingually—place one under your tongue. Do not swallow the tablet. Do not swallow until the tablet has dissolved. The tablet should burn slightly or "fizzle" under your tongue; if this does not occur, the tablet is not effective and you should get a fresh supply of tablets. It is ideal to take the nitroglycerin before your chest pain begins. If you know that a certain activity usually causes pain—for example, eating a large meal, attending a business meeting, engaging in sexual intercourse—take the tablet *before* undertaking the activity.
    Nitroglycerin dermal patches are applied daily. They can be placed on the chest, upper arm, upper thigh, or back. They should be placed in an area that is free of body hair, and the site of application should be changed slightly each day to avoid excess irritation to the skin.

(continued)

4. Sublingual *nitroglycerin* is an unstable compound. Do not buy large quantities at any one time, because it does not store well. Keep the drug in a dark, dry place; in a dark-colored *glass*, not plastic, bottle; in a bottle with a tight lid; in its own bottle, and *not* combined with other drugs.

5. Some side-effects of the drug that you should be aware of include the following:

Dizziness, lightheadedness	This often passes as you adjust to the drug. With sublingual nitroglycerin, great care should be taken: sit or lie down to avoid any dizziness or falls from the reaction to the drug. Change position slowly to help decrease the dizziness.
Headache	This is a common reaction. Over-the-counter (OTC) headache remedies are often of no help. Lying down in a cool environment and resting will often alleviate some of the discomfort.
Flushing of neck and face	This is usually a very minor problem, which passes as the drug's effects pass.

6. Tell any physician, nurse, or dentist who takes care of you that you are on this drug.

7. Keep this and all medications out of the reach of children.

8. Check with your nurse or physician before using any OTC medication. Drinking alcohol can increase the effects of the drug and can cause serious problems. It is advisable to avoid the use of alcohol while you are on this drug.

9. *Sublingual nitroglycerin* usually relieves chest pain within 3 to 5 minutes. If pain is not relieved within 5 minutes, another tablet can be used; if pain continues, another tablet can be taken within 5 minutes. A total of _____ tablets can be used. If the pain is still not relieved, call your nurse or physician or go to a hospital emergency room as soon as possible.

10. Do not stop using a *long-acting nitrate* without first checking with your nurse or physician.

Notify your nurse or physician at once if any of the following occur:

Blurred vision
Persistent or severe headache
Skin rash
More frequent or more severe
  angina attacks
Fainting

Guide to the nursing process: antianginal nitrates

Assessment	Nursing diagnoses	Intervention	Evaluation
Past history *(contraindications)*: Head trauma Cerebral hemorrhage Postural hypotension Evolving myocardial infarction Pregnancy Lactation *Allergies:* these drugs; tartrazine (certain preparations); others; reactions Medication history *(cautions)*: alcohol **Physical assessment** Neurologic: orientation, affect, reflexes Cardiovascular: BP, P, baseline ECG, orthostatic BP, peripheral perfusion Respiratory: R, adventitious sounds	Potential alteration in cardiac output Potential ineffective coping secondary to disease and restrictions Knowledge deficit regarding disease and drug therapy Potential for injury secondary to drug effects Potential alteration in tissue perfusion	Proper storage, preparation, and administration of drug Provision of comfort and safety measures: • Rest • Quiet, cool environment • Safety from falls and injury • Headache— medication, if appropriate Patient teaching regarding: • Disease • Drug • Storage • Administration • Cautions • Life style changes • Safety measures Provision of support and encouragement to deal with diagnoses, therapy, life style changes Provision of life support measures, if needed	Monitor for effects of drug: relief of pain, vital signs Monitor for adverse effects of drug: • Headache • Hypotension • Flushing • Orthostatic hypotension • Fainting Evaluate effectiveness of comfort and safety measures Evaluate effectiveness of patient teaching program Evaluate effectiveness of support and encouragement provided Monitor for drug–drug interactions: severe hypotension with *alcohol* Monitor effectiveness of life support measures, if needed

Summary of nitrate and nitrite adverse effects, cautions, and contraindications

Vasodilatory effects

Throbbing headache

Flushing

Rise in intraocular pressure (*caution* in patients with glaucoma)

Postural hypotension with episodes of dizziness, weakness, or faintness (alcohol may intensify these adverse effects)

Idiosyncrasy manifested by extreme sensitivity to the hypotensive effect may lead to pallor, perspiration, and collapse (nitrite syncope)

Reflex cardioacceleration (these drugs may be unsafe during the acute phase of a myocardial infarction)

Miscellaneous effects

Gastrointestinal disturbances: epigastric distress, nausea, vomiting

Drug rash; exfoliative dermatitis rare

Case study

Presentation

SW, a 50-year-old, white woman has a 2-year history of angina pectoris. She was given nitroglycerin (TNG) 0.15 mg, sublingual, to use in case of chest pain. For the past 6 months, SW has been very stable, experiencing little angina. This morning, following her exercise class, SW had an argument with her daughter, and experienced severe chest pain that was unrelieved by four TNG tablets taken over a 20-minute period. SW's daughter brought her into the emergency room, where she was given O₂ through nasal prongs and placed on a cardiac monitor, which revealed sinus tachycardia at a rate of 110. Her 12-lead ECG showed no changes from her last recording 2 years ago. Her chest pain subsided within 3 minutes of receiving 0.15 mg nitroglycerin sublingually. It was decided that SW should stay in the emergency department for several hours for observation. The diagnosis was an angina attack. What nursing interventions should be carried out while SW is a patient in the emergency room?

Discussion

SW's vital signs should be carefully monitored while she is a patient. Her response to the TNG should be recorded and discussed with the patient. Because SW reported taking four TNG before arrival at the hospital, it will be important to discuss the effects of the TNG with the patient. SW has had no angina for 6 months, so it is possible that the TNG she used was outdated. The proper storage of the drug should be reviewed with SW, as well as how to tell if it is effective. The disease process of angina pectoris should be reviewed with SW and her daughter (if appropriate). Measures that can be taken to decrease the cardiac workload should be discussed, as well as the precipitating factors that led to this attack. SW may need some help in reviewing her daily activities and organizing them to allow rest for her heart muscle. Because SW has been without angina for 6 months, she might find this attack very distressing. In addition, SW's daughter may experience guilt because their argument seems to have been the precipitating factor in this attack. Both women will need the opportunity to ventilate their feelings and to have all their questions answered. SW will need a great deal of support and encouragement to cope with her disease. The drug information should be given to SW in writing for quick reference in the future.

Following SW's recovery from this angina attack, the physician may order further cardiac studies to evaluate the status of SW's heart disease. If this is the case, SW will require further teaching and support. It seems, however, that SW's lack of therapeutic response to the nitroglycerin was a result of the age of the nitroglycerin and not a worsening of SW's condition.

Drug digests: nitrates

Erythrityl tetranitrate USP (Cardilate)

Actions and indications. This organic nitrate is slower in onset than nitroglycerin (5 minutes sublingually). Thus, it is *not* ordinarily used to abort an acute anginal attack. It may be taken prophylactically before expected physical or emotional stress to prevent anginal chest pains. (Maximum protective effects in such cases can be expected in about 30 to 45 minutes after taking a sublingual or chewable tablet.)

Oral tablets are taken during long-term treatment regimens.

Adverse effects, cautions, and contraindications. Headache is the most common side-effect during early days of treatment. A fall in blood pressure may cause dizziness, weakness, and other symptoms of cerebral ischemia. The drug should be used only with caution in patients who have had a recent cerebral hemorrhage.

Dosage and administration. The usual oral dose is 5 to 15 mg taken on arising, at lunchtime, in the late afternoon, and at bedtime. Such routine therapy may be supplemented by additional doses of sublingual or chewable tablets taken a few minutes before stress is anticipated. These dosage forms may be partially dissolved under the tongue for rapid action and then swallowed for more prolonged effects (up to 4 hours). Patients who develop tolerance may take a total daily dose of 90 mg or more.

662

Isosorbide dinitrate USP (Isordil; Sorbitrate)

Actions and indications. This organic nitrate is somewhat slower in onset than nitroglycerin (2 to 5 minutes when taken sublingually or as a chewable tablet). Its action lasts longer (1 to 2 hours by the latter routes and about 4 to 6 hours when an oral tablet is swallowed).

Taken sublingually, this drug is *effective* for treating an acute anginal attack and for preventing attacks when administered just prior to physical exertion. The oral form, which is not intended for use in the latter situations, is probably effective in the long-term prophylactic therapy of angina pectoris.

Adverse effects, cautions, and contraindications. Headache, sometimes severe and persistent, is the most common side-effect. Flushing may occur, as well as dizziness and weakness from postural hypotension. Caution is desirable in patients with glaucoma, and the drug is contraindicated in patients who are sensitive to its hypotensive effect. (A severe hypotensive response is marked by sudden nausea, vomiting, weakness, restlessness, pale, sweaty skin, and collapse—a reaction that can be increased if the patient has also taken alcohol.)

Dosage and administration. Sublingual and chewable tablets are taken in doses of 2.5 mg to 10 mg to abort an acute attack or for up to 1 or 2 hours of prophylactic protection. The dosage range of ordinary oral tablets is 5 to 30 mg taken three or four times daily (average dose, 10 mg). The duration of a single tablet's action is estimated to be 4 to 6 hours. Also available is a 40-mg sustained-action capsule claimed to provide effective action for 8 to 10 hours when administered orally every 6 to 12 hours. *This capsule should not be chewed.*

Nitroglycerin USP (glyceryl trinitrate)

Actions and indications. This is the prototype of the organic nitrates that act rapidly to abort an acute attack of angina pectoris when taken sublingually. It begins to act in about 1 minute, and in most cases pain is completely relieved within 3 minutes.

This drug is also often taken sublingually to prevent an anginal attack shortly before the patient is going to undertake physical activity or before anticipated emotional stress. The prophylactic effect lasts 5 to 15 minutes or longer.

Nitroglycerin is also available in oral form as conventional and sustained-action tablets and capsules for use in programs of long-term prophylaxis. Like other orally administered nitrates, it is rated only "possibly effective" for reducing the number and severity of daily anginal attacks and in lessening the need to take daily sublingual nitroglycerin tablets.

Like other nitrates, this drug relaxes all types of smooth muscle, but its antianginal effect is the result of its action on the walls of coronary arterioles and peripheral blood vessels.

Its vasodilator effect on healthy (*not* atherosclerotic) collateral coronary arteries may increase blood flow to ischemic areas of the myocardium. Systemic vasodilation results indirectly in a reduction in the work of the heart and in the heart muscle's consumption of oxygen.

Adverse effects, cautions, and contraindications. The patient should sit down or lie down after slipping a tablet under the tongue. This lessens the likelihood of postural hypotension and reflex tachycardia. Such hypotensive effects can cause feelings of faintness, weakness, and dizziness. Patients who are particularly sensitive may suffer a severe shocklike state of cardiovascular collapse called nitrite syncope. (This may also occur in patients who have been drinking alcoholic beverages before taking nitroglycerin.)

More common side-effects include a throbbing headache, flushing, nausea, and vomiting. Headache may be minimized by using the smallest dose effective for relief of anginal pain or by removing the tablet from under the tongue once the chest pain is relieved. Use of nitroglycerin in patients with an acute myocardial infarction has not been proved safe. It should be used with caution in patients with a history of stroke and in those with narrow-angle glaucoma.

Dosage and administration. Sublingual dosage for terminating an acute anginal attack must be individualized to gain relief with minimal side-effects. The required dosage ranges from as little as 0.15 mg to 0.6 mg or more. Special formulations are also available for administering this drug orally in capsules that release much larger doses (2 mg to 6 mg or more) over long periods of time; these are taken twice daily before breakfast and at bedtime. A 2% nitroglycerin ointment is also available that is said to produce prompt and prolonged effects following application to the skin of from 1 or 2 inches to as much as 4 or 5 inches. Transdermal pads are available in various doses for application once a day.

Pentaerythritol tetranitrate USP (Peritrate)

Actions and indications. This is an orally administered organic nitrate employed for sustained prophylaxis in the long-term therapy of angina pectoris. It is *not* used to stop acute attacks but is claimed to increase the collateral coronary circulation gradually. This is said to bring about improvement as measured by reduction in the number and severity of attacks and by a lessening in the daily need for sublingual nitroglycerin. However, it is at present rated only "possibly effective" for this purpose.

Adverse effects, cautions, and contraindications. Headache of the throbbing vascular type is common during the early days of treatment but usually lessens with continued treatment. Sensitive patients may continue to suffer severe headaches that require analgesic drugs for control.

The patient's skin may show transient flushing, but only the development of a persistent rash requires permanent withdrawal of this nitrate. Epigastric distress sometimes occurs early in treatment but tends to be transient. Caution is required in patients with glaucoma and in those with a recent history of stroke. Use of this drug during the first days following an acute myocardial infarction is not generally considered desirable.

The fall in blood pressure produced by this drug may cause feelings of faintness, weakness, dizziness, and other symptoms of postural hypotension. Patients who are hypersusceptible to the drug's generalized vasodilator effect may suffer a severe reaction marked by nausea, vomiting, restlessness, other signs of shock, and collapse. This is particularly likely to occur in patients who drink alcoholic beverages while taking the nitrate orally.

Dosage and administration. Treatment may be begun with 10 mg taken qid on an empty stomach. This may later be raised to 20 mg taken ¼ hour before or 1 hour after meals. Sustained-action tablets or capsules containing 30 mg to 80 mg are taken twice daily: one dose on arising in the morning, and the other 12 hours later.

Drugs used in the management of acute myocardial infarction

Myocardial infarctions strike about one million Americans annually, and about half of them do not survive. Many die instantly or within 4 hours without having received any treatment. However, most of those who live long enough to reach the coronary care unit (CCU) of a hospital recover. This section will discuss the use of drugs both in the routine management of uncomplicated acute myocardial infarction (AMI) cases and in the prevention and treatment of several common types of dangerous complications. Reference will be made to the chapters elsewhere in this textbook in which the various classes of drugs and individual agents are discussed in detail.

Uncomplicated cases

AMI patients who have no signs of heart failure when hospitalized and who develop no rhythm disturbances need relatively little drug treatment. Drugs are used mainly for relief of pain and anxiety and to help maintain bowel function. In addition, some physicians order anticoagulants and oxygen routinely for all cases.

Morphine (Chap. 51) is most commonly employed for relieving the patient's pain and restlessness. This is necessary, because pain and apprehension increase myocardial oxygen consumption. By promoting pain-free rest and comfort, morphine aids a major aim of treatment: reduction of cardiac workload and of the demands of the ischemic myocardium for oxygen. This helps to keep the size of the infarct from increasing and lessens the likelihood of rhythm disturbances.

Morphine is best administered intravenously in small divided doses of about 3 to 5 mg repeated at 5- to 10-minute intervals if pain persists and the patient shows no signs of excessive respiratory depression or hypotension. The IV route results in more predictable and readily observed effects, particularly in patients with poor peripheral circulation, in whom drugs may not be well absorbed from an intramuscular or a subcutaneous injection site. Intramuscular injections of any drug are also contraindicated for these patients because they result in an elevation of serum creatine phosphokinase (CPK) levels, and the serum CPK level is used to evaluate myocardial damage.

Meperidine (Demerol; Chap. 51) is sometimes employed for this purpose in doses of 50 mg to 100 mg. It is claimed to be less likely to cause constipation, because it has a weaker spasmogenic effect on gastrointestinal smooth muscle than morphine. Meperidine may also be preferred for asthmatic patients because it causes less bronchospasm. However, in these and in other patients with a history of chronic obstructive lung disease, the use of *any* potent analgesic requires caution because of its depressant effect upon the respiratory center.

Pentazocine (Talwin; Chap. 51) may be preferred to morphine for relief of chest pain in AMI patients with persistent hypotension. Unlike morphine, which tends to cause vasodilation (see below), this potent pain reliever raises peripheral resistance and arterial blood pressure in such patients when slowly injected into a vein. Although this avoids the further fall in pressure that administration of morphine might produce in such cases, the circulatory effects of pentazocine may prove undesirable in others. A pentazocine-induced increase in aortic pressure and

afterload might, for example, cause an undesirable rise in myocardial work and oxygen consumption in some patients.

Laxative drugs (Chap. 41) may be used to counteract constipation that occurs during bed rest and morphine administration. This is important not only for the patient's comfort but also because straining at stool can elicit a vagal response (Valsalva maneuver) along with a reflex sympathetic response, and these can cause cardiovascular instability. Milk of magnesia (30 ml twice daily) is the most commonly administered laxative for maintaining bowel function but mineral oil, which is also nonirritating, may be used instead. The stool softener dioctyl sodium sulfosuccinate (Colace) is now often also employed for this purpose.

The nausea or vomiting that is often set off by morphine injections is not actually a result of gastrointestinal irritation but is caused by stimulation of the central vomiting mechanism, the chemoreceptor trigger zone (CTZ). To prevent the circulatory instability that is sometimes set off by the stress of vomiting, a phenothiazine-type antiemetic such as prochlorperazine (Compazine) parenterally in doses of 5 mg to 10 mg may be administered to depress the CTZ (Chap. 41). However, these drugs tend to potentiate both the respiratory depressant and hypotensive effects of morphine. Thus, if the blood pressure tends to fall during combined treatment with these drugs, the patient may be put in a reverse Trendelenburg position and later doses of morphine should be reduced.

Potent analgesics are withdrawn when pain subsides, but *sedatives* (Chap. 45) are often substituted to keep the patient calm. Barbiturates and antianxiety agents of the benzodiazepine class such as chlordiazepoxide (Librium) and diazepam (Valium) are useful for this purpose. However, the personal reassurances of those caring for the patient are often most important for reducing apprehension about the outcome of the heart attack.

From the time of admission, the patient with an AMI must receive encouragement, support, and a great deal of teaching. Patients have been found to need the opportunity to ventilate their feelings, recount their heart attack experience, express their anger and fear, and be taught all about their disease, treatment, and rehabilitation. Patients who receive such total care have been found to return to their previous activities at a faster rate and to do better in obtaining a full recovery than patients who do not receive such care.

Anticoagulant therapy (Chap. 34) is often employed immediately after an AMI, but its value as a routine measure is controversial (see references). The injection of *streptokinase* directly into the coronary arteries to dissolve clots has proved successful if used during evolving MIs (Chap. 34). The other anticoagulant drugs do not dissolve a blood clot that has already formed in a vessel. Although, in theory, their use may prevent a coronary artery thrombus from enlarging, there is little evidence that these drugs actually help to reduce the size of the myocardial infarct. The real value of anticoagulants lies in their ability to prevent venous thrombi from forming and breaking off as emboli that may then lodge in lung vessels. However, use of these drugs to prevent thromboembolic episodes including pulmonary embolism is best limited to *selected* AMI cases.

Among the patients who are considered to run a high risk of thromboembolism following an AMI are those with a history of thrombophlebitis, peripheral vascular disease, or stroke. The use of these drugs may also be desirable in the elderly and in patients with congestive heart failure who must remain in bed for long periods after an AMI. However, in most other uncomplicated cases, patients who can begin walking within 3 to 5 days of their coronary attack do not require anticoagulation. That is, with early ambulation and the use of elastic stockings, most patients do not need to run the risk of hemorrhage that is always possible with these drugs. (Patients who develop pericarditis following an AMI are at particularly high risk of developing hemopericardium during anticoagulant drug therapy.)

In the selected AMI cases for which anticoagulant therapy may be warranted, the coumarin derivatives such as warfarin (Coumadin) are most commonly employed. Heparin was formerly reserved mainly for cases in which intravascular clotting had actually occurred as a complication of heart failure or cardiogenic shock. However, use of the low-dose heparin regimen (Chap. 34) has been advocated in AMI as well as pre- and postoperatively. Use of anticoagulants for this purpose requires all the usual precautions, including attention to possible drug interactions (Chaps. 4 and 34).

AMI patients, for example, often receive anticoagulants and sedative–hypnotics simultaneously. Chloral hydrate and its derivatives tend to intensify the effects of anticoagulants, and so their use may lead to unexpected bleeding unless the prothrombin time is carefully monitored whenever these sedatives are added to the patient's regimen. On the other hand, barbiturates, glutethimide (Doriden), and other drugs of this class tend to lessen the effectiveness of anticoagulants by stimulating development of drug-metabolizing enzymes (Chap. 4).

This interaction can, however, also lead to unexpected hemorrhage when the enzyme-inducing sedative drugs are discontinued. This can happen when anticoagulant therapy is continued at the same high dosage level that was required when the two types of drugs were being given together. Thus, when sedation is withdrawn, anticoagulant dosage must be adjusted downward with results of frequent prothrombin time tests used as a guide to restabilizing the circulating clotting factors at a safe and therapeutically effective level.

The question of whether to continue anticoagulant therapy following recovery from an AMI is even more controversial than that of whether these drugs

should be used routinely at the onset of an attack. Most authorities do not believe that prolonged therapy has been shown to prevent AMI recurrences or to reduce the long-term mortality rate. However, the results of some studies suggest that some types of patients may profit from long-continued postcoronary anticoagulant therapy. If these drugs are used in this way, all the necessary precautions in selecting patients and periodically monitoring their responses to drug treatment must be followed (Chap. 34). The experimental use of aspirin and of sulfinpyrazone for this purpose is discussed below (Recurrence prevention).

Oxygen therapy is beneficial for AMI patients who are suffering from hypoxia. This occurs in only about 10% of uncomplicated cases. Low-flow oxygen inhalation is now often ordered routinely, however, for all AMI patients for the first few days. The rationale for this is that, by raising the level of oxygen in ischemic myocardial tissues, it may be possible to salvage hypoxic cells that are still alive and thus limit the size of the infarct. However, because oxygen can have adverse effects in some patients—for example, those with chronic pulmonary disease and carbon dioxide retention—some authorities recommend its use only after checks of arterial blood gas levels indicate the presence of hypoxemia. In such cases, oxygen inhalation by means of a nasal catheter or face mask is employed to bring arterial oxygen levels back to normal. This is particularly useful in AMI cases that are complicated by heart failure or cardiogenic shock (see below).

Coronary vasodilator drugs such as sublingual nitroglycerin may prove useful for helping to reduce the size of the infarct, according to the results of studies in animals with experimentally induced occlusions. In theory, nitrates may have the same desirable effects after an AMI that they have in angina pectoris. However, because these drugs can also cause such adverse effects as hypotension and tachycardia, their use could be dangerous immediately after an AMI. Thus, the use of these and other vasodilator drugs is not now generally recommended during the first few days following a coronary attack. Of course, a patient who had been taking sublingual nitrates routinely before the AMI may resume taking them for relief of anginal pain once circulation has stabilized later in the postcoronary convalescent period. There is, on the other hand, no proof that the postcoronary administration of *oral* nitrates is useful for preventing AMI recurrences.

However, there *is* evidence that certain *β-adrenergic receptor blockers* can decrease the risk of reinfarction and reduce mortality when therapy is started in clinically stable patients 1 to 4 weeks after the original MI. Currently, timolol (Blocadren) and propranolol (Inderal) are the only drugs approved for this use in the United States, but metoprolol (Lopressor), as well as other β blockers available abroad (*e.g.*, alprenolol), have also been shown

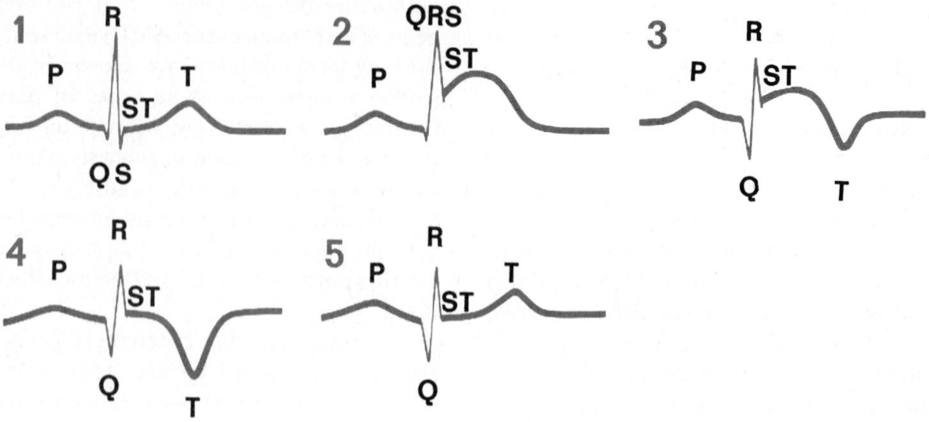

Figure 31-1. Sequence of the ECG following MI. (A) Normal tracing; (B) hours after infarction the ST segment becomes elevated; (C) hours to days later the T wave inverts and the Q wave becomes larger; (D) days to weeks later the ST segment returns to near normal; (E) weeks to months later the T wave becomes upright again, but the Q wave may remain large. (Blowers MG, Smith RJ: How to Read an ECG (rev ed). Oradell, NJ, Medical Economics, 1977)

to be effective. The mechanism of this beneficial effect is unknown.

AMI complications

Death rarely occurs in mild uncomplicated AMI cases or in those with mild arrhythmias that are detected and treated in the coronary care unit of a hospital. However, untreated arrhythmias may lead to death from ventricular fibrillation, even in patients with a relatively small infarct. Patients with a massive infarction that results in the loss of a large amount of the muscle mass of the left ventricle may suffer pump failure complications, including congestive heart failure with acute pulmonary edema and cardiogenic shock. This section will discuss the use of drugs in the management of various types of cardiac arrhythmias and in complications that are the result of mechanical failure of the heart.

Cardiac arrhythmias

Almost all AMI patients show some sort of cardiac irregularity when their ECG is monitored in the coronary care unit (Fig. 31-1). In that setting, the prompt detection and treatment of potentially dangerous dysrhythmias has resulted in a dramatic reduction in deaths from cardiac arrest. Unfortunately, most people whose hearts stop suddenly have little or no warning and get no treatment, because most sudden cardiac deaths occur within the first 4 hours or, in fact, within the first minutes of an attack. Many of them might be saved, however, by immediate measures such as cardiopulmonary resuscitation (CPR). Patients who can be kept alive by such so-called basic life

support measures long enough to reach the CCU, or who receive advanced life support measures from ambulance personnel, can now often be resuscitated. The long-term benefit of these measures is being seriously questioned. These measures and the role of drugs in CPR will now be briefly reviewed.

Cardiac arrest. The sudden cessation of an effective heartbeat takes two forms: ventricular fibrillation and ventricular asystole, or standstill. The latter does not often occur early in an AMI but may be the terminal event of such complications as severe heart failure and cardiogenic shock. In both types of arrest, the consequences of the heart's sudden loss of its ability to pump blood are the same: the blood vessels of vital organs such as the brain are no longer perfused with oxygenated blood, and their cells suffer irreversible damage within 3 to 6 minutes. Thus, immediate measures must be taken to keep blood flowing to the brain and to restore a spontaneous heartbeat, the goals of standard CPR technique.

Ventricular fibrillation, however, is best managed by electrical rather than mechanical means. This involves electrical defibrillation. Sometimes, though, neither electrical nor mechanical measures are effective for restoring a normal heartbeat and cardiac output. In such situations the adjunctive use of certain drugs may help to accomplish defibrillation or to overcome cardiac standstill.

The adrenergic drugs epinephrine and isoproterenol (Isuprel; Chap. 17) occasionally aid recovery from cardiac arrest of both the fibrillatory and asystolic types. In ventricular fibrillation, epinephrine sometimes makes electrical defibrillation more effective. Injected into the cardiac chambers in a 1:10,000 dilution, this drug helps to convert fine fibrillations to coarser waves that respond more readily to external countershocks.*

---

* One half of 1 ml (0.5 ml) of a 1:1000 solution is diluted to 10 ml with normal saline solution, and 3 ml to 5 ml are injected.

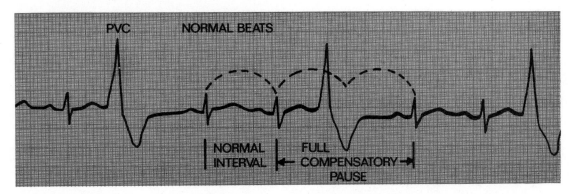

Figure 31-2. ECG for PVCs. Note that the PVCs come early in the cycle (premature) and are wider than the normal beat. (Blowers MG, Smith RJ: How to Read an ECG (rev ed). Oradell, NJ, Medical Economics, 1977)

In cardiac standstill, injection of several milliliters of the same solution sometimes helps to restore electrical activity and myocardial contractility. Isoproterenol is also useful for this purpose when 20 µg to 40 µg are injected rapidly in the form of a 1:50,000 dilution and followed by cardiac massage.* Calcium salts are also sometimes effective for increasing the response to electrical defibrillation and for strengthening myocardial contractility. Such soluble salts as calcium chloride, calcium gluconate, or calcium gluceptate are injected slowly into the heart or intravenously in doses of 3 ml to 10 ml of a 10% solution.

Metabolic acidosis, a condition that occurs when cells are deprived of oxygen and are forced to gain their energy from anaerobic metabolism, develops rapidly following cardiac arrest. Adrenergic drugs and electrical defibrillation are often ineffective during acidosis. Thus, this condition should be corrected by injecting 50 ml of sodium bicarbonate solution intravenously at the very start of treatment as a rapid bolus.† This alkalinizer may then be infused continuously throughout the resuscitation procedure or administered repeatedly at intervals of 5 or 10 minutes.

Various antiarrhythmic drugs are commonly administered both before and after the application of electrical countershock in efforts to restore a normal sinus rhythm and to prevent recurrences of ventricular fibrillation. Lidocaine (Xylocaine) is the drug most commonly employed for this purpose. It is first injected in an intravenous bolus dose followed by infusion of a dilute solution, as described below.

If the patient fails to respond to this drug and other standard resuscitative measures, such other agents as procainamide (Pronestyl), propranolol (Inderal), and

phenytoin (Dilantin) may be injected as IV bolus doses between shocks while the patient continues to receive external cardiac massage and application of assisted ventilation with oxygen. Reports of successful cardioversion following IV bolus doses of bretylium tosylate, after all other drugs and measures had failed, have led to the FDA's approval of this drug for use in terminating ventricular fibrillation and for preventing recurrences of further life-threatening ventricular arrhythmias (Chap. 30).

Ventricular tachyarrhythmias. The most common heart rhythm irregularities seen in ECG-monitored AMI patients are premature beats, or extrasystoles, also called premature ventricular contractions (PVCs; Fig. 31-2). This indicates that the ischemic hypoxic heart muscle is electrically unstable and vulnerable to more dangerous dysrhythmias, such as ventricular tachycardia and ventricular fibrillation (Figs. 31-3 and 31-4). Ventricular tachycardia with the heart beating at a rate of 150 to 200 beats/minute does not give the heart's chambers a chance to fill during diastole. This, in turn, reduces the cardiac output and the amount of blood flowing through the coronary arteries. As a result of the added myocardial ischemia and hypoxia, the heart may become even more likely to develop a fatal fibrillatory rhythm, or the infarct area may be enlarged.

Patients are monitored in the CCU for potentially serious PVC patterns. These include an increase of PVCs to more than six per minute, or repeated groups of two or more PVCs, especially when they originate at several different myocardial sites (multifocal PVCs). Most serious are PVCs that are so premature that they fall close to the start of the T wave of the preceding beat. The closer the PVC is coupled to the normal beat, the more likely it is to set off runs of tachycardia or to precipitate ventricular fibrillation (Fig. 31-5).

Patients who develop these arrhythmias are treated with drug therapy to prevent the development of more serious arrhythmias. The drug most commonly employed for this purpose is lidocaine (Xylocaine), which

* One milliliter of a 1:5000 solution (0.2 mg) is diluted to 10 ml with normal saline solution or 5% dextrose solution, and 1 ml or 2 ml are injected.

† Several dilutions are available; 50 ml of a 75% solution contains 44.6 mEq of bicarbonate.

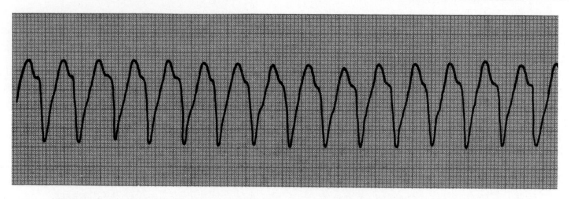

Figure 31-3. ECG for ventricular tachycardia. (Blowers MG, Smith RJ: How to Read an ECG (rev ed). Oradell, NJ, Medical Economics, 1977)

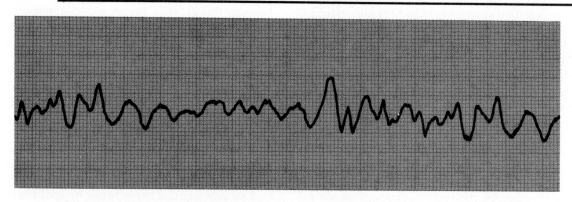

Figure 31-4. ECG for ventricular fibrillation. Note the complete distortion and irregularity of the complexes. Similar distortion may also be caused by the movement of the patient or by the monitor wires, so it is important for the nurse to rule out these possibilities. If the patient is alert, or if not alert and has a pulse, the rhythm is *not* ventricular fibrillation. There is no pulse in ventricular fibrillation. (Blowers MG, Smith RJ: How to Read an ECG (rev ed). Oradell, NJ, Medical Economics, 1977)

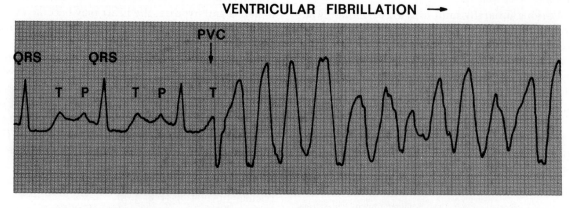

Figure 31-5. PVC causing ventricular fibrillation. When a PVC lands near the peak of the T wave (vulnerable period), it may precipitate fibrillation as shown. (Blowers MG, Smith RJ: How to Read an ECG (rev ed). Oradell, NJ, Medical Economics, 1977)

is said to offer several advantages over such other anti-fibrillatory agents as procainamide (Pronestyl) and quinidine, including a very rapid onset of action and a wider safety margin.

All these drugs depress automaticity in irritable ectopic foci—that is, they reduce the rate of spontaneous depolarizations in latent ventricular pacemaker cells (Chap. 30). However, lidocaine is less likely to cause the adverse effects that occur with other drugs of this class, such as a slowing of impulse conduction, a weakening of myocardial contractions, or a sharp drop in blood pressure. To ensure this, lidocaine must be titrated to the lowest, most effective dosage with close monitoring of the ECG to detect the heart's responses to drug therapy.

Lidocaine is administered in two ways: in single large, or bolus, doses and by continuous infusion of a more dilute solution.* In an emergency marked by dangerous PVC patterns or by actual ventricular tachycardia, a bolus dose of 50 mg to 100 mg is injected slowly over a 1- or 2-minute period. Often, the drug reaches therapeutic levels before the injection is completed, and the PVCs are successfully suppressed. Sometimes, because lidocaine leaves the bloodstream rapidly and is redistributed from the heart to other tissues, the PVCs soon recur. In such cases, a second bolus dose may be administered in about 5 minutes and repeated at intervals of 5 to 10 minutes, if necessary. However, no more than a total of 200 mg to 300 mg should be administered during an hour, because lidocaine can accumulate to toxic levels when its rate of administration exceeds its rate of elimination by the liver.

Continuous IV infusion of lidocaine at a rate of 1 to 4 mg/minute is employed to maintain the therapeutic level attained with single bolus doses until the patient's heart rhythm seems to have stabilized and signs of arrhythmias no longer appear on the ECG. The nurse adjusts the rate of infusion flow while constantly monitoring the patient's ECG for signs of overdosage as well as for absence of ominous PVC patterns. Ordinarily, the infusion rate can be gradually slowed to taper dosage downward before discontinuing parenteral administration entirely.

(Postcoronary patients who require antiarrhythmic drug therapy are usually maintained with oral doses of such agents as procainamide or quinidine.) However, if signs of cardiotoxicity develop, the infusion is stopped immediately.

These signs include the prolongation of the P–R interval and QRS complex on the ECG—signs of depressed cardiac conduction. Other signs and symptoms of systemic toxicity sometimes reported include drowsiness, dizziness or light-headedness, followed by confusion, disorientation, and agitation. Signs of motor system stimulation range from muscle twitching and tremors to convulsions of the type that occur with other local anesthetics (Chap. 14). Special care to avoid toxicity is required in patients with severe liver disease, because it may take them three times longer than normal to eliminate infused lidocaine.

Bradyarrhythmias and heart block. Many patients have a very slow pulse rate soon after onset of an AMI. This can be caused by sinus bradycardia—the result of reduced discharge of impulses by the sinoatrial (S-A) nodal pacemaker—or it may be the result of heart block of varying degrees, in which case the ventricles beat at a slower rate that is set by ectopic pacemakers (Fig. 31-6). Some patients with slow heart rates may require no circulatory support. Others, in whom bradycardia is accompanied by a severe drop in cardiac output and blood pressure, need prompt treatment to avoid possible cardiac arrest or enlargement of the infarct as a result of the poor perfusion of the coronary arteries with oxygenated blood.

Serious slow rhythms are best treated with a temporary pacemaker. However, atropine (Chap. 16) and isoproterenol (Chap. 17) are often useful for increasing the heart rate and cardiac output while the patient is being prepared for insertion of a transvenous pacemaker. Atropine, a drug that blocks the braking effect of vagus nerve impulses on the S-A and A-V nodes, is preferred for treating sinus bradycardia, and it may also be the first drug tried in heart block following infarctions of the inferior wall. Isoproterenol is preferred for sustaining patients with heart block after the more serious anterior wall infarcts until a pacing wire can be inserted into the ventricle. It is also employed if atropine fails to overcome sinus bradycardia.

Atropine sulfate is best injected in small intravenous doses (0.3 to 0.5 mg) repeated at intervals of 5 minutes, if necessary, to raise the patient's pulse to between 60 and 80 beats/minute. The total dose should not exceed 1 to 2 mg, because atropine overdosage can cause sinus tachycardia and other adverse effects (Chap. 16), including mental confusion in elderly patients and urinary retention in some male patients.

Isoproterenol is also potentially hazardous because overdoses tend to increase myocardial oxygen con-

---

* A 2% solution of lidocaine is used for treating cardiac arrhythmias. To administer the single large doses ("bolus" doses), a 5-ml ampule is employed. It contains a total of 100 mg of the drug (20 mg/ml). For continuous infusion, a much more dilute solution must be prepared to permit easier dosage adjustment. One way to do so is as follows:

1. Add the contents of a single 50-ml vial of the 2% solution to a 500-ml bottle of dextrose solution, from which 50 ml has been removed and discarded. The 500-ml dextrose solution bottle then contains a total of 1000 mg of lidocaine (there are 2 mg/ml of the diluted lidocaine solution).

2. A flow rate from a microdrip set adjusted to deliver 60 drops (1 ml)/minute then gives the patient 2 mg/minute of lidocaine. Reducing the flow rate to 30 drops, of course, delivers a dose of 1 mg/minute. Dosage may be adjusted to between 1 and 4 mg/minute, not only by altering the flow rate, but also by preparing solutions that are more or less concentrated than the one described above.

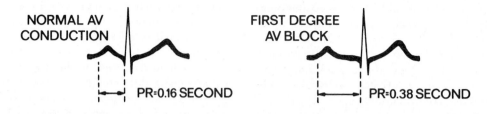

A

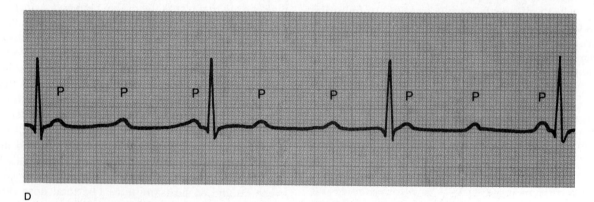

Figure 31-6. ECGs in heart blocks. (*A*) Normal A-V conduction and first-degree A-V block; (*B*) Mobitz 1 (Wenckebach) second-degree block: the PR interval becomes progressively longer until a beat is blocked with no conduction; (*C*) 2:1 second-degree block: one beat is conducted for each two P waves; (*D*) third-degree block (complete heart block): atria and ventricles are contracting independently. (Adapted from Blowers MG, Smith RJ: How to Read an ECG (rev ed). Oradell, NJ, Medical Economics, 1977)

sumption. This, together with the drug's tendency to stimulate ectopic pacemakers (Chap. 17) can lead to development of tachyarrhythmias, including fatal ventricular fibrillation. A very dilute solution containing only 2 μg/ml is dripped into a vein at an initial rate of only 1 to 2 ml/minute. The rate of infusion may be increased if necessary to raise the patient's heart rate to 60 to 70 beats/minute, and it should be reduced or discontinued if the rate rises suddenly to above 110 beats/minute or if the patient complains of chest pain. After the patient's recovery, isoproterenol may be taken prophylactically in sublingual form to prevent Stokes–Adams episodes. However, most patients with permanent heart block following recovery from an anterior wall infarct now usually have a permanent pacemaker implanted.

Pump failure complications

Before techniques for monitoring and treating cardiac arrhythmias in the coronary care unit became available, sudden development of ventricular fibrillation and cardiac arrest was the most common cause of death in patients hospitalized with an AMI. Now, with the remarkable reduction of inhospital deaths from this cause, the most common cause of death in this setting is pump failure. This sometimes results from structural damage that leads to rupture of papillary muscle or the septum separating the ventricles. More often the heart's reduced pumping power results in congestive heart failure complicated by acute pulmonary edema or in cardiogenic shock. The mortality rate from these complications is still very high, despite the advances in drug therapy that are reviewed here.

Heart failure and its treatments

Diuretics and digitalis. Mild failure is a common finding in hospitalized AMI patients. If an S_3 heart sound or signs of lung congestion develop, treatment with diuretics and digitalis may be required. Small IV doses (10 mg to 20 mg) of the high-ceiling diuretic furosemide (Lasix) may be effective for producing a moderate diuresis and symptomatic relief without causing such complications of excessive diuresis as hypovolemia and hypokalemia (Chap. 27). Later, oral diuretics may be required to prevent fluid from accumulating. These are more likely to remain effective and less likely to cause hypokalemic alkalosis and other electrolyte and acid–base imbalances when they are administered intermittently rather than daily.

If diuretics alone do not control congestion, digitalization may be required (Chap. 29). Physicians have often been reluctant to administer digitalis glycosides following an AMI because the hypoxic heart is sensitive to the cardiotoxic effects of these drugs, particularly when patients are also receiving diuretics that cause potassium loss. However, if hypokalemia is corrected and high doses

of digitalis are avoided, arrhythmias are unlikely to occur, particularly when the patient's response to each IV dose of a relatively rapid glycoside is closely monitored by ECG. Digoxin (Lanoxin) and deslanoside (Cedilanid-D) are most commonly employed for this purpose.

Vasodilator drugs. According to some authorities, digitalis glycosides are hazardous and produce a disappointingly small improvement in cardiac pumping function in patients with a massive myocardial infarction. They suggest, instead, that better results may be obtained by the use of adrenergic-type positive inotropic agents (Chap. 17) rather than digitalis. However, other cardiologists claim that such sympathomimetic drugs are also too dangerous for routine use, and should be reserved for use only in the desperately ill patients who have developed cardiogenic shock (see below). They recommend that various vasodilator drugs be employed, instead of positive inotropic agents of any type, to improve pump function and to permit the left ventricle to contract with less effort in patients with heart failure following an AMI.

Vasodilator drugs, such as sublingual nitroglycerin, are claimed to increase the cardiac output in this setting by their ability to cause a reduction in both preload and afterload, as previously described. However, this type of treatment is still experimental and is not yet recommended for routine use. When nitroglycerin, isosorbide dinitrate, or more potent agents such as sodium nitroprusside are employed for this purpose, the patient's hemodynamic responses must be carefully monitored. Obviously, too great a systemic vasodilator effect could cause an excessive decrease in venous return, cardiac output, and aortic pressure and thus interfere still further with coronary artery perfusion.

Acute pulmonary edema and its treatment. The mortality rate of AMI patients who suffer this most severe form of heart failure is high—about 25% to 30%—and, of those who also go into shock at the same time, almost all die. This syndrome may develop very suddenly—sometimes at the very onset of a coronary attack. Unless the patient is promptly and properly treated, acute pulmonary edema may end fatally in a few minutes. However, many patients respond rapidly when they are simply placed in an erect position and receive an injection of morphine. Others require management with further maneuvers and drugs. To understand how the various treatment measures are expected to help the patient with acute pulmonary edema, the pathogenesis of fluid formation in the lungs following left ventricular failure must be understood.

The main effect of a massive infarct in the left ventricle is a reduction in its ability to handle the load of blood that it is receiving from the right side of the heart by way of the pulmonary circulation. When the amount of blood pumped by each beat of the left ventricle—that is, its stroke volume—falls behind that pumped by the right ventricle, the volume of blood in the left chamber and the pressure within it at the end of the diastolic filling period are raised.

The increase in the end diastolic pressure of the left ventricle leads, in turn, to a rise in pressure in the left atrium and in the pulmonary veins and the venous capillaries. This increase in pulmonary venous pressure then forces fluid out of the capillaries and into the surrounding lung tissue. Fluid accumulates first in the narrow spaces, or interstices, between the capillary endothelium and the alveolar epithelium. Then it moves quickly from the interstitial spaces into the alveolar space, where it mixes with inhaled air and interferes with the vital exchange of oxygen for carbon dioxide.

The most immediate emergency measures are aimed at making it easier for the damaged left ventricle to handle the blood pouring into it from the left atrium and pulmonary veins. The load on the left ventricle can best be reduced by a combination of maneuvers and drugs that lessens the amount of blood being returned to the right side of the heart by way of the venous circulation. Among the mechanical *non*drug measures that are used to accomplish this are the following:

1. Putting the patient in an upright position—for example, raising the head of the bed or propping the patient up with pillows in bed or in an armchair, which tends to pool the blood in the extremities and decrease the venous return to the heart
2. Venesection (phlebotomy) to remove a pint to a quart of blood from the circulation
3. "Bloodless phlebotomy"—that is, reducing the volume of circulating blood by sequestering it in the extremities. This is done by impeding venous blood flow with rotating tourniquets through which pressure is applied to three of the four limbs for about 15 minutes. Tourniquet pressure is then rotated so that the venous circulation of the fourth, previously free, limb is cut off, and one of the other limbs is freed.

Morphine. This is one of the most effective of the various drugs that are also used to lessen the load on the left ventricle of the AMI patient who develops acute pulmonary edema.* The manner of its action is still uncertain, but it may be the result of this drug's depressant effect on the vasomotor center. This reduces the tonic discharge of vasoconstrictor nerve impulses to the veins and arteries, with resulting vasodilation. An effect brought

---

* Some authorities now claim that sodium nitroprusside (Chap. 28) is the preferred vasodilator drug for improving the performance of the failing left ventricle and thus for counteracting acute pulmonary edema.

about by dilation of the veins is a pooling of blood in the capacitance vessels and a decrease in venous return of blood to the heart. This lessening of the preload is accompanied by a reduction of the afterload. That is, dilation of the arterioles (resistance vessels) makes it easier for the left ventricle to eject its load of blood into the aorta. This combination of hemodynamic effects of morphine reduces pulmonary venous pressure and stops fluid from pouring into the lungs.

Morphine also helps to reduce the dyspnea that develops early in an attack when fluid leaking into the interstitial space stimulates nerve endings. This sets off rapid, shallow, labored breathing and a feeling of suffocation. Morphine helps both to calm the patient's anxiety and to stop the paroxysmal dyspnea. By restoring a more natural respiratory pattern, the drug also lessens the work of the respiratory muscles and reduces their waste of oxygen.

Morphine administration requires care, because overdosage could cause excessive depression of respiration or a drop in blood pressure to shock levels. Use of this drug is best avoided in patients with chronic lung disease who develop acute pulmonary edema from left ventricular failure following an AMI. In such cases and in right-sided heart failure in patients with chronic pulmonary artery hypertension, diuretic therapy is preferred to the use of morphine, meperidine, or other potent narcotic depressants of the central nervous system.

Diuretics. Potent rapid-acting diuretics (Chap. 27) are now available for relief of acute pulmonary edema in patients who do not respond promptly to morphine and to the other measures mentioned above. Intravenous administration of furosemide (40 mg), ethacrynate sodium (50 mg), or bumetanide (0.5 to 1 mg) results in peak diuresis, usually within 15 minutes. This leads to a reduction in total blood volume. In addition, these drugs may have a direct vasodilating effect on the veins and arteries that results in desirable hemodynamic effects similar to those described for morphine. As a result, dyspnea is often relieved, as are such other discomforts as cough and hemoptysis. Other signs of improvement are a lessening of the moist bubbling lung sounds (rales) that are heard all over the chest on auscultation of a patient with acute pulmonary edema, and the disappearance of the S_3.

Massive diuresis may, of course, be harmful for AMI patients and others with coronary or cerebral atherosclerosis. Too great a loss of fluid and of blood volume can cause a further reduction in aortic and coronary artery perfusion pressures that could lead to arrhythmias or to enlargement of the infarct area. Hemoconcentration as a result of dehydration makes some patients—particularly the elderly—prone to develop intravascular clots and such thromboembolic complications as stroke or pulmonary embolism. Acute hypotension and even shock are other possible complications of excessive diuresis. The mortality rate in AMI patients who suffer a combination of pulmonary edema and cardiogenic shock (see below) is close to 100%.

Digitalis glycosides. Digitalis is not ordinarily administered during the acute phase of pulmonary edema because the desired increase in cardiac contractile strength is relatively slow in onset. However, once the immediate emergency is over, the patient can be digitalized to prevent recurrences, especially if the pulmonary edema had been set off by a supraventricular arrhythmia complicating the AMI. Rapid digitalization within 24 hours with digoxin[+] or deslanoside will control the rapid ventricular rate in atrial flutter or fibrillation (Chap. 29) and so help to prevent pulmonary edema from forming again.

Oxygen. Inhalation of oxygen in high concentration is necessary to counteract the hypoxemia that develops when edema fluid accumulates in the alveoli and the air passages.

Aminophylline. When wheezing occurs as a result of increased airway resistance in acute pulmonary edema, aminophylline may prove particularly useful. It not only relaxes the constricted bronchial muscles, as it does when used for bronchial asthma (Chap. 40), but it also increases the contractile strength of the weakened left ventricle. A dose of 250 mg to 500 mg is injected at a very slow rate to avoid setting off rhythm irregularities in the damaged hypoxic heart.

Cardiogenic shock

This serious complication, which occurs in about 15% of hospitalized AMI patients, still leads to death in more than 80% of such cases. It results mainly from destruction of a large mass—40% or more—of the myocardial cells and the consequent reduction in cardiac contractile power and output. Another cause of reduction in cardiac output and resultant severe hypoperfusion of vital organs including the brain, kidneys, and heart muscle itself is the development of a very rapid ventricular or supraventricular arrhythmia. Cardiogenic shock from the latter cause may be prevented by electroconversion to sinus rhythm and by the use of certain antiarrhythmic drugs. Shock resulting from pump failure may be managed by mechanical assist devices such as the intra-aortic balloon pump and by surgical procedures for restoring myocardial blood flow. Here, however, the emphasis will be mainly on the use of adrenergic vasopressor drugs in the management of cardiogenic shock. (Details about these drugs such as their dosage, administration, and the manner in which their effects are monitored are found in Chapter 17.)

Adrenergic drugs. None of the available adrenergic drugs is ideal for all cardiogenic shock patients, and all can cause harm in some patients, particularly when administered in excessive amounts. Physicians differ in the drugs of this class that they prefer. Most have tended to choose the α- and β-adrenergic agonists levarterenol (Levophed) and metaraminol (Aramine). Most recently,

advantages have been claimed for dopamine (Intropin). The choice depends on evaluating the state of the patient's circulation as determined from appearance and other clinical signs, as well as from measurements of central venous pressure (CVP), pulmonary wedge pressure, arterial blood pressure, and urinary output, all of which must often be monitored by the cardiac care nurse.

Levarterenol and metaraminol. These drugs are often chosen when the patient's CVP and blood pressure remain low even after fluids have been infused to fill the vascular tree. This is thought to indicate the need for drugs with a vasoconstrictor component because the patient's own physiologic compensatory mechanisms have not been fully effective. Administered cautiously in low doses with constant monitoring, in the manner described in Chapter 17, these drugs are sometimes helpful in counteracting cardiogenic shock.

These vasopressors produce their beneficial effects by a combination of actions. Stimulation of cardiac (β_1-type) adrenergic receptors tends to increase the contractile strength of the still undamaged heart muscle cells. Stimulation of α-adrenergic receptors in the blood vessels tends to cause generalized vasoconstriction. This has two desirable effects. First, narrowing of the arterial tree results in a rise in arterial pressure, including a rise in intra-aortic pressure that, in turn, drives more blood through the coronary arterioles to the damaged myocardium. In addition, the drug-induced rise in peripheral arterial resistance causes a reflex reduction in the heart rate. This tends to antagonize any increase in heart rate that might be set off by the cardiac-stimulating effect of these sympathomimetic drugs, an effect that would be undesirable in an AMI patient who is already prone to develop dangerous arrhythmias.

Dopamine. This newer drug is now considered a desirable alternative to both other types of adrenergic drugs for treating cardiogenic shock. It is also useful in other clinical situations characterized by low cardiac output. Infused IV in moderate doses, dopamine increases cardiac contractile strength and output without being as wasteful of myocardial oxygen as is isoproterenol, and it does not cause excessive constriction of the peripheral blood vessels in vital organs, as levarterenol and metaraminol sometimes do. On the contrary, low doses of dopamine have a unique dilating effect on the arteries of the kidneys that helps to overcome oliguria and to produce a desirable rise in urine output.

Dobutamine. Some cardiologists have employed this adrenergic drug to treat pump failure following an acute myocardial infarction. They suggest that, when infused carefully with close monitoring, dobutamine (Dobutrex) can increase cardiac contractility and output without significantly raising the heart rate or myocardial oxygen demand. This drug has received FDA approval for use in other clinical situations that require strengthening of the decompensated heart (Chap. 17).

Nonadrenergic drugs. Other positive inotropic agents sometimes employed to increase cardiac contractile strength in shock cases include digitalis glycosides and the pancreatic hormone glucagon (Chap. 25). The adverse effects of digitalis on the damaged hypoxic heart are difficult to predict or control. Glucagon has been claimed to increase myocardial contractility and cardiac output without causing the dysrhythmias associated with digitalis intoxication (Chap. 29) and without the adverse effects of adrenergic drugs on cardiac rate, rhythm, and oxygen consumption. However, the usefulness and limitations of this hormone in treating pump failure syndromes still remain to be established at this time.

Recurrence prevention

Because atherosclerosis is a disease process that involves all the coronary arteries, patients who have recovered from an initial AMI are often prone to suffer a second heart attack during the following year. Sometimes this leads to sudden death from a fatal cardiac dysrhythmia. Thus, researchers have been looking for ways to prevent reinfarctions. One effort has been aimed at preventing coronary artery thrombosis by the prophylactic use of drugs such as aspirin, dypyridamole, and sulfinpyrazone, which are thought to interfere with platelet aggregation (Chap. 34). Another approach has involved the prolonged use of β blockers, as described earlier in this chapter. However, results of a well-controlled cooperative study suggest that prophylactic sulfinpyrazone taken daily may reduce the number of deaths from first-year postcoronary infarctions by about 50%. This could result in the saving of hundreds of thousands of lives annually, if further research confirms these findings.

In summary, this chapter has discussed the use of drugs in the management of the major coronary heart disease syndromes. When properly employed, the many potent drugs now available are useful for symptomatic relief and often also for counteracting life-threatening complications. However, none of these drugs can reverse the atherosclerotic lesions responsible for coronary artery disease.

The lipid-lowering drugs discussed in the next chapter may help to slow the progress of coronary atherosclerosis in some patients. However, authorities on preventive medicine suggest that the best approach is *not* pharmacologic in nature. They think that the most effective measure would be a mass effort to identify people who are at high risk of developing coronary disease. If reached early enough, these people might be taught to eliminate factors in their life styles that tend to increase their already high degree of risk. The nurse can often participate in public health educational efforts of this type, contributing to the achievement of a significant reduction in the currently high mortality rate of coronary heart disease.

References

Antianginal agents

Abrams J: Current status of nitroglycerin ointment in angina pectoris: A new look at an old drug. Angiology 28:317, 1977

Abrams M: Nitroglycerine and long-acting nitrates. N Engl J Med 302:1234, 1980

Aronow WS: Treatment of angina pectoris. Pharmacologic approaches. Postgrad Med 60:100, 1976

Braunwald E: Mechanisms of action of calcium-channel blocking agents. N Engl J Med 307:1618, 1982

Brogden RN et al: Metoprolol: A review of its efficacy in hypertension and angina pectoris. Drugs 14:321, 1977

Cohn JN (ed): Calcium-entry blockers in coronary artery disease, Part 2. Circulation 65:11, 1982

Conti CR et al: What is the role of coronary artery spasm in ischemic heart disease? Cardiovasc Clin 13:131, 1983

Frankel WS et al: What is optimal drug therapy in angina pectoris? Cardiovasc Clin 13:209, 1983

Frishman WH: Beta-adrenergic blockade in clinical practice. Hosp Pract 17:57, 1982

Goldstein RE: Is the use of long-acting nitrites beneficial in the patient with angina pectoris? (The negative side.) Cardiovasc Clin 8:149, 1977

Kay HB: Angina pectoris: Getting the most from drug therapy. Drugs 13:327, 1977

Needleman P, Johnson EM Jr: Vasodilators and the treatment of angina. In Gilman AG, Goodman LS, Gilman A (eds): Goodman and Gilman's The Pharmacological Basis of Therapeutics, 6th ed, pp 819–833. New York, Macmillan, 1980

Nitroglycerin patches: Med Lett Drugs Ther 26:59, 1984

Prichard BN: Propranolol in the treatment of angina. A review. Postgrad Med J 52(Suppl)4:35, 1976

Rangno RE: Stopping beta-blockers in patients with angina. Ration Drug Ther 15:1, 1981

Rodman MJ: Managing cardiac emergencies. RN 43:81, 1980

Rossi LP, Antman EM: Calcium channel blockers: New treatment for cardiovascular disease. Am J Nurs 83:382, 1983

Schroeder JS: Calcium and beta blockers in ischemic heart disease: when to use which. Modern Medicine 26:94, 1982

Vyden JK et al: Is the use of long-acting nitrites beneficial in the patient with angina pectoris? (The positive side.) Cardiovasc Clin 8:139, 1977

Drugs used for the treatment of AMI

Akhtar M: Management of ventricular tachyarrhythmias. JAMA 247:671, 1982

Chalmers TC et al: Evidence favoring the use of anticoagulants in the hospital phase of acute myocardial infarction. N Engl J Med 297:1091, 1977

Chatterjee K, Parmley WW: Vasodilator therapy for chronic heart failure. Ann Rev Pharmacol Toxicol 20:475, 1980

Cohn JN: Vasodilator therapy: Implications in acute myocardial infarction and congestive heart failure. Am Heart J 103:773, 1982

Cohn JN, Levine TB: Angiotensin converting enzyme inhibition in congestive heart failure. Am J Cardiol 49:1480, 1982

Gillespie TA et al: Effects of dobutamine in patients with acute myocardial infarction. Am J Cardiol 39:588, 1977

Goldberg AH: Cardiopulmonary arrest. N Engl J Med 290:381, 1974

Goldberg LI: Dopamine—clinical uses of an endogenous catecholamine. N Engl J Med 291:707, 1974

Goldberg LI: Newer catecholamines for treating heart failure and shock: An update of dopamine and a first look at dobutamine. Prog Cardiovasc Dis 19:327, 1977

Karch AM: Cardiac Care: A Guide for Patient Education. New York, Appleton–Century–Crofts, 1981

Meador B: Cardiogenic shock: Help break the vicious cycle. RN 45:38 (Apr) 1982

Modan B et al: The case for anticoagulants in acute myocardial infarction. Arch Intern Med 136:1230, 1976

Nevins MA, Lyon LJ: The treatment of acute myocardial infarction. Med Clin North Am 58:435, 1974

Russek HI: Anticoagulants should not be used routinely for acute myocardial infarction. Cardiovasc Clin 8:123, 1977

Singh BN: Beta-adrenoreceptor blocking drugs and acute myocardial infarction. Drugs 15:218, 1978

Streptokinase for acute coronary artery thrombosis. Med Lett Drugs Ther 25:33, 1983

Vedin JA, Wilhelmsson CE: Beta receptor blocking agents in the secondary prevention of coronary heart disease. Ann Rev Pharmacol Toxicol 23:29, 1983

Wessler S: Antithrombotic agents are indicated in the therapy of acute myocardial infarction. Cardiovasc Clin 8:131, 1977

Zellis R et al: Management of pulmonary edema. Ration Drug Ther 8:1, 1974

Chapter 32

Drugs
for reducing
elevated
plasma
lipid
levels

32

General considerations

The drugs discussed in this chapter act in various ways to affect the metabolism of the fatty substances called *lipids* and of lipid–protein complexes, or *lipoproteins*. These drugs reduce the level of serum lipids and of plasma lipoproteins by either interfering with the production of lipoproteins or by accelerating their catabolism, or breakdown, and excretion. Some drugs may act by a combination of mechanisms and, in some clinical situations, drugs with different mechanisms of action may be administered together to lower elevated plasma lipid levels by their combined effects on lipoprotein biosynthesis and elimination.

The lipid-lowering actions of these drugs—called *antilipemic* or *hypolipemic* agents—make them potentially useful for treating a group of metabolic disorders called *hyperlipidemias,* which are characterized by increased concentrations of such lipids as cholesterol and triglycerides in the circulation.* Because there is evidence that people with abnormally high levels of plasma cholesterol have a higher risk of developing coronary artery disease and other disorders in which atherosclerosis is the underlying pathologic lesion, scientific interest has focused on the questions of whether or not the long-term administration of antilipemic drugs can reduce the risk of death from heart attacks in patients who have high plasma cholesterol levels or in patients who have previously suffered an acute myocardial infarction (Chap. 31).

Before discussing the individual drugs of this class and their current status in the treatment of hyperlipidemia and coronary artery disease, the terms and concepts involved with the clinical uses of the antilipemic agents will be described. This will include discussion of the origin and function of plasma lipids and lipoproteins, their

properties, and how plasma levels of these substances are altered in the various classes of hyperlipidemias. The relation of these hyperlipidemic states to atherosclerosis and to coronary artery disease will be summarized before discussing the drugs used to lower plasma lipid levels.

Plasma lipids and lipoproteins

The main fatty substances found in the blood are classified as cholesterol and its esters, triglycerides, free fatty acids, and phospholipids (Table 32-1). Such serum lipids come both from the diet and from biosynthesis by the liver and by the cells of other body tissues. Because lipids are insoluble in water, they do not circulate in the free form in the bloodstream. Instead, the free fatty acid breakdown products of triglycerides are bound to serum albumin, and the other types of lipids are transported in the plasma after first being solubilized by binding to proteins that are synthesized in the liver. These plasma lipoproteins can be separated into several groups using ultracentrifugation to determine their densities and electrophoresis to determine their migratory behavior when subjected to an electrical field.

The different families of lipoproteins have been found to contain varying proportions of high-density proteins and low-density lipids. There are four major types of lipoproteins: (1) chylomicrons; (2) very low-density lipoproteins (VLDL), or prebeta lipoproteins; (3) low-density lipoproteins (LDL), or beta lipoproteins; (4) high-density lipoproteins (HDL), or alpha lipoproteins. It is helpful to understand the nature of these interrelated substances because variations in the amounts of lipoproteins present in the plasma of different patients determine the type of hyperlipoproteinemia and this, in turn, helps in the choice of treatment for the specific abnormality (Table 32-2).

Chylomicrons are formed in the intestine during the absorption of dietary fat. They are the largest of the lipoprotein transport complexes but also the lightest. This

---
* Other terms sometimes employed are *antihyperlipidemic* and *hypolipidemic* agents.

Table 32–1. Properties of plasma lipoproteins

Type of lipoprotein*	Physicochemical and other characteristics†
Chylomicrons	Largest and lightest of the lipoprotein complexes; made up mostly (80–95%) of triglycerides, with relatively little cholesterol, phospholipids, and protein; formed entirely from dietary fats during their absorption through the intestinal mucosa following a fat-containing meal
Very low-density lipoproteins (VLDL) (pre-beta-lipoproteins)	Second largest and lightest class of lipoproteins; made up of 50% to 65% triglycerides, 10% to 15% cholesterol, about 15% to 20% phospholipids, and about 5% to 10% protein; triglycerides that are carried in this form are biosynthesized in the liver rather than absorbed as such from foods—however, dietary carbohydrate is employed in the synthesis of these lipoproteins
Low-density lipoproteins (LDL) (beta-lipoproteins)	Formed from an intermediate-type lipoprotein (IDL) derived from the partial degradation of VLDL; third largest and lightest of the lipoproteins and contain about 45% cholesterol, 25% protein, 20% phospholipids, only 10% triglycerides; most of the total circulating serum cholesterol—50% to as high as 70%—is transported in this form, and an abnormally elevated LDL pattern is an almost certain sign that the plasma cholesterol level is also excessive
High-density lipoproteins (HDL) (alpha-lipoproteins)	Smallest and most dense, or heaviest, of the lipoprotein complexes; made up of about 45% to 50% protein, 30% phospholipids, about 20% cholesterol, and less than 10% triglycerides; HDLs are now thought to help clear cholesterol from body tissues, including the blood vessels; help to keep LDL cholesterol from being taken up by vascular smooth muscle cells; thus, this class of lipoproteins may serve a protective function against development of coronary heart disease

* Lipoproteins are classified in terms of the methods employed in measuring them. When separated by ultracentrifugation, their *density* is the most significant property. The lower the density, the higher the ratio of triglycerides and other lipids to the proportion of protein present. The electrophoretic classification as alpha, beta, and prebeta lipoproteins is based on the different behavior of the various lipoproteins when a drop of the patient's plasma is placed on filter paper and subjected to electrophoresis in the clinical laboratory. The differing electrical charges of the lipoproteins causes them to migrate at different rates in the electrical field, thus separating them into distinct bands on the paper strip.

† The different lipoproteins carry varying proportions of cholesterol, triglycerides, phospholipids, and proteins. The free fatty acid (FFA) breakdown products of neutral fat (triglycerides) are not transported as lipoproteins but are carried in combination with serum albumin to which they are bound.

is because they have a high concentration of triglycerides, or neutral fat, which has the lowest density of all the lipids. Chylomicrons are not normally present some hours after a person has last eaten a fat-containing meal. Their presence in the plasma of a patient who has fasted for 12 hours or more indicates a defect in the body's ability to handle dietary fat. (Serum that contains chylomicrons is cloudy and, when stored overnight in a refrigerator, it has a creamy layer on its surface, because the very light chylomicrons have floated to the top in the same manner as the cream in a bottle of milk that has not been homogenized.)

Very low-density lipoproteins are also very high in triglycerides. However, this lipid constituent differs from that of the chylomicrons in its origin, which is *not* dietary fat. The VLDL triglyceride is, instead, synthesized in the liver and is derived in part from dietary carbohydrate intake. Thus, although the source of this type of triglyceride-carrying protein complex is endogenous rather than exogenous, it can be reduced if present in excessive quantities by putting the patient on a low-carbohydrate diet.

Low-density lipoproteins are believed to be derived from the metabolic degradation of VLDLs through chemical steps that result first in the formation of a lipoprotein of intermediate density (IDL) and finally in particles (LDL lipoproteins) high—50% by weight—in cholesterol and low in triglycerides. Such LDLs account for the bulk of the cholesterol present in the plasma of a fasting patient, about 50% to 65%. LDLs are believed to carry cholesterol to the cells of the body that need it to make cell membranes and to the special endocrine cells that synthesize the adrenocortical steroids and sex hormones.

High-density lipoproteins contain a relatively large proportion of protein and a low amount of triglycerides. These particles are about 20% to 25% cholesterol, which has the highest density of all the lipids. HDLs are believed to carry cholesterol back to the liver from the body's cells. Research studies suggest that relatively high concentrations of HDL in a person's plasma are not only *un*related to any increased risk of developing coronary heart disease, but that their presence in excess may actually have a protective effect against the development of atherosclerotic lesions.

The hyperlipidemias or hyperlipoproteinemias

About 25% of all adults have abnormal elevations of one or another of their plasma lipids or lipoprotein complexes.

---

* Many authorities consider such so-called average or normal cholesterol levels actually to be abnormally high when compared with the values of 160 to 200 mg of cholesterol per 100 ml of plasma, which are common among people of various *non*-Western countries.

Often these reflect a family trait—that is, an inherited or genetically determined disorder in lipid or lipoprotein metabolism. Other primary hyperlipoproteinemias occur sporadically without any clear-cut evidence of any inherited metabolic abnormality and are probably of environmental, or dietary, origin. Sometimes the patient's abnormally elevated lipoprotein pattern can be traced to the presence of hypothyroidism, diabetes mellitus, or some other underlying disorder than can cause such secondary hyperlipoproteinemias.

Such patients were, at first, classified on the basis of the presence of increased levels of plasma lipids, such as cholesterol or triglycerides. People in this and other Western countries with plasma cholesterol levels above the average value of about 250 mg/100 ml have been called hypercholesterolemic.* Those with serum triglyceride concentrations above 150 to 200 mg/100 ml have been classified as having hypertriglyceridemia.

However, scientists can now classify patients on the basis of the specific types of lipoproteins that are elevated (Table 32-2). This translation of the hyperlipidemias into hyperlipoproteinemias permits a more spe-

Table 32–2. Types of hyperlipoproteinemias and their treatment*

Type	Nature of the lipid and lipoprotein abnormality	Other characteristics	Treatment
I	High levels of chylomicrons high in triglycerides of dietary origin not readily removed from the blood; HDL levels are low	Relatively rare; the result of an enzyme (lipoprotein lipase) deficiency; seen in infancy; marked by abdominal pain, pancreatitis; does *not* lead to atherosclerosis; *xanthomas* of eruptive type may develop	*No drug* is effective; *diet* low in fat (about 1 oz daily and about 30% of the total caloric intake); no restriction on carbohydrates, protein, or cholesterol; no alcohol; weight reduction
II—phenotype IIa	Hypercholesterolemia only; high LDL level; normal VLDL level	Relatively common, and a potential cause of atherosclerosis and premature coronary heart disease; xanthomas may develop in tendons of hands, feet, elbows, and knees together with xanthelasmas of the eyelids	*Dietary treatment:* limit intake of saturated fats and increase intake of polyunsaturated fats, and keep cholesterol intake as low as possible; *adjunctive drugs:* cholestyramine, colestipol, dextrothyroxine, niacin, probucol—clofibrate is used when triglyceride levels are high
II—phenotype IIb	Both hypercholesterolemia and hypertriglyceridemia; Both LDL and VLDL levels are raised		
III	High in IDL levels, also in LDL and VLDL levels; both cholesterol and triglyceride levels are elevated because of an abnormality that interferes	Not a common type, but it can lead to atherosclerosis and premature coronary heart disease; also to xanthoma tuberosum of elbows and knees and to	*Dietary treatment:* low cholesterol intake; use polyunsaturated rather than saturated fats; control carbohydrate intake but maintain high proteins while re-

(continued)

678

Table 32–2. Types of hyperlipoproteinemias and their treatment* (continued)

Type	Nature of the lipid and lipoprotein abnormality	Other characteristics	Treatment
	with the ordinary degradation of VLDL to LDL	xanthomas of the palms and fingers	ducing to ideal weight; *adjunctive drugs:* clofibrate is preferred, also niacin is used
IV	Hypertriglyceridemia and elevation of VLDL levels are prominent; cholesterol and LDL levels may be normal or slightly elevated when the VLDL levels are very highly elevated; low HDL levels	A common abnormality caused in part by excessive biosynthesis of triglycerides from dietary carbohydrates in the liver; can lead to atherosclerosis and premature heart disease; glucose intolerance and hyperuricemia may occur	*Dietary treatment:* control carbohydrate intake by keeping it to 40% of total calories; fat intake (30% of calories) should be mainly in form of polyunsaturated fat; alcohol and cholesterol intake should be limited; maintain protein intake while reducing to ideal weight; *adjunctive drugs:* clofibrate, gemfibrozil, and niacin are preferred
V	Hypertriglyceridemia from both dietary chylomicrons and VLDL because of slowed elimination of triglyceride-rich lipoproteins; HDL concentrations are low	A rare abnormality, *not* associated with atherosclerosis or premature heart disease; characterized by xanthomas, pancreatitis, glucose intolerance, hyperuricemia	*Dietary treatment:* keep fat intake low (30% of calories) and preferably in form of polyunsaturated fats; restrict cholesterol and carbohydrate intake and eliminate alcoholic beverages; *adjunctive drugs:* niacin, gemfibrozil, and clofibrate and, experimentally, norethisterone in women and oxandrolone in men

* *Primary hyperlipoproteinemias* may be familial (inherited or genetic) in origin or occur sporadically as a result of the life style—associated, for example, with obesity, a high-carbohydrate diet, or excessive alcohol intake. *Secondary hyperlipoproteinemias* can be caused by diseases such as diabetes mellitus, hypothyroidism, and the nephrotic syndrome, all of which should be treated specifically before employing low-fat diets or antilipemic drugs.

cific diagnosis of each patient's defect in lipid metabolism and transport. Such a classification into half a dozen subtypes helps, in turn, to determine the patient's prognosis. Most important, it allows the physician who has obtained an accurate laboratory diagnosis of the patient's disorder to select the type of dietary and drug therapy that is most likely to prove effective for reducing the high level of lipoproteins.

Type I hyperlipoproteinemia is characterized by an increase in the plasma chylomicron level, even when the patient is in the fasting state. This relatively rare condition is probably caused by lack of an enzyme, lipoprotein lipase, which normally removes chylomicrons by breaking down

their triglyceride content into free fatty acids and glycerol. This dietary type, or exogenous, hyperlipemia is not associated with any increased risk of atherosclerosis. Thus, it is desirable to differentiate this disorder from other high-triglyceride lipoproteinemias with a potentially more ominous prognosis. This is most simply accomplished by examining a sample of fasting plasma for the presence or absence of the creamy top layer that forms in chylomicron-rich serum that has been stored in the refrigerator overnight.

Type IIa hyperlipoproteinemia is marked by a high concentration of plasma cholesterol and LDL, and by normal, or only slightly elevated, triglycerides. In *type*

IIb, both the serum cholesterol (LDL) and triglyceride (VLDL) levels are raised above normal. In the first case, the chilled plasma sample is clear; in the latter, its appearance is slightly cloudy or turbid. Type II disorders are both common and potentially dangerous in terms of an increased risk of early development of coronary atherosclerosis. This is particularly true in the case of patients with familial hyperlipidemia, many of whom show signs of atherosclerosis before they reach the age of 30 years and have heart attacks before they become 50 years old.

Type III hyperlipoproteinemia can also lead to premature development of coronary heart disease, but fortunately it is not a common form of familial abnormality. This is characterized by the presence of lipoproteins of intermediate density (IDL) as well as by increased VLDL and LDL, which indicates that both triglyceride and cholesterol levels are elevated.

Type IV hyperlipoproteinemia is a commonly encountered lipid abnormality that can lead to premature vascular disease. It is marked by elevated levels of VLDL containing triglycerides synthesized in the liver in excessive amounts, particularly in those whose diet is relatively high in carbohydrates or who consume excessive quantities of alcohol. Such patients are often obese and sometimes have diabetes or, at least, an abnormally low tolerance for glucose.

Type V hyperlipoproteinemia is an uncommon disorder with some features of both types I and IV. Thus, for example, increased chylomicrons cause a creamy top layer to form in refrigerated plasma, and the presence of high triglyceride levels and VLDL produces cloudiness in the underlying liquid. Cholesterol levels are also elevated, but this condition is *not* associated with early development of atherosclerosis. HDL levels are normal (types II and III) or decreased (types I, IV, and V).

Atherosclerosis and its relationship to lipoprotein levels

Atherosclerosis, a form of arteriosclerosis, is characterized by a hardening or thickening of the arteries in which the vascular walls contain lipid deposits (atheromata). It is the cause of blood vessel diseases that are responsible for more disability and death than all other illnesses. More than 560,000 Americans are killed by this disease each year. The characteristic lesion, or atheromatous plaque, develops gradually in the large and medium-sized arteries of the heart, brain, kidneys, legs, and other sites. It is located within the arterial walls, and takes the form of a raised pearly gray mass of tissue. Although atheromata usually grow slowly and cause no symptoms during decades of progressive growth, they can finally cut off the flow of blood through the affected arteries. This leads to such complications of coronary heart disease, cerebral vascular disease, and peripheral vascular disease as acute

myocardial infarction, strokes, and intermittent claudication (Chaps. 31 and 33).

The basic mechanism of atherosclerosis and its relationship to plasma lipid levels is still uncertain. However, research results suggest that chronic hyperlipidemia sets off a complex series of events that starts with damage to the endothelium, the layer of epithelial cells that lines the inner surface of the arteries. Injury to the endothelium, which ordinarily provides a protective barrier that prevents constituents of the blood from making contact with vascular smooth muscle and connective tissues, exposes these subendothelial elements of the vessels to substances that can accelerate pathogenetic processes.

One hypothesis as to what then happens is that the arterial smooth muscle cells are stimulated to grow and divide by substances released from blood platelets that stick to the subendothelial connective tissue of the damaged vessels. The proliferating vascular smooth muscle cells may then begin to extract cholesterol from the plasma at an accelerated rate; and the presence of this lipid leads in turn to an increased accumulation of collagen-containing elastic connective tissue fibers. Such accumulations may account for development of the atheromatous mound made up of an inner core of cholesterol capped by fibrous scar tissue, which characterizes atherosclerotic lesions.

Relationship of hyperlipoproteinemias to atherosclerosis

Indirect evidence. Results of many types of epidemiologic studies indicate that people with abnormally high plasma cholesterol concentrations run a higher risk of suffering an acute myocardial infarction than do those with lower levels of plasma lipoproteins. The closely followed Framingham, Massachusetts study, for example, revealed that, over a 14-year period, middle-aged men with higher plasma lipid levels were much more prone to have heart attacks than those with low cholesterol concentrations. Similarly, people from families in which hypercholesterolemia was common showed a higher incidence of atherosclerosis and coronary artery disease (CAD). In addition to this and other types of indirect evidence, there is now direct evidence that early atherosclerosis can be favorably altered by measures aimed at reducing plasma lipid concentrations.

Direct evidence. Radiologists employing sensitive radiographic techniques obtained a series of repeat angiograms, which revealed the regression of atherosclerotic lesions in the femoral arteries of patients with types II and IV hyperlipoproteinemia when they were treated with appropriate diets and with combinations of antilipemic drugs. Inasmuch as the patients' atherosclerosis was in an early stage of development and did not involve the coronary arteries, it was not, of course, possible to predict whether similar treatment would be effective for protecting CAD patients who have more advanced, obstructive coronary artery lesions. However, a later study of 116 men with coronary atherosclerosis showed that diet and drug therapy slowed the progression of the deposits in the coronary arteries and, in some cases, actually shrank the deposits. This evidence adds strength to the already generally accepted positive relationship between hyperlipoproteinemia—particularly of the low-density (LDL), or high cholesterol, type—and the occurrence of an increased incidence of CAD and other forms of atherosclerosis.

The lipid hypothesis

These lines of evidence led to the hypothesis that lowering abnormally high serum cholesterol levels would decrease the incidence of heart disease in such people. Direct proof of the validity of this hypothesis was finally provided by a study of 3800 middle-aged men, begun, under sponsorship of the National Heart, Lung and Blood Institute (NHLBI) in 1971 and completed in 1984. When this study began, all subjects had elevated cholesterol levels (greater than 265 mg/100 ml) but no evidence of heart disease or hypertension. All subjects were instructed about a cholesterol-lowering diet but half were given cholestyramine, an antihyperlipidemic drug described below, and half were given a placebo. Almost immediately after the study began, the cholestyramine group was found to have lower plasma cholesterol levels. Compared to the placebo group, the cholestyramine group also showed a lower incidence of heart attacks, deaths from heart disease, symptoms of heart disease, and coronary bypass operations. Within the cholestyramine group, the reduction in the risk of heart disease correlated with the degree of compliance to the recommended drug regimen and with the degree of lowering of plasma cholesterol levels. Thus, these results provide a rational basis for recommending drug therapy to patients with very high cholesterol levels who cannot achieve lower cholesterol levels by dietary therapy alone.

Many questions remain unanswered, however. For example, an earlier study by the NHLBI, the Coronary Drug Project, had attempted to answer the question of whether patients who had already suffered a heart attack would be less likely to suffer a recurrence if their cholesterol levels were lowered by therapeutic means. This study revealed no evidence that the drugs used reduced the mortality rate of men who had survived earlier myocardial infarctions. In addition, the questions of why some patients with normal lipid and cholesterol levels

develop atherosclerosis and CAD, and what therapeutic interventions can benefit them, remain to be answered.

Another key question that should also be resolved before recommendations can be made about beginning long-term dietary and drug treatment programs in individual patients and in groups is whether the drugs are safe and free of discomforting side-effects that might make the subjects drop out of the program. Results reported at various stages of the Coronary Drug Project revealed the occurrence of potentially hazardous adverse effects from some drugs that failed to offer benefits that might have outweighed such risks. As a result, therapy with such hormones as *estrogens* and *dextrothyroxine* was discontinued long before the study was completed. Other drugs that continued to be tested to the end of the study were found to cause a higher incidence of certain adverse effects than were reported in patients receiving placebos. For example, as indicated in the discussions of individual drugs below and in the summary of adverse effects at the end of the chapter, patients taking *clofibrate* were much more prone to develop cholesterol gallstones (cholelithiasis) than those in the placebo group and, with *niacin* (*nicotinic acid*), the incidence of cardiac arrhythmias and of acute gouty arthritis was greater than in the placebo group. Side-effects of cholestyramine in the study completed in 1984 were minor. Bloating, constipation, and heartburn were reported by 65% of the men taking cholestyramine, but 45% of the patients taking placebo also reported these symptoms.

Treatment of hyperlipoproteinemia

Current status

Coronary artery disease

Results of this latest study provide impetus to the recommendation that, in patients with hyperlipoproteinemia, a vigorous attempt should be made to reduce these elevated levels. This is particularly true if the patient's parents or other relatives are known to have suffered heart attacks in their thirties or forties or died of CAD before the age of 50 years.

Dietary changes should always be instituted before drugs are prescribed. The most appropriate diet depends on the patient's specific type of hyperlipoproteinemia. In general, however, dietary measures include the following:

1. A reduction in foods containing saturated fats,* which tend to raise serum cholesterol levels, and a reduction in the daily dietary intake of cholesterol itself†
2. An increased intake of substances high in polyunsaturated fats, which helps to lower serum cholesterol levels‡

---

* Foods high in saturated fats include animal meats such as beef and pork, whole milk and cheeses made from it, butter, cream, and ice cream.

† Egg yolk is an example of a food rich in cholesterol.

‡ Fish, corn, soybean, safflower, and cottonseed oils and products containing them are high in polyunsaturated fats.

3. A reduction, in many cases, of the dietary intake of concentrated carbohydrate§

4. Restriction of the amount of alcohol consumed daily¶

It is also very often desirable for patients to reduce their body weight by limiting their caloric intake and by increasing their physical activity.

Only if diet alone is ineffective for lowering persistent hyperlipoproteinemia should drugs be added as a supplement. The choice of drug depends on the patient's particular hyperlipoprotein pattern and on the drug's relative safety and freedom from discomforting side-effects. As indicated in the discussions of individual drugs below, *clofibrate* is considered to be the most desirable drug for hypertriglyceridemia; it is relatively well tolerated, but has the potential to cause several forms of serious adverse effects. *Cholestyramine* is preferred for patients with hypercholesterolemia. However, this drug and *niacin* (*nicotinic acid*), which is sometimes combined with it, commonly cause gastrointestinal complaints. Patients taking any antilipemic drugs for long periods should be watched for signs of serious toxicity.

Xanthomas

The presence of lipid deposits of various types, within the skin, tendons, and joints is both a diagnostic sign of familial hyperlipidemias and an indication for dietary and drug treatment to remove these often unsightly and sometimes disabling lumps, nodules, and tumors. Patients with type I hyperlipoproteinemia, for example, sometimes develop sudden crops of yellow orange papules. Such eruptive xanthomas, which also appear occasionally in patients with other conditions marked by high triglyceride levels, are seen most often on the extensor surfaces of the arms, legs, and buttocks. A low-fat diet alone is often effective for control of such eruptions.

Type II hyperlipoproteinemia patients often have hard nodules in the tendons of their hands and feet—for example, in the Achilles tendon. These and yellowish tumors involving the elbows and knees—for example, the patellar tendon—also indicate the presence of hypercholesterolemia and LDL-type hyperlipoproteinemia. *Xanthelasmas*, yellowish plaques on or near the eyelids, are also often associated with high lipid levels, although they are sometimes also found in patients with liver disease or myelomas whose plasma lipid levels are within the normal range. The dietary measures previously described are most beneficial in such cases, but the addition of drugs such as cholestyramine and colestipol can sometimes help to hasten disappearance of such tumors.

Type III patients often have irregular yellowish plaques on their palms and fingers. These and tuberous xanthomas—large, hard yellowish nodules and tumors usually localized on the elbows and knees—often respond to treatment with clofibrate continued for as long as 1 year as a supplement to dietary therapy. Tuberous xanthomas also are frequent, but the eruptive type is relatively rare in patients with types IV and V hyperlipoproteinemia. The papular yellowish eruptions are readily cleared by dietary and drug therapies.

Individual antilipemic agents

Clofibrate

Action. This hypolipidemic drug is effective for reducing the plasma level of VLDLs in patients with elevated plasma triglyceride levels. In this respect, it acts more effectively than any of the other available antihyperlipidemic drugs (Table 32-3). This makes it particularly useful for types III and IV hyperlipoproteinemia, in which *hypertriglyceridemia* predominates (Table 32-2). It is less effective for treating the type IIa pattern, in which the cholesterol level *alone* is elevated. However, it is often administered in combination with one of the other drugs that are more effective for treating *hypercholesterolemia*.

Indications. As is the case with the other drugs of this class except cholestyramine, clofibrate (Atromid-S) has not yet been proved effective for reducing the incidence of illnesses associated with atherosclerosis, including CAD. In fact, patients on long-term therapy with this drug during the Coronary Drug Project tended to have a higher than normal incidence of pulmonary embolism and other thromboembolic disorders, as well as more frequent symptoms of coronary and peripheral vascular ischemia, such as angina and intermittent claudication. However, its continued use appears to have helped to clear up xanthomas—yellowish lipid deposits—from the skin over elbow and knee joints of patients with hereditary hyperlipidemias, and xanthelasmas of the eyelids have also sometimes disappeared as lipid levels were lowered.

Adverse effects. The most common side-effects of clofibrate include early nausea, abdominal distress, loose stools, and headache. Occasionally, patients taking clofibrate also complain of muscular aches, cramps, and weakness. Liver function tests occasionally show abnormalities, but the drug has not had to be discontinued because of hepatic toxicity. However, its use is undesirable in patients with a history of liver damage that has impaired hepatic function, and it is contraindicated in patients with primary biliary cirrhosis. The drug increases the incidence of cholelithiasis (gallstones); patients taking this drug have twice the risk of developing cholelithiasis that requires surgery. Rodents given higher than human doses for long periods of time have shown an increased incidence of benign and malignant tumors. Because of the markedly

---

§ Candy is a source of concentrated carbohydrate.

¶ Alcohol is handled in the body like a carbohydrate, and an excessive intake can markedly increase the level of triglyceride-rich VLDL.

Table 32–3. Antilipemic (hypolipemic) agents*

Official name	Trade name or synonym	Usual adult daily oral dosage	Comments
Cholestyramine resin USP	Questran	4 gm tid or qid before meals and at bedtime, taken as a suspension in liquid	A preferred drug for patients with type II hyperlipoprotein-emia with high cholesterol in the form of LDL
Clofibrate USP	Atromid-S	2 gm/day in two to four divided doses of 500–1000 mg	A preferred drug for reducing VLDL in patients with hypertriglyceridemia; less effective in reducing the level of elevated cholesterol present in the form of LDLs
Colestipol HCl	Colestid	15–30 g/day in two to four divided doses taken mixed with water or other fluids	Used to reduce elevated serum cholesterol levels in patients with hypercholesterolemia (high levels of LDL); no effect on triglyceride levels except possibly to occasionally increase them
Dextrothyroxine sodium USP	Choloxin	1–2 mg/day initially, with a gradual increase to 4–8 mg/day	Preferred to levothyroxine for use in hypothyroid patients with elevated cholesterol levels and cardiac disease; may also be used in patients with normal thyroid function and no evidence of organic heart disease
Gemfibrozil	Lopid	1200 mg/day in two divided doses ½ hr before the morning and evening meals	Used in lowering triglyceride and VLDL levels in patients with types IV and V hyperlipo-proteinemia; may increase HDL levels
Niacin USP	Nicotinic Acid	1–2 g tid with meals	Used to lower both plasma triglyceride and cholesterol levels in patients with abnormally elevated VLDL, IDL, and LDL levels
Probucol	Lorelco	500 mg bid with the morning and evening meals	Used mainly for reducing elevated cholesterol levels in patients with primary hypercholester-olemia (high levels of LDL)

* These drugs are used as supplements, or adjuncts, to appropriate dietary therapy of the various hyperlipopro-teinemias. None has been proved to be effective for benefiting patients with atherosclerosis and coronary heart disease by lowering the levels of serum cholesterol or other lipids.

increased incidence of gallstones, its potential for increasing the incidence of thromboembolic and ischemic disorders, and its potential carcinogenicity, clofibrate should be used only when clearly indicated, and should be discontinued promptly if elevated lipid levels fail to respond.

Drug–drug interactions. Clofibrate is thought to be able to displace certain acidic drugs from their plasma binding sites. This may be of clinical significance in patients who are being treated with coumarin derivatives such as *warfarin* and *dicumarol;* such patients should receive half the usual dose of these drugs and should be monitored frequently. This is because the interaction between these drugs may potentiate the action of the anticoagulant and cause unexpected bleeding.

Probucol
Action. This compound has proved effective for reducing elevated LDL levels and for lowering serum cholesterol levels in patients with primary type II hyperlipoproteinemia. It is not useful for treating cases in which the excessive plasma lipids are mainly triglycerides, because it does *not* consistently lower the level of VLDLs. Although it can be tried in patients with combined hypercholesterolemia *and* hypertriglyceridemia, probucol (Lorelco) must be discontinued if the level of *non*cholesterol lipids begins to rise markedly or stays persistently elevated despite dietary measures. When cholesterol levels have not been lowered after 4 months of therapy, the drug should be discontinued.

When added to the dietary (low-cholesterol) regimen of patients with serum cholesterol levels of over 250 mg/100 ml, this drug brings about a doubling of the degree of cholesterol lowering previously attained in about two out of three cases. The average reduction with combined therapy in successful cases is about 25%, compared to between 12% and 15% with diet alone. The recommended 1-g daily dose is best taken with the morning or evening meals (500 mg in the form of two 250-mg tablets with each meal), because its absorption is improved in the presence of food.

Adverse effects. The most common complaints involve the gastrointestinal system. Diarrhea develops in about 10% of patients, and flatulence, abdominal pain, nausea, and vomiting also sometimes occur early in the treatment regimen. Patients should be advised that such discomfort is usually only temporary so that they will not stop taking probucol before its gradual cholesterol-lowering effect becomes evident. In clinical trials, the drug had to be discontinued in only about 2% of patients. No adverse drug interactions with anticoagulants or oral hypoglycemic agents have been reported.

Niacin
Action. This vitamin of the B-complex group, also called nicotinic acid, is used as an adjunct to dietary therapy of hyperlipidemia. Its ability to lower elevated VLDL and LDL and thus to reduce both triglyceride and cholesterol levels is not related to its role as a vitamin but to other mechanisms of action that are still obscure. Administered orally in relatively large doses, it is effective in patients with types II, III, IV, and occasionally V hyperlipoproteinemia. However, the drug's ability to correct the serum lipid abnormalities in these disorders

that are said to make people more susceptible to atherosclerosis development has *not* been correlated with a corresponding decrease in the mortality rate from cardiovascular disease. The final report of the Coronary Drug Project suggests that niacin may have been slightly beneficial for protecting patients who had already experienced an acute myocardial infarction (AMI) against *nonfatal* recurrences.

Adverse effects. The most common complaint of patients taking large daily doses needed for effective treatment include heartburn, flatulence, and other gastrointestinal symptoms. These problems are lessened by taking the drug with meals.

These nicotinic acid products make the patient's skin become flushed and itchy at first, but these symptoms tend to lessen after a while. Thus, patients should be encouraged to try to bear these discomforts, and should be assured that these side-effects are likely to diminish and disappear.

On the other hand, because the Coronary Drug Project revealed long-term metabolic changes in some niacin-treated patients, they should be cautioned to come in periodically for blood tests to check plasma levels of glucose, uric acid, and liver enzymes. Caution is required in patients with diabetes, gout, active peptic ulcer, and liver disease. Although early flushing, pruritus and rash lessen with continued treatment, skin dryness often persists, and patients have occasionally developed hyperpigmentation disorders including acanthosis nigricans, a condition marked by diffuse skin discolorations, particularly in body folds.

Dextrothyroxine
Action. This optical isomer of the naturally occurring thyroid gland hormone lowers the LDL level without affecting the VLDL group to any degree, when it is administered in doses that do not stimulate general metabolism as much as do other thyroid derivatives. Dextrothyroxine (Choloxin) is considered particularly useful for treating younger patients with pure hypercholesterolemia—that is, the type IIa pattern of hyperlipidemia (Table 32-2)—especially when this occurs secondary to hypothyroidism.

Adverse effects. Early in the Coronary Drug Project, further administration of this drug to older men was discontinued when their death rate was found to be higher than that of a similar subgroup taking only a placebo. Patients also taking digitalis and diuretics and exhibiting conduction defects on the ECG appeared to be particularly susceptible to the adverse cardiac effects of dextrothyroxine. Later, after an average follow-up time of 36 months, this drug was discontinued in *all* patients, because its use was associated with a higher incidence of recurrent nonfatal myocardial infarctions and a greater overall death rate than in the placebo control patients.

The main advantage originally claimed for dextrothyroxine over levothyroxine and other thyroid hormones was that it was less likely to increase the body tissues' demands for oxygen. Such an increase in oxygen consumption makes the heart work harder, and is undesirable for patients with organic heart disease and cardiac irregularities. Despite this claimed advantage over other thyroid products, it is now apparent that dextrothyroxine must be used only with considerable caution in patients with coronary artery disease, particularly if their thyroid function is normal. This is because only slight overdosage might precipitate an attack of angina pectoris or even cardiac arrhythmias or congestive heart failure.

To avoid this danger, the drug's use should be limited largely to young patients who have *both* hypothyroidism and hypercholesterolemia, and little evidence of organic heart disease. Such patients begin treatment with very low daily doses that are raised only gradually. If a patient begins to experience heart palpitations or shows signs of nervousness and tremors, the drug is withdrawn and later begun again at a lower dose level. Diabetic patients are closely watched, because dextrothyroxine administration may increase their need for insulin or for the oral antidiabetic drugs. Like clofibrate and thyroid hormones, dextrothyroxine tends to potentiate the effects of anticoagulant drugs such as dicumarol and warfarin. The doses of these drugs must be reduced when dextrothyroxine is added to the patient's treatment regimen.

Gemfibrozil

Action. This newest drug of the group primarily lowers triglyceride levels, with a variable effect on total cholesterol levels. The VLDL fraction is lowered, and the HDL fraction may be increased. The increase of the HDL fraction may be beneficial in preventing atherosclerosis, although this has not been proven. Patients in whom the HDL fraction of lipoproteins is elevated have a lower incidence of CAD, while results of several studies have indicated that atherosclerotic patients have low HDL levels.

Gemfibrozil (Lopid) is indicated mainly for patients with very high triglyceride levels (type IV hyperlipoproteinemia) who have a risk of abdominal pain and pancreatitis and who do not respond to diet therapy alone.

Adverse effects. The most common adverse effects involve the gastrointestinal tract and include abdominal pain, nausea, diarrhea, vomiting, and flatulence. Headache, dizziness, and blurred vision have occurred. Depression of the hematopoietic system and liver function changes have been observed; therefore, blood counts and liver enzyme levels should be monitored periodically. Because gemfibrozil resembles clofibrate pharmacologically, there is concern that it will produce the same serious adverse effects as clofibrate, especially a higher risk of gallbladder disease and its complications. Rodents receiving gemfibrozil have developed liver and testicular tumors. Because of these potential adverse effects, gemfibrozil should be used only in patients for whom it is clearly indicated, and should be promptly discontinued if significant lowering of triglyceride levels cannot be demonstrated.

Cholestyramine resin

This is the only drug of the group that has been shown to reduce morbidity and mortality rates from heart disease in conjunction with its cholesterol-lowering effect.

Action. Cholestyramine resin (Questran), which reduces the plasma LDL and cholesterol levels, is preferred for patients with type II hyperlipoproteinemia. It is not suitable for treating patients whose hypercholesterolemia is accompanied by hypertriglyceridemia, because it not only has no lowering effect on IDL and VLDL levels, but may even increase them. Thus, it is *not* indicated for treating types I, III, IV, and V hyperlipoproteinemia.

Cholestyramine, a chemical that combines with bile acids in the intestine to form insoluble complexes that are then excreted in the feces, was first introduced for the relief of pruritus in patients with primary biliary cirrhosis and cholestatic jaundice (see Chap. 41) caused by partial biliary obstruction. However, the increased loss of bile acids, which would otherwise be reabsorbed and returned to the liver, was found to lead indirectly to a lowering of serum cholesterol levels. This occurs because the body then tries to replace the missing bile salts by breaking liver cholesterol down to form these substances, which are essential for aiding the absorption of the fatty substances in foods from the intestine.

Adverse effects. The main drawback of cholestyramine is that the drug has an unpleasant taste and must be taken in large amounts. It also causes heartburn, nausea, and constipation, which is usually mild and transient but can be severe enough to cause fecal impaction in elderly patients. Patients should be encouraged to continue taking the drug until the early gastrointestinal upset no longer occurs. Patients are told not to swallow the dry powder, because this might irritate or block the esophagus. Instead, it is mixed with liquids such as orange or apricot juice or with pulpy foods—applesauce, for instance. A temporary decrease in dosage and the supplemental use of a stool softener or dietary bran (Chap. 41) is recommended for older patients who develop constipation from cholestyramine. Some patients may require supplements of fat-soluble vitamins, such as injectable vitamin K, if bleeding tendencies or other signs of deficiency develop. This can occur because cholestyramine's binding of bile acids may interfere with normal absorption of fat. Thus, a water-miscible form of vitamins A and D should be given daily during long-term cholestyramine therapy.

Drug–drug interactions. The ability of cholestyramine to bind other chemicals is not limited to the bile acids alone. It can also prevent various other drugs that it may encounter in the intestine from being absorbed. Thus, these other medications should not be given at the same time. Instead, patients taking *oral anticoagulant drugs, phenylbutazone* and other antiarthritic agents, *phenobarbital, thyroxine,* and d*igitalis glycosides* should do so at the longest possible interval before or after administration of cholestyramine—generally, at least 1 hour before or 4 hours after the resin.

The ability of bile-binding resins to remove digitoxin from the body and thus shorten the period of poisoning by overdoses has been discussed in Chapter 29. Cholestyramine was reported to be effective for treating workers poisoned in a plant that manufactured the insecticide *chlordecone* (Kepone), which is excreted in the bile and eliminated in the stool. Cholestyramine binds chlordecone and prevents it from being reabsorbed from the intestine. Cholestyramine also binds the toxin produced by *Clostridium difficile,* the causative bacterium in antibiotic-related pseudomembranous colitis (Chap. 8). The oral antibiotic vancomycin can be lifesaving in this condition, but an ancillary role for cholestyramine is being investigated.

Colestipol

This drug, a bile-sequestering agent like cholestyramine, has similar actions, indications, and ability for causing drug–drug interactions. However, it has not yet been shown to have a beneficial effect on the incidence of CAD in patients whose baseline cholesterol level is increased. Its main advantage is that it is free of the fishy taste and smell of the other anion exchange resin. The tasteless, odorless, light powdery colestipol beads are mixed with water or other liquids such as milk, tomato or fruit juices, soups, or carbonated beverages.

Clinical results indicate that patients with primary hypercholesterolemia who took between 15 and 30 g of colestipol (Colestid) daily for periods of up to 5 years showed reductions in their cholesterol levels of between 15% and 30% because of the increased rate of LDL removal. The drug has no effect on serum triglyceride levels and, if these should rise above the original baseline level, treatment may have to be discontinued. Thus, before beginning treatment with colestipol, an attempt should be made for many months to control plasma cholesterol levels with an appropriate regimen of dietary change, weight loss, and treatment of disorders such as diabetes, hypothyroidism, the nephrotic syndrome, and other underlying causes of secondary hyperlipidemia.

Other hypolipidemic agents

Oral administration of the aminoglycoside-class antibiotic *neomycin* (Chap. 8) is known to cause a reduction in plasma cholesterol levels in patients with type II hyperlipoproteinemia. However, because of its potential ototoxicity and nephrotoxicity during long-term administration, this drug is not recommended for routine use. It is, instead, employed in selected cases in combination with one of the safer drugs such as niacin, when the antilipemic agents commonly used to lower plasma lipids have failed to do so.

Estrogens, which were once thought to be potentially useful for lowering plasma lipoprotein levels, have not proved effective for this purpose. Results reported in a progress report of the Coronary Drug Project, which suggested that estrogens caused complications in coronary patients, led to these drugs being dropped from the study at an early stage. The progestational steroid norethistorone has been employed in a limited number of patients with type V hyperlipoproteinemia. Its place in the treatment of women with this disorder is uncertain at present. It is interesting to note that women taking oral contraceptives mainly comprised of progestins had lower levels of HDL, the lipoprotein fraction considered by some authorities to be potentially beneficial in preventing atherosclerosis, whereas women taking oral contraceptives high in estrogens had higher levels of HDL.

Additional clinical considerations

The very recent evidence that lowering cholesterol levels of patients in whom they are markedly elevated can decrease the incidence of coronary artery disease and lower the mortality rate is an exciting development of this field. Combined with the other study results presented at the beginning of this chapter linking high cholesterol levels to atherosclerosis, it supplies cogent support to efforts to reduce high cholesterol levels, preferably by diet and, if this fails, by the judicious use of appropriate drugs. It is possible that, if high-risk patients are recognized early in the course of their disease, the atherogenic process could be stopped and reversed by putting them on a long-term preventive diet or on drug therapy. Such other cardiovascular disease risk factors as hypertension should also be controlled with the drugs discussed in Chapter 28 and by limiting the daily salt intake and reducing body weight. Patients should be advised to eliminate other risk factors by not smoking, getting regular exercise, and avoiding anxiety-provoking or stressful situations.

Because of the potential adverse effects of the currently available drugs, they should be reserved for those high-risk patients with documented hyperlipidemia. The patient needs to understand the disease, its potential complications, and the expected action of the drug prescribed. Because these drugs are used for prophylactic purposes, it is often difficult for a patient to tolerate the uncomfortable side-effects. It is also often difficult for the patient to make the dietary and life style changes that are recommended, and to agree to the large expense (estimated to be up to $600 monthly for some of the preparations) involved when no immediate benefits can be perceived. The patient will need continuity in the education program, support and encouragement to adapt to the drug therapy and to return for the necessary, periodic laboratory tests that will evaluate the effects of the drug therapy. The nurse responsible for the patient's teaching can use the changes in laboratory test results as a reinforcing incentive for the patient to continue with the prescribed medical regimen and to reinforce the teaching points regarding the disease and the drug therapy.

The patient needs to know how to prepare the drug. The drug should never be taken in the dry form; it can be mixed with soup, cereal, juices, or puréed fruits, such as applesauce. The drug should be hydrated for 1 to 2 minutes and then mixed thoroughly. If the patient is taking any other oral medications, it is advisable that they be taken 1 hour before or 4 to 6 hours after the antilipemic drug. Such spacing of medications can help to decrease some of the many possible drug–drug interactions.

Many uncomfortable gastrointestinal side-effects will decrease over time. The patient should be assured of this, but should be told to notify the nurse or physician if the side-effects become more severe or if they persist. Patients on prolonged therapy are at risk for developing deficiencies of the fat-soluble vitamins. These patients may require supplemental vitamins A and D. Patients on prolonged therapy may also develop bleeding tendencies secondary to decreased vitamin K absorption and to the subsequent decrease in synthesis of clotting factors. This problem is usually easily reversed by administration of vitamin K. The patient should be alert to the early signs of bleeding—bleeding while brushing the teeth, easy bruising, dark stools—to prevent serious problems from developing.

The patient teaching guide presents a summary of points to include in the teaching program of a patient on antilipemic drugs. The guide to the nursing process summarizes the clinical considerations to incorporate into the nursing care of a patient receiving these drugs.

Patient teaching guide: antilipemic drugs

The drug that has been prescribed for you belongs to a class of drugs called antilipemic agents. These drugs help to decrease the levels of certain lipids in the bloodstream. An increase in the serum level of these lipids has been associated with the development of many blood vessel diseases, including heart disease. The drug must be used in conjunction with a diet that is low in cholesterol and low in calories to be effective. The type of high lipid levels that you have is _____ . Your current blood level of these lipids is _____ . A normal range is considered to be _____ .

Instructions:

1. The name of your drug is _____ .

2. The dose that has been prescribed for you is _____ .

3. Your drug should be taken _____ times a day. The best time to take your drug is _____ . Never take the drug in the dry form. The drug should be hydrated for 1 or 2 minutes in a liquid—for example, soup, cereal, applesauce, juice—and then mixed thoroughly. It is often very helpful to take the drug with meals.

4. If you are taking any other oral medications, it is best to take the other drugs 1 hour before or 4 to 6 hours after taking this drug. This timing is important for preventing drug–drug interactions.

5. There are several side-effects of this drug, including the following:

GI upset: nausea, vomiting, heartburn, gas

Taking the drug with food often helps. These side-effects usually decrease over time as your body adjusts to the drug.

Constipation or diarrhea

If this problem becomes severe, consult with your nurse or physician for appropriate

(continued)

medication. This problem also often decreases over time.

6. Tell any physician, nurse, or dentist who is taking care of you that you are on this drug.

7. Keep this and all medication out of the reach of children.

8. You will need to have periodic blood tests to evaluate the effects of this drug on your blood lipid levels.

9. It is very important that you follow the diet prescribed for you while you are on this drug.

Notify your nurse or physician if any of the following occur:

Severe GI upset
Chest pain, difficulty in breathing
Bleeding gums, easy bruising
Rash, fever
Severe constipation

Guide to the nursing process: antilipemic drugs

Assessment	Nursing diagnoses	Intervention	Evaluation
Past history (*contraindications*): Pregnancy Lactation Biliary obstruction Abnormal GI function *Allergies:* these drugs; others; reactions Medication history (*cautions*): Many oral medications **Physical assessment** Neurologic: orientation, affect, reflexes Cardiovascular: P, auscultation, baseline ECG; if indicated, peripheral perfusion GI: bowel sounds, liver function Skin: lesions Laboratory tests: lipid series, liver function, clotting (with chronic therapy)	Potential alteration in bowel elimination Potential alteration in comfort Knowledge deficit regarding diagnosis and drug therapy Potential alteration in nutrition Potential noncompliance related to drug and side-effects	Proper preparation and administration of drug Provision of comfort measures: • Bathroom facilities readily available • Drug with meals • Small, palatable meals • Bowel program for constipation Patient teaching regarding disease, drug, side-effects, potential problems Support and encouragement to deal with disease, diet restrictions, side-effects, financial burden, frequent blood tests	Monitor for effectiveness of drug therapy: • ↓ Serum lipid levels • ↓ Skin lesions Monitor for adverse effects of drug: • GI problems • Vitamin deficiency • Bleeding tendency • Change in liver function • Rash, fever Evaluate effectiveness of patient teaching program Evaluate effectiveness of support and encouragement offered, and compliance to medical regimen Evaluate for possible drug–drug interactions: many possible

Summary of adverse effects of antilipemic drugs

Cholestyramine resin

Gastrointestinal: constipation, possible fecal impaction, exacerbation of hemorrhoids, abdominal cramps and pain, anorexia, flatulence, heartburn, nausea, vomiting, and steatorrhea

Clofibrate

Gastrointestinal symptoms: nausea, vomiting, flatulence, abdominal distress, loose stools

Increased incidence of cholelithiasis (cholesterol-containing gallstones), which requires surgery

Thromboembolism and ischemic disorders

Muscle aches, cramps, weakness

Headache, dizziness, fatigue

Anemia, leukopenia, cardiac arrhythmias

Colestipol

Gastrointestinal: constipation, diarrhea, flatulence, abdominal pain, nausea, vomiting (as for cholestyramine)

Idiosyncratic reaction: dizziness, chest pains, palpitations, syncope

Dextrothyroxine

Increased oxygen demand may precipitate angina

Extrasystoles, other cardiac arrhythmias: supraventricular tachycardia

Nervousness, insomnia, loss of weight, muscle tremors, headache, dizziness

Gemfibrizol

Gastrointestinal disorders: abdominal pain, diarrhea, nausea

Anemia, leukopenia

Liver function changes

Headache, dizziness, blurred vision

Niacin (nicotinic acid)

Transient flushing and itching; during prolonged therapy, skin dryness, hyperpigmentation, acanthosis nigricans.

Hyperuricemia and increased incidence of acute gout attacks; glycosuria, abnormal glucose tolerance

Abnormal liver tests and possible hepatotoxicity (these regress when the drug is discontinued)

Cardiac arrhythmias

Neomycin

Mild diarrhea; possible ototoxicity and nephrotoxicity in patients with poor renal function who fail to excrete the small amounts of the orally administered antibiotic that are absorbed systemically

Probucol

Mainly transient gastrointestinal symptoms: diarrhea, abdominal pain, flatulence, nausea, vomiting

Case study

Presentation

MM, a 55-year-old white businessman, was seen for a routine insurance physical examination. He was found to be obese, was a borderline hypertensive, smoked 2-packs of cigarettes daily, and was found to have a high blood cholesterol level. He described himself as a "workaholic." His family history revealed that both of his parents died of myocardial infarctions before the age of 50 years. The combination of these factors put MM at very high risk for coronary artery disease.

The primary medical regimen included decreased cigarette smoking, weight reduction, low-cholesterol diet, decreased salt intake, and an attempt to alleviate stressors. On a follow-up visit 4 weeks later, MM had succeeded in cutting his smoking down to one pack per day and had lost 7 lb, but no decrease was noted in his serum lipid levels. It was decided to refer MM for teaching and to start him on cholestyramine.

What nursing interventions are appropriate for this patient?

Discussion

MM's workaholic nature may make it very difficult for him to adjust to and accept all of the dietary and medical restrictions that he is being asked to incorporate into his life style. MM should receive extensive teaching about his disease, his risk factors—including the relationship of his parents' early deaths to his problems—and the goals of each of the aspects of the medical regimen. An explanation of the action and importance of each restriction may help MM to accept and comply with the restrictions. MM should be taught the proper preparation and administration of the drug, the side-effects that he can anticipate, and ways to cope with them. The need to incorporate diet restrictions with the drug therapy and the need to return for periodic blood tests should be emphasized. He should also be told the cost of the recommended drug therapy. MM will need a great deal of support and encouragement to cope with and adjust to all these restrictions. He will require continuity in his teaching program and supportive care. It might be helpful to refer MM to a dietician for help in incorporating his food restrictions into menus that are acceptable to his life style. The drug therapy does not guarantee that MM will not suffer CAD or its complications, but current studies seem to indicate that it may be helpful. If MM so desires, he has a right to the benefit of this drug to decrease his high-risk status.

References

Ahrens EH JR: The management of hyperlipidemia: Whether, rather than how. Ann Intern Med 85:87, 1976

Fisher WR et al: The common hyperlipoproteinemias: An understanding of disease mechanisms and their control. Ann Intern Med 85:497, 1976

Glueck CJ: Colestipol and probucol. Ann Intern Med 96:475, 1982

Grundy SM: Treatment of hypercholesterolemia. Am J Clin Nutr 30:895, 1977

Hansen RF: The efficiency of lipid-lowering drugs alone and in combination. Postgrad Med J 5:63, 1975

Harvengt C, Desager P: Colestipol in familial type II hyperlipoproteinemia: A three-year trial. Clin Pharmacol Ther 20:310, 1976

Havel RJ: Classification of the hyperlipidemias. Ann Rev Med 28:195, 1977

Havel RJ, Jane JP: Therapy of hyperlipidemic states. Ann Rev Med 33:417, 1982

Hunningshake DB: Pharmacologic therapy for the hyperlipidemic patient. Am J Med 74:19, 1983

Kane JP, Malloy MJ: Treatment of hypercholesterolemia. Med Clin North Am 66:537, 1982

Kolata G: Cholesterol–heart disease link illuminated. Sci 221:1164, 1983

Kolata G: Lowered cholesterol decreases heart disease. Sci 223:381, 1984

Levy RI: The effect of hypolipidemic drugs on plasma lipoproteins. Ann Rev Pharmacol Toxicol 17:499, 1977

Levy RI: Drugs used in the treatment of hyperlipoproteinemias. In Gilman AG, Goodman LS, Gilman A (eds): Goodman and Gilman's The Pharmacological Basis of Therapeutics, 6th ed, pp 834–847. New York, Macmillan, 1980

Levy RI et al: Treatment of hyperlipidemia. N Engl J Med 290:1275, 1974

Ryan IR et al: Long-term treatment of hypercholesterolemia with colestipol hydrochloride. Clin Pharmacol Ther 17:83, 1975

Salel AF et al: Probucol: A new cholesterol-lowering drug effective in patients with type II hypolipoproteinemia. Clin Pharmacol Ther 20:690, 1976

Scott PJ: Lipid-lowering drugs and coronary heart disease. Drugs 10:218, 1975

Yeshurun D, Gotto AM Jr: Drug treatment of hyperlipidemia. Am J Med 60:379, 1976

Chapter 33

Vasodilator drugs for peripheral and cerebral vascular disorders

33

General considerations

Other chapters of this section have discussed the pharmacologic effects and some important clinical indications of several classes of drugs that act in one way or another to dilate the body's blood vessels. Chapter 28 described, for example, how the *generalized* vasodilation induced by some types of antihypertensive drugs brings about a drop in the abnormally elevated blood pressure of hypertensive patients. Similarly, Chapter 31 described how the beneficial effects of nitroglycerin in angina pectoris stem mainly from the ability of that drug and other nitrates to dilate not only the coronary arteries, but also both the arterioles, or resistance vessels, and the venules, or capacitance vessels, of the *systemic* circulation.

This chapter, will deal mainly with the use of vasodilator drugs in attempts to increase the flow of blood through *specific* vascular beds—the vessels of the skin, skeletal muscles, and central nervous system. In theory, such *regional* vasodilation and the resulting rise in the rate of blood flow locally through poorly perfused tissues should result in relief of signs and symptoms that stem from ischemia. In practice, these drugs have not proved clinically effective for counteracting the painful and often disabling symptoms of skeletal muscle ischemia; nor, despite claims for improvement in mental functioning, have these drugs been proved beneficial for patients with impaired cerebral circulation. The response to vasodilator drugs is somewhat better in conditions caused by spasm of small arterioles in the skin.*

---

* Late in 1984 a drug long used in Europe received FDA approval for use in treating intermittent claudication, a painful impairment of circulation to the extremities. The drug, *pentoxifylline* (Trental), is claimed to represent a novel therapeutic approach to this problem, improving blood flow in the capillary microcirculation by a combination of actions that reduce erythrocyte and platelet aggregation and increase fibrinolytic activity.

Arterial diseases

As indicated in Chapter 32, atherosclerosis is the most common cause of coronary and cerebral vascular diseases. This lesion leads also to degenerative diseases of peripheral arteries such as those that carry blood to the muscles, skin, nerves, and other structures of the lower extremities. Although the effects of a reduction in the blood supply of the extremities are usually less dramatic and not as immediately deadly as a heart attack or stroke, these disorders—the *peripheral vascular diseases*—can have very serious consequences.

A severe reduction of the blood supply to a limb—which may come on gradually when the lumen of a major vessel is progressively narrowed by atherosclerosis, or with dramatic suddenness when a blood clot blocks the main channel completely—can cause so much injury to tissues that amputation becomes necessary. Even less severe degrees of diminished blood supply to the skin and muscles of a limb can have painful and, finally, disabling consequences. As the chronic forms of arterial or venous insufficiency advance, the patient may become too crippled to walk or to work with the hands. Often ugly skin ulcers or gangrene of deeper tissues develop and require eventual surgical intervention.

Other ischemic vascular disorders are not the result of organic damage to the blood vessels but are, instead, marked by *vasospasm*—constriction of the vessels as a result of excessive stimulation by nerve impulses reaching the vascular smooth muscle by way of the sympathetic nervous system. Raynaud's disease, a vasospastic disorder in which peripheral vessels tend to become reflexly constricted, especially on exposure of the body to cold or as a result of emotional upset, is an example of a functional arteriolar disorder of this type. It occurs mainly in young women and may, if uncontrolled, lead to painful ulcers on the fingertips and elsewhere. Unless delayed by vasodilator drug therapy, so-called trophic changes occur in the skin, which is often stretched tightly over the fingers. Such skin damage is relatively rare in a related condition called *acrocyanosis,* in which the skin of the patient's hands, feet, and legs turns blue and cold but without pain or permanent disability.

Vasodilator drug treatment of peripheral arterial disorders

An important objective of treatment with vasodilator drugs is to increase the blood supply to the poorly perfused tissues and thus supply the tissues with the oxygen and nutrients needed for normal function. Several different types of drugs that relax vascular smooth muscle are employed in attempts to correct the imbalance between the amounts of oxygen the tissues need and the insufficient quantities they are actually receiving.

In some clinical situations, this does seem to happen. In Raynaud's disease, for example, and in other conditions in which blood flow to the skin is reduced because the smooth muscle walls of the vessels have gone into spasm, drugs that relax the contracted muscles seem to open up the constricted channels and bring a better flow of blood to the skin. During the vasodilator drug's peak action, the skin often becomes flushed and warm, and numbness, tingling, and pain—if present—are relieved. Such relief is often relatively brief, because the action of most drugs is not of long duration.

Unfortunately, vasodilator drugs do not help even that much in arterial disorders in which the vessels have been damaged by degenerative atherosclerotic disease, because blood vessel walls made rigid by deposits of lipid plaques do not respond readily to the muscle-relaxing action of these drugs. Thus, for example, in thromboangiitis obliterans, or *Buerger's disease,* a condition in which the vessel walls have been damaged and hardened by arteriosclerosis and the vascular channels have been narrowed by organic obstructions bulging out from the walls, the administration of vasodilator drugs usually does little to increase blood flow to ischemic tissues.

Some physicians suggest that these drugs may be of benefit by dilating *collateral* blood vessels—alternate channels—that then deliver the needed blood. On the other hand, others argue that the dilating action of these drugs on undamaged blood vessels may sometimes actually serve to shunt blood away from the ischemic tissue areas that need it most. Thus, treatment of patients with chronic arterial diseases often depends not primarily on drugs but mainly on hygienic measures for maintaining a better arterial blood supply and for preventing breaks in the skin and other injuries that could allow microorganisms to enter.

Mechanisms of drug action
The drugs used to dilate blood vessels act in three main ways:

1. By reducing the number of nerve impulses that cause *vasoconstriction* when they arrive at vascular smooth muscle by way of sympathetic nervous system pathways
2. By acting through β_2-adrenergic receptors in vascular smooth muscle to cause *vasodilation*
3. By acting directly on the vascular muscle walls to *depress* the contractile mechanism that is not under sympathetic control

All such actions should theoretically cause the blood vessel smooth muscle to relax. This reduces the resistance to blood flow through the arterioles. As a result, the perfusion of blood through the previously ischemic tissues increases. In some cases—for example, with the drugs that block transmission of sympathetic vasoconstrictive impulses to the vessels of the skin—the increased blood flow brings about relief of signs and symptoms caused by ischemia. On the other hand, a drug-induced increase in the total blood flow through a limb does not necessarily produce relief of ischemic symptoms in most clinical situations.

The lack of proven effectiveness may be caused—as previously indicated—by a shunting of blood away from the disease-narrowed vessels in the ischemic area to those vessels that still can dilate and receive the greater amount of blood that is being delivered to the limb as a result of drug action. Another reason for failure of vasodilator drugs to relieve symptoms of ischemia is that the patient's blood vessels may already be maximally dilated as the result of a self-regulating blood flow mechanism that operates in muscular and central nervous system tissues.

Such so-called autoregulation occurs because of the release of local metabolites in ischemic tissues. For example, when working skeletal muscles are partially deprived of blood, the level of oxygen in their tissues declines, carbon dioxide and metabolic wastes accumulate locally, and tissue fluid acidity increases. Such local hypoxia, hypercarbia, and reduced pH cause the vessels to dilate to their maximum capacity. Thus, it is doubtful that the administration of vasodilator drugs, such as those that act on β_2 receptors or that act directly to depress the contractile mechanism, can bring about any greater blood flow to ischemic skeletal muscle areas than has already occurred as a result of the natural compensatory mechanism for counteracting local ischemia.

Types of vasodilators
The following discussion will consider various individual drugs of the several subclasses of vasodilators (Table 33-1). In each case, the current status of these drugs in

Table 33–1. Vasodilator drugs

Official or generic name	Trade name	Usual daily adult dosage and administration	Comments
Sympathetic blocking agents			
α-Adrenergic receptor blockers			
Ergoloid mesylates	Hydergine	1 mg orally or sublingually tid	Used to treat mental symptoms in the elderly; may act by a central mechanism rather than peripherally
Phenoxybenzamine HCl USP	Dibenzyline	10 mg, initially; later, after gradual increase, between 20 and 60 mg daily, route (orally)	See Drug digest, Chapter 18
Phentolamine mesylate USP	Regitine	5–10 mg in 10 ml saline solution, injected into area of norepinephrine extravasation	See Drug digest, Chapter 18
Phentolamine HCl USP	Regitine	50 mg, four to six times daily, route (orally)	See Drug digest, Chapter 18
Tolazoline HCl USP	Priscoline	10–50 mg qid; SC, IV, or IM	Dilates vessels also by a direct histaminelike action on smooth muscle
Ganglionic blocking agents			
Mecamylamine HCl USP	Inversine	2.5 mg initially; later 25 mg daily, route (orally)	See Chapter 18; used mainly to treat severe hypertension
Trimethaphan camsylate USP	Arfonad	Controlled continuous IV infusion	See Chapters 18 and 28; used mainly for treating hypertensive emergencies
β-Adrenergic agonists (β₂ receptor stimulants)			
Isoxsuprine HCl USP	Vasodilan	10–20 mg orally tid or qid; 5–10 mg IM, bid or tid	Drugs of this class dilate the vascular beds of skeletal muscles but not of the skin; some cerebral vasodilation may occur; isoxsuprine probably acts more as a direct vasodilator than through β_2 receptors
Nylidrin HCl USP	Arlidin	3–12 mg orally, tid or qid	
Direct-acting vasodilators			
Cyclandelate	Cyclospasmol	400–800 mg/day, orally, in two to four divided doses	Improvement, if any, occurs slowly only after long-term use
Ethaverine HCl	Ethaquin	100–200 mg orally, tid	Synthetic analogue of papaverine
Nicotinyl alcohol tartrate	Roniacol	50–100 mg orally, tid; or one 150-mg timed-release capsule, bid	Derivative of niacin (nicotinic acid)
Papaverine HCl USP	Cerespan; Pavabid	150 mg of sustained action oral form every 12 hr; 30–100 mg parenterally, including intra-arterial, q 3 hr as needed	See Drug digest

the management of various vascular disorders, in terms of their effectiveness or lack of efficacy and the potential adverse effects that may limit their usefulness, will be described.

Sympathetic blocking agents. Two types of drugs can block transmission of vasoconstrictor impulses to these blood vessel walls: the *α-adrenergic receptor blocking agents,* and the *ganglionic blocking agents.* Although drug-induced blockade of these types does tend to reduce transmission of excessive vasoconstrictor impulses, these drugs often produce various adverse effects that limit their usefulness. This is particularly true when attempts are made to employ these blocking agents in those chronic vascular diseases in which the vessels are partially blocked by physical obstructions to blood flow through skeletal muscles. Adrenergic neuron blocking drugs (Chap. 18 and 28) can also block sympathetic vasoconstrictor impulses, but their spectrum of adverse effects is so great that they are not indicated for use in this way.

Phenoxybenzamine (Dibenzyline; Chap. 18) is one of the best of the α-adrenergic blockers because it tends to produce a relatively prolonged peripheral vasodilator effect when taken by mouth. Administered in gradually increasing doses until full vasodilator effects are produced, this drug sometimes relieves vasospasm in the small arterioles of the skin of patients with Raynaud's disease, acrocyanosis, and other disorders that mainly involve the skin rather than the skeletal muscles. The resulting dilation of dermal arterioles may raise skin temperature and possibly prevent ulceration of fingertips, toes, and other parts in which blood vessels are abnormally constricted.

This drug is not very effective for increasing blood flow through ischemic skeletal muscle tissues in such peripheral vascular diseases as *intermittent claudication,* a condition characterized by attacks of pain in the patient's calf muscles while walking. This disorder responds best to *non*drug measures, including regulated exercises—for example, having the patient take several daily walks at a slow pace up to the point where pain develops. The length of the daily walks can gradually be extended, and other exercises that help to increase local collateral circulation can be added.

Phenoxybenzamine, like other α-adrenergic and ganglionic blocking agents, is not useful for treating Buerger's disease (see above). Attempting to increase local blood flow through skeletal muscle tissues and thus to relieve ischemic symptoms by raising the drug's dosage is undesirable, because this can then lead to dilation in systemic vascular beds more readily than in the partially occluded vessels of the affected limbs. This can cause dizziness and more severe signs of postural hypotension.

Elderly patients with generalized atherosclerosis as well as peripheral vascular disease must be carefully observed while taking this or other sympathetic blocking drugs. Generalized vasodilation may not only cause diz-

ziness, weakness, and fainting, but may even precipitate a stroke or a myocardial infarction in patients with severe cerebral or coronary atherosclerosis. Reflex tachycardia in response to a steep drug-induced fall in blood pressure might also set off an episode of angina or congestive heart failure in a patient on the borderline of cardiac compensation.

Tolazoline (Priscoline), a drug that produces vasodilation not only by α-adrenergic blockade but also by its histaminelike action (Chap. 39) and other possibly cholinergic actions, is also employed sometimes to relax vascular spasm and thus increase peripheral blood flow. The oral dosage form is no longer available in the United States. A drawback is this drug's tendency to stimulate secretion of gastric acid and thus cause epigastric distress, nausea, or vomiting.

This effect of the histaminelike and cholinergic components in the spectrum of tolazoline's actions makes its use in patients with gastritis or a history of healed or active peptic ulcer undesirable. Injections of this drug—which also has a sympathomimetic component—can set off cardiac arrhythmias, anginal chest pains, or a sudden rise in blood pressure. Thus, this drug should not be given to peripheral vascular disease patients who also have coronary artery disease or a history of a recent stroke.

Tolazoline is usually administered intravenously, intramuscularly, or subcutaneously. The intra-arterial route is also sometimes employed. Administered directly into the femoral, radial, or brachial artery by a special technique, the infused drug often causes flushing of the skin and a feeling of warmth, or even a burning sensation, all through the involved limb. This vasodilator effect may sometimes be useful following frostbite and against the vasospasm of Raynaud's disease and the Raynaud phenomenon of scleroderma. Its use may also help to relieve the burning pain of causalgia following peripheral nerve injuries and to prevent the development of trophic skin changes. It is, however, of little use for increasing blood flow through ischemic areas of lower limb skeletal muscles in patients with intermittent claudication. Patients with Buerger's disease and advanced arteriosclerosis obliterans may actually suffer a further decrease of blood flow in the ischemic area. The reason for this is that tolazoline, like other potent blocking drugs, may relax the smooth muscles of other arterioles more readily than the walls of damaged vessels. As a result, blood flow may be diverted into these newly opened channels and away from the tissues that need it most.

Phentolamine (Regitine; Chap. 18) is an α-adrenergic blocker that is now used mainly for diagnosis and treatment of pheochromocytoma rather than in peripheral vascular disease. However, its ability to dilate extremely constricted blood vessels is used in counteracting the local vasoconstrictor effect of *levarterenol* (Levophed; Chap. 17) when an infusion of that vasopressor drug accidentally leaks into the skin during treatment of a patient in shock. For that purpose, the affected area is infiltrated with phentolamine to prevent sloughing of the skin following local ulceration and tissue necrosis as a result of the powerful, prolonged ischemia that levarterenol can cause if its action is not counteracted by α-adrenergic blockade.

Ergoloid mesylates (Hydergine), a mixture of three natural ergot alkaloids that have been hydrogenated to reduce their characteristic vasoconstrictor effect (see ergotamine, Chap. 23 and ergonovine, Chap. 38) may produce peripheral vasodilation in some circumstances. This may be in part the result of depression of the medullary vasomotor center and partially caused by α-adrenergic blockade (Chap. 18). In this country it is not employed for treating peripheral vascular disease but is, instead, promoted for its possible effects against symptoms that may stem from impaired cerebral circulation. Its current status when used in the management of elderly patients and others with symptoms of possible cerebral origin is discussed below.

The ganglionic blocking agents—drugs that block transmission of vasoconstrictive impulses through the sympathetic ganglia (Chaps. 18 and 28)—produce vascular effects similar to those of the α-adrenergic blocking agents, and so they were once widely used in attempts to treat peripheral vascular diseases. However, these drugs are little used for this purpose in the United States today, mainly because their actions are diverse and difficult to control, and adverse systemic circulatory side-effects occur frequently. (Sympathectomy—the surgical removal of sympathetic ganglia in the lumbar region—is sometimes still employed instead of these sympathetic blocking drugs to improve blood flow to the skin of the legs in patients with partial femoral artery occlusions.)

β-adrenergic stimulant drugs. The arteriolar walls of the vessels that carry blood to the skeletal muscles contain mainly adrenergic receptors of the β_2 type. These receptors react to epinephrine released from the adrenal medulla in a way that results in relaxation of the vascular smooth muscle. This results in vasodilation and an increased blood flow through the skeletal muscles during stress. Thus, the use of certain synthetic sympathomimetic amines that also stimulate such β_2-type adrenergic receptors has been advocated for clinical use for relief of leg cramps and pain in patients with peripheral vascular diseases.

Two drugs of this class, *nylidrin* (Arlidin) and *isoxsuprine* (Vasodilan), are claimed to be β-adrenergic agonists and are claimed to bring about a marked increase in the amount of blood passing through the calf muscles of patients with intermittent claudication and other occlusive vascular diseases. They are said to do so without causing the degree of severe cardiac stimulation and hypotension that might occur with a more potent, nonselective β-adrenergic stimulant such as isoproterenol (Chap. 17). The vasodilator effects of isoxsuprine are not blocked by the β blocker propranolol; thus, its vasodilator effects are mostly exerted directly on smooth muscle. Nylidrin acts partly as a β-adrenergic agonist and partly directly. Nevertheless, isoxsuprine *is* a cardiac stimulant, and can produce the same types of adverse cardiac effects as isoproterenol. Orally administered nylidrin can cause nervousness, trembling, and occasional heart palpitations and postural hypotension.

Actually, there is no proof that the vasodilation that these drugs produce in the vascular beds of skeletal muscles of experimental animals and normal human subjects is beneficial for patients with the types of peripheral vascular diseases that cause ischemic leg pain during walking. As indicated previously, this may be because all the blood vessels that can still respond are already maximally dilated as a result of self-regulatory metabolic mechanisms, or because any drug-induced increase in *total* blood flow to the affected limb is not accompanied by better perfusion of the specific ischemic muscle areas that are most in need of a rise in flow rate.

Both of these drugs are also claimed to increase cerebral blood flow and thus to relieve symptoms that stem from insufficient flow of blood to brain areas served by atherosclerotic arterioles. Nylidrin has also been tried for the relief of ringing in the ears, hearing difficulties, and vertigo—symptoms that are thought to be caused by spasm of inner ear arterioles. There is little proof that this drug and others (see below) are really effective for relief of symptoms that are the result of cerebral or labyrinthine arterial insufficiency.

Direct-acting vasodilator drugs. Certain substances relax excessively constricted vessels by acting directly on their walls to reduce the tone of the smooth muscles and thus widen the arterial channels. The prototype of direct-acting muscle relaxants is *papaverine*[+] (Cerespan; Pavabid), a *non*-addicting opium alkaloid. Newer drugs of this type include derivatives of the B-complex vitamin niacin (nicotinic acid), such as *nicotinyl alcohol* (Roniacol) and *cyclandelate* (Cyclospasmol), a drug of a different chemical class.

Drugs of this type do not seem to be very effective when administered orally for peripheral vascular disorders. However, because facial flushing is seen with some of these agents, such as nicotinyl alcohol, patients may *feel* that the drugs are doing some good. Later, when flushing no longer causes such a positive placebo effect, patients may want to stop taking the drug. These patients should be encouraged to keep on taking their medication for as long as it is ordered, because short-term vasodilator drug therapy is of little use in these chronic conditions, and these drugs are relatively free of serious side-effects.

Papaverine, administered parenterally, does dilate arterioles by relaxing reflex spasm. However, large doses administered in this way may cause cardiac arrhythmias. In acute block of a major vessel by a blood clot, papaverine may sometimes be injected directly into the artery. However, most physicians now prefer to meet this emergency by blocking spinal ganglia with local anesthetics (Chap. 14) or by the use of thromboendarterectomy, embolectomy, or other vascular surgery following initial anticoagulant or thrombolytic drug therapy (see Chap. 34).

Effects of vasodilator drugs on cerebral circulation

Papaverine has also been injected IV following acute thrombotic strokes caused by clots forming in cerebral arterioles narrowed by atherosclerosis. The purpose of parenteral papaverine administration is to increase blood flow to the ischemic brain tissue areas. Although drug-induced reduction of cerebral vessel spasm is said to increase the flow of blood to tissues adjacent to the infarct area, it is doubtful that the increased perfusion at such sites is any greater than that which has already occurred naturally as a result of local ischemia, hypoxia, and carbon dioxide accumulation. In some circumstances, blood may even be directed away from the ischemic area. Thus, vasodilator drug therapy of stroke is not recommended.*

Senile dementia. Papaverine is also widely promoted and prescribed for treating elderly patients with mild to moderate degrees of the senile organic brain syndrome. Although the actual causes of the symptoms of mental deterioration that develop in some older people are largely unknown, and may be unrelated to compromised cerebral circulation, this disorder has been traditionally attributed to brain damage caused by a reduction in the blood supply to the cerebral cortex and related subcortical areas of the aged. Thus, the rationale for treatment with papaverine and other vasodilator drugs is that these agents may delay further damage by increasing the total amount of blood circulating through the brains of such patients.

This hemodynamic hypothesis relating mental impairment to inadequate circulation has been strongly challenged, as has been the assumption that relatively small, safe oral doses of papaverine and other vasodilators can relax cerebral vascular smooth muscle and thus increase the perfusion of brain tissue with oxygenated blood. Most neurologists doubt that the behavioral changes seen in elderly patients are caused primarily by cerebral atherosclerosis and ischemia, and pharmacologists doubt the efficacy of small doses of vasodilator drugs for increasing cerebral vascular blood flow.

Because all products of this type currently have DESI ratings (p. 15) of only "possibly effective," their manufacturers have been forced to conduct clinical studies

to provide further evidence of efficacy. Various results have been reported concluding that papaverine products and others containing cyclandelate, dihydroergotoxine, and other vasodilators help to improve "selected symptoms" in "selected cases," and that their long-continued use could help to delay further decline of mental and physical function in some patients. Such studies have been subject to severe criticism on various grounds by other authorities who feel that there is no convincing evidence that these vasodilator drugs are of any value for patients with senile dementia.

It certainly seems unlikely that any improvement reported in mental, physical, and emotional function, or in interpersonal social relationships, is the result of an increase in cerebral blood flow produced by small oral doses of these drugs. Thus, some proponents of these products have suggested that their supposed benefits may result from some still unknown mechanisms other than vasodilation. The improvement in memory, mood, and such symptoms as irritability and dizziness said to have been brought about by dihydroergotoxine, for example, has been attributed to a drug-induced improvement in neuronal metabolism by unexplained means. Similarly, relief of mental confusion and improvement in orientation and sociability said to have been produced by chronic papaverine administration has been explained in terms of a dopamine-blocking mechanism similar to that of the phenothiazines, haloperidol, and other antipsychotic drugs (see Chap. 46).

Alternatively, any improvement observed could be the result of a "placebo effect" or, more specifically, of an increase in the attention and expressions of concern that these patients most likely receive when they are put on drug therapy. Many studies of the efficacy of these drugs have not provided proper controls for such variables. Thus, the skeptical attitude that some researchers have expressed concerning the claims made for the above-mentioned products and others, appear to be justified. The nurse can best serve elderly patients who have some symptoms of senility by offering them strong psychological support. Ways in which the family can help by paying more attention to the patient's needs for good nutrition, companionship, and loving care can also be suggested. If adjunctive drugs are needed, the antidepressants and antipsychotics, administered in small doses (Chap. 46), or antianxiety and hypnotic drugs, administered intermittently (Chap. 45), seem superior to still unproved vasodilator drug therapy. The current increase in the geriatric population has resulted in an increase in the numbers of patients who exhibit signs of apparent decline in mental function. These range from such devastating diseases as senile dementia of the Alzheimer type (Alzheimer's disease) to more modest manifestations, such as more frequent lapses in memory. The increase in numbers of patients with these problems has stimulated interest in research on these patients and public interest in supporting such research. This has already led to new in-

* Other measures employed in the management of thrombotic stroke are discussed elsewhere. For example, the status of anticoagulant therapy in the various stages of stroke is taken up in Chapter 34, and the control of the cerebral edema with osmotic diuretics in Chapter 27 and with corticosteroids in Chapter 21.

formation about the groups of brain neurons that function abnormally and the brain neurotransmitter systems that are altered in some of these conditions (see references). Scientists are now using this knowledge as a rational basis for trying to devise new and effective drug therapy for some of these patients.

Venous diseases

Physiology and pathophysiology

The veins contain one-way valves that prevent blood from flowing backward when it is making its way back from the venous capillaries toward the heart. However, when these valves are stretched and become incompetent, gravity tends to pull some of the blood backward. This, in itself, does not interfere significantly with the venous return of blood to the heart, because there are so many venous pathways available. However, the increasing pressure within the distended veins tends to make their walls bulge outward in a way that may be disfiguring and painful.

Excessively engorged, dilated veins often cause discomfort—aching, cramping, and feelings of fullness, itching, and burning in the affected limbs. The development of this common condition—varicose veins—often stems from hereditary weakness of the venous walls. This may be aggravated by obesity or by the nature of a person's work—for example, standing for long periods at a job or lifting heavy loads. Pregnancy is another common cause, because distention of the uterus puts increased pressure on the veins of the lower limbs.

Treatment

Drugs are of only limited usefulness for treating varicose veins, and surgery is considered superior in most cases. Occasionally, however, chemicals may be employed to close off small superficial veins. The irritating substances employed for this purpose are called **sclerosing agents** (Table 33-2). *Sodium morrhuate injection* and *sodium tetradecyl sulfate* (Sotradecol) are among the most common chemicals used for obliterating segments of distended veins. They are injected carefully into a part of the vein that has been closed off from the general circulation, and the area is then kept clamped with compression bandages. The chemicals subsequently damage the inner lining of the collapsed veins, and this in turn leads to blood clot formation. Finally, after several weeks in which the patient continually wears elastic stockings over the bandages, the blood clots are converted to connective tissue. Once the inner surfaces become "glued" together by fibrous tissue, the varicose vein is firmly occluded or obliterated.

Care is required to avoid leakage of the sclerosing solution into the surrounding tissues, because extravascular spillages can cause pain, abscesses, and sloughing of necrotic tissues. Sometimes, the physician first administers a small test dose of these drugs to determine whether the patient is sensitive to them. Hypersensitization de-

veloping during a course of treatment can lead to allergic reactions, including anaphylaxis.

Phlebitis

Acute inflammation of veins with blood clot formation in the deep channels of the legs can cause a long period of disability or can result in fatal pulmonary embolism. The main groups of drugs used in the treatment of phlebitis, venous thrombosis, and pulmonary embolism are the anticoagulant, and thrombolytic agents discussed in Chapter 34. Prompt treatment with heparin injections followed by administration of the oral anticoagulants has helped to reduce the death rate from pulmonary embolism in patients with thrombophlebitis. The use of salicylates and anti-inflammatory agents such as phenylbutazone also tends to relieve local tenderness and edema in phlebitis when combined with watchful nursing care.

Many *locally acting* medications are used for control of the complications of phlebitis, including the deep ulcers that sometimes develop around the patient's ankles. The treatment of such stasis ulcers often involves soaks with astringent solutions, the use of local and systemic antibiotics to control infection, and application of enzyme-containing ointments to aid removal of skin debris and to speed healing.

Enzymatic debriding agents. The presence of surface debris and necrotic matter in dermal ulcers caused by venous stasis or by chronic arterial insufficiency tends to retard tissue repair. The topical application of proteolytic enzymes to clear away necrotic tissue helps to provide a clean layer of granulation tissue that serves as a base for epithelialization and optimal healing. Oral administration of proteolytic enzymes has not been proved effective as an adjunct to topical therapy.

There are a number of the enzymes employed in ointment or oral form for this purpose:

1. *Fibrinolysin* and *desoxyribonuclease,* which are available in combination as Elase powder and ointment, to which the broad-spectrum topical antibiotic chloramphenicol is sometimes added for treating infected lesions
2. *Papain,* a papaya plant enzyme, which is combined with urea and chlorophyll derivatives in Panafil ointment
3. *Trypsin,* available as an aerosol, and *chymotrypsin,* available in both oral and ointment forms
4. *Bromelains* (Ananase), a concentrate of proteolytic enzymes derived from the pineapple plant
5. *Sutilains* (Travase ointment) made up of proteolytic enzymes elaborated by *Bacillus subtilis*
6. *Collagenase* (Santyl ointment), derived from the fermentation of *Clostridium histolyticum*

Table 33–2. Drugs used in treating venous diseases

Official or generic name	Trade name	Usual adult dosage and administration
Sclerosing agents and adjuncts		
Adenosine phosphate (AMP)	Adeno; Cobalasine; Soraden	Adjunctive therapy in treating varicose vein complications (stasis dermatitis and varicose ulcer): 25–50 mg/day, IM only, or 50 mg three times a week until symptoms subside
Morrhuate sodium injection USP		For small- and medium-sized veins, 1–2 ml of a 5% solution; for large veins, 3–5 ml; multiple or repeated injections may be made
Sodium tetradecyl sulfate USP	Sotradecol	For small varicosities, 0.5–2 ml of a 1% solution; for large veins, up to 10 ml of a 3% solution, but usually only 0.5–2 ml in a single injection
Enzymatic fibrinolytic and proteolytic debriding agents		
Bromelains	Ananase	At first, 100,000 U orally qid; later, 50,000 U qid or 100,000 U bid
Chymotrypsin and mixtures, oral and ointment	Avazyme; Chymoral; Orenzyme; Biozyme (ointment)	Oral, one to two tablets qid; ointment, applied to lesions 1 to 3 times daily
Collagenase	Biozyme-C; Santyl (ointments)	Applied once daily or once every other day with a gauze pad or wooden tongue depressor
Fibrinolysin and desoxyribonuclease	Elase	Ointment applied as a thin layer one to three times daily; or gauze saturated with a solution and packed into the ulcerated area
Papain	In Panafil (ointment)	Applied to lesion once or twice daily and covered with gauze
Sutilains ointment USP	Travase (ointment)	Applied as a thin layer after cleansing and irrigating the wound area; repeated tid or qid
Trypsin	In Granulex (aerosol)	Applied at least twice daily; wound left open or covered with a wet bandage
Hydrophilic wound cleanser		
Dextranomer	Debrisan	Enough beads poured into a secreting wound to cover to a thickness of 1/8–1/4 inch, bandaged lightly

Most debriding agents, which are also employed in treating decubital ulcers, third-degree burns, and for other indications in addition to varicose ulcers, act in essentially the same way and require the same precautions for proper use. Skin surfaces should be kept clean and moistened with saline solution to ensure enzyme activity. Although their use together with topical antibiotics is desirable in infected wounds, antiseptics containing heavy metals such as silver or mercury should not be applied to the affected area because such substances and certain detergent antiseptics may inactivate the enzymes.

The enzyme collagenase is claimed to be unique, because it digests not only the denatured protein of dead skin tissues but also the still viable strands of collagenous connective tissue that anchor the necrotic tissue to the wound surface. Digestion of the undenatured collagen fibers is said to produce more complete debridement and more rapid healing.

Another unique approach employs *dextranomer* (Debrisan) a *non*enzymatic material that acts physically rather than chemically. This substance, which is not effective for *non*secreting wounds, is employed to pick up secretions from profusely draining skin wounds. Applied to such surfaces in the form of small spherical beads, this special type of hydrophylic dextran macromolecule avidly absorbs secretions by exerting a suctional force on exudates and tissue particles that tend to impede tissue repair.

Additional clinical considerations

As indicated, the effectiveness of vasodilator drugs for treating chronic circulatory disorders is doubtful, particularly when the patient's ischemic symptoms stem more from vascular obstruction than from reflex vasospasm. More effective than these drugs are other medical measures that the patient with chronic peripheral vascular disease should be taught to use routinely. Such treatment programs are intended to take the fullest advantage of the limited blood supply to the affected areas and, in that way, prevent the lesions from enlarging.

Patient teaching is essential for helping the patient to understand the disease and ways to cope with it. In addition to being encouraged to continue with regular drug therapy, these patients, who are most often at home rather than in the hospital, should be taught ways that they can care for themselves. There are some practical points that can be suggested:

1. *Keep the entire body warm at all times,* because chilling tends to cause reflex constriction of the peripheral blood vessels. Dress warmly if going out in cold weather.
2. *Do not apply local heat directly* to the affected parts. For example, never try to relieve ischemic foot pain by using a hot water bottle or a heating pad on the feet, because this can result in gangrenous ulcers.
3. *Avoid damage* to delicate ischemic tissues *by caustic chemicals* such as iodine or salicylic acid (in corn remedies). Instead, protect feet from chemical and mechanical injury by various means, such as gentle massage with lanolin and the use of soft sterile dressings. Potassium permanganate solution 1:5000 may be used as a foot soak to control fungus infections.
4. *Engage in light exercise, particularly walking* (within the limits recommended). This is desirable for maintaining muscle tone and for developing additional circulatory flow pathways.
5. *Rest in positions that aid blood flow.* For example, have the head of the bed raised so that blood will flow more readily to the lowered legs. Keep the legs elevated, if there are venous difficulties, because this tends to reduce edema and local tenderness and to aid venous return.
6. *Avoid clothing that constricts* the legs and thighs. Round garters and girdles that reduce arterial flow and cause excessive congestion of superficial veins are undesirable.
7. *Stop smoking,* because nicotine tends to make blood vessels constrict and thus reduces local tissue perfusion. Certain drug products, including several over-the-counter (OTC) preparations containing vasoconstrictive adrenergic drugs, such as ephedrine and amphetamines, should be avoided, as should headache remedies containing ergotamine.

In summary, although vasodilator drugs may offer relief of symptoms that stem from reflex spasm of cutaneous vessels, other measures may be even more important for improving the patient's circulation and preventing serious complications. Attentive nursing care of these patients to prevent breaks in the skin and to control fungal and other infections is very important, as is teaching the patient self-care at home to avoid developing the complications of peripheral vascular disease. Although these chronic conditions may only improve very slowly, if at all, proper patient care can be rewarding when it helps to lessen pain, heal ulcers, and prevent a limb from being lost.

Additional points specific to drug therapy that should be incorporated into the patient teaching program are included in the patient teaching guides for the specific chapters referred to in the text. The guides to the nursing process in these same chapters can be adapted for the care of the patient with peripheral vascular disease.

Summary of clinical indications for peripheral and cerebral vasodilators

The lengthy list of proposed clinical uses for vasodilator drugs does not indicate that these are effective therapeutic agents. On the contrary, their true clinical usefulness in most of these circulatory disorders is quite limited, and most are officially rated as only "possibly effective."

Peripheral vasodilation
Acrocyanosis and acroparesthesia
Arteriosclerosis obliterans
Buerger's disease (thromboangiitis obliterans)

Causalgia
Diabetic arteriosclerosis
Embolism and thrombosis, arterial
Endarteritis

Frostbite sequelae
Gangrene
Intermittent claudication
Nocturnal leg cramps
Raynaud's disease and phenomenon
Thrombophlebitis sequelae
Ulcers of extremities (and other types, such as decubital, diabetic, thrombotic, arteriosclerotic)

Venous or varicose ulcerations

Cerebral vasodilation
Cerebral arteriosclerosis marked by mood, memory, and behavioral changes
Inner ear disturbances marked by vertigo, dizziness, deafness, secondary to spasm or obstruction of labyrinthine circulation
Meniere's syndrome

Summary of adverse effects, cautions, and contraindications—vasodilator drugs

α-Adrenergic receptor blocking agents

Nasal congestion may aggravate respiratory infection. Increased gastrointestinal secretion and motility lead to diarrhea and peptic pain; caution in patients with peptic ulcer or gastroenteritis

Possible interference with male sexual function

Postural hypotension and reflex tachycardia: Feelings of fatigue, weakness, dizziness

Caution in patients sensitive to steep drops in blood pressure

Contraindicated in patients with severe cerebral or coronary atherosclerosis, compensated heart failure, and renal damage

Shock and circulatory collapse: Adrenergic vasopressors such as levarterenol may be employed if necessary, but epinephrine and other sympathomimetics with activity as β-adrenergic agonists are contraindicated.

β-Adrenergic agonists

Heart palpitations and hypotension occur *infrequently* with oral doses.

High doses, particularly by parenteral administration, should *not* be administered to patients with a history of recent myocardial infarction.

Drug rash (rare)—requires discontinuation
Nervousness and muscle tremors (rare)

Direct-acting vasodilator drugs

Gastrointestinal symptoms: anorexia, epigastric distress, nausea, diarrhea, or constipation
Cardiovascular effects: flushing, dizziness, vascular headache, diaphoresis (sweating), feelings of fatigue, weakness, drowsiness
Hypotension, tachycardia, and occasional cardiac arrhythmias make caution necessary in patients with severe coronary artery or cerebral artery disease.
Use with caution in glaucoma patients.

Case study

Presentation

MD is a 72-year-old independent widow who has lived in her home for 40 years. She is in good health for her age, with her only complaints being increasing weakness, fatigue, and leg cramping and pain with exercise. Physical exams in the past revealed that MD has arteriosclerosis with changes comparable to those of intermittent claudication. She has been taking cyclandelate (Cyclospasmol) for 4 years. It was prescribed by her family physician, who has since retired. MD wants to continue taking the drug, stating that she thinks that it makes her feel better. Her new physician agrees to continue the drug, and requests that a visiting nurse call on MD and carry out appropriate patient teaching activities in the home setting.
What points should be covered in MD's program?

Discussion

A home evaluation will allow the nurse to determine how MD can incorporate energy-conserving measures into her daily activities, as well as the best way for her to employ measures to help improve peripheral blood flow. MD can be taught to dress warmly, and to have blankets available when she is sitting in one spot. She needs to be instructed to keep her legs elevated when sitting for prolonged periods. She can be asked about the use of constrictive clothing and advised about how to avoid this. MD's supply of OTC medications can be evaluated, and she can be instructed about those that are contraindicated and advised about other preparations that would be safe. MD can be asked specifically about what measures she uses to relieve pain in her legs; this will provide the opportunity for patient teaching about the dangers of direct heat and caustic chemicals applied to the affected extremities. The nurse can help MD to find ways to incorporate exercise into her daily activities, and even to find ways so she can do more walking around her home. The drug therapy may or may not have physiologic effects on MD's vascular problem; psychologically, however, MD seems to need the drug. The visiting nurse can increase any effectiveness the drug may have by developing a trusting, caring relationship with the patient and by taking time to help her incorporate beneficial measures into her daily activities. Often this support and the nursing interventions involved are the most helpful nonsurgical therapy that is currently available for patients with peripheral vascular disease.

Drug digest

Papaverine HCl USP (Cerespan; Pavabid)

Actions and indications. The main action of this *non*analgesic nonaddicting opium alkaloid is its ability to relax all types of smooth muscle—vascular, bronchial, biliary, ureteral, and gastrointestinal. This drug is, however, rarely used today to relieve the colicky pain of visceral muscle spasm. It is, instead, promoted for use in geriatric patients, with claims that oral doses relieve various vague symptoms that might be attributed to cerebral ischemia. The improvement that is sometimes reported in patients with encephalopathy is supposed to result from increased cerebral blood flow following the drug's direct vasodilating action on cerebral vessels and a drug-induced decrease in cerebral vascular resistance. The drug's clinical efficacy when used for this purpose is doubtful.

The parenteral form of papaverine has been employed to counteract reflex coronary vessel spasm and cardiac arrhythmias in some cases of acute myocardial infarction and to bring about vasodilation in peripheral vascular disease. Injections have also been employed in the management of pulmonary embolism and for relaxing spasm in cerebral vessels, thus increasing blood flow to ischemic brain areas.

Adverse effects, cautions, and contraindications. The oral form of papaverine causes relatively few side-effects. These include flushing of the face, sweating, drowsiness, and such gastrointestinal symptoms as mild constipation, anorexia, nausea, and abdominal distress. Headache, dizziness, and malaise have been reported. Discontinue if jaundice and changes in liver function tests occur.

The injectable form of the drug can cause quinidinelike effects, including depression of cardiac conduction and lengthening of the refractory period. Its use is contraindicated in the presence of complete heart block, because it may produce premature ventricular contractions and paroxysmal tachycardia when atrioventricular conduction is depressed. Caution is also suggested in patients with glaucoma.

Dosage and administration. The usual oral dosage ranges from 100 to 300 mg administered three to five times daily. However, it is also administered once every 12 hours in specially prepared sustained-release capsules containing only 150 mg. These may be also administered at 8-hour intervals or in a dose of two capsules every 12 hours in some cases.

This drug may also be administered intramuscularly or as a slow (1- to 2-minutes) intravenous injection. Parenteral dosage is 1 ml to 4 ml of a solution containing 30 mg/ml. This may be repeated at 3-hour intervals, or—in the treatment of cardiac arrhythmias—as two doses given 10 minutes apart.

References

Branconnier RJ, Cole JO: Effects of chronic papaverine administration on mild senile organic brain syndrome. J Am Geriatr Soc 25:458, 1977

Cook P, James I: Cerebral vasodilators. N Engl J Med 305:1508, 1560, 1981

Coyle JT et al: Alzheimer's disease: A disorder of cortical cholinergic innervation. Science 219:1184, 1983

Drury DA: Foot care for the high risk patient. RN 45:46 (Nov), 1982

Freed MD et al: Prostaglandin E₁ in infants with ductus arteriosus-dependent congenital heart disease. Circulation 64:899, 1981

Greenwald BS: Neurotransmitter deficits in Alzheimer's disease: Criteria for significance. J Am Geriatr Soc 31:310, 1983

Kolata G: Clues to Alzheimer's disease emerge. Science 219:941, 1983

Needleman P, Johnson EM Jr: Vasodilators and the treatment of angina. In Gilman AG, Goodman LS, Gilman A (eds): Goodman and Gilman's The Pharmacological Basis of Therapeutics, 6th ed, pp 819–833. New York, Macmillan, 1980

Rao DB et al: Cyclandelate in the treatment of senile mental changes: A double-blind evaluation. J Am Geriatr Soc 25:548, 1977

Rhodes DJ et al: Treatment of varicose veins by compression and injection. Practitioner 208:809, 1972

Yesavage JA et al: Vasodilators in senile dementias: Review of literature. Arch Gen Psychiatr 36:220, 1979

Yesavage JA: Senile dementia: Combined pharmacologic and psychologic treatment. J Am Geriatr Soc 29:164, 1981

Zu-Xin W, Kampon S: Drugs used for the treatment of dementia. Ration Drug Ther 17:1 (May), 1983

Chapter 34

Drugs that affect blood coagulation

General considerations

Blood is able to remain in the liquid state as it flows freely through the arteries and veins, but it can quickly form a solid plug at the site of a break, cut, or tear in a blood vessel wall. This property of the blood—remaining as a fluid within the vascular system but being able to clot and thus stop bleeding following an injury—is the result of a changeable balance between anticoagulant and pro-coagulant substances in the circulating blood. This balance shifts in favor of the coagulation factors when a break in vascular integrity requires a *hemostatic* response to stop blood loss, but *intravascular* clotting is usually prevented by plasma factors that antagonize any tendency toward clot formation and that act to dissolve any small clots that do form.

Blood coagulation diseases
Pathologic changes in the dynamic equilibrium between the clotting and anticlotting components of this complex system, or in the blood vessels, can result in two types of diseases:

1. *Hemorrhagic disorders* marked by uncontrolled bleeding
2. *Thromboembolic disorders* which result in obstruction of blood flow

Both types of conditions call for quick action to avoid disability and death but, because bleeding disorders are less common than those caused by *thrombi* (blood clots) and *emboli* (clot fragments) that break off from thrombi and travel until they block an artery elsewhere in the body, the emphasis of this chapter will be on the drugs employed in the management of thromboembolic dis-eases. To understand how these drugs bring about their

therapeutically beneficial effects, the mechanisms by which blood clots form and dissolve must first be reviewed.

Blood coagulation physiology
Research has revealed how very complex the chemical reactions are that result in clot formation and resolution. In fact, hematologists still do not know all the functions of the many factors that take part in the blood clotting process. New information on blood clotting physiology has helped to clarify the nature of various hemorrhagic diseases and to aid in their diagnosis. However, to un-derstand how drug therapy affects blood coagulation, it is not necessary to know all the details of these complex interactions. To know what drugs do to help patients with blood clotting disorders, it is important to understand the main steps of the complex clotting process.

Blood coagulation steps
In simplest terms, blood turns from a liquid to a solid when a soluble plasma protein, *fibrinogen* (factor I), is converted to *fibrin*, an insoluble substance that precipitates out in solid strands (Fig. 34-1). These fibrin filaments trap the formed elements of the blood, platelets and red and white blood cells, to form a gelatinous mass—the throm-bus, or clot. This crucial conversion results from the prior formation of *thrombin*, a proteolytic enzyme that catalyzes the fibrinogen-to-fibrin reaction. Thrombin is not ordi-narily found in the circulating blood. It is formed from a pre-existing plasma protein precursor called *prothrombin* (factor II).

Understanding not only the final steps in clot formation, described above, but also some of the pre-ceding steps, helps to clarify how drugs act to prevent thromboembolism, and how some of the clinically im-portant aspects of these drugs differ. This sequence of steps is best presented by beginning with the initial event,

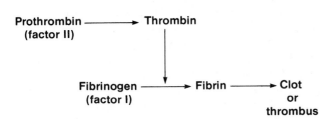

Figure 34-1. Steps in the clotting process.

injury to a blood vessel, that normally sets off the clotting mechanism.

When a blood vessel is injured and blood escapes into the tissues, five processes are initiated that act to decrease blood loss (Fig. 34-2):

1. The blood vessel constricts.
2. Loss of blood from the vessel into the surrounding tissues may increase extravascular pressure if the overlying tissue is intact and not distensible. If the injury is minor, this may compress the blood vessel.
3. Platelets in the blood will adhere to the vessel wall at the site of injury, and will adhere to one another, forming a platelet plug that is weak and needs reinforcement by fibrin from the clotting process, but that can, nevertheless, decrease blood loss rapidly (Fig. 34-3).

4. An *intrinsic pathway* that will lead to clot formation is activated. This pathway is called intrinsic because all the chemical substances are present in the blood itself. This reaction is slow, taking minutes to produce a clot.
5. An *extrinsic pathway* that also will lead to clot formation is activated. This pathway is called extrinsic because some of the substances (lipoproteins called *tissue thromboplastin*) are not in the blood but come from the cell membranes of the tissues at the site of injury. This mechanism can form a clot more rapidly—in seconds. The final steps of the intrinsic and extrinsic pathways are identical.

The first two processes will not be discussed further here. In cases of serious injury, they do not contribute significantly to hemostasis, and no drug described in this chapter acts on these processes.

The role of platelets. Blood vessel injury exposes the blood to collagen and to other substances under the endothelial lining of the blood vessel. This causes platelets in the circulating blood to adhere to the site of injury and to aggregate and form a platelet plug (Fig. 34-2). At the same time they release adenosine diphosphate (ADP), arachidonic acid, and other substances. ADP is a strong attractant for more platelets. Arachidonic acid causes further platelet adhesion and aggregation, and is a precursor of prostaglandins PGG_2 and PGH_2, from which throm-

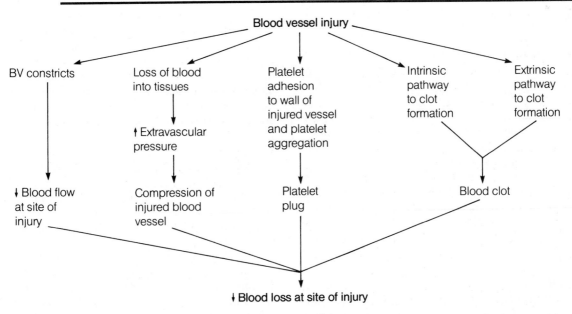

Figure 34-2. Hemostatic responses to blood vessel injury. (See Figures 34-3 and 34-4 for more details of the responses of platelets and the clotting processes.)

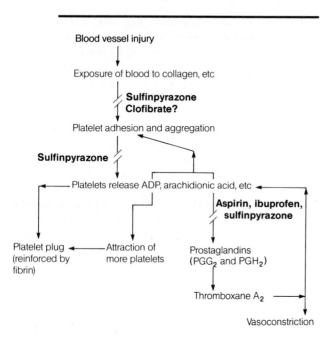

Figure 34-3. Details of platelet responses to blood vessel injury. The sites of action of some of the drugs that can influence these responses are shown in red.

boxane A_2 is formed. Thromboxane A_2 causes vasoconstriction and, like its precursor, arachidonic acid, stimulates platelet adhesion and aggregation. Thus, blood vessel injury sets off a series of processes that are self-reinforcing and result in a platelet plug at the site of injury. This plug is then reinforced by fibrin produced by the intrinsic and extrinsic pathways described below.

The intrinsic clotting pathway. As blood comes in contact with exposed structures such as collagen under the endothelium, a chemical substance in the blood called Hageman factor, or factor XII, is activated. Most of the blood clotting factors are referred to by a name as well as by a Roman numeral (Table 34-1), and the activated form of the factor carries a subscript *a*. Thus, activated Hageman factor is called factor XII_a.

Hageman factor plays an important role in initiating the clotting process. It also stimulates clot dissolution (see Fig. 34-5*B*), and participates in the inflammatory and immune responses (Chap. 36).

In the next step in the clotting process, activated Hageman factor activates factor XI, then a cascading series of precursor coagulant substances is activated, and each substance activates the next, until fibrin is formed and polymerized in the clot. Three of these factors, factors II (prothrombin), IX (Christmas factor) and X (Stuart factor), are synthesized in the liver by chemical reactions that require vitamin K.

The extrinsic clotting pathway. At the same time as the intrinsic pathway is operating, the extrinsic pathway

is activated (Fig. 34-4). A substance called tissue thromboplastin, which is *not* in the blood but rather is released from injured cells in the tissues, activates factor VII, another blood factor that is synthesized in the liver by a vitamin K-dependent chemical reaction. Factor VII_a activates factor X. It is at this step that the extrinsic pathway meets the intrinsic pathway.

The combination of platelet aggregation and fibrin formation leads to a clot that consists of a white core, or head, of platelets that is tied together with strands of fibrin. In addition to strengthening the platelet plug in the vessel wall, the fibrin filaments that overlie the platelet mass can also form a fresh clot that sometimes stretches back into the vascular channel to block blood flow. These large strands of clotted blood are seen clinically when IV lines are removed, and when venous strippings or endarterectomies are performed.

Anticlotting factors and clot resolution

The blood plasma also contains anticlotting substances that function to inhibit the reactions that might otherwise lead to obstruction of the circulatory channels by blood clots. One such substance, *antithrombin III*, inhibits the formation of thrombin and thus inhibits both fibrin and clot formation (Fig. 34-5*A*). Other plasma constituents act to break down the fibrin framework of blood clots. This process is carried out by a proteolytic enzyme called *plasmin*, or *fibrinolysin*. This substance does not exist as such in the circulating blood but is present as a precursor called *plasminogen*, or *profibrinolysin* (Fig. 34-5*B*). Just how plasminogen is converted to plasmin is unclear. The reaction may proceed spontaneously, but a number of factors are known to facilitate the conversion (Fig. 34-5*B*).

Plasmin is important in keeping blood vessels patent and functional. There are very high levels of plasmin in the lungs, which contain millions of easily injured capillaries, and in the uterus, which in pregnancy must maintain a constant blood flow to the developing fetus. The action of plasmin is evident in the female menstrual flow; clots do not form rapidly, but instead the uterine lining sloughs off and oozes blood slowly.

Drugs for treating thromboembolic and hemorrhagic disorders

Several types of drugs are employed to treat thromboembolic and hemorrhagic disorders. Each type acts at one or more steps in the sequence of clotting reactions in a manner that will be discussed in more detail below. At this point, some of these drug classes will be listed and the step(s) in the sequence at which they exert their effects on blood coagulation will be generally indicated.

Table 34-1. Blood clotting factors

Factor number	Synonym and comments
I	Fibrinogen—a soluble plasma protein synthesized in the liver that serves as the precursor of *fibrin*, the solid strands or filaments that form the framework of the clot
II	Prothrombin—a plasma protein produced in the liver in reactions involving vitamin K; serves as the precursor of *thrombin*, the proteolytic enzyme that acts on *fibrinogen* (factor I) to form *fibrin*
III	Thromboplastin—a lipoprotein released by injured body tissues; triggers reactions in the *extrinsic system* that convert *prothrombin* (factor II) to *thrombin* (Fig. 34-2)
IV	Calcium—ions required for various reactions that result in the activation of *prothrombin* (factor II) to generate *thrombin* and finally result in the formation of *fibrin*
V	Proaccelerin—a plasma protein (globulin) that speeds the rate at which *prothrombin* (factor II) is converted to *thrombin*
VII*	Proconvertin—a plasma protein produced in the liver in reactions that require vitamin K; speeds the extrinsic system reactions involving *thromboplastin* (factor III) and factor X that result in the conversion of prothrombin (factor II) to thrombin
VIII	Antihemophilic globulin (AHG), or factor (AHF)—a plasma protein that functions together with factor IX and a phospholipid released by blood platelets (platelet factor 3) in the intrinsic pathway reactions that activate prothrombin (factor II), absent in cases of classic hemophilia (hemophilia A)
IX	Christmas factor; plasma thromboplastin component (PTC)—one of the vitamin K-dependent factors that work together with factor VIII and platelet factor 3 in the presence of calcium ions in the *intrinsic pathway* reactions that speed the reaction of *prothrombin* (factor II) to *thrombin;* also called antihemophilic factor B
X	Stuart–prower factor—plasma factor produced in the liver in the presence of vitamin K; takes part in *both* intrinsic and extrinsic pathway reactions to produce a prothrombin-converting principle
XI	Plasma thromboplastin antecedent (PTA)—a plasma globulin that is activated by factor XII and then helps to speed the production of *thrombin;* also called antihemophilic factor C
XII	Hageman factor—a plasma factor that helps to trigger intrinsic system reactions; activates factor XI and may take part in inflammatory as well as clotting reactions; also called antihemophilic factor D
XIII	Fibrin stabilizing factor—a plasma component, which when activated by *thrombin* makes *fibrin* fibers stronger and able to form the gel that seals breaks in blood vessels

* Factor VI may be an unstable form of factor V, a labile accelerator globulin found in blood serum.

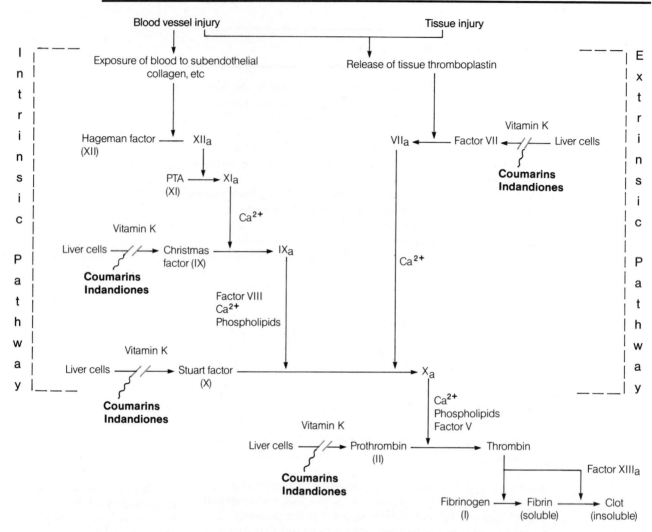

Figure 34-4. Details of the intrinsic and extrinsic clotting pathways. The sites of action of some of the drugs that can influence these processes are shown in red.

Drug classes

Anticoagulants. Two types of drugs act to prevent new clots from forming:

1. *Heparin* acts in the bloodstream to interfere directly with the functioning of several of the procoagulant factors involved in the conversion of prothrombin to thrombin, and it also prevents thrombin from reacting with fibrinogen to form fibrin (Fig. 34-5*B*). Heparin requires antithrombin III for its effectiveness in preventing clotting.
2. Drugs of the *coumarin* and *indandione* derivative classes do *not* act directly on the circulating clotting factors. Instead, these drugs act in the liver as competitive inhibitors of the enzymes that use vitamin

K in synthesizing new molecules of certain plasma clotting factors (factors II, VII, IX, and X; Fig. 34-4). Thus, these anticoagulants act indirectly and more slowly than heparin to prevent new clots from forming.

Thrombolytic agents. These are drugs that increase the rate of clot resolution. Two such agents, *streptokinase* and *urokinase,* act like natural kinase enzymes to activate plasminogen, the precursor of plasmin, the proteolytic enzyme that destroys the fibrin framework of clots (Fig. 34-5*B*).

Antiplatelet agents. Several types of drugs have been employed experimentally to prevent platelets from playing their part in blood coagulation. These substances, all of which were introduced for other purposes, were

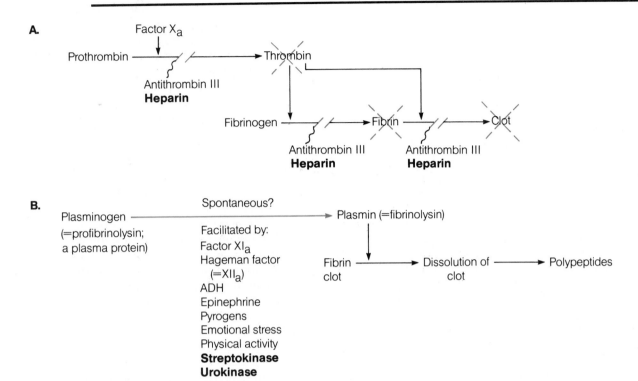

A.

Factor X$_a$

Prothrombin ——————→ Thrombin

Antithrombin III
Heparin

Fibrinogen ——————→ Fibrin ——————→ Clot

Antithrombin III   Antithrombin III
Heparin   **Heparin**

B.

Spontaneous?

Plasminogen ——————————————————→ Plasmin (=fibrinolysin)
(=profibrinolysin;
a plasma protein)

Facilitated by:
Factor XI$_a$
Hageman factor
  (=XII$_a$)
ADH
Epinephrine
Pyrogens
Emotional stress
Physical activity
Streptokinase
Urokinase

Fibrin ——————→ Dissolution of ——————→ Polypeptides
clot   clot

Figure 34-5. (*A*) Anticlotting process: prevents clotting. Antithrombin III (in plasma) inhibits the activity of Stuart factor (factor X$_a$) and thrombin; the drug, heparin, enhances the activity of antithrombin III. Steps in clot formation that are inhibited by heparin are indicated by —/ /—. (*B*) Fibrinolytic process: clots are dissolved. The step that is facilitated by the clot-dissolving drugs streptokinase and urokinase (and by other agents) is shown in red.

found to interfere with the reactions that cause platelets to aggregate at sites of arterial wall injury and in veins. They include *aspirin, ibuprofen, dipyridamole, dextrans,* and *sulfinpyrazone.*

Hemostatic agents. These are drugs used to stop bleeding. Some are natural clotting factors such as *thrombin* or *fibrin* that act when applied locally. Others act systemically when taken by mouth or injected. *Vitamin K,* for example, acts to aid in the biosynthesis of certain procoagulant factors in the liver when these are lacking in the blood plasma. *Aminocaproic acid* is used to prevent excessive amounts of plasmin from being formed. It acts by inhibiting various substances that activate plasminogen. It helps to control bleeding caused by rapid breakdown of fibrin and fibrinogen, and is used as an antidote when excessive doses of streptokinase and urokinase have been given.

Indications and contraindications for anticoagulant drug treatment

Status of therapy

Anticoagulant drugs have been used clinically for many years in the treatment of various types of thromboembolic disorders (see the summary of clinical indications at the end of this chapter). However, their usefulness for treating some conditions for which they have been employed has been questioned. The controversy over the clinical indications for anticoagulation is of considerable practical significance. These drugs can all cause serious, potentially fatal hemorrhage. Thus, it is not desirable to risk such bleeding in patients who are not likely to benefit from anticoagulant drug therapy. On the other hand, when properly employed in correctly selected patients, the anticoagulant drugs have been shown to lessen disability and to prevent deaths.

Indications

Before discussing the uses of the individual anticoagulant drugs, anticoagulant drug therapy for the treatment of various thromboembolic diseases will be briefly reviewed. Along with other pathologic conditions involving the cardiovascular system, these disorders, which are caused by clot formation in both veins and arteries and within the chambers of the heart, constitute the most common cause of death in this country. More than one million Americans die each year from diseases in which intravascular clotting of blood plays a major part. Thus, it is important to understand which types of thromboembolic diseases are likely to respond to anticoagulation and which types are more likely to be exacerbated than helped by these drugs.

Venous thromboembolism. Diseases caused by blood clots that form in the veins cause the hospitalization of more than 250,000 Americans annually. About 20% of these patients die of *pulmonary embolism,* the most dangerous complication of venous thrombosis.* Among the conditions that lead to formation of clots in the veins are *phlebothrombosis* and *thrombophlebitis.* The first of these is a *non*inflammatory disorder that results mainly from venous stasis, a slowing of blood flow that tends to cause fibrin to form behind the valves of the veins in the lower limbs. The clots that stick to the walls of the veins may then set off an inflammatory reaction within the blood vessel, leading to thrombophlebitis.

Thrombi may also form in the veins of the lower extremities when people are immobilized following hip or leg fractures or surgery, or when they suffer from chronic cardiac and lung diseases. Others at high-risk for thrombi include patients who undergo orthopedic procedures, particularly hip joint surgery. Clots also sometimes form in the pelvic or leg veins following gynecologic procedures or labor and delivery, particularly when obstetric complications have occurred, or when the patient has used birth control pills.

Anticoagulant therapy has proved to be remarkably beneficial for patients with acute thrombophlebitis. Prompt employment of heparin prevents the clot from extending from superficial veins into deeper, larger veins. This relieves local tenderness, edema, and pain, and it helps to prevent permanent disability from damage to the valves of the veins, as well as the complication of pulmonary embolism. Treatment with coumarin-type anticoagulants is started while the patient is heparinized and, once stabilized, it is continued for at least 6 weeks to prevent recurrences.

Selected patients also receive prophylactic anticoagulation to prevent pulmonary embolism from deep venous thrombosis in the various surgical, obstetric, and medical situations mentioned above. Use of these drugs for prophylaxis is limited to patients who are judged by their histories to have a high risk of thromboembolism. The need for anticoagulant drug therapy in most other cases can be obviated by early ambulation—that is, getting the patient out of bed and moving about as soon as possible. Postoperative and postdelivery patients are ambulated within hours of their procedure, which has greatly decreased the incidence of pulmonary embolism. The use of support stockings (Teds; Jobsts) and foot and leg exercises has also helped to prevent venous stasis in these patients, and has further decreased the incidence of complications.

When pulmonary embolism has actually occurred, it can also often be treated with anticoagulant drugs. Anticoagulant drugs do not, of course, dissolve the clots that have lodged in the lung artery. However, their use gives the body's own clot-resolving mechanisms a better chance of slowly removing the clot by preventing it from increasing in size while the patient is immobilized. Heparin is employed as soon as the disorder is diagnosed because of its prompt onset of action. The coumarin-type drugs are then used for several months or more to prevent recurrences of pulmonary emboli. (Agents of the thrombolytic class, discussed below, are employed in selected cases to hasten clot resolution and to reduce the need for embolectomy.)

Thromboembolism in heart disease. Patients with several types of cardiac disease are often considered as candidates for anticoagulant drug therapy. These include patients with *coronary artery disease,* particularly in the period immediately after the patient has suffered an acute myocardial infarction. Others for whom anticoagulants are often ordered include those with *chronic atrial fibrillation, rheumatic mitral valve disease,* and *congestive heart failure* with ventricular hypertrophy.

Acute myocardial infarction. The value of anticoagulant drug therapy in patients hospitalized with a myocardial infarction (MI) and in the postcoronary period continues to be controversial. Some authorities suggest that these drugs should be administered routinely to treat all patients who have had an MI, while others prefer to reserve anticoagulant therapy for selected high-risk cases, because they feel that the hazard of drug-induced hemorrhage could outweigh the advantages of these drugs in most patients with uncomplicated MIs.

Anticoagulants are administered in these cases to prevent thromboembolic complications, such as pulmonary embolism, stroke, and peripheral arterial occlusions. Among the MI patients considered likely to suffer such complications are those with pump failure leading to severe hypotension, shock, or congestive heart failure with pulmonary edema. Others who may be selected for anticoagulant drug therapy include those with a history of previous MI, venous thrombosis, pulmonary embolism, peripheral vascular disease, or stroke.

Postcoronary prophylaxis. The long-term usefulness of anticoagulant therapy is also controversial, because some studies have suggested that these drugs reduce recurrences of myocardial infarction, while others have offered no evidence that taking these drugs increases the survival rate. Those who believe that anticoagulant drugs do reduce deaths from coronary disease and thromboembolism recommend their use for periods ranging from several months to several years following the first acute coronary attack. Some say that continued anticoagulation is particularly useful for men under 55 years old who still suffer from angina pectoris or from acute coronary insufficiency. Patients who are placed on long-

---

*Some estimates place the number of pulmonary embolism fatalities from *all* causes at as many as 200,000 annually in the United States.

term treatment with these drugs must, of course, be free of the conditions in which their use is contraindicated, and all precautions for preventing bleeding episodes must be employed. Recent study results have led to the use of several antiplatelet drugs (*e.g.,* aspirin, ibuprofen; see below) instead of the classic anticoagulants in the post-MI period. These drugs seem to have fewer side-effects and have been found by some to be effective in preventing post-MI complications.

Cerebrovascular disease thromboembolism. The place of anticoagulant drugs in the treatment and prevention of strokes caused by cerebral arterial thrombosis and embolism is also uncertain. These drugs are, of course, *contraindicated* in strokes that are the result of cerebral hemorrhage. However, even when intracranial bleeding has been ruled out, the increased risk of drug-induced hemorrhage in some stroke patients makes the use of anticoagulants hazardous. The effectiveness of these drugs depends in part on the stage of the stroke at the time the patient is seen.

Completed stroke. Anticoagulants are of no value for limiting the size of a cerebral infarct once an acute stroke is completed. These drugs may even harm such stroke patients by causing hemorrhage. Once the patient has recovered, anticoagulant therapy may be started to prevent recurrences if the patient seems to be at risk for further cerebral thrombosis and embolism. However, it is more important to reduce the patient's blood pressure, both because hypertension is likely to lead to recurrences and because patients with high blood pressure have an increased risk of cerebral hemorrhage when taking anticoagulant drugs.

Progressive stroke. The administration of heparin to patients who are diagnosed as suffering from an *evolving* or *progressing* stroke is said by some authorities to help prevent the stroke from going on to completion. However, although anticoagulation may limit the amount of brain cell damage, there is no proof that it reduces the mortality rate. Patients in whom these drugs are employed must, of course, be free of other disorders that may make them prone to bleeding episodes during anticoagulant drug therapy.

Transient ischemic attacks (TIAs). Patients who suffer frequent symptomatic episodes caused by small cerebral thrombi and emboli are likely to suffer a massive stroke within months or a few years. The long-term administration of coumarin-type anticoagulants has been claimed to reduce the frequency of these attacks and to help prevent more serious strokes in some people. However, anticoagulant drug treatment has not been proved to reduce the mortality rate in these patients and, of course, the use of these drugs tends to increase the risk of cerebral hemorrhage.

Cerebral emboli. Anticoagulant therapy can be useful for preventing strokes in patients with diseases that increase the formation of clots that can be carried to the brain when they are dislodged from their site of origin. The heart valves and chambers are the most common sources of such emboli, which is why anticoagulant drug therapy is recommended for patients with rheumatic heart disease that has damaged the mitral valve. Anticoagulant prophylaxis is also justified for preventing strokes in patients whose damaged aortic or mitral valve has been replaced by a prosthetic heart valve, because thrombi tend to form on some of the synthetic substances used to make these valves. Porcine grafts (valves made from pig tissue) are not quite as likely to throw emboli, but the patients receiving these grafts are also often put on anticoagulants for a period of time.

As previously discussed, anticoagulants are indicated in MI patients when there seems to be a risk that clots may form and break loose. Such emboli are most likely to block cerebral arterioles when thrombi form on the walls of the left atrium or ventricle that has been damaged by an infarction. Similarly, clots that tend to form in an enlarged fibrillating left atrium may be dislodged and swept into the cerebral circulation to cause an incapacitating embolism. Most authorities seem to agree that long-term use of anticoagulants is useful for preventing cerebral emboli in patients with such chronic heart diseases. However, these drugs are almost always contraindicated in patients with bacterial endocarditis because the risk of cerebral hemorrhage is increased in this cardiac infection.

Other indications

Peripheral arterial thromboembolism. Massive clots that block the arterial blood flow to a limb and cut off the oxygen supply to its tissues can do so much damage that amputation becomes necessary. Prompt surgical removal of the arterial thrombus or systemic embolus (embolectomy) is the best treatment. However, heparin is usually injected intravenously in such cases to prevent further extension of the clot up and down the involved artery while the patient is being prepared for surgical thrombectomy or embolectomy.

Disseminated intravascular clotting (DIC). This syndrome is marked by both bleeding and by the formation of microthrombi in the small vessels of the kidneys, lungs, brain, and other organs. It occurs in many medical, surgical, and obstetric disorders as the result of tissue damage that releases thromboplastin into the bloodstream. As a result, the patient's clotting factors are used up and, because of excessive clotting, the patient can start to hemorrhage. The most important step in treating DIC is discovery and control of the underlying cause of tissue damage. However, heparin administration is also useful to prevent further clotting. Paradoxically, the prompt administration of heparin can stop bleeding in this disorder by its ability to interfere with the formation of the clotting which precedes the hemorrhaging.

Prevention of clotting of extracorporeal blood. Blood

that is withdrawn from the body for transfusion, sampling, dialysis procedures, or open heart surgery tends to clot quickly when it comes in contact with glass or with the surface of some other foreign substance. The addition of heparin to blood drawn for these purposes prevents it from clotting. The coumarin- and indandione-class anticoagulants cannot, of course, be employed for this purpose, because they do not act directly on blood components but only indirectly on their biosynthesis by the liver. Most extracorporeal blood is prevented from clotting by the addition of *citrate* ions, which combine with calcium in the blood and thus prevent the clot formation process. Once this blood is injected into a patient, the liver rapidly metabolizes the citrate, freeing the calcium, and the blood is free to clot again if needed.

Other uses: Warfarin is now being used as adjunctive therapy in small cell lung cancer.

Contraindications

The main danger in the use of anticoagulant drugs is hemorrhage. Bleeding is most likely to occur in people with illnesses that make them unusually susceptible to the effects of these drugs on the blood's ability to clot. Such patients may suddenly begin to bleed spontaneously, even when they receive ordinary doses that produce only the expected changes in plasma clotting activity. In other cases, bleeding results from overdosage—usually because of the patient's failure to follow instructions, or because of unanticipated drug–drug interactions.

Among the patients for whom any benefit from anticoagulation is outweighed by their increased susceptibility to hemorrhage are those with pre-existing blood disorders. The presence of blood dyscrasias and clotting abnormalities is ordinarily detected by the history, physical examination, and laboratory studies that must be performed before these drugs are ordered, and anticoagulant therapy is withheld in such cases. On the other hand, other disorders that can lead to bleeding may not be discovered until after the drugs are administered—for example, ulcerations and cancer of the gastrointestinal tract. Because the most common cause of death with these drugs is heavy gastrointestinal hemorrhage, anticoagulants are contraindicated in patients with peptic ulcer, ulcerative colitis, or carcinoma of the viscera.

Bleeding within the central nervous system is also serious. Thus, these drugs should not be employed in patients who have had a recent head injury or recent surgery on the brain, spinal cord, or eyes. The drugs are not given to patients with very high blood pressure or with subacute bacterial endocarditis—conditions that increase the risk of cerebral bleeding—and, of course, anticoagulants are not ordered for people who have suffered a hemorrhagic stroke. The drugs are also withheld from patients who are to have spinal anesthesia.

Other conditions that may make it necessary to use these drugs with extreme caution, if at all, include severe liver, kidney, or biliary tract disease. Patients with liver disease may have a deficiency of the hepatic enzymes needed to inactivate the coumarin-type anticoagulants, and they may lack the ability to biosynthesize plasma clotting factors normally, leading to excessive bleeding or even hemorrhage. Those with biliary tract obstruction may be excessively sensitive to the coumarin-type anticoagulant drugs because of their reduced ability to absorb vitamin K, the natural antagonist of these drugs. Patients with diarrhea may have difficulty in absorbing full doses of these orally administered anticoagulants, which may make it difficult to regulate dosage and may lead to variability in responsiveness to drug therapy.

Anticoagulants are also contraindicated during pregnancy and lactation. There is an increased risk of hemorrhage for the mother, and various fetal and infant deformities have been reported with their use.

Patients who cannot be counted on to cooperate should not receive these drugs for prolonged periods. Failure to take these drugs exactly as directed can lead to underdosage or overdosage, and patients who forget to return for the required periodic laboratory tests cannot, of course, be protected by early detection of the effects of improper dosage. Among those in whom these drugs are contraindicated for such reasons are chronic alcoholics, emotionally unstable or psychotic patients, or senile patients, unless they are being cared for by a reliable relative or are under professional care.

Anticoagulant drugs

Two types of anticoagulant drugs will be discussed in detail: heparin, an injectable, rapid-acting agent preferred for emergencies, and the coumarin derivatives and other orally administered drugs that are most commonly employed in long-term prevention of thromboembolic episodes.

Heparin

Source and chemistry. Heparin[+] is a strong organic acid found in many mammalian organs. It was first found in liver and took its name from *hepar*, the Greek word for that organ. It is also abundant in beef lung, which has served as a commercial source of heparin. However, it is now extracted mainly from the mucosal lining of pig intestine, freed of impurities, and standardized by biologic assay. Because heparin obtained from different sources can vary in strength, its dosage is designated not in milligrams but in standard USP units.

Mechanism of action. The exact way in which heparin lengthens the clotting time of whole blood is still uncertain. Because of its strong electronegative charge it reacts with a wide variety of the proteins that take part in the series of reactions that lead to clot formation. Heparin also activates a plasma protein anticlotting cofactor called antithrombin III, which is thought to prevent any already formed thrombin from reacting with fibrinogen to form the fibrin framework of blood clots. More important, perhaps, than the inactivation of preformed thrombin, is the fact that the heparin–cofactor interaction prevents thrombin from being formed in the first place. That is, it prevents such activated protease enzymes as factors IX, X, XI, and XII from participating in the complex reactions required to convert prothrombin to thrombin (Figs. 34-4 and 34-5A). In addition, there is evidence that heparin also inhibits activation of factor XIII, the fibrin stabilizing factor (Table 34-1). This prevents any fibrin that may be produced from forming a strong stable fibrin clot.

Because of its mechanism of action, heparin acts immediately when injected into the bloodstream. It is important to remember that heparin has no lysing activity—that is, it cannot dissolve any clots that have already formed.

Clinical indications. The immediate action of heparin accounts for its use in acute thromboembolic emergencies. Among the clinical situations in which heparin has proved highly effective is acute thrombophlebitis involving deep veins of the extremities. Its prompt parenteral administration prevents the venous clots from enlarging and emboli from breaking off. Heparin is also effective for treating patients with pulmonary embolism and for preventing recurrences of such embolic episodes. The administration of heparin in much lower doses than those required for *treating* venous thromboses has been found to be effective for *preventing* clot formation in high-risk cases. Thus, for example, this anticoagulant is being given prophylactically in small, safe doses to such clot-prone patients as elderly patients who are immobilized.

Heparin is also employed in cases of acute occlusion of systemic arteries by thrombi and emboli. Although embolectomy is required to remove such clots from the femoral and other arteries of the extremities, the immediate administration of heparin helps to prevent the clot from extending below and above the point of blood flow block while the patient is being prepared for surgery. Heparin may also be given to halt further clot formation in the involved cerebral arterial bed of patients with a progressing, or evolving, stroke. Although the ability of heparin to affect clot extension in coronary arteries has been questioned, the drug is undoubtedly useful for preventing thromboembolic complications following an acute MI, particularly if heart failure is also present. (See the summary at the end of the chapter for other clinical situations in which heparin is indicated.)

Adverse effects. The main danger of heparin administration is hemorrhage, which is more likely to occur with this immediate-acting agent than with the oral anticoagulants. Heparin-induced hemorrhage is best prevented by withholding heparin from patients with diseases that increase their susceptibility to bleeding. However, bleeding sometimes occurs in patients not previously known to have a condition that increases their tendency to bleed. A recent study suggests that otherwise normal women over 60 years old have a higher incidence of hemorrhage when receiving heparin. (See the Drug digest for other adverse effects of heparin.)

Laboratory control. To avoid bleeding episodes, the effects of heparin on clotting time of the patient's blood should be checked just before each dose is due. In the Lee–White test, the clotting time is kept at about 2.5 to 3 times the control value. Thus, if the patient's drawn blood clotted in about 10 minutes before treatment was begun, it should clot in no longer than 25 to 30 minutes during heparin therapy. When the test for partial thromboplastin time (PTT) is used, the clotting time is kept at 1.5 to 2.5 times the control value. If a blood sample taken more than 30 minutes before shows no sign of clotting, the next scheduled dose should be withheld. Patients receiving a continuous infusion of heparin should have their blood tested in this way or by other methods about every 4 hours.

Antidotal treatment. Most episodes of minor bleeding stop when heparin dosage is withheld or the drug is discontinued. If severe bleeding does develop, it can usually be controlled by administering a specific chemical antidote called *protamine sulfate.* This is a strongly basic substance that neutralizes heparin by combining with that acidic molecule and forming an inactive complex. The dose of protamine required for this depends on the amount of heparin that has been administered, and on the time that has elapsed since it was injected. One milligram of protamine neutralizes about 100 U of heparin. However, if 30 minutes have passed since the last intravenous dose of heparin, only about 0.5 mg of protamine should be given for every 100 U of the anticoagulant. If the heparin was administered subcutaneously, it is best neutralized by administering smaller doses of protamine periodically at intervals timed to the predicted time of entrance of heparin into the blood from the depot site.

Proper dosage of protamine is important because it is not a harmless substance. It should be infused at a slow rate—no more than 50 mg in any 10-minute period—because too rapid an injection can cause a steep fall in blood pressure. The drug can itself occasionally have a paradoxical anticoagulant effect, and can actually prolong the clotting time. Heparin overdosage can, however, also be counteracted by transfusions of whole blood or plasma, which supply new increments of clotting factors and thus dilute the excess heparin.

Disadvantages. The greatest drawback of heparin is that it has to be given parenterally. Because it cannot be taken by mouth, and because it has a short duration of action, the drug is unsuitable for long-term maintenance therapy of ambulatory patients. To keep heparin at effective anticlotting levels, it usually has to be administered by frequent intravenous injection, often using a heparin lock needle, or even by continuous infusion. This usually requires hospitalization, which adds further to the expense of administering a drug which is itself relatively costly.

The duration of action of heparin can be lengthened by administering the drug by deep subcutaneous injection. However, its absorption from subcutaneous abdominal fat pads is often erratic. Repository forms, in which heparin is suspended in substances such as gelatin, have the longest duration of action. However, because of the occurrence of tissue sloughing and the difficulty of bringing bleeding under control, these are rarely employed.

Drug–drug interactions. The effect of heparin will be increased if it is given with any other drugs that interfere with blood coagulation. *Digitalis, tetracycline, nicotine,* and *antihistamines* have been found to counteract partially the anticoagulant effect expected with heparin.

Coumarin derivatives and other oral anticoagulants

Drugs of two different chemical classes—derivatives of coumarin and indandione—differ from heparin in their manner of action and in being effective when taken by mouth. Those of the coumarin class, especially *warfarin*[+] and *dicumarol*[+], are widely used in this country (Table 34-2). Anticoagulants of the other chemical class are not commonly employed here, mainly because they sometimes tend to cause skin reactions and occasional liver or kidney toxicity. They are usually reserved for the rare patient who is sensitive to the coumarin-class anticoagulants.

Mechanism of action. All these drugs act in the same way: they interfere with liver cell biosynthesis of the plasma procoagulant proteins prothrombin (factor II) and of the related clotting factors VII, IX, and X (Table 34-1 and Fig. 34-4).* Thus, these drugs interfere with both the intrinsic and the extrinsic clotting pathways. These drugs act by preventing vitamin K from carrying out its physiologic function. As the competitive inhibitors of vitamin K exert their effect, the liver stops making molecules of the vitamin K-dependent clotting factors, and the levels of these protein substances in the blood gradually fall. Because the action of these drugs on the plasma clotting factors is indirect, therapeutic doses require about 1 to 4 days to produce the desired degree of anticoagulant activity.

Variability in response. People differ widely in their response to treatment with drugs of this class. Some—particularly elderly patients weakened by disease or by malnutrition, or patients with disease of the liver, pancreas or kidneys—are sensitive to small doses of coumarin drugs. Others require much larger amounts to bring their blood protein clotting factors down to the therapeutically desirable level. This may be because of their greater ability to metabolize these drugs to inactive substances. A particular patient's response cannot be predicted in advance and, in fact, dosage requirements may sometimes change during treatment. Often, illness marked by fever or diarrhea may decrease or increase dosage requirements, as may the addition of other drugs to the regimen.

Because of such individual variation, it is undesirable to administer the same standard dose to all patients. Instead, it is necessary to adjust each patient's anticoagulant drug dosage individually by monitoring the patient's response to therapy by tests performed daily in the hospital laboratory. Unless reliable facilities are available for following the patient's response and for adjusting drug dosage accordingly, treatment should not be undertaken. Long-term maintenance therapy must not be continued without checking the patient's response periodically. As indicated earlier, patients who cannot be depended on to return for such laboratory tests at specified intervals should not be maintained on anticoagulant drug therapy.

Laboratory control of dosage. The first and still most commonly employed test for monitoring the patient's response to coumarin and indandione derivative drugs is the Quick one-stage prothrombin time (PT) test. It measures the time, in seconds, required for a sample of the patient's plasma to clot when it is mixed with a tissue thromboplastin preparation and calcium under standardized conditions. Normally, clotting occurs in 11 to 13 seconds, because thrombin is formed by reactions that resemble those of the natural extrinsic mechanism (Figs. 34-2 and 34-4). However, this time becomes significantly lengthened as the drugs reduce and stop the biosynthesis of prothrombin and related procoagulation proteins. This reflects a fall in the circulating plasma clotting factors to below normal levels.

To attain a level of blood coagulability low enough to protect the patient against thrombosis without serious danger of bleeding, dosage is ordinarily adjusted to what is required to prolong the patient's PT to between 1.5 and 2.5 times normal. If, for example, the patient's PT was 12 seconds at the start of treatment, drug dosage may be stabilized at a PT of 24 to 30 seconds. This indicates a drop in the concentration of circulating procoagulant proteins to about 20% of normal—a level likely to prevent thromboembolic episodes in most patients. For full protection, some patients may require a further reduction in plasma clotting activity. However, the risk of hemorrhage is increased as the PT time is prolonged to three times normal—36 seconds, for example—and the concentration of clotting factors falls to 10% or less of the control value. (Some patients with a tendency toward bleeding may be stabilized at anticoagulant drug doses that lengthen the PT time to only 1.5 times normal—

---

* These drugs are commonly called hypoprothrombinemic agents. However, their action results in a reduction of plasma levels not only of prothrombin, but also of related clotting factors, some of which are even more sensitive to the inhibiting action of these drugs on their biosynthesis.

Table 34–2. Anticoagulant drugs of the hypoprothrombinemic type*

Generic or official name	Trade name or synonym	Total adult daily initial and maintenance dosages†	Comments‡
Coumarin derivatives			
Dicumarol USP	Bishydroxycoumarin	Initial loading dose: 200–300 mg first day, 25–200 mg second and third days; maintenance dose range: 25–200 mg daily	Onset: intermediate (24–72 hr); duration: long (4–6 days); see Drug digest
Phenprocoumon USP	Liquamar	Initial loading dose: 24 mg first day, 0.75–6 mg second and third days; maintenance dose range: 0.75–6 mg daily	Onset: slow (48–72 hr); duration: long (7 days or more), few side-effects
Warfarin sodium USP	Coufarin; Coumadin; Panwarfin	Initial loading dose: 40–60 mg average adult, 20–30 mg for elderly patients; maintenance dose range: 2–10 mg daily	Onset: intermediate (24–36 hours); duration: intermediate (2–4 days); see Drug digest
Warfarin potassium USP	Athrombin-K	Same as for sodium salt	Same as for sodium salt
Indandione derivatives			
Anisindione	Miradon	Initial loading dose: 300 mg first day, 200–300 mg second day, 100 mg third day; maintenance dose range: 25–250 mg daily	Onset: intermediate to long (48–72 hr); duration: intermediate (24–72 hr); dermatitis only side-effect reported, but others, typical of this chemical class, are possible
Phenindione USP	Hedulin	Initial loading dose: 200–500 mg first day, 100–200 mg second day; maintenance dose range: 50–150 mg daily	Onset: rapid (18–24 hours); duration: short (24–48 hr); hypersensitivity reactions include leukopenia and agranulocytosis, hepatitis and jaundice, nephropathy with albuminuria and edema, dermatitis, others

* Drugs listed are of the hypoprothrombinemia-producing type that act in liver as competitive antagonists of vitamin K.
† All doses are by *oral* administration; warfarin sodium is also available in form for parenteral administration. Maintenance dosage is determined by periodic prothrombin time determinations.
‡ Onset refers to time needed to reduce prothrombin activity to the therapeutic range (20% to 30% of normal). Duration refers to time required for prothrombin time to return to normal after the drug is discontinued.

only 18 seconds, for example—reflecting a fall in the concentration of clotting factors to only 30% or more.)

Antidotal treatment. The specific antidote for overdosage of oral anticoagulants is the form of vitamin K called *phytonadione*. Patients are often advised to carry tablets or capsules of this substance so that they can take a dose immediately if the physician tells them to do so when reached by telephone. Often this may be unnec-essary, because mild bleeding may stop when the next dose of the anticoagulant is skipped. In case of severe bleeding, on the other hand, such stopgap use of oral vitamin K is inadequate, and this antidote must be administered by vein. Ordinarily, this treatment will bring the plasma clotting factor concentrations and the PT time back to normal within a few hours. However, if hemorrhage is too severe to warrant waiting the several hours required for biosynthesis and passage into the blood of enough new procoagulant molecules, the patient may also be treated by transfusion of fresh whole blood, plasma, or blood fractions containing the already preformed clotting factors.

Drug–drug interactions. Many patients who take anticoagulants for long periods also receive other drugs at the same time. Some of these medications may alter the patient's response to anticoagulant therapy (Table 34-3). Drugs that cause an *increase* in activity of the oral anticoagulants may eliminate their narrow margin of safety and thus precipitate sudden episodes of bleeding. Drugs that *decrease* anticoagulant activity may make the patient more likely to suffer a thromboembolic episode by depriving him of the therapeutic benefits of these drugs.

This does not mean that patients taking anticoagulant drugs cannot be treated with other medications. It does mean that, whenever a new drug is added to a patient's regimen or one is discontinued, the patient's PT times must be monitored more frequently. Then, if a change in the patient's response to the anticoagulant

Table 34–3. Drug–drug interactions with oral anticoagulants

Mechanism of interaction	Drugs	Clinical response	Action
Displace anticoagulant from plasma protein sites	Salicylates, sulfonamides, sulfonylureas, triclofos, chloral hydrate, phenylbutazone, clofibrate	↑ bleeding tendency	↓ dose of anticoagulant
Inhibit liver metabolism of anticoagulant	Allopurinol, disulfiram, chloramphenicol, metronidazole, alcohol, cimetidine, phenylbutazone, sulfonamides, co-trimoxazole, sulfinpyrazone	↑ bleeding tendency	↓ dose of anticoagulant
Inhibit the absorption of vitamin K, reducing production of clotting factors	Tetracycline, penicillin, (most oral antibiotics)	↑ bleeding tendency	↓ dose of anticoagulant
Inhibit coagulation factors	Quinidine, quinine, salicylates, antimetabolites, alkylating agents	↑ bleeding tendency	↓ dose of anticoagulant
Inhibit platelet function	Salicylates, phenylbutazone, oxyphenbutazone, indomethacin, dipyridamole, sulfinpyrazone	↑ bleeding tendency	↓ dose of anticoagulant
Act as ulcerogenics	Corticosteroids, potassium products, salicylates, indomethacin, sulfinpyrazone	↑ bleeding tendency	↓ dose of anticoagulant
Unknown	Thyroid drugs, anabolic steroids, glucagon, danazol	↑ bleeding tendency	↓ dose of anticoagulant
Induce enzymes that metabolize anticoagulants	Barbiturates, griseofulvin, rifampin, phenytoin, glutethimide, carbamazepine	↓ anticoagulation effect	↑ dose of anticoagulant
Increase activity of coagulation factors	Oral contraceptives, estrogen, vitamin K	↓ anticoagulation effect	↑ dose of anticoagulant
Decrease absorption of anticoagulant	Colestipol, cholestyramine, antacids	↓ anticoagulation effect	↑ dose of anticoagulant

is detected, its dosage is adjusted downward or upward, depending on whether the drug interaction potentiates or antagonizes the effects of the anticoagulant.

Drug–drug interactions involving anticoagulant therapy are the most common of all those reported in the literature. Not *all* these reports have practical clinical relevance. However, medical personnel caring for patients taking anticoagulants should be aware of those prescription and *non*prescription drugs that are most likely to have significant effects on the patient's response to anticoagulant drug therapy. These are listed in Table 34-3, and are discussed with other drugs (as appropriate) throughout this text. Patients will require extensive teaching about the critical balance between their drugs and the clotting mechanism, and the importance of taking their drugs precisely as prescribed. They also need to be advised to avoid the use of over-the-counter (OTC) preparations and to check with their nurse or physician if any such remedies are needed.

Increased anticoagulant effect. Certain drugs, when given concurrently with oral anticoagulants, can increase the anticoagulant effect of the drug. Some drugs compete with the oral anticoagulant for plasma protein binding sites, releasing the anticoagulant to act in the liver (*e.g., salicylates, chloral hydrate*). Some drugs inhibit the liver metabolism of the anticoagulant, leading to increased levels of drug (*e.g., allopurinol, cimetidine*). Some drugs inhibit the absorption of vitamin K, further decreasing the production of clotting factors in the liver (*e.g., antibiotics*). Another group of drugs is known to increase the anticoagulant effect (*e.g., quinidine, thyroid drugs*), but the mechanism of these drug–drug interactions is not clearly understood.

If a patient is maintained on an oral anticoagulant and is started on one of the drugs known to increase the effect of the anticoagulant, the dose of the anticoagulant should be decreased accordingly to prevent excess bleeding. If, on the other hand, the patient has been stabilized on such a drug combination and the anticoagulant-enhancing drug is stopped, the dose of the oral anticoagulant will have to be increased to achieve the desired anticoagulant effect.

Increased bleeding tendency. Several drugs themselves act to interfere with clotting or to cause bleeding. When these drugs are taken concurrently with oral anticoagulants, they increase the risk of excessive bleeding. These drugs can act in several ways: by blocking coagulation factors (*e.g., salicylates, quinidine*); by inhibiting platelet aggregation (*e.g., sulfinpyrazone, salicylates*); or by producing bleeding gastrointestinal ulcers (*e.g., indomethacin, aspirin, corticosteroids*). Patients who are taking oral anticoagulants and any of these other drugs need to be carefully monitored for signs of bleeding, and clotting times should be determined frequently.

Decreased anticoagulant effect. Some drugs cause a decrease in the anticipated anticoagulant effect when given concurrently with oral anticoagulants. These drugs may induce the enzymes responsible for metabolism of the anticoagulant, thus decreasing the serum levels (*e.g., barbiturates, phenytoin*); they may increase the activity of procoagulation factors, making the dose less effective (*e.g., oral contraceptives, estrogen*); or they may decrease the absorption of the anticoagulant, resulting in lower than expected serum levels (*e.g., cholestyramine, colestipol*). These last two also bind vitamin K in the intestine and can cause bleeding in other patients; in patients on oral anticoagulants, the decreased drug absorption is of greater concern.

Patients receiving oral anticoagulants with any of these drugs will require an increased dose of the oral anticoagulant to achieve the desired therapeutic effect. If a patient has been maintained on a combination of these drugs, and one of the drugs is stopped, the patient will be at increased risk for excessive bleeding, and the dose of the oral anticoagulant will need to be decreased.

Because there are so many potential drug–drug interactions with the oral anticoagulants, whenever a drug is added to or withdrawn from the drug regimen of a patient receiving oral anticoagulants, the patient should be carefully monitored and evaluated for any change in blood coagulation.

Antiplatelet drugs

As noted earlier, platelets play an important part in setting off the series of reactions that cause a clot to form. Platelets in the blood that is passing over a damaged part of the inner lining of an arterial wall tend to adhere to the exposed smooth muscle and collagen fibers. The platelets that stick to the injured site of the vessel wall then release ADP, a substance that attracts still more platelets. The aggregating platelets form a white head, or core, from which a clotting factor is released that acts to form first thrombin and, finally, the fibrin threads that trap white and red blood cells. This type of clot, or platelet plug, stops vascular bleeding by sealing small breaks in the vessel wall. However, such so-called white clots can also be the basis of the thrombi that sometimes form in coronary, cerebral, and peripheral arteries.

Because of the danger of bleeding and of the other drawbacks of anticoagulant drug therapy for thromboembolic disorders, several drugs that interfere with platelet function have been used in efforts to prevent and treat various conditions of this type. All these agents were originally introduced for other therapeutic purposes, and their effects on platelet activity and the patient's bleeding time were first considered to be undesirable side-effects. Now, however, such drugs as *aspirin, ibuprofen, dipyridamole, dextrans,* and *sulfinpyrazone* are being employed experimentally to determine whether they can be administered in safe doses to prevent clot formation in patients who seem to be potential candidates for dangerous thromboembolic episodes.

These drugs appear to work by disrupting the balance between various factors that tend to cause platelet aggregation (thromboxane A$_2$, which is also a vasoconstrictor) and factors that naturally prevent platelet aggregation (prostacyclin; also called prostaglandin I$_2$). The latter substance is formed in endothelial cells (see Fig. 34-3).

Aspirin
A drawback of this widely used analgesic is its tendency to cause gastrointestinal bleeding in some users (see Chap. 37). One reason for aspirin-induced bleeding is the drug's ability to prevent platelets from aggregating, by irreversibly inhibiting the formation of thromboxane A$_2$ in platelets. It also blocks the release of ADP from platelet granules and thus stops the chain reaction that causes platelets to cohere and form the nucleus of a white arterial clot.

Because it can prevent formation of arterial thrombi, aspirin was employed experimentally to determine whether its daily use by patients considered at high risk for coronary or cerebral occlusion could prevent MI or stroke. The results of the studies have been inconclusive. The dosage used in the studies is now considered to be part of the problem. Low-dose aspirin appears to prevent platelet aggregation, as mentioned, while high-dose aspirin appears to inhibit the formation of both thromboxane A$_2$ and prostacyclin, negating any anticoagulant effect. Further studies are in progress to determine the dosage of aspirin that is actually the most therapeutic. Until conclusive results are obtained, many authorities recommend daily, low-dose aspirin for prophylactic purposes in high-risk patients.

Dipyridamole
This drug, introduced originally as a coronary vasodilator, has been administered alone and as an adjunct to oral anticoagulant drugs to prevent thromboembolic episodes. It possibly inhibits platelet aggregation by increasing the effects of prostacyclin. Dipyridamole (Persantine) has helped to protect patients with prosthetic heart valves from suffering strokes caused by platelet clots forming on these artificial valves, and breaking off and entering the cerebral circulation. The drug is also being investigated for use in preventing reinfarction and reducing the mortality rate after MI.

Sulfinpyrazone
This uricosuric agent (see Chap. 38) is claimed to be particularly effective for preventing TIAs when taken daily by patients prone to such episodes. It prevents thromboxane A$_2$ synthesis, thus leading to decreased platelet aggregation. Like the oral anticoagulants, this drug is said to reduce the frequency of such small strokes and the temporary loss of sensory or motor nerve function that follows. It is also claimed to have increased the ex-

pected survival rate when taken by patients who had previously suffered cerebral infarctions.

A widely acknowledged clinical trial appeared to have proved sulfinpyrazone (Anturane) to be able to reduce by about 50% the number of sudden deaths that occur in the first year after recovery from an initial acute MI. Patients in the placebo-treated group of a well-controlled cooperative study suffered sudden cardiac deaths at a rate of over 6%. Less than 3% of those in the patient group taking 200 mg of sulfinpyrazone qid died as a result of such reinfarctions during the same double-blind multicenter trial. Further results have not been as conclusive. Other studies have shown that the drug is effective in decreasing the mortality rate post-MI and in decreasing clot formation on prosthetic heart valves.

Ibuprofen
This drug is a nonsteroidal anti-inflammatory agent (see Chap. 38) that has been found to be a short-acting blocker of the synthesis of thromboxane A$_2$ in platelets, but does not also block synthesis of prostacyclin. Much research is being done on the effectiveness of ibuprofen (Motrin) for reducing the size of myocardial infarctions as well as for preventing post-MI complications.

Dextrans
The plasma volume expander *dextran 40* (see Chap. 54) is sometimes used to prevent deep vein thrombosis and pulmonary embolism. When used to prevent shock following major surgery, dextrans cause a prolongation of bleeding time and a tendency toward hemorrhage in patients with thrombocytopenia and hypofibrinogenemia. Studies of this adverse effect revealed that these drugs interfere with blood clotting in several ways when infused intravenously.

Dextrans have long been known to coat erythrocytes and thus to prevent red blood cells from forming rouleaux, or rows resembling stacks of coins. (The drugs are often used effectively for priming extracorporeal circulation devices, because this coating action protects blood cells.) This action, together with the reduction in blood viscosity brought about by these substances, accounts for their ability to prevent sludging of the blood and to improve its flow rate. Dextrans have been found to coat platelets also, thus interfering with their aggregation and with their function in setting off blood coagulation. In addition, dextrans inhibit blood clotting by forming complexes with fibrinogen (factor I) and with factors V, VII, and IX.

When used to prevent venous thrombosis and pulmonary embolism, dextran 40 is certainly less likely than the oral anticoagulants or heparin to cause hemorrhage; however, it is more likely to cause allergic reactions, including occasional anaphylactoid episodes. Thus, dextran 40 is approved for use in preventing thromboembolism only in patients undergoing surgical procedures with a high incidence of such complications. It appears to be especially beneficial for patients undergoing hip surgery.

Thrombolytic agents

The available anticoagulant drugs do not actually dissolve blood clots. Heparin and the oral anticoagulants only prevent new clots from forming, and they prevent already formed clots from enlarging and extending up and down the vessels. This gives the natural clot-resolving mechanism time to break up the clot gradually over a period of 1 week or more. If a thrombus is extensive, heparin alone may not give this relatively slow process enough help, and the large clot may be converted into a connective tissue mass that can do permanent damage to the vessel wall, or even obliterate the lumen completely. Thus, scientists sought and evaluated substances that appeared to be able to break down blood clots directly or to increase the rate of the natural clot-resolving process (Fig. 34-5*B*).

Two such activators of fibrinolytic activity have been introduced after undergoing cooperative clinical trials for several years. One of these thrombolytic agents is *streptokinase* (Streptase; Kabikinase), an enzyme obtained from β-hemolytic streptococci. Another enzyme, called *urokinase* (Abbokinase), because it was found first in human urine, is said to have certain advantages over streptokinase, especially a lack of antigenicity. The main disadvantage of both drugs is that they expose the patient to a greater risk of hemorrhage than does heparin. However, this risk is being reduced as physicians are learning how to use streptokinase and urokinase with proper precautions (see the summary of cautions and contraindications at the end of the chapter).

Current status

The benefits of thrombolytic therapy appear to outweigh the risks in only a limited number of clinical situations. Their primary indication at present is pulmonary embolism and, even in this very dangerous disorder, their use is reserved for only a minority of selected acute cases. These drugs are employed mainly in patients in whom lung vessel arteriography has confirmed the presence of massive obstructions in two or more lobar pulmonary arteries, particularly when this is accompanied by symptoms of circulatory instability. When thrombolytic drugs are promptly infused by vein in such cases, their use seems superior to heparin for bringing about rapid improvement. However, extensive studies have as yet failed to prove that these drugs actually decrease the number of deaths beyond what can be accomplished with heparin alone, and spontaneous bleeding is twice as likely to occur with these agents as when heparin is employed.

Streptokinase—but not, at present, urokinase—is also officially indicated for breaking up extensive blood clots in the deep veins of patients with acute thrombophlebitis. Its prophylactic use in such cases has not been proved to decrease the incidence of pulmonary embolism. However, its use seems to help avoid damage to the valves of veins deep in the extremities. This prevents development of chronic venous insufficiency and the postphlebitic syndrome, a condition that can leave patients with residual painful swelling of the limb and a tendency for stasis ulcers to form there. The use of streptokinase is considered to be particularly useful for younger patients with massive deep venous thrombosis extending above the knee.

Both of these thrombolytic substances are also approved for intracoronary infusion in patients with an evolving MI caused by coronary artery thrombosis, in whom a drug-induced breakup of the clot could, in theory, improve myocardial blood flow and limit the size of the infarction. Although intracoronary streptokinase has been shown to reopen obstructed coronary arteries, this therapy has not been shown conclusively to salvage myocardial tissue or reduce mortality. Results of studies with *intravenous* streptokinase in AMI patients are even less conclusive. The recent experimental use (by intracoronary infusion) of yet a third substance, a naturally-occurring *tissue plasminogen activator* (t-PA) that is produced in quantity by genetic engineering techniques, represents a potentially exciting development for the future treatment of patients with acute myocardial infarcts and strokes that are caused by arterial thrombi.

Other uses: These agents are also often used to clear arteriovenous (A-V) (streptokinase) and intravenous cannulas (urokinase) that have been occluded by clotted blood or fibrin. This helps to prevent surgical intervention in such cases, and to prevent the loss of IV lines in patients whose vascular status makes successful venipuncture difficult.

Drugs to control bleeding (hemostatic agents)

Drugs are not ordinarily an important means of dealing with bleeding. If someone's own clotting mechanism is functioning normally, the steps in the process are not accelerated by administering drugs or purified clotting factors. Mechanical measures such as gentle pressure or the use of ligatures or sutures are more helpful for hastening the clotting sequence and for halting the hemorrhage from a torn or cut vessel. However, there are two types of situations in which chemical substances from an outside source are employed to arrest bleeding:

1. Blood may continue to ooze persistently from tiny capillaries following surgery. In such a situation, locally active hemostatic substances may be applied to areas in which the tissues are too soft to be handled by mechanical means and the vessels are too small to be tied off or sewn.
2. Patients sometimes have a hereditary or an acquired defect in plasma protein

coagulation factors or in platelets. In such cases, the defective or deficient substance may be replaced or a *systemically active drug* may be administered to aid the failing hemostatic mechanism.

This section will describe first some of the substances applied topically to control capillary oozing. Then, some clinical conditions in which systemically active sub-

stances are employed to counteract abnormalities in coagulation factors, platelets, and blood vessels will be presented.

Locally active hemostatic agents

Two types of substances are applied topically to stem bleeding from small blood vessels in abraded and denuded tissue surfaces (Table 34-4). These are natural clotting factors, such as *thromboplastin, thrombin, fibrin,* and *fibrin-*

Table 34–4. Hemostatic agents

Generic or official name	Trade name	Usual adult dosage and administration	Comments
Systemically active agents			
Blood plasma clotting factors			
Antihemophilic factor, human	Hemofil; Factorate; Koate; Actif VIII	10 ml/min, IV	Highly concentrated; use small amount for hemophilia A
Factor IX complex, human	Konyne (factors II, VII, IX, and X); Profilnine; Proplex	20 ml (500 U)/wk, IV	Concentrated; used for treating hemophilia B
Anti-inhibitor coagulant complex	Autoplex; Feiba Immuno	10 ml/min, IV	Concentrated; used for hemophilia A
Prothrombogenic substances			
Menadiol sodium diphosphate USP (K_4)	Kappadione; Synkayvite	5–10 mg daily, orally or parenterally	Water-soluble form of vitamin K; does *not* need bile salts for absorption
Menadione USP (K_3)	Menadione	5–10 mg daily, orally	Insoluble vitamin K form; requires bile salts for absorption
Phytonadione USP*	AquaMEPHYTON; Konakion	1–25 mg orally, 10–50 mg IV, other parenteral routes	Vitamin K_1; fat-soluble form; more effective than water-soluble form
Antiheparin (heparin antidote)			
Protamine sulfate injection USP		50 mg IV; repeated as necessary after 10 min	1 mg neutralizes 90 U of heparin
Antifibrinolysin			
Aminocaproic acid USP	Amicar	5 gm orally or IV, followed by 1 g/hr; up to 30 g daily	Inhibits plasminogen activators and plasmin
Other			
Carbazochrome salicylate	Adrenosem salicylate	5 mg orally or IM; up to 10 mg/2 hr	Used to decrease capillary oozing postoperatively

Table 34–4. Hemostatic agents (continued)

Generic or official name	Trade name	Usual adult dosage and administration	Comments
Locally active hemostatics			
Absorbable gelatin sponge USP	Gelfoam	Topical	Can be left in place when wound is closed
Absorbable gelatin film	Gelfilm	Applied topically to brain, eye, and elsewhere	Absorbed in 1 wk to 6 mo
Microfibrillar collagen hemostat	Avitene	Applied dry to bleeding surface	Attracts platelets and causes them to adhere and aggregate
Oxidized regenerated cellulose	Novocell; Oxycel; Surgicel	Laid on bleeding sites in minimal amounts	Forms an artificial clot by a physical effect
Thrombin USP	Thrombinar Thrombostat	Used topically in solutions of various concentrations	Must *not* be injected

* **Warning:** Fatalities have occurred during and after intravenous administration of phytonadione.

ogen; and absorbable hemostatic substances that are not part of the natural clotting mechanism, such as *oxidized cellulose* and *absorbable gelatin sponge.*

Thrombin. This enzyme is used alone or in conjunction with fibrinogen or absorbable gelatin to control capillary bleeding during surgery. It is also used during skin grafting to help make wound edges adhere. In hemophilia it is often effective for stopping nosebleed, bleeding from a dental socket following tooth extraction, and hemorrhage from other accessible sites. Thrombin is not, of course, ever injected to stop bleeding from sites that cannot be reached by local application, because it could cause widespread intravascular clotting.

Thromboplastin has somewhat similar effects when applied locally during surgery. However, it finds its main clinical use in the prothrombin time test.

Oxidized regenerated cellulose. This is a form of specially treated surgical cotton (Surgicel) that reacts with blood to form an artificial clot. It can be packed into the abdominal cavity to control capillary bleeding following surgery on the liver, gallbladder, spleen, pancreas, or bowel. In such cases it is absorbed in a few days. On the other hand, it must not be implanted in fractures, because it interferes with bone regeneration and can cause cysts to form.

Absorbable gelatin. This may be employed in the form of sponges that are left in place when a surgical wound is closed. A film made of this material may be left in the brain following removal of a tumor or used to fill in defects of the dural membrane caused by a depressed skull fracture. A powdered form has sometimes been used

together with thrombin for control of massive bleeding within the gastrointestinal tract. A sterile form of the powder has also been employed in treating skin ulcers that are slow to heal.

These and similar substances seem to be free of adverse effects when applied topically to control capillary bleeding in the various surgical situations and medical conditions for which they are recommended.

Microfibrillar collagen hemostat. This is a topical absorbable hemostatic agent prepared by chemically treating the underlayer of the hides of cows or bulls to obtain purified collagen protein in the form of fine fibers. Applied dry to bleeding surfaces, the fluffy fibrils attract and trap platelets, which then aggregate to produce clotting within the fibrous mass. Pressure is briefly applied over the forming thrombus with a dry sponge for a brief period to stop capillary oozing and for a longer time (3 to 5 minutes) to control brisk bleeding. Excess fibers are teased away after bleeding ceases. Microfibrillar collagen hemostat (Avitene) is contraindicated for any patient allergic to bovine products.

Like other topical hemostatics, this substance is employed when ligatures alone cannot control bleeding and other ordinary procedures are impractical. The product is used during vascular surgery, in gynecologic procedures such as abdominal hysterectomy, and to control bleeding from such visceral organs as the spleen, stomach, liver, pancreas, and urinary bladder wall. It is claimed that, when packed firmly into cancellous bone to control oozing from its spongy surface, the fibers do not interfere with bone regeneration or healing or cause cysts to form, as is said to be the case with oxidized cellulose.

Systemically active hemostatic agents

Some people suffer repeated episodes of bleeding. Minor nosebleeds or bruise marks in the skin are most commonly caused by weakness of the capillary walls. Sometimes, however, serious bleeding may be caused by a lack of one of the blood factors required for normal clotting. Hemorrhagic disorders that develop during childhood are usually congenital—*hemophilia*, for example; other clotting factor deficiencies may occur in adults secondary to various medical disorders, or as a result of drug reactions—for example, drug-induced *thrombocytopenia*.

Transfusions of fresh whole blood or plasma help to replace the elements missing from the blood of patients with congenital or acquired bleeding disorders. Advances in separating specific clotting factors from blood have made it possible to administer only the substance that the patient lacks. Certain drugs can also be given that help to build up clotting proteins or to prevent their destruction.

This section will briefly discuss the treatment of a few important hemorrhagic disorders with specific blood components and drugs. The total management of patients suffering from these clinical conditions should be reviewed in an appropriate clinical management text.

Hypoprothrombinemia. Hereditary defects of prothrombin complex factors are very rare. However, if a person is deficient in vitamin K, a hemorrhagic disorder that is the result of a lack of the circulating factors that are synthesized in the liver by vitamin K-dependent reactions will develop. These factors include not only prothrombin (factor II), but also factors VII, IX, and X (Table 34-1 and Fig. 34-4). Hypoprothrombinemic bleeding usually responds readily to treatment with vitamin K preparations (Table 34-4).

Vitamin K. This substance is found so abundantly in foods, including the leaves of plants and vegetable oils, that any deficiency is rarely the result of a poor diet alone. It is also produced by bacteria in the intestinal tract that synthesize enough vitamin K to compensate for any dietary deficiency. Thus, a lack of this vitamin is usually the result of failure to absorb it because of an intestinal disorder or of failure to absorb it properly because of the presence of antagonists such as the coumarin and indandione drugs.

Two types of vitamin K preparations are available. *Phytonadione* (vitamin K_1) is the naturally occurring fat-soluble form. When given orally, it is absorbed only when bile is present. Thus, if administered by mouth to people with biliary obstruction or other disorders in which bile is lacking, it must be accompanied by bile salts. *Menadione* (vitamin K_3), a synthetically prepared substance, is also oil-soluble, but its water-soluble derivatives—the so-dium bisulfate and sodium diphosphate salts—do not require the presence of bile salts to be absorbed.

Therapeutic uses. The use of vitamin K as an antidote to overdosage with oral anticoagulants has already been discussed. The prompt response that occurs following administration of phytonadione has also been used to diagnose the cause of bleeding in those who have deliberately induced signs of hemorrhage by taking these drugs for *non*therapeutic reasons—that is, because of a behavioral disorder or with suicidal intent. Menadione derivatives should not be employed to counteract bleeding caused by anticoagulant drugs, because those forms of vitamin K are not nearly as effective as phytonadione for this purpose.

Newborn infants lack vitamin K for the first few days of life. The resulting hypoprothrombinemia may lead to bleeding from the intestine and other sites, including the brain. This hemorrhagic tendency may be increased in breastfed infants, because human milk contains less vitamin K than cows' milk. Infections requiring treatment with anti-infective drugs that interfere with the bacterial flora's being established in the intestinal tract may also precipitate such bleeding episodes. To avoid such hemorrhagic disease in the newborn, phytonadione injections are now sometimes administered routinely to all infants following delivery, or to the mother before the baby is born. Menadione is also effective, but its use in moderate doses has sometimes had toxic effects in premature infants and others.

Obstructive jaundice is often accompanied by bleeding, and hemorrhage may occur following surgery for biliary obstruction or fistula. Therefore, vitamin K should be given before biliary tract surgery, preferably by the parenteral route. Postoperatively, menadione may be administered orally, or phytonadione may be given by mouth together with bile salts until the natural flow of bile is re-established. If postoperative hemorrhage is severe, fresh blood or plasma may be administered to furnish the preformed procoagulant factors without waiting for their biosynthesis following vitamin K administration.

Malabsorption of vitamin K by patients with syndromes such as sprue and cystic fibrosis (mucoviscidosis) may lead to hypoprothrombinemic bleeding. Hemorrhage of this type may be prevented or corrected by bypassing the intestinal tract with parenterally administered vitamin K preparations. Injections of the vitamin are also employed for counteracting failure to absorb it following surgical removal of large parts of the intestine and in patients with ulcerative colitis and other inflammatory disorders of the intestinal tract. Patients receiving prolonged oral antimicrobial drug treatment, particularly while being fed intravenously, are also likely to develop hypoprothrombinemic bleeding unless vitamin K is added to their parenteral nutrition regimen.

Liver disease tends to interfere with the proper uptake of vitamin K. Because patients with hepatic cirrhosis or hepatitis, for example, may be unable to produce prothrombin complex factors despite adequate vitamin K dosage, these factors may have to be supplied already preformed in transfusions of fresh whole blood or plasma.

Hemophilia. This chronic hemorrhagic disorder results from a congenital lack of functional factor VIII, the antihemophilic factor (AHF). Children and others who have inherited an inability to produce a functioning form of this factor are subject to serious bleeding from even minor injuries. Bleeding into the joints (hemarthrosis) can cause severe pain and deformity. Hemorrhage into the central nervous system may produce disabling hematomas or death. Fatal exsanguination is possible following surgery or even dental extractions.

Treatment. Transfusion of plasma containing the missing factor is the main treatment for controlling hemorrhage. However, the amount of fresh or fresh-frozen plasma required to control bleeding following surgery or severe trauma is often so large that it tends to overload the patient's circulation. This can cause heart failure or cerebral edema. Today, however, there are also available concentrates of AHF that are effective when injected intravenously in much smaller quantities. Their use has reduced the risk of circulatory complications in hemophiliacs following surgical procedures.

One type of preparation now being employed is *cryoprecipitated* AHF, which is prepared by rapid freezing followed by thawing at hospital blood bank units. Also available commercially is *lyophilized* AHF, a dried preparation that can be reconstituted by gentle shaking with a suitable diluent. A typical commercial concentrate, *antihemophilic concentrate, human* (Hemofil) has about 60 times more factor VIII activity than blood plasma. It rarely causes the allergic reactions that may occur when animal blood concentrates are employed. However, as with all products prepared from human pooled plasma, there is a risk of hepatitis or of AIDS (acquired immune deficiency syndrome).

Anti-inhibitor coagulant complex (Autoplex; Feiba Immuno) is a new product available for the treatment of hemophilia. It is prepared from human plasma, and contains activated and precursor clotting factors in concentrated form.

These advances have greatly improved the prospect for patients with mild to moderately severe hemophilia, most of whom can now live a nearly normal life. Not only has their expected life span increased, but they are also spared once common chronic physical disabilities. Thus, it is more important than ever that hemophilic children and their parents receive counseling concerning how to cope with this hereditary disorder without suffering disabling emotional difficulties. Patients are, for example, advised concerning sports participation and

choice of vocation to guide them toward living as full a life as possible, consistent with their need to avoid hemorrhage-inducing injuries.

Christmas disease. This is a condition similar to hemophilia—it has been called hemophilia B—except that its cause is a functional deficiency of factor IX (Christmas factor; PTC). Thus, these patients do not respond to treatment with factor VIII concentrates. Fortunately, potent purified plasma concentrates of factor IX are also now available. One such product, *factor IX complex, human* (Konyne) contains factor IX together with the other vitamin K-dependent factors II, VII, and X. This concentrate stops bleeding by supplying the missing procoagulant factor without overloading the patient's circulation. However, it may sometimes be contaminated with hepatitis virus.

Hypofibrinogenemia and related disorders. A lack of the circulating plasma protein fibrinogen (factor I) can, of course, lead to bleeding because of failure to form the fibrin framework of clots. A deficiency of fibrinogen does not often occur as a result of a congenital inability to produce it, nor is failure of its biosynthesis by the diseased liver usually a significant factor in reducing the plasma level of fibrinogen. A fibrinogen deficiency severe enough to cause abnormal bleeding is most often the result of clinical conditions that cause it to be used up too rapidly. This seems to happen in such disorders because substances are released into the patient's blood that activate plasminogen, the precursor of plasmin. Excess production of this fibrinolytic enzyme then breaks down both fibrin and fibrinogen (see Fig. 34-5).

Fibrinolytic disorders. States of systemic hyperfibrinolysis may develop during the course of many medical, obstetric, and surgical situations. These include carcinomas of the prostate, stomach, lungs, and cervix; abruptio placentae (premature separation of the placenta) and amniotic fluid embolism; and surgical complications following heart surgery, nephrectomy, and prostatectomy. In all these conditions it is thought that tissue injury releases substances into the blood that set off the clotting mechanism and that this, in turn, precipitates a protective fibrinolytic reaction that goes too far in the opposite direction. The result of excessive fibrinolysis is a depletion of fibrinogen and other clotting factors that then leads to bleeding.

Aminocaproic acid (Amicar) has proved useful for treating bleeding that is definitely diagnosed as resulting from hyperfibrinolysis. This synthetic substance acts mainly by preventing plasminogen-activating kinases from stimulating production of plasmin, and it may also prevent any plasmin that *is* formed from acting to break down fibrin and destroy circulating fibrinogen. It has proven to be very successful in preventing recurrence of subarachnoid hemorrhage. This *antifibrinolytic agent* is also used to stop bleeding caused by overdoses of the thrombolytic agents streptokinase and urokinase. (Natural urinary urokinase probably is active in producing the severe hematuria sometimes seen after prostatectomy.) Aminocaproic acid must not be used to treat bleeding in conditions that are also marked by active clotting that is going on at the same time.

Disseminated intravascular clotting (DIC). This is a syndrome in which both bleeding and thrombosis may be found together. It can occur as a complication of many diseases, including severe infections that result in septic shock. In these disorders, local tissue damage releases procoagulant substances into the circulation that precipitate fibrin clot formation in small blood vessels of the brain, lungs, kidneys, and other organs. This continuing reaction often consumes excessive amounts of fibrinogen and other clotting factors as well as platelets, which can of course result in bleeding.

DIC treatment depends primarily on control of the disease state that induced it. Thus, for example, bleeding in septic shock may best be stopped by counteracting the shock state, and fibrinolytic bleeding following a miscarriage and retention of the dead fetus will subside after the products of conception have been evacuated. Transfusions of whole blood or infusions of the fibrinogen factor of human plasma may be employed to control severe hemorrhage. However, the use of blood and plasma factors sometimes results in serum hepatitis. In addition, administration of fibrinogen may set off further intravascular clotting in this complex condition. Paradoxically, the administration of the anticoagulant *heparin* to prevent the clotting phase also leads to control of hemorrhage in some cases by preventing the body from depleting its procoagulation factors.

Purpuric syndromes. Defects in platelet function and weakness of capillary walls are a common cause of hemorrhage in the skin, mucous membranes, and elsewhere. *Thrombocytopenia,* a reduction in the number of circulating platelets, is characterized by purpura, or hemorrhage into the skin. This may take the form of *petechiae,* pinpoint- to pinhead-sized bleeding spots, or *ecchymoses,* black and blue or purplish bruises caused by petechiae coming together to form larger masses of blood in the skin layers.

Thrombocytopenic purpura is not ordinarily responsive to drug therapy, and it is, in fact, commonly caused by sensitivity to certain drugs, including quinidine, sulfonamides, and thiazide diuretics. Most cases of drug-induced purpura clear up quickly after the drug is discontinued, and no other treatment is usually necessary. On the other hand, in other forms of purpura unrelated to drug exposure, patients do not readily make a complete recovery.

Corticosteroid drugs, administered in large doses, will often halt hemorrhaging in the autoimmune form of thrombocytic purpura. The steroids are thought to do so by strengthening the weakened capillary membranes and by bringing about an increase in circulating platelets. However, relapses are frequent following withdrawal of steroids to avoid toxicity. In such cases, splenectomy may be required for permanent remission. Episodes of severe hemorrhage are now best treated by transfusion of platelet concentrates rather than of whole blood.

Vascular fragility. Weak spots in capillary walls may allow blood to leak out into surrounding tissues. Various systemically active substances have been claimed useful for counteracting capillary oozing. However, their hemostatic activity has not been proved, and the best treatment for bleeding of this type is application of the local hemostatics previously discussed. Of course, in scurvy, a disease caused by chronic vitamin C deficiency, the administration of the vitamin (ascorbic acid) will counteract bleeding from the gums, nose, gastrointestinal and genitourinary tracts, and elsewhere. Ascorbic acid is ineffective for systemic hemostasis when bleeding is *not* caused by a vitamin C deficiency.

Similarly, although estrogen administration controls uterine bleeding that is the result of a deficiency of the female sex hormone, it has never been proved to be effective for control of capillary bleeding following tonsillectomy and the other surgical operations in which it has been employed as a systemic hemostatic. Other natural substances such as the bioflavonoids and various synthetic and semisynthetic chemicals that were formerly used as hemostatics and strengtheners of fragile capillary walls have been withdrawn from the market or are not now being promoted for this purpose.

Additional clinical considerations

The drugs that alter blood coagulation should never be used unless careful monitoring of blood coagulability can be done. The most significant problem with these drugs is hemorrhage; early detection of increased bleeding tendencies can prevent potentially dangerous blood loss.

Heparin should be avoided in patients who have certain conditions (*e.g.,* subacute bacterial endocarditis, SBE), or who are about to undergo procedures (*e.g.,* spinal tap, surgery, liver biopsies), that tend to cause blood loss. Heparin should never be given by IM injection because of the risk of bleeding into the muscle. The nurse who is responsible for heparin injections must take extra care to ensure that they are given SC and not inadvertently IM. Heparin is produced from animal sources, so patients need to be screened for allergies before heparin is given. Allergies to pork or beef products can result in allergic reactions to heparin from these sources. Heparin crosses the placenta and also crosses into breast milk. No studies have been done to determine the safety of the use of heparin during pregnancy and lactation, so the use of the drug at these times should be considered very carefully, and the benefits to the mother must outweigh the potential risk to the fetus or infant. Whenever a patient on a hospital unit is receiving heparin, it is the responsibility of the nursing staff to make sure that protamine sulfate is readily available on standby for emergency use.

The coumarin anticoagulants should never be given, in the hospital setting, until the patient's current PT test results are known. Some hospital medication sheets require that the PT results be recorded along with the daily dose of anticoagulant as a safety check to ensure that the PT is being monitored adequately. When an outpatient is maintained on an oral anticoagulant, the patient is responsible for having regular blood tests. It is sometimes recommended that such anticoagulants not be given to patients who will be unreliable in maintaining follow-up. Patients need to receive extensive teaching about the drug, and about the dietary, drug, and environmental factors that may alter their response to the anticoagulant. In addition, they should be taught about the side-effects of the drug and the signs that warn of toxicity, as well as about daily cautionary measures for their safety, and the problems they may encounter with injuries, dental work, or minor surgery. They need to incorporate all these considerations into their lives.

The coumarin anticoagulants should never be used during pregnancy. Some of the preparations contain tartrazine, and should be avoided in patients with tartrazine allergies. The coumarin anticoagulants have been shown to cause many side-effects, including alopecia, urticaria, dermatitis and skin rash, nausea and vomiting, anorexia, anemia, and a red orange, alkaline urine. Although these may not be harmful effects, they are often uncomfortable, and patients may need a great deal of reassurance.

Whenever a patient on a hospital unit is receiving an oral anticoagulant, phytonadione (vitamin K) should be readily available, on standby. In extreme cases, vitamin K can be administered as an IV preparation. This treatment will often bring the clotting factors into a normal range within a few hours instead of the many hours that may be needed with the oral preparation of vitamin K.

Certain precautions are also needed with the use of aminocaproic acid. This drug should never be given if there is a possibility that the patient has DIC, because fatal thrombus formation can occur. Aminocaproic acid should not be used in pregnant patients, or in patients with hepatic or renal disease or bovine allergies. The drug may cause infertility; any patients who are to be maintained on the drug should be aware of this possibility, and should be counseled appropriately. The drug can increase CPK (creatine phosphokinase) levels, and patients receiving this drug should have their CPK levels evaluated with this drug effect in mind.

The patient teaching guide presents a summary of the points that should be included when teaching a patient about the use of oral anticoagulants. Patient teaching may be one of the most important aspects of nursing care of these patients.

The guide to the nursing process summarizes the clinical aspects of the nursing care of a patient receiving anticoagulant drug therapy.

Patient teaching guide: oral anticoagulants

The drug that has been prescribed for you is called an anticoagulant. It works to slow the normal blood clotting processes in the body. In this way it can prevent harmful blood clots from forming. This type of drug is often called a "blood thinner." It cannot dissolve any blood clots that may have already formed. Your anticoagulant has been prescribed because _____ .

Instructions:

1. The name of your anticoagulant is _____ .

2. The dose of the drug prescribed for you is _____ . The dosage of the drug may have to be changed on occasion. Fever, change of diet, change of environment, or several other factors may change your need for the drug. It is important to write down any change of dose that is prescribed.

(continued)

3. Your drug should be taken once a day. The best time to take your drug is
   _____ .

4. *Never* change any medication you are taking—adding or stopping another drug—without consulting your nurse or physician. Many other drugs affect the way that your anticoagulant works; starting or stopping another drug can cause excessive bleeding or interfere with the desired effects of the drug.

5. Tell any physician, nurse, or dentist who is taking care of you that you are on this drug. You should carry or wear a medical alert tag, stating that you are on this drug. This will alert any medical personnel who might take care of you in an emergency that you are on this drug.

6. It is important to avoid situations in which you could be easily injured— for example, contact sports, shaving with a straight razor.

7. Some side-effects of this drug that you should be aware of include the following:

Stomach bloating, cramps	This often passes with time; if it becomes too uncomfortable, notify your nurse or physician.
Loss of hair, skin rash	This can be very frustrating and, if it becomes too uncomfortable, notify your nurse or physician.
Orange red discoloration of urine	This frequently occurs; if you fear it may be blood, simply add vinegar to the urine and the color should disappear, unless the color is caused by blood in the urine.

8. Avoid the use of any OTC preparations while you are on this drug. If you feel that you have a need for one of these preparations, consult with your nurse or physician.

9. You will need to have periodic blood tests to check on the action of the drug. It is very important to keep your appointments for these tests.

10. Keep this and all medications out of the reach of children.

Notify your nurse or physician if any of the following occur:

Unusual bleeding—such as when
    brushing your teeth, excessive
    bleeding from injuries, excessive
    bruising
Black or bloody stools
Cloudy or dark urine
Sore throat, fever, chills
Severe headaches, dizziness

Guide to the nursing process: anticoagulants*

Assessment	Nursing diagnoses	Interventions	Evaluation
Past history (*contraindications*): SBE	Potential for injury Knowledge deficit regarding drug therapy	Proper preparation and administration of drug Patient teaching	Monitor effectiveness of drug: PT time†
Hemorrhagic disorders	Potential alteration in	regarding:	PTT time‡
Tuberculosis	tissue perfusion	Drug	Monitor for adverse
Hepatic disease	secondary to loss of	Dosage	effects of drugs:
Gastric ulcers	blood	Cautions	• Excess bleeding
Renal disease		Warnings	• Loss of hair
Indwelling catheters		Blood tests	• Rash
Pregnancy†		Provide support and	• GI upset
Lactation†		encouragement to	• Guaiac stools
Diabetes		comply with drug	• Urinalysis
CNS trauma or surgery‡		cautions, frequent follow-up	• Bruising
Allergies: bovine products; tartrazine†; others		Provision of emergency measures as needed: Protamine sulfate on standby‡	Monitor for drug–drug, drug–diet interactions: change in effectiveness correlated with any change in drugs, diet,
Medication history: any drugs being taken—dosage		Vitamin K available† Provision of comfort and safety measures: No IM injections	environment Evaluate effectiveness of patient teaching: compliance with
		Avoidance of injury‡ Use of heparin lock	therapy Evaluate effectiveness of
Physical assessment		needle to avoid repeated injections‡	support and encouragement offered
Neurologic: orientation, reflexes			Evaluate effectiveness of comfort and safety
Cardiovascular: P, BP, peripheral perfusion baseline ECG			measures Evaluate effectiveness of emergency measures, as appropriate
Respiratory: R, adventitious sounds			
GI: liver function, quaiac stool			
Renal: urinalysis			
Skin: lesions, bruises			
Laboratory tests: Prothrombin time (PT)† Partial thromboplastin time (PTT)‡			

* The general principles of anticoagulant therapy are the same; points specific to heparin and oral anticoagulants are indicated. All other points refer to the use of both oral anticoagulants and of heparin.
† Specific to oral anticoagulants.
‡ Specific to heparin.

Summary of clinical indications for anticoagulants

Heparin only

Disseminated intravascular coagulation (DIC)

Arterial and heart surgery

Prevention of coagulation in blood transfusions, dialysis, extracorporeal circulation, laboratory blood samples

Heparin and hypoprothrombinemic agents

Treatment and prevention of venous thrombosis

Treatment and prevention of pulmonary embolus in patients at risk

Acute myocardial infarction: prevention of thromboembolic complications; prevention of recurrence (controversial)

Cardiac valvular disease and prosthetic cardiac valves: prevention of emboli

Cerebral thrombosis and embolism: transient ischemic attacks; evolving strokes (controversial)

Postoperatively: prevention of emboli and thrombosis in certain high-risk patients

Warfarin only

Adjunctive therapy for small cell lung carcinoma

Summary of cautions and contraindications: thrombolytic drug therapy*

Because there is a high risk of hematoma formation, avoid administering other drugs by IM injection during thrombolytic drug therapy.

Heparin and oral anticoagulants should not be employed concurrently with thrombolytic therapy. However, to prevent rethrombosis following termination of the thrombolytic agent infusion, heparin should begin to be infused after the thrombin time has decreased to a relatively safe level (less than twice the normal control value). Oral anticoagulants are also used as adjuncts at this point.

Because of possible hemorrhagic drug interactions, avoid the concurrent use of aspirin, indomethacin, phenylbutazone, or other drugs known to alter platelet function.

Patients should be closely observed for signs and symptoms of allergic reactions, particularly when their history indicates a predisposition to allergy. (Streptokinase, in particular, may be contraindicated in patients considered to be at high risk.) Discontinue immediately if severe reactions develop, and be prepared to treat with IV corticosteroids and antihistamines.

Thrombolytic therapy is usually avoided in patients in whom the risk of bleeding is considered unusually high or in whom the development of bleeding might be difficult to manage. The following are examples of such clinical situations:

1. Surgery, including liver or kidney biopsies and intra-arterial diagnostic procedures performed within the past 10 days (also frequent or extensive cutdowns, lumbar punctures, thoracentesis or paracentesis).
2. The presence of ulcerative wounds; ulcerative colitis, diverticulitis, bleeding lesions of the GI or genitourinary tracts; visceral or intracranial malignancies; chronic lung diseases with cavitation—for example, tuberculosis.
3. Possible presence of internal injuries as a result of recent injuries; pregnancy and the first 10 days of the postpartum period; recent cerebral embolism, thrombosis, or hemorrhage, or the presence of atrial fibrillation or other conditions in which there is a predisposition to cerebral embolism.
4. The presence of severe hypertension, subacute bacterial endocarditis, rheumatic valvular disease, renal insufficiency, acute or chronic liver disease, or uncontrolled hypocoagulable states caused by deficiency of a coagulation factor, thrombocytopenia, fibrinolysis, and other purpuric or hemorrhagic disorders.

* These conditions are relative rather than absolute contraindications. That is, thrombolytic agents may be employed when their benefits in a particular case appear to outweigh the risk of hemorrhage.

Case study

Presentation

GR is a 68-year-old white woman with severe mitral valvular disease. She has managed well with digitalis, a diuretic, and a potassium supplement for several years. On a recent clinic visit it was discovered that she had been experiencing periods of breathlessness, "palpitations," and dizziness. Tests revealed that GR was having frequent periods of atrial fibrillation, with a heart rate of up to 140. Because of the danger of emboli as a result of her valvular disease and the atrial fibrillation, GR was started on warfarin sodium (Coumadin).

How should this situation be evaluated, and what nursing care is required for this patient?

Discussion

GR's situation is complex. She has several chronic problems that could be contributing to her current situation. On her clinic visit a thorough patient assessment should be done, including a careful history to evaluate any change in medication or diet or any stress that might have altered the course of her disease. A complete physical examination should be done to evaluate the status of her valvular disease and congestive heart failure. Laboratory tests should include BUN, CBC, and determination of serum digitalis and potassium levels as potential causes of the atrial arrhythmias. If the patient's digitalis level is within normal limits, and her disease and drug therapy are being managed appropriately, the episodic atrial fibrillation may probably be a result of progressive mitral valve disease. In this case, an anticoagulant will be important to prevent emboli from forming as a result of the chronic atrial fibrillation. GR will need to receive extensive patient teaching about the drug therapy and about all the diet, environmental, and drug precautions that go with it. This is a good opportunity to review the patient teaching about valvular disease, congestive heart failure, and the drug therapy that GR is currently on. The patient will need to be cautioned about maintaining her drug regimen as prescribed with no alterations. She will need to be reminded not to take any OTC drugs without consulting her nurse or physician. GR should get a medical alert identification tag to alert any health-care professionals to her problems and therapy. The patient should be told that it is very important for her to return frequently for blood tests to evaluate her response to drug therapy. GR will also need support and encouragement to cope with this new drug and all its implications. A patient taking so many drugs and having such a chronic disease may have difficulty accepting one more drug, especially one with so many complications and precautions. Giving her a phone number to call if questions arise, as well as calling her to remind her when blood tests should be done, might help the patient to adapt better to the new demands. A patient, listening attitude can also go far in facilitating safe and effective anticoagulant therapy on an outpatient basis.

Drug digests

Dicumarol USP (Bishydroxycoumarin)

Actions and indications. This is the prototype of the oral anticoagulant drugs that act by interfering with the synthesis in the liver of the prothrombin complex plasma protein clotting factors. It causes a fall in these factors to therapeutic levels (20% to 30% of control levels) over a period of a few days. Thus, in treating acute conditions such as pulmonary embolism, it is administered together with heparin, which has a more immediate onset of action. Other conditions in which this drug may be administered immediately and then continued for several weeks or months after heparin is withdrawn include acute thrombophlebitis and phlebothrombosis, acute myocardial infarction,

and patients with atrial fibrillation both prior to and after attempts to convert to a sinus rhythm. Patients considered to have a high risk of developing thromboembolic episodes may be maintained on this drug for several years. In such cases, the relatively long duration of anticoagulant activity of this drug is said to aid in keeping the clotting factors in a stable state.

Adverse effects, cautions, and contraindications. Hemorrhage from overdosage is the main hazard; thus, dosage must be closely controlled in accordance with the results of periodic PT determinations. The drug should be discontinued at the earliest sign of bleeding, because its effects are cumulative

and relatively long in duration. Treatment is avoided in patients who tend to bleed readily because of concurrent disorders such as thrombocytic purpura, gastrointestinal tract ulcerative inflammatory and carcinomatous disorders, and subacute bacterial endocarditis. Its use is undesirable in patients with open wounds or in those who have had recent operations on the brain, spinal cord, and eye. It is contraindicated when spinal, regional, or lumbar block anesthesia is employed, when abortion threatens, and in hemorrhagic stroke.

Dosage and administration. Dosage is usually begun with 200 mg to 300 mg on the first day. However, because of variability in response, the subsequent doses required to reduce prothrombin to 25% of normal may range from 25 mg to 200 mg. During the initial adjustment period, daily blood tests may be done, and the drug is then administered only when prothrombin activity has risen above 25%. Following stabilization, PT determinations are made at moderate intervals.

Heparin sodium injection USP (Panheprin)

Actions and indications. This anticoagulant combines with a plasma protein to form a complex that acts immediately to interfere with blood clotting reactions. Thus, it is preferred for early prophylactic and therapeutic use in acute thromboembolic emergencies. There are a number of clinical situations in which it is valuable: for prevention of pulmonary embolism in patients with venous thrombosis and in the treatment of these conditions; as an adjunct to other measures following MI from coronary artery occlusion; in patients with a still evolving stroke to prevent cerebral thrombosis, to treat peripheral arterial embolism and prevent recurrences; in surgery of the arteries or of the heart; and in patients with atrial fibrillation who tend to produce emboli. In all these situations, heparin is employed to prevent clots from forming, or—if already formed—from extending. It *cannot* be expected to break up thrombi and emboli that already exist.

Adverse effects, cautions, and contraindi- cations. Hemorrhage is the main risk that must be avoided by proper selection of patients and by individualizing dosage in accordance with the patient's response. The drug should not be administered if facilities are not available for making frequent tests of the coagulation time of venous blood. Protamine sulfate should always be on standby when a patient receives heparin. It is also contraindicated in patients with thrombocytopenia and other blood dyscrasias or disorders that cause bleeding tendencies, including threatened abortion, gastrointestinal ulcers or GI tube drainage, and subacute bacterial endocarditis. Heparin should not be employed following ocular or neurologic surgery, and it is used only with caution late in pregnancy and early in the postpartum period.

Caution is required also in patients with a history of allergy, because hypersensitivity-type reactions sometimes occur. Urticaria (hives), chills, and fever are the most common signs, but bronchospasm, rhinitis, and even anaphylactoid reactions have been reported.

Dosage and administration. Heparin is best controlled when administered by IV drip of a diluted solution that is adjusted to deliver 20,000 to 40,000 U daily. It may also be given intermittently IV every 4 to 6 hours in doses of 5,000 U to 10,000 U.

A concentrated suspension containing 10,000 U to 12,000 U may be injected SC into fatty layers of the deep subcutaneous tissues of the lower abdomen, thighs, or hip area every 8 hours. It may also be administered IM in tissues of the thigh, buttocks, or arm. However, hematoma and tissue irritation are most common when this route is employed.

Clotting time is determined prior to each injection, or about every 4 hours when continuous IV infusions are employed. The therapeutic range is at about 2½ times the usual control value of 5 to 10 minutes.

Warfarin sodium USP (Coumadin; Panwarfin)

Actions and indications. This coumarin-type anticoagulant interferes with the synthesis of several clotting factors in the liver. Its therapeutic effects become evident in 24 to 36 hours and last from about 2 days to as long as 4 or 5 days after the drug is discontinued. It is indicated mainly for preventing the formation of venous clots, or their extension, in patients with thrombophlebitis or other conditions that could lead to development of pulmonary embolism and similar severe thromboembolic disorders. It is employed together with heparin for treating pulmonary embolism and for atrial fibrillation with embolization. It may also be used as an adjunct in managing acute MI following coronary occlusion and for treating transient attacks of cerebral ischemia.

Adverse effects, cautions, and contraindi- cations. Side-effects other than occasional allergic reactions are not common nor serious. However, hemorrhage is a constant threat that requires care in selection of patients for treatment and in the close control of dosage to avoid potentially serious episodes of spontaneous bleeding.

The use of this and other oral hypoprothrombinemic agents is contraindicated in patients with bleeding tendencies, including those with blood dyscrasias, gastrointestinal tract ulcerations, threatened abortion, and subacute bacterial endocarditis. It is not used in patients with cerebral aneurysms or hemorrhage or a history of recent neurosurgery. Severe hypertension and liver or kidney disease are other contraindications.

Caution is required in patients who may not follow instructions for taking this drug. Care is also required in elderly or disease-weakened patients and in those in a poor state of nutrition. Attention must be paid to what other medications the patient may be taking, because this agent may interact with other drugs in ways that alter the expected response to the dose level on which the patient is being stabilized.

Dosage and administration. Dosage is highly individualized, and must be adjusted in accordance with the results of PT determinations. A single oral or parenteral dose of 40 mg to 60 mg will produce a reduction of prothrombin activity to the 20% to 30% of normal that is considered to be in the safe therapeutic range. The initial dose for elderly or debilitated patients is 20 mg to 30 mg. Maintenance dosage for most patients ranges between 2 and 10 mg daily.

References

Anderson JL et al: A randomized trial of intracoronary streptokinase in treatment of acute myocardial infarction. N Engl J Med 308:1312, 1983

Anturane Reinfarction Trial Group: Sulfinpyrazone in the prevention of cardiac death after myocardial infarction. N Engl J Med 298:289, 1978

Breckenridge AM: Individual differences in the response to anticoagulants. Drugs 14:367, 1977

Chalmers TC et al: Evidence favoring the use of anticoagulants in the hospital phase of acute myocardial infarction. N Engl J Med 297:1091, 1977

Conley CL: Hemostasis. In Mountcastle VB (ed): Medical Physiology, 14th ed, pp 1137–1146. St. Louis, CV Mosby, 1980

Didisheim P et al: Actions and clinical status of platelet-suppressive agents. Semin Hematol 15:35, 1978

Editorial: Streptokinase. Br Med J 1:927, 1977

Frishman WH: Antiplatelet therapy in coronary heart disease. Hosp Pract 17:73, 1982

Green D, Smith NJ: Hemophilia. Current concepts in management. Med Clin North Am 56:105, 1972

Lewis HD, Jr et al: Protective effects of aspirin against

acute myocardial infarction and death in men with unstable angina: Results of a Veterans' Administration Study. N Engl J Med 309:396, 1983

Moncada S, Vane JR: Pharmacology and endogenous roles of prostaglandin endoperoxides, thromboxane A_2 and prostacyclin. Pharmacol Rev 30:293, 1979

O'Reilly RA: Therapy with anticoagulant drugs. Ration Drug Ther 8:1, 1974

O'Reilly RA: Anticoagulant, antithrombotic, thrombolytic drugs. In Gilman AG, Goodman LS, Gilman A (eds): Goodman and Gilman's The Pharmacological Basis of Therapeutics, 6th ed, pp 1347–1366. New York, Macmillan, 1980

Pitt B et al: Prostaglandins and prostaglandin inhibitors in ischemic heart disease. Ann Intern Med 99:83, 1983

Prescott S: The clinical role of antiplatelet drugs. Drug Ther 13:71, 1983

Ratnoff OD: Hemostasis and blood coagulation. In Berne RM, Levy MN (eds): Physiology, pp 411–436. St. Louis, CV Mosby, 1983

Rodman MJ: Thromboembolic disorders, part 1: Venous thrombosis. RN 39:79, 1976

Rodman MJ: Thromboembolic disorders, part 2: Arterial thrombosis and embolism. RN 39:61, 1976

Salem HH: Current status of anticoagulants. Drug Ther 13:57, 1983

Shafer K: Thrombolytic therapy: Current and potential uses. Drug Ther 13:95, 1983

Streptokinase for acute coronary artery thrombosis. Med Lett Drugs Ther 25:33, 1983

Swan HJC: Editorial: Thrombolysis in acute evolving myocardial infarction: A new potential for myocardial salvage. N Engl J Med 309:238, 1983

Walsh PN: Oral anticoagulant therapy. Hosp Pract 18:101, 1982

Wessler S: Prevention and treatment of thrombosis. Adv Intern Med 22:187, 1977

Wessler S: The anticoagulant dilemma—a prescription for its resolution. Am J Med Sci 274:106, 1977

Weykei D: Current status of anticoagulant therapy. Am J Med 72:659, 1982

Chapter 35

Drugs
for treating
deficiency
anemias

The blood

The previous chapters of this section have dealt mainly with drugs that improve the functioning of the circulatory system. Yet, the heart, arteries, veins, and capillaries are important only because of the vital fluid that they handle—*the blood*—because it is this life-giving liquid that brings to the brain and all other organs and tissues the oxygen and nutrients without which they could not survive. Blood is also essential, not only for nutrition and cellular respiration, but also for defending the body against infection.

Composition

There are two main components of this vital liquid tissue:

1. The *plasma,* a light yellow liquid containing proteins that play significant roles in protecting against infections and in fluid balance regulation
2. The *formed elements* of the blood—red blood cells, white blood cells, and platelets that are suspended in the plasma; the platelets, or thrombocytes, help to set off the series of reactions that results in formation of clots for plugging breaks in blood vessels (Chap. 34); the white cells, or leukocytes, make up one of the body's major defense mechanisms against invading microorganisms

This chapter is concerned mainly with the red cells, or erythrocytes, that transport oxygen from the lungs to all the tissues of the body. It will describe some substances that are administered when red blood cells are reduced below normal in number and when they become abnormal in their shape and size—disorders called *deficiency anemias,* or *nutritional anemias.* Other types of anemias, including *aplastic anemia,* which occurs as a result of bone marrow damage, and *hemolytic anemia,* which occurs as a result of circulating red cell destruction, are discussed in Chapter 5 and are mentioned among the toxic effects of the various drugs that can induce these blood disorders (see Index).

Erythrocyte production (*erythropoiesis*)

The myeloid tissue of the bone marrow, under the influence of the hormone erythropoietin, manufactures enormous numbers of red blood cells to make up for the millions destroyed every day (Fig. 35-1). By using the chemical elements released from the disintegrated red cells along with added substances supplied in the diet, the marrow factory builds new erythrocytes at a rate that keeps the blood count at a normal level. A normal erythrocyte has a life span of approximately 120 days. Senescent red blood cells are destroyed by hemolysis in liver, spleen, and bone marrow. The complicated processes of biosynthesis and maturation are aimed at building up the blood pigment *hemoglobin* and the *stroma,* the supporting structure that contains the hemoglobin molecules.

To make hemoglobin, the bone marrow requires dietary amino acids and other nutrients including vitamins and metals, of which the most important is *iron.* To form a stromal structure strong enough to resist too early destruction, the marrow requires minute amounts of the blood-building B-complex *vitamins* B_{12} (cyanocobalamin) and *folic acid.* Ordinarily, adequate amounts of all these essential substances are present in the diet and can be absorbed from the gastrointestinal tract. These elements are then used in the various steps of hemoglobin biosynthesis and for the several stages through which red cells are brought to maturity in the marrow before being released into the bloodstream.

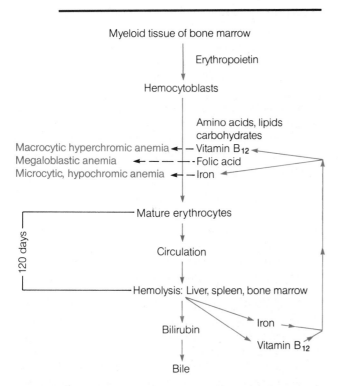

Myeloid tissue of bone marrow

Erythropoietin

Hemocytoblasts

Amino acids, lipids
carbohydrates

Macrocytic hyperchromic anemia ← — Vitamin B₁₂ ←
Megaloblastic anemia ← — — Folic acid
Microcytic, hypochromic anemia ← — Iron ←

Mature erythrocytes

120 days

Circulation

Hemolysis: Liver, spleen, bone marrow

Bilirubin   Iron

Vitamin B₁₂

Bile

Figure 35-1. Erythropoiesis. Red blood cells are produced in the myeloid tissue of the bone marrow in response to the hormone erythropoietin. The hemocytoblasts require various essential factors to produce mature erythrocytes. A lack of any one of these can result in an anemia of the type indicated opposite each factor. Mature erythrocytes survive for about 120 days, and are then lysed in the liver, spleen, or bone marrow.

The anemias

In some circumstances, the diet may not supply enough of a nutrient to meet a person's needs, or a substance present in adequate dietary quantities may not be absorbed in large enough amounts. Sometimes, abnormal losses of a nutrient may raise a person's requirements above what can be supplied by diet alone. In all such cases, continued deficiency of the nutrients needed for synthesis of hemoglobin and manufacture of healthy red blood cells results in an anemia of the *nutritional* or *deficiency* type.

People who take in less dietary iron than they lose each day suffer a gradual depletion of their total body stores of iron. Eventually, they form fewer red cells, and these erythrocytes are smaller and paler than normal and contain less hemoglobin. Patients with this type of *hypochromic microcytic anemia* may complain of feeling tired and weak and of having little appetite. Their relative lack of tissue oxygen may lead to headaches, dizziness, and even dyspnea (difficulty in breathing) after only mild exertion.

Other people may suffer the same types of vague nonspecific symptoms, but their blood and bone marrow

look quite different when examined under the microscope. The bone marrow of these patients is filled with large immature red cells, called *megaloblasts*. The circulating blood also contains an unusual number of these red cell precursors together with the abnormally large erythrocytes that they form, called *macrocytes*. Anemias of this type are called macrocytic, or megaloblastic or, because each of the reduced number of red cells is crammed with the red respiratory pigment hemoglobin, they are also sometimes called *hyperchromic macrocytic*. These abnormal red cells that have a relatively short life span are produced as a result of a deficiency of the B-complex vitamins cyanocobalamin (vitamin B₁₂) or folic acid.

These two types of anemia almost never occur together. Thus, each type needs to be treated by supplying only the specific blood cell-producing substance that is missing. Once the anemia is correctly diagnosed it can be quickly corrected by administering adequate doses of iron, *or* vitamin B₁₂, *or* folic acid in forms that can be absorbed and used in blood cell production.

It is not enough, however, to bring the patient's blood picture back to normal. It is also essential to determine the underlying cause in each case. Thus, for example, administering iron to a patient with internal bleeding may build up the hemoglobin levels while an undetected visceral malignancy goes undetected and continues to progress. Similarly, taking folic acid can correct the blood abnormality of a patient with undiagnosed pernicious anemia without improving the spinal cord lesions which are part of this disease, and this vitamin may, in fact, increase the severity of the neurologic symptoms.

Iron deficiency anemia

Iron metabolism. All body cells, not only red blood cells, require iron, but too much iron can cause cytotoxicity. Thus, the body has developed a system for keeping very close control over its total content of this metal. Iron balance is regulated mainly by an intestinal mechanism that limits the amount of iron that can be absorbed. Only enough iron to make up for the amount lost each day is allowed to pass through the intestinal mucosa.

Iron that enters the bloodstream is picked up by a plasma protein, called *transferrin* because it transports the metal to sites such as the liver, bone marrow, spleen, and other reticuloendothelial cells, where it is stored as ferritin and hemosiderin. Plasma transferrin also carries the iron from the spleen, where aged red cells are destroyed, back to the bone marrow for recycling into the hemoglobin of new erythrocytes. Ordinarily, most of the iron lost to the body is that which is contained in epithelial cells sloughed off from such body surfaces as the skin and the intestinal and urinary tract linings. This, and the small amount that is lost in sweat and other body secretions, amounts to about only 1 mg or less of iron daily.

Because of its ability to conserve its stores of iron, the body ordinarily needs to take in very little of the element to meet the demands of the bone marrow and all other cells. Because the same stores are used over and over again, only the 1 mg or less lost daily by excretion has to be made up from dietary sources. Although only a small percentage of the iron contained in even the best diet is absorbed, this is usually enough to keep most people in positive iron balance indefinitely. However, menstruating women may, in a few days, lose an amount of iron that is at least equal to that excreted by all other routes during the rest of the month. When this happens, the intestinal mucosal barrier is lowered, and allows from 2 mg to 4 mg of dietary iron to be absorbed daily to make up for the excessive loss.

Iron deficiency. Loss of blood from some internal source of bleeding is also a common cause of iron deficiency anemia among other adults, particularly men and postmenopausal women. However, those with abnormally increased iron requirements at various stages of life may also go into gradual negative iron balance. Although an inadequate diet is rarely a cause of iron deficiency in this country, some people may become anemic because of their inability to absorb enough of the metal—that is, because of gastrointestinal tract disease or some other pathologic malabsorption problem.

Indications for iron supplements

The question of which people require more iron than is available in the food they eat is a complex and controversial one. Although iron deficiency anemia is very common, most patients with abnormally low levels of hemoglobin have no significant symptoms. Some authorities even suggest that the prompt beneficial response that some people claim to feel soon after they start taking iron is simply a placebo effect. Nevertheless, most experts agree that there are some situations in which iron balance is so likely to be precarious that the supplemental administration of medicinal iron may be well warranted.

Pediatric patients. Infants between the ages of about 6 months and 2 years are particularly prone to developing iron deficiency. For the first few months of life, newborn babies can draw on the iron that they have accumulated from their mothers' stores while in the uterus. However, because they triple their birth weight and blood volume during the first year of life, infants cannot meet their bodies' demands for iron for very long. Full-term babies often develop symptoms of iron deficiency at about 6 months, and premature infants show signs of deficiency in about half that time. Because milk is a poor source of iron and the ability to absorb the iron from fortified baby cereal is quite variable, infants often develop iron deficiency anemia. When diagnostic tests indicate the presence of iron deficiency, such very young children should receive pediatric iron drops or even par-

enterally administered iron. Many pediatric vitamin preparations contain iron.

Pregnancy. Pregnant women cannot expect to meet their extra iron needs by dietary means alone. The growing fetus takes iron from the mother's stores, particularly during the last half of pregnancy. In addition, the mother herself needs more iron because her red blood cell volume increases by about one-third at the same time. Finally, of course, there is a further loss of iron during bleeding at the time of delivery. Thus, a woman who has had several pregnancies within a relatively few years may have markedly depleted her iron stores.

In such cases of definitely diagnosed depletion, the routine prophylactic use of iron seems justified. On the other hand, some authorities have questioned the practice of prescribing an iron preparation for *all* pregnant women. They claim that there is no evidence that the developing fetus fails to get all the iron it needs or that a woman with a relatively low hemoglobin level—for example, 10 g/100 ml compared to a normal 15 g/100 ml or so—suffers any significantly disabling symptoms. She may, in fact, be more discomforted by the adverse effects of iron salts than from her iron deficiency anemia. In any case, whether iron is administered only to selected pregnant patients or to all, some authorities suggest that it should be ordered only during the second and third trimesters, because this metal—like other drugs—could cause congenital malformations if taken during the embryonic and early fetal developmental stages of the first trimester.

Adolescence. The need for iron may double during the years of rapid growth that begin with puberty in both girls and boys. The chances of developing iron deficiency are greater in girls because of the monthly blood loss after they begin menstruating. Adolescent girls and other premenopausal women tend to lose between 14 mg and 28 mg of iron in the blood shed during even a normal menstrual period. This means that their added daily iron loss is about equal to the amount normally excreted by the usual routes—that is, 0.5 mg to 1 mg. Often, the extra iron is readily absorbed and assimilated from foods such as meats and dairy products eaten as part of a diet that also contains cereal grains, green, and yellow vegetables, and citrus fruits or tomatoes.

However, if (as is often true with teen-age girls) they neglect to eat an adequate diet, young women may readily suffer an iron deficiency. Obviously, if a girl had barely been in positive iron balance on a diet that supplied the 0.5 mg to 1 mg she needed as a prepubescent child, she will lose that precarious equilibrium when she both begins to menstruate regularly and enters a time of rapid growth and development. Even if she eats well and increases her food iron intake, she may not get quite enough dietary iron to meet her new needs. For this reason, some authorities have seriously suggested that so-called junk foods be fortified with iron.

Menorrhagia. Women with menorrhagia (an unusually heavy menstrual flow) are especially likely to become iron-deficient, as are those with metrorrhagia (bleeding at times other than the regular period). Often, such women may fail to consult a physician about their condition, because they think that it is normal for them. Thus, the nurse who gains such information in casual conversation with a woman may do well to suggest that she see a physician and have her hemoglobin level and red cell count checked. The character of the menstrual flow should be noted in taking the medical histories of all premenopausal women.

Gastrointestinal bleeding. Iron deficiency in adult men and in postmenopausal women is almost always caused by loss of blood from lesions that are most commonly located in the gastrointestinal tract. The possible presence of hidden hemorrhagic lesions must also be considered even in patients with more obvious possible causes of iron deficiency, such as a poor diet or unusually heavy menstrual blood loss. Peptic ulcer is the most common cause of chronic blood loss in young adults, even when the patient does not complain of abdominal pain. Often, in older patients, the cause of occult blood loss may be a carcinoma of the colon or the stomach that has not yet been diagnosed. Obviously, in such patients it is essential to determine the iron leak and, if possible, correct it as well as the iron deficiency anemia.

In summary, supplemental iron seems to be definitely needed by infants and by women in the latter half of pregnancy. Adolescents, particularly teen-age girls, and many women with normal or heavy menses are probably in borderline iron balance. Men, postmenopausal women, and others who are suffering blood loss from a bleeding lesion in the gastrointestinal tract or elsewhere will also profit from iron therapy, provided that the underlying cause of their bleeding is also found and eliminated.

Oral iron therapy

Patients whose iron depletion has progressed to a point at which hypochromic microcytic anemia is apparent cannot build up their hemoglobin levels by diet alone. To absorb enough of the element for rapid erythropoiesis, patients need to take large amounts of medicinal iron (Table 35-1). Most of the extra iron given by mouth never gets into the bloodstream at all but leaves the body in the feces. However, enough of the metal is absorbed to begin producing objective improvement within a week or two. Often, after a month or more of treatment, the patient's hemoglobin level has returned to normal. However, it may be many more months before the patient's depleted tissue reserves of iron can be raised to optimal levels, even after the cause of blood loss has been discovered and corrected.

Table 35–1. Iron-containing hematinic products

Official or generic name	Trade name or synonym	Dosage and administration
Selected oral iron compounds		
Ferrous fumarate USP	Ircon; Toleron	Recommended daily dietary allowances: adult men—10 mg; adult women—18 mg; during pregnancy and lactation—30–60 mg; replacement therapy: 90–300 mg elemental iron/day (6 mg/kg body weight/day)
Ferrous gluconate	Fergon	
Ferrous sulfate USP*	Iron sulfate hydrated	
Ferrous sulfate exsiccated USP	Feosol; Fer-In-Sol	
Parenteral iron product		
Iron dextran injection USP*	Imferon	IM or IV administration. Dose for correcting iron deficiency anemia by a single IV infusion is calculated as follows: $$0.3 \times \text{weight (lb)} \times \left(100 - \frac{\text{hemoglobin (g\%)} \times 100}{14.8}\right)$$ This formula gives the adult dose in milligrams of iron. Dividing by 50 gives the adult dose in milliliters.

* See also Drug digest.

Product selection. Hundreds of hematinic products are marketed by pharmaceutical manufacturers who claim unique superiority for their particular iron salt or formulation. Actually, the most effective products are also the least expensive ones—simple water-soluble iron salts such as ferrous sulfate[+], ferrous fumarate, and ferrous gluconate. These compounds present elemental iron in a form more readily absorbable than that found in many much more expensive products that are heavily promoted both to physicians and the public. These products are available over the counter, without a prescription. The main advantage claimed for these preparations is that they are less irritating to the gastrointestinal tract than the simple inorganic iron salts.

Actually, no single iron compound can be *both* the most readily absorbed and the least irritating, because any iron salt is absorbed only in proportion to the degree that it can be converted to soluble elemental iron in the gastrointestinal tract. Furthermore, the extent of local mucosal irritation produced by any particular product also depends on the amount of free (ionic or elemental) iron that the molecule releases. In practice, this means that the inexpensive iron salts such as ferrous sulfate are both the best absorbed and the most likely to cause gastrointestinal irritation, whereas the compounds that contain iron bound up into a complex molecule from which it is only slowly released will be both least well absorbed and less irritating.

The same is true of sustained-release and enteric-coated preparations, which are not recommended because the iron in such products is often not absorbed well enough by the mucous membranes lining the upper intestinal tract. Products containing various vitamins and trace metals also cost considerably more than simple iron salts, without increasing the absorption of iron or the effectiveness of this element for building up the patient's hemoglobin level and red blood cell count. Thus, because most patients are able to tolerate the simple salts when they are properly administered, such products should be suggested to the patient, and the patient should be instructed as to how to take them for best effects.

Administration of oral iron. Iron salts are best absorbed when taken on an empty stomach. However, they are also most irritating to the gastrointestinal tract when administered in this way. Patients who experience epigastric distress, nausea, or vomiting at the start of treatment may stop taking their medication. Thus, treatment is often begun with small doses taken right after meals. Then, the dosage is gradually raised, and the amount of food taken together with iron is reduced. If the patient does not complain of abdominal discomfort, diarrhea, or constipation, the medication may then be taken between meals for most complete absorption.

Patients who have difficulty tolerating iron at first need encouragement. They also need to be told that their stool may be colored red or black by an iron preparation, so that they will not be alarmed by the thought that this is a sign of gastrointestinal bleeding. To protect the teeth from staining by liquid iron preparations, the patient should be told to place the concentrated drops well back on the tongue, or to dilute the solution and sip it through a straw or drinking tube.

As indicated above, restoration of the anemic patient's iron stores often takes several months. Thus, patients should be encouraged to continue taking the prescribed daily dosage, even after they claim to feel entirely well. Often in such cases, periodic blood tests reveal that the patient's hemoglobin level has not actually improved. This could mean that blood and its iron content are still being lost to a greater degree than the iron is being replaced by the drug therapy. On the other hand, such so-called refractory anemia may be the result of the patient's failure to take the prescribed medication regularly in the recommended dosage. If a follow-up evaluation of the patient's status suggests this, treatment with an injectable iron product may be desirable.

Parenteral iron therapy

Most anemic patients tolerate oral iron well, and their hemoglobin rises at a steady rate. However, some types of patients may require iron by injection. These include the following types of cases: patients who refuse to take oral iron, or cannot be depended on to do so; those who have had extensive bowel surgery, or who suffer from ulcerative colitis or regional enteritis; and those who suffer from diseases that prevent oral iron from being absorbed. Although parenteral administration of iron does not result in more rapid correction of anemia, the patient's stores of reserve iron may be built up at a faster rate. This may be especially desirable for the rare patient with chronic bleeding that cannot be readily corrected.

The only currently available parenteral product, *iron dextran injection*[+] (Imferon), may be administered IM or by IV infusion over several hours. This product is reserved for patients whose iron deficiency anemia cannot be treated with oral iron, because both chronic and acute toxicity are possible when iron is administered by parenteral routes. Acute toxicity may be caused by an anaphylactic reaction or from overdosage leading to severe falls in blood pressure, sometimes to shock levels.

For IV administration, the total dose of iron that the patient requires must be calculated (see equation, Table 35-1). It is important to avoid overloading the patient's tissues with iron, a chronic disorder called *hemosiderosis*, which can in turn result in damage to the liver, heart, pancreas, and other organs—a condition called *hemochromatosis*, which also sometimes occurs in patients who have had too many blood transfusions. Although a specific antidote is now available for facilitating the removal of iron overload—the chelating agent *deferoxamine* *mesylate* (Desferal)—prevention is preferable to the prolonged treatment needed to hasten the excretion of excessive amounts of injectable iron.*

Accidental iron poisoning

Young children who ingest overdoses of an oral iron product may suffer acute iron toxicity. These salts can cause both local and systemic toxicity. The nausea, vomiting, and abdominal pain produced by the corrosive action of iron may be followed by a shocklike state. Death may occur from cardiovascular collapse within a few hours or after a delay of a day or so, during which the child may appear to be recovering.

In addition to symptomatic treatment with blood pressure-raising drugs, oxygen, systemic alkalinizers, and anticonvulsants, efforts are made to bind the iron in insoluble complexes and to remove it from both the gastrointestinal tract and the systemic circulation. If the child is seen soon after taking iron tablets, it may be desirable to induce vomiting or to wash out the stomach with sodium bicarbonate solution. Later, tissue erosion may make these measures too dangerous.

Deferoxamine, which converts both free and tissue-bound iron to a harmless chelate complex and carries it to the kidneys for excretion, can be used to bind and remove the iron from both the gastrointestinal tract and the bloodstream. However, as mentioned above in the discussion of chronic iron overload treatment, it is better to prevent acute iron toxicity than to have to treat the potentially fatal poisoning. Patients should be warned that iron preparations are not harmless and should be kept where children cannot reach the tablets, which often resemble brightly colored candies. The container should be of the "childproof" type that children cannot readily open, and it should be labeled "Keep out of the reach of children" to alert parents to the potential toxicity of these widely advertised products, which seem safe because they contain only natural nutrients found in foods.

Fortification of foods with iron

The average American diet contains about 6 mg of iron/1000 calories—an intake of about 15 mg of iron for people with a dietary intake of 2500 calories daily. Only about 5% to 10% of the iron contained in ingested foodstuffs is absorbed by normal adults. This quantity—between about 0.6 mg and 1.6 mg of iron—is enough to replace the daily iron loss and thus to meet the needs of adult men and postmenopausal women. Because other people with increased iron requirements assimilate about twice as much dietary iron as those with normal needs for the metal, the demands of most of these people can also usually be met by eating an ordinary diet, provided that blood is not being lost by internal bleeding.

However, because some people—for example, young, menstruating women with a daily dietary intake of only about 1500 calories—may not be able to satisfy their relatively high need for iron by eating an ordinary diet, some authorities recommend that foods be fortified with iron supplements to prevent iron deficiency. Other experts oppose lifting the current legal limit on the amount of iron that may be added to the flour used in making iron-enriched bread. They argue that men, most children, and others who have enough iron stored in their bone marrow, liver, and spleen may build up excessive levels of iron in these organs and suffer ill effects from iron overloading if they eat iron-fortified foods that they do not really need.†

To avoid an excessive iron intake with possible development of hemosiderosis and hemochromatosis, those who oppose raising the amount of iron added to commonly eaten foods suggest that such measures *not* be aimed at the entire population. They suggest, instead, that extra iron be taken only when a physician has determined that this is desirable for a particular person. In such cases, a single daily dose of an inexpensive soluble iron salt will be enough to meet the needs of even the group of young women at greatest risk who cannot assimilate enough iron from food alone.

Megaloblastic anemias

As indicated earlier in the general discussions of erythrocyte production and the anemias, a lack of vitamin B_{12} or of folic acid can lead to a type of anemia characterized by the presence in the circulating blood of abnormally large erythrocytes (macrocytes), and in the bone marrow of large immature red blood cell precursors (megaloblasts). Actually, the effects of a deficiency of cyanocobalamin or of folate are also seen in the formation of the other formed elements of the blood. Thus, the circulating blood of such patients also contains large platelets and polymorphonuclear leukocytes, and their bone marrow contains numerous enlarged "blasts," or germ cells, from which these abnormal thrombocytes and white blood cells are derived.

Megaloblastosis is believed to be the result of a slowing of the processes by which cell nuclei biosynthesize DNA. This, in turn, interferes with the cell's ability to divide at a normal rate, an effect that is not limited to the cells of the bone marrow but that also occurs in other rapidly dividing cells. Thus, for example, a lack of vitamin

---

* The Food and Drug Administration has approved the use of deferoxamine for treating chronic iron overload in children with Cooley's anemia (thalassemia), an incurable hereditary disorder that requires frequent transfusions of red blood cells with resultant accumulation of the cytotoxic metal in vital organs.

---

† The results of studies reported from Sweden, where enrichment of food with relatively large amounts of iron has been mandatory during the past 30 years, suggest that a somewhat higher incidence of hemochromatosis in men may be the result of iron fortification of food.

B_{12} can decrease the rate of epithelial cell formation in the tongue, and so cause a characteristic glossitis in which the tongue becomes smooth, sore, and sometimes red, raw, and even ulcerated. Interference with formation of the lining cells of the lower gastrointestinal tract presumably accounts for the diarrhea that often accompanies a dietary deficiency of folic acid.

Vitamin B_{12} deficiency

Vitamin B_{12} is one of the most potent biologically active substances found in nature. Only 1 μg—a millionth of a gram—must be absorbed from dietary sources to meet the body's daily need for vitamin B_{12}. Amounts much larger than that are available in liver, muscle meats, seafood, eggs, and milk. Thus, vitamin B_{12} deficiency is rarely the result—in this country, at least—of a lack of B_{12} in the diet. However, because B_{12} is absent in plants, vegetarians—especially those who eat no eggs, milk, or cheese as well as no meat—may occasionally become deficient. Even then, it takes several years for the body's stores of the vitamin to drop enough for signs of deficiency to appear.

The main cause of vitamin B_{12} deficiency is failure to absorb from the upper intestinal tract the tiny amount required to replace the little that is lost each day. This occurs because of the lack of a so-called intrinsic factor, a glycoprotein normally secreted by cells of the stomach mucosa, which is needed to aid in the absorption of vitamin B_{12} by the mucosal cells of the ileum. This factor is absent in patients who have had all, or even large parts, of the stomach removed. The vitamin taken in when animal protein foods are eaten cannot then get through the mucosal wall of the ileum and into the bloodstream. Some patients with intestinal disease, as well as those with gastric carcinoma or perforating peptic ulcer, who require subtotal gastrectomy or other massive surgical resection of the upper gastrointestinal tract, may also develop a gradual deficiency of vitamin B_{12}.

Pernicious anemia. This disease, the most common cause of vitamin B_{12} deficiency, stems from a steady reduction in the ability of the gastric mucosal cells to secrete intrinsic factor, until finally too little is produced to promote absorption of enough of the vitamin. This chronic condition is characterized not only by the blood cell and gastrointestinal tract abnormalities discussed above, and by the resulting feelings of fatigue and other symptoms seen in all anemias, but also by signs of damage to the nervous system. This occurs because vitamin B_{12} is needed for biosynthesis of the myelin sheaths of nerve cells.

Neurologic signs and symptoms. Peripheral neuropathy at first affects sensory function and may be manifested by complaints of numbness and tingling (paresthesias) in the hands and feet. Later, involvement of the motor fibers of peripheral nerves, the spinal cord, and other central nervous system areas can lead to motor incoordination, particularly while walking. The cerebral cortex may also be affected, with resulting mental abnormalities ranging from confusion to symptoms of psychosis.

History. Pernicious anemia was once an inevitably fatal disease, and it can still cause death from heart failure and progressive neurologic deficits if not detected and treated. Research studies of 60 years ago revealed that these patients could be kept alive by feeding them very large amounts of beef or pork liver. Later, these patients were treated with injections of liver extracts that were made increasingly potent in their concentration of the so-called extrinsic factor "antipernicious anemia principle." Finally, this protective and curative substance was found to be vitamin B_{12}, which was eventually isolated in pure crystalline form. Thus, there is now no need to use liver extract injections and run the risk of causing allergic reactions to the foreign protein. Instead, once pernicious anemia is diagnosed, the pure vitamin, which is completely free of toxicity and painless on injection, can be given. It is also inexpensive, because it can be prepared in large amounts by microbial synthesis.

Response to vitamin B_{12} therapy. Patients with pernicious anemia and others who fail to take in or absorb enough dietary B_{12} can have their symptoms completely reversed by receiving B_{12} by injection (Table 35-2). The form most commonly employed is a solution of the dark red crystals called *cyanocobalamin injection*[+] (Rubramin). Injected deep into the subcutaneous tissues or intramuscularly, the vitamin bypasses the mucosal barrier to its intestinal absorption. It is carried by the bloodstream to such sites as the bone marrow, intestinal mucosa cells, the nervous system, and all the other cells that need the vitamin to function normally.

Improvement in the patient's blood picture becomes apparent within a few days, with the entry of young red cells (reticulocytes) into the bloodstream. Large numbers of normal leukocytes and platelets are also seen as the megaloblastic cells in the bone marrow are brought to maturity by the availability of vitamin B_{12} and replace the immature forms of all the circulating blood cell types. Even before these favorable hematopoietic reactions are completed, the patient feels much better physically and mentally, and appetite improves as early as the first day of therapy.

In addition to this favorable hematologic response, the patient's digestive complaints—glossitis and diarrhea, for example—are largely eliminated. The sore tongue heals, and symptoms of intestinal irritation are lessened, as the mucosal epithelial cells lining the gastrointestinal tract are restored. The atrophied stomach cells do not recover their ability to secrete gastric acid and intrinsic factor. Similarly, although the milder symptoms of nervous system damage (numbness and tingling of the extremities, for example) soon disappear, and even the more severe motor symptoms may be relieved after

Table 35–2. Hematopoietic vitamins and related substances

Official or generic name	Trade name or synonym	Total daily dosage and administration	Comments
Cyanocobalamin crystalline, USP	Berubigen; Rubramin PC; vitamin B_{12}	Variable doses from 30–1000 μg, parenteral and oral	See Drug digest
Folic acid USP	Folvite; pteroylglutamic acid; Folacin; Folate	0.4–1.0 mg daily, parenteral and oral	See Drug digest
Hydroxocobalamin, crystalline, USP	AlphaRedisol; vitamin B_{12a}	30–1000 μg, IM	Claimed to be longer lasting than vitamin B_{12}
Leucovorin calcium USP	Citrovorum factor; folinic acid	1 mg daily, IM	In higher doses, used as antidote for overdosage with antifolic compounds and as leucovorin rescue in cancer chemotherapy
Liver injection	Pernaemon	Variable (IM only)	Contains vitamin B_{12} in crude form; may cause allergic reactions
Vitamin B_{12} with intrinsic factor concentrate	In various panhematinic products and oral liver preparations; Biopar Forte; Extralin	Variable	Orally effective but not as desirable as injections of B_{12} in pernicious anemia; intrinsic factor aids oral absorption of vitamin B_{12}

several months of continued treatment, little improvement can be expected in functions controlled by parts of the brain and spinal cord in which the neurons have already degenerated. However, further neurologic damage is arrested by B_{12} treatment.

Other indications. Patients whose vitamin B_{12} deficiency is not the result of the lack of intrinsic factor that leads to pernicious anemia will also improve when treated with cyanocobalamin. Even small oral doses are adequate, for example, for strict vegetarians whose megaloblastic anemia is caused entirely by prolonged dietary deficiency of vitamin B_{12}, and such people can, of course, *prevent* the anemia and other symptoms simply by taking a small daily supplement of this vitamin orally, if they choose not to eat even eggs or milk products. Those unable to absorb vitamin B_{12} because of some defect of the ileum are best maintained with parenteral preparations (see below) if their condition cannot be corrected surgically. Patients infected by the fish tapeworm parasite, which deprives people of dietary vitamin B_{12} are best treated with one of the anthelmintic drugs, niclosamide or paromomycin (Chap. 11). However, the adjunctive use of vitamin B_{12} helps to hasten their hematologic recovery.

Vitamin B_{12} is often prescribed for treating conditions that are not the result of a deficiency of this vitamin. People with symptoms similar to those observed in pernicious anemia patients and others with a definite B_{12} deficiency sometimes receive massive doses of the vitamin. It is highly unlikely that cyanocobalamin has any pharmacologic effects that would make it useful for patients who do not suffer from a B_{12} deficiency.

Although favorable reports have frequently appeared concerning the efficacy of B_{12} in nervous and mental disorders, there is no real proof of its value in these conditions. That is, the fact that B_{12} injections often clear up the numbness and tingling that pernicious anemia patients feel in their fingers and toes does not mean that this vitamin will help patients with paresthesias of the hands and feet that are not caused by a lack of dietary B_{12}. The same can be said of claims that B_{12} injections are sometimes of value in trigeminal neuralgia, multiple sclerosis, and some psychiatric conditions marked by mental defects and emotional upsets of the type that occur in pernicious anemia patients and others as a result of vitamin B_{12} deficiency. Fortunately, even when injected in massive doses, vitamin B_{12} causes no local or systemic toxicity. Thus, physicians who order injections of such large doses of this vitamin may be employing it as a harmless placebo while they seek the real cause and cure of the patient's condition.

Dosage and administration. The most effective form of vitamin B_{12} is a solution of the dark red crystals called cyanocobalamin injection (Berubigen; Rubramin). It is administered intramuscularly or into a deep subcutaneous site in the doses required to counteract acute symptoms and to build up body stores of vitamin B_{12} to normal and maintain them at that level. Recommended dosage schedules differ widely, depending on the severity of the anemia and its complications and other factors.

Patients severely ill with pernicious anemia may receive 100 to 1000 μg of cyanocobalamin daily during the acute phase of their illness. More commonly, doses of 30 μg daily for 7 to 10 days are considered adequate in most cases, because higher amounts are excreted without being used by the bone marrow. However, because of the safety of this substance, there is no harm in administering large doses. Thus, although some authorities claim that nothing is gained by giving amounts larger than 30 μg, it is customary to treat patients with spinal cord complications by administering about 10 to 30 times that dose daily for the first 1 or 2 weeks. This is often followed by similar weekly doses—for example, 250 to 500 μg IM—until the maximal degree of recovery has been attained.

Patients differ considerably in their ability to retain administered vitamin B_{12}. In some cases, total body stores drop to subnormal levels only 1 or 2 weeks after being restored to normal; other patients can go several months without requiring further replenishment. Generally, pernicious anemia patients require injections of at least 100 μg monthly to maintain normal levels of this vitamin. Some physicians inject five to ten times that amount at each visit.

It is important to make it clear to the patient and family that injections must be continued for the rest of the patient's life at the intervals specified by the physician. They should be helped to understand that, in most cases, the underlying defect that led to the B_{12} deficiency cannot be corrected. Thus, if the patient neglects to continue with treatment because of "feeling fine," the stores of B_{12} will inevitably slide to subnormal levels. Then, if the early warning signs of deficiency, weariness and malaise, are not heeded, the patient may suffer insidious damage to the nervous system without being aware that the disease is progressing to the point of irreversible spinal cord damage.

Other preparations. Hydroxocobalamin (vitamin B_{12a}) tends to produce high and longer lasting blood levels than cyanocobalamin after parenteral administration. Its longer retention in the body allows longer intervals between injections, an objective not yet accomplished with sustained-action, or depot type, preparations of cyanocobalamin. However, hydroxocobalamin has not proved to have any significant practical advantages over cyanocobalamin.

Oral treatment with vitamin B_{12} *alone* is effective only in the rare cases of megaloblastic anemia caused by a dietary deficiency of B_{12}. Patients with pernicious anemia require an oral preparation that also contains the intrinsic factor that they lack. However, even though tablets and capsules containing vitamin B_{12} combined with intrinsic factor concentrate are available, the use of such oral products for maintenance therapy in these patients is not considered desirable. Many patients who respond at first to oral products of this type tend to become resistant after some time and will relapse unless they receive injections. Thus, they are best reserved for patients who tend to bleed when they receive injections.

The large daily oral doses required to replenish body stores of vitamin B_{12} are actually more expensive than the injectable form of this vitamin. Patients can reduce the cost of therapy further if they or someone in the family can be taught to administer their B_{12} injections. However, because such patients are often elderly and victims of a chronic and incurable illness, they should be urged not to neglect periodic checkups for routine examination. This will still be true even if a cheap and completely dependable oral preparation is developed, or if one of the longer acting depot forms of vitamin B_{12} being currently tested lengthens considerably the time between injections.

Folic acid deficiency

Folic acid is a substance that is essential for cell division in all types of tissue. Dietary folate is converted in the body to a reduced form through the action of the enzyme dihydrofolate reductase. This metabolite, tetrahydrofolic acid, acts as a coenzyme in many biochemical reactions that lead to production of the purines and pyrimidines from which nucleic acids are finally biosynthesized. Deficiencies of folic acid appear first in those tissues that grow at the most rapid rates, including cancerous tissues, the bone marrow blood cell precursors, and the epithelial cells that line the gastrointestinal tract. That is why the *anti*folic drugs—chemicals that keep rapidly reproducing cells from using dietary folic acid—are useful in treating leukemia and other neoplastic disorders. It is also the cause of the toxic hematologic and gastrointestinal tract effects of these anticancer drugs (Chap. 12).

Most people have no difficulty in meeting their daily requirements for this B-complex vitamin—about 50 μg daily for adults. Leafy green vegetables such as lettuce, spinach, and asparagus, and foods such as milk, eggs, and liver, contain many times that much folate. However, deficiency may develop during malnutrition or during periods of increased demand for the vitamin, and in patients suffering from malabsorption syndromes, such as tropical or nontropical sprue and celiac disease.

Deficiency states. Malnutrition as a cause of folate deficiency is common in alcoholics and is often a factor in poor and elderly patients and in food faddists. Sometimes megaloblastic anemia occurs in women who have had several successive pregnancies, because of the increased demands on their folic acid stores by the growing fetuses. Infants fed on diets lacking in food folate sometimes develop megaloblastic anemia and diarrhea, particularly during periods of infection. Patients taking certain antiepileptic drugs for long periods sometimes develop a folate deficiency and a resulting megaloblastic anemia (Chap. 50). The antibacterial agent trimethoprim must be used with caution in patients low in folate, because it may block the production of tetrahydrofolic acid in human as well as bacterial cells (Chap. 8).

Symptoms. Patients deficient in folic acid develop a megaloblastic anemia that does not differ from that found in pernicious anemia. As in the latter disorder, gastrointestinal symptoms such as glossitis and diarrhea may also occur. Although people may show such signs of central effects of deficiency as forgetfulness, irritability, and insomnia, a lack of folic acid does not lead to the neurologic damage that results from a deficiency of vitamin B_{12}. This is probably because nerve cells do not reproduce themselves (vitamin B_{12} is probably needed for a metabolic step in the synthesis of nerve cell lipids such as myelin; folic acid is not needed in the synthesis of the myelin sheath lipids of neurons).

Response to treatment. Once a patient's megaloblastic anemia is definitely diagnosed as the result of folate deficiency, it can be readily reversed by oral or parenteral administration of crystalline folic acid. Patients who are not severely ill respond rapidly to as little as 0.1 mg administered by mouth. In practice, however, most hematologists start all patients on much higher doses of this *non*toxic substance. Orders for 5 to 15 mg daily are common, and although such large oral doses of *folic acid*[+] (Folvite) are adequately absorbed even in the presence of intestinal disease, the injectable sodium salt is often employed by the intramuscular or deep subcutaneous route in patients suffering from malabsorption syndromes.

Patients improve promptly both in how they feel and in their blood picture. Changes in the bone marrow from megaloblastosis to normoblastosis are seen within a couple of days, followed shortly by disappearance of macrocystosis in the peripheral blood that then begins to contain more and more normal red cells. Such symptoms as soreness of the mouth and tongue and diarrhea disappear, and the patient's improved appetite soon leads to a gain in weight. Improvement can be maintained with daily doses of 1 mg or less, but relapses are best prevented by providing a diet containing adequate quantities of food folates.

Folic acid is an entirely safe substance. However, its misuse by people who do not need it is not only unnecessarily expensive but also potentially dangerous for patients with pernicious anemia. This is so because small amounts of folic acid may bring the blood picture of these patients back to normal while their neurologic disorder continues to progress. (Folic acid cannot correct the neuronal myelin sheath damage that occurs as a result of vitamin B_{12} deficiency.) Thus, diagnostic tests are performed to exclude the presence of pernicious anemia before folic acid is prescribed for a patient with megaloblastic anemia.

Self-medication

The nurse should always advise patients not to try to treat themselves with *non*prescription antianemia products that contain mixtures of many different minerals and vitamins, including folic acid. The Food and Drug Administration now forbids the inclusion of more than 0.1 mg (100 μg) folic acid in *non*prescription products, because larger amounts may mask the presence of pernicious anemia and make its diagnosis difficult in patients whose real difficulty is a lack of vitamin B_{12}. The small amount of oral vitamin B_{12} that is offered in such so-called shotgun-type multivitamin and panhematinic products is not likely to protect the patient against progressive neurologic complications.

Patients should also be advised that they do not need supplements of this vitamin if their daily diet includes a piece of fresh fruit or a green, leafy vegetable. Its inclusion in products that contain iron only adds to their expense, because iron deficiency anemia rarely occurs together with the folic acid deficiency type and—as indicated earlier—inexpensive iron salts are available for treating that form of anemia. (Some heavily promoted *non*prescription products made up of complex combinations of minerals and vitamins cost 10 to 20 times as much as a simple ferrous sulfate tablet, which may be all the patient needs—if any medication at all is required.)

Additional clinical considerations

Most patients with deficiency anemias can be treated successfully. However, the key to successful treatment is a correct diagnosis of the cause of the anemia. When the nature of the deficiency has been determined, the specific missing substance can thus be administered, whether it is iron, folic acid, or vitamin B_{12}.

The patient should receive a thorough physical examination to determine the underlying cause of the anemia—for example, a nutritional deficit, a disorder that prevents the absorption of the needed element, or a disorder that causes excess loss of the elements. For immediate therapy, the patient can receive a supplement of the specific necessary nutrient that is deficient while the underlying cause of the problem is being corrected.

The public has a great need to be educated regarding the use of over-the-counter nutritional supplements. Unless a specific deficiency has been discovered, most people do not require supplemental vitamins and minerals. Self-medication with these compounds can mask serious problems, and in some cases can result in toxic levels of the supplement (*e.g.*, iron) accumulating in the body.

Iron is rather frequently used in clinical practice. The drug should not be given to patients with cirrhosis, peptic ulcer, ulcerative colitis, or regional enteritis, conditions that do not permit adequate absorption of the drug and that can be aggravated by the irritating iron preparation. IM use of iron should be avoided during pregnancy, because its safety for the fetus has not been established.

IM iron can stain the tissues and should only be given using the Z-track technique. Oral preparations can stain the teeth, and care should be taken to avoid contact with the teeth. Oral iron preparations should be taken on an empty stomach but, if gastrointestinal upset occurs, the drug can be taken with food or meals. Certain foods are known to bind iron, and should *not* be in the stomach at the same time as iron; these include milk, milk products, and eggs.

The oral iron preparations have been associated with all types of gastrointestinal upset. The sometimes severe constipation that may develop often requires additional interventions. Patients need to be alerted to the fact that stools will be a dark tarry color as long as they take the drug. They should be assured that this does not indicate gastrointestinal tract bleeding.

As mentioned above, iron can be very toxic. The drug should be kept safely away from children. The signs and symptoms of iron toxicity should be reviewed if any patient is on an iron preparation. These include weakness, drowsiness, lethargy, severe nausea and vomiting, abdominal pain or cramps, low blood pressure, weak pulse, tachycardia, bluish tint to lips, nailbeds, and palms and, in extreme cases, shock and coma.

Patients receiving vitamin B_{12} will need to know that they will require it for life. Family members can often be instructed in the proper technique for the IM injection of the drug. This instruction will need to include the proper storage and disposal of syringes, the rotation of injection sites, and advice about traveling with syringes. Many nurses and physicians use the patient's regular returns for B_{12} injections as an opportunity to evaluate the patient's physical status and the effectiveness of teaching programs. The safety of the use of vitamin B_{12} during pregnancy and lactation has not been established.

Drug–drug interactions

Vitamin C taken with iron can enhance the absorption of the iron. Iron absorption is decreased by the presence of *magnesium trisilicate antacids. Tetracycline* binds to iron and is not absorbed if taken with oral iron. Patients receiving both of these drugs should space the drugs at 2 to 4 hour intervals. *Phenytoin* levels are decreased if taken with folic acid, and seizure activity may be precipitated by inadequate phenytoin levels in epileptic patients. *Oral contraceptives* have been associated with decreased folate metabolism, and folic acid therapy may not be effective. Decreased vitamin B_{12} absorption has been associated with concurrent ingestion of *aminosalicylic acid, neomycin,* or *alcohol.*

The patient teaching guide summarizes points that should be included when teaching a patient receiving iron supplements. Similar guides could be developed for patients receiving vitamin B_{12} or folic acid. The guide to the nursing process summarizes clinical considerations to be incorporated into the nursing care of patients receiving iron supplements.

Patient teaching guide: iron supplements

The drug that has been prescribed for you is an iron supplement. Iron is a naturally occurring mineral found in many foods. The body uses iron to make red blood cells, which carry oxygen to all parts of the body. Supplemental iron needs to be taken when the body does not have enough iron available to make healthy red blood cells, a condition called anemia.

Iron is a toxic substance if too much is taken. You must avoid self-medication with over-the-counter preparations containing iron while you are on this drug. You will need to return for regular medical checkups while taking this drug to determine the effectiveness of the iron.

Instructions:

1. The name of the drug prescribed for you is _____ .

2. The dosage of your drug is _____ .

(continued)

3. Your drug should be taken _____ times a day. It is best to take the drug on an empty stomach (1 hour before or 2 hours after meals) with a full glass of water or fruit juice. If stomach upset occurs, the drug can be taken with food or meals. There are some foods that should not be taken with iron; these incude milk and milk products (such as cheese and ice cream) and eggs. The best times to take your drug are _____.

4. If *ferrous salts* have been prescribed, they may be dissolved in orange juice to improve the taste.

       Liquid iron preparations should be taken with a straw; this will prevent the iron from staining the teeth.

       If *iron drops* are being given, they should be placed far back on the tongue to prevent staining of the teeth.

5. Some side-effects of the drug that you should be aware of include the following:

Dark, tarry stools	The iron preparation stains the stools black; do not be concerned—the color will remain as long as you are on the drug.
Constipation	This is a frequent problem; if it becomes too uncomfortable, consult your nurse or physician for appropriate remedies.
Nausea, indigestion, vomiting	This problem can often be helped by taking the drug with meals.

6. Tell any physician, nurse, or dentist who is taking care of you that you are on this drug.

7. Keep this and all medications out of the reach of children. Because iron can be very toxic, seek emergency medical help immediately if you suspect that a child has taken this preparation unsupervised.

8. Because iron can interfere with the absorption of some drugs, do not take iron at the same time as *tetracycline* or *antacids*. If you are on these drugs, they will have to be taken at intervals when iron is not in the stomach.

Notify your nurse or physician if any of the following occur:

Severe diarrhea
Severe abdominal pain or cramping
Unusual tiredness or weakness
Bluish tint to lips or fingernails

Guide to the nursing process: iron supplements

Assessment	Nursing diagnoses	Interventions	Evaluations
Past history (*contraindications*): Cirrhosis Hepatic dysfunction Peptic ulcer Regional enteritis Ulcerative colitis *Allergies:* these drugs; tartrazine (certain preparations); others; reactions Medications history (*cautions*): Tetracycline Antacids **Physical assessment** Neurologic: reflexes, orientation, affect Cardiovascular; BP, P, peripheral perfusion Respiratory: R, adventitious sounds GI: bowel sounds, liver function, abdominal exam Skin: color, lesions	Potential alteration in bowel elimination Knowledge deficit regarding drug therapy Potential alteration in nutrition secondary to GI upset Potential alteration in tissue perfusion	Proper and safe administration of drug Comfort measures: • Bowel program • Drug given with meals • Rest Patient teaching regarding: • Disease • Drug • Side-effects • Cautions • Warnings Support and encouragement to cope with drug, blood tests, follow-up Provision of life support measures, if toxicity develops	Monitor for therapeutic effect of drug: blood tests Monitor for adverse effects of drug: • GI effects • Signs of toxicity Evaluate effectiveness of patient teaching program Evaluate effectiveness of support and encouragement offered Monitor for drug–drug interactions: ↓ tetracycline absorption with iron ↓ iron absorption with antacids Monitor for drug–diet interactions: ↓ iron absorption with milk, eggs Evaluate effectiveness of life support and detoxifying measures, if toxicity occurs

Summary of side-effects, cautions, and contraindications: iron salts

Side-effects

Oral therapeutic doses. Irritation to mucosa of stomach and intestinal tract tends to cause epigastric distress (with possible nausea and vomiting); abdominal cramps (with either diarrhea or constipation). Caution is required in patients with peptic ulcer, ulcerative colitis, regional enteritis, and other chronic gastrointestinal inflammatory disorders.

Oral toxic doses (acute poisoning in children). Nausea, vomiting, abdominal pain, diarrhea, with stools greenish and tarry as a result of mucosal damage and hemorrhage.

Lethargy, fast, weak pulse, low blood pressure, with possible circulatory collapse, pulmonary edema, coma, and death.

Parenteral therapeutic doses and overdoses. local: soreness, swelling, and brownish or bluish staining of skin at IM injection sites; possible pain, venous spasm, and phlebitis at IV injection sites; *systemic:* headache, dizziness, flushing, nausea; possible joint pain and swelling in arthritic patients or generalized pain in others; anaphylactic and hypotensive reactions.

Contraindications

Hypersensitive patients and those with any type of anemia *not* caused by iron deficiency because of the danger of hemosiderosis (iron overload disease). *Extreme caution* in patients with impaired liver function.

Case study

Presentation

LL, a 28-year-old white woman suffered a miscarriage 6 weeks ago. She lost a great deal of blood during the miscarriage, and underwent a D and C to stop the bleeding. On her 6-week follow-up visit, the physician found that LL had recovered physically from the event but that she was still very depressed over the loss. Her hematocrit was found to be 31, and she admitted that she had been very tired and weak. The physician offered her emotional support and gave her a supply of ferrous sulfate tablets with instructions to take one tid. When LL returned home, the envelope containing the tablets ripped, and she transferred the tablets to a decorative glass bottle that had once held multiple vitamins. LL left the bottle on the kitchen table as a reminder to take the tablets. The next day LL discovered her 2-year-old daughter eating the green tablets, and punished her for getting into them. An hour later, the toddler, P, was vomiting, complaining of severe abdominal pain, and becoming progressively lethargic. LL called the pediatrician, who immediately sent her to a nearby hospital emergency room and told her to take the remaining pills with her. At the emergency room, P was found to have a weak, rapid pulse (156), rapid shallow respirations (32), and a low BP (60/42). A diagnosis of acute iron toxicity was made. LL became distraught. She stated that she had no idea that iron could be dangerous; no one had told her this; and she knew that you could buy it over the counter in many preparations. How could it possibly be dangerous?

What nursing measures should be taken at this time?

Discussion

The most immediate concerns will involve supporting the child and detoxifying her. In cases of acute iron poisoning, the patient should be induced to vomit and then given eggs and milk. Once in a medical facility, gastric lavage is done using a 1% sodium bicarbonate solution. The lavage is considered safe only if done within the first hour after ingestion; beyond the first hour, there is increased incidence of GI erosion from the corrosive iron, and the lavage can be very dangerous. Because P was well beyond the first hour after ingestion, none of these treatments would be advisable. An iron chelating agent (*e.g.*, deferoxamine mesylate) should be given, and basic supportive measures should be taken to deal with the shock, dehydration, and GI damage.

LL will require a great deal of emotional support and encouragement. She is already depressed over the loss of her pregnancy and now must face serious illnes in another child, illness for which she might tend to blame herself. The nurse should try to locate a support person to be with LL while P is being treated. Once the situation has stabilized, LL will need extensive teaching about her drug and drug therapy. She should be assured that most people, unfortunately, do not take OTC or OTC-type drugs seriously, and are not aware of potential risks that they pose. She should be commended for calling the pediatrician and bringing P directly to the hospital. This unfortunate situation presents the opportunity, in addition, for staff inservice education specifically about the dangers of iron toxicity and, in general, about the vital importance for complete and adequate patient education before sending a patient off to start drug therapy at home. P's illness could have been avoided if the patient had received appropriate drug education about her iron tablets when they were prescribed for her.

Drug digests

Cyanocobalamin injection USP (vitamin B₁₂)

Actions and indications. This potent hematopoietic (blood cell-forming) substance produces prompt improvement of the symptoms of pernicious anemia and other megaloblastic anemias that are caused by a lack of vitamin B_{12}. Patients often feel better within 1 day; the bone marrow picture is completely converted from megaloblastosis to normoblastosis in 2 or 3 days; showers of reticulocytes appear in the peripheral circulation in 2 to 5 days and reach a peak before 2 weeks. The circulating macrocytes are completely replaced by normal erythrocytes after 1 to 3 months of treatment.

Vitamin B₁₂ also counteracts glossitis (inflamed tongue) and other GI symptoms such as constipation or diarrhea. Progressive neurologic deterioration is stopped, and minor neurologic symptoms such as paresthesias (numbness and tingling) of the hands and feet often improve promptly. Motor system derangements improve more slowly, or not at all, if irreversible damage has been done to the spinal cord or peripheral nerves. Neurologic disorders that do not stem from

a vitamin B₁₂ deficiency, such as trigeminal neuralgia and other neuropathies, and multiple sclerosis are *not* aided by cyanocobalamin injection. Similarly, although symptoms of cerebral malfunction secondary to B₁₂ deficiency may improve over a period of several months, symptoms of psychoses that do not result from a lack of this vitamin are *not* counteracted.

Adverse effects, cautions, and contraindications. Cyanocobalamin is remarkably free of systemic toxicity, and the virtually painless injections are not followed by any local reactions unless impurities are present. There are no known contraindications to vitamin B₁₂.

Dosage and administration. This substance is administered by deep subcutaneous or in-

tramuscular injection and occasionally by vein in various dosage schedules. In uncomplicated cases of pernicious anemia that respond to as little as 1 μg, it is customary to administer 30 to 100 μg daily for 1 week, followed by similar doses one to three times weekly until hematologic remission is complete. Patients *must* then receive 100 μg *regularly* for the *rest of their lives* at intervals ranging from every 2 weeks to every 4 months—usually once a month.

Patients with signs of neurologic damage customarily receive doses of 1000 μg weekly for several months, or for a year or more when symptoms do not improve. However, injection of such large amounts probably has no greater value than doses of only 100 μg to 250 μg.

Ferrous sulfate USP (Feosol; Fer-In-Sol)

Actions and indications. This inexpensive inorganic iron salt offers elemental iron in a form that is readily absorbable from mucosal sites in the upper intestine. It is useful for supplying iron required for the synthesis of hemoglobin in iron deficiency anemia. It also restores depleted iron stores in simple iron deficiency.

Adverse effects, cautions, and contraindications. Gastrointestinal irritation symptoms include epigastric distress with possible nau-

sea and vomiting, and abdominal cramps with either diarrhea *or* constipation. Caution is required in patients with peptic ulcer, ulcerative colitis, regional enteritis, and other chronic inflammatory disorders of the gastrointestinal tract.

Massive overdosage may cause local corrosion of the mucosa of the stomach and intestine leading to diarrhea with black tarry stools. Pulse may become weak and rapid with blood pressure falling to shock levels.

Dosage and administration. The usual daily dosage is one to four 300-mg tablets (60 mg to 240 mg of elemental iron). These are administered after meals to avoid gastrointestinal irritation but, for better absorption in patients who tolerate iron well, this salt may be administered between meals. Liquid forms, including an elixir, syrup, and drops, are also available.

Folic acid USP (Folvite; pteroylglutamic acid)

Actions and indications. This form of the B-complex vitamin is effective for treating megaloblastic anemias that develop as a result of folate deficiency. These occur sometimes as a result of failure to eat a diet adequate in natural food folates—for example, in alcoholics, elderly people and food faddists. Malabsorption syndromes such as tropical and nontropical sprue and celiac disease that result in reduced absorption of food folate are another cause of megaloblastic anemias that respond to treatment with this substance administered by injection or in large oral doses. This form of folate may also be useful for treating or preventing deficiency in those with especially high folate requirements—for example, during pregnancy, particularly in women who have had several successive pregnancies. It is also effective for treating

megaloblastic anemia in infants fed on diets lacking in food folate, particularly when diarrhea or infection increases their folate requirements.

Response of the bone marrow and blood is rapid, and favorable changes in megaloblastosis and macrocytosis are seen within 1 or 2 days. Patients very quickly feel better and their appetite improves, as does soreness of the mouth and tongue and diarrhea.

Adverse effects, cautions, and contraindications. Even massive doses of this vitamin cause no adverse effects. Its use is contraindicated in patients with pernicious anemia, because it can bring about a hematologic remission without any favorable effect on the neurologic complications of this condition. Thus, the use of folic acid may mask

pernicious anemia and make its diagnosis difficult. It is *not* to be used for treating antifol drug toxicity, which requires *folinic acid*.

Dosage and administration. Daily requirements of folic acid are much less than 1 mg, and deficiencies can be corrected by administering that amount orally or parenterally. However, folic acid is often administered in oral doses of 5 to 20 mg daily, and its sodium salt is injected intramuscularly or deep into a subcutaneous site in doses of 5 to 15 mg daily. Maintenance therapy of 0.1 mg to 1 mg is adequate for prophylaxis against folic acid deficiency, but keeping the patient on a proper diet containing such food sources of folate as fresh green leafy vegetables, liver, and yeast is the preferred prophylactic measure.

Iron dextran injection USP (Imferon)

Actions and indications. This injectable iron complex is effective for treating patients with iron deficiency anemia in whom oral iron therapy is undesirable. These include patients who cannot tolerate gastrointestinal irritation, or who are unable to absorb iron adequately through the intestinal mucosa. Patients who cannot be depended on to take oral iron, or who have continued chronic bleeding and require rapid replenishment of storage iron, may also require parenteral iron.

Adverse effects, cautions, and contraindi-

cations. Minor side-effects include headache, nausea, shivering, rash, and itching. Joints of rheumatoid arthritis patients may become red and swollen. Patients who have a history of hypersensitivity to parenteral iron or who react adversely to a small test dose should not be treated, because fatal anaphylactic reactions have resulted. Extreme caution is required in patients with impaired liver function.

Dosage and administration. To avoid iron overloading (hemosiderosis), the total dosage is calculated in terms of the patient's body

weight and hemoglobin level. The daily maximum dosage for average-sized adults is 5 ml (250 mg of iron) and proportionately less for smaller adults and children. Intramuscular injections are made into the upper outer quadrant of the buttocks by a technique (Z-track injection; see Chap. 3) intended to avoid leakage into subcutaneous tissues with soreness, staining, and inflammation at the injection site. Intravenous administration may also be employed in some selected cases.

References

Beal RW: Hematinics. I: Pathophysiological and clinical aspects. Drugs 2:190, 1971

Beal RW: Hematinics. II: Clinical pharmacological and therapeutic aspects. Drugs 2:207, 1971

Callander ST: Treatment of iron deficiency. Clin Haematol 11:327, 1982

Crosby WH: Who needs iron? N Engl J Med 297:543, 1977

Finch CA: Drugs effective in iron-deficiency and other hypochromic anemias. In Gilman AG, Goodman LS, Gilman A (eds): Goodman and Gilman's The Pharmacological Basis of Therapeutics 6th ed, pp 1315–1330. New York, Macmillan, 1980

Giorgio AJ: Current concepts of iron metabolism and the iron deficiency anemias. Med Clin North Am 54:1399, 1970

Goldberg L: Treatment of iron deficiency with parenteral iron. In Crosby WH (ed): Iron—A Symposium. New York, Medcom, 1972

Haut A: Iron deficiency anemia. Am Fam Physician 11:136, 1975

Herbert V: Oral iron therapy. In Crosby WH (ed): Iron— A Symposium. New York, Medcom, 1972

Herbert V: Anemias. Curr Concepts Nutr 5:79, 1977

Hillman RS: Vitamin B_{12}, folic acid, and the treatment of megaloblastic anemias. In Gilman AG, Goodman LS, Gilman A (eds): Goodman and Gilman's The Pharmacological Basis of Therapeutics, 6th ed, pp 1331–1346. New York, Macmillan, 1980

Hofferand AV (ed): Megaloblastic anemia. Clin Hematol 5:471, 1976

Mays T et al: IV iron–dextran therapy in the treatment of anemias occurring in surgical, gynecologic, and obstetric patients. Surg Gynecol Obstet 143:381, 1976

McCurdy PR: B_{12} shots. Flip side. JAMA 231:289, 1975

Modell C, Beck J: Long-term desferrioxamine therapy in thalassemia. Ann NY Acad Sci 232:201, 1974

Savin MA: A practical approach to the treatment of iron deficiency. Ration Drug Ther 11:1, 1977

Scott DE, Pritchard JA: Iron deficiency in healthy young college women. JAMA 199:897, 1967

Woodruff CW: Iron deficiency in infancy and childhood. Pediatr Clin North Am 24:85, 1977

Section 6

Drugs
that
modulate
the inflammatory
and immune
responses

The chapters of this section deal mainly with drugs that act in many ways to relieve signs and symptoms of inflammation and to alter the immune response. The inflammatory and immune responses to injury or invaders are vital natural responses that protect the body from some of the many stressors to which it is exposed. These responses release potent pharmacologically active chemicals that produce many beneficial and protective effects, but that also produce some of the signs and symptoms of disease (*e.g.*, fever) that may be excessive and deleterious in themselves. In addition, these responses sometimes go awry, mostly for reasons that are still largely unknown. Autoimmune diseases are examples.

Many drugs are available to alleviate the unwanted signs and symptoms of these responses. This section begins with a review of the inflammatory and immune responses to provide a background for understanding some drugs that directly affect these responses (Chap. 36). The chapters that follow describe the nonsteroidal anti-inflammatory drugs, some of which are more commonly called antipyretic–analgesic agents, which are used to manage many types of pain and fever (Chaps. 37 and 38), other anti-arthritis drugs that intervene in the inflammatory response (Chap. 38), antihistamines used in allergic disorders (Chap. 39), and drugs used to manage bronchial asthma and other forms of chronic obstructive pulmonary disease (Chap. 40).

Earlier chapters have already discussed other aspects of some of these drugs, and of others, that act on the inflammatory and immune responses. For example, the adrenal corticosteroids, which are used in acute exacerbations of arthritic and allergic disease, have been described in detail in Chapter 21. Chapter 12 described drugs used in the chemotherapy of cancer, many of which suppress the patient's immune system as a serious and unwanted side-effect. That chapter also indicated that therapeutic use can be made of this immunosuppresive property of some of these drugs: agents such as *azathioprine* (Imuran) and the recently approved drug *cyclosporine* (Sandimmune) are used to prevent rejection of renal and other organ transplants by the host's immune system.

The *exact* functioning of these responses is not yet completely understood, and new information is continually being obtained by research studies. The potential impact of manipulation of these mechanisms to alleviate suffering and disease is phenomenal, and makes the study of this somewhat complicated system very exciting.

Review of the inflammatory and immune responses

36

The human body is equipped with several barriers and defenses to protect it from external stressors. Whether these stressors are bacteria, viruses, or other foreign invaders; trauma, or merely extremes of environment, the defenses are basically the same.

The body's first line of defense is the skin, which acts as a physical barrier to protect the internal tissues and organs of the body. Glands in the skin also secrete chemicals that ward off many invaders. Finally, a whole array of bacteria, called the normal flora, live on the skin and destroy many potential invaders.

The mucous membrane that lines the gastrointestinal and respiratory tracts constitutes the next line of defense. The mucous membrane is not only a physical barrier, but it also secretes a sticky substance, mucus, that traps invaders and inactivates them for later destruction and removal. The respiratory tract is lined with cilia that move captured invaders toward the upper parts of the tract for removal by sneezes or coughs. Some invaders of the respiratory tract may reach the throat and be swallowed. Like many other foreign invaders that enter the gastrointestinal tract, they may be inactivated by the stomach acid. If an invader manages to get past these defenses, or if injury occurs to underlying tissues, the inflammatory response and, in some cases, the immune response, are activated to overcome the invader or to initiate reactions that lead to healing of an injury and return of the body to a homeostatic state.

The inflammatory response

The inflammatory response is the local response of the body to invasion or injury. Any insult to the body that injures cells or tissues will set into action a series of events and chemical reactions (Fig. 36-1). The cell injury causes the activation of a chemical in the plasma called *Hageman factor*. The role of Hageman factor (also called factor XII)

in initiating the intrinsic clotting process and fibrinolysis has already been mentioned in Chapter 34. Activated Hageman factor also activates the kinin system: it activates *kallikrein,* a substance found in the tissues, and this in turn causes *kininogen* to be converted to *bradykinin*. Activated kallikrein also sets off reactions that lead to the activation of the first component of *complement* (see below).

Bradykinin is very active pharmacologically. It causes vasodilation to bring more blood to the injured area; it increases capillary permeability, which allows blood proteins and white blood cells to escape into the injured tissue; it stimulates nerve endings and causes pain, which alerts the organism to the insult; and it activates an enzyme that releases *arachidonic acid* from cell membranes. This in turn leads to the synthesis of a number of arachidonic acid derivatives that also contribute to the inflammatory response. The identification of the mediators of the inflammatory response is a new and rapidly changing area of investigation; the present account should not be taken as either the final or the complete story of the inflammatory response. Among the arachidonic acid derivatives are two classes of chemicals, the *prostaglandins* (PGs) and the *leukotrienes* (LTs). PGI_2, like bradykinin, causes vasodilation; other PGs, in appropriate concentrations, produce vasoconstriction and in other ways oppose the inflammatory response. The leukotrienes, like the prostaglandins, differ in their properties; included among these is the ability to increase capillary permeability, to attract leukocytes (a process referred to as *chemotaxis*), and to cause neutrophils, one type of leukocyte, to become active phagocytes that engulf and remove foreign particles and debris at the site of injury. Some leukotrienes have also recently been found to be the "slow-reacting substance of anaphylaxis" (see Chap. 39).

At the same time that all this is occurring, *histamine* is released from mast cells in the injured tissues. Like bradykinin, histamine causes vasodilation, increases capillary permeability, and causes pain.

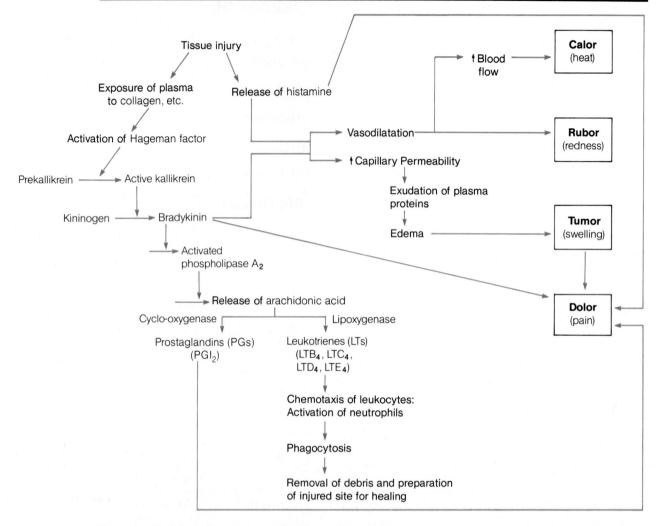

Figure 36-1. The inflammatory response in relation to the four cardinal signs of inflammation.

The clinical picture of inflammation may be described by four Latin words: *calor* (heat), *rubor* (redness), *tumor* (swelling), and *dolor* (pain). Figure 36-1 shows the origin of these signs and symptoms in relation to the events described above: redness and heat are produced by the increase in flow of warm blood to the area; swelling, by the increased capillary permeability, which leads to edema; and pain, by the actions of histamine and bradykinin on nerve endings, and by the pressure resulting from the swelling. These signs and symptoms are produced by various insults: lacerations, scratches of the skin, penetration of the skin by a splinter, or exposure of a part of the body to ionizing radiation or to extremes of temperature that cause frostbite or thermal burns.

Invasion of internal body structures by such organisms as bacteria or viruses produces the same set of responses. Although the signs and symptoms may appear in such cases to be different, careful study reveals that they are the same. For instance, a patient with viral or bacterial pneumonia will present with rales or fluid in the lungs produced by local vasodilation and by increased capillary permeability in the lungs; an increase in serum neutrophils produced by the activation of these white blood cells; pain produced by bradykinin and histamine, as well as by the swelling of tissues with edema fluid; and increased body temperature, or fever. This form of *calor* (heat) is actually produced in a different way from local heat at the site of an injury. Fever is produced by a substance released from macrophages in response to an invader. This substance has been called "endogenous pyrogen," but recent research has shown that it is a substance called an *interleukin*, a member of a class of hormonelike mediators (called *lymphokines*) produced by lymphocytes, neutrophils, and macrophages. This substance acts on neurons in the hypothalamus to "reset" the body's thermostat, thus raising body temperature. This increase in temperature acts as a catalyst for many of the body's chemical reactions that, when stimulated, help to fight against the invader.

Other chemicals can become activated when the inflammatory response continues, and it is their actions that can destroy local cells and tissues. Such destruction will release *lysosomal enzymes,* which destroy other cells and lead to increased release of destructive enzymes; a vicious cycle can consequently develop. Many inflammatory diseases are examples of these uncontrolled cycles. In fact, the signs and symptoms that health-care professionals see in many disease states are the result of the inflammatory response. Many of the drugs described in succeeding chapters act to break these cycles, allowing the body to respond more appropriately to the underlying problem.

The immune response

The next line of defense within the body is the immune system, which inactivates large molecules, called *antigens,* and destroys "nonself" cells. Because of its wide range of activities, this system is responsible for protecting the body from invaders, mutant cells, and old cells. This important function of protection from bacteria, viruses, and cancers also brings with it the problems of autoimmune diseases, transplant rejections, and some of the changes associated with aging. To understand the pharmacologic manipulation of the immune system, it is necessary to understand how this system normally functions.

T cells

Stem cells in the bone marrow give rise to two types of immature lymphocytes called pro-T cells and pro-B cells (Fig. 36-2). The pro-T cells leave the bone marrow and travel to the thymus gland (thus the name T cells), a bilobar gland located under the sternum, where they are somehow programmed to recognize "self." Some T cells become "helper T cells" and are responsible for potentiating the immune responses in the body. Other T cells become "suppressor T cells," and are responsible for turning off the immune responses when their work is done. T cells migrate to lymphatic tissue and various body tissues, where they monitor the body for the presence of "nonself" cells—for example, mutant cells, cells invaded by viruses, and aged cells. Some authorities estimate that the T-cell system protects the body from cancerlike mutant cells two or three times every day.

B cells

It is not known exactly where the pro-B cells are programmed to recognize specific antigens—possibilities include the bone marrow itself, or the liver or spleen. They are called B cells because, in chickens, they are programmed in an organ near the gastrointestinal tract called the bursa of Fabricius. Mammals do not have such an organ. Once programmed, these cells migrate to lymphatic tissue throughout the body where they are arranged in *clones,* or clusters of similarly programmed cells. Many researchers feel that humans are born with all the clones that they will ever have, which means that people are genetically equipped to deal with specific antigens and cannot develop specific defenses to any other antigens. If true, this would explain why certain allergies, diseases,

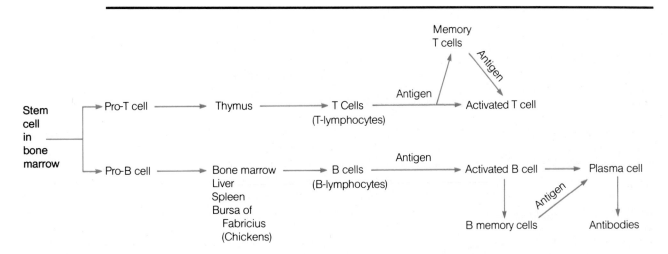

Figure 36-2. The components of the immune system. Bone marrow stem cells give rise to pro-T cells and pro-B cells, each of which is programmed to recognize a specific antigen and to react in a characteristic manner to this antigen.

and cancers tend to run in families. The B cells wait in these clones for exposure to their specific antigen, which triggers their activity.

Types of immunity

Humoral immunity

Each B cell recognizes a specific antigen. Antigens are large molecules with specific sites (*epitopes*) on the surface that react with appropriately programmed B cells. Once the antigen reacts with the B cells, the B cells in the clone can differentiate into *plasma cells,* which are antibody-producing cells, or into *memory cells,* which store the memory of the exposure to antigen and produce one type of *immunoglobulin* (antibody) called IgG, which is strong and long-lasting. The plasma cells, which are busily making antibodies, produce a type of immunoglobulin called IgM, which is made rapidly and has a short half-life. This system allows for a rapid and more vigorous response to the antigen if it should be encountered again. Clinically, this is seen most frequently in patients with repeated exposures to allergens, which elicit an immune response. Each exposure brings a greater and more intense reaction.

Once the antibody (Ab) has been produced, it combines with the antigen (Ag) to form an antigen–antibody (Ag–Ab) complex. In some cases this interaction will destroy, or *lyse,* the antigen. If the Ag is not destroyed, the formation of the complex will activate a cascading series of chemical reactions involving eleven factors, called the *complement system.* This series of reactions forms a tight ring of molecules around the Ag–Ab complex, a factor which could destroy the complex. It also generates

chemotactic factors that cause an aggressive inflammatory reaction at the site of the Ag–Ab complex, which allows the phagocytes to reach the area and destroy the invader, as in any inflammatory response (Fig. 36-3). These activities of the immune response are manifested clinically when the Ag–Ab complexes precipitate out of the blood into small capillary systems, such as those in the joints, skin, eyes, and kidneys. When the complexes precipitate into one of these areas, the area shows the four cardinal signs of the inflammatory responses: redness, swelling, heat, and pain. In the joints, this is manifested as arthritis; in the skin, as rashes, hives, or some other type of lesion; in the eye, as uveitis and vascular changes; in the kidneys, as progressive renal failure. Drugs can be given to block or suppress such deleterious immune or inflammatory responses. They alleviate the signs and symptoms of these responses, and some can prevent tissue damage from occurring as a result of prolonged inflammatory or immune responses.

Cell-mediated immunity

T cells do not produce antibodies (Fig. 36-4). Therefore, they do not depend on a supply of complement or on stored memory for their protective activity. The T cell, on recognition of a nonself cell, will respond in a number of ways: it may proliferate to form memory T cells, which can later respond with an accelerated activity against similar foreign cells; it may release lymphotoxins, powerful chemicals that destroy the foreign cell; it may release lymphokines that have chemotactic properties to attract macrophages and other phagocytes to the area to engulf and kill the foreign cell; it may release another lymphokine

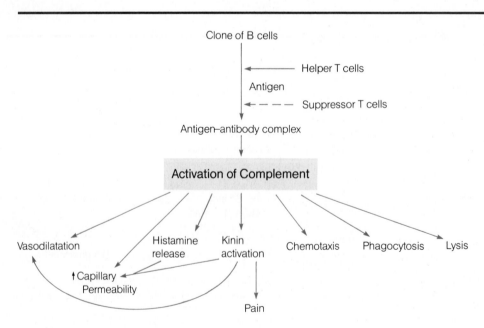

Figure 36-3. The humoral immune response.

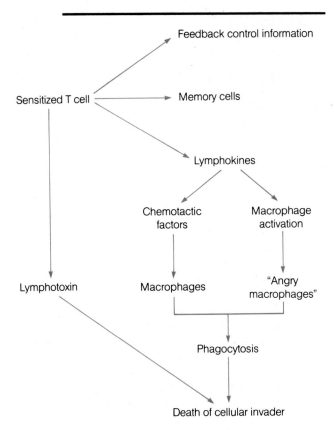

Figure 36-4. The cell-mediated immune response. Activation of a T cell by a "nonself" cell results in responses that destroy the foreign cell.

Thus, many drugs used to inhibit one part of the immune system or the inflammatory response will interfere with the body's response to invaders. Suppression of the inflammatory response, for example, allows antigens such as bacteria to enter the body and proliferate unchecked. Blocking T-cell activity removes the body's protection from cancerous cells, and also interferes with the control system of the humoral immune system.

References

Bullock B: Immunity. In Bullock B, Rosendahl P: Pathophysiology Adaptations and Alterations in Function, pp 109–136. Boston, Little, Brown & Co, 1984

Goetzl EJ: Leukocyte recognition and metabolism of leukotrienes. Fed Proc 42:3128, 1983

Goetzl EJ, Kaplan AP: Lipid and peptide mediators of inflammation. Fed Proc 42:3119, 1983

Kaplan AP: Hageman factor-dependent pathways: Mechanism of initiation and bradykinin formation. Fed Proc 42:3123, 1983

Samuelsson B: Leukotrienes: Mediators of immediate hypersensitivity reactions and inflammation. Science 220:568, 1983

that stimulates macrophages to become aggressive phagocytes called "angry macrophages" (because their activity is so aggressive); and, finally, it may send messages into a controlling loop that regulates the activation and suppression of the system. The exact control and function of this system is not clearly understood. However, it is known that the thymus gland produces hormones that influence the growth and activity of T cells, and that other cells in the body can suppress or excite T-cell activity. Future research should solve many of the mysteries of this system. It is known from clinical experience that T cells are responsible for tissue transplant rejection, for some aspects of the deterioration that accompanies aging, and for various autoimmune diseases. In each case the T cells, rightly (transplant cells) or wrongly (old or altered body cells), recognize the cells as foreign and destroy them. However, information on how to inhibit an undesirable or deleterious T-cell response selectively, without interfering with the cellular immune processes that protect the body against pathogens, is still very limited. Where it is known, the mechanism of action of the drugs discussed in the remaining chapters of this section will be described in terms of the events in the immune and inflammatory responses described here.

Chapter 37

Analgesic–antipyretics

General considerations

This chapter will describe the group of drugs most commonly used in this country. People do not need a prescription to obtain products made up of *aspirin*+, *acetaminophen*+, or combinations of these analgesics with other agents, such as caffeine and antacids (see Tables 37-1 and 37-2). This is desirable, because people should be able to purchase these relatively safe pain relievers without having to visit a physician for diagnosis of every ache and pain.

The main advantage of these drugs over the narcotic analgesics discussed in Chapter 51 is that they do not cause physical dependence. Even when taken daily for many months for relief of chronic pain, tolerance to their pain-relieving property does not develop. Another advantage is that therapeutic doses do not ordinarily cause drowsiness, euphoria, or other central nervous system effects.

For these reasons, this group is often referred to as the "nonnarcotic" or "nonaddicting" analgesics. Because they are effective mainly against pain of mild to moderate degree, they are also called "mild" or "weak" analgesics. All these terms are somewhat misleading, because they do not adequately indicate how very effective these drugs actually are for relief of the most common types of pain; that they *can* be abused; and that overdoses can produce serious toxicity—many children and adults are fatally poisoned each year. Thus, it seems best to characterize these drugs in terms of the two types of pharmacologic effects that are obtained with small therapeutic doses—that is, simply as analgesic–antipyretics.

Effectiveness

It is, of course, true that aspirin and similar analgesics are not nearly as effective against some types of severe pain as are the natural and synthetic opioids (see Chap. 51), which produce greater maximal analgesic effects. They

are not, for example, very effective for control of pain that stems from spasm of such visceral smooth muscles as the ureters or bile ducts (*e.g.*, in renal or biliary colic). Sharp pain from severe trauma or burns is also best managed with morphine or meperidine (Demerol) rather than with these analgesic–antipyretics. The analgesic–antipyretics work most effectively against pain that is associated with an inflammatory response.

This does not mean, however, that these nonnarcotic drugs are used only in minor illnesses or that the patient for whom they are ordered is not suffering. The physician may even use these analgesics to manage pain in cancer patients before turning to such drugs as codeine, meperidine, or morphine. Likewise, in chronically painful conditions such as Buerger's disease and rheumatoid arthritis, salicylates and similar agents are frequently used to provide pain relief. Because these drugs are available without a prescription, and because they are used so commonly by the public, patients for whom these drugs are ordered may feel that their pain has been underrated or that they have not been "taken seriously" by their physician. Thus, patient teaching should include reinforcement of the concept that these drugs are efficacious when used as directed, as well as dangerous when used in a greater than recommended dosage.

Abuse potential

Products containing aspirin, acetaminophen, and similar substances have a relatively low abuse potential compared to that of the potent narcotic analgesics, because these drugs do not tend to tranquilize or to produce other mental states that an abuse-prone person might want to seek habitually. However, some people with personality problems have abused over-the-counter (OTC) pain products of this type by continuing to take them in excessively high daily doses for prolonged periods. In such situations, these drugs, usually considered to be safe and nonaddicting, *can* cause serious chronic toxicity affecting such vital tissues as the kidneys, liver, and blood.

Self-medication

Although the self-administration of aspirin and similar antipain products is not ordinarily dangerous or addicting, people *do* need advice in choosing the product that is safest for them and best suited for relief of their pain. Unfortunately, the conflicting claims of the competing manufacturers of OTC analgesic products tend to confuse people instead of enlightening them. The Federal Trade Commission has, in fact, called many of the claims made for nonprescription pain-relief products misleading and deceptive. Thus, patients should be taught which substances are safe, effective and inexpensive, and which products are best suited to their own particular needs.

The salicylates

The salicylates, the most important group of nonaddicting analgesic–antipyretic drugs, are derivatives of salicylic acid, and include acetylsalicylic acid (aspirin), sodium salicylate, salicylamide, methyl salicylate, and many others (Table 37-1). Salicylate production has risen to over 40 million pounds annually, and Americans are said to take billions of aspirin tablets daily.

Hippocrates and other ancient physicians employed plants now known to contain natural salicylates. These include species of willow and poplar, and a species of *Gaultheria*, from which oil of wintergreen (methyl salicylate) is obtained. Extracts of willow bark came back into use for treating fevers late in the 18th century (the word *salicylate* is derived from *salix*, the Latin name for the willow tree). Synthetic salicylates were first prepared

Table 37–1. Analgesics and antipyretics*

Official or generic name	Trade name or synonym	Usual adult dosage and administration (oral, except as noted)
Salicylates and related drugs		
Aspirin USP	Acetylsalicylic acid	300–650 mg q 4 hr
Choline salicylate	Arthropan liquid	870 mg q 3–4 hr (5220–6960 mg/day maximum)
Diflunisal	Dolobid	250–1000 mg, at various intervals (1500 mg/day maximum)
Magnesium salicylate	Durasal; Magan	600 mg bid or qid (9.6 g/day maximum)
Methyl salicylate USP	Oil of wintergreen	Topical
Salicylamide	o-Hydroxybenzamide; Uromide	325–650 mg tid or qid
Salicylic acid USP	o-Hydroxybenzoic acid	Topical
Salsalate	Salicylsalicylic acid	325–1000 mg bid or tid
Sodium salicylate USP	Uracel 5	325–650 mg tid
Sodium thiosalicylate	Arthrolate; Tusal	IM: 100 mg q 3–4 hr × 2 days, then 100 mg/day for acute gout; 50–100 mg/day on alternate days for muscular pain; 100–150 mg q 4–6 hr × 3 days, then 100 mg bid
Para-aminophenol, coal tar, or aniline derivatives		
Acetaminophen USP	N-acetyl-*p*-aminophenol (in Tylenol); paracetamol	300–650 mg q 4 hr
Phenacetin	Acetophenetidin	150–300 mg bid
Pyrazolon derivatives		
Antipyrine		Topical (eye and ear)
Oxyphenbutazone USP	Oxalid; Tandearil	300–400 mg per day in divided doses
Phenylbutazone USP	Azolid; Butazolidin	300–600 mg per day in divided doses

* See also Chapter 38 for listing of other drugs with these actions, as well as with potent anti-inflammatory activity.

about 110 years ago. Aspirin itself was introduced at the turn of this century as a substitute for sodium salicylate, which has a disagreeable taste and causes a high incidence of gastrointestinal disturbance.

Pharmacologic effects

The salicylates act both centrally and peripherally to produce their varied therapeutic and toxic effects. Those most useful in treatment are the *analgesic–antipyretic* and *anti-inflammatory–antirheumatic* actions. The results of salicylate administration are dose-related to a large extent. Their pain-relieving and fever-reducing actions are readily brought by administration of low doses. Relatively large doses are required to bring about the anti-inflammatory action desired in rheumatic conditions.* Massive overdosage causes complex and potentially dangerous metabolic effects.

Analgesia

It is interesting to speculate whether aspirin, the most widely used of all analgesics, would have been discovered by today's drug screening methods in animals. In fact, laboratory tests for analgesic activity in human subjects do not reveal any consistently significant rise in the pain perception threshold after administration of salicylates. Nevertheless, several *clinical* studies have confirmed the effectiveness of aspirin for relief of pain in medical and surgical patients. In one study of patients suffering moderate pain caused by cancerous tumors, aspirin proved to be superior to all other nonprescription analgesics and more effective than various prescription products, including propoxyphene (Darvon) and codeine. It has also been shown to be effective for relief of pain following surgery and in the postpartum period.

In actual practice, small doses of aspirin—the amount contained in two 300-mg tablets—seem to be most effective for relief of mild to moderate pain that originates in the joints, skeletal muscles, skin, and connective tissues.

This dose is readily absorbed from the upper gastrointestinal tract to produce effective plasma levels in about 30 minutes. Relief of the general malaise of respiratory viral infections can be maintained by repeating this small dose every 2 to 4 hours. Similar small doses provide adequate relief of most types of headaches (Chap. 38), musculoskeletal pain, and other ailments, including dental discomfort. Severe arthritic disorders (see below, and Chap. 38) require larger doses to reduce inflammation. Most women do not experience significant relief from dysmenorrhea when they take salicylates, but some

---

* Large doses of salicylates also exert a *uricosoric* (uric acid-excreting) action. However, low doses interfere with uric acid excretion. Because of this dual dose–response, and because newer drugs are more efficacious, salicylates are rarely used for this purpose today in the treatment of gout (see Drug digest and drug treatment of gout, Chap. 38).

of the newer nonsteroidal anti-inflammatory drugs described in Chapter 38 are often very effective.

Occasionally, nurses may be asked which of the various heavily advertised analgesic products acts most rapidly and effectively. Despite the loud and conflicting claims that one or another headache remedy is most rapidly absorbed, the question of which one acts fastest is of no real clinical significance. When small doses of aspirin are being employed for relief of minor pain, as in most conditions, it matters little whether the salicylate is in solid or liquid form or whether it is administered alone or combined with other substances, including so-called buffer systems. All produce the desired pain relief in essentially the same relatively short time, and therefore the nurse is justified in recommending to almost all people the purchase of the least expensive product available— preferably, plain aspirin USP.

Site and manner of analgesic action. Aspirin and other salicylates have traditionally been believed to exert their pain-relieving effects by actions at sites within the central nervous system. Because these drugs do not cause drowsiness or other disturbances in consciousness or in mental functions and exert no significant effects on mood or emotional state, these central sites are believed to differ from those of the potent narcotic analgesics (Chap. 51). Thus, they are thought to act, not on the brain stem reticular-activating system, nor on the limbic system and the nervous pathways connecting these areas with the cerebral cortex (Chap. 44), but at other subcortical sites. The thalamus and hypothalamus have, for various reasons, been thought to be the primary sites of both the analgesic and antipyretic activity of aspirin and related drugs.

However, recent evidence concerning the role of prostaglandins and other arachidonic acid derivatives in inflammation (see below, and Chap. 36) has been interpreted to indicate that the peripheral actions of aspirin may play a primary part in producing pain relief. This may be of greater significance in explaining aspirin's effectiveness in pain associated with inflammation. One widely held view is that the salicylates act mainly by reducing the responsiveness of peripherally located pain receptors to stimulation by such substances as bradykinin and prostaglandin E_1 (see below). The ability of aspirin to lessen the sensitivity of nerve endings to the pain-producing effects of bradykinin has been linked to drug-induced inhibition of the enzyme cyclo-oxygenase, often referred to as prostaglandin synthetase (Fig. 36-1). This results in reduced formation of some prostaglandins, including prostaglandin E_1, a substance that is thought to sensitize the pain-responsive peripheral nerve endings to the action of bradykinin and other chemical mediators released locally by irritation, injury, and inflammation.

Antipyresis

The *antipyretic* (or fever-reducing) *effect* of the salicylates is often useful for making a febrile patient more comfortable. The salicylates do not reduce normal body temperature. There is some controversy as to the desirability of reducing fever. As noted in Chapter 36, elevated body temperature can facilitate some of the body's immune reactions. In any case, it is always important to ascertain the underlying cause of fever and, where possible, to treat the cause—for example, with specific anti-infective drugs, if this is appropriate. However, the use of salicylates, cool baths, and other measures for symptomatic relief are sometimes desirable. This is especially true in young children who sometimes run very high temperatures that make them excessively restless and irritable, and may even precipitate convulsions. Often, after an antipyretic dose of aspirin has brought the temperature down 1° or 2°, the sick child can relax and fall asleep.

The antipyretic effect of the salicylates helps the body rid itself of the excess internal heat that has accumulated in hyperpyrexia. Normally, body temperature remains remarkably constant as the result of a delicate balance between the amount of heat being produced and the amount being lost. This dynamic equilibrium is under the control of heat-regulating centers located in the hypothalamus, which transmit impulses to cutaneous blood vessels, sweat glands, and other peripheral structures. Infections and other illnesses may interfere with the functioning of these thermoregulatory centers in ways that allow enough heat to build up in the body to cause fever.

The salicylates and other antipyretics are thought to make this central thermostat more responsive to the high internal heat of fever. As a result, this hypothalamic center then sends out more messages of a kind that leads to dilation of cutaneous blood vessels and increased sweat gland activity. The excess heat is then removed by radiation, conduction, evaporation, and other physical means. Just how the salicylates do this is still not well understood. Some scientists believe that aspirin acts directly on the hypothalamic thermoregulatory center to reset it when an infection has caused it to be set too high.

More recent evidence indicates that, in some cases at least, fever is caused by a substance called *endogenous pyrogen*, now identified more precisely as *interleukin-1*, one of the family of *lymphokines* released by leukocytes in response to bacterial invasion. This pyrogenic factor is believed to be carried by the circulatory system to discrete areas of the central nervous system, including the thermoregulatory center where it stimulates the synthesis and release of prostaglandins. Many prostaglandins are pyrogenic; fever is a side-effect of those prostaglandins that are given systemically as abortifacients (Chap. 23). It has thus been postulated that salicylates lower fever by interfering with the synthesis of the prostaglandin (PG) intermediaries in the fever-producing process.

Anti-inflammatory antirheumatic action

Large doses of salicylates are often remarkably effective for controlling many manifestations of acute and chronic connective tissue inflammatory disorders. In acute rheumatic fever, the response to salicylates is sometimes quite dramatic. Not only are pain and fever relieved, but the inflamed joints are also benefited. Heat, redness, and swelling are reduced, and the patient can move his limbs more readily. Restoration of mobility helps to prevent or delay crippling, even though the salicylates do not actually halt the underlying disease process, and rheumatologists doubt that these drugs prevent cardiac damage. (The place of salicylates in the management of acute and chronic rheumatic conditions is discussed further in Chapter 38.)

Despite considerable study, the mechanism by which salicylates ease rheumatic joint symptoms is still not completely understood. It is known that the salicylates inhibit the enzyme cyclo-oxygenase, the first enzyme in the sequence of reactions by which PGs are synthesized from arachidonic acid (Fig. 36-1). It is also known that the ability of various anti-inflammatory drugs to inhibit this enzyme and to lower body levels of PG correlates well with their anti-inflammatory activity. As explained above, and in Chapter 36, the PGs are important mediators of inflammation, and augment the pain-producing and vasodilatory effects of bradykinin, another mediator of inflammation. Thus, the anti-inflammatory actions of salicylates are probably mostly attributable to their interference with the functioning of PGs and of bradykinin.

These and other effects on the basic biochemistry of inflammation may account for the suppression by salicylates of the signs of acute arthritis: redness, heat, swelling, pain, and reduced joint mobility. However, these drugs do not block the formation of leukotrienes, another class of arachidonic acid derivatives that contributes to the immune response (Fig. 36-1), and they do not affect the unknown causes underlying the pathologic processes involved in rheumatoid arthritis and rheumatic fever (Chap. 38).

Aspirin–platelet effects

Aspirin has long been known to lengthen the bleeding time of some patients, even when taken in only small analgesic doses. This was attributed primarily to a possible drug-induced reduction in the biosynthesis of prothrombin and related clotting factors, and its significance was interpreted mainly in terms of the possible harm that might come to patients with blood dyscrasias or a tendency toward gastrointestinal bleeding, and to those who were simultaneously receiving oral anticoagulant medications of the coumarin class (see Adverse Effects, below).

However, aspirin-induced prolongation of bleeding time is now known to stem mainly from its ability to interfere with platelet aggregation. This early step in the formation of intravascular blood clots—particularly in arteries with damaged inner linings and exposed collagen fibers—is believed to be blocked by the inhibitory effects of aspirin on the release of ADP (adenosine diphosphate) by the platelets, and by its interference with the formation of such chemical mediators of platelet aggregation as endoperoxides and thromboxanes (Fig. 34-1). This action of aspirin and its possible prophylactic function in patients known to be prone to thromboembolic episodes and, particularly, for possible prevention of strokes and recurrences of acute myocardial infarction, have been discussed in Chapter 34.

Adverse effects

The salicylates cause few ill effects when taken in the small doses usually employed for relief of minor pain. The much larger doses administered in acute rheumatic fever and chronic rheumatoid arthritis almost invariably cause discomfort that must be counteracted in various ways. Massive overdosage results in severe salicylate toxicity, which is often difficult to treat successfully and sometimes ends fatally.

The usual analgesic dosage of aspirin is well tolerated by most people. However, allergic hypersensitivity is not uncommon, and may lead to skin and gastrointestinal disturbances of some severity. Skin symptoms include redness, rashes, and urticarial (hives)-type reactions. Such edematous swellings can be extremely dangerous when they develop in respiratory tract mucous membranes. Asthmatic patients are especially susceptible to edema of the pharynx and larynx, and death from asphyxia has been reported in patients taking a single aspirin tablet (see Chap. 39).

Gastrointestinal disturbances

Gastrointestinal disturbances may be more common than was once suspected, after even small doses of salicylates. The mechanism by which these disturbances are produced is unclear, but the fact that other PG inhibitor drugs (Chap. 38) also produce this effect suggests that it may result from loss of protective PGs in the gastric mucosa.

Most people seem able to take one or two aspirins occasionally without any apparent stomach upset. Results of studies by gastroenterologists have established, however, that gastric bleeding from aspirin is fairly common. Bleeding in most patients taking repeated doses of aspirin for rheumatoid arthritis is relatively slight. Occult, or hidden, bleeding may be discovered only during a search for the cause of an iron deficiency anemia that develops in such a patient. Heavy overt bleeding is uncommon, and occurs mainly in patients with peptic ulcer, atrophic gastritis, or esophagitis. Salicylates should be avoided in such patients and used only with caution in patients with a history of hematemesis or even of heartburn.

Gastrointestinal distress is most likely to occur in patients receiving the very large daily doses of aspirin or sodium salicylate required for symptomatic relief of acute rheumatic fever and rheumatoid arthritis (Chap. 38). The usual daily dosage is 5 g to 10 g, administered in six doses of about 1 g to 1.5 g each. Directions for spacing salicylate dosage at 4-hour intervals day and night should be carefully followed to keep the drug at plasma levels that are effective but not toxic. Sometimes a patient

forgets to take a dose and then tries to make it up with extra medication, only to suffer stomach pain, nausea, and vomiting. Such symptoms can largely be avoided by taking the medication after meals or with milk and crackers rather than with water. Moderate amounts of sodium bicarbonate taken with the salicylates also help to allay stomach irritation, but the extra intake of sodium and the potential for systemic alkalosis may contraindicate this practice in certain patients.

Pharmaceutical products of several types are claimed to be less likely to cause gastric irritation than ordinary aspirin tablets. Enteric-coated tablets, for example, are less irritating than *non*coated tablets. However, the aspirin in such tablets is absorbed slowly and incompletely, or occasionally not at all. Most commonly, aspirin is combined with buffering agents such as aluminum glycinate and magnesium carbonate, the Dialminate of the proprietary product Bufferin. Results of some studies indicate that such buffering has reduced the frequency and severity of gastric distress in patients who had previously reacted adversely to straight aspirin products. Other scientists say that the addition of such buffering substances to aspirin serves no useful purpose. They claim that incorporating a tiny amount of alkali into an aspirin tablet does little to prevent stomach pain or bleeding in salicylate-sensitive patients. The difference in cost of these products can be enormous. The questionable value of these additional coatings and buffers should be considered if finances are a problem for the patient.

Aspirin presented in *solubilized form* is preferred for use in patients who regularly suffer from gastric irritation, dyspepsia, and bleeding. An aqueous alkaline solution in effervescent form tends to leave the stomach more rapidly than ordinary aspirin and there are, of course, no particles to lodge in the gastric mucosa to produce high local concentrations. However, proprietary products of the Alka-Seltzer type contain quantities of sodium that may be undesirable for some people, and they are relatively quite expensive. The use of such so-called "stomach-settling" alkalinizing products by patients who do *not* require the analgesic activity of salicylates has also been criticized as wasteful and potentially harmful.

Salicylism

Patients with acute rheumatic fever and others in whom the dosage of aspirin is being pushed should be watched carefully for other signs of early salicylism in addition to gatrointestinal upset. Dosage is usually raised until tinnitus (a ringing and roaring in the ears) occurs. When this toxic sign appears, the daily dosage is reduced—usually by about 10 grains (600 mg)—to a level that is effective yet tolerable. Continued administration of excessive salicylate dosage could lead to deafness and to blurring and dimness of vision, diplopia, and other signs of auditory and optic nerve damage resembling cinchonism, the syndrome caused by quinine and quinidine overdosage (Chaps. 10 and 30).

Salicylate poisoning

Salicylate poisoning occurs most commonly in preschool children who are both most prone to take massive accidental overdoses and most susceptible to dangerous drug-induced metabolic derangements. Acute intoxication is manifested by early signs of central nervous system stimulation, including a characteristically rapid respiration; later, complex acid–base imbalances and possible petechial bleeding may develop.

Hemorrhaging. Bleeding into the skin is caused in part by the anticoagulant action of salicylates, which act in this case like the coumarin-type drugs (Chap. 34) to reduce plasma prothrombin levels. (This is why patients on long-term anticoagulant therapy should be advised to consult their physician or nurse before taking salicylates.) As in overdosage of coumarin compounds, the antidote for hypoprothrombinemia is vitamin K. Thus, signs of bleeding may call for administration of phytonadione or a synthetic hemostatic substance with vitamin K activity. However, this will not counteract bleeding in patients with blood dyscrasias whose condition may be adversely affected by aspirin's tendency to reduce the stickiness of blood platelets. Such interference with platelet aggregation may prevent the formation of platelet plugs and thus prolong the bleeding time in some patients (see Chap. 34 and Fig. 34-2).

Acid–base imbalance. Much more difficult to treat are the complex biochemical imbalances that develop from salicylate overdosage. Most common in older children and adults is respiratory alkalosis. Infants, on the other hand, are very vulnerable to metabolic acidosis. Sometimes the patient swings between the two states or suffers from both simultaneously, and the physician must try to keep track of the fluid and electrolyte status by having frequent laboratory studies performed to check on blood acidity, serum carbon dioxide content, and serum levels of sodium and potassium as well as of salicylates. Dehydration as a result of excessive loss of body fluids is one factor that may produce a sharp rise in body temperature. Often, however, the high temperature that develops is a direct result of salicylate-induced stimulation of body metabolism. This has led some parents to administer more aspirin to feverish young children to reduce a paradoxical rise in their hyperpyrexia, which was actually induced by overdosage with the antipyretic drug.

Treatment. Intravenous fluids are used to correct acid–base imbalances and to keep the patient adequately hydrated. Parenteral solutions containing mixtures of physiologic saline solution, sodium bicarbonate, and dextrose are first administered to increase renal perfusion and to establish a urinary output. Solutions containing potassium and other electrolytes are then given as needed to restore ionic and acid-base equilibria.

Patients with severe acidosis may be given systemic alkalinizers such as sodium bicarbonate or sodium lactate solutions. These alkalinizers also increase the rate of renal excretion of salicylates. However, the sodium content of these solutions may be undesirable for patients with signs of heart failure. Thus, especially when hypokalemia is present, potassium salts may be used to alkalinize the urine.

An amine buffer, tromethamine (Tham), is also said to hasten salicylate elimination and to correct acidosis without adding sodium to the patient's system. Sometimes hemodialysis is used to lower dangerously high salicylate levels. When such equipment is not available, peritoneal dialysis with buffered isosmotic solutions of human albumin may be employed.

Other treatment measures include the use of calcium gluconate solution to stop tetanic spasms. Short-acting barbiturates may be given cautiously if convulsions occur. Respiratory depression may require artificial respiration and oxygen, but analeptics (see Chap. 47), which are seldom, if ever, indicated for *any* condition, should not be administered, because such stimulants are ineffective and may cause convulsions.

Prevention. Obviously, prevention of salicylate poisoning is more desirable than undertaking its difficult treatment. Public health nurses and those working in schools and elsewhere should take every opportunity to tell parents and older children that aspirin should not be given to small children without a physician's advice. The need to store salicylates properly should also be emphasized, and people with young children in the house should be advised to get rid of liniments containing oil of wintergreen, because methyl salicylate is the most toxic form of salicylate. The now mandatory use of containers that cannot be readily opened by youngsters should also help to lessen the incidence of salicylate poisoning, provided that the bottles are properly closed each time a therapeutic dose is removed. Remember that small children can be very adept at removing these bottle tops, and no one should feel safe with this drug around children. One of the best approaches to prevention is to teach children, from a very young age, to respect aspirin as a drug, not to call it "candy," and never to take it unless given to them by a parent or some other responsible adult.

Severe systemic effects of salicylates can often be prevented by emptying the patient's stomach as soon as possible. This may be done at home by inducing vomiting mechanically or with an emetic such as syrup of ipecac. If this fails, a physician may perform a gastric lavage or administer apomorphine subcutaneously (see Chap. 5).

Other salicylates

Various substances related to aspirin are claimed to be superior to the parent compound in one way or another. Choline salicylate is, for example, more water-soluble than aspirin and is claimed to cause less gastric irritation while being more rapidly absorbed. However, this and certain more exotic forms of salicylates do not seem to offer any significant advantages over aspirin that would warrant their higher cost.

Salicylamide, which is a component of some analgesic mixtures, also has little to recommend it as a partial replacement for a full dose of aspirin. It has a relatively rapid rate of absorption but is also rapidly eliminated without actually being converted to salicylate in the body. To retain its early analgesic effectiveness for several hours, this drug would have to be given in much higher doses than aspirin. Instead, the commercial products that contain salicylamide present it in relatively small amounts that are not likely to add any significant analgesic activity to that of the aspirin or other analgesic–antipyretic agents in the formulation.

Diflunisal (Dolobid) is a relatively new salicylate derivative. It appears to be more effective than aspirin in relieving the types of pain for which aspirin is effective, and it has a longer duration of action. It inhibits prostaglandin synthesis and is anti-inflammatory, but it is only weakly anti-pyretic. It shares most of aspirin's adverse effects and, like other forms of salicylates, is more expensive than aspirin.

Nonsalicylate analgesics

Other substances in addition to the salicylates possess properties that make them useful for relief of mild to moderate degrees of pain. Two of the earliest classes of chemicals synthesized—the para-aminophenols, or anilines, and the pyrazolons (Table 37-1)—were, like the salicylates, introduced as antipyretics late in the last century. Later, their analgesic action was recognized, and it is mainly for this purpose that some of them are still employed, either alone or in combination with salicylates.

Para-aminophenol (coal tar or aniline) analgesics

Actions and indications

Acetaminophen has become the most commonly employed drug of this class, having replaced phenacetin in essentially all headache products (Table 37-2). It is now often used alone as a substitute for aspirin in patients who are allergic to salicylates and who tend to wheeze or develop skin rashes when they take aspirin-containing products. Of course, atopic persons may also become hypersensitive to acetaminophen after a while. Similarly, although drop dosages of palatable liquid preparations are said to be safer than salicylates for febrile dehydrated children, acetaminophen is not free of acute toxicity when overdoses are taken. Clinically, acetaminophen is now con-

Table 37–2. Analgesic content of some combination products*

Product	Analgesic	Amount present (mg)	Other drug(s)
Alka-Seltzer	Aspirin	325	Sodium bicarbonate; citric acid
Anacin	Aspirin	400	Caffeine
A.S.A.	Aspirin	325	
Ascriptin	Aspirin	325	Aluminium hydroxide; magnesium hydroxide
Bromo-Seltzer	Acetaminophen	325	Sodium bicarbonate; citric acid
Bufferin	Aspirin	324	Aluminum glycinate; magnesium carbonate
Excedrin	Aspirin	250	Caffeine
	Acetaminophen	250	
P-A-C New Revised Formula Tablets	Aspirin	400	Caffeine
Vanquish	Aspirin	227	Caffeine
Caplets	Acetaminophen	194	Aluminum hydroxide; magnesium hydroxide

* The formulations of proprietary (over-the-counter) analgesic products are often changed without direct notice to the public.

sidered to be the analgesic–antipyretic of choice for children with viral infections or chicken pox. Aspirin use has been associated with the occurrence of Reye's syndrome, a potentially fatal complication of these infections involving the central nervous system and the liver. Although researchers cannot determine a direct link between aspirin use and the development of this syndrome, it is currently considered advisable to avoid the use of aspirin in these children. The increased use of acetaminophen may result in the more frequent appearance of acetaminophen toxicity. Hepatic necrosis has occurred in people who have ingested large amounts of acetaminophen (see below).

Acetaminophen may be preferred to aspirin in certain other clinical situations. It is less likely, for example, to cause gastric mucosal irritation, erosion, and bleeding. Thus, its use in patients with severe gastritis or active peptic ulcer may be more desirable than the administration of aspirin. However, it is more expensive than aspirin and may not have any real advantage for most people, who do not feel any stomach discomfort after taking one or two aspirin tablets with an amount of water adequate for readily dissolving the solid particles of the salicylate.

Acetaminophen does not interfere with blood clotting. Unlike aspirin, it does not affect platelet aggregation, prothrombin synthesis, or fibrinogen function. Thus, it may be preferred for use as an analgesic by patients with blood dyscrasias and by those taking anticoagulant drugs. However, like other drugs of this chemical class, acetaminophen may cause hemolytic anemia in patients sensitive to para-aminophenols (see below).

Acetaminophen may also be preferred to aspirin in patients with gout who require an analgesic for various other painful disorders. Unlike aspirin, which in small doses may interfere with uric acid excretion, acetaminophen does not antagonize the effects of the uricosuric agent probenecid (Chap. 38). The main disadvantage of this drug and of the others of this class in treating gout and rheumatoid arthritis is that they lack an adequate anti-inflammatory action. Acetaminophen is only a weak inhibitor of PG synthesis; this probably accounts for its lack of anti-inflammatory action, but it does not explain the mechanisms of its analgesic and antipyretic actions. Its inadequate anti-inflammatory action means that acetaminophen cannot be substituted for salicylates in the treatment of acute rheumatic fever even though, in theory, the danger of development of salicylism could be reduced if part of the high aspirin dosage were replaced by such para-aminophenols as acetaminophen and phenacetin.

Phenacetin (acetophenetidin) was, until recently, frequently found in combination with aspirin in remedies widely used by the public for relief of head, joint, and muscle pains and for dysmenorrhea. Phenacetin has analgesic and antipyretic activity of its own, but part of its effects are attributable to the action of its primary metabolite, acetaminophen. Although phenacetin is still available, mainly in APC formulations that contain codeine (see below) and are available only by prescription, it has been replaced by acetaminophen in virtually all OTC analgesic preparations in the United States.

The addition of mild opiate-type analgesics such as codeine or oxycodone to phenacetin or aspirin is rational drug therapy, because the two classes of analgesics cause different types of toxicity and produce analgesia by different mechanisms of action. Thus, unlike caffeine, the other component of the common APC (aspirin–phenacetin—caffeine) formulation, codeine adds desirable analgesic and sedative actions that increase the effectiveness of phenacetin, aspirin, and acetaminophen. The small amount of caffeine traditionally employed in such pain-relieving fixed-dosage combinations adds little if anything to the effectiveness of these products (see also the discussion of drug combinations for treating tension headaches, Chap. 38).

Acute and chronic toxicity

Analgesics of this chemical class seem quite safe when taken occasionally for relief of minor pain or fever. However, chronic toxicity affecting mainly the blood and kidneys has been known to develop in people who became habituated to the daily use of headache remedies containing certain of these drugs and who continued to take large amounts for long periods. Reports have appeared concerning acute liver damage and hepatic failure following the deliberate or accidental ingestion of acetaminophen in massive overdoses.

Injury to the liver is thought to result from the accumulation of a toxic metabolite of acetaminophen. The small amounts of this substance formed from ordinary therapeutic doses are inactivated by glutathione present in hepatic cells. However, large doses lead to production of more of the metabolite than can be bound by this sulfur-containing compound, and the excess binds to liver cell macromolecules to cause irreversible damage. Death of the hepatocytes often leads to central lobular necrosis. Initial anorexia, nausea, vomiting, and epigastric pain in the first few days after overdosage may be followed by late encephalopathy, coma, and death.

Results of animal studies suggest that the prompt administration of cysteamine can protect against liver damage. Oral administration of the sulfur-containing compound acetylcysteine (Mucomyst—140 mg/kg body weight, then 70 mg/kg q4 hr for 17 doses) as a 5% solution (see Chap. 40) reportedly has helped human victims of acetaminophen toxicity to recover. However, the most important measure is the immediate emptying of the stomach by gastric lavage, or by an emetic such as syrup of ipecac, followed by activated charcoal (Chap. 5). If acetylcysteine is to be given, it is important to remove any activated charcoal that may have been given previously because the charcoal will adsorb the acetylcysteine and prevent its absorption from the gastrointestinal tract.

Methemoglobinemia. This sometimes occurs when some part of the blood pigment hemoglobin is converted to methemoglobin by the oxidizing action of these drugs. *Acetanilid*, another drug of this group, is no longer employed because it has so great a propensity to cause methemoglobinemia. Because this abnormal blood pigment cannot carry oxygen to the tissues, the patient may suffer symptoms similar to those of anemia. The skin and fingernails may become bluish in color (cyanosis), and the patient may complain of dyspnea and chest pains. Sometimes, persons habituated to headache remedies such as the old formulation of Bromo-Seltzer, which contained acetanilid, kept taking the product to relieve head pain that was actually being *caused* by the drug-induced hypoxia.

The condition is readily reversed if it is detected early enough and the drug is withdrawn. Thus, patients who have a history of taking self-prescribed analgesics for pain should be assessed for signs of cyanosis. An ashen grey color of the skin, lips, and nail beds should be grounds for suspicion. The diagnosis may be confirmed by a spectroscopic examination of the patient's blood.

Hemolytic anemia. This is another blood dyscrasia sometimes seen in patients using phenacetin. This condition, in which red cells are destroyed and release their hemoglobin, may lead to acute kidney failure. It usually results from prolonged overdosage of these drugs. However, hemolytic anemia may occur when sensitive people whose red cells lack glucose-6-phosphate dehydrogenase take relatively small amounts of headache remedies containing phenacetin and other drugs. The condition is best treated by having the patient stop taking all drugs and by infusing fresh whole blood containing undamaged erythrocytes to replace those that have been destroyed.

Nephrotoxicity. The chronic abuse of products containing phenacetin has resulted in kidney damage, including papillary necrosis. Carcinoma of the urinary tract has also been reported. Such reports led to replacement of phenacetin by acetaminophen in almost all proprietary pain relief products. Actually, however, it has not been shown that the abuse of acetaminophen could not cause nephritis and, in fact, it is now believed that chronic abuse of any mixture of analgesic drugs can lead to nephrotoxicity. None of these drugs should be taken for longer than 10 days unless the patient is being observed by a physician or nurse.

Pyrazolon derivatives

This group includes the analgesic–antipyretics *antipyrine* (phenazone) and *aminopyrine,* which were introduced late in the last century, *phenylbutazone* (Butazolidin), and *oxyphenbutazone,* a metabolite of phenylbutazone that is given as a drug (Table 37-1). Aminopyrine is no longer used in

the United States (see below), and antipyrine is used only topically. Phenylbutazone and oxyphenbutazone are available only by prescription. All these agents exert excellent anti-inflammatory effects. However, because they can occasionally cause bone marrow toxicity, these drugs, unlike the agents discussed earlier, are not widely used in this country for relief of minor pain.

Aminopyrine has been the cause of cases of agranulocytosis that have ended fatally. Sensitized persons who take even a small dose of this drug may suffer a sharp drop in leukocyte count, which exposes them to fulminating infections. These usually begin with a severe sore throat characterized by breakdown of the mucous membranes and ulcerations. The number of patients hypersensitive to aminopyrine is statistically small. However, if the drug were as widely available as aspirin, the incidence of drug-induced agranulocytosis would be alarmingly high. It is this adverse effect of aminopyrine that has led to the discontinuation of its use in the United States.

Unlike aminopyrine, which rarely offers any advantage over aspirin, the related compounds phenylbutazone and oxyphenbutazone sometimes benefit some patients with chronic joint disorders that have not responded to salicylates. The use of these drugs in cases of gout, ankylosing spondylitis, and arthritis is discussed in Chapter 38.

Other analgesics

Certain centrally acting skeletal muscle antispasmodics, including *carisoprodol* and *orphenadrine* (Chap. 48), have been claimed to exert a weak analgesic action as well as to relieve pain by relaxing muscle spasms. Any direct analgesic activity in such preparations is probably supplied by the salicylates and similar drugs with which these muscle relaxants are often combined.

Other drugs with analgesic–antipyretic and anti-inflammatory activity that are used mainly in the treatment of rheumatoid arthritis—for example, the older drugs phenylbutazone and indomethacin, and the newer nonsteroidal anti-inflammatory drugs ibuprofen, fenoprofen, mefenamic acid, naproxen, sulindac, and tolmetin—are discussed in the following chapter.

Additional clinical considerations

The many effects of the salicylates make them very useful and important drugs in clinical practice. The ready availability of these drugs, however, and their frequent use for minor complaints, has given them the reputation of not being "real" drugs. If a salicylate is prescribed for a patient, the patient will need reassurance, encouragement, and teaching to help understand the drug, its actions, and its benefits. The patient who does not believe that a "real" drug has been ordered is unlikely to comply with the drug order. The very important placebo effect associated with the use of any drug, as well as its pharmacodynamic effects, will be lost in such a case. Overcoming the drug's reputation can be a major challenge.

Children need special attention when given salicylates. Many children are given these drugs for minor complaints—irritability, slight fever, vague discomforts—and they may regard the drug as "candy" or as something that "makes it all better." Unfortunately, aspirin can be very toxic, even fatal, to children. It is an important aspect of patient education to teach children and adults to respect all drugs, and especially these, for their therapeutic benefits as well as their potential toxicity. Proper drug storage should be stressed if children are in the home.

If the salicylate is prescribed as an antipyretic, the patient should be carefully monitored for response to the drug. Frequent monitoring and recording of vital signs is an important aspect of the drug therapy. After the onset of the antipyretic effects of the drug, the patient may perspire profusely and need frequent changes of linen. A tepid sponge bath may help not only to increase the patient's comfort but also to help lower the temperature. Other measures may also be taken as adjuncts to the drug therapy, including alcohol baths and application of cool wet cloths to hasten heat loss. During this rapid fall in temperature, it is important to keep the patient from becoming chilled, and to monitor fluid loss and maintain hydration.

Whenever a salicylate is prescribed for its analgesic effects, the patient's response to the drug should be noted. Additional nursing interventions should also be used to help decrease the patient's discomfort, including environment control, support, and positioning. In the hospital setting, it is very important to remember that, even though these drugs are OTC preparations, they can only be dispensed to patients with the appropriate legal prescription.

Severe allergic reactions have been reported with the use of salicylates. Aspirin sensitivity seems to be more prevalent in patients with asthma or nasal polyps, but should be considered with any patient who has a history of drug allergies. Patients with tartrazine dye sensitivity

or sensitivity to other nonsteroidal anti-inflammatory agents may have a cross sensitivity to aspirin.

The nursing staff should review the signs and symptoms of aspirin toxicity any time that a patient is receiving salicylates. If early signs and symptoms are detected, more dangerous toxicity can be avoided. Gastrointestinal upset is a very common side-effect of salicylate therapy. Taking the drug with food as well as with a liquid often helps. Research results have not consistently supported the claim that buffering or coating the tablet has any beneficial effect, but this helps some patients. Bleeding tendencies may be increased secondary to aspirin's effects on platelet function and on prothrombin synthesis (the latter occurs with high doses only; see Chap. 34). Patients also need to know that they may bruise more easily.

Drug–drug interactions

Because of the effects of salicylates on clotting, patients taking *oral anticoagulants* may need a decrease in dosage of oral anticoagulant if they are taking salicylates. There is evidence of increased risk of gastrointestinal ulcer if salicylates are taken with *steroids, phenylbutazone,* or *alcohol.* The uricosuric effect of *probenecid* and *sulfinpyrazone* is decreased if these drugs are taken with salicylates. *Methotrexate* levels are increased if this drug is taken with salicylates, which interfere with its protein binding and elimination. *Antacids* can affect the absorption of salicylates. Salicylate toxicity is increased if given concurrently with *furosemide;* patients taking these two drugs should have a lower dosage of the salicylate. Aspirin may inhibit the diuretic effect of *spironolactone.*

Many OTC preparations contain salicylates. Patients need to be cautioned about the use of OTC preparations while on salicylates to avoid inadvertent toxicity.

The patient teaching guide presents a summary of points that should be incorporated into the teaching program of a patient receiving salicylates. The guide to the nursing process summarizes the clinical considerations needed in the nursing care of a patient receiving salicylates.

Patient teaching guide: salicylates

The drug that has been prescribed for you is called a salicylate (or aspirin). Salicylates have many effects in the body. They are used to lower fever, to decrease pain, and to relieve the signs and symptoms of inflammation. This drug has been prescribed for you to treat _____ .

Instructions: 1. The name of the drug that has been prescribed for you is _____ .
If your drug is aspirin (acetylsalicylic acid), many OTC preparations with different costs are available. One preparation is likely to be as good as any

(continued)

other; you don't have to pay a high price for a well-known brand name product.

2. The dosage of the drug that is prescribed is ———————————— .

3. You should take the drug ——————— times a day. The best time to take your drug is ————————— . If the drug causes stomach upset, you can take the drug with food or milk.

4. Only take the drug as prescribed. Do not take more than has been prescribed for you.

5. Some side-effects of the drug that you should be aware of include the following:

GI upset, heartburn, nausea.   Taking the drug with food may help.

Easy bruising, gum bleeding.   These are related to aspirin's effects on blood clotting; if they become severe, notify your nurse or physician.

6. Avoid the use of other OTC drugs while you are on this drug. Many of these drugs contain aspirin, and serious overdosage can occur. If you feel that you need one of these preparations, consult with your nurse or physician for the best possible choice.

7. Keep this, and all medication, securely out of the reach of children. This drug can be very dangerous for children.

Notify your nurse or physician if any of the following occur:

Ringing in the ears
Dizziness, confusion
Abdominal pain
Rapid breathing
Nausea, vomiting

Guide to the nursing process: salicylates

Assessment	Nursing diagnoses	Interventions	Evaluation
Past history (*contraindications*): Hemophilia Bleeding states Chronic renal failure Hepatic failure	Potential alteration in breathing patterns if toxic levels develop Potential alteration in comfort: pain Knowledge deficit	Proper storage and administration of drug Provision of comfort measures: • Drug with food if GI tract upset	Monitor for therapeutic effect of drug: relief of presenting symptoms Monitor for adverse effects of drug: GI upset

(continued)

Assessment	Nursing diagnoses	Interventions	Evaluation

Pregnancy
Lactation
Children with chicken pox, influenza
Allergies: any salicylates; tartrazine; others: reactions
Medication history
  cautions:
  Oral anticoagulants
  Methotrexate
  Furosemide
  Antacids
  Steroids
  Phenylbutazone
  Alcohol
  Probenecid
  Sulfinpyrazone
  OTC drugs
 	
Physical assessment
Neurologic: reflexes cranial nerves, affect
Cardiovascular: P, BP, perfusion
Respiratory: rate, depth
GI: bowel sounds, liver function
Skin: lesions
Other: T, bleeding times
	regarding disease, drug therapy
	Potential sensory–perceptual alterations if toxic levels develop
		• Further measures to reduce pain, T, or inflammation
		Patient teaching regarding:
		  • Disease
		  • Drug
		  • Dosage
		  • Cautions
		  • Toxic signs and symptoms
		Support and encouragement to deal with disease and drug therapy
		Provision of life support and stabilizing therapy if toxicity develops
			↑ Bleeding
			Monitor for toxic effects of drug:
			  • Ringing in ears
			  • CNS changes
			  • ↑ R
			  • Acidosis
			Evaluate effectiveness of patient teaching program
			Evaluate effectiveness of support and encouragement offered
			Evaluate effectiveness of life support and maintenance therapy, as indicated
			Monitor for drug–drug interactions:
			  ↑ Bleeding with oral anticoagulants
			  ↑ GI ulcers with steroids, alcohol, phenylbutazone
			  ↑ Uric acid levels with probenecid, sulfinpyrazone
			  ↑ Methotrexate toxicity
			  ↑ Salicylate toxicity with furosemide, OTC drugs
			  ↓ Diuretic effect with spironolactone
			  ↓↑ Effect with antacids

Summary of the pharmacologic actions and therapeutic uses of the salicylates

Pharmacologic action

  Analgesic: Especially for pain originating in the joints, muscles, teeth, head, skin, connective tissues.

  Antipyretic: Reduces fever.

  Anti-inflammatory and antirheumatic actions.

Clinical uses

  Headache, toothache, arthritis and related musculoskeletal conditions, general malaise

  Respiratory viral illnesses, such as influenza and the common cold

  Acute rheumatic fever, acute and chronic rheumatoid arthritis and osteoarthritis, and related rheumatic disorders

Summary of the side-effects and toxicity of the salicylates and of acetaminophen

Salicylates

Allergic hypersensitivity. Skin, gastrointestinal, and respiratory effects of varying severity may develop suddenly.

Early salicylism. Gastrointestinal upset including nausea, vomiting, pain, gastric bleeding; tinnitus, partial deafness, diplopia, dizziness, drowsiness, lethargy, mental confusion.

Salicylate poisoning. Central stimulation may lead to convulsions, followed by respiratory and cardiovascular failure; stimulation of respiratory center causes hyperpnea, which in turn leads to respiratory alkalosis; fever; metabolic acidosis and disturbances such as *hyper-* or *hypo*glycemia and hypokalemia may also occur; bleeding disorders caused by hypoprothrombinemia or thrombocytopenia may develop.

Acetaminophen and related drugs

Hepatic toxicity and failure

Hematologic effects include methemoglobinemia marked by cyanosis, headache, chest pain, and dyspnea; also hemolytic anemia, which may lead to hematuria, anuria, and acute kidney failure.

Nephritis with papillary necrosis may develop in patients who abuse these drugs.

Case study

Presentation

GS, a 20-year-old college student, was seen in the University Health Service with complaints of nausea, slight feelings of "indigestion," a feeling of lethargy and drowsiness, slight dizziness, and occasional ringing in both ears. A physical exam was unremarkable except for a respiratory rate of 26 and a pulse of 110. History revealed that GS was a full-time student who was feeling somewhat overwhelmed. She reported that all the reading, the lectures, and the "whole place in general" were giving her headaches, which seemed to have subsided over the past few days, while the presenting complaints became progressively worse. GS denied drug use.

What are the appropriate nursing actions that should be taken?

Discussion

GS has all the signs and symptoms of salicylism. Further information should be elicited from GS regarding what actions she took to get rid of her headaches. Many people do not consider aspirin to be a drug. It is so readily available and so widely used that many people forget about its use or do not consider it as a medication to be reported. On further questioning, GS stated that she had been self-medicating with aspirin, two or three tablets prn, approximately 12 a day; that she took Alka-Seltzer to relieve the indigestion that she had developed; and that she had taken two or three Vanquish each day to "calm" her nerves. GS said that she did not know what ingredients were in the Alka-Seltzer and Vanquish. She also stated that she didn't think it necessary to mention these OTC drugs because they weren't prescribed; they were just available "remedies."

The OTC drugs GS used all contain aspirin. GS has taken enough of these preparations to have developed aspirin toxicity (salicylism). Salicylism can present with signs and symptoms that range from nausea, vomiting, gastrointestinal upset, tinnitus, and diplopia to dizziness, drowsiness, lethargy, confusion, and hyperpnea. Salicylism can progress to severe acid–base disturbances, coma, and even death. The severity of GS's toxic reactions will have to be evaluated immediately, and appropriate supportive measures should be taken. If GS stabilizes and her acid–base balance seems to be within a safe range, she may recover completely with no intervention other than total withdrawal from salicylates.

Once GS has recovered, the source of the headaches should be determined. GS may need to have an ophthalmologic examination, she may need counseling to cope with the stresses of college, or she may have an underlying medical problem that requires attention. She will need extensive teaching about the use of OTC preparations. This should include points to consider in choosing an OTC preparation, evaluation of the ingredients, and avoiding combinations of OTC preparations with similar ingredients. Alternative approaches to her complaints should be discussed. The signs and symptoms of aspirin toxicity should be reviewed and written down for GS. She should receive support and encouragement to cope with her underlying stresses as well as her current state of health.

Although aspirin offers many therapeutic benefits, its toxic side-effects occur frequently when the drug is taken in excess. Public education programs need to point out the risks as well as the benefits of OTC drugs, and health-care professionals need to be on the alert for inadvertent drug toxicity from OTC use.

Drug digests

Acetaminophen USP (APAP; Tempra; Tylenol)

Actions and indications. This metabolite of phenacetin is an effective analgesic and antipyretic, but it has little or no anti-inflammatory activity. It may be substituted for aspirin to relieve mild to moderate pain (but not in the management of rheumatic disorders) for patients who are hypersensitive to salicylates or who have low tolerance for the irritating effects of aspirin on the gastrointestinal mucosa.

It is also preferred to aspirin for relief of pain in gout patients who are taking probenecid or other uricosuric drugs that might be antagonized by salicylates. This drug does not seem to have the platelet-aggregating or prothrombin-prolonging effects of aspirin, and thus it may be preferable for pain relief in patients with hemorrhagic disorders or those who are receiving anticoagulant therapy.

Adverse effects, cautions, and contraindications. Ordinary doses cause few side-effects. This drug has rarely been reported to cause the types of renal damage, hemolytic anemia, and methemoglobinemia that have been recorded for the related drugs phenacetin and acetanilid. However, such adverse effects should be watched for; further administration of the drug would be contraindicated in those who showed symptoms of these disorders. Similarly, the drug is discontinued if such signs of hypersensitivity as skin redness, itching, or urticaria occur.

Accidental or deliberate massive overdosage has caused severe illness and death from acute hepatic necrosis and other complications, such as hypoglycemia and metabolic acidosis.

Dosage and administration. The usual adult dose is 300 to 600 mg repeated in 4 hours; for children 6 to 12 years old, half this dose is employed, and youngsters 1 to 6 years old receive only 60 to 120 mg at 4- to 6-hour intervals, if necessary.

Aspirin USP (Acetylsalicylic acid)

Actions and indications. Aspirin is the prototype of the salicylates and of mild analgesics with antipyretic and anti-inflammatory activity. It is very widely used for relief of pain that arises in connective tissues of the muscles, joints, and other skeletal system structures. Among the disorders for which it is most commonly employed are headache, toothache, neuralgia, and myalgia, and for reducing fever and malaise accompanying the common cold and other minor viral respiratory infections.

Larger doses are useful in rheumatic disorders for reducing inflammatory reactions, with relief of joint pain, swelling, and tenderness, and with a resulting increase in mobility. It is effective for both acute flares, including rheumatic fever signs and symptoms, and in the long-term maintenance therapy of chronic rheumatoid arthritis. Lower doses relieve the pain of osteoarthritis. Although large doses increase the excretion of uric acid, smaller doses have the opposite effect and actually antagonize the effects of more potent uricosuric agents such as pro-benecid. Because of this and the fact that other more potent anti-inflammatory agents are preferred for suppressing acute gout attacks, aspirin should *not* be used in this disorder.

Low doses of aspirin prevent blood platelets from aggregating. Thus, the drug is being employed prophylactically in men who have suffered transient ischemic attacks (TIAs) or strokes due to platelet emboli (benefit in women has not been shown), and it is being employed experimentally for the prevention of coronary thrombosis and pulmonary embolism in patients who seem prone to develop coronary thrombosis or lung infarct from venous thrombosis.

Adverse effects, cautions, and contraindications. Ordinary doses of aspirin cause complaints of epigastric distress in some patients. Moderately high doses can cause nausea, vomiting, and gastrointestinal bleeding if measures are not taken to minimize mucosal irritation. Large doses are potentially ulcerogenic and should not be employed in patients with active, or even possibly with healed, peptic ulcer.

The continued administration of high doses may result in signs and symptoms of salicylism, or mild salicylate intoxication. These include tinnitus (ringing and other noises in the ears), visual blurring, dizziness, drowsiness, and mental confusion, in addition to the usual gastrointestinal disturbances. Acute intoxication from massive doses can cause severe acid–base disturbances in children. Metabolic acidosis superimposed on respiratory alkalosis can lead to convulsions, coma, and fatal cardiovascular collapse and respiratory failure.

Dosage and administration. Aspirin is most commonly taken for pain relief in oral doses of 300 to 600 mg that may be repeated in 2 to 4 hours. In rheumatic disorders, much larger doses ranging from 3.6 to 10 g daily are required to maintain a therapeutic plasma level of between 25 and 35 mg/100 ml, the therapeutic range for anti-inflammatory activity. The drug should be administered with meals, milk, or snacks, or with large amounts of water.

References

Aspirin products. Med Lett Drugs Ther 23:65, 1981

Beaver WT: Mild analgesics: A review of their clinical pharmacology. Am J Med Sci 250:597, 1965; 251:576, 1966

Diflunisal (Dolobid): Med Lett Drugs Ther 24:76, 1982

Done AK, Temple AR: Treatment of salicylate poisoning. Mod Treat 8:528, 1971

Flower RJ, Moncada S, Vane JR: Analgesic–antipyretics and anti-inflammatory agents; drugs employed in the treatment of gout. In Gilman AG, Goodman LS, Gilman A (eds): Goodman and Gilman's The Pharmacological Basis of Therapeutics, 6th ed, pp 682–728. New York, Macmillan, 1980

Flower RJ, Vane JR: Inhibition of prostaglandin biosynthesis. Biochem Pharmacol 23:1439, 1974

Hill JB: Salicylate intoxication. N Engl J Med 288:1110, 1973

Inglefinger FJ: The side effects of aspirin. N Engl J Med 290:1196, 1974

Karch AM: Aspirin: Miracle drug or potential problem. J Prac Nurs 30:25, 1980

Koch–Weser J: Acetaminophen. N Engl J Med 295:1297, 1976

Leonards JR, Levy G: Gastrointestinal blood loss during prolonged aspirin administration. N Engl J Med 289:1020, 1973

Moertel CG et al: Relief of pain by oral medications: A controlled evaluation of analgesic combinations. JAMA 229:55, 1974

Prescott LF: Analgesic nephropathy: A reassessment of the role of phenacetin and other analgesics. Drugs 23:75, 1982

Settipane GA: Adverse reactions to aspirin and related drugs. Arch Intern Med 141:328, 1981

Sutton E, Soyka LF: How safe is acetaminophen? Some practical cautions with this widely used agent. Clin Pediatr 12:692, 1973

Toxicity of nonsteroidal anti-inflammatory drugs. Med Lett Drugs Ther 25:15, 1983

Chapter 38

Drugs used in the management of rheumatic disorders and chronic headache

38

This chapter will describe several groups of drugs. It will first discuss *nonsteroidal anti-inflammatory drugs* (NSAIDs), which are used to treat rheumatoid and other forms of arthritis, including gout. A second group of drugs, sometimes called *remission-inducing agents,* or *slow-acting antirheumatic drugs,* is used to treat rheumatoid arthritis that has not responded well to NSAIDs; this group includes such diverse substances as gold salts, quinine-type antimalarials, and immunosuppressive drugs of the type used in cancer chemotherapy. A third group of drugs is used *prophylactically* to manage patients who suffer recurrent episodes of *gout.* The fourth and last group of drugs considered in this chapter is used to treat or prevent migraine-type headaches.

General considerations

More than 20 million Americans suffer symptoms of one form or another of rheumatic disease. These are inflammatory or degenerative disorders that affect mainly the musculoskeletal system—that is, such structures as joints, muscles, ligaments, tendons, and bursae. However, some conditions that are marked mainly by joint and soft tissue pain, stiffness, and soreness are actually systemic connective tissue diseases that may also result in damage to the heart and blood vessels.

There are more than 100 different chronic and acute disorders in this class of conditions that the layman often lumps together with the catchall term "rheumatism." This chapter will cover in detail the drug treatment of only three disorders: *rheumatoid arthritis, rheumatic fever,* and *gouty arthritis.* These three disorders will provide the basis for explaining the main principles of the management of all acute and chronic rheumatic ailments—principles that can also be applied to other disorders that will be barely mentioned or will be discussed only briefly,

such as *osteoarthritis, ankylosing spondylitis, tendinitis, bursitis, fibrositis,* and *myositis.*

This section will describe the application to rheumatic disease treatment of two classes of drugs that are taken up in detail elsewhere in the text: the salicylates (Chap. 37) and the corticosteroids (Chap. 21). Other drugs with anti-inflammatory, analgesic–antipyretic, uricosuric, and other actions applicable to treatment of these disorders are discussed here for the first time.

Rheumatoid arthritis

This disease, which afflicts more than 5 million Americans, is characterized by chronic inflammation of the synovial membranes, a layer of loose connective tissue that lines the joints and secretes a lubricating fluid. The specific cause of the persistent inflammation is unknown. However, a widely held theory is that the inflammation is a result of a synovial tissue response to autoantibodies, and that rheumatoid arthritis is thus an autoimmune disease.

No drug now available can cure the disease by counteracting its still unknown primary cause. Instead, drug treatment is aimed at suppressing inflammation. This prevents the release locally within the joint of lysosomal enzymes and other substances such as bradykinin and prostaglandin E—chemicals that cause inflammatory tissue injury. Thus, anti-inflammatory drug therapy provides relief of joint pain, swelling and tenderness, heat, and redness. These drugs may also delay the progressive damage to the joint capsule, in which cartilage and other connective tissues are destroyed and replaced by fibrous scar tissues.

Salicylate therapy
The salicylates, especially *aspirin,* are still the cornerstone of conservative medical management of this disorder.

Some other available drugs—the corticosteroids, for example—are more potent than aspirin, but they are also much more likely to cause adverse effects during long-term therapy. All other antirheumatic drugs are also much more expensive than aspirin—a fact that must be considered in this chronic disorder and also in osteoarthritis, a degenerative joint disease that afflicts many elderly people with limited incomes.

Unfortunately, many arthritic patients find it hard to believe that this familiar nonprescription pain reliever is the safest and usually the most effective drug for treating chronic joint disorders. Scorning salicylates and seeking some "miracle cure" for an incurable condition, people who can least afford it often spend large sums of money for medications that are much less useful than aspirin, or they even buy worthless drugs, devices, and dietary regimens.

The nurse can help to direct such people away from the fraudulent purveyors of money-wasting remedies. Every opportunity should be taken to encourage patients to continue with the aspirin-based conservative program that their physicians have planned. Arthritis sufferers who may be impatient with the slow progress that they seem to be making should be assured that aspirin alone *can* control arthritis in most cases. They should be urged not to demand treatment with steroids or other potentially toxic drugs, but to continue taking aspirin in the highest daily doses that they can tolerate.

For full anti-inflammatory effectiveness in rheumatoid arthritis, aspirin must be taken in much larger amounts than are adequate for ordinary analgesia. Patients should, in fact, be told to continue taking large daily doses, even when they are not having much pain. This is because the peripheral anti-inflammatory action exerted by large doses of aspirin helps to keep the disease under control and prevents sudden acute flares.

To minimize gastrointestinal disturbances, therapy usually begins with relatively low daily doses that are gradually raised to the maximum that the patient seems able to tolerate. This requires at least 12, and often as many as 18, 5-grain tablets daily, divided into six doses of two or three tablets. As indicated in Chapter 37, each dose should be taken after meals or with a snack of milk and crackers.

For patients who complain of stomach symptoms and who can afford the extra expense, various products that present salicylates in the form of an effervescent alkaline solution may help to minimize drug-induced irritation. However, patients who do not suffer much gastric discomfort from aspirin or who cannot afford the more expensive brand name products can be advised to buy large bottles of an inexpensive brand of plain unbuffered aspirin and to take each dose with plenty of water. The tablets may be broken into small pieces or crushed to make them more soluble, thus minimizing the chance

that small erosive particles may lodge in the folds of the mucosal lining.

Nonsteroidal anti-inflammatory drugs

Most patients with rheumatoid arthritis respond to treatment with aspirin taken regularly in high daily doses. However, salicylates alone may not be able to control a very active inflammatory process in some patients. Others may be unable to tolerate more than relatively low doses of aspirin, or they may be unable to take it at all because of salicylate sensitivity that results in allergic reactions. In such cases alternative anti-inflammatory drugs are prescribed (Table 38-1).

The corticosteroids, which were hailed with great enthusiasm when first introduced, are not now considered the drug of choice as an early alternative to salicylates. Although they are often rapidly effective, the long-term employment of steroids can lead to so many complications (Chap. 21) that most rheumatologists prefer to try almost all other available antirheumatic drugs before very reluctantly turning to systemically administered steroid drugs. Thus, when aspirin alone is inadequate, nonsteroidal anti-inflammatory drugs (NSAIDs) are often added to the patient's regimen. Aspirin and the other salicylates may actually be included appropriately in the group of drugs called NSAIDs; salicylates have the same fundamental mechanism of action and generally cause the same types of adverse effects. However, many drugs that are newer than aspirin produce a higher ceiling analgesic effect and cause more serious toxicity.

Older NSAIDs

Phenylbutazone[+] (Azolid; Butazolidin) was the first drug of this type to be introduced. It proved to be a potent antirheumatic agent that could control acute inflammatory reactions. However, its long-term use in a chronic disorder such as rheumatoid arthritis is often accompanied by adverse reactions and dangerous complications. These include not only gastrointestinal upset, hemorrhage, and peptic ulcer, but also possible bone marrow depression leading to serious blood dyscrasias. Elderly patients are particularly likely to develop adverse reactions, including edema as a result of drug-induced sodium and water retention.

For these reasons, phenylbutazone and its metabolite, *oxyphenbutazone* (Oxalid; Tandearil) are not ordinarily administered to patients with a history of blood dyscrasias, peptic ulcer, or cardiac and renal disorders. Patients are instructed to return for frequent blood checks during the period of continued treatment with doses that have been adjusted down to the smallest effective level. They must be told to report such signs and symptoms as sore mouth or throat, fever, weight gain, stomach pain, or black tarry stools—all signs of potentially severe toxicity.

Table 38–1. Nonsteroidal anti-inflammatory drugs (NSAIDs) used in the management of arthritis and gout*

Official or generic name	Trade name	Usual adult dosage†	Maximum daily dose (mg)	Indications
Fenoprofen calcium	Nalfon	300–600 mg tid or qid	3200	Rheumatoid and osteoarthritis; mild to moderate pain
Ibuprofen	Advil; Motrin; Nuprin	300–600 mg tid or qid	2400	Rheumatoid and osteoarthritis; moderate pain; 1° dysmenorrhea
Indomethacin USP	Indocin	See Drug digest	200	Rheumatoid and osteoarthritis; acute gouty arthritis; bursitis; tendinitis
Meclofenamate sodium	Meclomen	200–400 mg/day in three or four equal doses	400	Rheumatoid and osteoarthritis
Mefenamic acid	Ponstel	Initially, 500 mg, followed by 250 mg q 6 hr	1000	Not approved for use for longer than 1 week; moderate pain; 1° dysmenorrhea
Naproxen	Naprosyn	250–375 mg bid	1000	Rheumatoid and osteoarthritis; acute gout; tendinitis; bursitis; mild to moderate pain; 1° dysmenorrhea
Naproxen sodium	Anaprox	275 mg bid	1100	See naproxen, above
Oxyphenbutazone USP	Oxalid; Tandearil	300–400 mg/day, in divided doses		Rheumatoid and acute gouty arthritis; acute attacks of bursitis and tendinitis
Phenylbutazone USP	Azolid; Butazolidin	See Drug digest		See oxyphenbutazone, above
Piroxicam	Feldene	20 mg/day in single or divided dose	20	Acute and chronic rheumatoid and osteoarthritis
Sulindac	Clinoril	150 mg bid	400	Acute and chronic rheumatoid and osteoarthritis; acute gouty arthritis; bursitis
Tolmetin sodium	Tolectin	400 mg tid	2000	Acute and chronic rheumatoid arthritis; juvenile rheumatoid arthritis

* The salicylate and corticosteroid drugs used in arthritis are listed in Tables 37-1 and 21-1, respectively.
† Dosage depends on use. Maintenance dosage for rheumatoid arthritis is given. When used for mild to moderate pain, a lower dose of some agents may be adequate; for acute episodes, a higher initial dose of some agents may be desirable.

Indomethacin[+] (Indocin) is a somewhat safer drug than phenylbutazone, but it does cause side-effects of some severity in many patients, especially at the start of treatment. About one of four patients complains of central nervous system symptoms, including headaches, vertigo, light-headedness and, occasionally, mental confusion. These reactions make it undesirable for the patient to drive during the early weeks of treatment. About 10% to

15% of patients taking indomethacin are forced to discontinue the drug because of headaches and other central nervous system symptoms.

As is the case with aspirin, phenylbutazone, and the other NSAIDs, indomethacin often causes epigastric distress. Although this may be minimized by giving the drug after meals or with a glass of milk, some patients must stop taking the drug because of continuing nausea, indigestion, burning stomach pain, and diarrhea. The drug is contraindicated in patients with active peptic ulcers, and is employed only with caution in those with a history of ulcerative gastrointestinal disease.

Indomethacin, phenylbutazone, and oxyphenbutazone are all best reserved for control of the *acute* phases of rheumatic disorders rather than for long-term maintenance therapy. Their use in high doses for a few days in attacks of acute gouty arthritis (see below) is quite effective and relatively safe. These drugs are also useful for control of *ankylosing spondylitis,* a rheumatic disorder that attacks the small joints of the spinal column and causes it to be bent like a bow or to become completely rigid. Because these drugs appear to be more effective than salicylates for slowing the progress of this chronic crippling condition, they are sometimes preferred to salicylates despite their greater toxicity. However, their long-term employment requires frequent laboratory tests and clinical observation to detect early signs of adverse effects, as described above and in the Drug digests.

A recent use of indomethacin, which is still not officially approved, is the production of what has been called a "pharmacologic closure" of a patent ductus arteriosus in premature infants. This is an alternative to surgical closure. Closure has occurred within 24 to 30 hours in most neonates given a single dose of 0.3 mg/kg body weight, or several doses of 0.1 mg/kg by enema or orogastric tube. Administration of this drug to pregnant women is contraindicated because it could cause prenatal closure of the duct and increased neonatal morbidity.

Newer NSAIDs

Various NSAIDs that are safer than the three drugs described above are now available. The first of these to be introduced, *ibuprofen* (Motrin) was rapidly followed by other, safer alternatives to aspirin: *fenoprofen calcium* (Nalfon), *naproxen* (Naprosyn), *sulindac* (Clinoril), and *tolmetin sodium* (Tolectin). The following were introduced more recently: *meclofenamate sodium* (Meclomen), *mefenamic acid* (Ponstel), *piroxicam* (Feldene), and *zomepirac sodium* (Zomax).* These drugs show some individual differences, such as time of onset and duration of action, that reflect differences in their pharmacokinetics. Naproxen, pyroxicam, and sulindac have the advantage of having relatively long half-lives. Because of their slow elimination rate these drugs produce prolonged anti-inflammatory activity, and thus need to be taken only twice a day. Piroxicam may be effective when taken only once a day. This makes patient compliance more likely than with the other drugs,

which must be taken more frequently to maintain symptomatic relief.

Indications. Some of these drugs are approved for use only in arthritic conditions, while others—for example, fenoprofen, ibuprofen (now available as a low-dose OTC drug—Advil; Nuprin), mefenamic acid, naprofen, and zomepirac—are approved for use as general analgesics for managing mild to moderate pain that is not necessarily related to inflammation of the joints and of the musculoskeletal system. Mefenamic acid and zomepirac are approved only for use as general analgesics. Three of these agents—ibuprofen, mefenamic acid, and naproxen—are approved for use in managing the pain of primary dysmennorhea (Chap. 23), which has recently been associated with high endometrial levels of prostaglandins, especially $PGF_{2\alpha}$. These three drugs have been found to be more effective than aspirin in decreasing the intensity of dysmenorrhea probably because, for an unknown reason, they are more effective than aspirin in inhibiting the action of the uterine cyclo-oxygenase enzyme. Other NSAIDs are also effective in this disorder, but these three have an appropriate time course and a low incidence of adverse effects, and have been studied the most.

Group characteristics. The main advantage claimed for all these new drugs is that they cause fewer complaints of gastrointestinal upset than aspirin when used in doses that are equally effective for relief of joint inflammation. The incidence of epigastric distress with these drugs is said to be only 50% that of aspirin, and they rarely have to be discontinued because of such complications as gastrointestinal bleeding or ulceration. Patients unable to tolerate the gastrointestinal side-effects of aspirin have sometimes been safely switched to one or another of these new antirheumatic agents. However, patients prone to develop hypersensitivity-type reactions to aspirin should not be treated with these drugs.

Adverse gastrointestinal effects. Despite the lower incidence of gastrointestinal distress with these drugs, some patients *have* suffered hemorrhage and peptic ulceration similar to those that occur more often in patients taking salicylates. Thus, patients with a history of aspirin-induced bleeding must be closely observed during transfer from salicylate therapy, and these drugs are usually best taken with meals in the same manner as the other orally administered antirheumatic drugs. Their administration to patients with an active peptic ulcer should be avoided, because—despite their claimed superiority—these drugs do possess potentially ulcerogenic activity.

Mechanism of action. Like aspirin, phenylbutazone, and indomethacin, the newer NSAIDs inhibit cyclo-oxygenase, the enzyme that catalyzes the production of prostaglandins from arachidonic acid. Their antirheumatic activity probably stems from the resulting reduction in the level of prostaglandins in the arthritic joints. However, a similar drug-induced deficiency of this prosta-

---

* Zomepirac sodium (Zomax) was voluntarily removed from the market in 1983 after several people died following severe allergic reactions to the drug. The drug company removed Zomax to re-evaluate the drug warnings and package inserts.

glandin in the gastric mucosa may also account for the ulcerogenic activity of antirheumatic drugs. As indicated in the forthcoming discussion of peptic ulcer treatment (Chap. 41), prostaglandin E may play a part in protecting the mucosa of the stomach and duodenum from the erosive effects of gastric acid. Thus, the same biochemical action that accounts for the desired effect of all NSAIDs in arthritis may be linked to their adverse effects on the gastrointestinal mucosa.

Other adverse effects. All these new drugs have been studied to determine the extent to which they can cause adverse effects similar to those reported with earlier NSAIDs. These drugs have all produced hypersensitivity reactions. Because of the possibility of cross sensitivity, they should be used with great caution in patients who have shown allergic reactions to aspirin or to other NSAIDs. All have reportedly produced central, sensory, and other side-effects of a type similar to those seen with indomethacin and other antirheumatic drugs. Although the incidence of these drug-induced disturbances is relatively low, patients must be observed for signs of toxicity that may require reduction of dosage or even discontinuing further treatment with these drugs.

At least two of the new drugs, fenoprofen and naproxen, can cause drowsiness severe enough to make driving hazardous. Thus, patients should be cautioned against engaging in activities that require alertness and motor coordination until they have taken these drugs long enough to know that they will not suffer from somnolence, dizziness, headache, or other symptoms involving the central nervous system. They should also be told to report any blurring of vision that may develop during long-term therapy. As with various other antirheumatic drugs, periodic ophthalmologic examinations are recommended to detect any adverse ocular effects. Fenoprofen has not been established as safe for use in patients with hearing impairment.

Because these drugs are eliminated from the body primarily by renal excretion, they should be used cautiously in patients with impaired renal function. Untoward renal effects of the drugs are also more likely in these patients. Fenoprofen, like indomethacin, appears to be more commonly associated with urinary tract problems than the other drugs.

Although one NSAID (benoxaprofen) was marketed only briefly before hepatic toxicity forced its withdrawal, serious hepatic toxicity is infrequent with these drugs.

Drug–drug interactions. After absorption, these acidic drugs become bound to plasma proteins. Thus, as is the case with phenylbutazone, they can displace molecules of other acidic drugs from plasma binding sites. This action increases the pharmacologic activity of such drugs, which includes the *coumarin-type anticoagulants, hydantoin-type antiepileptic agents, sulfonylurea-type oral hypoglycemic* agents, and *sulfonamides.* (See Chapter 4 and discussions elsewhere of the individual drugs for further details concerning the clinical significance of such drug–drug interactions.)

Attempts to obtain greater relief of arthritis with reduced toxicity by combining these nonsteroid–nonsalicylate drugs with aspirin have not proved successful. Some patients receiving such combinations seem, in fact, to have suffered increased gastrointestinal side-effects. In addition, the concomitant administration of aspirin has tended to increase the rate of renal excretion and thus reduced the plasma levels of fenoprofen, naproxen, and the sulfide metabolite of sulindac, which is believed to be responsible for that drug's antirheumatic activity. Although combinations with aspirin are not currently recommended for these reasons, patients who are receiving gold salt injections (see below) sometimes obtain further symptomatic relief when oral doses of sulindac or other drugs of this class are added to their treatment regimen.

Summary of current status. These drugs are much more expensive than aspirin and have generally not proved to be more effective than salicylates for relief of rheumatoid arthritis. Aspirin may, in fact, be preferable for relief of acute flares, because ordinary doses of these drugs often require several weeks to bring about their optimal effects. However, patients who suffer severe gastrointestinal upset from salicylates may be more willing to continue taking one or another of the nonsalicylate anti-inflammatory agents. When they do so for several weeks, they may be gratified to find that joint pain is lessened and joint mobility is improved. Periods of early morning stiffness may also be shortened, particularly in patients who have so few stomach complaints that they can take their first dose of the day on arising, without waiting until after breakfast.

The anti-inflammatory effectiveness of these drugs is not limited to rheumatoid arthritis alone. Some are also indicated for relief of the pain and stiffness of osteoarthritis, a degenerative joint disease that often develops with advancing age and sometimes follows injury to the knee, hip, and other joints in younger people (see Table 38-1). Some have produced favorable results in both these types of arthritis, as well as in ankylosing spondylitis and acute gout.

Isoxicam (Maxicam) is an investigational NSAID that is similar to piroxicam but that can be given once daily while still maintaining therapeutic effectiveness. It has been found to have no significant side-effects. This drug may offer many advantages for patients with rheumatic disorders.

Other drugs

This group of drugs includes agents of diverse chemical structure, many of which have other indications as their primary use. These drugs often must be given for several months before benefit is seen; hence, they are sometimes called *slow-acting antirheumatic drugs* (Table 38-2). They

Table 38–2. Miscellaneous drugs used in the management of arthritis and gout

Official or generic name	Trade name	Usual adult dosage and administration
Slow-acting antirheumatic drugs		
Aurothioglucose	Solganal	See Drug digest
Azathioprine	Imuran	Initially, 1.0 mg/kg body weight/day in 1 or 2 doses, PO; may gradually increase to 2.5 mg/kg/day; if no improvement after 12 wk, discontinue therapy.
Chloroquine phosphate	Aralen	250 mg/day, PO
Gold sodium thiomalate USP	Myochrysine	10 mg IM, initially; increasing to 50 mg weekly, to a total dose of 1 g
Hydroxychloroquine sulfate	Plaquenil	400–600 mg/day, PO
Penicillamine	Cuprimine; Depen Titratabs	Initially, 125–250 mg/day, PO, gradually increased to 1000–1500 mg/day; if no improvement after 3–4 months, discontinue therapy
Agents for gout		
Allopurinol USP	Zyloprim	See Drug digest
Colchicine USP		See Drug digest
Probenecid USP	Benemid	See Drug digest
Sulfinpyrazone	Anturane	Initially, 200–400 mg/day, PO, in two divided doses; maintenance, 200–800 mg/day in two divided doses

are sometimes also called *remission-inducing agents* because they are occasionally effective in halting the progressive degenerative changes that have not responded to more conservative therapy.

Gold salt therapy

Chrysotherapy—treatment with a course of gold salt injections such as *aurothioglucose*[+]—sometimes suppresses the rheumatic process in patients whose condition appears to be becoming progressively worse despite several weeks or months of salicylate-based conservative management. An advantage of these drugs is that, unlike other antirheumatic agents, they do not cause gastrointestinal pain, bleeding, or ulceration. Thus, they may also be employed in patients who do not tolerate the gastrointestinal irritation that occurs with high doses of aspirin or of other oral anti-inflammatory agents.

Because of the potential toxicity of chrysotherapy, it is best employed by rheumatologists who have had considerable experience in its use. These physicians often use gold salts early in the management of patients who have not been responding well to salicylates to prevent rapidly progressive destruction of cartilage, synovial scarring, and joint deterioration. These drugs are more effective if used early in the course of the disease, but consideration of their toxicity, combined with the knowledge that spontaneous remissions sometimes occur, make the decision to use these drugs early in the disease difficult.

Because objective improvement may require a slow buildup of the drug in the body, the patient often continues to receive salicylates during the first weeks to relieve joint pain and inflammation. Finally, however, more than 50% of patients treated with gold salts show some benefits, and even total remissions occur in some cases for variable periods.

Treatment must be discontinued if no improvement is noted after 4 months to avoid accumulation of the heavy metal to toxic levels. During the entire treatment course patients are watched closely for signs of toxicity, including pruritic skin rashes. Although an early itchy dermatitis may make it necessary to discontinue treatment, some patients may be able to resume the treatment course without further ill effects after the early skin symptoms subside. More dangerous reactions such as renal damage or blood dyscrasias are guarded against by urinalyses and blood tests that are performed before each weekly injection in the series is administered.

Auranofin (Ridaura) is an investigational oral gold compound. Clinical trials have shown that long-term use of this oral compound results in therapeutic gold levels with few toxic effects. The most frequent toxic effect reported was diarrhea. The availability of an oral gold salt may improve patient compliance with gold therapy, and may provide an improved method of managing rheumatoid arthritis with this type of therapy.

Antimalarial drugs

Chloroquine (Aralen) and, more commonly, *hydroxychloroquine* (Plaquenil; see Chap. 10) also sometimes benefit arthritic patients who have not profited from treatment with salicylates alone. Improvement appears only slowly, and many months of treatment may be needed for remission in those patients who respond at all. However, the time lag may be lessened by loading the patient's system with relatively large doses at the start of treatment. Later in the treatment course dosage is reduced by half, and the patient is watched closely for signs of cumulative toxicity.

These drugs cause minor side-effects in many patients, including gastrointestinal disturbances, headache, and skin eruptions, although these are less likely with hydroxychloroquine. Patients must be examined by an ophthalmologist at the start of treatment and at frequent intervals thereafter to detect changes in the cornea or retina. Deposition of these drugs in the cornea may cause complaints of visual disturbances such as blurring and the appearance of halos around lights. However, this is relatively harmless and disappears within a few months after these drugs are withdrawn. Much more serious are signs of retinal edema, because retinal lesions have resulted in blindness.

Immunosuppressive drugs

Certain cytotoxic antineoplastic drugs such as *cyclophosphamide* (Cytoxan) and *azathioprine* (Imuran; Chap. 12) have been employed experimentally in the management of severe, rapidly progressive rheumatoid arthritis. Azathioprine is now approved by the FDA for this purpose. The use of these drugs in arthritis was originally based on the concept that this is an autoimmune disease, and that these drugs block antibody biosynthesis. However, this has not been proved to be the reason for any benefits that these drugs produce; the real reason for their effectiveness may be a nonspecific anti-inflammatory effect.

The use of azathioprine has helped to halt joint erosion in some cases. Like gold salt therapy, onset of benefit is slow—usually 6 to 8 weeks—and may outlast the treatment period. However, use of the drug puts the patient at risk of developing cancer, especially lymphomas and leukemia, and serious infections. Nausea, vomiting,

alopecia, and pancreatitis also occur. Thus, the use of this drug should be reserved for patients who have failed to respond to other drugs, including gold and corticosteroids. Dosage must be carefully adjusted in accordance with each individual response, and patients must be closely monitored to detect early signs of toxicity (see also cautions, Chap. 12).

Another immunosuppressive drug used in cancer chemotherapy, *methotrexate*, has been found to be useful for treating psoriatic arthritis.

Penicillamine

Penicillamine (Cuprimine), a chelating agent introduced originally for treating a rare neurologic disorder (Wilson's disease, or hepatolenticular degeneration), has shown promising results when employed in some resistant cases of rheumatoid arthritis. Like the gold salts and antimalarial drugs, its beneficial effects come on slowly, but sometimes a long-lasting remission results. Gastrointestinal upset, skin eruptions, and albuminuria are among the adverse effects reported. Patients hypersensitive to penicillin are likely to prove allergic to this derivative. Patients must be observed carefully for signs of hypersensitivity that may require withdrawal of this drug.

Corticosteroid therapy

Systemic steroids

Rheumatoid arthritis. When they were first introduced, the corticosteroids were viewed with great hopes as a "cure" for rheumatoid arthritis. Unfortunately, the dramatic relief often brought about by administration of these drugs was not accompanied by arrest of the joint disease. In fact, some authorities believe that the use of these steroids sometimes accelerates destruction of joint tissue. Nevertheless, when properly employed, these potent anti-inflammatory agents may prove very valuable for patients in whom their use appears justified for socioeconomic reasons or because of development of systemic complications.

Thus, rheumatologists usually try to hold corticosteroid therapy in reserve, until these drugs are judged to be absolutely necessary to prevent the patient from becoming incapacitated and losing his livelihood as a result of crippling by rheumatoid arthritis. As indicated above, corticosteroids are never used in chronic rheumatoid arthritis until the advancing condition no longer responds to more conservative management with salicylates and other less dangerous drugs, together with a carefully planned program of rest, exercise, and physical therapy.

Other indications. Patients for whom steroids may also be indicated include those who tend to suffer from persistent fever, peripheral nerve damage (polyneuropathy), and inflammation of the arteries of various organs (arteritis or vasculitis). The latter systemic complication most commonly involves the skin of the arthritic patient's legs and leads to chronic ulcerations that can become gangrenous. However, vasculitis associated with the rheumatoid process may also occur in various viscera, such as the kidneys or even the heart and central nervous system. In such cases corticosteroids may be administered in massive doses, much as they are in acute life-threatening episodes of the related collagen disease systemic lupus erythematosus (SLE).

Dependence. Patients with severe, unremitting joint pain that requires continued use of narcotic analgesics for control are sometimes put on corticosteroid drug therapy to prevent addiction. However, steroids seem more likely than codeine to cause both psychic and physical dependence. That is, some patients become habituated to the mood-uplifting effect that they feel while taking steroids, and most patients develop characteristic signs and symptoms when steroids are withdrawn too rapidly. These include feelings of fatigue, muscle aching and weakness, loss of appetite, and emotional depression. In addition, too rapid a reduction in dosage can cause an acute flare-up of arthritis. Thus, those patients who have benefited from these drugs are often unwilling to give them up, especially when withdrawal leads to a return of pain even more intense than that previously experienced.

Dosage schedules. Patients who require corticosteroids are started out on only small doses—for example, 5 mg, 7.5 mg or, at most, 10 mg of *prednisone* or *prednisolone.* This does not replace the patient's previous regimen but is added to the salicylates, NSAIDs, gold salts, or antimalarials and, of course, such physical measures as heat, hydrotherapy and splints are continued. The aim of steroid therapy is not to relieve all the symptoms completely, but only to keep the patient relatively comfortable, encourage mobility and increased activity, and thus help reduce progressive crippling.

Patients are watched for signs of spontaneous remission of the active disease process. When this occurs, an attempt is made to reduce daily steroid dosage very gradually or even to withdraw these drugs completely to minimize the risk of adrenal suppression and other types of chronic corticosteroid toxicity (Chap. 21). Patients who complain of discomfort even during slow tapering of steroid dosage may be given increased amounts of salicylates and other safer antirheumatic drugs to help tide them over. A rise in dosage of such adjunctive drugs is also desirable when patients are being switched from a program of several doses daily to one of the intermittent dosage schedules described in Chapter 21.

Arthritis patients do not respond very well to *alternate day therapy* (ADT), because they tend to develop increasingly severe joint symptoms on the second, or "off," day of this schedule. To avoid loss of control of the condition with a possible subsequent acute flare-up,

patients for whom an intermittent dosage schedule seems advisable to avoid hypercorticism and adrenal suppression are best first converted from multiple daily doses to a single daily dose.

Such a total dose is best administered all at once in the early morning hours. This is desirable not only because morning administration mimics the natural diurnal rhythm of adrenal cortex secretion, but also because most arthritic patients suffer from morning stiffness, which is likely to be relieved by taking the large dose at that time. Of course, some patients on this schedule will complain of pain late at night, when the effects of the morning dose have largely worn off. It would be inadvisable to give them an additional dose of steroids at that time, because that would tend to depress production of corticotropin by the pituitary gland and this, in turn, would suppress synthesis and secretion of endogenous adrenal corticosteroids. Instead, the patient should take a hot bath at bedtime, use a heating pad, and take a high nighttime dose of aspirin or of some other NSAID.

Intra-articular steroid therapy

Sometimes, when a patient still has a few painfully inflamed joints after an otherwise positive response to salicylate-based conservative therapy, corticosteroids may be injected directly into the involved joints. Sterile aqueous suspensions of such steroid esters as *triamcinolone acetonide* (Kenalog) or *triamcinolone hexacetonide* (Aristospan) often provide prolonged relief of pain—2 to 4 weeks after each injection. Because the microcrystalline suspensions are relatively insoluble, they tend to be retained within the joint and are absorbed so slowly that systemic side-effects rarely occur.

Occasionally, a patient may suffer a paradoxical brief *increase* in joint swelling and pain several hours after such an injection—a so-called postinjection flare. Ordinarily, however, local pain is markedly relieved within 24 hours of the injection. Any persistent increase in pain and inflammation may signal the presence of joint infection. If such septic arthritis is suspected, a sample of synovial fluid should be drawn and tested for the presence of pathogenic microorganisms. A positive diagnosis requires immediate antimicrobial drug treatment to avoid joint destruction. This is continued for a week or more after swelling and other evidence of an active infection have subsided.

Intra-articular injection of any one joint must be employed sparingly, because too frequent administration may lead to joint destruction. In part this is a direct effect of the steroid, similar to that which occurs in some arthritic patients on prolonged oral steroid therapy. That is, the bony margin of a joint—particularly a weight-bearing joint such as the head of the femur—may begin to break down (aseptic necrosis), possibly because steroids intensify osteoporotic processes that are already present. Another reason is that some patients tend to become too active following dramatic relief of their pain. Thus, they must be warned to keep their physical activity limited for the first 7 or 10 days following an intra-articular injection to avoid possible bone compression, fracture, and joint destruction.

Steroid suspensions are also injected locally in such other rheumatic disorders as acute and subacute bursitis, tendinitis, and osteoarthritis. Oral corticosteroids are not ordinarily administered at all to patients with osteoarthritis. However, when this condition is especially severe and limited to only one or two weight-bearing joints such as the hip or knees, steroids may be injected directly into the inflamed joints. Sometimes a single injection of a relatively long-lasting steroid salt or ester may give relief lasting for several weeks without causing any systemic side-effects.

Corticotropin (ACTH) in rheumatic disorders

Corticotropin (Chap. 20) has sometimes been employed in rheumatoid arthritis. One possible advantage over corticosteroids is that this pituitary hormone, which stimulates production of endogenous steroids by the patient's own adrenal glands, does not cause suppression of adrenal function. Another possible advantage is less likelihood of osteoporosis or muscle weakness than when potent synthetic steroids such as triamcinolone are employed for prolonged periods.

Actually, however, any advantages of corticotropin are outweighed by the fact that it must be administered by injection. Because of its relatively short half-life—even when injected intramuscularly in repository form—corticotropin must be injected daily. This is, of course, an inconvenience in treating chronic rheumatoid arthritis. Another drawback is that repeated injection of foreign protein may lead to allergic sensitization and to possible anaphylaxis in some patients. Thus, this drug is now used mainly for control of pain and inflammation in acute gouty arthritis attacks and other acute rheumatic disorders that respond to treatment with only a few injections.

Additional clinical considerations

Rheumatoid arthritis is a chronic, painful and debilitating disease. Rheumatoid arthritis presents a nursing challenge to help the patient cope with the disease and the drug therapy. Aspirin is still the primary drug of choice for treating this disease. As discussed above, the psychological effect on the patient of taking "plain aspirin" for such a painful disease can cause a major problem with compliance, and therefore with the effectiveness of therapy. Careful and thorough patient teaching about the disease

process and the drug actions, along with a great deal of support and encouragement, can be very important in promoting patient compliance and increasing drug effectiveness. The arthritic patient can also be encouraged to use other measures to help increase drug effectiveness—for example, heat, resting joints, maintaining adequate nutrition, exercise as tolerated, and avoiding stress and fatigue.

The other NSAIDs have proven to be very useful for treating rheumatoid arthritis in patients who are sensitive or nonresponsive to aspirin therapy. Patients need to be cautioned to take the drug only as prescribed, and not to increase dosage or to self-medicate with these preparations. There are numerous adverse effects associated with these drugs, and patients must be followed closely and evaluated for adverse effects. Before giving any NSAID, a careful patient history should be taken to determine the presence of any allergies. Acute anaphylactic reactions have occurred with many of these drugs, and seem to occur more frequently in patients with a hypersensitivity to aspirin or to some other NSAID. Careful screening of patients can help to prevent the serious reactions and deaths that have occurred.

All the drugs discussed for the treatment of rheumatoid arthritis and rheumatic disorders (see below) are contraindicated in pregnancy and lactation. The benefit-to-risk ratio must be carefully considered if a pregnant woman requires one of these drugs. Women of childbearing age should be advised to avoid pregnancy while on any of these drugs. Lactating mothers should be advised to use another means of feeding the baby if any of these drugs are used.

Other drug–drug interactions

Indomethacin has been associated with many drug–drug interactions. It decreases the effectiveness of *furosemide, thiazide diuretics, hydantoins,* and *β-adrenergic blocking drugs. Lithium* can be increased to toxic levels when given with indomethacin; if these drugs are given together, the lithium dosage should be decreased and the patient should be carefully monitored. *Probenecid* inhibits the renal excretion of many drugs. A patient on probenecid and on any other drug should be carefully evaluated for signs of drug toxicity.

The patient teaching guide summarizes the points that should be incorporated into the teaching program of a patient receiving NSAIDs. The guide to the nursing process summarizes the clinical aspects that should be incorporated with the nursing care of a patient on NSAIDs. Guides for the application of the nursing process to the care of patients receiving other drugs used in the treatment of rheumatic disorders (see below) can be developed in a similar manner.

(*Text continues p. 780*)

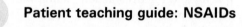

Patient teaching guide: NSAIDs

The drug that has been prescribed for you is called a nonsteroidal anti-inflammatory drug. Drugs of this group work in the body to decrease inflammation and to relieve the signs and symptoms of inflammation—for example, pain, swelling, heat, tenderness, and redness. This drug has been prescribed for you to treat

_____ .

Instructions:

1. The name of your drug is _____ .

2. The dosage that has been prescribed for you is _____ .

3. The drug should be taken _____ times a day. The best time to take your drug is _____ . If gastrointestinal upset occurs when you take your drug, it can be taken with food or milk.

4. Some side-effects of the drug that you should be aware of include the following:

Nausea, vomiting, abdominal discomfort	Taking the drug with food often helps this problem. If it persists or becomes intolerable, consult with your nurse or physician.
Constipation, diarrhea	These may decrease over time. If they persist, consult with your nurse or physician for appropriate treatment.
Drowsiness, dizziness, blurred vision	Avoid driving, performing delicate tasks, or operating dangerous machinery if you experience any of these problems.
Headache	If this becomes a problem, consult your nurse or physician for appropriate treatment. Do not self-medicate with aspirin or other analgesics.

5. Keep this and all medication out of the reach of children.

6. Tell any physician, nurse, or dentist who is taking care of you that you are on this drug.

7. Avoid the use of over-the-counter preparations while you are on this drug. If you feel that you need one of these drugs, consult with your nurse or physician.

8. Take this medication only as prescribed; do not increase the dosage.

(continued)

Notify your nurse or physician if any of the following occur:

Sore throat, fever
Rash, itching
Weight gain, swelling in ankles or
 fingers
Changes in vision
Black or tarry stools

Guide to the nursing process: NSAID

Assessment	Nursing diagnoses	Interventions	Evaluation
Past history *(contraindications)*: Ulcerative GI disease Peptic ulcer Renal dysfunction Blood dyscrasias Hearing impairment (fenoprofen) Hepatic dysfunction Pregnancy Lactation Allergies: aspirin; other NSAIDs; others: reactions Medication history *(cautions)*: Sulfonamides Hydantoin Probenecid Oral anticoagulants Oral hypoglycemics Phenobarbital (fenoprofen) Furosemide (indomethacin) Thiazides (indomethacin) β-adrenergic blockers (indomethacin) Lithium (indomethacin) **Physical assessment** Neurologic: affect, reflexes, peripheral sensation	Potential sensory-perceptual alteration, secondary to CNS effects Potential alteration in comfort, secondary to GI upset, headache Knowledge deficit regarding drug therapy Potential ineffective gas exchange, secondary to hypersensitivity reaction	Safe and appropriate administration of drug Provision of safety and comfort measures: • Drug given with meals • Measures for GI upset, headache • Safety provisions if dizziness or visual disturbances occur Patient teaching regarding: Drug Cautions Side-effects Warnings Support and encouragement to cope with disease, therapy, and side-effects Provision of emergency and life support measures in cases of acute hypersensitivity	Monitor for therapeutic effects of drugs: decrease in signs and symptoms of inflammation Monitor for adverse effects of drugs: • GI upset • Liver function changes • CNS effects • Congestive heart failure • Renal and urinary tract dysfunction • Blood dyscrasias • Visual changes • Rash • Asthma • Anaphylactic reactions Evaluate effectiveness of patient teaching program Evaluate effectiveness of support and encouragement Monitor for drug–drug interactions: ↑ toxicity of oral anticoagulants, oral hypoglycemics, sulfonamides, hydantoin ↓ effectiveness with aspirin

(continued)

Assessment	Nursing diagnoses	Interventions	Evaluation
Cardiovascular: BP, P, peripheral perfusion auscultation GI: bowel sounds, liver, stool guaiac Skin: lesions Blood tests: CBC, liver function, BUN, creatinine			↓ effectiveness of furosemide, thiazide diuretics, β-adrenergic blockers (indomethacin) ↑ toxicity of lithium (indomethacin) ↑ effectiveness with probenecid Evaluate effectiveness of emergency and life support measures, if needed

Rheumatic fever

This disease develops in a small proportion of patients who have previously had acute pharyngitis caused by group A β-hemolytic streptococci—a so-called strep throat that was not treated with adequate doses of penicillin or other effective anti-infective drugs (Chap. 8). Acute rheumatic fever develops within weeks of even a mild infection as the result of an *immune response* in a person sensitized by exposure to streptococcal antigen, or possibly because of autoantibodies formed during the infection. At the time of the rheumatic fever attack, the patient may have no detectable streptococci in the throat and is rarely suffering from an infection. Thus, the most important immediate treatment measure is the administration of salicylates, and sometimes corticosteroids, in large doses to control inflammation of the joints and other tissues, especially those of the heart.

Salicylates

Aspirin alone is almost always fully effective for reducing the patient's high fever and for relief of severe, acute polyarthritis, usually within 24 to 48 hours after therapeutic blood levels have been reached. To attain optimal plasma levels of salicylate—25 to 35 mg/100 ml of plasma—adults must take aspirin in doses of at least 6 to 8 g daily, and a 50-lb child requires at least 60 mg/lb. These high doses may cause signs of gastrointestinal and central nervous system toxicity in some patients.

To minimize gastric irritation, nausea and vomiting, or other signs, symptoms, and complications, the total daily dose of aspirin is divided into six doses, each of which is given with plenty of fluid after the patient has eaten some food. Some part of the total dose may be given in the form of enteric-coated tablets to avoid irritation of the upper gastrointestinal tract mucosa. The amount of alkali in buffered aspirin tablets is probably too small to reduce stomach irritation significantly. Taking 1 tsp of sodium bicarbonate with each dose of aspirin may be of some benefit, but that much alkali may increase the rate of renal excretion of salicylate and thus lower its level in the serum below that required for optimal therapeutic activity.

For full effectiveness, aspirin dosage is often pushed to the point of minor salicylate toxicity (salicylism; Chap. 37). A complaint of ringing in the ears (tinnitus) may be used as an early sign that the limits of safe salicylate dosage have been reached; a slight reduction in aspirin dosage should then be made to avoid serious metabolic toxicity while maintaining therapeutic effectiveness.

Corticosteroids

Steroids are administered under the following circumstances:

1. When effective salicylate levels cannot be attained because the patient suffers epigastric distress while taking less than the required daily doses of aspirin
2. When even full doses of aspirin do not completely control the patient's polyarthritis and fever
3. When the patient shows signs of *acute carditis*—that is, myocarditis, endocarditis, or pericarditis

Steroids are particularly effective for suppressing inflammation of heart tissues and thus counteracting cardiac arrhythmias or signs of congestive heart failure. However, although their use during acute myocarditis may be lifesaving, it is still uncertain that steroids prevent damage to the endocardium of the heart valves and the later development of chronic mitral or aortic stenosis. In any case, relatively large doses—for example, 40 mg or more of prednisone daily (or for a child, 1 mg/lb)—often control the signs and symptoms of the acute rheumatic fever attack in 2 or 3 days. No significant toxic effects occur when steroid dosage is then gradually reduced while salicylate therapy is maintained.

Anti-infective drugs

As indicated earlier, patients suffering an attack of acute rheumatic fever do not ordinarily have acute pharyngitis at the same time, and a throat culture taken during the attack may reveal no group A β-hemolytic streptococci. Nevertheless, high doses of procaine penicillin G are often injected, or oral penicillin G or V administered, while salicylates and steroids are being employed. This is done to eliminate any streptococci that may still persist in hidden foci and that might emerge to cause reinfection when the patient's resistance is reduced during the rheumatic illness and as a result of steroid administration. As indicated in Chapter 8, penicillin—or erythromycin or a sulfonamide in patients allergic to penicillin—may then be continued indefinitely to prevent recurrences of rheumatic fever, which increase the likelihood of rheumatic heart disease.

Gout and gouty arthritis

General considerations

Gout is a metabolic disorder marked by *hyperuricemia*, abnormally high levels of uric acid in the blood. This biochemical abnormality may cause no clinical signs and symptoms, or persistently high plasma uric acid may lead to potentially serious complications, which include the following:

1. Attacks of *acute gouty arthritis*
2. Development of *chronic gouty arthritis*, a disorder that can lead to joint destruction and permanent disability
3. *Gouty nephropathy*, kidney disease caused by uric acid deposits that can lead to impairment of renal function and even finally to renal failure

Acute and chronic gouty arthritis can be better controlled today than any other type of rheumatic disorder. As a result of advances in our understanding of the underlying causes, drugs have been developed that can keep gout patients free of the clinical complications of hyperuricemia. To understand the rationale for use of the several types of drugs available for treating gout, the factors involved in development of hyperuricemia and gouty joint inflammation must be understood.

Pathogenesis of hyperuricemia

Uric acid is formed by the metabolism of nucleoproteins from two sources: the body's own cells and cell-rich foods.

The nucleic acids from these cells are first converted to the purine bases hypoxanthine and xanthine. An enzyme, xanthine oxidase, then catalyzes the metabolic breakdown of these purines to uric acid.

Most uric acid produced in this way is eliminated in the urine as sodium urate. However, the clearance of urate by the kidneys is not an efficient process, because most of the urate filtered from the blood by the renal glomeruli is then reabsorbed by the tubules through which the filtrate passes. Thus, even though the renal tubules also actively secrete uric acid, the balance between production, filtration, and secretion favors a buildup of uric acid in the blood.

Blood ordinarily contains uric acid in a concentration of about 3 to 5 mg/100 ml of serum. However, in some people, the serum level of uric acid stays persistently at levels above 7 mg/100 ml, which is considered to be the upper level of normality. This may occur as a result of a genetic or familial factor that leads to an abnormal increase in uric acid production or to a decrease in the renal excretion of uric acid, or both. The plasma urate level of people with genetic, or *primary*, hyperuricemia may be elevated to a point beyond its ability to remain in solution in body fluids. As indicated below, the solid deposits that then form account for gouty arthritis and other complications.

*Non*genetic factors also sometimes lead to a similar imbalance between the biosynthesis and elimination of uric acid. Such *secondary* hyperuricemia may occur, for example, in patients with neoplastic diseases such as acute and chronic leukemia, in which very large numbers of cells are formed and destroyed with production of excessive amounts of nucleoproteins, purine bases, and uric acid, or in patients treated with certain antineoplastic drugs that rapidly destroy large numbers of tumor cells (Chap. 12). On the other hand, secondary hyperuricemia and gout may be the result of reduced renal excretion caused by kidney diseases such as glomerulonephritis. Certain diuretic drugs that interfere with the tubular secretion of uric acid can also cause secondary gout (Chap. 27).

Pathogenesis of gouty inflammation

The solubility of urates in tissue fluids is limited. When this saturation limit is exceeded, microcrystals of sodium urate are precipitated. Needlelike crystals settle out in the joints, kidneys, ear lobes, and other soft tissues as deposits called tophi. These foreign bodies attract leukocytes that attempt to engulf and phagocytize them, which sets off a series of biochemical reactions that may account for the signs and symptoms of gouty arthritis.

Leukocytes that are damaged during phagocytosis release large amounts of lactic acid, and enzymes leak from their intracellular lysosomes. The increase in local acidity further reduces the solubility of uric acid in the fluids of the joint, with a resulting increase in formation of urate microcrystals that attract still more leukocytes. The lysosomal enzymes released from the leukocytes damage or destroy joint tissues and provoke a further inflammatory reaction. The interaction between urate crystals and phagocytes also triggers the biosynthesis of bradykinin, another chemical mediator of inflammation (see Chap. 36).

Drug therapy for acute and chronic gout

Three types of drugs are employed in the treatment of acute and chronic gout:

1. Drugs for controlling the acute inflammation of an attack
2. Drugs for increasing the excretion of uric acid by the kidneys (*uricosuric* agents)
3. Drugs for reducing the production of uric acid

The regular use of the two types of drugs that affect uric acid metabolism is intended to prevent recurrences of gout attacks. Early administration of certain specific anti-inflammatory agents at the first warning sign often terminates an acute attack that develops despite prophylactic treatment.

Treatment of an acute attack

Most people who have hyperuricemia never develop painful joints or kidney stones. Often, however, after a minor injury or perhaps with no warning at all, crystals of a uric acid salt may form in a joint and set off an excruciatingly painful inflammatory reaction. The attack usually affects a single joint, usually in the big toe, but often in the ankle, instep, heel, or hand.

If the attack is not treated with anti-inflammatory drugs, the intense pain lasts for days and requires narcotics for relief. With rest, the inflammation subsides gradually in about a week. Later attacks occur more frequently and last longer. Finally, in chronic gout, many joints may stay inflamed and painful, and their movement is severely impaired.

Anti-inflammatory drugs. *Colchicine*[+] is a drug specific for aborting acute attacks of gouty arthritis (Table 38-2). Although it has no anti-inflammatory effect in other rheumatic disorders, colchicine is very effective for suppressing inflammation and pain in gouty joints when taken promptly in adequate doses. The way in which this drug, which has been used for hundreds of years, exerts its specific effect in acute gouty arthritis is only now being understood.

Mechanism of action. Colchicine stops the chain reaction that occurs when urate crystals form in a joint. The drug prevents polymorphonuclear leukocytes from migrating into the joint and attempting to engulf the foreign bodies. It also prevents any leukocytes that get into the joint from releasing lactic acid and lysosomal enzymes. Thus, no more microcrystals precipitate in the joint fluids, and production of the destructive enzymes that can damage joint tissues ceases. Bradykinin biosynthesis also ceases.

Administration. Patients who are prone to develop frequent recurrences of acute gout should carry a supply of colchicine tablets to take promptly when they feel the first twinge of typical joint pain. Sometimes two 0.6-mg tablets may be enough to stop any further symptoms. More often, additional doses of 0.6 mg must be taken at intervals of 1 to 3 hours to halt the attack. If treatment is delayed too long, larger doses are needed that may lead to development of diarrhea, nausea, vomiting, and abdominal pain that require treatment with paregoric or antiemetic drugs and discontinuation of further colchicine dosage.

Attacks that do not respond to oral doses that the patient can tolerate are sometimes treated by injecting colchicine intravenously. Although this makes gastrointestinal upset less likely, the total dose must be limited to avoid possible peripheral neuritis and bone marrow or kidney damage. To prevent vein irritation and painful infiltration into surrounding soft tissues, the drug should be well diluted with saline solution and injected into the tubing of a running solution.

Some specialists now prefer to use other anti-inflammatory drugs that they consider to be as effective as colchicine and relatively free of adverse effects when used for brief periods against acute gout. Among these are *phenylbutazone, indomethacin, sulindac,* and *corticotropin.* Intra-articular injections of corticosteroids are also useful for suppressing an acute attack that fails to respond to colchicine. Such steroid suspensions are deposited in large affected joints after excess synovial fluid has been drawn off.

Most acute gout attacks are quickly brought under control by phenylbutazone or indomethacin within 24 hours, when the patient starts taking these drugs in the higher than ordinary doses required at the start of treatment. Although the serious toxicity sometimes seen during chronic administration of these drugs does not occur when they are taken for only a few days, some side-effects are still possible. Phenylbutazone causes gastric distress in some patients, and indomethacin causes headache and dizziness in addition to epigastric pain. Both drugs are best taken after meals, and their high first-day dosage should be gradually reduced on each subsequent day and discontinued entirely within 1 week.

The nurse should see that the patient understands and follows the instructions for taking these drugs and that other measures are also carried out. Bed rest is desirable during the attack, for example. However, once the pain is completely relieved, and the affected joint can bear weight, the patient should be encouraged to walk about. Exercise of pain-free joints is necessary to avoid muscle weakness and atrophy.

Prophylactic treatment of chronic gouty arthritis

Chronic gouty arthritic processes can continue in the absence of acute attacks. Continued deposition of uric acid crystals may disable the patient by destroying cartilage, joints, and bone epiphyses. Thus, although continued administration of small daily doses of colchicine helps to lengthen the periods between acute attacks, other drugs are needed for preventing tophaceous structural changes in the intervals between attacks. Acute attacks can now be prevented by proper use of drugs that keep blood and tissue levels of uric acid below 7 mg/dl. The drugs most commonly employed for this purpose are the uricosuric agents *probenecid*[+] (Benemid) and *sulfinpyrazone* (Anturane).

*Uricosurics.*Probenecid and sulfinpyrazone, a derivative of phenylbutazone that has a greater uricosuric action than the parent compound but none of its anti-inflammatory action, both act in essentially the same way to prevent uric acid that has entered the lumen of the renal tubules from being reabsorbed into the blood. Thus, greater amounts of uric acid are eliminated in the urine, the concentration of plasma urates falls gradually to normal levels, and the size of the tophaceous deposits is gradually reduced. Sulfinpyrazone is more potent than probenecid but causes a greater amount of gastrointestinal upset, and may even reactivate peptic ulcers in susceptible patients.

Administration. Probenecid and sulfinpyrazone are occasionally given together, and their administration with colchicine or with other anti-inflammatory drugs does not cause adverse interactions. However, patients should not take aspirin together with probenecid or sulfinpyrazone, because salicylates tend to interfere with the ability of these drugs to eliminate uric acid. Patients who require an analgesic should take a nonsalicylate such as acetaminophen (Chap. 37).

Precautions. The drug-induced movement of uric acid from deposits in tissue back into the blood may at first increase the number of acute attacks. Thus, to prevent such flare-ups during early treatment, probenecid is commonly prescribed in combination with small amounts of colchicine. To prevent precipitation of uric acid in the urinary tract during its increased excretion as a result of the action of these drugs, certain precautions are necessary:

1. The uricosuric drugs are given in repeated low doses at first, rather than in single high doses.
2. Fluids are forced to produce a large volume of less concentrated urine.
3. The solubility of the uric acid in this dilute

urine may be further increased by alkalinizing it through concurrent administration of small amounts of sodium bicarbonate or potassium citrate several times daily.

Allopurinol. This drug differs from the uricosuric agents in the way by which it lowers serum levels of uric acid. It does so by interfering with the formation of uric acid rather than by increasing its renal excretion. Thus, allopurinol[+] (Zyloprim) ordinarily *lowers* the amount of uric acid that appears in the urine, an effect that makes it particularly useful for patients who are prone to form frequent stones during renal excretion of large amounts of uric acid (hyperuricosuria).

Mechanism of action. Allopurinol reduces the production of uric acid by inhibiting the enzyme *xanthine oxidase.* This prevents the last in the series of steps by which cellular nucleoproteins, nucleic acids, and purines are broken down to uric acid. Specifically, the later steps that are inhibited involve the conversion of the purine base hypoxanthine to xanthine and of xanthine to uric acid. Allopurinol is itself converted to alloxanthine, or oxipurinol, a metabolite that also exerts a long-lasting inhibitory effect on xanthine oxidase and thus adds to the desired reduction in uric acid production.

Indications. Allopurinol is especially useful for patients with kidney damage caused by deposits of urates in the kidney tissues and in urinary tract passages. Allopurinol is preferred to uricosuric drugs in such patients, not only because it lessens the amount of uric acid eliminated in the urine, but also because patients with gouty nephropathy often do not respond well to treatment with uricosuric drugs, which require relatively normal renal function for full effectiveness. Thus, this drug can be substituted for probenecid or sulfinpyrazone in such patients as well as in the rare patients who cannot tolerate either uricosuric agent because of allergic hypersensitivity.

Allopurinol may also be the first choice for treating hyperuricemia that occurs secondary to diseases that lead to overproduction of urates. It helps to prevent urates from being deposited in the joints, kidneys, and soft tissues of patients with blood dyscrasias and neoplasms—for example, polycythemia vera rubra, lymphomas, leukemias, and multiple myeloma—particularly when the malignant cell masses are undergoing rapid destruction as a result of radiation therapy or cancer chemotherapy (Chap. 12).

Precautions. As is the case with uricosuric drugs, flare-ups of acute gouty arthritis can occur at the start of allopurinol treatment. This is a reult of drug-induced mobilization of tissue urate deposits that may then recrystallize in joints. Thus, it is best to begin with low doses that are raised weekly. The simultaneous administration of small doses of colchicine or indomethacin is sometimes also recommended. The patient is advised to drink enough fluid to produce at least 2 liters of urine daily, and a systemic and urinary alkalinizer is also sometimes taken to keep in solution the increased amounts of xanthines that are excreted when allopurinol therapy prevents these purines from being broken down to uric acid.

Drug–drug interactions. Because of its complex metabolic effects, allopurinol may affect the actions of other drugs that are present in the body at the same time. It may, for example, prevent *oral anticoagulant drugs* from being metabolized by liver enzymes at the usual rate. Thus, if a drug such as dicumarol is part of the patient's regimen, the addition of allopurinol therapy should be accompanied by checks of any effect that it may have on the prothrombin time. Similarly, because allopurinol possibly increases the level of iron in the liver, patients should not take *iron salts* at the same time.

Allopurinol-induced inhibition of the enzyme xanthine oxidase may interfere with the metabolic degradation of drugs that are inactivated by this enzyme. This is particularly important in patients who are being treated with the antileukemic drug *mercaptopurine*. Its dose must be reduced to about one-third to one-quarter of the usual dose when allopurinol is added to the patient's regimen to prevent secondary hyperuricemia. The same is true for the immunosuppressive agent *azathioprine*, which is converted to mercaptopurine in the body. Failure to reduce dosage of these cytotoxic drugs could lead to dangerous depression of the bone marrow and to other typical toxic effects of these antimetabolites (Chap. 12).

Drug combinations. Allopurinol can be combined with all other drugs used in gout treatment, including colchicine, probenecid, and sulfinpyrazone. Its use in combination with probenecid, for example, may be required to reduce the size of large pools of uric acid that cannot readily be eliminated by use of the uricosuric drug alone. Some studies have suggested that probenecid may reduce the effectiveness of allopurinol by increasing the elimination of its active metabolite alloxanthine (oxipurinol). However, this has not really proved to be a drawback and, in many patients, the combination seems to be more effective than either drug alone for removing large urate deposits from chronically gouty joints and thus increasing their mobility. It is, of course, important to follow all the precautions employed when probenecid alone is being administered (see above).

Allopurinol, unlike the uricosuric drugs, *can* be taken together with salicylates without reducing its effectiveness. Thus, patients can take not only the relatively small doses of aspirin needed for relief of headache or other nongout pain but also the much larger doses required for anti-inflammatory activity. Large doses of aspirin also exert a uricosuric effect. However, as indicated above, the more potent uricosuric drugs are preferred for those patients who are likely to profit from a combination of drugs of that class with allopurinol.

Such a combined attack on hyperuricemia and on resistant tophaceous uric acid tissue deposits is especially effective, and is proving helpful to patients with severe gouty arthritis whose high uric acid production had previously prevented complete control of their condition. With the simultaneous administration of low daily doses of colchicine to prevent acute inflammatory reactions, most patients who are promptly treated with combinations of antigout drugs have an excellent prognosis. The nurse can confidently assure patients with gout that their condition is the best controlled of all the rheumatic disorders.

Chronic headache

The causes of headache

The nerve cells of the brain itself are insensitive to pain-producing stimuli. However, headache can result from stimulation of various cranial structures surrounding the brain. Arteries coursing through the membranous coverings of the brain contain pain-sensitive nerve endings. When these *intracranial* arteries are distended, signals are sent by way of afferent fibers to brain centers that translate them into pain that can be felt. Similarly, nerve impulses that arise in such *extracranial* structures as the skin, muscles, and blood vessels of the scalp and neck become a source of head pain when they reach the brain's pain-perceiving centers.

Headache is the most common complaint of patients seen by physicians. More than 50% of patients who consult a general practitioner report having headaches. The incidence of headache is even higher among patients seen by such specialists as neurologists and psychiatrists. Thus, one of a physician's main tasks is to determine the cause and significance of headache. The cause may be a minor functional disturbance of a temporary nature, but headache can also reflect an unresolved emotional conflict or the presence of an organic intracranial lesion.

Almost everyone has a headache at some time, either when coming down with a cold or other viral respiratory illness or as a result of a transient period of emotional tension. Such occasional headaches are of minor significance. They ordinarily need neither special medical diagnosis nor intensive drug treatment. On the other hand, patients who complain of chronically recurring headaches should be adivsed to visit a physician for proper diagnosis.

Organic causes

Such patients need a careful work-up to find the underlying disturbance. Occasionally, for example, headaches indicate the presence of intracranial structural changes caused by brain tumors, or serious cerebral vascular disorders such as aneurysms or angiomas. Ocular disturbances such as glaucoma may first be made manifest by headaches. Other organic disorders marked by the occurrence of frequent headaches include hypertension, chronic sinusitis caused by infection or allergy, and pressure on nerves in the region of the cervical spine.

Psychological causes

Headaches are usually not a sign of organic disease, but rather stem from psychophysiologic reactions to stressful situations. Some persons, for example, cannot express emotions such as anger. Sometimes such patterns of over-controlled behavior established in childhood seem to precipitate reactions in skeletal muscles and in vascular smooth muscles that result in periodic, incapacitating head pain. Personality factors of this type appear to play a part in the most common types of chronic headaches: *tension*, or *muscular contraction*, headaches, and *vascular* headaches.

Tension, or muscular contraction, headaches

The physiologic mechanism responsible for the development of these so-called tension headaches is a sustained state of contraction of the muscles of the neck and scalp. The tensing of these muscles often results from an unconscious reaction to stress—much as setting the jaw when reacting to a situation that calls forth a fighting response. Recurring headaches of this type may also be the result of other factors. For example, persons whose occupations require them to keep the head in a set position—for example, in typing or watch-repairing—may develop muscle tension headaches.

Nondrug treatment

Often such a headache problem can be solved by a simple physical change in work routine. Even when the main cause of a patient's headaches is emotional, with muscle tension stemming from psychological pressures, *non-pharmacologic* measures may relieve discomfort. Often, the nurse can suggest some safe, everyday measures such as gentle massage of the back of the neck, neck and back exercises, and setting aside some time for a quiet rest period or even for taking a warm relaxing bath. Sometimes it may be helpful to point out to a patient that such "pampering" is safer than the chronic use of drugs.

Pharmacotherapy

Despite the fact that drugs do not cure recurrent headaches and can be abused, drug therapy does have an important role as part of a total program for managing patients with chronic tension headaches. Thus, while the physician is trying to track down the sources of emotional stress that are triggering the patient's headaches, drugs may be ordered to help relieve head pain or to reduce the frequency of the painful episodes. Similarly, during attempts to resolve emotional conflicts in the patient's life situation by formal or informal psychotherapeutic techniques, drugs may be prescribed for their palliative effects when headaches develop.

Choice of products. The safest and simplest drugs for occasional adjunctive use in such cases are the mild analgesics discussed in Chapter 37. As indicated previously, the best procedure is to have the patient take a full dose of a single analgesic—preferably *plain aspirin* if, as is true for most people, this salicylate is tolerated. Patients sensitive to salicylates should receive a full dose of *acetaminophen* alone rather than a complex mixture of drugs.

Combinations. In theory, administering combinations of these drugs in fractional doses rather than full doses of each should reduce their adverse effects. In practice, however, there is no proof of lessened toxicity and, in fact, a person sensitive to one of the drugs in such fixed-dose combinations could suffer an allergic reaction that would not have occurred if a full dose of only the one analgesic to which he was not sensitive had been taken.

Similarly, such combinations are no more effective than full doses of aspirin or acetaminophen taken alone. There is also no reason to believe that the small dose of caffeine traditionally added to such analgesic combinations actually makes them more effective for pain relief. Although larger doses of caffeine may add to the effectiveness of ergotamine against migraine attacks (see below), the doses of 60 mg or less contained in most proprietary headache preparations—much less than in a cup of coffee—do not add to the effectiveness of the analgesics with which they are combined.

On the other hand, the addition of weak opiate-type analgesics such as *codeine* or *oxycodone* to aspirin, acetaminophen, or phenacetin may produce more effective pain relief than is obtainable with the latter drugs alone. The reason is that these opiates act centrally at a different site and in a different manner from the analgesic–antipyretics. Thus, the resulting supra-additive effect may be beneficial against unusually severe headaches.

Dependence. Such combinations should be ordered sparingly because the routine use of opiate analgesics—even one such as codeine, with relatively little abuse potential—is undesirable in the treatment of chronic conditions, including recurrent tension headaches. Actually, some people with chronic headaches tend to become psychologically dependent on various remedies, even when the drugs involved are not opiates. That is, they begin to take aspirin indiscriminately, alone or combined with phenacetin and caffeine, for relief of headache. As with anything else that produces a feeling of relative well-being, such tablet-taking soon becomes a habit, and the habitual ingestion of large amounts of even these relatively safe drugs can have serious results (see Chap. 37).

Careful patient education is needed to help patients realize the potential dangers of self-medication and the possible development of toxicity. Patients should be able to recognize the signs and symptoms of analgesic toxicity, as well as the limits of self-medication, and at what point they should consult with their physician or nurse. Thorough patient education can help to prevent serious problems from developing.

Other components. Various prescription products for tension headaches contain sedatives such as a barbiturate or an antianxiety agent with muscle-relaxing properties, such as meprobamate (see Chap. 45). In theory, this should add to the effectiveness of the analgesic drugs in the combination. Although sedation does not significantly raise the threshold for pain perception, it does tend to reduce the patient's emotional reaction to head pain, however, and relaxation of the contracted scalp and neck muscles should reduce the source of the pain. In practice, the small doses of sedative and muscle-relaxing drugs contained in such fixed-dosage combination products have not been proved effective for these purposes. Occasionally, however, the administration of a drug such as diazepam (Valium) in adequately large doses may help to relieve tension headaches in someone who does not respond to analgesics alone.

Depression

Most patients with tension headaches manage to control their symptoms reasonably well by modifying somewhat their responses to stress and by using the simple physical and pharmacologic measures mentioned above. Sometimes, however, muscle contraction headaches are only one symptom of a severe depressive syndrome. These patients should not be treated symptomatically with mere analgesics and sedatives, or even with superficial psychotherapeutic supportive measures. Instead, such patients with serious psychological conflicts should be referred to a psychiatrist. If this specialist believes in the use of any drugs at all for treating recurrent tension headaches, an antidepressant drug such as amitriptyline (Elavil) alone or in combination with a major tranquilizer such as perphenazine (Trilafon) will probably be ordered.

Vascular headaches

Headaches that develop as a result of dilation of the intracranial and extracranial arteries are less common but much more severe than tension, or muscle contraction, headaches. Vascular headaches are sometimes classed as migraine and *non*migraine types.

Nonmigraine headaches

In nonmigraine headaches the physician tries to find the underlying cause and deals with it directly rather than only through the use of analgesic and sedative drugs. For example, if cranial vasodilation stems from infection and fever, the remedy may be an antibiotic rather than aspirin alone. Similarly, even in more chronic conditions such as essential hypertension, the hypertensive vascular head-

aches with which the patient commonly wakens in the morning are best dealt with by controlling high blood pressure with antihypertensive agents (Chap. 28).

Migraine headaches

This term is used to describe several different types of symptom complexes that have in common the periodic development of severe throbbing headaches on one side of the head. Some authorities suggest that this unilateral head pain is only the most prominent symptom of true migraine, which is a constitutional disorder that can cause widespread disturbances involving various other systems including, in particular, the gastrointestinal and central nervous systems. Some patients, in fact, suffer periodic attacks of what are called migraine equivalents or variants, the main symptoms of which are varied changes in abdominal function and mood.

Migraine headaches are sometimes classified on the basis of differences in the pattern of individual attacks and in the patient's life history: classic migraine, common or ordinary migraine, and cluster headaches. In all three types the pain mechanism is the same. The pain is mainly the result of arterial dilation. Pulsations of the arteries with each heartbeat that drives blood up the carotid arteries distend the cranial and extracranial blood vessels. This is thought to stimulate pain-sensitive nerve endings in the smooth muscle walls of the arteries.

In addition, certain substances are believed to be released locally that play a part in the development and perpetuation of migraine attacks. One of these is a polypeptide called *neurokinin* that resembles—and may, in fact be—*bradykinin*, which can cause both vasodilation and stimulation of pain receptors. *Serotonin* also seems to be involved in setting off some of the local tissue changes seen in patients during migraine attacks. Sometimes, in the late stages of an attack, a tension-type headache is superimposed on the vascular headache, perhaps because the patient involuntarily contracts skeletal muscles and keeps the neck stiff in trying to avoid moving the head.

Treatment of an acute attack. Migraine patients are fortunate in having available a relatively specific agent for treating acute attacks: the ergot derivative *ergotamine tartrate*+ (Gynergen). This drug is an α-adrenergic receptor blocker and a serotonin receptor blocker. It acts mainly to contract the smooth muscle walls of the branches of the external carotid artery. This action on dilated, pulsating cranial arterioles directly counteracts the mechanism thought to cause the pain of vascular headaches. Interruption of vasodilation and distention stops any further stimulation of pain-sensitive nerve endings, and probably prevents leakage of inflammatory substances into the area. This often leads to dramatic relief of the attack.

Administration of ergotamine. A great deal is now known about how best to give ergotamine. More than 90% of patients can be helped by prompt administration of an adequate dose; failure to halt an attack is usually the result of giving too little of the drug too late. Thus, headache specialists advocate the use of full doses of ergotamine. First, the lowest dose of ergotamine needed to abort the attacks is determined. Then the patient is taught to take that amount as soon as an attack is felt to be coming on. At first, the patient takes the drug by mouth in divided doses—usually two 1-mg tablets at once, and then another 1-mg tablet every half hour up to a maximum of 6 mg (Table 38-3). Once a patient knows how much ergotamine it takes to abort the attacks, that entire amount may be taken at once, and then the patient may rest quietly in a darkened room for a few hours.

Other preparations. Although the oral route is the most convenient way to take ergotamine, it has certain drawbacks that sometimes limit its usefulness. Absorption of ergotamine from the gastrointestinal tract is relatively slow and unpredictable, even when there is no food in the patient's stomach. The delay of over 30 minutes in onset of action may allow a classic-type migraine headache, which can build up to peak severity very soon after the first prodromal symptoms appear, to become full blown. Thus, the more rapidly absorbed *sublingual* tablets (Ergomar; Ergostat) or the aerosol inhalation form of the drug (Medihaler Ergotamine) may be preferred in such cases.

Another difficulty in taking ergotamine orally is that the vomiting that often accompanies migraine attacks may cause loss of the drug before it can be absorbed. Inhalation or sublingual administration of ergotamine avoids such failure to absorb the full dose.

Cluster headaches. This type of unilateral vascular headache may be a variant of migraine, but it differs from classic and common migraine in the pattern that the attacks take. As the name suggests, attacks tend to come in clusters, sometimes as many as 20 a week. Each attack comes on suddenly, often during sleep, and the patient may pace the floor in agony until relief is obtained. It begins with a brief period of burning discomfort, often in the orbit of one eye, and then builds up to a steady, boring, throbbing pain on one side of the temple, jaw, and occipital region.

This condition is also called *histamine cephalalgia*, because it is believed to be associated with local release of histamine. Although, at the height of the headache, the eye on the affected side may be red and watery and the nostril runny or stuffy, these symptoms do not respond well to treatment with antihistaminic drugs, including

Table 38–3. Drugs used for the treatment and prevention of migraine and related types of headaches

Official or generic name	Trade name	Usual adult dosage and administration	Indications
Dihydroergotamine mesylate	D.H.E. 45	1 mg IM q 1 hr (maximum dose 3 mg); IV maximum dose: 2 mg/attack, 6 mg/week	To abort migraine-type headaches rapidly or when other routes are not feasible
Ergotamine tartrate	Gynergen	Two to six 1-mg tablets PO/attack	Treatment of migraine-type headaches
	Ergomar; Ergostat	Three 2-mg sublingual tablets q 30 min (maximum dose: three tablets/day, five tablets/wk)	
	Medihaler Ergotamine	One aerosol inhalation q 5 min (maximum dose: six inhalations/day)	
Methysergide maleate	Sansert	4–8 mg/day PO (drug must be withdrawn for 3–4 wk after 6 months)	Prophylaxis of severe migraine-type headaches
Propranolol HCl	Inderal	Initially, 80 mg/day PO in divided doses, or one sustained-release tablet/day; may gradually increase to 160–240 mg/day	Prophylaxis of migraine-type headaches

those having a strong antiserotonin component such as cyproheptadine HCl.

The most appropriate treatment for these rapidly developing attacks is the IM injection of *dihydroergotamine mesylate* (D.H.E. 45), a chemical and pharmacologic relative of ergotamine, whose effects begin about 15 minutes after IM injection. Quick control of the excruciating pain of cluster headaches is very important, for, although the pain often ends as suddenly as it began within 1 or 2 hours, some patients have been driven to suicide by such continued attacks of severe head and face pain.

Adverse reactions to ergotamine treatment. Ergotamine toxicity (ergotism; Chap. 23) is said to develop in only about one in every 10,000 patients who take the drug in the doses recommended for treating an acute attack. However, because of the seriousness of overdosage, the amount administered during a single attack is usually limited to 6 mg, and no more than 10 mg is the recommended weekly maximum intake of ergotamine.

Side-effects. Nausea and vomiting, which are the result of central stimulation rather than of irritation of the gastrointestinal tract, occur frequently. When the drug is given orally, it is often combined with belladonna-type antispasmodics, barbiturates such as pentobarbital, or antiemetics such as cyclizine (Chap. 41). If vomiting persists, a phenothiazine-type antiemetic (*e.g.,* chlorpromazine) may be administered.

More serious than these gastrointestinal complaints are signs of peripheral vasoconstriction, such as sensations of coldness, numbness, and tingling in the toes and fingers. The leg muscles may become painfully cramped as a result of ischemia caused by partial shutdown of circulation. Such potentially dangerous reactions are said to occur only rarely in most patients. However, the possible occurrence of excessive vasoconstriction makes the use of ergotamine undesirable in patients sensitive to any substance that reduces local blood flow.

Contraindications. Ergotamine is contraindicated in peripheral vascular diseases such as intermittent claudication (Chap. 33) and in various other vascular diseases marked by atherosclerosis. Patients with a history of coronary disease, for example, may complain of chest pains similar to those of an attack of angina pectoris; in hypertensive patients blood pressure may rise as a result of drug-induced generalized vasoconstriction. The drug is not given to patients with sepsis and liver or kidney disease. Because of its potential oxytocic effect on the uterine musculature, ergotamine is contraindicated during pregnancy. (For a discussion of the treatment of acute ergot toxicity, see Chapter 23.)

Other antimigraine agents. Isometheptene, a drug free of the adverse effects and contraindications of ergotamine, has reportedly proven to be effective for relief of vascular headaches in some patients. Because it does not stimulate uterine muscle contractions, it can be employed during pregnancy. Isometheptene is an adrenergic,

or a sympathomimetic, drug that is thought to exert a relatively specific constricting effect on branches of the external carotid artery when administered in small oral doses that have little or no vasoconstrictor effect on peripheral arterioles or on the systemic circulation. However, caution is required in patients with severe hypertension.

This drug is available in combination with mild analgesic and sedative drugs for both treating and preventing vascular headaches. It is not considered as dependable as ergotamine for suppressing severe migraine attacks, but the isometheptene-containing combination may be more effective than ergotamine against headaches that have a muscle tension as well as a vascular component.

Caffeine is commonly combined with ergotamine in products for treating vascular headaches, just as it is a component of tension headache products that contain such mild analgesics as aspirin and acetaminophen. There is some evidence that its presence may increase the effectiveness of ergotamine, possibly by raising the rate and completeness of its absorption or by adding to its cranial vasoconstrictor effect. The actual value of caffeine in vascular headaches has been questioned, as is the case when it is combined with mild analgesics (see above).

Prevention of acute attacks

Ergotamine. Although authorities agree that ergotamine is an effective drug for *treating* acute attacks, the question of its effectiveness for *preventing* attacks is quite controversial. Some say that they have found the drug useful for preventing headaches and harmless when it is taken daily in recommended doses. Others argue that ergotamine is of no value for preventing attacks and that its daily use could lead to habituation or, because of its peripheral vasoconstrictor effects, to arterial insufficiency.

People who have only occasional isolated migraine attacks—most patients with classic and common migraine—do not require a prophylactic drug in the intervals between their infrequent attacks. However, patients who suffer frequent severe attacks that interfere with their ability to work or function normally would clearly benefit from a safe and effective prophylactic drug.

Methysergide. This drug appears to be more effective than ergotamine for *preventing* all types of vascular headaches, including the cluster, or histamine cephalalgia, type. Although methysergide (Sansert) blocks the effects of serotonin, a substance believed to play a part in vascular headaches, the beneficial effects of the drug have not been clearly linked to its serotonin-antagonizing property. However, experience indicates that about 50% of patients with frequent, severe vascular headaches who take this drug regularly report improvement. That is, they seem to suffer fewer headaches, and those that do occur appear to be less severe and more readily controllable.

Patients taking methysergide must be followed quite carefully to avoid an unusual type of complication:

the development of inflammation followed by fibrosis in some body tissues. One such reaction—retroperitoneal fibrosis—occurs in pelvic area connective tissues and can lead to urinary tract obstruction. Similar lesions in lung tissue can lead to pleuropulmonary complications, and fibrotic thickening can also occur in cardiac valves and around major arteries. However, if symptoms caused by fibrotic phenomena are detected and the drug is discontinued, the growths readily regress in most cases.

Most side-effects of methysergide are minor and tend to disappear during continued treatment. Some of these are similar to those that occur when ergotamine is administered during migraine attacks. For example, the epigastric distress, nausea, and vomiting sometimes seen with ergotamine are likely to occur early in treatment with methysergide. To minimize such gastrointestinal side-effects, the drug is ordinarily taken with meals. Patients sometimes start on one tablet a day, taken at bedtime with food or liquid. Then, a second dose is added at breakfast and, after several days of observation, postluncheon and, finally, after-dinner doses are added to the regimen.

The patient who has been stabilized on the smallest dose that is both tolerated and effective for reducing headache frequency is examined regularly during a 6-month course of methysergide therapy and during a recommended drug-free interval of several weeks between courses. For example, intravenous pyelography is employed to detect any evidence of fibrosis affecting the ureters, and chest x-rays are taken if there is any reason to suspect that a lung lesion may be developing.

Patients are warned to report any signs of vasospasm, such as cold or numbness in the hands, cramping leg pains, or constricting chest pain. These reactions are most likely to occur in patients who already have some tendency toward vascular obstruction. Thus, methysergide is, like ergotamine, contraindicated in peripheral vascular disease and phlebitis. Evidence of arteriosclerosis or of coronary artery disease or severe hypertension also indicates that this drug should be avoided.

Propranolol (Inderal) was first observed to prevent migraine attacks in patients who were being treated for angina pectoris with this β-adrenergic blocking agent (Chap. 31). This serendipitous observation led neurologists to try propranolol in some of their patients who suffered frequent, intractable vascular headaches of this type. This use of propranolol was finally given FDA approval. When taken in daily doses of 80 to 160 mg, propranolol is significantly more effective than placebos, and its prophy-

lactic use reduces the number of headaches in most patients by more than 50%. A few patients have reportedly become entirely free of migraine headaches when continuous propranolol therapy was employed and, in some cases, the benefit outlasted the duration of therapy. On the other hand, headaches became more frequent than before treatment when propranolol was withdrawn from some patients. This could be prevented by maintaining these patients on lower daily dosages of 30 to 60 mg. It is now recommended that therapy be withdrawn gradually over a 2-week period when termination is desired.

The mechanism of propranolol prophylaxis is uncertain. Some scientists speculate that it acts to prevent reactive vasodilation in the arterioles of the extracranial vascular bed by blocking β-adrenergic receptors in the blood vessels, but some other β blockers are ineffective. Recently it has been suggested that the use of propranolol to prevent reinfarction in patients who have already suffered one myocardial infarction may be a result of the ability of propranolol to block calcium channels. It is interesting to note that the calcium channel blocker verapamil HCl (Chaps. 30 and 31) has been found in one study to be helpful in preventing migraine attacks. Perhaps blockade of calcium channels may be involved in the antimigraine effect of propranolol.

Experimental prophylactic agents. Several drugs considered to be safer than either ergotamine or methysergide have been reported to reduce the frequency and severity of migraine headaches in some patients subject to many attacks each month. Because many antimigraine measures were at first highly praised, and then later proved to be no more useful than placebos, caution is necessary before any new therapy is accepted as useful.

Clonidine (Catapres), an antihypertensive drug (Chap. 28), has also reportedly reduced the number of severe headaches in a majority of migraine patients taking small prophylactic doses of 50 to 100 µg daily.* Results of some studies suggest that, even after these patients stopped taking this drug, the frequency of their headaches remained low. On the other hand, some investigators have found clonidine to be no more effective than a placebo.

Cyproheptadine (Periactin), an antihistaminic drug with antiserotonin activity (Chap. 39), has been reported effective for reducing vascular headaches in about 50% of patients in whom it has been tried. Paradoxically, some patients who are not depressed are also helped by drugs used to treat depression—for example, monoamine oxidase inhibitors and tricyclic antidepressants (Chap. 46), both of which can *elevate* serotonin levels at synapses.

Additional clinical considerations

The treatment of chronic headache can be complex and difficult. Prevention is the most desirable approach. Once a severe headache has occurred, it is difficult to alleviate the pain. Most patients learn to recognize the early signs

---

* Clonidine has also been reported to relieve the distress of withdrawal from opioids such as heroin and methadone. Unlike the latter drug, which is used in detoxification and maintenance therapy in opioid-dependent patients (Chap. 53), clonidine does not cause physical or psychological dependence while suppressing the signs and symptoms of opioid withdrawal. In this respect it resembles propranolol, which is also being used experimentally for this purpose.

and symptoms of an impending headache, and should be taught to take their medication at this stage and, if possible, to rest until such feelings have passed. Patients need to learn to carry their medication with them at all times and to be prepared to deal with a headache if it should occur. Some patients can benefit from relaxation or stress reduction techniques, or from exercise. Other patients cannot discover ways to prevent or alleviate headaches. All these patients need support and encouragement to deal with this extremely painful disease. When an acute

headache occurs, and the patient can seek medical assistance, analgesia, control of environmental stimuli, and support will be required. The patient should know that a nurse is readily available, because many patients are in so much pain that they cannot move or respond effectively.

The patient teaching guides and guides to the nursing process of other chapters summarize the clinical points that should be considered with the drugs used to treat chronic headache.

Summary of adverse effects and contraindications of ergotamine

Minor side effects

Nausea and vomiting; occasionally diarrhea

Early signs and symptoms of ergotism

Numbness and tingling of the fingers and toes
Localized skin edema and itching
Transient tachycardia and bradycardia

Serious signs and symptoms of ergotism

Pain, cramps, and weakness in the muscles of the extremities
Extremities cold, pale, or cyanotic
Reduced or absent peripheral pulses
Thrombophlebitis, vascular spasm, possible gangrene

Chest pains, ECG changes, and possibly myocardial infarction
Somnolence, confusion, stupor, and coma
Rarely, trismus and convulsions

Contraindications

Peripheral vascular diseases
Coronary heart disease
Hypertension
Severe arteriosclerosis
Liver or kidney function impairment
Sepsis
Pregnancy

Case study

Presentation

NI, a 37-year-old female schoolteacher, was admitted to the emergency department in acute distress: BP 160/88, P 110, R 24, diaphoretic, pale, eyes tightly closed. NI had reportedly been acting strangely at work; she was somewhat disoriented, and her speech was slightly slurred. She was found, shortly after these observations, slumped on the floor near her desk. She managed to tell a colleague that she was having a severe headache, and an ambulance was called. NI was monitored, given meperidine hydrochloride (Demerol) and kept in a cool darkened room until her headache was relieved. NI was then thoroughly evaluated for possible etiologies of headache. It was determined that NI was suffering from migraine headaches. By history, it was found that NI experienced severe headaches about once every 6 months. The headaches were usually preceded by a period of light-headedness, slurred speech, and disorientation that occurred 1 to 2 hours before onset of the headache. NI had been experiencing more frequent migraine headaches over the past few months, with each one being more severe. It was determined that NI should be given ergotamine (Ergostat) 2 mg sublingually, and followed in the headache clinic.

What teaching considerations should be included in NI's nursing care?

Discussion

NI should be evaluated for the presence of any condition that would contraindicate ergotamine therapy: pregnancy, peripheral vascular disease, hepatic or renal disease, hypertension, thrombophlebitis. She should then receive patient teaching regarding the nature of her disease and the mechanisms of drug action. She should also be instructed in the use of sublingual tablets. The timing of drug use should be carefully explained. NI should be encouraged to talk through her experiences surrounding the headaches. Signs and symptoms that seem to occur preceding her headaches should be pointed out, and NI should be encouraged to be alert for the occurrence of these and to take the Ergostat as soon as any of them occur. She can take up to a total of five tablets for any one attack. The adverse drug effects that might occur should also be discussed and written down—numbness and tingling in toes or fingers, muscle pain, weakness, and nausea. NI should be encouraged to discuss her feelings about her disease. The necessity for treating migraine headaches before they become severe should be stressed. NI should be encouraged to carry her medication with her at all times, and should be encouraged to avoid excess stress and to decrease environmental stimuli when she feels that a headache is coming on. NI may require a great deal of support and encouragement to cope with her diagnosis and drug therapy. The severity of her most recent migraine was probably very frightening for NI. All the information given to NI should be written down for future reference, and she should be given an appointment for a follow-up visit to evaluate her response to drug therapy as well as the effectiveness of the teaching program and support offered.

Drug digests

Allopurinol USP (Zyloprim)

Actions and indications. This drug reduces the production of uric acid. This leads to a lowering of the level of uric acid in both the blood and the urine. Gout patients with kidney damage and those who tend to form uric acid kidney stones are particularly likely to benefit from the drug's ability to reduce uric acid in the tissues without increasing its concentration in the urine.

The drug is also employed to prevent hyperuricemia and uric acid nephropathy in patients with neoplastic diseases. Such patients are particularly susceptible to secondary gout and kidney stone formation when they are treated with radiation or antineoplastic drugs. Thus, in addition to its use in primary gout, allopurinol is employed to prevent a rise in plasma uric acid levels and subsequent precipitation of uric acid in the tissues of patients suffering from polycythemia, leukemias, lymphomas, and other malignancies.

Adverse effects, cautions, and contraindications. Skin rashes, mostly morbilliform, are the most common adverse effect. More serious types of dermatitis, chills and fever, and gastrointestinal disturbances may also result from idiosyncratic reactions to this drug. Drowsiness that may make driving dangerous sometimes occurs. Tests of liver function should be performed periodically to detect early signs of hepatotoxicity. Iron salts should not be administered simultaneously because of the possibility that iron may be deposited in the liver. The simultaneous administration of colchicine is desirable to prevent any increase in acute attacks at the start of treatment with allopurinol.

Dosage and administration. Treatment is begun with low doses—100 or 200 mg daily—to reduce gout attack flare-ups. This is increased gradually to 200 or 300 mg a day in mild cases or 400 to 600 mg for more severe gout. These amounts are divided into two or three doses that are taken after meals. A high fluid intake is also desirable during intensive therapy to prevent nephropathy.

Aurothioglucose USP (Solganal)

Actions and indications. This gold salt often brings about remissions in patients with rheumatoid arthritis that has not responded to a regimen of salicylates and conservative measures. A course of treatment is most effective when administered in the early stages of the disease and least effective when joint damage is well advanced. Recurrences are common, but the patient may respond well to additional courses administered whenever the disease becomes active again. Although this drug often halts progressive joint deterioration temporarily, x-rays indicate that joint damage continues to occur and is eventually as advanced as with other antirheumatic drug treatment.

Adverse effects, cautions, and contraindications. Various types of reactions are common, mostly in the early stages of treatment. Patients must be closely observed and questioned, and urinalyses and blood counts must be done frequently during treatment. The most common indication of approaching toxicity is pruritus and redness of the skin. Inflammation of the mucous membranes of the mouth may also occur. Such signs of dermatitis or development of stomatitis or glossitis require withdrawal of gold salts. However, treatment may be begun again at lower dose levels a few weeks after relatively mild reactions clear up.

Treatment should be discontinued immediately, if any clinical or laboratory signs of bone marrow, kidney, or liver damage develop. Chrysotherapy is contraindicated in patients with a history of blood dyscrasias, kidney or liver disease, severe diabetes, marked hypertension, or allergic skin disorders. Gold salts should not be administered together with other antirheumatic drugs—such as phenylbutazone—that are known to depress bone marrow function.

Dosage and administration. Various types of courses are employed depending in part on the response of the patient. A typical schedule of IM injections of this oily suspension is the following: First week, 10 mg; second and third weeks, 25 mg; then 50 mg at weekly intervals, until a total of 750 mg to 1000 mg has been given. Then, if remission has occurred without signs of toxicity, the 50-mg dose may continue to be administered every 3 or 4 weeks for many more months. Some rheumatologists stop chrysotherapy at the end of a year; others recommend its continued use in doses that keep the plasma level of gold at 0.3 mg/100 ml.

Colchicine USP

Actions and indications. This drug is specific in the treatment of gout. It acts to suppress inflammation and relieve pain while aborting acute attacks of gouty arthritis when it is administered early in the attack and in adequate doses. Although it does not affect uric acid metabolism, colchicine also helps to prevent or reduce the frequency of acute recurrences. For this purpose, it is often administered in small daily doses together with a uricosuric agent such as probenecid.

Its presence when treatment with a uricosuric agent or allopurinol is being initiated helps to prevent these drugs from setting off acute attacks in the early stages of their administration for prophylactic purposes. Similarly, prophylactic administration of colchicine makes it easier to bring an acute attack under control with therapeutic doses of the same drug, if an attack should occur.

Adverse effects, cautions, and contraindications. Oral doses often cause gastrointestinal irritation leading to diarrhea as well as nausea and vomiting. Thus, caution is required in patients with peptic ulcer or other chronic gastrointestinal disorders. Administration by the intravenous route is less likely to cause GI symptoms. However, the danger of other toxic effects, including kidney damage, may be increased in cases of overdosage. Shock may occur as a result of damage to blood vessels and severe hemorrhagic gastroenteritis. Caution is required in the elderly, in patients in a weakened state, and in those with cardiovascular disease. Long-term therapy may cause bone marrow damage or peripheral neuritis.

Dosage and administration. Acute attacks may be treated by oral administration of one or two 0.6-mg tablets as soon as the first warning signs appear, followed by one such tablet every 1 or 2 hours until pain is relieved or diarrhea develops.

When the intravenous route is employed, an initial dose of 1 mg or 2 mg is followed by 0.5 mg every 3 to 6 hours up to a total dose of not more than 4 mg in 24 hours. Care is required to avoid leakage of the solution into the subcutaneous or muscular tissues, because this can lead to pain and necrosis.

For prophylaxis during the intervals between attacks, smaller oral doses are employed, ranging from 0.5 or 0.6 mg one to four times weekly to once or twice daily.

Ergotamine tartrate USP (Gynergen)

Actions and indications. This ergot alkaloid is relatively specific for control of all types of acute vascular headache attacks, including the classic migraine and cluster types. It acts by constricting dilated cerebral arterioles and thus reduces their pain-producing pulsations. The addition of caffeine is claimed to potentiate ergotamine's vasoconstrictor effect. This drug is *not* recommended for long-term use for prophylactic purposes, and it should not be taken daily for longer than 1 week.

Adverse effects, cautions, and contraindications. Nausea, vomiting, epigastric distress, and diarrhea may occur with large doses administered by any route. More serious are signs of peripheral vasoconstriction, including paresthesias of the fingers and toes, muscle cramps, and possibly chest pain. Overdosage for prolonged periods can lead to blood vessel damage and gangrene.

This drug is contraindicated in patients with peripheral vascular diseases such as Buerger's and Raynaud's diseases and intermittent claudication. It should also not be taken by patients with coronary vascular disease or hypertension. Its use is avoided in pregnancy and in the presence of liver or kidney disease. Hypersensitive patients who develop localized edema and itching should discontinue use of this drug.

Dosage and administration. This drug is most effective when administered at the first sign of an attack. It may be administered orally, as an aerosol by inhalation, and by the buccal and sublingual routes.

Oral administration of 1 mg or 2 mg may be followed by additional doses every half hour. Maximum dosage for a 24-hour period is 6 mg; 10 mg is the most that should be taken this way in any 1 week.

Sublingually or by the buccal route, one 2-mg tablet is employed, and two more may be taken at half-hour intervals, if necessary.

Aerosol inhalation of 0.36 mg may be repeated up to six times in 24 hours.

Indomethacin USP (Indocin)

Actions and indications. This potent nonsteroidal anti-inflammatory, analgesic–antipyretic drug is employed to reduce pain, swelling, and tenderness of joints in moderate to severe rheumatoid and degenerative joint disorders that have not responded to safer drugs such as the salicylates. These conditions include active rheumatoid arthritis in both chronic and acute stages, ankylosing spondylitis, osteoarthritis of the hip, and acute gouty arthritis.

Adverse effects, cautions, and contraindications. Gastrointestinal reactions are marked by nausea, anorexia, vomiting, epigastric distress, and abdominal pain, and diarrhea. The occurrence of these symptoms may require discontinuing the drug to avoid gastrointestinal bleeding, ulcerations, and possible perforation or stenosis with obstruction.

Central nervous system reactions are marked by a high incidence of headache, drowsiness, dizziness, and light-headedness. If headache persists, the drug should be discontinued. Patients should be advised not to drive a car if the drug reduces their mental alertness or interferes with motor coordination. Mental confusion and psychological disturbances may occur in some cases.

Sensory disturbances including tinnitus and rarely deafness are sometimes reported. Blurring of vision may be an indication of ocular disturbances involving the cornea or the retina. Their occurrence warrants a thorough ophthalmologic examination. This may be desirable periodically even in patients without eye symptoms when they require prolonged therapy.

Dosage and administration. This drug is best given with food or immediately after meals in the smallest dose effective for symptomatic relief. Patients with most disorders responsive to treatment are started on 25 mg two or three times daily. This dose is raised in weekly increments of 25 mg, until a total daily dose of 150 to 200 mg is reached. This may be raised by 25 mg daily during acute flares of rheumatoid arthritis, or the dose may be reduced rapidly if severe adverse reactions develop.

In acute gouty arthritis, treatment is begun with 50 mg tid, but this large dose should be rapidly reduced and then discontinued as pain is relieved and joint tenderness and swelling subside during the next few days.

Phenylbutazone USP (Azolid; Butazolidin)

Actions and indications. The potent anti-inflammatory action of this drug accounts for its usefulness in carefully selected cases of rheumatoid disorders. Although the drug also has analgesic, antipyretic, and uricosuric actions, other safer agents are preferred for simple pain relief, fever reduction, and increasing the excretion of uric acid.

This drug is most valuable for symptomatic relief in cases of rheumatoid arthritis not controlled by salicylates, cases of ankylosing spondylitis not responsive to indomethacin, and acute gout attacks not controlled by colchicine. The drug's actions in relieving joint pain or tenderness, swelling, heat, and redness help the patient to maintain mobility.

This drug is also effective in cases of venous thrombosis in which acute inflammation plays a part, such as superficial thrombophlebitis.

Adverse effects, cautions, and contraindications. This drug can cause several types of severe side-effects, particularly in elderly patients and in those with various diseases that increase susceptibility to toxicity. Thus, patients must be carefully selected, observed frequently, and instructed to report development of various symptoms that may signal the onset of potentially dangerous adverse reactions.

Patients on long-term therapy must receive regular blood studies to detect changes in the formed elements. Sometimes hematologic disorders develop even despite such precautions. Use of this drug is contraindicated in patients with a prior history of blood dyscrasias.

Gastrointestinal distress is common and may lead to bleeding and possible ulceration and perforation. Patients with a history of persistent dyspepsia as well as those with gastritis or ulceration should not receive this drug. Its use in patients with cardiac decompensation, hypertension, and other cardiovascular, renal, and liver disorders is also contraindicated.

Dosage and administration. Dosage varies depending on many factors in each patient's situation. Initially, adults with most rheumatoid disorders receive between 300 and 600 mg daily tid or qid, with each dose taken immediately before or after meals or with a glass of milk. Administration should not be continued for more than 1 week if no benefit is seen. If improvement does occur, dosage is reduced to the smallest amount that will maintain relief.

In acute gouty arthritis, higher doses are administered for a period of a week or less—for example, 400 mg initially followed by 100 mg every 4 hours until joint inflammation subsides. In acute thrombophlebitis, daily doses of 600 mg are administered for 2 or 3 days, after which the dose is reduced to 300 mg for the final few days of treatment.

Probenecid USP (Benemid)

Actions and indications. This drug acts on renal tubular reabsorptive and secretory functions, which account for its two main types of clinical indications. The drug's most common use is as a uricosuric agent—a drug for increasing renal excretion of uric acid and thus reducing hyperuricemia in gout patients.

It is also often administered together with penicillin G, ampicillin, and other penicillins to raise the levels of these antibiotics in the plasma and tissues and to prolong their anti-infective effects in treating resistant cases of gonorrhea and other severe infections that require maintenance of prolonged bactericidal activity.

Adverse effects, cautions, and contraindications. This drug is *not* effective for treating acute gout, and its use may in fact sometimes set off an attack. (This is best avoided or treated by the simultaneous administration of colchicine.) If an analgesic is required for minor pain, acetaminophen should be employed, because aspirin and other salicylates act to antagonize the uricosuric effect of probenecid.

This drug is ordinarily well tolerated. However, hypersensitivity reactions, including pruritic rashes, fever, and even anaphylaxis, have occurred; the drug is contraindicated in patients with a history of hypersensitivity or of drug-induced hemolytic anemia. Headache and gastrointestinal upset are reported occasionally but are less frequent than with the other major uricosuric agent, sulfinpyrazone.

Dosage and administration. Treatment is started only after an acute gout attack has subsided. Initially, only 0.25 g is administered twice a day for 1 week. Later, this is raised to 0.5 g bid, or to still higher levels (up to 2 g daily) in patients with impaired kidney function. It is important to force fluids to prevent uric acid crystals from forming. Sometimes administration of systemic alkalinizers such as sodium bicarbonate or potassium citrate is also recommended to increase the solubility of uric acid in the urine and thus avoid urate stones.

As an adjunct to penicillin therapy, a total daily dosage of 2 g is recommended for most adult patients; children's dosages are calculated from body weight and body surface factors.

References

Chan WY: Prostaglandins and nonsteroidal anti-inflammatory drugs in dysmenorrhea. Ann Rev Pharmacol Toxicol 23:131, 1983

Cooper SA: New peripherally acting oral analgesic agents. Ann Rev Pharmacol Toxicol 23:617, 1983

Curry HLF et al: Comparison of azathioprine, cyclophosphamide, and gold in the treatment of rheumatoid arthritis. Br Med J 3:763, 1974

Dromgoole SH et al: Rational approaches to use of salicylates in treatment of rheumatoid arthritis. Semin Arthritis Rheum 11:257, 1983

Flower RJ, Moncada S, Vane JR: Analgesic–antipyretics and anti-inflammatory agents; drugs employed in the treatment of gout. In Gilman AG, Goodman LS, Gilman A (eds): Goodman and Gilman's The Pharmacological Basis of Therapeutics, 6th ed, pp 682–728. New York, Macmillan, 1980

Jaffe IA: D-Penicillamine. Bull Rheum Dis 28:948, 1977

Kantor TG (ed): Symposium: Pharmacology, Efficacy, and Safety of a New Class of Anti-Inflammatory Agents: A Review of Piroxicam. Am J Med 72:1 (Feb), 1982

Lance JW: Migraine: Current approach to prevention and treatment. Drugs 19:306, 1980

Lewis JR: New antirheumatic drugs. JAMA 237:1260, 1977

Mongan E et al: Tinnitus as an indication of therapeutic serum salicylate levels. JAMA 226:142, 1973

Raskin NH: Pharmacology of migraine. Ann Rev Pharmacol Toxicol 21:463, 1981

Rastegar A, Thier SO: The treatment of hyperuricemia in gout. Ration Drug Ther 8:1, 1974

Rodman MJ: Relief for rheumatic disorders. Part 1: Rheumatoid arthritis. RN 39:75, 1976

Rodman MJ: Relief for rheumatic disorders. Part 2: Gout and gouty arthritis. RN 39:71, 1976

Rodnan GP: Treatment of gout and other crystal-induced arthritis. Bull Rheum Dis 32:43, 1982

Sigler JW et al: Gold salts in the treatment of rheumatoid arthritis. A double-blind study. Ann Intern Med 80:21, 1974

Toxicity of nonsteroidal anti-inflammatory drugs. Med Lett Drugs Ther 25:15, 1983

Wilkinson M, Orton D: Some observations on use of ergotamine tartrate. Headache 20:159, 1980

Chapter 39

Antihistamines
and
other drugs
in the
management
of allergy

The nature of allergy

More than 35 million Americans are said to suffer from allergic disorders. The term *allergy* refers to the tendency of some people's tissues to react in an abnormal way when they come in contact with various ordinary substances that are part of the everyday environment. Most of these people are *atopic*—that is, they have inherited an immune system deficiency that results in their reacting differently from other people to the presence of substances foreign to the human body.*

One common type of allergic immune injury is called *type I hypersensitivity* (Chap. 5). It is involved clinically in producing such disorders as allergic rhinitis or nasal allergies, including hay fever, bronchial asthma, and urticaria or hives. This type of allergic hypersensitivity is also the cause of *anaphylactic* reactions that come on within minutes after exposure to a foreign substance and can quickly end fatally.†

This chapter will describe the drug therapy of these types of type I allergic illnesses.‡ To understand the ways in which drugs are used to prevent or relieve symptoms of these allergies, immunologic factors that set off the chain of events that results in such symptoms should be recognized. Many new developments have occurred in the branch of immunology that is concerned with allergy.

---

* The term *atopy* means "strange," or "out of place."

---

† Type I hypersensitivity is also called the "immediate" or "anaphylactic" type.

---

‡ Allergic disorders of other types are discussed in Chapters 5 and 43, and elsewhere.

Immunologic basis of allergy

As indicated in Chapter 36, the human immune system can recognize and react to substances that do not belong to the body. These substances, or *antigens,* stimulate the production of *antibodies,* specific proteins that help to defend the body against bacteria, viruses, and other invaders. However, this defensive response to the presence of foreign substances can sometimes be abnormal in ways that *cause* clinical disorders, including allergic diseases of several types.

One such immune disorder is set off when atopic people are exposed for the first time to the foreign proteins of plant pollens, mold spores, foods, and various other substances. These people react to such antigens, or *allergens,* by producing unusual amounts of an antibody type that is ordinarily present in the blood plasma in extremely small amounts. This protein, which was once called *skin-sensitizing antibody* (SSA), or *reagin,* is now known to belong to the *immunoglobulin E* (IgE) family of antibodies.

These circulating IgE antibodies become attached to the surfaces of leukocytes in the blood and mast cells in the connective tissues of blood vessels in the skin and other organs. Later, when these previously sensitized cells are re-exposed to the same type of antigen, the molecules of the foreign substance combine with the IgE antibodies attached to the cell surfaces. The resulting antigen–antibody reaction leads to the release of certain chemical substances, called *autacoids,* from the sensitized mast cells and basophils.

Among the several substances of this type that are bound within these cells in a biologically inactive form are histamine, bradykinin, prostaglandins, chemotactic factors, and the *slow reacting substance of anaphylaxis* (SRS-A), a member of the chemical family called leukotrienes (see Chap. 36). When freed by the antigen–antibody reaction, histamine and other autacoids become pharmacologically active. That is, they react with specialized receptors on the cells of target tissues such as specific blood vessels in the skin, mucous membranes of the respiratory tract, and smooth muscles of the bronchi in the lungs.

Pharmacologic reactions of this type between endogenously released autacoids and target tissue receptors bring about the clinical signs and symptoms of such specific allergic disease states as urticaria, rhinitis, angioneurotic edema, and anaphylactic shock states. Thus, for example, such *chemical mediators* of allergy as histamine, bradykinin, and SRS-A all cause contraction of the smooth muscle walls of the bronchial tubes—an effect that accounts for the wheezing and respiratory distress of bronchial asthma (Chap. 40). Similarly, the vascular effects of histamine (described below) and of bradykinin account for local redness and swelling of the skin, edema in subcutaneous tissues and mucous membranes, and the generalized drop in blood pressure sometimes seen in the other allergic disease states.

Histamine

Histamine is found in bound form in most body tissues. Its concentration in the skin, lungs, and gastrointestinal tract is particularly high. This may be because its release in free form aids in the body's inflammatory defense of such exposed tissues against injury. Actually, despite its wide distribution in body tissues, the role of released histamine in normal physiology is still uncertain. However, it is known that histamine plays a most important part in regulating the secretion of stomach acid (Chap. 41).

On the other hand, the pathophysiologic effects of histamine in the *immediate*, or *anaphylactic*, type of allergic disorders is readily apparent. That is, many of the signs and symptoms of such illnesses stem from the effects of histamine on small blood vessels, bronchial and gastrointestinal smooth muscles, exocrine glands, and other target tissues of hypersensitive people. These pharmacologic effects of free histamine occur when its molecules combine with specialized receptors on the cells of responsive tissues.

Histamine receptors

Histamine is now known to act on two different types of receptors, called H_1 and H_2. The contractile effect of histamine on smooth muscles of the bronchi and the gastrointestinal tract is brought about by the response of H_1-type receptors in these tissues. Secretion of hydrochloric acid by gastric glands results from their response to the activation of H_2 receptors by histamine. Both the H_1 and H_2 types of receptors are thought to be involved in the complex cardiovascular system responses to released histamine. The antihistamine drugs discussed in this chapter are all H_1 receptor blockers. Cimetidine (Tagamet), ranitidine (Zantac), and other drugs that are now being used and clinically tested in the treatment of acid peptic diseases (Chap. 41) are antagonists of the action of histamine on H_2-type receptors.

Vascular effects

The most important effects of freed histamine in humans are those that result from the response of the small vessels that make up the microvasculature. Small arterioles in the skin, mucous membranes, and elsewhere dilate, and the tissues through which these vessels run become engorged with blood. In addition, plasma proteins and fluid leak out of the capillaries to cause further edema in the surrounding tissues.

These local circulatory effects that play such an important part in the symptomatology of allergic rhinitis, urticaria, and angioneurotic edema are the result of the relaxant action of histamine on vascular smooth muscle and of the effect of histamine action on the endothelial cells that line the capillaries and postcapillary vessels. The profound fall in systemic blood pressure that occurs in acute anaphylactic reactions also stems from the hemodynamic effects that follow these vascular effects of histamine.

In such cases the loss of plasma proteins from the circulation, together with the reduced resistance of the arterioles, results in a steady fall in blood pressure. If blood continues to pool in the peripheral vessels, the venous return to the heart is reduced. This leads in turn to decreased cardiac output, despite reflex responses that increase the rate and contractile strength of the myocardium. The resulting reduction in blood flow to the brain can cause loss of consciousness and failure of nervous control over respiration and other vital functions.

Bronchial effects

Smooth muscles, other than those of the small arterioles, are contracted by contact with released histamine. This is most significant in the bronchioles, which are constricted, with a resulting reduction in vital capacity. This action of histamine is thought to contribute to the breathing difficulties of the patient with bronchial asthma. However, other substances released simultaneously during an antigen–antibody reaction also account for the respiratory embarrassment. For example, SRS-A exerts a potent constricting action on the bronchioles.

Exocrine gland effects

Exocrine glands of the gastrointestinal and respiratory systems, and others (*e.g.*, the lacrimal glands) are stimulated by histamine. The parietal cells of the stomach, which secrete hydrochloric acid, are most powerfully activated. This action, together with the contractile effects of histamine on smooth muscle of the gastrointestinal tract, probably plays a part in producing the epigastric distress, nausea and vomiting, and diarrhea that are often the first warnings of an oncoming anaphylactic reaction. The sensitivity of the gastric glands to injected histamine is the basis for a commonly employed test of stomach secretory function. The use of histamine, its analogue *betazole*, and other gastric secretory stimulants is discussed in more detail in the final chapter of this text (see Chap. 56, Drugs Used for Diagnosis).

Antihistamine drugs

Manner of action in allergic states

The effectiveness of these drugs for relief of symptoms in several allergic disorders stems from their ability to compete successfully with histamine molecules for the H_1 receptor sites of target tissues. When administered prior to an expected allergic reaction or early in its course, these histamine-antagonizing drugs occupy the H_1 receptors. This drug–receptor reaction does not set off any pharmacologic action. Instead, because many of the histamine molecules freed in allergen–antibody reactions cannot combine with the already occupied receptors, this endogenously released chemical mediator of allergy is prevented from initiating its expected effects.

Drugs of this class are more effective for relief of signs and symptoms of some allergic disorders than of others. These *competitive inhibitors* (Chap. 4) of histamine activity are best able to block the *vascular effects* of the natural amine. Thus, by occupying H_1 receptors in the small blood vessels of the skin and mucous membranes, the antihistamine drugs can often prevent the effects of histamine on these tissues. Such symptoms as the itchy skin wheals of urticaria, the subcutaneous swelling of angioneurotic edema, and the edematous congestion of the nasal mucosa in allergic rhinitis are often relieved by moderate doses of drugs such as *diphenhydramine*[+] (Table 39-1).

On the other hand, when massive amounts of histamine are released explosively—such as in severe local and systemic allergic reactions of the anaphylactic type (see below)—the antihistamine drug molecules cannot displace the more numerous histamine molecules from the receptors with which this autacoid is reacting to cause acute signs and symptoms. In such cases, treatment with these competitive antagonists is far less successful than is the administration of epinephrine, which is a physiologic antagonist of histamine—that is, a drug that acts promptly by another mechanism, activation of β-adrenergic receptors, to produce effects exactly opposite to those of histamine.

Allergic signs and symptoms that are *not* the result of a histamine reaction with H_1 receptors are also not readily prevented or reversed by treatment with antihistamine drugs. The relative ineffectiveness of these drugs for relief of bronchial asthma symptoms (Chap. 40) presumably results from their inability to block the effects of SRS-A, which plays an important part in producing bronchospasm in this disorder.

Similarly, antihistamine drugs that are competitive inhibitors of histamine at H_1 receptors are not ef-

Table 39–1. Antihistamine drugs

Official or generic name	Trade name	Usual adult single oral dose (mg)
Azatadine maleate	Optimine	1 or 2
Brompheniramine maleate USP	Dimetane	4
Carbinoxamine maleate USP	Clistin	4–8
Chlorpheniramine maleate USP	Chlor-Trimeton	4
Clemastine fumarate	Tavist	1.34–2.68
Cyproheptadine HCl USP	Periactin	4
Dexchlorpheniramine maleate USP	Polaramine	2
Diphenhydramine HCl USP	Benadryl	50
Diphenylpyraline HCl	Hispril Spansules	5
Methdilazine HCl USP	Tacaryl	8
Phenindamine tartrate USP	Nolahist	25
Promethazine HCl USP	Phenergan	25
Pyrilamine maleate USP		25–50
Trimeprazine tartrate	Temaril	2.5
Tripelennamine citrate USP	PBZ	50
Tripelennamine HCl USP	Pyribenzamine HCl	25–50
Triprolidine HCl USP	Actidil	2.5

fective for reducing excessive secretion of stomach acid. This response to physiologically and pathophysiologically released histamine is the result of the reaction of this autacoid with H_2-type receptors in gastric gland cells, and thus it is not prevented by drugs that block only H_1 receptors. Reduction of gastric acid secretion requires the use of drugs that compete with histamine for H_2 receptors (Chap. 41). Certain systemic effects of histamine on the circulatory system are also thought to be better blocked by these H_2 receptor antagonists than by the traditional antihistamine drugs.

Other pharmacologic effects

The antihistamine drugs do not cause any changes in physiologic functions through their blocking action on histaminergic receptors. However, in addition to preventing histamine from exerting its effects, these drugs can produce various effects of their own on both peripheral tissues and the neurons of the central nervous system. Some of these secondary effects are therapeutically useful not only in treating allergy symptoms but also in the management of many other clinical conditions.

Certain central effects of the antihistamine drugs are more important clinically than their histamine-blocking action. Thus, these drugs are used for purposes other than allergy treatment. Some, such as *dimenhydrinate*, are employed mainly to manage motion sickness and other conditions marked by nausea, vertigo, and vomiting (Chap. 41). Others, including *orphenadrine* as well as its relative *diphenhydramine*, are used for treating patients with parkinsonism (Chap. 49). The sedative–hypnotic actions of some of these drugs have led to their being advocated as substitutes for the barbiturates in the management of anxiety and insomnia (Chap. 45). In fact, the first drugs introduced as major tranquilizers (Chap. 46) were originally discovered and developed in the search for new antihistaminic agents for treating allergy.

None of these secondary effects of antihistamine drugs on the central nervous system involves their ability to block the effects of histamine. Similarly, the local anesthetic effect exerted by some of these chemicals when they are applied topically (Chap. 43) is not the result of histamine antagonism. Some of these drugs do, however, have atropinelike activity. Such anticholinergic actions (Chap. 16) account for certain of their peripheral and central side-effects (see below, and the summary at the end of this chapter), as well as for some of the therapeutically useful effects of antihistamine drugs in other disorders in addition to allergy (see above).

Adverse reactions and toxicity

Side-effects and precautions. The most common side-effect of antihistamine drugs is their tendency to cause drowsiness. This action is more marked with some chemical classes of antihistamines than with others. Certain H_1 receptor antihistamines (*e.g., terfenadine, mequi-*

tazine, and *astemizole*), said to be free of sedative effects, are being investigated in the United States and are available elsewhere in the world. However, sedation can occur in some patients with almost any of the drugs currently available in the United States. Thus, patients should be told not to drive if they become sleepy when they begin to take a new allergy medication, nor to engage in other activities that require alertness and motor coordination.

They should also be told to inform their nurse or physician if they experience sleepiness or ataxia, rather than simply to stop taking the medication. Other antihistamines that may prove less likely to cause drowsiness can then be tried. Patients should also be warned that alcoholic beverages, barbiturates, and other sedatives may add to the sedative effects of the antihistamine.

Toxicity. Children who accidentally ingest large amounts of antihistamine drugs, which are sometimes in the form of a pleasantly flavored cough syrup or cold capsules, may suffer acute poisoning. In such cases flushing, dilated pupils, and other atropinelike signs and symptoms are seen. Early sedation is followed by restlessness, increasing irritability, and muscular twitching. Occasionally, convulsive seizures may develop and, finally, coma, cardiovascular collapse, and respiratory failure may occur.

Treatment of poisoning by antihistamine products that have not been removed by vomiting or gavage is difficult because of this odd mixture of central depressant and stimulating features. It may be further complicated by the presence of salicylates and adrenergic drugs in the cold capsule. Prevention is, of course, the best approach to the problem. The nurse can make parents aware that these seemingly safe products, so widely advertised on television and elsewhere, contain potentially dangerous drugs and should be stored where young children cannot reach them.

If convulsions occur during the management of a case of antihistamine overdosage, diazepam (Valium; see Chap. 45) may be administered. This is usually preferable to administering even a short-acting barbiturate such as thiopental because diazepam is less likely to cause coma and respiratory failure.

Vasopressors may be required to treat hypotension. The use of a mechanical respirator may be required for ventilating the patient if the breathing becomes too slow and shallow. The use of analeptic drugs (Chap. 47) to stimulate respiration in such situations is considered undesirable, because these central nervous system stimulants may precipitate convulsive activity in an unconscious victim of antihistamine drug overdosage.

Management of allergy

One approach to the management of allergy is to employ drugs that act in one way or another to relieve the discomforting symptoms of these disorders. Among the drugs used for such symptomatic treatment are the *an-*

tihistamine drugs discussed above, in the Drug digests for individual drugs, and in the summaries at the end of this chapter; the *adrenergic*, or *sympathomimetic* drugs (Chap. 17); and the *corticosteroids* (Chap. 21). Before discussing the manner in which these and other pharmacologic agents are employed in the management of several typical allergic disorders, a *non*drug form of allergy treatment will be briefly described.

Immunotherapy

This form of treatment, also called desensitization or hyposensitization, has been employed most widely in the management of respiratory allergies such as allergic rhinitis and bronchial asthma. It is intended to modify the abnormal reactivity of the respiratory and other tissues of atopic persons. This involves administering repeated injections of dilute extracts of the specific substance to which a person is hypersensitive—ragweed pollen, for example—in an attempt to make the patient immune to the allergen when it is encountered in the environment.

The effectiveness of such inoculations has been questioned by some who suggest that there is little evidence that patients really profit from the prolonged treatment. However, most allergists believe that immunotherapy is worth trying in allergy patients whose symptoms cannot be well controlled by drug therapy alone, and reports have revealed objective evidence of bodily changes that offer a scientific basis for this treatment.

A series of injections is now believed to bring about an increase in the level of *immunoglobulin G* (IgG) antibodies in the serum of treated patients. These are called "blocking antibodies" because their presence is thought to prevent the reaction between antigens that enter the system and the specific IgE molecules against it that are fixed to sensitized mast cell and leukocyte surfaces. As a result, less histamine and other autacoid molecules are released when the patient actually comes in contact with the allergen in the environment—for example, the ragweed pollen in the air during the hay fever season. This is said to account for the subjective improvement that many patients report after a course of immunotherapy is administered prior to the start of the season in which they ordinarily suffer allergy symptoms.

Immunotherapy is an expensive procedure that is often inconvenient for the patient and can sometimes cause discomforting or even dangerous reactions. Thus, it is best reserved for use in selected cases—for example, patients with recurring severe symptoms that are poorly controlled by symptomatic treatment with antiallergy drugs alone. The following discussions of the management of various clinical allergies will deal only with drug therapy.

Allergic dermatoses

Acute and chronic urticarias (hives, nettle rash) are marked by development of red, raised, often intensely itching wheals. When the wheals appear suddenly and are wide-spread over the body, parenteral administration of epinephrine or of an injectable antihistamine drug is often rapidly effective for relief. Orally administered antihistamines help to control symptoms of the successive crops of wheals that sometimes develop after the first wave has faded. Chronic urticaria is less readily relieved than the acute type. It is best managed by identifying the causative allergen—often a food—and eliminating it.

Allergic contact dermatitis is also the result of sensitization. Here, however, the sensitizing substance is something that comes in contact with the skin. Some dermatologic symptoms that result from subsequent exposure are the result of histamine release; other symptoms are those of delayed hypersensitivity, a type of allergic reaction that is not entirely mediated by IgE antibodies and by the subsequent release of autacoids. However, certain antihistaminic drugs offer some relief, even when the dermatologic symptoms, including pruritus, are not caused by histamine.

The antipruritic effect of certain antihistamines here is thought to result mainly from their effects on the central nervous system rather than on the skin. Among the oral antihistamines that are most effective are those with a relatively strong sedative component, such as *diphenhydramine* (Benadryl). Other antipruritics that may be useful here and in other skin disorders with symptoms that have both a histamine and *non*histamine component are hydroxyzine (Atarax; Vistaril), an antihistaminic that is also a minor tranquilizer (Chap. 45) and the phenothiazine-type antihistaminic tranquilizers trimeprazine (Temaril), and methdilazine (Tacaryl).

Atopic dermatitis is a chronic allergic skin disorder in which oral antihistamines are sometimes employed even though histamine is not thought to be the cause of most symptoms. Here, too, the relief of itching that these drugs sometimes provide probably stems mainly from a central antipruritic action rather than from peripheral antagonism of histamine. The use of topically applied corticosteroid drugs for symptomatic relief of this condition is discussed in Chapter 43.

Topical anesthetics are sometimes employed for relief of itching in contact dermatitis but their use in chronic allergic disorders such as atopic dermatitis is considered undesirable, because allergy-prone patients can become sensitized to these substances. This is true even of antihistaminic drugs with local anesthetic activity, such as *tripelennamine*[+] (Pyribenzamine), which can cause skin sensitization and contact dermatitis when applied topically in such cases. Thus, this drug and other antihistaminics such as *cyproheptadine* (Periactin) are best taken orally for relief of itching in allergic and nonallergic dermatoses through their combined central antipruritic and peripheral histamine-antagonizing effects.

Angioneurotic edema

This allergic syndrome is marked by fluid accumulation in subcutaneous tissues rather than in the skin itself. The edema develops in such sites as the eyelids, lips, hands, and feet, or sometimes the genitalia. Such localized swellings are not painful or pruritic and are usually only temporarily disfiguring rather than dangerous. However, local urticarial lesions, or "giant hives," can quickly cause asphyxia when they develop in the glottal tissues of the larynx. Thus, angioedema should be treated promptly with subcutaneous injections of epinephrine, as described below in the discussion of drug treatment of acute systemic anaphylactic reactions.

Acute anaphylactic reactions

People sensitized to drugs, insect venom, or other allergens sometimes suffer sudden dramatic reactions on reexposure to the sensitizing substance. The explosive release of endogenous chemical mediators of anaphylaxis can cause serious symptoms to develop, sometimes within seconds. The victim may then die within a few minutes as a result of respiratory failure or circulatory collapse, unless prompt and effective treatment counteracts the effects of histamine and the other substances that are released in the antigen–antibody reaction.*

Treatment. The most rapidly effective drug for reversing the symptoms of sudden severe allergic emergencies is *epinephrine* (Chap. 17). It is most commonly administered subcutaneously in a dose of 0.3 ml of a 1:1000 solution. The injection site should be massaged to speed the drug's absorption. Similar injections can be repeated at intervals of 15 or 20 minutes during the first hour of treatment and later at less frequent intervals. However, if the patient has suffered circulatory collapse, which would prevent absorption of this drug from deep subcutaneous or intramuscular sites, it must be administered by slow intravenous injection. For this purpose, 1 ml of the 1:1000 solution is diluted to 10 ml with saline solution to make a 1:10,000 concentration.

Epinephrine usually relieves respiratory distress by its relaxant effect on bronchial smooth muscle, which counteracts severe, sustained bronchospasm and improves pulmonary ventilation. It also causes constriction of small blood vessels in various vascular beds. This helps to stop fluid from leaking out into the skin, subcutaneous tissues, mucous membranes of the tongue, throat, and larynx—an action that overcomes asphyxial laryngeal edema.

Patients who have suffered shock as a result of primary vascular collapse may not respond with an adequate rise in blood pressure when treated with epinephrine alone. Other adrenergic drugs that may prove more effective for this purpose are the vasopressors *levarterenol* and *metaraminol* (Chap. 17). Administered together with fluids to counteract hypovolemia and with the same monitoring procedures employed during their use in cardiogenic shock (Chap. 31), these drugs often

raise the mean arterial pressure of patients in anaphylactic shock.

Other less effective or slower acting drugs that may be employed as adjuncts to epinephrine and the other adrenergic drugs include the antihistamines and corticosteroids. The intravenous administration of *diphenhydramine*, for example, helps to relieve late symptoms such as skin itching and redness, after the more rapid-acting and more effective adrenergic drugs have prevented the early development of serious respiratory and circulatory symptoms. Large intravenous doses of soluble steroids such as *hydrocortisone sodium succinate, prednisolone phosphate,* or *dexamethasone phosphate* (Chap. 21) help to increase the responsiveness of the bronchial smooth muscles and the cardiovascular system to stimulation by circulating catecholamines and other adrenergic stimuli.

Prevention. Every effort should be made to prevent acute allergic reactions from occurring. Patients who are to receive penicillin or other drugs that are known to cause hypersensitivity in some people should be asked whether they have ever suffered reactions to them. Patients with a history of allergic disorders such as asthma may also be especially susceptible to allergic drug reactions. They and patients who have received an injection of an allergenic extract should be kept under observation for 20 to 30 minutes before being allowed to leave the clinic or office.

A kit containing equipment for emergency treatment should be kept available. Its contents include tourniquets and ice packs for delaying further absorption of allergens from injection sites, an endotracheal tube and a tracheotomy set for maintaining an airway, an oxygen tank, and the needles, syringes, and other materials needed for administering the drugs required for aiding the patient's respiration and circulation.

Drugs of the antihistamine and corticosteroid classes are sometimes employed prophylactically in attempts to prevent allergic reactions. Antihistamines have, for example, been given before blood transfusions, prior to the administration of immune sera, and combined with penicillin in parenteral products. Although such pretreatment may control some of the minor symptoms of reactions to these substances, it does not prevent more serious reactions such as respiratory embarrassment or circulatory collapse. It may, in fact, cause these life-threatening allergic emergencies to appear without warning by masking such early warning signs as skin itching and redness.

Corticosteroid drugs are often preferred for allergy reaction prophylaxis. Administration of prednisone for several days after the first signs of serum sickness or other delayed hypersensitivity reactions may, for example, help to suppress the late appearance of fever and joint pains—signs and symptoms that are not prevented by antihistamines. Patients seriously ill with life-threatening infections such as subacute bacterial endocarditis, who require treatment with penicillin or other antibiotics to

---

* Similar severe life-threatening reactions sometimes occur in which it is not possible to prove prior sensitization. Such possibly *non*immunologic reactions—to aspirin or iodinated contrast media, for example—are called anaphylact*oid.*

which they are allergic, are sometimes pretreated with corticosteroids to suppress possible severe hypersensitivity reactions to the anti-infective agents. They are, of course, closely observed during treatment, and emergency drugs and equipment are kept ready for use if needed to treat a severe reaction.

Rhinitis

The mucous membrane lining the nose often becomes inflamed as a result of antigen–antibody reactions or in response to exposure to infectious viruses and *non*allergenic irritants. The symptoms of acute rhinitis include sneezing, running nose (rhinorrhea), and a congestion of the nose and sinuses that causes a feeling of discomforting nasal stuffiness and headache. In chronic, or perennial, rhinitis, continued inflammation of the nasal mucosa may make it more susceptible to repeated infections and lead to formation of polyps, which may project into the air passages and block them completely.

The main types of drugs employed for symptomatic relief of rhinitis are the *antihistamines,* the *sympathomimetic amines,* or adrenergic nasal decongestants (Chap. 17), and the *corticosteroids* (Chap. 21). These drugs are more effective for control of acute rhinitis symptoms than in chronic cases. If used in excess, they can cause adverse effects locally on the already inflamed mucosa or produce systemic side-effects. In the following discussion of drug treatment in several acute and chronic rhinitis syndromes, the usefulness and limitations of these types of agents will be emphasized, together with the measures that must be employed to gain their benefits while minimizing potential toxicity.

Seasonal allergic rhinitis (pollinosis; hay fever)

This form of nasal allergy is set off at certain seasons of the year when people sensitized by previous exposure to plant pollens again inhale the specific allergen. The pollen protein combines with IgE antibodies bound to the surface of nasal cells, and the reaction results in the release of histamine molecules. The actions of histamine on tissues of the nose, throat, and eyes account for the familiar signs and symptoms of hay fever.

Antihistamines. The histamine-antagonizing drugs are effective for aborting symptoms of seasonal rhinitis in four out of five patients. Relief is most likely early in the season when the drugs are taken every day in the largest doses that the patient can tolerate without becoming drowsy. If one drug of this class causes discomforting side-effects in the doses needed to control symptoms, the patient may be switched to another that is less sedating.

When pollen counts are heavy and larger amounts of histamine are being released in the nasal and ocular tissues, antihistamine drug therapy becomes less effective. This is especially true late in the pollen season when the long-continued actions of histamine on the tis-

sues tend to cause congestive changes in the mucosa of the nose and the paranasal sinuses. Sympathomimetic amines and corticosteroid drugs may then be added to the patient's treatment regimen for brief periods to provide relief of nasal congestion and sinus headache.

Sympathomimetic amines. As was discussed in more detail in Chapter 17, some drugs of this class are effective for relief of nasal congestion when applied topically or when taken by mouth alone or combined with an antihistamine drug. These adrenergic drugs cause rapid, intense constriction of the dilated blood vessels in the congested nasal mucosa when they are applied directly to the nose. This opens the obstructed nasal air passages and blocked sinuses, and the patient obtains prompt relief of nasal stuffiness and headache.

For best results, nose drops containing sympathomimetic amines should be used for only a few days and applied properly to prevent the solution from trickling down into the throat and being swallowed. Instruct the patient to tilt the head back, insert the drops, and keep the head tilted back for 2 to 3 minutes.

Drugs of this type are less effective for relief of nasal congestion when taken by mouth. However, this route of administration is preferred for prolonged use during the hay fever season because it does not lead to rebound congestion, as is the case with the topically applied products. Taken in doses high enough to bring about nasal vasoconstriction, these drugs produce few sympathomimetic type side-effects in most patients with pollinosis. However, patients with a history of heart disease, hypertension, hyperthyroidism, and diabetes mellitus may suffer serious reactions. Thus, these systemically active sympathomimetic drugs are used with caution, if at all, in such cases.

Corticosteroid drugs. These are also available in topical and oral dosage forms for control of seasonal allergic rhinitis symptoms. Patients whose nasal congestion is no longer well controlled with antihistamine–decongestant combinations often obtain relief from acute symptoms with short courses of corticosteroid drugs. At the height of the pollen season, these patients may inhale an aerosol of dexamethasone (Decadron Phosphate Turbinaire) a few times daily to suppress inflammation of the nasal mucosa. Two other corticosteroids are also now available for intranasal topical use: *beclomethasone dipropionate* (Beconase; Vancenase) and *flunisolide* (Nasalide). When any of these products is employed sparingly for short periods, the small amount of corticosteroid absorbed systemically is not likely to cause toxicity.

Although orally administered corticosteroid drugs can cause many adverse effects when taken over long periods (Chap. 21), their short-term use for treating hay fever is generally considered to be safe. One method of administration is to give a steroid such as *prednisone* or *methylprednisolone* in a so-called stepdown or countdown dosage schedule. For example, a large loading dose may be given on the first day of a week of treatment, followed by a series of steadily diminishing doses during the next 5 days. The protective effects of such a safe, short course of steroids are claimed to last for as long as 4 weeks or sometimes for the rest of the period in which the patient is exposed to pollen.

Cromolyn. This drug has been used for many years by patients with asthma to prevent acute attacks induced by inhalation of antigen (Chap. 40). It acts as a mast cell stabilizer and prevents the release of histamine, SRS-A, and other autacoids. Recently, cromolyn sodium (Intal) has been marketed in the form of a nasal spray (Nasalcrom) for use by patients with allergic rhinitis. It has been found to be effective in reducing the symptoms of patients whose rhinitis is caused by an allergic reaction. Little of the drug is absorbed systemically when administered in this way, and the drug is well tolerated, although transient local reactions (*e.g.,* nasal irritation) have occurred. Antihistamines and sympathomimetic drugs may be used with cromolyn.

Perennial allergic and vasomotor rhinitis
Patients sometimes suffer chronic inflammation of the nasal mucous membranes, which causes congestion and rhinorrhea in all seasons rather than in a single season. In perennial rhinitis of the allergic type, an atopic person may be exposed continuously to an allergen, and the sensitized tissues respond with an antigen–antibody reaction that releases histamine and other autacoids throughout the year. Often, in such cases, the allergen is a food, such as milk, chocolate, or cola drinks.

In other cases, no allergen can be shown to be the cause of the patient's continuous nasal congestion. Such *non*allergic perennial rhinitis may be set off by various stimuli including inhalation of tobacco smoke, house dust, or perfumes. Recurrent attacks are also triggered by changes in temperature or emotional stress. Because the resulting vasodilation may be related to an autonomic nervous system imbalance, this condition is called vasomotor rhinitis.

Symptomatic management of both types of perennial rhinitis with drugs is much more difficult than in seasonal rhinitis. Treatment with antihistamine drugs, for example, is less successful than in hay fever. Although these drugs are commonly administered in combination with oral adrenergic decongestants, the histamine antagonists are not very effective for relief of congestion in the chronically inflamed nasal mucosa. The antihistamines may, however, offer some relief of rhinorrhea, because the anticholinergic, or atropinelike, action of these drugs may help to dry a running nose.

The continued use of topically applied vasoconstrictor–decongestant drugs is considered to be undesirable in perennial rhinitis. This is because patients tend to become habituated to these drugs in their eagerness to obtain the prompt relief that topical application at first

produces. Patients find that they require the drops at more and more frequent intervals, without realizing that it is the residual late vasodilator effect of these vasoconstrictors that is the cause of their increased nasal congestion. Finally, such overuse of decongestant drugs causes development of a chronic nasal congestive condition called *rhinitis medicamentosa.*

Treatment of this condition requires the total withdrawal of topically applied adrenergic decongestant drugs. This is, of course, accompanied by considerable discomfort. A short course of oral corticosteroids (as described above) may be prescribed to relieve the symptoms, or topical corticosteroids may be ordered for a few weeks. No more than two sprays of the aerosol in each nostril three times daily should be used. This sometimes helps to reduce the size of large nasal polyps that might otherwise require surgical removal to relieve obstruction of the nasal passages.

The continued use of orally administered corticosteroids is, of course, contraindicated in perennial rhinitis because of the toxic effects and complications that are likely to develop during long-term systemic steroid therapy (Chap. 21). Although topical corticosteroid therapy is safer and offers considerable relief during acute flare-ups of these nasal inflammatory disorders, it should be employed intermittently rather than continuously. This is because enough of the inhaled drug can be absorbed systemically over a period of several weeks or months to cause suppression of adrenal gland function. Thus, the daily dosage of these sprays should be gradually reduced whenever the patient's perennial rhinitis seems to go into spontaneous remission.

Infectious rhinitis (the common cold)
Infection by many types of viruses, including rhinoviruses, is a common cause of acute rhinitis. As indicated in Chapter 7, no drugs are available to cure upper respiratory tract infections by a direct attack on their viral cause. However, several classes of drugs can be used for relief of common cold symptoms, most of which resemble those occurring in acute allergic rhinitis (see above).

Symptoms. As everyone knows all too well from frequent personal experience, a cold often begins with a feeling of pharyngeal discomfort. Soon after, sneezing begins. The nose reddens and runs, and its membranes become swollen in a way that makes nasal breathing difficult. If the nasal congestion progresses up into the paranasal sinuses, a frontal headache and facial area tenderness may develop. Systemic symptoms include muscle and joint aches, mild fever, lethargy, and malaise. A dry hacking cough often develops in the late stages of the cold.

Symptomatic treatment. The reason for listing this dismal catalogue of familiar discomforts is that management of the common cold with drugs is best discussed in terms of the control of each of its specific symptoms. Ideally, a person should take a drug product that contains only one ingredient, or at most two or three, each of which is aimed at a single symptom. Instead, many products offered for self-medication are packed with many more ingredients that are intended to relieve every possible cold symptom. Because all the symptoms of a cold seldom occur at once, such over-the-counter cold remedies are irrational and excessively expensive.

Among the drugs that may be effective for relief of cold symptoms when taken in adequate doses are the following: *analgesics* for relief of headache and facial pain or muscle and joint aches; *antihistamines* for sneezing and rhinorrhea; *sympathomimetic* drugs for relief of nasal and sinus congestion; and *antitussives* to suppress coughs.

Pain and discomfort. Nonnarcotic analgesic–antipyretics such as *aspirin* or *acetaminophen* (Chap. 37) are useful for relief of sore throat, headache, and the muscle aches, malaise, and mild fever that often accompany the common cold. These drugs are best purchased and employed singly rather than as a component part of a multiple-ingredient product. The amount of aspirin contained in a "combination of ingredients" product can cost the consumer 20 times as much as when the same dose is taken separately. The addition of aspirin to a mixture of antihistamines, decongestants, and cough remedies does not make the aspirin any more effective for relief of aches, pains, soreness, or fever and, of course, if a consumer has none of these symptoms, but only a running or blocked nose, there is no need at all for the aspirin that is contained in such combination-type cold products.

Sneezing and rhinorrhea. *Antihistamine* drugs are effective for relief of these symptoms when they occur early in the course of acute seasonal rhinitis. This has led to the use of these drugs to relieve similar symptoms that are caused by reaction of the nasal tissues to infection by cold viruses. However, most authorities maintain that the antihistamine drugs have never been shown to be effective for prevention or cure of the common cold, or even able to stop the sneezing or dry the running nose in a respiratory virus infection. Symptomatic improvement, in such cases indicates—according to the experts—that the patient actually had an allergic rhinitis rather than a cold, an infection in which there is no proof that histamine is released or that it plays any part in producing symptoms.

Despite this authoritative view, many people judge from their personal experience that taking an antihistamine *has* helped to dry their watery nasal discharges and to reduce the frequency of sneezing—for a while, at least. Although objective evidence of this is lacking, the patient's subjective evaluation may be correct in many cases. The pharmacologic basis for the feeling that nasal secretions are dried by antihistamine drug treatment is the fact that many of these drugs also possess anticholinergic activity—that is, they have an atropinelike effect.

Atropine and other belladonna alkaloids are themselves a common component of products that are employed for self-medication of the common cold. The small doses that the FDA permits in such products are not likely to prove effective for relief of a running nose. However, when an allergist or other physician orders atropine in adequate doses, this drug does relieve rhinorrhea and reduce sneezing. Patients should, of course, be watched for signs of side-effects, and the drug should not be ordered for patients in whom it is contraindicated (see Drug digest and summary, Chap. 16).

Nasal congestion. As indicated earlier in this chapter, certain sympathomimetic amines (Chap. 17) are very effective for relief of nasal and sinus congestion, particularly when applied topically as liquid nose drops, aerosolized sprays or inhaled vapors. Applied for only a few days at intervals of at least 4 hours, most of these adrenergic drugs are not likely to cause significant rebound congestion.

Among the most long-lasting of the nasal decongestants is *oxymetazoline*[+] (Afrin), which needs to be applied only twice daily. Such infrequent application is not likely to cause rebound vasodilation as a result of overuse. *Ephedrine* and *phenylephrine* (Neo-Synephrine; Chap. 17) are also effective and do not cause more than a brief transient rebound congestion when low concentrations are applied occasionally for relief. *Naphazoline* tends to cause more late congestion than the other drugs of this class.

Taken orally, phenylephrine and ephedrine do not produce as intense a degree of vasoconstriction as when they are applied topically, and the risk of their causing restlessness, nervousness, and insomnia is increased. Oral *pseudoephedrine* (Sudafed) is said to be less stimulating to the central nervous system and is claimed to cause few cardiovascular side-effects. However, although this drug and *phenylpropanolamine* (Propadrine) are said to be safer when taken by normal people in oral therapeutic doses, their use in this way can cause adverse effects in patients with hypertension and other cardiovascular disorders, and in those who are sensitive to the central effects of sympathomimetic amines.

Coughs caused by colds

The common cold is often accompanied by a cough that is caused by irritation of the throat and upper respiratory tract tissues. This type of cough usually requires no specific treatment, because it stops when postnasal drip and other cold symptoms subside. Occasionally, however, specific medication for suppressing the cough reflex may be employed to control a dry, hacking cough for a few days.

Antitussive drugs suppress coughing in two main ways (Table 39-2). Some act by depressing the central nervous system or, more specifically, the cough center in the medulla oblongata. Others act peripherally to reduce stimulation of cough receptors in the throat, larynx, trachea, and lungs. The centrally acting antitussives most commonly employed for reducing unproductive coughs caused by virus infections are *codeine* and *dextromethorphan*[+]

Table 39–2. Drugs used in the management of coughing

Official or generic name	Trade name or synonym	Usual adult antitussive dose (mg)
Centrally acting antitussives		
Narcotic antitussive-analgesics		
Codeine USP	Methylmorphine	10–20
Codeine phosphate USP	Methylmorphine phosphate	10–20
Codeine sulfate USP	Methylmorphine sulfate	10–20
Hydrocodone bitartrate USP	Dihydrocodeinone; Dicodid; in Hycodan	5
Nonnarcotic antitussives		
Benzonatate USP	Tessalon Perles	100
Caramiphen edisylate	In Bay-Ornade	10–20
Chlophedianol HCl	Ulo	25
Dextromethorphan HBr USP	Romilar	10–30
Diphenhydramine HCl	Benylin; Noradryl; Robalyn	25
Levopropoxyphene napsylate USP	Novrad	100
Noscapine	Tusscapine	15–30
Peripherally acting antitussives		
Expectorants, demulcents, and vehicles		
Acacia syrup		
Ammonium chloride USP	In Tossecol Expectorant	90
Calcium iodide	In Calcidrine Syrup	150
Glycyrrhiza syrup	Licorice Syrup	
Guaifenesin USP	Glyceryl guaiacolate; in Robitussin	100
Honey USP		
Hydriodic acid syrup		5
Iodinated glycerol	Amonidrin; Organidin; Ipsatol	60
Potassium guaiacolsulfonate USP	In Codimel Expectorant	100
Potassium iodide USP		300
Terpin hydrate USP	In Terpin Hydrate with Codeine	85
Tolu balsam syrup		
White pine syrup		
Wild cherry syrup USP		

(Romilar). The antihistamine, diphenhydramine, is also now approved for this use and is available as an OTC preparation (Benylin) and by prescription. Peripherally acting drugs used for this purpose include *guaifenesin*[+] (*glyceryl guaiacolate*) and *terpin hydrate*. The usefulness and limitations of the centrally and peripherally acting antitussives will now be briefly discussed.

Central cough suppressants

The drugs that act to depress the medullary cough center and thus to reduce its sensitivity to sensory nerve impulses arriving from irritated pharyngeal, laryngeal, and other respiratory tract tissues are sometimes subdivided into two types: the narcotic and the nonnarcotic antitussives (Table 39-2). The drawbacks of the more potent narcotic analgesic-antitussives, such as the opioids *morphine, methadone,* and *hydrocodone,* discussed in Chapter 51, make their use totally inappropriate for treating coughs caused by colds. However, other less potent narcotics are considered both safe and effective for this purpose.

Codeine is the most commonly employed cough suppressant of this subclass. It is relatively free of the drawbacks of morphine and other opium derivatives and synthetic opioid antitussives when taken in the small doses effective for cough relief. It does not, for example, depress the patient's respiration, nor does it depress the cough reflex so strongly that productive coughing is prevented. (The danger of drugs that do so is discussed in the following chapter, which deals with the management of patients with chronic obstructive lung disorders.)

Although large doses of codeine can cause respiratory depression and various side-effects involving the central nervous and gastrointestinal systems, these rarely occur with the low doses required for cough control. Thus, only a patient especially sensitive to codeine is likely to become light-headed, dizzy, drowsy or excited, or to complain of headache, abdominal discomfort, nausea and vomiting, or constipation. Similarly, opiate dependence is not really a problem when codeine is taken for only 1 or 2 weeks, because this opium alkaloid has low dependence-producing liability.

Dextromethorphan is the most widely used of the nonnarcotic antitussives. It seems comparable to codeine in cough suppressant effectiveness and, because it may have a more selective effect on the cough center, it is claimed less likely to cause the types of side-effects that are sometimes seen with codeine. The fact that it is "nonnarcotic" does not really make it superior to codeine-containing cough medications, as television commercials for dextromethorphan-based cough products suggest. This drug is as capable as codeine of being abused by some people, but psychological dependence following use as cough suppressants is not a problem with either drug. Massive doses of both drugs can cause depression of respiration. Although no deaths from dextromethorphan overdosage have been reported, the nurse should suggest to parents that products containing this drug be stored out of reach of children—a warning that is proper with all cough and cold products.

Diphenhydramine is also an effective centrally acting antitussive. The primary side-effect of antitussive doses is sedation, although overdoses of these antihistamine cough syrups may cause all the problems described above for drugs of the antihistamine class.

Peripherally acting antitussives

Several types of substances are available that are intended to lessen irritation of the respiratory tract or to make cough receptors in these tissues less responsive to the stimuli that ordinarily set off the cough reflex (Table 39-2). These include the topical anesthetic *benzocaine,* a common ingredient of throat lozenges, another anes-

thetic, *benzonatate,* which dampens the cough reflex by its effect on stretch receptors in the respiratory passages, and drugs of the class called *expectorants* that act to stimulate increased secretion of a natural lubricant, respiratory tract fluid (RTF).

Expectorants are employed in the common cold for a somewhat different purpose than in the management of chronic obstructive lung diseases (Chap. 40). In patients with a dry cough caused by irritation of the inflamed membranes of the throat and upper respiratory tract, products containing an expectorant such as guaifenesin (glyceryl guaiacolate) are claimed to relieve the irritation and the cough by promoting the production of a fluid that protects the mucosa. This demulcent (soothing) effect is thought to help lessen the number of unproductive cough volleys.

Actually, there is little proof that any of the expectorants promoted for this purpose really increase the production of such a soothing fluid—at least, in the small doses that are considered safe for inclusion in over-the-counter cough products (Table 39-2). Thus, rather than take a drug that acts—if at all—after being swallowed, it seems simpler to reduce coughing from pharyngitis by sucking on a candy cough drop.

The sugary spicy confection tends to stimulate a flow of saliva, which acts as a natural demulcent to protect the dry or inflamed membranes. Then, too, the person sucking on a cough lozenge is keeping the mouth shut, thus preventing further drying of the membrane through the evaporation of moisture. The addition of a topical anesthetic such as benzocaine or some other medication adds little to the effectiveness of such lozenges.

Cough syrups containing such flavorful substances as wild cherry and licorice are of limited effectiveness. Little of their local demulcent–protective action in the throat persists once these sugary solutions are swallowed, and they do not, of course, reach the parts of the respiratory tract below the epiglottis. Thus, such syrups are used mainly as pleasantly flavored vehicles for other peripherally acting drugs, such as the expectorants.

Of course, a cough that stems from inflammation that has spread to lower levels, such as the larynx, cannot be stopped by local measures of this type. Thus, in laryngitis, tracheitis, and bronchitis, a more effective though potentially more toxic expectorant such as *potassium iodide* may be preferred. As indicated in the next chapter, high doses of such a drug, taken together with plenty of fluid, may help to lessen the frequency of cough by increasing the flow of respiratory secretions and thus reducing the local dryness, inflammation, and irritation.

Additional clinical considerations

Patient teaching is an extremely important aspect of the care of patients with allergies. The patient needs to know exactly what is causing the allergy, the signs and symptoms of the allergic response, and ways to avoid or decrease the intensity of the allergic reaction. Patients should be taught to avoid exposure to allergens, if at all possible. Keeping house and automobile windows closed and using an air conditioner and air filter can minimize the exposure of a patient with pollen allergies. Patients should be encouraged to avoid both physical and emotional stress as much as possible, because fatigue and tension may aggravate the signs and symptoms of allergies.

The patient will also need to know the adverse effects that can be expected with the drugs that are used to treat the signs and symptoms of the allergic reaction. Safety measures will need to be taken if the central nervous system effects of dizziness and drowsiness occur with antihistamine use. The atropinelike side-effects of the antihistamines can be uncomfortable for the patient. Many comfort measures can be used to help the patient cope with these: frequent mouth care, sugarless lozenges to help the dry mouth, voiding before taking the medication. The respiratory tract secretions may become very thick. This effect can make breathing difficult, which can be serious for patients with obstructive pulmonary diseases. If thickened secretions become a problem, the patient can be encouraged to drink plenty of fluids (if not contraindicated) and to use a humidifier or, if that is impossible, to place pans of water around the house to increase the humidity in the room air. The patient should be encouraged to report any unusual or different reactions to the antihistamine. Patients may become refractory to the effects of antihistamines over time, and switching to another class of antihistamines for a while may restore the patient's responsiveness to drugy therapy.

Care should be taken to evaluate the patient before ordering an antihistamine. Because of the atropine-like effects of antihistamines, several underlying medical conditions are contraindications for the use of these drugs: narrow-angle glaucoma, gastrointestinal obstruction or stenosis, bladder obstruction, and prostatic hypertrophy. The use of antihistamines is contraindicated in pregnancy unless the potential benefits outweigh the risks to the fetus. Antihistamines are contraindicated in nursing mothers—the drug is excreted into breast milk, and can cause serious problems for the baby. The lactating mother should choose another method of feeding the baby if these drugs must be taken. Elderly patients and small children are more likely to develop severe central nervous system effects, and should be monitored carefully.

Drug–drug interactions

Antihistamines have additive, depressant effects if given concurrently with *alcohol* or with other *central nervous system depressants* (e.g., sedatives, tranquilizers, anti-anxiety drugs, analgesics). *Epinephrine's* effects are enhanced by antihistamines. *Monoamine oxidase* (MAO) *inhibitors* prolong and intensify the anticholinergic effects of the antihistamines, and the two types of drugs should not be given concurrently. *Over-the-counter* (OTC) preparations contain several drugs that have additive effects with the antihistamines. The patient should be instructed to avoid these preparations and to consult with the nurse or physician if it is felt that one of these preparations is needed.

The patient teaching guide summarizes the points to include in teaching a patient on antihistamine therapy. The guide to the nursing process summarizes the clinical considerations to incorporate into the nursing care of a patient receiving antihistamines.

Patient teaching guide: antihistamines

The drug that has been prescribed for you is called an antihistamine. Drugs of this class are used to treat the signs and symptoms of various allergic reactions. Your drug has been prescribed to treat _____ . Because these drugs work throughout the entire body, many systemic effects can occur with their use—for example, dry mouth, dizziness, and drowsiness.

Instructions:

1. The name of your drug is _____ .

2. The dosage of your drug is _____ .

3. Your drug should be taken _____ times a day. The best times to take your drug are _____ _____ _____ . It is best to take the drug on an empty stomach. If stomach upset occurs, however, it can be taken with food.

4. Take the drug only as it has been prescribed. Do not increase the dosage if symptoms are not relieved. Consult with your physician or nurse if this occurs.

(continued)

5. Some side-effects of the drug that you should be aware of include the following:

Drowsiness, dizziness	Observe caution if driving; avoid operating dangerous machinery; use caution if performing delicate tasks.
GI upset	Taking the drug with food will often alleviate this problem.
Dry mouth	Frequent mouth care or sucking on sugarless lozenges may help.
Thickening of mucus, difficulty in coughing, "tight" chest	Using a humidifier, or placing pans of water throughout the house to increase the humidity of room air, may help alleviate this problem.

6. Keep this and all medication out of the reach of children.

7. Tell any physician, dentist, or nurse who is taking care of you that you are on this drug.

8. Avoid the use of OTC preparations while you are on this drug. If you feel that you need one of these preparations, consult with your nurse or physician.

9. Avoid the use of alcoholic beverages while you are on this drug. The combination of these can cause excessive drowsiness.

10. Use this drug only as prescribed. Do not give this drug to anyone else, or take similar preparations that have not been prescribed for you.

Notify your physician or nurse if any of the following occur:

Difficulty in breathing
Rash, hives
Difficulty in voiding
Abdominal pain
Visual changes
Disorientation, confusion

Guide to the nursing process: antihistamines

Assessment	Nursing diagnoses	Interventions	Evaluation
Past history (*contraindications*): GI obstruction GI stenosis	Potential ineffective airway clearance secondary to thickened secretions	Appropriate and proper administration of drug Provision of safety and comfort measures:	Monitor for therapeutic effect of drug: relief of symptoms Monitor for adverse *(continued)*

Assessment	Nursing diagnoses	Interventions	Evaluation

Bladder obstruction
Prostatic hypertrophy
Narrow-angle
  glaucoma
Pregnancy
Lactation
Allergies: *antihistamines;*
  tartrazine (some
    preparations);
    others; reactions
Medication history
  (*cautions*):
    MAO inhibitors
    Epinephrine
    Alcohol
    CNS depressants
 	
Physical assessment
Neurologic: affect,
  orientation,
  coordination
Cardiovascular: BP, P,
  perfusion
Respiratory: R,
  adventitious sounds,
  nares
GI: bowel sounds,
  abdominal exam
Genitourinary: urinary
  output
Skin: lesions
Others: CBC, glaucoma,
  tonometry (if appro-
priate)
	Potential decrease in
	  cardiac output
	Knowledge deficit
	  regarding drug
	  therapy
	Potential sensory–
	  perceptual alteration
	Potential alteration in
	  urinary elimination
	  patterns
	Potential alteration in
	  comfort secondary to
	  GI upset, dry mouth
		• Safety measures if
		  dizziness and
		  drowsiness occur
		• Drug with food
		• Mouth care
		• Sugarless lozenges
		• Void before drug
		  (if prostatic
		  hypertrophy
		  present)
		• Increase humidity, if
		  necessary
		Patient teaching
		  regarding allergy,
		  drug, cautions,
		  warnings
		Provision of emotional
		  support and
		  encouragement to deal
		  with allergy and with
		  drug therapy
			effects of drug:
			• GI symptoms
			• CNS symptoms
			• Respiratory
			  secretion thickening
			• Urinary retention
			• Glaucoma
			Evaluate effectiveness of
			  patient teaching
			  program
			Evaluate effectiveness of
			  comfort and safety
			  measures
			Evaluate effectiveness of
			  support and
			  encouragement
			  offered
			Monitor for drug–drug
			  interactions:
			  ↑ Epinephrine effects
			  ↑ Antihistamine effects
			    with *MAO* inhibitors
			  ↑ CNS effects with
			    alcohol, CNS
			    depressants

Summary of clinical indications for antihistamine drugs

Histamine antagonism and antipruritic
  Seasonal allergic rhinitis (hay fever; pollinosis)
  Perennial and vasomotor rhinitis
  Allergic conjunctivitis
  Urticaria (hives), acute and chronic
  Contact dermatitis, including poison ivy
  Dermographism (skin writing wheals)
  Physical allergy (such as a cold)
  Insect sting allergic reactions, mild and local
  Reactions to blood, plasma, serum, and drugs
      (for relief of pruritus and mild angioedema)
  Acute anaphylactic reactions: as an adjunct fol-
      lowing epinephrine and other more im-
      mediately effective measures

Selective central nervous system depression
  Insomnia: for sedative–hypnotic effects
  Anxiety and psychomotor excitement: especially
    in *some* hyperactive, emotionally disturbed
    children
  Preoperative and postoperative sedation
  Postoperative and postanesthetic nausea and
    vomiting: for antiemetic effects
  Motion sickness prevention and treatment
  Parkinson's disease: mild cases in elderly patients
  Parkinsonism, drug-induced: extrapyramidal
    motor reactions to phenothiazines and other
    antipsychotic drugs

Summary of adverse effects and cautions: antihistamine drugs*

Central nervous system depression

Drowsiness, dizziness, disturbed motor coordination and difficulty in concentrating may occur during the first few days of treatment. Caution patients against driving or engaging in other potentially hazardous activities; also against drinking or taking other sedatives, hypnotics, or tranquilizers.

Central nervous system stimulation†

Restlessness, nervousness, confusion and, occasionally, insomnia may occur.

Convulsions, following tremors, have occurred in children taking large overdoses; death has sometimes resulted.

Atropinelike peripheral effects

Dryness of the mouth, nose, and throat; thickening of mucous secretions may lead to tightness in the chest, wheezing, and dyspnea in asthmatic patients.

Vision may be blurred.

Urination may be difficult.

Constipation or diarrhea, nausea, epigastric distress, heartburn, and vomiting may occur.

Hypersensitivity reactions

Sensitized patients may develop skin eruptions and other signs and symptoms of allergic reactions, including anaphylactic shock.

Cardiovascular effects of parenteral administration

Hypotension, heart palpitations, and irregularities with faintness, weakness, sweating, and pallor

* The several different chemical classes of drugs that act to antagonize histamine may differ in their other pharmacologic effects. Thus, the drugs may not *all* produce the same side-effects.
† CNS stimulation is most likely to occur in drugs with a strong anticholinergic (atropinelike) component.

Case study

Presentation

EN, a somewhat frantic mother, called the doctor's office regarding her 14-year-old son, D, who suffers from seasonal allergies to various pollens. The pollen season arrived early this year and D was having severe problems with constant watery discharge from his nose and eyes, swollen eyes, difficulty in breathing and sleeping, and feeling "generally miserable." He started taking his Chlor-Trimeton decongestant (pseudoephedrine and chlorpenirame maleate), which had been prescribed each spring for the past few years, but his symptoms were not adequately relieved and his mood was "intolerable." EN reported that he was fatigued, grouchy, and "nervous." The family and child were unable to cope any further with the disease or the drug therapy.

What appropriate actions should be taken with this mother and son?

Discussion

EN should be encouraged to bring D in for evaluation. Several things could have happened since the drug was first prescribed a few years ago—new allergies, underlying illness, drug–drug interactions—that were not present earlier. D should be evaluated for all these factors. People do become resistant to antihistamines after a period of time, and D may just need to have his antihistamine changed to another one. The central nervous system effects may be a result of the drug. D is also at a very awkward stage in his life as far as psychological development is concerned. Feeling miserable and looking "puffy" can be very discouraging and upsetting for a teen-ager. EN and D will need support and encouragement to cope with the disease and the drug therapy. Several different antihistamines may need to be tried to find one that will provide D with adequate symptomatic relief and minimal central nervous system effects. D may require further sensitivity testing to determine if new allergies have developed, and may need to consider the possible benefit of desensitization injections. Careful history will need to be taken before this is done to determine all exposures and to rule out the use of any other drugs. OTC preparations are readily available for the treatment of allergy-related symptoms, and inadvertent overdosing could easily occur. EN and D should receive careful patient teaching regarding allergies, mechanisms of reactions, the drug therapy, and cautions that should be observed while on the drug therapy. Possible ways to decrease exposure to the responsible allergens and to cope with the allergy should be explored. Such allergies are very uncomfortable and frustrating, and the patient and family will require consistent support and counseling to deal with them.

Drug digests

Dextromethorphan HBr USP (Romilar)

Actions and indications. This synthetic opioid is the prototype of centrally acting nonnarcotic antitussive drugs. It acts selectively to depress cough center nerve cells and to raise their threshold of responsiveness to sensory impulses from the throat and respiratory tract. This makes it useful for control of coughs that occur during acute viral infections of the upper respiratory tract and in other conditions marked by a dry, hacking, unproductive cough that is set off by local irritation and inflammation.

Adverse effects, cautions, and contraindications. This drug is well tolerated and causes few, if any, side-effects when taken in therapeutic doses. It is claimed less likely than codeine to cause such opiate-type adverse effects as drowsiness or constipation. Very large overdoses can cause respiratory depression, but no deaths have been reported.

Although this drug is called *non*narcotic and does not cause physical dependence, it can be abused. Abuse can cause intoxication marked by hallucinations and bizarre behavior.

Like other centrally acting antitussives, it should be used only cautiously in patients with chronic bronchitis and other pulmonary obstructive disorders. Suppression of the cough reflex in such situations can be harmful, because it interferes with the patient's ability to clear mucous secretions from the bronchial passages. Use of this drug should not be continued without diagnostic measures to determine the cause of any cough that persists for a week or more.

Dosage and administration. The oral dosage range for adults is 10 to 20 mg every 4 hours or 30 mg every 6 to 8 hours. For children 6 to 12 years old, the dosage is half of the adult dose, with not more than a total of 60 mg in 24 hours. Children between 2 and 6 years old should receive no more than one-quarter of the adult dose, or no more than 30 mg daily.

Diphenhydramine HCl USP (Benadryl; Benylin)

Actions and indications. This is a prototype antihistaminic agent, but it also has several other actions that make it useful for treating other disorders in addition to allergy.

Among the allergic disorders for which this drug offers symptomatic relief are the following: seasonal rhinitis (pollinosis or hay fever); perennial allergic and vasomotor rhinitis; urticaria and angioedema; reactions to insect stings; and, following epinephrine or other more immediately effective measures, in the management of anaphylactic reactions. It may also be used to prevent or treat allergic reactions to blood or plasma in patients with a history of previous reactions. Because of other central and peripheral effects, this drug has also been advocated for the following clinical uses: as a sedative in treating insomnia; an antiemetic for prevention and treatment of motion sickness; an antiparkinsonism agent in mild cases; and for control of extrapyramidal reactions caused by certain antipsychotic drugs. It also has an antitussive effect that makes it useful in the control of nonproductive coughs associated with the common cold.

Adverse effects, cautions, and contraindications. The most common side-effect is drowsiness. This may make driving dangerous, and patients should be told not to use machinery that might be a hazard to one who is not completely alert. Patients should not drink alcoholic beverages or take other central depressant drugs that might have additive effects with diphenhydramine. Large overdoses may cause confusion, restlessness and, in young children, convulsions, coma, and death.

The atropinelike effects of this drug make it undesirable for treating asthmatic attacks, because the patient's bronchial secretions may be made excessively dry and thick. Such anticholinergic activity may also contraindicate its use in patients with an enlarged prostate or other genitourinary or GI tract obstructive disorders, and in narrow-angle glaucoma.

Dosage and administration. The usual oral dose for adults is 50 mg tid or qid; for children it is 12.5 mg to 25 mg at similar intervals. However, dosage is adjusted in accordance with the response of the child, and *total* daily oral dosage may vary from 12.5 to 300 mg. This drug may also be injected intramuscularly or intravenously in adult doses of 10 mg to 100 mg, up to a total of 400 mg daily. Children's dosage is calculated on a body weight or body surface area basis—for example, 5 mg/kg per 24 hours or 150 mg/m²/24 hours, qid.

Guaifenesin USP (glyceryl guaiacolate)

Actions and indications. This expectorant agent is used to increase the production of respiratory tract fluid (RTF) in patients with coughs caused by various acute and chronic respiratory disorders. In patients with chronic obstructive lung diseases, the RTF that this drug stimulates is supposed to decrease the viscosity of thickened mucous secretions. This helps the patient with chronic bronchitis, bronchial asthma, or emphysema to cough more productively and thus expel more sputum from the respiratory tract.

The drug-induced increase in a more fluid secretion is also thought to be helpful for patients with a dry, hacking cough caused by inflammation and irritation of the respiratory tract mucosa. This accounts for the common use of this expectorant for relief of cough associated with acute viral infections of the upper respiratory tract. Thus, it is employed in managing coughs caused by the common cold, laryngitis, tracheitis, acute bronchitis, bronchiolitis, and croup.

Adverse effects, cautions, and contraindications. This drug is well tolerated and causes few, if any, side-effects when administered in the small doses that are ordinarily employed. Much higher doses could be expected to cause nausea and, possibly, vomiting. Although inhibition of platelet aggregation has been reported experimentally, this does not seem likely to occur in clinical practice. Use of this drug may interfere with laboratory tests for chemicals present in excess in cases of carcinoid syndrome and pheochromocytoma. The drug is contraindicated only in patients known to have become hypersensitive to it.

Dosage and administration. The average adult dose is 100 to 200 mg every 3 or 4 hours. However, a higher dosage range of 200 to 400 mg every 4 hours is recommended for greater effectiveness. The total dose for 24 hours should not exceed 2400 mg. Dosage for children of various ages is reduced proportionately.

Oxymetazoline HCl USP (Afrin)

Actions and indications. This sympathomimetic amine exerts a potent, long-lasting constricting action on the small arterioles of the nasal mucosa when applied topically. In patients with allergic or infectious rhinitis, this vasoconstricting action produces prolonged (4 to 8 hours) nasal decongestion. This may be helpful for patients whose sleep might otherwise be disturbed by blocked nasal passages.

This treatment may help to relieve headache caused by obstruction of the paranasal sinuses, because it favors drainage of secretions through the ostia of the sinuses. It may also decrease congestion in the area of the eustachian ostia and thus help to prevent or treat middle ear infection.

Adverse effects, cautions, and contraindications. Rebound congestion is *not* common when drops or sprays containing this drug are employed for brief treatment periods and applied at the recommended intervals. However, excessive use over long periods could cause drug-induced nasal congestion. Other local side-effects may include mild, transient stinging or burning and sneezing followed by dryness of the nasal mucosa.

Little of this drug is absorbed systemically when it is applied properly. However, headache, light-headedness, and insomnia are possible central nervous system effects of overdosage. Heart palpitations are possible, and although adverse cardiovascular effects are unlikely, caution is required in the following situations: patients with coronary heart disease; hypertension; hyperthyroidism; diabetes mellitus; and those who are receiving medications of the monoamine oxidase (MAO) inhibitor type.

Children under 6 years old should not be treated with this drug, and its safety for the fetus when used by pregnant women has not been established. However, hypersensitivity to this drug and other chemicals in its preparations is the only contraindication.

Dosage and administration. Two to four drops of a 0.05% solution are instilled in each nostril in the morning and at bedtime with the patient in the lateral head-low position. A nasal spray of the same concentration may be squeezed into each nostril two or three times with the patient bending his head forward and sniffing briskly.

Tripelennamine HCl USP (Pyribenzamine)

Actions and indications. This prototype antihistamine drug is used for symptomatic relief of upper respiratory allergies such as hay fever and for dermatologic allergic reactions of the urticarial and contact dermatitis types. It is used occasionally for control of cough in asthmatic children with excessive respiratory tract secretions, but it is generally considered undesirable for patients with bronchial asthma. It is sometimes administered by injection as part of the emergency treatment of severe allergic (anaphylactic) reactions, but epinephrine is the most important agent for immediate use in such situations.

Adverse effects, cautions, and contraindications. Drowsiness is a common side-effect, and dizziness, confusion, and excitement sometimes occur. Such central symptoms may be most severe in patients also taking sedatives or hypnotic drugs, or drinking alcoholic beverages. Patients who react in this way are cautioned against driving or engaging in other activities that require alertness. Epigastric distress, nausea, mouth dryness, and difficulty in urination may occur but are rarely severe enough to require discontinuing the drug.

Dosage and administration. The usual oral adult dose is 50 mg taken once or twice daily, but dosage may range between 25 and 600 mg or more daily, depending on individual need and tolerance. The drug may be administered intramuscularly or by slow intravenous injection of 25 mg for rapid control of severe drug and transfusion reactions.

References

Black JW et al: Definition and antagonism of histamine receptors. Nature 236:385, 1972

Boyd EM: A review of studies of expectorants and inhalants. Int J Clin Pharmacol Ther Toxicol 3:55, 1970

Buissert PD: Allergy. Sci Am 247:86 (Aug), 1982

Chodosh S et al: Expectorant effect of glyceryl guaiacolate. Chest 543, 1973

Connell JT: Effectiveness of topical nasal decongestants. Ann Allergy 27:541, 1961

Cromolyn sodium nasal spray for hay fever. Med Lett Drugs Ther 25:89, 1983

Douglas WW: Histamine and 5-hydroxytryptamine (serotonin) and their antagonists. In Gilman AG, Goodman LS, Gilman A (eds): Goodman & Gilman's The Pharmacological Basis of Therapeutics, 6th ed, pp 609–646. New York, Macmillan, 1980

Feinberg SM: The antihistamines: Pharmacologic principles in their use. Pharmacol Physicians 1:1, 1967

Ginsburg R et al: Histamine receptors in the human heart. Life Sci 26:2245, 1980

Lockey RF, Bukantz SC: Allergic emergencies. Med Clin North Am 58:147, 1974

Norman PS: Specific therapy in allergy. Med Clin North Am 58:111, 1974

Patterson R: Rhinitis. Med Clin North Am 58:43, 1974

Rodman MJ: Drugs for allergic disorders. Part 1: Anaphylaxis and asthma. RN 34:63, 1971

Rodman MJ: Drugs for allergic disorders. Part 2: Pollinosis, perennial rhinitis, dermatitis. RN 34:53, 1971

Samuelsson B: Leukotrienes: Mediators of immediate hypersensitivity reactions and inflammation. Science 220:586, 1983

West S et al: A review of antihistamines and the common cold. Pediatrics 56:100, 1975

Chapter 40

Drugs used for respiratory tract obstruction

40

Chronic obstructive pulmonary disease

Chronic disorders of the respiratory tract have become a common cause of disability. An estimated 15 million Americans suffer from the three most common conditions—*chronic bronchitis, bronchial asthma,* and *emphysema.* These syndromes differ in their causes but share one common characteristic: airway obstructions block the free flow of air out of the patient's lungs.

Coughing, wheezing, and shortness of breath are common discomforting symptoms of chronic obstructive pulmonary disease (COPD). The patient's dyspnea can become progressively worse, and lead to a chronic buildup of carbon dioxide in the blood, acidosis, and electrolyte imbalance. These patients are prone to develop frequent respiratory infections that can precipitate into sudden episodes of acute pulmonary failure, congestive heart failure, and even cardiac arrest.

These diseases can be kept from progressing to such serious life-threatening stages when they are detected in their early stages and the patient is put on a program of long-term maintenance management. Thus, this chapter will first describe the use of drugs and other measures employed routinely to slow the progress of the various chronic obstructive pulmonary diseases. Then, it will describe how drugs are used in the management of such emergencies as severe asthma attacks, status asthmaticus, and acute respiratory failure.

Long-term maintenance management

As is the case in any chronic disease, what the patient does for himself on a daily basis is more important than anything that the physician or nurse can do during occasional visits to the clinic. Various self-care measures do not involve the use of drugs. In chronic bronchitis, which most often results from cigarette smoking, the condition can often be reversed in its early stages if the patient simply stops smoking. Patients with bronchial asthma can reduce the frequency of recurrent acute attacks by protecting themselves against exposure to the allergens that react with antibodies in their sensitized respiratory tract tissues (Chap. 39). Emphysema patients can be taught to breathe more efficiently so that the act of breathing becomes less exhausting.

Bronchial hygiene. Patients must be taught to employ regular measures included in a pulmonary toilet program—for example, postural drainage, hydration, cupping, rebreathing—that are aimed at keeping the airway open. By doing so daily in a routine way, patients can help to counteract the pathophysiologic mechanisms that cause airway obstruction. This results in relief of discomforting symptoms and helps to prevent the dangerous acute complications of these disorders.

The drugs and pulmonary toilet used in home maintenance programs help to keep the patient's respiratory tract clear in the following ways:

1. They widen the air passages by relaxing the bronchial smooth muscles that are often in a state of contraction.
2. They help to clear mucus that tends to accumulate in the disease-narrowed bronchi and bronchioles.
3. They reduce swelling of the inflamed and congested mucous membranes that line the bronchi and bronchioles.

Bronchodilator aerosols
Sympathomimetic amines. The most important single measure in bronchial hygiene is the daily inhalation of an aerosol containing an adrenergic bronchodilator drug (Table 40-1). As indicated in more detail in Chapters 13 and 17, sympathomimetic amines, including *isoproterenol*

(Text continues p. 814)

Table 40–1. Some drugs used in respiratory tract obstruction

Official or generic name	Trade name or synonym	Usual adult dosage and administration	Comments
Bronchodilator drugs			
Adrenergic type (see also Table 17–4)			
Albuterol (Salbutamol)	Proventil; Ventolin	2–4 mg oral, or two aerosol inhalations	Less likely than isoproterenol to cause cardiac stimulation; β_2 selective agonist
Ephedrine sulfate USP		25–50 mg oral	Best for treating and preventing mild attacks of bronchospasm
Epinephrine USP	Adrenalin; Sus-Phrine; Vaponefrin	0.2–0.5 mg SC or IM as 0.2–0.5 ml of a 1:1000 solution; 0.1–0.3 ml of a 1:200 solution SC; 1:100 solution for inhalation	Injections best for treating acute asthmatic attacks; inhalation of mists useful for rapid relief of mild attacks
Ethylnorepinephrine HCl USP	Bronkephrine	0.6–2.0 mg SC	Used to treat acute attacks; α, β_1, and β_2 agonist
Isoetharine HCl	Bronkosol; Bronkometer	Dosage varies with aerosol form and severity of attack	Less likely than isoproterenol to cause cardiac stimulation; β_2 selective agonist
Isoproterenol HCl or sulfate USP	Isuprel; Norisodrine	Inhalation of 1:100 or 1:200 solution; sublingual, 10–15 mg	Effective for mild to moderately severe asthmatic attacks; β_1 and β_2 agonist
Metaproterenol sulfate	Alupent; Metaprel	Two or three inhalations every 3 or 4 hours; or 20 mg orally tid or qid	Less likely than isoproterenol to cause cardiac stimulation; β_2 selective agonist
Terbutaline sulfate	Brethine; Bricanyl	5 mg orally tid at 6-hour intervals; or 0.25 mg SC—no more than 0.5 mg within a 4-hour period	Less likely than isoproterenol to cause cardiac stimulation; β_2 selective agonist
Theophylline or methylxanthine type			
		Dosage should ideally be individualized and adjusted on the basis of serum theophylline level; 10–20 μg/ml is therapeutic range	
Aminophylline USP	Theophylline ethylenediamine; Somophyllin; Phyllocontin	250 mg oral; 250–500 mg rectal; 250–500 mg by slow IV infusion of dilute solution	IV for acute bronchospasm and status asthmaticus; oral and rectal for milder attacks and prevention
Diphylline	Dilor; Lufyllin; Neothylline	Up to 15 mg/kg oral; 250–500 mg IM	Claimed to be less irritating and better absorbed than theophylline

Table 40–1. Some drugs used in respiratory tract obstruction (continued)

Official or generic name	Trade name or synonym	Usual adult dosage and administration	Comments
Oxtriphylline USP	Choline theophylline; Choledyl	200 mg oral	Claimed to be less irritating and better absorbed than theophylline
Theophylline anhydrous USP	Elixophyllin; Slo-Phyllin; Theo-Dur	100–200 mg oral	Now available in forms claimed to be 100% bioavailable, even in the form of sustained-release capsules or tablets
Theophylline sodium glycinate USP	Synophylate	330–660 mg oral	Effective alone or combined with ephedrine for relief and prevention of mild to moderate bronchospasm

Expectorants

Ammonium chloride USP	In Tossecol Expectorant	90 mg oral	Most of these drugs act mainly by irritating the gastric mucosa to produce reflex stimulation of the flow of respiratory tract fluids
Guaifenesin USP	Glyceryl guaiacolate; in Robitussin	100–200 mg oral	
Iodinated glycerol	Amonidrin; Organidin; Ipsatol	60 mg	
Potassium guaiacolsulfonate USP	In Codimal Expectorant	100 mg oral	See Drug digest
Potassium iodide USP		300 mg oral	
Terpin hydrate USP		85 mg oral	May act directly on bronchial secretory cells

Mucolytic agent

Acetylcysteine USP	*N*-Acetylcysteine; Mucomyst	1–10 ml of 20% solution or 2–20 ml of 10% solution by nebulizer; 1–2 ml of 10% or 20% solution by instillation	May cause bronchospasm in patients with bronchial asthma

Adrenocorticosteroids

Beclomethasone dipropionate	Beclovent Aerosol; Vanceril Aerosol	Two inhalations, 84 μg, tid or qid	Use causes no systemic side-effects and permits reduction in dosage of systemic steroids or their gradual complete elimination
Dexamethasone sodium phosphate aerosol USP	Decadron Phosphate Respihaler	Three inhalations, 252 μg, tid or qid	Causes some systemic toxicity

(continued)

Table 40–1. Some drugs used in respiratory tract obstruction (continued)

Official or generic name	Trade name or synonym	Usual adult dosage and administration	Comments
Hydrocortisone sodium phosphate USP	Hydrocortone Phosphate	15–240 mg/day IV or IM	Used in life-threatening emergencies such as status asthmaticus
Hydrocortisone sodium succinate USP	Solu-Cortef	100–500 mg IV or IM	
Methylprednisolone sodium phosphate USP	Solu-Medrol	10–40 mg IV	
Prednisolone sodium phosphate USP	Hydeltrasol	4–60 mg IV	
Triamcinolone acetonide	Azmacort	Two inhalations, 200 µg, tid or qid	New inhalation product used to prevent attacks of bronchial asthma

Miscellaneous drugs

Atropine sulfate	Dey-Dose Atropine Sulfate	Dilute with saline and administer by nebulizer tid or qid	New inhalation product used short-term to prevent and treat bronchospasm
Cromolyn sodium	Disodium cromoglycate; Intal	Inhale contents of one 20-mg capsule qid	Used to prevent attacks, not to treat them

and *epinephrine,* relax spasm of the bronchial wall smooth muscles, thus widening the narrowed air passages. This not only reduces dyspnea but also makes it easier for the patient to cough up mucous secretions.

Various devices are available for delivering adrenergic aerosols to their site of action in the lungs. These include bulb nebulizers and oral inhalers that release measured amounts of a liquid spray and—for patients so severely blocked that they cannot take a deep breath—pump-driven nebulizers and intermittent positive pressure breathing (IPPB) machines. For best results, patients who are to use oral nebulizers should be advised to inhale the mist deeply and then to hold their breath for several seconds before exhaling slowly through pursed lips. Each series of oral inhalations is repeated for only the number of times directed—usually two or three times with aerosols that release a measured amount of drug with each puff.

No matter which device is used, each patient must learn to adjust the bronchodilator drug dosage to his individual needs. The patient is taught not to overuse the aerosol but to inhale the smallest amount that will provide relief, and to do so no more often than necessary. Often, this may be on arising in the morning, then in the late afternoon, and finally in the evening, some time before bedtime. In no case should the procedure be repeated more often than about every 3 or 4 hours.

One reason for avoiding overuse is that tolerance tends to develop. The resulting reduction in effectiveness may then lead the patient to seek relief by using larger amounts. Repeated inhalation of sympathomimetic bronchodilators in excessive amounts can actually lead to a paradoxical rebound bronchospasm, and to development of the typical adverse cardiac and central effects of this drug class (Chap. 17). Thus, patients are advised to call their physician if they fail to get relief of bronchospasm from their usual dosage of the bronchodilator.

Heart palpitations and tachycardia can occur with these drugs, because their molecules occupy and react with β_1-type adrenergic receptors on cardiac muscle cells as well as with the β_2-type receptors of bronchial smooth muscle (Chap. 17). Adrenergic drugs that have a more selective action on β_2-type receptors have been introduced. These agents cause fewer cardiac side-effects than the standard drug *isoproterenol,* which stimulates both β_1 and β_2 receptors. (Deaths from sudden cardiac arrest have occurred in countries in which isoproterenol was available in highly concentrated inhalants that were abused by asthma patients; the aerosol propellant, a halogenated hydrocarbon, may have contributed to these deaths.)

Among the drugs that have a more selective β_2 action when inhaled by COPD patients are *metaproterenol sulfate* (Alupent; Metaprel), *albuterol* or *salbutamol* (Proventil; Ventolin), and *isoetharine* (in Bronkosol and Bronkometer). *Terbutaline sulfate* (Brethine; Bricanyl) is also somewhat selective for β_2 receptors. However, despite their greater affinity for the lungs than the heart, all can cause adverse cardiac effects, and so they must be used with considerable caution in COPD patients who also have coronary heart disease or other disorders that can be made worse by overdosage with sympathomimetic drugs.

Atropine. The status of a new inhalation form of atropine (Dey-Dose Atropine Sulfate) and an investigational inhalation anticholinergic drug, *ipratropium bromide* (Atrovent) as bronchodilators for managing patients with asthma and other obstructive pulmonary diseases is described on page 346 (Chap. 16).

Mucus control and removal

Pathophysiology. The respiratory tract contains cells that secrete protective mucoproteins. Normally, a layer of mucus covers the respiratory tract membranes and helps to trap dust particles, bacteria, and other foreign matter. Several mechanisms move the mucus stream containing this material upward toward the pharynx, from which it can then be expectorated or removed by swallowing. Most important in eliminating debris-laden mucus is the cough reflex discussed below, but ciliary activity and bronchial smooth muscle movements also help to keep the airway clear.

Many COPD patients are handicapped by an inability to handle the mucus produced in the respiratory tract. Chronic irritation by cigarette smoke, polluted air, or recurrent infection and inflammation increases the amount of mucus that is secreted. The secretions are also abnormally thick and sticky and thus cannot be readily removed by coughing and other protective mechanisms.

Chronic retention of viscous bronchial secretions accounts for several typical complications of COPD. *Non*productive coughing in attempts to clear almost immovable masses of mucus is a source of further irritation to the mucous membranes and leads to episodes of bronchospasm and wheezing. The smooth muscle walls weaken, and sections of the bronchioles become widely dilated (*bronchiectasis*). The cilia also become less active as the bronchioles become dilated and the mucus is not moved upward in the respiratory tract. The mucus also serves as a culture medium for pathogenic bacteria and infections are frequent, since sacs or pockets of pus form in the weakened bronchial walls.

Sometimes the retained mucopurulent plaques become dried out and form hardened plugs that completely block individual bronchioles. This interferes with expiration, because air containing carbon dioxide is trapped behind the mucous plugs. In some cases of chronic bronchitis, trapped air pressing on the delicate walls of the alveoli, or air sacs, breaks down their elastic

fibers. This leads to *emphysema*, a condition characterized by enlarged but nonfunctional air spaces and by a loss of the elastic recoil of the lung. The resulting chronic expiratory difficulties make the patient dyspneic and prone to episodes of acute respiratory failure.

Mucus control measures. The routine removal of mucus by the COPD patient can help to reduce breathing difficulties and slow the progressive respiratory tract damage that can lead to acute complications. The best way to keep the airway clear of excessive mucus is to reduce the viscosity of the secretions, so that they can be more readily removed by postural drainage and productive coughing following the use of a bronchodilator aerosol. How best to accomplish this is controversial. The adjunctive use of the expectorant and mucolytic drugs discussed below can sometimes be helpful for promoting sputum-producing coughing. However, many authorities believe that the simplest and safest way to loosen the thickened secretions is to liquefy them by local and systemic administration of water.

Local hydration is best carried out just after the air passages have been widened with bronchodilator drug inhalations. After employing an aerosol mist for this purpose, the patient may inhale steamy vapors from a simple device such as a "hot pot" water heater or kettle. Patients with more severe degrees of obstruction by mucus may use mechanical devices that deliver moisture in more efficient ways. An ultrasonic vaporizer, for example, breaks water particles into a mist of fine droplets. These penetrate deep into the lungs, where they help to liquefy tenacious secretions in sacs and other hard-to-reach recesses. *Systemic hydration* may also help to keep the sputum thin, so patients should be encouraged to drink large quantities of water, if not contraindicated by other medical conditions such as congestive heart failure or renal disease. It should be noted that even these measures may be inadequate. Some authorities believe that there is no conclusive evidence of benefit from the use of nebulizers or from the ingestion of large quantities of water.

Expectorants and mucolytic agents

The main mechanism for removing mucus is the *cough reflex* set off by the stimulus of mucus accumulating at sensitive sites in the bronchi, trachea, or pharynx. Nerve impulses travel from these peripheral receptors by way of afferent fibers of the vagus and glossopharyngeal nerves to the cough center in the medulla oblongata. Certain nerve cells in this brain stem area respond to these stimuli by sending out motor messages by way of efferent fibers. These impulses then cause contractions of the diaphragm and of the muscles in the chest and abdominal wall. At the same time, the vocal cords and epiglottis close shut over the top of the respiratory tree. When they snap open again an instant later, the air that had been confined and compressed within the passages is hurled forth at close to hurricane wind velocity. This helps to eject the mucous mass that had precipitated the reflex by irritating the sensitive receptors.

Expectorant drugs. The *expectorants*—the term means, literally, "out of the chest"—are supposed to make coughing more productive by stimulating the secretion of the natural lubricant fluid of the lower respiratory tract. This flow of natural secretions also helps to liquefy any thick mucous masses that may plug the narrow bronchioles. By decreasing the viscosity of such mucous plugs, the drug-induced secretion of fluid aids in removing mucus from the chest. Administration of a drug such as *potassium iodide*[+] may make it easier for patients with bronchial asthma to cough up the dry, hardened mucus blocking the bronchial tubes. In addition, the reduced tenacity of respiratory tract secretions increases the efficiency of the ciliated mucous blanket and the bronchiolar muscle peristaltic activity that also act to move thickened secretions toward the pharynx from the depths of the respiratory tract.

Mechanism of action. The expectorants do not enter the respiratory tract immediately on being swallowed. Instead, they act by one or both of two main mechanisms to stimulate the flow of respiratory tract fluid:

1. Some substances, ammonium chloride, or other strongly saline substances, irritate the stomach lining. This sets off the same sort of reflex activity that occurs during nausea. That is, nerve impulses pass to the medullary area to stimulate the reflex secretion of bronchial fluids and saliva.
2. Other agents are thought to act after being absorbed into the bloodstream. Substances such as guaifenesin and terpin hydrate are then excreted into the sputum by the bronchial glands. In the process of being eliminated by this route, they are thought to stimulate secretion of fluid by the mucosal glandular cells.

Some expectorants such as potassium iodide, which also appears in the sputum after being swallowed, are thought to act by a combination of both mechanisms.

Status. As indicated in Chapter 39, the small doses of expectorants employed in over-the-counter (OTC) products are not considered very effective. However, high doses of certain prescription-type expectorants such as inorganic iodide salts may sometimes be effective for liquefying hardened mucous casts, provided that the body fluids have first been fully restored and that the patient continues to receive fruit juices or milk with each dose. This measure also helps to disguise the saline taste and to lessen gastric irritation caused by iodides and large doses of most other expectorants, including ammonium chloride and ipecac.

Potassium iodide is still the most popular drug of this class, despite the introduction of organic iodide compounds that are claimed to be less irritating to the stomach. All the iodides are, however, undesirable for patients who are sensitive to them. Such sensitivity may become manifest as an acnelike skin eruption, which may spread from the sebaceous areas and become a generalized, potentially fatal furunculosis. Thus expectorants containing potassium iodide or iodinated glycerol should be withdrawn if a skin eruption appears shortly after treatment is started. A mumpslike painful swelling of the parotid gland also sometimes develops early in treatment, but it is less likely to occur if the patient has been receiving plenty of fluids. Hypothyroidism has also occurred.

Mucolytic agents. Certain substances act locally to help liquefy thickened sputum when they are brought into direct contact with the mucous masses by inhalation of aerosols or instillation of solutions. *Acetylcysteine* (Mucomyst), a drug that breaks up mucus by its chemical action, is sometimes nebulized into a face mask and inhaled several times daily. It is claimed to give relief to some COPD patients with abnormally viscid secretions. However, some asthmatic patients have suffered episodes of bronchospasm while inhaling the mist. If this happens, they should stop the treatment immediately and employ their adrenergic bronchodilator aerosol. Some authorities suggest that such reactions can be prevented by the addition of a drug such as isoproterenol to acetylcysteine prior to its being nebulized and inhaled by means of various devices (see Management of Respiratory Emergencies, below).

Other measures

It is important for COPD patients to avoid drugs that tend to dry respiratory tract secretions. Thus, although atropine and antihistamines have actions that may, in theory, be beneficial for asthmatic patients, the *systemic* administration of these drugs is usually considered undesirable in most cases, because these drugs may make mucus harden and form plugs that then block small bronchioles. The same is true of various other drugs that possess an anticholinergic component—for example, the phenothiazine-type antipsychotic agents and the tricyclic antidepressants (Chap. 46). However, some of the new *aerosol* forms of anticholinergic drugs that are available in the United States and abroad appear to be relatively free of the undesirable drying effect and other drawbacks of systemically administered atropine and other belladonna alkaloids (Chap. 16). The status of these anticholinergic aerosols in the treatment of asthma is described on page 346.

Other drugs to be avoided by COPD patients are the potent centrally acting narcotic analgesics, such as morphine, hydromorphone, and methadone (Chap. 51). These potent analgesic drugs reduce the capacity to cough to such an extent that secretions are not cleared adequately from the lower respiratory tract. The accumulating secretions may then prevent the lungs from expanding properly or may cause them to collapse at some points (*atelectasis*). This is one reason why the nurse often has to make special efforts to induce coughing in postoperative patients who have received such potent analgesics.

These drugs have various effects that account for their being *contraindicated* in such chronic obstructive diseases of the pulmonary passages as bronchial asthma, bronchiectasis, and emphysema. One such effect is that these potent antitussives tend to interfere with ventilation of the lungs by depressing the respiratory center almost as readily as they do the cough center.

In addition to this, and because they prevent the patient from coughing productively by excessively depressing the cough reflex, morphine and its relatives may have various adverse effects on other parts of the natural protective mechanism of the respiratory tract. For example, they may slow the activity of the cilia—hairlike processes that keep the mucous covering moving up toward the pharynx. The mucous stream may then stop flowing and become dried out, thus permitting microorganisms to penetrate into the underlying tissues. At the same time, the bronchial smooth muscle, which ordinarily contracts in a series of upward-sweeping peristaltic movements, may be sent into spasm by these drugs. The end result of all these adverse actions may be formation of hard mucus plugs in the constricted bronchiolar tubes and increased difficulty in breathing.

Codeine (Chap. 39) and *hydrocodone* are occasionally used in small doses for relief of coughing in COPD patients whose paroxysms are interfering with rest or who seem likely to rupture an emphysematous cyst if their coughing is not eased. Although these drugs are related to morphine and hydromorphone and are less effective antitussives than those more potent agents, they are relatively free of the main drawbacks of the latter. Codeine does not, for example, usually depress the respiratory center significantly, nor is it likely to suppress the cough reflex completely. Thus, although codeine reduces the reactivity of the cough center to some of the incoming afferent impulses, enough sensory stimuli still break through to permit productive coughing.

Prophylaxis against infection

It is important for COPD patients to try to avoid respiratory infections. Infection, of course, causes the respiratory tract mucous membranes to become inflamed and congested. This aggravates bronchial blockage in chronic bronchitis, and can lead to further loss of alveolar tissue in patients with emphysema. Often, in asthmatic patients,

a respiratory infection sets off a severe attack of the type that can lead to status asthmaticus (see below).

Intermittent antibiotics.

Patients are often told to keep at home a supply of a prescribed broad-spectrum antibiotic, such as *ampicillin* or a *tetracycline*. These are not intended for use against an ordinary cold, because virus infections do not respond to treatment with anti-infective drugs. However, the patient is instructed to watch for signs of bacterial infection such as a change in the color and character of the sputum that is coughed up. Thus, if the patient's sputum turns purulent and there is increased difficulty in bringing up the material by coughing, the patient should promptly begin taking the antibiotic.

Both types of broad-spectrum antibiotics are effective against the bacterial pathogens most likely to cause respiratory infections (Chap. 8). Thus, their use as previously directed for 2 or 3 days ordinarily controls the infection. The sputum becomes less viscid and easier to evacuate. The patient should, of course, continue to employ the usual regimen of bronchodilator, expectorant, and mucolytic drugs and other measures for facilitating the liquefaction and drainage of mucopurulent secretions.

Continuous prophylaxis

Some authorities recommend the daily use of prophylactic doses of these antibiotics, particularly during periods of cold weather, even when there is no evidence of a bacterial infection. Others argue that such prolonged use is not desirable, because it may lead to the emergence of resistant bacterial species and strains that can cause difficult to control superinfections. Such continuous prophylaxis is probably best suited for selected high-risk patients— for example, elderly and disease-debilitated patients or those who have a history of disease of the right side of the heart secondary to their respiratory disorder (cor pulmonale). In such cases, and in COPD patients who have been subject to frequent acute attacks of bronchitis, the continuous daily administration of antibiotics during the winter months may prevent the sudden development of bronchopneumonia and respiratory or cardiac failure.

Ordinarily, patients who employ either intermittent or continuous anti-infective drug prophylaxis do not require sputum cultures or sensitivity testing. However, if the patient develops an infection that fails to improve after 48 hours of broad-spectrum antibiotic therapy, the specific pathogen responsible for the infection should be identified, and its susceptibility to drug treatment should be determined.

Bronchial asthma attack: prevention and treatment

Up to now, this discussion has centered on aspects of long-term drug treatment that apply to *all* types of chronic obstructive airway disorders. Discussion will be limited here to the drug therapy of bronchial asthma. First, the daily maintenance management of mild or moderate asthma will be described, and then the management of more severe asthma and the emergency treatment of status asthmaticus will be presented.

Oral bronchodilator drugs

Two types of drugs are commonly administered orally for relief of asthmatic wheezing and shortness of breath: adrenergic or sympathomimetic drugs such as ephedrine that, unlike isoproterenol and epinephrine, resist inactivation in the gastrointestinal tract; and drugs of the methylxanthine or *theophylline* type, of which the prototype is *aminophylline*[+]. Some of these agents are also administered rectally as suppositories or as retention enemas.

Adrenergic bronchodilator drugs

Ephedrine is the drug most commonly taken by mouth to relax bronchospasm and keep patients with mild asthma comfortable. A single oral dose often prevents wheezing for 2 to 4 hours. However, with continued use, the drug tends to become less effective. Higher doses tend to stimulate the central nervous system and to cause symptoms similar to those produced by the related drug, amphetamine (Chap. 47). Peripheral side-effects typical of this drug class (Chap. 17) are not ordinarily discomforting with small therapeutic doses. However, the cardiovascular effects could be hazardous for an asthma patient who has heart disease or hypertension.

Terbutaline (Brethine; Bricanyl), a drug with an even more persistent duration of action than ephedrine, and *metaproterenol* (Alupent; Metaprel; see above), an agent to which tolerance does not develop as readily as with ephedrine, are both available in tablets and other dosage forms to produce bronchodilation and to help prevent mild wheezing from becoming more severe. *Albuterol* (Proventil; Ventolin) and *isoetharine* (Bronkosol; Bronkometer) are also used in oral or inhalation dosage forms. These four sympathomimetic drugs are less likely than ephedrine to cause cardiac stimulation. However, despite their greater affinity for the β_2-type adrenergic receptors in bronchial smooth muscle, they can also cause cardiac side-effects by β_1-(cardiac) receptor stimulation, especially in higher dosage. Thus, their use requires the same caution as when ephedrine is employed. These drugs also cause central side-effects similar to those of ephedrine.

Another adrenergic bronchodilator drug, *pseudoephedrine* (Sudafed), is said to cause less nervousness, insomnia, and muscle tenseness or tremors than the other drugs of this class that are administered by mouth to counteract bronchospasm and wheezing.

Methylxanthine bronchodilators

Theophylline and its derivatives are administered orally or rectally during the long-term maintenance management

of bronchial asthma (Table 40-1). These drugs are effective bronchodilators to which tolerance does not readily develop. However, patients' responses to therapy with methylxanthine derivatives have sometimes proved very variable. One reason for this is that some oral products do not disintegrate and dissolve readily in the gastrointestinal tract and, because of such bioavailability problems, they are not reliably absorbed from the upper gastrointestinal tract. Other derivatives contain relatively low proportions of anhydrous theophylline, the active agent. Another reason is that there are great individual differences in the rates at which people metabolize theophylline and its derivatives.

Aminophylline, oxytriphylline (Choledyl), and other double salts and complexes of theophylline with basic substances are claimed to be more soluble and absorbable, and thus more likely to attain therapeutically effective levels in the blood plasma and the bronchioles. The more rapid and complete absorption of these alkaline salts has also been claimed to reduce gastrointestinal tract irritation. However, newer forms of the parent compound, anhydrous theophylline—for example, microfine crystals formulated in tablets that are more readily soluble than earlier products—seem to be completely absorbable and to cause no more local irritation of the upper gastrointestinal tract. In fact, irritation may be more likely with highly alkaline double salts or with hydroalcoholic solutions of theophylline than with the fully bioavailable tablets.

It is now recommended that theophylline derivatives be taken without food to ensure complete absorption and full effectiveness. One reason for this is that such side-effects as anorexia, nausea, and vomiting stem mainly from stimulation of the central emetic mechanism (Chap. 41) rather than from local gastrointestinal irritation. Such side-effects, which occur when plasma levels of these drugs exceed the therapeutic range, are also often seen even when aminophylline is administered by the rectal route in suppository form or following injection of excessive amounts.

The most important factor in ensuring effectiveness and safety when these drugs are employed is careful titration of dosage. As indicated above, some patients metabolize theophylline very rapidly while others are slow metabolizers. Thus, therapeutic dosage has been found to vary from as little as 400 mg in 24 hours for slow metabolizers to as much as 3400 mg in the same period for rapid metabolizers. Obviously, the routine administration of a standard dose of a theophylline-type drug will provide too low plasma levels to produce bronchodilation in some patients and lead to development of signs and symptoms of cumulative toxicity in others.

The variability in dosage required to bring about optimal responses to theophylline therapy makes it necessary to watch patients closely for clinical signs of asthma improvement and for signs and symptoms of adverse drug effects. This is especially true when some of the newer sustained-release preparations are used. Fortunately, the development of accurate tests for measuring the serum levels of theophylline can aid as a guide in adjusting dosage of these drugs to the optimal levels required by different patients. It is now known, for example, that theophylline must attain a serum concentration of *at least 10 µg/ml* to bring about its beneficial bronchodilator effects. Similarly, as plasma levels rise *above 20 µg/ml*, there is a progressive increase in such adverse effects as nausea, diarrhea, vomiting, and headache. Signs of the most serious toxicity—convulsive seizures and cardiac arrhythmias—rarely occur at serum concentrations below 40 µg/ml but such life-threatening complications of theophylline therapy can sometimes develop without the prior warning of the early gastrointestinal signs and symptoms that ordinarily develop at lower plasma levels.

Various dosage regimens are recommended for attaining the maximal therapeutic effects of theophylline with the fewest adverse effects. Some authorities suggest starting patients off with a relatively high oral loading dose and then maintaining them at lower doses administered four times daily. Other authorities prefer to start patients off at a moderate dose that is then gradually increased at intervals of 2 to 3 days, until an optimal daily dosage is attained in terms of both freedom from clinical bronchospasm symptoms and attainment of blood levels that correlate with the desired therapeutic response.

Patients who metabolize theophylline slowly are stabilized at relatively low doses administered at less frequent intervals. Those who eliminate theophylline rapidly require larger doses taken more frequently, or they may do better when treated with a timed-release preparation that provides a prolonged therapeutic effect. Provided that the product is one of proven reliability, which makes the drug bioavailable at a sustained rate of release that ensures its steady absorption, these patients need take their medication at intervals of only about 8 to 12 hours, rather than by the much more frequent administration schedule they would require with ordinary tablets or liquids. The availability of these long-acting oral products has led to a reduction in the popularity of aminophylline suppositories for preventing nocturnal dyspnea.

Individualization of dosage is particularly important in asthmatic children, because toxicity has sometimes occurred even when seemingly safe doses have been employed. Apparently, young children are sensitive to the central stimulating effect of theophylline. They some-times tend to become restless and agitated after receiving only moderate doses. Fatalities have been reported following the administration of aminophylline rectal suppositories. Death occurred after severe bloody vomiting, dehydration, fever, convulsions, and cardiovascular collapse.

Because rectal use can cause local irritation, it should not be employed regularly. It should, instead, be reserved for children and others suffering occasional severe dyspneic distress during the night when an injectable bronchodilator may not be available. In such a situation, administering a solution of theophylline monoethanolamine or of aminophylline in the form of a retention enema is preferred to insertion of a suppository, from which these drugs are often erratically absorbed as compared to the complete and rapid absorption of the liquid form from the rectal mucosa, when the patient can retain the enema without leakage.

Fixed dosage combinations

Products containing theophylline and ephedrine combined with a barbiturate to reduce the central stimulating effects of both drugs are widely available and commonly employed. In theory, combinations of adrenergic and methylxanthine drugs should have synergistic bronchodilator effects.* In practice, it is probably better to administer each drug separately for greater effectiveness and safety. Some research results suggest that these standard dose combinations are no more effective than adequate doses of either drug administered alone at dose levels determined by individualizing dosage, and their routine use in fixed dosage combinations could lead to cumulative toxicity from one or another of the components. Results of other studies indicate that the addition of ephedrine to the regimen of a patient who is responding adequately to theophylline alone will not lead to a better bronchodilator effect but may, instead, cause increased central nervous system stimulation leading to the toxic effects described above.

Management of severe asthma

Many cases of asthma can be controlled with immunotherapy (Chap. 39) and with a program of self-care that includes the drugs and measures described above. Unfortunately, some patients fail to improve, and their condition becomes progressively worse. In such cases, several other types of treatment may be tried to control severe asthma symptoms and slow progressive disability, including the following:

1. *Injections of sympathomimetic drugs,* instead of aerosols or oral adrenergic and methylxanthine bronchodilators
2. Oral or aerosol *corticosteroid* drugs
3. *Cromolyn sodium,* a prophylactic drug that stabilizes the membranes of mast cells and

---

* Both drugs are thought to act by raising intracellular levels of *cyclic AMP*. As indicated in Chapter 17 sympathomimetic amines do so by increasing the rate at which this cyclic nucleotide is biosynthesized. The methylxanthines inhibit the intracellular enzyme *phosphodiesterase*, which catalyzes the breakdown of cyclic AMP. Because both drugs produce the same biochemical effect, but by different mechanisms, their combined bronchodilator effect should, in theory, be greater than that of either drug alone.

inhibits the release of histamine, slow-reacting substance of anaphylaxis (SRS-A), and other autacoids when the patient's respiratory tract is exposed to antigens.

This section will describe significant points concerning each of these types of drug therapy.

Epinephrine injection

This is considered to be the most effective drug and route of administration for patients who no longer obtain adequate relief from oral bronchodilators or from aerosols containing isoproterenol or other inhalable sympathomimetic amines, including epinephrine itself. One reason for the superiority of subcutaneously injected epinephrine over the inhaled form is that it reaches the lungs by way of the bloodstream, even when the presence of large amounts of mucous secretions and plugs prevents inhaled particles from reaching the reactive receptors of bronchial smooth muscle cells. An additional advantage of epinephrine over inhaled isoproterenol is that it reduces bronchial mucosal congestion by constricting dilated blood vessels. (Isoproterenol tends to dilate such vessels further and thus may increase local congestion, even though it is as effective a bronchodilator as epinephrine.)

Two forms of epinephrine are available: aqueous solutions that are rapidly absorbed, and oily or aqueous suspensions that are slower in onset of action but offer more prolonged duration of the drug's bronchodilator-decongestant actions when that is desired. A single dose of 0.3 ml of a 1:1000 aqueous solution of epinephrine is often rapidly effective when injected subcutaneously and the injection site is massaged to facilitate absorption. (This is the same preparation employed in the management of anaphylactic reactions described in Chapter 39.)

Sometimes the effects of such an aqueous injection wear off rather quickly, and symptoms return. In such cases these injections may be repeated—at 20-minute intervals at first, but after the first hour no more often than every 2 hours—or a 1:200 suspension (Sus-Phrine) may be employed at intervals of 4 hours or more to maintain prolonged bronchodilation. Patients who no longer respond to epinephrine injections should be hospitalized and receive the emergency management described below. One reason for this is that repeated administration of epinephrine may lead to cardiac arrhythmias in hypoxic patients with severe asthma.

Terbutaline (see above) is available in an injectable form, which may be safer than epinephrine is such cases because of its more specific effect on β_2 (bronchial) adrenergic receptors. However, as indicated previously, this and similar sympathomimetic drugs *can* cause cardiac arrhythmias in patients who have heart diseases that make them susceptible to the stimulating effects of all adrenergic drugs on β_1 (cardiac) receptors. Patients who do not re-

spond well to two successive doses of terbutaline should be given no more of this drug for at least 4 hours to avoid cardiac stimulation.

Corticosteroids in chronic asthma

Patient selection. Patients whose condition appears to be worsening in spite of intensive treatment with bronchodilators and with the other antiasthmatic drugs described previously sometimes have oral corticosteroids added to their regular regimen. Because of the hazards of long-term steroid therapy (Chap. 21), these drugs are employed only after careful evaluation of the patient's condition has demonstrated no contraindications to the continued use of steroids. Signs such as development of rib cage deformities in asthmatic children or of other disabilities that are interfering with the respiratory function of older patients also indicate that the use of corticosteroids is justified.

Dosage adjustment. Often the decision to employ these drugs is made during a period of severe illness. Patients first seen during an acute asthmatic episode are usually started on high doses—for example, 60 mg of prednisone daily. After a week or two, when the patient's breathing difficulties have improved, the daily dosage is gradually tapered down to about one-third of the initial amount. After keeping the patient at this dose level for a while, further attempts are made to reduce steroid dosage to the minimum amount needed to halt the progress of the disabling effects of the disease—usually 10 mg or less of prednisone.

It is *not* desirable to maintain the patient at a dose level that can completely relieve wheezing and other discomforting symptoms. Patients may become habituated to the relatively high doses needed to provide full symptomatic relief. Lower maintenance doses make it easier to reduce steroid dosage further whenever the patient's condition improves, and their use may then be discontinued entirely.

Withdrawal of steroids. Patients often resist attempts to wean them away from steroids. The nurse can facilitate the weaning by explaining why it is so important to reduce the dosage of these drugs. The patient will need encouragement and emotional support when the asthmatic symptoms seem to worsen as the daily steroid dosage is reduced. Pointing out the improvement in appearance that results from lower steroid dosage (and subsequent lessening of cushingoid-type toxicity signs), as well as the lessening of other side-effects, often helps the patient to cope with this difficult dosage adjustment period.

Intermittent dosage. To lessen the likelihood of such adverse steroid effects, dosage schedules have been devised that are aimed at minimizing the suppressant effect of steroids on the pituitary and adrenal glands. The most commonly employed of these intermittent dosage plans involves switching the patient from a program of several daily divided doses to a regimen in which the whole day's dosage is taken at once with the morning meal.

A similar plan is *alternate day therapy,* a method in which the total steroid dosage for 2 days is administered early in the morning every other day (Chap. 21). Although such schedules seem safer for many asthmatic patients, some become quite uncomfortable in the last part of the 48-hour period between doses of the drugs such as prednisone that are used for this purpose. This is particularly likely to occur when the patient is being switched from divided steroid dosage to the alternate day therapy plan. Here too, the nurse encourages the patient to cope with the return of some of the asthma symptoms during the dosage adjustment period.

Inhalational steroids. Attempts have also been made to reduce or eliminate oral steroid dosage by substituting a steroid that could be inhaled. It was hoped that delivering a high level of a drug locally would produce beneficial respiratory effects without causing systemic toxicity. However, the first aerosol that was marketed, *dexamethasone sodium phosphate inhaler* (Decadron Phosphate Respihaler), proved disappointing. Enough of this steroid was often absorbed systemically from the lungs to suppress adrenal function and to cause signs of typical metabolic toxicity.

Beclomethasone dipropionate (Vanceril Inhaler), a more recently introduced product, appears to be a more effective and safer steroid for topical application. This seems to be because low doses exert a local therapeutic effect, and the small amounts that are absorbed are rapidly eliminated. Thus, the typical adverse systemic effects of steroids do not occur. It is not known whether this drug has any long-term adverse local effects on lung tissue. This preparation frequently causes fungal infection of the mouth or throat, which can be readily controlled with topical antifungal antibiotics (Chap. 9).

Unlike bronchodilator aerosols, this inhalant is *not* intended for rapid relief of wheezing and breathlessness. When treatment is begun in patients who have had no previous steroid therapy, it may take a week or two for any improvement at all to be noted. Thus, other types of treatment, including bronchodilator drugs, should be continued. Patients who have been using oral steroids can have their daily dosage gradually reduced if they respond to beclomethasone inhalation. Some younger patients who had required only relatively small daily doses of oral steroids may be able to discontinue them entirely and use only the inhaler along with their nonsteroid antiasthma medications.

It is important to remember that substitution of inhaled steroids for systemic steroids may unmask symptoms of other allergic disorders that had been kept under control along with the asthma symptoms. Thus, for example, allergic rhinitis, conjunctivitis, or dermatitis may flare up when systemic steroid dosage is reduced. This is because the inhalant's effects are exerted only in the lungs and not in the nose, eyes, skin, or other tissues.

Patients transferred from systemic to inhaled steroids may feel worse even though their respiratory function improves. This may be caused by the syndrome that tends to occur when steroids are withdrawn too rapidly (see Steroid withdrawal, Chap. 21). Even more serious is the possibility that an asthmatic patient who has been switched to an inhalant after long use of oral steroids may be subject to episodes of acute adrenal crisis. Such patients should be warned to resume high oral doses of steroids if they suffer a respiratory infection that sets off a severe asthma attack. Other stressful emergencies may also require large oral or injectable doses of supplementary steroids.

Cromolyn

Cromolyn sodium (Intal) is a drug that sometimes helps to *prevent* attacks of asthmatic wheezing and coughing when it is added to a regimen of other drugs and measures that have not been entirely successful in controlling severe asthma symptoms. Although it is inhaled orally like bronchodilator aerosols, this drug is *never* used to *treat* acute asthmatic attacks. Instead, it is employed regularly on a daily basis as part of long-term programs for managing severe asthma, which include use of bronchodilators, expectorants and mucolytics, antibiotics, and anti-inflammatory corticosteroids.

Clinical response. Improvement is often noted after 2 to 4 weeks in which the drug is inhaled four times daily at regular intervals. Patients find that they suffer fewer attacks of wheezing and breathlessness during the day and at night. They tend to cough less but more productively. Their need for frequent use of bronchodilator drugs is lessened, and corticosteroid dosage can often be reduced. (Steroid withdrawal—as indicated above and elsewhere—must be carried out very gradually to avoid a flare-up of asthma or an adrenal crisis.)

Adverse effects. This drug should be discontinued if no improvement is seen after several weeks of use. Some asthmatic patients suffer attacks of bronchospasm when they inhale the finely powdered drug. If this cannot be prevented by prior inhalation of a bronchodilator aerosol, or if the patient shows signs of becoming hypersensitive to cromolyn, it should also be withdrawn. The drug causes few direct adverse effects, but some patients suffer allergic reactions. Skin wheals and rashes and even occasional angioedema and anaphylaxis have been reported.

Mechanism of action. This drug produces its prophylactic effects in a way that is different from all other antiasthmatic drugs. It apparently prevents release of such chemical mediators of allergic reactions as histamine and SRS-A. As indicated in Chapter 39, these autacoids are ordinarily released from previously sensitized mast cells and basophils when a foreign substance to which an asthmatic person is allergic (an allergen) combines with immunoglobulin E (IgE) antibodies on the cells' surfaces. By preventing the release of these potent autopharmacologically active chemicals, cromolyn prevents their molecules from reacting with bronchial and vascular smooth muscle target tissues. Thus, bronchospasm and mucosal congestion do not occur.

Administration. Cromolyn comes in a capsule containing a fine dry powder that is to be inhaled from a special type of inhaler. Obviously, the patient must be made aware that cromolyn capsules are not intended to be taken orally and swallowed. The patient should also be instructed as to how the inhaler has to be used for best results. As with other oral inhalants, the patient is told to press his lips tightly around the mouthpiece, and then to tilt his head backward and inhale the powder from above with a quick, deep breath, which is held for several seconds after removing the inhaler from the mouth. Some patients with impaired breathing may find this procedure difficult, but they should be encouraged in keep repeating it until all of the capsule's contents have been inhaled. Cromolyn also comes as a solution to be dispensed from a power-driven nebulizer equipped with a face mask.

As indicated in Chapter 39, a new nasal aerosol form of this drug (Nasalcrom) has recently been marketed for use by patients with allergic rhinitis. An oral drug said to act similarly to cromolyn is in use abroad and under investigation in the United States for use by asthmatic patients. This drug, *ketotifen fumarate* (Zaditen) would be especially advantageous for patients who develop bronchospasm when inhaling cromolyn. This drug does cause sedation and drowsiness, however, as well as other systemic toxic effects.

Management of respiratory emergencies

Status asthmaticus
Most acute attacks of asthma can be quickly controlled by inhalation, or subcutaneous injection, of potent sympathomimetic bronchodilators such as isoproterenol, metaproterenol, terbutaline, albuterol, isoetharine, or epinephrine. Sometimes, however, an asthmatic patient who suffers a respiratory infection or who has failed to follow the self-care program may be precipitated into a series of increasingly prolonged attacks. In such severe acute exacerbations of chronic asthma, the patient's bronchoconstriction may become continuous, because it fails to respond even to frequent epinephrine injections. This life-threatening complication, *status asthmaticus,* requires hospitalization—preferably in a respiratory intensive care unit (RICU)—to prevent possible respiratory failure.

General nursing care
An asthmatic patient who arrives at the hospital after suffering repeated severe attacks is as acutely ill as his appearance indicates. His pale face often mirrors fright, as the patient struggles to draw air through bronchi that are narrowed by smooth muscle spasm and clogged with thick tenacious secretions. Relief of the patient's distress requires prompt medical action and intelligent nursing care.

Sedative drugs are sometimes employed in small doses to help relieve anxiety and fear. However, depressant drugs may further reduce the rate and depth of the patient's already inadequate breathing. Certain nursing measures, such as support, encouragement, and careful explanations, can help to minimize the need for sedative and antianxiety drugs.

When administering medication, the nurse can often add to a drug's effectiveness by expressing confidence that it will shortly relieve the symptoms. Sympathetic and skillful nursing care is often more effective than drugs for reducing anxiety. Among the nursing measures that help to lessen apprehension are simply staying with the patient and listening to his personal concerns, or ensuring that the patient has a call bell readily available and answering it promptly if he rings.

Correction of physiologic abnormalities
Patients in status asthmaticus have usually become severely dehydrated and possibly hypoxic, hypercapnic, and acidotic during the several days of increasingly severe attacks that may occur before they seek admission to a hospital. These abnormalities should be corrected before the administration of potent drugs is attempted. The patient's refractoriness to injected epinephrine may, for example, be related to the acidotic condition, and repeated injections can cause cardiac arrhythmias in the presence of poor myocardial oxygenation. The ineffectiveness of inhaled isoproterenol or epinephrine may be secondary to dehydration, which leads to drying out of the patient's copious secretions. These then tend to prevent bronchodilator mists from getting through the clogged airway.

Rehydration. Before treating the bronchospasm itself, the physician usually orders medication that thins the tenacious bronchial secretions so that the patient can clear the lungs by coughing productively. The first step for loosening such secretions is to administer intravenous fluids to compensate for those probably lost in the days prior to hospitalization. When the patient can drink again, oral fluids may be forced, if not contraindicated by other conditions.

Once the patient has been rehydrated, *expectorant drugs* are administered to stimulate the secretion of respiratory tract fluids. Inorganic iodide salts have been traditionally employed for this purpose, and sodium iodide is still sometimes administered by slow IV drip. However, in hospitalized patients, mechanical measures for removing hardened mucous plugs may be preferred following direct application of a mucolytic agent (see above, and Table 40-1).

Mucus liquefaction. Substances that act locally to liquefy mucous masses are also sometimes employed to open blocked passages. These include detergents and other wetting agents that are intended to draw water into the thickened mucus in order to thin down these secretions. Other chemicals such as acetylcysteine break down the mucus chemically. Unfortunately, the irritating properties of this substance limit its usefulness for routine use in asthmatic patients.

Even when used in *non*asthmatic patients with obstructive pulmonary diseases such as emphysema and chronic bronchitis, administration of these substances is not always effective. Bulb atomizers and ordinary nebulizers may not deliver enough of the vaporized solution into the bronchioles. However, hospitalized patients are sometimes helped when an oxygen stream is used to pick up a mucolytic mist that is then pumped deep into the lungs by an intermittent positive pressure apparatus.

Patients close to asphyxia because of bronchus-blocking plugs may benefit from having the drug solutions instilled directly into the tracheobronchial tree. In such cases sterile solutions are instilled through an endotracheal tube, tracheostomy, or bronchoscope. After about 20 minutes of direct contact with the mucous plugs, the solution and the dissolved material are removed by mechanical suction or postural drainage.

With any drug that produces an increased volume of thinned sputum, prompt removal of the liquefied secretions is important to prevent the patient from drowning in his own fluids. Elderly and weakened patients must be closely watched and encouraged to cough productively.

Acidosis correction. Two types of acidosis tend to develop during status asthmaticus and in other COPD patients who are in respiratory distress:

1. *Respiratory acidosis,* which results from persistent hypoventilation of the alveoli and a consequent rise in the level of blood carbon dioxide, the source of carbonic acid
2. *Metabolic acidosis,* which occurs secondary to hypoxia and a shift to anaerobic metabolism

Respiratory acidosis is best corrected by measures that restore adequate pulmonary ventilation and lead to removal of the retained carbon dioxide. In the past, attempts have been made to stimulate the patient's respiratory center by carefully infusing an analeptic drug (Chap. 47) by vein. Drugs such as *doxapram hydrochloride* and *nikethamide* are said to help the patient blow off excess carbon dioxide and clear bronchial secretions by stimulating more effective coughing.

Other authorities deny that these drugs are beneficial for COPD patients. They claim that these central stimulants cause muscular contractions that use up precious oxygen and actually increase carbon dioxide production. They suggest that the best way to restore adequate ventilation and correct respiratory acidosis is by the measures already described for reducing the viscosity of the sticky sputum, so that the airway-clogging secretions can be removed by mechanical measures and chest physiotherapy. Mechanical ventilation (see below) may also be required to correct respiratory acidosis.

Metabolic acidosis results from the buildup of lactic acid, the main metabolite of anaerobic cellular activity. The body's bicarbonate reserve is reduced in neutralizing the lactic acid, and the loss of base leads to acidemia. Before attempting treatment with bronchodilator drugs, metabolic acidosis should be corrected by careful intravenous infusion of a systemic alkalinizer.

Sodium bicarbonate is preferred for counteracting the loss of alkaline reserve. It acts more promptly than *sodium lactate,* which has to be metabolically converted to bicarbonate. *Tromethamine injection* (THAM solution), a buffer that combines with hydrogen ions to form bicarbonate, is also employed occasionally. Care is required to avoid overdosage with these systemic alkalinizers, because metabolic alkalosis may occur, and the resulting low level of carbon dioxide—the natural respiratory center stimulant—can lead to further depression of ventilation.

Bronchodilators

Once physiologic abnormalities have been corrected and pulmonary passages have been partially cleared of mucus, the patient in status asthmaticus may again respond to inhaled or injected epinephrine. However, if epinephrine still fails to relax bronchospasm, or if the doses required for bronchodilation tend to cause nervousness, tremors, tachycardia, or cardiac dysrhythmias, the physician may order parenteral administration of *aminophylline.* The intravenous route is preferred for this nonadrenergic bronchodilator because its intramuscular administration can cause prolonged local pain.

Aminophylline is often effective in patients refractory to sympathomimetic amines. It not only relaxes bronchial smooth muscle spasm in the manner discussed above but may also stimulate the respiratory center. The latter effect is similar to that of parenterally administered caffeine, a close chemical relative among the methylated xanthines (Chap. 47). These effects are best brought about by IV administration of a relatively large loading dose followed by lower maintenance dosage.

This drug is administered by slow intravenous infusion—about 250 to 500 mg every 15 minutes—the amount depending, in part, on whether the patient had previously been taking an oral theophylline preparation. Too slow an infusion may fail to maintain the plasma level required for therapeutic activity; too rapid an infusion may cause cardiovascular or central nervous system toxicity. Although aminophylline can increase cardiac muscle strength (see the discussion of its use in treating acute pulmonary edema in Chapter 31), it can cause dangerous cardiac dysrhythmias when administered too rapidly or in overdoses to hypoxic COPD patients. (Overdosage with aminophylline may also cause a profound fall in blood pressure as a result of generalized vasodilation, because this drug relaxes smooth muscles of the blood vessels as well as of the bronchioles.)

If the initial aminophylline injection produces plasma levels of 15 to 20 $\mu g/ml$, marked relief of persistent bronchospasm is usually observed and the patient's labored breathing is improved. A slow continuous IV drip may be then employed to maintain the drug's plasma concentration at therapeutic levels, or the initial IV dose may be repeated three or four times daily until oral or rectally administered doses become adequate for control of a milder degree of wheezing. Finally, the patient who responds once more to a test dose of epinephrine may be maintained on aerosolized sympathomimetic amines.

Corticosteroids

Water-soluble steroid esters such as *hydrocortisone sodium succinate* (Solu-Cortef), *methylprednisolone sodium succinate* (Solu-Medrol), and *dexamethasone sodium phosphate* (Decadron Phosphate) are often infused intravenously in very high doses during the first day of status asthmaticus treatment. These drugs do not produce any immediate dramatic improvement, because they do not have an immediate direct bronchodilator effect. However, large doses of steroids seem to play a part in restoring the asthmatic patient's responsiveness to the bronchodilator action of epinephrine and other sympathomimetic amines. After 12 to 24 hours, bronchial congestion is markedly reduced as a result of the anti-inflammatory effect of the corticosteroids.

The typical metabolic and endocrine toxicity that is seen during long-term steroid therapy (Chap. 21) does not occur, even when 1 or 2 g of hydrocortisone or equivalent doses of other steroids are administered for a few days. However, patients with a history of hypertension, peptic ulcer, or emotional disturbances should be observed carefully for signs of flare-ups of these disorders during even short-term emergency treatment of severe asthma with high steroid dosage. In any case, steroid dosage is reduced rapidly to maintenance levels or discontinued entirely after a few days.

Acute ventilatory failure

Patients with advanced asthma or chronic bronchitis and emphysema sometimes suffer episodes of acute respiratory failure. These often tend to develop with little outward warning when the patient gets a respiratory infection that is not well controlled by broad-spectrum antibiotics. Because clinical signs of oncoming ventilatory failure are not very reliable, the physician often orders blood gas studies of serial samples of arterial blood. If the tests reveal oxygen levels below 50 mm Hg and a steady rise in the already chronically high blood carbon dioxide level, the patient requires carefully controlled oxygen therapy.

Controlled low-flow oxygen. Oxygen inhalation must be begun immediately to counteract hypoxemia. However, raising the arterial oxygen level too rapidly can be harmful in COPD patients. This is because hypoxia is the main stimulus to breathing in patients who have lived with chronic high levels of CO_2 and who no longer respond to these high CO_2 levels. The removal of this hypoxic drive with uncontrolled oxygen inhalation can lead to further reduction of pulmonary ventilation. The resulting rapid rise in arterial carbon dioxide levels can then cause narcosis, coma, and respiratory arrest.

This can be avoided by delivering the oxygen at a carefully controlled low rate of flow. Improved flowmeters now allow delivery of as little as 1 liter of oxygen per minute. This is enough to prevent a progressive rise in carbon dioxide (hypercapnia) and yet, in most cases, to supply enough oxygen to raise the blood content of this vital gas to a safer level. Patients whose hypoxemia cannot be counteracted by low concentrations of oxygen and who require a mixture with higher oxygen content must be watched closely for clinical signs of rising carbon dioxide retention.

The most common sign of an excessive buildup of carbon dioxide in COPD patients is drowsiness. Sometimes, however, hypercapnia causes increasing irritability and mental confusion. When this is coupled with the natural apprehension of the patient with severe dyspnea, the physician—or the nurse who has a prn order—may assume that the patient requires sedation. Although, as indicated earlier, small doses of sedative drugs can be helpful for allaying anxiety and fear when combined with emotional support, these drugs should not be used when determinations of arterial blood gases show that the blood contains high carbon dioxide levels. These drugs, and other depressants such as potent narcotic analgesics, are contraindicated in such COPD patients, because their use can quickly lead to respiratory arrest.

Assisted and controlled ventilation. The previous statement does not apply to patients who are being ventilated artificially by mechanical devices. Patients whose breathing becomes progressively weaker despite use of all the drugs and measures described above often require assisted ventilation. Mechanical ventilation is a very uncomfortable and frightening experience for the conscious patient. Sometimes it is desirable or necessary to use heavy sedation to prevent the patient from fighting the machine, thus permitting efficient respirations. The high doses of *diazepam* (Valium), *pentobarbital* (Nembutal), or even *morphine* employed for this purpose are, of course, not a threat to the patient's respiration once the machine is helping the patient to breathe, but high doses of pentobarbital could depress the patient's cardiovascular system.

Total control of ventilation is sometimes required in respiratory emergencies. This is desirable, for example, when mucous plugs are to be removed with the aid of bronchoscopy or when mucolytic chemicals are instilled by way of an endotracheal tube. In such situations the anesthesiologist, who is part of the RICU team of skilled physicians, nurses, and technicians, may administer *halothane* (Chap. 52) to anesthetize the patient lightly. Neuromuscular blocking drugs such as *succinylcholine* (Chap. 19) may also be employed to paralyze the respiratory muscles while the apparatus takes over the task of breathing for the patient.

Additional clinical considerations

The chronic obstructive pulmonary diseases are progressive and eventually debilitating. The patient who has COPD has several requirements: frequent and careful medical evaluation; a great deal of teaching to help the patient learn to adjust his life style to the limitations of the disease and to perform the many procedures that can be beneficial to his condition; and support and encouragement to deal with his diagnosis, therapy, and prognosis. The nursing care of these patients is very challenging and complex.

The sympathomimetic drugs used to treat COPD have been discussed in Chapter 17. The corticosteroids, which are used in severe cases of COPD and asthma, were discussed in Chapter 21. This discussion will concentrate on the overall nursing care of patients with COPD and asthma, and on the additional aspects involved when xanthine derivatives are used.

Prevention is the goal of therapy for asthmatics and COPD patients. Patients need to know what precipitates acute attacks, and should be encouraged to avoid such factors—for example, allergies, stressful events, crowded environments. Patients should also be encouraged to stop smoking and to avoid areas with high concentrations of smoke or other irritants. Drugs used for prophylaxis should be taken regularly, before an acute attack occurs. The patient and a significant other should be aware of the actions of the drugs and their proper use and administration.

As discussed earlier, the proper administration of inhalants is very important. Each inhaler comes with specific instructions for its use, and patients should be advised to consult the package insert before using a different inhaler. Each one is slightly different, and care should be taken not to administer the wrong dose inadvertently.

Patients and their significant others should know what actions should be taken if an acute attack occurs,

such as epinephrine injections or theophylline retention enemas. Patients should also be advised to wear or carry a medical alert tag. It is important for medical personnel who may take care of a patient with COPD in an emergency situation to be aware of the condition and any drug therapy that the patient might be on.

The adverse effects of the xanthine derivatives are the basis for their being contraindicated in several medical conditions. Cardiac disease, severe hypertension, congestive heart failure, and peptic ulcer can all be exacerbated by the use of xanthine derivatives. Pregnancy is another contraindication, because birth defects have been associated with the use of these drugs. Theophylline readily crosses into the breast milk, and can cause toxic reactions in nursing infants. If a lactating mother requires theophylline to control her pulmonary disease, she should nurse the baby just before taking a dose of theophylline, when blood levels are lowest; a different method of feeding the baby might well be considered.

Drug–drug interactions

Theophylline has been associated with numerous drug interactions. The effects of theophylline are decreased by *cigarette* and *marihuana smoking*, and by *phenobarbital*, all of which induce the hepatic metabolism of the drug. Patients who take phenobarbital or smoke will require greatly increased doses of theophylline to achieve a therapeutic level of the drug, and these patients should be taught about such interactions. They should be told to consult with their nurse or physician if any change in their smoking habits or phenobarbital use should occur. The serum levels of theophylline are increased by *cimetidine, erythromycin, influenza virus vaccine, troleandomycin,* and *furosemide*. Patients taking theophylline concurrently with any of these will require a decreased dosage of theophylline to avoid toxicity. Theophylline decreases the effects of *phenytoin*; seizure activity may result. Theophylline increases *lithium* excretion, decreasing its effectiveness. Theophylline and *β-adrenergic blocking agents* may be antagonistic; if a patient is receiving these drugs concurrently, the effects should be carefully evaluated. *Caffeine*, which is also a xanthine, adds to the adverse effects of theophylline; therefore, caffeine and products containing caffeine should be avoided by patients on theophylline. Many *over-the-counter* (OTC) preparations contain drugs that can increase the adverse effects of theophylline and cause toxic reactions. Because patients may be inclined to self-medicate with such cough, cold, or allergy preparations, it is very important to caution patients to avoid using OTC drugs while on theophylline.

The patient teaching guide summarizes the points that should be included in teaching a patient receiving an oral xanthine derivative. The guide to the nursing process summarizes the clinical aspects that should be incorporated into the nursing care of a patient receiving xanthine derivative therapy.

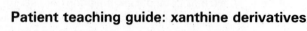

Patient teaching guide: xanthine derivatives

The drug that has been prescribed for you belongs to a class of drugs that are called bronchodilators. They work by relaxing the airways, helping to make breathing easier and to decrease wheezes and shortness of breath. To be effective, the drug must be taken exactly as prescribed.

Instructions:

1. The name of your drug is ———————————————— .

2. The dosage of the drug that has been prescribed for you is ———— .

3. Your drug should be taken ———— times a day. The drug has to be taken around the clock to be effective at all times of the day. The best times to take your drug are ————————————— .

4. The drug should be taken on an empty stomach with a full glass of water. If gastrointestinal upset occurs, the drug can be taken with food. Do not chew the enteric-coated or timed-release capsules or tablets—they have to be swallowed whole to be effective.

5. Some side-effects of the drug that you should be aware of include the following:

GI upset: nausea, vomiting, heartburn	Taking the drug with food often helps this problem.
Restlessness, "nervousness," difficulty in sleeping	The body often adjusts to these effects over time; avoiding other stimulants, such as caffeine, may help.
Headache	This often goes away over time; if it persists, consult with your physician or nurse for appropriate therapy.

6. Keep this and all medications out of the reach of children.

7. Tell any nurse, physician, or dentist who is taking care of you that you are on this drug.

8. Many foods can change the way that your drug works; if you decide to change your diet, consult with your nurse or physician.

9. Some side-effects of the drug can be decreased by avoiding foods that contain caffeine or other xanthine derivatives—for example, coffee, cola, tea, or chocolate—or by using them in moderate amounts. This is especially important if you experience such effects as nervousness, restlessness, or sleeplessness.

10. Cigarette smoking affects the way that your body uses this drug. If you change your smoking habits, such as increasing or decreasing the number

(continued)

of cigarettes you smoke each day, consult with your nurse or physician regarding the possible need to adjust your drug dosage.

11. It is very important to have regular medical care while you are on this drug to evaluate the state of your lung disease as well as your response to the drug therapy.

Notify your nurse or physician if any of the following occur:

Vomiting
Severe abdominal pain
Pounding, fast, or irregular
    heartbeat
Confusion, unusual tiredness
Muscle twitching
Skin rash, hives

Guide to the nursing process: xanthine derivatives

Assessment	Nursing diagnoses	Interventions	Evaluation
Past history (*contraindications*): Peptic ulcer Gastritis Renal dysfunction Hepatic dysfunction Coronary disease Pregnancy Lactation Allergies: these drugs; others; reactions Medication history (*cautions*): Cigarette smoking Phenobarbital Cimetidine Erythromycin Troleandomycin Flu virus vaccine Furosemide Sympathomimetic drugs Oral anticoagulants Digitalis Phenytoin Lithium β-adrenergic blockers Caffeine	Potential alteration in comfort: pain, secondary to GI effects Potential alteration in cardiac output, secondary to cardiac effects Knowledge deficit regarding drug therapy Potential sensory-perceptual alteration secondary to stimulatory effects Potential ineffective rest-activity pattern	Safe and appropriate administration of drug Provision of comfort and safety measures: • Drug with meals • Rest periods • Quiet environment • Dietary control of caffeine • Headache therapy, if necessary Patient teaching regarding: • Disease • Drug • Dosage • Cautions • Warnings Support and encouragement to cope with disease and drug therapy Provision of supportive measures if toxicity should develop	Monitor effectiveness of drug therapy: relief of respiratory difficulties Monitor for adverse effects of drug: • GI upset • CNS effects • Cardiac arrhythmias • Rectal irritation (if suppositories) Evaluate effectiveness of patient teaching program Evaluate effectiveness of support and encouragement offered Monitor for possible drug–drug interactions (several possible) Evaluate effectiveness of supportive measure, if needed

(continued)

Assessment	Nursing diagnoses	Interventions	Evaluation

Physical assessment

Neurologic: orientation,
    affect, reflexes,
    coordination
Cardiovascular: P, BP,
    baseline ECG,
    peripheral perfusion
Respiratory: rate,
    adventitious sounds,
    reserve
    GI: bowel sounds,
    liver function
    abdominal exam
Skin: lesions, color

Case study

Presentation

RL has a medical diagnosis of chronic bronchitis. He has been stabilized on theophylline for the past 3 years. He has been labelled as noncompliant to medical treatment because he continues to smoke cigarettes, two packs per day (2 PPD), knowing that he has a chronic and progressive pulmonary disease. He was referred to the nursing staff for patient teaching. His attending physician stated that he felt that the patient was the type who could benefit from some intense, personal attention, and RL subsequently received an in-depth, personalized teaching program. After several teaching sessions, it was felt that RL finally had an understanding of his problem and the treatment. RL agreed that he would try to stop smoking, or at least cut down to ½ to 1 PPD.

Three days after the last teaching session, RL presented in the emergency department with complaints of dizziness, nausea, vomiting, confusion, and "grouchiness." Physical exam findings included a pulse of 96 with occasional to frequent PVCs.

What probably happened to RL, and what nursing interventions should be taken at this point?

Discussion

RL felt bad enough to come into the emergency room, so the primary nursing intervention would be to make him comfortable and to alleviate his anxiety. Because of his chronic pulmonary disease and the current cardiac abnormalities, RL should be closely monitored and frequently evaluated for potentially serious complications. Blood gas levels should be determined, as well as serum theophylline levels. Because RL was seen only 3 days earlier with no apparent problem reported, his current state would seem to be the result of an acute process. RL's presenting signs and symptoms are classic signs of theophylline toxicity. Once RL has been stabilized, a careful history should be taken to determine what factors could have precipitated toxicity. In RL's case, the serum theophylline levels were elevated considerably. He stated that he had not changed his theophylline dosage or his diet in any way. He did admit that he had cut down his smoking from 2 PPD to ½ PPD for the past 3 days. He stated that he had not been feeling well for 2 days, but that he thought it was related to his need for cigarettes. He was determined, however, to follow through on his decision to cut down or stop smoking. Unfortunately, cigarette smoking stimulates the liver enzymes that inactivate theophylline. Patients who smoke cigarettes and are stabilized on theophylline require higher than usual doses of theophylline to achieve a therapeutic effect. If the patient reduces the level of cigarette smoking, theophylline levels quickly rise and the patient, like RL, develops the signs and symptoms of theophylline toxicity.

RL now presents a real nursing challenge. His efforts to comply with the medical regimen have finally been successful—he cut down his smoking—but the results have been unpleasant. RL will need a great deal of encouragement, support, and patient teaching. He will need to understand the delicate balance involved in his drug therapy, and should have the signs and symptoms of toxicity written down for him for easy reference.

This case can also be used as a good educational program for the staff. It is often difficult to remember all the intricate variables that can influence a patient's response to drug therapy. Every opportunity to review these aspects of drug therapy can be beneficial, not only for the patient involved, but also for other patients who may receive this drug in the future.

Drug digests

Aminophylline USP (theophylline ethylenediamine)

Actions and indications. This solubilized form of theophylline is the xanthine derivative most commonly employed clinically. The most important of its several pharmacologic effects is its ability to relax bronchial muscle spasm. This bronchospasmolytic effect is employed in the management of both chronic and acute asthma. Administered alone or in combination with ephedrine and a barbiturate, aminophylline often has a prophylactic effect that reduces nighttime attacks in children and others.

In patients with status asthmaticus unresponsive to treatment with epinephrine and other adrenergic bronchodilators, the slow intravenous administration of aminophylline sometimes affords almost immediate relief of dyspnea. This drug is sometimes administered in the same manner to patients with left ventricular failure and acute pulmonary edema. Here, the drug's cardiac stimulating effect may increase cardiac output, and the resulting decrease in pulmonary pressure relieves lung congestion and dyspnea.

Adverse effects, cautions, and contraindications. The most common side-effects are the result of gastrointestinal irritation that may cause epigastric distress, nausea, and vomiting. Intestinal bleeding and reactivation of healed peptic ulcer may occur. Overdosage may also be marked by signs of central stimulation, including restlessness, irritability, and insomnia. Children have sometimes suffered delirium, convulsions, persistent bloody vomiting ("coffee grounds" vomitus), and cardiovascular collapse following toxic doses of aminophylline. Too rapid intravenous administration may also lead to a severe drop in blood pressure and circulatory collapse.

Dosage and administration. Aminophylline is readily absorbed when administered orally, rectally, or parenterally. Oral dosage for adults in about 130 to 250 mg tid or qid. Rectal dosage for adults is about 300 mg up to tid, and for children 50 to 100 mg up to tid by suppository or retention enema.

For intravenous administration, doses of 250 mg to 500 mg are injected slowly over periods of 10 to 20 minutes. Although the drug may also be administered intramuscularly, local irritation may cause prolonged pain at the site of injection.

Potassium iodide USP

Actions and indications. This inorganic iodine salt is used mainly as a mucolytic expectorant that helps to cause a more productive cough in the management of chronic obstructive respiratory disorders, including bronchial asthma, bronchiectasis, and chronic bronchitis. It is thought to loosen retained sputum and to reduce the viscosity of these thickened secretions, which tend to form plugs within the bronchial tubes. It may do so by diluting the viscous sputum with aqueous respiratory tract fluid. The drug's irritating effect on the gastric mucosa is believed to set off a reflex that results in stimulating the flow of this natural lubricant. This effect is more likely to occur in patients who are kept well hydrated by drinking copious quantities of fluid.

Adverse effects, cautions, and contraindications. The irritating effect of moderate doses of this salty substance may cause epigastric distress, nausea, vomiting, and diarrhea. Prolonged intake of large doses may result in iodism, or chronic iodide poisoning. This may give the appearance of a heavy head cold, because it often begins with a sore throat and is followed by excessive secretion of the nasal and lacrimal glands and congestion of the chest. The rhinorrhea, pharyngitis, and laryngitis are sometimes preceded by stomatitis, in which the mouth soreness is accompanied by a brassy burning taste.

Sensitivity to iodides may be manifested by a painful swelling of the parotid glands that begins within a day or two of the start of treatment. Acneiform skin lesions may also appear after 4 to 7 days. Other eruptions, drug fever, and even anaphylactic reactions have also occurred in hypersensitive patients. Iodides may affect thyroid gland function and interfere with the interpretation of thyroid function tests. This drug is contraindicated in patients with tuberculosis.

Dosage and administration. Potassium iodide is administered orally in doses of 300 mg diluted in a liquid vehicle such as syrup, or in the form of a saturated solution containing 1 g/ml. This dose is usually ingested qid, but a total dose of up to 2 g may be administered if it is required and tolerated. Each dose should be administered with a glass of water or milk to reduce gastric irritation and to keep the patient well hydrated.

References

Bardana EJ: Modern aspects in diagnosis and treatment of the asthmatic patient. Clin Notes Resp Dis 15:3, 1976

Blancher GC: Caring for the patient with advanced emphysema. RN 37:41, 1974

Brogden RN et al: Sodium cromoglycate: A review of its mode of action, pharmacology, therapeutic efficacy and use. Drugs 7:164, 1974

Brogden RN et al: Beclomethasone diproprionate inhaler: A review of its pharmacology, therapeutic action, and adverse effects. I. Asthma. II. Allergic rhinitis and other conditions. Drugs 10:166, 1975

Clark TJ: Choice of drug treatment in asthma. Pharmacol Ther 17:221, 1982

Dolonich J, Hargreave FE: Strategies in the control of asthma. Med Clin North Am 65:1033, 1981

Flenley DC: New drugs in respiratory disorders. Br Med J 266:995, 1983

Greenberger PA: Theophylline. Ration Drug Ther 14:1, 1980

Harvey LI et al: Beclomethasone diproprionate aerosol in the treatment of steroid-dependent asthma. Chest 70:345, 1976

Hendeles L, Weinberger MW: A guide to oral theophylline therapy for the treatment of chronic asthma. Am J Dis Child 132:876, 1978

Hyde JS et al: Metaproterenol in children with chronic asthma. Clin Pharmacol Ther 20:207, 1976

Jacobs MY et al: Clinical experience with theophylline. JAMA 235:1983, 1976

Leifer KN, Wittig HJ: The beta 2 sympathomimetic aerosols in the treatment of asthma. Ann Allergy 35:69, 1975

Lieberman J: The appropriate use of mucolytic agents. Am J Med 49:1, 1970

Mazullo JM, Sundaresan PR: Treatment of chronic obstructive pulmonary disease. Ration Drug Ther 7:1, 1973

Nett L: Respiratory Care: A Guide for Patient Education. New York, Appleton–Century–Crofts, 1984

Pifafsky KM, Ogilvie RI: Dosage of theophylline in bronchial asthma. N Engl J Med 292:1218, 1975

Pontopiddian H et al: Acute respiratory failure in the adult. N Engl J Med 287:690; 743; 799, 1972

Richardson HB: Symptomatic treatment of adults with bronchial asthma. Med Clin North Am 58:135, 1974

Rodman MJ: Drugs used for chronic airway obstruction. RN 37:45, 1974

Rodman MJ: Drugs for acute respiratory failure. RN 38:49, 1975

Settipane GA et al: Adverse reactions to cromolyn. JAMA 241:811, 1979

Tager I, Speizer FE: Role of infection in chronic bronchitis. N Engl J Med 292:563, 1975

Webb–Johnson DC, Andrews JL: Bronchodilator therapy. N Engl J Med 297:476; 758, 1977

Weinberger M, Hendeles L: The pharmacological basis of bronchodilator therapy. Ration Drug Ther 11:1, 1977

Weissman G: The eicosanoids of asthma. N Engl J Med 308:454, 1983

Section 7

Drugs
used in
the management
of common
medical
conditions

Chapter 41

Drugs acting on the digestive system

Gastrointestinal (GI) disorders are among the most common of human ailments. The cause and cure of certain chronic GI conditions—ulcerative colitis, for example— still elude medical science. Fortunately, however, many types of drugs are now available to relieve the distress of acute and chronic GI disturbances as well as to retard the progress and reduce the complications of the chronic stomach and intestinal illnesses.

In this chapter, various types of agents employed to counteract common symptoms such as nausea, vomiting, painful spasms, burning sensations, bloating, belching, and diarrhea will be discussed. Special emphasis will be placed on the antacids and antispasmodics employed against the acid–peptic disorders, which are said to affect as many as 10% of the population of the United States. In addition, drugs used to treat motion sickness and other conditions, which are not actually GI ailments but manifest themselves, in part, in stomach upsets, will also be taken up here.

However, not all drugs that have desirable or adverse effects on the GI tract will be discussed in this chapter. The cholinergic drugs, which are among the most potent stimulants of gastrointestinal motility, are discussed in Chapter 15. Although the effects of opiates (Chap. 51) and anticholinergic agents (Chap. 16) on the GI tract will receive some mention here, their actions are discussed more fully elsewhere in this text, as are the actions of the corticosteroids (Chap. 21), which can both cause and relieve GI symptoms.

Acid–peptic disease

The gastric glands in the mucosal lining of the stomach contain parietal cells that secrete *hydrochloric acid* and chief cells that synthesize and store the proteolytic enzyme precursor *pepsinogen*, which is converted to *pepsin* in the pres-

ence of hydrochloric acid. Ordinarily, the mucous membrane that lines the stomach and the organs leading into and out of it—the esophagus and duodenum—resists irritation and digestion by the gastric acid–pepsin digestive juice. One of the main reasons for such resistance is that the surface of the fundus and body of the stomach contains cells that secrete large quantities of viscid mucus. This thick secretion coats and protects the stomach lining against irritation and digestion.

Sometimes, however, people do suffer discomfort and actual physical damage caused by the irritating and erosive action of their own gastric digestive juices on the mucosa of the esophagus, stomach and, most commonly, the first few inches of the duodenum. Among the minor ailments that result from excess gastric acidity is pyrosis or, as it is commonly called, "heartburn." The distress of this condition, often described as a "burning" or "warm" feeling in the epigastrium, is probably caused by acid stomach juices bubbling up (refluxing) into the lower esophagus to irritate its mucosal lining. If long continued, such acid irritation from gastroesophageal reflux may lead to the chronic inflammation of peptic esophagitis. In the related condition, gastritis, the inflammation of the stomach lining is not necessarily caused by acid. However, the sourness, bloating, and belching— symptoms sometimes called "indigestion" or "dyspepsia"—are often relieved by measures for neutralizing gastric acid.

Peptic ulcer

The most serious of the acid-related GI disorders is peptic ulcer, a condition in which localized areas of the stomach and duodenum become eroded by the corrosive action of acid gastric juices. Sometimes only the mucosal lining is eaten away, and the tissues may in time be repaired by the body's own healing processes. In some cases, however, the crater may deepen and extend down through the underlying layers of connective tissue and smooth muscle. This may cause some occult bleeding that can be detected only by special tests. On the other hand, if the erosive process finally breaks through a large blood vessel, massive hemorrhaging may occur, and perforation of the stomach or duodenal wall could lead to peritonitis. Either of these conditions can cause circulatory collapse and death.

Pathogenesis

Just why some people develop peptic ulcer while others do not is still not well understood. Research results suggest that some people may be genetically predisposed to develop peptic ulcers when they are exposed to certain environmental triggering factors. It has been found, for example, that people with high plasma levels of a substance called pepsinogen I pass this trait on to 50% of their children, and that such offspring are prone to develop duodenal ulcers. Their siblings—the 50% who did not inherit the genetic trait, do not suffer from this disease.

Hydrochloric acid and pepsin must always be present for an ulcer to form. However, this does not mean that ulcers occur only when these substances are secreted in excessive quantities. *Gastric ulcers* sometimes develop in people with normal amounts of acid secretion. *Duodenal ulcer* patients often do produce two to four times as much acid as is normal. However, hypersecretion even higher than that is sometimes seen in persons who have no sign of an ulcer.

Thus, it is now thought that ulcers develop as the result of an imbalance between the amount of acid that is being secreted and the various factors that are thought to be responsible for mucosal resistance to digestion by acid and pepsin. These include not only the production of protective mucus and the rapid neutralization of acid by alkaline secretions in the upper duodenum, but also other still largely unknown factors or substances that help to set up a protective barrier to the diffusion of acid secretions back through the underlying layer of epithelial cells. *Prostaglandin E* may, for example, be such a natural biochemical that plays a part in protecting the mucosa.

Hormonal and psychologic factors also have a role in determining whether or not ulcers develop. Emotional conflict, for example, is considered to be a cause of ulcer formation in some people with certain personality traits. However, the way in which psychological stress produces ulcers is not known. Similarly, the manner in which certain drugs and other substances lead to peptic ulcer production is still uncertain.

Alcohol, caffeine, and nicotine should be avoided by ulcer patients, because these substances stimulate increased secretion of gastric acid. However, most so-called ulcerogenic drugs do not increase acidity but seem, instead, to act by reducing mucosal resistance. Aspirin (Chap. 37) and nonsteroidal anti-inflammatory drugs (Chap. 38) seem to act, in part at least, by blocking a mucosa-protecting prostaglandin. Corticosteroid drugs may exert their ulcerogenic effects (Chap. 21) by interfering with the biosynthesis of various protective substances, including prostaglandins, that the mucosa requires for healing the mucosal lesions that are constantly being made by acid–pepsin digestive action while these erosions are still small.

Some people do suffer frequently recurrent ulcers that are the result of pathologic hypersecretory disorders. The *Zollinger–Ellison syndrome*, for example, is caused by pancreatic tumor cells that secrete large amounts of gastrin, a powerful stimulant of gastric acid secretion. This hormone, which is ordinarily released by stomach and duodenal cells in response to various types of stimuli, is—together with acetylcholine released by vagal nerves (Chaps. 13 and 15) and with mucosal histamine (Chap. 39)—a cause of both natural and excessive gastric acid secretion.

Medical management

The main objective of peptic ulcer therapy is to relieve peptic pain and bring about eventual healing by neutralizing gastric acid or by reducing the rate and volume of its secretion by the gastric glands. Neutralizing or reducing the amount of acid present both relieves the boring, burning, or gnawing sensation and, in time, allows natural healing of the ulcer to take place. The pain of the ulcer may be caused by the hydrochloric acid impinging on nerve fibers in the base and margin of the ulcer; this, in turn, produces reflex spasm of the surrounding smooth muscles. The ulcer itself is the result of the digestive action of the proteolytic enzyme pepsin on the gastric or duodenal mucosa. However, hydrochloric acid is required for this enzyme's catalytic action, which occurs most efficiently when the *p*H of the gastric contents falls between 1.0 and 2.0.

Several classes of drugs are commonly employed to relieve peptic pain and to hasten healing of the ulcer. These include the neutralizing antacids and two types of antisecretory agents: the anticholinergic, or parasympathetic blocking, drugs (Chap. 16), and a new class called H_2 receptor blockers that act by antagonizing histamine, a potent stimulant of gastric acid secretion. No drugs are yet available for specifically inhibiting gastrin, the strongest stimulant of stomach acid secretion. However, several drugs aimed at raising the resistance of the gastric and duodenal mucosa to acid–peptic action are under investigation or are already marketed abroad, and one (sucralfate), has recently been marketed in the United States.

Antacid therapy

Status. Antacids are an unglamorous group of inorganic chemicals that have been the mainstay of ulcer therapy because they can neutralize secreted stomach acid (Table 41-1). Because as many as 50% or more of ulcer

Table 41–1. Drugs used to treat peptic ulcer and other upper gastrointestinal tract problems*

Official or generic name	Trade name or synonym	Usual adult dosage and administration	Comments
Antacids			
Aluminum compounds			
Aluminum carbonate gel, basic	Basaljel	Two capsules or tablets; 10 ml of regular or 5 ml of extra strength suspension	Used to treat nephrolithiasis, and as antacid
Aluminum hydroxide gel USP	Amphojel	300–600 mg	See Drug digest
Aluminum phosphate gel	Phosphaljel	15–30 ml	Does not cause phosphate deficiency
Dihydroxyaluminum aminoacetate USP	Robalate	1–2 g	Available as tablets
Dihydroxyaluminum sodium carbonate USP	Rolaids Antacid	334–668 mg	Relatively rapid action; in part, systemically absorbable
Calcium compounds			
Calcium carbonate USP	Alka-2; Amitone; Tums	0.5–2 g	See Drug digest
Magnesium compounds			
Magnesium carbonate USP	—	500 mg–2 g	Liberates some carbon dioxide during slow neutralization of acid
Magnesium hydroxide USP	Milk of magnesia	Antacid: 600-mg tablet or 5–10 ml liquid; laxative: 1.8–3.6-g tablets or 15–30 ml liquid	See Drug digest for milk of magnesia
Magnesium oxide USP	Par-Mag; Uro-Mag	250–1500 mg	Same properties as the hydroxide
Magnesium trisilicate USP	—	1–14 g	Lowest in neutralizing capacity of the magnesium compounds
Mixtures of aluminum and magnesium compounds†			
Aluminum hydroxide and magnesium hydroxide tablets	Aludrox; Creamalin; Maalox	—	—
Aluminum hydroxide, magnesium hydroxide, and calcium carbonate	Camalox	—	—
Aluminum hydroxide and magnesium trisilicate	A-M-T; Neutracomp	—	—
Magaldrate USP	Riopan	400–960 mg	A complex hydroxymagnesium aluminate compound
Miscellaneous			
Sodium bicarbonate	Baking soda; Soda Mint	0.3–2 g	See Drug digest

Table 41–1. Drugs used to treat peptic ulcer and other upper gastrointestinal tract problems* (continued)

Official or generic name	Trade name or synonym	Usual adult dosage and administration	Comments
Histamine-2 (H₂) receptor blockers			
Cimetidine	Tagamet	300 mg PO qid with meals and at bedtime; may also be given IM and IV	Used to inhibit gastric acid secretion
Ranitidine	Zantac	150 mg PO bid	
Other drugs			
Metoclopramide	Reglan	10 mg PO qid, ½ hr before meals and at bedtime	Used to treat diabetic gastric stasis
		2 mg/kg body weight as dilute IV infusion administered slowly ½ hr before cisplatin administration, then q 2 hr for two doses, and q 3 hr for three doses	Used to prevent nausea and vomiting from cisplatin chemotherapy
Sucralfate	Carafate	1 gm PO qid, 1 hr before meals and at bedtime, for up to 8 wk	Used to promote healing of gastric and duodenal ulcers

* See Tables 16-1, 16-2, and 16-3 for anticholinergic parasympathetic blocking drugs also used sometimes in managing such conditions as peptic ulcer.
† Products similar to these mixtures, or with the addition of other substances such as calcium carbonate, magnesium carbonate and trisilicate, and simethicone, include Camalox, Di-Gel, Gelusil M, Mylanta I and II, Silain-Gel, and Win-Gel.

patients report relief of pain when they receive only a placebo, it has been difficult to prove statistically that antacids are superior to placebos in this respect. However, it seems clear enough from clinical experience that when they are properly employed in adequate doses, antacids *are* effective for relieving peptic pain. Studies in which the ulcer healing process was watched with repeated endoscopic visualizations also appear to prove that the administration of antacids in adequate daily doses for an average of 6 weeks brings about complete healing in a much higher proportion of patients than does placebo treatment.

Product selection. Antacid products can be purchased without a prescription and, as a result, the public is subjected to much advertising that can only be confusing and is often also misleading. Patients with peptic ulcer require a treatment regimen quite different from that of people who have only occasional transient episodes of stomach distress following overindulgence in food and alcoholic beverages. Thus, for example, a product containing an antacid ingredient for rapid relief in "settling a sour stomach" or "getting rid of gas pains" may be undesirable for a peptic ulcer patient who must take antacids in large daily doses for long periods.

In such patients, it is important to understand that no antacid is ideal in all respects, and that they all can cause adverse effects. The most serious toxicity is that which can occur when a patient with poor kidney function absorbs antacid ingredient ions into the systemic circulation and then fails to eliminate them. Thus, it is important for the nurse to know which antacids tend to be systemically absorbed, and what their effects may then be. In addition, because the most common reason for noncompliance is distress caused by the local actions of antacid in the bowel, it is important to know what effect each type of antacid is likely to have on the ulcer patient's bowel function. These and other considerations are taken up in the following discussions of individual antacids.

Individual antacids

Sodium bicarbonate. This commonly available household substance—*baking soda*—has high acid-neutralizing capacity. A teaspoonful or less is rapidly effective for alkalinizing the gastric contents. Thus, when used only occasionally for relief of a discomforting feeling of epigastric fullness or a burning sensation following over-indulgence in food or drink, it usually offers some symptomatic relief. However, this soluble, absorbable antacid has too short a duration of action, and it is very readily absorbed into the systemic circulation. These properties make its use in peptic ulcer therapy undesirable.

One reason for the short duration of effect of sodium bicarbonate[+] is that alkalinization of the gastric contents tends to decrease the time it takes for the stomach to empty its contents into the duodenum. This is undesirable because sodium bicarbonate, like other antacids, is effective only as long as it can come into contact with secreted acid. Thus, once this substance has been swept out of the stomach and past the first few inches of the duodenum, its usefulness comes to an end.

Not only is the neutralizing action of sodium bicarbonate short-lived, but it also seems often to be followed by an actual increase in acid secretion. This so-called *acid rebound* may be the result of an effort by the gastric glands to compensate for the actual alkalinity (*p*H higher than 7) produced by sodium bicarbonate. This and its short duration of antacid action make extremely frequent administration of huge amounts of bicarbonate necessary to keep ulcer pain under control. This, in turn, could overload the bloodstream with bicarbonate in amounts greater than the patient can eliminate, if kidney function is poor.

Systemic alkalosis. Ordinarily, the kidneys compensate for any rise in plasma alkalinity by increasing the rate of bicarbonate removal. If, however, kidney function is too impaired to get rid of the extra load of alkali, an insidious metabolic alkalosis may develop. This condition probably often goes unrecognized. The accumulation of excessive blood alkali may be accompanied by various vague signs and symptoms involving the GI, neuromuscular, and central nervous systems. The patient tends first to lose his taste for food, and this is often followed by nausea, vomiting, and an increase in stomach pain. There may be increased irritability and dizziness, headache, and muscular pain. Later, muscle twitching and cramps may occur; the patient may become increasingly weak and finally lapse into a fatal coma.

Electrolyte imbalances. People with poor kidney function may also suffer disturbances that stem from excessive retention of sodium and, in some circumstances, of calcium (an ingredient of other antacids; see below). Failure to eliminate absorbed sodium adequately can lead to edema and even precipitate congestive heart failure in cardiac patients who are close to decompensation. For this reason, people over 60 years of age (when renal func-

tion begins gradually to decline) should probably take no more than 2 tsp of sodium bicarbonate daily, and its use in younger persons should be limited to only twice that amount.*

Systemic electrolyte disturbance of another type is sometimes observed in ulcer patients taking large quantities of sodium or calcium carbonate and other alkalinizers combined with milk. This condition, called *Burnett's milk–alkali syndrome,* tends to occur most commonly in patients with kidney function impairment. The excess calcium precipitating out in the renal tissues may cause still further kidney damage, which leads, in turn, to alkalosis, potassium loss, and increased nitrogen retention in the blood and tissues.

Calcium carbonate. This inexpensive substance—*precipitated chalk*—was formerly widely used and recommended, because it exerts a potent, rapid, and (compared to sodium bicarbonate) relatively prolonged acid-neutralizing effect. Its only drawback appeared to be its tendency to cause constipation when employed alone over prolonged periods. However, this can be counteracted by combining it with a magnesium-containing antacid with mild laxative action.

It is now believed that calcium carbonate[+] may have two previously unrecognized drawbacks. First—as is true with *all* the antacids generally classed as "nonabsorbable" or "nonsystemic"—it is known that enough of the cation *can* be absorbed to produce adverse effects, particularly in patients with impaired renal function. In addition, the administration of this substance has been found to be followed by significant hypersecretion of acid 1 or 2 hours after intake of 1 tsp or less. This type of acid rebound seems to differ from that caused by sodium bicarbonate, because it appears to result from a direct stimulating effect of calcium ions on cells that secrete the potent acid-stimulating hormone gastrin.

A portion of the calcium carbonate reacts with stomach acid to form calcium chloride, a soluble salt that can be systematically absorbed in small amounts. This may lead to hypercalcemia in some patients and, particularly when they are also taking milk or cream, to the previously mentioned milk–alkali syndrome. Such systemically absorbed calcium can also precipitate out in the urine as kidney-damaging renal calculi. Thus, although the occasional use of a product containing this ingredient is harmless, its chronic use in peptic ulcer patients is potentially dangerous in some situations.

Magnesium-type antacids. *Magnesium hydroxide[+]* (milk of magnesia) is a prompt and potent neutralizer of gastric acid with a moderately prolonged action, provided that gastric emptying time is slowed by the presence of food in the stomach or by the motility-reducing action of other drugs. It does not seem to cause acid rebound or systemic alkalosis. Its main drawback is that the doses required for intensive therapy of acute ulcer cases often produce a laxative as well as an antacid effect. To coun-

* Other antacids in addition to sodium bicarbonate contain some sodium. This can be of clinical significance for patients who must maintain a low daily sodium intake. Information concerning the sodium content of many marketed antacid products is available from various sources.

teract this diarrhea-producing effect, magnesium hydroxide is frequently combined with calcium carbonate (above) or aluminum hydroxide (below), both of which tend to have a constipating effect when taken alone.

Magaldrate (Riopan) is a single chemical entity that has the same effects as the physical mixtures of magnesium and aluminum hydroxides. That is, it reacts with gastric acid to form salts of both elements, which then exert their buffering antacid effects without causing either constipation or diarrhea. This acid-consuming compound also contains relatively lower amounts of residual sodium than products made by mixing together two separate magnesium and aluminum preparations.

Magnesium trisilicate has relatively low acid-neutralizing capacity as compared to magnesium hydroxide or oxide and magaldrate. It has been claimed to exert a protective effect because it forms a jellylike mass of silicon dioxide that coats the ulcer crater. However, it is doubtful that this and substances of similar gelatinous consistency that are occasionally added to antacid mixtures, such as *sodium carboxymethylcellulose*, actually reduce local irritation or prevent acid from penetrating to the naked nerve endings in the eroded mucosal lining.

Magnesium antacid compounds have been classed as "nonabsorbable" or "nonsystemic," but enough of this ion is absorbed to produce systemic toxicity in patients with severely impaired kidney function. In such cases, the accumulation of magnesium in the central nervous system can cause coma and respiratory depression. Thus, lethargy and drowsiness in such patients should be noted and reported, because these may be early signs of hypermagnesemia. Absorption of the trisilicate salt has occasionally led to kidney damage from silica stone formation in the renal tubules of patients taking large doses during long-term ulcer therapy.

Aluminum hydroxide gel. This antacid does not cause acid rebound or alkalosis. However, it does not have high acid-neutralizing capacity, and the large daily doses that are required cause constipation unless it is combined with milk of magnesia or given alternately with it. This form of aluminum tends to bind dietary phosphate in the bowel and then to remove it in the stool before it can be absorbed. This can lead to bone demineralization and osteomalacia (softening of bones) in people already in poor phosphate balance. Calcium tends to move from the bones to the bloodstream, and this, along with absorbed unbound dietary calcium, raises blood and urine levels of that element. Such hypercalcemia and hypercalciuria increase the risk of stone formation in renal tissues.

Aluminum hydroxide[+] has been used deliberately to bind dietary phosphate and thus to prevent hyperphosphatemia and phosphate stone formation in patients with poor kidney function. However, analytical chemistry techniques have revealed that such patients can absorb significant amounts of aluminum administered in this form

or as aluminum carbonate, phosphate, or aminoacetate. The accumulation of aluminum in the central nervous system has caused neurotoxicity and an encephalopathic syndrome marked by dementia and by other neurologic signs and symptoms.

Other aluminum-containing antacids. *Aluminum phosphate gel* can be used without concern that dietary phosphate will be lost. However, it is a relatively ineffective neutralizer of gastric acid, and its use in patients with renal insufficiency could lead to hyperphosphatemia and urinary phosphate stone formation. *Dihydroxyaluminum aminoacetate* is claimed to be as effective as aluminum hydroxide and less constipating than the latter. *Dihydroxyaluminum sodium carbonate* is converted to aluminum hydroxide and gives off carbon dioxide when it reacts with gastric acid. This bicarbonatelike reaction offers rapid but brief acid neutralization, while the buffering effect of the newly formed hydroxide lasts for a somewhat longer time.

In summary, antacids vary in their acid-neutralizing potency and in their potential for producing adverse local and systemic effects. Low potency need not be a drawback if the antacid is administered in doses that are adequate for counteracting the individual patient's acid production. Adverse effects on bowel function such as constipation and diarrhea can be minimized by combining two or more drugs with antagonistic effects on intestinal motility—such as mixtures of magnesium and aluminum hydroxides, the basis for some of the most popular products for treating peptic ulcer. Single agents such as sodium bicarbonate or calcium carbonate are safe and effective for occasional use for minor acid–peptic symptoms, but their tendency to cause alkalosis in some patients following their systemic absorption makes them an unwise choice for long-term therapy of more serious chronic acid–peptic disease cases.

Other locally acting agents. Various substances that do not themselves neutralize gastric acid are sometimes added to antacid combination products. The rationale for doing so seems reasonable enough but, in practice, none of these added ingredients has been proved to add advantageous properties to the antacid mixture. The status of some of these substances will be briefly discussed here, before we conclude with a discussion of points that the physician, nurse, and patient should consider during the administration of anatacid combination products for treating peptic ulcer.

Simethicone is a silicone with an antifoaming action that is supposed to help relieve symptoms that stem from air or "gas" trapped in the upper GI tract when it is added to suspensions of aluminum and magnesium hydroxides to free trapped gas from the stomach. However, as indicated below, there is no evidence that this action actually relieves upper abdominal distress caused by stomach acidity and gas. *Alginic acid* is a substance that reacts with sodium bicarbonate to form a foam when tablets are chewed that contain both these substances in combination with antacids. The foaming mixture is then claimed to coat and protect the mucosa of the lower esophagus against acid reflux from the stomach. Such products have not been proved to be more effective for relief of gastroesophageal reflux symptoms than antacids alone (see Heartburn and Peptic Esophagitis, below). *Oxethazaine* is a topical anesthetic that has been added to suspensions of aluminum and magnesium hydroxides to help reduce the reflex spasm of gastrointestinal smooth muscle that is set off by gastric acid impinging on sensory nerve endings; however, its usefulness for this purpose has not been proved.

Additional clinical considerations

Antacid dosage and frequency of administration depend, in part, on the severity of the patient's pain and the seriousness of the condition. Patients hospitalized with an acute peptic ulcer require relatively large doses administered often enough to keep all of the gastric acid that is being produced completely neutralized. Patients with less severe pain and with less likelihood of developing such complications as hemorrhage and perforation can be maintained at lower antacid dosages. Administration is then timed mainly in relation to meals and other periods during which acid secretion is heightened.

Intensive care of patients with active ulcers is carried out with several classes of drugs in addition to antacids, including the antisecretory drugs discussed below. During the first week or two after an acute attack, moderate doses of antacids may be administered a dozen or more times daily. (The mixtures of magnesium and aluminum salts are most commonly employed.) The patient with an acute bleeding ulcer may require almost continuous medication. Sometimes an antacid suspension is dripped steadily into the stomach through an intragastric tube. During the acute phase, the patient may require frequent feedings and 24-hour antacid therapy. The patient will also require a great deal of emotional support and encouragement to cope with the pain, as well as with the lack of rest caused by the constant interruptions. Formerly, patients were often managed with the "Sippy diet" alternating milk and cream and antacids around the clock. Evidence now indicates that this regimen, because of the milk products used, may well have increased gastric acid secretion, interfered with ulcer healing, and caused such side-effects as the milk–alkali syndrome mentioned above.

The patient's responses to therapy must be observed and recorded to detect early signs of local or systemic side-effects. For example, the frequency of bowel movements and the appearance of the stools is noted to check for signs of magnesium-induced diarrhea or for constipation from the excessive effects of aluminum antacids or of calcium carbonate. Patients with a history of cardiovascular–renal disease should have daily fluid intake and urine output recorded to ensure that fluid is not being retained and that there is an adequate output of dilute urine. This helps to prevent the formation of calcium or phosphate kidney stones.

Ulcer patients with renal insufficiency are also watched for systemic signs of accumulation of magnesium, aluminum, calcium, or sodium ions. These include lethargy, fatigue, muscle weakness, bone pain and weight gain, as well as more serious central effects ranging from stupor to coma or dementia. The nurse also checks on what other medications the patient may be taking. This is not because other drugs interfere with the effects of antacids, but because these alkaline buffers often tend to affect the absorption of other medications.

Drug–drug interactions. As indicated in Chapters 4 and 8, a patient who must take *tetracycline-type antibiotics* orally for an infection may fail to improve when simultaneously receiving frequent doses of antacids. This occurs because the presence of calcium, magnesium, and aluminum ions in these products tends to bind these antibiotics into complexes that cannot readily be absorbed. The absorption of *oral iron salts* for treating anemia may also be impaired by simultaneous antacid therapy, and this may also be true of *warfarin, digoxin, isoniazid, phenytoin, corticosteroids, quinidine,* and other weakly acidic drugs such as *sulfonamides* and several other agents that are used in treating urinary tract infections, which are less readily absorbed when the GI contents are alkalinized. In general, because antacids change gastric *p*H and thus can influence the absorption of all oral drugs, it is best not to give other oral drugs within 1 or 2 hours of antacid administration.

Self-care. After the condition improves and less frequent medication, observation, and emotional support are required, the patient can be taught to take over much of his own treatment, as he will have to do at home during the period of several more weeks that it will take for the ulcer to heal. To help the convalescent assume this responsibility, a bedside supply of antacid tablets or suspension should be furnished, and the patient told how to take them. If antacid tablets are to be used, the patient should be advised to chew them thoroughly before swallowing or to suck them slowly. (Of course, this should not be done with other medications such as some anticholinergic drugs that have a bitter taste and mouth-drying effect.) If one of the more effective liquid suspensions is employed, the patient should be instructed to shake the bottle each time before pouring the dose, and to wash it down the esophagus and into the stomach with a little water. If the disposable cups are not calibrated, a clearly marked measuring cup should be furnished to ensure ease in pouring an accurate dose, even when the patient's eyesight is poor.

As part of the preparation for leaving the hospital, the duodenal ulcer patient should be shown how to arrange the antacid medication schedule around his own particular pattern of hypersecretion. Most patients with duodenal ulcers secrete gastric acid in greatest amounts about 1½ hours after meals and during the night. Thus, they should take adequate doses of antacids at these times of highest vulnerability—usually 1 hour after each meal and at bedtime. Some patients need an additional dose 3 hours after meals and whenever they are awakened by pain during the night.

The nurse should stress the importance of taking each daily dose at the proper time, and of maintaining the proper schedule for the 4 to 8 weeks of home treatment. The patient should be cautioned about using over-the-counter (OTC) preparations or relying on fad diets; indeed, new ulcer treatments are being tested, but these will require a prescription when they become available, and so the physician should be consulted instead of switching to some OTC product. There are several environmental factors that are known to increase gastric acid levels—for example, nicotine, caffeine, large meals, stressful situations—and the patient should be encouraged to avoid these factors to help decrease gastric acid levels further. The patient teaching guide summarizes factors that should be incorporated into the teaching program for patients receiving antacids.

Patient teaching guide: antacids

The drug that has been prescribed for you belongs to a class of drugs called antacids. These drugs work in the stomach to buffer or counteract the stomach acid. In addition to certain foods, many other factors increase stomach acid, such as nicotine (cigarette smoking), caffeine, and anxiety. You will help your situation if you can cut down or eliminate these other factors. The antacids are most effective if taken exactly as directed.

Instructions:

1. The drug that has been ordered for you is _____ .

2. The dosage that has been prescribed is _____ .

3. Your drug should be taken _____ times a day. The best times to take your drug are _____ , _____ , _____ . (As your ulcer heals, it may only be required 1 to 3 hours after meals and at bedtime.)

4. If *tablets* have been ordered, chew them thoroughly and then follow with a full glass of water.
   Suspensions should also be followed with a full glass of water.

5. Some side-effects of the drug that you should be aware of include the following:

Diarrhea	If this becomes too uncomfortable, consult with your nurse or physician.
Constipation	If this occurs, consult with your nurse or physician so that appropriate measures can be taken.

6. Antacids can interfere with the absorption of many oral drugs. It is best not to take any other oral drugs within 1 or 2 hours before or after your antacid.

7. Avoid the use of any other antacids while on this drug. If you feel that you need one of these preparations to supplement your prescribed drug, it is important to consult with your nurse or physician.

(continued)

8. Keep this and all medications out of the reach of children.

9. Take this medication exactly as prescribed for best results.

Notify your nurse or physician if any of the following occur:

> Swelling in ankles, fingers
> Decreased urination
> Difficulty breathing
> Lethargy, weakness, fatigue
> Flank pain

Gastric antisecretory agents

Anticholinergic drugs

Current status. Drugs of this class have been commonly employed together with antacids for treating peptic ulcer (see Chap. 16). However, their effectiveness has been a subject of controversy. That is, the cholinergic blocking agents have never actually been proved to be more helpful for healing ulcers than adequate antacid treatment alone. Their regular use has not been shown to prevent ulcers from recurring, nor has the development of bleeding, perforation, or other complications proved to be less likely to occur.

In theory, these drugs, which block the effects of the acetylcholine released by vagus nerve endings in gastric secretory cells, should reduce the amount of acid produced and thus lessen the digestive action of pepsin on the mucosa of the upper GI tract. In practice, ordinary doses of the natural belladonna alkaloids and the synthetic anticholinergic agents do not eliminate acid secretion. It is necessary to administer these drugs in doses that cause their numerous discomforting and sometimes dangerous side-effects to lessen the level of gastric acidity produced when food is eaten or to reduce the amount of gastric acid secreted during the night.

The effects of the anticholinergic drugs on GI smooth muscle are much more marked than their actions on secretory cells. For example, they may relax spasm of visceral muscles and thus relieve pain produced reflexly when gastric acid stimulates sensory nerve endings in the ulcer crater. These drugs also reduce GI motility, an effect that sometimes tends to prolong the effects of concurrently administered gastric antacid compounds. By prolonging the time required for the stomach to empty its contents, the vagus-blocking anticholinergic drugs allow the ingested alkalinizing and buffering agents to interact for a longer period with the acid that is secreted into the stomach. However, this same slowing of gastric emptying that permits the antacids to neutralize acids more efficiently may also be a source of danger for some patients. Those with partial pyloric obstruction caused by a stenosing ulcer may, for example, suffer complete blockage and gastric retention.

Dosage and administration. For full effectiveness, these drugs must be administered in the highest doses that the patient is willing and able to tolerate. This has to be determined for each patient by beginning with small doses that are then gradually raised at least to the point at which such minor side-effects as mouth dryness and slight blurring of near vision occur. Dosage titration with drops of belladonna tincture has been recommended, because drop dosage with this relatively inexpensive natural alkaloid preparation permits more accurate determination of the amounts needed to produce therapeutically desired effects with the fewest drug-induced discomforts. Later, if a synthetic anticholinergic agent is preferred, the patient may be switched to an equivalent dose of such a drug.

Anticholinergic drugs are best administered during the day about $\frac{1}{2}$ hour *before* meals. This allows the drug to be absorbed better and to reach its peak antisecretory effects by the time that ingested food is stimulating a high flow of gastric acid. As previously indicated, the reduction in GI motility that these drugs produce extends the duration of the desired neutralizing effects of the antacids that are administered an hour or so *after* meals. Thus, despite clear-cut evidence, it is possible that the combined effect of both drugs may be better for producing ulcer healing than antacids alone.

The ulcer patients most likely to benefit from anticholinergic drug therapy are those who have persistent pain during the night when the empty stomach secretes large amounts of acid that is not being buffered by food. In such cases, the patient may take a bedtime dose at least double that which has been taken before meals during the day. The patient does not suffer the expected adverse effects while asleep and, if the drug has a long enough duration of action, will not be wakened by acid-induced pain. On awakening in the morning, all but the most minor side-effects will have disappeared, because the drugs will have been largely eliminated by that time.

Synthetic anticholinergic drugs such as glycopyrrolate (Robinul) and isopropamide (Darbid) are claimed to have a more potent and prolonged action than the natural alkaloids. Their longer lasting effects may make these drugs more useful for reducing nocturnal

840

gastric secretion. These drugs have not been shown less likely to cause peripheral side-effects than atropine and the other natural alkaloids. However, those synthetic drugs that have a quaternary ammonium group in their chemical structure do not cause the adverse central effects of atropine and other tertiary amines, because their molecules do not pass through the blood–brain barrier (Chap. 4). Thus, they may be preferred for elderly patients and others who tend to become confused and disoriented or even suffer a psychosis from atropine overdosage.

In summary, the anticholinergic-type antisecretory–antispasmodic drugs have to be administered in high doses to produce effects that are of any benefit to peptic ulcer patients. Their lack of selective action on gastric acid-secreting cells and on GI smooth muscles leads to numerous adverse side-effects. These drugs are most useful as adjuncts to intensive antacid therapy of patients hospitalized with active severe ulcers. They are also of some use in ulcer patients who suffer continuous nocturnal pain from chronic recurring ulcers. The drugs are least useful for prolonged daytime use, because patients too often fail to comply with instructions for taking their medication in the full doses that tend to cause discomfort. The limited role of anticholinergic drugs in peptic ulcer therapy may become reduced still further because of the introduction of a new class of antisecretory agents. Chapter 16 presents the patient teaching guide as well as the guide to the nursing process for patients receiving these drugs.

Histamine$_2$ (H$_2$) receptor antagonists

Cimetidine (Tagamet) was the first of a new class of antisecretory drugs to be introduced in this country; *ranitidine* (Zantac) was the second (Table 41-1). Drugs of this type act by blocking the action of histamine at receptors in the acid-secreting parietal cells of the gastric mucosal glands. The conventional histamine antagonists used in allergy treatment (Chap. 39) are ineffective for inhibiting gastric acid secretion. It is thought that this is because the histamine receptors at this site are different from those in vascular, bronchial and other smooth muscle cells (H$_1$ receptors). Thus, these gastric cell receptor sites (and others in atrial and uterine muscles that are not blocked by the standard antihistamines) are called H$_2$ receptors.

The role of histamine in the physiologic regulation of gastric acid secretion is still uncertain. However, histamine has long been known to exert a powerful secretory effect on gastric cells when administered as a diagnostic agent (Chap. 56). Its gastric secretory action is somehow related to both that of the acetylcholine released by vagus nerve stimulation (Chaps. 13 and 15) and that of the hormone gastrin, which acts in several phases of gastric acid secretion, including that which occurs when ingested food enters the stomach.

Effects. These competitive inhibitors of histamine at H$_2$ receptor sites have proved to be remarkably effective for reducing basal gastric acid secretion and that induced by various gastric secretory stimulants, including food and chemicals such as caffeine and the diagnostic agents betazole and pentagastrin (Chap. 56). A single 300-mg dose of cimetidine can, for example, reduce basal acid secretion by more than 90% for over 4 hours in patients with duodenal ulcer. The same dose administered at bedtime suppresses nocturnal secretion to an equal extent overnight. Taken with meals, cimetidine reduces meal-stimulated acid secretion by about two-thirds during peak secretion times. (This compares with a reduction of only 25% by maximally tolerated doses of the standard synthetic anticholinergic drug propantheline.) Ranitidine appears to be equally effective. It is more potent than cimetidine (thus, doses are lower) and may cause fewer adverse effects (see below).

Clinical efficacy. Cimetidine has proved to be remarkably effective for relief of peptic pain and for production of *duodenal* ulcer healing. Patients report prompt relief of daytime and nocturnal pain to an extent greater than that obtainable with rest and placebos alone. Between 70% and 90% of patients have been proved ulcer-free after short-term (4 to 8 weeks) treatment when studied endoscopically. This is a rate of healing much higher than has ever been attained with rest and antacid therapy alone. Healing of *gastric* ulcers has also been high, and the drug has been approved for short-term treatment of benign gastric ulcers.

Among other patients who have responded favorably are those with the Zollinger–Ellison syndrome, a condition caused by gastrin-secreting pancreatic tumors and resulting high gastric acid secretion. Ranitidine as well as cimetidine is approved for this use. In this and other pathologic hypersecretory conditions such as mastocytosis and multiple endocrine adenomas, most patients receiving relatively large oral or intravenous doses of cimetidine had complete symptomatic relief or showed marked improvement. In some studies of patients with these disorders that once required total gastrectomy, all ulcers were healed with no signs of relapse or recurrences during many months of continued treatment. Both cimetidine and ranitidine have been used preoperatively to prevent aspiration of gastric acid, and both have been used to treat reflux esophagitis.

Adverse effects. Unlike the case with the anticholinergic-type antisecretory agents, these H$_2$ receptor antagonists cause only relatively minor and transient side-effects when administered in recommended doses. These complaints—mild diarrhea, dizziness, rash, and muscle pains—have occurred in only about 1% of patients treated with cimetidine. A few patients have developed mild gynecomastia or neutropenia. Some patients with the Zollinger–Ellison syndrome who have been treated with high doses have become impotent, but normal sexual function was restored when the drug was discontinued. No evidence of drug-induced bone marrow depression has been found. Confusional states have occurred in the elderly, especially in those with organic brain syndrome or impaired hepatic or renal function.

Cimetidine has been reported to induce changes in cardiovascular function in some circumstances. When administered in high IV bolus doses for control of GI bleeding, the drug has caused episodes of bradycardia and hypotension. Thus, to avoid a sudden precipitous drop in blood pressure, it seems safest to dilute the contents of a 2-ml vial with 100 ml of a compatible IV diluent solution and to infuse it slowly over a period of 15 to 20 minutes.*

Although there is less experience with ranitidine, it appears to cause fewer adverse effects. Headache, malaise, and nausea occur infrequently. Mild leukopenia and thrombocytopenia have also been reported, but were not clinically significant and did not lead to discontinuation of ranitidine therapy. Of potentially greater concern are reports of elevated serum enzyme levels, which suggest that ranitidine may cause hepatotoxicity.

Drug–drug interactions. Cimetidine reduces the hepatic metabolism of many drugs, including *oral anticoagulants, phenytoin, β-adrenergic receptor blockers, lidocaine,* and *theophylline.* The half-life of *benzodiazepines* (*e.g.,* diazepam, chlordiazepoxide; Chap. 45) is also prolonged, and the toxicity of *carbamazepine,* an antiepileptic drug (Chap. 50) is increased. The dosage of these drugs should be reduced when given concomitantly with cimetidine. *Cigarette smoking* is said to interfere with the inhibition of nocturnal gastric acid secretion by cimetidine. So far, ranitidine appears to be less involved in these drug–drug interactions. This is as expected, because ranitidine does not significantly interact with the hepatic microsomal drug-metabolizing enzyme system.

Dosage and administration. The recommended adult dose of cimetidine is 300 mg to be taken orally four times daily, once with each meal and at bedtime. Patients with the Zollinger–Ellison syndrome may require double the ordinary dose—that is, 2400 mg daily, administered orally or by vein. This drug can be taken at the same time that food is being eaten, because its antisecretory effect—although slowed in onset—is not interfered with, and patients are most likely to remember to take their medication when it is ordered for use at mealtimes. Although cimetidine itself raises gastric *p*H, patients should also continue to take antacids to help lessen gastric acidity.

Ranitidine is effective in lower dosage: 150 mg, or even 100 mg, twice a day, orally. In Zollinger–Ellison syndrome, more frequent doses may be needed.

Both these drugs should be given with caution and in reduced dosage to patients with decreased renal function.

In summary, published reports concerning this new type of antisecretory agent are uniformly favorabe in terms of both its efficacy for producing pain relief and ulcer healing and its lack of significant adverse effects. These drugs have revolutionized the therapy of duodenal ulcers. Cimetidine, the older drug, has become the largest selling prescription drug in the United States and has set worldwide drug sales records. An earlier, equally effective drug of this class, called metiamide, was never marketed in this country because it was occasionally found to cause agranulocytosis. Gastroenterologists hope that the two drugs currently marketed will not be found to cause bone marrow depression or to have other serious, chronic toxic effects.

Other ulcer medications

Sucralfate. Sucralfate (Carafate; Table 41-1) is a complex of aluminum hydroxide and sulfated sucrose. It was used for many years in Japan before being introduced in the United States. Its mechanism of action in promoting the healing of duodenal and gastric ulcers is not fully understood, but it appears to combine with proteins at the ulcer site to form a coating that resists the digestive action of both hydrochloric acid and pepsin. Because it acts locally and is only slightly absorbed into the systemic circulation, it is quite free of systemic adverse effects. Constipation is the most frequent complaint. The drug should be taken on an empty stomach. Antacids may be used by patients on sucralfate, but it is recommended that they be taken at least $\frac{1}{2}$ hour before or after sucralfate. Sucralfate can interfere with the absorption of oral tetracyclines.

Sedatives. Various other drugs are used either routinely or experimentally in the management of peptic ulcers. Some act by reducing acid secretion, and others by increasing mucosal protective factors. The most widely employed adjunctive drugs—sedatives and antianxiety agents—have never been proved to have either of these actions. However, sedatives such as *phenobarbital* and antianxiety agents such as *chlordiazepoxide* (Librium) may help to promote rest, which should be part of every regimen for healing ulcers and preventing their recurrence.

These drugs do nothing to alter the underlying disease process or to change the personalities of patients whose emotional responses to stress may play a part in precipitating an ulcer attack. However, to the extent that tension tends to set off increased gastric acid secretion and smooth muscle spasm in some patients, these anxiety-reducing drugs may be of some help. The pain of ulcers may also be somewhat less upsetting to patients who are more relaxed emotionally when taking these drugs.

Carbenoxolone. This antiulcer drug, a derivative of licorice, has been widely used abroad but is still on trial in this country. It is thought to act locally in the stomach to increase the factors that play a part in protecting the gastric mucosa against digestion by acid and

---

* Cimetidine injection remains stable at normal room temperature for 48 hours after dilution with sodium chloride injection (0.9%), dextrose injection (5% or 10%), lactated Ringer's solution (5%), or sodium bicarbonate injection.

pepsin. One way it seems to do so is by stimulating the biosynthesis of glycoproteins by mucosal cells. The treated cells themselves are said to have a 50% increase in their life span. The increased production of gastric mucin may be the main reason for this drug's proven ability to promote the healing of *gastric* ulcers. Its ability to prevent recurrences of stomach ulcers or to promote healing of duodenal ulcers has not yet been demonstrated.

A drawback of carbenoxolone (Biogastrone) is its tendency to cause fluid retention and potassium loss in some patients, particularly those with impaired kidney function and the elderly. These patients must be monitored carefully to avoid development of hypokalemia, hypertension, and congestive heart failure. Adverse effects of these types are thought to be caused by this drug's potentiating effect on the renal tubular action of the mineralocorticoid hormone aldosterone (Chap. 21). If they occur, they may be counteracted by administering the diuretic spironolactone (Chap. 27). However, that aldosterone antagonist cannot be employed routinely to prevent fluid–electrolyte imbalance, because it interferes with the therapeutic effect of carbenoxolone. A thiazide diuretic may be used to counteract any tendency toward sodium and water retention, but serum potassium levels must continue to be closely monitored, because this diuretic can cause a further loss of potassium when administered together with carbenoxolone.

Prostaglandins. Several natural prostaglandins and some synthetic analogues have been tested for treating peptic ulcers. Their use is based on the theory that a reduction in prostaglandins normally present in gastric mucosa may be a cause of ulcer formation. Several orally administered synthetic prostaglandin analogues, including the dimethyl derivative of prostaglandin E_2 (DMPG), have proved to be able to suppress basal and histamine-stimulated gastric acid secretion. Others are believed to exert a protective effect on the GI mucosa that helps to relieve epigastric pain and speeds the healing of peptic ulcer. A drug-induced deficiency of natural prostaglandins brought about by aspirin and by the nonsteroidal anti-inflammatory drugs, which act by inhibiting prostaglandin synthesis, is believed to be responsible for the ulcer-producing effects of many drugs used for treating arthritis (Chaps. 37 and 38).

Heartburn and peptic esophagitis

Most people who occasionally suffer the symptom they call "heartburn" or "sour stomach" are readily relieved by taking a dose of an antacid product, which rapidly neutralizes the gastric acid that has been regurgitated into the lower esophagus from the stomach. Occasionally, however, patients with hiatus hernia or some other mechanical defect that interferes with normal motility of the upper GI tract may suffer from the chronic reflux of acid–peptic gastric contents into the esophagus. This can lead to peptic esophagitis, an inflammatory disorder of the esophageal mucosa, which may cause it to erode or swell and results in narrowing of the lower esophagus.

One cause of this and other esophageal disorders may be the malfunctioning of a specialized band of smooth muscle located close to where the esophagus joins the upper, or cardiac, opening of the stomach. Weakness of this so-called lower esophageal sphincter (LES) and a reduction in the pressure it exerts to prevent gastric acid regurgitation may be responsible for many cases of chronic pyrosis and peptic esophagitis, spasm, and strictures. Thus, drug treatment has been aimed at increasing LES pressure when the condition is not controlled by antacids, cimetidine, diet, and various mechanical measures that help to reduce gastroesophageal reflux.*

One way of raising sphincter pressure in patients with reflux esophagitis is by subcutaneous administration of *bethanechol* (Urecholine), the cholinergic smooth muscle stimulant discussed in Chapter 15. Administered subcutaneously in small doses, this drug has proved to be effective for abolishing gastric acid reflux in most patients with peptic esophagitis in whom it has been employed experimentally in clinical trials. A drawback of bethanechol, however, is its tendency to increase the flow of gastric acid secretions.

Metoclopramide (Reglan; Table 41-1), a drug recently approved for use in diabetic gastric stasis (delayed gastric emptying), which exerts a potent stimulating effect on upper GI tract smooth muscle without simultaneously increasing gastric acid secretion, is also reported to be effective for symptomatic relief of reflux esophagitis. Administered orally or parenterally a few minutes before each meal and at bedtime, this drug increases the tone of the lower esophageal sphincter and speeds the emptying of the stomach into the duodenum. This drug, which has also been employed in Europe for relief of nausea and vomiting associated with gastritis, has sometimes proved to be helpful for relief of heartburn in pregnant women, and it is being used to prevent nausea and vomiting in cancer chemotherapy with cisplatin and other agents. It is also used to facilitate small bowel intubation and to stimulate the GI passage of barium during radiologic studies. It is being investigated as a drug to improve lactation; in doses of 30 to 45 mg/day, it increases milk secretion, perhaps by increasing serum prolactin levels. Like the phenothiazines and other dopamine receptor blockers (Chap. 46), it produces sedation and sometimes extrapyramidal signs and symptoms (*e.g.*, restlessness, parkinsonism).

Additional clinical considerations

As discussed in the section on antacids, many complex factors are involved in the care of the peptic ulcer patient.

---

* Actually, antacid therapy is thought to help tighten the LES indirectly when it acts to neutralize free gastric acid.

These patients need to avoid environmental factors that increase gastric acid secretion. They will also need support and encouragement to cope with the diagnosis and drug therapy and any life style changes that they may be asked to make. Dietary therapy for these conditions is no longer considered to be therapeutically effective, and patients are usually advised simply to avoid foods that cause them discomfort. The H_2 receptor blockers are especially helpful in allowing these patients to self-select their diet.

The safety of these drugs for pregnant or nursing women has not been established. As with many drugs, these preparations should only be used during pregnancy and lactation if the benefit for the mother outweighs the potential risk to the fetus.

The patient teaching guide summarizes points to incorporate into the teaching program of a patient receiving an H_2 antagonist. The guide to the nursing process summarizes the clinical considerations that should be incorporated into the nursing care of a patient on these drugs.

Patient teaching guide: histamine-2 antagonists

The drug that has been prescribed for you is called a histamine-2 antagonist. This drug works to decrease the amount of acid produced in the stomach. It is used to treat conditions that are aggravated by excess acid. Your drug has been prescribed to treat _____ .

Instructions:

1. The name of your drug is _____ .

2. The dosage of the drug prescribed is _____ .

3. You should take your drug _____ times a day. Cimetidine should be taken with meals and at bedtime. Ranitidine does not need to be taken with meals.

4. Some side-effects of the drug that you should be aware of include the following:

Diarrhea	This usually becomes less severe with time.
Dizziness, headache	These usually go away as your body adjusts to the drug; if they become severe, consult with your nurse or physician.

5. Keep this and all medications out of the reach of children.

6. Tell any nurse, physician, or dentist who is taking care of you that you are on this drug.

7. If your physician has ordered an antacid, take it exactly as directed. Otherwise, avoid the use of over-the-counter medications while you are on this drug. Many of these preparations contain drugs that could interfere with this drug's effectiveness.

8. If you are on other drugs along with cimetidine, do not vary your drug schedules. If something should happen to change the other drugs that you are taking, consult with your nurse or physician.

(continued)

9. It is important to have regular medical follow-up while you are on this drug to evaluate your response to the drug.

Notify your nurse or physician if any of the following occur:

Sore throat, fever
Unusual bruising or bleeding
Confusion
Muscle or joint pain

Guide to the nursing process: histamine-2 antagonists

Assessment	Nursing diagnoses	Interventions	Evaluation
Past history (*contraindications*): Pregnancy Lactation Renal failure Hepatic failure Allergies: reactions Medication history (*cautions for cimetidine*): Anticoagulants Phenytoin β-adrenergic blockers Lidocaine Theophylline Benzodiazepines Morphine Carbamazepine Digoxin **Physical assessment** Neurologic: orientation, affect Cardiovascular: pulse, baseline ECG GI: liver, abdominal exam, normal output Skin: lesions Blood tests: CBC, liver and renal function	Potential alteration in comfort: headache Potential alteration in bowel elimination: diarrhea Knowledge deficit regarding drug therapy Potential sensory-perceptual alteration: dizziness	Safe and effective drug administration Provision of comfort and safety measures: • Headache relief • Safety if dizziness occurs Patient teaching regarding: • Disease • Drug • Cautions • Warnings Support and encouragement to cope with disease, drug, and other therapies	Evaluate effectiveness of drug therapy: • Pain relief • Ulcer healing Monitor for adverse effects of drug: • GI problems • Dizziness • Headache • Change in renal function • Change in liver function Evaluate effectiveness of patient teaching program Evaluate effectiveness of support and encouragement offered Monitor for drug–drug interactions (documented with cimetidine): ↓ effectiveness of oral anticoagulants; phenytoin; β-adrenergic blockers; lidocaine; theophylline; benzodiazepines; carbamazepine; digoxin ↑ CNS effects with morphine

Case study

Presentation

WT, a 48-year-old traveling salesman, had experienced increasing epigastric discomfort over a 7-month period. When he finally sought medical care, it was determined that WT had a duodenal ulcer. For relieving his discomfort initially, WT was started on Riopan. He was also started on cimetidine, 300 mg qid. WT was then referred to the nurse for patient teaching, with an appointment for medical follow-up in 3 weeks.

What are the appropriate nursing interventions for WT at this time?

Discussion

WT's complete physical exam was unremarkable except for his duodenal ulcer. Because he is otherwise a healthy man, WT may have difficulty coping with his diagnosis and the changes it may bring to his life style. WT will need a great deal of patient education regarding his disease, including possible causative factors and measures that he can take to decrease his discomfort and further problems with the ulcer: small, frequent meals; decreasing his cigarette smoking; cutting down on stimulants of acid secretion such as caffeine products and alcohol; learning to cope effectively with stress and anxiety-producing situations. WT should also be assigned consistently to one nurse who can offer him support and encouragement and help him to develop a trusting relationship with the health-care system. WT will need to learn, over time, what his limits are and what foods and activities precipitate problems; this often requires a joint nurse–patient effort. Bland diets and other restrictions have been found not only to be of little therapeutic benefit but also to add stress. Allowing the patient control over his activities, with guidance, has been found to be the most useful approach to ulcer therapy. WT should also receive thorough instructions regarding his drug therapy. Of particular concern will be spacing of his two drugs. The antacid and cimetidine doses should be spaced 1 to 2 hours apart. A schedule could be developed to help WT to remember when each of the drugs should be taken. When the pain has been relieved, WT may no longer require the antacid therapy. He should be cautioned about self-medicating with other antacids while he is on this drug. Any increase in discomfort should be reported to his nurse or physician. The possibility of dizziness developing as a side-effect to the cimetidine therapy should be discussed with WT. If he drives as a traveling salesman, this could be a serious problem. Usually, this side-effect will pass with time. WT should also be encouraged to have regular follow-up visits to evaluate his medical condition, his response to drug therapy, and the effectiveness of the patient teaching program and the support being offered.

Summary of adverse local and systemic effects of antacids

Gastrointestinal side-effects

Diarrhea: as a result of laxative effect of magnesium-type antacids

Constipation: as a result of calcium and aluminum antacid compounds

Acid rebound: hypersecretion of gastric acid in response to excessive alkalinization of stomach contents

Flatulence: eructations from release of carbon dioxide from sodium bicarbonate and calcium carbonate

Nausea and vomiting: from astringent action of aluminum compounds

Systemic toxicity

Metabolic alkalosis: from systemic alkalinizers such as sodium bicarbonate or calcium carbonate

Electrolyte imbalance: edema from retention of sodium in sodium bicarbonate and in other antacids

Renal calculi formation: calcium in antacids may precipitate out of urine in kidneys

Bone demineralization: binding of dietary phosphate by aluminum hydroxide may cause phosphate deficiency leading to osteomalacia, or softening of the bones

Hypermagnesemia: patients with impaired renal function may accumulate magnesium ions in the central nervous system, leading to lethargy, drowsiness and deeper degrees of CNS depression, including coma

Hyperaluminemia: patients with impaired kidney function can accumulate aluminum in the CNS, leading to an encephalopathic syndrome marked by dementia and neurologic signs and symptoms

Drug digests

Aluminum hydroxide gel USP (Amphojel)

Actions and indications. This nonabsorbable antacid reacts slowly with hydrochloric acid to form aluminum chloride and other compounds including aluminum phosphate, which is then eliminated in the feces. The neutralizing action of the dried gel is relatively low compared to that of the liquid suspension. This chemical also has adsorbent, astringent, and demulcent properties, but their value in ulcer treatment is uncertain. In addition to its use alone or combined with magnesium compounds for relief of peptic pain, aluminum hydroxide is also sometimes used in the management of patients who tend to form phosphate-type kidney stones (nephrolithiasis).

Adverse effects, cautions, and contraindications. This compound does not cause metabolic alkalosis, and its potential for systemic toxicity is relatively low. However, high daily doses taken for long periods by a person eating a phosphate-poor diet might mobilize phosphate from the bones and result in osteomalacia, a softening or bending of the bones.

GI side-effects—possibly from its astringent action—include occasional nausea and vomiting and frequent constipation. Administration with magnesium hydroxide tends to counteract constipation.

Dosage and administration. Dose of the solid gel is 300 to 600 mg several times daily before meals in tablets that are chewed before being swallowed. Dose of the liquid suspension ranges from 5 ml to 40 ml, depending on the concentration. The latter dose, diluted with water, may be administered by intragastric drip in severe cases. It should not be taken at the same time as tetracycline-type antibiotics or anticholinergic drugs, because its adsorbent action interferes with their absorption.

Calcium carbonate USP

Actions and indications. This is the least expensive antacid and one that has high neutralizing activity, which is relatively rapid and prolonged. It is best administered in combination with magnesium compounds or alternated with them. Relatively frequent administration of high doses is required for full effects in reducing peptic activity in ulcer patients.

Adverse effects, cautions, and contraindications. Local GI side-effects include constipation most commonly, flatulence and belching sometimes, and nausea rarely. Constipation is counteracted by administration of magnesium hydroxide, as is the occasional formation of fecal concretions.

Systemic absorption of some calcium occurs. However, hypercalcemia is not significant, except possibly in patients with kidney dysfunction. It is contraindicated in such patients because metabolic alkalosis is possible, particularly when large amounts of milk or cream are also being taken. It is also contraindicated in patients with a history of kidney stones, because it can cause hypercalciuria and calcium calculi.

Dosage and administration. The usual oral dose is 0.5 to 2 g taken with water several times daily before meals. However, amounts as high as 2 to 4 g every hour may be needed in severe cases to keep gastric acidity below the level at which the enzyme pepsin stays active.

Milk of magnesia USP (magnesia magma)

Actions and indications. This aqueous suspension of magnesium hydroxide is employed both as an antacid and as a saline laxative. As an antacid, it reacts rapidly with gastric acid to neutralize large amounts. A residue remains for a time to combine with acid that continues to be secreted by the stomach. It is most commonly administered clinically in combination with aluminum hydroxide and calcium carbonate for treatment of hyperacidity in acid–peptic disorders, including peptic ulcer.

Adverse effects, cautions, and contraindications. The doses required for continuous acid neutralization are high enough to cause catharsis. Thus, diarrhea occurs commonly, unless administered together with astringent or constipating aluminum hydroxide and calcium carbonate, or given alternately with them.

The small amount of magnesium absorbed does not cause significant metabolic alkalosis or systemic toxicity. However, its use is contraindicated in patients with severe renal impairment, because systemic accumulation of magnesium may cause CNS depression marked by drowsiness, stupor, coma, and possible respiratory paralysis or circulatory collapse.

Dosage and administration. Milk of magnesia is given in doses of as little as 5 ml or as much as 30 ml four or more times daily, depending on the degree of severity of the acid–peptic disorder being treated. Doses between 15 ml and 30 ml are likely to have cathartic effects.

Sodium bicarbonate USP (baking soda)

Actions and indications. This soluble, absorbable alkalizer is widely used for the rapid relief of hyperacidity symptoms. It is an ingredient of the once widely used Sippy powders, but it is not now often prescribed for peptic ulcer treatment because of its too brief action, systemic absorption, and possible adverse effects.

Adverse effects, cautions, and contraindications. The release of carbon dioxide in the immediate reaction with hydrochloric acid causes belching and stomach distention. This may be dangerous for patients with a peptic ulcer that is close to the point of perforation. This compound, when taken in excess, is systemically absorbed and then excreted by the kidneys. It is contraindicated in patients with renal insufficiency because of possible development of metabolic alkalosis and of edema.

Dosage and administration. Oral doses of 0.3 g to 2 g are taken for relief of gastric hyperacidity at frequent intervals.

Drugs that affect intestinal motility

Aspects of digestive system physiology

The several layers of smooth muscle that comprise the alimentary tract contract mainly in response to local reflexes mediated by nerve plexuses located in the intestinal walls. These intrinsically innervated movements are modified by extrinsic impulses from both divisions of the autonomic nervous system (Chap. 13) and, to some extent, by locally released hormones. The nature of these contractions by the circular and longitudinal muscle fibers varies, as do the functions of the resulting movements.

Of the several types of complex muscular contractions that churn, mix, and move the stomach and intestinal contents along, the most important is *peristalsis,* a series of coordinated contractions and relaxations. In the small intestine, these wavelike movements go on at a slow steady rate that allows time for food to be digested and assimilated and for fluids to be absorbed. In the large intestine, peristaltic activity takes place only periodically at an irregular rate.

During periods of inactivity, fluid absorption continues, so that the liquid chyme is gradually converted to a semisolid mass by the time it reaches the transverse colon. Occasionally, strong peristaltic contractions shift this mass ahead for a considerable distance along the descending colon. Finally, one of these movements forces the fecal matter into the rectum, distending it and setting off the reflexes that lead to the desire to defecate. However, the defecation reflex can be inhibited because the skeletal muscle fibers of the outer anal sphincter are under voluntary control.

Ordinarily, people in good health who follow a regular routine are for the most part unaware of all these activities in the gut, and bowel movements occur at a rate normal for each person, whether it is several times a day or only once every two or more days. People vary widely in the time it takes for food to be digested and for its residues to leave the intestinal tract. Most of the nutrients and fluid from a meal are absorbed from the small intestine in a few hours. However, indigestible particles require at least a day and sometimes several to make their way to the rectum, from which they leave the body during the act of defecation.

Abnormal patterns of intestinal motility

Many physical and mental factors can interfere with the normal pattern of rhythmic movements. Dietary changes, nervous tension, infection, and drugs can all accelerate or slow down the rate of peristaltic activity. This then leads to such abnormalities in the frequency of defecation and in the nature of the stools as diarrhea and constipation.

Diarrhea results when the intestinal contents are rushed through the bowel too rapidly, so that the person is discomforted by many fluid movements daily. Constipation occurs when a person's intestinal sluggishness causes relatively few, infrequent, and incomplete movements.

Constipation

This common digestive tract disorder has many causes. Occasionally organic disorders are the cause of constipation, but much more common are mental and emotional states that lead to habitual behavior patterns deleterious to normal bowel movements. These include undesirable dietary habits, habitual inhibition of the defecation reflex until it loses normal sensitivity, and the misuse of laxative (cathartic) drugs.

Cathartics, or laxatives, are drugs used to bring about emptying of the bowel. A drug-induced increase in peristaltic activity is desirable in various clinical situations. For example, powerful parasympathomimetic or cholinergic drugs (Chap. 15) such as *bethanechol* and *neostigmine* are sometimes employed to induce evacuation of the bowels in postoperative and postpartum patients with intestinal atony and abdominal distention. Another drug approved for use in preventing postoperative paralytic ileus is *dexpanthenol* (dextro pantothenyl alcohol), which is given in a dose of 250 or 500 mg IM or IV immediately after surgery. Other surgical and medical patients also sometimes profit from administration of more gently acting cathartics for overcoming constipation. Actually, however, few patients with chronic constipation require more than brief treatment with laxatives and, when used at all, these drugs are only adjuncts to such more fundamental measures as proper diet and exercise.

The laxative habit

Many people believe, mistakenly, that they must have a bowel movement every day, and they suffer distress when they fail to do so. Often the type of person who becomes unduly upset when he fails to move his bowels tends to treat himself with cathartics in a way that leads to chronic constipation. This is what happens: First, the person takes a cathartic that stimulates peristalsis strongly enough to empty the entire intestinal tract. This prevents the colon from filling normally for several days. Because the desire to defecate arises only when the lower colon becomes packed with a fecal mass, the normal stimulus that sets off the defecation reflex is lacking, and so a day or two may pass without a bowel movement. This alarms the bowel movement-oriented person and often leads to taking a still stronger cathartic to overcome the drug-induced constipation.

Instead of restoring the "normal regularity," which is so prized by those who prepare TV commercials for these products, the continued use of cathartics soon makes it difficult for the laxative abuser ever to achieve a natural movement: he comes to depend on the drug's action rather than on the natural defecation reflex. Such dependence is both psychological and physical and, in one sense, does not differ a great deal from what takes place when people become addicted to drugs that act on the central nervous system.

What can the nurse do to help prevent such cathartic addiction? First, people with intestinal complaints should be advised to see a physician. Even though most constipation is caused by poor dietary and living habits, a sudden change in bowel function sometimes signals the presence of intestinal pathology. Once such organic lesions have been ruled out, the patient should be advised to follow a program aimed at correction of the causes of chronic constipation, thus re-establishing normal bowel movements.

Management of constipation

Among the most important treatment measures for constipation are education, behavioral therapy, and dietary changes. These are intended to replace the patient's faulty habits with others that foster the establishment of better bowel patterns. The nurse can play an important part in the instruction of patients as to what constitutes a proper diet and adequate fluid intake.

Diet. Researchers have intensified their study of the role of dietary fiber in maintaining health and preventing disease. Some suggest that diets too low in indigestible fiber residues may be responsible not only for constipation and such other intestinal disorders as diverticular disease and the irritable bowel syndrome (see Acute and Chronic Diarrhea, below), but also, indirectly, for the most common illness of Western civilization: coronary heart disease. Not all scientists accept these conclusions, some of which may have fostered a wave of fiber faddism. However, there is no doubt about the value of eating foods high in fiber as part of a program aimed at correcting constipation.

Some of the several types of fiber found in unrefined whole grain and in various fruits and vegetables have a high water-absorbing capacity. Coarse bran, for example, can take up to six times its weight of water as it passes through the intestinal tract, and even fine bran can hold two or three times its weight of fluid. This helps people on high-fiber diets to produce soft, bulky stools twice as heavy as the firm, hard scanty stools passed by people who eat only low-fiber refined foods.

A first step in the dietary management of constipation is having the patient take a daily handful of bran with raisins or cooked fruit to which flavoring, sweeteners, and a small amount of milk are added. During the first week of such added dietary fiber, the patient may complain of flatus. The daily dose of bran can then be increased to two handfuls, and this, plus such foods as carrots and beets, prunes and figs, and other peristaltic stimulants should become part of the permanent diet. The patient is advised to drink adequate quantities of water to ensure the sponging effect of the fiber as it sweeps through the gut.

Drug therapy. Patients whose constipation is

seen to stem from habituation to cathartics have to be withdrawn from these drugs. As in any other addiction, this is likely to lead to what has with some justice been termed a "withdrawal syndrome" because of the patient's complaints of discomfort. These are usually treated symptomatically, with aspirin for headaches and general malaise and perhaps, mild stimulants to overcome lethargy, weakness, and mental depression.

More important than antianxiety drugs is advice intended to counteract some common misconceptions about bowel movements that tend to cause anxiety. Patients must be assured, for example, that there is no "normal" number of daily bowel movements and that they are in no dire danger if they fail to defecate on any particular day. They should be taught not to suppress their awareness of the sensory stimuli that indicate fecal fullness in the rectum but that they should, instead, go to the toilet and make the appropriate voluntary movements that relax the anal sphincter and contract the muscles of the abdomen. Patients with chronic constipation may need to set aside a particular time each day, usually in the morning right after breakfast, to allow for uninterrupted toileting.

As indicated above, the patient with a laxative habit is also often put on a diet that includes foods that leave a bulky residue. These, taken together with plenty of fluids, help to build up the intestinal contents, so that normal defecation reflexes can be initiated. The attainment of this objective is sometimes aided by the judicious use of one type of nonirritating laxative. Bulk-producing substances, such as psyllium seeds, methylcellulose and similar, hydrophilic (literally, "water-loving") colloids, sometimes help to form a bulkier stool (Table 41-2). Taken daily with plenty of water, they act much as do the natural fibers in fruits, whole grain, and vegetable foods such as carrots, beets, and cabbage. These colloid laxatives are gradually discontinued after a few weeks, when the patient's bowels have begun to function normally. If the patient succeeds in learning to live under less emotional tension and in establishing proper dietary and toilet time habits and patterns, there should be no further need for cathartics.

Of course, it is not always wise or easy to try to change a patient's habits. Thus, if an elderly patient has been taking a daily mild laxative or stool softener in which he has great faith, the nurse should not be overzealous in urging him to give up his medication. The psychological effect of the drug may be as important as its physical effects.

Similarly, other patients may regularly use a mild bulk-producing laxative or stool softener with no obvious ill effects. Even in cases of obvious cathartic abuse, it is best to proceed slowly and gently. The patient who senses the sympathetic support of the nurse and physician may then more willingly follow their advice for rehabilitating his misused bowel.

Table 41–2. Classes of laxative or cathartic drugs

Official or generic name	Trade name or synonym	Usual adult dose
Drugs that stimulate peristalsis on contact with the colon		
Bisacodyl USP	Dulcolax	10–15 mg
Cascara sagrada aromatic fluidextract USP	—	5 ml
Cascara sagrada extract USP	—	325–650 mg
Cascara sagrada fluidextract	—	1 ml
Castor oil USP	—	15–30 ml
Danthron USP	Dorbane	37.5–150 mg
Phenolphthalein USP	Ex-Lax; Feen-a-Mint Gum	30–195 mg
Senna, senna syrup, senna concentrate	Senokot	Depends on preparation; consult manufacturer's recommendations
Sennosides A and B USP; calcium salts of sennosides A and B	Glysennid; Nytilax	12–24 mg
Drugs that stimulate peristalsis by increasing physical bulk		
Saline or osmotic cathartics		
Lactulose	Chronulac	10–20 g (15–30 ml of syrup)
Magnesium citrate solution USP	Citrate of Magnesia	240 ml
Magnesium sulfate USP	Epsom salt	15 g
Milk of magnesia USP	Magnesia magma	1.8–3.6-g tablets or 15–30 ml liquid
Sodium phosphate USP		4–8 g
Sodium phosphate and biphosphate	Phospho-Soda	20–40 ml
Hydrophilic colloids and indigestible fibers		
Methylcellulose USP	Cologel	5–20 ml
Psyllium hydrophilic mucilloid	Metamucil	1 tsp, rounded, in water (other preparations are given in different dosages)
Drugs that act by altering fecal consistency		
Emollient or lubricant cathartics		
Mineral oil USP	—	5–30 ml

Table 41–2. Classes of laxative or cathartic drugs (continued)

Official or generic name	Trade name or synonym	Usual adult dose
Fecal softeners (surface-active or wetting agents)		
Dioctyl calcium sulfosuccinate USP; docusate calcium	Surfak	240 mg
Dioctyl potassium sulfosuccinate; docusate potassium	Dialose; Kasof	100–300 mg
Dioctyl sodium sulfosuccinate USP; Docusate sodium; DSS	Colace; Doxinate	50–240 mg
Poloxamer 188	Alaxin	480 mg

Classes of laxatives, cathartics, and related medications

The routine ordering of bowel evacuation by harsh cathartics has declined as physicians recognized their un-
desirability and turned to more natural measures for
maintaining bowel function. However, some clinical situations do call for the use of drugs that induce defecation
or that, at least, alter the consistency of the stools. Before
discussing these clinical indications, which are summarized
at the end of this section along with the contraindications
for cathartics, the classification of these drugs will be
described (Table 41-2). Cathartic drugs act in several ways
to speed the passage of the intestinal contents through
the GI tract. Some substances act chemically to stimulate
intestinal smooth muscles to contract more forcefully and
frequently. Other agents cause an increase in intestinal
bulk, which acts as a mechanical stimulus to the motor
activity of the gut. The effects of other laxatives are exerted less on the GI tract itself than on its fecal contents.
That is, they soften hardened masses and ease their passage through the lower portion of the large intestine.
The choice of drug for each of the various situations in
which a laxative appears to be indicated depends on where
in the intestine these drugs act, and on their speed and
degree of thoroughness.

Stimulant laxatives
Drugs of this class induce peristaltic activity when they
or their breakdown products contact the intestinal wall
directly. The exact mechanisms by which drugs of the
several subgroups exert their effects is still uncertain,
despite considerable study and speculation. It is not
known, for example, whether the intestinal actions of
these contact cathartics is the result of a generalized irritation of the mucosa or of a specific stimulating effect
on intrinsic nerve cells in the plexuses that mediate local

motor reflexes. Some scientists have, in fact, suggested
that these drugs act not by directly stimulating intestinal
motility but by interfering with reabsorption of fluid by
the epithelial cells of the small intestine's mucosal lining.
They may do so by damaging the villi responsible for
fluid and electrolyte absorption.

Anthraquinones. Cathartics of this class, including cascara, senna, and rhubarb, contain plant principles
that are converted to peristalsis-stimulating chemicals in
the large intestine. Danthron, a free anthraquinone, requires no conversion. These drugs travel through the
small intestine and by way of the bloodstream, after absorption, to reach the large intestine. Their action therefore requires 6 or 8 hours or more, because it takes that
long for the anthraquinone derivatives to build up in the
large bowel in sufficient amounts. Thus, they are best
given at bedtime in order to bring about a bowel movement in the morning.

Cascara[+] and *senna* are considered to be the most
dependable of these plant products for producing a single
soft or semiliquid stool when desired. However, the solid
and liquid oral forms of these drugs are not suitable when
the rapid emptying of the entire GI tract is desired. They
are used, instead, to aid evacuation of the lower bowel
in bedridden patients and in others for whom a slow,
steady action is considered more suitable than prompt
purgation.

The rectal insertion of a suppository containing
a senna concentrate produces a more prompt evacuation
of the lower bowel—within ½ to 2 hours. Thus, it may
be used shortly before bowel emptying is desired prior
to sigmoidoscopy and other diagnostic procedures, instead
of being administered in the afternoon or evening before
intestinal or urologic radiography, as is the case with
orally administered anthraquinones. Senna products are
said to cause more griping pain than cascara.

Phenolphthalein and its chemical relatives. This

synthetic substance exerts most of its stimulant action in the colon after being broken down to an irritant principle by bile salts and alkali in the upper small intestine. It is a common component of many proprietary laxative preparations, including some of the most popular chocolate and gum medications. These forms of phenolphthalein are often eaten by children in large amounts, but severe toxicity is rare and is limited mainly to a dehydrating diarrhea. However, hypersensitivity reactions are not uncommon. These often take the form of a characteristically colorful dermatitis. Sometimes the itchy, burning patches blister and become ulcerated; occasionally the involved patches of skin stay pink or purplish for many months and, long after the condition has cleared up, identical lesions may appear in the same places on subsequent exposure to the drug—a so-called fixed eruption.

Bisacodyl[+] (Dulcolax) is a chemically related compound with a similar action on the large intestine. It may be given by mouth at night to produce a morning bowel movement. The drug is also available in suppository form for faster action. Rectal administration brings the chemical in contact with the mucosa and stimulates contraction of the colon within a few minutes. It has been employed in this way in preparing the lower bowel for proctoscopy or for radiographic examination and in other situations in which enemas are ordinarily administered. (In general, it may be noted that enemas—which will not be taken up here because of the *non*pharmacologic nature of such substances as tap water or soapsuds—are effective for evacuating the lower bowel without causing colicky contractions of the small intestine or being absorbed systemically.)

Castor oil. This product, pressed from the beans or seeds of a common ornamental plant, is a bland non-irritating oil that is converted by an enzyme-catalyzed reaction in the upper intestine to a substance that is said to be responsible for stimulating peristaltic motility. This irritant, ricinoleic acid, sets in motion contractions of the small intestine before it is absorbed and metabolized in the manner of other fatty acids. The contractions continue down into the large bowel to produce a relatively prompt and complete catharsis as compared to the slower, more limited and less drastic laxative actions of other stimulants.

The occasional use of castor oil[+] is considered to be harmless and clinically useful in some situations. Thus, for example, castor oil is still used in certain hospital procedures, although much less often than it once was. Castor oil is still employed prior to x-ray examination of abdominal organs, for example, to empty the intestine and thus eliminate interfering shadows. It is usually given on an empty stomach in the late afternoon so as not to interfere with digestion or with sleep. It should never be taken at bedtime because its strong action, which occurs 1 or 2 hours after ingestion, will cause a restless night.

The habitual use of castor oil is certainly undesirable. It causes the type of complete evacuation of both the small and the large bowel that leads to a period during which there is no natural stimulus to defecation. Thus, its frequent use can, in the manner previously indicated, lead to production of chronic constipation.

Saline or osmotic cathartics

Among the most rapid-acting and powerful of cathartics are various salts that are given in solution in large amounts of water. They produce their effects by increasing the bulk of the intestinal contents, thus distending the colon and stimulating contractions by a mechanical rather than a chemical action. Because they often act in only an hour or two, salts such as *magnesium sulfate* (Epsom salt) are preferred for clearing the entire intestinal tract in cases of poisoning. In general, they are used whenever a complete purge is desired—in worm treatments, for example, or to obtain stool specimens. They are usually given in the morning or in midafternoon, never in the evening.

The salty taste of some of these drugs makes them unpalatable. Thus, Epsom salt should be given in cold fruit juices to mask the taste. Magnesium citrate is available in a lemon-flavored carbonated liquid that is pleasant-tasting but relatively expensive. Various salts are often presented as extemporaneously prepared effervescent liquids, which also have greater palatability but are more costly. Some of these salts (*e.g.*, sodium phosphate) are also given by enema—in the form of Phospho-Soda, for example.

The more concentrated solutions exert greater osmotic activity but also cause more nausea. Thus, the salts are given as well-diluted isotonic solutions when only their cathartic action is desired. Sometimes hypertonic solutions are employed to reduce edema by pulling fluid from the blood and into the gut by an osmotic action. Less concentrated solutions not only are adequate for catharsis but are actually preferred. Taken on an empty stomach, such solutions pass the pylorus more readily and enter the intestine, where the unabsorbed ions retain enough fluid to initiate peristaltic activity.

Ordinarily, so little of these salts makes its way through the semipermeable intestinal membrane that there is not much chance of systemic toxicity. Poisoning has occurred, however, when the patient's kidneys were functioning poorly and thus failed to clear absorbed magnesium ions from the circulation. Accumulation of magnesium may cause coma as a result of the central nervous system depressant effect of this ion. The sodium-containing cathartic salts are undesirable for treating edematous patients with cardiovascular disorders. A *non*saline osmotic substance, *lactulose*, has received approval for general laxative use, in addition to its previously approved indication for use in the management of portal–systemic encephalopathy.

Other bulk-producing laxatives

Another type of mechanically acting cathartic is quite different from the saline type in actions and uses. This group includes the hydrophilic colloids and other indigestible fibers, mentioned earlier as useful adjuncts in the treatment of chronic constipation. Natural substances such as psyllium seed extracts, or semisynthetic materials such as methylcellulose, produce their desired action by forming a bulky jellylike mass in the intestine. This resembles the food residues that normally stimulate peristalsis and defecation in its effects.

These bulk formers are the most natural and least irritating of laxatives. They should not, however, be taken habitually any more than the harsher cathartics that cause passage of more stools. Patients should be told never to take these products without water. This is important, not merely because their effectiveness depends in large part on their ability to absorb enough fluid to make a gelatinous mass. When swallowed dry, these fibers, seeds, and granules may pick up just enough moisture in the esophagus to swell and obstruct that food passageway. Thus, these materials are to be both mixed with water and followed by plenty of fluid.

Emollient or lubricating laxatives and other fecal softeners

It is often desirable to make defecation easier, not by stimulating peristalsis but by changing the consistency of the patient's stool. This is generally accomplished with liquid petrolatum or with surface-active agents.

Liquid petrolatum (mineral oil). This indigestible oil, which does not add to the patient's caloric intake, is much more widely used in oral form for lubricating and softening the stool. It is employed mainly for patients with hemorrhoids or other painful anal lesions and for others who must avoid straining at stool. By coating the fecal contents, mineral oil also tends to reduce fluid absorption from the feces and thus prevents their becoming excessively dry.

For people who dislike the feel of the plain oil on the tongue, flavored emulsions may be employed. However, such products are relatively expensive, and their use may favor systemic absorption of the oil. Thus, the nurse may suggest sucking an orange slice to cut the oily aftertaste of plain oil products. Liquid petrolatum is best taken at bedtime and not with meals, because it may interfere with the absorption of fat-soluble vitamins. Loss of vitamin K in this way could make a patient more sensitive than previously to treatment with anticoagulant drugs. (See Drug–Drug Interactions, Chap. 4, and Table 4-1.)

Occasional use of a mineral oil enema for relief of fecal impaction avoids some of the disadvantages of oral administration. Rectal use prevents possible interference with food digestion and with absorption of vitamins A, D, E, and K. It avoids the possible aspiration of the liquid into the lungs by children and elderly or debilitated patients with resulting lipid pneumonia, and systemic absorption does not occur (see above and below).

However, following hemorrhoidectomy, healing may be delayed by excessive use of mineral oil enemas, as well as by seepage of orally administered liquid petrolatum. (Leakage leading to soiling of clothes or bedding is an adverse esthetic effect of liquid petrolatum.)

Surface-active agents. Certain inert chemicals that act like detergents are also used to soften the stool. *Dioctyl sodium sulfosuccinate* (DSS)[+], the most widely used of these substances, is available for oral administration and in enema form. It is thought to act by reducing the surface tension of the fecal contents of the rectum, which permits water and fatty materials to penetrate and produce a more moist and bulky mass. This action occurs when wetting agent solutions are administered as retention enemas; however, there is some doubt that small oral doses have the desired effect, and there is evidence that suggests that this fecal softener acts by stimulating the secretion of sodium and water into the intestinal lumen while decreasing chloride absorption.

The surface-active agents, which in themselves seem safe enough, are sometimes offered in proprietary combinations with irritant cathartics, which are considered much less desirable for long-term use. Thus, for example, a combination of DSS with the anthraquinone laxative danthron is said to have led to liver damage on chronic administration. It may also be undesirable to administer mineral oil together with these wetting agents, because they may tend to facilitate passage of the inert oil through the intestinal mucosa. Once the liquid petrolatum, which is ordinarily unabsorbable, gets into the tissues, it cannot be eliminated and may act as a foreign body in the lymph nodes, liver, and spleen.

Indications for cathartics

Physicians order laxatives far less frequently than in the past. There are, however, some clinical situations in which it is considered desirable to induce defecation with drugs or to alter the consistency of the stool. Most of the few conditions in which the use of cathartics is considered valid have been mentioned during the discussion of the several classes of laxatives and cathartics. These and other acceptable clinical uses will be briefly summarized at this point.

Cardiovascular disease. Patients who have suffered an acute myocardial infarction or who are found to have an aneurysm may be endangered by strenuous efforts to evacuate hard or impacted fecal masses. Thus, laxatives containing mineral oil or other lubricating and emollient laxatives or a stool softener such as DSS are often ordered to avoid having the patient strain at stool, which raises blood pressure and tends to cause adverse reflex effects on cardiac function.

Anorectal lesions. Patients with *hemorrhoids* or other anorectal lesions should not strain to remove retained feces. Thus, measures for promoting a soft stool that can be passed without pain are desirable. These include the regular use of the lubricating type of laxatives and the wetting agents or stool softeners.

Diagnostic procedures and surgery. Cathartics are employed as adjuncts to various diagnostic or surgical procedures—before abdominal operations or the administration of general anesthesia prior to other surgery, for example. Sometimes the entire intestine is emptied before taking abdominal x-rays to prevent shadows cast by gas and feces from interfering with the visualization of visceral organs and structures. At other times only the colon need be cleared—for instance, for proctosigmoidoscopy. Cathartics are not, however, a substitute for the colonic irrigations that must be given before surgery on the colon itself.

Anthelmintics. The treatment of intestinal worm infestations with anthelmintics sometimes requires administration of a cathartic both before and after therapy (Chap. 11). Some anthelmintics act more effectively when the bowel has first been cleared; other medications for killing worms are potentially toxic to the patient if too much is absorbed. These are often swept out of the GI tract by a cathartic as soon as they have had time to do their work on the worms.

Chemical poisoning. In cases of poisoning by ingested chemicals, poisons that have passed the pylorus and can no longer be eliminated by gastric lavage are often flushed from the intestine by purgative drugs (Chap. 5). This tends both to reduce local tissue damage by corrosive chemicals and to limit the systemic absorption of other toxic agents. Laxatives are also sometimes given routinely with constipating drugs, such as ganglionic blockers.

Pre- and postpartum care. Mild laxatives may be briefly employed occasionally in late pregnancy without concern about setting off reflex contractions of the uterus. They may also be used, preferably in suppository form, in preparation for delivery. Here, however, they should not be administered within 1 or 2 hours of the expected onset of second-stage labor. Laxatives are sometimes employed judiciously as part of postpartum (and postoperative) care to bring about a return of normal bowel movement regularity.

Bed-ridden patients. People confined to bed often tend to become constipated. This is understandable, because lack of exercise, loss of appetite, and the effects of illness and of the drugs used to treat it—narcotic pain relievers such as codeine, morphine, and meperidine, for example—all act to reduce intestinal motility. For this reason, it was once a regular practice for the physician to order milk of magnesia, cascara, or some other cathartic for all hospitalized patients.

Such routine use of cathartics is, for reasons previously discussed, no longer considered desirable. The nurse is in the best position to recommend and implement a bowel training program that makes only minimal ad-

junctive use of the mildest laxatives for the briefest possible time.

Among the most important of the measures that help to avoid the need for cathartics is seeing that the patient is taken to the bathroom or is given the opportunity to use a bedside commode at a regular time each day. This is now often possible and permissible because of the current emphasis on early ambulation. Without the need to use the bedpan, the patient can assume a more normal and comfortable position and should be encouraged to do so. He should also be left alone, if possible, because lack of privacy often inhibits defecation.

Another desirable development is the fact that patients often not only are allowed to get out of bed but also are encouraged to begin eating a regular, varied diet, including fresh fruits and vegetables, shortly after surgery if their condition permits, instead of being kept on liquids for days as they once were. Of course, to avoid constipation, it is also important to keep the patient well hydrated by such measures as the use of intravenous fluids postoperatively when this seems desirable or necessary, and by encouraging oral fluid intake.

Contraindications to cathartics

Cathartics should never be used habitually as a routine measure for inducing a daily bowel movement. Such use not only leads to chronic constipation but may produce local and systemic disturbances. The habitual use of purgatives and stimulants of intestinal motility has been responsible for many cases of chronic colitis and other intestinal disorders that are the direct or indirect result of continued irritation of the intestinal mucosa. In addition, repeated purgation can result in dehydration and cause electrolyte imbalances similar to those that result from severe diarrhea caused by GI infections.

More serious than the effects of the long-term misuse of cathartics is the damage that can be done by giving even a single dose of a cathartic to a person with an acute abdomen. The drug-induced increase in GI motility in the presence of an acute surgical abdomen may lead to perforation of the inflamed intestinal wall. Such rupture of the appendix, for example, may then spew pathogenic bacteria into the abdominal cavity.

Before the advent of antibiotics and other modern anti-infective drugs, the death rate from peritonitis in patients who had taken cathartics for treating painful cramps was very high. Even today peritonitis is a serious condition. Thus, people should be warned never to medicate themselves with cathartics when they have abdominal pain and cramps or are nauseated and vomiting. These drugs are never given before adequate diagnosis has ruled out appendicitis, enteritis, ulcerative colitis, diverticulitis, or the presence of organic obstructions.

In summary, laxatives are more likely to cause chronic constipation than to cure it. Thus, although some of these drugs are still used in some such cases, even the bulk-producing laxatives are best employed only briefly as adjuncts to measures more likely to correct the cause. If the cause is found to be cathartic abuse, withdrawal of these drugs becomes the primary corrective measure. However, other than in the presence of an acute abdomen, there is little harm in the occasional use of a mild laxative or enema to evacuate the bowel for various valid clinical purposes, particularly in a hospital setting under medical or nursing supervision.

Additional clinical considerations

As indicated, the abuse of laxatives can cause serious problems for some patients. Educational programs regarding the effects of laxatives, as well as normal bowel function and healthy ways to maintain it, are needed to decrease the abuse of laxatives.

Nurses in the hospital setting should remember that many of the stressors of hospitalization can cause constipation—for example, anxiety, lack of privacy, dietary changes, or scheduling of activities. The hospitalized patient should be assessed for early signs of constipation, and a bowel training program should be started at the earliest opportunity. A patient admission history should include questions regarding laxative use. Chronic laxative users can develop problems readily when the stresses of hospitalization are combined with the sudden withdrawal from laxatives. If a laxative is used, the patient should be evaluated for response to the drug, and this should be noted in the medical record.

The fat-soluble vitamins—A, D, E, and K—may not be adequately absorbed if a patient is taking mineral oil. A patient on prolonged mineral oil therapy should be evaluated for any of these vitamin deficiencies.

Laxatives should be used cautiously in pregnancy; castor oil, mineral oil, and bisacodyl tannex should not be used at all during pregnancy. Danthron and cascara are passed into the breast milk, and these laxatives should be avoided by the lactating mother.

Allergic reactions have occurred with these drugs, including facial swelling, rash, and discomfort. Some preparations contain tartrazine and should be avoided by patients with tartrazine sensitivity.

These, like all medications, should be kept out of the reach of children. Chocolated and candy-coated laxatives can be very appealing and toxic to small children.

Summary of indications and contraindications: cathartics

Indications

Prevention of fecal impaction in bedridden patients

Reduction in straining at stool: in patients with cardiovascular complications, such as aneurysm, embolism, and myocardial infarction; in patients with hemorrhoids and other anorectal lesions

Emptying the GI tract prior to diagnostic procedures such as abdominal roentgenography and proctosigmoidoscopy

Removal of ingested poisons from lower GI tract

Adjunctive use in anthelmintic therapy

Adjunctive use in correction of constipation

Contraindications

Habitual use for forcing bowel movements in constipation

Acute appendicitis and other causes of abdominal pain and cramps, including regional enteritis, diverticulitis, and ulcerative colitis

Pregnancy, late in third trimester

Drug digests

Bisacodyl USP (Dulcolax)

Actions and indications. This substance produces peristaltic activity on contact with the mucosa of the colon. It may be administered orally to bring about effects within 6 hours or rectally for rapid action—in about 15 to 60 minutes. Because the drug acts by setting off local as well as segmental reflexes, it may produce satisfactory effects even in paraplegic and other patients with spinal cord injuries.

Other clinical indications for this laxative include acute and chronic constipation, preparation of patients for abdominal and other surgery, for delivery, and for abdominal radiography, during postoperative and postpartum care, and in other situations in which a laxative or enema is indicated.

Adverse effects, cautions, and contraindications. As with other laxatives, this drug should not be used in patients with an acute surgical abdomen or in the presence of still undiagnosed GI pain. The drug's action may occasionally be accompanied by cramps or by a burning sensation in the rectum following insertion of the suppository form. Continued use of that form may cause mild proctitis. The suppository is not employed in the presence of an anal fissure or ulcerated hemorrhoids.

Dosage and administration. Two 5-mg tablets may be swallowed but not chewed, crushed, or taken with antacids, because this affects the enteric coating. One 10-mg suppository is inserted at about the time a bowel movement is desired. Combinations of tablets and suppositories are also employed.

855

Cascara sagrada USP

Actions and indications. This is probably the mildest of the anthraquinone class of irritant cathartics. It acts mainly in the large intestine, where its active constituent is liberated. The resulting peristaltic effect results in formation of a single soft stool in about 6 to 8 hours after it is taken orally. It is preferred for patients who do *not* require rapid, complete purgation. These include bedridden patients, and particularly those who should not strain at stool because of possible cardiovascular complications.

Adverse effects, cautions, and contraindications. Preparations of this plant produce few adverse effects other than diarrhea if taken in excess. Nursing mothers should not take these products, because the active constituents that are absorbed into the bloodstream may then reach the mother's milk and affect the infant. Patients should be told that their urine may be colored brown or red by constituents that are excreted by the kidneys. Those taking the drug for prolonged periods may show discoloration of

the colonic and rectal mucosa, but this is reversible when the drug is discontinued, as it should be after normal bowel activity is established.

Dosage and administration. The oral dose of about 300 mg is obtainable by taking 5 ml of the official Aromatic Cascara Fluidextract USP or 1 ml of the Fluidextract USP. Cascara Sagrada tablets (325 mg) are also available; the usual dose is one or two tablets. All are best taken at bedtime to bring about a formed bowel movement in the morning.

Castor oil USP

Actions and indications. This is a bland oil that is believed to break down in the small intestine to form an irritant cathartic principle called ricinoleic acid. It produces a relatively prompt and complete emptying of both the small and large bowels. Thus, it is employed in various situations in which rapid evacuation of the intestinal contents is desired. These include purges in the hospital on the day prior to x-ray examinations of the abdominal viscera, and removal of drug or food poisons from the intestine.

Adverse effects, cautions, and contraindications. This drug seems to be free of adverse systemic effects, and the diarrhea that may result from overdosage is self-limited, because the cathartic is itself removed from the bowel by its own action. The oil has a taste that most people find unpleasant. This can be disguised by taking castor oil with iced carbonated beverages or fruit drinks. It is also available as a pleasant-tasting pharmaceutic emulsion.

Dosage and administration. The adult dose is from 15 ml to 30 ml, and that for children is 5 ml to 15 ml. For full effects, the oil is best administered on an empty stomach. It should not be given at bedtime, because it commonly produces one or more copious watery bowel movements within 2 to 6 hours after oral administration.

Dioctyl sodium sulfosuccinate USP (Docusate Sodium; DSS; Colace; Doxinate)

Actions and indications. This chemical has physical properties that help to produce a softer stool, which is then more readily passed. It exerts a gradual surface tension-reducing effect that permits better penetration of a hardened fecal mass by fluid in the lower intestine. It is administered alone or as an adjunct to other laxatives, such as those of the stimulant type.

Adverse effects, cautions, and contraindi-

cations. This compound causes few side-effects, but occasional cramps may develop when it is administered in combination with other cathartics. It should *not* be taken with mineral oil because its presence may possibly increase the systemic absorption of liquid petrolatum through the intestinal mucosa. High concentrations applied locally by the rectal route may be irritating and could in-

terfere with the healing of hemorrhoids or surgical wounds.

Dosage and administration. The usual daily dose for oral administration to adults is 50 to 200 mg, and 10 to 40 mg for children in the form of a syrup or in fruit juice or milk. Higher doses may be needed at first to hasten the drug's full effects, which often do not develop for 1 or 2 days.

Drugs used in the management of diarrhea

Acute and chronic diarrhea

As indicated in the earlier discussion of intestinal motility, diarrhea is a symptom that develops as a result of abnormally rapid peristaltic activity. The watery, unformed stools characteristic of diarrhea are the result of the rapidity with which the chyme or liquid digestive mass is rushed through the intestine. Ordinarily, most fluids in the intestinal contents are reabsorbed into the blood by way of the large bowel wall. However, excessive peristaltic activity permits little time for such absorption by the colon and, as a result, unusually liquid stools are passed.

Acute diarrheal disease can quickly lead to extreme dehydration and to loss of vital electrolytes. This occurs most dramatically in cholera, a bacterial disease that can lead to the loss of 1 liter of electrolyte-containing fluid in a single hour. Unless patients are rapidly rehydrated, blood volume depletion can result in shock, metabolic acidosis occurs from bicarbonate loss, and cardiac arrhythmias that follow elimination of excess amounts of potassium in the so-called rice water stool can lead to death.

Fortunately, such severely dehydrating diarrhea is relatively rare. Diarrhea is most commonly an acute

but self-limiting symptom, because it helps to rid the intestinal tract of the irritant substances or the infective viruses or bacterial enterotoxins that are the most common causes of acute diarrhea. In most cases of acute nonspecific diarrhea, the immediate cause of intestinal irritation is so readily eliminated that there is no need for the underlying disease to be determined. In chronic diarrhea, on the other hand, the specific cause of a patient's persistent diarrhea may be very difficult to discover and remove—as, for example, in diarrhea of psychogenic origin.

Substances employed for symptomatic relief

In any case, even when the cause of diarrhea cannot be readily found and specifically treated, it is usually possible to give the patient some symptomatic relief. Certain systemically acting drugs often help to reduce intestinal hypermotility. These agents include the opiates (Chap. 51), which act directly on the intestinal smooth muscle to slow excessive peristaltic activity, and the anticholinergic drugs (Chap. 16), which relax spasm caused by parasympathetic nervous system stimulation.

Various locally acting substances are also said to provide relief of diarrhea by their physical effects on the intestine and its contents. Some physicians doubt that these chemicals actually duplicate their test tube actions within the intestinal tract. However, these substances are safe and inexpensive. Thus, they are widely employed as vehicles for the systemically active agents, on the assumption that, if nothing else, they may provide desirable placebo effects for the distressed patient.

This section will describe some substances that are claimed to act locally in the intestine and some of those that exert their effects on intestinal peristaltic activity and smooth muscle spasm following systemic absorption. This will be followed by a description of the applications and limitations of these and other drugs in the treatment and prevention of certain clinical conditions in which acute or chronic diarrhea is the main manifestation.

Locally acting substances

Adsorbents, astringents, and demulcents. Among the most commonly employed of the antidiarrheal drugs are *kaolin* and *pectin*, agents often given together several times daily in acute cases of diarrhea. Kaolin, an aluminum silicate clay, is an *ad*sorbent, a substance that can hold on its surface other chemicals with which it comes in contact (Table 41-3). This, it is thought, is responsible for its ability to pick up, bind, and remove bacteria, toxins, and other irritants from the intestine. It is also claimed to form a coating over the mucosa, which both protects it against irritation and filters out toxins that might otherwise be absorbed into the blood. The pectin component of such products is a plant derivative that is said to provide a demulcent or soothing effect on the irritated bowel lining in addition to aiding in adsorption.

Table 41–3. Drugs used to treat diarrhea

Official or generic name	Trade name or synonym	Usual adult dose	Comments
Locally acting antidiarrheal drugs			
Activated attapulgite	Rheaban; in various combination products	2–5 g	Adsorbent
Bismuth subgallate	Devrom; in various combination products	200–400 mg	Adsorbent–protective
Bismuth subsalicylate	Pepto-Bismol	500–600 mg	Adsorbent–protective
Kaolin mixture with pectin USP	Kaopectate	60–120 ml	Adsorbent–protective
Polycarbophil	Mitrolan	1–1.5 g	Hydrophilic–absorbent used to treat constipation or diarrhea associated with irritable bowel syndrome or with diverticulosis
Systemically active drugs			
Antiperistaltic opiates (see also Chap. 51)			
Opium tincture, deodorized	—	0.6–1.5 ml	
Paregoric tincture USP	Camphorated tincture of opium; in Brown Mixture	5–10 ml	
Antiperistaltic Opioid Derivatives			
Diphenoxylate HCl USP	In Lomotil and other preparations, in combination with atropine	5 mg	
Loperamide HCl	Imodium	2 mg	
Belladonna alkaloids and synthetic antispasmodics			
See tables in Chapter 16			

Attapulgite, a silicate clay like kaolin, is claimed to be several times more effective than the latter in its endotoxin adsorbing action. It comes in the form of an ultrafine powder said to offer a vast surface area. (The particles in 1 lb of powder, it is claimed, could cover 13 acres of surface!) A heat-treated form, *activated attapulgite* (Rheaban), possesses an increased adsorptive capacity. It is sometimes suspended in alumina gel, a substance with adsorbent, demulcent, and astringent properties of its own.

Recent evidence indicates that a suspension of *bismuth subsalicylate* is effective in *preventing* diarrhea in travelers (see also below, Prophylaxis against travelers' diarrhea). However, the doses necessary are so high as to be inconvenient to carry or to take (one 240-ml bottle/day) and, although the drug seldom causes adverse effects, it could increase serum salicylate concentrations to toxic levels in patients taking high doses of other salicylate preparations—for example, for arthritis. Thus, the use of bismuth salts for diarrhea is far from ideal.

Other substances, including activated charcoal and salts of such minerals as magnesium and aluminum are rarely employed in antidiarrhea mixtures. Valuable as it is in treating drug poisoning, activated charcoal does not seem to be very effective for treating diarrhea. The magnesium and aluminum preparations are more effective as antacids than for control of diarrhea.

Hydroabsorptive substances. Several of the substances used as bulk-producing laxatives are also sometimes employed in products for the relief of simple self-limiting diarrhea. The rationale for this seeming paradox is that these hydrophilic substances can absorb some of the excess fecal fluid. The previously mentioned *pectins* act, in part, in this manner, as do *psyllium seed mucilloids.*

Polycarbophil (Mitrolan) is claimed to have certain advantages over other hydrophilic absorbents. It does not swell in the stomach to cause an uncomfortable feeling of fullness. It is said to exert its water-binding action only on reaching the alkaline medium of the small intestine and colon, where it is said to absorb about 60 times its weight of water.

Systemically acting substances

The locally acting drugs described above are the basic ingredients of most antidiarrheal products that are sold OTC directly to the public. Actually, certain systemically active antiperistaltic–antispasmodic agents, most of which require a prescription, are much more effective for reducing the frequency of watery or loose bowel movements and for relieving the accompanying abdominal spasms (Table 41-3). These fall into two classes: derivatives of opium, or synthetic substances with similar actions on the GI tract; and derivatives of belladonna and synthetic anticholinergic antispasmodic drugs.

Opiate antiperistaltic preparations and related drugs. The natural alkaloids of opium—including mor-

phine, codeine, and papaverine—act directly on the intestinal musculature and glands in several ways that cause constipation (Chap. 51). This action is, of course, considered to be an undesired side-effect when these drugs are employed for the relief of pain. However, the antiperistaltic and antisecretory effects of the opiate alkaloids, and their ability to interfere with the propulsive activity of parts of the gut by their spasmogenic effects, are the basis for the therapeutic use of opium preparations such as paregoric and tincture of opium in the management of acute simple diarrhea.

In such cases, relatively low doses of these preparations—amounts small enough, in some situations, to permit their inclusion in nonprescription products in combination with kaolin, pectin, and other locally acting substances that serve as a vehicle—lessen hyperperistaltic activity and delay passage of the intestinal contents long enough to allow reabsorption of electrolyte-containing fluids by the bowel. In other cases, the recommended doses of these drugs in proprietary preparations are inadequate for relief of acute diarrhea; and larger oral doses are ordered, or an injection of morphine may even have to be given to stop an acute diarrheal state that has brought a patient to the brink of collapse.

The central side-effects of large doses of opiates and their potential for being abused constitute a drawback to the use of these drugs, particularly in the management of chronic diarrhea. Two derivatives of the synthetic opioid meperidine, or pethidine (Demerol), are relatively free of both central effects and abuse potential, while retaining the antidiarrheal activity of the opiates. The first of these drugs, *diphenoxylate HCl*[+] (in Lomotil), has been long-established as effective for relief of acute and chronic diarrhea. A similar drug, *loperamide HCl* (Imodium; REASEC outside the United States) has also been introduced, which is claimed to have even less abuse potential when used for long-term therapy of disorders that cause chronic diarrhea. However, because studies performed in primates have shown this drug to cause morphine-type dependence (Chap. 53), caution is required when it is used in human patients with a history of drug abuse. Caution should also be used in ordering diphenoxylate for such patients, although atropine has been added deliberately to diphenoxylate preparations to discourage abuse.

The adverse effects and toxicity of loperamide are essentially similar to those described in the Drug digest for diphenoxylate, except that the product does not contain atropine, and so it does not produce the typical side-effects of that drug in children or in others who are sensitive to anticholinergic agents.

Belladonna-type and synthetic antispasmodic drugs. The belladonna alkaloids atropine, hyoscine, and hyoscyamine (Chap. 16), the quaternary derivative homatropine methylbromide, and certain synthetic anticholinergic and similar antispasmodics such as dicyclomine

(Bentyl), thiphenamil (Trocinate), and mepenzolate (Cantil), among others, are sometimes employed to suppress peristaltic activity and spasm of the colon in patients with conditions that cause acute or chronic diarrhea. Administered in adequate doses—more than those permitted in *non*prescription products—the belladonna derivatives may help to lessen the frequent passage of loose stools and relieve discomforting smooth muscle spasm.

The doses of these drugs required for relief of diarrhea and intestinal spasm almost invariably cause the characteristic side-effects of anticholinergic drugs (Chap. 16). Thus, they must be employed with caution, if at all, in patients with other disorders that make them especially sensitive to the side-effects of cholinergic blocking agents. Patients with ulcerative colitis may suffer paralytic ileus and toxic megacolon if treated with large diarrhea-reducing doses that eliminate all types of intestinal motility.

These drugs are frequently combined with phenobarbital or other sedatives and antianxiety agents. Although rest and relaxation are desirable in acute diarrhea and supportive psychotherapy is often part of the management of patients with chronic diarrhea, most authorities doubt the effectiveness of sedatives added to antispasmodics in such fixed dosage combination products.

Treatment of acute infectious diarrhea

Acute diarrhea often develops as a result of ingestion of food or water contaminated by viruses, bacteria and, less frequently, amebae or other protozoan parasites. Most such enteric illnesses do not last more than a day or two and do not really require any treatment other than rest and taking liquids to replace the fluids lost with watery diarrhea. However, because of the discomfort and inconvenience of acute diarrheal attacks, people naturally want to take some sort of medication to alleviate their symptoms.

Symptomatic relief

Most authorities do not believe that it is desirable to employ antiperistaltic drugs to suppress diarrhea. The main reason for this is their view that diarrhea is the intestine's main defense mechanism for ridding itself of the enterotoxins most often responsible for mucosal irritation. Thus, they argue that the use of drugs that slow peristaltic activity tends to prolong the diarrheal illness. In cases of bacterial enteritis and dysentery caused by gram-negative enteropathogens such as *Shigella* and *Salmonella* species and some toxicogenic strains of *Escherichia coli* that can also invade the intestinal mucosa, the patient's febrile illnesses may be made even worse by the use of opiates, diphenoxylate and loperamide, and other antiperistaltic–antispasmodic agents.

Despite these authoritative opinions, some feel that there is little harm in administering moderate doses of antiperistaltic and antispasmodic drugs to relieve discomforting abdominal cramps and to lessen the number of loose bowel movements in cases that appear to be simply an acute nonspecific infectious diarrhea. For such symptomatic relief, diphenoxylate in doses of 2.5 to 7.5 mg every 3 or 4 hours or loperamide in doses of two 2-mg capsules followed by one capsule after each unformed stool may be prescribed. Those who prefer the traditional remedies may order 1 or 2 tsp of paregoric several times daily to control acute diarrhea or even 10 to 15 drops of tincture of opium taken at appropriate intervals. Atropine may be administered in doses of close to 1 mg orally or parenterally to relieve abdominal cramps. Such opiate and belladonna preparations are also often added to suspensions of kaolin, pectin, and other locally acting agents.

Anti-infective drugs. The question of whether to employ anti-infective drugs for treating and preventing acute infectious diarrhea is also a matter of continuing controversy. Most authorities feel that such agents should not be used routinely for the treatment of the commonly encountered acute diarrheal disorders. One reason is that the enteric viruses that are a common cause of acute febrile diarrheas are resistant to any available anti-infective drugs. Another reason for not administering these drugs is that most bacterial diarrheas subside spontaneously within a day or two, and those that do not should be treated only after the causative organism has been identified and the anti-infective drug to which it is most sensitive has been determined by laboratory tests.

Nevertheless, although many physicians will take a culture when a patient's diarrhea and fever continue for several days, they often then begin treatment immediately with a broad-spectrum antibiotic such as *ampicillin* or *tetracycline* while waiting for the results of the laboratory tests to come back. These antibiotics are likely to be effective against most strains of the most common bacterial enteropathogenic species responsible for diarrhea, including shigellae, salmonellae, *Vibrio parahaemolyticus*, and certain invasive and noninvasive *E. coli* strains. On the other hand, nonabsorbable and other sulfonamides are no longer used in this way, because so many sulfa-resistant bacterial strains have emerged. *Trimethoprim–sulfamethoxazole* (co-trimoxazole) may, however, be effective in preventing diarrhea caused by certain bacteria (see below).

If laboratory reports indicate the presence of salmonellosis, whether to use anti-infective drugs is decided mainly on the basis of the severity of the diarrhea and on the degree of systemic toxicity. Mild to moderate salmonella gastroenteritis may not have to be treated with anti-infective drugs at all, because these agents have not been shown to affect the course of the disease. Such cases may be managed adequately with only fluid and electrolyte replacement therapy.

On the other hand, when bacteremia is present or suspected—particularly in infants and debilitated patients—the antimicrobial agents to which the infecting *Salmonella* strain seems most susceptible in laboratory sensitivity tests are ordered. As indicated in Chapter 8, chloramphenicol may be preferred to ampicillin for treating bacteremia and severe dehydrating diarrhea when tests indicate that the *Salmonella* organism responsible is most sensitive to that antibiotic. The addition of trimethoprim to the sulfonamide sulfamethoxazole (co-trimoxazole) has proved to make an effective combination for treating such cases.

Prophylaxis against travelers' diarrhea*

Travelers to foreign countries often have their trips disrupted by several days of GI illness marked by diarrhea, abdominal cramps, nausea and vomiting, and sometimes headache and fever. In the past, the exact cause of travelers' diarrhea was uncertain, and it was sometimes attributed simply to the change in diet—for instance, to the presence in foods of cooking oils with a laxative effect. However, there is evidence that the most common cause is infection by certain strains of *E. coli* that produce an enterotoxin that sets off peristaltic activity.

This has revived interest in the question of whether people planning foreign travel should arm themselves with a preparation containing anti-infective drugs that they would then take daily during the trip to ward off GI infection and the inconvenient, demoralizing diarrhea that follows. Expert opinion is divided concerning the desirability of routine prophylaxis of this type. Some authorities warn against drug-induced toxicity, possible difficulty in treating any actual infections that do develop, and the fact that taking daily prophylactic doses of antimicrobial drugs might cause the emergence of resistant strains of enteropathogens. Others believe that the benefits of prophylaxis for most travelers outweigh the risks.

Among the antibiotics claimed to be most effective for preventing severe degrees of diarrhea are the tetracycline derivative *doxycycline* (Vibramycin) and the combination *trimethoprim–sulfamethoxazole* in double strength (Bactrim DS; Septra DS). The dosage of doxycycline recommended for this purpose is 200 mg on the first day of travel, followed by 100 mg daily for 3 weeks. One double-strength tablet of trimethoprim–sulfamethoxazole is taken daily. The adverse reactions, cautions, and contraindications described for these drugs in Chapter 8 also apply to this use.

As mentioned earlier, large doses of bismuth subsalicylate suspension (Pepto-Bismol) are also effective, but inconvenient. The dose is 60 ml, four times daily. The mechanism by which this drug prevents the enterotoxin of *E. coli* from causing diarrhea is unknown.

Whether or not a patient and physician decide that a prescription for prophylactic antimicrobial drugs should be given before departure, the person planning

a trip should be warned about the need to be careful about what is eaten and drunk while away. Fresh fruits and vegetables, for example, should be eaten only after being peeled, and unpeeled fruits or lettuce should first be washed in a chlorinated solution. Mineral waters or other beverages that are bottled are best, and other drinking water and milk should be boiled. Ice in beverages should also be avoided, because it may have been made from contaminated water. Shellfish should generally be avoided, and only food that has been cooked thoroughly and recently should be eaten. Restaurants with obviously poor sanitary practices should be shunned—for example, if refrigeration seems lacking, personnel do not appear concerned with personal hygiene, or the premises are infested with flies.

In summary, the most conservative approach to prevention of diarrhea while traveling should be based on efforts to employ caution in where one dines and in what one eats and drinks. People whose purpose in traveling to a foreign country is so important that they are unwilling to depend on such hygienic measures alone—for instance, athletes who are determined to confine their running to the track—may come supplied with a prophylactic antimicrobial preparation for daily use during their visit and for a week or so after their return home. If diarrhea develops despite all nonmedicinal precautions and drug prophylaxis, symptomatic relief may be sought with antiperistaltic-antispasmodic drugs and antinauseants (see below) and with kaolin-pectin-type preparations, although simple bed rest and replacement of lost fluids and electrolytes may really be all that is required. Finally, travelers with diarrhea and fever that persist for several days should consult a locally recommended physician who may prescribe specific antimicrobial therapy.

Treatment of chronic diarrhea

Diarrhea that persists or recurs at frequent intervals occurs in many different circumstances. Often, a patient who has frequent small stools followed by periods of constipation may have no organic GI lesions at all. However, before dismissing the patient's condition as psychogenic, the nurse or physician should advise a thorough examination by a gastroenterologist or other internist to rule out carcinomas of the colon or rectum, which are among the most common types of cancer. Other organic diseases such as regional ileitis (Crohn's disease) and ulcerative colitis require specific therapy, ranging from the use of anti-inflammatory corticosteroids to surgery. Sometimes surgery of the GI tract is itself a cause of diarrhea—for example, following such procedures as vagotomy, gastrectomy, or ileostomy. Radiation therapy often causes diarrhea as well as nausea and vomiting (see below). In all these disorders, the judicious use of antispasmodic and antiperistaltic drugs can offer considerable relief while efforts are being made first to find the cause of the diarrhea and then to eliminate it with specific therapy.

---

* Diarrhea is said to afflict 25% to 50% of the 1¼ million Americans who visit Mexico annually. It is also quite common in travelers to other foreign countries, including citizens of other countries who travel to the United States.

The GI disturbance called by such varied names as the irritable colon syndrome, spastic colitis, and mucous colitis, among others, is thought to be related to the patient's response to stress in the life situation. In such people, emotional tension is thought to cause intensified cholinergic nerve activity, with a resultant increase in the motility of the colon. By blocking acetylcholine, the neurotransmitter released by cholinergic nerves, the belladonna extracts, and synthetic antispasmodics such as dicyclomine (Bentyl), mepenzolate (Cantil), methscopolamine bromide (Pamine), propantheline (Pro-Banthine), and thiphenamil (Trocinate) often relieve this functional bowel disorder. The anticholinergic and other antispasmodic agents are frequently combined with phenobarbital or other sedatives and tranquilizers that tend to relieve the tension that is thought to cause, as well as accompany, the diarrhea of the irritable bowel syndrome. Rest and relaxation are important aspects of the treatment of these patients and others with functional GI disorders, which often improve when they receive reassurance and emotional support from a physician or a nurse who shows a personal interest in them and their plight.

Some patients require formal psychotherapy as well as drugs. Such support sometimes helps these patients to overcome their distressing symptoms. It often provides the patient with an opportunity to talk about his worries and concerns and may, perhaps, help the patient to recognize possible relationships between his emotional problems and intestinal symptoms.

Antispasmodic and other drugs may also be useful adjuncts to more specific measures in patients with diarrhea, abdominal spasms, and rectal tenesmus, or straining, that occur in such organic intestinal disorders as Crohn's disease, ulcerative colitis, and diverticulitis. However, their use in excessive doses carries the risk of causing intestinal atony in elderly or debilitated patients. Suppression of all intestinal motility in patients with severe ulcerative colitis can produce paralytic ileus or aggravate it to the point of causing toxic megacolon, a serious obstructive complication.

Thus, because of these possible complications and the numerous other potential side-effects of the anticholinergic drugs in the doses required for control (Chap. 16), many gastroenterologists prefer such safer measures as administering hydrophilic bulk-producing agents such as psyllium mucilloids. Opioids may also be employed occasionally to control especially severe diarrhea and spasms but, because of the potential abuse-producing properties of morphine, meperidine, codeine, and deodorized tincture of opium, chronic diarrhea control is best accomplished with daily doses of diphenoxylate or loperamide. These drugs are equally effective for rapid relief of diarrhea, and their long-continued use in lower doses then often helps to keep corticosteroid dosage low in the long-term management of chronic inflammatory bowel disorders. Loperamide has also proved to be useful for reducing the volume of discharges from ileostomies, thus helping to lessen nighttime soiling and aiding in maintenance of personal hygiene.

Additional clinical considerations

All the adverse side-effects of the atropine drugs (Chap. 16) can occur with many of these drugs. Patients should receive all the education and comfort measures that are used for atropinelike drugs while they are receiving antidiarrheal agents. Patients should not receive antidiarrheal drugs for any prolonged periods of time. Diarrhea that persists for prolonged periods should be evaluated for the underlying cause.

The abuse potential of loperamide and the opium derivatives has already been discussed. Patients who receive these drugs should be cautioned not to exceed the recommended dosage. These patients also need to know that they may experience drowsiness, dizziness, or both while taking these drugs. They should be warned to avoid driving and not to operate dangerous or delicate machinery while on these drugs.

The safety of the use of antidiarrheal drugs during pregnancy and lactation has not been established. These drugs should be avoided during pregnancy and lactation unless the potential benefits outweigh the possible risks involved.

Diarrhea is a common, usually benign, disorder that can occur as a response to dietary changes, viruses, drugs, or emotional stress. Nursing care of patients with diarrhea should include hydration, positioning for comfort, ready access to bathroom facilities, environmental control, and often bowel rest (e.g., avoidance of milk, spices, heavy meals, high-carbohydrate or high-protein meals). Drug therapy with antidiarrheal drugs is best reserved for the patient with severe discomfort or debilitating diarrhea.

Drug digest

Diphenoxylate HCl USP (in Lomotil)

Actions and indications. This chemical relative of the synthetic narcotic analgesic meperidine (Demerol) is employed for its antiperistaltic action as an adjunct in the management of diarrhea. It is effective for reducing the number of daily stools in chronic functional and inflammatory intestinal disorders without causing development of opiate-type dependence in patients who do not take doses larger than those recommended as effective for slowing intestinal motility. It may also be employed for control of acute diarrhea of varied etiology, except for cases known to be caused by infectious organisms that invade the intestinal mucosa or by certain antibiotic drugs.

Adverse effects, cautions, and contraindications. Because of its relationship to a dependence-producing opioid, caution is recommended in patients with a history of drug abuse who may attempt to take excessive amounts to achieve central subjective effects. To discourage such efforts to abuse it, each tablet contains a small subtherapeutic dose of atropine that causes discomforting side-effects in those who deliberately exceed the recommended dosage. Some side-effects of the product—particularly in children and in patients with Down's syndrome—are those typical of atropine. Ordinary doses of diphenoxylate cause only occasional drowsiness and constipation. However, overdoses can cause lethargy, coma, and respiratory

depression that must be managed like other cases of opioid intoxication, including repeated administration of the narcotic antagonist naloxone (Chap. 51).

As is the case with meperidine, this drug should be used with extreme caution in patients with severe liver disease, because its use could lead to hepatic coma. Similarly, its simultaneous use with monoamine oxidase inhibitors might cause hypertensive crisis. Patients with acute ulcerative colitis should be closely observed for signs of abdominal distention, because toxic megacolon has sometimes occurred in treating such patients

with drugs that delay intestinal transit time. This drug is contraindicated in cases of pseudomembranous colitis caused by the antibiotics lincomycin and clindamycin.

Dosage and administration. The recommended adult dose is 20 mg daily for initial control of diarrhea, divided into doses of 5 mg qid. Later, this may be reduced to as little as 5 mg daily. Lower doses are recommended for children from 2 to 12 years of age—for example 4 ml (2 mg) of a liquid preparation three to five times daily. The drug is contraindicated in children under 2 years old.

Antiemetic drugs

Nausea and vomiting

Nausea is one of the most commonly reported symptoms. This feeling of being "sick in the stomach," or nausea, is often followed by retching and vomiting, the complex reflex act by which the stomach's contents are ejected. Vomiting serves a useful purpose when it removes toxic irritants from the stomach before they can be absorbed into the systemic circulation. (The use of emetics to induce vomiting and thus to help rid the stomach of ingested poisons has been discussed in Chapter 5.)

Unfortunately, vomiting occurs most often in situations that do not require emptying of the stomach. Thus, there is no protective value in the vomiting that is part of the body's response to certain types of motion. Similarly, the nausea of early pregnancy does not serve as a useful warning signal in any way, and vomiting that persists may actually endanger the mother by causing a severe fluid–electrolyte imbalance and by interfering with her nutrition.

The stimuli that set off the vomiting reflex may originate not only in the GI tract but anywhere in the body. Such stimuli may be physical, chemical, or psychological. Thus, it is not surprising that nausea and vomiting should be part of the picture in so many clinical conditions, ranging from minor infections to metastatic carcinoma. The physician therefore first tries to determine the *cause* of the vomiting and then takes steps to eliminate it, if possible.

Once the cause has been recognized, however, symptomatic relief is desirable to reduce the patient's discomfort and to prevent the possibly dangerous consequences of persistent vomiting. Sometimes relief requires only simple nursing care measures, such as providing a quiet, restful environment and seeing that the patient gets ice to suck or a cold carbonated drink or hot tea to sip. On the other hand, effective antiemetic drugs, which act by dampening hyperactive vomiting reflex activity, may also be ordered.

Reflex vomiting mechanisms

Vomiting, like most other reflexes, requires the presence of receptors that react to stimuli and send nerve impulses centrally by way of afferent pathways. Such sensory stimuli may stream in from anywhere in the body, including not only the mucosa of the GI tract but also the labyrinth of the inner ear, as well as the cerebral cortex and other brain areas involved in emotional responses. Another group of nerve cells located in the brain stem—the chemoreceptor trigger zone (CTZ)—also relays afferent impulses toward the vomiting center.

The center that receives these incoming impulses and reacts by transmitting messages to the muscles involved in the vomiting act is located deep in the medulla oblongata. It lies near the nerve nuclei that control cardiovascular, respiratory, and other autonomic functions. Thus, when this area is being bombarded by excessive numbers of nerve impulses from overexcited receptors anywhere in the body, some of these impulses spill over onto these adjacent areas. This accounts for signs and symptoms such as salivation, sweating, pallor, and slowing of the heart rate in the nauseated, vomiting person.

Drug treatment

All the drugs used in the management of nausea and vomiting act by reducing hyperactive reflex activity in one way or another. Some do so by dulling the reactivity of the receptors to stimuli, thus lessening the rate at which impulses pass centrally from peripheral sites such as the stomach. Others make the chemoreceptor trigger zone less sensitive to emetic chemicals circulating in the bloodstream or to nerve impulses arriving at this relay station from motion receptors in the inner ear. Occasionally, the threshold of the vomiting center itself may be raised by drugs that depress its neurons.

The drugs used in the management of nausea and vomiting may be classified as *locally acting* and *centrally acting* (Table 41-4). Substances of the first type include topical mucosal anesthetics, antacids and adsorbents, demulcent–protective agents, and drugs that reduce dis-

Table 41—4. Centrally acting antiemetic drugs

Official or generic name	Trade name	Route of administration	Usual adult antiemetic dosage	Indications
Antidopaminergic drugs				
Phenothiazines				
Chlorpromazine HCl USP	Thorazine	Oral Rectal IM IV infusion	10–25 mg q 4–6 hr 50–100 mg q 6–8 hr 25–50 mg q 3–4 hr 25–50 mg	Nausea and vomiting, especially drug-induced; intractable hiccups
Perphenazine USP	Trilafon	Oral IM IV	8–16 mg/day in divided doses 5 mg 5 mg, slowly	Nausea and vomiting, especially drug-induced; intractable hiccups
Prochlorperazine maleate USP	Compazine	Oral Rectal IM IV	5–10 mg tid or qid 25 mg bid 5–10 mg q 3–4 hr 5–10 mg	Severe nausea and vomiting
Promethazine HCl USP	Phenergan	Oral Rectal IM IV infusion	25 mg bid 25 mg bid 12.5–25 mg 25 mg	Nausea and vomiting associated with anesthesia and surgery; motion sickness
Thiethylperazine maleate	Torecan	Oral Rectal IM	10 mg 10 mg 10 mg	Nausea and vomiting
Triflupromazine HCl USP	Vesprin	Oral IM IV	20–30 mg/day 5–15 mg q 4 hr 1–3 mg/day	Severe nausea and vomiting
Nonphenothiazine				
Metoclopropamide	Reglan	IV infusion	2 mg/kg body weight ½ hr before cisplatin administration, then q 2 hr for two doses and q 3 hr for three doses	Nausea and vomiting associated with cisplatin cancer chemotherapy
Anticholinergic drugs				
Antihistamines				
Buclizine HCl	Bucladin-S Softabs	Oral	50 mg bid	Motion sickness
Cyclizine USP	Marezine	Oral IM	50 mg q 4–6 hr 50 mg q 4–6 hr	Motion sickness
Dimenhydrinate USP	Dramamine	Oral IM IV	50–100 mg q 4–6 hr 50 mg 50 mg	Motion sickness

(continued)

Table 41–4. Centrally acting antiemetic drugs (continued)

Official or generic name	Trade name	Route of administration	Usual adult antiemetic dosage	Indications
Diphenhydramine HCl USP	Benadryl	Oral IM IV	25–50 mg tid or qid 10–50 mg; max. dose: 400 mg/day	Motion sickness
Meclizine HCl USP	Antivert; Bonine	Oral	25–50 mg q 24 hr 25–100 mg q 24 hr in divided doses	Motion sickness Possibly effective in vertigo associated with vestibular disease
Nonantihistamines				
Scopolamine HBr USP	Triptone	Oral	0.25–0.8 mg	Motion sickness
Scopolamine, transdermal	Transderm-Scōp	Trans-dermal	1 patch q 3 days	Motion sickness
Trimethobenzamide HCl	Tigan	Oral Rectal IM	250 mg tid or qid 200 mg tid or qid 200 mg tid or qid	Nausea and vomiting
Miscellaneous				
Benzquinamide HCl	Emete-Con	IM IV	50 mg repeated after 1 hr and then q 3–4 hr 25 mg	Nausea and vomiting associated with anesthesia and surgery
Dexamethasone	—	Unofficial use to prevent vomiting associated with cisplatin administration for cancer chemotherapy		
Diphenidol	Vontrol	Oral	25–50 mg q 4 hr	Labyrinthine vertigo (Meniere's disease and labyrinthitis)
Hydroxyzine HCl	Atarax; Vistaril	IM	25–100 mg	Pre- and postoperative, pre- and postpartum anxiety and emesis (see also Chap. 45)
Δ^9-Tetrahydrocannabinol; Δ^9-THC	—	Investigational drug available from the National Cancer Institute only in states that permit its use to prevent nausea and vomiting from cancer chemotherapy		

tention of the stomach by retained gases (*e.g.*, simethicone and the carminatives).

The centrally acting antiemetics may be further subdivided into three categories:

1. Antidopaminergic drugs, both phenothiazines and nonphenothiazines (the term "phenothiazine" refers to a chemical structure that these drugs have in common, and they also share certain pharmacologic properties. Many are used to treat mental illness and psychoses; see Chap. 46)

2. Anticholinergic drugs, both antihistamines (*i.e.*, H_1 histamine receptor blockers; Chap. 39) and nonantihistamines

3. Miscellaneous drugs, which do not belong in any of the above categories

Locally acting agents

Vomiting caused by local irritation of the GI tract is usually self-limited because, once the stomach rids itself of the troublesome irritant, the source of the difficulty is gone, and the mucosal receptors stop sending their distress signals centrally. In some cases of acute gastroenteritis, however, the inflamed membranes continue to bombard the vomiting center with messages that trigger nausea and vomiting. Drugs that reduce the reactivity of these receptors may be helpful in overcoming these manifestations of stomach upset while the patient's condition is being gradually cleared up by other measures aimed at removing its cause.

Topical anesthetics. Various local anesthetics are sometimes administered orally in an attempt to raise the threshold of receptor responsiveness to local irritants. Among the topically active agents sometimes taken by mouth to reduce the number of afferent impulses originating in the GI tract are *benzocaine* and *procaine.* It is doubtful, however, that these short-acting substances have much effect on vomiting. The longer acting local anesthetic, *lidocaine,* is available as a viscous solution that is said to control severe reflex vomiting for several hours when taken orally in 1-tbsp doses. Another agent, *oxethazaine* (Oxaine M Suspension), which is suspended in an antacid alumina gel, is said to afford prolonged topical anesthesia because it is present in an adherent coating that protects the irritated gastric mucosa.

Other agents. Other commonly employed antinauseants that are claimed to work for some people include *Coca-Cola syrup* and a product with essentially similar properties, *phosphorated carbohydrate solution* (Emetrol). These liquids are taken in 1-tbsp doses without any other fluids. Although there is little scientific evidence of how they act, these substances are said to relax GI muscle spasms by a local effect, thus reducing afferent impulses to the vomiting center.

The psychological effects of some agents used for stomach upset should not be ignored. Although scientific proof of their effectiveness is usually lacking, the placebo response is often a desirable one. Thus, if a patient who takes something occasionally to "settle the stomach" believes that it is doing some good, this confidence in the medication that he finds to be helpful should not be shattered.

Centrally acting antiemetics

The most effective drugs for prevention or relief of nausea and vomiting depress passage of nerve impulses in brain pathways. The first drugs used to depress the central parts of the vomiting reflex mechanism were the *barbiturates,* and other *sedative–hypnotics,* and *scopolamine (hyoscine),* a belladonna alkaloid with central depressant effects (Table 41-4). Because of their side-effects, the sedative–hypnotic drugs have been largely replaced by other more specific antiemetic agents. A new transdermal dosage form has renewed the popularity of scopolamine for the treatment and prevention of nausea and vomiting associated with motion sickness.

Antidopaminergic drugs. Many of the major tranquilizers, or antipsychotic agents, also possess potent antiemetic activity (Table 41-4). They seem to act mainly by reducing the responsiveness of nerve cells in the CTZ to circulating chemicals that cause vomiting.

Indications. The ability of the *phenothiazines* and of *metoclopramide* (Reglan), another antidopaminergic drug (see also Table 41-1), to block stimulation of the CTZ by drugs, hormones, and toxins, as well as nerve impulses, may account for the effectiveness of these drugs in the following types of conditions:

1. *Hyperemesis gravidarum,* or excessive vomiting of pregnancy
2. *Cancer,* particularly patients being treated with irradiation and antineoplastic chemotherapeutic agents
3. *Postoperative vomiting*
4. *Vomiting secondary to severe infections,* such as meningitis, or with uremia, hepatitis, or gallbladder disease

The phenothiazines are *not* usually considered to be very useful for treating the nausea, vertigo, and vomiting of motion sickness.

Adverse effects. Most adverse effects of phenothiazines that occur in treating mental illness (see Chap. 46) are unlikely to occur with the relatively small doses employed for relief of vomiting. However, even a single injection of a drug such as *prochlorperazine+* (Compazine) sometimes sets off muscle spasms, motor restlessness (akathisia), and other signs of extrapyramidal motor system reactions. Children and young adults are especially susceptible. Thus, even a relatively safe drug such as *thiethylperazine* (Torecan) is not recommended for children under 12 years old. These drugs are prescribed in the smallest doses effective for relief of vomiting, and the parents should be advised not to give children a higher dose than that ordered. *Metoclopramide* (Reglan), a new drug with centrally acting antiemetic properties (among its other effects on GI motility; see Table 41-1), has been employed successfully abroad for relief of nausea and vomiting in patients with gastritis, and it is now approved for use in the United States to prevent nausea and vomiting in patients receiving chemotherapy with cisplatin. Metoclopramide has also caused acute dystonic reactions in children similar to those that commonly occur with small doses of the phenothiazine-type antiemetics.

Precautions. Among the reasons for exercising caution in administering phenothiazines to vomiting children is the unconfirmed suspicion that these drugs may contribute to the development of Reye's syndrome in children suffering from a viral illness of unknown etiology. Children who already have this serious, potentially fatal disease could be made worse by the administration of centrally acting antiemetic drugs. The course of the disease could, for example, be unfavorably altered by a possible drug-induced increase in the child's susceptibility to encephalopathy and to fatty degeneration of the liver.

The extrapyramidal reactions to antidopaminergic drugs could also be mistaken for signs of Reye's syndrome or of some other primary disease. Thus, these drugs should be used only when the patient's vomiting is prolonged and when the reason for it is recognized, rather than in simple uncomplicated vomiting or in more severe vomiting, the cause of which has not yet been properly determined.

The phenothiazine antiemetics are effective for relief of postoperative vomiting that may threaten the success of surgery—for example, in patients who have had eye operations or extensive abdominal incisions. Although phenothiazines are often administered *preoperatively* for various purposes, their routine use before the operation to reduce later vomiting is considered unwise when weighed against the possible adverse effects of these depressant drugs, including sudden drops in the blood pressure of the anesthetized patient. Thus, if these drugs are to be administered at all, they are best injected shortly before the patient is going to waken from anesthesia. Two of these drugs, chlorpromazine and perphenazine, are given to treat intractable hiccups. They are often given intravenously when used for this purpose. Whenever any of the phenothiazines is administered by this route, it must be given slowly to avoid precipitous falls in blood pressure.

Anticholinergic drugs. The effectiveness of the first modern antiemetic drug, *dimenhydrinate*[+] (Dramamine), was discovered accidentally. This agent, which is a close chemical relative of the antihistaminic agent diphenhydramine (Benadryl; Chap. 39) was first tested for efficacy in treating allergic reactions. A patient who was susceptible to motion sickness noted that she did not become carsick on the trolley ride home from the clinic to which she went for treatment of hives with this drug. The physicians to whom she reported this were quick to follow up the lead. They tested dimenhydrinate on soldiers making a rough midwinter ocean voyage to Europe during World War II and found the drug to be a relatively effective antinauseant, with fewer side-effects than the belladonna derivatives and barbiturates previously employed.

Later, other drugs were introduced that were said to have an even lower incidence of side-effects such as drowsiness, mouth dryness, and visual blurring. These include the H_1 receptor antihistamines *cyclizine* (Marezine) and *meclizine* (Bonine). The latter is claimed to have an especially long duration of action—a single small dose is said to produce prophylactic effects against motion-induced nausea for up to 24 hours.

These drugs, *trimethobenzamide* (Tigan), and *scopolamine* all have anticholinergic properties and are thought to act mainly by blocking transmission of nerve impulses along the long nervous pathways passing from the inner ear to the vomiting center by way of the vestibular portion of the eighth cranial nerve, the vestibular

nuclei, the cerebellum, and the CTZ. This is said to account for their special effectiveness in motion sickness and in ailments such as labyrinthitis, Meniere's disease, and the dizziness and nausea that often follow surgical procedures involving the inner ear.

In all these conditions, receptors within the inner ear that involve maintaining body balance are overstimulated by motion, inflammation, or trauma. As a result, unusually large numbers of nerve impulses are relayed centrally from these receptor sites. Impulses passing to various nerve nuclei set off the sickening sensation of dizziness or giddiness called vertigo, as well as nausea and vomiting.

These drugs are thought to act mainly by their ability to interrupt transmission of such impulses from the labyrinth of the inner ear to the various responsive central sites. However, the fact that they sometimes cause drowsiness indicates that sedation may also play a part in reducing the patient's sensitivity to disturbing impulses. Thus, people who intend to drive or operate delicate machinery should be told that these centrally acting antihistaminic–anticholinergic agents may tend to reduce their alertness.

Drowsiness need not be a drawback in patients who do not have to stay alert. In fact, the sedative effect of some nonphenothiazines and the calming or tranquilizing effect of the phenothiazines may even add to their effectiveness as antiemetics in certain clinical situations. This is because these drugs reduce the anxiety and tension that are often involved in making patients susceptible to other stimuli that set off vomiting.

Other agents. *Diphenidol* (Vontrol), a drug that is neither a phenothiazine nor an antihistamine, is claimed to be effective for control of nausea, vomiting, and vertigo caused by labyrinthine disturbances such as Meniere's disease and middle and inner ear surgery and in other clinical conditions. However, its use is limited to hospitalized patients or to others who can be continuously observed. The reason for this is that the drug has sometimes caused confusion, disorientation, and hallucinations.

Benzquinamide HCl (Emete-Con) is claimed to have advantages over phenothiazines in the prevention and treatment of postoperative nausea, retching, and vomiting. It does not, for example, set off extrapyramidal motor system reactions or potentiate the depressant or hypotensive effects of other drugs employed in anesthesia. However, when administered by vein, this drug has sometimes set off a sudden rise in blood pressure and transient cardiac arrhythmias. Thus, it is best injected intramuscularly, particularly when patients are also receiving other preanesthetic medications with cardiovascular actions.

Actually, the use of this drug and other antiemetics postoperatively should be limited to those patients in whom vomiting might adversely affect the desired result of the surgery or cause particular harm to the patient.

Wherever possible, it is best to avoid administration of antiemetic drugs that have many and varied central and peripheral pharmacologic effects in addition to the control of vomiting. If at all possible, nonmedical measures should be employed to prevent nausea and vomiting.

An investigational drug, *domperidone* (Motilium), is being studied in the United States for its effectiveness in treatment of nausea and vomiting associated with the use of cytotoxic chemotherapy. This drug is available in Europe. Domperidone blocks dopamine receptors in the CTZ. It has few reported side-effects, and, because it is claimed not to cross the blood–brain barrier, it is expected to cause fewer extrapyramidal reactions than other antidopaminergic antiemetics.

As discussed in Chapter 12, Δ^9-*tetrahydrocannabinol* (Δ^9-THC), the active component of marihuana, is available in states that permit its use to qualified physicians from the National Cancer Institute for preventing the nausea and vomiting associated with cancer chemotherapy. A synthetic derivative, *nabilone* (Cesamet), is now used in other countries and is expected to be approved soon in the United States.

Dexamethasone and *methylprednisolone*, corticosteroids (Chap. 21), are used unofficially as antiemetics in patients receiving chemotherapy with cisplatin and other anticancer drugs. The mechanism by which marihuana derivatives and corticosteroids produce antiemetic effects is unknown.

Additional clinical considerations

Many drugs are available to prevent or treat nausea and vomiting. All are more effective at *preventing* than *treating* nausea and vomiting. Thus, the first dose of antiemetic drugs used in conjunction with anesthesia and surgery should be given before the anesthetic wears off, antiemetic drugs used in conjunction with cancer chemotherapy should be begun before the chemotherapeutic drug is given, and drugs given for motion sickness should be taken before travel as well as at appropriate intervals later if the trip is prolonged. When vomiting has begun and oral medication is unfeasible, many of these preparations are available as rectal suppositories or in parenteral dosage forms.

Although many of these drugs may be effective in managing the vomiting of pregnancy ("morning sickness"), their use in pregnant women, like the use of *all* drugs, should be avoided, if possible, because of the risk of harm to the fetus. For many years Bendectin, a combination of doxylamine succinate and pyridoxine HCl (vitamin B_6), was used successfully to treat the nausea associated with early pregnancy. Conflicting and controversial research studies have associated this drug with possible teratogenicity. While denying claims that the drug is unsafe, the manufacturer stopped producing it in 1983 because lawsuits and the associated adverse publicity made it economically infeasible to continue marketing the drug.

The nurse should always be aware of the strong psychological factors involved in nausea and vomiting. Comfort measures are very important for these patients. Noxious environmental stimuli—for example, odors, noise, vibrations—can aggravate the patient's symptoms. The patient should have ready access to an emesis basin or bathroom, clean, comfortable, and odor-free surroundings, and a great deal of support and encouragement. The nauseated patient should not be expected to eat routine meals but should be offered small frequent meals—usually consisting of anything that the patient thinks he can eat. Frequent mouth care, sips of ice water, and a cool face cloth can also be very comforting for the nauseated patient. Careful attention to these factors can facilitate the therapeutic effectiveness of the antiemetic drugs and lessen the patient's discomfort.

Drug digests

Dimenhydrinate USP (Dramamine)

Actions and indications. This antiemetic agent was tested originally as an antihistaminic agent for allergy but is employed mainly for its central nervous system action against motion sickness symptoms. In addition to preventing and relieving seasickness, airsickness, and so forth, this drug is used in various medical and surgical conditions marked by vestibular dysfunction. Such conditions include Meniere's syndrome, labyrinthitis, and streptomycin toxicity. The drug is also claimed to control nausea and vomiting in pregnancy and following anesthesia.

Adverse effects, cautions, and contraindications. Side-effects are few, except for drowsiness in some patients. People who intend to operate vehicles or other motorized machinery are warned that their efficiency may be impaired.

Dosage and administration. Adults may take 25 to 50 mg every 6 to 8 hours orally. If tablet or liquid forms cannot be retained, the drug may be administered parenterally, especially when prompt action is desired. Children may receive from 25% of the adult dose to the full amount, in some cases.

Prochlorperazine maleate USP (Compazine)

Actions and indications. This potent phenothiazine tranquilizer is used not only in psychiatry but also as an antiemetic in medicine, surgery, and obstetrics to control nausea, retching, and vomiting. It is believed to act by blocking the effects of circulating emetic chemicals on the chemoreceptor trigger zone (CTZ). Thus, it is probably more effective than the nonphenothiazine antiemetics against vomiting caused by radiation and nitrogen mustard therapy of cancer, uremia, hepatitis, infections, and drugs such as anesthetics and narcotics. It is probably not as effective against motion sickness.

Adverse effects, cautions, and contraindications. The drugs of this class are used with caution in children and avoided in pregnant women because of the high incidence and severity of side-effects caused by extrapyramidal motor system stimulation. Prochlorperazine and other drugs of its class are reserved for cautious use in cases of hyper-remesis gravidarum not readily controlled by other measures. It is used during labor and postpartum but is not given in eclampsia. Children receive the lowest effective dosage, and parents are cautioned not to exceed the prescribed dosage.

Dosage and administration. Treatment is begun with the lowest dose of this drug and adjusted in accordance with the patient's response. Dosage for antiemesis is much smaller than the amounts often required by psychotic patients. The drug is administered orally, and parenterally in single doses of 5 mg to 10 mg, and rectally in single 25-mg doses. Children's dosage is calculated on the basis of body weight, especially when the drug is to be administered parenterally (for example, 0.06 mg/lb body weight by deep intramuscular injection).

Digestants and related drugs

Digestion and indigestion

To be used by the body, food must be broken down into simple soluble molecules that can be absorbed into the blood and enter into cellular metabolic reactions. The many mechanical and chemical processes to which food is subjected in the mouth, esophagus, stomach, and intestines comprise *digestion*. The terms *indigestion* and *dyspepsia* are not as readily defined. They are usually used by laymen to describe any one of a number of vague abdominal symptoms, including feelings of flatulence or bloating, burning epigastric pain, and acidic belching.

Gaseousness. Some people are perpetually bothered by "gas" and uncontrollable burping. However, gastroenterologists remain unconvinced that the upper abdominal distress that develops soon after eating—what people call "gas pains"—is actually caused by gas. On the other hand, these authorities do agree that feelings of lower abdominal fullness, bloating, and pressure several hours following food intake can sometimes be caused by accumulations of gas in the transverse colon and elsewhere in the large bowel. This is particularly true when poor intestinal muscle tone prevents gas from moving past the points at which the gut makes sharp bends just beneath the liver on one side and the spleen on the other (the hepatic and splenic flexures).

Most medications that were formerly employed for relief of fancied and true gas pains are now known to have little, if any, actual value as carminatives or flatus-expelling agents. Peppermint and various other volatile oils, for example, have never been shown to be useful for this purpose—except possibly by a placebo effect—when taken in the form of alcoholic solutions, or spirits, or when added to water, powders, or other pharmaceutical forms of medication. Similarly, simethicone, a more modern antiflatulent that is a common ingredient of heavily promoted products, has not been proved to be effective for relief of the stomach distress that some people suffer soon after eating.

However, when simethicone is taken in large enough doses, it may help to relieve the bloating and abdominal pain and cramps that occur in the flexure-type flatulence syndromes mentioned above. The patient must take between 400 and 500 mg daily divided into several doses, preferably after each meal and at bedtime. Such relatively large amounts of this surface-active defoaming agent are said to be free of any harmful effects, even when used regularly by patients with chronic digestive disorders. Patients with acute postoperative abdominal distention often respond only to treatment with the potent cholinergic peristalsis-producing drugs bethanechol and neostigmine (Chap. 15), and to the physical and mechanical measures also described in that chapter.

Replacement therapy

Most symptoms of GI distress are caused by organic lesions or functional reactions to emotional stress. Only rarely are they caused by an actual lack of the chemical substances secreted into the GI tract during the digestive processes. However, many pharmaceutical preparations containing *digestive enzymes, bile salts,* and sources of *hydrochloric acid* are marketed for the management of indigestion (Table 41-5).

Most people who take such products do not actually have any deficiency of digestant chemicals, and the pharmaceutical digestants are usually present in amounts too small to substitute for any actual lack if it existed. However, a relatively few patients—mostly elderly or suffering from organic digestive tract ailments or the aftereffects of GI surgery—do have a deficiency of one or

Table 41–5. Digestants and related drugs*

Official or generic name	Trade name
Amylase	—
Betaine HCl	—
Cellulase	—
Dehydrocholic acid USP	Decholin
Glutamic acid HCl	Acidulin
Lipase	—
Ox bile extract	—
Pancreatin USP	Pancreatin Enseals; Viokase
Pancrelipase USP	Cotazym
Papain	—
Pepsin USP	—
Prolase	—
Protease	—

* Some of these substances are available alone (trade names given); most are in preparations that are mixtures, and dosage will depend on the preparation and specific use.

more digestive chemicals. In such cases, the administration of such substances in adequate amounts constitutes a rational form of replacement therapy.

Hydrochloric acid

A deficiency of gastric acid occurs in various conditions, including pernicious anemia (Chap. 35) and stomach cancer, as well as in some elderly people and others who have no such serious diseases. Oddly, patients with an almost complete absence of free hydrochloric acid (*achlorhydria*) may have few GI complaints, whereas others with a relatively small deficiency of gastric acid (*hypochlorhydria*) may be bothered by bloating and other symptoms of dyspeptic distress.

Hydrochloric acid itself is no longer administered. Instead, drugs that are sources of hydrochloric acid, such as *betaine hydrochloride* and *glutamic acid hydrochloride* (Acidulin) are given, alone or in combination with digestive enzymes. These are powders that, when taken in capsules or tablets, release hydrochloric acid in the stomach. They do not yield large quantities of free acid but offer a safe, convenient, and often adequate treatment in many cases of gastric achlorhydria.

Digestive enzymes

Pepsin. The hydrochloric acid is provided to furnish an optimal medium for the action of pepsin, the gastric enzyme that begins the breakdown of proteins into smaller fragments. Some patients with gastric achylia lack both acid and pepsin. Thus, this enzyme is often administered alone or combined with sources of hydrochloric acid to aid the digestion of patients with gastric hypoacidity or anacidity. Actually, however, pepsin is not ordinarily lacking, even in patients with achlorhydria and, in any case, the proteolytic enzymes of the pancreas and intestine can break down protein, even when it has not previously been acted on by pepsin.

Pancreatic enzymes. The juice secreted into the duodenum by the pancreas contains enzymes that can attack starches (amylases) and fats (lipases) as well as the enzymes trypsin and chymotrypsin, which aid in the breakdown of the polypeptide products of peptic digestion to amino acids. Many digestant products that are available contain these enzymes in the form of *pancreatin,* a substance prepared from hog pancreas. The amounts of pancreatin usually present ordinarily are not adequate for aiding digestion.

Pancrelipase (Cotazym) is a more concentrated mixture of pancreatic enzymes that is recommended for replacement therapy in patients whose pancreas has been surgically removed. Others with an enzyme deficiency that results in the patient's failing to gain weight may profit from treatment with products of this type. These include children with cystic fibrosis and patients with chronic pancreatitis or pancreatic duct blockage secondary to neoplastic disease.

Bile salts and other choleretics

Bile is secreted by liver cells, stored and concentrated in the gallbladder, and released into the duodenum by way of the common bile duct. Bile, although it contains no enzymes, plays an important part in the digestion of fats and is essential for absorption of the fat-soluble vitamins— A, D, E, and K.

Natural bile contains organic acids that are, in part, combined into complex salts—for example, *sodium glycocholate* and *sodium taurocholate.* These bile salts have detergent properties that account for their ability to aid in fat digestion and absorption. That is, they act like soaps to lower the surface tension of the large fat globules in food and break them down into tiny droplets. This emulsifying effect exposes a much larger surface area of the lipids to attack by pancreatic lipases. By this enzymatic action, the solubilized fat is rapidly converted to readily absorbable fatty acids.

Bile salts are sometimes useful as replacement therapy for patients with partial biliary obstruction or biliary fistulas, and after cholecystectomy or other surgical operations on the biliary system that have led to a deficiency of natural bile. In such patients, administration of natural bile salts in the form of *ox bile extract,* for example, aids in the digestion of fat and in absorption of fatty acids and fat-soluble food factors. It is also claimed to have a mildly stimulating effect on the smooth muscle of the GI tract that helps to keep peristaltic activity normal.

Choleretic activity. Bile salts have other pharmacologic effects in addition to those discussed above. For example, after they have been absorbed from the GI tract they tend to stimulate the liver to secrete increased quantities of whole bile. This so-called *choleretic* action is believed to serve little useful purpose in therapy.

However, certain substances that stimulate an increased flow of a thin, fluid bile seem to have some clinical usefulness. One of the best of these *hydrocholeretics,* as the agents that promote secretion of dilute bile are called, is *dehydrocholic acid,* a semisynthetic substance produced by oxidation of natural cholic acid. It is used to help flush out the biliary tract when it is only *partially* obstructed by mucus and small stones. This is supposed to keep the bile passages free of infections and calculi.

Chenodiol or *chenodeoxycholic acid* (Chenix), a natural constituent of human bile that has been prepared synthetically, has recently been approved for the treatment of selected patients with gallstones of the cholesterol type. It is thought that this substance may prevent cholesterol in gallbladder bile from becoming supersaturated and crystallizing out. The results of some studies suggest that gallstones still in a radiolucent, or noncalcified, state disappear in some patients taking the drug orally for long periods. Other patients, whose stones did not dissolve, showed improvement of their nonspecific dyspeptic or epigastric symptoms. This drug offers an alternative to surgery in some patients with gallstones who are at risk of surgical complications as a result of age or systemic disease. However, it could cause serious hepatotoxicity, and it may contribute to colon cancer. It causes a high incidence of diarrhea. Thus, it should be given only after due consideration of the risk-to-benefit ratio.

Another drug has recently been approved for use in patients who suffer from another type of lithiasis, or "stone" (calculus) formation. *Sodium cellulose phosphate* (SCP; Calcibind) is used to prevent the formation of nephroliths ("kidney stones") in patients who show a certain type of excessive calcium absorption. This drug binds dietary and secreted calcium in the GI tract and reduces urinary calcium levels, thus decreasing the likelihood that calcium salts will precipitate out in the urine.

Cholagogues

When fatty food enters the first portion of the small intestine, a hormone called *cholecystokinin* is released and causes the gallbladder to contract and force its contents into the duodenum. This hormone and other substances that stimulate evacuation of the gallbladder are called *cholagogues*. They have little or no therapeutic value but are sometimes employed in the diagnosis of cholelithiasis to obtain samples of the gallbladder's contents for microscopic examination. Among other substances used for this purpose are *olive oil* and *magnesium sulfate*. Taken on an empty stomach, the latter relaxes the tonically contracted sphincter of Oddi, the ring of smooth muscle that normally prevents bile from flowing out of the common bile duct into the duodenum.

Sincalide (Kinevac), a synthetic substance with the same actions as cholecystokinin, is said to have several advantages over the usual procedure for promoting gallbladder contraction and evacuation by having the patient eat a fatty meal. Injected by vein, this potent octapeptide produces prompt effects that reach a peak in 5 to 15 minutes. This compares favorably with the 40 minutes or more required for similar contractions following ingestion of a fatty meal, olive oil, or other substitutes for fatty food.

Sincalide is used to prepare the gallbladder for postevacuation radiography and also to obtain samples of bile and pancreatic secretions for chemical and cytologic analysis. For this purpose, it is sometimes injected following an infusion of *secretin*, an enteric hormone that also increases production of both bile and pancreatic secretions containing digestive enzymes (see above) and bicarbonate. The aspirated secretions can then be studied for various purposes, including a search for cells of cancers of the pancreas (see Chap. 56).

Drugs for liver disease complications

The most serious form of chronic liver disease is *cirrhosis*, a condition that develops as the result of progressive de-

struction of hepatic tissues and the liver's own attempts to repair the damage. This condition has many causes, including chronic alcoholism (Chap. 53), exposure to hepatoxic chemicals or to drugs to which a person is hypersensitive (Chap. 4), and acute viral hepatitis. The cirrhotic patient's presenting symptoms stem in part from the nature of the primary cause and partly from the complications that arise as the result of loss of liver parenchymal cells and their replacement by fibrous connective tissue and nodules of regenerating hepatic cells.

Ascites, the most common complication of chronic liver disease, is discussed in Chapter 27, Diuretic Drugs, because judiciously employed diuretic therapy is the primary method of removing fluid from the abdominal cavity in which it accumulates, mainly as a result of disease-induced blockage of blood flow through the liver. Here, discussion will center on the use of drugs in the management of several other complications, including *portal hypertension* and the GI bleeding that is its frequent result, and *hepatic encephalopathy*, a brain disorder that develops as a result of disordered neurochemistry caused by liver malfunction.

Portal hypertension

Blood flows through the liver from two sources: the *hepatic artery*, which carries oxygenated blood from the heart and maintains the nutrition of liver tissue, and the *portal venous system*, which carries blood from the GI tract, spleen, and pancreas into the liver. The flow of blood through the portal circulation is often partially blocked in chronic cirrhosis. Such blood flow obstruction leads to a rise in pressure in the portal system and in the veins of the various visceral organs that have circulatory connections with the liver.

Bleeding esophageal varices. In the presence of chronic portal hypertension, the collateral vessel anastomoses between the portal and systemic veins become enlarged and varicosed. A buildup of pressure in the collaterals between the spleen and the esophagus, for example, causes esophageal varicosities that bulge out into the lumen through which food passes from the mouth to the stomach. Eventually, irritation by swallowed food or alcohol can cause the esophageal mucous membrane to break down, and the dilated blood vessels beneath it to rupture. This results in massive internal bleeding and hematemesis, which must be promptly controlled to prevent further potentially fatal complications.

Management of GI hemorrhage from esophageal varices and other sources such as bleeding peptic ulcers in cirrhotic patients can be carried out by mechanical and surgical measures or by drugs. In addition, efforts are made to maintain the patient's circulatory volume and to correct any liver disease-induced blood coagulation defects. Transfusion of fresh whole blood is probably best for restoring both the blood volume and the clotting factors that the patient lacks. However, to avoid overloading the circulation, an infusion of fresh frozen plasma or of some of the new blood fractions now available may be employed (Chap. 54).

Vasopressin injection (Chap. 20) is often infused intravenously to control continued GI bleeding. By constricting blood vessels of the splanchnic vascular bed, this substance may help to lower portal vein pressure and to hasten the formation of blood clots that help to stop flow from the points of vascular leakage. However, when administered by vein, vasopressin may also constrict the coronary arteries, an effect that can cause further myocardial ischemia and chest pain in patients with coronary heart disease. Other possible systemic side-effects include increased GI motility and reduced production of urine.*

Some authorities have recommended that vasopressin be slowly infused directly into the superior mesenteric *artery* through a catheter placed there under x-ray guidance soon after bleeding is discovered. Administered intra-arterially, the drug immediately reaches high local concentrations in the blood flowing through the liver and adjacent organs. This promptly reduces portal venous system pressure in about 50% of patients treated—a higher proportion than respond to the intravenously administered drug. Thus, bleeding from esophageal varices is often stopped without the cardiac, renal, and other adverse systemic effects that can occur when vasopressin is given by vein.

Hepatic encephalopathy

Patients who suffer GI bleeding as a result of cirrhosis and ruptured esophageal varices sometimes slide swiftly into a stuporous or comatose state. This *acute* encephalopathic state is thought to occur because the protein in the blood that passes down into the lower intestine is broken down by bacteria into nitrogenous substances that are poisonous when they enter the blood and are carried to the brain. Thus, attempts should be made to lavage retained blood from the stomach with iced saline solution.

Often, however, in patients with *chronic* cirrhosis, changes in brain function develop so slowly that their relation to liver disease goes unrecognized. These patients may show only minor changes in personality and behavior, and only a gradual deterioration of mental functioning. This may sometimes be diagnosed as a psychosis and lead to their being institutionalized if the central signs and symptoms are not recognized as being the result of liver disease. However, these mental changes—and, indeed, even comatose states—can be reversed if the cause is

recognized and the patient is treated with appropriate medications that are now available.

Management

A first step in the prevention of severe hepatic encephalopathy is to place the patient on a low-protein diet. The extent of dietary protein restriction depends on the degree of severity of the patient's condition. This measure and others, such as cleansing enemas and the administration of saline cathartics, are intended to limit the availability of the substances that are the sources of such potentially toxic metabolites as ammonia and various biogenic amines. Ordinarily, these nitrogenous substances, which are formed in the intestine, are detoxified by the liver when carried to that organ from the intestine by the portal circulation. However, in cirrhotic patients, such toxins often tend to be shunted into the systemic circulation and carried to the brain.

Antibacterial drugs. Another common approach to the problem of toxin formation in the large intestine is to attempt to eliminate the colonic bacteria that convert urea and the amino acids of proteins into ammonia and other toxic metabolites. Most commonly employed for this purpose are orally administered aminoglycoside antibiotics such as *neomycin, kanamycin,* or *paromomycin* (Chap. 8). Because these drugs are poorly absorbed from the upper intestinal tract, they tend to reach high antibacterial concentrations in the colon without causing systemic toxicity.

In patients with poor kidney function, however, the small amounts of these antibiotics that are absorbed can accumulate to toxic levels in the eighth cranial nerve and the kidneys. This is most likely to occur in patients who are also receiving potent diuretics such as furosemide or ethacrynic acid for treating hepatic ascites and edema (Chap. 27).

Lactulose. This drug, a synthetic derivative of lactose, was introduced for reducing blood levels of ammonia in patients with portal–systemic encephalopathy, including some who were not helped much by antibacterial drug treatment or were unable to tolerate it. Taken orally in the form of a syrup, lactulose (Cephulac) passes through the upper GI tract without change, because it is a disaccharide that is not digested nor absorbed into the systemic circulation. However, when the intact lactulose molecules reach the large intestine, the colonic bacterial enzymes convert it to lactic acid and other low-molecular weight organic acids.

Drug-induced acidification of the colonic contents tends to prevent the passage of ammonia from the intestine to the blood and the brain.† Ammonia is trapped in the more acid medium in the form of the ammonium ion, which does not move through the membranes of the intestine. In addition, ammonia that is already in the blood tends to migrate back into the now more acid intestinal lumen in which it, too, forms the nonabsorbable

---

* Vasopressin is the *antidiuretic hormone* (ADH) produced physiologically by the posterior pituitary gland.

---

† *Alkalosis* induced by some of the diuretics (Chap. 27) administered in the management of hepatic ascites has an opposite effect on movements of ammonia between the intestine and the brain.

ammonium ion and is evacuated with the fecal contents of the bowel.

Large initial doses of this drug help to lower hyperammonemia by 25% to 50%. This leads to improvement in the mental state of most patients and increases their ability to tolerate larger amounts of dietary protein. Drug dosage can then be reduced to a lower level for the long-term maintenance therapy that is aimed at preventing recurrences of encephalopathic episodes.

The most common side-effect of the large early doses of lactulose is diarrhea. The development of loose stools is an indication that dosage should be reduced. Later, when the initial large hourly doses are lowered to smaller amounts taken three or four times daily, the patient produces only two or three soft stools a day. Other GI side-effects include flatulence and occasional abdominal cramps.

Pruritus. Patients with partial biliary obstruction often suffer episodes of intense itching. This occurs because bile acids back up into the blood and become deposited in the skin. Reabsorption of the bile pigment bilirubin may also occur and cause cholestatic jaundice in some cases.

One approach to the problem of pruritic jaundice is to prevent the reabsorption into the blood of bile acids, which were previously released into the intestine by the gallbladder. This can be accomplished by having patients take large oral doses of the anion exchange resin *cholestyramine*. This substance, which is also employed to lower cholesterol levels in patients with pure hypercholesterolemia (Chap. 32), mixes with the bile in the intestine and binds the bile acids into an insoluble complex that is then excreted in the feces. This results in a gradual reduction in serum bile acid levels and in relief of itching.

This medication is best taken in a two-portion dose just before breakfast and immediately after that meal. The bile salts that have accumulated in the gallbladder overnight and are discharged into the intestine during the meal are bound by the cholestyramine resin and then eliminated. Patients with primary biliary cirrhosis, who require more intensive and prolonged therapy, can get rid of even more bile acids by going with little or no lunch and then taking another large dose of cholestyramine at dinnertime to take up the bile that enters the intestine after accumulating in the gallbladder between breakfast and the evening meal. (See also Chapters 4 and 32 for other considerations in timing the administration of this drug in relation to others.)

References

Acid–peptic disease therapy

Aagaard GN: Drug spotlight on antacids and anticholinergics. Ann Intern Med 82:587, 1975

Bonaparte B: Gastrointestinal Care: A Guide for Patient Education. New York, Appleton–Century–Crofts, 1981

Brogden RN et al: Ranitidine: A review of its pharmacology and therapeutic use in peptic ulcer disease and other allied diseases. Drugs 24:267, 1982

Harvey SC: Gastric antacids and digestants. In Gilman AG, Goodman LS, Gilman A (eds): Goodman & Gilman's The Pharmacological Basis of Therapeutics, 6th ed, pp 988–1001. New York, Macmillan, 1980

Henn RM et al: Inhibition of gastric acid secretion by cimetidine in patients with duodenal ulcer. N Engl J Med 293:371, 1975

Hollander D et al: Inhibition of nocturnal acid secretion in duodenal ulcer patients by an H-2 histamine antagonist—cimetidine. Dig Dis Sci 21:361, 1976

Hunt RH: Use and abuse of H_2 receptor antagonists. J Roy Coll Physicians Lond 16:33, 1982

Ippoliti AF et al: Cimetidine versus intensive antacid therapy for duodenal ulcer. A multicenter trial. Gastroenterology 74:393, 1978

Isenberg JI: H-2 receptor antagonists in the treatment of peptic ulcer. Ann Intern Med 84:212, 1976

Ivey KJ: Anticholinergics: Do they work in peptic ulcer? Gastroenterology 68:154, 1975

Lewis JR: Carbenoxolone sodium in the treatment of peptic ulcer. A review. JAMA 229:460, 1974

Longstreth GF et al: Cimetidine suppression of nocturnal gastric secretion in active duodenal ulcer. N Engl J Med 294:801, 1976

McCallum RW et al: Controlled trial of metoclopramide in symptomatic gastroesophageal reflux. N Engl J Med 296:354, 1977

McCarthy DM: Peptic ulcer: Antacids or cimetidine. Hosp Pract 14:52, 1979

Petersen WL et al: Healing of peptic ulcer with an antacid regimen. N Engl J Med 297:341, 1977

Ranitidine (Zantac): Med Lett Drugs Ther 24:111, 1982

Rodman MJ: Current and coming treatment of peptic ulcers. RN 40:74, 1977

Rodman MJ: A fresh look at OTC drug interactions: Antacid preparations. RN 46:84, 1983

Romankiewicz JA, Reidenberg MM: Current status of cimetidine in acid–peptic disorders. Ration Drug Ther 15:1, 1981

Spiro HM: Pharmacology, clinical efficacy, and adverse effects of sucralfate, nonsystemic agent for peptic ulcer. Pharmacotherapy 2:67, 1981

Sucralfate for peptic ulcer—a reappraisal. Med Lett Drugs Ther 26:43, 1984

Drugs with cathartic action

Binder HJ: Pharmacology of laxatives. Ann Rev Pharmacol Toxicol 17:355, 1977

Burkitt DP: Dietary fiber and disease. JAMA 229:1068, 1974

Cooke WT et al: Laxative abuse. Clin Gastroenterol 6:659, 1977

Danhof IE: Pharmacology, toxicology, clinical efficacy, and adverse effects of calcium polycarbophil, enteral hydrosorptive agent. Pharmacotherapy 2:18, 1982

Donowitz M, Binder HJ: Effect of dioctyl sodium sulfosuccinate on colonic fluid and electrolyte movement. Gastroenterology 69:941, 1975

Dreiling DA, Fischl RA, Fernandez O: Dulcolax (bisacodyl), a new nonpurgative laxative. Am J Dig Dis 4:311, 1959

Ewe K: Physiological basis of laxative action. Pharmacology 20 (Suppl 1):2, 1980

Fingle E: Laxatives and cathartics. In Gilman AG, Goodman LS, Gilman A (eds): Goodman & Gilman's The Pharmacological Basis of Therapeutics, 6th ed, pp 1002–1012. New York, Macmillan, 1980

Klibinger H et al: Drugs increasing GI motility. Pharmacology 25:61, 1982

Medical news: Fiber. JAMA 238:1715, 1977

Metoclopramide (Reglan): Med Lett Drugs Ther 24:67, 1982

Morgan JW: The harmful effects of mineral oil (liquid petrolatum) purgatives. JAMA 117:1335, 1941

Rodman MJ: The use and misuse of cathartics. RN 21:48; 49, 1958

Snape WJ et al: Metoclopramide to treat gastroparesis due to diabetes mellitus: Double-blind controlled trial. Ann Intern Med 96:444, 1982

Taylor I, Duthie HL: Bran tablets and diverticular disease. Br Med J 1:988, 1976

Antidiarrheal drugs

Awouters F et al: Pharmacology of antidiarrheal drugs. Ann Rev Pharmacol Toxicol 23:279, 1983

Donta SI: Gastroenterologists on the move: The nature of traveler's diarrhea. N Engl J Med 294:340, 1976

Du Pont HL et al: Symptomatic treatment of diarrhea with bismuth subsalicylate among students attending a Mexican university. Gastroenterology 73:715, 1977

Du Pont HL et al: Prevention of traveler's diarrhea: Prophylactic administration of subsalicylate bismuth. JAMA 243:237, 1980

Editorial: New strategies for treating watery diarrhea. N Engl J Med 297:1121, 1977

Galambos JT et al: Loperamide: A new antidiarrheal agent in the treatment of chronic diarrhea. Gastroenterology 70:1026, 1976

Gangarosa EJ: Recent developments in diarrheal diseases. Postgrad Med 62:113, 1977

Gorbach SL et al: Traveler's diarrhea and toxicogenic *Escherichia coli.* N Engl J Med 292:1933, 1975

Goulston K: Diagnosis and treatment of the irritable bowel syndrome. Drugs 6:237, 1973

Mainguet P et al: Long-term survey of the treatment of diarrhea with loperamide. Digestion 16:69, 1977

Matesche JW et al: Chronic diarrhea: A practical approach. Med Clin North Am 62:141, 1978

Merson MH et al: Travelers' diarrhea in Mexico. N Engl J Med 294:1299, 1976

Netchvolodoff CV, Hargrove MD: Recent advances in the treatment of diarrhea. Arch Intern Med 139:813, 1979

Northfield TC: Ulcerative colitis and Crohn's colitis. Differential diagnosis and treatment. Drugs 14:198, 1977

Rodman MJ: Diarrhea: Think twice before giving medications. RN 43:73, 1980

Sack DA et al: Prophylactic doxycycline for travelers' diarrhea. N Engl J Med 298:758, 1978

Satterwhite TK et al: Infectious diarrhea in office practice. Med Clin North Am 67:203, 1983

Sinatra F et al: Cholestyramine treatment of pseudomembranous colitis. J Pediatr 88:304, 1976

Singleton JW: Current therapy of inflammatory bowel diseases. Drug Ther (Hosp) 7:93, 1982

Travelers' diarrhea. Med Lett Drugs Ther 23:107, 1981

Van Hees PAM et al: Effect of sulphasalazine in patients with active Crohn's disease: Controlled double-blind study. Gut 22:404, 1981

Weiss BD: Traveler's diarrhea: Update 1983. Am Fam Physician 27:193, 1983

Antiemetic drugs

Barbezat GO: The vomiting patient: Rational approach. Drugs 22:246, 1981

Belleville JW, Bross IDJ, Howland WS: Postoperative nausea and vomiting: Evaluation of antiemetic drugs. JAMA 172:1488, 1960

Borison HL, Wang SC: Physiology and pharmacology of vomiting. Pharmacol Rev 5:193, 1953

Boyd EM: Antiemetic action of prochlorperazine (Compazine). Can Med Assoc J 76:286, 1957

Chinn HI, Smith PK: Motion sickness. Pharmacol Rev 7:33, 1955

Codero JF: Is Bendectin a teratogen? JAMA 245:2307, 1981

Gralla RJ: Antiemetic efficacy of high-dose metoclopramide: Randomized trial with placebo and prochlorperazine in patients with chemotherapy-induced nausea and vomiting. N Engl J Med 305:905, 1981

Graybiel A et al: Prevention of experimental motion sickness by scopolamine absorbed through the skin. Aviat Space Environ Med 48:1096, 1976

Hoskins DW, Kean BH: Drugs for travelers. Clin Pharmacol Ther 4:673, 1963

Lazlo J: Treatment of nausea and vomiting caused by cancer chemotherapy. Cancer Treat Rev 9 (Suppl B):3, 1980

Lutz H, Immich H: Antiemetic effect of benzquinamide in postoperative vomiting. Curr Ther Res 14:178, 1972

North WC et al: Factors concerned with postoperative emesis and its prevention with thiethylperazine. JAMA 183:656, 1963

Rodman MJ: Drugs for gastrointestinal distress. RN 28:49, 1965

Trumbull R et al: Effect of certain drugs on the incidence of seasickness. Clin Pharmacol Ther 1:280, 1960

Winters HS: Antiemetics in nausea and vomiting of pregnancy. Obstetr Gynecol 18:753, 1961

Digestants and related drugs

Chenodiol for dissolving gallstones. Med Lett Drugs Ther 25:101, 1983

Hoffman AF: Gallstone-dissolving drugs: New approach to old disease. Drug Ther 12:57, 1982

Iser JH et al: Chenodeoxycholic acid treatment of gallstones and analysis of factors influencing response to therapy. N Engl J Med 293:378, 1975

Isselbacher KJ: Chenodiol for gallstones: Dissolution or disillusion? Ann Intern Med 95:377, 1981

Sargent EN et al: Cholecystokinetic cholecystography: Efficacy and tolerance study of sincalide. Am J Roentgenol 127:276, 1976

Tint GS et al: Ursodeoxycholic acid: Safe and effective agent for dissolving cholesterol gallstones. Ann Intern Med 97:351, 1982

Drugs for liver disease

Bossone CM: The liver: A pharmacological perspective. Nurs Clin North Am 12:291, 1977

Conn HO et al: Comparison of lactulose and neomycin in treatment of chronic portal–systemic encephalopathy: O double-blind controlled trial. Gastroenterology 73:573, 1977

Fenster LF: Therapy of cirrhosis of the liver. Ration Drug Ther 10(4):1, 1976

Maddrey WC, Weber FL: Chronic hepatic encephalopathy. Med Clin North Am 59:937, 1975

Martin FL: How to salvage a bleeding cirrhosis patient. RN 43:59, 1980

Petlin AM, Carolan JM: How to stop a GI bleed. RN 44:43, 1981

Popper H: Pathologic aspects of cirrhosis. Am J Pathol 87:238, 1977

Rodman MJ: Controlling chronic liver disease. RN 38:79, 75, 1976

Drugs used in the treatment and diagnosis of eye disorders

42

More than 50% of our population is plagued to some extent by impaired vision. Most of these ocular defects can be readily corrected with eyeglasses or contact lenses. More than a million Americans, however, are completely sightless and two million more are all but blind. Among the many causes of blindness in addition to accidental injury and congenital abnormalities are various diseases, including diabetes complications (Chap. 25), cataracts, and glaucoma.

This chapter will describe some of the most important drugs used to control glaucoma and ocular inflammatory disorders, as well as agents employed in the diagnosis of eye defects and as adjuncts to the surgical correction of cataracts and other conditions. Most of these belong to drug groups discussed elsewhere in this book. However, emphasis here will be on the particular agents of each class that are reserved mainly for use in ophthalmic therapy.

Nurses can do a great deal to advise patients in the proper use of drugs that are prescribed in eye disorders. They can perform an important public service by influencing people to give up self-medication for eye discomforts and by suggesting that they have their eyes examined by an ophthalmologist. Although eye medications that are available without a prescription are harmless—except to people sensitive to some of their ingredients—they are ineffective in such specific conditions as ocular infections and allergy, and are useless in such serious disorders as cataracts and glaucoma. Many people who suffer from chronic glaucoma, for example, can be spared the gradual but inevitable loss of vision if the condition is detected early through a simple test—*tonometry*, a quickly performed and painless procedure to determine the pressure within the eye.

Glaucoma

Glaucoma comprises a number of disorders that have in common an abnormally high intraocular pressure. The buildup of excessive pressure within the eye leads to progressive loss of vision resulting from damage to the optic nerve. Once a diagnosis of glaucoma is made, the physician tries to limit the extent of nerve fiber destruction and atrophy by ordering treatment measures that are aimed at lowering the intraocular pressure. Such treatment may be surgical, medical, or a combination of both, depending on the type of glaucoma with which the patient is afflicted.

Types of glaucoma

Normal intraocular pressure (below 20 mm Hg) reflects the presence and push of fluids that form naturally within the eye. Aqueous humor, one of the fluids that is secreted by cells of the ciliary processes, enters the posterior chamber of the eye and then passes through the pupil into the anterior chamber of the eye (Fig. 42-1). It drains out of the anterior chamber through the trabeculae in the anterior chamber angle, enters the canal of Schlemm, and ultimately passes into the venous circulation. The processes of secretion and reabsorption go on all the time; normally, the amount of fluid that is secreted equals the amount that drains away. Any abnormality that interferes with the normal functioning of this ocular hydraulic system, so that more fluid enters the eye than can leave it, leads to an increase in intraocular pressure.

Secondary glaucoma

Sometimes, such a rise in pressure within the eye occurs during an infection as a result of inflammatory processes that close off the drainage channels. This type of *secondary*

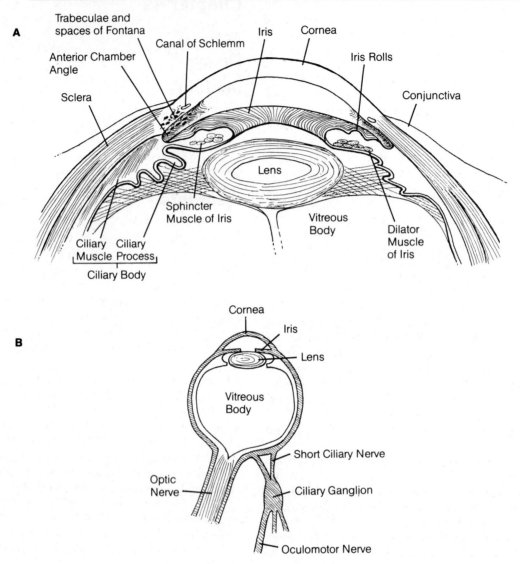

Figure 1. (*A*) The eye in cross section. An attack of glaucoma can occur when the folds of the iris and the ciliary processes crowd into the angle and block the outflow of fluid from the eye; (*B*) innervation of the eye.

glaucoma usually responds to treatment with *corticosteroid* and *anti-infective agents.* Once this and other temporary causes of a mechanical drainage block have been eliminated, secondary glaucoma usually clears up promptly. On the other hand, glaucoma that occurs as a result of such mechanical factors as dislocation of a lens or from its loss or absence (aphakic glaucoma) usually requires surgical correction as well as medical measures.

Primary glaucoma

A more common cause of glaucoma is some basic structural defect in the anterior chamber of the eye. Such so-called *primary glaucoma* takes two forms: the *narrow-,* or *closed-angle* type, and the *wide-,* or *open-angle* type. The angle referred to is the space between the base of the

iris and the place at which the cornea contacts the scleral coat, or outside layer, of the eye (Fig. 42-1). This angle contains the canal of Schlemm, a large outflow channel, and the spaces of Fontana—a meshwork of smaller openings also called the trabeculum, or the trabecular meshwork. Fluid normally filters through perforations in these layers of connective tissue and flows out of the angle by way of the main channel leading to venous outlets on the eyes' surfaces.

Narrow-angle glaucoma. Some people are born with shallow angles, which can be detected with an instrument called a *gonioscope* that allows the ophthalmologist to look directly into the angle of the anterior eye chambers by means of a mirror. Circumstances sometimes cause a narrow angle to become even more crowded, resulting in partial or complete blockage of fluid outflow and in a sharp rise in intraocular tension. Pressure following sudden angle closure can rapidly go from nearly normal to levels so elevated that permanent damage may develop within hours of onset of an attack.

A common cause of excessive crowding of the angle, leading to acute blockage, is dilation of the pupil. When this window in the iris widens, the folds of that colored curtain roll back into the already narrow angle and cut off fluid outflow (Fig. 42-1). This is why *acute attacks* are sometimes set off by emotional disturbances, in which sympathoadrenal discharge leads to pupillary dilation. For this reason *mydriatic* (pupil-dilating) drugs such as *atropine* are *always contraindicated* in glaucoma patients with a previously discovered narrow angle.

The nurse should make every effort to reduce the chance of a mydriatic drug solution being instilled accidentally into the eye of a patient with narrow-angle glaucoma by labeling the patient's chart and Kardex. The pupillary dilation and blockade of the drainage canals by the thickening root of the iris and by the relaxing (or paralyzed) ciliary muscle that result from the use of these drugs can set off an acute glaucoma attack (Fig. 42-1). This is not only extremely painful but can lead to permanent blindness, unless the high intraocular pressure is promptly reduced by surgical or medical measures (see below).

Paradoxically, strong miotic agents such as the long-acting anticholinesterase drugs discussed below can also trigger an angle-closure attack in narrow-angled eyes. These drugs do so by their powerful actions on the iris and on the muscles that control lens movements. This leads to tight contact between the back of the iris and the front of the lens, and prevents the aqueous fluid formed in the posterior chamber from reaching and passing out of the pupil, through which it ordinarily enters the anterior chamber. Such drug-induced *pupillary block* traps the fluid behind the iris and pushes it forward against the trabecular meshwork, thus closing the corneoscleral angle.

Open-angle (chronic simple) glaucoma. In this form of glaucoma, the angle of the anterior chamber is normally deep, or wide. It is thought, however, that the network of pores in the sclerocorneal structure somehow becomes blocked, thus reducing the rate of drainage into Schlemm's canal. In any case, intraocular pressure gradually increases. This often occurs so slowly and painlessly that most persons are unaware of any loss of vision until late in the course of the disease. By that time, steady pressure on the optic nerve may have irreversibly injured large numbers of axons. These axons will then no longer conduct visual impulses, and visual defects occur. This insidious form of the disease is a far more common cause of blindness than narrow-angle glaucoma.

Approximately 50,000 people in this country are completely blind from chronic simple glaucoma. Another 150,000 have lost the sight of one eye and live in fear of total blindness. An estimated one million more—mostly people over 40 years old—have this condition without being aware of it. The *routine use of mydriatic drugs is contraindicated* in patients of this age group, because these agents may precipitate acute attacks in these especially susceptible people. Such attacks are similar to those seen in narrow-angle glaucoma. However, patients with previously diagnosed open-angle glaucoma who are under treatment with the medications discussed in the following section, are not likely to suffer sudden angle closure if they must be treated simultaneously with systemically acting drugs that dilate the pupils, such as the anticholinergic drugs employed in peptic ulcer (Chaps. 16 and 41) and before general anesthesia (Chap. 52).

Drug treatment

Early detection is important because the longer the process goes on, the greater is the extent of visual loss. However, the progress of this blinding disease is often halted by drug treatment or by a relatively simple surgical procedure called *iridectomy*, in which a new drainage channel for intraocular fluid is made by cutting out a part of the iris.

The ophthalmologist must differentiate between narrow-angle and open-angle glaucoma, because treatment in the two conditions is usually quite different. Open-angle glaucoma is often controlled for long periods by the use of *miotic agents*, drugs that constrict the pupil. In narrow-angle glaucoma, on the other hand, treatment with miotics is a stopgap measure prior to surgery, which is the best treatment for most such patients. The weak miotics discussed in the next section do not offer adequate control of pressure in narrow-angle glaucoma, and the more powerful drugs of this type may sometimes cause a paradoxical *rise* in pressure in these patients.

Miotic drugs

Manner of action. The drugs most commonly employed to increase the rate of fluid drainage in glaucoma are the miotics (Table 42-1). These are mainly *cholinergic agents* (Chap. 15) that directly or indirectly cause the sphincter muscles of the iris and of the ciliary body to contract. This pulls these structures away from the angle and seems to open up the meshwork of small channels that drain into Schlemm's canal. Constriction of the pupil also tends to thin the iris and pull its folds and its root out of the angle. These and other local ocular actions lead to the desired reduction in intraocular pressure in cases of acute angle-closure glaucoma. The manner by which miotics bring about improvement in open-angle glaucoma is still uncertain. These drugs are thought to increase outflow facility in such cases by somehow opening or widening previously closed or narrowed trabecular channels.

Table 42–1. Miotics

Official or generic name	Trade name or synonym	Usual adult dosage and administration	Comments
Short-acting parasympathomimetic drugs			
Acetylcholine chloride, intraocular	Miochol Intraocular	0.5–2 ml of 1:100 solution	Used during cataract and other types of eye surgery to produce brief miosis
Carbachol, intraocular	Miostat Intraocular	0.5 ml of 0.01% solution	
Carbachol, topical	Carbacel; Isopto Carbachol	One or two drops of 0.75–3.0% solution; one to four times daily	Substitute for pilocarpine in some circumstances
Pilocarpine HCl USP	Isopto Carpine; Pilocar	One or two drops of 0.25–10% solution; one to six times daily	See Drug digest
Pilocarpine ocular therapeutic system	Ocusert Pilo-20; Ocusert Pilo-40	One sustained release unit in each eye; replace once a week	
Short-acting anticholinesterase compounds			
Physostigmine salicylate USP	Isopto Eserine	Two drops of 0.25% solution up to qid	See Drug digest
Physostigmine sulfate	Eserine Sulfate	0.25% ointment for application as needed, up to tid	For use mainly at bedtime
Long-acting anticholinesterase compounds			
Demacarium bromide USP	Humorsol	One or two drops of 0.125% solution once or twice daily or less often	See Drug digest
Echothiophate iodide USP	Phospholine Iodide	One drop of 0.03–0.25% solution once or twice daily	See Drug digest

Types of miotics. These drugs can be classified as *direct-acting* cholinergic drugs and as *indirect-acting,* or *anticholinesterase,* agents (Table 42-1). The latter type of drugs (Chap. 15) brings about an increased local concentration of the neurotransmitter acetylcholine by inhibiting the activity of cholinesterase, the enzyme that promptly destroys it. The resulting accumulation of acetylcholine at postganglionic cholinergic neuroeffectors in the iris and ciliary body causes these smooth muscle ocular structures to contract.

Although *acetylcholine* is not usually considered to be a drug, it *is* available as an ophthalmic preparation for use as a miotic during eye surgery. Its very brief duration of action makes it unsuitable for use to treat glaucoma. Other direct-acting drugs such as *pilocarpine+* are used to manage glaucoma, but they are relatively short-acting and must be instilled repeatedly. Most of the cholinesterase inhibitors—for example, *demecarium+* and *echothiophate+*—produce much longer muscle-contracting effects. Although their prolonged effects are often desirable in selected cases of chronic glaucoma, these potent miotics can cause many local and systemic side-effects (see below). Thus, the less efficient but better tolerated agent pilocarpine may be more widely useful than these more potent miotics.

Indications for use

Narrow-angle glaucoma. Miotics are used in the management of all forms of glaucoma, including *acute* *angle-closure attacks.* In such emergencies, prompt treatment is required to prevent such complications as peripheral anterior synechias—permanent adhesions between the iris and the cornea, which can develop in a matter of hours—and complete blindness, which can occur within a few days if the continued high pressure upon the head of the optic nerve is not reduced. Among the milder miotics employed for this purpose, pilocarpine is still the preferred agent.

The ophthalmologist instills one or two drops of a 2% to 4% solution of this drug into the affected eye repeatedly. This is ordinarily effective for breaking the attack before ocular structures can become clogged with exudates. However, if treatment has been delayed too long, and the sphincter muscle of the iris has become paralyzed, instilling pilocarpine at frequent intervals will not work in the dilated eye. That is, the miotic may then be unable to make this iris muscle contract in the manner required to cause miosis and pull the structure away from the blocked trabecular meshwork.

In such situations it is undesirable to flood the eye with more and more of the miotic, because this can cause both local ocular complications and systemic cholinergic-type toxic signs and symptoms. Instead, it is probably best to reduce the intraocular pressure with hyperosmotic agents such as oral glycerin or the intravenously administered carbonic anhydrase inhibitor-type and osmotic-type diuretics (see below). Often, after these drugs have rapidly reduced the intraocular pressure, the iris sphincter regains its responsiveness to pilocarpine. When this combination of drugs has lowered the pressure sufficiently, the eye surgeon can then safely perform an *iridectomy,* the definitive procedure that provides a cure for narrow-angle glaucoma.*

Other miotics occasionally applied instead of pilocarpine or in alternation with it are the synthetic cholinergic drug *carbachol* and the relatively mild anticholinesterase-type alkaloid *physostigmine*[+] (eserine). Although these drugs may add to the ocular congestion and cause some systemic effects if absorbed, they are relatively safe for use in angle-closure cases compared to the much more powerful prolonged inhibitors of cholinesterase also available.

The latter long-acting anticholinesterase compounds—*demecarium* and *echothiophate*—are *not* ordinarily administered in narrow-angle glaucoma or used to reduce the rise in pressure that often develops during inflammatory eye disorders (*e.g.,* secondary glaucoma of iritis). Their powerful and prolonged contracting action on the sphincter of the iris and ciliary body may cause congestion and push these muscles against other ocular structures in ways that can actually *decrease* the outward flow of fluid from the overcrowded angle. In addition, these cholinesterase inhibitors dilate the ocular blood vessels, which can lead to an increase in *fluid formation,* another factor in the paradoxical and potentially dangerous rise in intraocular pressure that these drugs may set off in eyes with narrow angles.

Open-angle glaucoma. Miotics remain the mainstay of medical therapy in chronic simple glaucoma, and pilocarpine is by far the most commonly employed drug of this class. Ophthalmologists who detect ocular hypertension by tonometry, together with ophthalmoscopic evidence of optic disc damage and some loss of visual field, usually initiate a trial of treatment with pilocarpine eye drops. The patient is instructed to instill drops of a 1% solution in only one eye at least twice daily for 7 to 10 days and then to return for a re-examination.

If tonometric measurements indicate an adequate drop in intraocular pressure of the treated eye—for example, a drop from 26 mm Hg to 20 mm Hg or less—the same regimen is also ordered for the other hypertensive eye. On the other hand, to control the elevated ocular tension, it may be necessary to raise the concentration of pilocarpine drops to 2% or more and to increase the frequency of administration to four times daily, preferably at 6-hour intervals. Concentrations higher than 4% are available but seem to be more irritating and no more effective than the 4% drops, though they may produce a more prolonged miotic–hypotensive effect.

A safer way of prolonging the therapeutic effects of pilocarpine has recently come into use for treating selected cases of chronic glaucoma. This involves a new system for delivering this drug at a steady rate for much more prolonged periods. It employs a different principle: membrane-controlled drug release. A commercial product called Ocusert Pilo-20 or Pilo-40 is a plastic device slightly larger than a contact lens, which contains a core reservoir of pilocarpine surrounded by synthetic polymeric membranes. When the waferlike disc is placed under an eyelid (in the upper or lower conjunctival cul-de-sac, but *not* in contact with the cornea), the drug begins to diffuse from the membranes into the film of tears over the eye. Delivery of the drug continues at a constantly controlled rate of 20 to 40 µg/hour for a period of 7 days.

The main advantage claimed for this ocular therapeutic system over the use of pilocarpine drops, which deliver an initially high drug level that then drops off rapidly, is its more constant control of intraocular pressure. Use of the programmed delivery device is claimed to result in a 24-hour response, which keeps pressure at low levels even in the early morning hours when

---

* During an angle-closure attack in one eye, the unaffected eye is also often treated if its angle is narrow although still not closed. Pilocarpine drops may, for example, be applied prophylactically to the other eye at much less frequent intervals than the minute-to-minute applications being employed simultaneously in the more intensive treatment of the eye with the completely closed angle. Most ophthalmologists prefer to perform an iridectomy on the second eye also, rather than to continue prophylactic miotics for a prolonged period, because experience has shown that that eye will sooner or later also suffer an angle-closure attack if not treated surgically.

internal eye pressure reaches its highest levels of the day in untreated patients and in those who last instilled their pilocarpine drops at bedtime. Another advantage is that patients need to remember to replace these units only once weekly. In addition, the myopia or nearsightedness that frequently follows pilocarpine drops is minimal in patients who employ the ocular system. Because the milder myopia is constant—rather than quite variable, as during drop therapy—it can be readily controlled by corrective lenses, including the contact type, which can be worn over the cornea even while the Ocusert system stays under an eyelid. (Patients are ordinarily unaware of the object's presence after the first week of use.)

Alternative miotics sometimes substituted for pilocarpine include the direct-acting cholinergic or parasympathomimetic agent *carbachol* and the anticholinesterase-type alkaloid *physostigmine* and its salts (Table 42-1). These offer few significant advantages over pilocarpine, and are employed mainly in patients who have developed hypersensitivity to the prototype drug or who have become unresponsive to it. Actually, allergic reactions to physostigmine occur even more commonly than with pilocarpine. Thus, some physicians reserve it for use mainly in an ointment form, which when applied at bedtime tends to produce prolonged ocular effects during the night after the effects of the pilocarpine drops have worn off.

Strong long-acting anticholinesterase-type miotics such as echothiophate have various disadvantages that limit their usefulness to the minority of chronic open-angle glaucoma patients whose condition worsens despite treatment with pilocarpine and other standard drugs, such as epinephrine drops and carbonic anhydrase inhibitors. Sometimes a switch from pilocarpine to one of these cholinesterase inhibitor agents brings about control of intraocular pressure in open-angle glaucoma patients who might otherwise have required surgery to open their ocular filtration channels. (Such filtration surgery is more complicated and potentially hazardous than peripheral iridectomy, the curative operation for narrow-angle glaucoma.) Fortunately, some patients who have to discontinue treatment with these potent drops because of such drug-induced ocular complications as development of lens opacities or iris cysts are found to have regained their responsiveness to pilocarpine and to other safer, standard antiglaucoma drug therapy.

Adverse effects. Most miotics cause some degree of discomfort on initial use. The physician tries to avoid local irritation by ordering dilute solutions initially and by increasing the strength gradually as needed. However, even the lowest concentrations that control intraocular pressure are likely to cause some annoyance. For example, the patient may complain of darkened vision, a natural result of the diminished amount of light entering the constricted pupils. The patient may also become myopic (nearsighted) because of the stimulating action of these drugs on the ocular muscles that control movement of the lens.

Contraction of the ciliary muscle, another expected and desired action of cholinergic eye drops, is often a source of inconvenience or pain. For instance, distant vision becomes blurred. This stems from spasm of accommodation, a condition caused by the sustained contraction of the ciliary muscles. When these lens-controlling muscles fail to relax, the suspensory ligaments around the lens loosen. The lens becomes more globular and is forced forward. It is then fixed for near vision and fails to flatten out as it must to bring distant objects into focus. Long-continued contraction of the ciliary muscles by the potent cholinesterase inhibitors often leads to aching in the eye, brow, and head.

These strong miotics can also cause serious changes in ocular structures during long-term therapy, including possible retinal detachment. Iris cysts can develop and grow large enough to interfere with vision. Prolonged use has led to development of lens opacities and, particularly in elderly patients, to cataracts that can cause a loss of visual acuity and require removal. As was previously discussed, possible miosis-induced pupillary block and intraocular congestion can also cause angle-closure glaucoma.

The stimulating effect of anticholinesterase-type miotics on skeletal muscles sometimes causes the eyelids to twitch. Occasionally, enough of these drugs is absorbed into the systemic circulation to cause signs and symptoms similar to some of those that occur in myasthenic patients in cholinergic crisis or in persons exposed to certain poisonous insecticides. Thus, the nurse should assess glaucoma patients for complaints of salivation, nausea and vomiting, and abdominal cramps or diarrhea.

To avoid adverse effects on other body organs and systems from such potent drugs as the cholinergic miotics discussed above or from atropine, measures must be taken to minimize the systemic absorption of drug solutions that are instilled in the patient's eyes. This is best done by applying slight pressure to the inner canthus. This area near the nose contains the lacrimal ducts, through which the solution may otherwise rapidly run into the upper respiratory tract and be absorbed into the bloodstream. Keeping the patient's lids apart for several seconds while applying such pressure tends to retain the drug solution on the surface of the eye and to prolong the action on eye structures. Anyone administering these drugs should wash his hands immediately, because these drugs may be absorbed from the mucosa of the mouth or nose if a drug-contaminated finger inadvertently contacts these areas.

Adrenergic agents

In some patients with open-angle glaucoma, intraocular pressure cannot be controlled completely with miotics, and certain sympathomimetic, or adrenergic, agents must be used (Table 42-2). Instillation of such substances as *epinephrine bitartrate*⁺ and *phenylephrine* shortly after the use of a miotic such as pilocarpine often produces an additive drop of pressure within the eye. Epinephrine is effective in some early glaucoma cases, even when used alone without concomitant miotic or carbonic anhydrase inhibitor drug therapy.

It may seem odd that a cholinergic and an adrenergic drug should have additive effects, because they are usually antagonists. Indeed, the adrenergic drugs *do* tend to dilate the pupil (Chap. 17), whereas miotics constrict it. However, it is the effect of adrenergic drugs on the ocular *blood vessels* rather than on the iris that accounts

for most of their therapeutically desirable effects in glaucoma.

Topical administration of epinephrine constricts the vessels of the eye. This is thought to reduce the rate at which aqueous fluid is formed within the eye. In addition, the outflow of fluid may be increased by adrenergic drugs in a manner that is not well understood. In any case, the *reduced* fluid *inflow* brought about by these drugs, together with the miotic-induced *increase* in *outflow*, helps to lower the intraocular pressure further. The miotic is always administered first to counteract any mydriatic action of the adrenergic drug. The latter pupil-dilating action, which tends to force the root of the iris into the

Table 42–2. Adrenergic and adrenergic blocking drugs

Official or generic name	Trade name	Usual adult dosage and administration	Comments
Adrenergic mydriatics and ocular decongestants			
Dipivefrin HCl	Propine	One drop of a 0.1% solution bid	Enzymes in the eye release epinephrine from this preparation; claimed to penetrate better than other epinephrine preparations
Epinephrine bitartrate USP	Epitrate	One drop of a 1% solution bid	See Drug digest
Epinephrine borate USP	Epinal; Eppy	One drop of a 0.25–2% solution bid	Claimed more stable and less irritating than other epinephrine salts
Epinephrine HCl	Epifrin; Glaucon	One drop of a 0.25–2% solution bid	More potent than the bitartrate salt. A 0.1% solution is used as a vasoconstrictor and mydriatic
Hydroxyamphetamine HBr USP	Paredrine 1% Ophthalmic	One or two drops of a 1% solution	Produces pupillary dilation lasting a few hours
Naphazoline HCl USP	Naphcon Forte; VasoClear	One drop of a 0.012–0.1% solution	Used for relief of itching and burning and for removing redness
Phenylephrine HCl USP	Neo-Synephrine Ophthalmic	One drop of a 0.125–10% solution	See Drug digest
Tetrahydrozoline HCl USP	Visine	One drop of a 0.05% solution	Used for reducing signs and symptoms of eye irritation
Adrenergic receptor blocking agent			
Timolol maleate	Timoptic	One drop of a 0.25 or 0.5% solution bid	A β-adrenergic blocking agent for use in open-angle glaucoma; aphakic glaucoma, secondary glaucoma, and ocular hypertension

angle, is especially undesirable in narrow-angle glaucoma. Thus, the use of adrenergic drugs is contraindicated in such cases.

The topical application of epinephrine often causes a stinging sensation in the eye. It is desirable to warn the patient of this in advance and to assure him that the discomfort will not last long and usually does not occur at all with continued treatment. Sometimes, however, prolonged use of sympathomimetic drug solutions results in redness, itching, and burning of the eye. Such acquired sensitivity makes it necessary to discontinue the use of the adrenergic drug. On the other hand, the blanching effect on the conjunctiva of dilute solutions of certain sympathomimetic drugs accounts for their presence in some over-the-counter (OTC) products promoted to "get the red out"—that is, to reduce redness caused by irritants and allergens.

Allergic reactions to epinephrine can sometimes be controlled by cautious administration of topical corticosteroids to reduce inflammation without causing a rise in intraocular pressure. Solutions that become discolored should be discarded, because their continued use may account for development of both hypersensitivity and deposit of pigments in ocular structures during prolonged epinephrine therapy. Some ophthalmologists claim that the borate salt of epinephrine is best for avoiding both oxidative breakdown product formation and the initial stinging that occurs more commonly with the bitartrate and hydrochloride salts.

Adrenergic blockade

A number of drugs that reduce sympathetic nerve impulses to ocular structures have been employed experimentally in both open-angle and narrow-angle glaucoma and in other ocular disorders. These include the adrenergic nerve blocking agent guanethidine (Chaps. 18 and 28), α-adrenergic blockers such as dibenamine and tolazoline (Chap. 18), and the β-adrenergic blocking agent propranolol (Chap. 18). Despite occasional reports of their effectiveness in reducing intraocular pressure when applied topically or administered parenterally, none of the above drugs has received FDA approval for use in the treatment of glaucoma. However, the FDA has approved the use of one β-adrenergic blocker in open-angle glaucoma, and an α-adrenergic blocker, thymoxamine, is used abroad.

Timolol maleate (Timoptic), a β-adrenergic blocking agent, is available in the form of ophthalmic solutions in concentrations of 0.25% and 0.5% (Table 42-2). Patients with chronic open-angle glaucoma are started out on one drop of the weaker solution applied to each eye twice daily. If the reduction in intraocular pressure is not sufficient, the stronger solution is instilled in the same manner. Once a satisfactory lower level of pressure is achieved, dosage of this long-acting drug may be reduced to one drop once a day in each eye. On the other hand, if the condition is not completely controlled, the patient can also be treated with pilocarpine or epinephrine eye drops and with a systemically administered carbonic anhydrase inhibitor drug.

This drug is said to be both more effective and better tolerated than pilocarpine and epinephrine. That is, drops of this β blocker are claimed to produce a greater decrease in intraocular pressure than either of the other drugs without causing the characteristic dimming and blurring of vision of pilocarpine or the ocular stinging that commonly occurs with epinephrine. Timolol also ordinarily causes no systemic side-effects. However, because the heart rate may be reduced slightly, glaucoma patients who have a history of severe cardiac disease should have their pulse rate checked before each instillation. In general, this ophthalmic preparation should be employed with caution in patients who suffer from disorders in which the systemic use of β-adrenergic blocking agents would be contraindicated (Chap. 18).

The exact mechanism by which blockade of β-adrenergic receptors in ocular structures reduces intraocular pressure is uncertain. This drug's therapeutic effects appear to result mainly from a reduction in the formation of aqueous humor. However, results of some studies suggest that the ease with which fluid leaves the eye—the outflow facility—is also increased. Because of its lack of effect on pupil size or accommodation and the absence of local side-effects other than occasional mild irritation, use of this ophthalmic preparation has also been recommended in patients with ocular hypertension who show no signs of optic nerve damage—a group of *non*glaucomatous patients that ophthalmologists have often been reluctant to treat with miotics or adrenergic drugs. It is also employed in cases of secondary glaucoma following trauma and inflammation and in aphakic glaucoma—that which develops in patients who lack a lens. Timolol is not yet recommended for angle-closure cases, however.

Thymoxamine (Opilon), an α-adrenergic blocking agent available abroad, has reportedly proved to be useful in the medical management of acute angle-closure glaucoma. Applied topically in a 0.5% concentration, this drug causes the pupil to constrict by cutting off sympathetic nerve impulses to the radial (dilator) muscle of the iris. This can help to break an angle-closure attack in eyes in which the sphincter muscle of the iris is ischemic and not readily responsive to the miotic action of pilocarpine. In other eyes, thymoxamine and pilocarpine administered together exert synergistic miotic effects that pull the peripheral iris musculature out of contact with the trabecular meshwork of the angle. Thymoxamine has also been employed to counteract pupillary dilation caused by the diagnostic use of drops of the α-adrenergic agonist phenylephrine (Chap. 17).

Carbonic anhydrase inhibitors

Sometimes intraocular pressure continues to rise, despite combined treatment with cholinergic miotics and adrenergic vasoconstrictors. This is especially likely to happen during an acute attack of glaucoma. The excruciating pain of this condition was formerly relieved only by morphine, followed by mandatory surgery. Now the pressure is often controlled by administering a carbonic anhydrase inhibitor such as *acetazolamide* (Chap. 27) or *dichlorphenamide*[+] (Table 42-3).

Drugs of this class were introduced as diuretics for treating edema but have been largely replaced for that purpose by the newer, thiazide-type diuretics. They are, however, uniquely useful for reducing the rate at which fluid is secreted into the eye. This is thought to result somehow from their ability to inhibit the activity of the enzyme carbonic anhydrase (CA), which apparently plays a role in the control of ocular fluid formation as it does in urinary acid secretion.

In an emergency acetazolamide is given by vein while miotics such as pilocarpine and physostigmine are being applied topically in repeated attempts to constrict the pupil. Often this reduces the intraocular pressure within a few minutes, and the effect may be sustained by additional oral doses. The oral route is employed during the long-term treatment of chronic simple glaucoma.

The adverse effects of these drugs are of two types. Some signs and symptoms are secondary to the dehydration and excessive electrolyte loss that follows continued diuretic therapy. These include such gastrointestinal effects as anorexia, nausea and vomiting, and nervous system difficulties including dizziness, headache, drowsiness, mental confusion, and numbness and tingling of the skin in various areas.

Other toxic reactions seem to be of the sulfonamide sensitivity type. These include blood dyscrasias such as agranulocytosis and thrombocytopenia, and skin rashes. Patients should be watched for early signs of these conditions, which require discontinuance of CA inhibitor drug therapy. The drugs are not employed in patients with acid–base imbalances or kidney and liver difficulties. Potassium salt supplements may be required to overcome drug-induced hypokalemia.

Adjuncts to ocular surgery

Most cases of narrow-angle glaucoma sooner or later require surgery. Even though acute attacks usually respond to treatment with the combinations of drugs described above, the condition tends to worsen with each attack that causes adhesions to form in the angle. When performed early as an elective procedure, a peripheral iridectomy is relatively simple and usually successful.

Hyperosmotic agents. In patients who require an emergency iridectomy, the high intraocular pressure must be reduced to safer levels. This is sometimes brought about by the intravenous administration of the *osmotic diuretics mannitol* and *urea* or by the oral administration of *isosorbide* (Chap. 27; Table 42-4). Because of various adverse effects of these parenteral drugs, some ophthalmologists employ high oral doses of a 50% *glycerin* solution preoperatively. This is said to bring about a prompt drop in the intraocular pressure of most patients.

All these drugs act by increasing the osmotic pressure of the blood plasma to a point above that of the aqueous humor and the vitreous body of the eyes. Fluid within the eye then follows the osmotic gradient into the hyperosmotic plasma. The loss of fluid leads to a reduction in intraocular pressure, which when combined with the

Table 42–3. Carbonic anhydrase inhibitors

Official or generic name	Trade name	Usual adult dosage and administration	Comments
Acetazolamide USP	Diamox	Orally 250 mg bid to qid; parenterally, IV, 500 mg followed by 250 mg every 4 hr	See Drug digest, Chapter 27
Dichlorphenamide USP	Daranide; Oratrol	Initially 100–200 mg orally; later 25–150 mg tid for maintenance	Claimed less likely to cause metabolic acidosis than other drugs of this class
Methazolamide USP	Neptazane	50–100 mg orally bid or tid	Claimed to penetrate into the eye more readily than other drugs of this class and less likely to cause kidney stones

Table 42–4. Hyperosmotic agents

Official or generic name	Trade name	Usual adult dosage and administration	Comments
Systemic drugs			
Glycerin USP	Glyrol; Osmoglyn	1–1.5 g/kg body weight of a 50% or 75% solution orally in normal saline solution, fruit juice, or cola beverage	Most convenient agent for use in acute angle-closure glaucoma; can cause nausea and vomiting
Isosorbide	Ismotic	1.5–2 g/kg body weight of a 50% solution poured over cracked ice and sipped	Claimed to cause little nausea and vomiting compared to glycerin, and safer for use in diabetic patients
Mannitol USP	Osmitrol	1.5–2 g/kg body weight of a 15%, 20%, or 25% solution given IV over a 30-min period	Claimed safer and more useful than urea for IV use to reduce intraocular pressure rapidly
Urea USP	Ureaphil	1–1.5 g/kg body weight of a 30% solution by slow IV injection	Reduces intraocular pressure rapidly; can cause thrombophlebitis and, if extravasated, tissue necrosis can occur
Topical ophthalmic preparations			
Glucose	Glucose-40 Ophthalmic	40% ointment	Used to reduce corneal edema
Glycerin	Ophthalgan Ophthalmic	One or two drops	
Sodium chloride, hypertonic	Various	One or two drops of 2% or 5% solution; 5% ointment	

actions of topically instilled miotics and an intravenously administered CA inhibitor helps to break the attack. Later, after the ocular inflammation has subsided, surgery can be safely performed on the softened eye.

Patients receiving such hyperosmotic agents tend to become dehydrated and thirsty. They must not have anything to drink, because that would tend to counteract the desired ocular hypotensive effect. The patient's thirst may be allayed by giving small amounts of cracked ice to suck on. The glycerin solution may be made more palatable by mixing it with fresh orange juice or a cola drink. This helps to prevent the nausea sometimes induced by concentrated glycerin. (Nausea and vomiting also often occur in response to the severe pain of an angle-closure attack or from systemic absorption of repeatedly instilled pilocarpine.) Isosorbide is made more palatable by pouring it over cracked ice.

Oral glycerin solutions are also used in preoperative preparation of patients who are to undergo cataract surgery. A cataract is a cloudiness of the lens most commonly seen in elderly patients but often also found in children and young adults. There is no medical treatment for this condition, and surgical removal of the opaque lens is usually recommended as soon as the condition begins to interfere with vision. In such cases the intraocular pressure is not usually high. However, surgery is safer when the pressure within the eye is reduced *below* normal.

The operation for cataract removal is relatively simple and highly successful. When recommended by an ophthalmologist, patients should be encouraged to undergo the procedure rather than to hope in vain for some new medical treatment. (Charlatans have sometimes taken advantage of people's fears of eye surgery by selling them prolonged, expensive, and useless drug therapy.) Drugs that produce proper anesthesia and fight infection have, of course, proved to be valuable in increasing the safety and success of surgery for cataracts.

Another agent, the enzyme α-chymotrypsin (Alpha Chymar), has simplified removal of some types of cataracts. This proteolytic enzyme dissolves the lens ligaments or zonules, a procedure that is particularly desirable in young patients with relatively resistant ligaments. The area is washed with a weak solution of the enzyme to loosen the cataract so that it can be lifted or suctioned out without mechanical manipulation. Removal of the lens without force is said to shorten convalescence. Recent advances in laser eye surgery may soon replace all other forms of cataract removal.

Topical hyperosmotic agents are also used to reduce corneal edema from various causes. This treatment is sometimes used to facilitate examination or surgery when edema is present.

Local anesthetics. Ocular surgery is usually carried out under local anesthesia. Some procedures require retrobulbar infiltration anesthesia (Chap. 14), but others can be carried out solely by surface anesthesia with topically applied agents (Table 42-5). In any case, retrobulbar anesthesia for orbital surgery is more readily accomplished after the conjunctiva and cornea are first desensitized by topical application of local anesthetics. In addition to their use during iridectomy and in cataract anesthesia, surface anesthetics are employed prior to removal of foreign bodies and sutures, and for facilitating such diagnostic procedures as tonometry and gonioscopy.

At one time, *cocaine* was most commonly used for ocular surface anesthesia, but it has been largely replaced by drugs that have fewer local and systemic side-effects. *Benoxinate, proparacaine HCl* (Ophthaine), and *tetracaine* (Pontocaine) are examples of such widely accepted agents. Benoxinate is combined with fluorescein, a dye that stains corneal abrasions, conjunctival lesions, and foreign bodies differentially and facilitates their detection. All three anesthetics produce relatively rapid anesthesia of short duration. With proparacaine, for example, enough anesthesia develops within 30 seconds of instillation of a drop or two to permit placement of a tonometer on the eye surface and measurement of intraocular tension. The relatively short effect (15 to 20 minutes) of these drugs is said to reduce the risk of corneal irritation and keratitis in short procedures; for longer procedures, adequate depth and duration of anesthesia is maintained by repeated instillation.

Unlike cocaine, these better suited ocular anesthetics do not cause much early stinging, burning, tearing, or redness, and dryness and pitting (stippling) of the corneal epithelium do not develop later. Cocaine's sympathomimetic action causes the radial muscle of the iris to contract, with resultant pupillary dilation, which can, of course, precipitate an acute attack of narrow-angle glaucoma. The more ideal ocular topical anesthetics do not affect pupillary size or intraocular pressure.

Ocular inflammation

The eyes, like other body tissues, become inflamed when irritated by allergy, infection, trauma, or exposure to toxic chemicals. Ocular inflammation is not only discomforting but can result in blindness. Inflammatory reactions in some structures, such as the conjunctiva, usually clear up readily without residual effects. However, the cornea and certain parts of the inner eye such as the iris and the ciliary body may be so badly damaged by inflammatory swelling and scar tissue formation that blindness results.

Before treating an eye inflammation, the physician tries to determine its cause. Some reactions—for example, most conjunctival inflammations—subside spontaneously. Potent medication administered here merely to "do something" may only irritate the eye fur-

Table 42–5. Topical ophthalmic anesthetics

Official or generic name	Trade name	Usual adult dosage and administration
Benoxinate HCl	In Fluress, a combination of an anesthetic agent and a disclosing diagnostic agent, fluorescein sodium	
Proparacaine HCl	AK-Taine, Ophthaine	One or two drops of a 0.5% solution
Tetracaine base	Pontocaine Eye Ointment	½–1-inch applied in lower conjunctival sac
Tetracaine HCl	Pontocaine	One or two drops of a 0.5% solution

ther or even interfere with its natural defenses against disease. When the specific cause has not been determined, simple *saline irrigation* or, at most, mild *antiseptic–astringent solutions* such as boric acid or zinc sulfate are considered to be the safest and least expensive remedies.

Certain more modern medications have helped to save the sight of many patients who might once have been left blinded by serious inflammatory eye disorders. The most useful of these drugs are the *corticosteroids*. They are most commonly employed in combination with *antibiotics* and other *anti-infective agents,* or with *antihistamine drugs.*

Corticosteroid therapy

Administration. Once the physician decides to employ steroid drugs to suppress inflammation in an ocular structure, the type of preparation best suited for the particular condition must be chosen. If the inflamed tissues lie close enough to the surface to be seen without special instruments, *topically applied steroids* are used (Table 42-6). Deep-seated disorders—for example, conditions involving structures behind the iris, such as choroiditis and optic neuritis—require administration of *systemic* steroid medication orally or by injection. Occasionally, to avoid systemic steroid side-effects, the ophthalmologist

Table 42–6. Drugs for ocular inflammation and infection

Official or generic name	Trade name	Dosage forms available
Topical ophthalmic corticosteroids		
Dexamethasone sodium phosphate USP	Decadron Phosphate Ophthalmic	0.05% ointment or 0.1% solution
Fluorometholone	FML Liquifilm Ophthalmic	0.1% suspension
Hydrocortisone acetate USP	Hydrocortisone acetate Ophthalmic	1.5% ointment
Medrysone USP	HMS Liquifilm Ophthalmic	1.0% suspension
Prednisolone acetate USP	AK-Tate; Econopred Ophthalmic; Pred Mild Ophthalmic; Pred Forte Ophthalmic; Predulose Ophthalmic	0.12–1% suspension
Prednisolone sodium phosphate USP	AK-Pred Ophthalmic; Inflamase Forte Ophthalmic; Metreton Ophthalmic	0.125–1% solution
Topical ophthalmic anti-infectives		
Bacitracin USP	Baciguent Ophthalmic	500 U/1-g ointment
Chloramphenicol USP	Chloromycetin Ophthalmic	1% ointment; 0.5% solution
Chlortetracycline USP	Aureomycin Ophthalmic	1% ointment
Erythromycin USP	Ilotycin Ophthalmic	0.5% ointment
Gentamicin	Garamycin Ophthalmic; Genoptic Ophthalmic	0.3% solution and ointment
Idoxuridine (IDU) USP	Dendrid; Herplex Liquifilm; Stoxil	0.1% solution; 0.5% ointment
Natamycin	Natacyn	5% suspension
Neomycin sulfate USP	In Neosporin Ophthalmic with Polymyxin B	
Oxytetracycline and polymyxin B sulfate USP	In Terramycin with Polymyxin B Sulfate Ophthalmic	0.1% or 0.25% solution
Sulfacetamide sodium USP	Bleph-10 Liquifilm; Isopto Cetamide; Sodium Sulamyd	10–30% solution and 10% ointment
Sulfisoxazole diolamine USP	Gantrisin	4% solution and ointment
Tetracycline	Achromycin Ophthalmic	1% suspension and ointment
Tobramycin	Tobrex Ophthalmic	0.3% solution and ointment
Trifluridine	Viroptic	1% solution
Vidarabine	Vira-A; ARA-A	3% ointment

may anesthetize the inflamed eye and make a retrobulbar injection of a steroid drug reservoir to reduce severe inflammation in these posterior chamber structures. Similar injections can be made under the conjunctiva (subconjunctival) to treat anterior segment inflammation resistant to topically applied steroids.

Systemic administration of high doses of corticosteroids or of corticotropin (ACTH) for a few days often relieves pain and discomfort dramatically. More important, steroids suppress the adverse early and late effects of ocular inflammation. By preventing the proliferation of tiny new blood vessels that leak edema fluid, these drugs reduce the swelling that can severely distort eye structures. They also interfere with fibroblast formation and thus lessen late scarring and synechiae (the adhesions that tend to form between parts of the eye pressed together by inflammation). These inflammation-suppressing actions of the steroids in such sight-threatening disorders as posterior uveitus, choroiditis, optic and retrobulbar neuritis, and sympathetic ophthalmia have done much to help reduce the incidence of blindness.

Adverse effects. Although high steroid doses are relatively safe for short periods, long-term use of these drugs for chronic intraocular inflammatory disorders can cause serious side-effects (see Chap. 21). The ophthalmologist who undertakes the treatment of a smoldering infection of the internal eye has to weigh the dangers of prolonged systemic steroid therapy against the chance that the patient may be blinded if the drugs are withheld. If long-term steroid administration is chosen, the same precautions are required as in other serious, chronic conditions of a nonocular nature that are treated with steroids.

Topical application of steroids rarely produces reactions. High local concentrations can be attained in the anterior chamber of the eye without causing systemic steroid side-effects. However, because long-term use of topical steroids for external eye infections sometimes raises the intraocular pressure, frequent tonometric checks are advised. (Ordinarily, steroids *prevent* the types of adhesions or synechiae that may lead to secondary glaucoma.)

Such steroid-induced elevation of intraocular tension appears to occur most commonly in patients with an inherited predisposition toward development of open angle glaucoma. Thus, if a patient's family history suggests that he may be prone to develop such a rise in pressure, topical steroids should be used for as brief a period as possible in the management of external eye inflammation. Some authorities recommend the use of certain steroids such as medrysone (HMS Liquifilm Ophthalmic) and fluorometholone (FML Liquifilm Ophthalmic), which are claimed less likely to cause corticosteroid-induced glaucoma than the more potent anti-inflammatory agents betamethasone and dexamethasone.

Other adverse ocular effects of corticosteroids include corneal perforation in diseases that tend to cause thinning of the cornea, and clouding of the lens. These complications occur not only with topically applied steroids but also with orally administered drugs. Some patients with *non*ocular disorders have proved prone to develop posterior subcapsular cataracts during long-term steroid therapy of chronic inflammatory disorders. Thus, for example, patients receiving prolonged steroid therapy for rheumatoid arthritis (Chap. 38) should be examined periodically for early signs of steroid-induced corneal clouding or cataracts.

Anti-infective therapy

The eye is subject to infection by bacterial, viral, fungal, and other pathogens. Infection of the outer eye may cause only minor discomfort marked by redness and edema of the outermost tissues and possibly a purulent exudate, or an infection advancing rapidly into the cornea and the structures of the inner eye can lead to irreparable damage and permanent loss of vision.

Fortunately, most serious ocular infections of the type that were once a leading cause of blindness can now be controlled by anti-infective drug therapy. All inner eye infections and, in fact, all but the most superficial external eye infections are best treated by oral or parenteral administration of the most appropriate anti-infective agent. The use of such systemic antibacterial drugs as the *penicillins* and *tetracyclines* has been discussed in Chapter 8, as was systemic *sulfonamide* therapy for trachoma and other ocular infections. Here, only topical ophthalmic therapy of bacterial and viral infections will be discussed (Table 42-6).

Bacterial infections. Among the anti-infective drugs most commonly applied topically for treating bacterial infections of the external eye are the antibiotics *neomycin, polymyxin, bacitracin, gentamicin,* and *chloramphenicol,* and the sulfonamides *sodium sulfacetamide* and *sulfisoxazole diolamine.* Most are available alone or combined with corticosteroids in sterile ophthalmic solutions, suspensions, or ointments. In minor infections, these products alone are instilled into the conjunctival sac or are applied to the outer tissues of the eye and adjacent structures. For more serious ocular infections, topical therapy is used as a supplement to systemic therapy (see Chap. 8).

In acute infections of the conjunctiva and cornea, eye drops are applied very frequently at first—for example, as often as every 15 to 30 minutes or, at least, once every hour or two. Later, as the infection subsides, suspensions or ointments may be applied at less frequent intervals. However, it is desirable to continue topical applications for 2 or more days after the eye appears normal to prevent a recurrence of the infection. Long-term therapy should be avoided, if possible, to prevent infections by fungi and other organisms that are not susceptible to antibacterial therapy. Long-continued topical application can also cause sensitization of ocular tissues and the later occurrence of allergic reactions.

The combined use of corticosteroids with topical antibacterial agents often helps to control inflammation and prevent eye-damaging complications (see above). However, preparations containing topically applied corticosteroids in combination with antibacterial drugs are contraindicated when eye infections are caused by fungi, tubercle bacilli, or viruses such as vaccinia, varicella, or herpes simplex (see below). Their use in acute *purulent* blepharitis (lid infections) and conjunctivitis is also contraindicated. Infections involving the posterior segment of the eye should be treated with systemic rather than topical antibiotics and steroids. The risk of steroid-induced glaucoma and cataracts (see above) must always be considered.

Viral infections. Three antiviral drugs (Chap. 7) are now available for topical application in the treatment of eye infections caused by herpes simplex virus types 1 and 2. *Idoxuridine* (IDU; Dendrid; Herplex; Stoxil) has been in use for many years for treating herpes simplex keratitis, a recurrent viral infection of the cornea that can lead to loss of vision caused by accumulations of scar tissue. *Vidarabine* (Vira-A), a more recently introduced topical antiviral agent, is sometimes effective in infections caused by herpes simplex strains that are resistant to IDU, and it may also be useful for patients whose ocular tissues have been sensitized by frequent applications of IDU. *Trifluridine* (Viroptic) has uses similar to those of vidarabine; in addition, it is sometimes effective in infections that are resistant to the other two drugs.

These substances act by interfering with the early steps in the synthesis of viral DNA (Chap. 7), thus preventing new virus particles from being formed within invaded eye cells. They are ineffective against viruses that have a nucleic acid core of RNA, nor do they work in bacterial, fungal, or chlamydial—for example, trachoma—infections. Thus, they should be used only after the eye infection has been diagnosed as definitely caused by herpes simplex. This is best done by slit lamp examinations that reveal the characteristic dendritic or geographic lesion that this virus produces in the corneal and conjunctival tissues.

Idoxuridine therapy should be intensive at first with hourly applications all through the day. The patient may have to be wakened during the night to continue the treatment at 2-hour intervals. The longer lasting vidarabine ointment requires application every 3 hours. Trifluridine is administered every 2 hours while the patient is awake up to a maximum of nine doses a day. Later, when evidence of re-epithelialization of the lesions is seen, the applications can be made at longer intervals. Treatment is continued for several days to a week after healing seems complete to prevent recurrences. The question of whether to employ topical corticosteroids concurrently is controversial. If these anti-inflammatory agents are used, patients should be closely observed for signs of spread of the virus infection into deeper tissues, as well as for the other steroid-induced ocular complications discussed above. Trifluridine has been given concurrently with many other ophthalmic drugs without evidence of adverse interactions; however, it is important that idoxuridine not be given concurrently with boric acid solutions, because irritation may result. All three of these drugs have mutagenic potential. They should be considered as being potential carcinogens, and should be used accordingly. Dendrid and Stoxil solutions and trifluridine require refrigeration.

Fungal infections. Intraocular mycotic infections are difficult to diagnose before they have evoked severe inflammatory reactions. These cannot be safely controlled by corticosteroid drugs, and the available antifungal antibiotics do not penetrate into the eye when applied topically in *nonirritating* concentrations. Intraocular injections of amphotericin B are locally toxic, and intravenous injections of that fungistatic antibiotic causes systemic toxicity (Chap. 9). An ophthalmic ointment containing nystatin is sometimes effective for treating keratomycosis, but many months of topical administration may be required to clear up the infection. A more recently introduced antifungal antibiotic, *natamycin*, or *pimaricin* (Natacyn), is said to be safer and more effective than the agents previously available for treating fungal keratitis, conjunctivitis, and blepharitis.

Ocular allergy therapy

Allergic eye disorders marked by itching, burning, and tearing are often treated with corticosteroids combined with antihistamine agents. The latter type of drug reduces the effects of free histamine released in ocular tissues by the antigen–antibody reaction (Chap. 39). The steroids help to control the exudative phase of the reaction—for example, the pale milky edema of allergic conjunctivitis is counteracted. Combined treatment with a topical steroid such as *prednisolone phosphate*[+] or *acetate* and an antihistamine drug such as chlorpheniramine often relieves the ocular symptoms of hay fever and of seasonal eye allergies such as vernal conjunctivitis, blepharitis, and keratitis.

Chemical burns of the eye

Corticosteroids are sometimes successfully employed in some types of chemical and heat burns to reduce scarring and to prevent the cornea from becoming opaque. However, steroids and all other medication are not nearly as important in chemical burns as is quick, copious, and continuous irrigation with water (or any other available bland liquid).

Industrial nurses are often called on to meet such emergencies or to advise workers on what to do in case of eye injury. Although first-aid manuals often list neutralizing agents for counteracting acid or alkali burns, time should not be wasted trying to obtain such substances. Instead, each eyelid should be gently pulled away from the eyeball and each pouch made in this way thoroughly irrigated to remove all traces of the irritant. It is important, too, to look closely for any particles—of plaster or lime, for example—and to remove them carefully.

Later, to prevent adhesions from forming during healing of denuded areas, boric acid or some other bland ointment may be placed between the lids. Other medications are applied sparingly, if at all, because they tend to delay healing. Topical anesthetics and antibiotics, for example, are not used routinely but only to treat pain and infection, and are usually promptly discontinued when no longer necessary. Painful inflammation of the iris following an alkali burn can sometimes be dramatically relieved by use of cycloplegics such as atropine, employed in the same manner as in treating iritis and iridocyclitis caused by other eye disorders.

Atropine is preferred when the physician wishes deliberately to induce prolonged rest, relaxation, and even paralysis of the sphincter muscles of the iris and the ciliary body. This is often desirable in treating inflammatory disorders of the inner eye to help relieve painful reflex spasm of these smooth muscle structures. It also tends to prevent contact and subsequent formation of adhesions between these and other ocular structures, such as the lens and cornea. (Sometimes, combinations of shorter acting mydriatic–cycloplegic drugs are alternated with miotics in an effort to break up adhesions that have begun to form.)

Ophthalmologic diagnostic aids

Mydriatic–cycloplegic agents

The ophthalmologist often employs drugs to facilitate examination of the structure and function of the patient's eyes. The agents most commonly employed for such purposes are the anticholinergic drugs (Chap. 16), which are applied topically to produce *mydriasis* and *cycloplegia*. *Atropine*, the most potent agent of this type, has been largely replaced for diagnostic purposes by other agents such as *cyclopentalate*[+] and *homatropine*[+] and by a more recently introduced anticholinergic drug, *tropicamide* (Mydriacil; Table 42-7).

The main advantage of these drugs over atropine is that their disabling effects on vision wear off much more rapidly. With the long-lasting cycloplegic action of atropine, the patient's near vision may be blurred for days; on the other hand, a drug such as tropicamide, which—in low concentrations at least—has little or no cycloplegic activity, permits the patient to read and to see close objects normally within a few hours. Thus, these drugs, or certain adrenergic mydriatics such as *hydroxyamphetamine* and *phenylephrine*[+] (Chap. 17), are preferred when the ophthalmologist wants to produce *only* mydriasis to examine internal eye structures.

However, for attaining the degree of cycloplegia required for refractive purposes, cyclopentolate and homatropine are usually preferred. Their effects on accommodation are ordinarily neither too transient nor too prolonged. However, it is important to explain to the patient that near vision may remain somewhat blurred

Table 42–7. Anticholinergic mydriatic–cycloplegic agents

Official or generic name	Trade name	Usual adult dosage and administration	Comments
Atropine sulfate USP	—	One or two drops of 1% solution	Prolonged duration of action
Cyclopentolate HCl USP	Cyclogyl Ophthalmic	Two drops of 0.5% solution or one drop of 1.0% solution	Relatively brief action
Homatropine HBr USP	Homatrocel Ophthalmic	One or two drops of 2–5% solution	Relatively brief action
Scopolamine HBr USP	Isopto Hyoscine Ophthalmic	One or two drops of 0.25% solution	Moderate duration of action
Tropicamide USP	Mydriacyl Ophthalmic	One or two drops of 0.5% solution for mydriasis; one or two drops of 1% solution repeatedly for cycloplegia	Rapid onset and brief duration of action

for the rest of the day. Also, the patient should be advised to wear dark glasses when outdoors to avoid discomfort caused by sunlight that enters the dilated pupils, which cannot constrict reflexly as readily as usual.

All these anticholinergic drugs are contraindicated in patients with glaucoma, and eye drops containing them are never used routinely without the doctor's permission, particularly in patients over 40 years old. Children tend to be quite susceptible to the systemic action of atropinelike drugs. Thus, special efforts are made to prevent topically applied drugs of this type from being absorbed. The nurse should be alert for signs of local hypersensitivity and systemic toxicity induced by these drugs.

Despite the danger that uncontrolled use of anticholinergic or sympathomimetic mydriatics may set off an angle-closure attack, such drugs are sometimes employed deliberately for diagnostic purposes in some patients with narrow-angle eyes. The purpose of such so-called provocative tests is to determine whether eyes with narrow angles but normal intraocular pressure and normal vision are likely to suffer a sudden spontaneous attack of angle closure. If the test proves positive, the ophthalmologist may advise the patient that it would be desirable to have a prophylactic peripheral iridectomy performed.

Drops containing cyclopentolate, or sometimes phenylephrine or hydroxyamphetamine, are instilled in one eye after measuring its intraocular pressure. If a second reading an hour later reveals a pressure rise of 8 mm Hg or more, and gonioscopy indicates that the narrow angle is now completely closed, the test is considered positive. Pilocarpine drops are then administered to reverse the drug-induced mydriasis and to produce miosis.

Although such provocative tests are not likely to set off an uncontrollable attack of acute glaucoma, most ophthalmologists prefer to employ physiologic rather than pharmacologic measures for inducing mydriasis. These include keeping the patient in a dark room for an hour or more, or having the patient assume a prone position for at least a half hour. Both these tests can provoke angle closure and rises in intraocular tension but are said to be safer and more sensitive than the tests in which mydriatic drugs are used.

Disclosing dyes

Certain dyes are often applied topically to stain ocular tissues and thus disclose the presence of local damage. *Fluorescein sodium*, for example, enters the cornea but leaves a greenish yellow stain only on those areas in which there is a break in the epithelial coat. Thus, it is used to find foreign bodies, locate abrasions, and reveal the characteristic branching pattern of a herpes simplex lesion on the cornea. The dye is also used as part of other diagnostic procedures, including applanation tonometry, and in contact lens fitting.

Although fluorescein and other dyes such as *rose bengal* are themselves harmless, bacterial contamination of their solutions can cause infection. Thus, freshly prepared solutions for individual use are preferred to stock solutions for general use, which might become contaminated with *Pseudomonas* and other pathogenic organisms. Sterile filter paper strips impregnated with fluorescein are available for insertion into the space under the lids. Left in place for a few seconds and then flushed out with sterile saline solution, these fluorescein papers leave a greenish discoloration on denuded areas that can be readily detected by the examiner.

Additional clinical considerations

Ophthalmologists administer drugs directly into the eyes and systemically such as by the oral and intravenous routes. They sometimes employ methods for continuous irrigation of the eyes and special types of local ocular injections, such as insertion of medications subconjunctivally and beneath the connective tissue layer called Tenon's capsule (subtenon's injections), as well as by the retrobulbar route (injections behind the eyeball). However, the most common method by which patients themselves employ ocular medications is by topical application. The nurse must often instruct patients in the proper use of eye drops, ointments, and other dosage forms that are prescribed for use at home, such as irrigations.

To avoid loss of the medication and to lessen the likelihood of local irritation, the patient should be taught how to instill eye drops and how to apply ophthalmic ointments. One or two drops are placed carefully in a sac made by gently everting the lower lid, instead of dropping the drug directly on the sensitive cornea. The patient then closes his eyelids gently instead of squeezing them tightly together. Ointments are squeezed in a thin ribbon onto the inner surface of the lower lid, which is then gently massaged.

All equipment for administering ophthalmic medications, including droppers, tubes, or plastic containers, must be sterile. The tip of the tube or dropper should not touch the eye, because the container could then become a vehicle for the spread of infection. To prevent the container from being thrust into the patient's eye if he moves, it is good practice to support your hand by placing a finger on the patient's forehead. Many hospitals permit patients to keep their bottles of eye drops on the bedside stand. The nurse responsible for medicating the patient may still be responsible for administering the drugs as well as for recording their administration. Allowing patients to keep their own bottle helps to eliminate confusion, errors, and potential cross contamination among patients when all drugs are kept in a central area.

In administering ophthalmic products, it is important to read the label carefully and to comply with all instructions for storage. Physostigmine solutions, for example, should be stored in a cool place and protected from light to reduce the rate of deterioration. Solutions should be checked before they are used, because physical changes may make them ineffective or irritating. Cloudy or discolored solutions may have to be discarded. (For example, physostigmine tends to turn pink or red, epinephrine turns brown, and phenylephrine becomes cloudy.)

Glaucoma patients who are being switched from pilocarpine drops to a continuous delivery system such as Ocusert should be asked to read the patient package insert (PPI) and then to ask questions concerning any points about which they are uncertain. Sometimes, nurses have the responsibility of showing the patient how to insert and remove these devices. One way to do this is to talk your way slowly through the procedure, inserting a unit for the patient. It is very helpful to have a significant other observe the procedure to learn to insert the unit, in case the patient is unable to do so, for any reason. The patient can be taught to first wash his hands, and then be shown how to locate the plastic unit by pulling down his lower lid and touching its top with his finger and moving it slightly. This helps to provide confidence in the ability to locate, adjust, and remove the small object. After becoming used to wearing the waferlike disc— within a week or less usually—the patient ordinarily is no longer aware of it, except when checking for its presence on awakening each morning to be sure that it has not slipped out during the night. If it has fallen out onto the eyelid, cheek, or pillow—as it occasionally does—the patient should simply wash it off with water and reinsert it.

Although ophthalmic medications, if administered properly, should not be absorbed systemically, it should be remembered that systemic absorption *can* occur. Therefore, underlying medical conditions that are contraindications to systemic administration of these drugs should also be considered to be cautions when these drugs are used as ophthalmic preparations. Generally speaking, patients should not experience any adverse effects from the ophthalmic drugs. Some medications may sting or cause some initial discomfort when they are administered. Patients should know that this is to be expected, and that it will pass within a few minutes.

The most difficult aspect of the care of patients using ophthalmic drugs is the appropriate administration of the preparation. Patients should receive thorough teaching regarding drug administration to ensure that the appropriate dose is effectively applied. The nursing staff and patients should periodically review administration technique.

The patient teaching guide summarizes key points to include when teaching a patient to use ophthalmic medications.

Patient teaching guide: ophthalmic medications

The drug that has been prescribed for you comes in the form of eyedrops. It is important to administer these drops precisely as directed. The points to remember in administering eye drops are the following:

Eye drops:

1. Wash your hands thoroughly before putting in your eye drops.

2. Lie down or tilt your head backward.

3. Gently pull down the lower eyelid.

4. Drop _____ drops inside the lower lid while looking up at the ceiling—do *not* touch the dropper to your eye, your finger, or to any other surface; the dropper should stay clean.

5. Release the lower eyelid and try to keep the eye open for 30 seconds. Try not to blink; do *not* close your eyes tightly or blink too often after administration.

6. Keep finger pressure on the inner corner of your eye, next to the bridge of the nose, for at least 1 minute to prevent the medication from draining out of the eye.

7. Never rinse off the dropper; if it becomes contaminated, get a new one.

(continued)

8. Never use eye drops that look cloudy or have changed color.

9. If you are using more than one type of eye drop, allow at least 5 minutes between the administration of different types of eye drops.

10. This drug may sting for a short time after it has been given.

11. Notify your nurse or physician if any changes occur in your vision or if you experience any eye discomfort.

The drug that has been prescribed for you comes in the form of an ophthalmic ointment. It is important to use the drug precisely as prescribed. The points to remember in administering this drug are the following:

Ophthalmic ointment:

1. Wash your hands thoroughly before putting in your eye ointment.

2. When you first use the ointment, squeeze out a small portion of ointment and discard it—this part may be too dry to use.

3. Warm the tube in your hand for a few minutes before use; this will make the ointment more liquid and easier to apply.

4. Lie down or tilt your head backward.

5. Gently pull down your lower eyelid.

6. Squeeze a small ribbon of ointment along the inner edge of the lower lid—do *not* touch the tip of the tube to the eye, your finger, or any other surface; the tip of the tube must stay clean.

7. Close your eye and roll the eyeball in all directions, gently massaging the eyelid—this will help to carry the drug to all parts of the eye.

8. If you are using more than one type of ointment, wait at least 10 minutes before using another ointment.

9. This medication may sting for a short period of time after administration, and your vision may be blurred for a short period of time after using the drug.

10. Notify your nurse or physician if any changes occur in your vision, or if you experience any eye discomfort.

Summary of adverse effects of drugs employed in the management of glaucoma

Topically applied cholinergic miotics

Early ocular effects

Stinging sensation, lacrimation, redness, and possible pain

Darkening and dimming of vision, particularly in poor light

Blurring of vision and accommodative myopia (near-sightedness)

Browache, headache; eyelid twitching

Possible pupillary block leading to paradoxical ocular hypertension (if this occurs, counteract it with an adrenergic mydriatic drug; avoid use of strong miotics in most narrow-angled eyes until after a peripheral iridectomy has been performed)

Possible retinal detachment (use with caution in patients with a prior history of this condition)

Late ocular effects (particularly with potent long-acting miotics)

Allergic conjunctivitis and dermatitis

Conjunctival thickening

Nasolacrimal duct and canal obstruction

Cysts on the pupillary margin of the iris

Lens opacities progressing to cataracts

Signs and symptoms of systemic absorption

Nausea, vomiting, abdominal cramps, diarrhea (caution in patients with peptic ulcer and spastic gastrointestinal disturbances)

Bronchoconstriction with wheezing and chest tightness (caution in patients with bronchial asthma)

Bradycardia and hypotension (caution in patients with a recent myocardial infarction)

Salivation, sweating, lacrimation

Respiratory muscle weakness (succinylcholine should not be used as a muscle relaxant in general anesthesia)

Possible mental effects

Topically applied adrenergic drugs

Local ocular effects

Stinging and lacrimation

Initial blanching, sometimes followed by reactive hyperemia

Pigmented deposits may appear on lids, conjunctiva, and cornea

Mydriasis may cause angle closure in eyes with narrow angles

Systemic signs and symptoms

Heart palpitations, tachycardia, extrasystoles

Rise in blood pressure, possibly potentiated in patients taking tricyclic and monoamine oxidase (MAO) inhibitor-type antidepressant drugs (caution in patients with hypertension, heart disease, hyperthyroidism, cerebrovascular arteriosclerosis, and diabetes)

Topically applied β-adrenergic blocking drugs

Local ocular effects

Mild ocular irritation (discontinue if caused by hypersensitivity)

Systemic effects

Resting heart rate is reduced by a mean three beats/minute. This effect may be additive with that of oral drugs of this class being taken for heart disease; thus, check the heart rate of such patients.

Caution is recommended in treating patients in whom systemic use of β-adrenergic blocking agents is contraindicated (severe degrees of heart block, heart failure, sinus bradycardia, bronchial asthma).

Carbonic anhydrase inhibitors (oral and parenteral)

Gastrointestinal

Anorexia, nausea, vomiting, vague abdominal distress

Nervous system

Headache, drowsiness, malaise, mental confusion

Paresthesias: numbness and tingling of hands and feet and around the mouth

Urinary tract and metabolic

Frequent urination at first

Hypokalemia, hyperuricemia

Ureteral colic from renal calculi

Hypersensitivity-type reactions

Agranulocytosis and thrombocytopenia; aplastic anemia

Skin eruptions; exfoliative dermatitis

Hyperosmotic agents (oral and parenteral)

Diuresis, dehydration, and thirst (patient should not be permitted to drink water while the medication is working)

Headache, sometimes severe, as a result of cerebral dehydration

Nausea and vomiting

Arm pain (during IV urea infusion)

Thrombophlebitis (following IV urea infusion)

Local tissue necrosis and sloughing (possible if urea solution extravasates)

Central nervous system stimulation leading to hyperactivity, confusion, disorientation, and possible convulsive seizures

Drug digests

Cyclopentolate HCl USP (Cyclogyl)

Actions and indications. This anticholinergic agent is applied topically to the eye to bring about rapid mydriasis and cycloplegia of relatively short duration. This offers an advantage over atropine in diagnostic ophthalmology, because the patient recovers normal vision within 1 day compared to the relatively prolonged blurring of near vision produced by atropine. This drug has also been used therapeutically to produce reflex paralysis of ocular muscle structures in the management of iritis, iridocyclitis, choroiditis, and keratitis.

Adverse effects, cautions, and contraindications. Caution is required to avoid accidental application of eye drops containing this or other anticholinergic drugs to the eyes of individuals with a narrow ocular angle, because mydriatics may precipitate an acute glaucoma attack in such people. The solutions should be used with caution, in any case, in those—particularly elderly patients—whose intraocular pressure has not been measured by tonometry.

Care should be taken to minimize systemic absorption, especially when drops of a more concentrated solution are applied to the eyes of young children. This has resulted in signs and symptoms of central and peripheral atropinelike toxicity, for which treatment with physostigmine may be required.

Dosage and administration. Ophthalmic solutions of several strengths are available. Two drops of a 0.5% solution or one drop of a 1% solution are usually effective for cycloplegia. For darkly pigmented irises and in other relatively resistant eyes, a 2% solution is used.

Demecarium bromide USP (Humorsol)

Actions and indications. This anticholinesterase-type cholinergic drug exerts a long-lasting miotic action when applied topically to the eye. Its use reduces intraocular pressure for 12 hours to several days in the eyes of patients with primary open-angle glaucoma that has not responded adequately to treatment with shorter acting miotics. The drug is also sometimes employed in secondary glaucoma that occurs following removal of the lens (aphakia) but never in glaucoma secondary to iritis or other ocular inflammatory disorders. It is sometimes used for treating the inturning squint of children with accommodative convergent strabismus or esotropia.

Adverse effects, cautions, and contraindications. Demecarium is contraindicated in acute narrow-angle glaucoma, because it can cause a further *rise* in intraocular pressure as a result of actions that add to local congestion and interfere with the free flow of fluid within the eye (pupillary block). Other local effects in addition to redness include blurring and dimness of vision and difficulty in accommodating for distant vision. Spasm of the ciliary muscles may cause browache, eye pain, and headache, and some eyelid twitching may develop. Chronic use may lead to cyst formation along the inner margin of the iris.

Dosage and administration. Treatment is started with the lowest effective concentration and maintained at the longest possible intervals. One drop of a 0.125% solution may be instilled only once or twice a week or as often as every 12 hours. Measures for minimizing systemic absorption should be employed to avoid abdominal cramps, bronchoconstriction, and other adverse cholinergic effects.

Dichlorphenamide USP (Daranide; Oratrol)

Actions and indications. This carbonic anhydrase inhibitor is used mainly to reduce intraocular pressure in glaucoma rather than as a diuretic for treating edematous disorders. Administered alone, or together with topically applied miotics, it often produces a prompt fall in intraocular pressure. This is thought to be brought about by a reduction in the rate at which fluid is secreted into the chambers of the eye.

Adverse effects, cautions, and contraindi- cations. Side-effects involve mainly the GI tract and nervous system. Loss of appetite, nausea and vomiting, dizziness, headache, mental confusion, and fatigue are sometimes seen. Paresthesias—numbness and tingling of fingers and toes, lips, and anus—are reported occasionally. Watch patients for signs of hypersensitivity, including red, itchy skin rash or hives. Agranulocytosis and thrombocytopenia have been reported. Potassium salts may be administered to counteract any indications of hypokalemia. The drug should not be used in patients with acid–base imbalance or renal or hepatic insufficiency.

Dosage and administration. Patients with open-angle glaucoma are often maintained on doses of 25 to 50 mg, one to three times daily. Larger doses—100 mg to 200 mg— may be needed in initiating therapy and especially during an acute attack.

Echothiophate iodide USP (Phospholine Iodide)

Actions and indications. This potent cholinergic drug of the type that acts by inhibiting the enzyme acetylcholinesterase exerts a very prolonged miotic effect. Instillation of a single drop of a dilute solution has effects that last for 4 days or more. It is used mainly to maintain intraocular pressure at close to normal levels in selected cases of chronic simple glaucoma that are not adequately controlled by treatment with the standard, short-acting miotics. It is only occasionally employed in the few patients in the *non*-congestive subacute or chronic stages of narrow-angle glaucoma for whom surgery is considered unsafe or in some cases that have already been treated by iridectomy. Other indications are aphakic and other types of secondary glaucoma not accompanied by intraocular inflammation. Children with inward deviation of one eye may respond to treatment when the squint is caused by accommodative difficulties (concomitant esotropia).

Adverse effects, cautions, and contraindications. This miotic is contraindicated in acute congestive cases of angle-closure glaucoma and in cases of secondary glaucoma in which acute inflammation is present—in iridocyclitis, for example. It is used with caution in patients such as those with myasthenia gravis who are taking other anticholinesterase-type drugs by systemic administration. Surgical patients should not receive succinylcholine as a muscle relaxant if test results indicate that the long-term use of echothiophate has significantly reduced the plasma levels of cholinesterase-type enzymes. Early local side-effects, including eye redness, dimness and blurring of vision, and brow ache, tend to lessen and disappear with continued treatment. Long-term treatment tends to cause development of iris cysts in some children and lens opacities (cataracts) in some adult glaucoma patients. Patients should be watched for such signs and symptoms of systemic absorption as GI spasm, nausea, vomiting, and diarrhea, salivation and sweating, and bronchospastic wheezing. The drug should then be discontinued temporarily.

Dosage and administration. This drug is instilled in the lowest concentration and at the least frequency that will ensure 24-hour control of intraocular pressure. In early cases, a single drop of a 0.03% solution may be instilled at bedtime and in the morning, or sometimes only once daily or every other day. Higher concentrations (0.06%, 0.125%, or 0.25%) are usually required by patients whose high intraocular pressure is no longer responsive to pilocarpine and other short-acting miotics.

Epinephrine bitartrate USP (Epitrate)

Actions and indications. Applied topically as a 2% ophthalmic solution, this substance reduces the rate at which aqueous humor is formed and may also improve outflow of fluid in some cases. Thus, used alone or in combination with a miotic, with or without a carbonic anhydrase inhibitor, this drug helps to control the intraocular pressure of patients with chronic simple (open-angle) glaucoma.

Adverse effects, cautions, and contraindications. Stinging commonly occurs on initial instillation of the drops. The conjunctiva is at first blanched but may then become reddened as a result of reactive hyperemia. Allergic reactions resulting in local irritation, tearing, and burning may make it necessary to discontinue therapy occasionally. Prolonged use may lead to pigmented oxidative breakdown products being deposited in conjunctival cysts, the lids, and the cornea. Gonioscopy should be performed before use, and this drug should not be employed if the eyes are found to have a narrow angle, because its mydriatic action may cause angle closure in such cases. Systemic absorption may lead to such effects as heart palpitation, tachycardia, extrasystoles, and other signs of sympathetic stimulation. Thus, caution is required in patients with heart disease, hypertension, hyperthyroidism, diabetes, and cerebrovascular disorders.

Dosage and administration. One drop is usually instilled twice daily, but frequency of instillation may vary from several times daily to only once every 2 or 3 days, depending upon the patient's response.

Homatropine HBr USP (Homatrocel)

Actions and indications. This ancholinergic agent brings about both mydriasis and cycloplegia. It has the advantage of wearing off more rapidly than atropine when employed as a diagnostic agent in ophthalmology. However, for therapeutic purposes, the more prolonged and complete cycloplegia produced by atropine is preferred—for example, in the treatment of keratitis and uveitis.

The mydriatic action of this agent is useful for examining ocular structures in the fundus and elsewhere. The cycloplegic effect is employed in measuring errors in refraction, because the partial paralysis of accommodation prevents involuntary reflex responses that interfere with measurement.

Adverse effects, cautions, and contraindications. This drug is contraindicated in patients with narrow-angle glaucoma, in whom its use may precipitate angle closure and an acute attack. It is used with caution in patients over 40 years old, who may be more subject to unexpected rises in intraocular pressure produced by mydriatics.

Dosage and administration. One or two drops of a 2% to 5% solution is used to produce mydriasis and cycloplegia. Topical administration of the 2% solution several times at 10-minute intervals may be necessary for maintaining cycloplegia.

Idoxuridine USP (IDU; Dendrid; Herplex; Stoxil)

Actions and indications. This is an antiviral chemotherapeutic agent specifically indicated in the treatment of herpes simplex keratitis. Topical application in infections that are limited to the corneal epithelium often checks such infections. Responses are less favorable in more deeply localized infections.

Idoxuridine may be combined with antibiotics to control secondary infections by bacteria. Its use in combination with corticosteroids is ordinarily contraindicated in *superficial* keratitis, because such steroids may accelerate the spread of the herpes simplex virus to deeper structures. However, some ophthalmologists employ such combinations of topical idoxuridine and systemic steroids cautiously for treating deep-seated virus infections of the eye.

Adverse effects, cautions, and contraindications. Some local irritation and edema of the eyes and lids have been reported after instillation of solutions of idoxuridine, but these may be manifestations of the condition being treated rather than side-effects of the drug. The simultaneous use of boric acid solutions is undesirable, because it can cause irritation in the presence of idoxuridine.

Dosage and administration. Idoxuridine is available in ophthalmic solutions and ointments. One drop of the solution is placed in each infected eye every hour during the day and every 2 hours at night, until definite improvement occurs. The ointment should be instilled only about every 4 hours. Treatment with these ophthalmic products is continued at reduced dosage for several days after the corneal lesions seem to have healed.

Phenylephrine HCl ophthalmic solution USP (Neo-Synephrine)

Actions and indications. This sympathomimetic drug produces rapid, moderately prolonged vasoconstriction and mydriasis when a drop is applied to the eye in various concentrations. A 10% concentration is used alone or with miotics in the management of chronic open-angle glaucoma to reduce elevated intraocular pressure. A 2.5% solution is employed as a diagnostic agent in a provocative test for potential angle block in patients with narrow-angle glaucoma. It may also be used together with an anticholinergic cycloplegic drug prior to refraction procedures and alone for facilitating ophthalmoscopic examinations and retinoscopy. The 10% solution is sometimes used to free or prevent posterior synechias in patients with uveitis.

Adverse effects, cautions, and contraindications. The 10% solution tends to cause stinging and lacrimation, which may be prevented by prior instillation of a drop of a topical anesthetic. Systemic absorption of a solution of that strength can occasionally cause a rise in blood pressure. Thus, caution is required in patients with a history of severe hypertension and signs of advanced arteriosclerosis. Vasopressor responses may be potentiated in patients taking tricyclic and monoamine oxidase inhibitor-type antidepressant drugs. Except for use in the provocative test, phenylephrine is contraindicated in patients with narrow-angle glaucoma, and caution is required in using it to treat wide-angle and secondary glaucomas.

Dosage and administration. One drop of the 10% solution or one or two drops of the 2.5% solution are employed for most procedures. One or two drops or an eye cup half-filled with well-diluted solution may be employed for relief of redness from minor eye irritation.

Physostigmine salicylate (and sulfate) USP (Eserine)

Actions and indications. The salts of the alkaloid produce miosis, spasm of accommodation, and a reduction in intraocular pressure when applied topically to the eye. These effects make the drug useful in the management of primary open-angle glaucoma. It is also instilled alternately with pilocarpine in the emergency treatment of acute attacks of narrow-angle glaucoma. This helps to reduce angle closure and intraocular pressure prior to definitive surgical intervention (iridectomy). Physostigmine is occasionally applied topically to counteract mydriasis induced by anticholinergic drugs, and it may be administered parenterally to counteract symptoms of central toxicity produced by atropine, scopolamine, and similar anticholinergic agents.

Adverse effects, cautions, and contraindications. Local side-effects include conjunctivitis and contact dermatitis as a result of irritation and allergic sensitivity. This is most likely to occur if partially decomposed salt solutions are employed. Thus, darkened solutions should be discarded.

Some blurring and dimming of vision may occur early in treatment, and long-term use may lead to development of follicular cysts of the conjunctival space. Eyelid twitching and headache may also occur.

Dosage and administration. One or two drops of 0.25% solution are instilled in each eye several times daily in primary open-angle glaucoma. In acute angle-closure attacks, one or two drops of a 0.25% solution may be applied alone or alternately with pilocarpine very frequently until the angle opens. Physostigmine sulfate is available as a 0.25% ointment for application at bedtime to produce an intense, prolonged effect.

Pilocarpine HCl (and nitrate) USP (Almocarpine; Pilocar)

Actions and indications. The salts of this alkaloid are the most commonly employed miotics used in the early management of primary open-angle glaucoma. Solutions penetrate the cornea rapidly and produce their maximal reduction in intraocular pressure in about 30 to 60 minutes. Its effects are of relatively short duration (about 4 to 8 hours) and tend to lessen as tolerance develops. Thus, this drug is administered in higher concentrations and at more frequent intervals during long-term maintenance therapy. Pilocarpine is also instilled repeatedly to open the angle prior to surgery for acute closed-angle glaucoma or for congenital glaucoma. It is sometimes employed to shorten atropine-induced mydriasis and cycloplegia, and is used alternately with atropine to prevent adhesions from forming between the iris and the lens.

Adverse effects, cautions, and contraindi-

cations. Pilocarpine produces fewer side-effects than most miotics. However, too frequent instillation of high concentrations (above 4%) can cause conjunctival irritation and allergic sensitization. Systemic absorption may lead to salivation, sweating, epigastric distress, and cramps.

Dosage and administration. Treatment may be initiated with relatively weak solutions (0.25% to 2%) and raised as required to concentrations of 4% or more. (Solutions of up to 10% strength are available but are rarely more effective than the 4% dilution.) In

open-angle glaucoma, one or two drops are instilled every 6 to 8 hours at first and as often as every 2 hours later. For treating acute narrow-angle glaucoma, one or two drops are instilled in the affected eye every few minutes in attempts to open the angle.

Prednisolone sodium phosphate ophthalmic solution USP

Actions and indications. This salt and the acetate ester of the same synthetic corticosteroid are commonly applied topically as ophthalmic preparations because of their superior ability to penetrate into the anterior segment of the globe by way of the cornea. They are combined with anti-infective agents such as sulfacetamide or neomycin or with antihistaminics such as chlorpheniramine in the management of certain inflammatory disorders of external eye structures.

Among the infectious, allergic, and traumatic

inflammatory conditions in which such solutions or suspensions are employed are the following: blepharitis, conjunctivitis, keratitis, iritis, and iridocyclitis. Their use is supplemented with systemic corticosteroids in severe forms of these conditions.

Adverse effects, cautions, and contraindications. Both local and systemic steroids are contraindicated in the early stages of acute viral diseases of the cornea, including herpes simplex infections. They are not used in the presence of active tuberculosis of the front

of the eye or in fungal disease of the conjunctiva and lids.

Dosage and administration. Acute inflammatory disorders are treated by frequent instillation of two or three drops into the conjunctival sac—every hour or two during the day and somewhat less often at night. (Ophthalmic ointments applied at bedtime provide relatively prolonged anti-inflammatory action.) If the response is favorable, dosage may be reduced gradually, but it is not discontinued prematurely.

Sulfacetamide sodium USP (Sulamyd)

Actions and indications. This sulfonamide is available in an official (USP) ophthalmic ointment and solution for use in the prophylaxis and treatment of external eye infections, including blepharitis, conjunctivitis, and keratitis. It penetrates readily into ocular tissues without ordinarily causing irritation or allergic sensitization.

Adverse effects, cautions, and contraindications. The use of sulfacetamide in patients already sensitive to sulfonamides is undesirable and, if employed cautiously in such cases, this drug should be discontinued at the earliest sign of an allergic reaction.

Dosage and administration. The 10% oint-

ment is used mainly for styes or as an adjunct to the more frequent instillation of the solutions. The 30% solution is instilled (0.1 ml) into the conjunctival sac every 2 to 4 hours. Simultaneous systemic therapy with this drug or other sulfonamides is recommended in the treatment of trachoma.

References

Ellis PP: Ocular Therapeutics and Pharmacology, 6th ed. St. Louis, CV Mosby, 1981

Faigenbaum SJ, Leopold IH: Drug therapy in ophthalmology. Ration Drug Ther 8:1, 1974

Frauenfelder FT: Recent advances in ocular toxicology. In Srinivasan BD (ed): Ocular Therapeutics. New York, Masson, 1980

Friedrich RL: The pilocarpine Ocusert: A new drug delivery system. Ann Ophthalmol 6:1279, 1974

Katz I: Beta blockers and the eye: An overview. Ann Ophthalmol 10:847, 1978

Schwartz B: The glaucomas. N Engl J Med 299:182, 1978

Wettrell K: Beta adrenoceptor antagonism and intraocular pressure. A clinical study on propranolol, practolol, and atenolol. Acta Ophthalmol (Suppl) 134:1, 1977

Zimmerman T, Kaufman H: Timolol: A new drug for the treatment of glaucoma. Arch Ophthalmol 95:601, 1977

Zimmerman TJ et al: Advances in ocular pharmacology. Ann Rev Pharmacol Toxicol 20:415, 1980

Chapter 43

Drugs
used
in
dermatology

43

Skin diseases are among the most common medical disorders. The dermatologic manifestations of disease are not often dangerous or life-threatening. However, because of their visibility, skin lesions can be a source of embarrassment and unhappiness, and they often cause acute discomfort, pain, and even disability.

The nurse who knows the general principles of dermatologic drug therapy, as well as the specific properties of the various types of topically applied agents, can help people to cope more successfully with their skin problems by employing nursing care measures that make drug therapy more effective. The nurse can also advise people with chronic skin ailments to see a physician for diagnosis and treatment, instead of smearing themselves with remedies promoted in the mass media.

This chapter will discuss the different types of effects that drugs can have on the skin, and the application of those pharmacologically induced functional changes in the treatment of several of the most common of the more than 600 known skin ailments. However, before discussing drug actions on the skin and the management of specific dermatologic disorders, the structure and function of the skin will be reviewed briefly. This will be followed by a description of the nature of the fundamental pathologic reaction patterns of the skin.

Anatomy and physiology of the skin

The skin is made up of a series of strata, or layers (Fig. 43-1). At the base is a layer of fatty subcutaneous tissue on which rests the *dermis*, or *corium*, which is made up mainly of connective tissues. On this layer is a thin cellular membrane, the *epidermis*, which consists of several strata; the most important of these are an inner layer of living cells called the *germinative stratum*, because it is the source of all the other epidermal cells, and the *stratum corneum*, a closely packed layer of flat, hard cells that have died during their gradual rise from the basal layer.

The epidermis contains two types of cells: those that manufacture a protein called *keratin,* which accounts for the hard, horny protective outer layer of the skin, as well as for the toughness of the hair and nails; and those that manufacture *melanin,* a dark pigment that accounts for skin color—the more melanin, the darker the skin. Only if the melanocytes fail to make any melanin at all is a person's skin truly colorless (albinism).

The epidermis is nourished by the underlying skin structures. The corium, or true skin, contains blood vessels, including the capillaries that carry nutritive materials and remove wastes. It is also supplied with a network of sensory and motor nerve fibers. In contrast to the keratin-containing epidermis, the corium is made up of bundles of fibers consisting mainly of another protein—collagen—through which run the blood vessels and nerves.

The sweat glands, sebaceous glands, and hair follicles originate in the epidermis and grow down into the corium. The sweat glands are of two types: the *eccrine* glands, which respond to heat by secreting a dilute, salty fluid into ducts that lead up to the surface of the skin; and the *apocrine* glands, which are not nearly so widely distributed, and which produce a different type of fluid under the influence of emotional stress. This milky secretion is odorless when it reaches the skin surface in the axilla and elsewhere, but bacterial decomposition of its chemical constituents produces its distinctive odor.

The sebaceous glands secrete a mixture of fatty substances known as sebum, which spreads out over the skin surface after reaching it by way of the hair follicles. The face and scalp contain many of these fat-secreting glands, whereas the palms and soles contain none. Excessive skin oiliness—seborrhea—is seen most frequently on the face and scalp and to a lesser extent on the chest and upper back. Oiliness is greatest during puberty, when androgenic hormones stimulate the sebaceous glands to

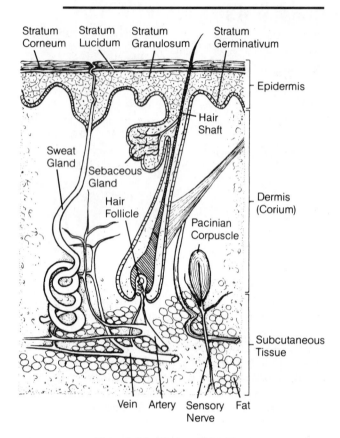

Stratum Corneum Stratum Lucidum Stratum Granulosum Stratum Germinativum

Epidermis

Hair Shaft

Sweat Gland

Sebaceous Gland

Hair Follicle

Dermis (Corium)

Pacinian Corpuscle

Subcutaneous Tissue

Vein Artery Sensory Nerve Fat

Figure 1. The histology of the skin.

heightened activity. The skin of elderly people is dry, because sebaceous function fails with age.

Pathologic reaction patterns of the skin

The hundreds of different dermatologic ailments are caused by varied combinations of functional or structural changes in one or more of the skin elements mentioned above. All the bewildering combinations of signs and symptoms of these skin disorders are the result of relatively few types of reactions. These include inflammatory responses to injury; acceleration, slowing, or even complete failure of a normal function; and changes in the growth rate of glands and other types of cells.

Inflammatory responses to trauma of all types are characterized by early redness and edema. Fluid may then accumulate in the dermis to form wheals, or it may collect within the epidermis as *vesicles* (blebs) and *bullae* (blisters). Sometimes pus is trapped in these raised, thin-walled areas and, when such *pustules* rupture, their contents form yellowish seropurulent crusts, or scabs, over the eroded areas. Deep erosions into the dermis in the form of denuding ulcers tend to develop into small pitted scars as they heal. When even deeper damage destroys the fatty subcutaneous tissue stratum, the destroyed areas

are replaced by overgrowths of fibrous connective tissue. Such scars may even become tumorlike *keloids.*

Abnormal growth rates of various skin elements and structures are often apparent. Sometimes, for example, the basal layer of epidermal cells develops daughter cells so rapidly that the dead cells of the stratum corneum pile up in high layers that come off in shreds, instead of just flaking off invisibly as they ordinarily do. This leads to *scaling,* or *desquamation,* a condition that varies in degree from formation of a relatively few light *dandruff* flakes to the disfiguring papulosquamous lesions sometimes seen in chronic *psoriasis.* This scaly skin debris may form dry and powdery flakes or thick, greasy plaques.

In other conditions, the outer layer of keratin-containing skin cells may be pressed into hard horny masses, such as *corns* or *calluses,* or viruses may mysteriously set off spurts of hyperkeratotic growth, resulting in crops of *warts.* Rarely, instead of such benign tumors, the uncontrolled growth of epidermal cells leads to epitheliomata or to malignant melanoma. Fortunately, hyperfunction of the basal cell melanocytes usually takes the form of *moles* and *freckles.* Failure of function in some of these cells occasionally results in loss of skin pigment in irregular patches, a condition called *vitiligo.*

Increased keratin formation at the mouth of the hair follicles combined with increased outpouring of sebum by the underlying sebaceous glands can plug the pores and lead to the characteristic lesions of *acne.* On the other hand, in some circumstances, these fat-secreting glands may atrophy. Similarly, the sweat glands often pour out excessive secretions that fail to evaporate. This then softens the skin and makes it subject to invasion by pathogenic microorganisms. In other circumstances many of the sweat ducts become blocked, resulting in the inflammatory epidermal reactions known as *prickly heat* or *miliaria.*

The skin in various parts of the body differs in its response to disease-producing stimuli. The skin in different regions varies in thickness, hairiness, oiliness, and the amounts of moisture that collect on its surface. Still, the generalizations made above about the structure of the skin and its basic responses to noxious stimuli should increase understanding of the different types of effects that drugs have on the skin.

Types of drugs acting on the skin

Many substances produce beneficial or harmful effects when applied topically to the skin. Broadly speaking, chemicals affect the skin in two main ways: they can *cause* varying degrees of irritation, and they can *prevent irritation* or *reduce inflammatory reactions* to skin injury (Tables 43-1 and 43-2). Although drugs that cause a mild degree of irritation are useful for treating certain skin symptoms,

Table 43–1. Glossary of terms used to describe the actions of drugs on the skin

Term	Definition	Term	Definition
Antieczematic	A general term for any drug used in treating eczema, which is itself a vague term denoting almost any type of chronic inflammatory skin condition, the cause of which is uncertain	Counterirritant	destroy tissues, including warts Chemical applied topically to the skin to produce irritation to relieve pain stemming from skeletal muscles or from visceral organs in various systemic diseases
Antihistaminic	A drug that antagonizes the effects of free histamine on the skin and its blood vessels, and thus relieves signs and symptoms of skin allergy	Demelanizing agent	A chemical employed to remove excessive skin pigment in the treatment of hypermelanosis (hyperpigmentation)
Anti-infective	A drug used to treat or prevent skin or mucous membrane infection by pathogenic microbes (*e.g.*, antimicrobials, antibacterials, antifungals, antiseptics)	Demulcent	A substance employed to coat the skin and mucous membranes; it provides mechanical protection against irritation of these surfaces
Anti-inflammatory	An agent used to reduce skin inflammation and relieve its signs and symptoms	Deodorant	A substance used to remove or mask disagreeable odors
Antiperspirant	A chemical claimed to reduce the local flow of sweat; it is usually also an astringent and deodorant	Depigmenting agent	See *demelanizing agent*, above
Antipruritic	An agent used to relieve pruritus, or itching; topically applied agents usually have local anesthetic properties	Depilatory	A chemical employed to remove hair
		Desquamating agent	A chemical used to cause shedding of epidermal scales (see *keratolytic*)
Antipsoriatic	A drug used in the treatment of psoriasis, including particularly skin irritants of the keratolytic and keratoplastic types	Detergent	An agent used to cleanse the skin; it usually also possesses antiseptic properties
Antiseborrheic	A chemical used to reduce the activity of the sebaceous glands or to remove greasy skin scales, including those of dandruff	Disinfectant	A chemical that destroys pathogenic microorganisms when applied to inanimate objects; in low concentration it may also be used on the skin as an antiseptic
Antiseptic	A chemical substance that kills microorganisms on the skin and elsewhere or prevents their growth	Dusting powder	An inert substance applied to the skin to protect the irritated surface or to absorb excessive moisture
Astringent	Chemical that acts locally to coagulate or precipitate protein; this action tends to contract tissues and thus to stop the flow of fluid secretions, including oozing, sweat, and blood	Emollient	An oily or fatty substance used to keep the skin soft and to prevent the evaporation of water and development of dryness
Caustic	A corrosive chemical used to	Enzymes, proteolytic	Biologic materials applied to the skin to speed the breakdown of necrotic tissues in ulcerated or burned skin areas (*i.e.*, for chemical debridement of dead tissue)

(continued)

Table 43–1. Glossary of terms used to describe the actions of drugs on the skin (continued)

Term	Definition	Term	Definition
Escharotic	A caustic or corrosive chemical that cauterizes or burns away tissue and causes scab or scar formation	Protectant	A substance used to protect the exposed skin or mucous membranes from irritation by mechanically covering them (see *demulcent, dusting powder, emollient*)
Hemostatic	A topically applied substance that stops bleeding from skin or mucosal surfaces	Pustulant	An irritant that causes formation of small pus-filled blisters
Irritant	A general term for locally applied drugs that induce inflammatory responses of various degrees, ranging from warmth and redness to blister formation (see *rubefacient, pustulant, vesicant*)	Rubefacient	An irritant that causes reddening of the skin as a result of local reflex vasodilation
		Scabicide	A chemical used to kill the burrowing mite that is the cause of scabies
Keratolytic	A substance that softens skin keratin so that epidermal scales are more readily loosened and removed (*i.e.*, a peeling or desquamating agent)	Sclerosing agent	An irritating substance employed to obliterate varicose veins by stimulating production of fibrous connective tissue
Keratoplastic	A substance believed to stimulate the growth of skin cells	Styptic	A topically applied substance that stops capillary oozing of blood by its astringent action
Melanizing agent	An agent employed to stimulate skin pigmentation in treating disorders marked by hypopigmentation (a pigmentation-stimulating agent)	Sunscreen	A chemical employed to absorb the burning rays of the sun and thus to protect the skin from sunburn
		Trichomonacide	A chemical employed to kill trichomonal protozoans, particularly *Trichomonas vaginalis*
Pediculocide	A chemical used to kill lice on the skin or in hair	Vesicant	A skin-irritating chemical that causes formation of blisters

the most important dermatologic agents are those that protect the irritated skin from further irritation and those that—like the topically applied corticosteroid drugs—reduce inflammatory responses in many skin disorders.

Topical corticosteroids

The availability of potent corticosteroids for local application has revolutionized the management of many common types of skin diseases. Products containing these substances account for half of all the orders and prescriptions that dermatologists and others write for relief of skin disease signs and symptoms. Before discussing their specific use in such conditions as atopic and contact dermatitis, psoriasis, and acne, this chapter will summarize the actions of these drugs, and describe how they must be employed for most beneficial results and least likelihood of adverse local or systemic reactions.

Actions. Applied topically to the skin in concentrations ranging from as low as 0.01% to 1%, all the various available corticosteroids can suppress inflammation, cause local vasoconstriction, and relieve redness and itching. Some, such as the esters of fluorinated steroids, exert much more potent *anti-inflammatory* activity than the natural glucocorticoid hydrocortisone. However, hydrocortisone, which is much cheaper than the synthetic steroids, can be equally effective when applied in relatively high concentrations. Another action of the corticosteroids is their ability to slow down the rate of cell division. This *antimitotic* property makes the drugs useful for treating skin disorders marked by increased epidermal cell proliferation, such as psoriasis.

Dosage forms. The effectiveness of locally applied steroids depends on their ability to penetrate through the stratum corneum and act on the underlying

Table 43–2. Dermatologic drugs

Agent	Uses	Agent	Uses
Substances that reduce the reaction of the skin to irritation		Calcium sulfide	Depilatory
		Calcium thioglycollate	Depilatory
		Chrysarobin	Keratolytic
Benzoin compound tincture USP	Protectant	Coal tar USP	Keratolytic
Bismuth subcarbonate USP	Protectant	Formaldehyde	Caustic; keratolytic
Calamine and calamine ointment USP	Protectant	Ichthammol	Keratolytic
		Podophyllin	Caustic; keratolytic
Camphor USP	Antipruritic	Resorcinol USP	Keratolytic
Cocoa butter USP	Emollient	Resorcinol monoacetate	Keratolytic
Collodion, flexible, USP	Protectant	Salicylic acid USP	Keratolytic
Cottonseed oil USP	Emollient	Selenium sulfide USP	Antiseborrheic
Dimethicone	Protectant	Silver nitrate USP	Caustic; keratolytic
Glycerin USP	Emollient–humectant	Sulfur, sublimed	Keratolytic
Hydrophilic ointment USP	Emollient	Sulfurated lime solution	Keratolytic
Lanolin USP and lanolin anhydrous USP	Emollient	Trichloroacetic acid	Caustic
		Zinc chloride USP	Astringent
Menthol USP	Antipruritic	Zinc oxide paste with salicylic acid	Astringent–keratolytic
Olive oil USP	Emollient	Zinc and potassium sulfates (white lotion)	Keratolytic–astringent
Ointment, white, USP	Emollient		
Ointment, yellow, USP	Emollient	Zinc sulfate USP	Astringent
Peruvian balsam	Protectant		
Petrolatum, hydrophilic, USP	Protectant	**Chemicals that affect the reaction of the skin to sunlight**	
Petrolatum, white, USP	Emollient		
Phenol, liquefied, USP	Antipruritic	Beta-carotene	Special sunscreen
Polyethylene glycol ointment USP	Protectant	Cinoxate	Chemical sunscreen
		Digalloyl trioleate	Chemical sunscreen
Silicone	Protectant	Dioxybenzone USP	Chemical sunscreen
Starch USP	Dusting powder	Ethylhexyl p-methoxycinnamate	Chemical sunscreen
Starch, glycerite	Emollient		
Talc USP	Dusting powder	Glyceryl p-aminobenzoate	Chemical sunscreen
Titanium dioxide USP	Protectant	Homosalate	Chemical sunscreen
Zinc, gelatin, USP	Protectant	Hydroquinone USP	Depigmenting agent
Zinc oxide USP	Protectant	Methyl anthranilate	Chemical sunscreen
Zinc stearate USP	Dusting powder	Methoxsalen USP	Repigmenting agent–photosensitizer
Zirconium oxide	Protectant		
		Monobenzone	Depigmenting agent
Chemicals that cause local irritation		Octyldimethyl-para-aminobenzoate	Chemical sunscreen
Alcohol, rubbing (ethyl and isopropyl) USP	Rubefacient	Octylsalicylate	Chemical sunscreen
Alum USP	Astringent–Antiperspirant	Oxybenzone USP	Chemical sunscreen
		Padimate A	Chemical sunscreen
Aluminum acetate USP	Astringent–antiperspirant	Padimate O (octyl dimethyl PABA)	Chemical sunscreen
Aluminum chloride USP	Astringent–antiperspirant	Para-aminobenzoic acid	Chemical sunscreen
		Petroleum, red, veterinary	Physical sunscreen
Aluminum subacetate USP	Astringent–antiperspirant	Titanium dioxide USP	Sunscreen (physical; opaque)
Anthralin USP	Keratolytic	Trioxsalen USP	Repigmenting agent
Cadmium sulfide	Antiseborrheic	Zinc oxide USP	Sunscreen (physical; opaque)
Calcium hydroxide USP	Astringent		

epidermal layers. Various vehicles, including creams, ointments, lotions, and aerosol sprays are employed for delivering these drugs to their sites of action (Table 43-3). Ointment bases seem best for producing prolonged local activity, and help to soothe skin that is excessively dry. Steroid creams are somewhat less effective but, because these vehicles disappear into the skin, patients often prefer them to the greasy ointments. Lotion vehicles also offer a cosmetic advantage and are preferred for application of corticosteroids to the scalp and to other hairy areas. Aerosol sprays are a convenient but somewhat wasteful way to apply these drugs to the skin and scalp.

Occlusive dressings. Penetration of a steroid such as hydrocortisone can be increased about tenfold by covering the area of application with an impermeable plastic. This prevents skin moisture from evaporating and retains body heat. As a result, the scaly outer layers of the skin are softened and the drug diffuses into the deeper parts of the epidermis and into the dermis. The plastic covering is kept on for several hours and is then removed to prevent prickly heat lesions (miliaria) and maceration that may make the skin more prone to microbial infections.

Adverse effects. *Systemic toxicity,* such as Cushingoid signs and symptoms and suppression of adrenal function (Chap. 21), is possible but actually occurs very rarely with topically applied steroids. Ordinarily, very little drug is absorbed into the systemic circulation. However, if a patient has had large inflamed areas of the skin covered with a potent corticosteroid for long periods, and particularly when occlusive dressings are employed, the risk of adrenal suppression is increased. If such a patient requires surgery, or suffers from some other form of stress, systemic steroid medication should be given to help prevent acute adrenal crisis.

Local side-effects—other than those that may occur with excessive use of occlusive dressings—are uncommon. Corticosteroids cause little or no local irritation or sensitization. However, because some of the substances contained in the vehicles may be irritating or sensitizing, patients may occasionally complain of skin burning or itching, and this can make it necessary to discontinue further use of the topical steroid product. These topical preparations are not intended for use in the eyes, and caution should be exercised to keep them out of the eyes.

Table 43–3. Some topically applied corticosteroids

Official or generic name	Trade name	Dosage forms				
		Aerosol	Cream	Gel	Lotion	Ointment
Amcinonide	Cyclocort		✓			✓
Betamethasone USP	Celestone		✓			
Betamethazone benzoate	Benisone		✓	✓	✓	✓
Betamethasone dipropionate	Diprosone		✓		✓	
Betamethasone valerate USP	Valisone		✓		✓	✓
Clocortolone pivalate	Cloderm		✓			
Desonide	Tridesilon		✓			✓
Desoximetasone	Topicort		✓	✓		
Dexamethasone USP	Hexadrol	✓	✓	✓		
Dexamethasone sodium phosphate USP	Decadron phosphate		✓			
Diflorasone diacetate	Florone		✓			✓
Flumethasone pivalate	Locorten		✓			
Fluocinolone acetonide USP	Fluonid; Synalar		✓			✓
Fluocinonide	Lidex		✓	✓		✓
Fluorometholone USP	Oxylone		✓			
Flurandrenolide	Cordran		✓		✓	✓
Hydrocortisone USP	Cetacort; Cort-Dome; Cortril	✓	✓		✓	✓
Hydrocortisone acetate USP	Cortef Acetate; Hydrocortone Acetate	✓	✓		✓	✓
Methylprednisolone acetate USP	Medrol Acetate					✓
Prednisolone USP	Meti-Derm		✓			
Triamcinolone acetonide USP	Aristocort; Kenalog	✓	✓		✓	✓

Rarely, the prolonged application of steroids to the face results in development of a rosacealike rash or an acneiform eruption. Sometimes a secondary infection occurs that requires concomitant treatment with a topical antimicrobial preparation (see below). However, if such an infection is not controlled by antibacterial or antifungal therapy, the topical corticosteroid should be discontinued. Such preparations may aid the spread of virus particles and therefore must never be used in the presence of chickenpox or cowpox lesions, or herpes virus infections.

Clinical indications. Some dermatologic disorders are more responsive than others to topical steroid therapy. Symptomatic relief occurs most readily—for example, in atopic and seborrheic dermatitis and in the nonweeping stages of contact dermatitis. Some skin areas are easier to treat than others—for instance, the thinner, more readily penetrated skin of the eyelids, face, scalp, scrotum, and groin. Areas of thickened skin such as the elbows, knees, palms, and soles require occlusive dressings to ensure adequate steroid penetration—for example, in treating the stubborn lesions of psoriasis (see below). Some disorders respond only to intradermal injection of corticosteroids directly into the lesions (see below, Acne: Topical Treatment—Corticosteroids).

Mechanical and physical protectives

Chemicals may *prevent irritation* of the skin or reduce pathologic reactions to skin-damaging chemical and physical factors. Some substances of this sort cover the skin mechanically; others act to make it softer, more pliable, and less subject to excessive dryness. Such topically applied agents soothe the skin. They either prevent loss of moisture or prevent irritating substances from contacting the skin. These protective chemicals come in the form of ointments, pastes, creams, lotions, and dusting powders. Sometimes they are added to bath water so that a protective residue forms on the skin. In general, such preparations are applied sparingly, otherwise they are both messy and wasteful.

Emollients are oily or fatty substances that are applied to the skin to keep it soft and to prevent or counteract dryness. Among the most important emollients are petrolatum and lanolin, substances that form the basis for many ointment bases that serve as vehicles for other soothing agents. These substances are most useful when applied to dry cracked skin, especially on the hands and feet. Other nongreasy ointments, such as hydrophilic ointment, are preferred for application to hairy areas. Pastes are not suited for hairy sites but are most useful for soothing subacute skin lesions, as are emulsion creams.

Dusting powders, including starch, talc, and stearates of magnesium and zinc, absorb moisture as it forms on the skin and reduce rubbing between adjacent irritated skin surfaces, or soothe diaper-irritated skin. Such skin surfaces are dried before the dusting powder is applied, because caking of powder leads to further irritation. Cornstarch and magnesium oxide are the constituents of an absorbable dusting powder used to lubricate surgeons' gloves.

Protective dressings are made of layers of gauze containing petrolatum, or bandages covered with a gelatin–zinc oxide jelly. Collodion, a viscous liquid containing pyroxylin dissolved in an ether–alcohol mixture, makes a flexible protective covering for sealing small wounds. Dimethicone, a water-repelling silicone oil, is sometimes used in ointment form to protect skin from external irritants such as soap, detergents, acids, and alkalis. It may also help to prevent diaper rash, bed sores, and chapping.

Local irritants

Drugs can *cause irritation* of varying severity. Depending on the degree of irritation and the extent to which it is kept under control, the actions of drugs may be mild and useful for treating certain skin symptoms, or they may be destructive and cause deep scarring. The extent to which chemicals induce inflammatory reactions when applied to the skin usually depends on how dilute or concentrated they are. A chemical may produce only faint redness—a rubefacient effect—in low concentration, whereas stronger solutions may lead to swelling and blistering, or vesication, and finally to a caustic, or corrosive, action that kills the tissue and results in scarring. Some drugs have only limited irritating properties, even when applied to the skin in full strength.

Astringents. These are chemicals that cause a slight protein-coagulating effect. Because the action is usually mild and the coagulum forms a protective film over the skin and mucous membrane surfaces, these drugs are hardly considered to be irritants at all. The aluminum salt solutions that are applied to oozing skin areas in poison ivy, athlete's foot, and acute eczematous states act in this way to aid in reducing inflammation. Other aluminum salts, however, such as aluminum chlorhydrate, may cause axillary skin irritation in some persons using antiperspirant and deodorant creams containing these substances. Similarly, some zinc salts have a desirable healing action when applied in dilutions with mild astringent activity, whereas stronger zinc solutions are dangerously irritating.

*Keratolytic agents.** These are the mildest skin irritants. Some, such as sulfur, tars, and ammoniated mercury, are so mild that there is even some doubt that they help to speed the rate of peeling of keratin-containing cells when they are applied in acne, seborrheic dermatitis, or psoriasis. On the other hand, the desquamating action of salicylic acid is quite clear-cut when it is combined in moderately high concentrations with resorcinol or other antifungal agents for treating athlete's foot, or when its keratolytic action is used to help remove corns and calluses. In fact, in peripheral vascular diseases or diabetes,

---

* Literally, keratin-dissolving.

self-medication with products containing such keratolytic substances is dangerous, because they are sufficiently irritating to cause skin ulcers if local circulation is poor.

Depilatories. These have somewhat stronger keratolytic action and are used for removing superfluous hair or, occasionally, instead of shaving in preparing patients for surgical procedures. Alkaline sulfides once used for this purpose have been largely replaced by mixtures of calcium and strontium hydroxides and calcium thioglycollate. The creams and lotions containing such substances are left on the skin for a specified time and are then removed by thorough washing to prevent irritation. Even so, some people's skin tends to redden before the hair shafts soften and dissolve. Patients who have a history of allergy are cautioned against trying out many new products of this type or, for that matter, *any* product, including even deodorants, that may contain potential skin sensitizers.

Caustics. These are corrosive chemicals that are sometimes carefully applied to destroy hyperkeratotic tissues. Substances such as glacial acetic acid, trichloroacetic acid, liquefied phenol, and podophyllin are sometimes used to destroy warts. Silver nitrate sticks are used on granulomatous tissues. In all such cases, care is required to see that these chemicals contact only the areas to be treated, and surrounding normal tissues must be protected.

Specific skin disorders

Dermatitis

Dermatitis is a general term that is used for all the varied dermatologic disorders in which inflammation occurs during the course of the condition. An inflammatory reaction, ranging from mild to severe, is the characteristic response of the epidermis to damage by chemical and mechanical irritation or by heat and ultraviolet radiation. Such injuries may cause skin changes ranging from only slight erythema, or redness, through formation of massive bullae, or blisters, with deep destruction in the underlying dermal layer. Usually these changes are temporary. If the patient does not scratch and rub the itchy areas or pick at the protective crusts that form over oozing blebs or blisters, the inflamed skin ordinarily heals completely.

The general purpose of all types of dermatitis treatment is to aid the natural recovery mechanisms. Dermatoses of quite different causes and with varied clinical courses are treated with many of the same types of topically applied agents, because the acute, subacute, or chronic stages of all types of dermatitis are essentially the same. Thus, the same drugs may be used to relieve itching, dry up oozing areas, or soothe and protect excessively dry cracked skin, no matter what type of dermatitis is encountered.

Acute contact dermatitis

This disorder results from exposure of the skin to chemical substances that elicit inflammatory responses. The reaction may range from a slight redness and itching to severe swelling and blistering of the skin. The chemical cause may be either a primary irritant or a substance to which a particular person has become allergic through prior exposure and sensitization. Although almost any chemical can cause allergic contact dermatitis, some substances are relatively stronger sensitizers than others.

One of the most familiar skin sensitizers in this country and some others is the plant called "poison ivy." Like its relatives of the *Rhus* genus, poison oak and poison sumac, it contains a sensitizing oil, called urushiol, to which most people react positively in skin tests. Exposure of the skin to this allergen leads to a dermatitis marked by the development of groups or lines of vesicles containing serous fluid.

Contrary to what is commonly supposed, the fluid from broken blebs is not a source of further quantities of allergen. Although the original allergen that was picked up on the fingers from contact with the plant itself may be quickly spread to parts of the body that the person touches or scratches, lesions that appear late in an attack of poison ivy may result from further exposure to the plant or may simply have developed more slowly because of local differences in skin susceptibility.

Treatment. Although various preparations of the active toxic principle extracted from *Rhus* leaves are available for the systemic treatment and prophylaxis of poison ivy, there is little evidence that these preparations are beneficial, and they may cause many uncomfortable and even dangerous adverse reactions. Thus, topical treatment and prevention of further exposure are the mainstays of therapy and prophylaxis.

Topical treatment is aimed primarily at relieving itching and thus stopping the urge to scratch. Scratching is undesirable, *not* because it "spreads the poison," but because pathogenic bacteria may enter breaks made in the skin by the fingernails. The secondary bacterial infections that frequently follow such scratching tend to prevent the skin from recovering its normal state of health.

Itching in the acute stage of contact dermatitis is best controlled with wet dressings followed by application of protective lotions. Evaporation of water from the compress has a cooling effect. Soaking the covering cloths with *aluminum acetate solution*[+] and *potassium permanganate solution*[+] adds their desirable astringent effects. This tends to aid drying of oozing areas and causes protective crusts to form over the weeping blebs and blisters.

Such solutions are applied for about 20 minutes, and the area is then daubed with a drying lotion that is shaken before use. The thin layer of skin protectant, such as zinc oxide, that is left on the denuded areas soothes the skin and relieves itching. The addition of phenol, menthol, or camphor to *calamine lotion*[+] adds to the antipruritic action of such preparations. In the later stages, when the skin may be dry and cracked, *calamine ointment* or some other greasy emollient substance may be used.

Topical steroid application is not very useful until the acute stage has subsided. Steroids do not penetrate the epithelium of vesicles and bullae and, when such blisters break, the flow of serous fluid simply washes away the drug. Later, however, when applied in the periods between wet dressings, creams containing hydrocortisone (some are now available without a prescription) or other steroids sometimes help to relieve inflammatory itching. However, topically applied steroids are not as necessary here as in other pruritic dermatoses, and may be too expensive to use if the eruption covers large areas of the body.

Systemic steroids are preferred in extensive and severe contact dermatitis. Large doses of these drugs, administered immediately and then rapidly reduced and finally withdrawn over a period of several days or a week, are indicated in the management of acute, self-limited conditions such as poison ivy. This type of steroid treatment is relatively safe, because it does not lead to hypercorticism or significantly depress adrenal cortical function, as is inevitably the case in more chronic conditions (see discussion of step-down dosage schedules; Chap. 21).

Later, when the acute stage has subsided, topical application of a *local anesthetic* cream containing benzocaine may be employed for relief of persisting pruritus (see discussion of topical anesthetics; Chap. 14). Some *antihistaminic* agents also exert *antipruritic* activity when applied topically—*tripelennamine*, for example. Orally administered antihistamines such as *cyproheptadine* (Periactin) and others may help to relieve itching by their central sedative effects.

Protection against further exposure. This is essential for recovery from an attack of contact dermatitis. Although creams containing certain chemicals, such as silicone oils (dimethicone), are claimed to offer some protection from contact irritants, elimination of the offending substance from the environment is a more effective measure. Persons with poison ivy should stay away from fields, gardens, or woods; if they do expose themselves, the skin should be washed repeatedly with a strongly alkaline soap solution followed by rinsing with alcohol.

Atopic dermatitis

This is a chronic skin condition that often appears in infancy and lasts through childhood into adult life. Like other chronic dermatoses that are often lumped under the vague term "eczema," its basic cause is unknown. There are indications that a predisposition to these skin lesions is inherited. Often the patient or members of the family suffer from hay fever, asthma, or a tendency toward urticarial reactions. Allergy is not always present, however. Similarly, although many patients with this condition seem to have psychological problems, it is not certain that psychological factors always play a part.

The lesions of this disorder do, however, seem to be the result of one primary condition—a skin that is extremely sensitive to stimuli that are interpreted as itchiness. Apparently either the sensory nerve network in the skin of these patients is excessively reactive, or their psychological makeup is such as to make them highly sensitive to afferent impulses of low intensity. In any case, slight sensations originating in the skin seem to be amplified and felt as pruritus and this, in turn, sets off bouts of scratching.

Scratching the skin with the nails seems to help suppress itching by substituting a stronger stimulus that breaks up the pattern of itch impulses traveling to the brain. However, scratching provides only temporary relief, and may even increase the hyperexcitability of the skin by setting free certain itch-producing proteolytic enzymes. Exactly how these protein-splitting enzymes precipitate itching is not well understood; they may act directly on the subepidermal receptors, or indirectly by releasing an itch-provoking agent from the protein of epidermal skin cells. In either case, patients with atopic dermatitis seem to be victims of an itch–scratch–itch cycle that subjects their skin to physical damage and secondary bacterial infections.

Treatment. Treatment of atopic dermatitis is based on the need to relieve itching and inflammation by means of topical and systemic medication. The most effective agents are *topical corticosteroids* in creams, lotions, or ointments. *Hydrocortisone* is the least expensive of these compounds, but *triamcinolone acetonide*[+] and other synthetic steroids such as *betamethasone valerate, benzoate and dipropionate* (Table 43-3) are more potent. However, corticosteroids can themselves cause allergic dermatitis, as can various substances used as vehicles in corticosteroid creams, ointments, sprays, and lotions.

Local anesthetic creams are employed to relieve itching, burning, and pain stemming from lesions of the skin and mucous membranes. Substances such as cyclomethycaine, lidocaine, pramoxine, and dimethisoquin (see Table 14-1) often provide relief by deadening sensory nerve endings in abraded skin. However, dermatologists do not advise the routine use of these drugs for long periods in patients with a definite history of allergy, because they are likely to become sensitized to them.

Claims are often made that such sensitization is unlikely with a particular product because it differs chemically from benzocaine, a well-known sensitizer, or because it is a so-called "non-caine" anesthetic. Actually, patients whose skins are predisposed to react to chemicals tend to develop allergic-type reactions to almost anything that is applied to the skin frequently. Thus, if any of these drugs are employed as antipruritics, including the antihistamine agents with local anesthetic properties, the patient's skin should be carefully watched for signs of allergic reactions.

Antihistamine drugs administered by mouth are considered more useful for relieving pruritis in atopic dermatitis than in contact dermatitis. This may stem, in part, from their ability to block histamine, serotonin, and other chemicals released in the tissues by antigen–antibody reactions, in much the same manner that antihistamine drugs act in urticaria. On the other hand, the role of these substances in atopic dermatitis is not always clear. Relief of pruritus by antihistamine drugs may be centrally mediated, much as is the drowsiness that often accompanies their use (Chap. 39).

In this regard, two antihistamine agents effective against itching—*methdilazine* and *trimeprazine*—are phenothiazine compounds with probable tranquilizing properties similar to those of the related drugs that are employed in emotional and mental disorders (Chap. 46). Thus, their effectiveness against pruritus in atopic dermatitis may stem from the ability to reduce the patient's perception of itch stimuli and to lessen emotional reaction to the type of psychological stressful situations that tend to precipitate itching and scratching in someone who is tense. This may also account for the antipruritic activity of a minor tranquilizer such as *hydroxyzine* (Chap. 45), which also possesses antihistaminic and anticholinergic properties, and of *cyproheptadine,* a central depressant that also has potent histamine and serotonin-antagonizing peripheral effects.

Seborrheic dermatitis

Seborrheic dermatitis is ordinarily one of the least severe dermatoses. In its mildest forms—ordinary dandruff, for example—hardly any inflammation is detectable. Instead, the main sign is an excessive scaliness of the scalp and of the skin around the ears, eyes, and nose. Such scales usually differ clearly from those of psoriasis, being greasy and yellowish rather than dry and silvery. Although the condition is never severely disabling (unless complicated by secondary infections), seborrheic itching is often annoying, and the unsightly scaling is sometimes embarrassing.

Treatment. The more severe forms of chronic seborrheic dermatitis are often treated with the same sort of irritant–keratolytic combinations that are employed against psoriasis (see below). Thus, antiseborrheic ointments containing coal tar, precipitated sulfur, resorcinol, and salicylic acid are often rubbed into the scalp at bedtime and kept on overnight. The head is shampooed the following morning. When such substances are used in lotion form, care is required to prevent them from running into the eyes and ears.

Ordinary soap and water or commercial cosmetic shampoos may be used for washing the head. Often, however, if the scales recur too promptly, special medicated shampoos are used. One of the most popular of these is *selenium sulfide*[+] detergent suspension. Selenium is similar to arsenic in toxicity when taken internally, and may irritate the eyes and sometimes increases the oiliness of the hair. Another antiseborrheic substance, cadmium sulfide, is available as a shampoo that is claimed not to cause systemic toxicity, conjunctivitis, or contact dermatitis.

Sunburn

Excessive exposure to sunlight can cause acute and chronic skin damage. The most common acute reaction is *sunburn,* which occurs when people stay in the late spring or summer sun too long, before their skin has built up a tolerance to the burning ultraviolet (UV) rays. Chronic overexposure to sunlight often has cumulatively damaging effects. It can lead to premature aging of the skin, or wrinkling, which results from sun-induced stretching of the connective tissues in the deeper (dermal) layers. Some people, particularly those with fair skin, develop precancerous and even cancerous skin lesions as a result of long-term overexposure to the sun.

Mild sunburn is marked by redness and swelling. In more severe sunburn, such erythema and edema are followed by vesication and desquamation—that is, by blistering and peeling, as in any second-degree burn. Such severe reactions are the result of UV ray damage of epithelial cells, with the resulting release of lysosomal enzymes and vasoactive autacoids that dilate dermal blood vessels and set off a typical inflammatory reaction (see Chap. 36).

The same invisible UV rays that can cause burning also induce a protective reaction when they reach the skin in small doses. Such short UV rays (in the range of 290 nm to 320 nm) stimulate the melanocytes to produce greater amounts of melanin granules. As these work their way up from the stratum germinativum and accumulate in the upper layers of the epidermis, they absorb increasing amounts of UV rays and prevent them from doing their damage.

To achieve this desirable *tanning* effect, it is important to expose the skin only gradually to the sun. People who go out into summer sunshine for the first time should be advised to avoid the sun at midday, when its burning rays are at their peak. Even in the late morning and afternoon hours, a first exposure should not exceed 15 minutes. The length of exposure can be increased to 30 minutes if the first exposure caused no more than slight erythema. Further gradual increases can be made in the following few days, depending on the person's response in terms of skin redness and tenderness.

Sunscreens. Most people with normal skin are not likely to follow this sensible advice about gradual exposure to summer sunshine when they go on vacation. Thus, they should be advised about which sunscreen products are most effective for preventing sunburn from overexposure. Some widely promoted "suntan" products contain only cocoa butter or liquid petrolatum and little or no sunscreen chemicals. Such emollients do *not* protect the skin from UV rays, even when combined with substances that stain the skin to give a cosmetic—not a natural—tan. Most sunscreen products available now have SPF (sun protection factor) ratings prominently displayed on their labels. This number indicates the amount of increased resistance to burning that the product provides, as compared to that of untreated skin. SPF ratings range from 2 (least protection against burning) to 15.

Chemical sunscreens that are applied over exposed skin act by absorbing UV rays in the burning range before their energy can damage skin cells. Products containing *para-aminobenzoic acid* (PABA) are considered best for preventing burning while permitting tanning (Table 43-2). An advantage of this substance is that it tends to build up in the stratum corneum. Because of this binding to skin keratin, it is not completely washed off when the person swims or sweats. (However, to obtain its best effects during early exposures, it is wise to reapply PABA lotions after each swim.) A disadvantage of this chemical is that it may stain bathing suits, towels, and clothing that contact it before it dries. Preparations containing PABA esters do not stain, but they are also more easily washed from the skin and require more frequent applications.

Certain other availabile sunscreen chemicals are intended to absorb *all* UV rays, including longer rays responsible for some of the total tanning effect. These are best for protecting the skin of people who are prone to suffer photosensitivity reactions when exposed to light, or who have had or are very susceptible to developing skin cancer. Of course, the best protection for such people is to stay out of the sun entirely and to keep the skin covered by clothing when they go outdoors. Opaque pigments such as *titanium dioxide* and *zinc oxide* can be applied as creams or pastes or combined with *red petrolatum* to provide a sunshade that blocks all light wavelengths.

Fortunately for those who cannot stay indoors during the day or who will not wear the white or greasy materials mentioned above, various products that are cosmetically more attractive are available for use when complete exclusion of all light rays is required. Sunscreens of this type belong to a chemical class called benzophenones and include *oxybenzone* and *dioxybenzone*. Another product claimed to block out all the sun's rays is a combination of methyl anthranilate with cinoxate. All are claimed to help prevent wrinkling and drying (senile elastosis), precancerous skin lesions (solar keratoses), and skin cancer. However, this has not been proved.

Special substances are sometimes employed to prevent sun-induced skin reactions in people with metabolic diseases that make them likely to react abnormally to light. Erythropoietic protoporphyria (EPP) is such a metabolic disturbance that lowers the skin's tolerance to sunlight, so that even a brief exposure leads to erythema, edema, pruritus, and various skin lesions. Ingestion of the natural vegetable pigment *beta-carotene* (Solatene) has been found to protect children and others with this disorder.

Taken for several weeks in doses that cause development of carotenodermia, a slight yellow pigmentation of the skin, this substance, which is not a sunscreen in people with normal skin, helps most EPP patients to double or quadruple the length of exposure to sunlight. Although the protective effect against photosensitivity reactions is not complete, people learn to determine their own safe limits of exposure. This substance is quite safe as compared to chloroquine and other antimalarial drugs, which may make patients with porphyria worse. (However, hydroxychloroquine has had some success in protecting patients with discoid and systemic lupus erythematosus from suffering light-sensitive eruptions.)

Photosensitivity reactions. Two types of reactions can occur in people whose skin is exposed to sunlight after sensitization by substances with which they have come in contact or have taken internally. One type—*photoallergic reactions*—resembles ordinary contact dermatitis (see above) except that the patient's eczematous papules appear mainly on areas of skin that have been exposed to sun, while areas that were covered by shirts, gloves or bathing suits show little or no signs of a similar eruption. Among common substances that act as photosensitizers that lead to later photoallergic reactions are coal tar derivatives, certain antiseptics that are sometimes added to antibacterial soaps, chemicals found in cosmetics, and certain plants.

Phototoxic reactions, the second type of photosensitivity, are characterized by a severe sunburn rather than by the papular rash that occurs in photoallergic reactions. People who have taken certain drugs sometimes suffer a sunburn that is quite exaggerated in terms of their relatively short later exposure to sunlight. Among such photosensitizing drugs are demeclocycline and other tetracycline-type antibiotics, phenothiazine-type tranquilizers, tricyclic antidepressants, thiazide-type diuretics, sulfonamide and sulfonylurea (antidiabetic) drugs, and the psoralens (see below).

Treatment. *Sunburn treatment* varies depending on the degree of severity and the extent of the burn. Some cases require only application of compresses made with cool tap water or a mildly astringent cooling liquid such as *aluminum acetate solution.* When larger areas are involved, the patient may be advised to take a tepid bath containing oatmeal, cornstarch, or some other colloidal skin-soothing substance. If blisters have developed and broken, aerosol sprays containing *corticosteroid* drugs may be applied to control local pain and itching. Later, *phenolated calamine lotion* and *zinc oxide* ointment may be applied for protection of the healing areas. (Products containing topical anesthetics, antibiotics, and antihistaminics are employed but are not very useful, and—as indicated earlier—they increase the risk of sensitization and allergic reactions.)

Photosensitivity reactions of both types may require administration of systemic (rather than topical) corticosteroids to control the severe sunburn reactions of phototoxicity or the widespread inflammatory eruptions of acute photoallergy. These are best administered by the step-down dosage described above and in Chapter 21. The patient must be started immediately on a high (30 mg to 40 mg) oral dose of a drug such as prednisone or prednisolone. Then dosage is gradually reduced by one 5-mg tablet daily. When dosage is down to one or two tablets, this can be continued for several more days on a daily or alternate-day basis. Aspirin for relief of pain (and possibly of inflammation) is the only other systemically active drug required. Topical therapy as described above for sunburn may also be used in phototoxicity reactions; topical treatment of photoallergy is similar to that of contact dermatitis (see above). The photosensitizing substance should be determined and eliminated to avoid future reactions.

The skin lesions of *solar keratoses* tend to develop in light-skinned people who are chronically exposed to sunlight. Because the cause of these premalignant lesions is exposure to the sun's rays and aging, the condition is sometimes also called actinic, or senile, keratosis. If the patient takes care to keep out of the sun, the lesions may stay unchanged for many years. Sometimes, however, they may grow and lead to development of squamous cell carcinoma.

The antineoplastic antimetabolite fluorouracil (Chap. 12) has proved effective for causing complete disappearance of most such solar keratosis lesions when applied locally in the form of a cream or solution (Efudex, Fluoroplex). The drug is taken up by the diseased skin tissues and sets up an inflammatory reaction marked by redness, blistering, and erosion of the lesion. Although these ulcerated areas fill in with healthy new epithelium within a month or two after treatment is completed, the skin at first seems much worse during the typical 2- to 4-week treatment course. There is often a certain degree of pain, burning, or itching at the site of application.

Thus, the nurse should encourage the patient to continue treatment despite physical discomfort and emotional distress. The patient can be assured that the unsightly appearance of the treated lesions will lessen in a month or two, and is cautioned to avoid exposure to sunlight during topical fluorouracil treatment. The patient is also warned to wash the hands immediately after applying the medication with a gloved hand or nonmetallic applicator. Special care is needed in applying the drug while treating solar keratosis lesions located close to the eyes, nose, and mouth.

Skin pigmenting and depigmenting agents

Several drugs are available for treating various skin disorders that are the result of a lack of melanin or an excess of this skin pigment. *Vitiligo*, a *hypo*pigmentation disorder marked by loss of melanin in scattered patches of skin, has been successfully treated with orally administered drugs of the psoralen type—*trioxsalen*[+] (Trisoralen) and *methoxsalen*[+] (8-methoxypsoralen; 8-MOP; Oxsoralen). However, full repigmentation may require several years of carefully regulated treatment. The use of methoxsalen followed by exposure to high-intensity, long-wave UV light in the management of severe psoriasis is discussed below.

*Hyper*pigmentation is managed by local application of chemicals such as *hydroquinone*[+] and *monobenzone.* Applied locally in lotion or ointment form to heavily freckled skin, these substances often lighten the spots. Similarly, in *melasma* or *cloasma*, a condition that sometimes develops during pregnancy or in women taking oral contraceptives, these depigmenting agents may lighten the darkened skin areas. Care is required to avoid removing melanin from normal skin. Contact dermatitis occasionally develops in sensitized persons.

Psoriasis

Pathogenesis. Psoriasis is one of a group of dermatoses called *papulosquamous* eruptions, which are characterized by raised scaly lesions. These disorders also include lichen planus and seborrheic dermatitis (see above), a much milder skin condition that is sometimes mistaken for psoriasis. However, in psoriasis, instead of a mild scaling of the skin and scalp, the characteristic lesion is a round reddish plaque that rises abruptly from normal unaffected skin areas. Each of these raised erythematous areas gives off large quantities of dry silvery scales.

The reason for such shedding of scales is that the epidermal cells of psoriatic skin grow and divide at a very rapid rate that is estimated to be between 10 and 100 times that of normal skin. The turnover time from the formation to the death of these cells is only 3 or 4 days, as compared to almost 30 days for the normal epidermal cells. Thus, the greatly increased number of dying cells accounts for the profuse production of powdery scales that are, of course, the dead cells of the stratum corneum layer of the hyperplastic epidermis.

Psoriasis affects an estimated five to six million Americans. Some cases are relatively mild, and the few scattered lesions are readily responsive to topically applied medications. In other cases the plaques spread swiftly over most of the body surface and stubbornly resist treatment with topical drugs. Sometimes the disfiguring plaques of such acute stages of psoriasis are coupled with a painfully disabling arthritis. The 5% of patients with psoriatic arthritis and others with extensive disease often require treatment with potentially toxic, systemically active chemotherapeutic agents such as methotrexate (see below and Chap. 12) rather than with topical therapy. Although the existing psoriatic lesions usually disappear under intensive therapy with any drugs that interfere with the rapid cycle of cellular replication, new plaques always appear before long. There is, at this time, no true cure for psoriasis.

Topical treatment. Mild cases of psoriasis can often be cleared up by application of preparations containing such substances as *coal tar+, anthralin+, salicylic acid+,* and *ammoniated mercury+.* Coal tar applications are often followed by exposure to UV light, because this combination tends to slow the rate of epidermal cell division. Often treatment with these traditional mild irritants is combined with topical corticosteroids.

Topical corticosteroids work best when the psoriatic lesions are located on thin-skinned areas such as the scalp, eyelids, or elsewhere on the face, and in skin folds. In such cases, a low-concentration cream, gel, or ointment of a potent fluorinated steroid such as betamethasone benzoate, dipropionate, or valerate is often effective when rubbed gently into the lesions two to four times daily. Occlusive dressings are seldom required, even with reduced strength products containing only 0.01% of the corticosteroid.

However, to penetrate psoriatic lesions on the thicker skin of such areas as elbows, knees, soles, and palms, steroids should be applied under occlusive dressings. A convenient form for covering scattered individual lesions is flurandenolide tape (Cordran Tape), which contains a potent corticosteroid distributed in a layer of adhesive polyethylene film. Plastic gloves, boots, or even whole body suits can also be put on over larger steroid-treated areas. These can be kept on for up to 12 hours but, because of possible systemic absorption, occlusion of large body surface areas should be limited to only a few hours daily. The treated skin areas should be cleansed and allowed to dry in the periods between treatments.

Intralesional injection of corticosteroids such as triamcinolone acetonide, hexacetonide, or diacetate often produces long-lasting remissions. Suspensions of such steroids infiltrated into unsightly psoriatic lesions at monthly intervals often eliminate unsightly plaques on the patient's arms, legs, and body. Because steroids are not systemically absorbed from these superficial injection sites, hypercorticism has not occurred. However, the high local concentrations of corticosteroids have sometimes caused shrinkage of the skin tissues at the injection site. Such pseudoatrophy is itself disfiguring but is only temporary.

Intensive topical therapy in a hospital setting is sometimes required for patients with severe extensive psoriasis. The special techniques employed in such cases vary from clinic to clinic. However, a typical therapeutic regimen includes the following:

1. Bathing the patient in a tub of lukewarm water containing 2 oz or 3 oz of a coal tar emulsion or solution
2. Exposure of the patient's whole body to UV irradiation in doses not quite strong enough to cause redness or discomfort; the exposure time should be less than half a minute at first, but the exposure to light can be increased gradually to 8 to 10 minutes
3. Application of a corticosteroid cream or ointment under occlusion
4. Washing to remove the steroid and excess scales

Sometimes, instead of a coal tar bath, the hospitalized patient is covered with an ointment or paste containing such substances as coal tar and salicylic acid, or anthralin. A permeable dressing is then applied to prevent staining of clothing or bedding. After varying periods, the dressing is removed, and the paste and adhering scales and crusts are washed off with peanut oil or some other light lubricating oil. The tar-free (but now photosensitized) skin is then exposed to UV light to suppress cell division in the lower layer of the epithelium.

These types of treatment—modifications of the Goeckerman and Ingram techniques—must be closely supervised by the dermatologist or by the nurse specialist. The materials must be prevented from contacting the patient's eyes, and the treated areas should not be exposed to direct sunlight. With some substances, such an anthralin, it may be necessary to protect normal skin from contact with the medicated cream, ointment, or paste and, because the systemically absorbed substance can cause kidney irritation, the patient's urine should be examined weekly for casts and for the presence of protein.

Systemic treatment. The *acute stages* of psoriasis may be made worse by applying the traditional irritating coal tar–keratolytic combinations to the rapidly spreading eruptions. Instead skin-soothing emollient baths followed by frequently applied lubricant ointments are ordered. This treatment keeps the skin hydrated and softened, while potent systemically acting agents are being administered in an attempt to control the condition. Among the systemically active substances employed for treating severe disabling cases of psoriasis that do not respond to topical therapy are corticosteroids and methotrexate.

Corticosteroids. These are sometimes employed systemically to control extensively spreading acute psoriasis. The high doses required often cause hypercorticism and, when the steroids are finally withdrawn, the condition may become worse than before. Continued use of corticosteroids in a chronic condition such as psoriasis is undesirable. Although the use of long-term steroids to control skin symptoms may be justified in potentially fatal conditions such as pemphigus and systemic lupus erythematosus, psoriasis is, after all, essentially benign and never fatal.

Methotrexate. This dangerous drug, previously employed only for treating leukemia, lymphosarcomas, and other malignancies (Chap. 12), began to be used in psoriasis during the 1960s. Deaths resulted from its use in this nonfatal disease, presumably because dermatologists and others who were not experienced in how to employ it properly did not take the required precautions. The FDA finally authorized its use in the management of this *nonneoplastic* disease in 1972 and set strict guidelines to ensure safe use.

Methotrexate[+] should be used only in severe cases of psoriasis that are making the patient increasingly disabled and that are not being adequately controlled by any other type of treatment. The patient's skin should be biopsied and studied to rule out any diagnosis other than psoriasis. The physician who undertakes treatment with this drug should be experienced in the use of antimetabolites, and should keep the psoriatic patient under constant observation during courses of methotrexate therapy.

The nurse who is in contact with patients taking this treatment should be familiar with the drug's adverse effects and the precautions that are required to keep toxicity to a minimum (see the Drug digests in this chapter and in Chapter 12). If the patient expresses fear of the high risks involved—of which he should have been fully informed by the physician—the nurse can assure him that the risks are reduced in his case because he had been selected for therapy on the basis of his general good health. The patient should be encouraged to come in regularly for all the necessary laboratory and physical examinations.

Photochemotherapy. A relatively new treatment technique has proved successful in completely clearing widespread psoriatic lesions from the bodies of many patients who have failed to respond to conventional therapy. This treatment is referred to as PUVA (psoralen plus UVA—that is, long-wave UV light). Patients take an oral dose of the photosensitizing drug *methoxsalen*, and 2 hours later are exposed to high-intensity, long-wave UV light. Between 12 and 20 treatments are needed for optimal results. The method is *not* a cure, and maintenance therapy has not prevented recurrences. Adverse effects, such as vomiting, headache, and generalized exfoliation, have occurred, as has aggravation of psoriasis. Whether an increased incidence of skin cancer occurs is still unclear, but this possibility, as well as the other adverse effects, indicate that this treatment should be reserved for severe psoriasis that has failed to respond to other measures.

Acne

Almost all adolescents suffer from one or another form of acne. About 50% of cases are of the mild noninflammatory type. This is marked mainly by increased skin oiliness and by the appearance of open comedones (blackheads) and closed comedones (whiteheads). These can usually be controlled by simple measures aimed at keeping the skin clean, dry, and free of excess oil.

Much more serious is the inflammatory form of acne, in which the skin may be covered by crops of persistent papules (red, raised areas) and pustules (pus-containing sacs, or pimples). In a small proportion of cases, skin nodules and cysts develop and lead to sterile, or to secondarily infected, abscesses. The resulting skin damage may cause permanent disfiguring scars and sometimes also affect the adolescent's personality development adversely.

The nurse can help young people with acne in several ways. Patient teaching about skin hygiene measures, diet, and nonprescription skin cleansers and medications can be given. When such measures and medications alone cannot control the condition, the nurse can recommend a competent dermatologist. The adolescent with severe acne will require a great deal of support and encouragement to cope with the chronic condition and with the alteration in body image. The nurse is often in the best position to provide this support. The patient may try many "cures" that are advertised in efforts to get rid of the disease. Frustration and discouragement are common problems, and the nurse may have a real challenge helping the patient to cope.

Pathogenesis. Several pathophysiologic factors contribute to acne lesion development. First, *androgens* (Chap. 24), secreted by the testes of boys or by the adrenal glands of both boys and girls, stimulate the sebaceous glands to grow and to increase their output of sebum. At the same time, the keratin-containing epithelial cells that line the wall of the hair follicle duct proliferate rapidly. As a result, dead keratin-containing cells tend to accumulate close to the duct outlets, or pores. This blocks the free flow of sebum to the surface of the skin. (These plugs, made up mainly of keratin and hardened sebum, are the comedones, or basic lesions of acne.)

Inflammatory acne occurs partly as the result of a reaction to the foreign bodies blocking the follicle and partly because of the production of irritating chemicals—free fatty acids formed when bacterial enzymes act on the sebum in the blocked follicles. These chemicals can injure the walls of the follicles and even cause them to break down. This releases the irritating fatty acids into the dermis, where they provoke inflammatory reactions.

The drugs and chemicals employed in the management of acne act in various ways to interfere with the chain of reactions that causes comedones to form and trapped sebaceous secretions to break down to fatty acids. Topical treatment is designed to prevent plugs from forming in the pores by removing keratin, reducing oiliness, and keeping the skin clean and dry. Systemic therapy is intended to reduce sebaceous gland activity and to lessen the numbers of skin bacteria that are the source of the lipolytic enzymes that break sebum down to fatty acids.

Topical treatment. Cleansing the skin well with warm soapy water helps to clear up minor types of non-inflammatory acne. Comedones are less likely to form when scrubbing removes keratin-containing scales, surface bacteria, and excess oil. The addition of antiseptics to make special "medicated" or "acne" soaps does not seem to offer any significant advantage over ordinary soap. However, the presence of small abrasive particles may help to keep the pores clear of small keratin plugs. *Polyethylene* granules and *aluminum oxide* particles are claimed to aid in the mechanical removal of keratin when added to soaps or to combinations of soapless cleansers with surface-active wetting agents. (Detergents are desirable for patients whose skin is sensitive to the fatty acids or alkali contained in soap.)

Keratolytic agents. These act chemically, rather than by a physical abrasive action, and are better for actually loosening comedones and for exerting a peeling, or desquamating, effect. Many traditional acne creams and lotions contain *sulfur, salicylic acid,* and *resorcinol*[+] in various vehicles to help remove occluding follicular plugs. *Benzoyl peroxide* also provides desquamating, drying, and antibacterial effects. It is said to be more effective than the older keratolytics, but it is also more irritating. It is used, at first, in lower concentrations that are built up gradually to greater strengths to avoid excessive irritation. Such products should not be used when acute inflammation is present, and further applications are discontinued if excessive stinging and redness develop.

Tretinoin. This acid derivative of vitamin A is also stronger than the traditional keratolytic agents. It has proved to be effective for treating moderately severe acne marked by many pustules and papules. Tretinoin (Retin-A) is applied only once daily as a liquid or in a cream or gel, preferably at bedtime. At first this treatment may make the patient's acne seem worse, because it tends to bring out underlying inflammatory lesions that were previously unseen. However, improvement usually becomes apparent in 2 or 3 weeks, or at most, after 6 weeks of therapy.

Treatment with tretinoin must be carefully controlled to avoid excessive irritation. It should not be begun until several days after other keratolytics have been discontinued, and it should not be used together with abrasive soaps or skin cleansers that are excessively drying. Patients should avoid exposing tretinoin-treated skin areas to sunlight because of increased likelihood of getting sunburned. The medication must be discontinued if the patient's skin proves excessively sensitive to it and becomes red, swollen or blistered, and crusted.

Corticosteroids. Tretinoin is not effective for treating most cases of severe acne marked by the presence of deep nodules and cysts. Such nodulocystic acne is best treated by injecting a suspension of a corticosteroid such as *triamcinolone acetonide* directly into the lesions. This often produces a dramatic reduction in the size of the cyst or nodule and eliminates the need for surgical drainage. It has made the traditional treatment of this type of acne with hot soaks or compresses of sulfurated lime solution (Vleminckx's solution) followed by application of zinc sulfate and sulfurated potash lotion (white lotion) almost obsolete.

Topical antibacterial agents. These are applied in two sets of circumstances in the treatment of acne: to prevent secondary infections by staphylococci and other pathogens, and to inhibit the growth of the nonpathogenic bacterium *Corynebacterium acnes,* which is believed to be responsible for converting the fat in sebaceous secretions to irritating free fatty acids.

Hexachlorophene[+] is an example of an antibacterial chemical employed to prevent infection by staphylococci and other gram-positive organisms that might invade open acne lesions. A 3% emulsion in a detergent cleanser (pHiso-Hex) is worked into a lather with water and used to cleanse the affected area. Among substances applied topically to lower free fatty acid levels by antiseptic action are *benzoyl peroxide* and the antibiotics *tetracycline HCl* (Topicycline), *meclocycline sulfosalicylate* (Meclan), *erythromycin* (A/T/S; Eryderm; Staticin), and *clindamycin* (Cleocin T). However, benzoyl peroxide is a potent irritant and a sensitizer that can lead to later allergic reactions, and the current status of topically applied antibiotics is uncertain.

The main advantage of administering tetracycline topically instead of orally, as described below, is its freedom from systemic side-effects. Favorable responses are somewhat less frequent with topical tetracycline (about 75%) than with oral tetracycline (over 90%). However, in those patients who do respond to daily applications of the liquid solution, it is equally effective for clearing up severe acne.

The only complaint commonly noted with topical application of this product is a brief stinging or burning sensation. This does not cause enough discomfort during the few minutes it lasts to warrant discontinuing the treatment. The treated skin of some light-skinned patients shows a yellowish tinge, but this can be removed by washing with water. One case of severe dermatitis reportedly developed in a patient exposed to sunlight after topical tetracycline treatment. However, this cleared up quickly with corticosteroid therapy.

Systemic treatment

Antibacterial therapy. Acne cases that do not respond to topical treatment alone are often controlled by oral antimicrobial drug therapy. Broad-spectrum antibiotics of the *tetracycline* type are most commonly employed. Low doses are taken daily for long periods to control the anaerobic organism (see above) that is believed to be responsible for the high ratio of free fatty acids to triglycerides in the sebum of acne patients. Such small doses seem to be free of most typical side-effects of tetracyclines. However, overgrowths of *Candida albicans* occasionally cause vaginitis, and photosensitivity reactions sometimes occur in patients taking *demeclocycline* and other antibiotics of this class. Thus, it may be desirable to discontinue these drugs during the late spring and summer, a time during which acne often goes into remission, perhaps because of exposure of the skin to the UV rays of the sun.

Patients who do not respond to tetracyclines alone may do so when treated simultaneously with topically applied tretinoin (see above). Others in whom tetracyclines are ineffective or not tolerated may improve when antibiotics of the *erythromycin* class are employed. *Clindamycin* has also been administered orally for this purpose but, because it can cause severe diarrhea and pseudomembranous colitis, it should not be given systemically for acne. The chemotherapeutic drug combination sulfamethoxazole–trimethoprim has also been reported to improve severe acne.

Isotretinoin. This oral vitamin A derivative was approved relatively recently by the FDA for use in treating nodulocystic acne. Unlike tretinoin (Retin-A; see above), isotretinoin (Accutane) is ineffective topically. Taken orally, isotretinoin is highly effective in clearing up cystic acne, usually within a month after treatment has begun, and produces remissions that sometimes outlast the course of therapy by months or years. It acts by inhibiting the sebum-producing activity of the sebaceous glands. This, in turn, decreases the concentration of the bacteria (*Propionibacterium acnes*) that are believed to be responsible for inflammation in acne.

The recommended dosage of isotretinoin is 1 mg/kg body weight/day divided into two doses. Treatment continues for 15 to 20 weeks. Almost all patients treated experience cheilitis (inflammation of the lips), dryness, itching and chapping of the skin and mucous membranes—the signs of hypervitaminosis A. Topical lubricants help to control these adverse effects, which disappear when treatment is stopped. Other more serious adverse effects also occur, including fetal abnormalities and abortions when the drug is used in pregnancy; central nervous system effects, including papilledema; corneal opacities; joint and muscle pains that can cause discontinuation of the drug; abnormalities of liver function; and elevated serum triglyceride levels and decreased high-density lipoprotein cholesterol levels (see Chap. 32). Thus, despite its efficacy in acne, this drug is contraindicated in pregnancy, and close monitoring of liver function serum lipid levels is recommended. As with all drugs, its benefit-to-risk ratio should be carefully evaluated before its use is begun.

Female hormone therapy. Estrogens are sometimes employed to counteract the stimulating effect of androgens on the sebaceous glands and thus reduce sebum production. This treatment cannot be used in boys because of possible gynecomastia or other feminizing effects. When used in selected cases of severe acne in young women, the same precautions against possible adverse effects of estrogen apply as when these hormones are used in older women at the menopause (Chap. 23), or when oral contraceptives are employed regularly to prevent pregnancy. Such estrogen–progestin combinations are, in fact, often prescribed for acne in young girls. Their cyclic use provides the added benefit of regularizing the patient's menstrual periods, but it may also expose susceptible girls to an increased risk of thromboembolic episodes.

Other measures. Patients can be assured that almost all cases of acne respond to therapy with topically applied keratolytic agents or to a combination of these with oral antibiotics or with other systemically acting drugs. The relatively few cases that are recalcitrant to pharmacologic therapy can be controlled by physical therapy. This includes graded doses of UV light or of x-rays that penetrate only into the superficial skin layers. Cryotherapy, the local use of extreme cold in the form of dry ice (solid carbon dioxide) applications or liquid nitrogen, is sometimes effective for treating deep, large acne cysts. Finally, after the disease has subsided, severe scars can be removed by dermabrasion, a physical operative procedure.

Infections of the skin

As mentioned in Chapter 36, the unbroken skin acts as an effective barrier against the invasion of pathogenic microbes. Most microorganisms among the transients that are always pouring onto the skin from the surrounding air do not survive for long. The outer layer of skin cells is low in moisture and relatively high in organic acids and apparently offers a hostile environment in which bacteria quickly dry out and die. Some species can survive and colonize in the skin; these residents then apparently prevent colonization by other species, including potential pathogenic invaders.

Sometimes, however, the natural resistance of the skin may be reduced. In such cases, pathogenic microbes—most commonly gram-positive bacteria such as staphylococci, but also fungi and other types of organisms—can set off skin infections. In addition, bacteria that break through the weakened skin defenses can then enter the blood and reach other organs such as the kidneys, bones, or brain.

When the host's defenses are weakened by injury or disease, even ordinarily harmless residents of the skin's bacterial flora can become pathogenic (Chap. 6). Such opportunistic microbial infections are especially common in patients with leukemia, diabetes, and various debilitating diseases. Patients taking high doses of corticosteroid drugs or broad-spectrum antibiotics for long-term treatment of chronic ailments are also subject to superinfections.

Prevention

Many products containing antiseptic chemicals are available for topical application to the skin and mucous membranes to prevent infection or, at least, to limit its spread (Table 43-4). Most commercial antiseptic products that are offered to the public for applying to cuts have little value. On the other hand, the proper use of skin antiseptics by medical personnel is an important part of patient care.

Among the purposes for which such anti-infective substances are employed are the following:

1. Reducing the numbers of pathogenic microorganisms on the hands of those responsible for patient care—surgical and nursery personnel, for example
2. Preoperative preparation of the patient's skin and postoperative care of the surgical wound
3. Prevention of infection in possibly contaminated cuts, scratches, and abrasions
4. Treatment of superficial infections of the skin and of the mucous membranes of such adjacent organs and structures as the vaginal tract, anorectal region, and eye (see below, and Chap. 42)

Skin cleansing and disinfection

The surgical patient is, of course, exposed to an unusual risk of infection. Wound infections following surgery cannot be eliminated entirely. Even if bacterial contamination from the environment could be prevented entirely, the effects of anesthesia, trauma, and other factors that shock the system and upset normal biochemical balances would so lower the tissues' defenses that organisms already present could become invasive. This should not discourage efforts to keep contaminating skin bacteria to a minimum; rather, it should spur greater effort in that direction.

Surgical scrubbing. The importance of cleansing the skin at the site of surgical incisions and the hands of attending medical personnel has been recognized since the discoveries of Pasteur and Lister during the 19th century. Despite the present availability of systemically active antimicrobial agents for prophylaxis against postoperative infections and the now frequent installation of laminar (one-way) flow ventilation systems to reduce airborne

bacterial contamination, antiseptic cleansing of the skin is still an essential part of preoperative preparation. In fact, experts on infection control feel that hand washing by hospital personnel is the single most important measure for controlling *nosocomial* (hospital environment) infection.

Hand washing and operative field scrubbing are done in many different ways and with a wide variety of antiseptic chemicals. Here, only a few of the substances used in such scrubs will be described, along with how these are best employed for full effectiveness and safety. Broadly speaking, such substances should have the following properties:

1. Rapid and persistent bactericidal activity against a wide range of pathogens, including particularly *Staphylococcus aureus* and *Pseudomonas aeruginosa*
2. A low level of adverse skin reactions, including both primary irritation and allergic contact and photosensitization reactions
3. No absorption through the skin that might result in systemic toxicity

Scrubbing the skin of the hands with *soap* and water and long-continued, vigorous friction for relatively prolonged periods is a standard preliminary procedure. Soap has little effect as an antibacterial agent, but as a detergent it removes such skin debris as keratin and natural fats. At the same time most of the contaminating bacteria contained in such surface substances is removed. Soaps and certain synthetic anionic surfactants, or "wetting agents," permit water to penetrate better and thus help to float out some of the flora that reside deep in the crypts, crevices, pits, and ridges of the skin.

Ethyl and isopropyl *alcohols* are often used to rinse residual soap from the skin. Both can kill bacteria but not their spores. For best results, a 70% concentration by weight of *ethyl alcohol*[+] is recommended, whereas *isopropyl alcohol* is used full strength. The longer these alcohols are in contact with the skin, the greater the germicidal effect. However, even briefly swabbing the skin with an alcohol-soaked cotton sponge just before inserting a hypodermic needle has some usefulness. This is because the solvent action of alcohol on the sebaceous secretions helps to clean the skin of surface bacteria.

The cleaning, drying, and hardening actions of alcohol may account for its ability to prevent bed sores in some patients prone to decubital ulceration. However, emollients are preferred if the skin is dry and may be irritated and become fissured from alcohol rubs. Alcohol rubs, of course, have other desirable effects. When massaged into the skin, alcohol is mildly irritating and aids the local flow of blood, as is seen in the increased redness

(Text continues p. 916)

Table 43–4. Topical anti-infective agents

Official or generic name	Trade name or synonym
Antibiotics	
Bacitracin USP	Baciguent
Chloramphenicol USP	Chloromycetin
Chlortetracycline HCl USP	Aureomycin
Colistin sulfate	In Coly-Mycin S Otic
Erythromycin USP	Ilotycin
Gentamicin sulfate USP	Garamycin
Neomycin sulfate USP	Myciguent
Polymyxin B sulfate USP	In many multiple antibiotic preparations
Tetracycline HCl	Achromycin
Antibacterial sulfonamides	
Mafenide acetate USP	Sulfamylon
Silver sulfadiazine	Silvadene
Chemical classes of other antibacterials	
Alcohols	
Ethyl alcohol USP	Ethanol
Isopropyl alcohol USP	Isopropanol
Cationic detergents (quaternary ammonium type)	
Benzalkonium chloride (BAC)	Zephiran
Benzethonium chloride USP	In combination products for diaper rash
Methylbenzethonium chloride USP	Diaparene
Dyes	
Gentian violet USP	Methylrosaniline
Iodine compounds	
Iodine tincture USP	
Poloxamer–iodine	Prepodyne
Povidone–iodine USP	Betadine; Isodine
Strong iodine USP	Lugol's solution
Mercury compounds	
Merbromin	Mercurochrome
Mercocresols	Mercresin
Phenylmercuric nitrate USP	Phe-Mer-Nite
Thimerosal USP	Merthiolate

Table 43–4. Topical anti-infective agents (continued)

Official or generic name	Trade name or synonym
Oxidizing agents	
Benzoyl peroxide USP	
Hydrogen peroxide solution USP	
Phenols and derivatives	
Hexachlorophene USP	pHisoHex
Silver compounds	
Silver nitrate USP	
Silver protein, mild, USP	Argyrol
Silver sulfadiazine	
Miscellaneous antibacterials	
Boric acid	
Chlorhexidine gluconate	Hibiclens
Nitrofurazone USP	Furacin
Antifungal antibiotics and chemicals	
Acrisorcin	Akrinol
Amphotericin B	Fungizone
Candicidin USP	Vanobid
Carbol–fuchsin solution USP	Castellani's paint
Ciclopirox ethanolamine	Loprox
Clotrimazole	Lotrimin; Mycelex
Econazole	Spectazole
Gentian violet USP	Genapex; Hyva
Haloprogin	Halotex
Iodochlorhydroxyquin	Vioform
Miconazole nitrate	Monistat-Derm
Nystatin USP	Mycostatin; Nilstat
Salicylic acid USP	
Tioconazole	tz-3
Tolnaftate USP	Aftate; Tinactin
Triacetin USP	Enzactin; Fungacetin
Undecylenic acid and salts	Desenex; Quinsana Plus
Scabicides and pediculicides	
Crotamiton	Eurax
Gamma benzene hexachloride USP	Kwell; lindane
Malathion	Prioderm
Antiviral agent	
Acyclovir (acycloguanosine)	Zovirax

of the skin surface. Such rubefacient and counterirritant activity often helps to relieve muscle aches and pains in a manner that may be more a psychological response than the result of the vasodilation itself. In addition, alcohol sponging is a desirable way to remove heat from the body surface by evaporation and thus temporarily reduce the body temperature of feverish patients.

Iodine[+] dissolved in diluted alcohol, which was introduced for use in preoperative skin preparation at the end of the last century, is still widely used for this purpose. The modern tincture of iodine irritates the skin less than the strong solutions that were previously employed. The iodine-stained skin site is swabbed with alcohol before the operative area is draped, because residual iodine may damage the epidermis. Some people are sensitive to even small amounts of iodine, and severe skin reactions may result.

Iodine has been combined with various organic substances to form complexes that release elemental iodine when in contact with the skin. These so-called *iodophors* are free enough of the irritating properties of iodine to be safely used on mucous membranes as well as on the skin.

Povidone–iodine[+] is employed for pre- and postoperative scrubbing by operating room personnel and on patients, and for general use as a general antiseptic in physicians' offices. Its claimed advantages include a lack of skin irritation, stinging, and staining.

Hexachlorophene, a phenol derivative, is an effective antibacterial agent that does not damage the skin in ordinary concentrations. The 3% detergent emulsion form is effective when employed regularly in surgical scrubbing. When it is to be used preoperatively, patients should be instructed to wash the area daily for 4 to 7 days to build up bacteriostatic residue on the skin. Such home scrubs with hexachlorophene-containing products are also recommended after surgery and for families infected by staphylococcal organisms. In such situations, patients should be told *not* to rinse the skin with alcohol, because this removes the hexachlorophene film from the skin that is being built up by the daily washings.

This substance was formerly added to many types of deodorants, cosmetics, and nonprescription drug products, including baby powders. It was removed from all such preparations after it was found to damage nerve tissue when absorbed through the skin. However, hexachlorophene is still available by prescription for acne treatment programs or other infection and prevention uses.

Phenol, the first substance to be used for preoperative skin disinfection and for prevention of post-surgical infection, is no longer used for this purpose. Concentrations effective for control of skin bacteria and fungi are too irritating for safe use on human tissues. However, low concentrations help to relieve itching when added to antipruritic lotions. Full-strength phenol is occasionally used for cauterizing tissue.

Quaternary ammonium compounds such as *benzalkonium chloride*[+] (Zephiran) have both antiseptic and detergent properties when used preoperatively in hand washing and for disinfection of the patient's skin. These surface-acting agents kill the common gram-positive and gram-negative pathogens, which are then removed from the skin along with sebum and keratin debris. However, it is important to remember that the antibacterial action of these *cationic* substances is almost completely neutralized by the presence on the skin of even small traces of soaps, which are *anionic* in nature. The surgical field is rinsed thoroughly with water and is then swabbed with alcohol before benzalkonium or some other cationic detergent antiseptic is applied.

Chlorhexidine gluconate (Hibiclens; Hibitane; Hibistat) is now available in this country after long use abroad. It is claimed to have all the properties previously indicated as being desirable in antimicrobial skin cleansers. Because it remains active in the presence of blood and does not delay wound healing, it has been advocated for use in cleaning superficial skin wounds. However, further evidence is needed before this chemical can be proved to be superior to other substances that are applied topically to lacerations, most of which have proved disappointing for one or another reason.

Cuts and abrasions

Most antiseptics offered to the public for treating cuts have little value. Some substances used for applying to breaks in the skin or irrigating lacerated areas may even interfere with the skin's natural defenses. Thus, most scratches and abrasions are best dealt with by washing the wound and the skin around it with soap and water.

Boric acid is now known to have only weak antibacterial and antifungal effects. It is harmless in ordinary concentrations. However, applied to the abraded buttocks of babies with diaper rash as a full-strength powder, boric acid has caused toxicity and death. In any case, the traditional use of this relatively ineffective antiseptic no longer seems to be desirable.

Mercurial compounds such as mercury bichloride, an inorganic form, are ineffective when applied to open wounds because they are inactivated in the presence of serum and tissue proteins. Organic mercurials such as *merbromin* (Mercurochrome) *nitromersol* (Metaphen), and *thimerosol* (Merthiolate) do not precipitate protein and are thus not as irritating as inorganic mercury. However, the tinctures, creams, and ointments containing these compounds, which are commonly used for preventing infection of cuts, abrasions, open wounds, and other denuded surfaces, are not now considered to be very effective for this purpose, and some are relatively strong sensitizers.

Silver salts, on the other hand, are highly germicidal in low concentrations. *Silver nitrate*[+] in a 0.5% solution is effective and nonirritating when applied to severely burned skin surfaces. A 1% solution is safe and useful for preventing ocular infection when instilled into the eyes of newborn babies who may have come into contact with their mother's vaginal gonorrheal infection. Unfortunately, this silver salt stains skin black and it is thus unpopular for routine use as a skin infection prevention measure.

In summary, most skin scratches and abrasions are best dealt with by washing the skin around the wound with soap and water, drying gently with a clean towel or tissue and, perhaps, covering the area with a simple dressing to keep out dirt and lessen local irritation. Such simple measures help the healthy skin's own natural defenses. Strong antiseptic solutions may injure healthy tissues and interfere with the body's own ways for preventing pathogenic organisms from becoming established in a break in the skin.

Bacterial skin infections

Bacteria that break through the skin's natural defenses can cause various primary and secondary infections. More than 90% of these are caused by staphylococci and streptococci. These gram-positive organisms are responsible for such pyodermas as impetigo, ecthyma, folliculitis, and cellulitis. These and other pathogens, including such gram-negative bacilli as *Pseudomonas* and *Proteus,* often also contaminate burns and cause the secondary infections that sometimes complicate acute and chronic dermatitis.

General treatment measures. Soaks and compresses containing no antiseptics are often useful for various purposes. Hot, wet applications help to localize boils in patients with furunculosis. Compresses can also be applied with gentle friction to help remove crusts and other skin debris in impetigo. If surgical debridement is necessary, it is best performed immediately after skin-softening soaks or following application of hot compresses. As previously indicated, the cool moist soaks that are employed to soothe sunburn and to dry oozing surfaces in contact dermatitis also help to harden the outer horny, or keratinized, layers of the skin. This acts to build up that barrier against further bacterial infection.

Patients who are prone to suffer from recurrent staphylococcal skin infections must have their skin very thoroughly yet gently cleansed after their boils or carbuncles are drained. Hexachlorophene-containing cleansers are still often used for bacteriostasis of such relatively small areas. However, these must not ever be applied to burns or large skin lesions, because this chemical has caused fatal neurotoxicity following its systemic absorption. The desirability of employing soaps and detergents containing this and other antiseptics has been questioned because of the possible development of contact dermatitis and photoallergy in some patients. Thus, some authorities advocate washing infected areas only with ordinary soap and warm water.

Antimicrobial drug therapy. Most of the metallic and other antiseptic substances commonly applied to the skin (Table 43-4) are ineffective for treating skin infections, because they tend to be inactivated by the serum and pus of suppurating lesions. However, some antibiotics available are applied topically in combinations that may possibly be effective in certain localized infections. Still, the most dependable type of antimicrobial treatment in dermatologic infections is the administration of systemically active antibiotics with the adjunctive use of various physical and surgical measures.

Systemic antibiotics are best reserved for use in patients who are feverish or who show other signs that their illness is not limited to the skin alone. Penicillin G or one of the penicillinase-resistant antistaphylococcal penicillins (Chap. 8) is preferred in such cases. Patients sensitive to penicillin can be treated with an alternative antibiotic, preferably erythromycin or a tetracycline, unless the pathogenic strain is shown to be resistant. Serious skin infections, such as streptococcal cellulitis (erysipelas) must be treated with whatever antibiotic proves to be most effective in susceptibility testing of the infecting organism, even if it turns out to be a potentially toxic one such as chloramphenicol.

Topical antibiotic therapy most commonly uses combinations of several antibiotics such as bacitracin, polymyxin B and its close relative colistin, neomycin, and sometimes gramicidin. One advantage claimed for such combinations is their broad antibacterial spectrum. Thus, for example, bacitracin is active against gram-positive coccal pathogens, and polymyxin B is active against *Pseudomonas* and other gram-negative rods. The two together are said to "cover" virtually all bacteria that are likely to cause skin infections.

Another possible advantage of such combinations is that these antibiotics are very rarely employed for treating serious systemic infections. Thus, if a patient were to become sensitized to an antibiotic such as neomycin, he would be less likely to need it in the future and yet have to be deprived of it, as might be the case with penicillin. The penicillins are, of course, relatively strong sensitizers, particularly when applied to the skin. Because of this and of the importance of continuing to have penicillins available for use in treating possible future systemic infections, these antibiotics are not used for topical therapy of skin infections. Single broad-spectrum antibiotics, such as chloramphenicol and gentamicin, which are not strong sensitizers, are sometimes preferred to the antibiotic combinations for topical treatment of certain specific skin infections.

Treatment of specific infections. Primary pyodermas such as impetigo, a superficial staphylococcal infection, and *ecthyma,* a similar but deeper invasion of the skin caused by a mixture of staphylococci and streptococci, may possibly respond to topical application of creams containing the antibiotic combinations mentioned above. It is important that the honey-colored crusts first be lifted off by soaks or with compresses. Because even a minor streptococcal skin infection of this type may sometimes be followed by acute glomerulonephritis, some authorities also recommend systemic treatment with penicillins or erythromycins when these bacteria are isolated from skin lesions.

Furuncles, or boils, particularly when they coalesce into *carbuncles* or come in recurrent crops, are also best treated with a systemic antibiotic chosen on the basis of culturing and sensitivity studies, rather than by topical therapy. Single isolated boils may be treated without systemic antibiotics. After hot compresses have helped to localize the infection, it is incised and drained. The area is then kept scrupulously clean with washes of 70% alcohol or of skin cleansers containing hexachlorophene and similar substances, as described above.

Otitis externa, an external ear infection such as swimmer's ear, is treated topically with otic solutions containing such antibiotics as polymyxin B, colistin, and neomycin, alone or combined with hydrocortisone to reduce local redness, itching, and edema in the ear canal. Such treatment should be stopped and systemic therapy employed if the ear infection fails to improve or tends to spread. Topical therapy should be discontinued after 10 days, in any case, because it may lead to local overgrowths of fungal organisms.

Although neomycin has the advantage of a broad antibacterial spectrum, it is the most sensitizing of the topically applied antibiotics. High local concentrations of neomycin can also cause ototoxicity in patients with a perforated eardrum. In such cases, and when otitis externa is accompanied by fever and swelling of local lymph nodes, injections of penicillin G are often administered, particularly when streptococcal or pneumococcal pathogens are the suspected cause of infection; gentamicin injections may be best when *Pseudomonas* infection is suspected. The only local measure employed is application of a 70% alcohol solution.

Severe infections following deep third-degree *burns* that destroy the entire skin thickness can lead to death from septicemia. Burn infections are best prevented and treated by topical application of such substances as *mafenide acetate* or *silver sulfadiazine,* or by parenteral administration of an aminoglycoside antibiotic such as gentamicin to prevent sepsis and septicemia (Chap. 8). However, topical care is only one aspect of acute burn care. Severely burned patients often require assistance of respiratory function, close attention to balance between IV fluid intake and elimination, management of pain with analgesics and sedatives, and systemic steroids to fight inflammation.

In accordance with the general principle of treating the most severe inflammatory reactions with the mildest measures, badly burned patients are kept immersed in tepid water for long periods and are transferred to talcum-powdered bed sheets. The burned parts of the body are protected, rested, and exercised only lightly to maintain the range of motion. Complete rest, rather than the use of chemical protectants, is the rule.

Fungal infections

As indicated in Chapter 9, these are caused by two main types of microorganisms: *dermatophytes,* several genera of fungi that burrow into the skin, hair, and nails to cause such conditions as athlete's foot (tinea pedis) or ringworm in such areas as the scalp (tinea capitis) and the groin (tinea cruris); and *Candida albicans,* a yeastlike fungus that invades not only the skin but also the mucous membranes of the mouth, vaginal tract, and anorectal area. It can also cause systemic infections.

Treatment of dermatophytic infections. The parasites responsible for these superficial fungal infections possess enzyme systems that can digest the keratin of the stratum corneum. This keratolytic action enables these fungi to invade the skin, hair, and nails. This leads to itchy and often unsightly lesions that are usually limited to a single specific area but may also spread over large sections of the skin.

Griseofulvin (Chap. 9) is the most effective treatment for most common dermatophytic infections. In most cases, itching and redness of the skin are relieved after a few days of treatment with this oral antifungal antibiotic; and, after a week or two, cultures no longer reveal any fungi. A course of 3 to 4 weeks of treatment will clear up most skin infections. However, 2 months or more may be required when the soles and palms are involved; and griseofulvin may have to be given for 6 to 12 months for clearing infections of the nails.

Topical application of creams, ointments, solutions, and powders containing various antifungal chemicals may also be employed during the period of oral griseofulvin administration. Among the older compounds of this type are certain fatty acids (and their salts) that are part of the skin's natural defenses. These substances, including undecylenic acid (and zinc or calcium undecylenate), are often quite effective for athlete's foot, but they are less useful for treating ringworm of the scalp and other fungal infections.

Several synthetic chemicals with a broader spectrum of antimicrobial activity have been introduced for topical application in tinea-type and other fungal infections (Table 43-4). Some, such as *clotrimazole, miconazole,* and *haloprigin* are effective against organisms that are resistant to griseofulvin—for example, *Malassezia furfur,* the organism responsible for tinea versicolor, a condition characterized by depigmented spots on the skin—as well as against the less resistant dermatophytes.

Clotrimazole and micronazole are also effective against candidal organisms resistant to griseofulvin and to the earlier topical therapies. Clotrimazole has been used successfully for treating perlèche, an inflammation of the skin at the corners of the mouth caused by *Candida albicans*. Miconazole is effective in cutaneous candidiasis as well as in dermatophytosis. A claim made for all these compounds is that they rarely cause the skin to become sensitized. However, if burning or other signs of sensitivity or chemical irritation occur, these medications may have to be discontinued.

Other topically applied substances are employed for relief of symptoms and to control conditions that favor the spread of fungal infections, rather than directly against the fungi. For example, *salicylic acid* is used for its keratolytic action in the classic combination with the antifungal agent *benzoic acid,* called *Whitfield's ointment.* Its keratin-softening action enables the antimicrobial benzoic acid to reach fungal organisms deep in the skin. *Carbolfuchsin solution*[+] contains substances that help to dry infected skin and thus indirectly stop further fungal growth, while other ingredients act directly on the fungus. *Formaldehyde* solution soaks are also sometimes ordered to reduce sweating of the feet and thus exert a desirable drying and deodorant action.

Treatment of candidal infections of the skin and vagina. *Nystatin, amphotericin B,* and *candicidin* are, as discussed in Chapter 9, the antifungal antibiotics most commonly applied topically in the treatment of cutaneous and vulvovaginal candidiasis. The latter condition has become increasingly common with the wide use of oral contraceptives, which produce changes in the vaginal pH and thus alter secretions that favor fungal growth. The antifungal agents clotrimazole and miconazole are also effective for treating this vaginal infection when administered as vaginal tablets or applied as a cream. Clotrimazole tablets, applied for 7 days, appear to produce a lower incidence of local burning, itching or irritation than the 2-week course with miconazole cream, but both are relatively safe drugs and rarely have to be discontinued.

If these drugs do not clear up the vaginal infection, the initial diagnosis is reconsidered, and other pathogens associated with vulvovaginitis, including *Hemophilus vaginalis* and *Trichomonas vaginalis*, are ruled out (see Chap. 8 for a brief discussion of topical sulfonamide therapy of *H. vaginalis* infections and Chapter 11 for a discussion of the current status of *metronidazole* in the management of *T. vaginalis* infections). As in the case of skin infections, adjunctive measures are employed to strengthen the body's own defenses—the use of mildly acidic douches, for example, or insertion of suppositories containing estrogenic substances.

Parasitic skin infections

Parasitic infestations by mites and lice lead to itching and to scratching that often results in secondary skin infections, which cause oozing and crusting of the skin and scalp. These conditions, called *scabies* and *pediculosis,* are highly communicable diseases that used to be associated with conditions of overcrowding and poor hygiene. Today pediculosis, in particular, is a major problem for the nurse working in the school setting. Affluent, clean, well-nourished children are just as susceptible to infestation with lice as are other children. The disease is so communicable that a child who brings the disease home from school often spreads it to the entire family. The school nurse must deal not only with the infestation but also with prevention by teaching children never to borrow combs or hats, and with anxious parents, who often have little information about the disease and misunderstand its implications.

Treatment. Safe and effective insecticides, including *malathion* (Prioderm), *crotamiton* (Eurax), *gamma benzene hexachloride*[+] (lindane; Kwell) and numerous combination products can quickly overcome these conditions. Scabies lesions, which are caused by the burrowing of a female mite in the stratum corneum of the skin, are found in the spaces between fingers, on the wrists, waistline, buttocks, axillae, and breasts. The tunneling mite can be seen with a magnifying glass when the upper layer of skin is lifted gently with a needle. Lice are not readily seen, but pediculosis is recognized by the presence of nits, or eggs, attached to the patient's hair or clothing.

Scabies and pediculosis are readily controlled by application of creams and lotions containing scabicides and pediculocides in regimens that also employ prolonged bathing in warm, soapy water and vigorous shampooing. It is also important, however, that combs and brushes be sterilized and that clothing and bedding be laundered, sterilized, or fumigated to avoid prompt re-exposure to the parasites.

Additional clinical considerations

In caring for the patient with a dermatologic problem, it is important to remember that the skin covers the entire body. The patient should be thoroughly assessed, and the location and description of the lesions should be recorded as a baseline for future reference. In determining the cause of the problem, the patient should be asked about all possible exposures of the skin to foreign substances, including any new or different skin contact—for instance, detergent, cosmetics, soap, lotion, unwashed clothes, perfume, or insect repellent.

Dermatologic problems can be a real challenge. They are often uncomfortable and sometimes embarrassing. Pharmacologic treatment often requires direct application of such substances as creams or ointments. The patient should be instructed in the proper application of the medication. Instruction should also include basic principles of hygiene and nutrition, which are essential for maintenance of proper skin integrity. The patient with infectious lesions will need to understand that the lesions are caused by an organism that can spread the lesions, and will need to know what precautions must be taken to protect other areas of his body, as well as people with whom he comes in contact.

Patients with a history of contact allergies are especially susceptible to developing sensitivities to new allergens with which they come in contact. These patients should be advised to use purified skin products and to

avoid switching products. They should be encouraged to stay with products that give them no adverse reactions.

As more is learned about the correlation between the increased risk of skin cancer and sun exposure, the use of sunscreens may become a primary public health issue. Education about the risks of sun exposure and the proper selection and use of sunscreens is an important aspect of the care of patients with a history of skin cancer. It should probably be incorporated into the general health teaching of all patients.

Skin lesions, although often self-treated by patients with various over-the-counter (OTC) preparations, can present a real health problem. As indicated earlier, the skin serves several important functions, and loss of skin integrity can result in a disruption of these functions.

Summary of types of topical skin preparations

Type of preparation	Physical properties	Usefulness
Ointments	Up to 10% of active ingredients dispersed in fatty bases such as petrolatum and lanolin, or in nongreasy bases	Best when applied to dry, scaly, or keratotic lesions; exert a prolonged protective action when applied at night; *not* suitable for use on hairy areas or on oozing surfaces
Pastes	Ointments into which powders are mixed, such as zinc oxide, starch, talc, and small amounts of tars, salicylic acid, and other medications	Possess a prolonged protective and occlusive action but are porous enough to permit heat to escape from the skin; *not* suited for hairy surfaces or on oozing areas
Creams	Active ingredients are incorporated into an emulsion-type base that vanishes when rubbed in, which has cosmetic advantages	Good for daytime use, particularly with potent active ingredients that are effective when rubbed into oozing denuded areas (*e.g.,* corticosteroids)
Lotions	Suspensions or solutions of active ingredients are applied liberally by brushing or daubing on the affected area, after shaking to disperse the ingredients	Protect and cool oozing areas in acutely inflamed dermatoses on the face and on hairy areas of the body
Liniments (emulsions)	Have a higher proportion of oil than ordinary lotions; various active ingredients may be added	Protect skin that is dry, cracked, or fissured
Paints	Liquids used to touch up small localized areas (*e.g.,* anogenital) or intertriginous surfaces (such as moist lesions between the toes or in the axillae)	Often have a desirable drying effect on moist areas at which two skin surfaces are in contact; sometimes stain and are messy
Powders	Materials in fine particles for dusting on surfaces (*e.g.,* inorganic substances such as talc)	Absorb moisture from large areas and exert a cooling or protective effect
Wet dressings, soaks, and compresses	Aqueous solutions of substances with mild astringent properties (*e.g.,*	Have a soothing, cooling, antipruritic effect when applied to areas of skin containing

aluminum acetate, potassium permanganate)

vesicles, pustules, and oozing serous fluids and debris, which are washed away (hot soaks and compresses are also employed to localize boils and cellulitis)

Baths — Starch, oatmeal, and other substances are dissolved or suspended in water and added to a bath in which the patient is immersed (medication such as coal tar or potassium permanganate may be added) — Useful for treating generalized acute inflammatory dermatoses to stop widespread itching and to soften psoriatic or keratotic lesions

Drug digests

Aluminum acetate solution USP (Burow's solution)

Actions and indications. This solution is used as a soak and as a basis for soothing wet dressings. It is employed in the treatment of acute inflammatory reactions of the skin serving mainly as a mild astringent. In undiluted form, it exerts a mild antiseptic effect and may be used as a gargle as well as on the skin.

Applied to oozing, or weeping lesions in acute contact dermatoses (e.g., poison ivy), acute fungal infections of the skin, and bacterial infections, especially in intertriginous areas, this solution helps to give some relief of itching and pain. Its cleansing and antiseptic actions also exert a favorable effect on the local environment that helps healing after opening of vesicles.

Adverse effects, cautions, and contraindications. The solution is said to be nonirritating and nonsensitizing. However, it should not be allowed to contact the eyes. When applied topically, evaporation should *not* be prevented by plastic coverings or other impervious materials.

Dosage and administration. The official 5% solution is diluted with 10 to 40 parts of water for use as a wet dressing that may be applied in cold, tepid, or warm form. Powder in packets and tablets is also available, from which solutions of the proper strength may be conveniently prepared for application to loosely bandaged areas every 15 to 30 minutes for 4 to 8 hours.

Ammoniated mercury USP

Actions and indications. This form of mercury is an insoluble compound that releases the free ion slowly in small amounts that have an antiseptic action on the skin without being excessively irritating. It is used in ointment form in impetigo and fungal infection of the skin, and as an ophthalmic preparation for application to the conjunctiva.

The official ointment is one of the mildest medications for accelerating the scaling and healing of dry lesions in chronic psoriasis. It may also be useful in pediculosis, pinworms, and pruritus ani.

Adverse effects, cautions, and contraindications. The continued use of ammoniated mercury in infants and young children is contraindicated, because toxic amounts of mercury may be absorbed through the skin in some rare circumstances.

Dosage and administration. A 5% and a 10% ointment are available for topical application to the skin.

Anthralin USP (Dithranol; Anthra-Derm; Lasan Unguent; Drithocreme)

Actions and indications. This is a synthetic substitute for the exfoliative plant principle chrysarobin. It has largely replaced the latter in the treatment of psoriasis, because its action on the skin is less irritating and more predictable, and it does not stain the skin or clothing as much as chrysarobin does. Anthralin is now believed to act by inhibiting certain enzymes involved in skin cell metabolism, with a resulting reduction in cell division in psoriasis. It has also been employed for its nonspecific stimulating action on the skin in such other dermatoses as seborrheic dermatitis and atopic dermatitis (eczema).

Adverse effects, cautions, and contraindications. Preparations containing this substance should not be used in the acute inflammatory stage of psoriasis but only on chronic, quiescent lesions. It should not be used in patients with kidney damage, and the urine should be tested weekly for such signs of renal irritation from absorbed anthralin as albuminuria and casts. Preparations should be kept away from the eyes, and normal skin areas should be protected by applying a petrolatum film. Discontinue if redness or other signs of irritation appear.

Dosage and administration. Anthralin is applied as an ointment for the skin or a scalp unguent in concentrations ranging from 0.1% to 1%, the lowest concentration being used first. It is applied to the affected areas with plastic gloves to protect the hands. If well-tolerated—no erythema or hyperpigmentation—a higher concentration (e.g., 0.25% or 0.5%) may be employed.

Benzalkonium chloride USP (Zephiran)

Actions and indications. This cationic-type detergent and antiseptic is effective against gram-positive and gram-negative bacteria. It is used preoperatively and on small wound surfaces for preventing and treating infections of the skin. Dilute solutions may be used for irrigating mucosal surfaces. Higher concentrations are employed for preserving the sterility of heat-sterilized surgical instruments and other operating room materials that are to be stored in a sterile state.

Adverse effects, cautions, and contraindications. To avoid inactivation when applied to the skin preoperatively, benzalkonium solutions should be used only after all soap has been rinsed from the skin site and it has been swabbed with alcohol. Dilute solutions are not ordinarily irritating, but irritation may occur if the skin is kept covered for long periods. Concentrated disinfectant solutions may have caustic effects. Absorption of irritating solutions from body cavities may result in skeletal muscle weakness.

Dosage and administration. A 1:750 dilution is used for disinfection of the patient's intact skin and the surgeon's hands. More dilute aqueous solutions (1:5,000–1:20,000) are ordinarily preferred for use on broken skin and on mucous membranes of the eye, vaginal tract, and urinary bladder.

Calamine lotion phenolated USP

Actions and indications. This lotion offers the protectant action of calamine and zinc oxide and the mild antipruritic action of a low dilution of phenol. It may be applied to the oozing lesions of poison ivy and of other contact dermatoses, or in acute exudative stages of fungal and bacterial skin infections. Other substances may be added to the basic lotion, including 1% camphor or menthol, which possess cooling and antipruritic actions that also relieve the discomfort of itchy, oozing eruptions. This lotion may be made more drying by the addition of alcohol, or it may be made more soothing by the addition of such emollients as glycerin and lanolin when the skin is scabby, dry, or fissured. (A petrolatum-based ointment may sometimes be preferred for such cases.)

Adverse effects, cautions, and contraindications. The use of this lotion in the presence of infection is not desirable, and its accumulation in excessive quantities in hairy areas may cause discomfort and irritation.

Dosage and administration. After *shaking*, the lotion is applied in small amounts to the affected areas. Frequent application with cotton pledgets or a brush is preferred to the occasional use of large amounts. A firm touch is used, because light dabbing may increase itching sensations.

Carbol-fuchsin solution USP (Castellani's paint)

Actions and indications. This alcohol–acetone solution of the antiseptic dye fuchsin, and such other antifungal agents as resorcinol, acetone, and phenol, is often effective against ringworm in interdigital areas and intertriginous sites. Painted between the toes, on the axillae, or in the anogenital region, the medication tends to dry the moist tissues and relieve itching.

Adverse effects, cautions, and contraindications. This solution is rarely irritating or sensitizing. However, it may cause excessive drying and thus add to the chronic fissuring if applied too frequently.

Dosage and administration. The solution should be applied with an applicator no more than once daily. It should be kept tightly closed to avoid evaporation and concentration of the solution. Care should be taken to avoid staining clothing. A fresh solution should be used, because deterioration occurs in a few weeks.

Coal tar USP (in numerous proprietary preparations)

Actions and indications. This substance, a thick fluid derived from the distillation of coal, is combined with zinc oxide paste and in various ointments and lotions. Applied to the skin in psoriasis, seborrheic dermatitis, and chronic eczematous or lichenified lesions, it is often effective for removing scales and plaques. In addition to this keratolytic action, coal tar is said to possess antiseptic, astringent, and antipruritic properties, among others.

The exfoliative effect of coal tar is increased when its application is followed by carefully regulated daily doses of UV irradiation. The patient then takes a long tub bath to remove the loosened scales (Goeckerman regimen).

Adverse effects, cautions, and contraindications. Prolonged use may lead to allergic sensitization. Exposure of the skin to direct sunlight should be avoided because of the photosensitizing effect of coal tar. Application to hairy areas may result in irritation and folliculitis. This substance has an odor that some may find unpleasant, and it tends to stain the skin and darken blond hair.

Dosage and administration. Coal tar is used in concentrations of 1% to 10%, and most commonly as a 1% dilution in zinc oxide paste (coal tar ointment), or as an alcoholic solution (Liquor Carbonis Detergens) for direct application or for use in bath water.

Ethyl alcohol USP (ethanol)

Actions and indications. Topically applied alcohol has several properties that make it useful for skin care and disinfection. It is used preoperatively in surgical scrub procedures to dissolve sebaceous secretions and to reduce the bacterial flora of the skin. It is also rubbed on the skin over sites at which parenteral injections are to be made.

Alcohol is the basis for skin rubs because of its mild rubefacient and counterirritant effects. Its skin cleansing, drying, and hardening effects may make it useful for preventing decubital ulcerations. The solvent properties of alcohol have been used for removing the plant oils responsible for poison ivy from the skin, and also for removing concentrated phenol that has been spilled on the skin.

Adverse effects, cautions, and contraindications. Alcohol is not very effective for disinfecting instruments, because it cannot kill bacterial spores (sterilization by heat is preferred). When applied to open wounds, it causes painful stinging, irritation, and protein precipitation. It has a dehydrating action that can cause excessive skin dryness. Allergic sensitization sometimes occurs.

Taken internally it can, of course, cause central nervous system depression, leading to signs and symptoms typical of alcohol intoxication. Young children may suffer from hypoglycemia following accidental ingestion or even after absorption from burn surfaces or skin lesions.

Dosage and administration. Alcohol is used in concentrations ranging from 50% to 95%. However, its antiseptic action appears to be most effective when a 70% solution in water is employed, because this dilution possesses the most efficient penetration.

Gamma benzene hexachloride USP (Lindane; Kwell)

Actions and indications. This parasiticide is effective for treating scabies and lice infestations. In pediculosis it kills the nits or eggs as well as the adult head and crab lice. This relieves itching and thus stops the scratching that is often the cause of secondary infections.

Adverse effects, cautions, and contraindications. Skin eruptions may occur in sensitized persons or as a result of direct irritation. This may require discontinuation of the product. Care should be used while shampooing to avoid contact with the eyes; if this occurs, the eyes should be thoroughly flushed out with water.

Repeated use should be avoided to prevent possible absorption of toxic quantities into the systemic circulation. Accidental ingestion has resulted in central nervous system stimulation and cardiac arrhythmias. In treatment of poisoning, oily gavage fluids and cathartics should be avoided and epinephrine should *not* be used.

Dosage and administration. A 1% cream and lotion are available for use on the body after the patient takes a hot, soapy bath and then dries the skin. In treating scabies, a thin layer is applied to the entire body surface and kept on for 24 hours before being completely washed off. If further treatments are needed, they are carried out at weekly intervals. For pediculosis, a thin layer of cream or lotion is left on hairy infested areas for 12 to 24 hours, and 1 oz of a 1% shampoo is rubbed vigorously into the wet hair of the head, which is then rinsed and dried.

Hexachlorophene USP (HCP; pHisoHex)

Actions and indications. This chlorinated diphenol antiseptic possesses potent bacteriostatic action against gram-positive organisms, especially strains of the staphylococcus. The 3% detergent suspension is employed as a presurgical hand scrub and for preparing the skin of the operative field.

It is also used by hospital nursery personnel for washing the hands just before and after handling each infant. However, its routine use for total body bathing of newborn infants to prevent staphylococcal infections is controversial. Some sources condemn its use for this purpose; others feel that the benefits outweigh its risks, provided that the hexachlorophene solution is rinsed off completely following the infant's bath.

HCP is available in prescription products for treating acne, impetigo, carbuncles, cradle cap, and other infectious and allergic dermatoses. It is no longer available for use in nonprescription consumer products such as soaps, deodorants, cosmetics, and toiletries.

Adverse effects, cautions, and contraindications. Systemic absorption from burn surfaces and the vaginal mucosa has caused central nervous system toxicity and death. Absorption through the intact skin of newborn monkeys has also caused nervous system lesions, and it is possible that enough may be absorbed through human skin to cause similar toxicity.

Dosage and administration. Detergent solutions (3%) are applied topically by various techniques as a surgical scrub or as an adjunct to other measures for preventing and treating skin infections. Regularly repeated use is needed to build up a residue sufficient for antibacterial action.

Hydroquinone USP (Eldoquin; Eldopaque)

Actions and indications. This depigmenting agent is believed to act by blocking an early step in the biosynthesis of melanin. Thus, it temporarily bleaches and lightens hyperpigmented skin areas. The drug is indicated for treating severe facial freckling, bleaching skin blemishes such as liver spots, and counteracting cloasma caused by oral contraceptives, pregnancy, or age.

Adverse effects, cautions, and contraindications. The patient's possible sensitivity should be determined before treating wide areas of skin to avoid generalized allergic reactions. The drug is discontinued if rash or signs of irritation develop. Preparations are not applied to irritated or sunburned skin, following use of a depilatory, or in the presence of prickly heat. Occasionally, depigmentation may not be uniform with only slight hypopigmentation in some areas and excessive melanin loss elsewhere.

Dosage and administration. A 2% ointment, cream, or lotion is applied to the affected area twice daily at 12-hour intervals and rubbed in well. A 4% concentration in a base that is opaque to light is applied without rubbing to cover the area for cosmetic purposes and to exclude UV light during the day. More rapid and dependable bleaching occurs when the treated area is protected from sunlight in this way.

Iodine USP

Actions and indications. This element is an effective antiseptic when applied to the skin in dilute solution. It is still often employed preoperatively to disinfect the skin of the surgical site. However, it is no longer recommended for direct application to cuts to prevent skin infections. Iodine, like chlorine, can be used to disinfect water that may be contaminated by bacteria or amebae.

Adverse effects, cautions, and contraindications. Topically applied alcoholic solutions of iodine tend to irritate the abraded skin. Iodine, used preoperatively, should be removed from the skin with alcohol to prevent possible irritation by residues remaining on the skin. It should not be used on those known to be sensitive to iodine.

Taken internally, strong iodine solutions may have a corrosive effect on the mucosa of the mouth and other alimentary tract areas. Ordinarily, only nausea, vomiting, and diarrhea result. However, death from circulatory collapse has sometimes occurred. Thus, it may be desirable to wash out the patient's stomach with a solution of starch, which acts to precipitate iodine. (Weak dilutions of iodine—1:250—may be safely employed as a gavage fluid for precipitating alkaloidal poisons.)

Dosage and administration. Tincture of iodine, a 2% alcoholic solution, is a form preferred for preoperative preparation of the skin but not for application to open wounds. Iodine solution (2% aqueous) and strong iodine solution (7% aqueous) are diluted to much lower concentrations and are applied to cuts and abrasions, but soap and water cleansing is now preferred. For disinfecting water, one to three drops of the tincture may be added to 1 liter of water.

Methotrexate (Amethopterin; MTX)

Actions and indications. This antineoplastic drug is used in the management of severe cases of psoriasis in which the patients are becoming disabled despite the use of all other forms of therapy. It acts as an antimetabolite that interferes with skin cell reproduction by inhibiting the enzyme responsible for reduction of dietary folic acid to the form required for DNA synthesis and cellular replication. This drug controls the psoriatic process, in which the rate of production of epithelial cells in the skin is very rapid compared to that of normal skin.

Adverse effects, cautions, and contraindications. Patients with psoriasis should not receive this drug if their history or laboratory and physical examination results indicate that they have a blood dyscrasia, or a severe liver or kidney disorder. Pregnant patients should not receive this drug, and women should take steps to prevent pregnancy for at least 8 weeks after a course of therapy with it, because congenital abnormalities or death of the fetus can occur.

Patients must be kept under constant observation during therapy to detect signs and symptoms of bone marrow depression and hematologic toxicity, and treatment must be stopped immediately if counts of blood cells drop suddenly or steeply.

Other common adverse reactions involve the alimentary system. These include ulcerative stomatitis, nausea, vomiting, abdominal distress, and diarrhea. However, hepatotoxicity has occurred without any of these earlier signs of gastrointestinal toxicity, and even without significant changes in the formed elements of the blood. Thus, liver function tests must be employed before beginning treatment and periodically during treatment.

Dosage and administration. Several types of schedules are in common use, all of which require individualizing dosage in accordance with the patient's weight and responses. There are three types of starting dose schedules based on an adult weight of 70 kg: (1) a single weekly dose of 10 mg to 25 mg may be administered orally, IV, or IM and adjusted upward until an adequate response to therapy is observed, but no greater than 50 mg per week; (2) oral doses may be given intermittently over a 36-hour period. These may be divided as follows: 2.5 mg for three doses at 12-hour intervals or four doses at 8-hour intervals; (3) daily oral doses of 2.5 mg for 5 days followed by a rest period of at least 2 days—doses may be raised in subsequent courses but should never exceed 6.25 mg per day, because this schedule may have a higher risk of causing hepatotoxicity.

After gradually adjusting the dosage in each of the above schedules to attain an optimal clinical response, the schedule is reduced to the lowest possible dose and to the longest possible rest periods. Topical antipsoriatic therapy should be employed in such situations.

Methoxsalen USP (Oxsoralen)

Actions and indications. This potent photosensitizing agent is used with UV light in regimens intended to bring about repigmentation of skin patches in vitiligo. It is effective for this purpose provided that the depigmented skin patches still contain melanocytes that can be activated.

This drug is also employed with careful brief exposures to UV light to increase the ability of light-sensitive patients to tolerate sunlight. It is being employed experimentally for treating cases of severe widespread psoriasis.

The drug itself interferes with epithelial cell synthesis of DNA and, when the drug is followed by exposure to special high-intensity, long-wave light, the replication of psoriatic epithelial cells is markedly reduced.

Adverse effects, cautions, and contraindications. This drug may cause stomach upset and such central side-effects as sleeplessness and irritability. However, the main danger is the possibility of severe blistering if the exposure to light is too long in the period after the drug has been taken. This is particularly likely when a solution of the drug has been applied to the patient's skin. Therefore, this is an office procedure employed only by the dermatologist and not by patients.

Dosage and administration. Two 10-mg tablets are taken about 2 to 4 hours before the patient is exposed to UV lights for periods of, at first, 5 minutes and later up to 30 minutes. A 1% lotion is applied once weekly and followed by only 1-minute exposure to UV light.

Potassium permanganate USP

Actions and indications. This oxidizing-type antiseptic and deodorant may be applied in dilute solution to weeping skin lesions in acute, exudative dermatoses, and in fungal or bacterial skin infections. These solutions also have a mild astringent action that aids drying of oozing areas in the acute vesicular stages of contact dermatitis.

Strong solutions are bactericidal and are used to disinfect organic matter. Very much weaker solutions are sometimes used internally as a vaginal douche or as a gavage fluid for oxidizing certain ingested poisons such as strychnine, for example.

Adverse effects, cautions, and contraindications. The purple crystals must be completely dissolved in adequate amounts of water to avoid irritant and caustic actions. Severe local trauma has occurred when undissolved tablets intended for solution have been inserted into the vaginal tract. The skin and dressings are stained by solutions of this substance.

Dosage and administration. Solutions ranging from 1:1,000 to 1:10,000 and higher are employed for various purposes. A 1:1,000 solution is used in poison ivy. A 1:10,000 solution is applied as a soak, wetting dressing, or in compresses for acute dermatoses. Tablets or crystals totalling 5 g to 15 g may be dissolved in 1 liter of water, which is then added to a tubful of water to serve as a bath in cases of generalized exudative dermatoses. (This makes a solution of about 1:50,000.)

Povidone–iodine USP (Betadine; Isodine)

Actions and indications. This topical antiseptic contains iodine in a complex with polyvinylpyrrolidone, from which it is released when it contacts the skin or mucous membranes to which the solution is applied. The iodine freed in this way is not as irritating to tissues as tincture of iodine.

This type of iodine preparation is often preferred for application to abraded or burned skin, for vaginal douching, and for mouth and throat swabbing. However, it is not considered as effective as iodine tincture as a surgical scrub for operating room personnel and for preoperative preparation of the patient's skin.

Adverse effects, cautions, and contraindications. Patients sensitive to other iodine products are likely to prove allergic to this compound also. Treatment should be discontinued if redness, swelling, or other signs of irritation develop.

Dosage and administration. There are a number of products available: an antiseptic solution for full strength application as a soak, spray, or paint, and as a surgical scrub; an aerosol for spraying on burns, wounds, and stasis, or decubital, ulcers; an ointment applied in prevention and treatment of bacterial and fungal infections, lacerations, and abrasions; a gargle for use following oral surgery and in stomatitis and Vincent's infection; and a douche and gel for use in the management of vaginal moniliasis, trichomoniasis, and nonspecific bacterial infections.

Resorcinol USP and resorcinol monoacetate

Actions and indications. This phenolic substance is a constituent of many proprietary dermatologic preparations. It exerts a mild irritant effect that helps to loosen and remove the outer layer of dead skin cells or scales. This keratolytic action is useful in the management of eczema, psoriasis, and seborrheic dermatitis. Its mild drying and peeling actions are also thought to be useful in the management of acne. Resorcinol has also been employed as an antibacterial in pyoderma and for fungal infections such as ringworm and athlete's foot.

Adverse effects, cautions, and contraindications. Higher concentrations of this chemical may cause skin irritation marked by excessive redness, dryness, and scaling. Topical use should be discontinued if signs of sensitization appear. Accidental ingestion by a child or excessive absorption through the skin may cause systemic toxicity involving the central and circulatory systems.

Dosage and administration. Resorcinol is applied topically in ointments, pastes, and lotions varying in concentration from 2% to 20%. It is frequently found in combination with sulfur and with salicylic acid in lotions and soaps. Resorcinol monoacetate, which releases resorcin at a slow rate, is said to exert a longer lasting effect and to be less likely to cause light hair to darken.

Salicylic acid USP

Actions and indications. Depending on the degree to which it is concentrated or diluted, this topical irritant can produce several different effects useful in dermatologic treatment. In higher concentrations it exerts a mildly caustic or strongly keratolytic action that aids in removal of warts, corns, calluses, and fungus-infested layers of skin keratin. Lower concentrations that are only mildly keratolytic may be useful in seborrheic dermatitis, psoriasis, and acne, especially when combined with coal tar, resorcinol, and sulfur.

Adverse effects, cautions, and contraindications. Caution is required in applying high concentrations of this chemical to the skin of people with poor peripheral circulation, including diabetics and patients with peripheral vascular disease. Overuse may cause inflammation and skin ulceration in such cases.

It should not be applied over wide areas for prolonged periods, because enough may be absorbed through the skin to cause signs and symptoms of salicylism.

Dosage and administration. Salicylic acid is compounded in concentrations of 1% to 40% in the form of ointments, powders, plasters, and lotions or solutions. Dilutions of 1% to 3% are used in seborrheic dermatitis, acne, and psoriasis. Somewhat higher concentrations (up to 6%) help to remove calloused or thickened epithelial tissue and permit penetration of the other agents with which it is combined—for example, the antifungal agent, benzoic acid in Whitfield's ointment. Removal of corns and warts may require still higher concentrations up to 40%.

Selenium sulfide USP (Selsun)

Actions and indications. This antiseborrheic agent, available in the form of Selenium Sulfide Detergent Suspension USP (a 2.5% suspension), is effective in the control of mild to moderately severe seborrheic dermatitis of the scalp. It is most successful against the dry form of seborrhea—that is, common dandruff marked by profuse, dry, powdery scales. It is also useful for tinea versicolor but *not* for scalp ringworm caused by *Microsporum audouini*.

Adverse effects, cautions, and contraindi- cations. The suspension should be prevented from contacting the eyes, because it may cause irritation, stinging, and conjunctivitis or keratitis. Avoid application to the genital area also. Although selenium is a toxic substance when taken internally, systemic absorption from the scalp is unlikely, except in the presence of extensive acute inflammatory lesions.

Dosage and administration. Control chronic seborrhea of the scalp with two treatments weekly of the following type. Massage 1 tsp or 2 tsp into the wet scalp and keep it in contact for 2 or 3 minutes. Then, after thoroughly rinsing the scalp, repeat the application.

For treating tinea versicolor, allow the suspension to remain in contact with the affected areas for 5 minutes and then rinse thoroughly. Repeat this procedure on each of the next 3 days. Further courses may be employed for treating recurrences.

Silver nitrate USP

Actions and indications. This silver salt is bactericidal in low concentrations. Higher concentrations have astringent and caustic actions. A 1% ophthalmic solution is employed routinely for preventing gonorrheal eye infections in newborn babies. (Prophylaxis of ophthalmia neonatorum is often required by state law.)

A highly local concentration of silver nitrate is sometimes attained deliberately by moistening a solid stick of the salt and applying it to tissues for caustic effect. This is sometimes used for removing warts and granulomatous tissues and for cauterizing wounds. Care is required to see that solutions of the proper strength are employed for the intended purposes.

Adverse effects, cautions, and contraindications. Silver nitrate solutions often cause a chemical conjunctivitis, and accidents in their use have resulted in cauterization of delicate eye tissues, with subsequent blindness.

Dosage and administration. The official 1% ophthalmic solution is available in wax ampules containing five drops for topical application to the conjunctival sacs of the eyes of infants. Solutions ranging from 1:10 to 1:10,000 concentration are sometimes ordered.

Triamcinolone acetonide USP (Aristocort; Kenalog)

Actions and indications. This potent topical corticosteroid provides prompt and often prolonged anti-inflammatory, antipruritic, and antiallergic effects in the management of many acute skin disorders, including atopic dermatitis, contact dermatitis, seborrheic dermatitis, neurodermatitis, exfoliative dermatitis, and sunburn, and also as an adjunct to other measures in the management of such chronic dermatoses as psoriasis, lichen planus, lichen simplex, and eczematous dermatitis.

Adverse effects, cautions, and contraindications. Local adverse reactions occasionally reported include sensations of itching, burning and dryness. Treatment must be discontinued if signs of irritation or of sensitization to any of the components of the steroid preparation appear. Failure to respond favorably in the presence of infection also requires discontinuation of steroid therapy until the infection is brought under control. Application is not made to the external ear canal if the patient's eardrum is perforated.

Products containing this or other topical corticosteroids are *not* applied in the presence of viral skin infections, including herpes simplex, vaccinia (cowpox), and varicella (chickenpox), or on tuberculous or fungal lesions. Any skin infection that cannot be controlled by concomitant treatment with antimicrobial drugs is a contraindication to the use of topical corticosteroids.

Systemic side-effects are rare but can occur when extensive skin areas are treated for long periods, particularly when occlusive dressings are employed. In such cases it is preferable to treat small areas in sequence rather than large areas simultaneously. Patients are observed for signs and symptoms of steroid withdrawal when topical medication of this kind is stopped.

Dosage and administration. Creams (0.025%, 0.1% and 0.5%), ointments (0.025% and 0.1% and 0.5%), and lotions (0.025% and 0.1%) are applied to the affected area bid to qid and rubbed in gently. When an occlusive dressing is also employed, the preparation is reapplied to leave a thin coating on the lesion, and the area is covered with a pliable, nonporous film of plastic material. The aerosol spray or foam should not be inhaled or allowed to contact the eyes.

Trioxsalen USP (Trisoralen)

Actions and indications. This photodynamic drug is used to produce repigmentation in vitiligo and to increase pigmentation and tolerance to sunlight in selected fair-skinned persons who fail to tan. Taken by mouth, the drug is thought to concentrate in the melanocytes located in the basal layers of the epidermis. There, when activated by UV light, it acts to stimulate production of melanin.

Adverse effects, cautions, and contraindications. The photosensitizing action of this drug during its first days of administration makes the patient's skin more subject to sunburn than usual. Thus, exposure to sunlight may be very carefully controlled to prevent severe reactions, which may result in skin damage.

This drug is contraindicated in patients with prophyria, lupus erythematosus, and other disorders marked by photosensitivity. High oral doses may cause epigastric distress. If this occurs, the dose is reduced, and the drug is taken after meals or with milk.

Dosage and administration. One or two 5-mg tablets are taken daily after a meal. The patient with vitiligo then waits 2 to 4 hours before exposing himself to a source of UV light or to fluorescent black light for a brief period to increase sunlight tolerance. The fair-skinned patient takes the drug 2 hours before exposure to sunlight or to UV light. The dose of the drug and the exposure time to light must be carefully controlled to produce a gradual increase in skin pigment and to avoid severe burning and injury to the skin.

References

Anderson TF, Voorhess JJ: Psoralen photochemotherapy of cutaneous disorders. Ann Rev Pharmacol Toxicol 20:235, 1980

Blaney DJ, Cook CH: Topical use of tetracycline in the treatment of acne. Arch Dermatol 112:971, 1976

Bond CA et al: Photochemotherapy of psoriasis with

methoxsalen and longwave ultraviolet light. Am J Hosp Pharm 38:990, 1981

Drugs for acne. Med Lett Drugs Ther 22:31, 1980

Fritsch WC: Therapy of impetigo and furunculosis. JAMA 214:1862, 1970

Isotretinoin (Accutane) for acne. Med Lett Drugs Ther 24:79, 1982

Lerman S et al: Potential ocular complications from PUVA therapy and their prevention. J Invest Dermatol 74:197, 1980

Phototherapy for psoriasis. Med Lett Drugs Ther 24:72, 1982

Robertson DB, Maibach HI: Topical corticosteroids. Int J Dermatol 21:59, 1982

Rodman MJ: Systemic and topical drugs for psoriasis and acne. RN 38:63, 1975

Stern RS et al: Risk of cutaneous carcinoma in patients treated with oral methoxsalen photochemotherapy for psoriasis. N Engl J Med 300:809, 1979

Sunscreens. Med Lett Drugs Ther 26:56, 1984

Update on isotretinoin (Accutane) for acne. Med Lett Drugs Ther 25:105, 1983

Section 8

Drugs acting on the central nervous system

8 This section will describe drugs that produce their primary effects by altering the functioning of nerve cells located in the brain and spinal cord—the central nervous system. These drugs have a greater variety of clinical uses than those acting on any other system. The description of these drugs is divided into four main parts:

1. Drugs that affect mental and emotional function and behavior
2. Drugs that are used in treating neurologic and musculoskeletal disorders
3. Drugs that are used to relieve and prevent pain
4. Drugs, including alcohol, that are abused.

The application of these drugs in the treatment of various clinical disorders will be described, as well as aspects of their chronic and acute toxicity. Several classes of centrally acting drugs are commonly abused by people who employ them for purposes that are not medically approved. The last chapter in this section will discuss the management of patients who use centrally acting drugs in this way, and the management of patients who are suffering from chronic alcoholism.

To understand how centrally acting drugs produce their therapeutically desirable and adverse effects, one must first be familiar with the normal functioning of the central nervous system. The introductory chapter that follows will review those aspects of the anatomy, organization, and physiology of this complex system that are most relevant to an understanding of the actions of these drugs. It will also introduce some general concepts of central nervous system pharmacology and indicate, in general terms, the chief differences among the various classes of centrally acting drugs.

Chapter 44

Introduction to the pharmacology of the central nervous system

44

The human brain is the most complex of all biologic mechanisms. Neuroscientists still lack real understanding of how the billions of brain and spinal cord cells work together to control the functioning of the body's other structures, organs, and systems. Chapter 13 has described the fundamental properties of nerve cells, the generation, conduction, and transmission of nerve impulses, and the transmission of these impulses, or action potentials, from one neuron to another or from a neuron to an effector organ cell.

This chapter will therefore begin by reviewing the gross anatomy of the central nervous system (CNS) and by stating some significant principles concerning the still incompletely understood functional relationships of various groups of nerve cells. This will provide the foundation for learning how drugs can disrupt normal functioning or correct abnormal activity in the circuits that control consciousness, sensory perception, intellectual and emotional function, and motor or behavioral responses, among other activities.

Functional organization of the central nervous system

The CNS includes the brain and spinal cord. Most drug effects that are called CNS effects are actually produced in the brain. Therefore, most of the discussion here will be about the brain.

The human brain has been called "the most complex organ in all creation." However, despite its anatomic and functional complexity, neuroscientists are continually filling in gaps in human knowledge of the neuroanatomy of the CNS, the functional relations between the various structures, and the manner in which the activity of one part affects that of others.

Anatomy of the brain

The brains of all vertebrate animals show certain basic similarities, despite their many differences and modifications, and are built along the same general lines. All contain an older, underlying portion that is connected by many nerve tracts to the more recently developed parts of the brain above and the even more primitive spinal cord below.

The brain has three major divisions—the *hindbrain*, the *midbrain*, and the *forebrain*—and each of these may be subdivided into other related groups of nerve cell bodies (nerve *nuclei*) and fiber *tracts* (Figs. 44-1 and 44-2). This chapter will review only those parts that will be referred to later as sites at which various drugs act to bring about important changes in CNS functions.

The hindbrain runs from the top of the spinal cord into the *midbrain*, or *mesencephalon*. It includes the *medulla oblongata* and the *pons*, the most primitive parts of the brain; these form the *brain stem*, a slender 3-inch stalk on which the cerebrum seems to be balanced. Above and behind the brain stem and connected to it by thick bundles of nerve fibers is the *cerebellum*. This organ, which lies in the lower, back part of the skull, works together with the brain stem and certain cerebral structures to coordinate the activity of the muscles that are concerned with maintaining resting posture and with the control of the body's balance during complex voluntary movements.

The forebrain is composed of the centrally located *diencephalon*, or tween-brain, which is flanked by the two cerebral hemispheres that make up the *telencephalon*, or end brain.

The diencephalon includes the *thalamus* and the *hypothalamus*, groups of nerve cells that connect with the cerebral cortex above and with various subcortical structures, including the brain stem. The thalamic nerve nuclei

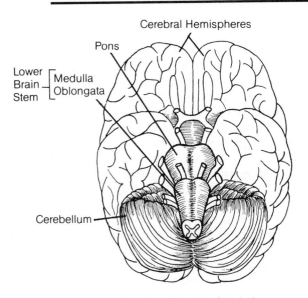

Figure 44-1. View of the underside of the brain.

serve as receiving and relay stations for sensations such as heat and cold, pain, touch, and muscle position sense. Some of these are sent directly to the appropriate receiving stations in the cerebral cortex; other sensory impulses are shunted to nerve cells in the core of the brain stem for further processing before being passed on to cortical areas. Other thalamic nuclei subserve a motor function.

The hypothalamic nuclei that lie below the thalamus help to make continuous adjustments in the control of body temperature, water balance, blood sugar levels, appetite, and sleep. They also seem to play a central part in the expression of emotions. The hypothalamus also plays an important role in autonomic nervous system function (Section 3) and endocrine function (Section 4, Chap. 20).

The cerebral hemispheres of the telencephalon—and especially their frontal lobes—have grown to relatively tremendous size in humans. Their outer layer, the *cerebral cortex,* is made up of masses of nerve cell bodies, the gray matter. This, the most recently evolved part of the brain, has buried beneath it the more primitive parts of the cerebral cortex—the *rhinencephalon,* or "nose brain," which in lower animals is concerned with the sense of smell. The cerebral cortical cells also cover over the subcortical structures of the diencephalon and the brain stem.

This folded cloak of cortical nerve cells contains not only the sensory neurons by which information about the environment is received, and the motor neurons through which we act on such information, but also the interneurons that comprise the machinery that plays so important a part in the mental processes that are thought to account for the intellectual superiority of human beings.

Embedded in the strands of subcortical whitish nerve fibers, or white matter, are still other masses of gray matter, the *basal ganglia.* These groups of nerve cells include the caudate, amygdaloid, and lentiform nuclei. These cells send out fibers that connect with other subcortical motor centers and are, in turn, connected with the motor area of the cerebral cortex. Together with the cerebellum, the basal ganglia make up an *extrapyramidal* motor system, which influences the functioning of the upper motor neurons of the motor cortex, and which—by way of its connections with the reticular core of the

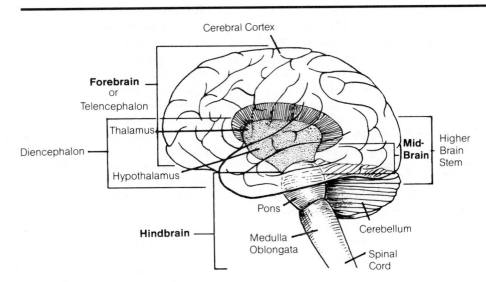

Figure 44-2. Median or midsagittal view of the brain.

brain stem (see below)—affects the activity of the lower motor neurons of the spinal cord.

The reticular formation is a network of neurons located in the core of the brain stem. It is made up of several different types of nerve cells scattered diffusely among a tangled mass of nerve processes (dendrites and axons) running from the top of the spinal cord up through the medulla, pons, and midbrain into the thalamus and hypothalamus. Located at a crucial crossroad for nerve tracts passing into and out of the brain, the reticular formation plays a very important part in the integration of both sensory and motor activity.

Such coordination by the reticular formation seems to involve first a filtering of sensory data, and then the selection of the appropriate motor response to fit the pattern of incoming information. All the main sensory pathways passing toward the cerebral cortex send collateral branches to the reticular formation, in which most of the 100 million sensory signals generated every second are filtered out.

Only the most significant messages are then relayed to the cerebral cortex. Such ascending impulses pass to all parts of the cerebral cortex by way of diffusely spreading polysynaptic nerve chains. Other reticular formation nerve cells send their signals downstream to modify the rate at which the spinal motor neurons fire their impulses out to the muscles. Thus, this neuronal "middleman" can help to cope with environmental changes by influencing muscular (and glandular) reactions to incoming messages, which it also helps to monitor.

Functions of the brain

The brain has several different types of functions, which it carries out through the interactions of nerve cells located at all levels. In general, however, all these varied activities serve the same broad purpose—coordinating the reactions of the person to a constantly changing external and internal environment. In this respect humans are not essentially different from lower animals, except that their cerebral cortex, with its innumerable interneuronal connections, is capable of an enormously increased number and variety of responses to environmental stimuli.

In reviewing some of the main activities of the brain in terms of the operation of certain of its functional systems, the systems involved in *sensory, motor, mental,* and *emotional* activities will be considered separately. However, these systems actually work together in many ways. That is, the various parts of the CNS do not operate independently but as a unit. Thus, although there is a tendency to speak of various drugs as acting at particular central sites, one should be aware that the same drug may cause changes in many different functions through its indirect effects on other parts of the brain. In addition, a drug may act at one dose level to affect only one area of the brain and one main function, while larger doses may

affect several functions in addition to the most sensitive one.

Sensory circuits and consciousness

Millions of sensory impulses—perhaps 100 million a second—are constantly streaming into the CNS from peripheral receptor outposts. Many of these messages reach specialized areas of the cerebral cortex by way of special sense organs in the eyes, ears, nose, and tongue. Other sensations stem from receptors and nerve endings in the skin and internal organs. Some receptors are specialized for reporting touch, pressure, heat, and cold, and pain; others—the proprioceptors—inform the brain of changes in the position of the body's parts.

Much of this stream of sensory data makes its way directly to terminals in the sensory, visual and auditory areas of the cerebral cortex. From there, signals are flashed to nearby associative cortical areas, where the data are analyzed to determine what messages should be sent to the motor cortex which controls voluntary movements.

However, more primitive parts of the brain also have a role in the handling of sensory messages. These include the thalamus, the hypothalamus, and the several parts of the brain stem. Neurophysiologic research studies have helped to clarify the role of the brain stem's reticular formation in the sorting and efficient processing of incoming sensations.

Certain studies that concentrated on the nature of what is called "consciousness" and on the wake–sleep cycles have revealed the role of the *reticular activating system* (RAS), the *ascending* portion of the reticular formation, which receives sensory stimuli by way of collateral fibers and then relays selected nerve impulses up to the cerebral cortex from the inner core of the brain stem. It is these signals, rather than those that pass to the sensory cortex by way of more direct pathways from the periphery, that help to keep the cortex awake.

Arousal of the cortex apparently depends on the spraying of a particular pattern of nerve impulses from the RAS to various cerebral cortical areas. However, the cortex itself also seems to have something to say about its own state of excitability. It feeds a continuous stream of impulses back down to the reticular formation in the brain stem and hypothalamus. These messages can both reduce and increase the activity of the RAS.

The control mechanisms involved in sleep are complex; however, it has been suggested that sleep is controlled neurologically in two ways:

1. A lessened input of external stimuli may deactivate the RAS and thus result in fewer facilitatory impulses passing upstream to stimulate the cerebral cortex.
2. Inhibitory impulses descending from the

cerebral cortex can depress reticular activity and thus induce sleep.

In any case, it is known that damage to the brain stem can cause coma of indefinite length. In addition, the central depressant drugs that produce sleep and anesthesia are believed to affect cerebral cortical functioning not by a direct action on the cortex but by their ability to interfere with the transfer of information between the tangled axons and dendrites of nerve cells located in the reticular activating system. The RAS then fails to send up to the higher cortical areas the specific patterned spray of signals that is required for maintaining consciousness. As a result, the anesthetized patient feels nothing, even though electroencephalographic evidence indicates that sensory impulses are continuously reaching the cerebral cortex by way of the direct sensory pathways.

Motor circuits for muscular activity

The sensory stimuli that enter the CNS set off responses that are mediated by motor and glandular cells. Muscular movements may be involuntary or purposeful. The simplest reflex contractions can be carried out in response to motor messages sent by the spinal cord alone, but voluntary acts require the planning and command functions of the cerebral cortex. In addition, muscular coordination calls for constant modification of the motor commands from above by the nerve cells of the cerebellum, basal ganglia, and reticular motor system.

Two main bundles of motor nerves in the brain influence the activity of the spinal motoneurons that finally send out the messages that make muscles move. One of these fiber tracts—the *pyramidal system*—originates in the cells of the motor cortex. Most of its fibers cross over to the opposite side of the spinal cord at a point in the base of the brain stem. The other nerve fiber bundles, which make up the *extrapyramidal system*, help in carrying out the complex automatic adjustments needed for maintaining balance and posture in response to constantly changing environmental situations. The extrapyramidal system also interacts with the upper and lower motoneurons to ensure the smooth performance of all voluntary movements.

Damage to the different parts of these motor systems can result in permanent muscular malfunction. Some drugs may temporarily interfere with the nervous control mechanisms for smoothly coordinated movements; other drugs may sometimes help to relieve neuromuscular disability. For example, certain tranquilizer drugs sometimes induce reversible disorders of the extrapyramidal motor system as an undesired side-effect; alcohol and other depressants may cause incoordinated motor activity or ataxia; still other chemicals can control disordered motor function. Certain centrally acting drugs can, for example, relieve the rigidity and tremors of the basal ganglia disorder Parkinson's disease. Others can reduce the writhing movements of athetosis and other manifestations of cerebral palsy, and the explosive neuronal activity responsible for epileptic seizures can be dampened by drugs that reduce the responsiveness of the cells that lie in the motor circuits.

Neuronal circuits for intellectual and emotional functions

The cerebral cortex is considered the seat of the higher intelligence of humans. Actually, however, no single site for intellectual activity has ever been localized in the cortex. Apparently, the type of behavior that is considered to be uniquely human depends on the neural connections between all the different areas of the cortex and between the cortex and certain subcortical sites. The latter include the hypothalamus and several groups of nerve cell bodies, or nuclei, which make up the subcortical part of the so-called limbic system. These structures, the amygdala, the hippocampus, and the fornix, form a closed nerve cell circuit together with the limbic lobe of the primitive "nose brain" cortex.

The more recently developed parts of the cerebral cortex—the neopallium—are connected with these lower centers by fiber tracts that run between the frontal lobes and the underlying subcortical areas. The cortex plays a major role in intellectual function such as learning, memory, judgment, and creative thinking. That is, it receives sensory data, stores this data in coded form, and then recombines all these bits of information in countless ways. The hypothalamic and limbic system nuclei seem to play a part in automatically selecting the program of behavior best suited to a particular situation. The two systems act together in translating thought into behavioral responses that are appropriate to the situations that must be dealt with.

These two interconnecting systems sometimes seem to influence one another in ways that are harmful to people. For example, under the influence of the frontal lobes of the cortex, which control the experiencing and expression of emotion, the subcortical areas sometimes seem to shower the visceral organs with messages that call forth psychosomatic symptoms. Conversely, excessive impulses ascending from the areas that control *responses* to emotion seem to play a part in disrupting cortically controlled mental or intellectual function.

Cutting the fiber bundles between the frontal lobes and subcortical areas, as in the psychosurgical operation known as a prefrontal lobotomy, brings about strange changes in the patient's personality and emotional reactions. For example, the patient does not seem to be disturbed by pain or by other previously upsetting stimuli. However, the general lack of emotional reactivity tends to leave the patient dull and apathetic.

Nonetheless, there are clinical situations in which

it seems desirable to break the circuits between cortical and subcortical areas and thus partially disconnect the patient's thought processes from his emotional responses. Various drugs seem to be able to affect the relationship between intellectual and emotional activity temporarily. As with lobotomy, people under the influence of these drugs may be benefited in some ways and hurt in others.

Morphine, for example, may prevent a patient from responding to pain even though he continues to feel it, perhaps because the drug performs a partial and reversible chemical lobotomy. People who become addicted to opiates often show the same lack of emotional drives that blunts the personality of the lobotomized patient. Similarly, the major phenothiazine tranquilizers that often offer symptomatic relief of mental illness symptoms—perhaps by their effects on the subcortical areas involved in emotional responses—may prove harmful if used only as a substitute for dealing constructively with emotional problems.

General pharmacology of the central nervous system

Mechanism of drug action

Ideally, it should be possible to demonstrate how drugs act on the nerve cells of various CNS structures to alter central nervous system functions. However, there is at present no single acceptable basis for adequately explaining precisely how and where drugs generally act to affect the functioning of the CNS.

Actually, this is not surprising, because the complicated nerve pathways involved in the control of many functions are still not completely mapped. In fact, the intimate details of the functioning of individual nerve cells are still obscure, as is the neurochemistry of synapses. Thus, one can hardly hope to explain exactly how drugs affect synaptic transmission and such fundamental properties of nerve cells as their excitability and conductivity, when these aspects of nervous function are not yet fully understood.

Nonetheless, enough is known to make some useful generalizations about the nature of drug action on the CNS. First, nervous tissue is characterized by excitability, and drugs may act by altering such neuronal irritability. Furthermore, and somewhat more specifically, the state of excitability of various nerve nuclei at any moment in time is the result of the sum of excitatory and inhibitory stimuli impinging simultaneously on the nerve cell membranes. Drug molecules can be considered to be a form of foreign intervention that alters the precarious balance between these facilitatory and inhibitory influences that ordinarily determines the degree of central neuronal excitability.

Cellular effects of drugs

How do drugs exert the cellular actions that result in changes in central function? Individual drugs no doubt act in many different ways to modify the various functions of individual nerve cells and of the nervous system as a whole. Here, however, it is sufficient to say that drugs may affect the following:

1. The metabolism
2. The cell membrane potentials of individual neurons
3. The manner in which nerve impulses are transmitted at the synapses between two or more neighboring nerve cells

Metabolic action. Some drugs may act by affecting the cellular respiratory *enzyme systems* responsible for the chemical reactions from which the nerve cell derives its energy. Because some of that energy is used to run the cell's "sodium pump," the drug could then affect the excitability of the nerve cell membrane in ways that increase or decrease the cell's activity as a receiver or sender of nervous signals. The antiepileptic drug phenytoin (Dilantin), for example, is thought by some to reduce the excitability of normal neurons in this way, so that the explosive discharges from groups of disordered nerve cells, or epileptic foci, fail to fire off abnormal activity in the cells of the rest of the brain.

Action on membrane potential. Drugs may act directly on the nerve cell membrane itself. The general anesthetics are thought to act, according to one theory, by preventing the changes in brain cell membrane permeability that normally occur at the point at which they are stimulated. The resulting alteration in the normal flow of ions into and out of the nerve cell is then thought to prevent the membrane from depolarizing and sending its signal down the axonal fiber. Local anesthetics are believed to act on peripheral nerve fibers in the same manner (Chaps. 13 and 14).

Action at synapses. Another way in which centrally acting drugs may produce their effects is through interference with the chemical processes that are involved in the transmission of nerve impulses at synaptic junctions. It is believed that the drugs that affect excitatory and inhibitory postsynaptic potentials do so in ways that are essentially similar to those of the drugs that act at peripheral junctional sites (Chap. 13). They may, for instance, act by imitating, blocking, or otherwise affecting the metabolism and actions of certain neurotransmitter chemicals localized in parts of the brain—acetylcholine, dopamine, norepinephrine, serotonin and γ-aminobutyric acid (GABA), for example. By altering the normal relationships of these and other neurochemicals at presynaptic (axonal terminals) and postsynaptic (dendritic and nerve cell body) sites, antipsychotic drugs (Chap. 46) such as the phenothiazine tranquilizers and antidepressant drugs may alter the rate of transmission of nerve impulses through various functional pathways in the CNS.

The sensitivity of central synapses to interference by foreign chemicals (*i.e.*, drugs and poisons) is thought to account for the fact that those areas in the brain that contain the most synaptic connections are the ones most susceptible to drug action. Thus, the ascending reticular formation, which is very rich in the number of interconnected nerve cells that it contains, is one of the first areas affected by many central depressant drugs. Very small doses of barbiturates or of general anesthetics such as ether can thus block the transmission of impulses from the reticular activating system to the cortex. As a result of their actions on this multisynaptic pathway, these drugs quickly cause a loss of consciousness and produce sleep and stupor, or narcosis.

On the other hand, drugs that act selectively at central nerve pathways with relatively few synaptic connections do not induce loss of consciousness or general depression as readily. They tend, instead, to interfere with specific functions, such as the emotional reaction to pain or other disturbing stimuli.

For example, the major tranquilizers that are used for treating mental illness symptoms such as restlessness and agitation may act mainly on the closed nerve circuits between the frontal lobes of the cortex and the subcortical nuclei of the nervous system. These limbic system structures contain relatively few linked neurons as compared to the more sensitive polysynaptic circuits of the RAS. This may account for the ability of these drugs to reduce excitement without causing excessive sleepiness or loss of consciousness.

Classification of centrally acting drugs

Despite such speculations, neuroscientists really do not know enough about the intimate actions of drugs on the CNS to categorize them on the basis of the ways in which they act. Even if it were possible to speak with more confidence concerning the exact sites and manner of action of drugs, such a classification would still have relatively little meaning. One reason for this is that drugs rarely act on only one group of central cells, or affect only a single functional nerve circuit system. Certainly, when a drug's dosage is raised, its effects usually tend to spread from the most sensitive central cells to involve many more resistant pathways and often the entire CNS, as well as peripheral organs.

Nevertheless, it is usually possible to administer drugs in amounts that allow their actions to be kept more or less localized at particular neuronal nuclei. This permits their use in the treatment of conditions marked by specific functional disorders. Thus, centrally acting drugs are commonly classified in terms of the main pharmacologic effect that it is desirable to elicit in the treatment of patients with various nervous disorders or emotional symptoms—for example, sedative, hypnotic, analgesic, or antiepileptic actions.

More broadly, of course, drugs may first be classified as central *stimulants* and *depressants*, and each of these groups may, in turn, be subdivided on the basis of whether their actions affect the entire CNS in the same way or whether they act differently at various sites. Some drugs seem able to stimulate specific central neuronal sites and to depress others, but most of the centrally acting drugs tend either to depress or to excite the entire central nervous system.

General depressants

Actually, the drugs that can depress all nervous tissue are never deliberately used in doses that would knock out nerve centers at every level of the CNS—the result of which would, of course, be catastrophic. They are, instead, administered in amounts calculated to induce just the degree of functional loss required in the treatment of clinical conditions of specific type. Fortunately, this is relatively easy to do, because drug-induced depression of the CNS follows a general pattern that is more or less predictable.

Generally speaking, these drugs first depress the most recently developed functions of the cerebral cortex, and the most primitive functions of the medullary centers are the last to fail. Thus, the first effects of drugs such as alcohol, ether, and the barbiturates are on the psychosensory and psychomotor functions of the cerebral cortex. Later, the subcortical and spinal centers that control muscle tone are depressed; finally, the brain stem centers responsible for respiration and other automatically controlled vital functions stop sending out their signals.

Sometimes certain centrally acting drugs of the general depressant type may seem to be causing stimulation of the CNS. Alcohol may, for example, appear to be producing excitement. Actually, however, such apparent stimulation always results from the drug's depressant action on the functioning of nerve cells somewhere in the brain. The depressed nerve cells are located in the inhibitory areas of the brain. As a result, the areas that are released from inhibitory control may send out their excitatory impulses at a more rapid rate. Such "pseudostimulation" (technically called "disinhibition") accounts for the uninhibited behavior of alcoholic intoxication and for the so-called excitement stage of general anesthesia. Increased activity of the CNS also occurs when depressant drugs are withdrawn abruptly from people who have been abusing them by taking large doses for long periods to the point of becoming physically dependent upon them.

Depending on the dose employed, the general depressant drugs can bring about every degree of depression from light sedation, through sleep, stupor or narcosis and, finally, deep coma, with loss of all reflex activity. Thus, depending on how they are used clinically, the general depressants are commonly classified as *sedatives, hypnotics,* and *general anesthetics* (Chaps. 45 and 52). Although many of these drugs can also prevent epileptic seizures, relax skeletal muscles, and relieve pain, they are not classified on the basis of these secondary pharmacologic actions. That is, these drugs are not ordinarily referred to as antiepileptics, muscle relaxants, and analgesics; these terms are reserved for those depressants that produce these effects primarily and in a more selective manner when used in safe clinical doses.

Selective depressants

Some drugs can alter certain central functions when given in doses that do not affect the functioning of the CNS in general. For example, those classified as *antiepileptics* can reduce epileptic seizure activity when administered in amounts that do not interfere with normal psychomotor or psychosensory function. That is, they are less likely to make the patient excessively drowsy or interfere with judgment, muscle tone, or finely coordinated movements.

Similarly, the selectively acting *potent analgesics* such as morphine can reduce the patient's reaction to severe pain without rendering him unconscious, and the *major tranquilizers* can calm the emotionally disturbed patient without inducing sleep. Other more or less specific CNS depressants include the lissive, or skeletal muscle *antispasmodic,* drugs, the *antiparkinsonism* agents, the *antitussives,* and *antiemetics,* as well as the *analgesic–antipyretic* agents. Some of these drugs have been discussed in earlier sections, and will not be described further in this section.

Some selective depressant drugs seem to stimulate certain central sites even as they depress others. Thus, an opiate pain reliever such as morphine may stimulate the vomiting center and the spinal cord, and some phenothiazine-type tranquilizers cause increased activity in extrapyramidal motor systems. Similarly, some of these drugs—the salicylate analgesic–antipyretics, for instance (Chap. 37)—may act peripherally as well as through a combination of central depressant and stimulating actions. The antiparkinsonism drugs often exert potent peripheral effects on various organs.

Central nervous system stimulants

Certain drugs act to increase the general excitability of the CNS. Although they are sometimes classified on the basis of the central sites that seem most susceptible to their stimulating action, the effects of most of these drugs tend to spread to all levels of the CNS when the dose is increased. For example, a so-called brain stem stimulant, such as doxapram, may stimulate not only brain stem

respiratory control mechanisms but also motor control areas throughout the CNS, including spinal motor centers.

Some central stimulants are somewhat more specific than others. Caffeine and the amphetamines mainly affect certain subcortical areas to produce increased cortical activity of the psychomotor type. Their effects do not spread to the spinal cord in humans, and thus typically spinal convulsive seizures do not occur even with massive overdoses. On the other hand, because the pharmacologic actions of caffeine and the amphetamines are not limited to the CNS, these drugs can cause frequent peripheral side-effects.

Most stimulants generally act in any of several ways to increase central excitability through their effects at excitatory synapses; however, some convulsant drugs are now known to act by lessening the effectiveness of central *inhibitory* influences. *Strychnine,* for example, stimulates increased activity of spinal centers by blocking the effects of the inhibitory neurotransmitter, glycine, which ordinarily tend to counteract many of the excitatory stimuli that are simultaneously reaching certain central nerve cells.

CNS stimulants do not ordinarily produce direct depression of the CNS, although theoretically they could do so by stimulating inhibitory areas without at the same time affecting excitatory sites equally. However, excessive drug-induced activity is often followed by a period of relative inexcitability of the CNS. This is particularly apparent after the occurrence of drug-induced convulsions, which are often followed by a period of postictal depression.

The CNS is of awesome complexity, and being aware of this, the student will develop a healthy respect for the drugs that can interfere with neuronal function. Fortunately, despite their manifold and seemingly mystifying mechanisms of action, these drugs can be used with safety and with great benefit to suffering patients.

The following chapters of this section will describe how these drugs are used to gain their desirable effects and what precautions are employed to avoid accidental overdosage leading to acute toxicity. The need to prevent the abuse of many of these centrally acting drugs by addiction-prone people will also be emphasized.

References

Bloom FE: Neurohumoral transmission and the central nervous system. In Gilman AG, Goodman LS, Gilman A (eds): Goodman and Gilman's The Pharmacological Basis of Therapeutics, 6th ed, pp 235–257. New York, Macmillan, 1980

Cooper JR, Bloom FE, Roth RH: The Biochemical Basis of Neuropharmacology, 4th ed. New York, Oxford University Press, 1982

Eccles JC: Understanding of the Brain, 2nd ed. New York, McGraw–Hill, 1977

Section 8
Part 1

Drugs
that affect
mental and
emotional
function and
behavior

Chapter 45

Sedative–
hypnotics
and
antianxiety
agents

45

This chapter will describe the use of drugs in the management of insomnia and anxiety. The drugs most commonly employed in these disorders and in various other medical and psychiatric conditions and surgical procedures fall into the following three classes:

1. The *barbiturates,* a class of synthetic chemicals that can be used to produce any degree of depression of the central nervous system. This chapter will describe only those barbiturates that are used primarily as sedatives, or drugs that calm nervous patients, and as hypnotics, or sleep-producing drugs (see Tables 45-1 and 45-2).
2. The *nonbarbiturate* sedative–hypnotics, drugs of several other chemical classes that—like the barbiturates—can reduce nervous tension and help to bring about sleep (see Table 45-3).
3. The *antianxiety agents,* or *minor tranquilizers,* newer drugs that are used mostly for treating patients with the same types of emotional, mental, and physical conditions for which the barbiturates and other classic types of sedative–hypnotics have traditionally been employed (see Table 45-4).

The barbiturates

The barbiturates, derivatives of barbituric acid, are general depressants of cellular activity in all body tissues, but the clinically significant effects result almost entirely from the ability of these drugs to depress all parts of the central nervous system. Hundreds of these substances have been synthesized since barbital (Veronal; no longer available for therapeutic use) and phenobarbital (Luminal), the

first of this class of compounds, became available shortly before World War I and were shown to be clinically useful. However, less than a dozen or so derivatives are in common use today, and the physician can obtain good results in most cases by knowing how to use only three or four of these versatile drugs judiciously.

The physician who has learned to pick the best barbiturate for a particular purpose and to employ it properly can produce any desired degree of depression from mild sedation to deep anesthesia (Table 45-1). Although all the barbiturates possess essentially similar pharmacologic effects, some are better suited than others for achieving different clinical goals. By selecting the best drug for producing a desired effect and by giving it in the right dose and by the most efficacious route of administration, these drugs can be used in the management of a wide variety of clinical conditions in addition to those requiring sedation and sleep (see Table 45-2).

Pharmacologic actions

Sedation and antianxiety effects. Sedation involves the loss of awareness and reactivity to environmental stimuli. Drowsiness is a frequent concomitant, and sleep is produced by higher doses of most sedative drugs, including the barbiturates. With the advent of the benzodiazepines (*e.g.,* diazepam—Valium) and some of the other newer drugs (see Table 45-4), it has been possible, to some extent, to separate sedative from antianxiety effects. Although drowsiness may be a desirable effect of a drug given preoperatively to allay anxiety, and psychomotor impairment may not create a serious problem for patient safety under those circumstances, both are clearly undesirable effects in a drug given to calm an ambulatory outpatient who is trying to maintain his activities of daily living.

Barbiturates produce sedation in the smallest effective doses. They reduce restlessness, irritability, and

Table 45–1. Barbiturate-type sedative–hypnotics*

Official or generic name	Trade name	Usual adult daily oral dosage range†	Comments‡
Amobarbital and amobarbital sodium USP	Amytal; Amytal Sodium	30–200 mg	Moderately long-acting; parenteral preparation available
Aprobarbital	Alurate	120–160 mg	Intermediate duration of action
Butabarbital sodium USP	Butisol	45–100 mg	Intermediate duration of action
Mephobarbital	Mebaral	90–400 mg	Used only as sedative or antiepileptic; long-acting
Pentobarbital and pentobarbital sodium USP	Nembutal; Nembutal Sodium	40–100 mg	Intermediate duration of action (see Drug digest); parenteral preparation available
Phenobarbital USP	Luminal	30–100 mg	Long duration of action (see Drug digest, Chap. 50); parenteral preparation available
Secobarbital and secobarbital sodium USP	Seconal; Seconal Sodium	30–100 mg	Short duration of action (see Drug digest); parenteral preparation available
Talbutal	Lotusate	120 mg	Used only as hypnotic; should not be administered longer than 2 wks; intermediate duration of action

* Barbiturates employed mainly as anticonvulsants are listed in Chapter 50, and those ultrashort-acting barbiturates used mainly in anesthesia appear in Chapter 52.
† Dosage varies widely and must be individualized for each patient. Here, the lower dose generally represents about twice the smallest single daytime sedative dose; the higher dose indicates the usual hypnotic dose. It is not unusual for each of the indicated doses to be doubled in some cases.
‡ Although barbiturates are commonly classified in terms of their duration of action, the distinction is of real clinical significance mainly with the long- and ultrashort-acting drugs. Individual differences in the way people metabolize the drugs classified as short- to intermediate-acting tend to blur any distinction between them.

nervousness, but also produce some degree of drowsiness and lethargy. The use of barbiturates (*e.g.*, phenobarbital, butabarbital) for daytime sedation of patients suffering the mental and physical discomforts of anxiety has declined considerably in recent years. It is now preferable to order one of the newer antianxiety drugs—in particular, one of the benzodiazepines (see Table 45-4)—for this purpose, because these drugs have greater efficacy, are safer, produce fewer adverse effects (including less physical dependence), and are involved in fewer drug–drug interactions.

Hypnosis. Administered at bedtime in doses about three or four times higher than those used for sedation during the day, the barbiturates produce a greater degree of central depression. Most patients who have had little previous exposure to these or to other depressant drugs fall asleep promptly. Once asleep, they usually stay asleep for 6 or 7 hours, even after such a relatively short-acting barbiturate as *secobarbital*⁺ (Seconal) has been metabolized and eliminated from the body. This and such other drugs of short to intermediate duration as *pentobarbital* and *amobarbital* are preferred to such long-

acting drugs as *phenobarbital* for treating occasional insomnia.

Here, too, the popularity of these barbiturates has declined in favor of *flurazepam* (Dalmane) and other benzodiazepines, which have a number of clinical advantages. Actually, all hypnotic drugs—barbiturates and *non*barbiturates, including this benzodiazepine—are equally effective for most patients when taken only occasionally, and no class of hypnotic drugs has any real advantages in efficacy over any other for long-term treatment of patients with *chronic* insomnia. As will be discussed later, the prolonged use of *any* hypnotic, or somnifacient, drug in such cases is undesirable (see below).

The drugs classified as sedative–hypnotics have a relatively selective action on the reticular formation in the brain stem (Chap. 44). Small doses deactivate this area, which is so important in maintaining consciousness and wakefulness. By blocking some of the nerve impulses that normally ascend to the cerebral cortex by way of the reticular activating system (Fig. 45-1), these drugs reduce excessive psychological activity and promote sleep. The effects of larger doses can, of course, spread to de-

Table 45-2. Pharmacologic actions and clinical indications: barbiturates

Pharmacologic actions	Clinical indications	Preferred compounds
Sedative	Anxiety state; excitement and restlessness; organic conditions involving gastrointestinal tract, cardiovascular system, endocrine system, and allergic reactions	Amobarbital; butabarbital; pentobarbital; phenobarbital
Hypnotic	Insomnia; preanesthetic medication (intermediate-acting drugs at bedtime; short-acting drugs 1 hr prior to surgery in larger dose)	Amobarbital; butabarbital; pentobarbital; secobarbital
Antiepileptic and anticonvulsant	Epilepsy (long-acting drugs); control of acute convulsions in eclampsia, tetanus, and overdoses of convulsant poisons (short-acting drugs)	Phenobarbital; mephobarbital; metharbital; thiopental; pentobarbital; amobarbital
Analgesia	Combined with salicylates and other analgesics, small doses are employed for headache, joint and muscle pain	Amobarbital; butabarbital; pentobarbital
Amnesia	In obstetrics to reduce memory of delivery pain, without necessarily relieving the pain itself or producing anesthesia	Pentobarbital
Anesthesia (general and basal)	Rapid, pleasant induction of anesthesia, prior to administration of other agents, or as sole anesthetic in short surgical operations and manipulative procedures	Thiopental; thiamylal; methitural; methohexital; hexobarbital
Miscellaneous	In neuropsychiatry for narcoanalysis, narcosuggestion, narcosynthesis, and narcotherapy	Thiopental; secobarbital; pentobarbital; amobarbital

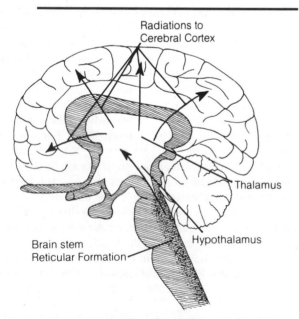

Figure 45-1. The reticular activating system. Diffuse impulses from this area excite cerebral cortical activity. Depression of impulse transmission in this polysynaptic system reduces alertness and wakefulness.

press other parts of the nervous system, including the spinal cord and the vital centers of the medulla oblongata.

Antiepileptic effects. Most barbiturates can prevent or control convulsive or motor seizures by reducing the responsiveness of normal neurons in the central nervous system to nerve impulses that reach them from an abnormal brain area that is rapidly discharging repeated stimuli. However, some barbiturates are better than others in this respect. As Chapter 50 will describe, the goal of antiepileptic therapy is to maintain patients both seizure-free and with as normal a life style as possible. When barbiturates are given to prevent and control seizures, they frequently cause drowsiness. Other drugs can sometimes control the patient's seizures without this side-effect. However, *phenobarbital* is still often useful for preventing grand mal epileptic seizures, and tolerance often develops to its sedating effects. *Thiopental*[+] (Pentothal; see Drug digest, Chap. 50) is the barbiturate of choice when a drug is needed to combat convulsions once they have begun; however, diazepam or other antiepileptic drugs are more often used. The anticonvulsant action of these and such other barbiturates as *mephobarbital* and *metharbital* will be discussed in Chapter 50.

Anesthesia. High doses of any barbiturate can produce loss of consciousness by blocking passage of nerve impulses from the reticular activating system to the cerebral cortex. However, here too, some barbiturates are preferred to others for clinical purposes. *Thiopental* and *methohexital* (Brevital) act very rapidly when injected intravenously, as do other ultrashort-acting barbiturates such as *hexobarbital* (Evipal) and short-acting agents such as *secobarbital*. (See Chapter 52 for further discussion of the use of barbiturates in anesthesia.)

Analgesia. None of the above drugs is ordinarily used alone during surgery, because they are not very effective for preventing responses to painful stimuli. As discussed in Chapter 52, thiopental and other ultrashort-acting barbiturates are used only as basal anesthetics to induce sleep rapidly and pleasantly. For preventing pain, other anesthetic substances such as nitrous oxide or halothane must then be inhaled. The sedative effect of moderate oral doses of barbiturates is said to reduce patients' emotional responses to painful stimuli (Chap. 51) when these drugs are combined with true analgesics. However, when administered without an analgesic, sedative doses of barbiturates sometimes set off episodes of excitement, confusion, and delirium. Rarely, in idiosyncratic patients, barbiturates may actually *cause* pain. This antianalgesic effect may occur when a barbiturate depresses neurons that ordinarily inhibit transmission of pain impulses in certain nerve pathways.

Disinhibition. A clinically more common example of the ability of barbiturates to release certain nerve cells from the influence of others that normally exert inhibitory activity is seen in the effect of these drugs on mental, emotional, and behavioral responses in various circumstances. This action is thought to account for the emotional lability and occasionally aggressive behavior of barbiturate abusers when they are in a state of mild to moderate drug-induced intoxication.

This loss of control is sometimes put to clinical use in psychiatry for diagnostic purposes and as an adjunct to verbal interviewing techniques and other therapeutic procedures. The use of this disinhibiting property of the short- and ultrashort-acting intravenous barbiturates will be briefly discussed in Chapter 52.

Amnesia. Forgetfulness sometimes follows the use of moderate doses of barbiturates. Barbiturate-induced amnesia and confusion may be a factor in leading to accidental overdosage and acute intoxication (see below).

Pharmacokinetics

Many points clinically significant for the safe and effective use of barbiturates depend on knowledge of how the body handles these drugs from the time they are administered until their molecules or those of their inactive metabolites are finally eliminated. How each drug is dealt with depends, in turn, on such physicochemical properties as lipid solubility and degree of ionization. As discussed in Chapter 4, these properties and the way in which a drug behaves in relation to the pH of body fluids determines its ability to move through biologic membranes, including those that make up the blood–brain barrier.

Absorption and distribution. Most orally administered barbiturates are absorbed from the upper gastrointestinal tract and enter the blood at about the same rate, once their dosage form is dissolved and its contents are dispersed over the absorptive mucosal surfaces. More important in determining the onset time of different drugs is the speed with which they penetrate into the brain. Thus, *secobarbital* has a much more rapid onset of action than *phenobarbital*, because its higher solubility in membrane lipids speeds its passage through the blood–brain barrier. Drugs such as *thiopental* and *methohexital* (Chap. 52) that have the highest lipid solubility also have an extremely rapid onset of action when delivered directly into the blood, from which they begin to pass immediately into the brain.

The duration of action of these drugs depends on the speed with which they leave the brain and are carried to other organs, including particularly the liver and the kidneys. As discussed in Chapter 4, the ultrashort duration of thiopental-induced anesthesia is the result of its rapid redistribution from the brain to fat, to lean muscle tissue, and finally to the liver. The long-lasting action of phenobarbital reflects, in part, the slowness of its removal from the brain, where it had accumulated only gradually after absorption. However, the final removal of phenobarbital and the end of its depressant effects depends, in the end, mainly on its *partial* breakdown by liver enzymes to inactive metabolites and, most importantly, on the excretion by the kidneys of those molecules that were not metabolized by the liver.

Liver enzyme action. The most significant site for initiating the breakdown of most barbiturates is the endoplasmic reticulum of the liver (Chap. 4). Enzymes located in this liver cell structure attack most barbiturate molecules and convert them to more water-soluble compounds that cannot re-enter the brain but *can* be more readily excreted by the kidneys. Thus, these oxidized barbiturate by-products are pharmacologically inactive and can be removed by such renal processes as glomerular filtration and tubular secretion—in most cases with little tubular reabsorption.

Renal elimination. This is a much slower process than the hepatic enzyme-catalyzed metabolic degradation of barbiturates. Thus, a barbiturate such as phenobarbital, which is in large part eliminated by the renal route, can be expected to exert a prolonged central depressant effect. As suggested in Chapter 4, this depressant action can be shortened by administering drugs that alkalinize the patient's urine. A greater proportion of the phenobarbital that appears in the glomerular filtrate is then in the ionized form. These ionized particles cannot be readily reabsorbed into the blood through the renal tubular membranes. Thus, more of the drug is eliminated in the urine, and the drug's level in the patient's blood and brain is lowered.

Clinical significance. These pharmacokinetic factors are also important in other aspects of the safe use of barbiturates. Obviously, it would be dangerous to order a drug such as phenobarbital for a patient with severely impaired renal function, because this drug could then not be readily eliminated by the kidneys and could accumulate to toxic levels in the brain. Similarly, secobarbital and all other barbiturates that depend on the liver for breakdown to metabolites that can then be more readily removed by the kidneys would be contraindicated in liver failure.

Patients with renal or hepatic insufficiency are, in any case, very sensitive to even small doses of barbiturates. Thus, these drugs are contraindicated in patients with uremia or severe liver cirrhosis. Patients who show signs of hepatic encephalopathy, including central excitement for example, should not be treated with barbiturates, because this could send them into hepatic coma (Chap. 41). These drugs must also not be administered to patients with status asthmaticus or severe emphysema, because their use in hypoxic, hypercapnic patients could lead to acute respiratory failure (Chap. 40).

Drug–drug interactions. Those involving barbiturates are also often based on pharmacokinetic factors. As discussed in Chapter 4, for example, phenobarbital and other drugs of this class stimulate an increase in the amount of drug-metabolizing enzymes in the livers of people who regularly receive such sedative-hypnotics. Such *enzyme induction* leads not only to an increased rate of degradation of the barbiturates, but also of various other drugs that are metabolized by the same hepatic microsomal enzyme system. As a result, the blood plasma levels of both the barbiturates *and* the simultaneously administered other drugs are lowered.

Such drug–drug interactions are of particular clinical significance when the drugs that are taken by the patient who is also receiving barbiturates are very potent and have only a relatively narrow safety margin. These include coumarin-type oral anticoagulant drugs such as *warfarin*, heart-stimulating digitalis derivatives such as *digitoxin*, and corticosteroid drugs such as *hydrocortisone*. In all cases, the barbiturate-induced increase in enzymatic activity leads to a reduction in the plasma concentrations of these drugs, with a resulting loss in their effectiveness.

In addition to possibly depriving the patient of the therapeutically desired effects of these drugs, such drug–drug interactions can lead to toxic reactions in some cases. For example, the presence of the barbiturate first increases the dosage requirements for the second drug. Then, if the barbiturate is discontinued and the level of liver enzymes falls back to normal, the continued administration of the second drug at the high level that was previously necessary can lead to toxicity. (See Chapter 34 for a further discussion of how the withdrawal of bar-

biturates from the regimen of a patient who had been taking them together with anticoagulant drugs can lead to an episode of dangerous bleeding.)

Other drug–drug interactions involving barbiturates are based, not on pharmacokinetic or metabolic factors, but on their potential additive effects with other depressant drugs. Thus, for example, patients taking barbiturates for daytime sedation should be warned not to drink *alcoholic beverages* because they may suffer excessive psychomotor depression. This may make it more dangerous for these patients to drive than if they had taken only the barbiturate. Similarly, special care is required to avoid respiratory depression in patients who receive barbiturates parenterally after they have already been treated with a *tranquilizing drug* or with a potent *narcotic analgesic.*

Adverse effects of barbiturates

When taken by most patients in the small doses recommended for daytime sedation or the somewhat larger doses needed to produce sleep, the barbiturates do not ordinarily cause severe side-effects or toxic reactions. However, some patients tend to react poorly to barbiturates (see the summary of adverse effects at the end of this chapter). The patient history should include questions about whether a patient has ever taken barbiturates, and what the response was. Being aware of a previous hypersensitivity reaction will alert the staff to potential problems with the patient.

Excessive sedation. Sometimes, patients treated with a long-acting barbiturate such as phenobarbital may waken feeling dazed, dizzy, and lethargic. Shorter acting drugs may also leave the patient drowsy and with a headache, especially when they have to be given repeatedly during a night of interrupted sleep. Such a "hangover" effect may make it dangerous for a patient to drive or to carry out any complex task requiring judgment and motor coordination. However, hospitalized patients are not usually harmed by some residual sedation from an intermediate- or long-acting barbiturate. The patient should be made aware of this effect, and assured that it is a normal response.

Excitement. Some patients, especially elderly people, tend to become excited instead of calmed when they are given sleep-producing doses of certain barbiturates at night. This paradoxical excitement seems most likely to occur with the short-acting compounds, such as secobarbital. Patients with arteriosclerotic brain damage, who often become confused and disoriented in the dark, are the most likely victims of this idiosyncratic reaction. However, other patients may also become restless and even delirious, especially if they are in pain or feverish.

The nurse should always keep a close watch on the patient who has become confused by barbiturates. Side rails may be put up to prevent patient injury, but cuffs or other restraints should not be applied because

Table 45–3. Other sedative–hypnotics

Official or generic name	Trade name	Usual adult daily oral dosage range*	Comments
Nonbarbiturate sedative–hypnotics			
Chloral hydrate USP	Noctec	250–1000 mg	See Drug digest
Ethchlorvynol USP	Placidyl	100–1000 mg	Rapid onset; short duration
Ethinamate USP	Valmid	500–1000 mg	Rapid onset; short duration
Glutethimide USP	Doriden	250–500 mg	See Drug digest
Methyprylon USP	Noludar	200–400 mg	Similar to secobarbital in onset and duration of action
Paraldehyde USP	Paral	5–30 ml	Also administered rectally and IM against acute convulsions (see Drug digest)
Triclofos sodium	Triclos	1500 mg	Metabolized to trichlorethanol, the same active metabolite that is formed from chloral hydrate
Benzodiazepines			
Flurazepam HCl USP	Dalmane	15–30 mg	Chemical relative of chlordiazepoxide and diazepam (Table 45-4; see Drug digest)
Lorazepam	Ativan	2–4 mg	Chemical relative of chlordiazepoxide and diazepam; used primarily as antianxiety agent (Table 45-4)
Temazepam	Restoril	15–30 mg	Chemical relative of chlordiazepoxide and diazepoxide and diazepam (Table 45-4)
Triazolam	Halcion	0.25–0.50 mg	Chemical relative of chlordiazepoxide and diazepam (Table 45-4)

* The lower dose is usually administered several times daily for daytime sedation; the larger dose represents either the total daily sedative dose or the highest single dose administered at bedtime for hypnosis.

this may make the patient even more restless and could result in injury to the patient. Instead, the nurse can often calm the patient and help him orient himself by putting on the bedside light and talking to him.

Allergic and idiosyncratic reactions. Hypersensitivity reactions involving mainly the skin and mucous membranes sometimes occur in patients taking barbiturates. However, these drugs are not considered to be strong sensitizers—like the penicillins, for example—and such allergic reactions tend to occur mainly in atopic patients with a prior history of urticarial or other skin eruptions, allergic rhinitis, or asthmatic attacks in response to various other drugs, foods, and environmental substances. Blood dyscrasias are rare, but a few patients may complain of persistent muscle or joint pains after treatment with barbiturates. Patients who prove truly sensitive to barbiturates may have to be treated with a nonbarbiturate sedative–hypnotic (see Table 45-3).

Acute intermittent porphyria is one of the few conditions in which barbiturates must never be administered. Patients with a personal or family history of this hereditary disorder should never take these drugs, because they could set off a severe, potentially fatal attack of the type that tend to recur periodically in these people. The barbiturates are thought to do so by an action that adds to the metabolic defect that makes it difficult for the bodies of these people to regulate the biosynthesis of heme and of other porphyrin compounds.*

---

* *Heme* is the iron-containing porphyrin compound that is responsible for oxygen transport when it is combined with the protein globin in the molecule of hemoglobin.

Barbiturates such as secobarbital stimulate the synthesis of the specific enzyme that is most important in the production of porphyrins. This results in the biosynthesis of more molecules of these compounds, which already tend to be present in excess. As a result, the patient may suffer a wide variety of painful and disabling physical and mental reactions. Signs and symptoms of a barbiturate-induced attack of acute porphyria include abdominal cramps, muscular weakness or paralysis and, sometimes, delirium caused by toxic psychosis.

Acute and chronic toxic effects

The main problem with the barbiturates is that some of the people most in need of their calming effects are also the very ones who are most likely to abuse the drugs and become tolerant to and physically dependent on them (see Chapter 53 for a discussion of these terms, and for a description of barbiturate tolerance and dependence). Many patients—epileptics, for example—often take small doses of barbiturates for years without running into difficulty of any kind, but some emotionally unstable people may get into trouble if these drugs are carelessly prescribed or administered. Also, emotionally depressed patients with chronic insomnia may sometimes save up sleeping pills and take a massive overdose for suicidal purposes.

Chronic toxicity. People who habitually receive barbiturates for medical purposes tend to take them in increasing amounts as tolerance develops. This in itself need not lead to chronic toxicity although, as indicated here and below, the practice is undesirable for other reasons. However, people who begin to abuse barbiturates, not for medical reasons but to keep on getting a "downer high," are likely to develop chronic physical and mental difficulties. In addition, people who continue to seek barbiturate-induced euphoria soon become physically dependent on these drugs and are prone to develop severe mental and physical reactions, including life-threatening convulsive seizures, when they are abruptly deprived of their accustomed daily intake. (For a further and more detailed discussion of chronic barbiturate toxicity and the measures necessary to prevent and treat it, see Chap. 53, General Depressant Abuse and Dependence.)

Acute toxicity. Barbiturate overdosage ranks as one of the leading causes of drug-induced deaths. It is the publicity given to "sleeping pill" suicides of people prominent in the entertainment world, political life, and business that has aroused public distrust and fear of these drugs. Accidental poisoning is not common but sometimes occurs in children who are attracted to brightly colored capsules kept in a bedside table or in some other readily accessible place. Also, adults may take too many capsules unintentionally, especially if they have been drinking alcohol.

It is said that sometimes an insomniac becomes confused from the effects of the first couple of capsules and, in this dazed and disoriented condition, downs the contents of an entire bottle without realizing it. Whether such "twilight zone automatism" is a common factor in barbiturate poisoning has been disputed. However, the nurse should advise the patient never to keep a sleeping capsule container by the bedside, nor should a person take barbiturates while under the influence of alcohol. Some physicians make it a practice never to write a prescription for a lethal dose of any hypnotic drug to be dispensed in one container.

Sleep-producing doses taken on a physician's order are ordinarily harmless, but only five to ten times this hypnotic dose can cause deep depression. Between ten and twenty times the therapeutic amount may produce stupor, coma, and death. Thus, an emotionally depressed patient who deliberately ingests a dozen or more sleeping capsules is going to need prompt and vigorous treatment if his life is to be saved. This is why physicians use great caution in prescribing barbiturates for patients who seem depressed and possibly suicidal.

Signs and symptoms of overdosage may be quite varied. Some patients may seem excited, instead of depressed, when first seen. Then, as in alcohol intoxication, they may become lethargic and lapse into stupor and coma. The chief danger, especially with large amounts of the quick-acting barbiturates, is that circulatory collapse or respiratory failure may occur rapidly. Patients who survive this stage and those who have taken long-acting barbiturates may go into a deep, prolonged period of central nervous system depression, during which they can develop pneumonia. This is most likely to occur in comatose patients who have lost their cough reflex, with the resulting accumulation of purulent secretions and the development of atalectasis.

Other complications include possible kidney failure, gastrointestinal bleeding, and extensive skin lesions. The patient may be feverish, or his body temperature may drop steeply. Signs of pulmonary edema—moist rales heard in the lower lungs, for example—may indicate the onset of congestive heart failure. Cardiac irregularities occur in some cases.

Treatment. Management of intoxication by barbiturates and other sedative–hypnotics is based on constant observation of the patient and aggressive use of the general supportive measures that were discussed in Chapter 5. The central nervous system stimulants, or analeptics (Chap. 47), which were once used to help rouse the patient and to stimulate respiration, are now rarely employed. However, vasomotor stimulants (Chap. 17) are still sometimes ordered to raise the patient's blood pressure and prevent shock if intravenous fluids alone fail to do so.

In addition to applying physical measures to support the patient's vital functions, the nurse must be ready to offer emotional support and to employ psychotherapeutic measures in the case of patients who have swallowed barbiturates in a suicide attempt. The nurse should develop a plan of nursing care that takes into account the fact that the patient may remain emotionally disturbed and may be even more depressed after failure of his suicide attempt. The patient requires emotional support as he faces the need to attack constructively the problems that had led him to take an overdose of barbiturates. The patient will need an opportunity to talk and react to his situation, and will most likely require a psychiatric referral.

Therapeutic uses

The clinical indications for the barbiturates are listed in Table 45-2, and have been mentioned briefly in the discussion of the applications of the various pharmacologic actions of these drugs. The current status of these drugs in the management of insomnia and of anxiety will be taken up later in this chapter. The barbiturates employed mainly as antiepileptics will be discussed in Chapter 50, Drugs for treating epilepsy, and the role of barbiturates as adjuncts to anesthesia and psychiatric procedures and as basal anesthetics will be discussed in Chapter 52.

Other sedative–hypnotics and antianxiety agents

Many drugs in addition to the barbiturates can produce sedation and sleep (Table 45-3). The older drugs of this group are often called *nonbarbiturate sedative–hypnotics*. Newer drugs are mainly in the chemical class of *benzodiazepines* and will be referred to by this chemical name. In addition, several H₁ antihistamines are available as OTC sleep aids.

Nonbarbiturate sedative–hypnotics

Some of these drugs, such as *chloral hydrate*⁺ (Noctec) and *paraldehyde*⁺, have been used for many years and have been largely replaced by the easier to administer barbiturates. Others are agents introduced rather recently with the hope that they would in turn replace the barbiturates.

Certain advantages are usually claimed for the newer nonbarbiturate depressants. Actually, however, there is little proof that they are safer or otherwise superior to the barbiturates. In fact, most of them seem weaker and generally less dependable than the short-acting barbiturates, which they were designed to supersede, and some, such as *glutethimide*⁺ (Doriden) may be more dangerous in overdoses.

Among the advantages often claimed for any new hypnotic are that it is less likely to have the following effects:

1. To be habit-forming and dependence-producing
2. To cause "hangover" or residual sedation

3. To cause "paradoxical excitement" in patients who are prone to react abnormally to depressant drugs
4. To prove toxic for patients with liver or kidney disease
5. To cause severe toxicity if taken in massive overdosage

Actually, most of these drugs are similar to the barbiturates in effectiveness and safety when taken by most people in small sedative–hypnotic doses, and all have essentially the same drawbacks as the barbiturates. Thus, for example, all these drugs can be abused to the point of producing the same general depressant type of dependence (Chap. 53) as that which occurs with barbiturates. Sudden withdrawal has resulted in psychoses and grand mal convulsions of the same types seen when barbiturates are withdrawn too quickly from people who have been taking large amounts for months for their euphoric effects.

It is also sometimes said that, because some of these drugs are detoxified relatively rapidly, residual sedation is rare. However, their short duration of action sometimes makes several doses necessary if the patient wakes repeatedly during the night. In such cases, "hangover" is as common as when the short-acting barbiturates are given in the same way. Others among the *non*barbiturate sedative–hypnotics are only slowly eliminated and exert as persistent a degree of drowsiness as do the long-acting barbiturates.

These drugs are no less likely than the barbiturates to cause excitement in elderly patients, those in pain, or emotionally upset people who react abnormally to light sedation. These drugs *are* relatively safe for patients with liver and kidney disease—but the same may also be said for the short-acting barbiturates when only small oral doses are administered for sedation and hypnosis.

In general, the short- to intermediate-acting barbiturates are still among the most useful sedative–hypnotics in the hospital setting and for occasional episodes of anxiety or insomnia in ambulatory patients. The newer nonbarbiturate hypnotics are preferred mainly for patients who have developed tolerance or, on the other hand, allergic hypersensitivity to the barbiturates. However, all these drugs have been prescribed less frequently since the advent of the benzodiazepines.

Nonprescription agents

Various products that contain the central depressant H₁ antihistamine drugs *diphenhydramine* or *pyrilamine* are available without a prescription (see Chap. 39). Many people find that these drugs are useful aids for relief of insomnia. They should be used only according to the manufacturer's directions, with special care not to exceed the recommended dosage or to use these drugs with alcohol or other central nervous system (CNS) depressants. Because they are anticholinergic, these preparations are contraindicated in people with asthma, narrow-angle glaucoma, or prostatic hypertrophy. They should not be used by pregnant or nursing mothers, or by children under the age of 12 years. Special cautions are needed to prevent accidental poisoning of children.

Benzodiazepine sedative–hypnotics and antianxiety agents

The benzodiazepines have considerable advantages over both the barbiturates and the other drugs, such as chloral hydrate and glutethimide, that are called nonbarbiturate sedative–hypnotics (see Table 45-3). The two original benzodiazepines, diazepam⁺ (Valium) and chlordiazepoxide⁺ (Librium), are generally used as antianxiety agents (see below), and not as sedative–hypnotics. However, *flurazepam* (Dalmane) and newer drugs of this group,

triazolam (Halcion) and *temazepam* (Restoril), are used as sedative–hypnotics and *lorazepam* (Ativan) is used both as a sedative–hypnotic and an anti–anxiety agent. The benzodiazepines have a wider safety margin between their hypnotic and lethal doses, produce fewer adverse effects, and are involved in fewer drug–drug interactions than either the barbiturates or the nonbarbiturate sedative hypnotics listed in Table 45-3.

The close to a dozen drugs of this chemical class now available here or abroad deserve some special discussion because of the frequency with which they are prescribed (Tables 45-3 and 45-4). An estimated one in ten Americans takes one or another of these drugs during any year. The enormous popularity, first of the prototype agent *chlordiazepoxide* (Librium), and later of its successor *diazepam* (Valium) for treating anxiety, and of *flurazepam* (Dalmane) in the management of insomnia, has led to the introduction of such other benzodiazepines as *clor-*

Table 45–4. Antianxiety agents

Official or generic name	Trade name	Usual adult daily oral dosage range	Comments
Benzodiazepines*			
Alprazolam	Xanax	0.75–4.0 mg	Rapid onset; short duration of action
Chlordiazepoxide USP	Libritabs; in Limbitrol	15–100 mg	Long duration of action
Chlordiazepoxide HCl USP	Librium	15–100 mg	See Drug digest; parenteral preparation available
Clorazepate dipotassium	Tranxene	15–60 mg	Long duration of action
Diazepam USP	Valium	6–40 mg	See Drug digest
Halazepam	Paxipam	60–160 mg	Rapid onset; long duration of action
Lorazepam	Ativan	2–6 mg	Rapid onset; short duration of action; parenteral preparation available
Oxazepam	Serax	30–120 mg	Rapid onset; short duration of action
Prazepam	Centrax	20–60 mg	Long duration of action
Others of miscellaneous chemical classes			
Chlormezanone	Trancopal	600–800 mg	Nonhypnotic antianxiety agent
Doxepin HCl	Adapin; Sinequan	75–150 mg	Tricyclic antidepressant (see Chap. 46)
Hydroxyzine HCl USP	Atarax	200–400 mg	Sedative–antihistamine (see Drug digest); parenteral preparation available
Hydroxyzine pamoate USP	Vistaril	200–400 mg	Sedative–antihistamine (see Drug digest)
Meprobamate USP	Equanil; Miltown	1200–1600 mg	See Drug digest

* Clonazepam, which is employed clinically only as an anticonvulsant in epilepsy, is listed in Table 50-2. Other drugs of this chemical class that are mentioned in the discussion of the benzodiazepines are not listed here because they are not yet available in this country.

azepate (Tranxene), *prazepam* (Centrax), *oxazepam* (Serax), and *lorazepam* (Ativan). More recently, *alprazolam* (Xanax), *halazepam* (Paxipam), *temazepam* (Restoril), and *triazolam* (Halcion) have been introduced either as sedative–hypnotics or as antianxiety agents. Alprazolam has been found to be effective in panic disorders, and is also being investigated for use in depression. *Clonazepam* is available for use as an antiepileptic drug. Other drugs of this chemical class are available abroad (*e.g., nitrazepam*—Mogadon) or are being investigated (*e.g., clobazam*—Frisium, and *quazepam*). Until recently, these drugs and some of the others in Table 45-4 were referred to as *minor tranquilizers,* a term intended to connote their sedative and anti–anxiety effects, and to distinguish them from the *major tranquilizers* used to treat psychoses (see Chap. 46). Use of this term has gradually declined as the number of benzodiazepines has increased, and as the name of this chemical class has become better known.

Advantages. All these structurally similar compounds possess essentially the same neuropharmacologic effects. Like the barbiturates, they produce sedation, hypnosis, and antiepileptic effects. There are two main advantages of these drugs over the barbiturates and other nonbarbiturate sedative–hypnotics:

1. When administered in small therapeutic doses, they produce the therapeutically desired reduction of disabling degrees of anxiety with less likelihood of causing excessive drowsiness and impairment of motor functions.
2. When taken in massive overdosage, they are less likely than the barbiturates to cause cardiovascular and respiratory depression, coma, and death. This safety factor seems to be the main reason for their popularity among the general practitioners who now prescribe them as freely as they once ordered barbiturates.

Precautions. Despite the first claimed advantage, daytime drowsiness is the most common side effect of these drugs. Such excessive sedation, and also dizziness, unsteadiness, and feelings of weakness occur most commonly in elderly and debilitated patients. An unexpectedly deep degree of depression may also occur in patients who happen to take other CNS depressant drugs simultaneously. Thus, in addition to being cautioned not to drive or to carry on other activities that require alertness when they first begin benzodiazepine drug treatment, patients should also be warned against drinking alcoholic beverages.

Although these drugs have a high safety margin and are remarkably free of adverse effects and drug–drug interactions (except for additive depression with other CNS depressants), they may cause physical dependence and produce a withdrawal syndrome (Chap. 53) when long-term use is discontinued. They should not be given chronically but, if a patient has been taking them for a prolonged period, especially in high doses, they should be gradually withdrawn to prevent a dangerous withdrawal syndrome, which may even include convulsions. Rebound insomnia may occur for several nights after use of these drugs as hypnotics has stopped. Daytime anxiety has occurred when triazolam is used as a hypnotic.

These drugs should not be taken during pregnancy, because an increased risk of fetal malformations has been associated with such use.

Pharmacokinetic factors. Despite claims for the superiority of each newly marketed benzodiazepine over earlier drugs of this class, all seem to be about equally effective and to have similar safety margins. The main differences among these drugs seem to be in the manner in which they are metabolized. Some, such as chlordiazepoxide, diazepam, and flurazepam, are either slowly eliminated or are converted to still-active metabolites that continue to exert long-lasting effects. Others, such as oxazepam and lorazepam, form inactive metabolites and are inactivated either quickly or over a period of intermediate duration.

The drugs with a longer duration of action tend to accumulate gradually in the patient's system, until a steady state (Chap. 4) is reached in about 1 week. This has both advantages and disadvantages. An advantage—of clorazepate and prazepam, for example—is that after the initial dosage adjustment period, a single daily dose taken at bedtime may continue to exert its antianxiety effect throughout the following day. Patient compliance is likely to be better with such a regimen, or when only a single supplementary daytime dose is needed, than when several daily doses are required.

One disadvantage of the slowly cumulative drugs is that they take a relatively long time to reach peak therapeutic effects. Thus, for example, flurazepam may not be as effective for producing sleep with the first few bedtime doses as it is likely to be later on, and when this drug, and diazepam also, are discontinued, they may continue to exert their depressant effects for several days. With oxazepam and lorazepam, on the other hand, peak plasma levels are quickly reached and the resulting therapeutic activity develops completely soon after therapy is begun. When these more rapidly eliminated drugs are administered, several daily doses may be required to maintain their effectiveness but, on the other hand, patients taking therapeutic doses of these drugs for long periods never accumulate excessive levels in the CNS.

The more slowly absorbed benzodiazepines, such as chlordiazepoxide, are less likely to be abused for their disinhibiting effects than those such as diazepam and oxazepam, which have a more rapid onset of activity. However, all these drugs can cause psychological dependence; therefore, patients whose history indicates that they have been prone to take alcohol and other drugs to excess should be closely observed to detect any tendency to take larger doses than were prescribed. With the more slowly eliminated benzodiazepines, patients who have taken doses large enough to develop physical dependence may be slow to develop withdrawal symptoms when they stop taking these drugs. However, when these finally occur after a week or so, the muscle cramps, tremors, agitation, and insomnia typical of barbiturate and other general depressant drug withdrawal (Chap. 53) can be quite discomforting, and convulsions can even occur following abrupt discontinuation of benzodiazepines.

Unlike the barbiturates, however, the benzodiazepines do not appear to produce the induction of increased levels of liver enzymes. Thus, their simultaneous use with coumarin-type anticoagulants and the other drugs mentioned above does not cause the therapy-complicating drug–drug interactions (Chap. 4) that sometimes occur during treatment with other types of sedative–hypnotics or following their withdrawal. The lack of effect on enzyme induction may also account for the fact that tolerance to flurazepam tends to develop more slowly than when patients are receiving other hypnotic drugs.

In summary, drugs of this chemical class are safer than the barbiturates and other sedative–hypnotics when taken in overdosage or when large doses are required for control of anxiety and agitation in certain clinical situations. They also have certain advantages over other drugs during routine daily use as antianxiety agents. However, the benzodiazepines should be employed judiciously, because they can be misused and abused with potentially serious consequences. It is difficult to determine whether any one of the many drugs of this class now available has any advantages over the others, including chlordiazepoxide, the first benzodiazepine, which is now available in relatively inexpensive form under its generic name. Some appear to cause less sedation when used to treat anxiety. Whichever drug is chosen, it should be administered with knowledge of the pharmacokinetic properties that determine the rate of its onset and duration of action and the extent to which it tends to accumulate in the body during long-term administration of therapeutic doses. This will ensure that therapeutic effects are attained and maintained without toxicity or even minor side-effects.

Other antianxiety agents

The increasing popularity of the older and the more recently introduced benzodiazepine derivatives has resulted in a reduction in the prescribing of other chemical classes of antianxiety agents. These include the propanediol carbamate derivatives, *meprobamate*[+] (Equanil; Miltown); and antihistaminic–sedative drugs such as *hydroxyzine*[+] (Atarax; Vistaril). These drugs possess central actions similar to those of the barbiturates and benzodiazepines. In addition, some exert secondary peripheral effects—at least, when administered to laboratory animals experimentally. It is doubtful that such secondary effects add to the effectiveness of these sedatives for the various clinical conditions in which a specific peripheral effect might prove to be therapeutically useful.

In treating peptic ulcer or other disorders marked by gastrointestinal spasm, for example, hydroxyzine has been claimed to exert a therapeutically desirable combination of antianxiety and smooth muscle relaxing effects. In practice, however, this drug has been made available in combination with a specific synthetic anticholinergic drug—a fact that suggests a lack of confidence in the ability of the drug's laboratory-proved antispasmodic action to be carried over to actual clinical use. Similarly, the central antiemetic activity of this drug and the central skeletal muscle relaxant effect of meprobamate are not likely to occur clinically when these drugs are administered in ordinary oral doses.

As mentioned in Chapter 18, the β-adrenergic receptor blocker *propranolol* (Inderal) is being investigated as an antianxiety agent. Many people have found it helpful in controlling stage fright and other forms of anxiety.

Additional clinical considerations

As discussed earlier, the anxiety and tension of everyday life is best managed by nonpharmacologic means. Patients can best benefit from support, encouragement, and help with learning how to manage their stress and cope with tensions. If an antianxiety drug is ordered, the drug therapy should be supported with comfort measures and other similar therapeutic measures. Because the benzodiazepines are the most widely used antianxiety agents today, a few points about these drugs will be summarized.

Elderly patients and patients with debilitating diseases that give them a decreased respiratory and cardiovascular reserve are more apt to develop adverse reactions to these drugs, including hallucinations, hypotension, dizziness, and fainting. If these patients need one of these drugs, they should receive a smaller than normal dose and be constantly monitored for adverse reactions to the drug. All patients should be assessed for therapeutic and adverse effects of the drug. Dosage may need to be adjusted to individual needs. As previously discussed, several underlying medical conditions are contraindications to the use of these drugs; these include psychoses, narrow-angle glaucoma, renal failure, hepatic failure, pregnancy, and lactation.

Patients should know the expected therapeutic effects and the possible adverse effects of these drugs. They also need to understand that the drug will be most effective if combined with other measures to decrease anxiety and to cope with stress. Many patients experience drowsiness and a change in alertness when started on the drug. Safety precautions should be discussed with all patients.

Patients should be told to avoid alcohol while on benzodiazepines, because the additive depressant effect can cause serious problems. If gastrointestinal upset occurs, the patient can be advised to take the drug with food. The patient should be cautioned to avoid taking the drug with antacids, which can decrease the absorption of the antianxiety drug. Patients also need to know that, if these drugs are taken over a long period of time, a dependence does develop. The drug should not be stopped suddenly but should be withdrawn gradually. Sudden withdrawal can result in seizures, irritability, insomnia, confusion, and other CNS effects. The patient teaching guide summarizes the points that should be in-

corporated into the teaching of a patient receiving benzodiazepines.

Drug–drug interactions. Several drugs are known to interact with the benzodiazepines. *Alcohol* and other *CNS depressants* have a combined depressant effect with these drugs. The patient should not receive these drugs concurrently. Increased drug effects are also seen with *phenothiazines, antihistamines, narcotic analgesics, barbiturates, monoamine oxidase (MAO) inhibitors,* and *tricyclic antidepressants. Cigarette smoking* may result in a decreased effect of the benzodiazepines.

The guide to the nursing process summarizes the clinical considerations that should be incorporated into the nursing care of a patient receiving benzodiazepines.

Patient teaching guide: benzodiazepines

The drug that has been prescribed for you is called a benzodiazepine. This type of drug is used to relieve tension or nervousness. The exact way that this drug works is not completely understood, but this group of drugs also relaxes muscle spasm, relieves insomnia, and helps in convulsive disorders. Your drug has been prescribed to treat _____ .

Instructions:

1. The name of your drug is _____ .

2. The dosage of your drug is _____ .

3. You should take your drug _____ times a day. The best times to take your drug are _____, _____, _____ . If stomach upset occurs, the drug can be taken with food.

4. Some side-effects of the drug that you should be aware of include the following:

   Drowsiness

   This happens to many people. It is important to avoid driving, operating dangerous machinery, or performing delicate tasks if this happens to you.

   Vision changes, slurred speech, unsteadiness

   These reactions usually pass after your body adjusts to the drug. Take extra care in your activities for the few days that these persist. If these reactions do not go away after 3 or 4 days, consult with your nurse or physician.

   Nausea, loss of appetite, vomiting

   Taking the drug with food often helps the GI upset. Do *not* take the drug with antacids.

   (continued)

Constipation or diarrhea

These reactions also often pass as the body adjusts to the drug. If they do not go away, consult with your nurse or physician for appropriate therapy.

5. Tell any physician, nurse, or dentist who is taking care of you that you are taking this medication.

6. Keep this and all medications out of the reach of children.

7. Avoid the use of over-the-counter preparations while you are on this drug. If you feel that you require one of these drugs, consult with your nurse or physician for one that is appropriate for use while you are on this drug.

8. Avoid the use of alcohol while you are on this drug. The combination of the two can cause serious problems.

9. If you are on this drug for a prolonged period of time, do not stop it suddenly. Your body will need time to adjust to the loss of the drug. The dosage will need to be gradually reduced to prevent serious problems from developing.

Notify your nurse or physician if any of the following occur:

Skin rash, itching
Fever, sore throat
Inability to sleep
Depression
Continued clumsiness, nervousness, irritability

If you are withdrawing from the drug, notify your nurse or physician if any of the following occur:

Trembling
Muscle cramps
Sweating
Irritability
Confusion
Seizures

Guide to the nursing process: benzodiazepines

Assessment	Nursing diagnoses	Interventions	Evaluation
Past history (*contraindications*): Psychoses	Potential for injury secondary to side-effects of drug	Proper and appropriate administration of drug Provision of comfort and	Monitor therapeutic effectiveness: decrease tension or anxiety *(continued)*

Assessment	Nursing diagnoses	Interventions	Evaluation
Narrow-angle glaucoma Renal failure Hepatic failure Pregnancy Lactation ↓ respiratory reserve Allergies: these drugs; others; reactions Medication history (*cautions*): Alcohol CNS depressants Phenothiazines Antihistamines Narcotics Barbiturates MAO inhibitors Tricyclic antidepressants Antacids Cigarette smoking **Physical assessment** Neurologic: orientation, affect, reflexes, state of anxiety Cardiovascular: BP, P, peripheral perfusion Respiratory: R, adventitious sounds GI: bowel sounds, normal function, liver function tests Renal: creatinine, BUN levels	Knowledge deficit regarding drug therapy Potential sensory–perceptual alteration secondary to drug effects Potential alteration in thought processes secondary to drug effects	safety measures: • Safety if drowsiness, dizziness, visual changes occur • Drug with food for GI upset • Appropriate therapy for constipation or diarrhea Patient teaching regarding drug therapy Support and encouragement to cope with stressors, anxiety and drug therapy; support to cope with drug withdrawal Life support measures if overdose occurs	Monitor for adverse effects of drug: • GI upset • Constipation • CNS effects • Cardiovascular depression • Renal failure • Depression Evaluate effectiveness of patient teaching program Evaluate effectiveness of support and encouragement offered Monitor for drug–drug interactions: ↑ effects with alcohol, CNS depressants, phenothiazines, antihistamines, narcotics, barbiturates, MAO inhibitors, tricyclic antidepressants ↓ effects with antacids, cigarette smoking Evaluate effectiveness of life support measures, if necessary

Clinical uses of antianxiety and sedative–hypnotic agents

The nature of anxiety

Anxiety is an emotional or a psychological response to real or imaginary troubles. It is marked mainly by unpleasant feelings of uneasiness, physical and nervous tension, and apprehension—that is, the feeling that something bad is about to happen. When these discomforting feelings are set off by a person's perception of a problem that is actually present, anxiety is normal. It can help in coping with problems by stimulating constructive actions to solve them.

On the other hand, if a person has no real reason to feel anxious, or if the anxiety reaction is excessive, it can be counterproductive and actually interfere with the ability to function effectively. The psychophysiologic effects of anxiety are similar to those of fear in many respects.* Both emotions may trigger central and autonomic nervous system and endocrine reactions that affect the functioning of somatic and visceral organs and systems. The resulting bodily reactions may be brief and subside quickly or, in chronic anxiety, long-lasting functional and organic changes may develop.

---

* Fear is an emotional response to a real, immediately dangerous situation. Anxiety is triggered by difficulties that a person expects to arise. The anticipated troubles may be real or imaginary. That is, anxiety may be precipitated by a person's correct assessment of a threatening life situation, or it may be set off by an unrealistic evaluation of the situation.

Among the discomforting symptoms of anxiety are a feeling of inner tremulousness that stems from increased skeletal muscle tone. Muscle tension in the scalp and neck is a cause of tension headaches (Chap. 38). Increased contraction of gastrointestinal smooth muscle may lead to painful spasms and, if persistent, to the constipation and diarrhea of the irritable bowel syndrome (Chap. 41). The anxious person's heart may pound rapidly and the blood pressure tends to rise. There may be a feeling of heaviness and tightness in the chest to which the person responds unconsciously by overbreathing. Hyperventilation leads, in turn, to loss of carbon dioxide, and the resulting respiratory alkalosis can cause such additional symptoms as dizziness and vertigo.

Anxiety can also interfere with a person's ability to think clearly, so that judgment becomes poor, just when the most difficult decisions may have to be made. Chronic anxiety can affect intellectual functioning to a degree that leads to mental illness. It is, in fact, often hard to tell whether a patient is suffering from severe simple anxiety or from agitated depression (Chap. 46).

Management of anxiety

A first step in the management of the anxious patient is to determine what is causing the symptoms and the degree of their severity. If the anxiety is actually a manifestation of emotional depression of more than a mild degree, a patient is not likely to respond to treatment with sedatives or antianxiety drugs, and may sometimes actually suffer a paradoxical increase in apprehension, tremulousness, and insomnia when treated with a drug such as diazepam instead of with a specific antidepressant drug. On the other hand, most patients with mild, transient anxiety precipitated by a stressful life situation probably do not need any drug treatment at all, and would respond to reassurance and counseling alone. However, because most general practitioners do not have time to listen to their anxious patients and to respond with such emotional support and advice, they are likely to prescribe an antianxiety agent (see summary of clinical indications at the end of this chapter).

The question of whether these drugs should be prescribed as frequently and freely as they are is a subject of continuing controversy. Some physicians favor nonpharmacologic measures for most patients with anxiety reactions that have been precipitated by stressful life situations. They feel that it is better for people to learn to deal with situational stress than to depend on what they disparage as a "chemical crutch." These physicians—often psychiatrists who write only a small percentage of the 100 million or more prescriptions that are ordered each year—claim that ours has become an "overmedicated society."

Obviously, however, most practitioners see little harm in prescribing antianxiety agents. Some agree that these drugs are often ordered for patients with only trivial complaints who do not really need such medication. However, they claim that these drugs are both effective and safe when prescribed for properly selected patients and when certain principles of dosage and administration are followed. Which patients should receive sedative or antianxiety drugs, and what should be done to minimize their misuse and prevent possible adverse effects?

Patient selection. These drugs are best employed in patients whose anxiety is causing physical and mental effects so discomforting or disabling that they find it difficult to carry on their normal activities. Often, for example, appropriate doses of these drugs will calm and relax patients suffering from situational stress. The drug-induced reduction in nervousness, irritability, and tremulousness helps these patients to concentrate on completing their daily activities. Whenever possible, these patients should also receive other forms of treatment ranging from simple reassurance to some form of psychotherapy.

Administration of these drugs can also be helpful in patients with organic and functional disorders that are aggravated during periods of excessive psychological tension. By reducing the emotional reactions responsible for aggravating symptoms of cardiovascular, gastrointestinal, and other somatic and visceral conditions, these drugs often offer some temporary symptomatic relief. They should be used only for brief periods, because there is no proof that their long-continued use favorably influences the course of even those cases of organic disease that are thought to be of psychosomatic origin.

In any case, dampening the emotional component of such disorders with sedatives or antianxiety agents is no substitute for more specific therapy. As previously indicated, the secondary peripheral and central effects claimed for some of these drugs—for example, antispasmodic, antihistaminic, and antiemetic effects—are not of much use in most functional and organic syndromes in which both physical and psychological discomfort occur. In such cases, the use of an antianxiety agent adjunctively does not go away with the need for cardiac drugs such as nitroglycerin for angina, antihypertensive agents for high blood pressure, bronchodilator antiasthmatic drugs, topical corticosteroids for neurodermatitis, or estrogen replacement therapy in women with menopausal symptoms.

The role of antianxiety drug therapy in patients with persistent, or chronic, anxiety punctuated by occasional acute anxiety attacks is also uncertain. Such patients, whose anxiety arises from unconscious, unresolved emotional conflicts, should receive psychotherapy. Some psychiatrists are opposed to the adjunctive use of drugs for symptomatic relief of anxiety. They argue that the patient is more likely to face up to problems in the life situation and to talk about them more openly when suffering from emotional distress than when he has been made more relaxed by an antianxiety agent.

Other physicians feel that drugs that relieve discomforting symptoms make it easier for the patient to discuss problems and to achieve rapport with the physician. They point out that the process of discovering the underlying sources of the patient's chronic anxiety by penetrating his ego defenses is often slow and painful. Thus, they say, the judicious use of an appropriate antianxiety agent can be a useful adjunct to sympathetic discussions of the situation while the patient is gradually gaining insight into his unhealthy ways of handling anxiety-provoking internal conflicts.

Other patients for whom the use of sedatives and antianxiety agents seems justified in some circumstances include those suffering from drug-induced panic reactions (Chap. 53), alcoholics in combative states of intoxication or suffering the effects of withdrawal and emotional upset during periods of abstinence (Chap. 53), and patients with mild degrees of mental depression for which antidepressant drug therapy does not seem warranted (Chap. 46), as well as those suffering from a moderately severe degree of agitated depression for whom an antianxiety drug may be administered in combination with an antidepressant. (Use of these drugs to allay preoperative apprehension will be discussed briefly later in this chapter and in Chapter 52.)

Drug choice and administration. Agents from any of the several chemical classes of drugs discussed earlier can produce relief of anxiety symptoms. The benzodiazepines can calm anxious patients without causing the degree of drowsiness seen when barbiturates are employed for the same purpose. Supposedly these drugs act more specifically on the limbic system, while the chief site of action of the barbiturates is on the reticular activating system.

This is said to account for their ability to reduce the patient's response to emotional stress without producing lethargy or impairment of motor performance. Some of the newer benzodiazepines are clearly superior to the barbiturates and to the older benzodiazepines in this respect.

Another significant reason for the popularity of the benzodiazepines is their much wider safety margin when taken in massive overdoses. Unlike the barbiturates, which can prove lethal when taken in doses as low as a dozen times that of the hypnotic dose, benzodiazepines rarely cause death from respiratory failure or cardiovascular collapse even when 100 or 200 times the therapeutic dose has been ingested.

Despite the relative safety of diazepam and its chemical relatives, they are quite able to cause acute intoxication. These drugs have, in fact, displaced the barbiturates as the most common cause of drug-induced coma in Canada and in some parts of this country. Contrary to what is commonly believed, deaths from diazepam overdosage *have* occurred, not only when this drug was taken with alcohol and other central depressant drugs,

but also when deliberately ingested alone in large amounts.

Similarly, although tolerance to the benzodiazepines tends to develop more slowly because of their low enzyme-inducing activity, patients who abuse these drugs do become dependent on them. The effects of chronic intoxication may not be as devastating as with barbiturates, but it *can* be disruptive. Thus, while the advantages of these drugs usually outweigh their drawbacks, and while there may be valid reasons for selecting a drug of this class over the older sedatives, it is important to employ all the traditional precautions for preventing the misuse and abuse of general depressants of the CNS (Chap. 53).

It is best, for example, to prescribe these drugs for short courses of anxiety therapy. They are best taken intermittently rather than continuously. Thus the patient is instructed to take these minor tranquilizers during an episode of peak anxiety—usually less than 1 week—and then to reduce the daily dose or to discontinue the drug entirely when the symptoms have abated. If symptoms return during a drug-free period, the drug may be begun again and continued for a while until the patient's condition improves.

Adjusting dosage in this way to periods of peak emotional stress helps to delay development of tolerance and lessens the likelihood of habituation and dependence. Adjusting each patient's dosage individually is also desirable to find the lowest dose for relief of anxiety without producing excessive daytime drowsiness. Once the total daily dose is determined, it is best to give most of it at bedtime. With the longer-acting benzodiazepines, such a regimen produces sleep and residual sedation on the following day. Often the desired antianxiety effect can be maintained with only a single supplemental daytime dose.

The nature of sleep and insomnia

An estimated 20 to 25 million Americans are said to suffer from sleeplessness either occasionally or chronically. As indicated in this chapter, many drugs are available for treating insomnia. About one of every five ambulatory patients for whom medication has been prescribed receives a hypnotic, and many of these patients continue to have the prescription renewed for long periods. Over 50% of hospitalized patients also receive sleeping medications routinely during their stay. As is the case with the use of sedatives and antianxiety agents, hypnotic drugs are undoubtedly prescribed for many patients who do not really need them and who may, in fact, be harmed by continuing to take them. Before discussing the proper indications for these drugs and the matters that must be considered in employing them with maximum effectiveness and minimal harm, it is appropriate to review briefly some aspects of what is known about sleep and wakefulness.

Sleep. Research studies performed in sleep laboratories have revealed a great deal about the nature of normal sleep. Such studies have shown that sleep is not a single state but rather is comprised of a series of stages that follow one another progressively through a clearly structured cycle, and that there is a series of such cycles during a night's sleep. Each cycle consists of two main types of sleep that are differentiated by changes that can be detected in brain waves on the electroencephalogram (EEG), in eye movements measured on the electro-oculograph (EOG), and in muscle tone changes measured on the electromyogram (EMG).

The type of sleep that takes up most of the total sleeping time is divided into four substages on the basis of differences in the frequency and size of the waves recorded on the EEG. It is sometimes called slow wave sleep to differentiate it from the other type, in which frequent fast waves are seen. Another difference noted in sleep of the second type is the presence of rapid eye movements (REM). REM sleep occurs at the end of each approximately 90-minute cycle of nonREM (NREM) sleep. Ordinarily, four or five REM periods develop during a night of mostly NREM sleep.

Despite a great deal of speculation, the actual functions served by each type of sleep are still not understood. Thus, for example, although people seem to be most deeply asleep in the third and fourth stages of NREM sleep, there is no proof that such slow wave sleep stages play a major part in the restorative and recuperative functions of sleep. People deprived of stage 4 sleep perform normally when awake and, in fact, this stage may be completely absent in elderly people.

Similarly, the role—if any—of REM sleep in determining a person's waking behavior is not really understood. Contrary to what was once thought, deprivation of REM sleep by awakening the person each time that stage is entered does *not* lead to adverse changes in behavior. People deprived of either REM or NREM sleep, or of both, can function effectively, if their total sleep time is still adequate for their needs. That is, the most important factor in determining whether a person feels rested after sleeping and performs daytime tasks well is the total amount of sleep, rather than the proportion of time spent in any particular stage or substage of sleep.

Insomnia. People vary greatly in the amount of sleep they need. In general, however, most people will feel fatigued and groggy when they get less than 4 hours of sleep a night. People who feel that way because they

have been abnormally wakeful and had relatively little sleep can be considered to be suffering from hyposomnia, or insomnia. This condition can occur sporadically in response to all sorts of physical and emotional factors— pain or anxiety, for example. Such occasional bouts of insomnia last only as long as the painful medical condition or the psychological stress that precipitated the sleeplessness.

Under some circumstances, such secondary insomnia can become chronic. Some people suffer from primary sleep disturbances, possibly caused by a neurologic or neurochemical defect, the nature of which is not understood. Such cases of primary insomnia are always chronic, as are those thought to result from prior negative conditioning. To treat chronic insomnia properly, it is very important to try to find the underlying causes. Unfortunately, most physicians find it much easier to write a prescription for a sleeping pill—elapsed time less than 1 minute—than to take time to make an accurate diagnosis of the real reasons for the patient's sleep disturbance.

Patients with insomnia generally show one of three main patterns of sleep abnormalities. In the most common form, patients have difficulty in falling asleep. Often the patient with such *sleep onset* type of insomnia may sleep well enough, once he finally falls asleep. Others may fall asleep readily enough but then awaken frequently during the night and find it difficult to get back to sleep again. Such *fragmented sleep* leaves them tired and irritable.* The most ominous pattern of insomnia is one that is marked by awakening in the early morning hours. This *early arousal* type of insomnia tends to develop in patients suffering from a major, or psychotic, endogenous depression (Chap. 46).†

Management of insomnia

The problem of how best to handle sleep disturbance problems will be considered on the basis of whether the patient's sleeplessness occurs as a sporadic episode that requires only occasional treatment for short periods, or whether there is a chronic sleep disorder. The main reason for approaching the subject in this way is that the occasional brief use of a hypnotic drug is both harmless and effective for producing sleep in most patients. However, the long-continued use of sleep-producing medications in chronic sleeplessness is generally ineffective and potentially harmful—that is, the drugs fail to do what the prescribing physician desires, and their long-term use leads to various adverse effects, including drug-induced, or drug-dependency, insomnia.

Occasional insomnia

Almost everyone has had a night when, for any of many reasons, it was difficult to fall asleep or when, having fallen asleep, he soon awakened and could not get back to sleep again. Ideally, during such a sporadic episode of sleeplessness, the person could simply rest, read, or oth-

---

* Results of sleep laboratory studies suggest that many people who complain of fragmented sleep and long frequent periods of wakefulness actually get much more sleep than they think they do. The reason for such so-called *pseudoinsomnia* is not well understood. Some such people may have the illusion that they "didn't sleep a wink" because most of their REM sleep time was spent dreaming that they were awake.

---

† Sleeplessness in patients with agitated depression of the exogenous type, including neurotic, rather than psychotic, cases usually suffer from insomnia of the sleep onset type.

erwise be occupied without worrying about the failure to fall asleep and stay asleep. Loss of a night's sleep is not harmful to health, and even several successive nights of fragmented sleep have no serious consequences, because such insomnia is self-limited, and the person finally falls into a deep sleep from cumulative fatigue.

Actually, however, such occasional bouts of insomnia are most commonly caused by some stressful situation that has triggered anxiety that interferes with the person's ability to sleep. The longer the troubled person lies awake worrying about what is bothering him, the more anxious and emotionally upset he is likely to become. This is particularly true of the hospitalized patient whose inability to sleep because of concern about his illness may be compounded by physical discomfort or pain. Although nonmedical measures may be useful to help the patient relax in such situations, there is no harm in reinforcing such efforts by having the patient take a prescribed hypnotic drug to help induce sleep.

Choice of drug. Almost all the available prescription hypnotics are equally effective for occasional use by patients who have not been habitually taking sleep-producing medications or alcohol, and single small hypnotic doses of all these drugs are safe for patients who have no underlying medical disorder that might contraindicate their use. (Even small doses of depressant drugs can be dangerous for patients with severe emphysema, who might be precipitated into respiratory failure, or for those with liver damage, who might suffer hepatic coma.) Flurazepam (Dalmane) is claimed to be effective for inducing and maintaining sleep in all the several types of insomnia mentioned above: difficulty in falling asleep, frequent awakenings during the night, and early morning awakening.* However, for occasional use during transient sleeplessness episodes, the less expensive barbiturates and nonbarbiturate hypnotics such as chloral hydrate and its derivatives are still considered to be useful and safe.

Because the barbiturates differ in the speed with which they take effect and the duration of their sleep-producing effects, physicians have been accustomed to choosing the compound that can best be tailored to each patient's sleep disturbance pattern. Patients who have trouble falling asleep may respond best to a rapid-acting sleep inducer such as secobarbital or pentobarbital. Those who drop off easily enough but then have difficulty staying asleep may be given a barbiturate of intermediate duration, such as amobarbital or butabarbital, as a sleep maintainer. To ensure a full night's rest, hospitalized patients may be given a long-acting sleep-sustaining agent such as phenobarbital, while ambulatory patients may receive a small supply of any of several available "repeat-

action" products that release a second dose of a short- or intermediate-acting barbiturate or a combination of them during the night.

Other considerations. Physicians often order hypnotics for all their hospitalized patients; and the nursing staff sometimes insists too rigidly that patients take the sleeping medication whether or not they wish to. Some patients can get along perfectly well without these drugs when they are made comfortable and relaxed by other means. Others, who could profit from a night of drug-induced sleep, refuse their medication because of their concern about the habit-forming effects of barbiturates and the dangers of these and similar drugs that they have heard about in stories about the "sleeping-pill menace." Careful assessment of the situation will facilitate the care of these patients.

A patient for whom a hypnotic has been ordered routinely but who does not really require it may benefit from control of environmental factors that favor rest and sleep. The position of the patient's bed should be properly adjusted, for example, and the room should be kept well ventilated and at optimal temperature. A warm drink or a light snack can be given. The patient can also be helped to feel more at ease in the strange environment if the nurse spends some time talking to him, offering him a back rub, and letting him talk and express his concerns before leaving. Even if the patient still appears to require medication after such measures, the drug is more likely to exert its desired relaxing effect when the patient has been prepared in these ways.

Patients who are afraid of becoming dependent on hypnotics but who obviously do need them to ensure their rest during hospitalization should be allowed to express their apprehension. However, the patient can honestly be assured that the stories he has heard or read about these drugs do not apply to his situation, and that brief exposure to barbiturates and to other sleep medications is not likely either to be habit-forming or to cause toxicity. He should be convinced, instead, that these medicines will help him to get the rest that he needs to regain his health. When the patient's alarm is allayed in this way, he will usually be willing to take the tablet or capsule, and the strong positive suggestion will also often actually increase the drug's desired calming, relaxing, and sleep-inducing effects.

Deciding what to do when the doctor has left a prn order is an important professional responsibility. It is necessary to assess *why* the patient has been unable to fall asleep or *why* he has awakened, rather than to administer another hypnotic dose routinely. Patients who are in pain do not respond well to hypnotics alone. The barbiturate or other hypnotic may be combined with a salicylate such as aspirin. Codeine or an even stronger analgesic such as meperidine (Demerol) may even be required for the patient whose sleeplessness stems from pain.

---

* Other benzodiazepines, such as diazepam and triazolam, which reach therapeutic levels in the brain more promptly, may be even better suited for occasional use than flurazepam.

It is always important to assess how patients react to hypnotic drugs and to act accordingly. Obviously, if the patient falls into a deep sleep after receiving a drug of supposedly short duration, he should not be awakened for the next scheduled dose. Likewise, if he seems unusually lethargic, the next dose should be withheld. As indicated earlier, patients with respiratory difficulties or with severe liver or kidney disease sometimes become deeply depressed after receiving apparently safe doses of a barbiturate or of a nonbarbiturate hypnotic.

As indicated previously, elderly patients—particularly those with brain damage secondary to cerebrovascular disease—sometimes tend to become excited, instead of calmed, when they receive hypnotics in the hospital. The night nurse listens for sounds indicating that such a paradoxically excited patient is awake and trying to get up. She may have to help him out of bed or even help him to remember where he is.

It is important to prevent the confused patient from falling or otherwise hurting himself. This may require putting up side rails, but other restraints are usually unnecessary. Instead, it is more desirable to stay with the patient and talk to him. Simply orienting the patient often helps to calm and relax the patient and to reorient him.

Chronic insomnia

Results of studies conducted in sleep laboratories with patients who took nightly doses of hypnotics for from 1 to 4 weeks have shown that almost all these drugs tend to lose their effectiveness after only 1 or 2 weeks of continued use. Flurazepam appears to be an exception in this regard, because it continued to retain its effectiveness in sleep laboratory studies lasting 28 days. However, despite this indication that tolerance to this benzodiazepine develops slowly, its use for prolonged periods—like that of the other hypnotics—is not generally recommended.

One difficulty with the continued use of hypnotics is that treated patients not only sleep as poorly as those insomniacs who have received no medication at all, but that they often sleep worse and have long periods of wakefulness and disturbing dreams and nightmares. This may occur as a result of REM rebound, a tendency of the drug-suppressed REM sleep to increase markedly when the dose that the patient has been taking becomes inadequate for inducing or maintaining sleep. REM rebound also occurs when hypnotic drugs that a patient has been taking continuously in increasing doses are abruptly reduced or discontinued. The resulting drug-withdrawal insomnia is thought to be a factor that contributes to the development of dependence on these drugs.

An advantage is also claimed for flurazepam in this respect. That is, there is some evidence that patients taking this hypnotic develop little REM sleep suppression during the first 1 to 3 weeks of treatment. REM rebound is also relatively slight when this drug is withdrawn, but rebound insomnia has occurred when this and other benzodiazepines were withdrawn abruptly after single nightly doses had been given.

Actually, flurazepam is quite as able to cause adverse effects as the barbiturates when it is administered on a regular basis. Thus, for example, the same pharmacokinetic factor that probably accounts for this drug's advantages can also be a cause of residual oversedation and other problems. That is, the lack of drug-induced sleep disturbances with flurazepam probably stems from the fact that it is converted to an active metabolite that is only slowly eliminated, and that continues to exert its gradually diminishing effects even after the hypnotic drug has been stopped for several days. However, if flurazepam is administered daily for several weeks, this same metabolite may accumulate to toxic levels. In elderly nursing home patients this has led to the insidious development of such signs and symptoms as ataxia, confusion, and hallucinations, which might be easily overlooked in institutionalized geriatric patients. Thus, like the barbiturates, flurazepam should be used only for brief periods or on an intermittent basis in patients who complain of chronic insomnia.

Advising the patient. In view of the fact that flurazepam and other benzodiazepines that are used as hypnotics—despite their advantages over older sedative–hypnotic drugs—are not considered desirable for long-term treatment, what advice can the nurse offer the patient who claims to suffer from chronic insomnia? The single most important suggestion to make is that a physician be seen who is willing and able to seek out the causes of the patient's sleep problem. In some areas, the nurse may be able to direct the patient to a sleep clinic in which specialists employ new diagnostic techniques to help determine the underlying causes of chronic insomnia.

Once a specific physical or psychological cause has been found, it may be possible to treat the patient with more effective drugs than the hypnotics that have proved so ineffective and potentially harmful—for example, antidepressants, if the patient is actually suffering from mental depression, or medications directed at previously unrecognized endocrine disturbances or cardiovascular and respiratory disorders. Some sleep specialists may even employ biofeedback training and various deconditioning and reconditioning measures.

The nurse can aid patients who do not have access to such optimal medical approaches by suggesting ways for them to try to induce sleep without sleeping medications. A patient can, for example, be taught to control the home environment in much the same way in which the nurse has tried to keep the hospital room free of sleep-disrupting factors. It should, in fact, be easier to ensure quiet and proper temperature and ventilation at home than in the hospital. The nurse can also help the patient to work out a bedtime regimen that reduces restlessness and promotes relaxation. The development of such a routine related to sleep is very beneficial.

Going for a walk or doing other light exercise

followed by a warm bath helps some people to fall asleep. Listening to music while reading may also be relaxing. In any case, a patient can be assured that loss of sleep by an otherwise healthy person has no serious physical consequences, according to authorities on sleep. Thus, it may be best not to be bothered when one occasionally fails to fall asleep and to try, instead, to find constructive ways to use the hours of wakefulness.

Patients who continue to require sleeping medication should be warned about the need for safe storage of such chemical substances. They should also be advised not to keep hypnotic capsules or tablets in a place that is readily accessible to children. Sleep capsules should not be kept in a bedside table or in an unlocked medicine cabinet, because they can attract toddlers who may then ingest the medication and suffer severe intoxication. The patient himself may, in some circumstances, waken in a dazed or disoriented condition, and take an excessive quantity of hypnotic medication if it is within too easy reach.

Miscellaneous uses of sedative–hypnotics and antianxiety agents

The effects of drugs that depress the nervous system depend in part on the excitability of this system. Thus, larger than ordinary doses may be needed to calm patients who are unusually anxious, apprehensive, or agitated. Often such doses are administered parenterally to produce their effects more rapidly and surely. The types of clinical situations that often call for parenteral administration of these drugs are summarized at the end of this chapter.

Preoperative sedation. The barbiturates and other drugs of this type are often ordered for patients who are to undergo surgery. Oral hypnotic doses are administered the night before surgery is scheduled, because the patient comes to the operating room in better physical and mental condition after a good night's sleep. Listening to the patient and answering questions about the procedure that is to be undergone also helps the patient to deal more effectively with anxiety about the next morning's operation.

On the morning of the operation, patients are likely to be particularly apprehensive. To reduce reflex nervous excitability, they usually receive a high hypnotic dose parenterally, alone or combined with morphine, meperidine, and other preanesthetic medications. The nurse should be sure that such medications are given on time so that the patient will arrive at the operating room in the best condition for undergoing anesthesia induction smoothly. (See Chapter 52 for further discussion of preanesthetic medication and the use of barbiturates for basal anesthesia.)

The patient who has been heavily sedated in this way must be kept from harm while waiting to go to the operating room for anesthesia and surgery. No smoking is allowed unless someone stays with the patient. Side rails may also have to be put up to protect the patient. Personal observation and communication are still the best means of making certain that the patient arrives for surgery feeling as relaxed and trusting as possible in this stressful situation. Taking the drug may in itself lead some patients to become fearful, because this step signifies the beginning of a period in which the patient temporarily becomes helpless and thus very dependent on others. If there is such a reaction, it is particularly important to stay nearby until the patient arrives in the operating room.

Sedation and amnesia during labor. Although these drugs are themselves not good pain relievers, they are sometimes administered to obstetric patients together with narcotic analgesics such as meperidine and alphaprodine. Because barbiturates combined with narcotics can cause excessive depression of respiration in both mother and baby, some do not approve of this use of these depressants.

Some antianxiety agents that are less likely than barbiturates to depress respiration may be substituted. There is some evidence that *diazepam* and *hydroxyzine* are effective in producing pain relief and forgetfulness of the obstetric procedure without causing breathing difficulties in the newborn babies. Use of these drugs permits—and, in fact, requires—reduction in dosage of narcotic analgesics. This may also be a factor in reports that labor was not unduly prolonged when these drugs were used experimentally for this purpose.

Acute psychotic reactions. The injectable forms of diazepam and chlordiazepoxide are sometimes used for quieting highly agitated patients. These drugs seem to be safer than the barbiturates for bringing severely excited patients under control. However, the hallucinations and delusions that may underlie a schizophrenic patient's behavior are not relieved. For this purpose, and for long-term therapy of mentally ill patients, the major tranquilizers or antipsychotic agents are preferred (Chap. 46).

Case study

Presentation   PP, a 42-year-old married mother of three teen-age sons, was seen in the outpatient department for a routine physical examination. Results were unremarkable except for BP 145/90, P 98, and an appearance of tension—jittering, avoiding eye contact, teary eyes. She stated that she was having a lot of difficulty dealing with "life in general." Her sons present her with many stressful times; her husband is very busy at work and doesn't have time to deal with home problems but is demanding when he is home; she is entering an early menopause and having trouble coping with the idea of menopause as well as with the side-effects of the hormonal changes; and she feels that she has no outlet for all her anger, tension, and stress. The physician assured PP that this is a common problem for women her age and prescribed Valium, 2 mg, qid for anxiety. PP is then referred to the nurse for patient teaching.

What nursing interventions would be appropriate for this patient?

Discussion

Because PP has just received a prescription for Valium, she should receive thorough patient teaching regarding the drug. She needs to be aware of the possible CNS effects of the drug so that appropriate safety measures can be taken if she has to drive or perform delicate tasks. She needs to know that she may feel more relaxed and less tense, but that with this may come a weakness and fatigue that could change her daily activities. She should be advised to take the drug with food if stomach upset occurs, but to avoid combining the drug with antacids. She should be cautioned to avoid the use of over-the-counter drugs and alcohol while on Valium, and should be encouraged to check with the nurse or physician if she feels that she needs one of these preparations. All the cautions and side-effects, along with the dosage information, should be written down for PP for easy reference.

To supplement PP's drug therapy, a good nursing assessment should be done to determine PP's coping behavior and support systems. She should be encouraged to discuss her feelings, and to explore what she identifies as stressors in her life. Alternate methods of coping can be explored with PP, and she should be offered support and encouragement to verbalize her feelings and to call if she needs additional encouragement. The antianxiety drugs do not "cure" the problem. PP may experience even more stress in her life if the depressant effects of the drug change her coping and behavior patterns while her environment does not change. Some busy practitioners prescribe antianxiety drugs to placate women who are faced with all the problems PP is encountering. Astute nursing care can facilitate the drug's effectiveness and can allow the patient to cope with her life situation once again. With such thorough patient care, the drug should only be needed for a short period of time, and hopefully many of the problems associated with long-term use can be avoided.

Summary of clinical indications for sedatives, hypnotics, and antianxiety agents

Small oral doses with sedative or antianxiety effects

1. Calm patients reacting to stressful life situations.
2. Reduce anxiety and tension states in psychoneurosis.
3. Dampen the emotional component in organic and functional disorders in which psychophysiologic reactions play a significant psychosomatic or somatopsychic role. For example,
   a. Gastrointestinal (*e.g.*, hypersecretion and hypermotility in peptic ulcer, pylorospasm, colitis)
   b. Cardiovascular (*e.g.*, palpitations, tachycardia, chest pains, and high blood pressure in angina pectoris; essential hypertension)
   c. Allergic (*e.g.*, skin eruptions and pruritus in neurodermatitis; wheezing, cough, dyspnea in bronchial asthma and other obstructive respiratory disorders)
   d. Menopausal symptoms (*e.g.*, nervousness, palpitations, headaches, sweating, "hot flashes") and menstrual disorders (including

premenstrual tension, dysmenorrhea)

e. Arthritis and other chronically painful conditions that are emotionally upsetting, and other musculoskeletal conditions or tension headaches that may be the result of emotional reactions to stressful situations

Higher oral doses with hypnotic effects

1. Induce sleep in patients with insomnia who have difficulty in falling asleep.
2. Maintain natural sleep in patients with insomnia who have difficulty in staying asleep.

3. Use as adjunct to analgesics in patients unable to sleep because of pain.
4. Ensure restful sleep on the night before surgery.

Parenterally administered doses for greater sedation

1. Reduce the patient's apprehension preoperatively and prior to various anxiety-provoking procedures.
2. Sedate the mother and produce amnesia during labor.
3. Control combative behavior in alcoholic intoxication.
4. Relieve acute anxiety, agitation, and delirium in alcoholic withdrawal syndromes.
5. Reduce agitation and control excessive excitement in acute psychotic and psychoneurotic reactions.

Summary of adverse effects of sedatives, hypnotics, and antianxiety agents

Side-effects of therapeutic doses

Central effects: Drowsiness, dizziness, headache, weakness; occasional paradoxical excitement.

Allergic and idiosyncratic reactions: Skin eruptions, including urticaria and erythematous rash; hematologic reactions, including occasional leukopenia, thrombocytopenia, and agranulocytosis

Effects of continued excessive dosage (chronic intoxication)

CNS Depression: Ataxia, vertigo, slurred speech, impaired thought and judgment; and ocular

disturbances, including diplopia, nystagmus, strabismus, and difficulty in accommodation

Withdrawal signs and symptoms in dependent persons

Nausea, vomiting, abdominal cramps; anxiety, restlessness, insomnia, confusional states, hallucinations and delirium; muscular twitching, tremors, cramps, and convulsive seizures of the grand mal epileptiform type

Effects of massive overdosage (acute intoxication)

Mental confusion, somnolence, stupor, coma; hypotension, shock, circulatory collapse; respiration slow, shallow; transient apnea, or possible respiratory failure

Drug digests

Chloral hydrate USP (Noctec)

Actions and indications. This is the oldest sedative–hypnotic drug and one that is still considered a relatively cheap, rapidly effective, and safe sleep producer. It is used alone in the management of insomnia or combined with potent analgesics during labor and for pre- and postoperative sedation.

Adverse effects, cautions, and contraindications. The undiluted liquid occasionally causes nausea and vomiting as a result of gastric irritation. Taken together with al-

cohol, this drug can cause an excessive degree of depression. Its use is contraindicated in patients with a history of severe hepatic, renal, or cardiac disease. Caution is required when this drug is added to the treatment regimen of patients taking anticoagulant agents, as well as when the sedative is removed from such regimens, because its presence in the body may affect the metabolism of the anticoagulants so as to cause unexpected bleeding episodes.

Dosage and administration. For daytime sedation oral doses of 250 to 500 mg are administered tid after meals. For hypnosis 500 mg to 1 g is administered at bedtime in most cases, but some patients may require up to 2 g. Capsules are taken with a full glass of fruit juice, ginger ale, or other liquid; syrups are diluted with a half-glass of the same fluids. The drug may also be administered rectally in suppository form.

Chlordiazepoxide USP (Librium), and chlordiazepoxide HCl USP (Librium HCl)

Actions and indications. This benzodiazepine is used to relieve anxiety and tension of varying degrees of severity in various psychiatric and somatic disorders, and preop-

eratively. Small oral doses taken alone or together with antispasmodics, coronary vasodilators, estrogens, and other specific drugs help to relieve symptoms of gastrointestinal,

cardiac, menopausal, and other organic or functional conditions. Higher oral and parenteral dosage helps to reduce apprehension preoperatively and to control states of acute agitation in psychoneurotic patients or in alcoholics, particularly during withdrawal states such as alcoholic hallucinosis and impending or active delirium tremens.

Adverse effects, cautions, and contraindications. Drowsiness, the most common side-effect, may make driving hazardous, so patients are cautioned not to engage in this and other activities that require complete alertness. Excessive sedation, ataxia, and confusion tend to occur most commonly in elderly or debilitated patients, for whom treatment is therefore initiated with small doses that are raised only gradually. Occasionally, paradoxical excitement is seen, par-

ticularly in hyperactive children or psychiatric patients. Caution is required in patients with suicidal tendencies who may take massive overdoses. (This can lead to coma and depression of vital functions, but the danger of fatal respiratory and vasomotor depression is much less than in intoxication by barbiturates.) The depressant effects of this drug are increased by alcohol and phenothiazines, so care is required in using this drug alone or combined with major tranquilizers for control of the combative or excited stage of acute alcoholic intoxication. Similarly, patients with paradoxical excitement from this drug should not be treated with barbiturates.

This drug may occasionally be abused by addiction-prone patients.

Dosage and administration. The usual adult dose for relief of mild to moderate anxiety is 5 to 10 mg tid or qid. More severe emotional upset may require 20 or 25 mg tid or qid by mouth. Severe anxiety in alcoholic patients and others is treated with repeated parenteral (IM or IV) administration of 50 mg to 100 mg, up to a total of 300 mg in any one 24-hour period. The daily dose for elderly or debilitated patients is initially 10 mg or less; this is gradually increased as tolerance develops.

Diazepam USP (Valium)

Actions and indications. This benzodiazepine possesses antianxiety, anticonvulsant, and antispasmodic properties. It is used for symptomatic relief of states of anxiety and tension and in neurologic and other disorders for control of seizures and skeletal muscle spasticity and spasm. Small oral doses are more useful for control of emotional upset than for relief of muscle spasm. Larger doses administered parenterally may be useful for reducing muscle spasticity in cerebral palsy and athetosis, for facilitating orthopedic manipulations requiring skeletal muscle relaxation, and for controlling recurring convulsions in status epilepticus, tetanus, and other seizure states. High doses are also useful for producing sedation and amnesia preoperatively and prior to such procedures as cardioversion, gastroscopy, and esophagos-

copy. Its use in labor is said to have advantages over barbiturates for both the newborn baby and its mother.

Adverse effects, cautions, and contraindications. The central depressant effects of the drug are most marked when it is administered parenterally, particularly in patients who are acutely intoxicated with alcohol or who have also received treatment with narcotics or barbiturates. When used IV, it is injected slowly to reduce respiratory depressant, hypotensive, and cardiac effects. This drug is contraindicated for patients with acute narrow-angle glaucoma. It may cause coughing and laryngospasm, and is thus not recommended for use as an adjunct to bronchoscopy and laryngoscopy. Although drowsiness and ataxia are the most common

side-effects, paradoxic reactions marked by excitement, insomnia, sleep disturbances, and muscle spasticity occur in some relatively rare cases. Patients are warned against drinking alcohol when taking this drug, and are cautioned against driving or engaging in other potentially dangerous activities.

Dosage and administration. Oral doses of 2 to 10 mg bid to qid are recommended for relief of anxiety and muscle spasm in most adults. However, elderly patients are started on only one or two daily doses of 2 mg, while alcoholic withdrawal may require 10 mg tid or qid by mouth, or 10 mg IM initially, followed by 5 mg to 10 mg more in 3 or 4 hours. Repeated IM or IV doses of 5 mg to 10 mg may be necessary to control acute agitation in other conditions also.

Flurazepam HCl USP (Dalmane)

Actions and indications. This drug, another benzodiazepine, is a chemical relative of the antianxiety drugs chlordiazepoxide and diazepam, and is employed as a hypnotic in all patterns of insomnia. Clinical and sleep laboratory studies indicate that it induces sleep rapidly in patients who have difficulty in falling asleep and that those who tend to waken during the night are less likely to do so and more likely to have an increase in their total nocturnal sleep time. One of several advantages claimed for this hypnotic is that tolerance is slow to develop during periods of as long as 1 month of nightly administration. However, prolonged use of this and other hypnotics is not recommended. The withdrawal of this drug after several successive nights of use is said not to be followed by a

rebound increase in dream time or by disturbed sleep.

Adverse effects, cautions, and contraindications. Daytime drowsiness, or "hangover," is claimed to occur only infrequently. However, elderly and debilitated patients have become drowsy, dizzy, and light-headed and have shown signs of motor incoordination or suffered falls. Patients should be warned against drinking alcoholic beverages or taking other drugs that can add to the depression caused by flurazepam. They should be cautioned against driving a car or attempting other tasks that require alertness after taking this drug. Overdosage has resulted in various degrees of central depression, including coma. However, fatalities from intoxication with this drug alone have not been reported.

Physical or psychological dependence does not develop when this drug is taken for brief periods in the recommended doses. However, people who have a history of drug abuse should receive only limited amounts of this drug at one time and few, if any, refill prescriptions. The increased risk of birth defects reported with other drugs of this chemical class has not been observed with flurazepam. However, this drug is probably best avoided by women during the first trimester of pregnancy when the risk of congenital fetal abnormalities is greatest.

Dosage and administration. The usual adult dose is 30 mg at bedtime. However, 15 mg may be adequate for many patients, and this dose is recommended for initiating therapy in elderly or disease-weakened patients.

Glutethimide USP (Doriden)

Actions and indications. This nonbarbiturate depressant drug is used for daytime, preoperative, and first stage of labor sedation, and in the management of insomnia. It has no advantages over the barbiturates except in patients hypersensitive to the latter hypnotics.

Adverse effects, cautions, and contraindications. Excessive sedation may occur in sensitive patients, and allergic hypersensitiv-

ity may result in skin rashes of several types. Blood dyscrasias and porphyria have also developed on rare occasions. Acute intoxication is similar to that caused by other depressants, but it is sometimes complicated by excitatory effects on motor systems that result in convulsions. Atropine-like effects such as dilated pupils, dry mouth, dysuria, and reduced peristaltic activity are also often seen following ingestion of toxic doses. The drug is used

with caution in patients prone to abuse drugs, because it has produced dependence.

Dosage and administration. Oral doses of 150 mg to 250 mg are administered tid after meals for daytime sedation. For hypnotic action 250 mg to 500 mg may be given at bedtime and repeated during the night, if necessary. Doses of 500 mg to 1.0 g are administered for preoperative sedation 1 hour before anesthesia and surgery.

Hydroxyzine HCl USP (Atarax) and hydroxyzine pamoate USP (Vistaril)

Actions and indications. This antianxiety agent is claimed also to possess several other peripheral and central effects in its spectrum of pharmacologic activity. These include antihistaminic, antiemetic, and antispasmodic effects on both skeletal and smooth muscles. These secondary effects are of little clinical significance. Thus, when the drug is employed as an adjunct in the management of organic disorders with an emotional component, it is commonly made available in combination with a more potent peripherally acting agent. For example, despite claims that this drug has an antisecretory effect, it is commonly combined with a more truly effective antisecretory–antispasmodic of the anticholinergic type when used as an adjunct in the treatment of peptic ulcer. Although the intramuscular solution for

parenteral use can calm acutely disturbed patients, this drug should not be used in the long-term management of psychotic patients. It is best employed as an adjunct to psychotherapy in neuroses and with other drugs in psychosomatic disorders.

Adverse effects, cautions, and contraindications. Drowsiness is common early in treatment. Higher doses can cause mouth dryness and, rarely, tremors, and convulsions. When hydroxyzine is administered preoperatively or as an adjunct in the management of labor, the dosage of narcotic analgesics such as meperidine must be reduced by up to half the usual amount, because this drug tends to potentiate the effects of narcotic analgesics, barbiturates, and other depressants. Patients taking oral doses are

warned not to drink alcoholic beverages. They should not drive a car or operate dangerous machinery when under the influence of this drug's sedative effect. Its use in early pregnancy is contraindicated, because high doses of the drug have caused abnormalities in animal fetuses.

Dosage and administration. Oral doses for adults range from 25 mg tid to 100 mg qid; thus, dosage is adjusted according to each patient's individual response. The parenteral solution is administered only intramuscularly, because it is now considered too irritating for intravenous or subcutaneous use. It is injected deep into large muscles in doses of 25 mg to 100 mg and is repeated every 4 to 6 hours if needed for control of acute excitement in emotional emergencies.

Meprobamate USP (Equanil; Miltown)

Actions and indications. This drug is used mainly for its sedative or antianxiety effect in many medical, psychiatric, and surgical disorders. In psychiatry, use of this drug for relief of anxiety and tension states affords support to alcoholic, neurotic, and some psychotic patients during psychotherapy. In medical conditions with an emotional component, including tension headache, cardiovascular, allergic, gastrointestinal, and menstrual disorders, this drug may be a desirable adjunct to more specific drugs and measures. Small oral doses administered in orthopedic, rheumatic, and neurologic conditions are not thought to be specifically effective for relaxing skeletal muscles. However, parenteral

administration of larger doses may be effective for relaxing painful muscle spasm—in tetanus, for example.

Adverse effects, cautions, and contraindications. Patients should be warned to avoid driving and other activities requiring alertness until development of tolerance leads to disappearance of the drowsiness that may develop at first. Other central depressant effects include dizziness, weakness, and headache. Chronic intoxication may be marked by slurred speech, ataxia, and vertigo. (To avoid development of dependence in patients with a history of alcoholism and addiction, dosage is carefully supervised.) Acute intoxication, which is particularly likely in patients

who have also been drinking, may result in stupor, coma, shock, and respiratory failure. (Patients with suicidal tendencies should also have dosage closely supervised.) This drug is contraindicated in patients with acute intermittent porphyria, in whom it may increase disease symptoms, and in those with a history of allergic or idiosyncratic skin and blood reactions to this drug.

Dosage and administration. The usual oral dose for adults is 400 mg tid or qid. A sustained-release capsule containing 400 mg may be administered bid (morning and bedtime) or in larger doses, depending on the patient's response.

Paraldehyde USP

Actions and indications. This rapid-acting sedative–hypnotic has been used mainly in the management of hospitalized alcoholic patients to prevent or to treat delirium tremens during withdrawal. It has also been employed to control convulsions in tetanus, status epilepticus, and other acute seizure states. It is occasionally used in labor and as a basal anesthetic.

Adverse effects, cautions, and contraindications. This liquid's unpleasant taste and

odor have not discouraged abuse of the drug by some alcoholics who have become dependent on it. When deprived of the drug, these addicts suffer the typical depressant drug withdrawal syndrome, including delirium tremens. Accidental overdosage results in deep depression that is sometimes complicated by metabolic acidosis. Decomposed paraldehyde containing high levels of acetaldehyde and acetic acid contaminants should not be used.

Dosage and administration. The usual oral dose is 5 ml to 10 ml, but as much as 30 ml may be needed by some patients. The liquid's taste is disguised by flavored syrups or fruit juices and by chilling it. It may be administered rectally for control of convulsions but must be well diluted with olive oil to reduce local irritation. IM or IV injection was employed in the past but is now considered inadvisable.

Pentobarbital sodium USP (Nembutal)

Actions and indications. This sedative–hypnotic of short to intermediate duration of action is used in small daytime doses to reduce nervous tension in patients with various psychiatric and medical conditions, including gastrointestinal, cardiovascular, and endocrine disorders (*e.g.,* hyperthyroidism, menopausal syndrome). A single larger dose is administered at bedtime in the management of insomnia. Still higher parenteral doses are used for inducing sedation or hypnosis prior to surgical and obstetrical procedures, for rapidly quieting acutely agitated psychiatric patients, and for producing narcosis in such psychotherapeutic techniques as narcoanalysis and narcotherapy.

Adverse effects, cautions, and contraindi-

cations. This habit-forming drug is not ordinarily administered to patients known to be addiction-prone, because it can cause psychological and physical dependence when abused. It is used with caution in patients with a history of hepatic disease and in patients who are simultaneously taking coumarin-type anticoagulant drugs. The drug is contraindicated in patients hypersensitive to barbiturates and in those with a history of porphyria. Overdosage results in respiratory depression and hypotension.

Dosage and administration. The usual dose for producing daytime sedation is 20 mg or 30 mg administered orally tid or qid. A single 100-mg morning dose of a slow-release preparation provides a similar effect. A capsule

containing 100 mg, or a 200-mg suppository, produces hypnotic effects in adult patients. (Dosage for children is reduced in accordance with their age and weight.) Intravenous administration of fractional doses is carried out slowly to avoid overdosage and respiratory depression, as well as hiccupping, coughing, and laryngospasm. Intramuscular injections at any single site are limited to 5 ml and are made deep into a large muscle mass such as the upper outer quadrant of the gluteus maximus. Usual adult dosage administered in this manner is 150 mg to 200 mg; IV dosage is 100 mg with increments as needed up to between 200 mg and 500 mg total dose.

959

Secobarbital sodium USP (Seconal)

Actions and indications. This short-acting sedative–hypnotic is best employed when a rapid relaxant or sleep-producing effect of relatively short duration is desired. Oral dosage forms are usually employed in the management of insomnia, but rectal administration is sometimes preferred in children and others for this and such other purposes as producing sedation prior to surgical operations and obstetric procedures.

An injectable form of secobarbital is employed to produce sleepiness in preparing patients for general, spinal, and regional anesthesia, and for intubation procedures. It is also often preferred to reduce apprehension in dental patients who are about to receive nerve block and before periodontal procedures. It may also be used for control of acute convulsions.

Adverse effects, cautions, and contraindications. The most common side-effect in patients hypersusceptible to the hypnotic effect of this drug is persistent drowsiness and lethargy, or hangover. Some patients, particularly the elderly or those in pain or weakened by chronic disease, may respond with paradoxical excitement or confusion. Overdosage may result in respiratory depression, especially if the patient has also ingested alcohol or received potent analgesics or other central depressant drugs.

Secobarbital should be used cautiously, if at all, in patients with severe liver disease and in those with a history of drug abuse. It should not be administered to patients with severe pain that has not been fully controlled by potent analgesics. Like other barbiturates, this drug is contraindicated in dyspneic patients with emphysema, status asthmaticus, or other chronic obstructive pulmonary disease. Patients with a history of latent porphyria as well as those who manifest signs and symptoms of this disorder must not receive this drug.

Dosage and administration. An oral dose of 100 mg or a rectal suppository containing 120 mg or 200 mg may be administered to adults at bedtime; for older children 60 mg to 120 mg is administered rectally; 60 mg or less is enough for this purpose in younger children, but those who are being prepared for ear, nose, and throat procedures may receive 4 or 5 mg/kg of body weight by rectal instillation of a solution.

Intramuscular or intravenous injections are made in amounts that vary with the degree of central depression desired and the age or physical condition of the patient. Total dosage of as little as 50 mg to no more than 250 mg is administered intravenously at a rate of no more than 50 mg/15 sec.

References

Alprazolam (Xanax). Med Lett Drugs Ther 24:41, 1982

Bellantuono C et al: Benzodiazepines: Clinical pharmacology and therapeutic use. Drugs 19:195, 1980

Blackwell B: Rational drug use in the management of anxiety. Ration Drug Ther 9:1, 1975

Greenblatt DJ, Allen MD, Schader RI: Toxicity of high dose flurazepam in the elderly. Clin Pharmacol Ther 21:355, 1977

Greenblatt DJ, Schader RI: Drug therapy: Benzodiazepines. N Engl J Med 291:1011, 1239 (Pts I & II), 1974

Greenblatt DJ, Schader RI: Clinical use of benzodiazepines. Ration Drug Ther 15:1, 1981

Greenblatt DJ, Schader RI, Koch–Weser J: Flurazepam hydrochloride: A benzodiazepine hypnotic. Ann Intern Med 83:237, 1975

Greenblatt DJ et al: Pharmacokinetic properties of benzodiazepine hypnotics. J Clin Psychopharmacol 3:129, 1983

Harris E: Sedative–hypnotic drugs. Am J Nurs 81:1329, 1981

Harvey SC: Hypnotics and sedatives. In Gilman AG, Goodman LS, Gilman A (eds): Goodman & Gilman's The Pharmacological Basis of Therapeutics, 6th ed, pp 339–375. New York, Macmillan, 1980

Hayes SL et al: Ethanol and oral diazepam absorption. N Engl J Med 296:186, 1977

Johnson LC, Chernik DA: Sedative–hypnotics and human performance. Psychopharmacol 76:101, 1982

Kales A, Kales JD: Editorial: Shortcomings in the evaluation and promotion of hypnotic drugs. N Engl J Med 292:826, 1975

Kales A et al: Chronic hypnotic drug use. JAMA 227:513, 1974

Kales A et al: Sleep laboratory studies of flurazepam: A model for evaluating hypnotic drugs. Clin Pharmacol Ther 19:576, 1976

Kales A et al: Insomnia and other sleep disorders. Med Clin North Am 66:971, 1982

Kosman ME: Pharmacokinetic drug interactions, sedative, hypnotic and antianxiety agents. JAMA 229:1485, 1974

Lasagna L: Drug therapy, hypnotic drugs. N Engl J Med 287:1182, 1972

Modell W: Updating the sleeping pill. Geriatrics 29:126, 1974

Morgan AJ: Minor tranquilizers, hypnotics, and sedatives. Am J Nurs 73:1220, 1973

Regestein QR: Chronic insomnia provokes more prescriptions than diagnoses. JAMA 237:1569, 1977

Triazolam—a new benzodiazepine for insomnia. Med Lett Drugs Ther 25:32, 1983

Chapter 46

Drugs used in the management of mental illness

46

One out of ten people in this country suffers from some form of mental or emotional illness. The previous chapter dealt with drugs used in the management of emotional disorders that are marked mainly by disabling degrees of anxiety. It described, for example, the properties of sedative–hypnotic and antianxiety drugs and their uses in the control of symptoms in patients suffering from psychoneurosis, psychophysiologic reactions, and psychosomatic ailments.

This chapter, will describe several other classes of psychopharmacotherapeutic agents that are used in the management of psychiatric disorders. These conditions—psychoses, such as schizophrenia, and affective, or mood, disorders, such as depression and mania—are considered to be more serious than those in which the main symptom is anxiety. The most important drugs employed in the symptomatic management of these major psychiatric illnesses are called *antispsychotic* agents, or *major tranquilizers,* and *antidepressant* drugs.

Before discussing the properties and uses of these and other psychoactive drugs, the nature of psychoses in general and schizophrenia in particular will be briefly reviewed.

The nature of psychosis

The term "psychosis" is defined in different ways by various authorities. A chief characteristic of psychotics seems to be a persistent inability to recognize reality. Patients, of course, differ in the degree to which their reality-testing ability is impaired. Some have *hallucinations*—that is, they hear voices or see objects when there are really no external sensory stimuli. Some suffer from *delusions*—that is, they have fixed systems of false beliefs that nothing can persuade them to give up. Reacting to the misperceptions of reality in the mind, psychotic persons may

behave in a bizarre manner. Sometimes, personality and behavior become so severely disorganized that patients cannot cope with the environment in which they have to function, and they must be hospitalized for their own protection as well as for the safety of others.

Etiology

Some types of psychoses have obvious organic causes. A person may be out of touch with reality, for example, because of chronic brain damage secondary to cerebrovascular disease, neurosyphilitic infection, or a head injury. An acute toxic psychosis can occur in people abusing amphetamine drugs or LSD (Chap. 53). Such a psychosis is usually transient, and the patient recovers after the drugs are eliminated from his brain. Similarly, the acute brain symptoms that accompany pellagra are reversible, and clear up when the patient's niacin-deficient diet is supplemented by high doses of this and other B-complex vitamins.

Actually, however, organic causes account for only a minority of mental illnesses. Most psychoses seem to be functional rather than organic. That is, there are no specific pathologic lesions that are detectable during brain surgery or at autopsy. Similarly, despite numerous biochemical theories of mental disease, in most cases no clear-cut neurochemical abnormalities can be detected by current methods of chemical analysis.

Schizophrenia

This is the most common of the functional psychoses. About 1% of the population—over two million Americans—are said to be schizophrenic and in need of treatment at some time in their lives. The disorder is not really a single specific disease but is rather various somewhat different symptom complexes or syndromes. Thus, there are, for example, such subgroups of schizophrenia as the so-called simple, hebephrenic, catatonic, and paranoid types.

All schizophrenics have certain primary symptoms in common:

1. *Disturbed thinking.* This may vary in severity from illogical ideation in a single sphere to total disorganization of thought processes. Thus, some paranoid patients may have normal intellectual capacity except for harboring delusions about certain subjects, while others may not make any sense at all because their ideas follow no meaningful order.
2. *Inappropriate affect.* Patients do not respond emotionally in a normal manner. Most often their emotional expression is flat and lifeless but sometimes, in hebephrenic schizophrenia, for instance, they may act silly and smile or laugh when nothing funny has happened.
3. *Autism.* Patients may seem so absorbed with their inner life that they pay no attention to the external world, and thus do not relate to other people.

The behavior of schizophrenic patients may take many forms, from mild ambivalence to severe psychomotor retardation or excitement. Catatonic schizophrenic patients may show periods of both stupor and excitement. That is, they may remain mute and immobile and retain the same position for hours, or they may suddenly explode into bursts of violent activity. (Signs and symptoms of psychomotor excitement and retardation are summarized in the summary of clinical indications for phenothiazines at the end of this section.)

Current status of schizophrenia treatment
The availability of antipsychotic drugs during the past 30 years has revolutionized the management of mentally ill patients. These drugs—also known as *neuroleptics* and *ataractics*—do not cure schizophrenia, but their actions are usually quite effective for suppressing such secondary symptoms as hallucinations and delusions and for controlling disturbed behavior. This has both brought about a great change in the atmosphere of mental institutions and has allowed patients to be released to re-enter the community more quickly.

The unique tranquilizing effect of these drugs (see below) contributed first to a reduction in the violent behavior that once characterized hospitals for chronically psychotic patients. Their use has done away with the need

for physical restraints such as straitjackets and for facilities such as pack rooms full of slabs and tubs for hydrotherapy. In addition, patients who were once merely kept in custody while their mental condition deteriorated now respond more readily to other types of treatment that truly speed their recovery and return to society. Thus, the number of patients confined in mental institutions has declined from over 500,000 in the mid-1950s to about 250,000 in the early 1980s.

Nurses are now better able to help psychotic patients in both the hospital and home environments. Because the effects of the antipsychotic drugs have helped make it easier to communicate with hospitalized patients who were once too agitated or too withdrawn to be reached, the nurse can interact with them in therapeutic ways that contribute to their recovery. After their release, patients must continue to take maintenance doses of their drugs. Here, too, the nurse can help to prevent relapses by checking to see that patients do not discontinue drug therapy. In addition, of course, the public health nurse has opportunities to interact with patients effectively on their periodic visits to the psychiatric clinic or when visiting their homes.

The next section of this chapter will describe in more detail the mental effects of antipsychotic drugs that account for their therapeutic value. It will also describe the secondary effects that often cause adverse reactions, and will review the measures that must be taken to minimize the harm that these potent drugs can do.

Antipsychotic drugs or major tranquilizers

Drugs of several different chemical classes have demonstrated an ability to relieve the symptoms of schizophrenia and of other psychoses and emotional disturbances (Table 46-1). Drugs of the following chemical classes are available for clinical use:

1. The phenothiazines
2. The butyrophenones
3. The thioxanthenes
4. The dibenzoxazepines*
5. The dihydroindolones
6. The rauwolfia alkaloids

Although the alkaloids of *rauwolfia* were the first of these drugs introduced for treating psychotic patients in the 1950s, they are not now used to any extent for this purpose because they are more likely than the phenothiazines and other antipsychotic drugs to produce hypotension, as well as emotional depression. They are employed today mainly in the management of hypertension (see Chap. 28).

On the other hand, compounds of the phenothiazine class, of which chlorpromazine was the first to

---

* Although the names of their chemical classes appear to be somewhat similar, the antipsychotic drugs of the dibenzoxazepine class are different from the antianxiety drugs of the benzodiazepine class described in the last chapter.

Table 46–1. Antipsychotic drugs or major tranquilizers

Official or generic name	Trade name	Usual adult daily dosage range
Phenothiazines		
Aliphatic subgroup		
Chlorpromazine HCl USP	Thorazine	30–1000 mg
Promazine HCl USP	Sparine	40–1000 mg
Triflupromazine HCl USP	Vesprin	60–150 mg
Piperazine subgroup		
Acetophenazine maleate USP	Tindal	60–120 mg
Carphenazine maleate USP	Proketazine	25–400 mg
Fluphenazine decanoate and fluphenazine enanthate USP	Prolixin Decanoate; Prolixin Enanthate	12.5–50 mg (every 2–3 wks)
Fluphenazine HCl USP	Permitil; Prolixin	0.5–20 mg
Perphenazine USP	Trilafon	12–64 mg
Prochlorperazine edisylate and prochlorperazine maleate USP	Compazine	15–150 mg
Trifluoperazine HCl USP	Stelazine	2–40 mg
Piperidyl subgroup		
Mesoridazine besylate	Serentil	30–400 mg
Piperacetazine	Quide	20–160 mg
Thioridazine HCl USP	Mellaril	150–800 mg
Thioxanthenes		
Chlorprothixene	Taractan	75–600 mg
Thiothixene	Navane	6–60 mg
Butyrophenone		
Haloperidol USP	Haldol	1–15 mg
Dibenzoxazepine		
Loxapine succinate	Loxitane	20–250 mg
Dihydroindolone		
Molindone HCl	Moban	15–225 mg

be introduced (at about the same time as the rauwolfia alkaloid reserpine), are still the most important group of antipsychotic agents. Because the phenothiazines are by far the most frequently employed drugs, only these drugs will be discussed in detail. Certain individual drugs from among the other chemical groups will then be briefly compared with the phenothiazine compounds that they most closely resemble.

The phenothiazines

History. Phenothiazine, the chemical from which the antipsychotic drugs of this class are derived, has little significant effect on the central nervous system. A derivative, *promethazine* (Phenergan) was originally introduced as an antihistamine (Chap. 39), but it was found to possess a central depressant effect that limited its daytime use in the management of allergy. However, because promethazine not only produced drowsiness but also potentiated the effects of other central depressants such as the opiates, it was employed as an adjunct to potent analgesic drugs in the preoperative and postoperative management of obstetric and other patients.

Chlorpromazine[+] (Thorazine), the prototype of today's antipsychotic drugs, was discovered in a further search for phenothiazines with properties that might be usefully employed in anesthesia. It was found to have the then unique property of making patients calm and unconcerned about what would usually be anxiety-provoking situations. At the same time, this drug did not produce any significant degree of the psychomotor depression that the barbiturates and similar sedative–hypnotics caused when employed as preoperative sedatives. This led to trials of chlorpromazine for reducing agitation in manic and in other mentally disturbed patients that proved its usefulness in the treatment of psychotic patients.

Chemistry. Once the effectiveness of chlorpromazine became apparent, chemists began to synthesize closely related congener compounds to discover relatives that might be more potent and cause fewer side-effects. The currently available derivatives are prepared by substituting various radicals (atoms or side chains) in the number 2 (R_2) or the number 10 (R_{10}) positions, or both, in the three-ring structure of phenothiazine (Fig. 46-1). These derivatives can be divided into three chemical subgroups that differ from one another to some extent in their pharmacologic effects:

1. The *aliphatic* or *dimethylaminoalkyl group* (*e.g.*, promazine, chlorpromazine, triflupromazine)
2. The *piperazine* subgroup (*e.g.*, fluphenazine, trifluoperazine, perphenazine)
3. The *piperidine* subgroup (*e.g.*, thioridazine, mesoridazine, piperacetazine)

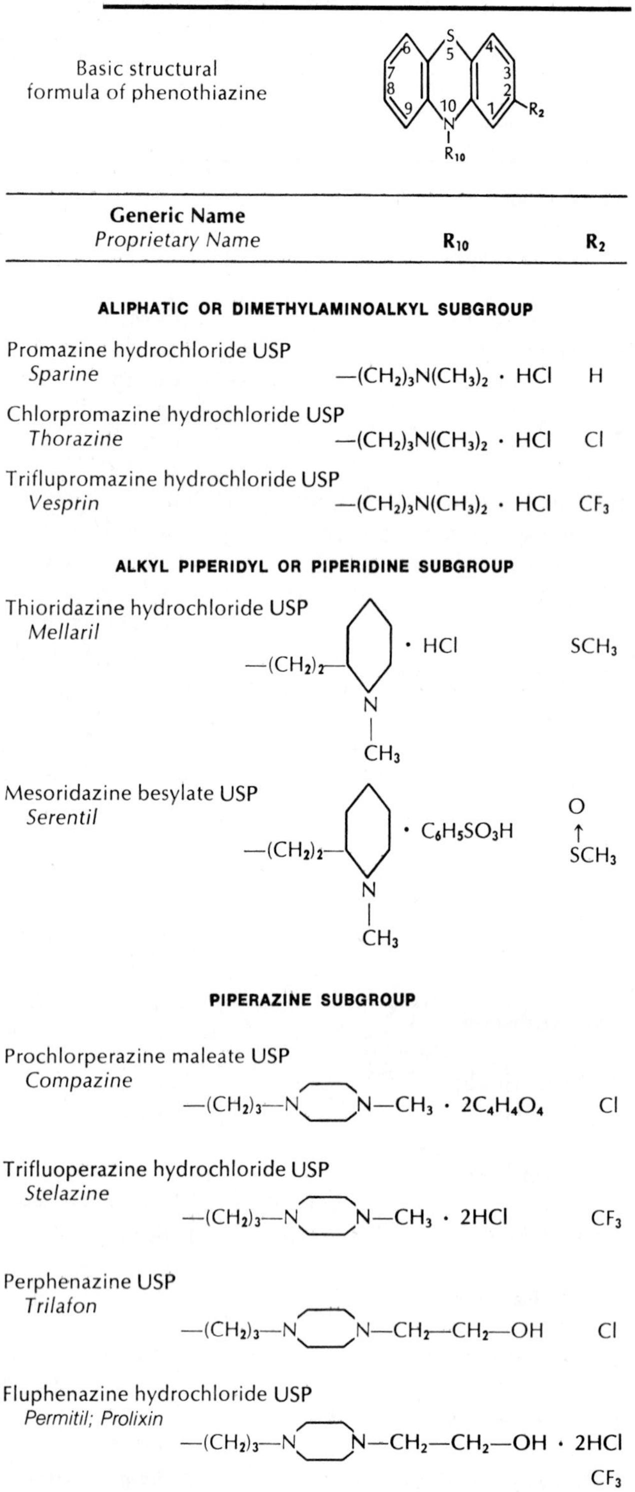

Phenothiazines of all three classes are essentially similar to the prototype chemical chlorpromazine in their effectiveness as antipsychotic agents. They differ from one another mainly in their potency and in the types of side-effects that they tend to cause. Thus, for example, drugs of the piperazine subclass are as effective in doses of a few milligrams as are doses of hundreds of milligrams of the derivatives of the other two subclasses. These piperazines are, however, much more likely to cause extrapyramidal motor system side-effects (see below). Phe-

| Basic structural formula of phenothiazine | | |

Generic Name *Proprietary Name*	R_{10}	R_2
ALIPHATIC OR DIMETHYLAMINOALKYL SUBGROUP		
Promazine hydrochloride USP *Sparine*	$-(CH_2)_3N(CH_3)_2 \cdot HCl$	H
Chlorpromazine hydrochloride USP *Thorazine*	$-(CH_2)_3N(CH_3)_2 \cdot HCl$	Cl
Triflupromazine hydrochloride USP *Vesprin*	$-(CH_2)_3N(CH_3)_2 \cdot HCl$	CF_3
ALKYL PIPERIDYL OR PIPERIDINE SUBGROUP		
Thioridazine hydrochloride USP *Mellaril*	$-(CH_2)_2 \cdots \cdot HCl$	SCH_3
Mesoridazine besylate USP *Serentil*	$-(CH_2)_2 \cdots \cdot C_6H_5SO_3H$	$\overset{O}{\underset{SCH_3}{\uparrow}}$
PIPERAZINE SUBGROUP		
Prochlorperazine maleate USP *Compazine*	$-(CH_2)_3-N \bigcirc N-CH_3 \cdot 2C_4H_4O_4$	Cl
Trifluoperazine hydrochloride USP *Stelazine*	$-(CH_2)_3-N \bigcirc N-CH_3 \cdot 2HCl$	CF_3
Perphenazine USP *Trilafon*	$-(CH_2)_3-N \bigcirc N-CH_2-CH_2-OH$	Cl
Fluphenazine hydrochloride USP *Permitil; Prolixin*	$-(CH_2)_3-N \bigcirc N-CH_2-CH_2-OH \cdot 2HCl$	CF_3

Figure 46-1. Some phenothiazine derivatives. Substitutions in the number 10 position account for the names of the subclasses. Substitutions of Cl or CF_2 in the number 2 position increase the antipsychotic potency of the phenothiazines.

nothiazines of the other two classes are more prone to produce oversedation and blockade of peripheral sites that are innervated by the autonomic nervous system.

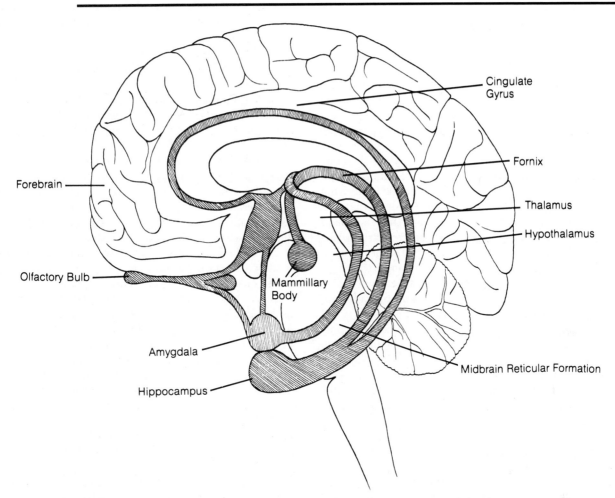

Figure 46-2. The limbic system—the rhinencephalon (nose brain) and related structures—is thought to constitute a neuroanatomic emotional circuit. The phenothiazines and other antipsychotic drugs are believed to act primarily by affecting the excitability of subcortical centers in this "anatomic substrate of the emotions." More specifically, much evidence now indicates that these drugs act by blocking limbic and cortical dopaminergic receptors that receive input from neurons in the mesencephalon (midbrain).

Pharmacologic effects. The phenothiazines can produce many different effects by their actions at several peripheral as well as central sites (see the summary at the end of this section). The peripheral actions on the cardiovascular system and various visceral organs are the cause of some of the side-effects commonly seen clinically (see the summary of adverse effects at the end of this section). The most characteristic and clinically significant effects of the phenothiazines involve their ability to alter the psychological functioning of mentally disturbed patients and to produce changes in their motor activity. Both of these central effects may stem from the same types of drug-induced neurochemical changes.

Mechanism of action. The exact mechanism of action of the phenothiazines and the other chemical classes of antipsychotic drugs is not fully understood at this time. However, there is evidence that these drugs affect the transmission of nerve impulses in certain central nervous system (CNS) pathways in which the transmitter is the catecholamine dopamine (Chap. 13). The most important of these dopaminergic pathways are the mesolimbic, mesocortical, nigrostriatal, and tuberoinfundibular pathways (Fig. 46-2).

The phenothiazines and other antipsychotic drugs are believed to act by blocking receptors that ordinarily respond to nerve-released dopamine.* This interferes with nerve impulse transmission in the four dopaminergic pathways mentioned above. Actions in the mesolimbic and mesocortical pathways are believed to be responsible for the therapeutic antipsychotic effects; actions in the nigrostriatal and tuberoinfundibular pathways

---

* The dopamine-sensitive receptor sites are enzymes of the *adenylate cyclase* class. As indicated in Chapter 13, the result of interactions between catecholamines and enzymes of this type is an increase in the intracellular level of the nucleotide, cyclic adenosinemonophosphate (cAMP). The manner in which higher levels of cAMP affect nerve cell function is not yet known.

are believed to be responsible for the adverse extrapyramidal and endocrine effects.

Psychological–behavioral effects. The phenothiazines cause two types of effects when administered to mentally disturbed patients. One of these, the so-called *tranquilizing* or *neuroleptic* effect, is a unique form of sedation. It comes on quickly and is particularly marked in patients receiving chlorpromazine and other phenothiazines of the aliphatic group. The other response, the so-called *antipsychotic* effect—a normalizing of thought, mood, and behavior—takes several weeks to develop. Some authorities suggest that this is the result of a direct influence that the phenothiazines exert on the underlying disease process in schizophrenia. Others deny that this effect is so specific and believe, instead, that the drugs act only to make patients more responsive to nonpharmacologic influences that account for their improvement.

Psychosedation. The behavioral changes that have been called the *neuroleptic syndrome* can be observed in both normal and disturbed persons soon after administration of an adequate dose of *chlorpromazine, thioridazine*[+] (Mellaril), and drugs of the same subgroups as these phenothiazines. These drugs produce a quieting or calming effect that differs in quality from that which follows administration of the barbiturates, the *non*barbiturate sedative–hypnotics, and the minor tranquilizers (anti-anxiety drugs). Among these differences in their depressant effects are the following:

1. Patients are made apathetic and indifferent to exciting environmental stimuli without suffering severe mental and motor impairment. That is, they can be more readily aroused than patients depressed by drugs such as barbiturates and meprobamate. Thus, they are more alert and responsive, and they can move about with better motor coordination following arousal.
2. Patients do *not* go through any preliminary excitement phase before becoming calm and quiet, as often occurs with alcohol, barbiturates, and similar depressants, nor do even very large doses result in severe respiratory depression, stupor, and coma, as occurs with the other depressants.
3. Psychological dependence rarely develops, presumably because patients do not feel the euphoric release of inhibitions often produced by the sedative–hypnotics and minor tranquilizers. People who are not anxious or agitated actually find the feelings that are induced by these drugs dysphoric. That is, normal persons often complain of feeling lethargic, lifeless, and lacking in spontaneity.

Patients show reduced motor activity, as occurs with the general depressants. Unlike the latter, however, the phenothiazines do *not* have good anticonvulsant activity. On the contrary, these drugs may increase susceptibility to seizures in epileptic patients and others, presumably because of their complex effects on extrapyramidal motor system nerve pathways (see below).

Antipsychotic effect. The usefulness of the phenothiazines seems to depend on more than their ability to calm anxious or acutely agitated patients. Their effectiveness in the treatment of acute schizophrenic reactions appears to involve actions other than their ability to quiet hyperactive patients and to control aggressive or combative behavior. This is why the term "tranquilizer" has been criticized as an inadequate description of the psychopharmacologic effects of these drugs.

One argument in favor of a more direct effect of these drugs on psychotic processes is seen in the response of some schizophrenic patients whose main symptoms are those of psychomotor retardation rather than excitement (see the list of psychiatric target symptoms in the summary of clinical indications at the end of this section). After several weeks of treatment with phenothiazines, including congeners of the piperazine group such as *fluphenazine*[+] (Permitil; Prolixin) or *trifluoperazine* (Stelazine) that cause relatively little sedation, some of these patients become less withdrawn, apathetic, and mute. Similarly, even after patients with symptoms of psychomotor excitement become tolerant to the sedative effects of *chlorpromazine* and *thioridazine*, their mental status may still continue to improve.

Just what these drugs may do to bring about and maintain improved thinking and behavior is uncertain. The first improvement in the primary symptoms of schizophrenia seems to occur in the affective sphere—that is, in the patient's emotional responsiveness. Patients whose excited or withdrawn behavior may reflect a fearful or hostile response to their misperceptions of reality often seem less disturbed by their hallucinations or delusions. They may still suffer from such secondary symptoms at first, but they seem to be less bothered by them. As one patient said, "I still hear my enemies' voices calling me names and threatening me, but I pay them no mind."

Later, as the patient continues to take these or other antipsychotic drugs, the hallucinations may disappear and he may give up his delusions. Improved intellectual functioning often follows, particularly if the patient receives psychotherapeutic support. That is, once the drugs have helped make the patient better able to interact constructively with others, it is important for professional counseling to be given. It is also essential that the patient continue to take the antipsychotic medications, because these drugs do not permanently correct the still unknown causes of schizophrenia.

Other central effects. In addition to the central effects discussed above, which presumably stem from actions in the limbic and ascending reticular activating systems (Fig. 46-2), the phenothiazines also affect other areas of the brain. Some of these result in pharmacologic effects that are undesirable, such as the responses of the extra-pyramidal motor system and of the hypothalamic–hypophyseal system, which are discussed below in the section on adverse effects. However, some central effects of the phenothiazines have been applied in areas of therapeutics other than psychiatry.

Antiemetic effects. Most phenothiazines—particularly those of the piperazine subgroup, such as prochlorperazine+ (Compazine; see Drug digest, Chap. 41)—exert a direct depressant effect on the chemoreceptor trigger zone (CTZ), the group of nerve cells that relays impulses to the medullary vomiting center. Prochlorperazine and perphenazine (Trilafon) are, for example, commonly used to prevent or overcome vomiting in various clinical conditions (see Chap. 41). All the phenothiazines, with the possible exception of thioridazine (Mellaril), are effective antiemetics.

The use of some of these drugs, often intravenously, to control intractable hiccups, has been described in Chapter 41.

Potentiating effects. An important CNS effect of the phenothiazines is their ability to intensify and prolong the action of other depressant drugs. The pain-relieving properties of the narcotic analgesics, for example, are potentiated by combining them with phenothiazines, especially those of the dimethylamine subgroup, such as chlorpromazine (Thorazine). This action is due partly to their ability to reduce the patient's emotional reaction to pain and partly to their action in somehow increasing the effect of the narcotic analgesic drugs on pain perception. This is often useful for patients in severe pain; however, the potentiating action of the phenothiazines on barbiturates, alcohol, and narcotics may sometimes cause deep sleep, stupor, and even coma.

Autonomic blocking effects. The phenothiazines also exert complex effects on the functioning of peripheral organs that receive nerve impulses from both divisions of the autonomic system (Chap. 13). In addition to effects that are the result of actions on central areas that integrate autonomic function, these drugs also often block the responses of cardiac, smooth muscle, and glandular cells to sympathetic and parasympathetic nerve impulses. More specifically, the phenothiazines and other antipsychotic drugs have varying degrees of anticholinergic, α-antiadrenergic, and antihistaminic activity. The resulting changes in the functioning of the heart, gastrointestinal system, and other organs are usually considered to be undesirable side-effects. Thus, these are discussed below in the section that deals with the adverse effects of the phenothiazines.

Clinical indications. The phenothiazines are most commonly employed clinically for control of symptoms such as anxiety and agitation in various psychiatric disorders (see the summary at the end of this section). These include alcoholism (Chap. 53) and affective illnesses such as mental depression and mania (see below). However, the most important application of these drugs in therapeutics is in the management of acute and chronic schizophrenia.

Acute schizophrenic reactions. The phenothiazines are most dramatically effective when administered by injection to control acutely agitated patients. For this purpose, chlorpromazine or one of the other drugs of the same sedating subgroup is usually preferred. Injected repeatedly in small doses—for example, 25 to 100 mg as often as once an hour for several hours—the aliphatic phenothiazines quickly control the hyperactive patient's restlessness and aggressive, assaultive, or destructive behavior. After the patient's excitement has subsided—usually within 48 hours—treatment is continued with daily oral doses for a period long enough to determine whether the drug will also help to improve primary schizophrenic symptomatology, such as thought and mood disturbances and autism.

Patients whose psychotic break came on suddenly, especially following some specific traumatic event in their life situations, are most likely to respond favorably to treatment with these and other antipsychotic drugs. Often, after about 3 weeks of therapy, the patient has improved enough to profit further from sociotherapy and psychotherapy, and is able to take part in occupational therapy and recreational activities. This is also a time in which the nurse can contribute to the patient's recovery by taking every opportunity to interact with him. Even in a large custodial institution, the nurse should view the time when administering medications as an opportunity for therapeutic intervention.

Chronic schizophrenia. These drugs are least likely to prove successful in patients who were hospitalized after a long gradual slide into mental illness. People who have lost all interest in such activities as school or job, and have few friends and poor intrafamily relationships, may not do well when treated with antipsychotic drugs alone. Some people with so-called simple schizophrenia who never received psychiatric treatment because their behavior was not bizarre enough to attract much attention, may retreat even further into a private autistic world when attempts are made to treat them with central depressant drugs.

On the other hand, chronically ill patients, including some who were considered to be hopelessly regressed, have sometimes responded to intensive therapy with relatively high doses of these drugs. The piperazine-type phenothiazines fluphenazine (Permitil; Prolixin) and trifluoperazine (Stelazine) have been preferred for this purpose, because these nonsedating ("activating" or "stimulating") drugs seemed to be most desirable for treating hypodynamic patients. However, high doses of chlorpromazine—for example, 2000 mg or more daily—

have also proved to be effective in patients with such symptoms of psychomotor withdrawal as apathy, seclusiveness, mutism, and catatonic posturing. Apparently, the antipsychotic action of all drugs of this class can help some chronic schizophrenics whose fear and hostility has led them to withdraw from human contact, as well as those patients whose psychotic reaction takes the form of violent excitement.

Maintenance therapy. As indicated earlier, one benefit of the phenothiazines has been their ability to help patients improve sufficiently to leave the hospital and return home in a relatively short time. However, only a small minority—as few as 15%—make a complete recovery and never return for further hospitalization. Often when subjected to the same stresses at home or at work that had led to their previous psychotic episodes, patients fail to cope with their problems. Thus, patients should continue to take antipsychotic drug medication and to receive psychotherapy or psychological counseling after discharge from the hospital.

Unfortunately, it has been shown that up to 50% of outpatients fail to take their drugs faithfully. This is the most common cause of relapse. Thus, the public health nurse who has occasion to visit patients in their homes should make sure that they are following instructions for taking their medication in prescribed doses. Patients who cannot be trusted to comply with advice for taking oral drugs sometimes receive IM injections of the long-acting enanthate or decanoate esters of fluphenazine. These slowly absorbed antipsychotic drugs usually exert their effect over a period of about 2 weeks. Outpatients are expected to return to the clinic for injections about twice a month. If they fail to return for follow-up injections, a public health nurse may give the injection on a home visit.

Other indications. Not all patients for whom the phenothiazines are ordered suffer from schizophrenia. These drugs are also useful for control of anxiety, restlessness, and agitation in patients with other psychiatric disorders. Medical and surgical patients may also benefit from the central effects of phenothiazines. Chlorpromazine, for example, is useful in the management of cancer patients, in whom it relieves anxiety, potentiates the action of narcotics, and reduces nausea and vomiting caused by drugs or irradiation.

Organic and toxic psychoses. The restlessness, confusion, and excitement seen in patients suffering from chronic brain syndromes are also controlled with phenothiazines. Both elderly patients with organic brain damage caused by cerebrovascular atherosclerosis and mentally retarded children are made calmer and quieter with these drugs. They are also useful for quick control of excitement and disturbed behavior caused by the effects of drugs such as LSD (toxic psychosis) and in acute alcoholic intoxication.

Alcoholic patients may also profit from phenothiazine administration during withdrawal states such as alcoholic hallucinosis and delirium tremens. Here, however, they are best combined with general depressants such as the barbiturates, paraldehyde, or chlordiazepoxide (Librium; Chap. 45); given alone, they are more likely to precipitate seizures.

Affective disorders. As indicated below, some emotionally depressed patients with symptoms such as sluggishness and lethargy may respond poorly to phenothiazines if their retarded state stems from one of the depressive syndromes (see summary at the end of this chapter) rather than from schizophrenia. On the other hand, emotionally depressed patients who show signs of agitation often profit from the addition of a phenothiazine such as perphenazine (Trilafon) to their antidepressant drug medication.

The manic phase of the manic–depressive psychosis can often be brought under control most rapidly with one of the more sedating types of phenothiazines. Slower acting lithium salts are administered simultaneously, and the phenothiazines are then usually discontinued once effective levels of lithium have been attained in the brain.

Psychoneurosis. Patients with relatively mild to moderate degrees of anxiety that causes discomforting nervousness or physical symptoms are sometimes treated with small oral doses of phenothiazines such as fluphenazine (Permitil; Prolixin) or acetophenazine (Tindal). Although low doses of the phenothiazines rarely cause severe side-effects, some patients occasionally develop severe hypersensitivity reactions (see below). Thus, many physicians now prefer to use one of the safer minor tranquilizers for control of anxiety and tension in patients with personality disturbances and in patients with conditions that seem to have psychoneurotic or psychosomatic components.

Adverse effects

Types of toxicity. The phenothiazines can cause many types of ill effects, particularly when these drugs must be administered to hospitalized patients in high doses for long periods (see the summary of adverse effects at the end of this section). Some side-effects of phenothiazines are the result of excessive actions on the CNS; others are the result of blockade of nerve impulse transmission by way of both divisions of the autonomic nervous system. Endocrine imbalances are occasionally brought about by continued administration of these drugs. Some side-effects are the result of allergic hypersensitivity rather than of the drugs' direct pharmacologic effects.

Central nervous system. The side-effects of the phenothiazines may be the result of either excessive depression or excessive stimulation. Depression manifested by drowsiness, dizziness, lethargy, and feelings of fatigue is more common with drugs of the aliphatic subgroup (*e.g.,* promazine, chlorpromazine) and the piperidyl subtype (*e.g.,* thioridazine) than with the piperazines (*e.g.,* fluphenazine, trifluoperazine). On the other hand, drugs of the latter type seem to be more likely to overstimulate the extrapyramidal motor system. That is, the effects of blockade of dopamine receptors in the nigrostriatal pathway are more readily seen. Thioridazine (Mellaril) seems to cause less extrapyramidal stimulation than other phenothiazines. This may be because it also has certain other central effects, especially central anticholinergic effects, that depress the basal ganglia. This helps to counteract its tendency to stimulate motor activity.

The most common symptoms of *extrapyramidal stimulation* can be grouped in three categories:

1. *Parkinsonism*—marked by a lack of activity, or akinesia, muscular tremors, rigidity, and other signs resembling those seen in Parkinson's disease
2. *Dyskinesia*—sudden involuntary contractions of muscle groups in spasms resembling convulsive seizures
3. *Akathisia*—extreme restlessness marked by increasing mental turbulence and motor activity (patients often complain of having "the jitters" or "restless legs")

These symptoms are best controlled by reducing the dose of the antipsychotic drug or by withdrawing it entirely. Once the symptoms have subsided, treatment may be begun again at a lower dose level. Patients may also receive daily doses of one of the centrally acting anticholinergic drugs that are employed in the treatment of Parkinson's disease (Chap. 49). These concurrently administered drugs—*benztropine* and *trihexyphenidyl,* for example—help to relieve the pseudoparkinsonism that occurs as a result of the blocking effect of the phenothiazines on dopaminergic pathways in the basal ganglia (see above).

It was once thought that motor disturbances were to be expected with antipsychotic drug dosage high enough to produce the desired therapeutic effects. This is now known not to be true, and many patients taking antipsychotic drugs improve without developing signs of extrapyramidal motor stimulation. Thus, it is *not* necessary for all patients on antipsychotic drug therapy to receive antiparkinsonism drugs routinely for prophylactic purposes. Patients who do not need such adjunctive antiparkinsonism medication should be spared their discomforting atropinelike side-effects, which can be especially severe when these drugs are given together with phenothiazines that cause similar side effects (see below). In addition, there is evidence that anticholinergic drugs can interfere with the absorption of some of the antipsychotic agents.

Persistent tardive dyskinesia. A fourth type of drug-induced neurologic disorder sometimes develops gradually in patients treated for several months or years with these or other antipsychotic drugs. This late-developing, or tardive, disorder differs from the three other syndromes in several other significant ways: the nature of the neurologic signs, the lack of symptomatic control or prevention with antiparkinson drugs; and the persistence and, in some cases, irreversibility of the symptoms. Tardive dyskinesia is marked primarily by abnormal repeated movements localized mainly around the mouth. The patient's lips may be pursed and the mouth puckered, with the tongue protruding in a rapid, rhythmic manner. Chewing movements may continue incessantly. In addition, some patients develop choreoathetoid movements resembling those seen in patients with Huntington's chorea or in Parkinson's disease patients who develop the late neurologic side-effects (called abnormal involuntary movements, or AIMs) of levodopa treatment (Chap. 49).

This disorder was once thought to be a relatively rare adverse effect that developed mainly in elderly women patients with organic brain disorders who had received years of massive dosage with phenothiazines. It is now known to occur more commonly than was previously suspected, and it may affect younger patients with no pre-existing brain damage after as little as 6 months of moderate dosage. All the phenothiazines are considered equally likely to produce tardive dyskinesia.

There is, at present, no known treatment for this most disabling of the drug-induced neurologic syndromes. It may be prevented if the medication is discontinued when early signs, such as a fine wormlike movement of muscle fibers in the tongue, are noted.

Autonomic effects. The phenothiazines exert complex effects on the functioning of organs that are innervated by the autonomic nervous system. Some of these effects are the result of drug action on central areas that integrate autonomic activity, but most occur because of blockade of both cholinergic and adrenergic nerve impulses at peripheral receptor sites in various organs (Chaps. 16 and 18). Side-effects of these types occur more commonly with drugs of the aliphatic subclass such as chlorpromazine, and of the piperidine group such as thioridazine, but cholinergic blocking effects are also sometimes seen with certain of the piperazines, such as trifluoperazine and fluphenazine.

Typical atropinelike side-effects include dryness of the mouth, blurring of vision, and constipation. A drug-induced reduction in sweating caused by the same anticholinergic mechanism may make some patients prone to suffer heat stroke during hot weather. On the other hand, α-adrenergic blockade of impulses to blood vessels may cause peripheral vasodilation, with heat loss from the skin and a drop in body temperature. Other side-effects caused by adrenergic blockade include nasal congestion and occasional interference with male sexual function—for example, failure of ejaculation.

The cardiovascular side-effects of chlorpromazine and of drugs of its subclass are also the result of α-adrenergic blockade and increased compensatory reflex responsiveness. Patients often complain of dizziness, weakness, faintness, and heart palpitations as a result of drug-induced postural hypotension and reflex tachycardia. Parenteral administration may sometimes intensify the fall in blood pressure, and direct cardiac depressant effects may add to the autonomic-type rhythm irregularities that these drugs occasionally cause. Injection of promazine (Sparine) to quiet an alcoholic may, for example, send the blood pressure plummeting. This hypotension occurs because the drug reduces vasomotor tone by cutting off some of the tonic vasoconstrictor nerve impulses passing to the arterioles by way of sympathetic nerve fibers. Promazine may also potentiate the depressant effects of alcohol and barbiturates in intoxicated patients and thus cause coma as well as falls both in blood pressure and in the rate and depth of respiration.

Sudden death has sometimes been reported in patients taking phenothiazines. Although the cause has not always been determined, some have suggested that these drugs may cause ventricular fibrillation or sudden cardiac arrest as a result of a quinidinelike effect (Chap. 30) of certain phenothiazine derivatives. Others think that these patients may be made subject to sudden seizures and that death may be caused by asphyxia from food aspirated into the air passages.

Endocrine effects. Some phenothiazines appear to be able to block the effects of the hypothalamic neurohormones that influence the release of anterior pituitary gland hormones. As indicated in Chapter 20, the hypothalamic hormone, prolactin release-inhibiting factor (PIF), may be dopamine, or dopamine may be a neurotransmitter in the pathway that controls PIF release. By blocking the dopamine receptors in this tuberoinfundibular pathway, the phenothiazines can cause elevated circulating levels of the anterior pituitary hormone prolactin. This is thought to account for the occurrence of milk secretion, or galactorrhea, in women who have been taking these drugs. Actions at this hypothalamic–hypophyseal site are also believed to be responsible for signs and symptoms of endocrine gland derangements, including delayed menstruation and ovulation, or even amenorrhea, false positive pregnancy tests in women, and breast growth (gynecomastia) in men. Patients also sometimes gain weight and show such signs as hyperglycemia and glycosuria.

Hypersensitivity-type reactions. Many reactions reported in patients taking phenothiazines are the result of individual hypersensitivity. There are several of these reactions, which occur most commonly with chlorpromazine.

Agranulocytosis. This and other types of blood dyscrasias may occur. Patients should be warned to report the occurrence of a sudden severe sore throat. If blood studies show a low white blood cell count, phenothiazines should be discontinued, and anti-infective drug therapy should be begun.

Cholestatic hepatitis. This is an obstructive type of liver disorder. Chlorpromazine-induced jaundice is caused by swelling of the walls of the canaliculi, the tiny bile channels within the liver. When these become blocked, the bile backs up into the blood. The condition usually clears up when the drug is discontinued. However, because the symptoms resemble those of more serious obstructive biliary disorders, such as bile duct stones or cancer of the pancreas, exploratory abdominal surgery may be required to eliminate the possibility that the patient's symptoms stem from such conditions.

Skin reactions. These range from mild urticaria to severe exfoliative dermatitis. Patients taking phenothiazines are advised to avoid excessive exposure to sunlight, which may play a part in both skin pigmentation and ocular changes that sometimes occur during long-term therapy. The skin discolorations and visual difficulties may be caused by melanin pigment deposited in the skin, eyes, and other organs of patients taking high doses of phenothiazines. Although the exact cause is still unknown, some authorities suggest that such phenothiazine-induced melanosis may be the result of the action of certain wavelengths of light on the drugs (and their metabolites) that have accumulated in the skin. In any case, whatever the mechanism by which it is brought about, the slate blue to deep blue black or purplish skin discolorations constitute a serious cosmetic problem. The nurse may be asked to help prevent such phototoxic reactions by keeping patients out of direct sunlight during the spring and summer months. The nature and significance of the ocular opacities are not well understood at present, but ophthalmologists suggest that all patients receiving prolonged treatment with high doses of phenothiazines be subjected to serial slit lamp studies periodically.

Additional clinical considerations

There is a wide margin of safety between the doses of phenothiazines needed to produce the therapeutic neuroleptic effects and those that could cause fatal overdosage. However, despite their low lethality, these drugs can cause many different types of adverse effects. These are not only discomforting for the hospitalized patient, but also play a part in the failure of outpatients to comply with the maintenance dosage regimen.

The observant nurse can help to minimize adverse drug effects of all types in mental patients by assessing and reporting unusual signs and symptoms. Thus, for example, patients may complain of drowsiness, dizziness, weakness, and faintness—particularly, early in treatment with aliphatic-type phenothiazines such as chlorpromazine. The drug's dosage should then be reduced temporarily to counteract the depression and postural hypotension produced by this drug.

The nurse can explain to the patient the true significance of drug-induced side-effects. Outpatients, for example, are sometimes alarmed by physical feelings that they may think are caused by a return of the perceptual distortions that were part of their illness. The nurse may be able to assure them that visual difficulties or other strange sensations that they may be experiencing are actually the result of temporary central and autonomic side-effects of their phenothiazine maintenance medication.

Similarly, the nurse's support and encouragement can help to reduce the patient's concern about the side-effects on sexual function sometimes set off by these drugs. Reduced sex drive and impotence in the male outpatient are ordinarily only temporary, and women with delayed menstruation, breast enlargement, and weight gain can be assured that these are drug-induced effects rather than signs of pregnancy.

Dosage and administration. As indicated in Table 46-1, the dosage range for phenothiazine drugs is very wide. Patients may, in fact, require doses much larger than those listed as "usual" in the table. For example, some patients on high dosage regimens have received as much as 3000 mg of chlorpromazine daily or 80 mg or more of fluphenazine or trifluoperazine. The dosage of any phenothiazine drug must be adjusted to meet the needs of the individual patient. Usually patients suffering from acute psychotic reactions require much larger doses than those with milder symptoms. After the psychotic crisis and its acute excitement have been controlled, dosage may be continued at high levels until the psychosis resolves. It is then gradually reduced to lower levels for long-term maintenance therapy.

The phenothiazines are effective whether administered orally or parenterally. The latter route is usually reserved for treatment of the more severely agitated patient who needs large doses. The intramuscular route is preferred to intravenous administration because the danger of sudden severe falls in blood pressure is decreased when phenothiazines are more slowly absorbed. Instructions for diluting solutions with saline solution should be followed carefully, and the solutions should be injected into a muscle, not into subcutaneous tissues, because such tissues are more subject to irritation than are muscular sites. Injections are best made slowly and deep into the muscle, and the usual precautions must be taken to see that a vein has not been entered accidentally. The physician may sometimes order the addition of procaine 2% to reduce pain.

Most patients are best maintained on oral dosage forms administered at bedtime. Taking the total daily maintenance dose at that time reduces the patient's

awareness of discomforting or somewhat disabling side-effects, such as dizziness and faintness, which are much less likely to occur when the patient is lying down. Drug-induced drowsiness is desirable at bedtime. A single daily dose is convenient and more likely to ensure the outpatient's compliance. Patients who fail to take even a single daily oral dose may require periodic injections of one of the available repository forms of fluphenazine.

Nonphenothiazine antipsychotic drugs
Drugs of several other chemical classes—some chemically similar to the phenothiazines and others quite different—exert clinically effective antipsychotic activity. These drugs are best employed in two types of clinical situations:

1. For patients with chronic schizophrenic symptoms that have not been completely controlled by any of the several prototype phenothiazines, the physician may order a trial of a drug of different chemical structure.
2. Patients who have shown hypersensitivity reactions to phenothiazine-type drugs may be transferred to therapy with one of the newer agents. Although the pharmacologically related adverse effects of these drugs are essentially similar to those of the phenothiazines, patients allergic to the latter can usually tolerate one of the structurally different antipsychotic agents.

Butyrophenones. *Haloperidol* (Haldol) is the only drug of this chemical class available for use in this country for psychiatric therapy.* This drug resembles the piperazine-type phenothiazines in its actions, indications, and adverse effects. Thus, for example, it is less likely to cause excessive sedation and hypotension than phenothiazines such as chlorpromazine, but extrapyramidal motor stimulation side-effects are more common than with chlorpromazine and are similar in incidence to those of fluphenazine and trifluoperazine. Thus, although haloperidol may be the first-choice drug of some physicians, its main use is as an alternative to phenothiazines for patients hypersensitive to drugs of that class.

One rare clinical disorder for which haloperidol is reportedly more effective than the phenothiazines and various other chemical and pharmacologic drug classes is the *Gilles de la Tourette* syndrome. This is a neurologic disorder in which patients exhibit bizarre behavior as well as neuromuscular symptoms. The disorder begins during childhood with involuntary twitching and jerking of the limb muscles and grotesque facial tics and grimaces. The child then begins to make coughing, throat-clearing, and even barking sounds. Involuntary short, loud screams and shouts may be heard, as well as the most pathognomonic feature: *coprolalia*—the compulsive use of foul language.

---

* The use of another butyrophenone, *droperidol*, in anesthesia will be discussed in Chapter 52.

Pharmacotherapy and psychotherapy have not helped youngsters who have this affliction. Psychotherapy may make it easier for the children, who are usually of normal intelligence, to adjust to their disorder and to avoid the deterioration of personality that often develops, but it does not significantly improve the primary symptoms that are neurologic in origin. The doses of *diazepam* and of the piperazine phenothiazines required for even partial reduction of neuromuscular symptoms usually cause excessive side-effects. Haloperidol, however, has sometimes produced immediate marked improvement when taken in moderate doses that are relatively free of extrapyramidal motor side-effects. The dosage is adjusted to the minimal amount that is both safe and effective for the long-term maintenance therapy that is necessary, because spontaneous remission of the Gilles de la Tourette syndrome has rarely been reported. Haloperidol and other antipsychotic drugs are also sometimes used to control the chorea of patients with Huntington's disease.

Thioxanthenes. Two drugs of this chemical class are available. *Chlorprothixene* (Taractan) resembles chlorpromazine in its chemical structure, and its pharmacologic properties are similar to those of the aliphatic phenothiazine subgroup. *Thiothixene* (Navane) is structurally and pharmacologically similar to drugs of the piperazine-type phenothiazines such as trifluoperazine. Each of these drugs may be substituted for the type of phenothiazine that it resembles in the management of patients who cannot tolerate drugs of the more commonly employed class. Although relatively free of some of the side-effects commonly seen with the phenothiazines, the thioxanthenes do not seem to be more effective for the treatment of any type of psychiatric disorder.

Dibenzoxazepines. *Loxapine* (Loxitane), the only drug of this class currently available clinically in the United States, resembles the phenothiazines in its pharmacologic actions and indications. Thus, it is useful in the management of manifestations of schizophrenia but can cause adverse central, autonomic and other effects similar to those of the phenothiazines. Most common during the first days of treatment are mild drowsiness and sometimes severe extrapyramidal motor symptoms, including dyskinetic reactions that can lead to convulsions in epileptic patients, even when they are also taking anticonvulsant drug therapy.

Clozapine (Leponex), a drug of this chemical class that is available in Europe and is being investigated in the United States, seems much less likely to cause extrapyramidal system stimulation. This may be because this drug—like thioridazine among the phenothiazines—also has high cholinergic blocking activity at central synapses of the basal ganglia. That is, it possesses a "built-in" effect similar to that of the antiparkinsonism drugs that are used adjunctively to reduce the neurologic symptoms of antipsychotic drug therapy. Fatal agranulocytosis has occurred in a few patients on this drug, so studies are proceeding cautiously.

Dihydroindolones. *Molindone* (Moban) is an antischizophrenic drug with pharmacologic effects similar to those of the piperazine group of phenothiazines, haloperidol, and thiothixene. It offers an alternative to these other antipsychotic agents when these neuroleptics either fail to help patients or cause intolerable side-effects. So far, various of the hypersensitivity-type side-effects seen with the phenothiazines—for example, ocular opacities—have not been reported. However, as expected, this drug causes early drowsiness and extrapyramidal motor reactions, and thus its use requires precautions similar to those for the phenothiazines (see the summary at the end of this section).

Diphenylbutylpiperidines. No drugs of this class are currently available in the United States but two, *pimozide* (Orap) and *penfluridol* are used in Europe. The first of these is undergoing clinical trials in this country. It appears to be as effective as other antipsychotic drugs in treating chronic schizophrenia, and appears to produce fewer sedative and autonomic effects, although the incidence of extrapyramidal reactions is typical of the other drugs. This drug is expected to be given orphan drug status for Gilles de la Tourette syndrome.

The choice of an antipsychotic drug

Efficacy. No single antipsychotic drug seems to be superior to any other in its ability to bring about recovery from schizophrenic symptoms. Thus, for example, the piperazine-type phenothiazines—despite their much greater potency—have not been proved to be more effective than the prototype, chlorpromazine. Although the latter must be administered in much larger doses, it is as able to help resolve acute schizophrenic reactions and maintain a patient in remission as the drugs that do so in very low doses.

All drugs appear to be equally effective, regardless of the nature of the patient's symptoms. It was once thought, for example, that the more sedating aliphatic phenothiazines were preferable for patients with symptoms of psychomotor excitement, and the less sedating, or even stimulating, piperazine phenothiazines were thought to be better for patients who presented with symptoms of psychomotor retardation (see the summary at the end of this section). Now, however, it is believed that both types of drugs are equally effective in any type of schizophrenic patient who is likely to respond at all to antipsychotic pharmacotherapy.

Despite the above generalization, some individual patients who do poorly when treated with one type of drug may respond when changed to another of somewhat different chemical structure. Unfortunately, there is no way of knowing in advance which drug is likely to be most effective for a particular patient. So, although a patient is usually started on the antipsychotic drug with which the physician has had the most experience, the patient may have to be switched to a totally different drug, such as one of the newer nonphenothiazine derivatives, if there is no response during a trial of several weeks with large doses of the first choice drug. A previously favorable response of a patient or a family member to a given drug may indicate that a favorable response is more likely with this drug.

Adverse effects. The most important criterion for determining which drug to select for treatment of an individual patient is susceptibility to side-effects. Thus, for example, if a patient is discomforted by heavy sedation or suffers hypotensive reactions to aliphatic phenothiazines, one of the piperazine-type drugs such as fluphenazine may be preferred. That drug, or its chemical congener trifluoperazine, may also be best for ambulatory outpatients because of the low incidence of sedative and autonomic blocking effects. On the other hand, patients who are prone to develop disabling extrapyramidal motor effects with the latter drugs may be better maintained with a piperidine derivative such as thioridazine.

Patients who have a history of hypersensitivity reactions when previously treated with phenothiazines may profit from treatment with haloperidol or with a more recently introduced drug such as loxapine or molindone. An advantage claimed for drugs of these classes is that they have not caused such adverse effects as skin pigmentation, deposition of particles in the lens and cornea of the eyes, and other reactions sometimes seen in patients taking phenothiazines in high doses for long periods. However, patients transferred to one of the newer drugs should be observed for similar changes, which are always possible.

Additional clinical considerations

Before using an antipsychotic agent, it is important to assess the patient for the presence of any underlying medical conditions that would be contraindications to, or cautions for, the use of these drugs. Such conditions include the following: coma or severely depressed central nervous system (CNS); bone marrow depression; hepatic failure; chronic obstructive pulmonary disease; Parkinson's disease; cardiovascular disease; severe hypotension or shock; glaucoma; epilepsy; peptic ulcer. The safety of antipsychotics during pregnancy and lactation has not been es-tablished. These drugs should be used during pregnancy only if the benefits outweigh the potential risks to the fetus. If a nursing mother requires the use of one of these drugs, a different method of feeding the baby should be established.

Several adverse effects can be seen with these drugs. The patient who is going to be maintained on these drugs for any prolonged length of time should be made aware of these adverse effects, and should be evaluated for their occurrence. These undesirable reactions include pseudoparkinsonism, drowsiness (usually passes after 1–2 weeks); changes in vision, hyperpyrexia, lactation and breast engorgement, dry mouth, constipation, and sensitivity to sunlight. The patient should be helped to cope with these uncomfortable side-effects. The possibility that the patient will develop tardive dyskinesia should be kept in mind by anyone caring for a patient who has been on these drugs for months or years. Early diagnosis of this condition and gradual dosage reduction, as discussed earlier in the chapter, may prevent the full-fledged development of this sometimes irreversible syndrome. The patient teaching guide summarizes the key points that should be included in teaching a patient who is receiving phenothiazine-type antipsychotic drugs.

Drug–drug interactions. Additive depressant effects are seen if these drugs are combined with other CNS depressants, such as *barbiturates, narcotic analgesics, anesthetics,* or *alcohol.* Increased anticholinergic effects are seen if combined with *anticholinergics. Phenothiazine* absorption is decreased with *antidiarrheal drugs* and *antacids.* Antipsychotic agents given with *guanethidine* block the antihypertensive effect of the drug. Phenothiazines and *propranolol* given concomitantly result in increased levels of both drugs. *Lithium* can interact with several of these drugs in various ways. Phenothiazines can increase serum *phenytoin* levels, leading to toxicity. *Caffeine* can counteract the antipsychotic effects of these drugs by some sort of reversal or physical incompatibility in the gastrointestinal tract.

The guide to the nursing process summarizes the clinical considerations that should be incorporated into the nursing care of a patient receiving phenothiazines.

(Text continues p. 978)

Patient teaching guide: phenothiazines

The drug that has been prescribed for you belongs to a family of drugs called the phenothiazines. These drugs are given to treat various mental and emotional conditions. The drug should be taken exactly as prescribed. Because this drug affects many body systems, it is important that you have regular medical evaluation.

Instructions:

1. The name of the drug prescribed for you is _____ .

2. The dosage of your drug is _____ .

(continued)

3. The drug should be taken _____ times a day. The best time to take your drug is at bedtime. The drug should best be taken with water.

4. Some side-effects of the drug that you should be aware of include the following:

Dizziness, fainting	If this occurs, change positions very slowly. This sensation often passes after 1 or 2 weeks.
Drowsiness	Use extreme care if this occurs. Avoid driving a car, operating heavy machinery, or performing delicate tasks.
Sensitivity to sunlight	The sunlight may hurt your eyes and injure your skin with less exposure than before. Protect your skin and wear sunglasses if you must be in the sun.
Pink or reddish urine	Do not be alarmed by this change; it does not mean that your urine contains blood. The drug causes some people's urine to change color.
Sensitivity to heat	Some people become very sensitive to heat and may suffer "heat stroke" while on these drugs. Monitor your temperature and be very careful in hot weather.
Constipation	Consult with your nurse or physician for appropriate therapy.

5. Avoid the use of alcohol or other depressants while on this drug. It is also best to limit your use of caffeine.

6. Avoid the use of over-the-counter medications while on this drug. If you feel that you require one of these drugs, consult with your nurse or physician.

7. Keep this and all medications out of the reach of children.

8. Tell any nurse, physician, or dentist who is taking care of you that you are on this drug.

9. Take this drug exactly as prescribed. If you run out of medicine, or find that you cannot take it for any reason, notify your nurse or physician.

Notify your nurse or physician if any of the following occur:

Sore throat, fever, rash
Tremors
Weakness
Visual changes
Unusual bleeding or bruising

Guide to the nursing process: phenothiazines

Assessment	Nursing diagnoses	Interventions	Evaluation
Past history (*contraindications*): Coma Bone marrow depression Hepatic failure Chronic obstructive pulmonary disease Parkinson's disease Cardiovascular disease Hypotension Glaucoma Epilepsy Peptic ulcer Pregnancy Lactation Allergies: *these drugs; tartrazine*—some preparations Medication history (*cautions*): Barbiturates Alcohol Narcotics Anesthetics Anticholinergics Antacids Antidiarrheal drugs Guanethidine Lithium Propranolol Phenytoin Caffeine	Potential for injury secondary to adverse effects Knowledge deficit regarding drug therapy Potential sensory-perceptual alteration Potential alteration in thought processes	Safe and appropriate administration of drug Safety and comfort measures provided: • Position changes—very slow • Avoidance of driving, hazardous activities • Protection from sun • Protection from hot weather • Comfort measures for atropinelike effects Patient teaching regarding drug therapy Support and encouragement to cope with diagnosis and drug therapy Life support measures in case of overdose	Monitor for desired therapeutic effect Monitor for adverse effects: • Tardive dyskinesia • Pseudoparkinsonism • ↑ skin pigmentation • Cardiovascular effects • Liver changes • Endocrine changes • Bronchospasm • Bone marrow depression Evaluate effectiveness of safety and comfort measures Evaluate effectiveness of patient teaching program Evaluate effectiveness of support and encouragement offered Monitor for drug–drug interactions: several possible Evaluate effectiveness of life support measures, if appropriate

Physical assessment
Neurologic: orientation, affect, reflexes, tone, coordination
Cardiovascular: BP, P, rhythm, perfusion
Respiratory: R, adventitious sounds
GI: abdominal, liver exam
Other: CBC, eye grounds

Summary of the pharmacologic effects of the phenothiazine-type antipsychotic drugs

1. Sedation (tranquilizing or calming effect): brings about a reduction in mild to moderate anxiety or in severe agitation
2. Antipsychotic: at first, reduces the patient's reaction to such symptoms of psychosis as hallucinations and delusions, and later helps to improve the patient's disturbed behavior
3. Potentiation of the effects of narcotic analgesics and of general depressant drugs
4. Antiemetic: control of nausea and vomiting
5. Autonomic blockade (see summary of adverse effects, below)

Summary of clinical indications for the phenothiazine-type antipsychotic drugs

Psychiatric indications

Schizophrenia: acute and chronic
Manic phase of the manic–depressive psychoses
Senile confusional states and psychoses
Childhood psychoses and mental retardation
Other chronic brain syndromes brought about by organic damage
Toxic psychoses caused by LSD, amphetamines, and acute alcoholic intoxication
Alcoholic withdrawal syndromes, including alcoholic hallucinosis, impending delirium tremens, and—in combination with general depressants—full-blown delirium tremens
Postwithdrawal long-term management of anxious–depressed alcoholics
Psychoneurosis (adjunct to psychotherapy)
Psychosomatic disorders (adjunct to specific drugs)

Psychiatric target symptoms
Psychomotor excitement
Agitation, mania, tension, anxiety, nervousness, restlessness, and confusion; hyperactive, aggressive, assaultive, destructive behavior.
Psychomotor retardation
Apathy, withdrawal, seclusiveness, mutism, autism, catatonic posturing, listlessness, lethargy of schizophrenic (not depressive) origin.
Other symptoms of psychosis:
Hallucinations, delusions, and other disturbances in thinking.

Some medical, surgical, and obstetric indications
Preanesthetic sedation
Postoperative vomiting control
In labor to reduce dosage of analgesics
In management of cancer patients to prevent vomiting induced by antineoplastic agents
Intractable hiccup

Summary of adverse effects of the phenothiazine-type antipsychotic drugs

Central nervous system side-effects

1. Drowsiness, lethargy, feelings of fatigue and weakness
2. Extrapyramidal motor system reactions:
   a. Pseudoparkinsonism: akinesia, masklike facies, shuffling gait, tremors, rigidity
   b. Akathisia: motor restlessness marked by feelings of inner tension or an inability to sit still or sleep
   c. Acute dyskinesia or dystonia: contractions of small muscle groups resembling tics and of large muscle groups resembling convulsions
   d. After use for months or years, persistent (tardive) dyskinesia: continued movements of the lips, tongue, and jaws may make speech and swallowing difficult; muscles of upper and lower extremities may twitch and jerk continuously

Cardiovascular and other autonomic reactions

1. Postural (orthostatic) hypotension: dizziness, weakness, fainting can be minimized by keeping the patient lying with head low and legs raised; development of shocklike state may require administration of vasopressor drugs, but *not* epinephrine

because of presence of α-adrenergic blockade.

2. Cardiac palpitations, changes in the electrocardiogram; possible sudden death caused by cardiac arrest
3. Anticholinergic (atropinelike) effects; dry mouth; blurring of vision; constipation, or possibly obstipation and paralytic ileus; urinary retention; failure of sweating followed by high fever
4. α-adrenergic receptor blockade: hypotension; nasal stuffiness; inhibition of ejaculation

Endocrine disorders

1. Menstrual irregularities, including amenorrhea and false positive pregnancy tests
2. Gynecomastia (breast engorgement) and lactation
3. Reduction in libido (sex drive)
4. Weight gain with increased appetite and edema
5. Hyperglycemia and glycosuria (also hypoglycemia)

Hypersensitivity-type reactions

1. Hematologic: blood dyscrasias reported include leukopenia and agranulocytosis;

hemolytic anemia; thrombocytic purpura; and pancytopenia

2. Hepatic: cholestatic jaundice in which laboratory tests of liver function give results resembling those of extrahepatic obstruction
3. Dermatologic: urticaria, contact dermatitis, photosensitivity, erythema, exfoliative dermatitis

Miscellaneous effects

1. Melanosis: skin pigmentation ranging from mild darkening to deep skin discolorations (slate gray to violet)
2. Ocular changes: deposits in conjunctiva, lens, and cornea may form star-shaped opacities; rarely, pigmentary retinopathy may impair vision
3. Abrupt withdrawal may be followed by nausea, vomiting, dizziness, and tremulousness.
4. Pregnant patients should receive this drug only when essential, because newborn babies have had hyperreflexia, extrapyramidal signs, and jaundice; offspring of drug-treated animals have shown signs of toxicity, including nervous system damage.

Drug digests

Chlorpromazine HCl USP (Thorazine)

Actions and indications. This prototype phenothiazine of the aliphatic type has many actions that make it useful not only in psychiatry but also in general medicine, surgery, and obstetrics. In managing labor, for example, its potentiating effect on analgesics, hypnotics and anesthetics permits the use of 25% to 50% of the usual doses of those drugs, with reduced risk of respiratory depression for mother and infant. Its antiemetic action helps to control nausea and vomiting following surgical anesthesia, in cancer patients receiving antineoplastic agents, and in many other conditions.

The drug controls moderate to severe anxiety in psychoneurosis, and it reduces severe agitation and other symptoms of psychosis in schizophrenia, in the manic phase of the manic–depressive psychosis, and in confused senile patients. In alcoholic withdrawal syndromes, including delirium tremens, it is best given combined with sedatives, hypnotics, or minor tranquilizers.

Adverse effects, cautions, and contraindications. Drowsiness and postural hypotension, marked by dizziness and faintness, are the most common early side-effects, particularly when the drug is injected. Both types of symptoms tend to disappear as tolerance develops in a week or two. Drowsiness may be diminished by administering small doses of dextroamphetamine; hypotension is counteracted—if severe—by administering vasopressor drugs. Extrapyramidal reactions resembling parkinsonism occur more frequently than do dystonic reactions. Akathisia, or motor restlessness, may also appear. These neuromuscular signs are ordinarily transient and readily reversible. However, long-lasting dyskinesia of the lips, tongue, jaws, and other areas sometimes persists indefinitely following high dosage with this and other phenothiazines, particularly in elderly patients with a history of organic brain damage.

Hypersensitivity-type reactions, including hematologic and hepatic disorders, are rare

but potentially serious. The blood dyscrasias include agranulocytosis, hemolytic anemia, and pancytopenia. Jaundice may develop as a result of obstruction of bile channels. It ordinarily fades after the drug is withdrawn but can occasionally become chronic. Caution is required in administering the drug to patients with a history of liver disease, and its use is not recommended in patients who have previously shown sensitivity to phenothiazines.

Dosage and administration. Doses differ very widely, depending on the purpose for which the drug is employed. They may range from 10 mg tid by mouth to 1000 mg or more administered IM. In general, dosage is begun with small amounts and increased gradually until psychiatric symptoms are controlled; dosage is then gradually reduced to a maintenance level that still offers effective control. Suppositories (25 mg or 100 mg) are available for control of vomiting in children and others.

Fluphenazine HCl (Permitil; Prolixin)

Actions and indications. This piperazine-type phenothiazine derivative has a highly potent and prolonged psychotropic action.

Low oral doses are used to control anxiety and tension states in psychoneurotic patients and in those with such somatic disorders as

tension headache, hypertension, premenstrual tension, gastrointestinal hypermotility and hypersecretion, and vomiting. Administered parenterally, the drug quickly controls agitated behavior in acute and chronic schizophrenia, the manic phase of the manic-depressive psychosis, senile psychoses, hyperactive children and patients suffering from organic brain damage or from mental deficiency. Long-term oral administration then often brings about behavioral changes as a result of a reduction in hallucinations and delusions.

Adverse effects, cautions, and contraindications. This drug has the potential for producing the various adverse effects reported for other phenothiazines. However, hypotensive reactions are relatively rare, drows-iness and lethargy are uncommon, and potentiation of alcohol and other depressant drugs is less likely than with other compounds of this chemical class. Extrapyramidal reactions are common and can be alarming. Sudden onset of hyperreflexia, dystonic contractions of large muscle groups, must be recognized as drug-induced rather than a manifestation of neurologic disease. Dyskinetic reactions of this type, including even opisthotonus and oculogyric crisis, can ordinarily be quickly controlled by administration of antiparkinsonism drugs (*e.g.*, benztropine). Long-term administration of large doses may produce a dyskinetic syndrome that persists after the drug is discontinued. Caution is required in patients with a history of convulsive disorders.

Dosage and administration. The usual daily dosage for adults ranges between 0.5 mg and 3 mg, administered as a single oral dose. However, psychotic patients often require 10 mg or more daily by intramuscular administration. Initial doses should be low, 1.25 mg, for example, and should be raised as needed to control symptoms. Once control is achieved, dosage is reduced to from 5 to 1 mg daily, administered by mouth.

Fluphenazine enanthate and fluphenazine decanoate

Long-acting parenteral forms of this phenothiazine are administered intramuscularly or subcutaneously in doses of about 12.5 to 50 mg every two to four weeks.

Thioridazine HCl USP (Mellaril)

Actions and indications. This piperidine-type phenothiazine is effective in psychiatric conditions marked by anxiety, tension, excitement, agitation, and manic states. After such symptoms are controlled, schizophrenic patients may have fewer hallucinations and show less delusional and other thought disturbances. The drug is also useful for control of agitation in senile patients and of hyperactivity in mentally retarded children. Small daily doses are employed for control of moderate anxiety in psychoneurotic and alcoholic patients and for severe anxiety in patients with mental depression manifested by agitation.

Adverse effects, cautions, and contraindications. Drowsiness is common early in treatment of patients receiving large doses, but lethargy lessens with continued treatment as tolerance develops. Patients are warned not to drive when they are not com-pletely alert mentally. They should not drink alcohol or take other depressant drugs together with this one. Cardiovascular side-effects include orthostatic hypotension and occasional electrocardiographic changes that have on rare occasions preceded sudden death, presumably from cardiac arrest. The drug is contraindicated in patients with severe heart disease and either hyper- or hypotension.

Extrapyramidal reactions are relatively rare, and are more likely to be of the pseudo-parkinsonism-akinesia type than of the dyskinetic and akathisia type. This drug has relatively little antiemetic activity, which may be an advantage, because it is less likely than other phenothiazines to mask this sign of possible brain tumor, GI tract obstruction, or drug overdosage. The drug may itself cause constipation and ileus, as well as such other signs of autonomic blockade as urinary retention, inhibition of ejaculation, nasal stuffiness, dry mouth, and blurred vision. High doses have caused reduced vision as a result of the deposit of pigment in the retina. Pigmentation has also been noted in the conjunctiva, sclera and cornea, and opacities have occasionally developed in the lens.

Dosage and administrations. The total daily dose for patients with moderate anxiety ranges from 20 to 200 mg. In the psychoses, this drug is commonly administered in doses ranging from 200 mg to 800 mg. For both types of patients, the initial relatively low doses are raised gradually to the point of optimal response. Thus the usual starting dose for psychoneurotic and similarly anxious patients is 25 mg tid; for psychotics, it is 50 to 100 mg tid. Doses for disturbed children also depend on the degree of severity of the condition as well as on the child's weight and age.

Drugs for treating affective disorders

The nature of affective disorders

The psychiatric term "affect" refers to the feelings—pleasant and unpleasant—that people experience when they respond emotionally to what they perceive taking place around them. Such feelings may be mild or strong but, taken all together, they help to determine their emotional and mental state at any moment and how they think and behave.

A person who is in one type of affective state for a few hours or several days is said to be in a "good mood" or a "bad mood." Normally, no mood lasts very long, and people rarely become ecstatically happy or extremely sad. Of course, everyone feels sad at times without necessarily being depressed, in the sense of suffering from a symptom of mental illness. Indeed, it would be most remarkable if people did *not* feel sad after the loss of loved ones and after other traumatic events that inevitably occur during the course of life.

However, in the *pathologic* mood states that are called affective disorders, the patient's highs or lows go far beyond what is customary in daily life situations. In manic–depressive illness, for instance, the patient's mood swings are much more intense and long-lasting than is considered normal. In addition, there is usually no apparent reason for such extreme reactions. In other types of depression, even if the event that precipitated the patient's reaction is known, the sadness and the behavior that stems from it seem to be quite out of proportion to the severity of the stressful incident that had occurred.

Depression

This affective disorder afflicts very many people in our society. An estimated eight million Americans each year require psychiatric treatment for moderately severe depression. Many millions of other people never get the treatment they need because their depression takes the form of physical signs and symptoms, alcoholism, or overeating to the point of gross obesity. Depression has been called "the most widespread, the most persistent, and the most frequently unrecognized emotional disorder that afflicts mankind—a condition that has caused more suffering than any other single disease."

Actually, despite the frequency with which it masquerades as something else, depression is relatively easy to diagnose. Among the depressive symptoms that most commonly indicate a condition needing treatment are feelings of fatigue, lack of interest in personal appearance, loss of appetite, and sleeplessness. The patient may suffer a loss of self-esteem and say such things as "I am nothing" or "I am worthless." Typically, he may become apathetic and lose interest in people or affairs that had formerly engaged his attention. The patient may, for example, withdraw from participation in activities and decisions both at work and at home, perhaps saying "Nothing seems worthwhile; nothing seems worth doing." Behavior cannot, however, be neatly categorized. Some patients may show mainly psychomotor retardation, a marked slowing down of all their activities; others may be in a state of psychomotor agitation, during which they move about constantly, complaining and voicing fears of impending disaster. (See the summary of signs and symptoms of depressive syndromes at the end of this chapter.)

Depression is probably not one disorder but several, each with different underlying causes. Psychiatrists use different terms to describe the various subtypes of depression. Some divide patients in terms of the target symptoms mentioned above—that is, as "retarded" or "nonretarded," or as "agitated." Others classify patients in terms of their degree of contact with reality as "psychotic" or "nonpsychotic," or as "neurotic." Perhaps the most common currently employed dichotomy is that between "endogenous" and "reactive," or "exogenous," depressions. As will be described later in more detail, making such distinctions in differential diagnosis has some relevance in selecting the most appropriate type of therapy.

Pathogenesis of depression:
The biogenic amine hypothesis

Largely on the basis of research with the drugs that are effective in managing depression, several slightly different hypotheses have been presented to describe a potential underlying biochemical abnormality in the brains of depressed patients. Almost all the drugs that produce significant therapeutic benefit alter the function of norepinephrine or serotonin, two chemicals known to be brain neurotransmitters. Psychomotor stimulants, such as amphetamine, release norepinephrine; monoamine oxidase (MAO) inhibitors interfere with the enzymatic breakdown of norepinephrine and serotonin; and different tricyclic antidepressants block the neuronal reuptake of norepinephrine or serotonin, or of both. The result of all these drug effects is an increase in the amount of one or both of these biogenic amine neurotransmitters present in syn-

apses. Furthermore, drugs such as reserpine, that deplete brain norepinephrine and serotonin, have been observed to cause a syndrome in humans and experimental animals that resembles depression.

Results such as these have led to the hypothesis that one or both of these neurotransmitters are deficient in the brains of depressed patients. Many studies have attempted to correlate urinary and cerebrospinal fluid levels of these neurotransmitters or their metabolites with the clinical status of patients. Attempts to show biochemical alterations that correlate with the onset of depression and with either spontaneous or therapeutically-induced recovery have not been as successful as many investigators had hoped. Biochemical analyses of the brains of suicide victims have similarly failed to pinpoint a biogenic amine (or any other) deficit. Furthermore, the time course of many of the drug-induced changes in neurotransmitter function does not correlate well with the time course of the clinical response of depressed patients to drug therapy: most of the biochemical changes occur quickly (within hours) after drug treatment has begun, whereas clinical response often requires weeks of therapy.

Nevertheless, the fact that the clinically effective drugs have in common an effect on these neurotransmitters continues to keep the biogenic amine hypothesis alive, and to stimulate research into the causes and cures of depression. In addition, making the association between increased levels of functional norepinephrine and antidepressant drugs can help you to learn and remember some of the more common adverse effects and drug interactions of antidepressant drugs.

Types of depression treatment

Broadly speaking, physicians can draw on three main types of therapy:

1. Psychotherapy
2. Electroconvulsive therapy (ECT)
3. Pharmacotherapy, which is the main concern of this book

There are several primary categories of drugs employed in the management of depression:

1. *Antidepressants* of two types: the so-called tricyclic drugs and those known as MAO inhibitors
2. *Antipsychotic* agents such as the phenothiazine-type major tranquilizers discussed earlier in this chapter
3. *Antianxiety* agents such as the benzodiazepines discussed in Chapter 45— for example, chlordiazepoxide (Librium)
4. *Psychomotor stimulants,* such as the amphetamines that are taken up in detail in Chapter 47

5. *Lithium carbonate,* a drug used mainly in manic states, but that is also apparently effective for preventing recurrences of some types of depressions

This chapter will next discuss in detail the three most important types of antiaffective drugs: the tricyclics, the MAO inhibitors, and lithium. Then it will indicate the current status of the use of these types of psychotherapeutic agents in relation to the several other classes of drugs and to the two other therapeutic modalities, psychotherapy and ECT.

Tricyclic antidepressants and trazodone

Mechanism of action. Drugs of this class are the most commonly employed antidepressants (Table 46-2). They are similar in chemical structure to the phenothiazine-type tranquilizers; one drug, *maprotiline,* actually has a four-ringed, or tetracyclic, structure (Fig. 46-3). It is pharmacologically similar to the tricyclics and therefore will be described here. Most of these drugs exert a sedative effect during the first days of their use in depressed patients. However, after several weeks of treatment, most patients respond in a manner different from that to the antipsychotic drugs. That is, about 60% to 70% of patients show a definite reduction in both main types of target symptoms after 2 to 4 weeks of treatment with tricyclic antidepressant drugs.

The exact mechanism by which these drugs bring about their effects is still uncertain. One view is that they act to overcome an imbalance in the brain among the several neurochemical substances that are thought to influence the state of people's moods. More specifically, the tricyclic compounds are believed to increase the amount of the neurotransmitter substances *norepinephrine* and *serotonin* (Chap. 13) that are available for sending signals from one neuron to another in certain parts of the CNS. These drugs act to keep molecules of one or the other neurotransmitter in central synapses for longer periods by interfering with the normal reuptake mechanisms that remove the released molecules of neurotransmitter from the synaptic cleft. However, as stated earlier, in most experiments this biochemical effect can be demonstrated considerably sooner after the onset of drug administration than the therapeutic effects that occur clinically.

Clinical indications. These drugs have proved to be effective in treating patients in all diagnostic categories of depression. That is, they offer relief of psychomotor retardation in patients with major psychotic depressions of both the endogenous and reactive types, and they are also often effective in anxious agitated patients with the types of somewhat less severe reactive depressions that are sometimes called psychoneurotic. (See the discussion below concerning the status of the use of these drugs and other treatment measures in the management of various categories of depression.)

One drug of this class, the prototype agent *imipramine*[+] (Tofranil), has another FDA-approved clinical indication. It is used to help prevent bed-wetting (enuresis) in children over 6 years old. It should be used only after possible organic causes have been ruled out, particularly in children who have such symptoms as urgency and frequency during the daytime. In about 25% of all cases, the use of this drug as an adjunct to various nondrug measures for bladder training is said to have helped enuretic children stay dry even after imipramine was gradually withdrawn.

Individual drugs. The two first tricyclic agents to be introduced, *imipramine* and *amitriptyline*[+] (Elavil) are still the most commonly employed. Many tricyclic drugs have been introduced since then, most with the claim of some advantage over the older drugs. Among such claims are that they produce less sedation; that they produce more sedation, which may be an advantage in *agitated* depressed patients or in those with sleep disturbances; that they have a more rapid onset of action; and that they are less anticholinergic and cause fewer atropinelike side-effects. Few of these claims are supported by convincing evidence. However, there *are* differences among these drugs: they *do* differ in their sedative properties. *Desipramine HCl* (Norpramine; Pertofrane) and *protriptyline HCl* (Vivactil) are less sedating and may be advantageous in overcoming the feelings of fatigue and indifference seen in patients whose depression takes the form of psychomotor retardation. *Trimipramine maleate* (Surmontil), *amitriptyline HCl* (Elavil), *doxepin HCl* (Adapin; Sinequan), *amoxapine* (Asendin), and the tetracyclic drug *maprotiline HCl* (Ludiomil), are *more* sedating.

Furthermore, maprotiline and *trazodone HCl* (Desyrel), a new drug that is chemically and pharmacologically different from any other antidepressant drug, but may act by blocking serotonin reuptake, cause fewer anticholinergic side-effects, and trazodone is less likely than the tricyclics to cause cardiotoxicity (see below). *Nomifensine maleate* (Merital), an investigational antidepressant that is chemically unrelated to the tricyclic antidepressants or to trazodone, also appears to cause fewer anticholinergic side-effects and less cardiotoxicity than the tricyclics. In addition, it is less epileptogenic. Like some of the tricyclics, it blocks norepinephrine reuptake. This drug is available in Europe. *Amoxapine,* a tricyclic that is also related chemically to the antipsychotic drug loxapine, has caused some of the extrapyramidal reactions (akathisia, dystonia, parkinsonism) that are typical of the antipsychotic drugs.

Adverse effects. Although therapeutic doses of these drugs seldom cause the severe toxicity sometimes seen with agents of the MAO inhibitor type, they can produce a wide variety of discomforting side-effects in about one out of four patients taking them (see the summary at the end of this section). These discomforting effects are mainly the result of autonomic blockade and CNS stimulation.

Table 46-2. Antidepressant drugs

Official or generic name	Trade name	Usual adult daily oral dosage*	Comments
Tricyclic drugs			
Amitriptyline HCl USP	Elavil	75 mg (100–300 mg)	See Drug digest
Amoxapine	Asendin	200 mg (150–300 mg)	Chemical relative of the antipsychotic drug loxapine
Desipramine HCl USP	Norpramine; Pertofrane	150 mg (25–300 mg)	Relatively rapid onset of action (3–5 days)
Doxepin HCl	Adapin; Sinequan	75 mg (25–300 mg)	Has marked antianxiety as well as antidepressant activity
Imipramine HCl USP	Tofranil	150 mg (100–300 mg)	See Drug digest
Imipramine pamoate	Tofranil-PM	75–150 mg	May be used on a divided dosage schedule or on a once-daily at bedtime basis
Nortriptyline HCl USP	Aventyl	150 mg (25–100 mg)	Claimed useful also for gastrointestinal psychophysiologic disorders and for childhood enuresis
Protriptyline HCl	Vivactil	30 mg (5–60 mg)	Claimed more potent and rapid in onset; its activating effect may cause increased anxiety in some patients
Trimipramine maleate	Surmontil	100 mg (100–300 mg)	More sedating than some tricyclics
Tetracyclic drug			
Maprotiline HCl	Ludiomil	150 mg (75–300 mg)	Long-acting; may cause fewer anticholinergic side-effects
Monoamine oxidase inhibitors			
Isocarboxazid USP	Marplan	30 mg (10–60 mg)	See Drug digest
Phenelzine sulfate USP	Nardil	30 mg (15–90 mg)	A potent antidepressant that can cause all the potential adverse effects of drugs of this class, requiring all the usual precautions
Tranylcypromine sulfate USP	Parnate	20 mg (10–60 mg)	See Drug digest
Miscellaneous agent			
Trazodone HCl	Desyrel	400 mg (150–600 mg)	A pharmacologically distinct drug; may act by blocking serotonin reuptake; does not cause anticholinergic side-effects
Lithium preparations			
Lithium carbonate	Eskalith; Lithane		Used as treatment and prophylaxis of manic–depressive disorders; dosage needs to be adjusted for the individual patient on the basis of serum lithium levels (1.0–1.5 mEq/liter) and clinical response; margin of safety is very low
Lithium citrate	Cibalith-S		

* Dosage range from lowest initial and maintenance dosage to highest doses for hospitalized patients is given in parentheses.

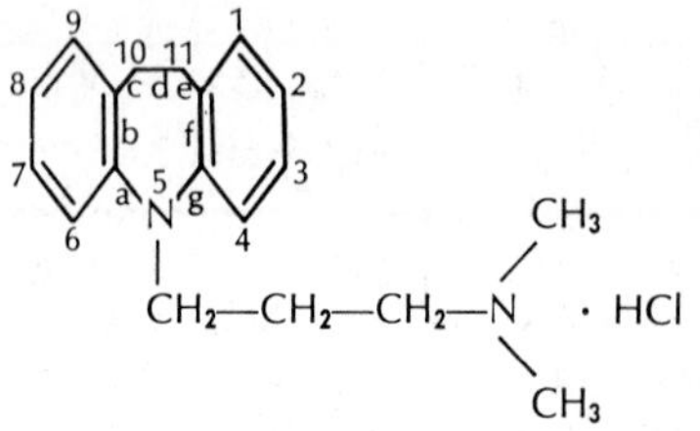

Imipramine

Desipramine (DMI, and others) is identical except that the side

N
|
chain is CH—CH—CH—NHCH (one of the methyl groups has been dropped and replaced by a hydrogen attached to N)

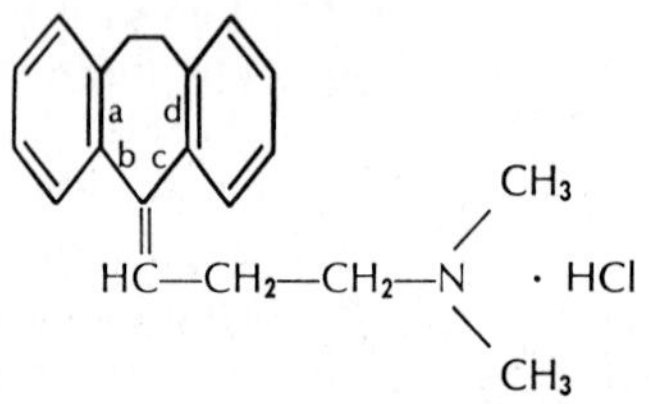

Amitriptyline

Nortriptyline (Aventyl) is identical except that the side chain is —CHCH—CH—NHCH (one of the methyl groups has been replaced by a hydrogen).

Figure 46-3. Chemical structure of tricyclic-type antidepressants. Note the structural resemblance of these useful psychotropic drugs to the phenothiazine structure (Fig. 46-1).

The autonomic side-effects are mainly of the anticholinergic or atropinelike type and include mouth dryness, blurring of vision, constipation, and delayed urination. This means that imipramine, amitriptyline, and their derivatives must be administered cautiously if at all to patients with a history of glaucoma and to elderly male patients with prostatic enlargement. These drugs can also cause tachycardia, and, paradoxically, excessive sweating. Hypotension, jaundice, and blood dyscrasias are rare. However, laboratory tests of the patient's liver function and blood picture may be ordered periodically during long-term maintenance therapy.

The CNS side-effects may take the form of either drowsiness or restlessness along with confusion, dizziness, and headaches. Depressed schizophrenic patients especially are likely to become unduly agitated when being treated with these psychostimulants, and may require phenothiazine tranquilizers or sedation with other agents. The imipramine-type agents are most likely to cause insomnia and nervousness, or mild muscle tremors and twitching. Caution is required in epileptic patients because of hyperreflexia induced by these drugs.

Treatment of toxicity. Depressed patients sometimes attempt suicide by taking large amounts of pre-

scribed tricyclic antidepressant medications. Children also occasionally ingest these drugs accidentally. The consequences of overdosage with these drugs can be quite serious and potentially fatal. Most dangerous are the rapid development of CNS and cardiovascular toxicity.

The central effects are an extension of the adverse effects that can, as described above, occur with therapeutic doses. Patients may pass swiftly from a drowsy state to stupor and light coma. This depressed state is interrupted periodically by muscle tremors and rigidity, by hyperreflexia, and by clonic convulsive spasms.

The most serious of the cardiovascular effects of overdosage is the development of irregularities in cardiac rate and rhythm. These include various combinations of tachycardias and conduction disturbances. Rapid cardiac arrhythmias may be mixed with electrocardiographic signs of atrioventricular (A-V) block and intraventricular conduction defects. Death may occur suddenly from cardiac arrest of the ventricular fibrillation type (Chap. 26, 30, and 31).

Treatment is aimed at controlling such symptoms as convulsions, while supporting the patient's cardiovascular and respiratory functions. Dampening of CNS excitability requires cautious parenteral administration of central depressant drugs. Diazepam[+] (Valium; see Drug digest, Chap. 45) is preferred for this purpose, because it is less likely than barbiturates to cause excessive respiratory depression. It may, in any case, become necessary to support the patient's respiration by artificial means such as inhalation of oxygen by way of a cuffed endotracheal tube or by mechanical ventilation of the lungs.

The patient's electrocardiogram (ECG) should be monitored and a transvenous pacemaker inserted for possible use if treatment with antiarrhythmic drugs fails to control serious cardiac irregularities. Lidocaine[+] (Xylocaine; see Drug digest, Chap. 30), propranolol[+] (Inderal; see Drug digest, Chap. 18) and phenytoin are sometimes administered intravenously under ECG monitoring to control ventricular and atrial tachyarrhythmias (Chap. 30). Physostigmine (Chap. 15), a drug that passes the blood–brain barrier, has been reported to reverse not only the peripheral atropinelike adverse effects, but most of the cardiovascular and CNS effects, including hyperpyrexia. However, the external application of cold packs is a safer means of reducing the extremely high body temperature that occasionally develops. IV fluids are safer than adrenergic vasopressor drugs for counteracting severe hypotension and preventing shock. However, care is required to avoid overloading the patient's circulation because of the danger of cardiac failure.

Obviously, prevention of tricyclic drug toxicity is preferable to attempting treatment of this difficult to manage emergency. Only relatively small amounts of antidepressant drugs should be prescribed if there is any possibility that the patient may use them for attempting suicide.

Monoamine-oxidase-type antidepressants

Mechanism of action. Drugs of this class were the first pharmacologic agents to prove effective for treating severe psychotic and psychoneurotic depressions (Table 46-2). Today, however, they are largely reserved for treating depressed patients who have failed to respond to one or more courses of the tricyclic-type antidepressants, which are less toxic and less likely to lead to dangerous drug interactions (see below). Another reason for initiating treatment with the tricyclics instead of the MAO inhibitors is that the latter can cause a biochemical imbalance that persists long after these enzyme-inhibiting drugs have been eliminated from the body. Thus, if the MAO inhibitor-type agents were tried first without success, the patient would have to wait at least 10 to 14 days before being safely switched to a tricyclic-type drug.

Inhibition of MAO is believed to be the basis for the gradual development of the antidepressant effect of these drugs. Because MAO is the enzyme mainly responsible for the intraneuronal inactivation of norepinephrine, drugs that interfere with MAO activity may lead to an increased level of that neurotransmitter in the brain, heart, and other organs. According to one view (described above), this accumulation of norepinephrine and of other biogenic amines, such as serotonin, in certain brain areas may account for the antidepressant effects of the MAO inhibitor drugs.

Clinical indications. These drugs are indicated for symptomatic relief of depressed patients who have proved difficult to treat with other drugs, psychotherapy, and sometimes even ECT. Among the patients who are said to benefit most often from treatment with an MAO inhibitor are those who are classified as suffering from severe depression of the endogenous and the neurotic, or reactive, types. Some schizophrenic patients with depressive symptoms are also said to do better on combinations of an MAO inhibitor with an antipsychotic phenothiazine-type tranquilizer than they do when treated with the tricyclic compounds.

One drug of the MAO inhibitor class, pargyline HCl (Eutonyl), is not employed for treating depression but is, instead, occasionally ordered for treating patients suffering from a moderately severe degree of hypertension (Chap. 28). Some of these drugs have been tried in the treatment of the relatively rare sleep disorder, *narcolepsy,* for reasons that are discussed in Chapter 47.

Individual drugs. The prototype drug of this class, iproniazid (Marsilid), was originally introduced for treating tuberculosis. Psychiatrists who noted its tendency to make many tubercular patients euphoric decided to try it in emotionally depressed patients. The drug proved dramatically effective for reducing signs of psychomotor regression and for providing relief of other symptoms of depression. Unfortunately, iproniazid, a hydrazine derivative, had to be withdrawn when it was found to cause hepatitis leading to severe liver damage in some patients.

Several of its successors were also withdrawn because of their toxicity, and there are at present only three drugs of this class available in this country (Table 46-2).

All seem to be equally effective and all, including the *non*hydrazine derivative *tranylcypromine sulfate*[+] (Parnate) cause similar side-effects (see the summary of adverse effects at the end of this chapter). Tranylcypromine, which was once removed from the market for a time after reports of toxicity and fatalities in elderly patients, is now not recommended for use in patients over 60 years old. It is reserved mainly for patients hospitalized with severe depressions, because its continued use requires close observation for cardiovascular side-effects. This age restriction does not apply to the other drugs of the MAO inhibitor type, *isocarboxazid*[+] (Marplan) and *phenelzine acid sulfate* (Nardil). However, both can cause the same types of toxicity as tranylcypromine, and their use requires the same kinds of precautions (see the summary at the end of this chapter).

Adverse effects. Hepatitis has not been a problem with the MAO inhibitors now available, including the two hydrazine derivatives chemically related to iproniazid. The most serious side-effects are, instead, those that involve a sudden fall or rise in blood pressure, particularly in elderly patients. Most common are such symptoms of postural hypotension as dizziness, weakness, and feelings of faintness. More dangerous, however, are episodes of hypertension, because these have sometimes resulted in hypertensive crises that have occasionally led to fatal brain hemorrhages. Patients taking these drugs should be observed closely for such signs and symptoms as severe headache, stiff neck, sweating, nausea, and vomiting, because these may be early warning signs of dangerous blood pressure increases.

Because of such possible adverse effects, the use of these drugs is contraindicated in patients with cerebrovascular disease, headaches, congestive heart failure, and pheochromocytoma. Their use in treating depressed patients who have very high blood pressure is not recommended. When caring for depressed patients taking MAO inhibitors, nurses should take frequent blood pressure readings so that these drugs can be quickly discontinued if hypertension, heart palpitations, or headaches develop.

These drugs also sometimes cause side-effects that are the result of blockade of autonomic nervous system receptors and of overstimulation of the CNS. The autonomic blocking effects include mouth dryness, constipation, blurring of vision, and cardiac palpitation. The central effects are seen in some patients who tend to become restless and hyperactive and who may, in fact, show symptoms of agitation to the point of mania. To avoid such increased anxiety and hypomanic reactions, MAO inhibitor-type antidepressants such as tranylcypromine are sometimes administered together with a phenothiazine tranquilizer (*e.g.,* trifluoperazine). Another

CNS effect that sometimes occurs is the development of muscle spasm and tremors. Thus, special caution is required to avoid convulsive seizures when depressed epileptic patients are treated with these drugs.

Interactions with drugs and foods. (See also Additional clinical considerations, below). Drugs of the MAO inhibitor class should not be used in combination with sympathomimetic and central depressant drugs, or with others that alter catecholamine metabolism in the peripheral and central nervous systems. Patients must also be warned against eating certain foods. This is because drug-induced inhibition of MAO in sympathetic and central adrenergic nerve endings and in the liver and gastrointestinal tract potentiates the actions of drugs such as amphetamines, methyldopa, and levodopa, and enzyme inhibition leads to reactions after eating certain foods that contain the amino acid *tyramine*. Also, drug-induced inhibition of the liver enzyme systems responsible for the metabolic breakdown of barbiturates, alcohol, and opioids such as meperidine (Demerol) may intensify the central effects of these depressants.

Patients taking this class of antidepressants, which cause increased accumulation of norepinephrine in nerve endings, should be told not to take over-the-counter (OTC) cold remedies or medications that may be prescribed by other physicians for treating allergic rhinitis or as adjuncts to low-calorie diets for weight reduction. All such products contain sympathomimetic drugs that can release the abnormally large amounts of norepinephrine stored in the terminations of adrenergic nerves in blood vessels and elsewhere in the body. This can lead to generalized peripheral vasoconstriction and to the sharp rises in blood pressure that cause hypertensive crises and intracranial bleeding.

Among foods that have a high content of tyramine as a result of bacterial breakdown of proteins during aging or fermentation processes are certain cheeses, pickled herring, chicken livers, sour cream, and canned figs. Drinks that should be avoided include Chianti wine, sherry, and beer. Coffee and other caffeine-containing beverages should be consumed only in moderate amounts. Inhibition of the enzyme MAO in the gastrointestinal tract favors the absorption of large quantities of tyramine, which would ordinarily be broken down before absorption, when foods containing this catecholamine are eaten. The absorbed substance then acts, like the sympathomimetic drugs mentioned above, to release the extra amounts of norepinephrine that have accumulated in nerve endings as a result of MAO inhibition at such sites.

Antidepressants of this class should not be taken in combination with those of the tricyclic type. Patients who have taken drugs of both types together have sometimes suffered very severe reactions, apparently because the MAO inhibitors potentiate certain atropinelike CNS and peripheral effects of the agents of the second class. People taking overdoses of the two types of drugs have

become delirious and developed high fever (up to 109°F, or 42.8°C); and muscular tremors, rigidity, and convulsive seizures, followed by collapse, coma, and death.

Patients who have not responded to a trial of tricyclic drug therapy should not begin to receive drugs of the MAO inhibitor type for at least a week to avoid such interactions, and only half-doses of these drugs are ordinarily ordered for the first week. The medication-free interval must be much longer if patients who first received a MAO inhibitor-type antidepressant are to be transferred to tricyclic-type drug therapy. Rest periods are also recommended when patients who have had an unsuccessful trial of one MAO inhibitor are to be switched to a second drug of the same class.

Treatment of toxicity. These drugs are sometimes taken deliberately in overdoses by depressed patients who are suicidal. Signs of intoxication may not appear for 12 hours or more after ingestion. Thus, if a patient is found to have taken an overdose, an effort should be made to prevent absorption of these drugs by gastric lavage or by induced vomiting. Once absorption has occurred, little can be done to hasten elimination, and the complex central and cardiovascular toxic effects are difficult to treat.

Effects that are similar to those of tricyclic drug toxicity may be managed in the same way. Convulsive seizures, for example, can be controlled with diazepam, and high fever is best reduced by applying ice packs or cold, wet towels externally. Repeated parenteral doses of chlorpromazine may be useful for control of hyperpyrexia as well as of agitated, hyperactive behavior.

The drug-induced development of hypertensive crisis requires treatment with rapid-acting antihypertensive agents to reduce pressure within the brain and to prevent pulmonary edema. Intravenous administration of the α-adrenergic blocking agent, phentolamine, or of ganglionic blockers such as pentolinium (Chap. 28), is recommended for this purpose. However, these drugs must be administered very cautiously to avoid an excessive drop in blood pressure, because hypotension can lead to death from circulatory collapse. Infusion of fluids and electrolytes may be required to maintain hydration and acid–base balance.

Lithium carbonate

Mechanism of action. This salt of the element lithium exerts central effects that lead gradually to control of acute episodes of mania in the manic phase of manic–depressive affective disorders. The drug does not depress the CNS in ordinary therapeutic doses. However, it reduces the characteristic excitement of the manic state and relieves the signs and symptoms of excessive mental and motor activity (see the summary of manic syndrome signs and symptoms at the end of this chapter).

The neurochemical effects of lithium carbonate[+] (Eskalith; Lithane; Lithonate) are not truly understood at this time, despite numerous speculative hypotheses. The lithium ion may act primarily to alter certain abnormalities in the transport of sodium and potassium ions through nerve cell membranes. This, in turn, may favorably affect the balance between such biogenic amines as norepinephrine and serotonin in the CNS areas that are involved in emotional responses. This may account for the stabilizing effect that the drug is said to exert in patients who are prone to both mania and depression.

Clinical indications. At present, lithium is used mainly to control manic episodes in the manic–depressive psychosis and to prevent their recurrence. It has proved highly effective for symptomatic relief of motor, mental, and verbal hyperactivity and aggressive or hostile behavior in patients with this specific illness. It does *not* dampen similar signs and symptoms in patients with other mental disorders, such as schizophrenia of the paranoid or catatonic subtypes or organic brain damage.

Lithium is also considered to be useful for preventing depressive episodes in patients who are subject to frequent recurrences. It seems most likely to do so in patients with so-called *bipolar* affective disorders—that is, in those who have recurrences of *both* manic and depressive episodes. Some psychiatrists have suggested that lithium may also be useful for prophylaxis of *unipolar* depressions—that is, in patients who suffer only cyclical depressive episodes, without intervening periods of mania. However, the efficacy of lithium in this subgroup of depressed patients has not yet been established, and lithium does not seem to be effective against other categories of reactive and endogenous depression.

Serum lithium levels. The dosage of lithium needed to control acute mania is close to that which can cause toxicity. Long-continued maintenance therapy at lower doses may also sometimes lead to gradual development of lithium toxicity. Fortunately, a simple laboratory procedure is available for determining the level of lithium in the patient's plasma. Such serum levels are an excellent index of whether the drug's dosage has reached the therapeutic range and is being maintained there, or whether toxicity is likely to occur from overdosage. Serum lithium determinations are essential for safe and effective lithium therapy. Patients who will not comply with a strict dosage regimen and frequent monitoring should not be started on lithium maintenance therapy.

The therapeutic plasma level of lithium for controlling manic episodes is between about 1.0 and 1.5 mEq of the ion per liter of plasma. This level can usually be attained in about a week of treatment with 1800 mg divided into three daily doses of 600 mg. Larger doses may be needed, because acutely manic patients are relatively resistant to lithium.

After the acute episode has been controlled and the patient's behavior normalizes, lithium may be administered for long periods at lower doses that prevent recurrences, with serum lithium levels of as little as 0.6 mEq/liter and rarely as much as 1.2 mEq/liter. This level can usually be maintained with a total daily dose of 900 mg to 1200 mg. This can be administered as a single daily dose or divided into three or four 300-mg doses.

In both the treatment of acute mania and the prevention of recurrences, the serum lithium level should not be allowed to rise above 1.5 mEq/liter. Above that level, clinical signs and symptoms of toxicity begin to appear. Lithium levels between 2.0 mEq/liter and 3.0 mEq/liter are associated with increasingly severe degrees of toxicity, including potentially fatal cardiovascular effects. Thus, even in relatively resistant acute manic patients, the serum lithium level should not be permitted to exceed 2.0 mEq/liter.

Adverse effects. Tremor, thirst, and polyuria are common adverse effects. Lethargy, slurred speech, confusion, and ataxia may signal the need for dosage reduction to avoid serious toxicity, such as convulsions, delirium, coma, and even death. Extrapyramidal reactions have also occurred.

With long-term therapy, hypothyroidism, sometimes irreversible, can occur (see Chap. 22). All patients should have their thyroid function monitored before and at intervals during lithium therapy.

Renal toxicity can be a serious problem. Lithium causes a nephrogenic diabetes insipidus that may become irreversible. Other adverse renal effects indicate that a patient's renal function, like thyroid function, should be evaluated before and during therapy.

The nurse should teach patients and their families to discontinue lithium treatment if gastrointestinal side-effects occur, or if the patient becomes drowsy or giddy and has some difficulty in moving about because of muscle weakness or motor incoordination. In such cases, the plasma lithium level should be checked. If this is not done, and the patient continues to take the drug, he may become restless and confused before lapsing into a stuporous or comatose state. This may be punctuated by sudden muscle spasms of the extremities and by epileptiform seizures. Comatose patients may also suffer respiratory complications, cardiac arrhythmias, hypotension, and circulatory collapse.

Treatment of toxicity. There is no specific antidote for lithium overdosage. The comatose patient's recovery depends mainly on good nursing care, including frequent changes in position, measures to support vital functions, and forced diuresis to increase excretion of the excess ion. The osmotic diuretics mannitol and urea are often effective for this purpose, as is hemodialysis. Other procedures that are said to help lower serum levels of lithium are the slow IV infusion of aminophylline several times daily, and alkalinization of the patient's urine by administration of such systemic alkalinizers as sodium bicarbonate or sodium lactate.

Precautions. Lithium salts were first recommended for mania in 1949, before any of the other modern psychotherapeutic drugs were available. Lithium was not, however, approved for this purpose until 1970. The reason for this delay was the occurrence—also in 1949—of an epidemic of deaths from lithium toxicity when the substance was marketed as a salt substitute for cardiovascular patients on low-sodium diets.

It is now known that these are exactly the types of patients who should *not* take lithium. That is, this drug is contraindicated in patients with heart and kidney diseases whose stores of sodium are depleted or who are dehydrated. Thus, patients who require treatment with diuretics that remove sodium and water should not ordinarily be treated with lithium.

All patients being stabilized or maintained on lithium should eat a diet containing normal amounts of salt and maintain a fluid intake of almost 3 quarts daily. If patients develop an elevated temperature and lose fluid through fever and sweating, or diarrhea, they should receive a salt supplement and drink more fluids, or they should at least stop taking their lithium medication temporarily. Loss of sodium through excessive perspiration, natriuresis (urinary sodium loss), or reduced sodium intake all reduce the renal clearance of lithium and can cause toxic levels of lithium to accumulate.

Choice of treatment for affective disorders

Depression is a potentially lethal disease. About two million Americans attempt suicide each year, and at least 40,000 of them succeed. An estimated half of these people are thought to have been suffering from one or another of the several clinical categories of depressive illnesses.

However, despite the possibility of death by suicide, depressed patients have a very good chance of recovering spontaneously as compared to those who suffer from schizophrenia and other mental illnesses. Once their condition has been diagnosed as depression, their recovery can be hastened by one or a combination of several effective treatment methods now available. Acute depressive reactions can be rapidly relieved, and even those patients whose condition is chronic can be prevented from having frequently recurring episodes of depression or mania.

Depending on the diagnosis, the physician decides on what type of treatment to employ, or whether any specific type of therapy is needed at all. Treatment may be initiated with ECT or with any of several varieties of psychotherapy or pharmacotherapy. Sometimes, a combination of two or more of these therapeutic modalities may be used.

The choice of therapy is most often based on the following types of factors:

1. Whether the patient's depression seems to stem from a specific event to which he is reacting, or whether the depression has no obvious cause

2. Whether the patient has a history of previous episodes and of a personality or character structure that may account for frequent recurrences, or whether the depression is an isolated event
3. Whether the patient's symptoms can be classified as mild, moderately severe, or of extreme severity
4. Whether the target symptoms are of the retarded or the agitated type (see the summary at the end of this chapter)

Even when all such information is available to a psychiatrist, the diagnosis of the patient's specific category of depression is not easy. Authorities often disagree as to which signs and symptoms are truly significant in determining the subtype of affective disorder from which a particular patient is suffering. Even when a clear-cut diagnosis is made, there is often disagreement about which type of treatment is best. However, despite such reservations, the following discussion will attempt to indicate what seems to be the consensus regarding the types of treatment that are currently preferred in the management of patients who are diagnosed as falling into one or another category of depression.

Reactive depressions

The vast majority of acute clinical depressions—perhaps 80% to 90%—can be traced to a specific stressful event to which the patient is reacting. Although some psychiatrists question the validity of dividing depressions into reactive (exogenous) and endogenous subclasses, making such a diagnosis does seem relevant to selecting the best type of treatment with which to begin. Patients with reactive depressions of mild to moderate degree are, for example, most responsive to *psychotherapy* or to other interpersonal supportive measures. They do *not* require ECT, and cases of reactive depression that develop in people judged to have a normal personality structure do *not* even need treatment with tricyclic or MAO inhibitor-type antidepressant drugs.

Other drugs may, however, be helpful for relief of the often painful or disabling symptoms that follow serious losses and disappointments, even in people with stable personalities. Although it is true that a person deeply saddened by the loss of a loved one, for example, needs mainly the emotional support of family and friends, psychotherapeutic drugs can help lessen such misery. Thus, the physician may order an antianxiety drug such as *chlordiazepoxide HCl*⁺ (Librium; see Drug digest, Chap. 45) or some other sedative to reduce daytime restlessness and distracting nervousness. Prescribing a hypnotic such as *flurazepam HCl*⁺ (Dalmane; see Drug digest, Chap. 45) or even a barbiturate in small amounts and for brief periods can help sleepless patients get the rest they require while "working through" their grief.

For patients whose depressive symptoms take the form of apathy, lethargy, and listlessness, small daily doses of *dextroamphetamine sulfate*[+] (Dexedrine), *methylphenidate*[+] (Ritalin; see Drug digest, Chap. 47) or other psychomotor stimulants (Chap. 47) may be beneficial. As indicated in Chapter 47, these drugs tend to exert a mild euphoretic or mood-elevating effect that helps some patients to regain interest in going on with their lives. The stimulants are best taken early in the day, in part because that is when the tired, dejected patient has the most difficulty in rousing himself to take up the type of daily activities and interrelationships on which recovery really depends. Another reason is that late afternoon or evening doses of amphetamines may cause insomnia. This and other drug-induced restlessness may be lessened when a psychomotor stimulant is given in combination with a barbiturate or other depressant drug, which may also help to lessen the depressed patient's anxiety.

An investigational drug, *bupropion HCl* (Wellbutrin), resembles the amphetamines in chemical structure and stimulant properties. Its mechanism of action is unknown, but it appears to be effective in many types of depression, and preliminary results indicate that sedation, anticholinergic effects, and cardiotoxicity are less common than with many currently available drugs.

Neurotic depressions

People who have a history of behavior that reflects emotional instability or unresolved internal conflicts often become depressed after personal setbacks that most people would not find very distressing. These people are prone to suffer recurrent episodes of *reactive* depression that are usually more distressing and prolonged than those discussed above. Sometimes, however, these patients improve with no treatment other than hospitalization and placebo medication.

Apparently, just being taken away from their familiar home environment is helpful, as is having an opportunity to relate to health-care personnel in the hospital setting. Of course, such so-called *milieu therapy* will not prevent these particularly vulnerable people from suffering further depressive episodes. Thus, the nurse should encourage patients whose recurrent bouts of depression arise from their chronic personality–character inadequacies to enter some form of intensive interpersonal therapy. Depressive patients with lifelong personality problems require intensive psychotherapy on an individual or a group basis to bring about lasting improvement.

Some psychiatrists feel that drugs are only a crutch for such psychoneurotic patients. However, most believe that the tricyclic antidepressants are often useful in such cases for the relief of distressing symptoms that interfere with psychotherapy. If these drugs fail to help, a trial of an MAO inhibitor agent may be worthwhile. All agree that in such cases the amphetamines should *not* be employed for several reasons. Such stimulants are not effective in moderately severe depressive states and, when dosage is raised, the patient's anorexia and sleeplessness may tend to intensify. Most important is the fact that an introduction to amphetamines may compound the problems of patients with personality disturbances. Instead of stopping the medication after a few weeks, they may continue to take larger doses on a regular basis for the euphoric effect.

The possibilities of drug abuse and dependence must also be considered before barbiturates are ordered for agitated-depressed patients. The newer antianxiety agents of the benzodiazepine class, such as chlordiazepoxide, offer some relief but can also be abused by these patients. Thus, phenothiazine-type antipsychotics such as thioridazine or fluphenazine are sometimes administered for relief of agitation, because these drugs—like the tricyclic and MAO inhibitor antidepressant drugs—do not offer euphoric effects that encourage abuse and development of psychological dependence.

Psychotic depressions

Some patients who first become depressed because of distressing events in their life situation soon lose touch with reality. That is, their mood disturbance becomes so severe that they develop delusions and other thought disorders and fail to grasp what is actually going on around them. Unlike patients with neurotic depression, those who suffer such a psychotic depressive reaction do *not* respond to hospitalization alone nor to opportunities for social interaction or even intensive psychotherapy.

In this respect, these patients are similar to those whose depression does not seem related to any specific precipitating event—that is, those with so-called endogenous depressions such as the *involutional melancholia* that occurs in older patients, or the *manic–depressive* psychosis. Such severe or major depressions—whether in reaction to external events (exogenous) or endogenous—require somatic or physical therapies. These include ECT and pharmacotherapy with antidepressant and antipsychotic drugs.

Drugs versus ECT. The physician's first decision in managing patients with psychotic depression is whether to employ drugs or ECT. Most prefer to begin with an antidepressant drug—usually one of the tricyclic compounds, unless the patient refuses to take or cannot tolerate medication, or is considered a high suicide risk. In such cases, ECT may be better because it is more rapidly effective than the drugs, which require several weeks for full effectiveness or may not prove effective at all.

Among the advantages claimed for drug therapy over ECT are the following:

1. Most patients and their families have an aversion to ECT and find the idea of taking medication more acceptable.
2. The family may also find it more

convenient for a patient who has not been hospitalized to take drugs, rather than have to accompany him to a clinic for each of the six to twelve shock treatments in the usual several-week course of ECT. The reason for this is that an ECT treatment often leaves the patient confused and with some temporary loss of memory. (Some psychiatrists claim that such transient mental impairment is rare when unilateral ECT is employed. This is a procedure in which the electrodes are applied to only one side of the patient's head, so that the current enters only the patient's *non*dominant cerebral hemisphere.)

3. Drugs are considered safer than ECT in patients who are properly supervised and taught to detect early signs of serious side-effects and to prevent potentially harmful drug interactions. Of course, the proponents of ECT deny that it is a dangerous procedure. They claim that it causes no permanent brain damage and that it is free of the serious circulatory effects that can occur during drug therapy. However, although ECT itself may have no serious effects, its use requires the intravenous administration of several potent adjunctive drugs. Thus, for example, to prevent possible fractures of vertebrae and long bones in convulsive spasms, patients are pretreated with the neuromuscular junction blocking drug succinylcholine, and with thiopental and atropine.

4. Drug therapy is less expensive than a course of ECT, which usually requires the presence of an anesthesiologist or other specially trained personnel equipped to perform endotracheal intubation and artificial respiration if the patient becomes apneic from the combined effects of the adjunctive drugs and the ECT.

Other considerations. ECT is effective in a higher proportion of depressed patients than drug therapy. It often affords more rapid, dramatic relief. However, because of various drawbacks of ECT that make drug therapy seem safer, cheaper, more convenient, and more acceptable to the patient and family, most physicians—particularly the *non*psychiatrists who see and treat the vast majority of depressed patients—prefer to initiate the treatment of most cases with antidepressant drugs.

ECT may be employed if a patient who cannot be hospitalized and kept under constant close observation is judged to be a high suicide risk. ECT is also generally kept in reserve for those cases in which depression is still severely incapacitating, after the patient has failed to respond to 4 to 6 weeks of treatment with adequate doses of each of the two main classes of antidepressant drugs, or cannot tolerate them.

Choice and use of drugs

There is no way of knowing in advance whether a drug selected for initiating treatment of a depressed patient is likely to prove effective. Despite claims that certain of the available drugs may be better for patients with one or another of the various subtypes of serious depressions, there is no proof at present that any single antidepressant drug is superior to any of the others for treating any particular category of depressed patients.

Tricyclic-type antidepressants are the first choice of most physicians. This class of drugs is generally considered to be somewhat safer than the MAO inhibitor-type antidepressants. For reasons discussed earlier, the latter drugs are generally reserved for use in patients who have failed to respond to a trial with one or more tricyclic compounds administered for at least 4 weeks in daily doses gradually adjusted to the most that the patient can tolerate.

The prototype tricyclics imipramine and amitriptyline are still the most commonly employed drugs. They are effective in both neurotic and psychotic depressions and against target symptoms of both the retarded and agitated types (see the summary at the end of this chapter). Occasionally, some physicians prefer doxepin (Sinequan; Adapin), or other more sedating tricyclics (see above) for anxious, agitated, depressed patients. Protriptyline (Vivactil) or some other less sedating tricyclic may be preferred for depressed patients who are withdrawn and anergic, because they may have an activating action that could help to rouse patients from their apathy even before the drug's full antidepressant effects develop.

Patients are best started out on a single small dose of one of the sedating tricyclics administered at bedtime. Dosage of most drugs is then raised rapidly by adding daytime doses.

The patient who does respond to the tricyclic drug may be maintained on it for several months to help prevent relapses. During this time, it may be desirable for the patient to take a single daily dose instead of the several doses into which the daily total had previously been divided. Imipramine pamoate (Tofranil-PM) is administered on a once-daily basis in capsules containing up to 150 mg, and amitriptyline is now available in 150-mg scored tablets, one of which may be taken at bedtime as the total daily dose. This has the advantage of improving the compliance of patients who might forget to take several daily doses. It also helps to eliminate the need for a hypnotic drug, and it makes the patient less aware of atropine-type and other side-effects of the tricyclic drugs.

Combination therapy. Some agitated patients may not be benefited, at first, by even the more sedating tricyclic antidepressants (see above). In such cases an antianxiety agent such as diazepam may be added to the patient's regimen. Some hostile patients may even require the addition of a major tranquilizer such as thioridazine or perphenazine.

Phenothiazine-type antipsychotic drugs of this type are also used in patients judged to have schizophrenic as well as depressive symptoms. Such borderline or *schizoaffective* patients sometimes tend to become more agitated when treated with a tricyclic alone. After the dosage of both drugs has been individually adjusted, patients may be switched to products that contain each drug in the same ratio that has been established by trial and error. Two such combination products, Etrafon and Triavil, contain amitriptyline and perphenazine in various fixed dosage ratios.

Phenothiazines are sometimes also administered in combination with lithium for control of acute mania. The reason for this is that lithium alone may require a week or more to become fully effective. Thus, while the patient is taking daily oral doses of lithium, intramuscular injections of chlorpromazine may also be given. If the drug combination does not quickly quiet the patient, ECT may be employed until the lithium treatment becomes effective.

Patients who are seen during an episode of depression that is actually the depressive phase of the manic–depressive illness may not do well on tricyclic therapy alone. Imipramine administration, for example, may actually set off a manic attack in such cases. Thus, the patient whose depression is known to be of the bipolar type may be better maintained on lithium alone or combined with a tricyclic antidepressant. Maprotiline, the tetracyclic drug, is also indicated for the treatment of depression in patients with manic–depressive illness.

Current status and future prospects

Treatment with tricyclic and MAO inhibitor-type antidepressants and with lithium is now often effective for relieving bouts of depression and for preventing their recurrence. Some psychiatrists suggest that drug therapy could be much more effective if it could be tailored to fit the specific subtype of depression from which each patient is suffering. This is now often very difficult, because the physician may not learn enough about the patient's illness from the history and signs and symptoms alone.

It is difficult, for example, to tell whether a patient is suffering from an acute, but single isolated episode of depression, or one of a series of recurrent unipolar depressions, or the depressive phase of a manic–depressive (bipolar) affective illness. However, each of these types of depression may have a different neurochemical cause. If so, each should respond best to those drugs or other somatic treatment measures that might act specifically to correct the underlying abnormality.

Some research psychiatrists have suggested that such specific therapy could be ordered if they had laboratory tests that could be used in the work-up of depressed patients, much as internists have for evaluating patients with various endocrine and medical disorders. Thus, they are seeking biochemical tests for differentiating between the several subtypes of clinical depression.

Experimental results suggest that it may soon be possible to do so by testing the depressed patient's blood or urine. Finding an abnormally high or low level of various metabolites of biogenic amines such as norepinephrine, dopamine, or serotonin might indicate that the patient's brain has an abnormal neurochemical content that is characteristic of a specific affective disorder. The patient might then be able to be treated on a rational basis rather than by the empirical—trial-and-error—method that must now be employed.

Additional clinical considerations

Before receiving any antidepressant drug, the patient should be given a psychiatric evaluation and should be assessed for underlying medical conditions that could be cautions or contraindications to the use of these drugs. Such conditions include acute cardiovascular disease, glaucoma, urinary retention, prostatic hypertrophy, hyperthyroidism, hepatic failure, renal failure, and pheochromocytoma. The safety of these drugs in pregnancy and lactation has not been established. The use of lithium during pregnancy has been associated with several congenital defects, particularly of the cardiovascular system. The use of any antidepressant in pregnant or nursing women should be discouraged.

Many systemic effects are to be expected when using the antidepressant drugs. The patient should be aware of the possibility of these effects so that the changes experienced will be reported and will, hopefully, not add to the patient's depression or inability to cope. These adverse effects include cardiovascular depression, reflex excitation ($\downarrow$ or $\uparrow$ BP, arrhythmias, congestive heart failure), or both; dry mouth; urinary retention; visual changes; restlessness; "anxiety"; insomnia; nightmares; drowsiness; fatigue; difficulty in concentrating; tremors; numbness; speech changes; photosensitivity; nausea, vomiting; loss of appetite; stomatitis. Nursing measures can be used to help make the patient more comfortable and better able to cope with some of these effects. Overall, however, the patient will require support and encouragement to cope with the many effects of these drugs. If elective surgery is to be done, antidepressant drugs should be stopped about 2 weeks before the surgery. If emergency surgery is needed, it is important that the patient's chart clearly state that the patient is on one of these drugs, and should clearly indicate the time of the last dose so that special precautions can be taken.

Drug–drug and drug–food interactions. Numerous drug–drug interactions have been reported.

Tricyclic antidepressants taken concurrently with:

Sympathomimetic drugs can increase their effect.

Alcohol, barbiturates, or *CNS depressants* can enhance their effect and lead to toxicity.

MAO inhibitors can cause hypertensive crises.

Guanethidine or clonidine can block their antihypertensive effect.

Quinidine or procainamide can produce dangerous additive effects.

Oral contraceptives can inhibit the effect of the tricyclic antidepressant.

MAO inhibitors taken concurrently with:

CNS depressants can lead to coma and death.

Tricyclic antidepressants or *other MAO inhibitors* can cause severe hypertensive crises.

Other *psychotropic drugs* can cause dangerous additive effects.

Antihypertensives can result in severe hypotension.

Insulin or *oral hypoglycemia drugs (sulfonylureas)* can have an additive hypoglycemic effect.

Sympathomimetic drugs or *foods containing tyramine* can cause severe hypertensive crisis.

Lithium taken concurrently with:

Urinary alkalinizers or *osmotic diuretics* will need to be taken in higher than usual doses because these drugs increase the excretion of lithium.

Other types of *diuretics* may lead to decreased renal excretion of lithium and the development of toxicity.

Nonsteroidal anti-inflammatory drugs reportedly increase the serum level of lithium, increasing the danger of toxicity.

Generally, it is important to remember that many OTC drugs contain sympathomimetics, and patients should be cautioned to avoid the use of OTC preparations while on an antidepressant drug. Alcohol also needs to be avoided.

The patient teaching guide summarizes points that should be incorporated into the teaching program of a patient receiving tricyclic antidepressants. Similar teaching guides can be adopted for patients receiving other antidepressants. The guide to the nursing process summarizes the clinical aspects that should be incorporated into the nursing care of a patient receiving tricyclic antidepressants.

Patient teaching guide: tricyclic antidepressants

The drug that has been prescribed for you is called a tricyclic antidepressant. Drugs of this group are used to treat certain mental or emotional disorders. To be effective, this drug needs to be taken exactly as prescribed.

Instructions:

1. The name of your drug is ———————————— .

2. The dosage prescribed for you is ———————————— .

3. The drug should be taken ———— times a day. The best times to take your drug are ———————————— . If dosage is increased, take the first increased dose at bedtime. If GI upset occurs, the drug can be taken with food.

4. Some side-effects of the drug that you should be aware of include the following:

Increased sensitivity to sun

Wear protective clothing, sunglasses, or sunscreens if out in the sun.

Drowsiness, dizziness, visual changes

Take care to avoid driving, operating heavy machinery, or performing delicate tasks while you are on this drug.

(continued)

Difficulty in sleeping, nightmares, dreams	This is a common reaction; if this becomes too uncomfortable, notify your nurse or physician.
Dry mouth, sore mouth	Frequent mouth care, sucking sugarless lozenges, and drinking plenty of fluids may help.
Loss of appetite, nausea, vomiting	Taking the medication with food may help.

5. Keep this and all medications out of the reach of children.

6. Tell any nurse, physician, or dentist who is taking care of you that you are on this drug.

7. Avoid the use of alcohol while you are on this drug.

8. Do not take any over-the-counter medications while you are on this drug. If you feel that you need one of these preparations, consult with your nurse or physician for an appropriate preparation that will not interact with this drug.

9. Do not stop taking this drug suddenly. If for any reason you can't take the drug, notify your nurse or physician.

Notify your nurse or physician if any of the following occur:

Chest pain
Difficulty in breathing
Difficulty in voiding
Dark urine, pale stools
Confusion, hallucinations
Rash

Guide to the nursing process: tricyclic antidepressants

Assessment	Nursing diagnoses	Interventions	Evaluation
Past history (*contraindications*): Cardiovascular disease Glaucoma Urinary retention Prostatic hypertrophy Hyperthyroidism Hepatic failure Renal failure Pheochromocytoma Pregnancy Lactation	Potential alteration in cardiac output Potential for injury secondary to adverse effects Knowledge deficit regarding drug therapy Potential sensory–perceptual alteration Potential alteration in comfort: GI upset	Safe and appropriate administration of drug Provision of comfort and safety measures: • Drug with meals • Safety measures if drowsy • Mouth care • Meal planning • Sleep measures Patient teaching regarding drug therapy	Monitor for therapeutic effectiveness of drug Monitor for adverse effects of drug: • CNS effects • Cardiovascular effects • Liver enzyme changes • Anticholinergic effects • GI upset *(continued)*

Assessment	Nursing diagnoses	Interventions	Evaluation
Allergies: *these drugs; tartrazine* (certain preparations); others; reactions Medication history (*cautions*): Sympathomimetics Alcohol Barbiturates CNS depressants MAO inhibitors Guanethidine Clonidine Quinidine Procainamide Oral contraceptives **Physical assessment** Neurologic: affect, mental status, reflexes, peripheral sensations Cardiovascular: baseline ECG, BP, pulse, peripheral perfusion, auscultation GI: abdominal exam Renal: normal output, prostate (if appropriate) Other: liver enzyme levels, CBC		Support and encouragement to deal with depression, drug therapy, and side-effects Emergency or life support measures to deal with toxic reactions, if needed	• Bone marrow depression Evaluate effectiveness of patient teaching program Evaluate effectiveness of support and encouragement offered Monitor for drug–drug interaction: many possible Evaluate emergency or life support measures if necessary

Case study

Presentation

BA, a 34-year-old white mother of two, has been treated repeatedly over the past 3 years for depression. She has undergone a 12-week course of ECT treatments, intense psychotherapy, and tricyclic antidepressants. BA was admitted to a private psychiatric hospital of her own volition when her depression became so severe that she felt she was no longer able to function and to care for her family. At this admission, BA was started on Nardil (phenelzine) and family therapy. Over a 2-week period, BA seemed to be progressing. She and her husband were able to communicate about her fears and concerns, and she stated that she was ready for discharge.

What particular instructions will BA require before discharge?

Discussion

With BA's repeated history of depression, one of her major instructional needs will be a definite schedule of follow-up visits and a telephone number she can call for help if she needs it. The MAO inhibitor phenelzine seems to be working for BA. She will, however, require a lot of patient teaching regarding this drug before she goes home on it. Particulars that need to be included are the following: this drug may cause drowsiness or blurred vision, and special safety precautions should be taken; dizziness can occur when changing position, so position changes should be made slowly; do not stop taking the medication suddenly; avoid the use of alcohol and over-the-counter medications while you are on this drug; do not take any other prescription drug while on this drug unless first discussing it with your nurse or physician; notify your nurse or physician if any of the following occur—headache, skin rash, dark urine, pale stools, unusual reactions. The dietary restrictions associated with MAO inhibitor use are more complex and should be written down in detail.

The patient needs to be instructed to avoid foods containing tyramine. Such foods include certain cheese and dairy products (blue, American, processed, Boursault, Brie, Camembert, cheddar, Emmenthaler, Gruyère, Stilton, and Roquefort cheese; sour cream, yogurt), meat and fish (meats with tenderizers, fermented sausages, herring—especially pickled, game meats), beverages (beer, ale, red wine—Chianti, sherry), fruits and vegetables (yeast, bananas, raisins, figs), and soy sauce. She should also be warned to avoid caffeine products, which can aggravate such reactions. BA should be advised to report any severe headache immediately.

The written instructions for this drug may be quite overwhelming to BA. The teaching should best be done by a nurse who is familiar with BA and with the therapeutic approach that works best for her. She will need support and encouragement to cope with all the cautions and restrictions associated with this drug therapy. A positive, helping attitude may mean a great deal in the effectiveness of this drug therapy.

Summary of signs and symptoms often seen in depressive syndromes*

Mood

Sad, dejected, downcast, irritable, tearful, and with loss of ability to find anything pleasurable or enjoyable.

Physiologic

Sleep disturbances: insomnia marked by early morning awakening; anorexia: loss of appetite and weight; loss of libido: decrease in sex drive; headache, abdominal distress, constipation, fatigue or feeling of weakness, and such signs of autonomic imbalance as cardiac palpitations, flushing, sweating.

Thought and behavior

Retarded depression features. Signs of psychomotor slowing such as slow speech in a low, weak, or whispered voice; apathy or indifference: loss of interest in the environment, family, work, personal appearance; failure to respond to questions; slow, deliberate or dragging gait and movements; unwillingness or inability to get out of bed and, in severely retarded cases, stupor.

Agitated depression features. Verbal and motor expressions of anxiety, such as pacing back and forth, wringing the hands, and complaining volubly of the above physical symptoms that may be seen as signs of cancer, heart disease, and other serious illnesses; preoccupation with possible tragedy and death; thoughts of personal inadequacy, lack of competence, guilt, hopelessness, worthlessness, hallucinations, delusions, and preoccupation with the idea of suicide.

* Depressed patients usually show a half-dozen or more of these signs and symptoms but never, of course, all of them.

Summary of signs and symptoms often seen in manic syndromes*

Hypomanic state

Mood. In high good spirits; friendly and warm toward others, but sometimes to a degree not warranted by the circumstances; optimistic, but sometimes too much so in view of the difficulties posed by the reality of the situation.

* Manic patients may not necessarily progress from minor levels of activity to the most intense degree of delirious mania noted here.

Speech. Talks with great glibness and facility; may move from one topic to another in a nonstop way because of distractibility.

Motor activity. Appears tireless and full of energy while moving about in what seems to be inexhaustible physical health and well-being.

Acute manic state

Mood. Good spirits become excessive to a degree that may disturb others; humor may become crude or blasphemous, because discretion and concern for the feelings of others may be lacking; if antagonized, may instantly become viciously angry.

Speech. Ideas may be expressed as rapidly as they enter his mind and thus his talk may be marked by flight of ideas and incoherence.

Motor activity. Extreme mobility, restlessness, and impulsive activity; if real situations pose difficult problems, may react with tears or aggressive behavior.

Delirious mania

Pressure of speech to point of complete incoherence; hallucinations and delusions make it difficult to keep contact with the patient and gain cooperation; constantly in a state of extreme purposeless activity which may lead to high fever and a state of exhaustion; incontinent; this state may end fatally if not controlled.

Summary of side-effects of antidepressant drugs

Tricyclic type (amitriptyline, imipramine, and others)
Autonomic side-effects
Mouth dryness, blurred vision, constipation, difficult urination
Fall in blood pressure in the standing position (postural hypotension) with resulting feelings of faintness, dizziness, and weakness
Localized sweating; male sexual function disturbances (impotence; delayed ejaculation); GI disturbances, including nausea and vomiting; headache

Central side-effects
Early feelings of drowsiness and fatigue followed by later signs of mental overstimulation (*e.g.,* restlessness, jitteriness, agitation; or hypomania, mania, confusion, hallucinations, and delirium)
Motor overstimulation marked by muscle twitching and tremors, hyperreflexia, and possibly convulsive seizures

Peripheral nerve effects
Sensory signs of neuritis with possible numbness and tingling (paresthesia) and ringing in the ears (tinnitus)

Hypersensitivity-type reactions
Obstructive jaundice; agranulocytosis; skin eruptions, including photosensitivity reactions

MAOI: Monoamine oxidase inhibitors (phenelzine; tranylcypromine)
Autonomic side-effects
Postural *hypo*tension marked by dizziness, weakness, and fainting; occasionally, *hyper*tension marked by severe headache, nausea, and vomiting
Mouth dryness, blurred vision, constipation and other GI disturbances; male genitourinary disturbances, including difficulty in micturition, delayed ejaculation, or impotence; localized sweating

Central side-effects
Euphoria sometimes leading to hypomanic and manic behavior; hyperactivity and hyper-reflexia; confusion, agitation, hallucinations, delirium; muscular twitching and tremors, and convulsive seizures

Hypersensitivity and other reactions
Skin reactions, including flushing, photosensitivity, and rashes; edema and weight gain

Summary of drugs that may interact adversely with monoamine oxidase inhibitor drugs

Other MAO inhibitor drugs, including agents *not* employed as antidepressants: for example, pargyline (Eutonyl) and furazolidone (Furoxone)
Tricyclic-type antidepressants and other dibenzazepine derivatives employed for other purposes: for example, carbamezepine (Tegretol) and cyclobenzaprine (Flexeril)

Potent narcotic analgesics such as meperidine (Demerol) and morphine; also, possibly, codeine and dextromethorphan
Other central depressant drugs such as alcohol, barbiturates, and general anesthetics
Sympathomimetic (adrenergic) drugs such as amphetamine, ephedrine; also cocaine and caffeine

Other drugs that affect catecholamine metabolism, including methyldopa and levodopa
Insulin and oral hypoglycemic agents
Antihypertensive drugs, including thiazide-type diuretics and guanethidine (Ismelin)

Antiparkinsonism drugs with central anticholinergic activity, including benztropine (Cogentin)

Drug digests

Amitriptyline HCl USP (Elavil)

Actions and indications. This antidepressant drug has a tranquilizing component that is claimed to make it particularly effective in cases of depression marked by anxiety and agitation. It also often brings about gradual improvement in such target symptoms of depressive syndromes as anorexia, insomnia, physical complaints including headache, and psychomotor retardation. It has been used with varying degrees of benefit in such types of depression as the depressed phase of the manic–depressive psychosis; involutional melancholia; certain reactive, neurotic, and schizoaffective depressions.

Adverse effects, cautions, and contraindications. Adverse reactions are the result of the drug's effects on central and autonomic nervous system activity. The drug's atropinelike (anticholinergic) effects include dry mouth, blurred vision, constipation, and urinary retention. Thus, it is contraindicated in glaucoma and in men with an enlrged prostate or other conditions that can lead to dysuria. Tachycardia, dizziness, faintness, and orthostatic hypotension may occur, and precautions are required against injury in falling.

The earliest central effect is drowsiness and impaired alertness, so patients are warned not to drive. Drinking alcoholic beverages is avoided, because this drug potentiates the depressant effects of alcohol. Later in therapy signs of central psychological and motor excitement may develop. These include jitteriness, confusion, tremors, and incoordination. Occasionally convulsive seizures, mania, and symptoms of schizophrenia may develop. These can be controlled by raising the dosage of anticonvulsant drugs in epileptics and by adding phenothiazines to the regimen of schizoaffective patients.

Dosage and administration. Most patients respond to oral doses of 25 mg tid. Some require intramuscular injections of 20 to 30 mg qid for the first 2 weeks. Most are maintained on oral doses of 25 mg bid to qid. Some need as little as 10 mg qid. Although most patients rarely need doses of over 150 mg daily, a few hospitalized patients may require up to 300 mg daily for therapeutic effects.

The drug is ordinarily not administered to patients who have been receiving MAO inhibitor-type antidepressants until about 2 weeks after the latter have been discontinued.

Imipramine HCl USP (Tofranil)

Actions and indications. This prototype antidepressant drug of the tricyclic class is particularly effective in endogenous depressions marked by psychomotor retardation. However, it is also often effective in other types of depression and against other target symptoms, including loss of appetite, insomnia, apathy, feelings of sadness and despair, headache, and other hypochondriacal or psychosomatic complaints. Patients with involutional melancholia or in the depressed phase of the manic–depressive psychosis respond more consistently than do those with depressions that are secondary to neurologic or psychiatric disorders, such as parkinsonism or schizophrenia.

Adverse effects, cautions, and contraindications. Adverse reactions are mainly the result of autonomic blockade and stimulation of certain groups of neurons in the CNS. Central excitation may be marked by agitation, disorientation, confusion, hallucinations, and hypomanic or schizophrenic reactions that require dosage reduction or discontinuation and the addition of antipsychotic-type tranquilizers. Motor signs may range from mild tremors to muscular incoordination, or even convulsions, particularly in cases of massive overdosage. (Extreme caution is required in patients with a history of convulsive seizures.)

Caution is also required in patients with glaucoma because of the drug's anticholinergic blocking effects on the ocular muscles of accommodation. Its possible effects on cardiovascular function, such as cardiac arrhythmias and orthostatic hypotension, require caution in patients with a history of heart disease and strokes. (It is contraindicated in patients with a history of recent myocardial infarction.)

Dosage and administration. Dosage is highly individualized, depending on the severity of the patient's illness and response to therapy. Patients who are hospitalized are often started on intramuscular doses of 100 mg. Oral doses are added every few days to a total of 200 mg. If required, a combination of intramuscular and oral doses totaling 300 mg daily may be reached after several weeks. In patients who respond, dosage is gradually reduced to the minimal amounts that remain effective. These levels may be maintained for months. Elderly patients and adolescents are started on and kept on lower doses (*e.g.*, 30 to 40 mg daily at first, then raised to no more than 100 mg daily).

Isocarboxazid USP (Marplan)

Actions and indications. This is an antidepressant drug that acts as an inhibitor of the enzyme monoamine oxidase in neurons and other cells. It is effective when administered alone or in conjunction with electroshock therapy of patients with moderate to severe depression. Among depressive states benefited are involutional and manic–depressive psychosis (depressive phase), as well as depressions developing secondarily to chronic physical and psychic illness.

Adverse effects, cautions, and contraindications. Although this drug is a hydrazine derivative and thus requires checks on liver function, jaundice has rarely developed. If this or laboratory test abnormalities appear, the drug is discontinued. Patients with poor hepatic and renal function are not ordinarily treated with this drug.

Orthostatic *hypo*tension is the most common side-effect. It may lead to dizziness and falling or to cardiac irregularities. Thus, the drug is contraindicated in patients with congestive heart failure. *Hyper*tensive crises may be set off if certain drugs (*e.g.*, sympathomimetic amines) or foods (*e.g.*, cheese, chicken livers), and beverages (*e.g.*, wine, beer) are ingested. This can cause severe headache and possibly fatal intracranial bleeding, particularly in elderly patients with cerebrovascular disease. This drug is contraindicated in patients with pheochromocytoma, a condition often marked by episodes of hypertension and tachycardia.

Central stimulation may cause excessive activity, hyperreflexia, tremors, muscle twitching and occasionally convulsions. Patients may become confused, jittery and hypomanic and, rarely, have hallucinations. This requires reduction of dosage or discontinuation of the drug.

Dosage and administration. Most patients are started on an oral dose of 30 mg daily, but this is adjusted in accordance with the patient's response. Because the drug's effects are cumulative, the dose is customarily reduced once a favorable response has developed (usually within 3 or 4 weeks). Patients are then maintained at a minimally effective dose—usually, 10 to 20 mg daily.

Lithium carbonate (Eskalith; Lithane; Lithonate)

Actions and indications. This lithium salt is specific for the control of acute manic episodes in patients with the manic–depressive psychosis. Its continued use may also be effective for preventing recurrences of the manic phase of this disorder, and for reducing the length and severity of any such episodes. The drug is not considered useful for control of mania or catatonic excitement in schizophrenia. It may be effective for preventing episodes of depression in bipolar affective disorders and in some subgroups of patients with unipolar depression.

Adverse effects, cautions, and contraindications. Adverse effects of various types occur as the serum level of lithium rises above the therapeutic range. Consequently, laboratory facilities should be available for frequent checks of serum lithium levels following the start of treatment and for periodic monitoring during prolonged maintenance therapy.

Early side-effects include mild nausea and thirst (which are transient) and a fine tremor that may continue even at lower doses. More serious when they develop during long-term treatment are such early signs of lithium toxicity as drowsiness, muscle weakness and incoordination, vomiting, and diarrhea. Patients and their families are taught to discontinue the drug and to report such signs to the doctor, who will then have the serum lithium level checked.

Severe toxic symptoms occur most commonly in patients with heart and kidney diseases who are being treated with sodium-eliminating diuretics. Thus, use of lithium is contraindicated in patients with cardiovascular or renal disease, particularly if their condition requires sodium restriction or diuretic therapy.

Severe toxicity is characterized by neuromuscular signs such as tremor, twitching, hyperreflexia, and clonic spasms; central stimulation marked by restlessness, confusion, and convulsive seizures, followed by stupor or coma; cardiovascular effects including cardiac arrhythmias and circulatory collapse.

Dosage and administration. Oral doses of 600 mg tid are employed to attain control of mania with serum lithium levels ranging from 0.5 to 1.5 mEq/liter. Later, dosage is reduced to 300 mg tid to maintain a level of 0.5 to 1.0 mEq/liter.

Tranylcypromine sulfate USP (Parnate)

Actions and indications. This antidepressant, which acts by inhibiting the enzyme monoamine oxidase, is ordinarily reserved for patients hospitalized with severe endogenous depressions who have failed to respond to other drugs and in whom electroconvulsive therapy is contraindicated.

The drug's energizing effects are sometimes unusually rapid in onset, but this may tend to increase anxiety in patients with agitated depressions. Thus, if used at all in such cases, this drug is combined with a tranquilizer of the phenothiazine type.

Adverse effects, cautions, and contraindications. Blood pressure is checked frequently, because postural hypotension is common early in therapy. More important, however, is the hazard of hypertensive crisis, because it can lead to fatal intracranial bleeding. Thus, this drug is contraindicated in patients thought to have sclerotic cerebral blood vessels, including people over 60 years old. Patients with cardiovascular disease or hypertension—particularly that resulting from pheochromocytoma—should also not receive this drug.

Patients are told to report the occurrence of frequent headaches, because occipital headache may be a sign that the drug should be discontinued. Patients are also warned not to medicate themselves with cold and hay fever remedies or with weight-reducing preparations, because these may contain pressure-raising sympathomimetic amines. Other drugs that are not ordinarily ordered for these patients include narcotic analgesics, antihypertensive agents, and antiparkinsonism drugs.

Patients should not drink alcoholic beverages or eat certain foods that have a high content of the catecholamine tyramine. These include varieties of strong or aged cheese, chicken livers, pickled herring, and canned figs.

Dosage and administration. Patients are started on oral doses of 20 mg daily for 2 weeks. This may then be raised to 30 mg daily by increasing the morning dose from 10 mg to 20 mg while keeping the afternoon dose at 10 mg. If the patient responds to treatment, dosage may be reduced to maintenance levels of 20 mg or even only 10 mg daily.

References

Baldessarini RJ: Schizophrenia. N Engl J Med 297:988, 1977

Baldessarini RJ: Drugs and the treatment of psychiatric disorders. In Gilman AG, Goodman LS, Gilman A (eds): Goodman & Gilman's The Pharmacological Basis of Therapeutics, 6th ed, pp 391–447. New York, Macmillan, 1980

Burks JS et al: Tricyclic antidepressant poisoning. JAMA 230:1405, 1974

DeGennaro MD et al: Antidepressant drug therapy. Am J Nurs 81:1304, 1981

Drugs for psychiatric disorders. Med Lett Drugs Ther 25:45, 1983

Fink M: Convulsive and drug therapies of depression. Ann Rev Med 32:405, 1981

Gallant DM, Simpson GM: Depression: Behavioral, Biochemical, Diagnostic, and Treatment Concepts. Spectrum Publications, 1976

Harris E: Antidepressants: Old drugs, new uses. Am J Nurs 81:1308, 1981

Harris E: Antipsychotic medications. Am J Nurs 81:1316, 1981

Harris E: Extrapyramidal side-effects of antipsychotic medications. Am J Nurs 81:1324, 1981

Harris E: Lithium. Am J Nurs 81:1310, 1981

Hollister LE: Current antidepressant drugs: Clinical use. Drugs 22:129, 1981

King DJ: Drug management of depression. Ir Med J 76:44, 1983

Rivera–Calimlim L, Hershey L: Neuroleptic concentrations and clinical response. Ann Rev Pharmacol Toxicol 24:361, 1984

Rodman MJ: Pathways to the cure of mental depression. RN 40:73, 1977

Rodman MJ: Controlling acute and chronic schizophrenia. RN 41:75, 1978

Rosal–Greif VL: Drug-induced dyskinesias. Am J Nurs 82:66, 1982

Snyder SH: Dopamine receptors, neuroleptics, and schizophrenia. Am J Psychiatr 138:460, 1981

Tosteson DC: Lithium and mania. Sci Am 239:164, 1981

Van Der Velde CD: Effectiveness of loxapine succinate in acute schizophrenia. Curr Ther Res 17:1, 1975

Van Praag HM: Depression. Lancet 2:1259, 1982

Chapter 47

Psychomotor and other stimulants of the central nervous system

47

Many natural and synthetic substances can stimulate the central nervous system (CNS). As indicated in Chapter 44, these drugs act by upsetting the delicate balance between the various excitatory and inhibitory neurons that continually influence the state of CNS excitability. Some drugs act by increasing the rate at which nerve cells send out impulses that excite other neurons. Other CNS stimulants are now known to act by blocking inhibitory transmitter substances. Such interference with the transmission of inhibitory nerve impulses, of course, causes the excitatory influences on various parts of the CNS to predominate.

Only a relatively few central stimulants have clinical applications compared to the large number of CNS depressant drugs that are in therapeutic use. The main reason for this is that these drugs are relatively lacking in *specificity*. That is, it is difficult to administer these drugs in doses that act selectively at the specific central target sites that it would be therapeutically desirable to stimulate. Thus, some stimulants can produce a desirable increase in the activity of the depressed respiratory center; however, at the doses that do so, the drugs may, at the same time, overstimulate other groups of motor nerve cells and thus cause harmful effects such as convulsive muscle spasms.

Other reasons for the limited usefulness of the CNS stimulants include the following:

1. Some produce undesirable *peripheral* effects at the doses needed to bring about the desired central actions.
2. Some can be *abused* in ways that result in development of dependence and addiction (Chap. 53).

Types of CNS stimulants

Drugs that increase the excitability of the CNS are commonly grouped on the basis of their *primary* sites of action and on their clinically significant pharmacologic effects (Table 47-1):

1. Cerebral, or psychomotor, stimulants
2. Brain stem stimulants, or analeptics
3. Spinal stimulants, or convulsants

Actually, however, this classification may give the misleading impression that these drugs possess more selectivity of action than they actually have. Although small doses of these drugs may stimulate some neurons before they affect others, their actions tend to spread swiftly to nearby, and even distant, parts of the neuraxis. Thus, for example, the drugs that are arbitrarily classified as psychomotor stimulants, such as the amphetamines and caffeine, can also stimulate the brain stem respiratory and vasomotor systems, thus exerting an analeptic action.

In addition, these so-called cerebral stimulants do not actually act on the cerebral cortex directly. They increase cerebral activity by stimulating subcortical sites such as the reticular activating system (Chap. 44). It is the increased number of impulses that then pass upward from this lower reticular arousal level that causes activation of cerebral cortical functions. Also, as indicated above, the *peripheral* actions of these drugs affect the total response of the patient. Thus the amphetamines, for example, affect the functioning of the heart and blood vessels, because they act not only centrally but also on α- and β-adrenergic receptors located in these organs (Chap. 13). In fact, the effects of *ephedrine*, a drug with central

Table 47–1. Central nervous system stimulants

Official or generic name	Trade name	Usual adult dosage and administration
Psychomotor (cerebral) stimulants		
Amphetamines		
Amphetamine complex	Biphetamine	One capsule containing appropriate predetermined dose/day for obesity or attention deficits
Amphetamine sulfate USP	Benzedrine	5–60 mg/day in divided doses; dose depends on use
Dextroamphetamine sulfate USP	Dexedrine	5–60 mg/day in divided doses; dose depends on use
Methamphetamine HCl USP (desoxyephedrine HCl)	Desoxyn; Methampex	5 mg before each meal for obesity; 5–20 mg/day for attention deficits
Nonamphetamines		
Caffeine USP	—	100–200 mg q, 4 hr
Caffeine and sodium benzoate USP	—	500 mg IM or SC
Citrated caffeine USP	—	60–120 mg
Methylphenidate HCl USP	Ritalin	10 mg bid or tid
Pemoline	Cylert	37.5–75 mg once daily
Analeptic agents (brain stem stimulants)		
Doxapram HCl USP	Dopram	0.5–1.5 mg/kg, IV
Nikethamide	Coramine	2–5 ml of a 25% solution, IM or IV (use governs dose)

stimulating activity, are so predominantly peripheral that it is not discussed in this chapter at all. (This drug was described in Chapter 17, Adrenergic, or sympathomimetic drugs.) When this drug is being used to produce clinically desirable peripheral actions, its central action is considered only as a cause of undesirable side-effects.

Psychomotor stimulants

Caffeine

This alkaloid, which is found in coffee beans, tea leaves, and kola nuts, produces mild mental stimulation and helps to overcome drowsiness and feelings of fatigue. These alerting and antidepressant actions probably account for the popularity of caffeine-containing beverages, and they play an important part in the few therapeutic applications of caffeine[+] in medical practice.

Chemically, caffeine is a derivative of xanthine and, like such other methylxanthines as *theophylline* (Chap. 40) and *theobromine*, it has peripheral as well as central effects. Caffeine can, for example, increase the heart rate, cause diuresis, and produce a prolonged increase in secretion of stomach acid. It also relaxes smooth muscle in most areas, including the vasculature, but is much less potent than theophylline in this respect and, unlike the latter related drug, caffeine is not clinically useful for overcoming bronchospasm in asthma.

Mechanisms of action. Caffeine, like the other methylxanthines, inhibits the enzyme phosphodiesterase, which metabolizes cyclic adenosine monophosphate (cAMP), and thus promotes the accumulation of this intracellular second messenger (see Chap. 13). It also increases the calcium permeability of sarcoplasmic reticulum; this effect may account for its skeletal muscle stimulatory ability.

Central effects

Caffeine can stimulate all parts of the CNS. However, the amounts ingested during ordinary drinking of the beverages containing it affect mainly the mental functions of the cerebral cortex. The effects of drinking coffee and tea have been extensively studied by psychologists. They have shown that small doses of caffeine increase the ability to maintain intellectual effort in the face of weariness.

This is probably the result of the psychological effect of caffeine in counteracting fatigue, boredom, and drowsiness. Although people seem somewhat more alert to sensory stimuli and react more rapidly and with a freer flow of ideas, it is doubtful that caffeine improves learning ability and memory. Caffeine-induced tremors may actually interfere with the efficiency of motor performance requiring coordinated muscular activity.

Moderate doses of caffeine can cause discomfort marked by restlessness, irritability and, in those who have not developed tolerance to it, sleeplessness. Higher doses—or even small doses in caffeine-sensitive persons—can cause ocular and auditory nerve disturbances such as flashes of light in the visual field and ringing in the ears. Often, chronically overdosed patients may be misdiagnosed as suffering from an anxiety reaction because of their nervousness, agitation, and rapid breathing and heart rates.

The coffee habit. Coffee is, of course, drunk in enormous quantities in this country. It is estimated that Americans annually consume about 2.5 billion pounds. However, it is hard to think of this dietary beverage as the cause of a "drug habit" and, indeed, for most people the degree of habituation, or psychological dependence, is so mild as to constitute no real problem. On the other hand, the adverse effects of overindulgence may be more common than is generally suspected. People who habitually drink too much coffee may suffer from cardiac irregularities and gastrointestinal upset, as well as restlessness. There is also evidence that they may often be irritable and have headaches when forced to go without their usual amounts of coffee.

Some research results suggest that people who regularly drink five or six cups of coffee a day—an intake of 500 to 800 mg of caffeine—may have twice as high a risk of suffering a heart attack. Other studies have shown no direct link between coffee drinking and myocardial infarction in people with no prior history of coronary heart disease. However, those who have already had a heart attack should limit their intake of caffeine, because in large amounts it can cause cardiac arrhythmias. If they find it stressful to give up the coffee habit, they should, at least, use decaffeinated coffee (2 to 4 mg per cup), instead of brewed coffee (100 to 150 mg per cup), or instant coffee (85 to 100 mg per cup). People with an active peptic ulcer should also not drink regular coffee, and even the decaffeinated type is best taken well diluted with cream.

Patients should be questioned about their coffee drinking patterns—the same applies to their intake of tea, cola drinks, and caffeine-containing headache remedies—before being put on tranquilizers for treating anxiety (Chap. 45). What appears to be anxiety may actually be caused by excessive intake of caffeine, and the symptoms should be relieved by removing that stimulant drug from the patient's diet rather than by giving a depressant drug.

Recent research by the FDA has shown that caffeine is teratogenic in rats. Although there is no evidence that this is true in humans, the FDA has suggested that pregnant women be advised to limit their consumption of coffee and other caffeine-containing beverages. Another recent research report implies that people who drink coffee, including decaffeinated coffee, may have a higher incidence of pancreatic cancer than those who do not.

Coffee and fatigue. The type of physical fatigue that ordinarily forces us to stop working is actually a warning signal intended to prevent us from unwisely using up our energy reserves. Fatigue is also often emotional in origin. That is, anxiety and tension, or feelings of futility, boredom, and aimlessness, may be the most significant source of habitual weariness. However, when chronic fatigue is fundamentally psychosomatic in nature, it will not be allayed by an endless round of coffee drinking or by taking tablets or capsules of caffeine or of the amphetamines. Drugs such as caffeine and amphetamine make it easy to ignore the sensation of tiredness but do nothing to replenish low energy stores. Thus, their habitual use may set up a vicious cycle marked by the various adverse effects mentioned above superimposed on those of physical exhaustion.

Therapeutic uses

Antidepressant. Caffeine is often the main, or sole, ingredient of various proprietary products that are promoted for allaying drowsiness. It seems wasteful for people to purchase such preparations for preventing themselves from dozing, when they can get at least as much caffeine in a cup of coffee. Unless someone is sensitive to the volatile oils in coffee or to the tannins in tea, it would seem more sensible to drink one of these beverages (while taking a break from work or driving) rather than to buy caffeine in tablet or capsule form promoted as a "no dozing" product.

People who have been drinking alcoholic beverages are sometimes urged to drink a cup of coffee before attempting to drive. The rationale for this advice is that the effects of the stimulant, caffeine, will counteract those of the depressant, alcohol. Although the advice to make the "one for the road" coffee instead of alcohol is well intentioned, it is probably unwise. Coffee is unlikely to sober an unfit driver sufficiently to make it safe for him to operate a motor vehicle. He might better be urged not to drive at all until the effects of the alcohol have entirely dissipated.

Caffeine has, however, been used in the treatment of acute alcoholic intoxication to stimulate the patient's depressed respiration and to speed arousal. *Caffeine sodium benzoate* is sometimes administered intramuscularly for this purpose.

Caffeine and headache. Caffeine is a common

ingredient of headache remedy products in which it is combined with aspirin and other mild analgesics (Chap. 37). It is usually present in a dose of only about 30 mg. Thus, even a two-tablet dose contains only about half the amount of caffeine in a cup of coffee. It is doubtful whether such small amounts taken orally have any pain-relieving property that adds to the effectiveness of the analgesics in such combination products. However, people who are heavy coffee drinkers and whose headaches when they are trying to taper off may be a symptom of a sort of caffeine withdrawal syndrome (see above) may obtain some added relief from the presence of caffeine in such products.

Caffeine is also often combined with ergotamine in products used in the management of migraine and other vascular headaches (Chap. 38). Here, caffeine—administered in doses of 100 mg per tablet—may, when several tablets are taken, add its relatively slight constricting action to the powerful vasoconstrictor effect of ergotamine on the dilated cranial and extracranial blood vessels. This is said to help relieve throbbing headaches by reducing blood flow through painfully pulsating cerebral and scalp blood vessels, and the same action may account for the relief of hypertensive headache when caffeine sodium benzoate is occasionally injected into a vein of a person with high blood pressure.

Neonatal apnea. Like theophylline, another methylxanthine, caffeine is used unofficially in the treatment of neonatal apnea. An initial dose of 10 mg caffeine/kg is followed by maintenance doses of 2.5 mg/kg/day.

The amphetamines

The drugs of this chemical class were first synthesized in a search for safer sympathomimetic drugs (Chap. 17). Scientists attempting to discover a synthetic substitute for the natural vasoconstrictor adrenergic drug ephedrine developed a series of related compounds that included amphetamine (Benzedrine), dextroamphetamine+ (Dexedrine), and methamphetamine (desoxyephedrine; Desoxyn). When these drugs were tested in laboratory animals and clinically, their peripheral effects on blood vessels and on bronchial smooth muscles turned out to be less powerful than their stimulating effect on the CNS.

This was first seen when amphetamine tended to rouse anesthetized animals to which it was administered in laboratory experiments. Later, when amphetamine was tried out clinically in nose drops for shrinking swollen nasal tissues, patients complained that, although the test product worked well enough, they had trouble falling asleep when they used the drops at night. A final indication of the central activity of these drugs was the discovery that some prison inmates and other people were removing the drug-impregnated paper from nasal inhalers and chewing it in order to get ''high''—that is, for the euphoria induced by the drug's central effects (see Chap. 53).

Pharmacologic effects

All the amphetamines possess certain psychopharmacologic effects that account for most of their therapeutic applications. All also act peripherally to bring about effects that are usually considered undesirable. The physician tries to choose the safest drug and to administer it in the minimal dose that will produce the desired primary effects on the CNS without overstimulating it and without causing discomforting cardiovascular or other peripheral side-effects.

Psychopharmacologic effects of two types form the basis for the various clinical uses of these drugs and for most of the central side-effects that are seen when they are taken in excessive amounts. One of these effects is an *increase in alertness and wakefulness.* The other is manifested by a *mood-elevating,* or *euphorigenic,* effect. Both effects are dose-related, in the sense that they become progressively more marked as the dosage is raised. Each of these actions will be described in further detail. However, it should be remembered that, with drugs that exert psychopharmacologic effects, the nature of a particular patient's response depends in large part upon his underlying personality, his mental state at the time the drug is taken, and the setting, or circumstances, in which the drug is taken.

The increase in alertness produced by small doses of amphetamines is believed, on the basis of electroencephalographic (EEG) evidence, to stem from the stimulating action on the reticular activating system (RAS). The evidence that appears on the EEG record of increased activity at this subcortical site manifests itself clinically in signs of stimulation of certain cerebral cortical functions. Thus, a person who might expect to feel sleepy and fatigued sometimes feels wakeful and willing to keep on working because he does not feel at all tired. If engaged in intellectual activity, ideas may seem to come more freely, and these thoughts may be expressed with more than ordinary ease. Some types of athletic performances are also reported to be improved by small doses of amphetamines.

The euphoric, or mood-elevating, effect is also one that is best elicited by doses so small that the patient hardly realizes that the feeling of well being is drug-induced. That is, these drugs are acting desirably when they gently evoke favorable attitudes toward tasks that need to be done, bring about an increase in a depressed and apathetic patient's self-confidence and initiative, and foster in the somewhat withdrawn person a tendency to become more outgoing in human relationships. The extension of this action to a point at which the patient feels excessively elated and so sanguine about his abilities and prospects that he gets grandiose ideas and expresses them with great garrulity is undesirable.

Adverse central effects. As the dose of these drugs is raised, the mild alerting and fatigue-fighting effect is replaced by less desirable signs of excessive cortical activity. The patient may become aware of an inner tension or irritability that is somewhat discomforting. He may find himself restless, nervous, and "jittery"—a term that he uses to describe his awareness of tremulousness caused by muscular as well as emotional tension. His earlier increased ability to concentrate and to express himself may give way to easy distractibility and to a sense of confusion. Thus, although he may be even more talkative than before, his increased loquacity may be marked by a flight of ideas that do not quite make good sense.

As indicated in detail in Chapter 53, the abuser of amphetamines becomes increasingly confused and hyperactive or hypomanic (see also the summary of signs and symptoms of manic syndromes, Chap. 46). With continued abuse of amphetamine-type drugs, their adverse effects on brain function are seen first in signs of marked agitation and apprehension and later in states of panic that may end in a toxic psychosis marked by delirium and visual and auditory hallucinations that elicit paranoid delusions.

Adverse peripheral effects. Cardiac arrhythmias, an increase in heart rate, and elevation of systolic and diastolic blood pressures are the most serious peripheral effects of overdosage or even of ordinary doses in hypersusceptible patients. Thus, caution is required in patients with even mild hypertension, and these drugs are contraindicated in those with severe hypertension. The therapeutically desired hypotensive effect of *guanethidine* (Chap. 28) in patients with moderate hypertension may be antagonized if they also receive amphetamines as part of a weight-reducing program.

Although a drug-induced loss of appetite is one of the effects of the amphetamines sometimes sought clinically, such anorexia with consequent loss of weight is undesirable when these drugs are being employed for other purposes, particularly in children. These drugs may dry the mouth and cause an unpleasant taste. Constipation and occasionally diarrhea may develop. The person's pupils may become widely dilated—a fact that makes these drugs contraindicated in patients with glaucoma.

Clinical indications

The alerting and mood-elevating effects of the amphetamines account for the former uses of these drugs in neurology, psychiatry, and general medicine. However, there is now public and professional concern with the abuse of these drugs, which has resulted in measures that have sharply limited their legitimate medical use.

The amphetamines are currently indicated mainly in the management of *hyperactivity* in children, in a relatively rare neurologic disorder called *narcolepsy,* as adjuncts to antiepileptic drugs to prevent excessive drowsiness, and as an adjunct to low-calorie diets for *obesity* (see the Summary of clinical indications at the end of this chapter). Some authorities are at present even pressing for the elimination of the last indication for these drugs.

The detailed discussion of the neuropsychiatric uses of the amphetamines, will be taken up after certain

other psychomotor stimulants that are used for the same purposes have been described. At this point, discussion of the clinical uses of the amphetamines will be limited to aspects of their current status in the management of obesity.

Obesity. These drugs tend, temporarily, at least, to lessen the patient's desire to eat. The exact way in which the amphetamines exert this so-called anorexigenic or anorectic action is disputed, but there seems no doubt that the appetite suppression that they produce is mainly central in origin (probably due to effects on the lateral hypothalamic feeding center and on the ventromedial satiety center) rather than the result of their peripheral effects on the gastrointestinal tract or of their effects on metabolism. Many authorities feel that the anorectic effect of the amphetamines is related, at least in part, to their mood-elevating action. That is, these drugs are thought to help people stick to a low-calorie diet, despite its discomforts, by making them feel better emotionally. These effects are probably related to the ability of amphetamines to release norepinephrine and dopamine from neurons in central pathways (including those in the hypothalamus) that use these neurotransmitters.

The usefulness of this psychopharmacologic effect is limited at best. Most patients soon tend to develop tolerance to the psychological lift that the amphetamines offer at first. If this happens after 4 to 8 weeks it is not advisable to raise the dose, because this may cause cardiovascular side-effects and lead to abuse by addiction-prone patients. Instead, it is best that the medication be discontinued for a few weeks. If drug treatment is then still indicated, it can be begun again following loss of tolerance during the period of abstinence.

Related sympathomimetic anorectics. The disadvantages and limitations of the older amphetamine drugs led to efforts to find safer and more effective appetite suppressants. The claims made for most of these drugs are that they cause fewer adverse central, cardiovascular, and gastrointestinal effects than the original amphetamines, and that they are less prone to be abused (Table 47-2). In general, however, these drugs share the same drawbacks as the amphetamines and require the same precautions if adverse effects are to be avoided.

Phenmetrazine (Preludin), for example, is quite capable of being abused to the point of psychological dependence by those who are prone to abuse psychomotor stimulants. Even the more recently introduced anorectics, such as *phendimetrazine, phentermine,* and *mazindol,* cause central and peripheral side-effects similar to those of the amphetamines. Thus, their use requires caution in hypertensive patients and in patients whose history suggests that they might abuse these drugs. These chemical and pharmacologic relatives of the amphetamines are also contraindicated in patients with severe hypertension, cardiac arrhythmias, and glaucoma.

One of the newer anorectic drugs, *fenfluramine* (Pondimin), differs from the others in producing central

Table 47–2. Anorexiant agents

Official or generic name	Trade name	Usual adult dosage
Amphetamines (see Table 47-1)		
Other sympathomimetic amines		
Benzphetamine HCl	Didrex	25–50 mg one to three times daily
Diethylpropion HCl USP	Tenuate; Tepanil	25 mg tid
Fenfluramine HCl	Pondimin	20 mg tid
Mazindol	Mazanor; Sanorex	1–2 mg one to three times daily
Phendimetrazine tartrate	Bontril; Plegine	17.5–70 mg bid or tid
Phenmetrazine HCl USP	Preludin	25 mg bid or tid
Phentermine HCl	—	8 mg tid

depression rather than stimulation. This sedative effect may make it more useful than the amphetamines for patients with the so-called "night eating syndrome," who have insomnia and tend to eat heavily late at night. On the other hand, drowsiness is a more common side-effect with this compound, and it has not yet been proved to be free of drug abuse potential or to be any more effective than the other drugs of this class when used for more than a few weeks.

Phenylpropanolamine, a sympathomimetic drug that is used as a nasal decongestant, is also available in several OTC preparations promoted as appetite suppressants (Acutrim, Dexatrim). Studies have found weight loss with this drug to be slight and maintained only for the duration of drug use. Patients using this drug have experienced the expected spectrum of adverse effects of a combined α- and β-adrenergic agonist (Chap. 17), as well as psychoses. Patients using this drug as an aid to weight loss should be appropriately warned.

A new narcotic antagonist (Chap. 51) is claimed to have anorectic properties, and is being investigated for this use as well as for use in rehabilitating those who habitually abuse narcotic analgesics. This drug, *naltrexone,* should be free of the major drawbacks of the currently available anorectics and, if proven effective and safe in other respects, could be of major importance in the treatment of obesity.

Other psychomotor stimulants

Methylphenidate[+] (Ritalin) is chemically related to the am-

phetamines and has similar pharmacologic properties and therapeutic uses, except that it is not promoted for use in obesity even though weight loss does occur. Many physicians favor this drug over dextroamphetamine for treating behavioral disorders in children, but there is no clear proof of its superiority in such cases. Drug interactions leading to adverse effects may occur if this drug is administered to depressed patients who are also receiving antidepressants of the monoamine oxidase (MAO) inhibitor or tricyclic types (Chap. 46), among other drugs. Because this drug may interfere with the metabolic breakdown of coumarin-type anticoagulants (Chap. 34), patients should have their prothrombin time checked periodically to determine whether a reduction in anticoagulant drug dosage is warranted.

Pemoline (Cylert) is a central stimulant that is chemically and pharmacologically different from the amphetamines and methylphenidate. It may act on central dopaminergic pathways. In ordinary doses, this drug does not cause cardiovascular side-effects. However, liver test abnormalities have been noted in some children taking the drug for several months for management of hyperkinetic syndrome or of minimal brain dysfunction (see below), which are the only clinical indications for this drug. Clinical improvement of hyperactivity in children with this condition is gradual, and is usually not noted until the third or fourth week of treatment.

Neuropsychiatric uses

Hyperactivity in children

Millions of American schoolchildren—an estimated 5% to 10%—show symptoms of a behavioral disorder that keeps them in trouble in the classroom from the time they enter the first grade until adolescence. This condition, which is called by several names, including *hyperkinetic reaction* or *syndrome* and *minimal brain dysfunction* (MBD), is characterized by persistent hyperactivity and such other signs as easy distractibility or inattentiveness, excessive restlessness, and a tendency to act impulsively.

Actually, these children are not necessarily any more active than normal children. Their difficulty is that they become unusually restless in situations that require them to sit still—for example, in a classroom, in church, or at the dinner table. This may be because the brain's nerve pathways that exert inhibitory control over motor activity are relatively immature. The exact cause of this dysfunction is not known, but the vast majority of children with a hyperactive behavioral pattern have no detectable areas of brain damage despite some slight EEG abnormalities.

Hyperactive children are a trial to their teachers, parents, siblings, and other children. Although they are usually of average intelligence, they perform poorly in school because of their inability to pay attention and to work at any task for a long enough period to complete it. Some children also suffer from neurologic deficits that impair their auditory and visual perceptions, which lead to additional learning disabilities. As a result of their poor performance in school and their interpersonal conflicts, some children suffer from secondary emotional disorders—depression, for example—or develop antisocial personality traits. These lead to adjustment difficulties as young adults, even after their early hyperactivity has stopped.

Stimulant drug therapy. Almost 2% of all elementary schoolchildren—several hundred thousand—are under treatment with such psychomotor stimulants as *methylphenidate* (Ritalin) and *dextroamphetamine* (Dexedrine). Parents and educators have expressed concern about such widespread use of drugs similar to those "uppers" that are commonly abused by several segments of the adult population (Chap. 53). Some have suggested that these drugs are possibly being used to keep children under control for the convenience of their teachers and parents, with possible harm to the children themselves. The nurse must often discuss the advantages and limitations of this form of treatment with concerned parents.

Status of stimulant therapy. Drug treatment should be employed only after a child has been carefully studied to diagnose the exact nature of the disorder. This is because not all children need drug therapy, and some may even be made worse when they receive stimulants. Although some parents who are seeking quick and relatively inexpensive solutions may put pressure on their physicians to prescribe these drugs, they should be tried only after the child's condition has not improved despite special educational measures and psychological therapy.

Published reports of the results of studies with stimulant drugs indicate that this treatment controls hyperactivity in about 70% of patients with the hyperkinetic syndrome or minimal brain dysfunction. Often, dramatic improvement is noted on the very first day of treatment. The child's teacher may report a marked reduction in the usual restlessness and an increase in attentiveness. The child does not appear drowsy or sedated. Instead, there seems to be a greater ability to channel normal activity into constructive learning tasks.

Stimulants alone do not, however, always produce complete remission of all symptoms of the hyperkinetic syndrome. They do not, for example, counteract emotional depression or benefit other aspects of the child's behavior that are of emotional origin rather than the result of neurologic immaturity. Thus, although these stimulants tend to lessen the child's overactivity and distractibility, other measures, to which these drugs are only an adjunct, must also be employed. These include psychotherapy, social measures, and—if the child has fallen far behind in school or continues to have learning problems—special remedial education.

Misconceptions. The nurse is often called on to counsel parents who have erroneous notions about these drugs. Occasionally, some tend to overmedicate their children because they cannot tolerate any restlessness at all. It may be useful to suggest to such parents that they adjust to the child's behavior to some degree, and that they should certainly not exceed the prescribed dosage or give the drug at unscheduled times. More commonly, parents are unnecessarily fearful of continuing this medication. They should be assured that these drugs do not create a craving or psychological dependence in children that will later lead to their becoming drug abusers in adolescence. They may be told that these drugs are not "narcotics" and that, although the drugs cause behavioral quieting or calming, they do not depress the child's central nervous system or leave him lethargic or "spaced out."

Mechanism of Action. The exact way in which these stimulant drugs paradoxically reduce hyperactivity is still uncertain. However, a current hypothesis is that they act by increasing the activity of the RAS, which may be underaroused in these neurologically immature children. This subcortical center then sends more impulses up to cerebral cortical inhibitory areas. The child's brain then gains control over the excessive motor and sensory system activity that produces restlessness and distractibility. This results *not* in any *decrease* in total activity but in an actual *increase* in the type of controlled and directed activity that leads to improved learning performance. Thus, in terms of their neuropharmacologic effects, these drugs do not really act paradoxically in these children; rather, they act in the same way that they do in adults.

Side-effects. Parents should be told in advance that these drugs may cause some side-effects. They should be told what to look for and what to report to the physician or nurse. This—like the allaying of misconceptions (above)—prevents the parents from becoming nervous and discontinuing medication at the child's first complaints. Occasionally the child may appear pale and complain tearfully of a headache or stomachache. More commonly, if the first doses are a bit high or are taken too late in the day, the child may not be able to fall asleep at the usual bedtime. However, such symptoms tend to be transient and can, in any case, be lessened by reducing stimulant drug dosage and by having the child take the main dose in the morning and a second one, if necessary, no later than noon.

Lack of appetite may be a longer lasting symptom during prolonged therapy. Children taking dextroamphetamine may not gain weight or grow in height at the expected rate for their age. The parents may make an extra effort to have the child eat a late snack before bedtime. If the child still fails to grow normally, this drug may have to be discontinued and replaced with methylphenidate, which has less of a suppressant effect on appetite, or by pemoline (Cylert), which is said to have the least effect of all the stimulants. Usually, the child's growth rate then rebounds rapidly to a normal level.

Treatment failure. Most children who are properly diagnosed and receive an adequate initial dose of dextroamphetamine or methylphenidate show prompt improvement within a few days at most. Pemoline must sometimes be administered for several weeks before its full effects become apparent. However, some children may fail to benefit even after the initial doses have been doubled and side-effects such as insomnia and irritability occur. Occasionally, stimulants may even make a child emotionally depressed or set off overt signs of psychosis. Thus, children taking these drugs must be closely supervised so that the stimulants can be promptly discontinued and some more appropriate drug substituted.

Other drugs. Ordinarily, such sedative drugs as phenobarbital make a child with minimal brain dysfunction *more* restless and uncooperative. However, there is some evidence that children whose restlessness does not respond to even large doses of stimulants may improve when they are switched to such antihistamine-type sedatives as *diphenhydramine* (Benadryl; Chap. 39) and *hydroxyzine* (Atarax; Chap. 45). The major tranquilizers *chlorpromazine* (Thorazine) and *thioridazine* (Mellaril) may help to reduce restlessness, although they do not lessen distractibility and may even impair the child's attentiveness. These antipsychotic drugs (Chap. 46) are best reserved for children who happen to be hyperactive but who are actually diagnosed as being borderline psychotic or mentally retarded.

More recently, the tricyclic-type antidepressant drug *imipramine* (Tofranil; Chap. 46) has been claimed to be more effective than stimulant drug therapy for some children. It may also be added to the regimen of the rare child who becomes emotionally depressed when taking stimulants. Imipramine may also be employed when bed wetting is a symptom, because it has been proved effective for treating nocturnal enuresis in children. This medication is best taken about an hour before bedtime in doses that range from 25 to 75 mg nightly in children over 12 years old.

No matter which drugs are employed, they should be discontinued at intervals to see if the child can get along without them. Summer school vacations are a good time to see whether the child's condition has improved. Often, it is found that the drug is not needed, except perhaps on rainy days or in other confining situations or those requiring the child to be on what adults consider "best behavior." Finally, after the child reaches puberty, stimulating drugs may be permanently discontinued.

Other disorders

Narcolepsy. This is a neurologic sleep disorder in which the patient is periodically overcome by uncontrollable drowsiness. Patients may be overwhelmed by a sudden desire to sleep anywhere and at any time. Such "sleep attacks" occur most commonly during an emotional reaction marked by surprise, anger, or laughter. Discovery of the alerting action of amphetamine

led to its use in this embarrassing and potentially dangerous condition.

This prototype proved to be effective for keeping narcoleptic patients awake and for preventing cataplexy, a sudden loss of muscle tone that often accompanies the onset of sleep in these patients. Today, dextroamphetamine is most commonly employed for this purpose, because the large doses that are sometimes required are less likely to cause cardiovascular side-effects. Methylphenidate is also effective and may be less likely to suppress the patient's appetite. Fortunately for the people whom treatment with these drugs helps to convert from social and occupational misfits to useful and productive citizens, tolerance to the wakefulness–stimulating action of these drugs does not seem to develop. Imipramine and MAO inhibitors are also effective and are being used; they must *not* be given concomitantly with amphetamines.

Epilepsy. Unlike narcolepsy, epilepsy is only rarely responsive to the central stimulating action of the amphetamines. However, these drugs are commonly combined with antiepileptic drugs, mainly to counteract their tendency to cause drowsiness. Thus, in the management of grand mal epilepsy, methamphetamine is often added to phenobarbital and phenytoin mixtures. Similarly, small doses are administered together with trimethadione to counteract the sedation occasionally produced by that drug in patients with petit mal epilepsy. Some children with petit mal seizures and other seizure states that develop during sleep may improve when treated with only a stimulant, such as dextroamphetamine or methylphenidate.

Parkinsonism. Patients with this disorder who cannot take levodopa (Chap. 49) may get some symptomatic relief from amphetamines alone or in combination with centrally acting anticholinergic drugs. Often, the distressing complication called oculogyric crisis, in which the patient's head is pulled back by neck muscle contractions and the eyes deviate upward in their orbits, responds to amphetamine drug treatment. Similarly, torticollis and other spastic complications of extrapyramidal motor system disorders (Chap. 48) are relieved by adding amphetamines to the patient's skeletal muscle relaxant regimen. The amphetamines often help to counteract both the physical depression produced by some of the centrally acting antiparkinsonism drugs and the emotional depression that afflicts many of these patients. Presumably, the slightly beneficial effect on the extrapyramidal symptoms of this disorder is a result of the ability of the amphetamines to release dopamine from the nigrostriatal dopaminergic neurons that are functionally deficient in such cases. Because these neurons contain lower than normal amounts of dopamine, it is not surprising that the amphetamines are not very efficacious.

Emotional depression. Emotionally depressed patients with relatively mild and temporary mood disturbances may be benefited by administration of amphetamines as an adjunct to psychotherapeutic support. Some patients, reacting to distressing events such as a death in the family, marital unhappiness or divorce, financial loss or prolonged unemployment, seem to lose their zest for life and their interest in their former goals. Often, suffering from so-called morning melancholia, they feel fatigued even after a night's sleep and seem unable or unwilling to rouse themselves to face another day.

Sometimes, in such cases of mild reactive depression, small daily doses of the amphetamines tend to speed the patient's recovery, especially with the help of people—whether professional, or friends and family—who are willing to listen and to offer sympathetic understanding. The drugs then seem to help make the patient brighter and more alert and attentive. His depressive apathy, lethargy, and listlessness are gradually overcome, and interest in participating in the normal activities of daily living is regained.

Patients with more severe degrees of emotional depression are not ordinarily helped by amphetamine therapy and may even be harmed by these drugs, because some people are prone to become dependent. These psychomotor stimulants tend also to increase the insomnia and appetite loss of those who are already sleeping and eating poorly. Thus, they are not employed for the more severe neurotic and psychotic depressive symptoms, which require the more specific antidepressant drugs (Chap. 46), electroshock therapy, and intensive psychotherapy.

Adjunctive medical uses

The mood-elevating effect of the amphetamines is sometimes helpful for patients suffering from various painful or disabling organic ailments. People with arthritis, for example, may be aided by the addition of small doses of amphetamines to their regimen of salicylates, rest, special exercises, and physical therapy. Although the amphetamines are neither analgesic nor anti-inflammatory, their favorable effects on the patient's emotional state make it easier to bear discomfort. Similarly, women with dysmenorrhea, premenstrual tension, or other menstrual disturbances often do better when an amphetamine is added to their antispasmodic, analgesic, or hormone medication. There is also evidence that the amphetamines may potentiate the analgesic action of morphine and other potent narcotics without increasing their undesirable depressant effects on consciousness, respiration, and cardiovascular function. Children suffering from nocturnal enuresis sometimes benefit from amphetamines and from the related centrally acting sympathomimetic drug ephedrine.

Analeptics (brain stem stimulants)

The Greek word *analeptikos* means *restorative*, and certain CNS stimulants that can restore consciousness to a patient deeply depressed by central depressant drugs were once used mainly for this purpose. At present, however, the main aim of therapy with these analeptic drugs—when they are used at all—is to stimulate the nerve cells of the patient's *respiratory center* when it is depressed following general anesthesia or in certain chronic disease states that sometimes lead to acute respiratory insufficiency.

General considerations

Mechanism of action. Drugs such as *doxapram*$^+$ (Dopram) and *nikethamide* (Coramine) act mainly to stimulate the vital centers located in the medulla oblongata. Thus, they tend to increase the sensitivity of the respiratory center neurons to the carbon dioxide that has built up to abnormal blood levels during the patient's period of respiratory depression. In addition, these drugs stimulate chemoreceptors in the carotid bodies of the neck vessels and at other peripheral sites. These receptors then send impulses to the CNS that provide a further drive for the respiratory center. These drugs also often raise the patient's blood pressure by stimulating the vasomotor center and by increasing cardiac output. Stimulation of the RAS causes increased numbers of nerve impulses to pass by way of ascending pathways to the cerebral cortex, thus stimulating various cortically influenced functions, including consciousness.

Current clinical status. Unfortunately, when these drugs are administered in the doses needed to produce these clinically desirable effects, they also stimulate other central sites. This can lead to convulsions, vomiting, and cardiovascular or respiratory difficulties. Thus, most authorities are now opposed to the routine use of analeptics for treating the clinical conditions in which these stimulants were once considered indicated. Even those anesthesiologists and others who still employ analeptic therapy do so only in carefully selected patients and with considerable caution.

Analeptic treatment of disorders marked by respiratory depression

Depressant drug overdosage

Patients suffering from intoxication by barbiturates, glutethimide (Doriden), alcohol, and other general CNS depressants were once routinely treated with brain stem stimulants such as *pentylenetetrazol, picrotoxin,* and *nikethamide,* as well as with the previously discussed psychomotor stimulants *caffeine sodium benzoate* and *amphetamine.* Administered intravenously, these central stimulants were intended to reduce the depth of drug-induced psychomotor and respiratory depression and to counteract circulatory collapse. However, depressant drug poisoning is now managed mainly by use of the supportive measures described in Chapter 5. Pentylenetetrazol and picrotoxin are no longer available for therapeutic use. These drugs and another convulsant, strychnine, which is also no longer available for therapeutic use, have been important in research on how the nervous system functions, and they are likely to continue to be useful in neurobiologic research.

Occasionally, nikethamide and doxapram, a drug with a relatively selective respiratory stimulating action, are still employed as adjuncts to the standard supportive and resuscitative techniques. After an adequate airway has been established, a drug such as doxapram may be cautiously administered by vein in the lowest dose likely to stimulate an increase in spontaneous respiration. Care is required in positioning the patient to avoid aspiration of gastric contents if the drug stimulates the vomiting center as well as the respiratory center.

Patients are also carefully monitored for signs of cardiac arrhythmias, skeletal muscle contractions, and increased deep tendon reflexes to adjust the rate of analeptic drug infusion downward or to discontinue it entirely, if necessary. Although the well-managed patient is unlikely to suffer convulsive seizures because of the relatively wide margin of safety of doxapram, the physician should have available—in addition to oxygen and resuscitative equipment—such IV anticonvulsants as diazepam and thiopental. If convulsive seizures occur, there is the danger that the neuronal depression that follows, even without treatment by IV anticonvulsants, will depress the patient's respiration further. This is another reason why most authorities do not recommend the use of these so-called analeptics.

Postanesthetic respiratory depression

Patients who have received various central and peripheral depressants before and during surgery sometimes suffer from drug-induced respiratory depression of varying degree postoperatively. Recovery room nurses try to encourage patients to breathe deeply as part of the pulmonary toilet regimen for preventing the development of atelectasis.

Although analeptics are not used routinely to aid postoperative recovery, some anesthesiologists now recommend the occasional use of doxapram to bring about a deep breath, or physiologic sigh, and thus to aid respiratory function in patients with poor tidal ventilation.

This drug is not very effective for stimulating respiration when it has been depressed by overdoses of opiate analgesic drugs or when apnea is the result of the residual effects of neuromuscular junction blockers (Chap. 19). Respiratory depression by potent narcotic analgesics is best treated with a specific narcotic antagonist such as *naloxone* (Chap. 51), and overdosage with a curariform neuromuscular blocking agent is best counteracted with a cholinesterase inhibitor such as *neostigmine* (Chap. 15).

It has also been suggested that the patient's response to a relatively specific respiratory center stimulant such as doxapram may aid in the differential diagnosis of postanesthetic respiratory depression. Thus, when the patient's hypoventilation is the result of residual curarization—that is, persisting partial depression by neuromus-

cular blocking agents such as *curare*—injection of the central respiratory stimulant will increase the breathing rate but *not* the respiratory minute volume. On the other hand, when the patient's poor breathing is caused by central depression rather than by peripheral respiratory muscle paralysis, the intravenous injection of a small bolus dose of doxapram will usually bring about a prompt, although often transient, increase in tidal volume. In the latter case, treatment with a continuous IV infusion of doxapram may be continued together with oxygen inhalation until spontaneous respiration has been re-established.

Chronic obstructive pulmonary diseases

Patients with chronic respiratory diseases such as pulmonary emphysema may occasionally benefit from very careful infusion of a respiratory stimulant when they suffer a superimposed episode of acute respiratory insufficiency (see also Chap. 40). In such cases, some physicians have reported that intravenous administration of the relatively specific respiratory center stimulant doxapram (Dopram) has helped to increase the depth of the patient's respiration and has improved the ventilation of the alveoli. The resulting decrease in arterial carbon dioxide levels is also said to help to rouse drowsy patients from their hypercapnic lethargy.

Other authorities claim that such drug-induced treatment of hypercapnia is counterproductive in chronic pulmonary disease patients. They argue that excessive drug-induced stimulation of respiration may make the muscles used in breathing work *too* hard. This makes them use up too much oxygen and permits the accumulation of even more of the carbon dioxide by-product of muscular effort. If analeptic therapy is used at all in such cases, the patient should continue inhaling oxygen to prevent oxygen debt from occurring. Arterial blood gas levels must be constantly monitored during the very careful analeptic drug infusion. The drug should not be administered for much more than 2 hours, and it must be discontinued entirely if it is decided to put the patient on a mechanical ventilator.

Another danger of these drugs—particularly in patients with bronchial asthma—is that their use may set off bronchospasm and laryngospasm. Their use in such cases is indicated only as a desperation measure in patients whose blood oxygen level has been raised too rapidly by improperly controlled oxygen inhalation (Chap. 40). In such cases, some authorities recommend a short period of analeptic drug infusion to help blow off the excess carbon dioxide that builds up as a result of oxygen-induced hypoventilation.

The *oral* use of respiratory stimulants for emphysema has not proved effective, and tablets of ethamivan, a drug that was promoted for daily long-term use in emphysema, are no longer marketed. In any case, none of these drugs can, of course, reverse the underlying cause of the patient's hypoventilation. That is, they cannot correct the obstruction caused by the breakdown of the walls of the alveoli, the millions of tiny air sacs that have lost their elasticity and, with it, the ability to expand and contract. At best, the carefully controlled intravenous administration of an analeptic may occasionally help to counteract temporarily some of the complications that result from the rapid, shallow breathing of patients with chronic obstructive pulmonary disease.

Convulsant drugs and poisons

Various natural and synthetic substances stimulate motor areas of the CNS so strongly that muscle groups are forced into violent contractions, or convulsive spasms. Alkaloids such as *strychnine* and *cocaine,* and the brain stem stimulants *picrotoxin* and *pentylenetetrazol,* can cause convulsions. *Tetanospasmin,* a substance produced by the pathogenic microorganism *Clostridium tetani,* is an extremely powerful convulsant toxin.

Neurophysiology of convulsive states
Poisons and toxins produce two types, or patterns, of muscular contractions—*clonic* and *tonic*—or a combination of both called an *epileptiform* convulsion because it resembles what is seen clinically in grand mal epilepsy (Chap. 50).

Clonic convulsive spasms are characterized by the occurrence of a quick series of alternating *contractions* and *relaxations,* first in one and then in another group of muscles. This *coordinated* muscular activity may appear to be *purposeful,* or cortically directed. Actually, the person reacting in this way has no control over the tics, twitches, and spasms that seem to start in the muscles on one side of the body and move to the other—that is, in an *asymmetric* pattern. Clonic convulsions are seen most commonly with small overdoses of the stimulants—including picrotoxin and pentylenetetrazol—that act primarily at brain stem centers.

Tonic convulsive seizures are much more dramatic, and even fearful, to see. They are characterized by the *sustained rigidity* of all muscle groups. Actually, the action of the more powerful of two opposing muscle groups predominates but, because the antagonists are also maximally contracted, coordinated muscular activity is impossible. Thus, in humans, the extensor muscles of the legs, back, and neck are the stronger and pull the person into a bowlike position, with the back arched and the body resting only on the head and heels (opisthotonos).

Such tetanic spasms are *symmetric*—that is, they occur in the muscles on both sides of the body simultaneously. Tonic muscular activity is also *uncoordinated,* so that no purposeful movements can be carried out. This happens because the opposing muscle groups (*e.g.,* the flexors), which would ordinarily be relaxed as a result of reciprocal inhibition, remain, instead, in a state of sustained contraction. Tonic convulsions are seen mainly following poisoning by spinal cord stimulants such as strychnine or tetanus toxin, but they may also occur with massive overdoses of brain stem stimulants such as pentylenetetrazol when the effects of these drugs spread to the spinal cord from their primary site of activity.

Neuropharmacology of convulsant drugs
Neurophysiologists and neurochemists now know a good deal about the ways in which various substances act to alter the balance between excitatory and inhibitory influences at CNS synapses (Chaps. 13 and 44). Actually, these scientists have often used drugs such as strychnine as a tool with which to probe the complex interrelationships between neurons located at different levels of the CNS. Thus, some of the facts that will be presented at the beginning of Chapter 48 concerning the *neurophysiology of movement* were first found as a result of neuropharmacologic studies.*

Some central stimulants cause convulsions by removing some of the inhibitory influences that normally impinge on central motor neurons. *Strychnine,* for example, is known to compete with the inhibitory neurotransmitter glycine, released by certain neurons at their synapses with central motor neurons and interneurons. By preventing this transmitter substance from producing inhibitory postsynaptic potentials on the postsynaptic neuronal membrane, this drug indirectly increases the level of postsynaptic neuronal excitability. Thus, incoming sensory stimuli produce exaggerated activity in polysynaptic reflex pathways and this, in turn, results in exaggerated muscle contractions and convulsive spasms. Because strychnine blocks postsynaptic inhibitory influences on the motor neurons of antagonistic muscle groups, both the agonists and the antagonists contract simultaneously to produce the tonic convulsive pattern described above.

Although strychnine is no longer used therapeutically, it is apparently still available in some areas as a preparation to poison rodents and other undesirable animal pests. Occasionally people are poisoned, either inadvertently or when they use such poisons in suicide attempts. Thus, this discussion has potential clinical application (see also below, Strychnine poisoning).

Tetanospasmin, the tetanus bacillus neurotoxin, also interferes with the postsynaptic inhibition process. However, it acts not by competing with glycine for receptor sites on the postsynaptic neurons, as strychnine does, but by preventing this transmitter from being released by the spinal interneurons that normally exert in-

---

* For a fuller understanding of how drugs elicit convulsive movements, it would be useful for students to read the introductory material in Chapter 48 at this time, which reviews such subjects as spinal reflexes and the supraspinal neuronal activities that influence them. The brief discussions of pyramidal and extrapyramidal motor systems in that chapter and in Chapters 13 and 44 should also be reviewed.

hibitory control over polysynaptic reflex activity. The end result is, of course, the same—that is, when the inhibitory influence of these tetanotoxin-poisoned cells is removed, central excitatory influences predominate, and the resulting simultaneous contractions of the antagonistic extensor and flexor muscles lock the victim's limbs into a state of convulsive spastic paralysis.

Picrotoxin and other convulsants block synaptic inhibition that is mediated by γ-aminobutyric acid (GABA), a different inhibitory neurotransmitter. Because these agents and pentylenetetrazol have no therapeutic value or toxicologic importance, they will not be considered further here.

Toxicology of convulsant drugs

As stated above, drugs such as strychnine, pentylenetetrazol, and hexafluorodiethyl ether (fluorothyl) no longer have any clinical usefulness. The occasional need to control convulsive seizures in children and others who accidentally ingest overdoses of drugs with central stimulating properties or who react to parenterally administered drugs with signs of motor center stimulation is of clinical concern, however. Among the medications that can cause convulsions in such circumstances are certain antihistamine drugs (Chap. 39) and local anesthetics (Chap. 14). The management of convulsive seizures by these and other drugs is discussed in those chapters and elsewhere in this book (see Index). The use of drugs and other measures in the management of tetanus is discussed in Chapter 48 and elsewhere. Here, poisoning by the prototype natural convulsant substance strychnine will be discussed because, as stated above, this type of poisoning does still occur.

Strychnine poisoning

Strychnine is a drug that has no place in modern therapy. It has been used as a respiratory stimulant, a digestive tonic, and an ingredient of cathartic combinations. Its usefulness, if any, is far outweighed by the danger of poisoning from accidental ingestion. Similarly, the use of strychnine in so-called mouse seeds or rat poison pellets and as a bait for field rodents is unjustified in view of the present availability of safer substances.

The incidence of strychnine poisoning has declined as preparations containing it have deservedly lost popularity; however, cases are still reported.

Signs and symptoms of strychnine overdosage come on quickly. Often, the patient begins to feel a tightness in the muscles of the face, neck, back, and legs. The patient is alert, anxious and fearful, and the reflexes become hyperactive. Then, quite suddenly, a slight stimulus may set off a violent convulsion. In a characteristic full-blown tonic seizure, the patient's back is arched and his face contorted into what seems a smile. Actually, the patient, who does not usually lose consciousness until becoming asphyxiated, can fully feel the extreme pain pro-

duced by the massive muscular spasms. Because such muscular activity tends to use up large quantities of oxygen at a time when the muscles of the diaphragm and the chest are in spasm, the patient quickly becomes hypoxic and cyanotic. Thus, management is aimed mainly at controlling convulsions and maintaining adequate oxygenation.

Total treatment requires not only the use of chemical antagonists to destroy any strychnine remaining in the stomach and pharmacologic antagonists to depress the overstimulated CNS, but also measures to support the patient's respiration and to prevent injury. Thus, for example, before pharmacotherapy is employed, an adequate airway must be ensured by removing mucous secretions from the patient's mouth, nose, and throat. Measures should be taken to prevent the patient from biting the tongue, damaging the teeth, or being hurt by thrashing about. Oxygen should be administered during the convulsions.

Control of convulsions requires the careful administration of depressant drugs in doses that produce muscle relaxation and light sleep without impairing respiratory center function. Intravenous injection of *diazepam*⁺ (Valium; Drug digest, Chap. 45) is now the preferred method for dampening convulsive spasms. This centrally acting antispasmodic (Chap. 48) and anticonvulsant (Chap. 50) is injected slowly at a rate of about 5 mg/minute to avoid development of cardiac arrhythmias or respiratory depression. Diazepam is much less likely than the barbiturates to depress the respiratory center. However, ultrashort-acting drugs of that class (Chaps. 45 and 52) such as thiopental (Pentothal) are also effective for convulsion control, and phenobarbital, administered intramuscularly, may help to prevent recurrence of convulsions. General anesthetics and neuromuscular blocking agents (Chap. 19) are also effective but are not usually needed for treating strychnine-induced convulsions.

Induction of vomiting by drugs or other measures is not considered desirable, because the procedure may precipitate convulsions. It is generally wise to try to keep all sensory stimulation to a minimum by putting the patient in a quiet, darkened, warm room. He should be constantly watched and protected from hurting himself in any way. If reflex activity begins to increase, the patient may require more of the sedative–anticonvulsant. Removal of the poison from the stomach by gastric lavage is more desirable, but this is best delayed until the patient's hyperreflexia has been blunted with anticonvulsant drugs, because the attempt to pass a stomach tube may set off convulsive seizures. The gavage solution is used in copious quantities to wash out all traces of strychnine before it can be absorbed. A solution of 1:10,000 potassium permanganate (100 mg/liter) is said to aid by destroying the poison chemically. Other chemical antidotes that may be employed include activated charcoal (Chap. 5), tannic acid, and diluted tincture of iodine.

Clinical status

Chemical convulsants have been used to precipitate seizures for diagnosing epileptic patients and they have been used, instead of electroconvulsive therapy (ECT; Chap. 46), for treating psychiatric patients. These uses have been superseded by other diagnostic procedures for epilepsy, and by ECT and antidepressant drugs for treating psychiatric patients.

Additional clinical considerations

The psychomotor stimulants should be used with caution in all patients. Because of the abuse potential of these drugs, they are prescribed in small amounts and the number of refills permitted is limited.

Several cautions and contraindications apply to the use of these drugs; these should be considered before any of these drugs is used. The overall effect of these drugs is stimulation. Several medical conditions can be exacerbated by such general stimulation and these are, therefore, contraindications to their use. These conditions include arteriosclerosis, cardiovascular disease, hypertension, hyperthyroidism, peptic ulcer, glaucoma, and diabetes mellitus. The safety of the use of these drugs during pregnancy has not been established. Birth defects have been associated with the administration of these drugs to pregnant experimental animals. The psychomotor stimulants cross into the breast milk and have been associated with neonatal problems. It is advisable, therefore, to avoid these drugs during pregnancy and lactation. This has special patient teaching implications, because caffeine is found widely in over-the-counter (OTC) preparations as well as in foods (chocolate) and beverages (coffee, tea, cola).

Patients who are taking psychomotor stimulants need thorough teaching regarding not only the side-effects and cautions of the drug but also the disease for which the drug was ordered. The patient being treated for obesity needs to understand that the drug therapy has to be combined with reduced caloric intake and increased exercise to be effective. Patients also need to be cautioned not to combine prescribed amphetamines with OTC appetite suppressants or "diet pills." Serious cardiac arrhythmias can result. Patients using these stimulants to overcome fatigue need to understand that the drug is not a substitute for sleep. They may still have impaired abilities and concentration while taking the drug, and appropriate caution should be used. All patients should be alerted to the possible adverse effects that can occur—for example headache, insomnia, dizziness, restlessness, euphoria, dry mouth, rapid heartbeat, gastrointestinal upset. Loss of libido and impotence have been reported with prolonged use.

The patient teaching guide summarizes key points that should be incorporated into the teaching program of a patient receiving psychomotor stimulants.

Drug–drug interactions

Patients taking psychomotor stimulants should never receive *MAO inhibitors*. In fact, the patient should be withdrawn from MAO inhibitors for at least 14 days before beginning these stimulants to avoid potential hypertensive crisis. *Antihypertensive* agents may not have the desired effect if given concurrently with one of these stimulants. *Insulin* requirements may change with amphetamine use. Methylphenidate may inhibit the metabolism of *oral anticoagulants, phenytoin,* and *phenylbutazone*. Patients receiving these drugs concurrently will require lower doses to achieve the desired therapeutic effect. *Sympathomimetics* and other stimulants in prescribed drugs, foods, and OTC preparations can have additive effects, and should be avoided.

The guide to the nursing process summarizes the clinical considerations that should be incorporated into the nursing care of a patient receiving psychomotor stimulants.

Patient teaching guide: psychomotor stimulants

The drug that has been prescribed for you belongs to a class of drugs called psychomotor stimulants. These drugs act to stimulate various parts of the nervous system to achieve such effects as appetite control or control of fatigue. Your drug has been prescribed to treat _____ .

Instructions:

1. The name of your drug is _____ .

2. The dosage that has been prescribed is _____ .

3. Your drug should be taken _____ times a day. The drug should be taken early in the day to avoid interruption of sleep. The best time to take your drug is _____ .

(continued)

4. Do not chew or crush sustained-release or long-acting tablets. This will inactivate much of the drug.

5. Some side-effects of the drug that you should be aware of include the following:

Restlessness, nervousness, jitteriness	These are common effects of the drug. Avoiding other stimulants, such as caffeine, can help.
Insomnia	Taking the drug early in the day can help. Rest periods during the day can reduce the feeling of fatigue.
GI upset	Taking the drug with food may help, as may eating small, frequent meals.
Loss of libido, impotence	If this occurs, consult with your nurse or physician.

6. Keep this and all medications out of the reach of children.

7. Tell any physician, nurse, or dentist who is taking care of you that you are on this drug.

8. Avoid the use of over-the-counter preparations while you are on this drug. If you feel that you need one of these preparations, consult with your nurse or physician to determine one that will be safe for use with this drug.

9. Take this drug exactly as prescribed. Do not increase your dose for any reason.

Notify your nurse or physician if any of the following occur:

Chest pain
Difficulty in breathing
Severe headache
Hallucinations
Tremors, restlessness

Guide to the nursing process: psychomotor stimulants

Assessment	Nursing diagnoses	Interventions	Evaluation
Past history *(contraindications)*: Arteriosclerosis	Potential alteration in cardiac output Knowledge deficit	Safe and appropriate administration of drug Patient teaching	Monitor therapeutic effectiveness of drug: weight, activity

(continued)

Assessment	Nursing diagnoses	Interventions	Evaluation

Cardiovascular disease
Hypertension
Hyperthyroidism
Peptic ulcer
Glaucoma
Diabetes mellitus
Pregnancy
Lactation
Allergies: these drugs;
  tartrazine (certain
  preparations); others;
  reactions
Medication history
  (*cautions*):
  MAO inhibitors
  Antihypertensives
  Insulin
  Oral anticoagulants
  Phenytoin
  Phenylbutazone
  Sympathomimetics
 	
Physical assessment
Neurologic: mental
  status, affect, reflexes,
  coordination
Cardiovascular: BP, P,
  peripheral perfusion,
  baseline ECG
Respiratory: R,
  adventitious sounds
GI: abdominal
Weight
	regarding drug
	  therapy
	Potential alteration in
	  nutrition
	Potential sensory–
	  perceptual alteration
	Potential sleep pattern
	  disturbance
		regarding disease and
		  drug therapy
		Support and
		  encouragement to deal
		  with disease and drug
		  therapy
		Provision of comfort and
		  safety measures:
		• Small meals
		• Rest
		• Environmental
		  control
		• Avoidance of
		  driving, dangerous
		  tasks
		• Slow position change
			Monitor for adverse
			  effects of drug:
			• Cardiovascular
			  effects
			• CNS changes
			• GI upset
			• Loss of libido
			Evaluate effectiveness of
			  patient teaching
			  program
			Evaluate effectiveness of
			  support and
			  encouragement
			  offered
			Evaluate effectiveness of
			  comfort and safety
			  measures
			Monitor for drug–drug
			  interactions:
			  Hypertensive crises
			    with *MAO inhibitors*
			  ↓ effect of
			    antihypertensives
			  ↑↓ effect of *insulin*
			  ↑ effect of *oral
			    anticoagulants,
			    phenytoin,
			    phenylbutazone,
			    sympathomimetics*

Case study

Presentation

Jeff is a 6-year-old boy who was seen in a diagnostic clinic at the request of his school. Jeff was noted to be easily distracted, to have a short attention span, to be emotionally labile and impulsive, and to be unable to sit still for any period of time. His teacher was frustrated and unable to cope with Jeff in the classroom. Following testing, it was determined that Jeff had an attention deficit disorder (sometimes called minimal brain dysfunction). It was decided that Jeff should try a course of methylphenidate (Ritalin) and should return in 6 weeks for evaluation.

What teaching points should be included in the initial teaching session with Jeff and his mother?

Discussion

Jeff's mother should meet with the behavior specialists who diagnosed his problem to review the tests that were done so that she has an understanding of Jeff's problems, as well as strengths that he may have. She will also need to know what other environmental, educational, and social programs should be instituted to help Jeff. Jeff's school will also need a full report on the results of the testing and the prescribed programs that will be most beneficial to Jeff. Jeff's mother should be advised to give him his last drug dose of the day in the early evening to help prevent insomnia. She can also be alerted to watch for signs of restlessness, loss of appetite, dizziness, and skin rash. Sometimes these effects can be alleviated by reducing the drug dosage. Jeff will require periodic CBCs while on long-term therapy. He will also need to be evaluated for growth and development, because severe weight loss can occur. Jeff and his mother will need support and encouragement to cope with his diagnosis and therapies. Neither the syndrome nor the mechanisms of the drug's beneficial effects is understood. The clinic nurse can do a great deal to facilitate the success of Jeff's therapy by contacting and developing a working relationship with his school nurse. In most cases, consistent and supportive care can result in a marked increase in attention span, which will help the child to fit into the school environment and to learn more effectively.

Summary of clinical indications for central nervous system stimulants

Psychomotor stimulants

Obesity: Adjunct to low calorie diets for brief periods (4 to 8 weeks)

Hyperactivity in children: hyperkinetic reaction or syndrome; minimal brain dysfunction

Narcolepsy: sleep attacks; hypersomnia

Miscellaneous: adjunct in epilepsy, parkinsonism, emotional depression, headache, dysmenorrhea, premenstrual tension, arthritis, and other physical conditions; depressant drug overdosage

Analeptics

Depressant drug overdosage

Postanesthetic respiratory depression

Chronic obstructive lung disease: episodes of acute hypercapnia in acute respiratory failure

Summary of side-effects and toxicity of psychomotor stimulants

Central nervous system side-effects and toxicity

Nervousness, restlessness, jitteriness, irritability, anorexia, insomnia, headache, dizziness, anxiety, tension, difficulty in concentrating, confusion, delirium, hallucinations, toxic psychosis with paranoid delusions

Peripheral side-effects and toxicity

Cardiac arrhythmias, tachycardia, chest pain, systolic and diastolic blood pressure elevation, dry mouth, constipation, nausea, vomiting, excessive sweating, pupillary dilation

Drug digests

Caffeine USP

Actions and indications. This alkaloid found in coffee, tea, and cola is a psychomotor stimulant that increases alertness and wakefulness. It is used by the public in beverages containing it and in solid dosage forms to overcome drowsiness and to counteract the depressant effects of alcohol. The injectable form is sometimes employed medically to hasten recovery from acute alcoholic intoxication. Caffeine is frequently combined with analgesics such as aspirin in proprietary headache remedies and with ergotamine in prescription products for treating migraine and hypertensive headaches.

Adverse effects, cautions, and contraindications. The adverse effects are mainly those caused by excessive CNS stimulation—for example, insomnia, nervous irritability, and tremors. However, heart palpitations may occur in some sensitive people and epigastric distress may be seen in others. Many people are both tolerant to and psychologically dependent on the caffeine in coffee. When deprived of the beverage, they may become irritable and have headaches.

Dosage and administration. A cup of coffee ordinarily contains 100 to 150 mg of caffeine, but tea and cola beverages contain considerably less. The amount found in pharmaceutic preparations (50 to 100 mg) is thus less than is available in a cup of coffee. For central stimulation of persons deeply depressed by alcohol or depressant drugs, caffeine sodium benzoate may be injected intramuscularly or subcutaneously in doses up to 500 mg.

Dextroamphetamine sulfate USP (Dexedrine)

Actions and indications. This psychomotor stimulant is now indicated mainly in the management of neurologic disorders such as narcolepsy and hyperkinetic behavior in children with the minimal brain dysfunction syndrome. It is also still used as an adjunct to low-calorie diets in the short-term treatment of obesity. It is sometimes added in small doses to prescriptions containing such depressant drugs as antihistamines and antiepileptics, but it should *not* be used to counteract symptoms of hangover caused by alcohol or barbiturates. It is now rarely used in the treatment of mental depression.

Adverse effects, cautions, and contraindications. Side-effects of central origin include restlessness, irritability, and insomnia and, in overdosage, muscle tremors, increased reflex activity, confusion and, possibly, panic states. Continued abuse of high doses can cause psychological dependence and possible paranoid reactions. The extreme fatigue and mental depression that follow abrupt withdrawal of this drug may be also an indication of physical dependence. It is contraindicated in patients with a history of having abused other drugs.

Adrenergic stimulation may cause cardiac palpitations and arrhythmias, a rise in blood pressure, and chest pains. The drug is contraindicated in patients with symptoms of cardiovascular disease and hyperthyroidism. It is not administered to patients who have been taking drugs of the monoamine oxidase inhibitor class.

Dosage and administration. The usual oral dose is 5 mg taken before meals, but daily dosage may range from 2.5 to 30 mg. Sustained-release capsules (Spansules) containing 5, 10, or 15 mg are taken in the morning and, occasionally, about 6 hours later.

Doxapram HCl USP (Dopram)

Actions and indications. This central stimulant increases respiratory tidal volume by stimulating the medullary respiratory center directly and secondary to its action on carotid body chemoreceptors. It may be used following anesthesia to cause deep breathing in the postoperative patient. It may also be used following drug-induced depression of the CNS to hasten arousal, return laryngeal and pharyngeal reflex activity, and stimulate respiration that is mildly to moderately depressed. Doxapram may also be employed in patients with chronic obstructive pulmonary disease who are hospitalized with acute respiratory insufficiency. In such cases, it may be tried as a temporary measure to prevent arterial carbon dioxide levels from rising while the hypercapnic patient is inhaling oxygen.

Adverse effects, cautions, and contraindications. This drug is used only when the patient's airway is not obstructed and *not* during mechanical ventilation. It can cause laryngospasm and bronchospasm, and it is contraindicated in acute bronchial asthma, pulmonary fibrosis, and other restrictive respiratory diseases, pulmonary embolism, and respiratory failure caused by neuromuscular disease or neuromuscular junction blocking drugs.

Doxapram commonly causes a rise in blood pressure and is contraindicated in patients with severe hypertension, heart failure, and coronary artery disease. Caution is required to avoid drug-induced cardiac arrhythmias in hypoxic patients. The drug is not recommended for epileptic patients, because it can cause hyperreflexia, muscle spasticity, and convulsions.

Dosage and administration. This drug may be administered by single and repeated intravenous injections or by intermittent intravenous infusion. A priming dose of 1 to 2 mg/kg may be injected IV, depending on the depth of the patient's depression, and repeated in 5 minutes and then every 1 or 2 hours until the patient awakens or the maximum dose of 3 g/day has been administered. (Repetitive doses are administered only if the patient responds to the first dose.) Patients who respond to the priming dose may be maintained on an infusion that delivers 1 to 3 mg/min (60 to 180 mg/hr), depending on the size of the patient and the depth of coma, until the patient awakens or up to a dose of 3 g.

Methylphenidate USP (Ritalin)

Actions and indications. This central stimulant is midway in potency between caffeine and amphetamine. Small or moderate oral doses may be useful for reducing hyperkinetic behavior in children correctly diagnosed as suffering from minimal brain dysfunction, for maintaining daytime wakefulness in patients with narcolepsy, and possibly the management of senile patients who are apathetic and withdrawn.

Addition of this drug to the regimen of patients who are made drowsy by depressant drugs such as antihistamines, anticonvulsants, and barbiturates may help to counteract their lethargy. Injections are sometimes used to speed recovery from barbiturate anesthesia. However, in treating acute poisoning by barbiturates, it should be used only if facilities are not available for proper supportive therapy.

Adverse effects, cautions, and contraindications. Overstimulation of the CNS causes nervousness and insomnia and, in massive overdosage, muscular tremors, twitching, and convulsions. High doses also produce adrenergic effects including cardiac palpitations and acceleration, hypertension, sweating, mydriasis, and mouth dryness. It is contraindicated in agitated patients and in those with glaucoma, and it is administered cautiously to alcoholic patients and others with a history of drug abuse.

Dosage and administration. Adult oral doses range from 15 to 60 mg daily, with an average of 20 to 30 mg, administered in two or three divided doses before meals. In children, treatment is initiated with 5 mg bid, and dosage is gradually raised, if necessary, up to 60 mg daily by gradual increments of 5 to 10 mg weekly.

References

Aranda JV et al: Pharmacological considerations in therapy of neonatal apnea. Pediatr Clin North Am 28:113, 1981

Franz DN: Central nervous system stimulants. In Gilman AG, Goodman LS, Gilman A (eds): Goodman & Gilman's The Pharmacological Basis of Therapeutics, 6th ed, pp 585–591. New York, Macmillan, 1980

Hardin JA, Griggs RC: Diazepam treatment in a case of strychnine poisoning. Lancet 2:372, 1971

Jackson G et al: Strychnine poisoning successfully treated with diazepam. Br Med J 3:519, 1971

Meyers TF et al: Low dose theophylline therapy in idiopathic apnea of prematurity. J Pediatr 96:99, 1980

Phenylpropanolamine for weight reduction. Med Lett Drugs Ther 26:55, 1984

Rall TW: Central nervous system stimulants (continued). In Gilman AG, Goodman LS, Gilman A (eds): Goodman & Gilman's The Pharmacological Basis of Therapeutics, 6th ed, pp 592–607. New York, Macmillan, 1980

Rodman MJ: Use and abuse of the amphetamines. RN 33:55 (Aug.), 1970

Rodman MJ: Drugs for acute respiratory failure. RN 38:49, 1975

Tan T-L et al: Current therapy of eating disorders II: Obesity. Rat Drug Ther 18(2):1, 1984

Zarcone V: Narcolepsy. N Engl J Med 288:1156, 1973

Section 8

Part 2

Drugs
used
in neurologic
and
musculoskeletal
disorders

Up to now the discussion of drugs affecting the functioning of the central nervous system has focused attention on agents that mainly alter emotional responses, mental states, and behavior in ways that are of therapeutic significance. The next three chapters will describe drugs that are useful clinically because of their effects on central motor control systems.

Drugs of this type are employed mainly for the symptomatic relief of neurologic disorders such as the *epilepsies, Parkinson's disease,* and such spastic disorders as *cerebral palsy.* However, some may also be ordered for treating musculoskeletal conditions marked by muscle spasm and pain. To understand the basis for the use of the several classes of drugs discussed in the chapters dealing with antiparkinsonism and antiepilepsy agents, the nature of the neurologic disorder will be discussed first in each case. To explain the rationale for the use of the centrally acting antispasmodic drugs, the neurophysiologic mechanisms by which muscular activities are normally controlled will be discussed first, and then the signs and symptoms of various disease states will be related to the nervous system pathology responsible for their characteristic neuromuscular malfunctions.

Some of the nervous system structures that make up the motor circuits controlling muscular activity have already been mentioned in Chapter 44. This section will add some further details to help explain how volleys of nerve impulses that originate in motor nerve nuclei of the central nervous system pass out to the skeletal muscles by way of complexly interacting nerve fiber tracts. Such detailed knowledge of the ways in which the motor systems normally function and of how various diseases disrupt the split-second timing of nerve transmission needed for muscular coordination is necessary to understand how the drugs discussed in this section act to reduce Parkinson's disease disability, prevent epileptic seizures, and relieve the crippling signs and symptoms of other neurologic and musculoskeletal disorders.

Chapter 48

Centrally acting skeletal muscle relaxants

General considerations

The neurophysiology of movement

The body's posture, balance, and movements from moment to moment are the result of a constantly shifting sequence of muscular contractions and relaxations. The motor messages that coordinate this muscular activity flow continuously from the central nervous system. As indicated in Chapter 44, the spinal motor neurons are influenced by nerve impulses from higher levels of the brain. Thus, it is necessary to discuss here both spinal reflex activity and the supraspinal influences that also contribute to the control of muscle tone and movement.

Spinal reflexes. The simplest circuits for regulating motor responses are located at the spinal level. For example, the stretch reflexes responsible for maintaining muscle tone involve only a single sensory neuron connecting with only one motor neuron. When a muscle spindle is stretched, sensory nerve impulses pass by way of afferent pathways into the posterior portion of the spinal cord by way of the dorsal root ganglia (Fig. 48-1). The endings of these sensory nerve fibers transmit their signals directly to motor neurons located in the anterior horn portion of the same segment of the cord. These motor nerve cells then send impulses back to the muscle fibers that cause them to contract.

Other spinal reflexes involve a third type of cell located within the spinal cord between the sensory and motor neurons. These *interneurons* relay sensory signals from peripherally located sensors, or proprioceptors, to motor neurons located at several spinal segments. Such *multineuronal,* or *polysynaptic, reflexes* permit more complex motor responses to stimuli from the tendons and other outlying musculoskeletal structures. In addition, the spinal interneurons integrate the sensory signals arriving at spinal cord segments from the skeletal muscles with other nerve impulses coming downstream from higher levels

of the nervous system. As a result, the motor neurons that are influenced in these ways send out patterns of impulses that can produce all the complex coordinated movements required for making postural adjustments and proper limb placements.

Supraspinal influences. The impulses that pass down to the spinal level from higher centers can both excite and inhibit the activity of the lower motor neurons located in the anterior horns of the spinal cord. Messages from motor areas of the cerebral cortex are constantly streaming down to the spinal reflex centers. In addition, other fiber tracts from nerve cell bodies that originate in such subcortical structures as the basal ganglia, the brain stem reticular formation, and the cerebellum also exert a modulating influence on the activity of spinal motor neurons. The cerebellum, for example, plays a part in coordinating the contractions of various muscle groups. This structure collects data concerning the body's position and the movement of its various parts at any moment. It then feeds information back to the motor portions of the cerebral cortex, and the motor cortical command areas then make the continuous corrections needed for the precise control of body movements.

Cortical control areas. The nerve impulses that set off consciously controlled movements originate in the cerebral cortex. One group of motor cortex neurons, the *pyramidal* (Betz) cells, send out fibers that form the *corticospinal,* or *pyramidal, tract.* Signals sent out by Betz cells on each side of the brain pass down fiber tracts that cross to the opposite side of the spinal cord to set off muscle contractions that control skilled coordinated movements made by the muscles on that side of the body.

The *extrapyramidal motor system,* made up of neurons in other cortical areas and at several subcortical levels, including the reticular formation and basal ganglia (and the cerebellum), is responsible for modulating unconsciously controlled muscle contractions. This system

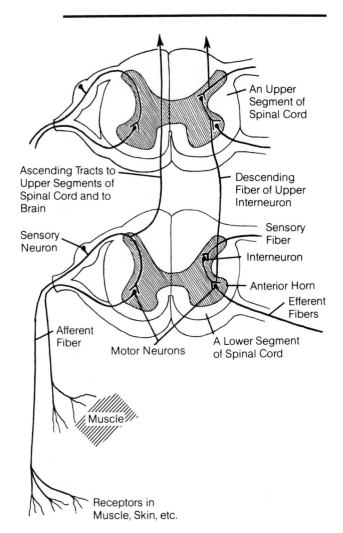

Figure 48-1. Polysynaptic reflex arc pathways. The neurospasmolytic drugs depress the interneurons in hyperactive reflex pathways (hyperreflexia). This reduces excessive reflex excitability and muscle spasm without affecting normal muscle tone.

Muscle spasm often results from injury to peripheral musculoskeletal system structures. Overstretching a muscle, wrenching a joint, or tearing tendons or ligaments, for example, can cause violent involuntary muscle contractions. These are the result of excessive reflex action at the spinal level set off by the streams of sensory impulses that pass into the nervous system from the injured parts. These messages are then passed by one or more interneurons to the spinal motor neurons. It is the excessive number of motor impulses passing to the periphery from these nerve cells that causes the painful muscle cramps. Often, the acute pain sets off further spasms. In chronic musculoskeletal inflammatory diseases such as arthritis, for example, pain is one factor responsible for the disabling spasm of the muscles around the affected joints.

Muscle spasticity stems from damage to neurons within the central nervous system rather than in the peripheral structures. The resulting muscular hypertonicity is permanent rather than temporary, and can readily lead to crippling contractures. Spasticity and such other hypertonic states of central origin as muscular rigidity, dystonia, and athetosis can be caused by injury to nerve cells at any of the various centers in the cerebrospinal axis that contribute to the control of muscle tone and to the coordination of complex movements. The signs and symptoms of such chronic neurologic disorders as cerebral palsy, multiple sclerosis, and paraplegia are quite varied, and differ according to which motor control areas have suffered disease-induced damage.

Spasticity can result from either an increase in excitatory (facilitatory) influences or a decrease in inhibitory impulses. The resulting imbalance in these reciprocal regulatory mechanisms makes muscle fibers respond to stretch in an exaggerated manner. Thus, for example, when the cells of the spinal reflex centers are released from their normal supraspinal inhibitory influences, they fire abnormally large volleys of motor nerve impulses to the skeletal muscles that they innervate. This leads to sustained contractions that sometimes affect both types of antagonistic muscle groups simultaneously, resulting in loss of coordinated motor activity and even in spastic paralysis.

helps the body to make automatic adjustments in posture and balance. It controls the crude motor activities that serve as a background against which the more precise movements controlled by the motor cortex and the pyramidal system may be performed.

Neuromuscular pathology

Injuries or poisons that interfere with the normal flow of nerve impulses between the brain and spinal cord and the skeletal muscles produce various signs and symptoms of abnormal muscle function. These may range from temporary minor muscle spasm following excessive activity to permanent flaccid or spastic paralysis. Before discussing the several classes of drugs that are used to relieve or prevent disordered muscular activity, it is necessary to review briefly the ways in which these abnormal muscle responses are brought about.

Drugs for relaxing muscle spasm and spasticity

Several different types of centrally and peripherally acting drugs can relax skeletal muscle spasms and spasticity. Curare and other neuromuscular blocking agents (Chap. 19) that interfere with transmission of motor nerve impulses to skeletal muscle fibers not only relax even convulsive spasms but can also produce complete paralysis. Local anesthetics, injected at specific spots in skeletal muscles, can relax spasm and, of course, spinal anesthesia (Chap.

14) can block conduction of all motor impulses in the peripheral nerves that innervate the muscles. The general anesthetics (Chap. 52) and other relatively nonselective depressant drugs (Chap. 45) such as the barbiturates can also bring about skeletal muscle relaxation. However, they do so usually only when administered in doses that also cause various degrees of depression of consciousness.

Centrally acting skeletal muscle relaxants

The class of compounds discussed in this chapter differ from other muscle relaxant drugs in their relatively greater selectivity for motor neuronal pathways. That is, they are better able than the barbiturates, for example, to bring about muscle relaxation without depressing consciousness or respiration. Although the exact mechanism of action of these *neurospasmolytic*, or *lissive*, drugs is uncertain, their site of action is thought to be at the spinal and supraspinal interneurons involved in the hyperactive polysynaptic reflex activity (Table 48-1). By depressing the activity of these interneurons, the centrally acting antispasmodics reduce the excessive reflex activity responsible for muscular hypertonicity, spasm, and spasticity. Ideally, these drugs do so when administered in doses that do not cause drowsiness, and they do not interfere with normal muscle tone. In practice, sedation is a common side-effect of adequate dosage, and high overdosage with these drugs can cause flaccid paralysis and respiratory depression.

Clinical uses. The available neurospasmolytic agents are used in two general types of clinical conditions:

1. *Musculoskeletal disorders* that are the result of local injury to or inflammation in

muscles, tendons, ligaments, joints, and other peripheral structures.
2. *Neurologic disorders* that are the result of disease or damage within the central nervous system (see the summary, at the end of this chapter).

Trauma or inflammation involving the *musculoskeletal system* causes abnormally large numbers of sensory impulses to arise at the peripheral structures. These enter the spinal cord by way of afferent pathways and are relayed by spinal interneurons to the motor cells located in the anterior horn of each spinal segment. These spinal motor neurons then send abnormally large numbers of nerve impulses back to the injured area. The excessive number of nerve impulses sets off sudden contractions in these muscle groups. Sometimes these painful spasms are the sensory source of still more afferent impulses, thus setting off a vicious cycle of spasm, pain, and still more painful spasm.

Neurospasmolytic drugs such as *diazepam*[+] (Valium; see Drug digest, Chap. 45), *methocarbamol*[+] (Robaxin), and *carisoprodol* (Soma; Rela) are often prescribed in oral doses or administered parenterally to reduce excessive polysynaptic reflex activity and thus relieve the painful muscle spasms occurring in acute musculoskeletal disorders. Actually, however, it is uncertain whether the relatively small oral doses ordinarily prescribed can produce relaxation of muscle spasm. Some authorities suggest that any relief of discomfort that occurs is the result of the effects of drugs such as diazepam on the patient's emotional state. That is, it may be the sedative, or antianxiety, effects of these drugs (Chap. 45) rather than

Table 48–1. Centrally acting skeletal muscle relaxants

Official or generic name	Trade name	Usual single oral adult dosage	Comments
Baclofen	Lioresal	5–20 mg	Used for spasticity in multiple sclerosis and in spinal cord injuries and diseases
Carisoprodol	Rela; Soma; Soprodol	350 mg	Claimed to have analgesic activity
Chlorphenesin carbamate	Maolate	400–800 mg	Relatively weak central depressant
Chlorzoxazone	Paraflex	250–750 mg	Available in combination with analgesics
Cyclobenzaprine HCl	Flexeril	10 mg	Used for acute muscle spasm for periods of only 2–3 wk
Diazepam USP	Valium	2–10 mg	Antianxiety agent also; see Drug digest in Chapter 45
Methocarbamol USP	Robaxin	750–1500 mg	Analogue of mephenesin carbamate, the prototype drug of this class
Orphenadrine citrate	Norflex	60–100 mg	Related to the antihistamine diphenhydramine (Benadryl)

their antispasmodic activity that account for the relief sometimes reported by patients with the common low back and cervical root syndromes, strains, sprains, bursitis, fibrositis, myositis, arthritis, and similar conditions.

Cyclobenzaprine (Flexeril), a more recently introduced antispasmodic that is chemically related to the tricyclic-type drugs used for treating emotional depression, is employed only for the short-term treatment of skeletal muscle spasm and pain that stem from acute traumatic and inflammatory disorders. It is claimed to be as effective as diazepam for producing prompt relief of spasm-induced pain and tenderness, and for increasing the range of motion required during daily activities when administered in doses that cause less central depression than diazepam.

Nonetheless, as is the case with other drugs of this class (see Adverse effects, below), drowsiness is the most common complaint and has been reported by about 40% of patients taking cyclobenzaprine. In addition, this drug has significant anticholinergic activity, which is the cause of side-effects similar to those of atropine (Chap. 16). These atropinelike actions make it necessary to employ cyclobenzaprine with caution, if at all, in patients with narrow-angle glaucoma or a history of hyperprostatism, and in those with heart disorders that might be adversely affected by a drug-induced increase in heart rate. Deliberate or accidental overdosage can cause signs and symptoms of central toxicity similar to those reported following suicide attempts with amitriptyline (Elavil) and other tricyclic-type antidepressants (Chap. 46).

Patients with chronic musculoskeletal conditions often profit more from physical therapy measures than from oral doses of muscle relaxant drugs. Moist heat, massage, traction, and bed rest are often more effective than drugs for treating an acute flare-up of low back pain and similar disorders. The patient should also learn how to prevent recurrences by avoiding the types of activities that tend to set off spasms, yet should not be afraid to engage in physical activity. In fact, after the flare-up has subsided, a program of regular exercises prescribed by the orthopedist should be followed.

The administration of adequate doses of the parenteral forms of diazepam or methocarbamol is often effective for relaxing moderately severe reflex spasm that stems from an acute injury. Injected intravenously or intramuscularly, these drugs sometimes aid in the reduction of dislocations or the setting of fractures. Their main advantage in such situations is that, even when large doses are injected, these drugs are less likely than the barbiturates, for example, to cause excessive central depression that results in loss of consciousness, coma, or cardiovascular and respiratory center depression. However, intravenous injections of even these relatively selective safer drugs must be made slowly and carefully to avoid too rapid an accumulation in the central nervous system, with resulting excessive depression. Care is also required during IV infusion to avoid leakage of hypertonic solutions of methocarbamol into the surrounding tissues.

Neurologic disorders are also often treated with parenterally and orally administered neurospasmolytic drugs. These drugs are thought to relieve spasticity by restoring the balance between inhibitory and excitatory nervous influences on muscle tone. A common characteristic of the conditions in which spasticity occurs is damage to those upper motor neurons that ordinarily send inhibitory impulses down to the lower motor neurons. Loss of these inhibitory controls leads to an excessive influence by those other supraspinal centers that exert an excitatory influence on motor activity. Drugs of this class are believed to depress these subcortical facilitatory areas selectively, as well as the spinal interneurons themselves. As a result of this drug-induced reduction in excitatory interneuronal activity, the hyperactive polysynaptic reflexes are dampened, and the exaggerated contractions of the skeletal muscle are relaxed.

Drugs of this class cannot, of course, repair disease-damaged neuronal pathways, and any relief of painful spasticity that they induce is only temporary. However, the adjunctive administration of neurospasmolytic agents may help spastic patients to profit from the physiotherapeutic measures that are so important in preventing permanent crippling and in slowing the rate of functional impairment in progressive neurologic disorders such as parkinsonism and multiple sclerosis. These drugs may also facilitate habilation and rehabilitation of patients with hemiplegia following a stroke, paraplegia resulting from poliomyelitis, or those disabled by cerebral palsy.

Baclofen (Lioresal), the most recently introduced drug for relief of spasticity, has been employed mainly in the management of patients with multiple sclerosis and spinal cord injuries. It seems to be most effective for reducing the rigidity of flexor muscles and for lessening clonus in such cases. The drug also lessens spasticity of the extensor muscles of the lower limbs, but loss of this reflex response sometimes tends to reduce some patients' abilities to balance and support themselves while standing, and it may even adversely affect their gaits and lessen their abilities to ambulate. Its use for treating muscle spasm associated with musculoskeletal disorders is not recommended, and its usefulness in other neurologic disorders such as Parkinson's disease, hemiplegia in stroke patients, and cerebral palsy has not yet been established.

Although it is claimed to be less sedating than diazepam, over 60% of patients taking baclofen in some studies have reported drowsiness. Other side-effects include dizziness, light-headedness, and headache. If signs of hypersensitivity develop, this drug should be discontinued only gradually, not only because abrupt withdrawal has led to a sudden return of severe spasticity, but also because hallucinations have been reported in such cases.

The following discussion of the usefulness and limitations of these drugs in treating patients with cerebral palsy may serve to indicate the current status of centrally acting antispasmodic drugs in the management of most chronic neurologic disorders.

Cerebral palsy. This condition is marked by a very wide variety of chronic motor dysfunctions. *Spasticity* of muscle groups in the lower and upper extremities occurs most frequently. However, muscular *rigidity*—the result of simultaneous contractions of opposing muscle groups—may predominate in some patients. Others, with damage to basal ganglia such as the corpus striatum, may suffer mainly from *athetosis.* This type of motor abnormality is marked mainly by slow wormlike writhing or twisting of the hands and arms and by other involuntary movements. In some cases the same patient may show several different types of neuromotor disabilities, including tremors and motor incoordination (ataxia of cerebellar origin), as well as spasticity, rigidity, or athetosis. The signs and symptoms of cerebral palsy are not, in fact, limited to motor systems, but may also sometimes include sensory and mental defects in brain-damaged children in whom intracranial injury has occurred in *nonmotor* areas.

Obviously, no one drug or class of drugs can be expected to relieve all of the many varied signs and symptoms of the cerebral palsy syndromes. The treatment of children with this disorder often requires many modalities in addition to drug therapy, including physical, occupational, and speech therapy, bracing, and orthopedic services or surgery. In general, neurospasmolytic drugs seem to be most beneficial when employed as adjuncts to these types of treatment in children with spasticity and athetosis.

When administered at first parenterally and later orally during prolonged maintenance therapy, drugs such as diazepam and methocarbamol produce both muscular and emotional relaxation. These effects are said by some authorities to improve the patient's response to the total, or global, comprehensive management program; other reports of adjunctive drug use suggest that these drugs are no better than a placebo or that drug-induced drowsiness limits their usefulness.

The favorable reports emphasize the fact that these drugs often help cerebral palsied children learn to take care of their personal needs. That is, as a result of drug-induced motor and mental relaxation, many children become better able to sit up, stand, or walk. They can then wash, dress, and feed themselves, and perform other functions that had previously been made difficult by their abnormal posture and movements.

Use of diazepam and similar spasmolytic agents is also said to make these and other patients with painful muscle cramps more willing to undertake physical therapy. Guided exercises are needed to prevent crippling contractures in palsied and other spastic patients. Because the manipulation of spastic movement-resistant limbs is so painful, patients with cerebral palsy, multiple sclerosis, hemiplegia, quadriplegia, or paraplegia often fail to cooperate. Following the parenteral administration of these drugs, however, to reduce muscle spasticity and the discomfort of forced manipulation, patients are often said

to benefit from more effective physiotherapy, in regard to increased muscle strength, mobility, and flexibility.

Although the sedative effects of the centrally acting antispasmodics may cause daytime drowsiness, they also often promote more restful sleep. Thus, children whose sleep is usually interfered with by painful muscle spasticity are often more alert than previously during the day. As a result, they are said to learn more readily than before and to respond better to occupational and speech therapies. An added indirect benefit of drug-induced sleep improvement is sometimes seen in the family of the spastic child. Nurses have noted an improvement in the emotional climate of the family when spastic children becomes less irritable and easier to manage. Another factor in creating a more pleasant atmosphere in the home is the hope offered the family by drug-induced improvement in the child's response to other forms of treatment.

Tetanus. This is an acute infection characterized by severe muscle spasms, and it is also sometimes managed by administration of neurospasmolytic agents, among other drugs, and biologic products (Chap. 55). The symptoms of tetanus stem from the effect of a potent toxin called *tetanospasmin* (Chap. 47), which is produced by bacteria that have entered the body through a break in the skin. This neurotoxin interferes with the functioning of the nerve cells that exert inhibitory influences in polysynaptic reflex pathways within the central nervous system. In particular, it prevents release of the inhibitory neutrotransmitter glycine. The resulting increase in reflex excitability leads to severe convulsive spasms.

Control of the patient's convulsions is the single most important treatment measure in tetanus. This not only helps make the patient more comfortable, but also promotes better pulmonary ventilation and prevents pneumonia and other potentially fatal respiratory complications. Several different types of central depressant drugs have been employed for this purpose, including general anesthetics, anticonvulsant barbiturates, and other sedative–hypnotic drugs. The difficulty in their use is that the doses required to reduce the reflex excitability often also cause excessive depression of the vital centers in the medulla that control breathing and circulation.

The centrally acting antispasmodics are safer in this respect because of their more selective depressant effect on the interneurons that exert excitatory influences on reflex activity. Administered parenterally, various drugs of this class, including methocarbamol, have helped to restore the balance between excitatory and inhibitory influences on the spinal cord, and have thus controlled the severe muscle spasms of tetanus. Unlike the nonselective central depressants, these drugs are usually effective in doses that do not cause unconsciousness or respiratory depression.

Injectable diazepam appears to be more effective in treating tetanus than are the other drugs of this class, and it seems to be safer in various respects. It is not, for example, irritating to the tissues or likely to cause thrombophlebitis, as is sometimes the case with methocarbamol. However, because too rapid intravenous injection of diazepam has occasionally caused cardiac arrest or periods of apnea, intravenous infusion of this drug is best done at a slow rate—2 minutes or more for administration of a fully effective dose.

Actually, skilled nursing care is the most important factor in management of patients with tetanus. Despite the usefulness of drugs of the neurospasmolytic type and other anticonvulsants, pharmacologic agents alone cannot prevent the complications that often occur during the weeks in which treatment is sometimes required. Many nursing measures are necessary to protect the patient from serious complications. This is particularly true if treatment with central nervous system depressants alone fails to control the tetanic spasms, and the patient is put on a long-term regimen of peripherally acting neuromuscular blocking agents such as tubocurarine (see Chap. 19).

Adverse effects. The centrally acting skeletal muscle relaxants are relatively safe drugs, particularly when administered in small oral doses. However, hypersensitivity reactions sometimes occur and must be watched for, and large overdoses can cause central depression similar to that seen with barbiturates, despite the much wider margin of safety of these selective neurospasmolytic agents (see the summary of side-effects at the end of this chapter).

Gastrointestinal upset. Gastrointestinal effects, including epigastric distress, nausea and vomiting, heartburn, and hiccups, cause occasional complaints. However, these are less likely to occur with the more potent drugs available today than with mephenesin, the prototype agent of this class, which is no longer available. Drugs such as diazepam, which are effective in only a tiny fraction of the doses required with earlier drugs, rarely cause gastrointestinal upset.

Signs of central depression. These signs, including drowsiness, are the most common side-effects of diazepam and similar muscle relaxants that are also minor tranquilizers or antianxiety agents. Thus, it is desirable to warn ambulatory patients not to drive a car, operate machinery, or undertake other tasks that require mental alertness when they begin taking diazepam, meprobamate, and related drugs such as carisoprodol. Although these drugs do not have a strong abuse potential, care is required in patients with a history of drug abuse because of the possibility that psychological or physical dependence might develop in addiction-prone patients during the prolonged use of these agents for treatment of a chronic disorder.

Parenteral administration is more likely to cause hypotensive reactions marked by feelings of weakness, dizziness, vertigo, and light-headedness. Thus, it is desirable that patients be kept in a recumbent position for 10 to 15 minutes following administration of methocarbamol. Motor incoordination is also most marked following injection of large doses. As has previously been indicated, intravenous infusions of diazepam should be made slowly to avoid adverse cardiovascular and respiratory depressant effects.

Local irritation. This makes intramuscular injection of some of these agents painful. Care is required to avoid leakage of methocarbamol into the tissues around veins, because thrombophlebitis may result. Sloughing of tissue at the injection site sometimes occurs. Thus, when this drug is administered intramuscularly, it is desirable to divide the total dose in two and to make separate injections into each of the gluteal areas. Once parenteral administration has brought about some relief, the patient is best maintained on oral doses.

Hypersensitivity reactions. A wide variety have been reported, but their incidence is not very high. Skin rash and pruritus are most common; other allergic manifestations such as wheezing are less frequent. Anaphylactoid reactions are rare. Carisoprodol has, on rare occasions, caused an unusual idiosyncratic reaction marked by alarming mental and muscular effects, including transient quadriplegia.

Dantrolene

This drug relaxes spastic skeletal muscles by a peripheral rather than a central action. However, it is appropriate to discuss it here in this chapter that deals mainly with centrally acting skeletal muscle relaxants. This is because this drug has made a distinct contribution to the management of spasticity in patients with various of the chronic neurologic disorders discussed above and listed in the summary of drug indications at the end of this chapter. (However, it is *not* used for treating muscle spasm that occurs as a result of the rheumatic and other musculoskeletal conditions, also listed in that summary.)

Site and mechanism of action. Dantrolene sodium (Dantrium) was the first of what may become a new class of muscle relaxants called direct-acting antagonists of muscle contraction. The drug, which at this time remains unique in the manner of its action, differs not only from diazepam and other centrally acting antispasmodics but also from such other peripherally acting drugs as curare and succinylcholine (Chap. 19). Unlike the latter neuromuscular blocking agents, dantrolene does not block the transmission of spinal motor nerve impulses at the neuromuscular junction in skeletal muscles, nor does it act at the surface of the muscle fiber membranes. Instead, this drug acts within each muscle fiber to prevent the release of calcium ions from the sarcoplasmic reticulum, a response to excitation of the fiber by nerve impulses that is a necessary step in activation of the contractile response.

Clinical indications. Dantrolene is indicated for patients with chronic neurologic disorders such as cerebral palsy and multiple sclerosis and for those who have suffered a severe stroke or spinal cord injury. By bringing about a sustained decrease in muscle spasticity and exaggerated reflex activity, the drug often lessens the patient's pain and helps to prevent deforming muscle and soft tissue contractures and the resulting permanent disabilities.

As is the case when diazepam and other centrally acting spasmolytic agents are employed, those who prescribe dantrolene for nerve-damaged patients start out by setting up specific goals that they hope to have the patient achieve during therapy. Improvement is measured in terms of the patient's increased ability to perform some simple activity of daily life such as washing, dressing, or feeding himself, which he could not quite do before taking the drug. The drug's dosage is gradually raised until the patient's performance of each function is the best that can be achieved. Other therapeutic goals include increased ability to perform exercises, maintain posture and balance, and use braces, and a reduction in the need for nursing care.

A main limitation of this drug is that it may tend to induce persistent weakness in *non*spastic muscles. This occurs, for example, in some patients with multiple sclerosis or athetoid cerebral palsy. In other cases, the drug-induced reduction in spasticity may be undesirable, because the patient's ability to remain upright and to maintain balance and mobility depends on certain of the muscles staying in a spastic state.

The drug is also indicated in the management, and perhaps in the prevention, of malignant hyperthermia, a syndrome triggered in susceptible persons by certain general anesthetics (*e.g.*, cyclopropane, halothane, methoxyflurane).

Adverse effects. The most common side-effects of dantrolene are central in origin. That is, although the drug's desirable effects are mainly the result of its action peripherally in skeletal muscles, it can also cause drowsiness, dizziness, and feelings of fatigue. It is claimed, however, that this drug causes less sedation than diazepam when each drug is administered in doses that are equally effective for reducing spastic clonus and hyperreflexia. In addition, such central depressant effects are said to be transient, and they can often be avoided entirely, even early in treatment, by beginning treatment with a low dose that is raised gradually until the lowest dosage level that can produce optimal improvement in the patient's performance has been attained.

Gastrointestinal side-effects include gastric irritation and bleeding, abdominal cramps, and diarrhea that is occasionally severe enough to make it necessary to discontinue treatment with dantrolene temporarily or permanently. The most serious adverse reaction to dantrolene is the possible development of liver damage in patients who have continued to take the drug for long periods, or who have used high doses even for short periods. Deaths from hepatitis have occurred in about one or two of every 1000 patients who were treated for longer than 2 months. Hepatotoxicity seems to develop most often in women over 35 years old who have also been taking estrogens. Thus, the drug is administered with particular care in such cases or in patients with a history of previous liver disease. Liver function tests are performed at the start of drug therapy and at regular intervals thereafter and, if abnormalities develop in such tests, the drug is almost always discontinued.

Cautions and contraindications. As has already been suggested, this drug is contraindicated in patients who show clinical or laboratory signs of active liver disease and in those spastic patients in whom spasticity seems to serve a useful function, such as helping to keep the patient in an upright posture or in maintaining balance while moving about. The drug is also undesirable for patients with breathing difficulties caused by respiratory center depression, and caution is required in patients with chronic obstructive pulmonary diseases such as emphysema. Its use in patients with severe heart disease also requires caution. Patients taking this drug should be warned against exposing themselves to sunlight to avoid possible development of photosensitivity reactions.

In summary, dantrolene appears to be a useful drug for adjunctive use in patients with neurologic disorders whose rehabilitation is interfered with by muscular spasticity and hyperreflexia. It seems to be as effective as diazepam in such cases, and less likely to cause excessive drowsiness or other signs of central depression than that drug. However, the possible development of hepatotoxicity and fatal hepatitis during long-term therapy can prevent the continued use of this valuable drug in the long-term management of some patients with chronic neurologic disorders.

Chymopapain

This drug, a proteolytic enzyme derived from the papaya plant, has been approved by the FDA since 1983 for treating those patients with herniated lumbar intravertebral discs and evidence of nerve compression, who have not responded to more conservative therapy. Chymopapain (Chymodiactin; Discase) is injected, by specially trained physicians, directly into the nucleosus pulposus of the affected disc, where it rapidly destroys the mucoprotein of the disc ("chemonucleolysis"). Thus, in successful cases, it relieves the severe and painful spasms of the lower back muscles, as well as the other neurologic consequences of nerve compression. The success rate of injections of chymopapain, compared to that of injections of placebo, has varied in different studies, but has been consistently higher. For example, in one study of patients with sciatica, 63% of the patients receiving injections of chymopapain were free of pain 6 months after the injection, compared to only 27% of patients receiving placebo injections.

The advantages of this procedure over surgical

techniques include a shorter hospital stay (usually only 24–48 hr after the injection), with concomitant lower cost, and more rapid recovery.

The procedure is not without risk, however. Chymopapain, like all enzymes, is a protein and thus can cause allergic reactions. Anaphylaxis, fatal in some cases, occurs in 0.4% to 1% of patients. Because chymopapain is present as an additive in some foods (*e.g.*, it is used as a meat tenderizer) as well as in the fruit of the papaya tree, and is used in making beer, some patients may have been sensitized before receiving the drug. Allergic reactions to papaya fruit and products, as well as previous injections of chymopapain, are contraindications to its use. All patients receiving chymopapain injections should have an IV line in place to facilitate the rapid injection of epinephrine if needed to treat angioneurotic edema or anaphylaxis.

In addition, serious adverse neurologic effects—paraplegia and cerebral hemorrhage—have occurred soon after injection in some patients. More common adverse effects, about which patients should be warned preoperatively, include back pain, stiffness, and soreness, which occurs in about 50% of patients.

Additional clinical considerations

Patients who require the use of skeletal muscle relaxants often require efficient nursing care to facilitate the therapeutic effects of the drugs. Such measures include positioning, skin care, application of braces, use of exercises, environmental control and, sometimes, additional pain relief measures. Patients with neuromuscular diseases who require long-term treatment need regular evaluation and a total care plan aimed at helping them to achieve their highest level of functioning.

In addition to the cautions and contraindications associated with these drugs that have already been discussed, it is important to remember that the safety of their use during pregnancy and lactation has not been established. Several of these drugs have been associated with fetal malformations in animal models, and all cross over into human breast milk. Because of this, it is recommended that these drugs be avoided entirely during pregnancy and lactation.

Patient teaching points covered with these drugs should include the side-effects and cautions discussed above. Patients who receive methocarbamol should also know that their urine may change to brown, black, or dark green as it stands. The patients need to know that this is an expected side-effect of the drug, and is not an indication of renal problems.

The patient teaching guide summarizes teaching points that should be incorporated into the teaching program of a patient receiving long-term therapy with dantrolene sodium.

Drug–drug interactions

Because these drugs have central nervous system depressant effects, they should not be used concurrently with other *CNS depressants,* (*e.g.*, alcohol, tranquilizers). Because of its anticholinergic effects, *cyclobenzaprine* should be used with caution in patients receiving *anticholinergic drugs.* The hepatotoxicity associated with *dantrolene* seems to occur more frequently if the drug is given concurrently with *estrogens.* Although an exact mechanism of action has not been established, this combination of drugs should probably be avoided.

The guide to the nursing process summarizes the clinical aspects that should be considered in the nursing care of a patient receiving dantrolene.

Patient teaching guide: dantrolene sodium

The drug that has been prescribed for you is a direct acting muscle relaxant. It is used to relax muscles that are clinically spastic. Because this drug could have serious effects on the liver, it is important that you receive regular medical evaluation.

Instructions:

1. The name of your drug is _____ .

2. The dosage that has been prescribed for you is _____ .

3. The drug should be taken _____ times a day. The best time to take your drug is _____ .

4. Some side-effects of the drug that you should be aware of include the following:

(continued)

Sensitivity to sunlight	Avoid exposure to the sun. Wear protective clothing and sunglasses. Use of sunscreens may help if exposure cannot be avoided.
Weakness, fatigue	Frequent rest periods and spacing of activities may help. If this becomes too severe, consult with your nurse or physician.
Drowsiness, dizziness	This is a frequent problem with this drug. Avoid driving, using hazardous equipment, and trying to perform delicate tasks if this side-effect occurs.
Diarrhea	This may subside over time. If the problem persists, consult with your nurse or physician.

5. Avoid the use of alcohol or other depressants while you are on this drug.

6. Keep this and all medications out of the reach of children.

7. Tell any nurse, physician, or dentist who is taking care of you that you are on this drug.

8. Take this drug exactly as prescribed. Regular, medical follow-up care is necessary to evaluate the overall effects of this drug on your body.

Notify your nurse or physician if any of the following occur:

Fever, chills
Rash, itching
Black, tarry stools
Yellow coloring to your eyes or
   skin

Guide to the nursing process: dantrolene sodium

Assessment	Nursing diagnoses	Interventions	Evaluation
Past history (contraindications): Severe cardiac disease Hepatic disease COPD Pregnancy Lactation	Knowledge deficit regarding drug therapy Potential sensory–perceptual alteration Potential for injury	Safe and appropriate administration of drug: (if IV, care to avoid extravasation) Patient teaching regarding drug therapy	Monitor for therapeutic effectiveness of drug: decreased spasticity Monitor for adverse effects of drug: • Liver enzyme level changes

(continued)

Chapter 48 Centrally acting skeletal muscle relaxants

Assessment	Nursing diagnoses	Interventions	Evaluation
Allergies: this drug; others; reactions Medication history (*cautions*): *Tranquilizers* *CNS depressants* *Estrogens* **Physical assessment** Neurologic: complete exam Cardiovascular: P, BP, perfusion Respiratory: R, adventitious sounds GI: liver, abdominal exam Skin: lesions Laboratory tests: liver enzyme levels		Comfort and safety measures: • Positioning • Skin care • Environmental control • Protection if dizziness or drowsiness occurs Support and encouragement to cope with disease and drug therapy	• Photosensitivity • Drowsiness, CNS problems • GI upset • Rash Evaluate effectiveness of patient teaching program Evaluate effectiveness of comfort and safety measures Evaluate effectiveness of support and encouragement offered Monitor for drug–drug interactions: Hepatic problems with *estrogens* CNS problems with *CNS depressants* (*e.g.,* tranquilizers, alcohol)

Case study

Presentation

LG, a 26-year-old white male, has had a diagnosis of cerebral palsy since shortly after birth. He is currently living in a community maintenance home with six other cerebral palsy victims under the supervision of two adult caretakers. Over the past few months, LG's spasticity has become progressively more severe, making it impossible for him to carry on his activities of daily living without extensive assistance. LG was evaluated in the clinic and it was decided to try a course of dantrolene therapy. The risks of hepatic dysfunction were discussed, and LG decided that the potential benefit was much more important to him at this stage in his life than the risks of hepatotoxicity. A baseline complete physical exam was performed, including liver enzymes. LG was started on 25 mg, tid, with a visiting nurse referral to evaluate his progress in 4 days.

What basic principles must be included in the nursing care plan for this patient as he is followed by the visiting nurse?

Discussion

On the first visit to LG's maintenance home, the visiting nurse will need to establish a relationship with LG and his caretakers. The step-by-step goals of therapy should be established and written down for future reference. The nurse will need to do a physical assessment of LG to establish baseline data of his disease and current functioning. A careful patient history should also be done to determine what parameters have changed since drug therapy was begun 4 days ago, as well as to determine LG's past functioning and his resources and limitations. If drug therapy has been helpful, the dosage may be slowly increased until the optimum level of functioning has been achieved.

The nurse will need to evaluate the effectiveness of the drug therapy and to confer with the patient's physician.

While evaluating the patient in his home setting the nurse can also evaluate the resources and limitations of the patient's environment, and can make appropriate suggestions for additional measures that could facilitate the drug therapy—for example, positioning, environmental controls, use of braces. The patient and his caretakers will also need a written list to alert them to drug cautions and warnings, and LG should have follow-up medical visits to evaluate liver enzyme levels as well as his total response to the drug therapy. There is no cure for LG's disease and the drug therapy, combined with other measures, is used to help him make the most of the strengths that he still has to achieve the highest level of functioning possible. This therapy involves a long-term commitment, and will be facilitated by a trusting and working relationship between the patient and all members of the health-care team.

Summary of clinical indications for centrally acting muscle relaxants

Musculoskeletal disorders (peripheral injury or inflammation)

Muscle strains as a result of excessive stretching or overuse

Sprains resulting from wrenched joints with stretched or torn ligaments

Whiplash injuries of the cervical spine processes; cervical root syndromes; herniated disk syndrome; low back syndrome; dislocations and fractures; arthritis, myositis, fibrositis, tendosynovitis, bursitis, and neuritis

Neurologic disorders (hypertonicity resulting from central nervous system disease and damage)

Cerebral palsy

Multiple sclerosis

Muscular dystrophy

Poliomyelitis

Amyotrophic lateral sclerosis

Hemiplegia

Quadriplegia

Parkinson's disease

Laminectomy

Spinal tumors

Tetanus

Summary of side-effects and toxicity of centrally acting muscle relaxants

Gastrointestinal

Small doses. Epigastric distress, nausea and vomiting, hiccups

Central nervous system

Moderate dosage. Drowsiness, dizziness, vertigo, light-headedness, headache (Ambulatory patients should not drive or operate dangerous machinery.)

Overdosage. Muscular incoordination (ataxia), loss of flexor reflexes, flaccid paralysis (including muscles of respiration), stupor, coma, respiratory failure

Cardiovascular reactions

Facial flushing, bradycardia or tachycardia, hypotension with feelings of faintness and weakness and possible syncope, shock

Miscellaneous reactions to various agents (allergic, idiosyncratic, and others)

Skin rashes, redness, itching, urticaria, angioneurotic edema, asthmatic breathing

Thrombophlebitis (methocarbamol)

Dependence: psychological and possibly physical (diazepam, carisoprodol, meprobamate, and others)

Extreme muscle weakness, transient quadriplegia, temporary blindness (carisoprodol idiosyncrasy)

Blurred vision, mouth dryness (orphenadrine)

Drug digest

Methocarbamol U.S.P. (Robaxin)

Actions and indications. This centrally acting skeletal muscle relaxant is used to relieve spasm and spasticity in various musculoskeletal and neurologic disorders. Oral doses are used mainly for depressing spinal interneurons, thus reducing the number of sensory impulses being relayed from peripheral muscle and joint areas to spinal motor neurons. The resulting interruption of excessive polysynaptic reflex activity relieves the spasm and pain associated with muscle strains, sprains, and such inflammatory musculoskeletal conditions as arthritis, bursitis, fibrositis, and myositis. Intravenous administration is effective for relief of spasm following whiplash injuries, herniated disk, and other cervical and lumbar nerve root syndromes. Spasticity, dystonia, rigidity, and athetosis are relieved in hypertonic states resulting from nervous system diseases, including multiple sclerosis and cerebral palsy.

Adverse effects, cautions, and contraindications. Drowsiness, dizziness, light-headedness, and nausea occur with oral dosage. In addition, parenteral administration sometimes causes incoordination and syncopal reactions as a result of bradycardia and hypotension. Intravenous administration may also lead to thrombophlebitis and intramuscular administration to formation of painful nodules and tissue sloughing. The drug is contraindicated in patients with a history of hypersensitivity to it, marked by skin rashes and fever. The parenternal form is contraindicated in patients with kidney disease because of the presence of a vehicle considered unsafe when renal impairment is present. Use of the drug in epileptic patients is not recommended.

Dosage and administration. Oral doses of about 6 to 8 g a day are used during the first few days of treatment and then reduced to about 4 g daily. Parenteral administration by the intramuscular route is best accomplished by dividing the 1-g dose into equal 500-mg amounts injected into each gluteal muscle. The usual total intravenous dose for adults is 1 g (10 ml) injected undiluted at a rate of no more than 300 mg (3 ml)/min. The total adult IV dose does not ordinarily exceed 3 g (30 ml) daily. In tetanus, this amount may have to be administered every 6 hours. Patients receiving the drug by this route are instructed to lie flat during the infusion and for 10 to 15 minutes afterward.

References

Bianchine JR: Drugs for Parkinson's disease: Centrally acting muscle relaxants. In Gilman AG, Goodman LS, Gilman A (eds): Goodman & Gilman's The Pharmacological Basis of Therapeutics, 6th ed, pp 475–493. New York, Macmillan, 1980

Chymopapain for herniated lumbar discs. Med Lett Drugs Ther 25:41, 1983

Merritt JL: Management of spasticity in spinal cord injury. Mayo Clin Proc 56:614, 1981

Rodman MJ: Drugs for treating tetanus. RN 34:43, 1971

Utili R et al: Dantrolene-associated hepatic injury: Incidence and character. Gastroenterology 72:610, 1977

Young RR, Delwaide PJ: Spasticity (Pts I and II). N Engl J Med 304:28, 96, 1981

Chapter 49

Drugs
for
treating
parkinsonism

49

The nature of Parkinson's disease

Parkinson's disease is a chronic progressive motor disorder that is the result of damage to neurons located in the basal ganglia of the brain. Parkinsonism is seen mainly in people past middle age. Some cases stem from cerebral arteriosclerosis; others are the result of drugs (the anti-dopaminergic drugs described in Chapter 46), chemical toxicity (chronic exposure to manganese; carbon monoxide poisoning), encephalitis, and other brain infections. However, the specific cause of most cases of Parkinson's syndrome is unknown, or idiopathic. The recent discovery that a chemical called MPTP (1-methyl-4-phenyl-pro-pionoxy-piperidine), a contaminant in the illicit synthesis of a heroinlike drug that was used by addicts, induces in humans and monkeys an irreversible syndrome that is indistinguishable from Parkinson's disease, is potentially a valuable clue to the identification of the etiologic agent of naturally occurring Parkinson's disease, as well as a clue to drugs that may provide prophylaxis or new approaches to therapy for this disease.

The signs and symptoms of parkinsonism are insidious in onset. Rhythmic tremors that are, at first, barely perceptible may be the first sign. Some muscle groups tend to become rigid, while others weaken. The patient makes very few spontaneous movements and these may be extremely slow and sluggish—a condition called *bradykinesia* or *akinesia*. Yet, if pushed even gently, the patient may not be able to stop his rapid progress forward or backward, and will fall down if not caught and supported.

These difficulties affecting the patient's posture, balance, and movements become progressively more pronounced. In addition, the patient in advanced stages of parkinsonism may drool, speech becomes slurred, and his face assumes a masklike expression. Despite the dullness of his appearance and his seeming unresponsiveness, the parkinsonism patient does not ordinarily suffer from intellectual impairment. He may, however, become deeply discouraged and emotionally depressed.

Thus, these patients need constant emotional support during the long years in which they are being treated in an effort to slow the rate at which they are becoming disabled. Until fairly recently, most patients became bedridden between 10 and 20 years after onset of the disease. New drugs, surgical procedures, and physical therapy measures now offer new hope of preventing complete disability. However, emotional support is still an important part of the treatment of Parkinson's disease.

Neuropathology of Parkinson's disease

Research in the 1960's revealed some aspects of the pathology within the extrapyramidal motor system (Chap. 44) that leads to the muscular malfunctions of Parkinson's disease. Scientists found that nerve cell bodies located in the *substantia nigra,* a midbrain nerve nucleus, show signs of degeneration. This loss of nerve cells results in reduction of nerve impulse transmission from the substantia nigra to the *corpus striatum,* one of the several basal ganglia located in the white matter beneath the cerebral cortex.

The lessening of impulses along this so-called *nigrostriatal pathway* has been linked to neurochemical changes in these brain areas. Specifically, a deficiency of the catecholamine *dopamine* (Chaps. 13 and 17) develops in both the nerve cell bodies of the substantia nigra and their axon terminals in the corpus striatum. One hypothesis is that this lack of dopamine leads to a neurochemical imbalance, in which central nerve cells that release *acetylcholine* (Chap. 13) exert an excessive influence on the corpus striatum. This, in turn, affects the functioning of other basal ganglia—the *globus pallidus,* for example—and of the cerebellar and cerebral cortical components of the extrapyramidal motor system.

This theory is probably an oversimplification of what actually occurs. However, it is useful for visualizing the ways in which the two major types of currently available antiparkinsonism drugs discussed below may act to exert their beneficial effects on the disabling motor difficulties of Parkinson's disease and related symptoms. Drug-induced parkinsonism is caused, not by degeneration of nigrostriatal neurons, but rather by blockade of dopamine receptors (phenothiazines) or depletion of neuronal dopamine stores (reserpine).

Management of parkinsonism

Although the primary concern of this chapter will be the antiparkinsonism agents, drugs are only one aspect of the total care these patients require. Drugs cannot, of course, cure a condition caused by damage and death of motor neurons deep in the brain, but in many cases they can relieve some distressing symptoms of this condition. Employed together with massage and other physical therapy measures, drugs may help to delay development of crippling deformities.

Even though drugs may offer only partial relief of symptoms and slow the progress of parkinsonism only slightly, their judicious use can often help attain a major objective of management—keeping patients active and able to care for themselves as long as possible. A drug-induced improvement in their ability to do some simple task on their own, unaided by others, often offers patients an important boost in morale.

Care of parkinsonism patients presents a challenge to even the most skilled and experienced nurse. Nursing care must include assisting patients with exercises prescribed for preventing deformity, encouraging them to take care of personal needs themselves, and instructing them and their families in administration of drugs for maximal effectiveness and minimal reaction discomfort. All these measures help patients maintain their will to keep active despite their illness. This is very desirable, because feelings of independence tend to counteract the despair that often assails people with this chronic neurologic condition.

Drugs used in the treatment of Parkinson's disease

Until fairly recently, only one class of drugs was available for adjunctive use in the management of parkinsonism—*the centrally acting anticholinergic agents*, including the natural belladonna alkaloids, synthetic atropinelike drugs, and agents with mainly antihistaminic activity but with secondary acetylcholine-blocking effects (Table 49-1). However, in 1970, the Food and Drug Administration authorized the introduction of *levodopa*, a new drug with properties entirely different from those of the traditional drugs. At present, levodopa is considered to be the drug of choice among available pharmacotherapeutic agents for treating parkinsonism. However, the administration of levodopa does not preclude the use of the still important anticholinergic-type medications. Thus, both types of antiparkinsonism agents will be described.

Natural and synthetic anticholinergic drugs

The first drugs introduced for relaxing muscle rigidity and relieving the other symptoms of Parkinson's disease were derivatives of plants of the deadly nightshade family, such a hyoscyamus and belladonna. More or less accidentally, the alkaloids atropine and scopolamine (Chap. 16) were found to help many patients. These anticholinergic agents are thought to act centrally to reduce the disorderly transmission of the impulses that are passing out to the skeletal muscles by way of extrapyramidal nerve tracts. Unfortunately, these drugs also have many undesirable peripheral actions, which are the result of blockade of parasympathetic nerve impulses to smooth muscles and glands. This results in many discomforting and even dangerous side-effects (see Chapter 16 and the summary of adverse effects at the end of this chapter).

Numerous synthetic chemicals (see Table 49-1 and Drug digests) have been developed for relaxing rigidity and reducing the tremors of parkinsonism. Like the natural substances, these somewhat safer drugs bring about their therapeutically desired effects through their central action. In fact, they have an even greater affinity for these central sites. Thus, their main advantage is that they are less likely to cause the undesired peripheral effects of atropinetype alkaloids. Nonetheless, these synthetics are themselves not entirely free of peripheral side-effects similar to those of atropine.

Side-effects. Atropinelike side-effects include dryness of the skin and mouth, constipation, dysuria, and blurring of vision. Some of these secondary actions may actually be beneficial for some patients. For example, the secretion-drying effect may be desirable for patients with postencephalitic parkinsonism who often tend to drool and sweat excessively. In other patients, however, atropinelike side-effects may precipitate severe reactions, including attacks of glaucoma and tachycardia. Elderly men, who often have an enlarged prostate gland that presses on the neck of the bladder, should be watched for signs of difficulty in urination brought on by the adverse effects that these drugs sometimes have on bladder function.

Behavioral changes. Certain of these synthetic anticholinergic drugs can produce behavioral changes. In some cases, these psychopharmacologic effects may be beneficial; in others, they may be harmful. For example, patients who tend to be tense and nervous may be calmed by the sedative action sometimes found when *diphenhydramine*[+] (Benadryl; see Drug digest, Chap. 39), *benztropine mesylate*[+] (Cogentin), or the natural substance *scopolamine* (hyoscine) is being used to treat their tremors. On the other hand, patients whose illness is marked by excessive sluggishness may do better when taking a drug such as *orphenadrine* (Disipal), which has, in addition, a mild cen-

Table 49–1. Drugs for treating parkinsonism

Official or generic name	Trade name	Usual adult daily dosage range	Comments
Synthetic anticholinergic and antihistaminic drugs			
Benztropine mesylate USP	Cogentin	0.5–6 mg	See Drug digest
Biperiden HCl and lactate USP	Akineton	2–8 mg	Similar to trihexyphenidyl
Diphenhydramine HCl USP	Benadryl	75–150 mg	See Drug digest, Chapter 39
Ethopropazine HCl USP	Parsidol	50–100 mg	Has properties of both trihexyphenidyl and diphenhydramine
Orphenadrine HCl USP	Disipal	150–250 mg	Similar to diphenhydramine
Procyclidine HCl USP	Kemadrin	10–20 mg	Similar to trihexyphenidyl
Trihexyphenidyl HCl USP	Artane; Tremin	6–10 mg	See Drug digest
Dopamine agonists			
Bromocriptine mesylate	Parlodel	2.5 mg/day in two doses; may increase gradually	Acts directly to stimulate striatal dopaminergic receptors
Other drugs			
Amantadine HCl USP	Symmetrel	100–200 mg	Antiviral agent; also effective as adjunct in parkinsonism
Carbidopa	Lodosyn	—	Dopa decarboxylase inhibitor available only to physicians for use with levodopa in patients who need different dosage adjustment than is available in the fixed ratio product
Levodopa USP	Dopar; Larodopa; Levopa; L-dopa	4–6 g	Amino acid precursor of dopamine; see also Drug digest
Levodopa and carbidopa	Sinemet	Dosage must be adjusted individually; dosage is usually initiated with one 25/100 tablet tid (75 mg carbidopa + 300 mg levodopa/day)	Carbidopa is a dopa decarboxylase inhibitor combined with levodopa in a ratio of 1:4 and 1:10

tral stimulating effect. (Amphetamine-type agents are also sometimes used to help overcome drowsiness and lethargy in parkinsonian patients with such symptoms.)

Obviously, these depressant and stimulating actions on the nervous system can be dangerous if allowed to go too far. Mental confusion, loss of memory, and disorientation may develop, especially in elderly patients with the atherosclerotic form of parkinsonism. The development of such signs should be watched for. They are usually relieved by a reduction in dosage. Such drug-induced effects may be difficult to distinguish from signs of the patient's illness; however, it is important to attempt to make this distinction, because such drug-induced signs may be the forerunner of serious drug-induced toxic psychosis.

Dosage and administration. As a rule, treatment is begun by administering small doses of the least toxic antiparkinsonism drugs. For elderly patients and others with low tolerance to the central effects of the synthetic atropinelike agents *diphenhydramine* (Benadryl) and of related antihistamines such as *orphenadrine HCl* (Disipal) are often preferred. However, these drugs are relatively ineffective for most patients, and must be administered in combination with one of the more potent centrally acting anticholinergic agents such as *trihexyphenidyl HCl*[+] (Artane).

Trihexyphenidyl is the preferred agent for initiating treatment in most cases. It is administered at first in a single small dose taken by mouth at bedtime. Dosage is then gradually raised in small increments at intervals of 5 or 6 days, until optimal effects are attained. The amount of the drug that produces maximal benefit with minimal toxicity must be adjusted for each patient individually. Some patients benefit from treatment with a total dose of only 1 or 2 mg daily, while others require doses of as high as 8 mg.

If even such high doses of trihexyphenidyl fail to provide full relief, or when tolerance develops to the effects of this drug or of its congeners, *biperiden* (Akineton) and *procyclidine* (Kemadrin), small amounts of *benztropine mesylate* (Cogentin) may be added to the patient's regimen. Administered at bedtime to patients unable to sleep because of muscle rigidity, spasm and pain, this drug's ability to relieve skeletal muscle spasms and its sedative effects often provide enough relief to allow the patient to rest. It also makes it easier for the patient to turn in bed and to arise in the morning. However, the potential peripheral and central toxicity of this drug is greater than that of most others.

Use in drug-induced extrapyramidal disorders. Drugs such as the phenothiazines, butyrophenones, and reserpine sometimes cause extrapyramidal motor system reactions when used in the management of psychosis or vomiting (Chap. 46). Acute dystonic reactions can usually be brought quickly under control by the parenteral administration of *benztropine, biperiden,* or *diphenhydramine.*

Patients under long-term antipsychotic drug treatment who begin to develop parkinsonism symptoms often benefit from the temporary addition of an antiparkinsonism drug to their regimens. After the added drug has reduced such drug-induced disturbances of tranquilizer therapy as dyskinesia and rigidity, it is gradually withdrawn. If reactions recur with continued tranquilizer therapy, treatment with the antiparkinsonism drug may be begun again, or dosage of the phenothiazine or other antipsychotic agent may be reduced. One reason for reducing tranquilizer drug dosage rather than continuing the patient on antiparkinsonism medications indefinitely is the possibility that these drugs may mask the symptoms of the permanent tardive dyskinesia that is now known to develop in 15 to 45% of patients on prolonged treatment with phenothiazine-type tranquilizers (Chap. 46).

Levodopa

Historical aspects. Advances during the 1960s in understanding catecholamine metabolism (see Chaps. 13 and 17) led to the suggestion that the basic biochemical lesion of Parkinson's disease might be a deficiency of dopamine in the corpus striatum. Attempts to treat the neurologic disorder with this catecholamine were unsuccessful, because it failed to pass the blood–brain barrier and enter the brain. Clinical investigators then tried administering *dopa* (dihydroxyphenylalanine), the immediate precursor of dopamine in the series of reactions that result in the biosynthesis of catecholamines in the brain and elsewhere in the body (Table 49-2).

Although the administration of this amino acid was followed by the improvement of many patients with parkinsonism, the very large doses of dopa that were needed for effectiveness often caused severe gastrointestinal upset. Later, the *levo isomer of dopa—L-dopa,* or *levodopa*—became available in a pure form that permitted treatment with only about half the daily dosage previously needed and with a resulting reduction in gastrointestinal side-effects.

The results of early controlled clinical trials with levodopa[+] (Dopar; Larodopa) indicated that about a third of patients showed marked improvement and that another third made moderate gains. This led physicians to demand that the drug be released for general use, even though it had not yet been fully evaluated. Because Parkinson's disease is an incurable affliction that had not been adequately controlled by the standard available drugs, the FDA in 1970 took the unusual step of approving the release of this drug before its long-term safety and effectiveness had actually been established by the types of studies ordinarily demanded. Levodopa is now marketed as Dopar, Larodopa and, combined with carbidopa (see below) in Sinemet.

Results of therapy. When levodopa passes the blood–brain barrier, it is enzymatically converted to dopamine in the terminals of nigrostriatal dopaminergic neurons. Most patients with symptoms secondary to a deficiency of dopamine begin to show signs of improvement within 1 or 2 weeks. Continued treatment of patients correctly diagnosed as parkinsonism sufferers results in maximal improvement after about 6 weeks of therapy. Many severely disabled patients handicapped by muscular rigidity and akinesia show marked improvement in their ability to move about in a more coordinated manner. Posture, balance, and ability to speak are also obviously improved in many cases, and there is often a reduction

Table 49–2. Steps in the biosynthesis of dopamine and other catecholamines

Substrate	Type of enzyme	Product
1. Phenylalanine (amino acid)	Hydroxylase	Tyrosine
2. Tyrosine (amino acid)	Hydroxylase	Dihydroxyphenylalanine (dopa)
3. Dopa (amino acid)*	Decarboxylase	Dopamine
4. Dopamine (catecholamine)	β-hydroxylase	Norepinephrine
5. Norepinephrine (catecholamine)	N-methyltransferase	Epinephrine

* The series of reactions ends with step 3 in the *substantia nigra;* steps 4 and 5 occur at other sites (see Chap. 13).

in salivation, sweating and skin oiliness (seborrhea). Tremor, which is usually controlled by the anticholinergic drugs, is probably the parkinsonian sign least helped by levodopa. Sometimes patients feel so well physically and mentally that they tend to exert themselves excessively. Thus, they must be cautioned against becoming too active too soon. In contrast to the marked or moderate improvement in most patients, some do not respond readily to treatment with levodopa, and others cannot tolerate effective doses of the drug.

Adverse reactions. The most common side-effects that occur early in treatment are anorexia, nausea, and vomiting (see the summary at the end of this chapter). These ill effects can usually be minimized by initiating treatment with relatively small doses—only 0.5 to 1 g daily, divided into three or four doses of only one 250-mg capsule taken with food.* Then, as the patient shows increased ability to tolerate the drug, the amount administered with each meal is gradually increased every few days. Ordinarily, it takes about 6 to 8 weeks for each patient to reach the individually adjusted dosage at which maximal improvement is exhibited, with side-effects so minimal that the patient is willing to tolerate them to maintain the gains that have been made in mobility.

During dosage adjustment and long-term treatment, patients must be closely observed for signs of cardiovascular, neurologic and psychiatric toxicity. Development of cardiac arrhythmias may, for example, make it necessary to discontinue treatment with levodopa. Patients with a history of a heart attack that has left them with cardiac arrhythmias are best hospitalized at the start of treatment, so that their cardiovascular responses can

be carefully monitored and intensive coronary care employed if necessary. Patients with high blood pressure may require a downward adjustment of their antihypertensive drug dosage, because levodopa tends to cause postural hypotension. (Hypertension, an effect theoretically more likely to be produced by a precursor of norepinephrine, also sometimes occurs.)

Some patients taking levodopa develop involuntary movements of the limbs. These usually resemble the types of movements seen in patients with the extrapyramidal motor system disorders called *choreas*—Huntington's (hereditary) chorea, for example, or Sydenham's chorea (St. Vitus' dance). Occasionally, the neurologic effects of levodopa overdosage take the form of dyskinesias—movement of the mouth, or massive muscle spasms of the neck or torso—and oculogyric crisis, in which the eyeballs roll up out of sight in the orbital socket. Ordinarily, these alarming signs and symptoms can be overcome by reducing the drug's dosage. Sometimes this results in a return of parkinsonism symptoms, but it is often possible to raise the dosage gradually to effective levels again without setting off the neurologic reactions.

Unfortunately, the incidence of drug-induced neurologic disorders seems to be increasing in patients who have been maintained on levodopa for several years. This may be because patients who have been on levodopa therapy for prolonged periods tend to respond abnormally to the cumulative actions of the drug in the nervous system. This long-term levodopa syndrome is marked mainly by the choreiform, dystonic, and other involuntary movements of the limbs, mouth and face described in the previous paragraph, referred to as AIMs (abnormal involuntary movements). As mentioned in Chapter 46, this syndrome resembles the tardive dyskinesia seen in patients on long-term therapy with antidopaminergic antipsychotic drugs.

* In actual practice, many physicians now start patients on the combination of levodopa and carbidopa (see below), because some of the dose-limiting adverse effects, especially nausea and vomiting, are less likely to occur.

In addition, however, a puzzling phenomenon has been reported in some patients. This is a sudden development of muscle weakness and loss of muscle tone called hypokinesia, or bradykinesia. A previously well-controlled patient may suffer a complete change in motor behavior within a few seconds. The patient first reports feeling "weak in the legs" or "heavy in the feet" and, often, moments later, may be unable to move at all. This switch happens so swiftly that it has been termed the "on–off" effect. The cause of such episodes of irregular responsiveness to levodopa is unknown.

Various psychological disturbances have also been reported. In most cases, these take the form of nervousness and insomnia, which can be readily controlled by adjunctive administration of sedatives and hypnotics. Sometimes, however—particularly in patients with a history of organic brain damage or mental disturbances—treatment with levodopa may cause suicidal depression or a frank psychosis marked by hallucinations, delusions, and assaultive behavior. Patients should be watched closely and precautions should be taken if their behavior becomes abusive, loud, or assaultive, because they may require restraint and withdrawal of the drug.

Interactions with other drugs. Patients who have been taking the standard *anticholinergic drugs* need not discontinue these agents when levodopa treatment is initiated. It may, however, be possible to reduce the dosage of drugs such as trihexyphenidyl or benztropine to better tolerated levels when the effects of levodopa begin to bring about improvement.

The effects of *adrenergic drugs* may be potentiated by levodopa. This is why it is usually undesirable to use levodopa to treat patients suffering also from severe bronchial asthma or emphysema—conditions that may require treatment with ephedrine, isoproterenol, or other *sympathomimetic amines* (Chaps. 17 and 40). Although levodopa was formerly administered experimentally with drugs of the *monoamine oxidase (MAO) inhibitor class* (Chap. 46) in an effort to potentiate the antiparkinsonism activity of levodopa and in the management of depressed parkinsonism patients, its use for this purpose is not now recommended. Instead, patients receiving MAO inhibitors must have these drugs discontinued at least 2 weeks before a trial of levodopa is begun to avoid possible episodes of hypertensive crisis.

As indicated in Chapter 46, the *phenothiazines, butyrophenones,* and other classes of *antipsychotic agents* can cause parkinsonism symptoms by blocking dopaminergic nerve pathways in the basal ganglia. Thus, the concurrent administration of antipsychotic drugs with levodopa can be expected to antagonize its therapeutic effects. If their use cannot be avoided, patients must be carefully observed to see whether signs of the patient's parkinsonism are returning. The same need for close observation applies to parkinsonism patients who take *tricyclic-type antidepressant drugs,* because these also sometimes tend to antagonize the therapeutic effects of levodopa.

Pyridoxine (vitamin B$_6$) forms a coenzyme that is required by dopa decarboxylase for catalyzing the conversion of levodopa to dopamine in both peripheral and central tissues (Table 49-2). This reaction takes place mainly in the peripheral tissues and very little of any administered dose of levodopa reaches its central site of action. Thus, if a patient takes a multivitamin preparation that contains pyridoxine, the peripheral enzymatic reaction may be so greatly increased that the amount of levodopa that enters the brain is too small to exert any antiparkinsonism activity.

To avoid reversal of the antiparkinsonism effect of levodopa in patients who require a vitamin supplement, a preparation (Larobec) has been made available that contains all the B-complex vitamins and ascorbic acid, but *not* pyridoxine. This preparation is available only by prescription. In addition, parkinsonism patients who receive levodopa in combination with the dopa decarboxylase inhibitor drug described in the following section *can* take pyridoxine, because this vitamin does *not* then tend to reverse the therapeutic effects of levodopa.

Levodopa with peripheral dopa decarboxylase inhibitor

Levodopa is now available in combination with a drug that prevents most of an administered dose of levodopa from being converted to dopamine in the peripheral tissues. This drug, *carbidopa* (Lodosyn), acts by inhibiting the enzyme dopa decarboxylase at peripheral sites only (Table 49-1). Because this inhibitor does not enter the central nervous system, it does not interfere with the desired enzymatically catalyzed conversion of dopa to dopamine at cerebral sites such as the nigrostriatal nerve pathway, in which there is a deficiency of this neurotransmitter. As a result of peripheral inhibition of the enzyme by these drugs, much more of an administered dose of levodopa is transported to its central site of action because very much less of it is converted into dopamine peripherally, where it is wasted because it cannot cross the blood–brain barrier.

Several fixed ratio combinations of levodopa with carbidopa are available. In addition, carbidopa is now available alone, but only by direct request of physicians to the manufacturer, for individualizing dosage of carbidopa with levodopa. (Carbidopa has no beneficial effects when administered alone.)

Advantages. The main advantage of administering levodopa in combination with carbidopa is that the daily dosage required for control of parkinsonism symptoms can be reduced by about 75%—from 8 g to 2 g, for example. The importance of this is that anorexia, nausea, and vomiting are much less likely to occur with these lower doses of levodopa. This not only allows more patients to tolerate levodopa therapy, but also makes it possible to reach optimal dosage much more rapidly than when the dose must be raised only very gradually in small periodic increments until the patient develops tolerance to the drug's nauseating effects. The combination also causes fewer cardiac arrhythmias than does levodopa alone. These are thought to result from the peripheral actions of dopamine and the other cardioactive catecholamines formed from it—norepinephrine and epinephrine—at cardiac β-adrenergic receptors (Table 49-2).

As suggested above, combining levodopa with a peripheral inhibitor of dopa decarboxylase permits pyridoxine to be taken without interfering with the antiparkinsonism effects of levodopa. This is so because, with the enzyme inhibited, the vitamin does not perform its function as a coenzyme in the peripheral tissues and cannot take part in the premature conversion of levodopa to dopamine at *extra*cerebral sites. Instead, more of the administered vitamin enters the brain, where its presence may actually *add* to the effectiveness of levodopa that has also arrived at its central site of conversion to dopamine in greater quantities than when it is administered alone.

Combining levodopa with carbidopa does *not*, however, decrease the central side-effects of the antiparkinsonism drug (these include postural hypotension, which is of central origin). In fact, the abnormal movements of the mouth, face, limbs, and trunk may develop at lower dose levels of levodopa. These and the adverse mental effects tend to come on more quickly and more intensely, and last longer than when levodopa alone is administered. Because such central side-effects may be more severe, patients receiving combination therapy must be carefully observed for early signs of drug-induced neurologic and psychiatric disturbances. An early sign of too high central levels of levodopa is development of muscular twitching in the eyelids (blepharospasm) and elsewhere. Dosage must then be reduced to avoid more massive involuntary muscular contractions. Patients must also be watched for development of signs of mental depression and suicidal tendencies and for such symptoms of psychosis as hallucinations and delusions, including paranoid ideation.

Dopaminergic agonists

An increasingly large number of patients whose parkinsonism symptoms were at first controlled by levodopa have begun to show signs of relapse despite its continued administration. This is thought to occur because neither levodopa nor any other drug can arrest the progress of the underlying neurologic disorder. Thus, as more and more nigral nerve cells die, and the content of the converting enzyme dopa decarboxylase in the striatal nerve termination decreases, it becomes increasingly difficult for administered levodopa to be changed to the dopamine that is responsible for inhibiting excessive muscular activity.

It is now possible to bypass the need to produce dopamine indirectly from levodopa. Instead, drugs that mimic the central effects of dopamine by stimulating the same dopaminergic receptors directly may be administered.

Bromocriptine (Parlodel), a derivative of ergot, appears to be the most effective of several such dopaminergic agonists that have been employed experimentally in the treatment of parkinsonism patients who are no longer responding well to treatment with levodopa alone. It is the only drug of its class now marketed in the United States, although others are under investigation. Bromocriptine has helped to reduce tremor, rigidity, bradykinesia, and gait disturbances in patients with advanced Parkinson's disease that appeared to be progressing despite initial optimal responses to treatment with levodopa–carbidopa combinations.

The side-effects of bromocriptine are similar to those of levodopa except that there seem to be fewer dyskinetic side-effects and more mental disturbances. The drug also seems to cause a higher incidence of orthostatic hypotension. Its continued efficacy beyond 2 years has not been established.

Bromocriptine also inhibits the release of prolactin, and is used to treat the amenorrhea–galactorrhea syndrome and to prevent physiologic lactation (Chap. 20).

Amantadine

This antiviral agent (Chap. 7) was accidentally found to benefit some patients with Parkinson's disease for whom it had been prescribed for prevention of Asian influenza. It apparently acts by releasing dopamine from striatal nerve terminals. This increases the number of dopaminergic nerve impulses and helps to relieve muscular rigidity. It may also act by blocking dopamine reuptake. In addition, as described in Chapter 7, it has anticholinergic properties. The drug acts even more rapidly than levodopa, but tolerance to its effects tends to develop. It is best administered in combination with levodopa.

Amantadine does not seem to cause serious side-effects. However, in elderly patients, its use—particularly in combination with centrally acting anticholinergic drugs—has led to the development of confusion and even hallucinations. Its use in patients with a history of psychosis or severe psychoneurosis requires caution. An unusual reaction to this drug is the development of ankle edema and other signs of a condition called livedo reticularis.

Additional clinical considerations

As described in detail in Chapter 16, the anticholinergic drugs produce many side-effects that are detrimental to patients with narrow-angle glaucoma, gastrointestinal obstruction or recent surgery, prostatic hypertrophy, urinary tract obstruction or recent surgery, cardiovascular disease, or cerebrovascular disease. The conversion of levodopa to catecholamines in the periphery is the cause of effects that make its use potentially dangerous or contraindicated in patients with peptic ulcer, previous myocardial infarction, cardiac arrhythmias, cerebrovascular disease, convulsive disorders, psychoses, glaucoma, or chronic obstructive pulmonary disease (COPD). As with many drugs, the safety of these drugs during pregnancy and lactation has not been established.

Patients who receive drugs as part of their medical regimen for Parkinson's disease will require extensive and continual teaching and support. The patient and a significant other need to know the adverse effects to anticipate (as stated above), and ways to make these effects more tolerable. The patient needs to be encouraged to seek regular medical care to evaluate his disease process; liver, renal, cardiovascular, and hematopoietic function; and ocular pressure in those patients who are likely to have glaucoma. The patient will require a great deal of support and encouragement to maintain as much independence as possible, to maintain social contacts and the benefits derived from them, and to stay active. The nursing care of the parkinsonian patient can be complex and frustrating as the disease progresses. The patient teaching guide summarizes the points that should be incorporated into the teaching program of a patient receiving levodopa.

A similar teaching guide can be developed for the anticholinergic drugs (see Chap. 16).

Drug–drug interactions

Levodopa has been associated with many drug–drug interactions (see Chap. 16 for anticholinergic-type drug–drug interactions). Whenever a patient is receiving levodopa and any other drug, the possibility of a drug–drug interaction should be considered if any unexpected drug response is noted. Some of the documented drug–drug interactions that occur with levodopa include the following: increased drug effects with *anticholinergic drugs, guanethidine, diuretics* used as *antihypertensives,* and *sympathomimetic drugs;* a decreased effect of levodopa is seen if given concurrently with *reserpine, benzodiazepines, phenothiazines, butyrophenones, phenytoin, papaverine,* and *pyridoxine* (vitamin B_6). The control of diabetic patients taking *oral hypoglycemic agents* may be adversely affected by the use of levodopa. The concurrent use of *MAO inhibitors* and levodopa is contraindicated because of the risk of hypertensive crises. MAO inhibitors should be stopped 14 days before levodopa therapy is started.

The guide to the nursing process summarizes the clinical aspects that should be incorporated into the nursing care of the patient receiving levodopa therapy.

Patient teaching guide: levodopa

The drug that has been prescribed for you is given to increase the levels of dopamine in certain areas of your brain. This has been found to decrease the signs and symptoms of Parkinson's disease. Often this drug is combined with carbidopa, which helps the correct levels of levodopa to reach the brain. All patients must have their individual dosage needs adjusted over time.

Instructions:

1. The name of your drug is ⸻⸻⸻ .

2. The dosage of the drug prescribed for you is ⸻⸻ .

3. The drug needs to be taken ⸻⸻ times a day. The best time to take your drug is ⸻⸻ . It is helpful to take the drug with food if stomach upset occurs.

4. Some side-effects of the drug that you should be aware of include the following:

Drowsiness, weakness, fatigue	If any of these happen to you, take precautions to avoid driving, operating dangerous machinery, or performing delicate tasks.
Dizziness, fainting	Changing position very slowly will help to alleviate this problem.

(continued)

Darkening of the urine, sweating	This is a normal reaction; do not be concerned.
Headaches, difficulty in sleeping	These usually pass as the body adjusts to the drug. If they become too uncomfortable, and persist, consult with your nurse or physician.

5. Keep this and all medications out of the reach of children.

6. Tell any nurse, physician, or dentist who is taking care of you that you are on this drug.

7. Vitamin B_6 interferes with the effects of levodopa. If you feel that you need a vitamin product, consult with your nurse or physician for something appropriate that does not contain vitamin B_6. Also, avoid eating large quantities of health foods that contain vitamin B_6. (This does not apply if you are taking carbidopa with levodopa.)

8. Do not overexert yourself as you start to feel better. Pace your activities.

9. Be sure to have regular medical check-ups to evaluate your body's response to the drug as well as the progress of your disease.

Notify your nurse or physician if any of the following occur:

Uncontrolled movements of any
  parts of your body
Chest pain
Heart palpitations
Depression or mood changes
Difficulty in voiding
Severe or persistent nausea and
  vomiting

Guide to the nursing process: levodopa

Assessment	Nursing diagnoses	Interventions	Evaluation
Past history (*contraindications*): Glaucoma Cardiovascular disease COPD Cardiac arrhythmias Peptic ulcer Psychoses Convulsive disorders	Potential ineffective coping secondary to diagnosis Potential for injury, secondary to disease and drug effects Knowledge deficit regarding drug therapy	Safe and appropriate administration of drug Comfort and safety measures: • Slow position changes • Safety if driving, performing dangerous tasks	Monitor for therapeutic effectiveness of drug Monitor for adverse effects of drug: • Liver changes • Cardiovascular changes • Renal changes • CNS effects

(continued)

Assessment	Nursing diagnoses	Interventions	Evaluation
Pregnancy Lactation Allergies: *these drugs;* *tartrazine* (certain preparations); others; reactions Medication history (*cautions*): Anticholinergics Guanethidine Antihypertensives Reserpine Benzodiazepines Phenothiazines Butyrophenones Phenytoin Papaverine Pyridoxine Oral hypoglycemics MAO inhibitors	Potential sensory– perceptual alteration secondary to drug effects	• Drug with food • Sleeping, headache measures Patient teaching regarding drug therapy Support and encour- agement to cope with diagnosis, drug therapy, and prognosis	Evaluate effectiveness of patient teaching program Evaluate effectiveness of support and encour- agement offered Monitor for drug–drug interactions: several possible
Physical assessment Neurologic: reflexes, affect, mental status, gait, peripheral controls Cardiovascular: BP, P, baseline ECG, peripheral perfusion Respiratory: R, adventitious sounds GI: abdominal exam Renal: bladder function (prostate) Laboratory tests: liver enzyme levels, CBC, BUN			

Summary of adverse effects of drugs used in treating Parkinson's disease

Belladonna alkaloids and synthetic drugs with atropinelike actions

Mouth dryness or xerostomia. May make speaking or swallowing difficult; may lead to loss of appetite and rarely to a mumpslike parotitis.

Blurring of vision caused by cycloplegia and pupillary dilation (mydriasis). May make reading difficult.

Constipation and, occasionally, nausea and vomiting

Urinary retention or hesitancy (dysuria)

Cardiac palpitations, tachycardia, and hypotension. Caution in patients with cardiovascular instability.

Skin dryness or anhidrosis. Lack of sweating may lead to fever with flushed, hot, dry skin and possible heat prostration in hot weather, particularly in chronically ill, elderly, or debilitated patients.

Central nervous system stimulation or depression. Drowsiness, muscle weakness, and ataxia caused by some of these drugs may make driving and other such activities dangerous; elderly patients with cerebral arteriosclerosis are particularly prone to reactions marked by mental confusion, memory lapses, disorientation, excitement, or agitation; visual hallucinations, and acute delirium also occur, and even a toxic psychosis is possible, particularly in mental patients.

Miscellaneous. In theory, at least, these drugs may *mask* toxic effects of cholinergic drugs in patients with myasthenia gravis, and of phenothiazine drugs (tardive dyskinesia).

Levodopa

Gastrointestinal disturbances. Loss of appetite, nausea, vomiting, abdominal pain, and diarrhea or constipation

Cardiovascular disturbances. Heart palpitation and possible increase in rate and rhythm; flushing; postural hypotension or occasional hypertension

Neurologic disturbances. Involuntary movements of the mouth, face, and head; dyskinetic reactions in large muscle groups, including the neck (torticollis); also possible oculogyric crisis and convulsions; sudden bradykinetic episodes ("on-off" phenomenon)

Psychological disturbances. Either euphoria and hyperactivity or depression with fatigue and drowsiness may develop; check patients for early signs of mental changes, because suicidal depression or hypomanic behavior with hallucinations and delirium have occurred.

Visual disturbances. Blurring of vision, pupillary dilation, double vision

Respiratory disturbances. Postnasal drip, hoarseness, cough; breathing pattern irregularities and feelings of pressure in the chest

Case study

Presentation

SS has been maintained on levodopa (Larodopa) for treatment of his Parkinson's disease. He has been doing fairly well. His daughter recently returned from her freshman year in college and started the family on a new "health" regimen, including natural foods and plenty of supplemental vitamins. His daughter was so enthusiastic about her new approach to life that everyone in the family joined in to give it a try.

SS soon developed severe nausea, anorexia, fainting spells, and palpitations. His parkinsonian symptoms returned, and were markedly restricting.

What probably happened to SS? What appropriate nursing interventions should be planned for SS?

Discussion

SS should be encouraged to come in immediately for medical evaluation. His signs and symptoms seem to reflect an increase in his parkinsonian signs and symptoms as well as an increase in peripheral dopamine-type reactions (*e.g.,* palpitations, fainting, anorexia, nausea). SS assured the nurse that he had meticulously taken his levodopa as usual, with no change. It will be necessary to determine if SS is losing his response to levodopa therapy (which reportedly occurs over time) or if something else has occurred to interfere with the effectiveness of the levodopa therapy. A careful review of SS's history shows that SS has been receiving large amounts of pyridoxine (vitamin B_6) in the vitamin preparations he was taking as well as in the natural foods that he has been eating. Pyridoxine helps to convert levodopa to dopamine before it has a chance to cross the blood–brain barrier and reach the areas of the brain where it is needed. As a result, SS has experienced a return of his parkinsonian symptoms in what he perceives as a more severe form than before. At the same time, the peripheral buildup of dopamine has led to the signs and symptoms of dopamine toxicity—cardiovascular stimulation and gastrointestinal upset and decreased activity. SS, after a thorough evaluation of his disease process, should be started back on levodopa therapy, beginning with small doses and building up to the lowest dosage that achieves the therapeutic effects. It might be wise to consider combining the levodopa with carbidopa (Sinemet) to prevent some of these problems from developing again. SS and his family will then require extensive patient teaching regarding the drug, the cautions and warnings to be aware of with this drug, and what happened to SS to cause these problems. The family will need a great deal of support and encouragement to understand and cope with what has happened. SS's daughter may feel guilty about what happened, and she should have the opportunity to discuss her feelings and to explore other aspects of proper nutrition and healthy foods. This situation can serve as a good teaching example for staff, as well as presenting them with an opportunity to review the drug therapy of Parkinson's disease and the risks and benefits of such fad diets.

Drug digests

Benztropine mesylate USP (Cogentin)

Actions and indications. This potent synthetic antiparkinsonism agent is used mainly as a supplement to other drugs to bring about greater symptomatic relief. It is also substituted for first-choice drugs to which patients are no longer adequately responsive. The drug's central anticholinergic effect relaxes skeletal muscle rigidity, cramps, and spasm. Relief of pain by this antispasmodic action together with the drug's sedative effect often helps patients with insomnia to sleep. Its long duration of action is also desirable, because patients taking this drug at bedtime are said to be able to turn in bed more easily and to arise more readily when they want to get up.

This drug is also employed for preventing and treating parkinsonism produced by phenothiazine-type antipsychotic agents, reserpine, and other drugs that induce extrapyramidal motor system reactions. Administered by vein in acute dystonic reactions,

it rapidly relieves such severe manifestations as torticollis (twisted neck) and oculogyric crisis; its use in this way is also desirable in patients with dysphagia who cannot take medication readily by mouth.

Adverse effects, cautions, and contraindications. Side-effects of the atropine type are common but not usually serious, because they can readily be controlled by reducing the dosage until tolerance develops. These effects, which include dry mouth, nausea, vomiting, nervousness, blurring of vision, and constipation, are usually only discomforting. However, hypersusceptible patients such as those with prostatic hypertrophy or a tendency toward gastrointestinal obstruction should be closely observed. Caution is also required in hot weather, when the drug's interference with sweating might lead to heat stroke in chronically ill patients. Narrow-angle glaucoma is a contraindication.

More serious effects of overdosage include

mental confusion, excitement, disorientation, and delirium. A toxic psychosis marked by visual hallucinations and delusions may be set off by high doses, particularly in mental patients or in elderly patients with cerebral arteriosclerosis.

Dosage and administration. Treatment is usually started with a bedtime dose of 0.5 to 1 mg. If necessary, additional doses of 0.5 mg are administered every 5 or 6 days, until the smallest dose needed for optimal relief has been reached. Although the usual total daily dose is only 1 to 2 mg, patients with postencephalitic parkinsonism often require and can tolerate 4 to 6 mg daily.

Acute drug-induced dystonic reactions are treated by administering 2 mg IV; less severe reactions usually respond to 1 mg (1 ml of the injection) administered IM. Parkinsonism developing during therapy with antipsychotic neuroleptic agents is usually relieved by oral doses of 1 to 2 mg bid or tid.

Levodopa USP (Dopar; Larodopa; L-dopa)

Actions and indications. Levodopa is at present the most effective drug for symptomatic treatment of idiopathic Parkinson's disease, postencephalitic and arteriosclerotic parkinsonism, and similar syndromes resulting from hypoxic damage to cerebral neurons—for example, following carbon monoxide poisoning or chronic intoxication by the metal manganese.

Levodopa relieves such symptoms as akinesia, tremors, and rigidity by counteracting a disease-induced deficiency of the central neurotransmitter substance dopamine. To do so, it must be transported into the CNS after its absorption into the bloodstream. In the cerebrum this drug is converted to dopamine in a neurochemical reaction that is catalyzed by the enzyme dopa decarboxylase in the presence of pyridoxal 5-phosphate, a coenzyme derived from the B-complex vitamin pyridoxine (vitamin B_6).

Adverse effects, cautions, and contraindications. The most common side-effect is nausea, often accompanied by anorexia and vomiting. Care is required in patients with

peptic ulcer to avoid bleeding in the upper GI tract, because use of this drug has occasionally led to hemorrhage and ulceration. Involuntary movements often appear in patients taking excessive doses, particularly in those who have been taking levodopa for prolonged periods. These movements may be mild or seriously incapacitating, and vary from minor twitching of small muscles of the face to massive and painful myoclonic spasms of the trunk and limbs. Some patients on long-term therapy suffer sudden episodes of movement slowing and near-motionless paralysis called bradykinesia, hypokinesia, or the "on–off" syndrome.

Serious mental disturbances may develop, particularly in patients with a history of psychosis. Patients must be watched for signs of depression, anxiety, confusion, and agitation, as well as for indications of hallucinations, delusions, and paranoid ideation or suicidal tendencies.

Cardiac arrhythmias and episodes of orthostatic hypotension may occur. Particular care is required in patients who have had a

myocardial infarction that has left them with various residual arrhythmias, and caution is also needed in patients who are being treated with antihypertensive drugs.

Levodopa is contraindicated in patients with narrow-angle glaucoma. It may be used cautiously in those with wide-angle glaucoma with frequent monitoring of the intraocular pressure. This drug is also contraindicated in patients with a history of melanoma or with suspicious, still undiagnosed skin lesions.

Dosage and administration. Treatment is usually begun with 0.5 to 1 g daily, divided into two or more doses, each of which is taken with food. The total daily dose is then gradually increased by amounts of no more than 0.75 g every 3 to 7 days, until a level of optimal antiparkinsonism activity is reached with doses that the patient can tolerate—usually no more than 8 g daily. When levodopa is administered with carbidopa (as Sinemet), the starting and optimal doses are usually only about 25% of those stated above.

Trihexyphenidyl HCl USP (Artane; Tremin)

Actions and indications. This synthetic atropinelike drug is mainly used for symptomatic relief of all forms of parkinsonism—idiopathic, atherosclerotic, and postencephalitic. The drug acts centrally to reduce skeletal muscle rigidity, lessen tremor, and counteract akinesia. It is said to exert a mild euphoric effect that aids in overcoming the mental depression often associated with this progressive neurologic disorder. The drug's peripheral anticholinergic effect may help to reduce excessive salivation (sialorrhea) and sweating (hyperhidrosis) that are often seen in Parkinson's disease.

This centrally acting antispasmodic is also used to prevent or correct the extrapyramidal motor system reactions sometimes set off in psychotic patients and others being treated with neuroleptic drugs, including phenothiazine and butyrophenone derivatives and rauwolfia alkaloids such as reserpine.

Adverse effects, cautions, and contraindications. This drug is generally considered to be the most desirable drug with which to begin treatment of parkinsonism because of its relative safety. However, minor side-effects occur in about 50% of patients treated, and severe side-effects are possible in some patients. Thus, measures should be taken to minimize discomfort and precautions employed to avoid toxic reactions in hypersusceptible patients.

Minor side-effects are mainly similar to those of atropine and include mouth dryness, blurring of vision, dizziness, constipation, and either drowsiness or nervousness and insomnia. Elderly patients with cerebral arteriosclerosis may show signs of mental confusion, agitation, and disorientation. Caution is required in patients with a tendency toward gastrointestinal or genitourinary tract obstruction, including elderly men with enlargement of the prostate. The drug may cause a dangerous rise in intraocular pressure in patients with narrow-angle glaucoma.

Dosage and administration. It is advisable to begin treatment with doses as low as 1 mg, particularly in patients over 60 years old. Dosage may then be built up gradually to levels optimal for each patient. This is usually done by increasing the dose by 2 mg at 3- to 5-day intervals. Most patients need a total daily dose of between 6 and 10 mg, but some may require as much as 15 mg. These dosages are divided into three or four parts, administered near mealtimes and at bedtime. (The drug is best given before meals to avoid excessive dryness of the mouth, or after meals when its action in reducing excessive salivation is desired.)

A sustained-release capsule containing 5 mg may be employed in the same total dose. These capsules are usually taken after breakfast and in the early afternoon.

References

Bianchine JR: Drugs for Parkinson's disease: Centrally acting skeletal muscle relaxants. In Gilman AG, Goodman LS, Gilman A (eds): Goodman & Gilman's The Pharmacological Basis of Therapeutics, 6th ed, pp 475–493. New York, Macmillan, 1980

Calne DB: Developments in the pharmacology and therapeutics of parkinsonism. Ann Neurol 1:111, 1977

Cotzias GC: Metabolic modification of some neurologic disorders. JAMA 210:1255, 1969

Fahn S, Calne DB: Considerations in the management of parkinsonism. Neurology 28:5, 1978

Granerus AK: Factors influencing the occurrence of "on–off" symptoms during long-term treatment with L-dopa. Acta Med Scand 203:75, 1978

Hoehn MM: Bromocriptine and its use in parkinsonism. J Am Geriatr Soc 24:251, 1981

Lewin R: Trail of ironies to Parkinson's disease. Science 224:1083, 1984

Lieberman AN et al: Treatment of Parkinson's disease with dopamine agonists: Review. Am J Med Sci 278:65, 1979

Lieberman AN et al: Use of pergolide, potent dopamine agonist, in Parkinson's disease. Clin Pharmacol Ther 32:70, 1982

Penney JB Jr, Young AB: Speculations on the functional anatomy of basal ganglia disorders. Ann Rev Neurosci 6:73, 1983

Weiner WJ et al: Drug holiday and management of Parkinson's disease. Neurology 30:1257, 1980

Chapter 50

Drugs
for
treating
epilepsy

50

The nature of epilepsy

Epilepsy is the most common of all neurologic disorders. An estimated 2% of the population suffer recurrent epileptic seizures of one type or another. Actually, this condition is not a single disease but rather several different syndromes that have one common characteristic: a sudden discharge of excessive electrical energy from nerve cells located at any of various areas within the brain. Some so-called *focal seizures* stem from a localized lesion—that is, from a focus of abnormal neurons located in the cerebral cortex or in a subcortical structure. More commonly, many different brain areas seem to explode (electrophysiologically) all at once to produce a *generalized seizure.*

The form that seizures take clinically depends in part on the location of the abnormal cells and also on the pathways that the initial volleys of nerve impulses take as they pass to other parts of the central nervous system. That is, the paroxysmal firing of abnormal neurons spreads to normal nerve tissues in the cerebral cortex or in deep-lying brain structures. These, in turn, send out synchronous nerve impulses in ways that disrupt the functioning of the cells which they innervate. These functional changes may be mainly motor in nature—resulting in convulsions, for example—or they may be sensory, psychic, or autonomic—that is, *non*convulsive seizures. Still other types of seizures produce only momentary lapses of consciousness, which may be hardly detectable by an observer.

Classification of seizures
Neurologists classify the epilepsies in several different ways. Traditionally, the most important subdivisions were *grand mal, petit mal, psychomotor,* and *focal motor* or *jacksonian* types of seizures. An international commission has now classified the epilepsies on the bases of both their

clinical and electroencephalographic characteristics: (1) *generalized* (unlocalized), and (2) *focal* (localized, at least at their onset). Generalized seizures are, in turn, subdivided into *convulsive* and *nonconvulsive* types, and focal seizures may be subdivided into *elemental* and *complex* symptom types (see the summary of types of epileptic seizures in Table 50-1; it is a modification of this modern classification of the epilepsies).

Classifying the type of epilepsy from which each patient suffers is considered very important, because an accurate diagnosis is necessary to choose the drug or combination of drugs best suited for each case. Once the type of seizure has been accurately determined, it is usually possible to control the condition with properly selected drugs. Often the epileptic patient can then lead a nearly normal life. Misdiagnosis, on the other hand, results in failure to control the patient's seizures. Sometimes patients with mixed seizures pose particularly difficult diagnostic and therapeutic problems. However, the most common cause of treatment failure is the patient's own unwillingness to take the drugs prescribed.

General considerations in antiepileptic drug therapy

Drugs have been developed that can reduce the number and severity of epileptic attacks (Table 50-2). These agents are often called *anticonvulsants.* However, convulsions do not occur in all types of seizures, and drugs such as neuromuscular junction blockers (Chap. 19) can stop convulsions but are not useful in managing the epileptic patient. Thus, the term "antiepileptic" is preferable for characterizing drugs that have *selective* antiseizure activity and that are therefore useful in managing epilepsy. Antiepileptic drugs are believed to act by reducing the re-

Table 50-1. Summary of types of epileptic seizures*

Generalized seizures (bilateral, symmetric)

Convulsive seizures
Major motor or tonic–clonic (*grand mal epilepsy*)
Minor motor or myoclonic, akinetic, and atonic
Infantile spasms or hypsarrythmia

Nonconvulsive seizures
Typical absence attacks (true *petit mal epilepsy*)

Focal (partial) seizures (localized at onset)

Elemental symptoms
Examples: localized, but possibly spreading to become a major motor seizure (*jacksonian epilepsy*); sensory seizures

Complex symptoms
Example: automatism or temporal lobe epilepsy (*psychomotor epilepsy*)

Miscellaneous seizures

Examples: autonomic seizure equivalents

* The epilepsies can be classified in several different ways. No one classification is accepted by all authorities.
  This classification, which is based on both clinical and electroencephalographic factors, is a modification of
  one proposed by an international commission. It differs from the traditional division of the epilepsies into
  grand mal, petit mal, psychomotor, and focal motor types.

sponsiveness of normal neurons to the sudden storms of nervous impulses arising at the focal disturbance sites, or by depressing the hyperirritable focus itself.

The goal of drug treatment in epilepsy is the complete control of seizures with doses that cause no adverse effects and interfere only minimally with the patient's life style. No drug can do this in all cases. To achieve maximal control of seizures with minimal side-effects and toxicity, the best drug or combination of drugs must be selected for the particular type of epileptic seizures to which the patient is periodically subjected. Patients are usually started on small doses of the drug considered to be the safest of those known to be effective for their type of epilepsy. The dose is then raised gradually at intervals of a few days or a week until the seizures stop or discomforting side-effects develop. If the first drug does not completely control seizures without causing toxicity, a second relatively safe and effective drug may be added to the patient's treatment regimen. Dosage of the combined drugs is then adjusted to meet the patient's needs and ability to tolerate the treatment. Occasionally a third drug is employed, either for its added antiepileptic effect or to counteract side-effects of the first two agents.

Sometimes, when such combinations of safe drugs still fail to control the patient's seizures, more toxic drugs may be tried. Some antiepileptic drugs can cause serious toxicity, including skin reactions, liver or kidney damage,

and blood dyscrasias (see the summary of side-effects and toxicity at the end of this chapter). Because patients may be taking these drugs for long periods of time without close supervision, they and their significant others must be taught to be alert for skin rashes and discolorations, sore throat, and fever. These may be the first signs of toxic drug reactions that necessitate withdrawal of the antiepileptic agent.

It is important, however, for drugs to be discontinued gradually, because too sudden cessation of medication may increase the number and severity of seizures. Usually control can quickly be reestablished by reinstituting the medication. Sometimes, however, abrupt discontinuance of antiepileptic drugs may precipitate status epilepticus, a succession of severe seizures that could end fatally.

Thus, in shifting a patient from one drug to another during the trial-and-error period, doses of the first drug are usually decreased gradually while doses of the new drug are raised gradually to an optimal level. The nurse can help in this situation by teaching the patient and his family the importance of his taking the medication exactly as prescribed. Cooperation between patient, physician, and nurse is necessary for complete success in seizure control.

Epilepsy was, in the past, viewed with fear and prejudice by some people. In recent years, public edu-

Table 50–2. Antiepileptic drugs*

Official or generic name	Trade name or synonym	Usual adult daily oral dosage range	Indications by type of seizure benefited				
			Grand mal and focal	Petit mal	Psycho-motor	Minor motor	Status epilepticus
First-line agents							
Diazepam USP	Valium	4–40 mg	+†	+†	+†	+	+
Ethosuximide USP	Zarontin	750 mg–1.5 g	–	+	–	+	–
Paramethadione USP	Paradione	900 mg–2.4 g	–	+	–	+	–
Phenobarbital USP	Luminal	100–400 mg	+	+†	+†	+†	+
Phenytoin USP	Dilantin	100–400 mg	+	–	+	+	+
Primidone USP	Mysoline	250–750 mg	+	–	+	+	–
Trimethadione USP	Tridione	900 mg–2.4 g	–	+	–	+	–
Second-line agents							
Acetazolamide USP	Diamox	8–30 mg/kg body weight	+†	+†	+†	+†	–
Carbamazepine	Tegretol	200–1200 mg	+†	–	+†	–	–
Clonazepam	Clonopin	1.5–2.0 mg	+†	+†	+†	+	–
Clorazepate dipotassium	Tranxene	22.5–90 mg	+	–	–	–	–
Corticotropin USP	ACTH	40–60 U	–	+	–	+‡	–
Dextroamphetamine USP	Dexedrine	5–15 mg	+§	+†·§	+§	+§	–
Ethotoin	Peganone	1–3 g	+	–	+	–	–
Mephenytoin USP	Mesantoin	100–400 mg	+	–	+	–	–
Mephobarbital USP	Mebaral	400–600 mg	+	–	+	+	–
Methamphetamine	Desoxyn	2.5–5.0 mg	+§	+†·§	+§	+§	–
Metharbital USP	Gemonil	100–400 mg	+	–	+	+	–
Methsuximide USP	Celontin	600 mg–1.2 g	–	+	+	+	–
Methylphenidate USP	Ritalin	10–60 mg	+§	+§	+§	+§	–
Phenacemide USP	Phenurone	1–3 g	+	–	+	+	–
Phensuximide USP	Milontin	1–3 g	–	+	–	+	–
Valproic acid	Sodium dipropylacetate; divalproex, sodium valproate; Depakene; Depakote	15–60 mg/kg body weight	+†	+†	+†	+†	–

* These are divided into first-line, or primary drugs (safest and most effective), and drugs of secondary importance, some of which may prove effective when some first-line drugs fail. Drugs of lesser importance used occasionally are not listed.
† Used mainly as an adjunct to other drugs in special cases.
‡ Used mainly against infantile spasms (hypsarrhythmia; various corticosteroid drugs may also be used for this purpose).
§ Used mainly as a psychomotor stimulant to counteract excessive drowsiness.

cation campaigns have done much to eliminate these fears and prejudices. Most epileptic patients can be controlled with drug therapy and lead normal, active lives. The patient and family will still need support and encouragement to cope with and adjust to the diagnosis and drug therapy, with all its implications.

Treatment of specific types of seizures

Grand mal epilepsy

Grand mal epilepsy is characterized by the periodic occurrence of a sudden severe generalized tonic–clonic convulsive seizure (see Chap. 47 for descriptions of different types of convulsions.) The seizure may be preceded by a brief aura—a warning that may take the form of flashes of light, special sounds, or other visual, auditory, or sensorimotor phenomena. In the next moment, the patient falls unconscious, sometimes with an involuntary cry. This is followed by a series of tonic convulsions, in which the limbs are rigidly extended or flexed, and the muscles of respiration fail to function usefully. Because breathing stops for a time, the person may become cyanotic. These symmetric spasms give way to a series of muscular tremors or jerks—the clonic convulsive phase—and then the patient begins to breathe again. Finally, the patient recovers consciousness and may then fall into an exhausted sleep.

Drug therapy

The drugs most commonly employed for preventing grand mal seizures are *phenobarbital*[+] (Luminal) and *phenytoin* (Dilantin). Other barbiturates occasionally used for this purpose are *mephobarbital* (Mebaral) and *metharbital* (Gemonil); other hydantoins occasionally used are *ethotoin* (Peganone) and *mephenytoin* (Mesantoin). Ethotoin is less efficacious than phenytoin and offers no advantage over phenytoin. Mephenytoin is sometimes of greater therapeutic benefit than phenytoin, especially in focal seizures, and it causes fewer central nervous system (CNS) side-effects. However, because it has caused serious hematologic and liver toxicity, and systemic lupus erythematosus, it should be used only after less toxic drugs have been tried. One such drug that is also recommended for focal seizures is a new benzodiazepine, *clorazepate dipotassium* (Tranxene). Patients with grand mal-type seizures who are not controlled by a combination of phenobarbital and phenytoin sometimes respond to *primidone* (Mysoline),

---

* One explanation of the mechanism by which phenytoin selectively protects against seizures is based on its ability to alter the permeability of brain cell membranes to certain ions. Evidence indicates that this drug reduces the sodium content of nerve cells, possibly by stimulating the metabolic "pump" by which all cells remove sodium from their interior when this ion tends to accumulate intracellularly in excess. This membrane-stabilizing ionic effect may counteract a characteristic property of rapidly stimulated synaptic connections called *posttetanic potentiation* (PTP) that is thought to contribute to the spread of seizure activity. By reducing PTP—which is the increased excitability that results from repeated high-frequency stimulation of synapses—phenytoin tends to stop the explosive chain reactions between loops of neighboring nerve cells.

It has been suggested that this property may make phenytoin useful in patients with certain types of emotional and personality disorders. However, this threshold-stabilizing effect is not limited to brain cells. Two painful peripheral nerve syndromes—*trigeminal neuralgia* and the lightning pains of *tabes dorsalis*—are believed to be benefited by this drug's ability to halt the progress of explosions of electrical energy. Similarly, this normalizing effect of phenytoin on excitable cell membranes may also account for the drug's effectiveness against certain cardiac arrhythmias (Chap. 30)

a drug structurally similar to barbiturates that is metabolized partly to phenobarbital.

Some physicians begin treatment of epilepsy, especially in children, by prescribing phenobarbital because of its relative safety as compared to that of other antiepileptics. Although fully effective doses of phenobarbital often cause drowsiness, this drug rarely causes any of the serious types of chronic toxicity sometimes seen with other antiepileptic agents (see the Summary of side-effects and toxicity at the end of this chapter). If phenobarbital fails to stop all seizure activity when administered in doses that the patient can tolerate, phenytoin may be added to the patient's treatment program while the dosage of the barbiturate is gradually reduced.

Most physicians prefer to begin therapy of motor epilepsy with phenytoin, because it is free of the sedative effect of phenobarbital and is effective in about three out of four patients with grand mal epilepsy. The freedom from CNS depression with properly adjusted doses of phenytoin probably stems from this drug's ability to stop the spread of abnormal neuronal activity without interfering with normal nerve cell responsiveness to stimulation. This relatively selective antiepileptic action of phenytoin against major seizures is thought to stem from its special ability to stabilize cell membranes that are being subjected to excessive stimulation.*

Dosage adjustment. Successful seizure control calls for careful adjustment of phenytoin dosage to meet each patient's individual needs. Patients vary widely in the rate at which they metabolize this drug. This means that, if all patients received the same dose at the same intervals, not enough of the drug would get into the brain of some patients to reach levels effective for controlling seizures, while in others the drug would accumulate to toxic levels within the nervous system.

Physicians treating problem patients of these types now often order laboratory tests to learn whether the administered doses of phenytoin, phenobarbital, and primidone are actually reaching therapeutically effective levels in the brain. The amounts of these drugs in the blood plasma can be measured accurately, and thus serve as an index of their concentrations in the central nervous system. If, for example, a patient's plasma shows a concentration very much less than the level of phenytoin known to be needed for control of seizures (10 to 20 μg/ml), an increase in daily dosage of the drug can be ordered.

On the other hand, when a patient seems sensitive to normal doses and shows such signs of central toxicity as nystagmus and ataxia, blood tests may reveal toxic levels of phenytoin (30 to 50 μg/ml). The drug dosage should then be reduced to below average amounts, and plasma levels should be monitored periodically during prolonged therapy to be sure that levels stay in a therapeutically effective nontoxic range.

Interactions with other drugs. Sometimes the simultaneous administration of other drugs alters blood and brain levels of antiepileptic drugs in ways that interfere with attempts to attain the aim of safe, effective seizure control therapy. Among the drug interactions (Chap. 4) that may lead to phenytoin intoxication, for example, are those involving the antituberculosis drugs *isoniazid* and *para-aminosalicylic acid,* the alcoholism treatment drug *disulfiram* (Antabuse), and the anticoagulants *dicumarol* and *warfarin.* All these drugs act to reduce the rate at which liver enzyme systems inactivate the antiepileptic drug. Thus, when an epileptic patient previously controlled by phenytoin requires the addition of one of these other drugs to the regimen, the dosage of phenytoin must be reduced to prevent it from rising to plasma and brain levels high enough to set off the nervous system syndrome characteristic of phenytoin overdosage (see the summary of side-effects and toxicity at the end of this chapter).

Chronic toxicity. The first-line drugs used in treating grand mal epilepsy are among the least toxic of the antiepileptics. Although CNS side-effects are common when the dosage of phenobarbital, phenytoin, or primidone exceeds what most patients can tolerate, these drugs rarely cause the types of dangerous reactions sometimes seen during long-term treatment with certain other antiepileptic agents (see below and the summary of toxic reactions). Nonetheless, some patients taking these drugs do develop hypersensitivity. Thus, patients must be watched for signs of sensitivity and they should be instructed to report symptoms of illness, because these may be drug-induced and require a reduction in dosage or withdrawal of the drug.

Skin reactions from phenytoin are usually mild and resemble the rashes of measles, scarlet fever, or acne. Often these disappear when dosage is reduced or the drug is temporarily discontinued, and they may not reappear during a later trial of the drug. Rarely, treatment may not be resumed because of the danger of more serious and potentially deadly dermatologic reactions. Occasionally, in women and girls, growth of facial hair may constitute a cosmetic problem during long-term treatment with phenytoin.

Gingival hyperplasia, a condition in which the gums grow over the teeth, is a more common disfiguring complication of phenytoin therapy. Although the swelling is painless when it first develops after several months of treatment, secondary inflammation (gingivitis) later leads to tenderness and bleeding that make eating difficult. Gingivitis may be prevented by meticulous oral hygiene to remove food particles, prevent dental plaque formation, and clear away calculi. Because care of this type is difficult to carry out in children who must wear dental braces, phenytoin is sometimes not administered during orthodontia. Often, patients must undergo periodic periodontal surgery for removal of overgrowths of hypertrophied gum tissues. Gingivectomy is also often followed by medical measures for controlling the unsightly condition, in-

cluding application of anti-inflammatory corticosteroids. However, if all these measures fail and this drug reaction continues to cause pain and embarrassment—particularly in teen-age patients—phenytoin may have to be discontinued even if the drugs that replace it are less effective.

Although serious blood dyscrasias are rare with phenytoin, phenobarbital, and primidone, all these drugs occasionally cause anemia of the megaloblastic type (Chap. 35). This blood disorder, which develops gradually in some patients taking antiepileptics for prolonged periods, can be readily detected by periodic blood studies. Fortunately, it is also readily reversible by small daily doses of crystalline *folic acid*+ (see Drug digest, Chap. 35) administered orally or by injections of folinic acid (calcium leucovorin; Chap. 12). Routine administration of these vitamin supplements for prophylactic purposes is not recommended for children on antiepileptic drug therapy. However, folic acid administration is particularly desirable when macrocytosis is seen in a pregnant patient, because the drug-induced folic acid deficiency may lead to fetal damage if not corrected. A similar deficiency may account for the peripheral nerve damage that occasionally develops in patients taking large doses of phenytoin for periods of a decade or more. The cause of lymph node hyperplasia that is another rare development of phenytoin treatment is unknown. Fortunately these disappear soon after the drugs that led to their development are discontinued, but they need to be evaluated to distinguish them from Hodgkin's disease, which has also been reported during prolonged phenytoin treatment.

Use in pregnancy. There is evidence to suggest that, although the vast majority of women being treated for epilepsy during pregnancy give birth to normal infants, the incidence of certain birth defects is two or three times higher in infants born to women who took phenytoin and phenobarbital during pregnancy. This does not necessarily mean that these drugs were the cause of the fetal defects, because the main hazard to the developing embryo or fetus is hypoxia following a major seizure.

Thus, in general, these and other antiepileptic drugs should *not* be discontinued during pregnancy, especially because to do so abruptly can cause an increase in the number of major seizures and even set off status epilepticus (see below). However, the possibility of gradually withdrawing antiepileptic medication prior to or during pregnancy in individual patients who have only mild infrequent seizures may be considered. Epileptic women who wish to become pregnant need extensive teaching and counseling about the risks to the fetus of maintaining or reducing the dosage of their antiepileptic medication, and they should participate in the decision about their drug therapy.

Status epilepticus.

Most grand mal seizures last only a few minutes and, even though the patient may become cyanotic, he is in no danger of respiratory failure. No drugs are needed to terminate the attack, so, instead of leaving the patient to look for an antiepileptic drug, the nurse should remain to protect the patient from injury. Sometimes, however, one convulsion may be followed by another without the patient's regaining consciousness between attacks. Such continuous major seizure activity, called *status epilepticus*, requires prompt treatment with parenterally administered anticonvulsant drugs to avoid possible exhaustion, respiratory failure, and death.

The older depressant drugs used for controlling status epilepticus—for example, phenobarbital, paraldehyde, and even ether—are often effective but are also potentially dangerous, because they must sometimes be administered in doses that could cause coma and respiratory arrest. Thus, the parenteral forms of *phenytoin* and of *diazepam*[+] (Valium; see Drug digest, Chap. 45), which often can control continuous seizures without causing excessive depression, are now often preferred in this emergency. However, both these safer anticonvulsant drugs must be injected slowly over a period of several minutes to avoid possible cardiovascular toxicity.

One difficulty in using parenteral phenytoin for this purpose is that its anticonvulsant action is slow to develop when administered at the rate and dosage ordinarily recommended. To speed the drug's onset of action, some neurologists have suggested that it be infused rapidly IV in relatively large doses. However, this has occasionally resulted in hypotensive reactions and even in cardiac arrest in some cases. (See Chapters 29 and 30 for a discussion of the cardiac effects of phenytoin.) Although this danger may be minimized by monitoring the patient's cardiac responses on the electrocardiograph, many neurologists now consider diazepam to be the drug of choice for treating status epilepticus because of its greater safety margin and more rapid onset of action.

Ordinarily, diazepam is remarkably reliable for promptly halting the continuous seizures of status epilepticus. Sometimes, repeated injections or intermittent infusions are necessary in resistant cases and, occasionally—particularly in recurrent seizures resulting from acute cerebral disease rather than chronic epilepsy—even massive doses of diazepam may fail to control convulsions. Administration of this drug in too high doses in an effort to stop such resistant seizures is also quite able to cause cardiac arrest and respiratory failure. Thus, drug treatment of this dangerous emergency is best managed by an anesthesiologist with equipment for monitoring heart action and for maintaining the patient's respiration artificially while oxygen is administered through an airway.

Petit mal epilepsy (absence seizures)

Petit mal epilepsy occurs mainly in children and tends to disappear as they grow up. Attacks are characterized not by convulsions but by brief lapses in consciousness. The child may suddenly stop what he is doing and stare blankly for a few seconds. Such trancelike states may happen dozens of times a day and may interfere with learning. Sometimes, the patient also has a tendency toward grand mal seizures, which may predominate in adult life.

Other patients suffer from certain variations of the simple or pure petit mal epilepsy. These variants, the Lennox–Gastaut syndrome and so-called minor motor seizures, which are marked either by sudden brief muscular contractions (*myoclonic* seizures) or by a sudden loss of muscle tone that makes the child fall down (*akinetic*, or *drop*, attacks), do not respond very well to treatment with the drugs that are effective in the *non*convulsive, or so-called absence, seizures of classic petit mal epilepsy.

Drug therapy

Two main classes of chemicals are effective for control of classic petit mal absence seizures. One class, the succinimides, including *ethosuximide*[+] (Zarontin), *phensuximide* (Milontin), and *methsuximide* (Celontin), is considered safer for long-term use than the oxazolidinedione class that includes *trimethadione*[+] (Tridione) and *paramethadione* (Paradione). *Diazepam* (Valium) is often effective for both pure petit mal and its so-called variants, the minor motor seizures of the myoclonic and akinetic types. Another benzodiazepine derivative, *clonazepam* (Clonopin), is also being employed to treat absence seizures and petit mal variants.

Treatment is best started with ethosuximide, a drug that combines both safety and effectiveness against most petit mal seizures. For patients with mixed forms of epilepsy, phenobarbital may be added to avoid setting off major seizures; sometimes phenytoin may have to be added to ethosuximide for the same purpose. Ordinarily, adequate doses of ethosuximide succeed in controlling seizures in three out of four petit mal patients and in benefiting most of the rest. Trimethadione may prove effective for those who do not respond to treatment with the first-choice drug. Some patients profit from treatment with paramethadione, which is said to produce fewer side-effects than its relative; others are best controlled by a combination of these two oxazolidinedione derivatives.

Chronic toxicity. Some side-effects of these first-line drugs such as sedation, nausea and vomiting, and photophobia are not serious. They either diminish as tolerance develops or can readily be controlled. For example, dark glasses help to lessen discomfort from the day blindness or glare phenomenon that sometimes occurs in patients taking trimethadione. This condition, in which outdoor objects often seem to be covered with ice or snow, does not lead to optic nerve damage. On the other hand, other adverse effects including hypersensitivity reactions that affect the bone marrow and other vital organs are potentially very dangerous.

To detect the onset of serious adverse effects at an early stage, various measures are routinely employed in patients taking trimethadione and paramethadione, and even in those being stabilized on safer drugs such as ethosuximide and diazepam. Before beginning treatment with these and other antiepileptic drugs, laboratory studies of the patient's blood and liver and kidney function are often ordered. The information obtained in this way serves as a baseline against which the results of later studies can be compared periodically during the course of prolonged treatment. Thus, for example, the onset of bone marrow depression in a patient taking trimethadione may be detected by a steady drop in the white blood cell count (leukopenia), or routine urinalyses may show increases in the presence of protein (albuminuria) that may make it necessary to discontinue trimethadione therapy.

Because some serious reactions may come on suddenly during the periods between these laboratory studies, patients and their families should be told to report certain types of signs and symptoms promptly. Severe sore throat accompanied by fever can, for example, be the first indication of the blood dyscrasia agranulocytosis. If a patient reports such signs or symptoms, a differential blood count may be ordered to determine whether the neutrophils have fallen to an abnormally low level. Similarly, if the patient reports bruiselike skin marks or other signs of bleeding, platelet counts may be ordered to detect the presence of thrombocytopenia. Abnormal decreases in all the formed elements of the blood, including red blood cells, and low hemoglobin levels may indicate that drug-induced bone marrow damage is leading to development of aplastic anemia. In such cases these drugs are immediately discontinued, despite the danger of setting off increased seizure activity.

Petit mal variants. Although the electroencephalograms (EEGs) of children with myoclonic and a-kinetic seizures sometimes superficially resemble the EEGs of pure petit mal, drugs such as trimethadione and ethosuximide are often ineffective for seizure control. Children with these drug-resistant forms of epilepsy often suffer severe injury, including skull fractures, when they suddenly drop to the floor or ground as a result of postural control loss. (Often, they must wear padded helmets to prevent serious injury.) This has led to trials of many types of drugs, some of which seem effective to a varying extent in some of these cases.

Diazepam (Valium) and chemically related benzodiazepine agents, including *chlordiazepoxide* (Librium; Chap. 45), clonazepam (Clonopin), and a drug of this class

called *nitrazepam* (Mogadon) that is widely used abroad in seizure control, have been reported to be useful for treating these cases of myoclonic and akinetic epilepsy. Administered in doses that do not cause excessive drowsiness and lethargy, diazepam and clonazepam have often proved to be particularly effective for many cases of myoclonia. In those cases that require diazepam in doses that do induce drowsiness, the addition of dextroamphetamine (Dexedrine; Chap. 47) often counteracts the sedation; sometimes, substituting ethosuximide for part of the diazepam dosage brings about control in doses of the drug combination that the patient can tolerate. An important advantage of diazepam and clonazepam is that these drugs do not cause the types of chronic toxicity that sometimes develop with the first-line drugs for petit mal and its variants (see above). Thus, treatment may be maintained for long periods in patients with minor motor seizures and pure petit mal with little danger of blood, liver, kidney, or skin reaction development. Unfortunately, tolerance tends to develop to the antiepileptic activity of most benzodiazepines after several months of therapy. This requires increased dosage with a greater chance of toxicity.

Valproic acid (Depakene), one of the newest antiepileptic drugs to receive FDA approval, is used in treating absence seizures, including petit mal epilepsy.* It is useful in both simple absence seizures, marked only by brief periods of clouding of consciousness, and in complex absence seizures, in which muscle contractions also occur. This drug also is useful when used as an adjunct to the standard drugs employed in the management of grand mal, psychomotor, and focal motor types of epilepsy.

Nausea, vomiting, and diarrhea are the drug's most common side-effects, but these and other gastrointestinal complaints may be avoided by beginning with small daily doses that are given with food and then gradually raised to higher levels. Drowsiness and motor incoordination sometimes occur, particularly when valproic acid is combined with phenobarbital, a combination that may also occasionally lead to signs of neurologic toxicity.

Of greater consequence, however, are the reports of serious and even fatal cases of hepatotoxicity, which have occurred in the first 6 months of therapy. Liver function tests should be performed before beginning treatment and at frequent intervals during therapy. Nonspecific symptoms such as lethargy, malaise, nausea, loss of appetite, and jaundice, as well as loss of seizure control, may precede hepatotoxicity, and the patient should be alerted to report these. In addition, platelet counts should be done periodically to detect early development of thrombocytopenia.

Other measures

Some patients with minor motor seizures and petit mal epilepsy have required treatment with a ketogenic diet for control of their condition. Apparently, the acidic ke-

* Physicians and the public previously had to apply pressure on the FDA to speed the approval procedure for drugs that appeared particularly effective for patients in desperate need of them. For example, it required forceful testimony by groups of neurologists to obtain FDA clearance for levodopa long after its outstanding effectiveness in Parkinson's disease was proved. Similarly, psychiatric associations had to force FDA action on lithium carbonate's approval, when its usefulness for treating manic–depressive illness was amply apparent.

tone bodies produced by this diet exert metabolic effects that reduce susceptibility to seizures. Diuretic drugs of the carbonic anhydrase inhibitor class (Chap. 27), such as acetazolamide (Diamox), may produce similar acidifying and dehydrating effects on the body. Thus, these drugs are sometimes employed instead of the expensive, unpalatable, and difficult-to-prepare ketogenic diet; occasionally, a combination of drug and diet therapy is used to bring about the degree of metabolic acidosis needed to gain control over minor motor seizures in preschoolage children. However, one problem with using acetazolamide is that tolerance to its beneficial effects often develops quickly.

Sometimes, psychomotor stimulants such as the amphetamines and methylphenidate (Chap. 47) benefit some children with petit mal and other seizures, including those that seem to be activated by deep sleep during the night. Occasionally, potentially more dangerous drugs, such as the antimalarials quinacrine and chloroquine (Chap. 10) must be employed in an effort to control akinetic-type seizures. Infants with massive myoclonic spasms resistant to treatment with all other drugs sometimes improve with courses of corticotropin (ACTH; Chap. 20), or of cortisone (Chap. 21).

Psychomotor seizures (temporal lobe epilepsy)

Psychomotor seizures are characterized by changes in behavior. These usually take the form of automatic repetitions of some pattern of movements. (The patient may, for example, go through the motions of lighting a cigarette, starting a car, or completing some other series of acts in a stereotyped manner.) On the other hand, these acts may sometimes become bizarre and, by attracting public attention and comment, bring difficulty with the law, which may regard the patient as a psychiatric case. These seizures are often the most difficult both to diagnose and to treat.

Drug therapy

The drugs most commonly employed for control of psychomotor seizures are the same as those considered to be most effective for grand mal epilepsy—combinations of phenytoin with phenobarbital or with primidone. Primidone is particularly useful as a substitute for phenobarbital if that drug or the other long-acting antiepileptic barbiturates make a sensitive patient's seizures worse, as sometimes happens.

Sometimes, if phenytoin also fails or has to be discontinued because of skin rashes, overgrowths of gum tissue, or ataxia, one of its chemical relatives, mephenytoin or ethotoin, may be substituted. As described earlier in the chapter, ethotoin is not very efficacious and mephenytoin causes serious adverse effects.

Carbamazepine[+] (Tegretol), a drug that was first introduced for treating trigeminal neuralgia, has also proved to be useful for preventing psychomotor and grand mal seizures. It may be added gradually to the regimen of patients whose psychomotor seizures have not been well controlled by phenytoin, phenobarbital, or primidone. Often, after dosage of these relatively ineffective drugs has been reduced or even discontinued, some patients may be maintained successfully on carbamazepine alone. An added advantage claimed for this drug is that it causes less excessive sedation than the other antiepileptics.

The main drawback of carbamazepine is its tendency to cause bone marrow depression in some patients. For this reason, complete blood counts are taken before beginning treatment and at frequent intervals following the start of therapy. The drug must be discontinued if various of the formed elements of the blood fall below certain minimal levels—for example, if the leukocyte count drops to less than 4000/mm^3 of blood. Failure to do so has led to development of agranulocytosis and fatal aplastic anemia in a few cases. On the other hand, some patients who developed drug-induced leukopenia had their white blood cell counts return to normal despite the continued use of carbamazepine by physicians who felt that the drug's benefits for patients with previously uncontrolled psychomotor seizures outweighed the risk of a severe blood dyscrasia.

As a last resort in uncontrolled cases of psychomotor epilepsy, the physician may decide to use an even more dangerous drug, *phenacemide* (Phenurone). When patients with severe seizures that are unresponsive to safer drugs are transferred to phenacemide therapy, many measures for detecting toxicity in its earliest stages are taken.

The patient usually has to be hospitalized during the first weeks of treatment while the drug's dosage is being adjusted to a safe and effective level. He is observed closely for the appearance of signs indicating possible drug-induced toxicity on the liver, brain, or bone marrow.

Jaundice is, of course, an indication of possible hepatic damage by the drug; it may be preceded by anorexia, nausea, and vomiting or followed by fever and general malaise. Early CNS side-effects may include headaches, insomnia, and restlessness in some cases, and apathy in others. The latter is more serious, because a loss of interest may signal the start of emotional depression. The drug is often withdrawn in such cases, because some psychomotor epilepsy patients have committed suicide while taking phenacemide.

Laboratory reports of differential blood counts and liver function tests also aid in monitoring the patient's responses to this dangerous drug. However, complaints of a sore mouth or throat can alert the health-care team to the presence of possible agranulocytosis in the period between blood studies.

Miscellaneous seizures

Not all patients who suffer seizures have epilepsy. In some cases, convulsions may be the first sign of a brain tumor or of some other acute and progressive brain disorder. On the other hand, convulsive seizures may be the result of temporary and readily reversible disturbances. Fever, for example, sometimes sets off seizures in young children. These febrile seizures can usually be prevented by prompt treatment with aspirin and phenobarbital. Newborn babies may convulse because of a deficiency of the B-complex vitamin pyridoxine, which will promptly stop the seizures when infused intravenously. These infants and those with seizures traced to a deficiency of calcium (hypocalcemic tetany) may then be maintained on diets supplemented by the required vitamin or mineral.

Patients who have become physically dependent on alcohol, barbiturates, or other general depressants (Chap. 53) sometimes suffer one or more seizures when they are withdrawn from the high doses that they have been taking. When the condition is correctly diagnosed, it is safest to stabilize the patient on adequate doses of a barbiturate such as pentobarbital (Nembutal) or phenobarbital. The drug is then very gradually withdrawn over a period of several weeks. Similarly, alcoholic patients in whom impending delirium tremens develops may be prevented from suffering seizures by substituting a general depressant drug such as paraldehyde or chlordiazepoxide (Librium) and then slowly tapering it.

An incapacitating condition called *postanoxic intention myoclonus* sometimes develops in people who have recovered from an episode of prolonged respiratory arrest. For example, some drug abusers who remained hypoxic for too long following a heroin overdose or barbiturate intoxication have been left subject to such seizures and to other disabling motor system dysfunctions. Their incapacitating loss of motor coordination is most marked when they attempt to write or perform other simple motor acts that trigger myoclonic convulsive spasms.

Some such cases have reportedly improved under treatment with clonazepam, a drug previously reported to be very useful for children with hereditary progresive myoclonic epilepsy. Even better results—an improvement in terms of 50% fewer seizures in over 60% of patients have been reported with treatment in which clonazepam was administered together with a combination of the amino acid L-5-hydroxytryptophan (L-5HTP) and the peripheral enzyme inhibitor carbidopa (Lodosyn).*

---

* Carbidopa inhibits the enzyme L-aromatic amino acid decarboxylase in peripheral tissues. Its use to treat parkinsonism in combination with the amino acid levodopa is discussed in Chapter 49. In that case and in the management of myoclonus, the concurrent use of carbidopa permits more of the therapeutically active amino acid to escape peripheral destruction and reach its central site of action. L-5HTP is now available to physicians through a treatment IND under the FDAs orphan drug program. (See pages 14 and 17)

Additional clinical considerations

The total care of a patient who has been diagnosed as having an epileptic disorder involves a great deal of patient teaching, support, and encouragement. The patient and significant others need to understand the nature of the illness and its implications. The patient can be helped to recall the events surrounding any seizure activity, including signs and symptoms that could represent an "aura," as well as environmental stressors that could have precipitated the events. By understanding his illness in these ways, the patient can become more involved in its management. He will need the opportunity to ventilate his feelings and to ask questions. This type of support will need to be continued throughout the patient's long-term therapy.

Once an antiepileptic drug or combination of drugs has been selected and the patient has been stabilized on the optimal dosage, he will need extensive teaching about the drug(s), as well as appropriate cautions and warnings. To be effective, all the antiepileptic drugs must be taken continually in the prescribed dosage. The patient needs to understand how important this scheduling of medications is to therapy. In some cases it is helpful to prepare a calendar with boxes for the patient to mark off each dose, or to place single doses of the drug in commercially available long-term dispensers. The patient needs to know that the medication cannot be stopped suddenly, and should be advised to call the nurse or physician immediately if anything occurs that prevents his taking the medication.

The patient also needs to be aware of all the adverse effects that can be anticipated with the drug, as well as the cautions that warn of toxicity, and to have these written down for reference. It is advisable to tell the patient to avoid the use of any other drugs—prescription or over-the-counter—until the nurse or physician has been consulted. Many drug–drug interactions may occur with these drugs, so consultation before using any other drugs can help to avoid both toxicity and the return of seizures. The patient should be cautioned to tell any nurse, physician, or dentist who is taking care of him that he is on this drug. The patient should also be advised to wear a medical alert tag to alert any healthcare professional who may care for him in an emergency situation that he is an epileptic on specific drug therapy, so that appropriate measures can be taken.

Patients receiving antiepileptic drugs must be encouraged to receive regular medical follow-up. These drugs are potentially toxic, and the patient should be evaluated for any developing toxicity. The patient needs to know the importance of such regular follow-up, and that blood tests will be required with each visit.

The patient teaching guide summarizes the key points that should be included when teaching the patient who is receiving antiepileptic drugs. Specific teaching points for each drug should be incorporated into a written teaching guide for the patient.

The safe use of these drugs in pregnancy has not been established. In fact, many of these drugs have been associated with specific syndromes of fetal malformation. A phenytoin syndrome has been clearly identified; valproic acid has been associated with an increasing incidence of spina bifida; oxazoladinediones (*e.g.,* trimethadione) have been associated with various fetal malformations. Other antiepileptics have not been proven safe, although specific deformities may not have been identified. The woman who is stabilized on an antiepileptic and who decides to become pregnant needs to know the risks involved, and she should be counseled by her neurologist and obstetrician. An antiepileptic should not be stopped suddenly, because the risks of seizure activity and its adverse effects on the mother and fetus are too great. The woman's antiepileptic drug may be slowly withdrawn, and a somewhat safer drug may be started. If a woman becomes pregnant while on one of these drugs, she will need to know the risks involved and her available options. All the antiepileptics cross into breast milk, and thus pose a risk for the neonate. Women receiving these drugs should be advised to select another method of feeding their babies.

Drug–drug interactions

As already mentioned, these drugs have the potential for several drug–drug interactions. Phenytoin, in particular, is a widely used drug that has been associated with many such interactions. Because this drug is used frequently, some of these interactions will be briefly reviewed.

Drugs that increase the effects of phenytoin include *coumarin anticoagulants, disulfiram, phenylbutazone, isoniazid, chloramphenicol, cimetidine, sulfonamides,* and *salicylates.* If a patient who has been stabilized on phenytoin is started on any of these drugs, the dosage of phenytoin will have to be reduced to avoid toxicity. The effects of phenytoin are decreased by *barbiturates, carbamazepine, folic acid, alcohol, CNS depressants, antacids, calcium gluconate, oxacillin,* and *antineoplastic drugs.* If a patient receiving phenytoin is started on any of these drugs, the dosage of phenytoin will need to be increased to suppress seizure activity. Phenytoin is known to decrease the effects of *dicumarol, disopyramide, quinidine, prednisolone, dexamethasone, corticosteroids, oral contraceptives, digitoxin,* and *furosemide.*

The guide to the nursing process summarizes the clinical aspects that should be incorporated into the nursing care of a patient receiving phenytoin. Similar guides can be developed for each of the other antiepileptic drugs.

Patient teaching guide: antiepileptics

The following general points should be incorporated into the teaching plan, which should also include specifics about the patient's particular illness and the details of the drug(s) selected for him.

Instructions:

1. The scheduling of this drug is very important. The drug must be taken regularly, as prescribed, to be effective.

2. Do not stop taking this drug suddenly. If, for any reason, you are unable to take your drug, notify your nurse or physician at once.

3. It is advisable to wear a medical alert tag so that anyone who takes care of you in an emergency situation will know that you are on this drug.

4. Tell any nurse, physician, or dentist who is taking care of you that you are on this drug.

5. Keep this and all medications out of the reach of children.

6. Do not take any other drug—including prescription drugs, over-the-counter drugs, or alcohol—without first consulting with your nurse or physician about the safety of the use of that drug while you are taking this antiepileptic.

(continued)

7. If you become pregnant or decide to become pregnant while you are on this drug, it is very important that you discuss it with your nurse and physician.

8. Record and report any seizure activity that occurs while you are taking this drug.

9. It will be very important for you to receive regular medical follow-ups while you are on this drug. Your regular examination will probably include a blood test.

10. Be aware of the signs and symptoms of toxicity that should be reported to your nurse or physician.

Guide to the nursing process: phenytoin

Assessment	Nursing diagnoses	Interventions	Evaluation
Past history (contraindications): Hepatic failure A-V block Bone marrow suppression Myocardial insufficiency Hypotension Pregnancy Lactation Allergies: these drugs; others; reactions Medication history (cautions): Oral anticoagulants Disulfiram Phenylbutazone Isoniazid Chloramphenicol Cimetidine Sulfonamides Salicylates Barbiturates Carbamazepine Folic acid Alcohol CNS depressants Antacids Calcium gluconate Oxacillin	Potential alteration in bowel elimination Knowledge deficit regarding drug therapy Potential alteration in nutrition secondary to gingival hyperplasia Potential sensory–perceptual alteration Potential alteration in thought processes Potential alteration in comfort: headache, joint pain	Safe and appropriate administration of drug Provision of safety and comfort measures: • Rigorous oral hygiene • Pain relief for headache, arthralgia • Drug given with food if GI upset occurs • Safety if dizziness and drowsiness occur Patient teaching regarding drug therapy Support and encouragement to cope with diagnosis and drug therapy Life support measures, if overdose occurs	Monitor for therapeutic effects of drug: control of epilepsy Monitor for adverse effects of drug: • CNS changes • Cardiovascular depression • Gingival hyperplasia • Enlarged lymph nodes • Hematologic depression • Skin rash • Increased blood sugar level • Hepatic changes • GI upset Evaluate effectiveness of patient teaching program Evaluate effectiveness of safety and comfort measures Evaluate effectiveness of support and encouragement offered Monitor for drug–drug interactions: many possible

(continued)

Assessment	Nursing diagnoses	Interventions	Evaluation
Antineoplastic agents Disopyramide Quinidine Steroids Oral contraceptives Digotoxin Furosemide **Physical assessment** Neurologic: orientation, affect, mental status, reflexes, EEG (if appropriate) Cardiovascular: P, BP, baseline ECG, peripheral perfusion GI: abdominal exam, normal function; mouth—mucosa, gingiva, teeth Skin: lesions Laboratory tests: blood sugar, liver function, CBC and differential, urinalysis			Monitor effectiveness of life support measures, if necessary

Summary of general principles of antiepileptic drug therapy

1. Treatment is started with a single drug selected for its known effectiveness in controlling the type of seizures to which the patient is subject, and for its relative safety in long-term treatment.
2. *Small doses*—usually about one-third of the average daily dose—are administered at first, and dosage is gradually raised at intervals of 5 to 7 days, until the patient's seizures are controlled or significant side-effects occur.
3. If the drug is effective but causes minor signs and symptoms of overdosage, its dosage is slowly reduced to a level that the patient can tolerate; if seizures are not completely controlled by safe doses of a single drug, a second relatively safe drug is gradually added to the patient's regimen.
4. In adjusting the dosage of a drug or combination of drugs to the needs of each individual patient, various clinical and laboratory aids are used:
   a. The patient or family keeps a record, charting the number of seizures that occur during drug treatment to determine whether attacks are actually occurring less frequently.
   b. The blood levels of certain of the drugs are checked and dosage adjusted as necessary to attain optimal plasma levels and clinical control of seizures.
   c. Treatment is continued at the highest dose the patient can tolerate and for a long enough trial period (at least 2 weeks) before deciding to discontinue therapy and switch to another drug.
5. Drugs are discontinued only gradually while another drug is being gradually substituted. Patients are also warned never to discontinue drug therapy abruptly, because this can set off episodes of status epilepticus.

Case study

Presentation

JM is a high school senior who had his first major seizure in school 2 months ago. During class one day, JM suddenly slumped to the floor and suffered a grand mal convulsion.

JM's fellow students were frightened and did not know what to do for him. Fortunately, his teacher had observed such seizures before and was able to protect Joe from injury. She was also able to explain the significance of what they had seen to the students who had observed JM's seizure.

JM's illness was diagnosed as grand mal epilepsy, idiopathic type (*i.e.,* of unknown cause). His physician prescribed phenytoin (Dilantin) and phenobarbital. However, his seizures have not yet been entirely controlled, even though he tends to be a bit drowsy during the day at the dose levels of the drug combination that he is taking. JM has had three more seizures since the first one—one at school and two at home. His parents and teacher realized later, in retrospect, that just before each seizure occurred, JM was involved in situations that created considerable nervous tension. JM is being seen in the clinic for evaluation of his drug regimen and for referral to the nurse for patient teaching.

Considering JM's situation, what key aspects should be included in his nursing care?

Discussion

A primary goal of JM's first teaching session should be the development of a trust relationship between JM and his family and the nurse who will be responsible for his care. JM is at a sensitive stage of development, and will no doubt require a great deal of support and encouragement to accept this diagnosis and its implications and to cope with this change in his self-concept. He will need to feel free to verbalize his feelings and anger and to ask questions that will help him to deal with his situation. JM's family will also need encouragement and support to cope with the diagnosis. They will need to learn about JM's therapy, and how to help him when seizures do occur. As the nurse learns more about JM and his response to the diagnosis and drug therapy, it will be appropriate to contact and work with JM's school nurse to facilitate his adjustment in this very critical aspect of his life.

The nurse should help JM to recount the situations surrounding his seizures. Working together, specific incidents or environmental activities that seem to precipitate the seizures might be determined. If specific stressful events are determined, JM will need to be helped to find ways to avoid or to cope with these events.

JM and his family will need teaching about epilepsy and what is known about the disease and its prognosis. In many communities there are support groups that help patients and their families learn to live with the disease. All the details of drug therapy should be discussed and written down for future reference by JM, his family, and the school nurse. In particular, JM should be alerted to the need for meticulous oral hygiene, the importance of avoiding the use of *any* other drugs until it has been discussed with his nurse or physician, the advisability of wearing a medical alert tag, the importance of taking the medication regularly as prescribed and not stopping it suddenly, and the importance of regular medical follow-up and evaluation, including blood tests.

JM's illness is a chronic one. His teaching program must be continued and updated for several years. The period of drug adjustment and evaluation will be the most trying time for JM and his family, and it will be a critical time for developing a trusting and supportive relationship with the health-care team. The nurse is in the crucial position to support the patient throughout this period and to provide the important foundation for successful therapy.

Summary of side effects and toxicity of antiepileptic drugs*

Drug type	Type of adverse reaction					
	Gastrointestinal	Dermatologic	Nervous system	Hematologic	Hepatic and renal	Miscellaneous
Hydantoins						
Phenytoin Mephenytoin Ethotoin	Anorexia; epigastric distress; nausea and vomiting	Rashes of measles and scarlet fever and acne-like types; hirsutism or hypertrichosis; Stevens–Johnson syndrome with mephenytoin	Unsteady gait (ataxia); slurred speech (dysarthria); double vision (diplopia); nystagmus, tremors, lethargy	Megaloblastic anemia; other blood dyscrasias with mephenytoin	Liver and kidney damage, especially with mephenytoin	Gingival hyperplasia (overgrowth of gum tissue); pseudolymphoma; cardiac arrhythmias and arrest; lupus erythematosus with mephenytoin
Oxazoladinediones						
Trimethadione Paramethadione	Epigastric distress; nausea and vomiting; hiccups	Minor rashes also but exfoliative dermatitis, and Stevens–Johnson syndrome (erythema multiforme)	Drowsiness	Neutropenia; thrombocytopenia; agranulocytosis; aplastic anemia	Hepatitis; nephrosis	Photophobia (hemeralopia or blindness) marked by the "glare phenomenon"; pseudolymphoma; lupus erythematosus
Succinimides						
Ethosuximide Methsuximide Phensuximide	Anorexia; nausea and vomiting; hiccups	Minor skin eruptions	Drowsiness, lethargy, fatigue; headache, dizziness; diplopia and ataxia rare	Rare leukopenia and other blood dyscrasias	Rare nephropathy or hepatitis	Occasional behavior disturbances; psychological aberrations, or psychoses
Phenacemide						
	Anorexia; nausea; vomiting; abdominal discomfort	Minor and major skin reactions	Personality changes; insomnia, restlessness; apathy and withdrawal; toxic psychosis; suicidal depression	Bone marrow changes resulting in agranulocytosis and aplastic anemia	Hepatitis (watch for jaundice and darkening of the urine); nephropathy	Fever; general malaise; sore throat; bruise marks, and other signs of infection or bleeding

Drug	Gastrointestinal	Dermatologic	Hematologic	Hepatic/renal	Neurologic	Other
Primidone	Nausea and vomiting	Measleslike skin rash	Rare megaloblastic anemia or leukopenia	Rare signs of liver or kidney involvement	Drowsiness, dizziness; headache, ataxia	General malaise
Barbiturates Phenobarbital Mephobarbital Metharbital	Nausea and vomiting	Rashes resembling measles or scarlet fever; rarely, exfoliative dermatitis or erythema multiforme	Rare megaloblastic anemia and other blood disorders	Rare signs of liver or kidney involvement	Drowsiness, dizziness; headache, lethargy; rarely, restlessness or excitement	Weakness and paralysis in patients with *porphyria*, in whom these drugs are contraindicated
Benzodiazepines Clonazepam Diazepam	Anorexia; nausea; mouth dryness; constipation or diarrhea	Rare rashes; hair loss; hirsutism	Rarely blood disorders, such as anemia, leukopenia, thrombocytopenia	Rare liver or kidney involvement manifested by transient liver function test abnormalities; urinary retention or incontinence	Drowsiness, headache; ataxia, fatigue; rarely, paradoxic excitement	Rapid IV injection of diazepam can cause cardiac and respiratory failure; blurred vision, diplopia, nystagmus
Carbamazepine	Anorexia; nausea and vomiting; epigastric distress; mouth dryness	Minor skin eruptions, but also possible exfoliative dermatitis or Stevens–Johnson syndrome	Leukopenia; thrombocytopenia; agranulocytosis; aplastic anemia	Rare liver or kidney involvement manifested by liver function test abnormalities; jaundice; also acute urinary retention and oliguria	Drowsiness, dizziness, headache; lethargy, disturbed coordination, and involuntary movements	Muscle and joint aches, leg cramps; fever and chills; blurring of vision, diplopia
Valproic acid	Nausea; vomiting; epigastric distress; diarrhea	Minor skin rashes	Thrombocytopenia; prolonged bleeding time	Fatal hepatoxicity has occurred	Drowsiness; occasional increased aggressive behavior and hyperactivity	Uncertain

* See the discussion in the text of use in pregnancy, which applies not only to phenytoin and to phenobarbital but to all antiepileptic drugs.

Drug digests

Carbamazepine USP (Tegretol)

Actions and indications. This drug is effective for control of certain partial and generalized epileptic seizures, for preventing the pain of trigeminal neuralgia and glossopharyngeal neuralgia attacks and, reportedly, for halting hiccup attacks that have not responded to other measures.

It has proved to be particularly beneficial for patients with psychomotor epilepsy that has not responded to standard drug therapy. It is also sometimes effective for patients with grand mal epilepsy or with mixed seizure patterns, whose disorders have not been brought under adequate control by such first-line drugs as phenytoin, phenobarbital, or primidone.

Adverse reactions, cautions, and contraindications. Some side-effects are relatively minor and can be minimized by initiating treatment with low doses that are then raised gradually. These include drowsiness, dizziness, nausea, and vomiting during the early stages of therapy. Although sedation is said to be less heavy than with the barbiturates, patients should be cautioned about the hazards of driving or operating machinery and performing other possibly dangerous tasks. Depression of bone marrow with resulting reductions in the formed elements of the circulating blood is the most serious potential adverse effect. Leukopenia, agranulocytosis and fatal aplastic anemia have been reported. Pretreatment blood counts are performed to establish a baseline against which the results of frequent further tests are compared. Leukopenia below 4000/mm^3, platelets below 100,000/mm^3, and erythrocytes less than 4 million/mm^3 are indications that the drug should be discontinued.

Development of abnormalities in liver function tests or of active liver disease requires discontinuation of drug therapy. Periodic eye examinations should be performed, particularly in patients with elevated intraocular pressure. Adverse drug interactions may occur with monoamine oxidase inhibitors, which should not be administered concurrently.

Dosage and administration. On the first day of epilepsy treatment a total dose of 200 mg is administered, and for trigeminal neuralgia the initial daily dose is 100 mg. These are administered in two divided doses with food. Dosage is then increased in small increments up to a maximum (in most cases) of 1200 mg daily, divided into three or four doses administered with meals.

Ethosuximide USP (Zarontin)

Actions and indications. This drug is preferred for first trial in petit mal epilepsy, because it is both effective for suppressing three-cycle/second spike and wave activity and is relatively safe for long-term use compared to drugs of other chemical classes. It is also used against other minor motor seizures, including the akinetic and myoclonic types.

In patients with mixed minor and major seizures, this drug is administered in combination with anticonvulsants that can control conditions that are *not* helped by succinimide drugs—for example, grand mal, psychomotor, and focal motor epilepsy. When this drug is added to the regimen of patients with such seizures, the anticonvulsant drug dosage on which they were previously stabilized may have to be raised to prevent loss of seizure control.

Adverse effects, cautions, and contraindications. Early gastrointestinal side-effects include loss of appetite, epigastric distress, hiccups, nausea, and vomiting. Central adverse effects include drowsiness, lethargy, fatigue, and reduced motor coordination; patients are warned against driving and engaging in other activities that require unimpaired alertness and motor control. Use of this drug is contraindicated in patients with a history of hypersensitivity reactions to this drug and its chemical relatives—for example, severe skin reactions or blood dyscrasias.

Hematologic, hepatic, and other adverse reactions are relatively rare compared to their occurrence with certain older antiepileptic agents. However, blood counts should be performed periodically to detect early falls in the formed elements of the blood. Liver function tests should also be performed. This drug should be administered only with extreme caution to patients with known liver or kidney insufficiency.

Dosage and administration. Children between 3 and 6 years old are started on a dose of 250 mg a day; those over 6 receive 500 mg daily. It is suggested that the dose then be raised by 250 mg a day about once a week, until complete control is achieved. However, dosage is usually limited to 1 g in younger children and rarely exceeds 1.5 g in older children or adults.

Phenobarbital USP (Luminal)

Actions and indications. This long-acting barbiturate is the preferred anticonvulsant compound of that class for prevention of epileptic seizures. It is particularly effective for grand mal, focal motor, and psychomotor epilepsy when administered alone or combined with phenytoin. Some patients with petit mal epilepsy improve, but in others with variants of petit mal more frequent seizures may develop.

The sodium salt of phenobarbital is effective for control of acute convulsive states, including status epilepticus and eclamptic convulsions in patients with pregnancy toxemia. It is also used for preoperative and postoperative sedation and occasionally for controlling agitation and bringing about sleep in manic patients with various types of psychoses (though it has largely been replaced by the phenothiazines for this purpose).

Adverse effects, cautions, and contraindications. This drug is considered to be safer than other anticonvulsants for the long-term management of chronic epilepsies, because serious toxicity involving the bone marrow, liver and kidneys is rare. Skin rashes resembling measles and scarlet fever develop occasionally in patients hypersensitive to barbiturates and, like other drugs of that type, it is contraindicated in patients with porphyria.

Phenobarbital is considered to be somewhat less safe than such other antiepileptics as phenytoin and diazepam for control of acute, recurring convulsions, because its tendency to accumulate may lead to excessive degrees of depression. This is particularly true in patients with impaired ability to excrete the drug by way of the kidneys. The drug is contraindicated in patients with nephritis, and is used only with caution in patients severely weakened by pulmonary and other diseases. Excessive hypnotic doses produce "hangover," or residual sedation, marked by drowsiness, lethargy, headache, and nausea. Chronic overdosage may lead to delirium, ataxia, and stupor.

Dosage and administration. In epilepsy, dosage varies with the need and tolerance of the patient but, for adults, it generally ranges between 100 and 200 mg daily in two divided oral doses. For daytime sedation, smaller oral doses of 16 to 32 mg administered bid or tid are adequate. A single dose of 100 mg is administered orally at bedtime for producing sleep in insomnia; larger hypnotic doses—200 to 300 mg—may be administered for preoperative sedation. Higher doses may be administered parenterally as needed for control of acute convulsions or extreme excitement, but the total dosage injected subcutaneously, IM, or IV should not exceed 600 mg in one 24-hour period.

Phenytoin USP (Dilantin)

Actions and indications. This antiepileptic is effective orally for preventing grand mal and other major motor seizures and psychomotor epilepsy. It is also sometimes effective in minor motor (myoclonic and akinetic) epilepsy. The drug has also been advocated for treating trigeminal neuralgia and migraine headache.

The parenteral form is employed in treating status epilepticus and other recurrent convulsive states. It is also used prior to neurosurgical procedures to protect the patient against seizures during surgery. It is also useful for control of rapid cardiac arrhythmias, including tachycardia in digitalis intoxication.

Adverse effects, cautions, and contraindications. This drug is best given during or after meals to reduce local irritation and resulting gastric distress, nausea, and vomiting, or constipation. A common oral side-effect is development of gingival hyperplasia—unsightly swelling of the gums. This may be minimized by frequent cleansing of the mouth, but occasional surgical excision of the tissue overgrowths may also be required. Other hypersensitivity reactions include morbilliform skin rashes; megaloblastic anemia may develop with long-term use, but serious blood dyscrasias are rare.

This drug does not cause sedation in ordinary doses, but excessive amounts may cause various signs and symtoms of central nervous system toxicity. These include lethargy, slurred speech and staggering gait (dysarthria and ataxia), and mental confusion. Nystagmus may be noted, and patients may complain of double vision, dizziness, and headache. Massive overdosage can result in coma, apnea, and death from respiratory depression. Too rapid intravenous administration may result in cardiac arrest.

Dosage and administration. Initial oral adult doses of 100 mg tid are later adjusted to levels optimal for each patient. Maintenance of seizure control may be attained with as little as 100 mg daily or require as much as 600 mg total daily dosage.

Children are started on oral doses of 5 mg/kg body weight daily, divided into three doses. They may then be maintained on doses ranging from 3 to 8 mg/kg administered in several pediatric dosage forms including suspensions containing 30 or 125 mg/5 ml.

The parenteral form is injected IV at a slow rate (no more than 50 mg/min) in doses ranging from 150 to 250 mg. It may also be administered IM in doses of 100 to 200 mg.

Primidone USP (Mysoline)

Actions and indications. This antiepileptic drug is used alone, or combined with phenytoin, for preventing grand mal, focal, and psychomotor seizures, including cases resistant to other antiepileptic agents. In general it serves as a substitute for phenobarbital, which it resembles chemically, and it is safer than phenacemide, another secondary or back-up drug reserved for refractory cases of various types of epilepsy.

Adverse effects, cautions, and contraindications. Common early side-effects include drowsiness, dizziness, headache, and ataxia. These may be minimized by building up the dosage slowly. Occasionally, nausea and vomiting and a measleslike rash may develop. Rarely, megaloblastic anemia may occur, but this can be overcome by administering small doses of folic acid. Routine laboratory tests at regular intervals are recommended to detect blood changes, including leukopenia. However, serious toxicity rarely occurs.

Although effects of this drug on the fetus are uncertain, the drug is used in pregnant women when its ability to control convulsions is believed to be worth the risk. Some babies born to mothers taking primidone have had hemorrhages as a result of hypoprothrombinemia. Thus, pregnant women taking this drug should receive daily doses of vitamin K during the last month and at delivery to prevent development of coagulation defects. Use of the drug may have to be discontinued in nursing mothers if the baby becomes excessively lethargic.

Dosage and administration. Daily dosage for adults usually ranges between 750 mg and 1.5 g. Treatment is commonly begun with 250 mg administered at bedtime for 1 week. During the second week, this dose is administered twice daily. A third dose is added daily during the following week and, in the fourth week, the patient receives 250 mg qid if needed for full control of convulsions. Doses may be increased up to 2 g daily if required for control, and if the patient can tolerate such large amounts. Children are started and eventually stabilized on half the daily adult dosage.

Trimethadione USP (Tridione)

Actions and indications. This was the earliest drug for treating petit mal epilepsy. However, it is now reserved for patients whose seizures have not been brought under control by drugs with less potential for producing serious hypersensitivity-type reactions. It is not useful for grand mal and other major motor seizures, but it may be combined with adjusted doses of phenytoin and phenobarbital in the management of patients with mixed seizures. It is also occasionally helpful for minor motor seizures of the myoclonic and akinetic types.

Adverse effects, cautions, and contraindications. Some early side-effects such as drowsiness and stomach distress tend to lessen as tolerance develops with continued treatment. Others, such as the characteristic type of photophobia—hemeralopia, or day blindness—are also reversible with reduced dosage. However, skin rashes require that this drug be discontinued because of possible severe skin reactions, such as the Stevens-Johnson syndrome and exfoliative dermatitis. Other dangerous adverse reactions that must be watched for include blood dyscrasias, hepatitis, and the nephrotic syndrome. Laboratory tests of the patient's blood and urine and tests of liver function should be made frequently. Falls in neutrophils below 2500/mm³, increasing albuminuria, and the appearance of jaundice all indicate that this drug should be discontinued. Patients and their families are instructed to report signs and symptoms such as sore throat and fever, bleeding from nose and gums, dark urine, or other early warnings that the drug should be discontinued to avoid serious drug reactions. An increased incidence of fetal malformations has been reported in babies born to women taking trimethadione.

Dosage and administration. Treatment of adults is initiated with doses of 300 mg tid and then increased by 300 mg at weekly intervals until seizures are controlled or toxicity occurs. The usual dosage ranges from 900 to 2100 mg daily. Children's dosage is gradually increased to optimal levels of effectiveness and tolerance after starting with 150-mg doses.

References

Browne TR: Therapy of status epilepticus. Compr Ther 8:23, 1982

Bruni J, Wilder BJ: Valproic acid: Review of new antiepileptic drug. Arch Neurol 36:393, 1979

Bruya MA et al: Epilepsy: A controllable disease. Part 1. Classification and diagnosis. Part 2. Treatment. Am J Nurs 76:388, 396, 1976

Cereghino JJ et al: Carbamazepine for epilepsy. Neurology 24:401, 1974

Delgado–Excueta AV, Bayorek JG: Status epilepticus: Mechanisms of brain damage and rational management. Epilepsia 23 (Suppl 1):529, 1982

Drugs for epilepsy. Med Lett Drugs Ther 25:81, 1983

Eadie MJ: Plasma level monitoring of anticonvulsants. Clin Pharmacokinet 1:52, 1976

Freeman JM: Febrile seizures: Concensus of significance, evaluation and treatment. Pediatrics 66:1009, 1980

Hart RG, Easton JD: Carbamazepine and hematological monitoring. Ann Neurol 11:309, 1982

Penry JK et al: The use of antiepileptic drugs. Ann Intern Med 90:207, 1979

Penry JK, Porter RJ: Epilepsy: Mechanisms and therapy. Med Clin North Am 63:801, 1979

Rall TW, Schleifer LS: Drugs effective in the therapy of the epilepsies. In Gilman AG, Goodman LS, Gilman A (eds): Goodman & Gilman's The Pharmacological Basis of Therapeutics, 6th ed, pp 448–474. New York, Macmillan, 1980

Reynolds EH: Chronic antiepileptic toxicity: A review. Epilepsia 16:319, 1975

Reynolds EH, Shorvou SD: Single drug or combination therapy for epilepsy. Drugs 21:374, 1981

Richens A: Interactions with antiepileptic drugs. Drugs 13:266, 1977

Singer WD et al: Effect of ACTH therapy upon infantile spasms. J Pediatr 96:485, 1980

Spero L: Epilepsy. Lancet 2:1319, 1982

Thurston JH et al: Prognosis in childhood epilepsy: Additional follow-up of 148 children 15 to 23 years after withdrawal of anticonvulsant therapy. N Engl J Med 306:831, 1982

Section 8

Part 3

Drugs used for relief and prevention of pain

The next two chapters deal with drugs employed mainly to prevent or relieve relatively severe acute and chronic pain. These drugs act in the central nervous system (in the brain and possibly in the spinal cord) to alter the ways that pain impulses from the periphery are processed centrally. Drugs that block the conduction of pain impulses into the CNS—that is, local anesthetics—were described in Chapter 14. Drugs that act on the peripheral and central nervous systems are not the only types of drugs that relieve pain.

Drugs discussed elsewhere in this book also relieve pain. They do so by counteracting conditions that cause pain at the points at which they arise. Thus, for example, nitroglycerin and other coronary artery vasodilator drugs (Chap. 31) relieve the chest pains of angina pectoris by their actions on blood vessels. The pain of vascular headaches such as migraine is relieved by ergotamine (Chap. 38), which appears to act by constricting excessively dilated cranial and extracranial arteries. The antispasmodic drugs derived from belladonna (Chap. 16) reduce pain arising in the upper gastrointestinal tract by relaxing its smooth muscle walls or by lessening gastric acid secretion (Chap. 41).

Before beginning to discuss the several classes of pain-relieving drugs taken up in this section because of their effects on the CNS—the potent narcotic analgesics and general anesthetics—this introductory section will review briefly some aspects of the neurophysiologic mechanisms involved in the perception of pain sensation and in people's reactions to it. The nurse should know something about the extremely complex neurologic basis for the pain experience, not only because such knowledge permits better understanding of pain-relieving drugs, but also because such information leads to better understanding of the need for psychological measures in managing patients who are suffering pain.

Neurophysiology of pain

Peripheral systems

Pain is produced by damage to tissues that leads to the liberation of various chemical substances in the vicinity of nearby nerve endings. It has not been proved that these nerve endings contain chemoreceptors specifically sensitive to such substances and responsive to them in ways that would permit their properly being called "pain receptors." However, there is ample evidence indicating that locally produced chemical substances such as *bradykinin* and *prostaglandins* are associated with the production of pain (see Chap. 36).

Two types of small-diameter fibers within peripheral sensory nerves, A_δ and *C fibers,* are believed to respond to stimulation by generating and transmitting nerve impulses that give rise to pain sensations. Impulses from the skin, subcutaneous tissues, muscles, and deeper visceral structures are conducted by these afferent branches back to their nerve cell bodies located in sensory ganglia called the dorsal root ganglia. These are located just outside the dorsal, or posterior, horn of the spinal cord (Fig. A). They send their efferent fibers into the dorsal horn, where the axons synapse with the second nerve cell in the pain pathway—that is, the first centrally located neuron.

Other peripheral sensory nerve fibers—the large-diameter A_α fibers—also enter the dorsal part of the spinal cord and synapse with neurons located there. However, these larger and more rapidly conducting afferent fibers do not conduct impulses associated with pain sensation. When stimulated, their nonpain impulses that transmit touch sensation tend, in fact, to reduce the ability of A_δ and C fibers to send their pain signals to the second neuron in the series. That is, the ability of the dorsal horn neurons to receive and transmit pain sensation im-

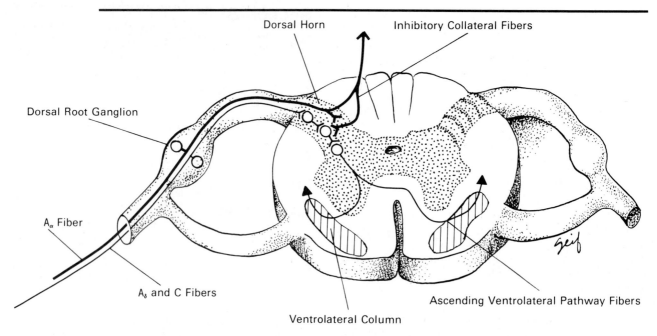

Figure A. Cross section of a spinal cord segment that is receiving afferent fibers from a peripheral spinal nerve. Small diameter A_δ and C fibers transmit pain impulses, and large diameter A_α fibers transmit other sensations. All fibers enter the dorsal horn by way of the dorsal root ganglion. A_α fiber collaterals inhibit transmission of pain impulses to dorsal horn cells.

pulses upward to the brain is influenced by inhibitory as well as excitatory impulses entering this spinal cord segment from peripheral sites.

Central neural mechanisms

Pain and other sensory impulses are transmitted from dorsal horn cells to higher parts of the neuraxis by several different ascending pathways (Fig. B). Some fibers project upward to the thalamus, where they synapse with various groups of nerve cells, or nuclei, that, in turn, relay pain impulses to nerve cells in the cerebral cortex. However, this spinothalamic nerve tract is not the only sensory pathway that plays a part in pain production, and neither the dorsal horn cells nor the thalamic cells are the simple relay stations that they were once thought to be. Contrary to the long-held view that compared the transmission of pain sensations to a direct line telephone system, it is now known that these and other sensory impulses are subject to modification at every point in their passage along the neuraxis from the peripheral receptors to the somatosensory and other cerebral cortical areas.

Modulation of sensory messages occurs first in the dorsal horn of the same spinal cord segment at which the afferent impulses enter. Here, according to the "gate control" hypothesis, certain spinal interneurons influence sensory functioning at the very first synapse in the pain pathway. These interneurons, in effect, control sensory impulse traffic at the point where the impulses begin their ascent. This gate mechanism is further modulated at higher segments of the spinal cord and at supraspinal levels.

It is now known that nerve impulses *descending* from neuraxis levels above the spinal cord exert a constant influence on those *ascending* in the several sensory pathways. Thus, for example, the cerebral cortex is not only a receiver of nerve impulses relayed from the thalamic nuclei, but also a sender of signals back to the same subcortical and spinal areas (Fig. C). Such impulses from the cortex influence nerve cell functioning in the gray matter of the midbrain, the thalamus, the reticular formation of the brain stem, and other associated relay stations, including those that send fibers all the way down the dorsal horn column of the spinal cord or dorsolateral tract.

What is the significance of this? One important clinical implication is that the participation of the highest level of the human brain, the cerebral cortex, can influence how much pain is perceived as well as how people feel about it and how various bodily functions are affected by it. This explains, for example, why pain can be made better or worse by psychological and emotional factors. Thus, anxiety and fear can provoke a pain experience that is marked by greater pain and suffering and, conversely, whatever the physician or nurse can do to reduce the patient's nervousness and apprehension will have a favorable influence on his total pain experience.

These new concepts of local and higher level inhibitory processes also help to explain how hypnosis acts to prevent pain and why placebos and other forms of suggestion work to prevent pain in many cases. Similarly, the gate control theory provides some insight into why stimulation of acupuncture points at a distance from the source of pain often exerts an influence on pain perception, and why such remedies as the application of heat and cold and massage help to inhibit perception of pain stimuli. The theory is also being applied to the control of pain by electrical stimulation, biofeedback mechanisms, and better use of the various types of pain-relieving drugs.

The next two chapters will focus only on pharmacologic pain relief measures. The drugs described act by affecting central neural mechanisms of the pain pathways. The potent narcotic analgesics act at specific central sites in ways that increase inhibitory influences on pain perception and decrease emotional reactions to perceived pain. The general anesthetics also act centrally but, unlike the potent narcotic analgesics, which suppress pain perception and reaction without causing loss of consciousness, drugs of this class cause heavy clouding of consciousness and, usually, complete elimination of all awareness. Even though anesthetized patients may not be aware of feeling any pain, however, enough noxious stimuli often get

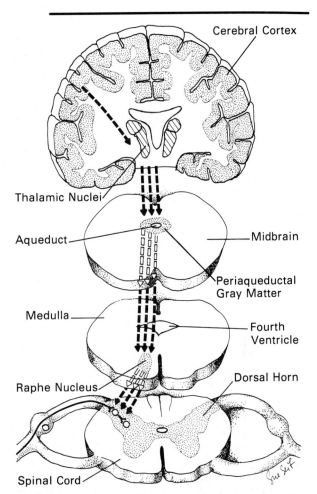

Figure C. Descending inhibitory neural pathways from supraspinal sites influence lower ascending system structures, including the dorsal horn neurons that are the first central cells to receive pain impulses from the periphery. Modulation of sensory impulses at this first synapse and others lessens the number of pain impulses that ascend to the thalamus and the somatosensory and frontal cortex areas.

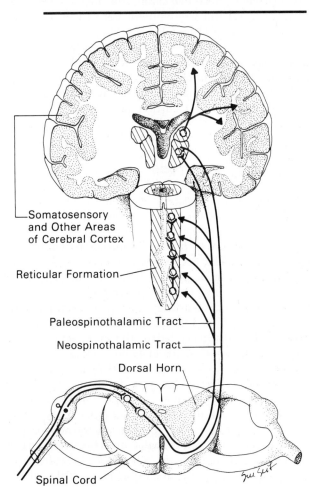

Figure B. The spinothalamic system is one of several ascending sensory pathways that play a part in pain impulse transmission. One spinothalamic tract runs to thalamic nuclei that then relay fibers to the somatosensory cortex. Another spinothalamic tract sends collateral fibers to the reticular formation and to other structures from which further fibers project to the thalamus that finally influence the hypothalamus and limbic system, as well as the cerebral cortex.

through to the central nervous system to set off reflex responses that may be harmful.

Among the drugs that exert peripheral actions are the local anesthetics (Chap. 14) that interfere with the conduction of pain impulses in the sensory nerve fibers and other sites outside the central nervous system. These sites include the "pain receptors" in the ends of afferent nerves and the sensory nerve fibers of the nerve cell bodies that run to the dorsal root ganglion and beyond to the roots of the spinal nerves at the point of their entrance into the cord. Local anesthetics have been described already in the section of the book that deals with the pharmacology of the periperal nervous system. Increasing evidence that aspirin, acetaminophen, and other mild analgesics act mainly on the most peripheral mechanisms for pain reception—for example, by their effects on bradykinin and prostaglandins biosynthesis—has led to the discussion of these drugs elsewhere (Chap. 37), rather than here with the drugs that act on the central nervous system.

Chapter 51

Narcotic analgesics and antagonists of narcotics

Analgesics are drugs that can relieve pain when administered in doses that have little, if any, effect on other functions of the central nervous system. Several other classes of drugs—alcohol, sedative–hypnotics, and other nonselective depressants of all parts of the CNS, including the general anesthetics—can also relieve pain. However, to do so they must be given in amounts that tend to interfere with the patient's consciousness and cause mental confusion, stupor, or total unconsciousness.

Analgesics are commonly classified in terms of both the degree of pain severity that they can control and the extent to which they can cause dependence and addiction. Neither classification is entirely satisfactory, and it would be better to divide these drugs on the basis of where and how they act to bring about reduced perception of pain sensation and lessened reaction to it. Perhaps recent advances and current research may soon make this possible.

At present, however, analgesic drugs are still divided into two main classes: those that relieve only mild to moderate degrees of pain and that are commonly considered to be nonaddicting, and those that can relieve severe degrees of pain but that are also moderately or strongly addictive—the narcotic analgesics. Drugs of the first type—also called nonnarcotics—include aspirin, acetaminophen, phenacetin, and other analgesic–antipyretics. The latter, because a large component in their pain-relieving activity is peripheral rather than central, have been taken up, not in this section, but in Chapter 37.

This chapter will present the narcotic analgesics, most of which are quite potent in their ability to relieve severe pain. These potent analgesics are also called *opioids* because the first of them came from the opium plant, and later drugs of this type were also derived from opium, or—even when they are prepared synthetically—exert pharmacologic effects that closely resemble those of opium and its natural and semisynthetic derivatives. Here, the opium alkaloids will be taken up first, and followed by discussions of the synthetic narcotic analgesics and of drugs that can counteract their effects—the narcotic antagonists. Finally, the chapter will indicate how these and other drugs and measures are best employed in the management of acute and chronic pain in various clinical situations.

Opium and its analgesic alkaloids

The poppy plant, *Papaver somniferum,* is the source of opium, a substance used since ancient times for relieving pain. However, the effects of powdered opium and of liquid preparations such as laudanum and paregoric were often undependable because of differences in the alkaloid content of the crude plant extracts. Then, early in the last century, a young German pharmacist, Friedrich Serturner, succeeded in isolating a pure plant principle which he called *morphine,* for Morpheus, the Greek god of dreams. This discovery led to the extraction of other crystalline opium alkaloids including *codeine,* and to the preparation of substances such as *heroin* and other semisynthetic derivatives, drugs made by chemically treating the natural opiate alkaloids. Heroin is not used clinically in this country (it *is* used abroad) but other semisynthetic modifications of morphine, codeine, and the nonanalgesic natural opium alkaloid thebaine are effective for relief of moderate to severe pain. These include *hydrocodone, hydromorphone, oxycodone,* and *oxymorphone* (Table 51-1).

Morphine analgesia
Despite the later development of potent synthetic pain relievers, morphine—the prototype opioid—is still the

Table 51–1. Narcotic analgesics and narcotic antagonists

Official or generic name	Trade name or synonym	Usual adult dosage range	Comments
Potent narcotic analgesics with high dependence-producing potential			
Alphaprodine HCl USP	Nisentil	20–60 mg	Short duration (see Drug digest)
Codeine phosphate and sulfate USP	Methylmorphine	15–60 mg	Opium alkaloid for mild to moderate pain; low abuse potential (see Drug digest)
Fentanyl citrate USP	Sublimaze	0.05–0.1 mg	Very potent analgesic and respiratory depressant
Heroin	Diacetylmorphine	2–8 mg	Not used clinically in United States (abuse drug)
Hydromorphone HCl	Dilaudid	2–4 mg	More potent than morphine
Levorphanol tartrate USP	Levo-Dromoran	2–3 mg	More potent and longer acting than morphine
Meperidine HCl USP	Demerol; pethidine	50–100 mg	Less sedating and spasmogenic than morphine (see Drug digest)
Methadone HCl USP	Dolophine	2.5–10 mg	Less euphoric than heroin; now used in management of heroin dependence (see Drug digest)
Morphine sulfate USP	—	5–20 mg	Prototype opium alkaloid (see Drug digest)
Opium alkaloids	Pantopon	5–20 mg	Mixture of purified opium alkaloids
Oxycodone HCl	—	5–10 mg	More potent and more dependence-producing than codeine
Oxymorphone HCl USP	Numorphan	1.0–1.5 mg	Potent, rapid onset, moderate duration
Less potent and less dependence-producing narcotic analgesics			
Propoxyphene HCl USP	Darvon; dextropropoxyphene	32–65 mg	About half as potent as codeine but even less likely to produce dependence in normal use
Propoxyphene napsylate USP	Darvon-N	100 mg	Most effective when combined with aspirin (see Drug digest)
Narcotic agonist–antagonist analgesics			
Butorphanol tartrate	Stadol	1–4 mg	More potent than morphine
Nalbuphine HCl	Nubain	10 mg/70 kg body weight	Potency similar to morphine
Pentazocine HCl and lactate USP	Talwin; Talwin NX	30–50 mg	Tolerance develops only slowly to therapeutic doses; can produce dependence in abusers (see Drug digest)
Nonnarcotic (phenothiazine) analgesic			
Methotrimeprazine USP	Levoprome	10–30 mg	Does not produce dependence or respiratory depression, but its usefulness is limited by orthostatic hypotension and sedation

(continued)

Table 51–1. Narcotic analgesics and narcotic antagonists (continued)

Official or generic name	Trade name or synonym	Usual adult dosage range	Comments
Narcotic antagonists			
Levallorphan tartrate USP	Lorfan	1 mg IV	Partial agonist
Naloxone HCl USP	Narcan	0.4–2.0 mg parenterally	Pure antagonist (see Drug digest)
Naltrexone HCl†	—	—	Similar to naloxone but with longer duration of action

* The natural opium alkaloid codeine is an exception, but is included here for convenience.
† This is an experimental drug of considerable clinical promise; other, still experimental, antagonists include cyclazocine and propiram (see text).

drug most widely employed for relief of severe pain. The nurse who learns the actions and uses of *morphine sulfate*⁺ ("MS") should then find it easy to compare any newly introduced synthetic drug with this prototype in terms of their similarities and differences. The nurse may also be better able to evaluate claims for advantages of new drugs when the value and limitations of this morphine salt are understood.

Morphine and its natural, semisynthetic, and synthetic relatives relieve pain in three main ways:

1. They reduce the patient's perception of pain by raising the pain perception threshold.
2. They change the patient's reaction to pain by reducing the unpleasant emotional response that pain evokes.
3. They can produce sleep despite the presence of trauma that can cause severe pain.

Relatively small doses of morphine can dull the ability to perceive pain without significantly altering mental functioning. The drug is especially effective against continuous dull pain of moderate intensity originating in the smooth muscles of the internal hollow organs.

Despite this effect of morphine on pain perception, the patient can still feel sharp, stabbing pain following fractures, extensive burns, and other traumata. However, the patient who is under the influence of morphine may not mind this pain even when aware of it. This alteration in the patient's response to pain is one of the most characteristic and important effects of morphine and other narcotic analgesics.

Although morphine analgesia is not necessarily accompanied by drowsiness, the drug does often have a hypnotic action. Such a sleep-producing effect is sometimes desirable for patients whose rest is disturbed by their pain. It is especially important for some pain-tossed patients, such as those who have suffered a myocardial infarction or other condition that requires complete rest and relaxation. On the other hand, excessive drug-induced sedation is undesirable in patients who need to remain ambulatory and active in spite of pain.

Sites and mechanisms of action. Scientists have recently made rapid progess toward solving the problem of how morphine produces its potent analgesic effects. Advances in this field during the 1970s began with the discovery on brain cell membranes of receptor sites highly specific for opioid molecules. An area of the midbrain and of the limbic system contains neurons that are rich in such opioid receptors. This has led to the current view that these drugs activate natural neural mechanisms that function to reduce the perception of pain and the emotional reaction to pain.

As indicated in Chapter 44 and in the introduction to this section, the higher levels of the neuraxis are now known to exert descending inhibitory influences on lower levels of the ascending pain pathways. It is thought that morphine reduces pain perception by activating certain midbrain neurons located in the gray matter that borders on the third ventricle and the narrow channel, or aqueduct, that connects it with the fourth ventricle. These periventricular and periaqueductal nerve cells then fire impulses at a more rapid rate down to another group of nerve cells, the *raphe nucleus* (Fig. C, introduction to this section), which relay the inhibitory impulses to the dorsal horn neurons that are the first CNS cells to receive pain stimuli from peripheral sites.* This, of course, prevents many pain signals from continuing their ascent to the thalamus, brain stem, and related supraspinal nerve centers, and consequently the perception of pain is reduced.

Morphine may also alter limbic system function in a manner that inhibits the characteristically unpleasant emotional response to pain. It may do so by performing the physiologic function of certain endogenous substances in limbic system neurons that also produce analgesia when they bind to the opiate receptors. These *endorphins,* endogenous morphinelike substances, or shorter peptide fragments of this class called *enkephalins,* are present in the brain and pituitary gland and may function as inhibitory neurotransmitters or modulators of the emotional reaction to pain.† Administered opiates may act like these natural substances to bring about their typical state of indifference to the pain impulses that are perceived at cerebral cortex sites.

Other effects. In addition to analgesia, morphine and related drugs produce various other central and peripheral effects. Some of these account both for their therapeutic usefulness in certain nonpainful conditions and for the side-effects and toxicity sometimes seen during their administration. Although the many natural, semisynthetic, and synthetic narcotic analgesics differ in the degree to which therapeutic doses produce these other actions, all share these properties to at least some extent. Thus, a description of some of the many pharmacologic properties of morphine can serve to explain the effects sometimes seen with most other drugs of this class.

Subcortical and spinal centers. These seem to be both depressed and stimulated in ways that produce characteristic effects. Small doses of morphine, for example, depress the medullary cough center. Consequently, morphine is sometimes employed to suppress coughing. It is usually preferable, however, to use related drugs that are less likely to depress the closely related respiratory center.

Codeine⁺ is the opioid alkaloid most commonly employed for treating coughs caused by colds. As is indicated in more detail in Chapter 39, the use of codeine as an antitussive in such cases has various advantages, including the fact that it is likely to cause dependence. Thus, morphine and other potent antitussives such as *hydromorphone HCl* (Dilaudid) and *methadone*⁺ (Dolophine) are best reserved for patients with rib fractures or bronchial carcinoma and other conditions marked by both cough and moderate to severe pain.

Stimulation of the central vomiting mechanism. This mechanism, located in the medulla, is often stimulated and causes vomiting (Chap. 41) following administration of opioids. Nausea, dizziness, and vomiting are most likely to occur in ambulatory patients. Other signs of central stimulation are the restlessness and excitement seen in some patients, instead of the expected sedation. The characteristic pupillary constriction produced by these drugs is the result of stimulation of the oculomotor nucleus, the cranial nerve nucleus that is the source of the parasympathetic innervation of the eye (Chap. 13).

Gastrointestinal effects. Morphine produces these effects as the result of complex actions directly on the smooth muscles and glands of the digestive tract. The combination of decreased peristaltic motility, increased spasticity of sphincters and other bowel sections, together with lessened glandular secretion, often results in constipation. Actually, of course, this "side-effect" is desirable for treating diarrhea. Thus, *paregoric* (camphorated tincture of opium) is commonly employed for this purpose (Chap. 41).

The *biliary tract* pressure may actually be increased when morphine is administered for relief of spastic pain caused by gallstones blocking the biliary duct. Thus, morphine is commonly combined with an antispasmodic in treating biliary colic. The opium alkaloid *papaverine,* which is not an analgesic and also not addicting, is often used for its direct relaxing effect on the spastic smooth muscle. (Atropine also is employed to counteract the natural and morphine-induced smooth muscle spasm in this condition, as well as in renal colic caused by stones in the urinary tract.)

Cardiovascular effects. Such effects of morphine are minor compared to the depression of respiratory function that occurs with clinical as well as toxic doses. The heart's rate and rhythm are hardly affected at all, and the drug may be safely administered even to patients who have suffered an acute myocardial infarction. In such cases the calming effect of morphine tends to produce an indirect reduction in the work of the heart that is therapeutically beneficial (Chap. 31).

The direct and indirect effects of morphine on blood vessels have clinical significance in some situations. The drug causes peripheral vasodilation that may lead to postural hypotension, dizziness, weakness, and fainting in ambulatory patients. On the other hand, morphine-induced dilation of both veins and arteries may account for the drug's therapeutic effect in patients with heart pump failure and pulmonary edema. As discussed in more detail in Chapter 31, this indirectly aids left ventricular function and helps to stop the seepage of fluid from pulmonary venous capillaries into the lungs.

---

* The word *raphe* means a seam. This group of nerve cells is located on the line just below the cerebral aqueduct that divides this cerebral gray area into two symmetric parts.

---

† The actual physiologic role of the endorphins is not completely understood at this time, nor is it certain what role this class of substances may play in the pathophysiology of various disorders with which they have tentatively been linked, including schizophrenia, epilepsy, and narcotic drug addiction.

Morphine also causes cerebral blood vessels to dilate. This is not a direct effect of the drug on these blood vessels but one that occurs because of the buildup of carbon dioxide in the blood as a result of respiratory depression. That is, the resulting increase in cerebrospinal fluid pressure and intracranial pressure is caused by the action of CO_2 on the brain's vessels rather than by the action of morphine at this site or on the vasomotor center.

Side-effects and contraindications. In addition to the drowsiness, nausea and vomiting, and constipation commonly encountered with morphine, numerous other side-effects are seen, especially in people who are hypersensitive to opiates. Patients often feel flushed, warm, dizzy, and light-headed. Some occasionally become excited, restless, and even delirious, instead of calm and sedated. This paradoxical reaction seems to be more common in women and elderly patients.

Older patients and those debilitated by chronic diseases may be more sensitive to the depressant effects of morphine, and thus require relatively small doses. Also, patients with breathing difficulties are given smaller amounts of morphine. In bronchial asthma, emphysema, and other lung disorders, morphine may cause contractions of the muscles of the respiratory tree. This, together with the drug's depressant effect on the respiratory center, may tend to reduce pulmonary ventilation to dangerously low levels.

Morphine is undesirable in patients with head injuries, because it tends to increase intracranial pressure and mask signs of this complication. For the same reason, it is usually withheld from patients who have been injured during a bout of acute alcoholic intoxication, because its use may precipitate delirium tremens (Chap. 53). Similarly, patients in a state of shock should normally not receive narcotics, because these drugs could cause a further drop in cardiac output and blood pressure. However, if severe pain is contributing to the shock, morphine or some other narcotic analgesic may be given intravenously.

Acute toxicity. Morphine overdosage produces severe depression of respiration. Breathing becomes markedly slowed, shallow, and irregular as the respiratory center fails to respond to relatively high blood concentrations of carbon dioxide. Respirations may slow to only four per minute or may be characterized by alternating periods of apnea and hyperpnea (Cheyne–Stokes breathing).

The nurse, of course, should note any unusual decrease in the depth and rate of respiration before breathing difficulties become very advanced. Other early signs of opiate poisoning include constriction of the pupil to pinpoint size and deep sleep or stupor. This triad of responses (respiratory depression, severe sedation, and pinpoint pupils) is almost diagnostic for narcotic analgesic overdose when an unidentified patient is brought into the emergency room with these presenting signs and symptoms. Later, the patient may pass into coma and, as

hypoxia becomes more severe, asphyxial dilation of the pupils may develop. The progressive anoxia causes the skin, which is at first flushed, warm, and wet with sweat, to become cyanotic or lividly mottled, cold, and clammy. Death is usually the result of respiratory failure. Occasionally, circulatory collapse develops before breathing stops and, rarely, terminal convulsions occur.

Respiratory depression is sometimes seen postoperatively in patients who received moderate doses of opioid analgesics among other depressant drugs employed during a prolonged surgical operation. Newborn infants whose mothers have received narcotic analgesics late in labor sometimes show depression of depth and rate of pulmonary ventilation. Acute toxicity has occurred in nontolerant persons who have taken a dose of *methadone* intended for a person in a methadone maintenance program (Chap. 53). Fatalities have occurred in children who accidentally swallowed a take-home dose of methadone that they found in the refrigerator dissolved in what looked like orange juice.

Fatalities are common in heroin addicts despite the high degree of tolerance that they develop. In many cases, death occurs with greater suddenness and with different signs than when overdoses of opioid medications have been taken. For example, massive pulmonary edema, rather than respiratory failure, is the most common finding in fatalities from heroin mixtures that have been ''mainlined,'' or injected intravenously. The exact cause of this so-called acute heroin syndrome is uncertain. Some authorities have even suggested that the sudden flow of fluid into the lungs is not caused by a heroin ''OD,'' or overdose, at all but by the presence of contaminants, including quinine, in the crude mixture that the addict injected into the vein. Others attribute such sudden deaths to circulatory collapse as a result of an anaphylactoid reaction in an addict who has developed hypersensitivity to heroin or to one of its diluents or contaminants. In any case, the swiftly fatal reaction is much more difficult to treat successfully than the slowly developing type of opioid toxicity.

Treatment. In the relatively rare cases of oral methadone overdosage, it may be desirable to administer a charcoal mixture or to wash the stomach with solutions of alkaloid precipitants (*e.g.*, tannic acid) or oxidizers (*e.g.*, potassium permanganate, 1:5000 dilution). If a dosage error is discovered shortly after subcutaneous injection of morphine, application of a tourniquet or of ice may delay full absorption of the drug long enough for the body's detoxifying mechanisms to destroy a good part of the overdose.

In actual practice, however, most measures are directed at combating advancing respiratory depression. This first requires the maintenance of an open airway and application of assisted or controlled ventilation. This is then followed by parenteral administration of the narcotic antagonist *naloxone* (Narcan), which is now consid-

Chapter 51 Narcotic analgesics and antagonists of narcotics

ered to be the safest and most effective drug for reversing respiratory depression induced by overdosage of morphine and related narcotic analgesics (see below). The response to injection of this drug and of other antagonists appears promptly when the patient's depressed respiration is the result of a narcotic overdose but not when barbiturates or other central depressants are responsible.

Because the therapeutic effects of the antagonist may wear off while the toxic effects of the narcotic continue, patients must be observed for signs of returning depression. In cases of overdosage by a long-lasting narcotic such as methadone, many repeated injections of naloxone may be required over a period of 1 to 3 days. When a mother appears to have received an excessive dose of *meperidine HCl*[+] (Demerol) or of some other narcotic before her baby has been delivered, it is best to prevent neonatal depression by administering naloxone to her when the baby is about to be born. If this is not done, and the newborn has not received the antagonist by way of the placental circulation, a very small dose (see Drug digest) of naloxone may be injected into the baby's umbilical vein. This is usually quite effective for improving pulmonary ventilation, provided that the infant's poor respiration was caused by a narcotic and not by complications of delivery or by other drugs.

Chronic toxicity or opiate addiction. The nature of opiate-type dependence (in terms of such aspects as how abuse of these drugs leads to dependence, the nature of the opiate withdrawal syndrome, and the treatment and rehabilitation of the addict) will be discussed in Chapter 53. Here, only some measures to minimize the development of dependence during clinical use will be described.

Dependence prevention. Pain often can be adequately controlled with nonnarcotic analgesics, sedatives, tranquilizers, or oral doses of codeine, which has a relatively low addiction liability. Such agents are sometimes alternated with the more potent analgesics. In any case, it is preferable to give opiates in the smallest dose that will produce the desired degree of relief and at irregular intervals. An exception to this is the management of severe pain in terminally ill cancer patients; here, adherence to a strict "by-the-clock" oral dosage regimen using a narcotic analgesic alone, or in combination with, for example, a phenothiazine or alcohol (Brompton cocktail and related potions) has been found to be the best treatment. Narcotics should, of course, never be administered routinely merely to keep the patient comfortably sedated, so that he will keep quiet and make few demands.

On the other hand, analgesic drugs should not be withheld for fear of causing addiction if the patient's condition indicates the need for these drugs. Thus, narcotics should be avoided in such chronic conditions as arthritis, but their long-term use in patients with severe pain from terminal cancer is completely justified despite the danger of addiction. The nurse should not withhold prn narcotics when such patients experience excruciating pain but should administer them at the specified intervals.

The nurse should be able to recognize the patient who typically tends to rely on potent analgesics for relief of anxiety rather than actual pain. Such a patient may, for example, complain of pain in the incision postoperatively long after most other patients with similar conditions no longer require analgesics. Counseling may be desirable to help the patient become aware of the anxiety and to develop insight. By helping the patient deal more effectively with problems, such aid may reduce the desire for medication.

All health-care professionals have the responsibility of seeing that narcotic drugs, hypodermic syringes, and needles do not fall into the hands of addicts. Drugs that cannot for some reason be used (*e.g.*, because of contamination) must be disposed of, after a notation in the narcotic record has been made, usually signed by two staff members. Disposable needles and syringes should be rendered unusable before being discarded, and should not simply be thrown into the trash where they can readily be picked up by addicts.

Synthetic opioid analgesics

Morphine and codeine and the semisynthetic agents prepared by chemically altering these natural opiate alkaloids have various disadvantages. Their adverse effects on the nervous system and gastrointestinal tract often limit their usefulness. The constant need to consider the danger of addiction is another drawback.

Consequently, chemists have been searching for some time for safer analgesics that would be equally effective against severe pain but free of the limitations and dangers of the older drugs. Several different chemical classes of synthetic analgesics have been prepared. Although no highly potent pain-relieving agent has proved to be entirely free of addiction liability, there is evidence that the chemists may finally be approaching this goal.

Some scientists suggest that there may be—among the descending CNS pathways that inhibit pain—a neural mechanism that does not depend on the presence of endorphin, or opiate, receptors for impulse transmission. Such opiate-independent inhibitory pathways could be activated by drugs to relieve pain without causing the tolerance and the dependence that is characteristic of the opiates and that, apparently, also occurs with the natural and synthetic enkephalins that have been studied.

In any case, various synthetic narcotic analgesics now available possess some advantages that may make them more desirable than morphine for some patients. In the following discussion, the advantages claimed for some of these synthetic analgesics will be emphasized. Actually, however, all these drugs can cause side-effects and toxic reactions similar to those of morphine, and all are addicting to varying degrees.

Side-effects and toxicity

Central nervous system. An advantage claimed for several of the synthetic agents is their ability to produce analgesia with less of the drowsiness, dizziness, and disorientation sometimes seen when morphine is employed. This may make the less sedative synthetic analgesic *meperidine* (Demerol), for example, better for the management of pain in patients whose treatment requires that they remain ambulatory.

Actually, whether these side-effects and others such as nausea and vomiting occur depends more on the patient's physical condition than on the particular drug employed. Thus, it is well to remember that postoperative patients are likely to experience faintness, dizziness, and nausea on early ambulation. This may be caused not only by analgesic medication but also by the physical and emotional effects of surgery. The patient should be assisted when getting out of bed and carefully observed while walking, so that assistance can be provided, if necessary, to prevent fainting and injuries from falls.

Sedation. Some sedative and somnifacient action may, of course, be desirable in certain painful situations. Thus, when meperidine is employed as an adjunct to anesthesia, it is often desirable to reinforce its analgesic action with promethazine (Phenergan), barbiturates, or other tranquilizers and sedative–hypnotics to allay apprehension before the operation and to reduce restlessness after it. However, some authorities have suggested that adding the sedative effects of these drugs may not provide better pain relief than meperidine alone and may, in fact, exert an *antianalgesic* effect.

Respiratory depression. Morphine often reduces pulmonary ventilation, and most of the newer synthetic analgesics have been introduced with claims of superiority in this respect. Here too, however, any advantage of this type is relatively limited, and caution is required to prevent respiratory depression with all these drugs. In general, the more potent a drug is as an analgesic, the greater is its ability to reduce the rate and depth of the patient's respiration. That is, all share similar margins of safety, despite differences in their milligram-for-milligram potency.

Thus, for example, *fentanyl* (Sublimaze), is so potent that a dose of 0.1 mg is equal to 100 mg of morphine in analgesic strength. However, because this synthetic narcotic is 80 to 100 times more potent than morphine, its use requires even closer observation of the patient to avoid development of severe respiratory depression and apnea. All the precautions required with morphine in patients who are especially susceptible to respiratory depression—for example, those with chronic obstructive pulmonary diseases or with increased intracranial pressure—must be maintained when fentanyl is employed. For instance, narcotic antagonists and equipment for resuscitating apneic patients must always be available when fentanyl is employed for pain relief or in the procedure called *neuroleptanalgesia* (see below).

In the presence of severe pain, patients can tolerate larger doses of opioids without having their respiration become deeply depressed. However, if the pain subsides spontaneously, the previously administered drug may cause marked respiratory depression. For example, if a long-acting opioid such as *methadone* or *levorphanol tartrate* (Levo-Dromoran) is employed to prevent sudden sharp pain prior to procedures such as the setting of a fracture or the passing of a cystoscope, the drug's action continues long after the painful manipulation has been completed, and deep depression may develop.

On the other hand, with a drug that wears off comparatively quickly, such as *alphaprodine HCl*[+] (Nisentil), the patient's respiration tends to return to normal more rapidly. Similarly, in the event of overdosage requiring treatment with narcotic antagonists, respiratory depression can be overcome more readily when the analgesic employed was one of short duration of action. (Of course, for pain that is steady and long-continued—as in patients with malignancies and other chronically painful conditions—long-acting analgesics such as the synthetics mentioned above and morphine may be preferred despite their tendency to produce prolonged respiratory depression.)

Peripheral side-effects

Constipation. This common side-effect of morphine is claimed to occur less frequently with several of the synthetic narcotic analgesics, including *meperidine* and *hydromorphone HCl* (Dilaudid). This may make these drugs a better choice for bedridden patients, who tend to become constipated more readily than those who are ambulatory. On the other hand, these drugs are not as effective as paregoric or other preparations containing the natural opiate alkaloids for managing patients who have diarrhea.

Smooth muscle spasm. Meperidine, the first of the synthetic drugs to be developed, was found in the course of a search for drugs that could relax smooth muscles. The drug is said to exert an antispasmodic action, but this effect is not dependable enough to make it especially useful for patients with bilary or renal colic. Although the drug may be somewhat less spasmogenic—and, thus, less likely to raise biliary or ureteral pressure—than morphine, it must be supplemented with more potent spasmolytics such as atropine and papaverine when used as an analgesic in these conditions. (Similarly, the spasmolytic action of meperidine on the bronchial smooth muscle is probably too slight to give it any real advantage over morphine in patients with asthma and other pulmonary difficulties.)

Addiction. Most of the newer synthetic analgesics were prepared with the hope that they would prove less likely to cause dependence and addiction. However, all can be abused by people whose personalities predispose them to addiction. All require the precautions previously discussed if addiction is to be prevented during their prolonged use in chronically painful conditions.

Some authorities have expressed doubt that the chemists who are trying to develop better synthetic analgesics can ever succeed in separating analgesic potency from addiction liability. They claim that any drug that can make the pain experience acceptable to suffering patients is also bound to be abused by people who want to escape from their emotional pain in coping unsuccessfully with life's harsh realities.

Several synthetic analgesics have been marketed with claims that they are "nonnarcotic" or "nonaddicting." It is true that most of these drugs have less potential for producing dependence than morphine and narcotic analgesics of similar potency. However, they have not been proved safer than codeine in this regard, and all have been abused to some extent by people who are prone to become psychologically dependent on drugs. With the possible exception of *pentazocine*[+] (Talwin), the degree to which these drugs tend to produce physical dependence appears to be related to their potency as analgesics.

Narcotic analgesic drugs with lower dependence-producing potential

Propoxyphene HCl[+] (Darvon) does not produce dependence when administered in doses that are effective for relief of mild to moderate pain—amounts about twice as high as those required for codeine. The drug has been widely prescribed, perhaps because it was believed to be as effective as codeine and free of that drug's disadvantages. Actually, propoxyphene can be abused and, in such cases, both psychological and physical dependence have developed. Similarly, when administered in doses equal to codeine in pain-relieving effectiveness, it causes central and gastrointestinal side-effects that resemble those of codeine and other opioids.

This analgesic is available in combination with aspirin, aspirin and caffeine, and acetaminophen. These combinations are more effective than propoxyphene alone, because the presence of the analgesic–antipyretic drugs offers an additive analgesic effect and, in the case of aspirin, the added advantage of anti-inflammatory activity. However, this drug and its combinations are more expensive than codeine and various codeine–analgesic-antipyretic combinations, and they offer no advantages over the latter. Thus, propoxyphene products are probably best reserved for patients who cannot tolerate codeine.

This drug is related to the narcotic analgesic methadone, and overdosage leads to similar serious signs and symptoms. Respiratory depression is treated with naloxone or other narcotic antagonists, and with the same supportive measures as are employed in acute opioid toxicity (see above). Because convulsive seizures also often occur in most cases of severe poisoning by propoxyphene, cautious administration of diazepam or other anticonvulsants may be necessary.

Narcotic agonist–antagonist analgesics

Three drugs, *butorphanol tartrate, nalbuphine HCl,* and *pentazocine*, which have both narcotic agonist and antagonist properties, are now available in the United States. These drugs have less abuse potential than such drugs as morphine or meperidine, and various authorities state that two of them (pentazocine and nalbuphine) have less abuse potential than even codeine or propoxyphene. However, both these drugs have caused physical dependence and the typical narcotic analgesic withdrawal syndrome (see Chap. 53).

All three drugs can produce analgesia approximately equal to that of morphine, although some evidence indicates that pentazocine may be less effective in severe pain. All three drugs also produce the same adverse effects as MS; these are reversed by the narcotic antagonist naloxone. In addition, these drugs produce disturbing psychotomimetic reactions. Pentazocine and butorphanol raise arterial resistance, thus increasing myocardial work and oxygen demand; this property makes them contraindicated in patients who have suffered an acute myocardial infarction.

In addition to being narcotic agonists, these drugs are narcotic antagonists. The clinical significance of this is that, if administered to a patient in pain who has been treated with a narcotic agonist, they may *increase* the intensity of the patient's pain by reversing any residual analgesic effect from the agonist. Thus, caution must be exercised in replacing such drugs as MS or meperidine with one of these drugs. Furthermore, these drugs can precipitate a withdrawal syndrome in patients who are physically dependent on narcotic analgesic agonists.

Nonnarcotic (phenothiazine) analgesic

Methotrimeprazine (Levoprome), a phenothiazine derivative, is, like the injectable form of pentazocine, as effective as the potent narcotic analgesics for relief of moderate to severe pain. Unlike the latter drugs, it does not cause development of dependence or depress respiration and the cough reflex. Unfortunately, it cannot be used in ambulatory patients with chronic pain because it often causes feelings of weakness, faintness, and dizziness—the result of orthostatic hypotension.

This drug's use is limited largely to control of acute pain in surgical and obstetric patients. Administered preoperatively, it helps to reduce the patient's apprehension and anxiety. Smaller doses are used for postoperative analgesia, because this drug may potentiate the residual effects of general anesthetics. The solution employed for intramuscular injection is irritating. Thus, it is recommended that injection sites be rotated. The drug should not be given subcutaneously or intravenously.

Narcotic antagonists

Drugs of this class can prevent and reverse respiratory depression and other pharmacologic effects of the narcotic analgesics (Table 51-1). They are used clinically in the treatment of acute opioid toxicity (see above), in the diagnosis of opioid overdosage, and experimentally in the diagnosis and treatment of opioid addiction (Chap. 53). The individual antagonists differ somewhat in their mechanisms of action in ways that are significant for determining their usefulness in various clinical situations.

Mechanism of action. These drugs bring about their antagonistic effects on respiratory depression and other opioid-induced reactions by their ability to prevent morphine, meperidine, and other opioid molecules from remaining on the opioid receptor sites of neurons and other responsive cells. Their molecules displace the opioid agonists by competitive inhibition (Chap. 4). As a result of such displacement from their binding sites on nerve cells, the opioid molecules can no longer continue to exert their depressant effects.

Naloxone HCl+ (Narcan) and the experimental narcotic antagonist *naltrexone HCl,* are almost entirely "pure" antagonists. That is, they act only on the opioid receptors that are occupied by opioid molecules and, when naloxone or naltrexone displaces the opioids and occupies these receptors, these drugs do not exert any agonistic, or pharmacologic, actions of their own. *Naloxone* (Nalline), the first available antagonist, which is no longer marketed, and *levallorphan tartrate* (Lorfan), on the other hand, do exert some agonistic activity when they occupy opioid receptors. Thus, when administered to patients who have not taken any narcotic drug, these antagonists, which are also *partial agonists,* can cause depression and other effects similar to those of morphine and other opioids.

In addition, levallorphan, like the agonist–antagonists, pentazocine, butorphanol, and nalbuphine, and the experimental antagonist *cyclazocine,* also acts at other central sites in addition to opioid binding sites. This presumably accounts for the fact that hallucinations and other effects that resemble those of the psychotomimetic drugs (Chap. 53), rather than the opioids, sometimes occur following their administration. A third type of antagonist, typified by the experimental drug *propiram,* is also a partial agonist. That is, this group causes morphinelike pharmacologic effects when administered in the absence of opioids. However, they differ from nalorphine and levallorphan in *not* causing hallucinations and other psychotomimetic effects, presumably because their agonistic

as well as their antagonistic actions are limited only to opioid receptors.

Clinical applications. Naloxone is now preferred to levallorphan because naloxone is a pure antagonist. This is particularly true for clinical situations in which the cause of a patient's respiratory depression is uncertain and not definitely known to be the result of narcotic drug overdosage. If, for example, a patient's deep respiratory depression has actually been caused by barbiturates or other nonnarcotic drugs, the administration of levallorphan is likely to increase the depth of depression. Similarly, a newborn infant with respiratory difficulties caused by a traumatic delivery rather than by narcotics administered to the mother might be made worse when treated with levallorphan.

Naloxone would not be effective if tried in such cases. In fact, its failure to reverse respiratory depression is an indication that the condition was caused by something other than narcotic drug overdosage. However, because it is a pure narcotic antagonist, largely lacking in any pharmacologic effects, naloxone would not make the depression deeper, if it had been caused by barbiturates, anesthetics or other depressant drugs, or if apnea in a newborn infant was the result of trauma during a difficult delivery.

The main drawback of naloxone is its relatively short duration of action in comparison to that of morphine, methadone and other narcotics. However, this drawback can be overcome by administering repeated doses, whenever the patient's previously antagonized depression appears to be returning during the period of observation. Two antagonists that have been employed experimentally mainly in the management of addiction (Chap. 53)—cyclazocine and naltrexone—do have a longer duration of action. This property may lead to the clinical use of naltrexone to provide prolonged antieuphoric effects for patients who might be tempted to inject themselves with heroin during rehabilitation treatment.

Additional clinical considerations

The potent narcotic analgesics are employed for the relief of acute and chronic pain in a wide variety of clinical conditions (see the summary at the end of this chapter). These drugs should be used in ways that will reduce the patient's pain most effectively while keeping unwanted side-effects to a minimum.

Acute and chronic pain have quite different physiologic and psychological characteristics. Consequently, the factors that must be taken into consideration in administering narcotic analgesics to patients with each type of pain are also different. Thus, the following discussion, which applies the facts previously set forth concerning these drugs to actual clinical situations, is divided into two parts: first, aspects of the use of potent narcotic analgesics against acute pain, and second, some significant clinical considerations in the use of these drugs in patients with chronic pain.

Control of acute pain

Acute pain commonly accompanies surgery or other trauma and medical disorders that are marked by tissue injury. It tends to subside as the damaged tissues are gradually repaired by natural healing processes. Because acute pain can lead to various complications, health-care personnel should not hesitate to administer narcotic analgesics in adequate doses, provided that appropriate precautions are taken.

Pain and diagnosis

Pain is, of course, an important symptom that aids in diagnosing the nature of a patient's illness. Thus, potent analgesics are ordered only after the cause of acute pain has been determined. It would not, for example, be desirable to administer opiates for relief of acute abdominal pain until the possibility of acute appendicitis had been ruled out. These drugs might mask the pain and make diagnosis difficult, with the result that the patient might suffer a ruptured appendix. Similarly, it is not advisable to administer analgesic drugs that have been ordered for one painful condition to relieve pain that may develop suddenly from another source.

Thus, for example, if a patient for whom analgesic drugs were ordered during the postoperative period after abdominal surgery were to develop severe pain in a leg, the previously ordered drugs should not be routinely administered. Instead, the reason for the pain in the extremity should be determined. This could be the result of a developing thrombophlebitis, which requires specific therapy rather than mere pain relief.

Postoperative pain relief

Surgical patients may require potent analgesics when the anesthetic wears off. However, narcotics are not given routinely to all postoperative patients. The physician usually decides whether the patient requires medication following surgery after first considering various factors, including the type of general anesthetic that has been employed (Chap. 52). For example, patients who have been anesthetized with *halothane* (Fluothane) or *enflurane* (Ethrane) are more likely to require analgesics after their rapid recovery than those who have been given an anesthetic with long-lasting residual analgesic effects, such as *methoxyflurane* (Penthrane).

Patients in whom surgery has been performed under a balanced anesthesia procedure (Chap. 52) that included large doses of narcotics will also not require additional postoperative opioid analgesia. On the contrary, because their respiration may remain depressed, these patients may need a narcotic antagonist such as naloxone. In such situations, the antagonist must be administered in the minimal dosage necessary for improvement of pulmonary ventilation. Too high an initial dose of naloxone can reverse the desired residual analgesia as well as the patient's respiratory depression. This can expose the patient to sudden extreme pain.

On the other hand, some cardiac surgeons claim that when naloxone is administered in appropriate doses to morphinized patients, its use eliminates the need to maintain the patient on a mechanical ventilator, while permitting persistence of the opioid-induced analgesia for several days postoperatively. This has made it possible to use morphine alone as an anesthetic for high-risk open heart surgery patients, for whom it is the preferred means of preventing operative pain because of its relative lack of depressant effects on cardiovascular function. Naloxone administered in low doses at 3-hour intervals restores respiration to normal soon after the patient reaches the recovery room, and then keeps him alert and able to cooperate in his own care, while remaining relatively free of pain for several days postoperatively without administration of further narcotic analgesics.

Another important factor in determining the degree of postoperative pain and the patient's probable need for narcotic analgesics is the type of surgery that has been done. Operations performed at certain sites are particularly likely to be followed by severe pain and, in some cases, complications secondary to pain-induced autonomic and somatic reflexes. Major joint surgery such as total replacement of a hip can cause excruciating postoperative pain. Operations on the spinal vertebrae and related back structures, or anorectal surgery, are often followed by painful reflex spasm of the skeletal muscles.

Surgical operations that involve the walls of the chest or abdomen and their viscera cause dull, diffuse pain and reflex spasm of related smooth and skeletal muscles. Following cholecystectomy or thoracotomy, for example, these muscles, incuding the diaphragm, often go into reflex (involuntary) spasm and splinting. In addition, the patient often suffers reflex bronchospasm. These reactions and the patient's failure to breathe deeply, move, or cough for fear of making the pain worse can lead to such postoperative complications as atelectasis and pneumonitis.

In such patients, administration of adequate doses of narcotic analgesics is desirable, because this helps to prevent hypoventilation and the decrease of 50% or more in ventilation that is common on the first postoperative day. However, these drugs can themselves, of course, cause impairment of ventilation by their ability to depress the respiratory center and dampen the cough reflex. In addition, morphine and many of the related opioids sometimes cause bronchoconstriction. The resulting retention of secretions and blockage of bronchioles can cause air behind the block to be absorbed with collapse of a lobe of the lung. Thus, it is very important to titrate each patient's narcotic dosage to the minimally effective amount needed to relieve some of the pain without setting off opioid side-effects.

Of course, as previously indicated, the administration of opioids must sometimes be avoided entirely in patients with certain pre-existing disorders. Thus, for example, these drugs can be particularly hazardous for patients with pulmonary disease, including those with bronchial asthma, emphysema, or cor pulmonale. The resulting retention of carbon dioxide in such patients may send them into a comatose state. Patients with liver damage may also be precipitated into coma by these drugs, which depress the central nervous system and respiratory center. Patients with head injuries may suffer an increase in intracranial pressure as a result of a drug-induced buildup of carbon dioxide that leads to cerebral vasodilation.

Excessive narcotic drug dosage also tends to aggravate gastrointestinal complications that are the result of reflex responses to abdominal surgery. Such visceral reflexes result in increased sympathetic nervous system influences on the gastrointestinal tract that cause inhibition of its activity, leading to distention, constipation, nausea, and vomiting. As indicated earlier, the opioids have peripheral and central effects that can also cause decreased intestinal motility and emesis.

In addition, these depressant drugs can, when given in excess, decrease the patient's physical activity and prevent him from becoming ambulatory. The dangerous result of this on the patient's pulmonary function may be the same as when pain has not been relieved by adequate narcotic dosage and the patient fails to move because of fear of causing more pain. In both cases, blood clots in the veins of the legs may also develop, which could lead to serious thromboembolic complications.

Administration. Proper administration of opioid analgesics can not only keep patients comfortable but can also prevent serious postoperative complications while these drugs, when improperly employed, can cause or intensify several of the same complications. Thus, these drugs should never be administered routinely but with due regard for each patient's physical condition and need for narcotic medication. When the decision to administer these drugs is made, it is then very important to adjust their dosage and frequency of administration to each patient's specific needs. Pain is managed best and with the least total amount of analgesic drug if treatment is begun before the level of pain becomes severe, and if dosage is adequate to prevent the pain from becoming severe.

One of the best ways to titrate opioid dosage is to administer these drugs by slow intravenous injections of several small doses. Thus, for example, when morphine

is injected in doses of only 2 or 3 mg or meperidine is injected in doses of only 15 to 25 mg at intervals of about 20 minutes, the desired degree of analgesia is achieved with greatly reduced total dosage and a resulting reduction in opioid-induced adverse effects. This is because patients vary widely in their need for narcotics, depending on the degree of severity of their pain and their ability to tolerate it, their age, and their underlying physical condition.

When these drugs are administered subcutaneously or intramuscularly, pharmacokinetic factors are a further cause of differences in the response of patients. Such factors as the rate of blood flow to and from the injection site help to determine the time it takes for the drug to become effective or whether it will take effect at all. This is particularly important for patients who are in shock and in whom the peripheral circulation is sluggish. Such a patient may not respond to several subcutaneous doses; then, if blood pressure is brought back to normal by other therapeutic measures, several doses of the potent analgesic drug may be rapidly absorbed at once and send the patient into deep depression. Thus, for prompt pain relief in such cases without the danger of delayed toxicity, the drug should be given by slow injection into a vein.

The recovery room nurse is often required to judge whether a postoperative patient will need a narcotic and, if so, how much. Later, the nurse on the unit who has been given a prn order for a narcotic may have to determine whether a dose of the drug should be omitted. This requires experience and good judgment. The skilled nurse recognizes from carefully assessing the patient whether he is uncomfortable and in need of the ordered analgesic, or, on the other hand, whether he is excessively sedated and would be better off with the drug withheld.

It is good practice to be particularly observant after the first two doses of the narcotic. The length of time during which the patient's pain seems to be relieved should be recorded on the chart. Often, this differs considerably in duration from the 3 or 4 hours at which administration of these drugs is most commonly spaced. To produce steady analgesia and avoid periods of either pain or excessive depression, it is best to give each successive dose of these drugs regularly about 30 minutes before the predicted end of the activity of the previous dose, as determined by the patient's initial responses.

When medication is ordered, it should be given promptly; minutes can seem like hours to the patient in pain. If the dose ordered by the physician does not relieve the patient's pain, the nurse should let the physician know this. Similarly, if the medication makes the patient so somnolent that he cannot be readily aroused, this too should be reported so that a reduction in dosage can be ordered. Idiosyncrasy to narcotics is not uncommon; therefore, patients receiving analgesics should be closely observed for any unusual reactions.

The nurse should be alert for signs of strain and tension, and should ask the patient whether he is experiencing pain. Some stoical patients pride themselves on never complaining. However, the skilled nurse recognizes their discomfort from such clues as a slight frown or tightness of the lips, and takes prompt action to relieve it.

Some patients are so fearful of becoming addicted that they will refuse even a single dose of analgesic medication. The nurse should try to discuss the patient's fears with him to help him accept the drugs that have been ordered. On the other hand, medication should not be forced on a patient who refuses it despite explanation and reassurance. The patient may once have been addicted to narcotics, and consequently may be rightly fearful of reactivating that condition.

Unfortunately, some physicians are themselves excessively concerned about the addiction potential of opioid analgesics. As a result, they often order these drugs in doses that are inadequate for relief of acute pain and at too long intervals. If the nurse reports that the patient continues to complain of pain, the unwarranted concern about dependence on these drugs may be confirmed, and the physician may be unwilling to raise the dose or to decrease the interval between doses. Actually, authorities on pain control feel that the first concern in cases of acute pain should be to keep the patient comfortable, and that the chance of triggering true addictive behavior is very small. Although some patients may become physically dependent on narcotics while in the hospital, very few of these will ever develop drug-seeking or "addictive" behavior once they recover and have been discharged from the hospital. (As indicated below, the development of tolerance and dependence in cases of *chronic* pain *does* deserve constant consideration.)

Psychological factors. The need for narcotic analgesics can often be reduced by offering the patient psychological support and attending to physical comfort. A personal word of reassurance and such measures as a soothing back rub, a change of position, or even straightening the patient's bedclothes may help to lessen the pain. Instituting a program of counseling and diversional activities has also been found to reduce the amount of narcotics required markedly.

It is also important to prepare surgical patients properly concerning what to expect during an impending operative procedure and in the postoperative period. Such instructions, offered by the surgeon, anesthesiologist, or nurse, help to reduce anxiety and aid in the establishment of the patient's own defenses. This, in turn, tends to "close the gate" to some of the stream of sensory impulses that would otherwise be perceived as pain. The resulting reduction in the transmission of pain-producing impulses often reduces the need for narcotic analgesics or other psychotropic drugs.

Preoperative drug use

The preoperative use of opioids for their antianxiety or sedative effects is not as frequent as it once was, because many physicians now prefer to use antianxiety drugs such as parenteral *hydroxyzine* (Atarax; Vistaril) or *diazepam* (Valium) for this purpose. This is a result of such disadvantages of the narcotic analgesics as their previously mentioned tendency to cause nausea, vomiting, and constipation.

In addition, these drugs sometimes cause confusion and even perceptual distortions in some patients who are being prepared for anesthesia and surgery. In fact, many patients suffer dysphoria from opioids, perhaps because they do not like to feel that they are losing control, even temporarily, of their ability to care for themselves. Such patients may find the early phase of their response to these preoperative medications anxiety-provoking until the drug produces sufficient effect to overcome this apprehension.

Neuroleptanalgesia, a newer form of preoperative preparation, does, however, have advantages in some cases. This is a state of reduced awareness of pain produced by administering a neuroleptic agent in combination with a potent analgesic. Under the influence of this drug combination the patient is kept quiet, pain-free, and yet completely cooperative during various diagnostic and neurosurgical procedures that require consciousness. If necessary for performing major surgical anesthesia, the patient who has been prepared in this way may then inhale a nitrous oxide–oxygen mixture to induce and maintain a state of general anesthesia.

Innovar, a clinically available combination of this type, contains *droperidol* (Inapsine), a neuroleptic of the butyrophenone-type (Chap. 46) in combination with the potent synthetic analgesic *fentanyl citrate* (Sublimaze). Fentanyl is, as indicated earlier, about 100 times more potent than morphine, and its analgesic action is potentiated by the presence of droperidol, a drug that induces a state of detached calmness. This combination is particularly useful for elderly and other low-risk surgical patients, because it has little adverse effect on cardiovascular function.

A disadvantage of this neuroleptic combination is its tendency to produce depression of respiration. As is true of all potent analgesics, the pain-relieving potency of fentanyl is matched by an equally powerful depressant effect on the patient's respiratory center. In addition, this drug often induces skeletal muscle rigidity that may further interfere with the patient's breathing. Sometimes the drug-induced mental detachment may last for a relatively long time after a minor operative procedure has been completed.

(For further discussions of the control of acute pain in the preoperative, intraoperative, and postoperative periods by the administration of narcotic analgesics, general and local anesthetics, and other drugs, see Chapters 14 and 52.)

Control of chronic pain

Chronic pain that has persisted for weeks, months, or longer, and has proved refractory to routine medical measures, is obviously a much more difficult problem to cope with than acute pain. Unlike acute pain, which is usually related to surgical or other trauma or to a readily diagnosed medical disorder, the cause of chronic pain may not be immediately apparent. Even when painstaking diagnostic procedures succeed in establishing its etiology, chronic pain may be much more difficult to manage than acute pain. Often this is because chronic pain is related to personality problems that are not directly related to the disease-related source of pain.

Chronic pain that seems out of proportion to what appears to be its cause, and that does not respond to treatment, is now best dealt with in a special pain clinic or pain control unit (PCU) of a general hospital, in which a multidisciplinary team approach may be employed for its diagnosis and therapy. Personnel skilled in many different disciplines participate in the search for the cause of the patient's prolonged suffering. Frequently, it is necessary to search for factors other than those revealed by even complete physical examinations supplemented by neurologic and radiologic diagnostic techniques. Sometimes, for example, patients are interviewed under drug-induced hypnosis in a search for hidden psychological factors responsible for chronic pain. Often double-blind studies are conducted comparing placebos and real analgesics or diagnostic nerve blocks. The patient is visited at 15-minute intervals to evaluate the effects of the drugs or the placebos.

Drug use considerations

Patients in chronic pain react differently to drugs than those suffering acute pain. This may be because the psychological factors involved in chronic pain are much more complex than the natural anxiety that influences the patient experiencing acute pain. As indicated above, once the cause of acute pain has been diagnosed and the narcotic drug dosage needed for its safe and effective control has been individually determined, there is no reason to withhold these potent pain relievers for fear of fostering dependence on them. In cases of chronic pain, on the contrary, patients have often already been taking excessive amounts of narcotics and other medications, and some already show the effects of drug abuse.

Thus, when the cause of such a patient's persisting pain is still uncertain, it may be necessary to discontinue all drugs gradually and to take measures aimed at changing the patient's medication-taking habits and behavior. Whenever possible, it is desirable to employ nondrug measures for control of chronic pain, to the extent that such psychological, neurosurgical, electrical, or other measures prove even partially effective.

It is not appropriate here to discuss in detail the current status of the nonpharmacologic pain control measures that appear quite promising. Instead, discussion will be limited mainly to considerations that relate to the proper use of potent narcotics and other analgesics and psychotropic drugs. Emphasis will be on how to delay the development of tolerance and dependence on opioids in patients with cancer and other chronically painful disorders.

The administration of narcotics may not be indicated at all in some chronically painful conditions. Thus, for example, patients with painful disorders that are rarely fatal, such as rheumatoid arthritis, do not ordinarily receive narcotic analgesics other than codeine, occasionally, for control of their joint pains, which are best relieved by nonaddicting analgesic–anti-inflammatory agents (Chaps. 37 and 38). On the other hand, narcotics are not withheld in cases of terminal cancer for fear of causing psychological dependence. The main concern here should be with employing these drugs in a manner that will maintain their pain-relieving effectiveness for as long as possible.

Physical dependence and tolerance to the opioids are inevitable when these drugs are administered regularly. Development of dependence in patients with terminal cancer is sometimes unavoidable. However, tolerance is a more practical problem because these drugs can, in time, lose their analgesic effectiveness. To avoid a situation in which even very large doses may not control the patient's pain, the potent narcotic analgesics are often held in reserve. Another problem in using narcotic analgesics chronically is that, although tolerance develops to their analgesic and respiratory depressant effects, tolerance does not develop to the gastrointestinal effects. Constipation may become a serious problem as the dosage is increased to maintain pain relief.

Patients may be started on aspirin or acetaminophen at first, because these drugs are effective for control of moderate pain. An antianxiety agent such as diazepam (Valium) or hydroxyzine (Atarax; Vistaril) may be added to these nonnarcotic analgesics. The addition of propoxyphene HCl (Darvon) to a combination of this type is claimed to offer analgesia superior to that of aspirin alone.

When these nonaddictive drugs fail to control the patient's pain, oral doses of codeine or such other opioids as hydrocodone that have relatively low dependence-producing effects may be employed. If further pain relief is required, the physician may first administer oral doses, and finally injections, of the somewhat more potent, low addiction potential analgesic pentazocine (Talwin), to which tolerance and dependence develop much more slowly than with the opioids (see above).

If narcotics become necessary, they are often

given at irregular intervals rather than on a predetermined regular schedule. If the nurse has a choice, an ordered dose of a potent opioid should be replaced with a nonaddictive analgesic or tranquilizer when the patient's pain seems to have subsided. Narcotics should not be administered routinely in anticipation of pain or for their sedative effects.

Of course, the nurse should not withhold prn narcotics when the patient is actually experiencing excruciating pain. The purpose of all these delaying tactics is to slow tolerance development so that the opiates will retain their effectiveness when the patient needs them most. The main duty of all health-care personnel is to keep the patient comfortable rather than to prevent physical or psychological dependence.

Psychological dependence on opioids occurs in only a minority of patients. The observant nurse can often detect the addiction-prone patient. Often there is a history of alcoholism or abuse of other drugs. The nurse notes whether the patient's complaints of pain or discomfort seem warranted by the nature of the disorder. If his demands for drugs are greater than those of most patients in similar circumstances, the health-care team should discuss the situation.

It may be decided that a patient's complaints are related to a reactive depression (Chap. 46). It is natural for patients made miserable by chronic pain to suffer feelings of hopelessness, helplessness, and despair. Many suffer progressive physical deterioration from pain-induced loss of sleep and appetite. They often become so preoccupied with their pain that they lose interest in other people and in maintaining social activities and employment. In such cases, antidepressant drugs such as *amitriptyline HCl* (Elavil) and other tricyclic agents (Chap. 46) may prove helpful when administered alone or combined with a major tranquilizer such as the phenothiazines, *chlorpromazine HCl* (Thorazine), *thioridazine HCl* (Mellaril), or *perphenazine* (Trilafon).

In addition to administering drugs of this type, which help to reduce the patient's emotional reaction to his physical discomfort, the nurse can help to lessen the patient's need for narcotic analgesics by employing the measures previously described for making patients more comfortable physically, and by offering support and encouragement to the patient.

The patient's response to the drug should be recorded, along with his vital signs before and after drug administration. Because these drugs are controlled substances, each institution has its own guidelines for the proper recording of these substances, and the nurse is responsible for knowing and complying with these regulations.

There are several underlying medical conditions that are contraindications to the use of narcotic analgesics. These include head injury, increased intracranial pressure, chronic obstructive pulmonary disease (COPD), hy-

potension, hepatic failure, renal failure, thyroid disease, severe gallbladder disease, and delirium tremens. All these conditions can be exacerbated by the effects of the narcotic analgesics. The safety of the use of these drugs in pregnancy has not been established and they should be avoided, if at all possible. If given to the mother shortly before delivery, the neonate may be born with respiratory depression.

Drug–drug interactions

These drugs have been associated with several drug–drug interactions. Reduced dosage of narcotics should be used in patients who are also receiving *general anesthetics, antihistamines, phenothiazines, barbiturates, tranquilizers, sedative–hypnotics,* and *tricyclic antidepressants,* all of which also depress CNS function. The analgesic effect of *morphine* is increased by *chlorpromazine* and *methocarbamol.* The depressant effects of morphine are increased by *chloral hydrate, glutethimide, β-adrenergic blockers,* and *furazolidone.*

Meperidine should never be given concurrently with *monoamine oxidase* (MAO) *inhibitors,* and should not be used in patients who have recently received MAO inhibitors. Unpredictable and even fatal reactions have occurred when these two drugs were combined. *Methadone* blood levels are reduced by concurrent use of *rifampin* and *phenytoin.* Withdrawal reactions have occurred when one of these drugs has been given to a patient on methadone.

Patient teaching about the narcotic analgesics should be incorporated into the overall teaching program about the patient's disease, trauma, or medical procedure. Some key points about the drug therapy that should be incorporated into the teaching program are included in the patient teaching guide.

The guide to the nursing process summarizes the clinical aspects that should be incorporated into the nursing care of a patient receiving narcotic analgesics.

Nonpharmacologic measures for chronic pain control

In spite of all efforts to employ potent analgesics and other drugs, including local anesthetic nerve blocks (Chap. 14), some patients with chronic pain soon fail to obtain adequate relief from drugs alone. In such situations, various other procedures—some well established, others in experimental stages—are now available. These include such neurosurgical procedures as anterolateral cordotomy, dorsal rhizotomy, and cingulotomy. Among measures that employ electrical stimulation are those involving transcutaneous and percutaneous techniques and the implantation of devices into the spinal cord and brain. Needle therapies include not only acupuncture but also osteopuncture and injections into special trigger zones.

Psychological measures involve operant conditioning and behavior modification, biofeedback and relaxation training, psychotherapy, and placebo therapy.

Nurses who decide to specialize in pain control will receive training and education in these areas when they participate in the teaching programs that are now being developed. The PCU nurse will, it is hoped, soon have a place among clinical nurse specialists similar to that of coronary care unit nurses and intensive care unit nurses.

Patient teaching guide: narcotic analgesics

The following points should be incorporated into the general teaching program of a patient who is receiving narcotic analgesics for the relief of pain.

Instructions:

1. This drug has been prescribed to relieve your pain. *Do not hesitate* to use this drug if you feel uncomfortable. It is important to use the drug before the pain becomes severe, when it will be much more difficult to treat.

2. If GI upset occurs, this drug can be taken with food.

3. Constipation is a common problem with these drugs. Your nurse or physician will suggest an appropriate bowel program to help alleviate this problem.

4. This drug often causes drowsiness, dizziness, or visual changes. If this occurs, use caution if driving, operating machinery, or performing delicate tasks. If this happens in the hospital, the side rails may be left up on your bed for your protection.

5. Other measures may be taken to make this drug more effective—for example, positioning, controlling the environment, and relaxing. Your nurse will help you to receive the most benefit from the drug.

Guide to the nursing process: narcotic analgesics

Assessment	Nursing diagnoses	Interventions	Evaluation
Past history (*contraindications*):	Potential alteration in cardiac output	Safe and appropriate administration of drug	Monitor for therapeutic effectiveness of drug: pain relief
Head injury	Potential ineffective coping secondary to CNS effects	Provision of safety and comfort measures:	Monitor for adverse effects of drug:
Increased intracranial pressure		• Safety if dizziness and drowsiness occur	• Respiratory depression
COPD	Potential for injury secondary to drug effects		• Cardiovascular depression
Hypotension		• Positioning	
Delirium tremens		• Environmental control	• CNS effects
Hepatic failure	Knowledge deficit regarding drug therapy		• Dry mouth
Renal failure		• Measures to relieve constipation	• Constipation
Severe gallbladder disease	Potential sensory–perceptual alteration		• Arrhythmias
Addison's disease		Support and encouragement to cope with pain and	• Urinary retention
Thyroid disease			• Rash
Pregnancy			

(continued)

Assessment	Nursing diagnoses	Intervention	Evaluation
Allergies: these *drugs;* *tartrazine* (some preparations); others; reactions Medication history (*cautions*): Other narcotics General anesthetics Antihistamines Phenothiazines Barbiturates Tranquilizers Tricyclic antidepressants Chlorpromazine (MS)* Methocarbamol (MS)* Chloral hydrate (MS)* Glutethimide (MS)* β-adrenergic blockers (MS)* Furazolidone (MS)* MAO inhibitors (meperidine) Rifampin (methadone) Phenytoin (methadone)		drug therapy Patient teaching regarding drug therapy Life support, if necessary, for adverse response	Evaluate effectiveness of safety and comfort measures Evaluate effectiveness of patient teaching program Evaluate effectiveness of support and encouragement offered Monitor for drug–drug interactions: many possible Evaluate effectiveness of life support measures, if necessary
Physical assessment Neurologic: mental status, affect, reflexes Cardiovascular: P, BP, peripheral perfusion Respiratory: R, depth, rhythm GI: abdominal exam, normal output Renal: output Skin: lesions, color, temperature Laboratory tests: liver function, renal function			

* MS refers specifically to morphine sulfate.

Summary of main pharmacologic actions and therapeutic uses of opiates and opioids

Analgesic, sedative, tranquilizer, hypnotic

These CNS actions account for the effectiveness of these drugs against even very severe pain, including that caused by acute smooth muscle spasm and chronic bone disease. Among the conditions in which potent analgesics are employed are acute coronary attacks; biliary and renal colic; trauma caused by fractures or extensive

(continued)

burns; intractable pain of malignancies; control of post-operative pain; preanesthetic sedation; short diagnostic and operative procedures in orthopedics, urology, ophthalmology, rhinology, and laryngology; obstetric analgesia.

Antiperistaltic, antisecretory, and spasmogenic

These peripheral actions on gastrointestinal muscles and glands account for the usefulness of opiate alkaloids in diarrhea, dysentery, and various other gastrointestinal conditions, including peritonitis.

Antitussive

The depressant action of many of these drugs on the medullary cough center mechanism accounts for their usefulness for decreasing the frequency of coughing. Morphine, methadone, and dihydromorphinone are preferred for coughs accompanied by pain, following rib fractures, or in lung cancer or tuberculosis. Less addicting and less depressant antitussives such as codeine and hydrocodone can control lesser coughs, including those caused by dryness and irritation of the respiratory tract mucosa in the common cold.

Summary of opiate side-effects and toxicity

Central nervous system side-effects and toxicity

1. Drowsiness, clouding of consciousness, and inability to concentrate; occasionally, especially in women or elderly patients, paradoxical excitement marked by nervousness, restlessness, and even mania may develop (Excitement is more common with codeine or meperidine overdosage and may progress to convulsions or to disorientation, delirium, or hallucinations.)
2. Light-headedness, dizziness, nausea, and vomiting are central in origin, and are more common when patients are ambulatory; skin may become warm, flushed, and itchy
3. Respiratory depression may occur, especially in elderly and debilitated patients and in those with certain pre-existing disorders
4. Circulatory collapse: may be the result of severe hypoxia, or direct central and peripheral vasomotor depression

Peripheral side-effects

1. Gastrointestinal tract smooth muscle movements are slowed, and muscle tone increased to the point of spasm. These actions and others, including reduced secretions, lead to constipation, a side-effect to which the addict does not develop tolerance
2. Biliary and urinary tract muscle is also made spastic, and increased choledochal pressure may lead to rupture of *diseased* gallbladder and duct tissues; spasm of the bladder sphincter may act to interfere with urinary flow
3. Bronchiolar constriction by morphine is undesirable for asthmatic patients; small doses of meperidine are less likely to cause contraction of bronchial muscles

Case study

Presentation LM, a 25-year-old white male, was in a serious automobile accident and suffered a fractured pelvis, a fractured left tibia, and a fractured right humerus, along with numerous contusions and abrasions. For the first 2 days following surgery to reduce the fractures, LM was heavily sedated. As healing progressed, LM was maintained on IM injections of morphine sulfate, every 4 hours, prn for pain. LM requested the morphine every 2 to 3 hours and became very agitated by the end of the prescribed 4 hours. LM's physician decided to switch him to meperidine, given for a few days IM every 4 hours, and then given orally as a prelude to progressively weaning him from the narcotic. Concern was expressed by the physician that LM might become dependent on narcotics over the extended period of time it would take him to recover from his injuries.

What nursing care considerations related to drug therapy should be incorporated into LM's care plan?

Discussion

In assessing LM's response to drug therapy, it is readily apparent that the morphine was not providing the desired therapeutic effect. Numerous research studies have shown that, in general, the dosage of narcotics prescribed for pain relief provides inadequate analgesic coverage. It could be that the dose of morphine ordered is not sufficient to relieve LM's pain. Because of the physician's concern about LM's dependence on narcotics, it is unlikely that the dosage will be increased. It is possible that other measures could be taken to relieve LM's pain and to facilitate the therapeutic effectiveness of the drug therapy. LM may be very anxious about his injuries and fearful of impending pain, asking for the medication early to ensure that he receives it on time; he may be uncomfortable with his dependent situation and his anxiety may be contributing to his perception of pain. LM's nurse should first spend some time with LM to determine the nature of his pain. Other therapeutic measures can be tried to relieve LM's pain (e.g., environmental control, positioning) and to relieve his anxiety, which can accentuate pain perception. Reassurance, comfort measures, responding quickly to his requests, and often just being available can relieve a great deal of a patient's anxiety and thus facilitate other pain relief measures. Changing from morphine to meperidine may provide increased relief in some cases, because people respond differently to different drugs. In LM's case, the drug of choice could have been either drug, because he does not have any underlying conditions that would contraindicate the use of either. Meperidine has the advantage of being available in an oral form, facilitating frequent administration. The health-care team should discuss the benefits of narcotic analgesia versus the potential risks of dependence on the drug in this case, and should let LM know what the results of this discussion are and the rationale behind the scheduling of the drug therapy that is chosen. Involving LM in his care in such a way may further decrease his anxiety and facilitate the therapeutic effectiveness of the narcotic. LM's injuries are extensive and a coordinated, long-term approach to control of his pain should be developed.

Drug digests

Alphaprodine HCl USP (Nisentil)

Actions and indications. This narcotic analgesic has a relatively rapid onset and short duration of action. This makes it useful for preventing pain and discomfort during procedures such as cystoscopy, minor surgery of the eye, nose, and throat, and orthopedic manipulations. When used in obstetric analgesia, this drug's short duration tends to minimize depression of respiration in the newborn infant.
Adverse effects, cautions, and contraindications. This drug's depressant effect on

respiration may be intensified in patients who are also receiving barbiturates, phenothiazines, and general anesthetics. Its dose should be reduced in such cases. Excessive depression is best managed with the narcotic antagonist *naloxone HCl* (Narcan), particularly if depression develops during obstetric analgesia shortly before delivery. After delivery, the same antagonist may be injected into the baby's umbilical vein to counteract any residual respiratory depression caused

by administration of this analgesic to the mother. Alphaprodine is not considered desirable in the management of chronically painful disorders. The frequent administration required would tend to increase the likelihood of development of dependence.
Dosage and administration. The usual dose range is 0.4 to 1.2 mg/kg body weight SC or 0.4 to 0.6 mg/kg IV. Early doses are about 60 mg SC or 30 mg IV. The IM route is **not** recommended.

Codeine phosphate USP (methylmorphine)

Actions and indications. This and other salts of the opium alkaloid have central analgesic and antitussive effects when taken orally in adequate doses. Codeine is most often combined with aspirin for producing additive effects that relieve pain of mild to moderate intensity. It also reduces the frequency of cough volleys by raising the threshold of the cough reflex center to afferent impulses that arise in irritated or inflamed areas of the

respiratory tract mucosa. Its sedative effect may also reduce the patient's concern about his coughing.
Adverse effects, cautions, and contraindications. This drug causes little respiratory depression and fewer of the discomforting side-effects that occur with morphine and other more potent opioids. Because of this and its relatively low dependence-producing potential, codeine is preferred for cough

control and pain relief in most clinical situations in which it is adequately effective. The usual oral doses cause few side-effects, but some patients may become constipated or complain of nausea, epigastric distress, dizziness, and drowsiness. Large overdoses rarely depress respiration severely, but may cause confusion, agitation, and other signs of central excitement, including delirium and convulsions.

Dosage and administration. Oral doses of 30 mg are required for relief of pain and are administered every 4 hours. Oral and subcutaneous administration of up to 60 mg may increase the extent of the drug's analgesic effectiveness. For cough relief, doses of 8 to 15 mg are taken orally several times daily.

Meperidine HCl USP (Demerol; Pethidine)

Actions and indications. This synthetic strong analgesic is somewhat less effective than morphine against moderate to severe pain and has a slightly shorter duration of action. However, it is useful for relief of pain following a coronary occlusion and in conditions marked by spasm of visceral smooth muscle, such as biliary or renal colic. Although it is less likely than morphine to cause GI spasm, it does not actually have an antispasmodic effect in ordinary doses.

Meperidine is also used as an adjunct to anesthesia, preoperatively and sometimes during the surgical procedure, and for producing obstetric analgesia. In such situations it is often combined with sedative drugs such as promethazine, scopolamine, diazepam, or barbiturates.

Adverse effects, cautions, and contraindi- **cations.** The most common side-effects, particularly in ambulatory patients, are dizziness, light-headedness, sweating, flushing, nausea, and vomiting. Occasionally, patients may feel extremely weak and become mentally confused, disoriented, or agitated.

Meperidine must not be used in patients who have recently been taking MAO inhibitor drugs, because severe reactions have been reported in such cases. Caution is also required in patients taking the tricyclic-type antidepressant drugs. Dosage must be reduced for patients who are also receiving other CNS depressants, including barbiturates, phenothiazine-type tranquilizers, and general anesthetics

Like other potent analgesics, it is used only with extreme caution, if at all, in patients with head injuries or other conditions that cause an increase in intracranial pressure, in bronchial asthma or other chronic obstructive pulmonary diseases, and in elderly or debilitated patients. This drug's weak atropinelike action may make its use undesirable in patients with supraventricular tachycardias or prostatic hypertrophy. The drug produces dependence of the morphine type.

Dosage and administration. The usual range of dosage for adults is between 50 and 150 mg administered orally or parenterally every 3 or 4 hours. For preoperative purposes and obstetric analgesia, only parenteral routes are employed—usually IM, sometimes SC, and occasionally by slow IV administration of fractional doses or by continuous infusion.

Methadone HCl USP (Dolophine)

Actions and indications. This strong synthetic analgesic and antitussive drug is as effective as morphine for relief of pain and coughing. It is slower in onset, longer in duration, and less sedating than morphine. It is not ordinarily used for preanesthetic purposes nor in obstetric analgesia, in which its long-lasting depression of respiration of the fetus is undesirable.

Methadone is used in two ways in the management of addiction: to suppress the abstinence syndrome in patients who are being withdrawn from heroin or other narcotics; and to maintain patients who have been withdrawn from heroin in a state of minimal craving for the illicit narcotic and unresponsive to the euphoric effect of heroin.

Adverse effects, cautions, and contraindications. Side-effects include drowsiness, dizziness, mouth dryness, nausea, vomiting, and constipation. Overdosage may result in stupor or coma, deep respiratory depression, cardiac slowing or arrest, and hypotension or cardiovascular collapse. Symptoms are of long duration, and repeated injections of the available narcotic antagonists are required to prevent recurrences of respiratory depression and other toxic effects. This drug can cause morphine-type dependence.

Caution is required in patients taking other depressant drugs or the drugs used for treating mental depression, including the MAO inhibitors, because of potentially dangerous drug interactions. This drug is used with extreme caution, if at all, in patients suffering an acute asthma attack or with head injuries.

Dosage and administration. The usual adult dosage for relief of pain ranges from 2.5 to 10 mg every 3 or 4 hours orally or by injection (IM or SC). For cough relief the adult dose is 1 to 2 mg every 4 to 6 hours. Dosage for stabilizing addicted patients is variable.

Morphine sulfate USP

Actions and indications. This opium alkaloid is the prototype of the potent narcotic analgesics that can relieve severe degrees of pain. It is effective for this purpose against pain of visceral origin such as that caused by reflex spasm of the smooth muscle of the biliary ducts and ureters in biliary and renal colic. It also relieves the sharp pain from injuries, including fractures and burns.

This drug's sedative effect is desirable in patients who have suffered a coronary occlusion and also when the analgesic is employed as preanesthetic medication to bring about easier induction of anesthesia and recovery with minimal excitement. Morphine-induced sedation and peripheral vasodilation are the actions thought to account for its effectiveness in patients with acute pulmonary edema and failure of the left ventricle. It also has antitussive and antiperistaltic effects.

Adverse effects, cautions, and contraindications. Common side-effects include drowsiness, dizziness, light-headedness, sweating and flushing, nausea and vomiting, and constipation. Patients who are ambulatory are warned that morphine may impair their ability to drive a car or to perform other potentially dangerous tasks that require alertness and good judgment.

Overdosage results in respiratory depression, particularly in elderly or disease-weakened patients. Others likely to suffer a dangerous decrease in ventilation include patients with chronic obstructive pulmonary diseases, particularly during acute attacks of bronchial asthma or emphysema. Poor ventilation with resulting hypoxia and hypercarbia leads, in turn, to dilation of cerebral vessels and to an increase in intracranial pressure. If this condition already exists—in patients with head injuries, for example—morphine can cause a marked exaggeration of the already high cerebrospinal fluid pressure. Thus, its use is usually contraindicated in such cases.

It must also be employed cautiously in patients with severely impaired liver or kidney function and certain endocrine disorders. For example, patients with cirrhosis of the liver, hypothyroidism (myxedema), and Addison's disease may sometimes be deeply depressed by relatively low doses of morphine. The drug's spasmogenic effect on smooth muscle of the urinary tract may lead to urinary retention and dysuria in patients with prostatic hypertrophy or urethral strictures.

Dosage and administration. Morphine is **not** ordinarily administered orally but is instead injected subcutaneously in doses of about 10 mg/150 lb of body weight for effects that reach peak levels in about 1 hour and last about 4 hours. For more rapid action and more certain absorption, smaller doses are diluted with saline solution and injected slowly by vein.

Naloxone HCl USP (Narcan)

Actions and indications. This drug is a pure narcotic antagonist. That is, it has no pharmacologic activity of its own but acts only to reverse the depression produced by excessive doses of morphine, methadone, heroin, and other natural and synthetic narcotics. Administered in small parenteral doses, naloxone readily counteracts deep respiratory depression, raises blood pressure that has dropped secondary to severe hypoxia, and antagonizes other opioid effects. This drug is so effective for reversing opioid effects that its failure to do so suggests that the patient's depression is the result of overdosage by other depressant drugs or has been caused by other medical conditions. Thus, it is used for the differential diagnosis of opioid overdosage. Its ability to unmask signs of the opioid withdrawal syndrome means that it may also be useful for diagnosing physical dependence on narcotics, but it is rarely used specifically for this purpose.

Adverse effects, cautions, and contraindications. Naloxone administration requires caution in those known to be physically dependent on narcotics, because it may set off an acute withdrawal syndrome that is oc-

casionally more dangerous than the degree of respiratory depression that it reverses. The same applies to the newborn infants of mothers suspected of being narcotic addicts. Patients who improve should continue to be observed, because depression may return when the effects of the antagonist wear off and those of the longer acting narcotic continue. Other resuscitative measures, such as maintenance of an open airway, must not be neglected.

Dosage and administration. For treating narcotic overdosage a 1-ml ampule containing 0.4 mg (400 µg) is injected IV, IM, or SC. This dose may be repeated IV at intervals of 2 to 3 minutes until the desired degree of respiratory function improvement ap-

pears. If several such doses fail, the patient's depression probably has some other cause. Smaller doses are employed in patients with postoperative respiratory depression so as not to reverse therapeutically desirable postoperative analgesia. The same is true for suspected narcotic addicts to avoid nausea, vomiting, sweating, and a rise in blood pressure, or other signs and symptoms of withdrawal.

The usual dose for newborn infants whose respiration is depressed by narcotic analgesic drugs administered to the mother during labor is 0.01 mg/kg body weight IV, IM or SC. A 2-ml ampule containing 0.02 mg/ml (20 µg) is available for this purpose. Dosage may be repeated in the manner stated above.

Pentazocine HCl and lactate USP (Talwin)

Actions and indications. Both forms of this analgesic are indicated for relief of moderate to severe pain. The oral salt (HCl) is similar to codeine in potency and in its relatively low potential for producing dependence. It is the preferred form for use in chronically painful conditions, because it is less likely to be abused or to produce dependence. The injectable form (lactate) can produce a degree of analgesia equal to that of morphine when administered in doses several times that of the natural opioid. This parenteral form is preferred for short-term use, including employment as a supplement to other pain-relieving medications prior to and during surgical anesthesia.

Adverse effects, cautions, and contraindications. The most common adverse effects are nausea, vomiting, dizziness and lightheadedness, and drowsiness. Constipation

and euphoria occur infrequently and, rarely, patients have hallucinations and become disoriented and confused. Respiratory depression resulting from overdosage can best be counteracted by naloxone, but other narcotic antagonists are **not** effective. Caution is required in patients with bronchial asthma and other chronic obstructive pulmonary conditions and in those whose respiration is already depressed.

Because the parenteral form has been abused to the point of dependence development by patients with a history of drug abuse, such patients should be closely observed when receiving either form of this drug for long periods. This drug possesses slight narcotic antagonist activity and can cause opioid-type withdrawal symptoms when added to the regimen of patients taking methadone as maintenance therapy of narcotic addiction.

Dosage and administration. Single injections should not exceed 30 mg IV or 60 mg IM. Subcutaneous injections should be avoided because of possible tissue damage and, even when the drug is injected intramuscularly, the injection sites should be rotated to minimize local irritation. Total daily dosage should not exceed 360 mg.

For patients in labor, a single IM dose of 30 mg is often adequate. If the intravenous route is employed, dosage is reduced to 20 mg and repeated at 2- or 3-hour intervals if necessary.

The usual oral dose is 50 mg, but 100 mg may be employed if needed. These doses may be administered every 3 or 4 hours, but the total daily dose should not exceed 600 mg.

Propoxyphene HCl USP (Darvon) and propoxyphene napsylate NF (Darvon-N)

Actions and indications. This chemical relative of methadone is used for relief of mild to moderate pain. It is about half as potent as codeine but can control pain equally well when given in twice the dose of the opiate. Unlike the latter, it is not subject to narcotic law restrictions. The effectiveness of propoxyphene is about equal to that of aspirin, and a combination of the two drugs is said to produce a better analgesic effect than that of either drug administered alone.

Adverse effects, cautions, and contraindications. This drug is classified as *non*addicting, but it can produce psychological and physical dependence of the morphine–codeine type when abused. Similarly, massive overdosage causes toxicity similar to that of codeine and other opiates, including convulsions, coma, circulatory collapse, and respiratory failure.

Ordinary doses may cause drowsiness, dizziness, and headache or, occasionally, ex-

citement and insomnia. Psychomotor impairment may make driving a car hazardous. Epigastric pain, nausea, vomiting, and constipation are also among the minor adverse effects.

Dosage and administration. The hydrochloride salt is administered orally in doses of 32 or 65 mg; doses of the napsylate salt range from 50 to 100 mg. Both are usually given tid or qid in combination with aspirin or with aspirin, phenacetin, and caffeine.

References

Basbaum AI, Fields HL: Endogenous pain control systems: Brain stem spinal pathways and endorphin circuitry. Ann Rev Neurosci 7:309, 1984

Bonica JJ: Neurophysiologic and pathologic aspects of acute and chronic pain. Arch Surg 112:750, 1977

Drug treatment of cancer pain. Med Lett Drugs Ther 24:95, 1982

Foley KM: The practical use of narcotic analgesics. Med Clin North Am 66:1091, 1982

Friedman FB (ed): Clinical controversies. PRN analgesics: Controlling the pain or controlling the patient? RN 46:67, 1983

Goldstein A: Opioid peptides (endorphins) in pituitary and brain. Science 193:1081, 1976

Halpern LM: Analgesic drugs in the management of pain. Arch Surg 112:861, 1977

Isler C: New approach to intractable pain. RN 38:17, 1975

Jaffe JH, Martin WR: Opioid analgesics and antagonists.

In Gilman AG, Goodman LS, Gilman A (eds): Goodman & Gilman's The Pharmacological Basis of Therapeutics, 6th ed, pp 494–534. New York, Macmillan, 1980

Lawrence RM, Lawrence EB: The pain control nursing program. In Bonica JJ, Albe–Fessard D (eds): Advances in Pain Research and Therapy, Vol 1. New York, Raven Press, 1976

Marx JL: How the body inhibits pain perception. Science 195:471, 1977

McCaffrey M et al: Undertreatment of acute pain with narcotics. Am J Nurs 76:1586, 1976

Newburger PE, Sallan SE: Chronic pain: Principles of management. J Pediatr 98:180, 1981

Pert A: Mechanisms of opiate analgesia and the role of endorphins in pain suppression. Adv Neurol 33:107, 1982

Pflug AE, Bonica JJ: Physiopathology and control of postoperative pain. Arch Surg 112:773, 1977

Rodman MJ: How to coax maximum pain relief from standard drugs. RN 43:83, 1980

Rogers AG: What to expect from the most common analgesics. RN 46:44, 1983

Urca C et al: Morphine and enkephalin: Analgesic and epileptic properties. Science 197:83, 1977

Chapter 52

General
anesthetics

52

General anesthetics are central nervous system depressants that are used to bring about loss of pain sensation and consciousness. Their use permits painful surgical procedures to be performed without the patient's being aware of discomfort or even reacting with reflex movements. The modern anesthesiologist administers anesthetics and other drugs in ways that produce minimal changes in the patient's vital functions. Properly employed, these potent drugs are safe for producing the brief loss of consciousness needed for minor procedures or even for the deep anesthesia required for performing lengthy major operations.

General considerations

History
Before the first general anesthetics came into use about 130 years ago, the only agents available for alleviating the pain of the surgeon's knife were opium extracts, alcoholic beverages, and various plant products with only weak central depressant effects.

These substances were neither safe nor effective. Their safety margin was so slim that respiration might readily fail if the patient were given amounts large enough to maintain unconsciousness all through the operation. Smaller, safer doses of opiate–alcohol–belladonna mixtures might succeed only in putting the patient into a stuporous fog from which the painful stimuli of surgery readily aroused him. Often, it took several husky assistants to hold down the struggling delirious patient, while the surgeon worked as swiftly as possible to complete the painful task.

Then, in the decade 1840 to 1850, several simple organic chemicals came into use for the relief of surgical and obstetric pain. First, nitrous oxide, an inorganic gas first prepared in the previous century, was shown to induce analgesia deep enough to permit painless dental surgery. (The substance, also called "laughing gas," had previously been used only to amuse the public, because inhaling small amounts often caused delirium.)

At about the same time, inhalation of the vapors of two volatile liquids, ethyl ether and chloroform, was proved capable of producing a state of unconsciousness deep enough to block out the pain of extensive surgical procedures. For the first time patients could be kept completely free of pain for as long a time as the surgeon needed for performing a lengthy, complicated operation.

After World War I, new general and local (Chap. 14) anesthetics were introduced, and many advances were made that increased the safety of inhalation anesthesia. Although various new anesthetics have been introduced, no single agent has all the characteristics of the ideal drug (see the summary, at the end of this chapter). Thus the trend has been to employ combinations of anesthetics—both general and local with various adjunctive drugs to keep the patient in a physiologic state as close to normal as possible.

Balanced anesthesia
The lack of any single anesthetic that is ideally suited for use in every patient and in all surgical situations has led to the concept of balanced anesthesia. This involves the use of several different types of drugs to counteract the disadvantages of various potent anesthetics and to make the most of the desirable properties of less potent agents such as nitrous oxide (see Table 52-1, below, for the advantages and disadvantages of individual anesthetics).

The drugs employed for this purpose include such nonanesthetic central nervous system depressants as the sedative–hypnotics and antianxiety agents such as diazepam, phenothiazines and other neuroleptic and antiemetic drugs, and the potent analgesics morphine, meperidine, and fentanyl, among others.

In addition, the general anesthetics and other

central depressant drugs are also supplemented by certain peripherally acting agents. These include atropine and other anticholinergic drugs and the neuromuscular blocking agents employed to aid in producing skeletal muscle paralysis, including succinylcholine and *d*-tubo-curarine, among others. The judicious use of two or more of these different types of drugs usually allows the anesthesiologist to achieve the various objectives of general anesthesia more readily and safely than is possible with any single anesthetic drug alone.

Objectives of general anesthesia

The potent general anesthetics can produce several clinically useful pharmacologic effects. The anesthesiologist tries to use these drugs to achieve these effects safely. Thus, the goals of general anesthesia are the safe attainment of the following effects:

1. *Analgesia,* or sensory block, the loss of pain perception.
2. *Unconsciousness* or a state in which the patient is unaware of what is going on and is later totally unable to recall what took place (amnesia, or loss of memory). Actually, it is possible to employ ether and certain other general anesthetics in amounts that produce analgesia *without* complete loss of consciousness, but these drugs are rarely used in this way clinically.
3. *Block of reflexes,* peripherally, to reduce various involuntary responses that might adversely affect the patient's respiratory, cardiovascular, and gastrointestinal functions. Thus, for example, efforts must be made to minimize reflex breath-holding, laryngospasm, or bronchospasm, to prevent cardiac arrhythmias, and to reduce salivation, vomiting, and postoperative abdominal distention.
4. *Neuromuscular junction or motor block.* Block of the spinal reflexes that maintain muscle tone is often desirable during abdominal surgery. Only the most potent general anesthetics depress these reflexes so completely as to cause abdominal muscle relaxation without, at the same time, dangerously depressing the brain's centers for control of breathing.

Types of anesthetics

The general anesthetics are administered mainly by inhalation. Some, such as *nitrous oxide*[+] and *cyclopropane*[+] (Trimethylene) are gases. Others, including *ether*[+] and *halothane*[+] (Fluothane) are volatile liquids that give off vapors at room temperature. Still others, such as the rapid-acting barbiturates *thiopental sodium*[+] (Pentothal) and *methohexital sodium* (Brevital), are introduced into the bloodstream by intravenous or rectal administration.

These substances are sometimes classified in terms of their potency and safety under conditions of clinical use. A potent anesthetic produces all the objectives of general anesthesia with relative safety. *Ether,* for example, induces full, or complete, surgical anesthesia when inhaled in low concentrations that do not prevent the patient from also inhaling adequate amounts of oxygen at the same time. *Nitrous oxide,* on the other hand, is a less potent substance that produces full anesthesia only when the gas is given in such high concentration that the amount of oxygen in the mixture is reduced below safe levels.

Similarly, the barbiturates cannot be safely administered in doses that can produce complete anesthesia. Nevertheless, despite its relatively weak anesthetic properties, nitrous oxide is now the most commonly employed inhalation anesthetic, and the intravenous administration of short-acting barbiturates is the most widely used measure for producing *basal anesthesia,* a state of unconsciousness that is achieved rapidly and pleasantly prior to administration of one of the more potent anesthetics and other agents that can bring about sensory and motor block more safely.

The following discussions will take up first the pharmacology of the inhalation anesthetics and comment on the properties of individual general anesthetics. It will then discuss the various intravenously (and rectally) administered anesthetic drugs, and the applications of drugs from both groups in clinical situations together with nonanesthetic adjunctive drugs.

The pharmacology of the inhalation anesthetics

These anesthetics produce a progressive depression of the central nervous system (CNS). The degree of depression depends on the concentration of the drug in the CNS. This, in turn, depends on the dynamic balance between the rates at which the gas or vapor is taken up from the alveoli by the blood, transported past the blood–brain barrier, and redistributed by the blood and eliminated by the lungs.

Pharmacokinetic aspects

To produce anesthesia, an inhaled drug's molecules must attain a critical concentration in the various regions of the CNS. The rates at which the levels of anesthesia (see anesthetic syndrome, below) are attained depend on such factors as the rate of delivery of the gas or vapor into the lungs, its uptake by the blood, and its initial distribution and later redistribution (Chap. 4). The portion of delivered drug in the CNS at any moment is what determines the degree of anesthesia. Most of the drug's molecules that are in the body at any time after inhalation begins are, of course, *not* in the CNS but are distributed in the much greater mass of tissue outside the CNS where they do not have any effect in maintaining clinical anesthesia.

As soon as the first breath of volatile anesthetic reaches the bronchioles and alveoli, it begins to pass into the capillaries lining the pulmonary membranes in this, the terminal portion of the respiratory tree. This transport from lungs to bloodstream occurs because gases tend to diffuse from areas of higher concentration (*e.g.*, the alveoli) into those in which their concentration is lower (*e.g.*, the arterial capillaries). When continuous administration of volatile vapors keeps the partial pressure of the anesthetic in the lungs at a high level, the amount of the drug in the arterial blood leaving the lungs for the heart, brain, and other organs rises rapidly.

The drug's concentration in the brain builds up quickly because of the abundant blood supply and the high affinity of anesthetics for fatty tissues, including the lipoids of the nervous system. Even in concentrations too low to affect the functioning of other organs, these depressants begin to disrupt the highly sensitive neuronal pathways and the activities that these nerve cells control.

Each portion of anesthetic carried to the brain by the arterial circulation soon leaves it by way of the venous blood, which redistributes the drug to other body organs. Some is stored temporarily in the body's fat stores, but almost all of the volatile anesthetic is eventually excreted in the exhaled air. By balancing the amount of anesthetic that is entering the patient's lungs from an outside source against the quantity of anesthetic that the venous blood is delivering to the lungs for elimination, the anesthesiologist can control the drug's concentration in the brain and consequently keep the patient at any desired level of anesthesia.

When it is desirable to lighten the plane of anesthesia, or to terminate it entirely, the anesthesiologist simply stops the flow of vapor into the patient's lungs. This leads to a reversal of the diffusion gradient and to a lightening of the anesthesia. That is, the anesthetic moving "downhill" from the brain into the venous blood is no longer being replaced by new increments coming in through the lungs and arteries. The level of depressant drug in the nervous system drops, the neurons recover from their reversible narcosis, and the functions that these nerves control begin to return. The emergence from anesthesia may be slow or rapid, depending on how much of a particular anesthetic had been inhaled by the patient, the rate of its redistribution to other tissues, and finally on the rate at which it leaves the blood by way of the lungs.

Sites and mechanism of action. Exactly how the anesthetics arriving at the brain depress neuronal function has not yet been determined. It is known that lipid-soluble substances, such as general anesthetics, tend to reach the nerve tissues most readily, but this reveals nothing about what they do there to disrupt nerve cell activity. Fortunately, the disruptive effect of these drugs on the physicochemical and neurophysiologic properties of the neurons is reversible, and complete recovery of function occurs when their molecules are eliminated from the nerve tissue.

No single one of the many mechanisms that have been proposed to explain how anesthetics affect the physical or biochemical properties of nerve cells can explain what actually causes the pharmacologic effects that occur clinically. This may be, of course, because there is no mechanism common to all depressant drugs, and different agents may act in various ways. Thus, it may well be that some anesthetic gases act on nerve cell membranes to alter their physical properties, while the vapors of other substances may act by interfering with nerve cell oxidative processes through their inhibitory effects on the essential enzymatic reactions required for metabolic, or energy-producing, functions to proceed normally.

The neural basis for the progressive depression of the CNS is somewhat better understood. As indicated in Chapter 44, the part of the brain most sensitive to anesthetics is the reticular activating system (RAS), the midbrain neuronal network that relays sensory impulses to all parts of the cerebral cortex, thus maintaining consciousness. Doses of anesthetics too small to exert any direct depressant effect on other parts of the nervous system disrupt the stream of impulses that ascend constantly from this area to the cerebral cortex. This interferes with the functioning of the higher centers, awareness of sensory perceptions is diminished and distorted and, finally, consciousness is lost.

As the concentration of anesthetic increases, other areas of the nervous system are progressively depressed. This produces a characteristic pattern of altered reflex activity because first the higher and then the lower nervous centers are knocked out. However, the depression from above downward temporarily bypasses the medulla oblongata to affect first the reflex centers in the spinal cord, which lies beneath it. This "irregularity" in the pattern of descending depression is what makes it possible for the anesthetic to produce profound muscular relaxation without paralyzing the vital respiratory and cardiovascular centers of the medulla.

The anesthetic syndrome

As each succeeding area of the CNS becomes depressed, certain signs and symptoms—the "anesthetic syndrome"—appear (see the summary at the end of this chapter). These have been grouped arbitrarily in ways that help the anesthesiologist determine how deeply depressed the patient is at any time. Nurses, too, should know these signs so that they know what the patient's condition is as they observe it during induction, in the operating room, and in the recovery room where the nurse's care of the patient during the immediate post-operative period is so important.

The anesthetic syndrome described in the following section is based on what commonly occurs when ethyl ether is employed. The pattern of stages and planes varies somewhat when various other anesthetics such as the barbiturates or the fluorinated anesthetics are used, and the administration of preanesthetic medication as part of a balanced anesthesia procedure may alter the pattern in various ways.

Stages and planes of general anesthesia

The anesthetic pattern is commonly broken into four stages that reflect fairly clear-cut differences in the patient's condition. The third stage, and sometimes the first, are further subdivided into "planes," based on finer distinctions in the patient's state. The first two stages comprise the induction period; the third stage is the one in which most surgical procedures requiring skeletal muscle relaxation may best be performed; the fourth is a stage of undesirably deep depression.

When basal anesthesia with rapid-acting barbiturates is employed, induction may occur so quickly that

signs of the first two stages are scarcely seen. During recovery from deep anesthesia, reflex activities return in reverse order from that in which they were lost. (The effects of ether anesthesia on respiration, pupil size, eyeball activity, and other important reflex signs are summarized in Figure 52-1.)

Stage I: Early induction. This stage extends from inhalation of the first breath of anesthetic vapor until the patient loses consciousness. Progressive disruption of higher cortical activities causes a clouding of consciousness marked by feelings of floating, numbness, and the loss of pain sensation. This analgesic state has long been considered to be adequate for dental surgery and obstetric procedures but it was formerly deemed dangerous to do more extensive surgery at this level because of the possibility that the patient might pass from this stage with its dreamlike disorders of sight and hearing (visual and auditory hallucinations) into the delirium and excitement of stage II (see following section). Actually, however, various major operations, including cardiac surgery, have been performed under first-stage ether analgesia. The patient, properly premedicated to minimize the danger of delirium, is first taken down to a deeper level of anes-

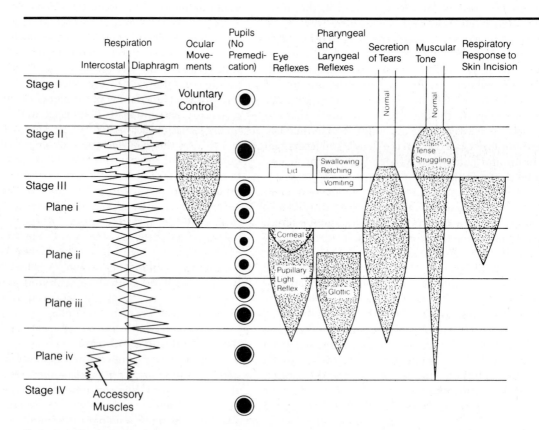

Figure 52-1. The signs and reflex reactions of the stages of anesthesia. The wedge-shaped areas indicate (1) the variability from person to person and (2) the variability of the disappearance of the signs in the several planes of anesthesia. These descriptions apply only to a nonpremedicated patient and to diethyl ether anesthesia. Similar signs are used to judge the depth of anesthesia with other agents, but some signs may not occur with other agents and the sequence may be different. (Gillespie NA: Curr Res Anesth Analg **22:**275, 1943)

thesia, which is then gradually lightened until he can hear and respond to commands. However, the patient feels no pain during the operation and remembers nothing of it later.

Stage II: Delirium or excitement. This stage lasts from the time that the patient loses consciousness until the first plane of surgical anesthesia is entered (see following section). In this stage, subcortical and other lower neurons are released from inhibitory control by higher cerebral centers, resulting in release reactions that account for the signs of excitement seen clinically.

It is important to remember that the patient is not responsible for his actions during this excitement stage. He is actually unconscious, even when he may be thrashing about restlessly or laughing, crying, or swearing.

No surgical procedures are ever attempted in this stage of anesthesia. Instead, every effort is made to help the patient pass as quickly as possible through this dangerous stage and down to the deeper planes of surgical anesthesia. Many of the mechanical as well as the pharmacologic and nursing measures employed preoperatively (see below) are intended to help ease the patient through this period without harm. Thus, for instance, the anesthesiologist sees to it that the patient is secured by straps, even before anesthesia is begun, so that he will not harm himself by becoming restless and thrashing about during this stage. Similarly, the patient's stomach must be empty when entering the anesthesia room because all the reflexes, including the gag reflex, become hyperactive during induction, and it is at this time that the patient is most likely to vomit and aspirate food particles. (The chances of inhaling gastric contents are increased during recovery also, before swallowing and cough reflexes have fully recovered; thus, the proper positioning of the patient for emesis is important to minimize this danger.)

Stage III: Surgical anesthesia. As the concentration of anesthetic in the CNS rises, the nerve cells that were temporarily released from inhibition become depressed. As their hyperactivity ceases, certain characteristic signs occur.

The third stage of anesthesia begins when the patient stops struggling and his breathing becomes regular again in rhythm and depth. This stage may be artificially divided into four planes, based on changes that can be detected in the patient's respiration, pupillary and eyeball movements, and reflex muscular responses as the degree of anesthesia deepens.

Respiration changes are most informative and important to the anesthesiologist. Breathing is most nearly normal in the first two planes. Increasingly shallow breathing, caused by depression of the spinal nerves that control the muscles of the rib cage, marks entrance into the third plane of stage III. The diaphragm contracts more strongly to compensate for the failing intercostal muscles; its downward pressure makes the abdomen heave heavily and, at the same time, the movements of the

patient's chest, or thorax, are diminishing. When thoracic breathing ceases entirely and even abdominal breathing begins to grow shallow and irregular, the patient has descended to the dangerous fourth plane of surgical anesthesia.

Eye signs are also informative to the anesthesiologist. The eyeballs, which roll or "rove" about as the patient is entering plane 1, grow gradually less active until they finally become fixed and motionless at the top of plane 2. (This diminishing eyeball activity reflects increasing depression of the midbrain's oculomotor center.)

The pupils, which were widely dilated during the excitement stage, return to normal in the first plane of this stage. They tend to contract in plane 2 but then dilate progressively as inadequate pulmonary ventilation in the lower plane of this stage causes an asphyxial oxygen lack. (Premedication with atropine and morphine alters these pupillary responses, but the experienced anesthesiologist can, of course, still learn something of the patient's status from the eye signs.)

By the bottom of plane 2 or early in plane 3, the eyelid no longer contracts in a wink when the cornea is touched and, a little later, light flashed in the patient's eye fails to cause pupillary constriction. Loss of these reflex signs indicates that the patient is down deep enough for any procedure and should be taken no deeper.

The *skeletal muscles* of the extremities and, later, of the abdomen become increasingly relaxed as spinal reflex centers no longer react to the stimuli that normally set off tonic contractions. Loss of these reflexes (by the bottom of plane 2) allows the surgeon to cut through the abdominal wall without setting off powerful contractions. In some surgical situations, it is desirable to supplement this action of the anesthetic with that of a peripherally acting neuromuscular blocking agent (see below). The paralysis of these muscles by such a combination of central and peripheral effects facilitates abdominal surgical and exploratory procedures.

Stage IV: Medullary paralysis. Spontaneous breathing stops at the beginning of this deepest stage of anesthesia. Unless the anesthetic is withdrawn and resuscitative measures applied, the heart soon fails, blood pressure falls from shock level to zero, and the patient dies. Deaths of this type need never occur; attention to the signs of anesthesia should prevent the patient from ever being carried below the third plane of the previous stage. When volatile agents are employed, the still functioning circulation will carry the anesthetic from the brain to the lungs, from which it may be removed by artificial respiration. Administration of oxygen by mechanical means may then help revive the patient.

The anesthesiologist is equipped to maintain pulmonary ventilation mechanically if breathing stops. For some surgical procedures, the patient's respiratory movements are purposely stopped with skeletal muscle blocking drugs, and assisted or controlled breathing is temporarily employed. Ordinarily, however, the anesthesiologist avoids the use of general anesthetics for depressing the patient's respiration, because this can lead to an acid–base imbalance or be followed by collapse of the cardiovascular system.

Recovery. As indicated earlier, the anesthesiologist can control the level of anesthesia by balancing the amount of anesthetic that is being inhaled against that which is being eliminated by the lungs. When it is desirable to lighten anesthesia or to terminate it entirely, the flow of gas or vapor going to the patient's lungs is simply stopped. As the anesthetic level at the various nerve centers falls, the depressed nerve cells regain their activity.

The functions that these neurons control then return at a rate that depends on how much anesthetic has been administered and on how long and how deeply the patient has been anesthetized. During recovery from deep anesthesia, the patient's reflexes return in the reverse order from that in which they were lost (Fig. 52-1). The excitement stage during recovery is not dramatic. However, it is important that the patient be properly positioned to avoid aspiration of gastric contents as a result of vomiting before protective gag reflexes have returned.

Individual anesthetics

The individual anesthetic drugs differ from one another in several of their central depressant properties, including their ability to produce analgesia and skeletal muscle relaxation. They also differ in several of their peripheral effects, including the extent to which they may adversely affect cardiac function. Thus, the anesthesiologist tries to select the anesthetic or combination of drugs best suited to the physical condition of the patient and to the surgical operation that is to be performed.

The general anesthetics are used in two main ways:

1. To produce complete anesthesia, in which patients are kept in planes of deep surgical anesthesia for prolonged periods during which major surgery is performed, and
2. To produce basal anesthesia, a state of light anesthesia, in which various minor surgical and diagnostic procedures are carried out. In such states of basal narcosis the patient feels little discomfort and is not aware of what is going on.

This section, will briefly discuss some of the main properties of individual drugs, even though anesthetics are rarely used alone today. The advantages and disadvantages of each drug are summarized in Table 52-1, and several are also discussed in the Drug digests.

Potent inhalation anesthetics

The substances most able to produce complete anesthesia with safety are the volatile liquids *ether* and *halothane,* and

the gas *cyclopropane.* Various fluorinated hydrocarbons related to halothane, including *methoxyflurane, enflurane,* and *isoflurane,* are also effective for achieving full anesthesia. They have the advantage of being nonflammable and nonexplosive.

Malignant hyperthermia or hyperpyrexia. Fairly recently, a rare but often fatal complication has been identified as developing in certain patients exposed to some of these potent, lipid-soluble inhalation anesthetics. This complication is characterized by various signs of increased metabolism, including tachycardia, rapid respirations, and elevated body temperature. It appears to have a genetic basis, and is sometimes associated with abnormal muscle function that can be detected by muscle biopsy. When this complication occurs, the anesthetic must be discontinued immediately and measures taken promptly to reduce body temperature and support vital functions. Dantrolene sodium (Dantrium; Chap. 48), a directly acting skeletal muscle relaxant, is given IV to treat this emergency and orally, for several days before surgery, as prophylaxis in susceptible patients.

Ether. Diethyl ether, one of the first substances to be employed for general anesthesia, has properties that helped to make it the most widely used all-purpose anesthetic during the long period when anesthesiologists favored use of a single agent rather than combinations of anesthetics.

The relative safety and efficacy of ether stems in part from the potency of its vapors, which produce full anesthesia even when inhaled in low concentrations that permit administration of oxygen in amounts comprising as much as 95% of the mixture. Another factor in its relatively wide safety margin is the fact that its irritating action on the respiratory tract mucosa causes a reflex stimulation of the respiratory center. Ether is also unique in possessing a peripheral curarelike blocking effect on skeletal muscle, which helps to produce excellent abdominal relaxation. Most important is the fact that, even when patients are maintained in deep anesthesia during prolonged operations, ether causes relatively little harm to nonnerve tissues, including the liver, kidneys, and heart.

Gastrointestinal disturbances are fairly common after operations in which large amounts of ether are employed. Postoperative nausea and vomiting occur in a high percentage of such cases. Such upsets are said to be less frequent when the patient has inhaled high oxygen concentrations simultaneously; when it seems severe enough to endanger the patient, vomiting may be counteracted by administration of one of the potent phenothiazine-type antiemetics. Postoperative distress from retention of gastrointestinal fluids and gases is sometimes blamed on ether's antiperistaltic effects, but such intestinal stasis may actually be the result of prolonged surgery, especially when the abdomen has been opened and the intestines handled during laparotomy. Paralytic ileus is

Table 52–1. Characteristics of individual anesthetics

Official or generic name	Trade name, synonym, or chemical name	Chemical or physical characteristics	Comments concerning clinical status	
			Advantages	Disadvantages
Inhalation anesthetics				
Cyclopropane USP	—	Cyclic hydrocarbon gas; flammable and explosive	See Drug digests	
Enflurane	Ethrane	Volatile liquid; fluorinated hydrocarbon	Rapid induction and recovery; pleasant odor; good muscle relaxation; nonflammable and nonexplosive	Analgesia not great; cardiac arrhythmias possible; respiratory depression may develop rapidly, together with EEG abnormalities
Ether USP	Ethyl ether; diethyl ether	Volatile liquid; flammable and explosive	See Drug digests	
Ethylene		Gas with an unpleasant odor; flammable and explosive	Rapid induction and recovery; good analgesia; not toxic to heart, lungs, liver, or kidneys	Not potent enough for full anesthesia; must be supplemented by potent analgesics and other depressant drugs
Halothane USP	Fluothane	Volatile liquid; halogenated hydrocarbon	See Drug digests	
Isoflurane	Forane	Volatile liquid; halogenated methyl ethyl ether	Good muscle relaxation; nonflammable; nonexplosive	Pungent odor; newest inhalation agent; experience with its use is limited
Methoxyflurane USP	Penthrane	Volatile liquid; halogenated methyl ethyl ether	Very potent anesthetic with prolonged analgesic effect; nonflammable and nonexplosive	Slow induction; prolonged recovery from anesthesia; deep respiratory depression and hypotension at levels required for muscle relaxation; fatal liver and kidney damage has occurred
Nitrous oxide USP	Nitrogen monoxide	Gas with little odor or taste; nonflammable but can support combustion when mixed with ether and other flammable substances	See Drug digests	
Intravenously and rectally administered anesthetics (basal anesthetics)				
Etomidate	Amidate	0.2% solution for IV use only	Relative absence of cardiopulmonary effects when used for inducing anes-	Venous pain on injection; myoclonic muscle movements

(continued)

Table 52–1. Characteristics of individual anesthetics (continued)

Official or generic name	Trade name, synonym, or chemical name	Chemical or physical characteristics	Comments concerning clinical status	
			Advantages	Disadvantages
			thesia; onset and recovery times similar to those with thiopental	
Fentanyl citrate and droperidol	Innovar	Solution for injection	Neuroleptanesthesia or neuroleptanalgesia; usually does not produce loss of consciousness	Hypotension, respiratory depression, and skeletal muscle rigidity can occur
Ketamine HCl USP	Ketalar; Keta-ject	Solution for IV and IM administration	Produces a dissociative state in which patient seems to be conscious but is unaware of pain in minor surgical and diagnostic procedures	May cause delirium or hallucinations during recovery; requires supplementation with muscle relaxants, nitrous oxide, and other agents for major surgery
Methohexital sodium USP	Brevital sodium	Barbiturate solution (1%) for IV use	Rapid onset of hypnosis, with recovery of consciousness more rapid than with thiopental	Can cause respiratory depression and apnea; can cause laryngospasm, particularly in asthmatic patients; *not* a good analgesic or skeletal muscle relaxant
Thiamylal sodium USP	Surital sodium	Barbiturate solution (2.5%) for IV use	Similar to thiopental in its rapid onset and ultra-short recovery time	Similar to thiopental in its adverse effects on respiratory system and lack of analgesic or skeletal muscle relaxant properties
Thiopental sodium USP	Pentothal sodium	Barbiturate solution (2.0% and 2.5%) for IV use and 40% for rectal administration	See Drug digest	

treated by administration of peristaltic stimulants such as neostigmine or vasopressin (Pitressin), and by physical measures such as application of heat to the abdomen.

Although ether is almost never used now in modern, fully equipped medical centers, it has several properties that make it a favorable anesthetic for use in emergencies under less optimum conditions. Its relative safety and lack of organ system toxicity have been described above. It can also be administered (open drop method) without the complex metering equipment that many of the newer anesthetics require, and it has a wide margin of safety—that is, concentrations somewhat in excess of those needed for anesthesia can be administered briefly without serious adverse effects. It is, however, flammable and explosive, and appropriate precautions are essential.

Cyclopropane. This potent anesthetic gas is administered together with adequate amounts of oxygen by means of the closed system method. Inhalation of the gas for only 2 or 3 minutes induces surgical anesthesia with minimal struggling. Muscular relaxation is good but may require supplementation with neuromuscular blocking drugs in some cases. It does not cause nearly as much nausea as ether postoperatively, nor does it irritate the lining of the respiratory tract during induction.

Although cardiac arrhythmias can occur during

cyclopropane anesthesia, it is considered to be a relatively safe drug when the patient is properly ventilated and closely observed. It is, in fact, often chosen for patients in poor physical condition, because it can maintain blood pressure at stable levels and because high concentrations of oxygen can be inhaled along with it. The decline in its use has occurred not from any lack of efficacy compared to other anesthetics nor from any greater potential toxicity but because of concern about possible accidents. Its safe use requires special precautions to prevent sparks from static electricity, because the gas is highly flammable, and its mixtures with oxygen are explosive.

Fluorinated anesthetics. Halogenation of hydrocarbons and ethers helps to make them nonflammable and nonexplosive. Chloroform, the first halogenated hydrocarbon anesthetic, is rarely used today despite these advantages. However, other compounds with high chemical stability but without the potential toxicity of chloroform are commonly employed because of their relative safety and efficacy.

Halothane (Fluothane) is the most widely used of the fluorinated compounds and is, in fact, the most commonly employed potent inhalation anesthetic. Its popularity stems from its many advantages over ether, cyclopropane, and other older agents. Halothane vapors produce rapid, pleasant induction of anesthesia and, because its effects are readily reversible, recovery is also rapid. The vapors do not irritate the respiratory mucosa nor cause increased salivary or bronchial secretions. Halothane is a preferred anesthetic for asthmatic patients, because it tends to dilate the bronchi. Nausea and vomiting do not ordinarily occur following recovery.

Despite these advantages, halothane falls short of being the ideal anesthetic. In addition to its lack of ability to produce adequate relaxation of abdominal and other skeletal muscles, the drug has several disadvantages that can lead to serious complications. The potency of halothane is so great that patients may pass quickly into states of very deep depression of respiration. Thus, a specially calibrated vaporizer is employed to keep the concentration of vapor being delivered to the patient within safe limits. Further, the anesthesiologist should have thorough training in the measures necessary to minimize potential toxicity, including the sharp sudden drops in blood pressure that sometimes develop as a result of adverse effects on cardiovascular function.

Hypotension occurs mainly as a result of a drug-induced reduction in cardiac output and, in part, because of peripheral arterial dilation. Halothane has a greater tendency than ether to depress myocardial contractility, but it is less likely to cause cardiac tachyarrhythmias than either chloroform or cyclopropane. The latter arrhythmias are best prevented by keeping the patient well oxygenated and by avoiding a buildup of carbon dioxide. Premedication with atropine helps to prevent bradycardia and hypotension during halothane induction, and ad-

ministration of catecholamines such as epinephrine is employed only very cautiously.

Some anesthesiologists experienced in employing halothane sometimes put its potentially adverse effects to good clinical use. They may, for example, deliberately use its hypotensive effect to reduce blood pressure and thus minimize bleeding during certain surgical procedures. Similarly, although halothane can cause relaxation of the uterus so excessive as to lead to uncontrolled hemorrhage following evacuation of the uterus, this action of the drug is sometimes useful in the management of special obstetric situations such as breech and version deliveries and manual removal of the infant or the placenta. Halothane is contraindicated for routine use in obstetric anesthesia, however, because the myometrium may then not respond to oxytocics such as ergot alkaloids and posterior pituitary extracts (Chap. 23).

The use of halothane anesthesia has in relatively rare instances been associated with development of hepatitis and with death from hepatic necrosis in about 50% of such cases. Hypersensitivity reactions to halothane of this type occur in only 1 in 10,000 patients to whom halothane is administered for the first time but in about 7 in 10,000 patients who are repeatedly exposed to this anesthetic, especially when any earlier administration has been accompanied by postanesthetic fever, jaundice, and elevation of white blood cells. Thus, many anesthesiologists avoid using halothane for several successive procedures within a brief period to guard against possible development of hepatic hypersensitivity reactions, and they generally employ another anesthetic for patients with a history of liver disorders.

Methoxyflurane (Penthrane) is the most potent available anesthetic—that is, it produces anesthesia at lower inhaled concentrations—but it is employed much less often than halothane. Unlike the latter, it produces induction of anesthesia quite slowly, and full recovery is also prolonged. It is customary to employ basal anesthetics such as nitrous oxide or thiopental (see below) for more rapid induction, prior to administering this anesthetic for maintaining surgical levels of anesthesia, and adjunctive neuromuscular junction blocking agents are recommended during anesthesia. Morphine and other opiates should not be administered preoperatively, because their use is not only unnecessary but may lead to rapid development of respiratory depression and apnea when this anesthetic is then inhaled. The long-lasting residual analgesia with methoxyflurane also makes narcotics unnecessary in the early postoperative period.

This anesthetic is much less likely than halothane to cause cardiac arrhythmias, and it has no adverse effects on uterine contractions when used during delivery. However, its use has occasionally been followed by liver necrosis, particularly in patients who have had previous exposures to it or to other halogenated anesthetics. Thus, it is best not repeated within a month of prior administration, and its use is contraindicated in patients who reacted to this and other halogenated anesthetics with an episode of fever or jaundice.

Renal failure following prolonged exposure to methoxyflurane is the most serious type of potential toxicity associated with this anesthetic. Patients' urinary outputs must be monitored following anesthesia to detect the production of a large volume of urine with a low specific gravity. Such polyuric kidney dysfunction resembles the disorder diabetes insipidus (Chap. 20). To reduce the possibility of renal injury, this anesthetic should not be employed during long-lasting procedures, nor in the large amounts required for skeletal muscle relaxation when the drug is not supplemented by peripherally acting relaxants. It should not be used in patients taking tetracycline for infection, because fatal kidney toxicity has resulted from concurrent use of the two drugs. Methoxyflurane may also increase the adverse renal effects of potentially nephrotoxic antibiotics such as the aminoglycosides, polymyxins, and amphotericin B (Chaps. 8 and 9).

Enflurane (Ethrane), a more recently introduced fluorinated anesthetic, has not so far been reported to cause renal or hepatic injury, and it does not cause the bradycardia or other signs of cardiovascular depression that sometimes occur with halothane. However, like other halogenated anesthetics, it sensitizes the myocardium to the fibrillating effects of epinephrine in animals. Thus, use of that and other potent catecholamines is not recommended during enflurane anesthesia.

Like halothane, this anesthetic produces rapid induction of anesthesia, usually followed by quick recovery. It can be used for prolonged procedures that require profound muscular relaxation, including cholecystectomy and total gastrectomy. In such situations, anesthesia is maintained with lower concentrations of enflurane than were necessary for induction to avoid depression of respiration and of the circulation. Inhalation of too high concentrations of this anesthetic can also cause such signs of central motor system stimulation as twitching movements in the muscles of the jaw, neck, and extremities. To avoid this, the anesthesia should be lightened when signs of seizure activity are detected on the electroencephalogram. The lower concentration of the anesthetic should then be supplemented with a small dose of a peripherally acting skeletal muscle relaxant to maintain the desired degree of relaxation required during prolonged abdominal surgery.

The newest of the fluorinated ethers, *isoflurane* (Forane), is claimed to be much less likely than halothane and related drugs to cause cardiac arrhythmias, even when epinephrine is administered during anesthesia. It is also said not to cause the type of increased CNS excitability seen with high concentrations of enflurane. Surgical anesthesia is accompanied by good skeletal muscle relaxation, and peripherally acting relaxants are markedly potentiated in the presence of isoflurane.

Basal anesthetics

Various substances are available that can produce complete anesthesia only when given in doses that may cause deep respiratory or cardiovascular depression. Other central depressant drugs lack the ability to produce one or another of the components of complete anesthesia, even at the highest dose levels. Despite their inadequacies in comparison to the potent inhalation anesthetics discussed above, however, some of these substances—in particular, nitrous oxide and thiopental sodium—are among the most important drugs employed in modern anesthesiology.

Administered alone (whether by inhalation, injection, or the rectal route), these drugs produce one or more of the effects desired in an anesthetic, and these effects can be employed to produce unconsciousness or to relieve pain in various procedures. In addition, the anesthesiologist often builds on the drug-induced basal state by administering other drugs that supply components of full anesthesia that the first drugs may lack. In this way, it becomes possible to perform any surgical procedure while maintaining the patient in the higher planes of anesthesia and with greater safety than when potent inhalation anesthetics are employed to produce degrees of surgical anesthesia deep enough to depress skeletal muscular and other reflexes.

Intravenously administered barbiturates and nonbarbiturate depressant drugs have several advantages over inhalation anesthetics. Most important is their ability to produce rapid, smooth, and pleasant loss of consciousnss. The patient's recovery also occurs quickly and without the discomforting effects that often accompany arousal from inhalation anesthesia. Injected in appropriate doses, these drugs are not likely to cause excessive depression of vital functions. On the other hand, inadvertent overdosage can be very dangerous.

The volatile anesthetics are considered safer than those given by vein, because the anesthesiologist can more readily control the elimination of any excess drug. As soon as signs of overdosage are recognized, the mask can be removed from the patient's face. As long as the patient is still breathing and the blood is circulating, each exhaled breath rids the body of some of the anesthetic, and the amount in the brain begins to fall promptly to safer levels. Unlike the volatile anesthetics, which are almost always excreted chemically intact, the injectable or "fixed" anesthetics must be broken down by the body's own detoxifying mechanisms. Thus, the elimination of an overdose cannot be influenced by the anesthesiologist and takes much longer than the exhalation of volatile substances through the lungs.

The ultrashort-acting barbiturates are by far the most commonly employed agents administered by vein to produce unconsciousness, and thiopental is still the most widely used of these drugs. However, *methohexital* (Brevital) is claimed to offer certain advantages, including more rapid recovery of consciousness. Neither drug is a good analgesic, nor do they produce adequate skeletal muscle relaxation. Thus, after producing prompt loss of consciousness, IV administration of these drugs is frequently followed by inhalation of a nitrous oxide–oxygen mixture for reducing the patient's reflex responsiveness to painful stimuli. When muscular relaxation is required, it can be achieved by having the patient inhale a potent anesthetic such as halothane in much smaller amounts than would ordinarily be needed, or a peripherally acting neuromuscular blocking agent such as succinylcholine or *d*-tubocurarine may be used intravenously for this purpose following the IV barbiturate and inhalation of the anesthetic gas or volatile vapors.

As indicated earlier, despite their convenience, the IV barbiturates can cause serious systemic and local complications. The most immediately serious reaction is respiratory depression and even sudden apnea as a result of too rapid injection or use of too highly concentrated solutions, which then cannot be readily removed from the bloodstream. Thus, these drugs should be employed only when equipment for establishing an airway is available—an endotracheal tube and laryngoscope, for example—and when apparatus for suctioning and for mechanical ventilation is at hand.

Care is also required to prevent concentrated IV solutions from leaking into tissues outside the vein or from being injected into an artery. Thiopental sodium solutions are highly alkaline and can cause severe pain and damage to surrounding tissues that are inadvertently infiltrated. Occasionally, even the relatively resistant vein lining may be injured and become inflamed, but phlebitis is rarely followed by thrombosis and embolism. Much more serious is the damage that may result from an intraarterial injection, a rare accident but one that can cause arterial spasm, ischemia, and thrombosis that could lead to gangrene. Emergency measures must be promptly applied to prevent these local complications when the patient's reaction suggests that the solution has entered the brachial artery instead of the intended vein.

Other indications. In addition to being useful for basal anesthesia, the rapidity with which these ultrashort-acting barbiturates take effect also makes them valuable in the emergency treatment of acute convulsive states (Chaps. 47 and 50, and elsewhere). Convulsions caused by overdoses of CNS-stimulating drugs such as strychnine or of the local anesthetics can, for example, often be brought to a quick halt by the careful intravenous administration of thiopental-type agents. However, intravenously administered *diazepam* (Chaps. 45 and 48) is increasingly preferred in such situations because of its wider safety margin—that is, it can control convulsions without causing the excessive depression of respiration sometimes produced by barbiturates.

Thiopental is often used in psychiatry as part of the premedication procedure of patients who are to receive electroconvulsive therapy (ECT) for mental depression or schizophrenia (Chap. 46). Some psychiatrists also use IV barbiturates as disinhibiting drugs in the interviewing procedures known as "narcoanalysis" and "narcosynthesis." These are methods sometimes employed in psychiatric emergencies such as conversion hysteria to facilitate reaching the roots of a patient's emotional difficulties and to help him deal more effectively with them. The drug is injected slowly with the patient counting, until his speech becomes an indistinct mumble and then suddenly stops completely. This indicates that a stage of light surgical anesthesia has been reached. The slow infusion is then stopped, and the injected drug begins to be redistributed from the brain to other body tissues (Chap. 4). As the effects of the drug wear off, the drowsy patient becomes able to understand and respond to questions and, because the defenses are down, may say things that are usually suppressed. The interviewing psychiatrist tries to uncover previously hidden material that will help in making a diagnosis and in deciding on the direction that further psychotherapy should take. Psychiatrists who employ these techniques must be trained in the emergency resuscitative measures mentioned earlier, or—as is often the case when patients are being prepared for ECT—an anesthesiologist should be present to carry out intubation and artificial respiration if airway occlusion or apnea develops.

Rectal administration of thiopental and other barbiturates and nonbarbiturates is sometimes employed to produce basal narcosis, particularly in children.

Other nonbarbiturate anesthetics

Ketamine (Ketalar; Ketaject) is a nonbarbiturate injectable anesthetic. It is used both for induction prior to administration of more potent anesthetics and alone to prepare patients for minor surgical and diagnostic procedures. It produces profound analgesia and a peculiar mental state in which the patient appears to be awake and yet is unaware of what is taking place. This anesthetic state has been called *dissociative anesthesia*, because the patient seems disconnected from reality rather than asleep.

Injected slowly in the small doses adequate for induction and for carrying out painful or discomforting procedures, ketamine does not depress respiration or the cardiovascular system. Actually, the heart rate tends to increase, and blood pressure becomes elevated during induction. This offers an advantage over thiopental for patients with low blood pressure but may contraindicate the use of this anesthetic for those with a history of stroke or of severe hypertension.

Ketamine seems especially suited for use in infants and children who require repeated painful procedures such as changes of burn dressings, debridement of burn tissues, and skin grafts. It may also be employed for adults who must undergo discomforting diagnostic procedures such as pneumoencephalography or cardiac catheterization. It may even be used in preparing patients for cardiac surgery and for abdominal operations, but in such cases ketamine should be supplemented by a potent inhalation anesthetic such as halothane.

One drawback of this anesthetic, which is chemically related to the hallucinogenic drug *phencyclidine* (a veterinary anesthetic no longer manufactured because it became a human drug abuse problem), is that some patients become confused or excited and behave irrationally when emerging from anesthesia with this drug. To minimize reactions of this type, it is best to avoid stimulating the patient in any way during the recovery period. Preoperative administration of morphine or other opiates and postoperative administration of diazepam or of the butyrophenone-type neuroleptic agent droperidol (Chaps. 46 and 51) also help to prevent vivid dreams or hallucinations during recovery. Use of this agent is probably best avoided in patients with a history of chronic alcoholism. Outpatients should be released only after complete recovery from the anesthesia, and they should be accompanied home by a responsible adult.

Neuroleptanesthesia is a deeper extension of the state of neuroleptanalgesia that was described in Chapter 51. It is brought about by rapid IV drip administration of Innovar, which is then followed by inhalation of nitrous oxide–oxygen or more potent general anesthetics for maintaining surgical levels of anesthesia. Sometimes IV or IM injection of this droperidol–fentanyl combination is followed by administration of local anesthetic agents (Chap. 14).

Patients should be kept under close observation for 24 hours after the procedure. Although this light type of anesthesia is recommended for elderly, debilitated, and other low-risk patients, it can cause apneic periods. In addition to the usual equipment and measures for respiratory resuscitation, a narcotic antagonist such as naloxone should be readily available for repeated injection to counteract the effects of fentanyl, the potent narcotic component of the Innovar combination.

Etomidate (Amidate) is the newest of the nonbarbiturate intravenous agents to be approved for use in the United States (it has been used abroad for many years). It is ultrashort-acting and is used for inducing anesthesia. Advantages claimed for it include fewer adverse cardiopulmonary effects. It lacks analgesic activity and has caused pain on injection, as well as myoclonic muscle movements.

Earlier inhalation anesthetics that were once widely used in the same manner as nitrous oxide or the IV barbiturates but that are now rarely employed for induction of anesthesia or for brief pain relief include ethylene, trichloroethylene, vinyl ether, and ethyl chloride. Only ethylene is still used, and even that is used only rarely. The most common sequence of anesthetics and adjuncts used today is the following:

1. IV barbiturate induction, and
2. Nitrous oxide–oxygen inhalation for analgesia, followed if necessary by
3. A neuromuscular junction blocker such as succinylcholine, and
4. Inhalation of halothane, ether, or a fluorinated ether in relatively low concentrations

Additional clinical considerations

In addition to basal anesthetics, most patients still receive various nonanesthetic drugs intended to make the induction of surgical anesthesia proceed more smoothly. Centrally acting depressant drugs are employed to reduce natural preoperative anxiety and to put the patient in a state of emotional and mental relaxation. Certain other drugs that act at peripheral sites are used to reduce adverse reflex responses to the anesthetic and the surgical procedure.

Central depressant premedication

Various types of depressants are employed to help the patient remain calm and relaxed before being subjected to anesthesia and surgery. Patients who are fearful and apprehensive tend to struggle against going under anesthesia during induction. Those who have been properly premedicated with *sedative–hypnotics, antianxiety agents,* or other drugs with a tranquilizing component tend to slip more smoothly into a state of surgical anesthesia when they then inhale relatively low concentrations of a potent general anesthetic.

Preparing the patient mentally begins the night before the scheduled operation with administration of a hypnotic dose of a benzodiazepine (*e.g.,* flurazepam; Chapter 45), a short-acting barbiturate such as *pentobarbital* or *secobarbital,* or a *non*barbiturate sleep producer such as *chloral hydrate.* This is intended to give the patient a good night's rest before undergoing the stress of surgery.

Personal contact between the patient and medical and nursing personnel also helps to attain this objective. In many hospitals, the anesthesiologist visits the patient the night before surgery to give some explanation of what to expect. The patient may be told what type of anesthesia he will receive and how it will be administered. In addition to learning these facts, the patient gets an opportunity to see the anesthesiologist in person, instead of meeting for the first time in the operating room. This helps to develop the patient's confidence in the surgical team, and also affords the anesthesiologist the opportunity to assess the patient personally before administering the anesthetic. In this way, the most appropriate drug or combination of drugs can be individually planned.

Research has shown that patient teaching before surgery is an important aspect of total patient care. The patient needs to know the technical aspects of the procedure, but also what he will feel, what he will be expected to do after surgery, and an estimated time frame for the expected progress of recovery. Sharing this information with the patient has been shown to decrease anxiety, facilitate anesthesia, and decrease recovery time and the need for postoperative analgesia. Many institutions provide standardized, routine preoperative programs for all elective surgery patients. It is also important to remember that the patient undergoing emergency surgery needs the same information.

In the morning, about an hour before anesthesia and surgery, patients receive preanesthetic sedation. The dose should be high enough to prevent fear and apprehension but not so heavy as to depress the patient too deeply, because this could delay recovery after anesthesia. Some physicians prefer injectable antianxiety agents for this purpose, rather than barbiturates. For example, *hydroxyzine* (Atarax; Vistaril) may be administered intramuscularly, and *diazepam* (Valium) is also commonly employed to help patients go under the anesthetic more readily and to emerge from anesthesia with reduced restlessness and confusion.

These drugs are now often administered together with *regional* (e.g., *spinal* or *caudal*) anesthesia to reduce discomfort and anxiety during the procedure. They are also useful in obstetrics to smooth the course of labor and delivery. *Diazepam*, for instance, does not depress respiration in the mother or newborn baby as the narcotic analgesics do. Thus, its use reduces the dosage of *meperidine HCl* (Demerol) or *morphine* needed for pain relief.

Narcotic analgesics of this type have other disadvantages, including production of postoperative vomiting and depression of the cough reflex. They should not be employed routinely but only when the patient is expected to experience postoperative pain. This may occur with *halothane* (Fluothane) and *enflurane* (Ethrane), anesthetics that wear off quickly and leave little residual analgesia. Potent analgesics are often unnecessary when *ether* or *methoxyflurane* (Penthrane) has been employed because of the prolonged analgesic effects of these anesthetics.

Phenothiazine-type tranquilizers are also sometimes used preoperatively either alone or to potentiate the analgesic effects of *meperidine HCl* (Demerol) and other opioids. In addition to calming the patient, these drugs exert an antiemetic effect. However, drugs such as *chlorpromazine* (Thorazine), *promazine* (Sparine), and *triflupromazine* (Vesprin) may make the patient's blood pressure drop during anesthesia. Thus, many anesthesiologists now prefer to use these drugs *post*operatively to control actual vomiting, rather than to use them routinely as preoperative prophylaxis.

The preoperative use of combinations of tranquilizers such as the neuroleptic agent droperidol and the potent narcotic analgesic fentanyl to achieve the preoperative state called neuroleptanalgesia is discussed in the previous chapter, and the supplementation of these drugs with inhalation and regional anesthetics to produce neuroleptanesthesia was taken up above.

Peripherally acting premedication

Anticholinergic drugs (Chap. 16)—mainly atropine, scopolamine and, more recently, glycopyrrolate (Robinul)—are used for two main purposes:

1. To reduce excessive salivation and tracheobronchial secretions of the type that an anesthetic such as *ether* tends to stimulate strongly
2. To counteract the heart-slowing effects of vagal stimulation of the type caused by *halothane* during induction, or as a result of reflexes that are set off by the manipulation of internal organs in some types of surgical procedures

In addition, scopolamine produces central sedative and amnesic effects that are considered desirable in some clinical situations.

These drugs are not administered routinely, but only with anesthetics that are known to cause excessive secretions and bradycardia. This is because they not only produce unpleasant mouth dryness and blurring of vision, but can also cause restlessness and mental confusion, particularly in elderly patients or those suffering severe pain. They are also contraindicated in children with fever and in patients with coronary heart disease, cardiac arrhythmias, or thyrotoxicosis, who may react adversely to the increase in heart rate that these drugs tend to cause. Glycopyrrolate is claimed to cause less tachycardia than atropine, and—because it does not pass the blood-brain barrier—it is said not to produce the undesired central effects of the natural belladonna alkaloids.

Other adjunctive drugs. The anesthesiologist makes use of these and other peripherally acting medications to cope with situations that arise during surgical procedures and in the postoperative period. Anticholinergic drugs, for example, may be used to counteract laryngospasm and bronchospasm and to prevent aspiration of stomach acids into the lungs, a complication that could lead to cardiac arrest. The antiarrhythmic drugs procainamide, lidocaine, and propranolol (Chap. 30) are sometimes employed to overcome ventricular tachycardia and other rapid, irregular rhythms that can develop during anesthesia and operative procedures—for example, following sensitization of the myocardium to epinephrine and other catecholamines in patients who have been anesthetized with a halogenated hydrocarbon or with cyclopropane.

Neostigmine and other anticholinesterase-type cholinergic drugs (Chap. 15) are sometimes used to counteract the effects of the curare-type neuromuscular blocking agents (Chap. 19), which, as has been indicated, are often used to bring about skeletal muscle relaxation while the patient is maintained in a state of relatively light surgical anesthesia. These and other cholinergic drugs may also be useful for overcoming postoperative weakness of visceral smooth muscles. For example, they are sometimes administered to patients suffering from abdominal distention and urinary retention. By stimulating the smooth muscles of the intestine and the urinary bladder to resume their stalled peristaltic activity, these drugs help to relieve the discomfort caused by retained gases and wastes.

Postanesthesia measures

The frequency of these complications and those caused by the cholinergic drugs can be reduced by various nursing measures instituted in the postanesthetic period. In the immediate postoperative period, the patient is usually positioned on his side with no pillow and with the head of the bed flat. This position facilitates the drainage of secretions and helps to decrease the risk of aspiration of secretions and vomitus, if vomiting should occur. In some cases, the patient will need to be suctioned mechanically if the secretions are copious and the consciousness level returns slowly to normal.

The patient's vital signs should be monitored frequently to detect any adverse response to the anesthesia or the surgery. Early signs of hemorrhage (*e.g.,* tachycardia, blood pressure changes), or of respiratory problems (*e.g.,* rales, increased respiratory rate) can be detected and immediate therapeutic action taken to prevent more serious complications from developing.

Comfort and safety measures should be provided and continued until the patient has fully recovered from the effects of the anesthesia. Such measures include temperature control, skin care measures, protection from falls (use of side rails is often hospital policy), analgesia to alleviate postoperative pain, pulmonary toilet (turning, deep breathing, vigorous coughing, cupping, and postural draining, if needed) to facilitate the removal of respiratory secretions that have accumulated during anesthesia, control of environmental stimuli, early ambulation and movement to decrease the risk of the complications associated with immobility, positioning to alleviate abdominal pain and flatus, and early measures to facilitate voiding and return of bowel function. All these nursing interventions should be incorporated into the total care of the patient, with specific activities focused on the interventions appropriate for each patient's particular needs.

The patient teaching guide summarizes the points that should be incorporated into the preoperative teaching program of a patient who is to receive a general anesthetic. Such a teaching program should be designed to meet the needs of each individual patient as determined by the underlying medical conditions and the surgery being performed. The patient will also need support and encouragement to cope with the procedure and the recovery process. As mentioned earlier, research has shown that effective patient teaching, and the support offered through teaching programs, have decreased the complications of surgery, facilitated anesthesia, and improved patient recovery.

Patient teaching guide: preoperative considerations with general anesthesia

The following points should be incorporated into the overall preoperative teaching program, which is designed around each patient's specific needs.

1. Procedure
   a. Type of surgery being performed
   b. Details of procedure, especially site of incision
   c. Implications for normal function
   d. Anticipated length of procedure

2. Medications
   a. Preoperative medications: when they will be given and route; what reaction the patient should expect (*e.g.,* dry mouth, drowsiness); other related procedures (*e.g.,* use of side rails, environmental controls)
   b. Anesthesia: when it will be given and route; what reaction the patient should expect (*e.g.,* dizziness, floating, loss of consciousness); other related procedures (*e.g.,* positioning, intubation, monitoring)

3. Postoperative measures
   a. Where the patient will regain consciousness

(continued)

b. Pain to anticipate
c. Tubes, stitches, clips, dressings, etc., to anticipate
d. Positioning for safety reasons
e. Frequent monitoring to assess recovery
g. Need to turn, cough, deep breathe
h. Need for early ambulation
i. Need for measures to facilitate return of bladder and bowel function
j. Medications that will be available, and when to ask for them
k. Comfort measures that will be used to alleviate discomfort
l. Anticipated progress of recovery

Summary of the characteristics of an ideal general inhalation anesthetic

The anesthetic should possess physical properties that make it nonflammable and nonexplosive:

1. It should not react chemically with the alkali used for absorbing carbon dioxide in closed anesthesia systems.
2. It should not have a corrosive effect on metallic equipment or damage rubber or plastic materials.
3. It should be chemically stable when stored indefinitely in clear glass containers without the need to add any stabilizers.

The vapor or gas should *not* be irritating to the respiratory mucosa or skin, and the patient should *not* be aware of any pungent, unpleasant odor in the few moments before losing consciousness.

Induction of the surgical stage of anesthesia should occur rapidly and easily. The excitement stage should be brief and free of excessive psychomotor activity, salivation, or bronchial secretions of the type that cause pharyngeal and laryngeal hyperreflexia, marked by coughing, gagging, laryngospasm, or bronchospasm.

The anesthetic should be potent enough to produce full anesthesia (unconsciousness, analgesia, and skeletal muscle relaxation) when inhaled in a low concentration that allows inhalation of oxygen in adequate amounts at the same time.

Recovery of consciousness should be rapid after the anesthetic is discontinued. The patient should *not* be confused, excited, disoriented, or subject to hallucinations. Thought processes should be lucid, and there should be no discomforting feelings such as dizziness, heaviness, headache, grogginess, or pain. Nausea and vomiting should not occur, and appetite should return promptly.

The anesthetic should not adversely affect vital functions during induction or prolonged maintenance of deep surgical planes:

1. It should *not* cause cardiac depression or arrhythmias, even when catecholamines such as epinephrine are administered, but both heart rate and blood pressure should remain stable.
2. The rate and depth of respiration should *not* become excessively depressed but, if this does occur, it should be easy for the anesthesiologist to take over the respiration with mechanical ventilation measures.
3. It should not adversely affect brain metabolism or set off electroencephalic abnormalities and seizure activity.

The anesthetic should have no adverse post-anesthesia effects on such vital organs as the liver and kidneys (*i.e.*, it should not be hepatotoxic, nephrotoxic, or adversely affect other parenchymatous organs, metabolic processes, or laboratory tests).

Summary of the stages and planes of anesthesia (the anesthetic syndrome)*

Stage I: Early induction
Consciousness becomes progressively clouded.
The patient's awareness of sensory stimuli is disrupted:
Sight, hearing, and other perceptions are distorted

Feelings of floating and numbness
Analgesia (loss of pain sensation) may be profound with some anesthetics (*e.g.*, ether; methoxyflurane†)
Complete loss of consciousness marks the end of this stage.

Stage II: Delirium or excitement

Patient is unconscious but may show signs of psychomotor excitement, which are the result of drug-induced depression of inhibitory areas of the CNS.

Respiratory and cardiovascular reflexes may be hyperactive.

No surgical procedures are carried out. Efforts are made to minimize excitement and to protect the patient from injury.

Stage III: Surgical anesthesia

Begins with a change from irregular to regular breathing and a loss of eyelid reflexes.

Artificially divided into four planes to indicate an increasing depth of anesthesia:

Plane 1. Eyeball movements; regular breathing

Plane 2. Eyeballs fixed; breathing less deep or full; skeletal muscle tone reduced

Plane 3. Chest breathing shallow; abdominal respiration deeper; no wink response when the cornea is touched

Plane 4. Chest breathing stops; abdominal breathing becomes increasingly shallow.

Stage IV: Medullary paralysis

Respiration ceases; cardiovascular collapse may occur if respiratory arrest is not corrected by resuscitative measures.

* This classic (Guedel) pattern applies mainly to ether anesthesia. It varies somewhat when other anesthetics are employed (*e.g.,* the first two stages are scarcely seen when anesthesia is induced with a rapid-acting barbiturate, and the response to methoxyflurane follows quite a different pattern).

† Guidelines developed for this drug include five levels of deepening anesthesia. Analgesia and loss of consciousness occur at level 3, which is similar to stage III. However, analgesia also is evident earlier, while the patient is still conscious (*i.e.,* at level 2, which corresponds to stage I of the classic pattern).

Drug digests

Cyclopropane USP (Trimethylene)

Actions and indications. This potent gas can promptly produce complete anesthesia. Recovery is also rather rapid. It has a relatively wide safety margin when inhaled in amounts that provide good analgesia and adequate muscle relaxation. It can be used prior to every type of surgical operation and is said to be particularly useful for patients in shock because of the stability of the blood pressure. (The pressure may even rise slightly because of sympathetic nervous system stimulation.)

Adverse effects, cautions, and contraindi- cations. Postoperative headache is common, as is nausea and vomiting. Delirium may also develop during recovery, but can be prevented by pretreatment with a potent analgesic. Respiratory acidosis sometimes occurs and this, in turn, may lead to vasodilation, a fall in blood pressure, and reflex tachycardia.

Cardiac irregularities may be precipitated by the administration of epinephrine or other catecholamines and adrenergic vasopressor drugs, particularly if patients are not adequately oxygenated, or if carbon dioxide levels have been allowed to rise. This gas is flammable and explosive.

Dosage and administration. The gas is administered by means of a closed or semiclosed system provided with carbon dioxide-absorbing chemicals. Induction of anesthesia may require 15 to 30 vol% of gas, which may then be reduced to lower levels for maintaining adequate analgesia. The gas may have to be supplemented with a neuromuscular blocking agent when a lower volume percent is employed. Atropine premedication is desirable.

Ether USP (ethyl ether; diethyl ether)

Actions and indications. This is a potent general anesthetic that produces excellent analgesia and skeletal muscle relaxation when inhaled in low concentrations. Analgesia sufficient for the performance of major surgery can be achieved with low blood and brain levels that have little or no effect on vital functions. Other safety factors include the following: (1) the drug can stimulate respiration reflexly and thus antagonize its direct depressant effect on the respiratory center; (2) it stimulates the sympathetic cardioacceleratory mechanism, which counteracts the drug's direct depressant effect on the myocardium; (3) ether does not sensitize the heart to epinephrine or other catecholamines, so cardiac arrhythmias rarely occur during ether anesthesia; (4) it is not toxic to liver tissues.

Adverse effects, cautions, and contraindi- cations. Ether is irritating to the respiratory mucosa and stimulates the flow of bronchial and salivary secretions. This tends to interfere with inhalation of the vapors and to slow further an induction period that is relatively prolonged because of the drug's relatively high solubility in blood. (Ether is flammable and explosive.)

Recovery from ether anesthesia is also relatively slow, and postoperative nausea and vomiting are common. Gastrointestinal tone and motility are decreased postoperatively, and urinary output is reduced during anesthesia. The dosage of adjunctive neuromuscular blocking agents should be reduced to avoid prolonged paralysis. Caution is required in patients receiving high doses of antibiotics such as kanamycin, polymyxin, and colistimethate, which possess neuromuscular blocking properties.

Dosage and administration. The amount needed to produce anesthesia varies with the age and condition of the patient and the depth of anesthesia required for the surgical procedure that is to be performed. Higher vapor concentrations (10 to 15 vol%) are employed during induction than are required for maintenance of anesthesia (5 vol%). The blood level for analgesia is as low as 10 to 15 mg%, but between 80 and 100 mg% is required for maintaining surgical planes of anesthesia.

Halothane USP (Fluothane)

Actions and indications. The vapors of this nonflammable liquid produce rapid induction of anesthesia with little excitement, respiratory tract irritation, salivation, nausea, or vomiting. It tends to produce bronchodilation rather than bronchospasm. It may be used to lower blood pressure deliberately to produce a bloodless surgical field. Its relaxant effect on the uterine musculature may be useful in some obstetric situations.

Adverse effects, cautions, and contraindications. Halothane often produces hypotension and bradycardia, and occasionally causes cardiac arrhythmias, particularly in the presence of epinephrine and other catecholamines. Neuromuscular blocking agents of the tubocurarine type may intensify the fall in blood pressure while use of succinylcholine may add to the drug's heart-slowing tendency.

Liver damage may occur, particularly if this anesthetic is employed repeatedly over a short period of time. Patients who develop fever and vomiting after exposure to halothane should not be anesthetized with it again, because fatal hepatic necrosis has occurred in such cases. Relaxation of the uterine musculature may inhibit normal labor.

Dosage and administration. A special vaporizer is employed to control the concentration of vapors delivered to the lungs. Surgical levels of anesthesia are induced by administering a 2 to 2.5% concentration of the vapors in a stream of nitrous oxide–oxygen mixture. This is then reduced to a level of 0.5 to 1.5% for maintenance of anesthesia. Atropine premedication is desirable to prevent bradycardia. Intravenous barbiturates administered for basal narcosis reduce the concentration of halothane required for induction.

Nitrous oxide USP (dinitrogen monoxide; N_2O)

Actions and indications. This inorganic gas has only low potency when inhaled alone, and thus must be supplemented by more potent anesthetics and by other adjunctive drugs to attain the objectives of complete anesthesia. However, high concentrations inhaled for a brief period produce analgesia and unconsciousness (plane 1, stage III anesthesia) within 1 or 2 minutes. Recovery occurs rapidly after brief exposure to the unsupplemented gas.

Inhalation of nitrous oxide mixed with an equal concentration of oxygen is commonly employed prior to dental surgery, and similar mixtures of 65:35 N_2O–O_2 combinations are employed in obstetrics during the second stage of labor. Its use prior to inhalation of more potent anesthetics such as halothane, ether, and methoxyflurane permits employment of low concentrations of the latter anesthetics during prolonged procedures.

Adverse effects, cautions, and contraindications. Hypoxia can occur with concentrations above 65 to 70% if these are maintained for more than brief periods. Hypoxia may also occur during recovery following prolonged use of nitrous oxide if the patient breathes only room air. Thus, patients should inhale 100% oxygen for the first 5 to 10 minutes after inhalation of nitrous oxide is stopped. Prevention of hypoxia is particularly important in patients with sickle cell anemia, hypertension, and ischemic heart disease. When used for brief periods in low to moderate concentrations, this gas does not cause nausea, vomiting, salivation, or respiratory tract irritation, and it has no adverse effects on the heart, liver, or kidneys.

Dosage and administration. Nitrous oxide is inhaled together with oxygen through a tight face mask. Concentrations of nitrous oxide should not ordinarily exceed 80%, even for brief procedures. During more prolonged procedures, mixtures containing as little as 20% nitrous oxide may be employed, provided that the patient has been premedicated with adequate doses of such adjunctive drugs as ultrashort-acting barbiturates, opioid analgesics, or neuroleptic agents such as phenothiazines or the butyrophenone droperidol.

Thiopental sodium USP (pentothal sodium)

Actions and indications. This rapid-acting barbiturate produces sleep within 1 minute when injected intravenously in a hypnotic dose. Recovery from a single such dose is also rapid with this ultrashort-acting barbiturate. However, repeated doses may accumulate in the body's fat depots, resulting in prolonged unconsciousness.

Thiopental does not produce complete general anesthesia, because it does not possess good analgesic or skeletal muscle relaxant properties. It is used alone only for maintaining the patient in an unconscious state while certain procedures of short duration (15 minutes) are being carried out. It is most commonly employed to produce basal narcosis prior to administration of a more potent general anesthetic, or in combination with nitrous oxide–oxygen mixtures and narcotic analgesics or regional anesthetics.

In addition to its use in anesthesia to induce light levels of depression, thiopental is sometimes employed in the emergency management of drug-induced convulsions. It has been employed in psychiatry in the procedures called narcoanalysis and narcosynthesis.

Adverse effects, cautions, and contraindications. Overdose may result in respiratory center depression and cardiac arrhythmias. Thus, resuscitative equipment, including oxygen and an endotracheal tube for maintaining an open airway, must always be available. The drug also sometimes causes coughing, bronchospasm and laryngospasm, particularly in patients with asthma in whom it must be employed with caution, if at all. It is also relatively contraindicated in patients who may suffer prolonged central depression, myxedema, and increased intracranial pressure.

Dosage and administration. For induction of anesthesia, the drug is injected IV in a dose of 2 or 3 ml of a 2.5% solution (50 to 75 mg), followed by further intermittent injections at intervals of 30 to 60 seconds as needed. The average amount required for adult men is 200 to 400 mg, and for women and children 150 to 300 mg.

The drug is also available in a form for rectal administration in doses ranging from 1 g/75 lb of body weight to 1 g/50 lb. The total dose for children should not exceed 1 g, and for adults of even above average weight, no more than 3 or 4 g is administered by this route.

References

Conahan TJ: New intravenous anesthetics. Surg Clin N Am 55:851, 1975

DiPalma JR: Use of the newer anesthetics. RN 36:47 1973

Dykes MHM, Bunker JP: Hepatoxicity and anesthetics. Pharmacol Physicians 4:1, 1970

Eger EI: Isoflurane. Semin Anesth 1:1, 1982

Elliott E et al: Ketamine anesthesia for medical procedures in children. Arch Dis Child 5:56, 1976

Etomidate for induction of anesthesia. Med Lett Drugs Ther 25:71, 1983

Gronert GA: Malignant hyperthermia. Anesthesiology 53:395, 1980

Linde HW et al: The search for better anesthetic agents: Clinical investigation of Ethrane. Anesthesiology 32:555, 1970

Marshall BE, Wollman H: General anesthetics. In Gilman AG, Goodman LS, Gilman A (eds): Goodman & Gilman's The Pharmacological Basis of Therapeutics, 6th ed, pp 276–299. New York, Macmillan, 1980

Mazze RI et al: Renal dysfunction associated with methoxyflurane anesthesia. JAMA 216:278, 1971

Mazze RI et al: Methoxyflurane metabolism. Anesthesiology 44:369, 1976

Ramamurthy S et al: Glycopyrrolate as a substitute for atropine: A preliminary report. Anesth Analg (Cleve) 50:732, 1971

Rapper EM: The pharmacologic basis of anesthesiology. Clin Pharmacol Ther 2:141, 1961

Rodman MJ: Drugs used in anesthesia. RN 33:53, 1970

Salem MR: Therapeutic uses of ganglionic blocking drugs. Int Anesthesiol Clin 16:171, 1978

Smith NT, Miller RD, Corbascio AN (eds): Drug Interactions in Anesthesia. Philadelphia, Lea & Febiger, 1981

Stanley TH: High-dose narcotic anesthesia. Semin Anesth 1:21, 1982

Ward CM et al: An appraisal of ketamine in the dressing of burns. Postgrad Med 52:222, 1976

Section 8
Part 4

Alcoholism
and
drug
abuse

Chapter 53

Alcoholism
and
drug
abuse

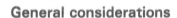

53

General considerations

The use of drugs for nonmedical purposes is very common in American society. People take drugs without medical supervision for various reasons, and drug-taking behavior patterns differ in ways that often determine the seriousness of drug misuse or abuse. Some young people, for example, experiment with drugs only occasionally out of curiosity or because of peer group pressure to do so. The vast majority do not get deeply involved with drugs as a result of such exposure, but some continue to take one or more drugs in increasing doses to a degree that leads to severe physical and social disability.

The spread of drug abuse to younger groups has been one of the startling phenomena of the 1970s and 1980s. Once limited to certain relatively small subcultures, the use of drugs to get "high" has reached epidemic proportions. Now, not only college-age young people but many at the high school and junior high school levels are regularly involved with various drugs.

This indiscriminate use of drugs by youngsters may turn out to be only a passing fad. More probably, however, drug abuse will continue to be a major public health and social problem. This seems likely because so many people in our society are turning to drugs for escape and for the transient relief of tension that some drugs offer. This has, of course, been true in all times and places. However, no other era has offered such a variety of potent drugs that could alter people's moods, perceptions, and behavior.

The nurse's role
The nurse has an important part to play in helping people and communities to cope with problems arising from the improper use of drugs. Some nurses have a greater responsibility than others—for example, those involved in specific programs aimed at detoxifying and rehabilitating addicts, and nurses in school and pediatric clinic settings who instruct others about the dangers of drug abuse. However, *all* nurses should know the pharmacologic facts and be aware of the social issues that are involved so that they can work with other professionals—physicians, social workers, teachers, and clergy—in handling the personal and public health problems that arise from drug abuse.

Useful information
Drug abuse is an extremely complex problem to which there is no simple solution. Many professionals are concerned with the problems posed by drug misuse. To answer all questions that arise, a person would have to be an authority not only in pharmacology and medicine, but also in the behavioral sciences, such as psychology and sociology, and in such specialties as law and criminology. Often, in fact, the various experts find themselves in violent disagreement when they have to work together. Controversy and disagreement seem to mark most efforts to deal with the medical, legal, and social aspects of drug abuse.

Nevertheless, the nurse who often is called on to help by instructing people and by answering their questions about drug problems has an opportunity to make a valuable contribution. This chapter is intended to furnish a general foundation on which the student can build, and thus acquire the detailed knowledge needed in the role of counselor on personal and community drug abuse problems. After first indicating certain significant aspects of these problems while defining some of the commonly employed terms, this chapter will describe the several most common types of abused drugs:

1. The potent narcotic analgesics—drugs derived from opium, such as heroin and morphine, and synthetic drugs with similar actions

2. The general depressant drugs, including alcohol, the barbiturates, and other sedative–hypnotics and antianxiety drugs, and various inhalable vapors

3. The psychomotor stimulants, including cocaine, the amphetamines, and related drugs

4. The hallucinogens or psychotomimetics, such as LSD, mescaline, and others

5. Other drugs that defy easy classification, such as the cannabis derivatives— marihuana and hashish—and the belladonna derivatives.

More detailed discussions of the pharmacologic effects of the first three of the above drug groups, which have medical applications in the drug therapy of various disorders, will be found in Chapters 51, 45, and 47, respectively, and elsewhere in the text (see Index).

Here, however, the emphasis will mainly be on the effects of these drugs when they are being misused and abused. For each drug class, the following types of information will be furnished:

1. The acute effects—what a person feels when under the influence of each of these drugs and the behavior when intoxicated

2. The chronic effects—the physical and mental changes, including medical and psychiatric complications that may result from long-term misuse of drugs

3. The management of the patient suffering from the acute and chronic intake of and withdrawal from excessive amounts of the various types of abused drugs

The nurse who knows these facts about the effects of the most widely abused drugs will be able to teach people more effectively and be better able to answer most questions asked by concerned parents and others. However, to gain perspective on the controversial public issues that arise, the nurse must continue to read widely about the many and varied aspects of the drug abuse problem.

Definition of terms

Before studying the various classes of abused drugs, it is important to know the meanings of the commonly employed terms. Unfortunately, the disagreement and controversy that characterize so many aspects of the drug abuse problem extend even to the very meanings of the words used to describe the various degrees of involvement with drugs. In the discussion that follows, examples will be used whenever possible to explain more clearly the meaning of various terms and the problems that arise in their use.

Drug misuse refers mainly to the improper use of common medications in ways that can lead to acute and chronic toxicity. This type of drug taking is caused by ignorance rather than by any desire to get "high." However, the unsupervised use of self-administered *non*prescription-type medications can lead to various types of harmful consequences. For example, people who think that they cannot have a bowel movement unless they take a daily laxative soon suffer from chronic constipation caused by their misuse of strong cathartic drugs (Chap. 41). Chronic misuse of headache remedies has also led to gastrointestinal bleeding and kidney damage (Chap. 37).

Substances that are not usually medicines at all are also widely used and misused. Alcoholic beverages, for instance, are used by an estimated 75 million Americans. Most people who indulge in social drinking suffer no harm from this drug, which is merely a mild sedative or tension reliever in small doses, but even a person who usually takes care to control alcohol intake may sometimes misuse this chemical with consequences that are unpleasant (*e.g.*, hangover, vomiting) or even dangerous (*e.g.*, automobile accidents). Thus, even the occasional use of a chemical for either medicinal or recreational purposes exposes a person to risks resulting from its potential for misuse.

Drug abuse goes well beyond mere misuse. The term is rather hard to define, because its meaning depends in part on what most people in a particular society think is abusive in another person's pattern of drug-taking behavior. In general, however, people become concerned when they realize that someone is taking too much of a drug, either continually or periodically. A person who drinks alcoholic beverages and shows signs of being even moderately intoxicated at times when most people expect him to be sober—at work, for instance—may be considered a drug abuser. So may someone who goes on frequent sprees or binges, even though he may function more or less normally most of the time.

A person is most likely to be labeled a drug abuser when the substance that is chronically used to excess is *not* one that most other people use for recreational purposes. Thus, the behavior of a person who drinks too much alcohol may be tolerated in our society, but the behavior of another person who takes several tablets of a prescription-type medication such as a barbiturate to reach the same state of intoxication will commonly be labeled drug abuse. However, until recently, people who smoked cigarettes excessively were not the objects of scorn, let alone labeled "abusers," even though their need to feel the effects of nicotine could cause lung damage and lead to the development of other clinical disorders. The attitude of society toward cigarette smokers has recently begun to change from acceptance to actual hostility, in part because of the belief that nonsmokers can be harmed by exposure to tobacco smoke. (Evidence is accumulating that supports this belief.) The change over time in what society considers to be drug abuse is another indication that the term lacks precise and absolute definition.

Drug dependence denotes a further stage in an abuser's involvement with the drug that has been taken continuously or periodically. Different drugs cause dependence of varying types and degrees. In general, however, it can be said that the drug-dependent person has lost the ability to keep his drug intake under control. As a result, such a person finds it hard to function when not under the influence of the drug. At the same time, the large doses of some drugs that may be taken tend to disrupt mental and physical functioning to a degree that makes it difficult to behave in a socially acceptable way. Drugs can cause either *psychological* or *physical* dependence, or dependence of both types together.

Psychological dependence of the most severe type is marked by a craving for the feeling that the drug produces. The user's compulsive desire to experience the pleasurable state that the drug induces is so great that all other goals and sources of satisfaction are often given up. Some psychiatrists have suggested that people who can become drug-dependent to this degree must be suffering from a personality disorder to begin with. However, no one knows why some emotionally or psychologically disturbed people become drug-dependent while others do not, and there is reason to think that some drugs may set off dependence-producing behavior in some seemingly stable people.*

Habituation is a term now often used to denote a much milder degree of psychological dependence. Anyone can form a habit of this type with one chemical or another—the caffeine in coffee, for example. A person who has such a habit simply feels better when taking the chemical than when not taking it, and so tends to continue taking it even when aware that its use may be detrimental to health. Thus, cigarette smokers may be unhappy about the chronic cough and other symptoms of their habituation to nicotine without being willing to give up the habit. However, unlike the case in more severe degrees of psychological dependence, most people habituated to nicotine *can* stop smoking without experiencing truly severe mental and emotional discomfort.† Similarly, a person may habitually take a barbiturate or other prescribed hypnotic, because he thinks that he won't sleep well without it. However, if the physician decides to discontinue the drug, the patient—if he has a more or less normal personality and average emotional stability—does not show the type of compulsive drug-seeking behavior that characterizes the truly dependence-prone person.

Physical dependence is a state that develops in people who have been taking certain drugs continuously. The term implies that an abstinence or withdrawal syndrome (see below) will occur when prolonged use of the drug is abruptly stopped. Physical dependence is particularly likely to occur in those who have become tolerant to the desired drug effect and who take increasingly greater doses to gain the feeling that they seek. Taking the drug in large amounts for varying periods of time tends to produce biochemical changes, particularly in the tissues of the nervous system. These nerve cells soon seem to require the drug's presence to keep functioning normally. When the person is deprived of the drug, and its level in the body begins to drop, the resulting malfunctioning of various systems sets off a series of discomforting signs and symptoms.

The *withdrawal syndromes* that then develop differ depending on the *type* of drug on which the person has become physically dependent, and on the *amount* of the drug that the drug abuser has been taking continually over a period of time. Thus, an opiate-dependent person suffers a characteristic pattern of ill effects when the drug is withdrawn, which is different from the typical abstinence syndrome that develops when a physically dependent barbiturate abuser is deprived of the drug. Also, the discomfort caused by withdrawal of either type of drug is mild in a person who has been steadily taking only relatively low doses; it may be quite severe in a person who has been taking high doses of the same drug for a longer time.

Addiction is a term that has been used in so many different ways that it is no longer very meaningful. Some call a drug addicting when it can cause physical dependence manifested by a withdrawal syndrome when it is discontinued. Others consider a drug to be addicting when people taking it tend to lose control over their intake and become obsessively involved in drug-seeking behavior. Such a compulsive degree of psychological dependence is indeed an important characteristic of addiction. In fact, drug abusers who have undergone drug withdrawal and who are no longer physically dependent tend to relapse readily, because they are still psychologically dependent.

Actually, however, in discussing drug abuse of the type formerly referred to as addiction because of such elements as compulsive use to satisfy a craving or to avoid physical discomfort, total involvement in drug-seeking and drug-taking behavior, and the high frequency of relapse, it is now thought to be least confusing to use the

---

* It is relevant to note that not only human beings but also experimental animals (*e.g.*, rodents, primates, of many species), given access to drugs that humans seek, will work to obtain the drug—for example, they will press a bar in their cage to release a dose of drug from a drinking tube—and will sometimes even give themselves lethal doses of certain drugs in this way to satisfy their apparent craving.

---

† The subject of habitual cigarette smoking will not be dealt with further in this chapter. Many references have been made throughout this book to adverse effects of cigarette use on disease states, and to drug–cigarette smoking interactions. The difficulty that some people experience in giving up cigarette smoking is perhaps underscored by the recent FDA approval given to nicotine-containing chewing gum (Nicorette) to aid patients in medically supervised behavioral modification programs to stop smoking.

general term *dependence*. Because drugs differ in the types of dependence they cause, the type of drug dependence that is meant can then be specified. Thus, drugs will be described as causing *dependence of the opiate type*, or *dependence of the barbiturate type*, or *dependence of the amphetamine type*. Such usage also helps to describe the dependence-producing potential of any *new* drug more specifically than simply saying that it is "addicting." It is important to remember, however, that not all drug dependence leads to compulsive drug-seeking behavior. Thus, as pointed out in Chapter 51, most patients who become physically dependent on narcotic analgesics while hospitalized do not seek to continue the drug experience when they are withdrawn from the drug and discharged from the hospital.

Table 53-1 summarizes the characteristics of dependence on the major classes of drugs described in this chapter.

Opiate-type dependence

Addiction to the potent narcotic analgesics (Chap. 51) is commonly considered to be the most serious form of drug abuse. *Heroin* is the opiate alkaloid with the widest illicit use. *Morphine* and the synthetic analgesic *meperidine HCl* (Demerol) are sometimes used by persons—including physicians, nurses, and pharmacists—who have ready access to medical supplies. There has been a rise in the abuse of cough medicines containing *codeine* and related antitussives by youths seeking "kicks." The spread of experimentation with "hard" drugs to younger and younger groups has caused considerable alarm. Many middle-class families now need advice on how to handle the heroin problem of a child who has become dependent on this drug. The nurse should acquire the information necessary to offer such counseling.

Types of effects

Subjective effects. Which effects that people feel after taking opiates account for the compulsive craving that some people develop for heroin and related drugs? Oddly, most people find their initial experience with opiates unpleasant. They may complain of feeling dizzy and mentally foggy, their skin feels hot and itchy, and frequently they become nauseated and vomit. This dysphoria may be enough to prevent most experimenters with heroin from ever trying it again. However, others tend to overlook the drug-induced discomforts and concentrate instead on subjective effects that they find pleasurable, or euphoric.

The main psychopharmacologic effect sought by people who take opiates in excess is a drowsy relaxed feeling, frequently called "goofing off," "getting high," or "going on the nod." Shortly after taking a subcutaneous injection ("skin popping" or "joy popping"), the heroin addict "takes off" and drifts dreamily in a state between sleep and waking. Personal problems and conflicts seem to cease to exist, because the drug deadens anxieties. Like the related narcotic analgesics that are used for relief of physical pain, heroin can make a person indifferent to stressful situations that would ordinarily produce feelings of fear and panic. The drowsy, dreamy state that the drug usually produces makes it hard for a person to stay concerned about any personal problems that may have been worrying him.

Psychological dependence. What type of people find these feelings so gratifying that they continue to take opiates to stay "high" and not "come down"? Despite various psychodynamic formulations offered by psychologists, there does not seem to be any single opiate dependence-prone personality. One of the most widely held views is that some people who experience the subjective effects of heroin as pleasurable become dependent on the drug because its effects help them to escape from conflicts in their life situations that they find intolerable. They enjoy the drug-induced feeling of pleasurable relaxation and relief of anxiety, depression, and frustration.

This sort of self-medication to treat symptoms of pre-existing emotional conflict is a factor that favors continued drug taking. In psychological terms, the opiates are potent *positive reinforcers* of drug-taking behavior because of their unsurpassed ability to relieve psychological as well as physical pain (Chap. 51).

Another type of positive reinforcing effect that some users seek when they inject heroin directly into a vein ("mainlining") is a sudden surge of physical ecstasy called a "rush," "blast," "jolt," or "buzz." They describe this feeling, which comes when a concentrated dose of heroin rapidly reaches the central nervous system, in terms usually reserved for sexual orgasm: an initial pleasurable sensation centered in the lower abdomen that then radiates swiftly throughout the rest of the body. This is then followed by the much more prolonged lethargic state.

Tolerance. To keep getting these highly prized effects, the heroin abuser has to take larger and larger doses as the body becomes increasingly tolerant to the drug. Addicts often develop a relatively high level of resistance to the effects of opiates compared to the only moderate tolerance found when alcohol or barbiturates are chronically abused. Whereas 60 mg of morphine may prove toxic to most normal people, addicts can take several grams of opium alkaloids daily without suffering from severe toxicity. It is, however, possible for the addict to kill himself by administering doses of these drugs that exceed even his high degree of tolerance (see Acute toxicity, Chap. 51).

The exact nature of how tolerance to opiates develops is still uncertain. An increased ability to metabolize these drugs plays only a minor part. Instead, true tissue, cellular, or pharmacodynamic tolerance seems to

Table 53–1. Characteristics of different types of drug dependence

Agents	Psychological dependence	Physical dependence	Withdrawal syndrome	Tolerance
General depressants				

Alcohol
Sedative-hypnotics
  Barbiturates
  Glutethimide
  Methyprylon
  Chloral hydrate
  Paraldehyde
Minor tranquilizers
  Meprobamate
  Chlordiazepoxide
	Mild to strong; develops slowly	Develops slowly but to marked degree	Varies in intensity with duration and amount of drug intake; potentially severe and most dangerous; characterized by convulsions; deaths not uncommon	Irregular and incomplete; little tolerance to adverse effects of high doses; cross-tolerance among members of group

Narcotic analgesics				
Natural opiates Synthetic derivatives of opiates Synthetic opiate-like drugs	Strong; develops rapidly	Early development which increases in intensity, paralleling increase in dosage	Severe symptoms but not life-threatening; may be precipitated by administration of narcotic antagonist	Striking degree of tolerance to all but effects on pupil and gastrointestinal tract; cross-tolerance with other opiates or opiate-like drugs
Psychomotor stimulants				
Amphetamines	Mild to strong	Low degree	Mild	Marked but incomplete; cross-tolerance with amphetamine-like agents but not with cocaine
Cocaine	Strong	None	None	None
Psychedelics				
LSD	Variable	None	None	Marked
Marihuana	Mild to strong	None	None	Low degree developed to high doses
Phencyclidine	Mild to strong	Mild (but still questionable)	Mild but prolonged (still questionable)	Low degree to both behavioral and toxic effects

(Reproduced, with permission, from Levine RR: Pharmacology: Drug Actions and Reactions, 3rd ed., Boston, Little, Brown & Co, 1983) be much more significant than such drug-disposal tolerance (Chap. 4). However, none of the various speculative explanations of how the brain's neurons adapt to the presence of opiates can account fully for all the phenomena involved in the rapid development of tolerance to larger and larger doses. One commonly held view is that when opiate molecules occupy cellular receptors more or less continuously, the cells biosynthesize an increased number of opiate receptors. These added cellular sites can bind still more molecules of these drugs.

Physical dependence. Those who become tolerant to opiates and continue to take them in increasingly higher doses become physically dependent. That is, the presence of the drugs in the central nervous system is actually *required* for the neurons to function normally in regulating various body functions.

The biochemical basis for physical dependence on drugs is still obscure, as is its relationship to tolerance. In the case of the opiates, it is thought that the same cellular changes in the central nervous system that lead to the ability to withstand the drugs' actions may also be involved in the development of physical dependence on these agents.

Although scientists are still not sure how physical dependence to opiates develops, there is no doubt about what happens when an opiate-dependent person is deprived of the drug. As the level of these depressants in the person's system drops, a marked increase in the activity of many previously depressed functions begin to develop. *Rebound hyperexcitability* of previously depressed neurons is thought to account for the characteristic signs and symptoms of the opiate withdrawal syndrome. One explanation of its cause is that the continued presence of opiates in the system leads to a cutback in biosynthesis of the endogenous morphinelike substances called *endorphins* by the brain and anterior pituitary gland (Chap. 13). The withdrawal, or abstinence, syndrome that then develops is—according to this hypothesis—attributed to the drug-induced deficiency of these natural substances, which normally react with the same receptors as morphine, heroin and other opiates.

Opiate withdrawal syndrome. The withdrawal of opiates and other potent narcotic analgesics is marked by many signs and symptoms of autonomic nervous system hyperactivity as well as by increased central nervous system excitability. This begins about 12 to 18 hours after the last dose during "cold turkey" treatment—abrupt abstinence without the aid of any medication. The effects of withdrawal (see the summary of major drug withdrawal syndromes at the end of this chapter) are somewhat stereotyped and vary mainly in their degree of severity. This in turn depends on how much drug the addict had been taking daily; that is, on the degree of physical dependence on the drug.

The physical discomfort that develops when a person is deprived of opiates that he has been taking in excess for a prolonged period tends, of course, to make it more difficult for him to stop abusing these drugs, even if he makes an effort to do so. That is, the withdrawal syndrome is another negative factor that reinforces such positive factors as the euphoria that the psychologically susceptible person feels when beginning to take the drug. Actually, however, the pangs of withdrawal are less important in perpetuating addictive behavior than people have been led to believe by dramatizations.

Many people assume that the opiate addict's main reason for continuing to take drugs is the desire to avoid the physical suffering brought on by abstinence. Authorities on addiction to opiates, however, say that the highly diluted heroin available on "the street" does not cause a great degree of physical dependence or a truly severe withdrawal syndrome. They claim that the ordinary opiate withdrawal syndrome is no worse than what most people experience when they have a case of the "flu." They argue that the difficulties of so-called cold turkey withdrawal are overrated, and that the heroin addict's abstinence agonies are part of a purposeful bid for sympathy. In any case, the person who goes back on narcotics soon after release from a drug treatment center does so for *psychological* rather than physical reasons, because he is, obviously, no longer physically dependent and is not suffering from withdrawal sickness without the narcotic.

Diagnosis of opiate addiction

The best evidence of narcotic addiction is, of course, the appearance of the pattern of signs and symptoms typical of abstinence. This syndrome ordinarily begins to develop and reach its peak a dozen or more hours after the opiate-dependent person had the last "fix." However, the syndrome can rapidly be precipitated in its most severe form by an injection of a narcotic antagonist such as *naloxone* or *levallorphan* (Chap. 51). Bringing about the sudden onset of the full-blown withdrawal syndrome in this way to prove dependence is *not* necessary, and may be not only needlessly cruel but dangerous.

Narcotic antagonists are, instead, sometimes administered in relatively minute doses to determine if a person has recently had a dose of the drug. This dose of antagonist, which has no effect of its own on the person's pupils, is enough, however, to bring about a characteristic pupillary dilation in those whose pupils are even slightly constricted from a previously self-administered narcotic drug. Actually, the presence of pinpoint pupils alone, the result of the central miotic action of morphine and heroin (Chap. 51), is by itself a conspicuous sign of the presence of opiates in a person's system. This is an effect of narcotic analgesics to which tolerance does not appear to develop.

Another sign of drug-taking is that the skin on the inner aspects of the arms of "mainlining" addicts is usually marked by "tracks." These raised and discolored areas running along the course of the veins are the scars of old sores and abscesses. The presence of fresh punctures is, of course, a sign that the person has had an injection fairly recently. This can be confirmed by positive test results for opiates in the urine.

Treatment of opiate addiction

Detoxification

The process of ridding the patient's body of heroin is the first step in treatment. It is ordinarily carried out in a hospital unit but may sometimes be done on an out-patient basis. Depending on the degree of the patient's physical dependence, the abstinence sickness may be mild or severe. In either case, good nursing care is needed to keep the patient comfortable during this detoxification period.

Drugs of various types are often employed to minimize the patient's discomfort during detoxification. *Methadone*, a synthetic narcotic, is often employed for this purpose. Its use to suppress the signs and symptoms of withdrawal from heroin is based on the phenomenon of *cross dependence*—that is, on the ability of one opiate to substitute for another on which a person may be dependent. The reason for substituting a temporary methadone dependence for a previous heroin dependence is that methadone is eliminated much more slowly, and thus its withdrawal causes a much milder abstinence syndrome than that of heroin withdrawal.

Physicians in the different institutions that use methadone for heroin detoxification may employ any of several different dosage schedules. The addicts sometimes tend to be demanding and manipulative and often exaggerate the extent of their physical dependence to continue satisfying their opiate craving with methadone, which is itself, of course, an addicting drug. Because of this, scheduling and dosage plans must be determined and carefully followed by all members of the health-care team. In any case, once the patient has been stabilized on a dose of methadone that keeps him comfortable, the dosage is gradually reduced and finally discontinued entirely in a few days.

Nonopiate-type drugs to aid relief of symptoms are also sometimes ordered. These include salicylates for muscular pain, sedative–hypnotics such as *phenobarbital* for anxiety and insomnia, and antianxiety or tranquilizing drugs such as *chlordiazepoxide* (Librium) or *chlorpromazine HCl* (Thorazine) for agitation. These drugs, usually ordered on a prn basis, should be administered whenever they seem to be needed. *Clonidine HCl* (Catapres), a centrally acting antihypertensive drug (Chap. 28), is being investigated for use in withdrawing patients from methadone and other narcotic analgesics. Preliminary evidence indicates that it rapidly decreases the signs and symptoms of withdrawal but sometimes causes hypotension.

Clinical considerations. During withdrawal, the patient is especially sensitive to the attitudes of others. At this time of physical discomfort and psychological distress, he needs emotional support and encouragement. This can be given by developing a supportive relationship, and by listening to him, answering questions, and allaying his fears. Recovery is a long and often discouraging process. The patient will need continuity in the support, encouragement, and education that is offered.

Measures should be taken to make the patient comfortable and to allay fears. A back rub helps to relax cramped and aching muscles. Chills are counteracted with warm blankets and heating pads, set at a safe temperature and observed often to prevent burns. Once the patient's early nausea and vomiting have subsided, frequent and small but nourishing meals should be given.

Keeping these patients from obtaining drugs illicitly while they are under medical care is usually a nursing responsibility. In following the security measures of the institution, the nurse is often in the position to observe and confront visitors. The patient should understand the rules and how they are enforced to avoid any unpleasant experiences.

Firmness is necessary in dealing with persons who abuse drugs. These patients frequently test the limits set by nurses and other staff members. Thus, an attitude of supportive listening is not to be confused with laxity or indulgence. In many instances patients who abuse drugs have not experienced others' caring about them, and they need a firmness of approach to assist them not only to develop their own self-control but also to show them that someone cares what they do.

Participation of other patients in the treatment program is widely practiced through such measures as group therapy and the group's role in developing rules for the community of patients. An important aspect of the nurse's role involves working not only with individual patients but also with groups of patients through such measures as leading or coleading group discussions.

Rehabilitation

Detoxifying the patient does not, of course, do anything to alter the underlying emotional difficulties that led him to take drugs in excess in the first place. Then, to quiet the uneasiness that he may feel when deprived of drugs, the abuser may try every sort of subterfuge in an effort to obtain depressant drugs. The rehabilitation of opiate addicts, consequently, is by far the most difficult part of the whole treatment procedure. The rate of recidivism in opiate addiction in the past has been estimated to be over 90%. Thus, if merely detoxified and released from confinement, the addict may soon return to his drug-seeking and drug-taking behavior. He may commit crimes continuously to get the large sums of money needed to support his habit. In time, the addict's round of criminal activities leads to arrest and prison—a pattern repeated again and again. In many cases the addict ends up in the morgue, a victim of accidental or deliberate overdosage or of hepatitis, endocarditis, tetanus, or other medical complications.

Methadone maintenance programs. Methadone, discussed above as an aid to detoxification therapy, has also been widely employed as a pharmacologic adjunct to routine rehabilitative measures. In these programs methadone is not discontinued as it is at the end of the ordinary detoxification procedure. Instead, after the drug has been given in doses high enough to control the heroin abstinence syndrome, its dosage is adjusted individually to the amount that is required to develop tolerance. Some patients may need as much as 120 mg of methadone daily.

Such large doses do not prevent the properly stabilized patient from functioning normally. That is, once tolerance to methadone has been acquired, the patient on a methadone maintenance program can carry on ordinary activities without showing drowsiness, confusion, euphoria, or other effects of the opioid.* Most important are the effects of methadone on the person's responses to heroin.

Methadone has two effects in addition to preventing the patient from suffering abstinence sickness:

1. It blocks the compulsive craving for heroin, the so-called heroin hunger that tends to drive detoxified opiate addicts back to drugs.
2. It prevents the addict from feeling the euphoric effects of heroin. That is, most addicts cannot get high on heroin while they are being maintained on high doses of methadone.

According to evaluations of the results of various methadone maintenance programs, most patients have been able to stay off heroin. Their response to such other rehabilitative measures as vocational training and group psychotherapy is said to be better than when methadone is not employed as a pharmacologic adjunct. Many hardened addicts with long histories of involvement in crimes related to drug-seeking behavior have made a successful social adjustment when maintained on methadone. Freed from the need to satisfy their craving, these people can stop the vicious cycle of stealing, prostitution, and other types of antisocial behavior. Many are now working, going to school, and rehabilitating themselves in other ways.

However, methadone maintenance has various drawbacks that critics of these programs have been quick to point out. Most addicts are not really "cured." Some begin to abuse barbiturates, alcohol, amphetamines, and cocaine. Another disadvantage is that the patient must make almost daily visits to the clinic, where he is kept under observation while taking the drug dissolved in fruit juice. Although this is desirable during the first phase of treatment, it becomes burdensome when the patient is working or caring for a family.

To avoid this difficulty, patients are often given a 2-day take-home supply of methadone. Unfortunately, such supplies are sometimes diverted to illicit use. Some patients have, for example, sold their methadone tablets to other addicts, who then dissolve the drug in water and inject themselves to get high, just as they would with heroin. One way to avoid this problem would be to develop a longer acting drug that would keep the patient free of withdrawal symptoms for several days after it is taken at the clinic. *Acetylmethadol* (Acemethadone) is an experimental drug with long-lasting methadonelike effects, which, it is hoped, will make it unnecessary to give patients take-home supplies.

Another approach to the problem of illicit diversion of methadone is to mix it with the narcotic antagonist naloxone in a ratio of 20 parts of the narcotic to one part of the antagonist. Combination tablets of this type have the same effects as methadone alone when dissolved and taken *orally.* That is, the small naloxone content has no effect. However, if an attempt is made to inject a solution made from the tablets to get "high," the *injected* antagonist sets off the opiate withdrawal syndrome. Thus, this combination is claimed to prevent the parenteral abuse of methadone and discourage its illicit diversion.

Narcotic antagonists. Such drugs as naloxone have also been used alone. These nonaddicting drugs can block the euphoric effects of heroin that a patient may then try to inject. However, unlike methadone, such narcotic antagonists do not eliminate the patient's craving for heroin. In addition, the currently available drugs have only a short duration of action. Thus, unless a patient is already highly motivated toward abstinence, he needs to miss only one day's dosage of the antagonist to regain his sensitivity to the euphoric effects of heroin.

Naltrexone, a new experimental narcotic antagonist, has been shown to block the effects of injected heroin, methadone, and other narcotics for at least 48 hours. The drug, which has few effects of its own, has been used in several ways to treat thousands of heroin users and addicts. In one program it was employed immediately after patients had been detoxified with the aid of methadone. After that drug was withdrawn, the patient received naltrexone regularly to prevent readdiction. Continued use of this long-acting drug is claimed to prevent patients who try to take an occasional dose of heroin from feeling its effects, and thus to prevent both psychological and physical dependence. Patients still require counseling, though, to maintain their motivation to stay on naltrexone and to remain both detoxified and rehabilitated.

---

* This characteristic of physical dependence of the narcotic analgesic type is not shared by physical dependence of the barbiturate type; that is, patients who are physically dependent on such substances as barbiturates or alcohol cannot generally take enough of such drugs to prevent a withdrawal syndrome without losing their ability to function normally in society.

Drug-free programs. Many authorities on the rehabilitation of narcotic addicts do not approve of the use of drugs such as methadone or the antagonists. They claim that such pharmacologic adjuncts are only a chemical crutch that—in the case of methadone, at least—merely substitutes one addicting drug for another. They feel that this is particularly undesirable in the case of teenage users of heroin, who should be weaned from addicting drugs rather than maintained on them. They advocate, instead, that adolescents and other opiate addicts participate in drug-free programs.

Those who operate such rehabilitative programs, including Narcotics Anonymous and Synanon, try to get the drug abuser to take a realistic look at himself and his life situation. The leaders of these groups are usually themselves former addicts who have suffered the same types of experiences as the patient. Thus, knowing how an addict may delude himself and others, these counselors do not err in the direction of excessive permissiveness. This is apparent both during the detoxification process, which is carried out "cold turkey" in such facilities, and later in the rehabilitation processes. Many of these facilities use group confrontation and support techniques to promote the rehabilitation process. These methods are not successful for all patients, but have proven to be very successful for others.

Prevention of opiate addiction

The measures that nurses must employ to prevent development of opiate dependence in patients receiving potent narcotic analgesics have been discussed in Chapter 51. Nurses in various other settings within their communities can play an important role in educating young people and others about the nature of drug abuse. Working together with teachers, social workers, physicians, and others, nurses can help to reduce experimentation with drugs such as codeine and thus help to prevent opiate dependence-prone people from becoming dependent on more potent drugs of this type.

Health-care professionals, who have ready access to these drugs, must be cautious to avoid self-medication with these drugs. Even occasional self-treatment of this type could lead to the habitual use of a dangerous drug, and eventually to disastrous dependence on it.

Drug abuse is not limited to those who lack adequate information on the physical damage that drugs can do; this is apparent from the high incidence of addiction among medical personnel. Many professionals function perfectly well and maintain a high level of competence as long as they can obtain enough of the drug—problems arise when the drug is no longer available. When this happens, the professional resembles any other patient withdrawing from an opiate.

Thus, the nurse must be alert to the unusual situation in which a colleague may be stealing narcotics or other drugs from the stores of the unit. Someone may, for example, be substituting falsely labeled solutions or tablets for drugs that have been taken for personal use. Sometimes there may be an indication of this when several patients fail to obtain relief of pain after routine administration of morphine, meperidine (Demerol), or some other potent analgesic. This could be because sterile saline solution has been used to replace the actual narcotic drug in the labeled vial or because an inert tablet—resembling codeine or hydromorphone (Dilaudid), for example—has been substituted for the actual analgesic. In such cases, most institutions have clear guidelines that should be followed.

General depressant abuse and dependence

The most widely abused of all substances are not the opiates but the drugs that are classed as general depressants of the central nervous system. These drugs, which—as their name suggests—are able to depress *all* parts of the CNS, include the following:

1. Sedative–hypnotics and other antianxiety agents (Chap. 45)
2. Ethyl alcohol
3. General anesthetics (Chap. 52) and certain volatile solvents that have somewhat similar effects

The abuse of inhalation anesthetics such as ethyl ether is relatively uncommon, but the effects of ether intoxication resemble those of both ethyl alcohol and the volatile solvents that are discussed in the next two sections of this chapter. Here, the nature of abuse of such sedative–hypnotics as the barbiturates and antianxiety agents such as the benzodiazepine class—*chlordiazepoxide* (Librium) and *diazepam* (Valium)—will be discussed.

Sedative–hypnotics and antianxiety agents

Pattern of general depression
All the substances of this class can produce a progressive depression of the CNS. Although individual drugs vary in the rapidity in which they bring about their effects on the functions controlled by the nervous system, all produce the following pattern of effects as their doses are raised:

1. Sedation—a reduction in anxiety, tension, and alertness
2. Impairment of mental and motor function marked by drowsiness, lethargy, incoordination, and sleep
3. Deepening stupor with decreased responsiveness to stimuli, including pain
4. Coma and death from respiratory and circulatory failure

Still another effect is often seen before sleep and stupor. This is a period of excitement, confusion, and clouded consciousness. In this stage, the person's behavior becomes unpredictable but is most often boisterous and disorderly, behavior similar to that sometimes exhibited by people who are intoxicated by alcohol. Sometimes, particularly when vapors are being inhaled, the most marked changes are in a person's *sensory perceptions*. As some people may know from the experience of "going under" after a few whiffs of an anesthetic such as ether, vision, hearing, and other sensations may be markedly distorted in this stage.

Patterns of abuse and dependence

People begin to take these drugs to excess when they find that barbiturates such as *secobarbital* (Seconal), *pentobarbital* (Nembutal), and *amobarbital* (Amytal), which have a rapid onset of action, quite dependably bring on feelings that they find pleasurable or satisfying in one way or another. Some seek the sleepy, almost stuporous, state that these drugs can produce to get relief from chronic anxiety about aspects of their life situation with which they find it difficult to cope. Their drug-induced impairment of psychomotor function is reflected in a lack of alertness, slowed mental processes, and sluggish movements.

Other people discover, as they develop tolerance to the hypnotic, or sleep-producing, effects of these barbiturates and such other drugs of this class as *glutethimide* (Doriden) that they actually feel exhilarated. This feeling is often accompanied by the same sort of uninhibited behavior that is brought about by alcoholic intoxication. Alcohol is, in fact, often taken in combination with barbiturates, meprobamate, glutethimide, and other drugs of this class to increase the feeling of exhilaration. Occasionally other drugs, such as stimulants of the amphetamine type, are combined with barbiturates or taken alternately to counteract each others' excessive effects.

People who attain this state of drug-induced disinhibition may become boisterous and unruly. Often they are irritable and tend to act out their hostile feelings. In general, they show the same lack of judgment and motor incoordination as that seen in people in a moderate state of alcoholic intoxication. In fact, when you see a person who looks and acts drunk but whose breath has no odor of an alcoholic beverage, you should consider the possibility of his being under the influence of barbiturates or other sedative–hypnotics and tranquilizers.

The nature and degree to which people become involved with depressant drugs also resembles the ways in which different people abuse alcohol. Some—usually teen-agers and young adults—go on only occasional sprees. Others—most commonly middle-class and middle-aged people who were first introduced to these drugs by way of a drug prescription for anxiety or insomnia—gradually begin to take larger and larger daytime doses that keep them in a state of chronic inebriation. For members of the drug culture, barbiturates may be only one group in a "smorgasbord" of other drugs, ranging from heroin through cocaine to LSD, that they take for "kicks" as part of a life style that revolves around steady drug taking.

The prognosis for peole who follow these patterns of abuse of barbiturates and the other drugs of this class is more serious, leading as it does to daily, almost total involvement in drug-seeking and drug-taking behavior. Like the alcoholic, this type of drug abuser may become unkempt in appearance. If he has been injecting himself with highly alkaline barbiturate salt solutions as "street" users sometimes do, his skin may be scarred or abscessed. Often his hands tremble and his reflex responses and eye signs are abnormal. However, because he usually eats better than the alcoholic, he does not ordinarily suffer from malnutrition and show the resulting signs of more severe neurologic damage that are so often seen in the chronic alcoholic. The barbiturate abuser's life style and muddled mental state make him especially subject to accidental injury or death from falls, fires, or automobile accidents.

Tolerance and physical dependence

People who take barbiturates and other depressants repeatedly and continuously tend to develop a high but limited degree of tolerance. That is, like alcoholics, they can often function quite well without showing signs and symptoms that most people would recognize as those of depressant drug intoxication, even when they have taken several times the ordinary sleep-producing dose. However, when an abuser takes only slightly more than the upper limit of his tolerance—which, with his drug-induced loss of judgment, he can readily do—he may suffer a severe and often fatal degree of central nervous system depression.

Poisoning, resulting in coma and death from respiratory and circulatory failure, is a common occurrence in habitual barbiturate abusers. Sometimes this happens when the mentally confused person accidentally takes too many capsules and exceeds his tolerance. Severe toxicity is particularly likely to occur if he has also been drinking heavily. Occasionally an abuser may, in a fit of depression, deliberately take an overdose of barbiturates. He may not necessarily wish truly to commit suicide, but death may come before medical assistance is summoned. (See Chapter 45 for a discussion of the management of barbiturate poisoning.)

Physical dependence. This develops fairly rapidly in people who take daily doses of barbiturates that keep them mildly or moderately intoxicated. How great their degree of dependence becomes depends on how high a dose has been taken and for how long a time. Mild but regular intoxication with moderate doses tends to make a person physically dependent after a few weeks or months; heavier abuse can lead to dependence in less than 2 weeks. Such a person may suffer a severe withdrawal syndrome that is different from the opiate withdrawal pattern and potentially more dangerous. This is because the abuser who is abruptly deprived of his drug may suffer from convulsions and delirium. As in the case of the alcoholic with the "DTs," agitation and restlessness may lead to physical exhaustion and circulatory collapse if the withdrawal excitement is not brought under control.

Withdrawal symptoms. These are most commonly first manifested by signs of restlessness and increasing anxiety and nervousness. These emotional reactions, which resemble the "jitters" of alcoholic withdrawal syndromes (see below), are also often accompanied by neuromuscular features resembling the "shakes" that occur in alcoholics who are deprived of that drug. These include mainly muscle weakness with tremulousness and coarse tremors. Occasionally, a strongly drug-dependent person, who is brought into the hospital after an accident, may suffer a severe grand mal seizure before any such prodromal signs have appeared.

Because such barbiturate abusers are often unwilling or unable to give an accurate history, the nurse should be alert for early signs of an abstinence syndrome. In patients who have been taking high doses of relatively rapid-acting and short-acting barbiturates, these begin to appear about 12 hours after their last dose. Patients who had, at first, appeared to be recovering from a state of intoxication, become irritable, complain of nausea and weakness, and may vomit. By the next day they have often become increasingly confused and disoriented.

Withdrawal treatment. Such patients should not be allowed to leave their beds, because they may suffer blackouts from postural hypotension and injure themselves in a fall. Their mounting agitation and tremulousness should, instead, be promptly controlled by the administration of depressant drugs of this same class in doses that quickly return the patient to the customary state of intoxication. That is, the patient should receive a drug that not only suppresses withdrawal symptoms but actually produces mild intoxication again as indicated by such signs as slurred speech, ataxic gait, and drowsiness.

The standard drugs most favored for stopping further signs of withdrawal illness are the barbiturates *pentobarbital* and *phenobarbital*. Some authorities prefer the former because of its more rapid onset; others prefer phenobarbital, because this long-acting barbiturate provides a more constant blood level and more prolonged stabilization of the patient's state. Sometimes, however, when the patient reveals the name of the specific drug that has been abused, this drug is administered instead of one of the barbiturate substitutes with similar effects.

Once the patient is stabilized at a level of mild inebriation and has been maintained in that state for 1 or 2 days with doses adjusted to individual needs, the slow process of reducing daily dosage is begun. Because of the risks of too rapid withdrawal, the patient is carefully observed for signs of both withdrawal and intoxication during the very gradual dosage reduction procedure. If the patient shows such signs of abstinence as anxiety, tremors, and restlessness, the daily dosage of the abused drug or its pharmacologic equivalent is raised just enough to suppress these signs and symptoms. On the other hand, if signs of drug intoxication develop, the next scheduled dose of the depressant drug is omitted.

Total detoxification takes much longer with general depressant drugs than does the opiate withdrawal procedure, because the abuser of barbiturates and similar drugs is in much more danger than the patient who is dependent on heroin. The stabilization and dosage reduction periods are particularly prolonged in patients who have been abusing chlordiazepoxide (Librium) or diazepam (Valium) and who are being treated with these drugs. This is because these benzodiazepine-type antianxiety agents are only very slowly eliminated from the body. Thus, instead of beginning to show withdrawal symptoms within hours of being deprived of their drug, as is the case with barbiturate abuse, people who have been taking chronically excessive doses of these widely misused tranquilizers may show no effects for 3 to 5 days and may not suffer a seizure until more than a week after abrupt withdrawal.

Rehabilitation

Rehabilitation of patients dependent on nonnarcotic depressant drugs is as difficult as that of the alcoholic. This is understandable, because these people usually have the same sort of emotional problems, and these drugs produce essentially the same type of pharmacologic "solutions" for them as alcohol does. (Often, as previously indicated, patients may be dependent on both alcohol and barbiturates, or on both barbiturates and opiates.) If patients in the *postdetoxification* period require pharmacologic as well as psychological support, they should not, of course, receive sedatives or tranquilizers to relieve their anxiety or agitation. Instead, drugs that do not seem likely to be abused—phenothiazine-type tranquilizers, for example, or antidepressant drugs (Chap. 46)—should be employed.

Preventing sedative drug abuse

Most people who receive barbiturates for medical reasons feel no compulsion to raise the daily or nightly dose. However, some people, particularly alcoholics, tend to abuse these and other sedatives, hypnotics, and tranquilizers when they are exposed to these drugs. Thus, physicians try to avoid prescribing these agents to addiction-prone patients. If one of these drugs is chosen for controlling the patient's anxiety or for sleeplessness, the amounts prescribed should be limited, and the patient should be kept under close observation as long as the medication is being employed.

The nurse plays an important part in preventing abuse of these drugs by patients who are prone to become dependent on them. Such patients, as well as elderly people who are often forgetful, need to be carefully observed when taking sedatives, hypnotics, and tranquilizers. Nonhospitalized patients have to be instructed in how to deal with the problem of preventing dependence on drugs that are readily available to them when they are at home. The teaching program for any patient who is receiving a drug with abuse potential should incorporate information on the potential hazards involved, as well as the benefits of drug therapy. Patients should feel free to ask questions and to voice any concerns that they may have about this issue.

Alcohol and alcoholism management

Two out of three Americans drink alcoholic beverages. Most drink only moderate amounts and rarely become intoxicated. However, others drink heavily enough, at times, to get into trouble in one way or another. Even a small amount of alcohol can cause physical consequences, ranging from a hangover to death in an automobile accident. Among those in the 10% or more of our population who regularly drink to excess are many millions whose compulsion to continue drinking creates serious problems for themselves and others.

Alcoholism is one of this country's most serious public health problems. It is impossible to calculate the costs of this devastating and most common form of drug addiction. This disease often leads to liver damage, neurologic disorders, and other medical complications. It is a frequent cause of crimes of violence and of family disruptions that affect the futures of young children.

Problem drinking is now known to exist at every level of society. It has become increasingly clear that there are probably as many women as men who drink to excess. Women with drinking difficulties may keep their secret hidden for longer periods, but the consequences of a mother's alcoholism may be even more damaging to a family's stability than drinking by the father.

Although the social consequences of chronic alcoholism cannot be taken up here, the nurse is often involved professionally with patients who have this disease and with their families. To carry out responsibilities most effectively, the nurse needs to know what effects alcohol has on the brain and on the body. Complete and effective care of the alcoholic patient requires an understanding of the acute and chronic changes produced by this substance.

Pharmacologic actions of alcohol on the CNS

The central nervous system is most sensitive to the depressant effects of ethyl alcohol. This substance is similar to the barbiturates and to general anesthetics such as ethyl ether (Chap. 52) in the pattern of progressive CNS depression that it can produce. Contrary to common belief, alcohol is *not* a stimulant, and the drinker's excited behavior actually stems from depression of the brain areas that ordinarily exert inhibitory control over psychomotor activity and behavior.

The effects of alcohol on the functioning of the CNS are related largely to the level of alcohol in the blood (Table 53-2). The concentration of alcohol in the blood at any time after it is ingested depends on many factors, including not only the total amount taken in but also how the body handles the alcohol (see the section on alcohol metabolism, below). The drinker's behavior depends in large part on the amount of alcohol that is accumulating in the brain. However, people do vary in their ability to tolerate similar levels of alcohol in their brains. Such tissue, or pharmacodynamic, tolerance (Chap. 4) accounts for the fact that some heavy drinkers can continue to function without appearing to be intoxicated despite blood and brain alcohol concentrations that would totally disrupt a novice drinker's behavior.

The following discussion of the effects of alcohol on centrally controlled functions will attempt to correlate behavior with the blood alcohol level (Table 53-2). For such purposes, the blood level of alcohol is expressed in the number of milligrams of alcohol per milliliters of blood—that is, in mg%. Such expressions are of medicolegal significance in determining whether a person is legally fit to drive a car. However, as with any other substance that exerts psychopharmacologic effects, alcohol causes behavioral effects by actions on intellectual function and emotional response that are less readily predictable or measurable than are its effects on reflex responses, reaction times, and motor coordination.

Thus, a margin for error must be allowed in relating the following generalizations concerning blood alcohol content and behavior to the actual responses of any specific person at a particular time.

Low blood alcohol levels. Drinking even a relatively small quantity of alcohol that produces only low levels in the brain results in reduced nervous tension—that is, a sedative or tranquilizing effect. However, even this relaxed feeling and the increase in self-confidence that often accompanies it are an indication of alcohol's ability to affect the highest functions of the cerebral cortex. In neurologic terms, it may be said that this sedative effect reflects the action of alcohol on the reticular activating system (RAS; see Chap. 44), with a resulting release of some aspects of behavior from the inhibitory control of the cerebral cortex.

Practically speaking, the effects of drinking an amount of alcohol that can raise the level of alcohol in the blood to about 50 mg%—2 or 3 oz of whiskey (Table 53-3)—are generally considered socially and medically beneficial for many people.

Social drinking. Psychologists suggest that people drink socially because alcohol helps to reduce self-consciousness and to relieve feelings of inner tension. As a

Table 53–2. Blood alcohol levels and effects on CNS function*

Blood level	Possible behavioral change(s)
20–30 mg%	Slight impairment of psychosensory function
30–50 mg%	Some impairment of judgment and motor coordination may occur; this level is *not* considered to be legal evidence of "impaired ability" to operate a motor vehicle in the United States, but in some European countries it is illegal to drive with even this level of blood alcohol
50–150 mg%	Varying degrees of impairment of fine motor coordination and judgment; delayed reaction time. Drivers with blood alcohol concentrations between these levels may be required to take tests of gross motor coordination to determine their fitness to drive
	The 100 mg% level is now considered to be evidence of "impaired ability" to operate a motor vehicle—a chargeable offense in some states
150–250 mg%	Moderate intoxication marked by progressive deterioration of higher cortical functions. Levels above 150 mg% are considered to be prima facie evidence of "driving while under the influence of alcohol" in most of the United States
250–400 mg%	Marked intoxication characterized by increasing difficulty in maintaining motor function and by a high degree of uninhibited behavior. The drinker may be boisterous or belligerent and may be involved in violent incidents or accidents
400–600 mg%	Severe intoxication results in a stuporous state from which arousal is difficult
600–800 mg% and above	Coma and death from respiratory or cardiovascular failure or complications are likely to occur at these levels

* The blood alcohol content (BAC) correlates with the concentration of alcohol in the brain and—within limits—with its effects on functions controlled by the CNS. However, individual behavior varies depending on such factors as the drinker's tolerance and the "set" and "setting," as well as on whether the BAC is rapidly rising or gradually dropping.

result of increased self-confidence, a person with a blood alcohol level approaching 50 mg% often tends to lower some socially acquired defenses. Thus, things may be said or done in social situations that would ordinarily not be said or done. Presumably, this is because judgment and inhibitory controls have been affected by the depressant effect of alcohol on nerve pathways that play a part in intellectual function.

Ordinarily, in our society, people tend to be rather shy and subdued when in the company of strangers. This is because they have learned to inhibit their natural drives in response to the demands of society. When the effects of this blood level of alcohol on the brain begin to appear, the normally or excessively inhibited person tends to lose some of his capacity for critically evaluating himself and his relationships with others. This, of course, makes it easier for casual acquaintances to communicate.

(This action of alcohol as a social lubricant may be as beneficial as sociologists say, but alcohol-released social spouting can also be considered unacceptable—especially to those whose blood alcohol content is still at a substantially lower level.)

Caution must, of course, be exercised in attempting to predict changes in human behavior at this low level of alcohol, because circumstances may alter cases. For example, environmental factors—what psychologists call the "setting"—may make the same person react differently at various times. When partying with jovial companions, the imbiber may be gay and a bit boisterous. In sedate company, or when alone, the same person may merely become drowsy from the same amount of alcohol.

Therapeutic uses. The euphoric sedation that often accompanies blood alcohol levels between 30 and 50 mg%, together with the rise in pain threshold that occurs, accounts for some of the medical uses of alcohol. Such tranquilizing and analgesic actions, rather than this drug's direct effects on the heart and blood vessels, are thought to be responsible for any benefits felt by patients with cardiovascular disorders.

The use of alcohol as a "nightcap" may help a restless person to fall asleep. However, its habitual use as a *hypnotic* in this manner may be harmful to people prone to abuse depressant drugs. Of course, alcohol is safe enough when used only occasionally for this purpose. For example, a person suffering from a heavy cold does no harm when following the time-worn practice of getting into bed after taking a warm alcoholic drink and one or two aspirin tablets. The *diaphoretic* (sweat-inducing) action of the combination may help to lower a mild fever, although alcoholic sponge baths—applied *externally*—are better for this purpose. Actually, the main advantage of the alcoholic drink is that it makes the patient with a head cold drowsy and helps him to rest.

Higher blood alcohol levels. A person who takes a little alcohol may feel better as a result of its relaxant action. However, when alcohol is ingested in amounts that make the blood and brain concentrations rise rapidly to still higher levels, its beneficial effects begin to be outweighed by behavioral changes that may be socially harmful. These reflect both a blurring of the drinker's judgment and a diminished ability to perform finely coordinated movements.

Driving. At first, these effects may be manifested merely by an excessive increase in self-confidence and by signs such as a seemingly accidental difficulty in lighting and holding a cigarette. Later, as blood alcohol levels rise toward 100 mg%, the drinker's diminished ability to evaluate reality and restrain his impulses, coupled with increasing clumsiness, may make it dangerous to drive a motor vehicle. At a blood alcohol level above 0.1%, most people are mildly intoxicated and legally unfit to drive. Actually, however, much lower levels of alcohol can cause enough reduction in judgment and skilled motor abilities to make it unsafe for a person to drive. Thus, in view of the disrupting effects of alcohol on these important CNS functions, *no one should attempt to drive while still feeling any effect at all, even from moderate drinking.*

States and countries vary greatly in the maximum level of blood alcohol that is permissible for operating a motor vehicle without a penalty. In the United States, drivers with a blood alcohol content (BAC) less than 50 mg% are usually not considered to be in violation of the law. In some other countries, driving with a BAC of even 30 mg% is a punishable offense.

Signs of intoxication. The extent of a person's motor impairment with a BAC of 50 to 100 mg% may not be very great. It may be manifested only by slightly slurred speech and by a tendency to bump into things while brushing by them, rather than by overt staggering. However, when combined with the drinker's tendency to act

Table 53–3. Alcohol content of beverages*

Beverage and type or source	% alcohol by volume	Proof†
Neutral spirits	90–95	180–190
Vodka (from neutral spirits)	40–55	80–110
Gin (from neutral spirits)	40–45	80–110
Whiskey (from cereal grains)	40–45	80–110
Rum (from molasses)	40–55	80–110
Brandy (from wine)	40–55	80–110
Wine (table, light)	10–12	
Wine (dessert)	15–22	
Beer (light)	3–6	
Ale	6–8	
Cider (hard)	8–12	

* The amount of a beverage taken within a brief period of time can be related within limits to the level of alcohol likely to be attained in the blood and brain and to the probable behavior of the person.

For example, 1 oz of a concentrated beverage such as 100-proof whiskey, taken all at once on an empty stomach, might produce a blood alcohol level of 20 mg% (0.02%) within half an hour. Similarly, 2 to 3 oz of whiskey could produce a blood level of 0.05% alcohol; 8 oz (half a pint) 0.15%; 16 oz (1 pint) 0.30%, etc. However, such factors as the amount and type of food eaten before and during drinking; and the pattern of drinking—for example, slow sipping or rapid gulping—also influence the amount of alcoholic beverage required to produce a particular blood alcohol level.

† *Proof* is the standard of strength for alcoholic liquors. The proof figure in this country is always twice the percentage of alcohol by volume. The term is said to stem from an old test for the alcohol content of whiskey. If gunpowder on which the whiskey was poured ignited, this was "proof" that the whiskey contained at least 50% alcohol.

impulsively or foolishly, and delayed reaction times, motor incoordination of this degree markedly increases the chances of being involved in an accident. Thus, unwise drinking is the cause of serious injury and death as a result of falls, fires, and industrial accidents, as well as those involving drivers and pedestrians who have been drinking.

Most people with a 150 mg% blood alcohol level, and just about everyone with 200 mg%, may be considered to be moderately intoxicated, and those with 300 mg% are markedly intoxicated. People who have ingested enough alcohol to have blood levels this high show many signs of rapidly progressive deterioration of higher cortical functions. This appears in the form of increasingly uncontrolled behavior as a result of the release from both emotional and motor inhibitory controls. The person at this stage of an alcoholic episode may become belligerent and pugnacious, or he may have a crying or laughing "jag." At the same time, he tends to have increasing difficulty in locomotion, marked at first by a staggering gait, then by trouble in simply trying to stand and, finally, by falling and being unable to get up.

The drinker's uninhibited behavior may lead to

his involvement in violence, in which *he* is the one likely to be injured because of his inability to defend himself. When the blood level of alcohol is at around 300 mg%, the person's state of excitement may be similar to that of a patient in the second stage of anesthesia (Chap. 52), in the sense that he, too, is not truly conscious of what is going on and is really not responsible for his words and actions. Thus, it does little good to reason with the acutely intoxicated person, because he is not likely to understand. Instead, he should be kept from harming himself and, in some cases, hospitalized and treated with tranquilizing medication and other medical measures.

Toxic and lethal blood levels. People with blood alcohol concentrations of 400 mg% are no longer a behavioral problem; they have entered a stuporous state from which they cannot be readily aroused. Although the drinker can no longer bend an elbow to take in any more liquor, the continuing absorption from the gastrointestinal (GI) tract of alcohol ingested earlier may cause him to lapse into coma. As the blood level rises above 500 mg%, the alcoholic's breathing becomes shallow and slow, and the circulation may come close to collapse. Death from respiratory paralysis and shock usually occurs with blood levels of 600 mg% and above.

A person who collapses in an alcoholic stupor outdoors in winter may freeze to death if not found. This occurs, in part, because alcohol depresses the brain's centers for regulating body temperature. Body heat is then rapidly lost, because the vessels of the skin tend to remain dilated instead of constricting reflexly. Even if found in time, the stuporous or comatose alcoholic may die of hypostatic pneumonia or as a result of a severe complicating bronchopulmonary infection. Also, head injuries or cerebral edema as a result of brain hypoxia may sometimes prove fatal.

Pharmacokinetics of alcohol

Many factors affect the level of alcohol attained in the blood and brain at any time after a person begins to drink. As is true with any drug (Chap. 4), the alcohol concentration depends on the rate and completeness of such processes as its absorption into the blood, its transport to the tissues of the CNS and its redistribution to other parts of the body and, finally, its metabolic breakdown and elimination. The amount of alcohol in the blood and brain at any given moment is the result of a constantly shifting balance between these processes.

This section of the chapter will attempt to relate what is now known about the body's handling of ingested alcohol to both the behavioral effects discussed in the previous section and to the next topic—the management of acute intoxication and chronic alcoholism. Knowledge of some of the factors that determine how quickly alcohol gets into the blood, how it is carried to the brain, and how it disappears from the body will also increase understanding of what behavioral effects to expect in a person who has ingested alcohol under known conditions.

Absorption. Alcohol is a rapidly absorbed substance, because it requires no digestion and diffuses readily through the GI mucosa. About 20% of the ingested alcohol is absorbed from the stomach, but the bulk of any drink makes its way into the bloodstream only after it enters the small intestine. The CNS effects of a concentrated alcoholic drink can often be felt very quickly when taken on an empty stomach, because absorption begins immediately and reaches a peak in as little as 20 minutes.

The period required for absorption may, however, be considerably delayed when the stomach contains a moderate amount of food. The presence of food tends to dilute the alcohol in the stomach and to interfere with its absorption from that site. More importantly, milk or other fat- and protein-containing foods tend to slow the rate at which the stomach empties into the small intestine. The duodenal mucosa is the point at which the alcohol content of a drink is most quickly and completely absorbed. Because more of the alcohol can be detoxified during such delayed absorption, its concentration in the blood and brain remains relatively low, and its effects on the CNS are less marked. Similarly, sipping a drink slowly over a period of time results in lower blood alcohol concentrations and fewer CNS effects than are likely to occur when the same amount of alcohol is downed all at once.

Distribution. Once the alcohol enters the capillaries of the duodenal mucosa it diffuses from the blood into all the body's tissues, where it mixes with their water content. The better a tissue's blood supply, the more rapidly does its concentration of alcohol build up. Thus, the level of alcohol in the brain quickly comes into balance with that of the blood. Later, tissues that receive proportionally less blood or contain less water finally take up their full share of the alcohol. Redistribution to secondary storage sites tends to draw some of the alcohol away from the brain and thus aids in the sobering up process, provided that no further drinking is done.

Metabolism. By far the most important factor in the reduction of brain levels of alcohol is the body's ability to burn up, or oxidize, the alcohol in the tissues. Between 90 and 95% of all the alcohol absorbed is broken down to carbon dioxide and water in a series of three enzymatically catalyzed steps. Most of the remaining alcohol leaves the body unchanged by way of the breath and urine.

The first steps in the metabolic breakdown of alcohol take place largely in the liver. Two enzymes catalyze the conversion of alcohol, first to *acetaldehyde* and then to *acetate.* Ordinarily, the second step immediately follows the first, so that there is little or no accumulation of acetaldehyde. However, sometimes—for example, after the prior administration of certain drugs that suppress the activity of the oxidative enzymes (see below)—acetaldehyde may build up to toxic levels.

Rate of oxidation. The speed of oxidation of alcohol to acetaldehyde—the first step in the metabolic series—determines the rapidity with which alcohol disappears from the body. The rate of this reaction, which may vary from person to person and even in the same person at different times, has been calculated for the average man weighing 150 lb to be about 10 ml/hr, or 7 g/hour. This is the amount of alcohol contained in about ⅔ oz of whiskey, 3 to 4 oz of a light wine, or 8 to 12 oz of beer (Table 53-3). This means that, because alcohol is metabolized at the same slow steady rate no matter how much has concentrated in the body's tissues, it takes a drinker almost a full day to eliminate the alcohol in a pint of whiskey. This has some practical significance in the treatment of acute intoxication (see below).

Caloric content. The third and final step in the metabolism of alcohol takes place in all the cells of the body. Here, the acetate derived from alcohol is fed into the cellular system for obtaining energy from foodstuffs. This is the Krebs tricarboxylic acid cycle, the main chemical pathway used by the body's cells to burn the acetate fragments from foods and produce energy while giving off water and carbon dioxide as waste products. Seven calories are produced for every gram of alcohol that is oxidized in this way. This is more energy than is obtained from an equal weight of carbohydrate or protein food, and nearly as much as is obtainable from fat. Thus, alcohol can—up to a point—take the place of food as a source of energy. It does not, however, contain other essential food factors such as vitamins, minerals, or amino acids— a fact that often has serious consequences for the health of alcoholics who fail to eat even a minimally adequate diet while drinking large quantities of distilled spirits.

Thus, although the heavy drinker can satisfy a large part of the daily energy requirements by alcohol intake alone, the nutritional result may be compared with that of trying to subsist solely on pure cane sugar, which also is a source of calories only. Many of the chronic alcoholic's ailments are the result of prolonged malnutrition and a consequent lack of the food factors that are needed to keep liver, nerve, and other body tissue in good health.

Another consequence of practical significance is the development of obesity in some drinkers. Those who drink even moderately *without reducing normal food intake* are likely to put on weight, because the calories from alcohol are added to those derived from dietary carbohydrates, fats, and protein. Certain beverages—beer, for example—contain substances with food value in addition to their alcohol content. Thus, obesity is all the more likely to occur in people who consume large quantities of such beverages and eat heartily at the same time.

Management of alcoholic patients

People who have been drinking heavily are often hospitalized for emergency and long-term treatment. Some acutely intoxicated patients are brought to the emergency room following an injury incurred in an accident. They may be combative and hyperactive or may be in a coma. Others may be obviously intoxicated, but their main dif-

ficulties may stem from other causes, including withdrawal symptoms, which often develop when injury or illness cuts short a prolonged drinking bout. Each of these states requires different treatment measures.

Acute alcoholic excitement: Sedation. The intoxicated patient who is admitted in a hyperactive state must be quieted to prevent exhaustion or self-injury. This was once done with repeated injections of barbiturates, such as phenobarbital or amobarbital, or with paraldehyde. However, these potent depressants can cause coma and respiratory paralysis when their effects are added to those of the alcohol that may still be in the process of being absorbed. Thus, the use of such sedative–hypnotics has largely been abandoned in favor of somewhat safer depressants such as the benzodiazepines (Chap. 45) and the phenothiazines (Chap. 46).

Some physicians prefer to control combative, destructive, or violent behavior with an injection of one of the more sedating phenothiazines, such as promazine (Sparine) or chlorpromazine (Thorazine). These drugs also have an antiemetic action that helps to prevent nausea and vomiting. However, care is required in administering these drugs, because they may potentiate the depressant and hypotensive effects of alcohol. For example, intramuscular injections of promazine should be made with the patient recumbent, and he should be kept lying down to prevent dizziness and fainting, leading to possible injury.

The benzodiazepine drugs chlordiazepoxide (Librium) and diazepam (Valium) are also often used for calming intoxicated patients, because they do not cause postural hypotension. However, intramuscularly administered chlordiazepoxide has a rather slow and erratic absorption and, although both drugs are more rapidly effective when given by vein, IV injection of the irritating solutions is difficult in struggling patients. Care is required if the acutely intoxicated alcoholic shows depression of vital signs, because administration of these depressants can lead to apnea and cardiac arrest.

Alcoholic stupor and coma

Stupor. Patients admitted in an alcoholic stupor usually need little or no drug treatment. Nothing is gained by attempting to rouse the patient with an injection of a central stimulant such as caffeine sodium benzoate (Chap. 47), if breathing is satisfactory. The patient should be left to sleep off the effects of the excessive alcohol intake, while the body gradually metabolizes and eliminates it. The stuporous patient can be examined to see that there is no head injury and no respiratory infection, or other possible complications of heavy drinking such as gastrointestinal bleeding.

If the patient is seen soon enough, the stomach may be emptied by cautious gastric lavage to avoid further absorption of ingested alcohol and possible deepening of depression. Measurement should be made of the BAC on admission and at later intervals. When the BAC is relatively low—300 mg%, for instance—but the patient becomes comatose, barbiturates or other depressant drugs may also have been taken. Patients in coma from alcohol alone or alcohol combined with barbiturates, glutethimide, or other sedative–hypnotics require support of vital functions.

Coma. The main danger in comatose patients is possible development of hypostatic pneumonia, respiratory failure, or cardiovascular collapse. Pneumonia is best prevented by keeping the patient's airway and lungs clear. Suctioning helps to avoid accumulation of secretions, and the patient should also be turned frequently. At the present time, analeptics are not often employed to stimulate the alcoholic patient's respiration. Although such drugs as doxapram (Chap. 47) do increase the depth and rate of respiration, these benefits are usually outweighed by the risk of drug-induced convulsive seizures, cardiac arrhythmias, and vomiting.

Mechanical ventilation of the patient's lungs is desirable during periods of respiratory depression. Oxygen is not necessary except in severe hypoxemia. If the patient is breathing spontaneously but in a slow and shallow manner, 5% carbon dioxide can be inhaled periodically to deepen the respirations. Other general supportive measures include IV fluids to maintain blood volume and prevent shock. Thiamine and other B-complex vitamins, electrolytes, and minerals, including magnesium, and glucose may be added to counteract possible effects of malnutrition or dehydration and hypoglycemia.

Increased alcohol elimination. Attempts are sometimes made to speed the rate at which alcohol is being removed from the body. As indicated earlier, alcohol is eliminated at the same slow rate whether the BAC is relatively low or very high. In patients with a BAC above 600 mg% it would, of course, be desirable to speed the destruction of the alcohol in the body and thus lower its level in the blood and brain.

Alcohol may sometimes be removed more rapidly by hemodialysis and peritoneal dialysis—particularly when patients are believed to have also taken other dialyzable drugs—when the benefits of these procedures appear to outweigh their risks. Diuretic therapy does little to eliminate significantly larger amounts of alcohol. However, the osmotic–dehydrating diuretics urea (Ureaphil) and mannitol (Chap. 27) may sometimes be employed for another purpose: the reduction of increased intracranial pressure in patients with cerebral edema. Injected intravenously, hypertonic solutions of these substances draw fluid from the brain into the bloodstream and remove it by way of the kidneys.

Alcohol withdrawal symptoms

People who continue to take in more alcohol each day than their bodies can metabolize soon become physically dependent on this addicting drug. When they are suddenly deprived of alcohol—during hospitalization following an accident, for example—they suffer withdrawal syndromes of varying degrees of severity (see the summaries at the end of this chapter). Sometimes symptoms develop even while an alcoholic is still drinking a great deal—for example, when vomiting from gastritis prevents enough alcohol from being absorbed to maintain the brain concentration required to prevent the withdrawal syndrome.

The degree of severity of withdrawal depends mainly on how heavily the alcoholic has been drinking and for how long. Symptoms may range from merely a mild hangover through a state of agitation and tremulousness to potentially fatal delirium tremens (the "DTs"). If the discomforts of a hangover are indeed withdrawal phenomena, as some authorities suggest, physical dependence on alcohol can be said to develop even in those who drink only occasionally. Actually, however, hangovers that sometimes occur even in social drinkers are probably the result of physiologic imbalances brought about by overindulgence in alcoholic beverages.

"Hangover." Aftereffects of even moderate drinking that often develop several hours after the drinking has stopped include a throbbing headache, heartburn and nausea, and feelings of fatigue, mental dullness, and irritability. These "morning after" symptoms cannot be attributed to any single cause, although they have been associated with many factors, including the presence in some alcoholic beverages of *congeners*—other alcohols, organic acids, and oils produced following fermentation and during aging in storage barrels. Similarly, despite the endless number of recommended hangover remedies, there really is no known specific cure. The best treatment measure is rest in a quiet, darkened room. Simple analgesics may help to relieve a pounding headache. However, aspirin may further irritate an already upset stomach.

Serious syndromes. Withdrawal from alcohol is marked by increased nervous system excitability. Unmasking of the compensatory neurophysiologic changes that develop in the CNS during drinking leads to signs and symptoms of sensory and psychomotor stimulation. These include, first, the development of anxiety and tremulousness within a few hours of the last drink. Increasingly severe tremors and hyperreflexia may be followed after a day or so by a convulsive seizure. Finally, after several days of increasing confusion, disorientation, and even hallucinations, the alcoholic may develop the DTs. Patients with "the shakes," as they call the tremors of mild to moderate withdrawal, are best treated with general depressant drugs that substitute for the alcohol that is leaving the patient's system. The aim of this type of replacement therapy is to reduce restlessness without making the patient excessively lethargic or too groggy to move about without staggering or falling. After the patient is stabilized, the depressant drug is very gradually withdrawn.

Some physicians still prefer paraldehyde for this purpose; others substitute pentobarbital for alcohol.

However, *chlordiazepoxide*[+] (Librium; see Drug digest, Chap. 45) is now the drug most commonly used to quiet the agitation and tremulousness of these patients and to ensure rest and sleep. These drugs are themselves withdrawn when the patient's symptoms are controlled to avoid development of dependence.

Chlordiazepoxide is best given in an initial large loading dose, because its onset of action is relatively slow in lower doses. Dosage is then reduced on each succeeding day to avoid the gradual accumulation to toxic levels of chlordiazepoxide and its active, slowly eliminated metabolites. The related drug diazepam[+] (Valium; see Drug digest, Chap. 45) is more rapid in onset but, because it is also more rapidly eliminated, several daily doses are required for relief of acute alcohol withdrawal symptoms.

For the complication that alcoholics call "the horrors" and psychiatrists call alcoholic hallucinosis, phenothiazine-type tranquilizers or haloperidol (Chap. 46) are often added to the patient's regimen. These major tranquilizers, or antipsychotic agents, help to dampen the patient's fearful response to the auditory and visual hallucinations. However, unlike the benzodiazepines, these drugs do not prevent convulsions, and their use may, in fact, set off seizures in susceptible patients.

The convulsions that may occur during the second withdrawal day are best controlled by diazepam, which is more rapidly effective than phenytoin sodium (Dilantin). However, slow intravenous infusion of large doses of the latter drug may be best for alcoholic patients with a prior history of epileptic seizures. Such patients may then be kept on a daily regimen of oral phenytoin for control of the underlying neurologic disorder (Chap. 50). *Non*epileptic patients do not need to continue to take anticonvulsant medications after the first few withdrawal days, when the danger of seizures is past.

Delirium tremens is the most serious form of alcohol withdrawal, because it can cause death in 15% of patients. However, patients who are hospitalized during the early stages of withdrawal and managed in the manner discussed above rarely reach this stage. The 5% of patients who develop DTs during withdrawal must receive vigorous treatment to control their severe agitation and prevent death from exhaustion, dehydration, and circulatory collapse. The measures used in the general management of this disorder include not only deep sedation with substitute-type sedatives such as the benzodiazepines, barbiturates, and paraldehyde or chloral hydrate, and infusions of fluids, electrolytes, glucose, and vitamins (see the summary at the end of this chapter), but also extremely skilled and competent nursing care. The nurse must always explain every procedure carefully before performing it, even when only feeding or bathing the patient or taking his temperature and blood pressure. There should be no use of physical restraints, because this may only increase the patient's struggles. A firm but gentle manner may help to lessen fear and keep the patient relatively quiet. The room should be kept well lighted at night, and environmental stimuli should be controlled. The patient should be constantly observed, if at all possible.

Long-term rehabilitative treatment

As with other addictions, withdrawing and stabilizing the patient after a prolonged drinking bout is only the beginning of treatment. When an acutely intoxicated patient is hospitalized, the patient's sobriety is brought about by others. However, to stay sober, the patient alone must take the responsibility for abstaining from alcohol. Helping him to do so is the most difficult and, in the long run, the most decisive aspect of treatment.

Unfortunately, although some alcoholics seem normal except for their excessive drinking, most suffer from emotional disorders of one type or another. Thus, most patients could profit from psychotherapy of the underlying depression or neurosis that commonly accompanies chronic alcoholism. Even if this is not undertaken, pharmacotherapy for relief of discomforting symptoms is desirable to prevent the patient from seeking to relieve them with alcohol.

Psychopharmacologic agents. Tranquilizing agents are used during the detoxification period to reduce the patient's nervousness, irritability, insomnia, and tremulousness. Daytime doses of chlordiazepoxide (Librium) or other benzodiazepine-type antianxiety agents, such as oxazepam (Serax) and clorazepate (Azene; Tranxene) and bedtime doses of barbiturates, chloral hydrate, or flurazepam[+] (Dalmane; see Drug digest, Chap. 45) are commonly employed for this purpose. However, long-term use of these drugs is not considered desirable during the later rehabilitation period. This is because alcoholics often abuse other depressant drugs also, and may become addicted to them. Thus, for example, some alcoholics formerly became addicted to the barbiturates, paraldehyde, chloral hydrate, and other sedative–hypnotics with which they were being treated. Today, addiction to meprobamate, glutethimide, and other modern tranquilizers and sedatives is common among former alcoholics.

Other anxiolytic drugs are sometimes employed because addiction-prone patients, including alcoholics, do not tend to abuse them. Antihistamine-type sedatives such as hydroxyzine (Atarax; Vistaril) and diphenhydramine (Benadryl) are among the anxiety-relieving agents that do not seem to lead to psychological or physical dependence, but these are considered to be less effective drugs than the benzodiazepines mentioned above. More effective psychotherapeutic drugs that do not cause dependence are the major tranquilizers and antidepressant drugs.

The phenothiazine-type tranquilizers, including thioridazine HCl[+] (Mellaril; see Drug digest, Chap. 46), trifluoperazine (Stelazine), and fluphenazine HCl[+] (Permitil; Prolixin; see Drug digest, Chap. 46) are often employed for this purpose. However, serious hypersensitivity reactions sometimes develop during long-term use of this drug class (see summary, Chap. 46). Thus, these and other antipsychotic drugs are probably best limited to those alcoholics who have also been diagnosed as schizophrenics.

The tricyclic antidepressant drugs, including amitriptyline, are commonly prescribed for control of anxiety in recovering alcoholics when their nervousness is thought to stem from an underlying depressive state. Lithium carbonate has also been prescribed for those alcoholic patients who are believed to be subject to bipolar depressions or to manic–depressive psychosis. All patients receiving such drugs should, ideally, also be receiving individual, group, or family therapy. The nurse should know what resources are available in the community to offer emotional support or psychotherapy to the alcoholic patient who needs help.

Some physicians have advocated the use of the *non*psychotherapeutic β-adrenergic blocking drug propranolol (Inderal; Chap. 18) for relief of anxiety-induced symptoms in alcoholic patients, among others. It is thought to act centrally at limbic system sites, as well as at peripheral adrenergic receptors, to relieve symptoms that stem from central and sympathetic nervous system hyperactivity. These include not only heart palpitations and the other rapid irregular cardiac rhythms for which this drug is most commonly ordered (Chap. 30), but also the tremulousness that develops during withdrawal and in the posthospitalization recovery period.

Deterrent drugs. No one can make the alcoholic stop drinking. However, the nurse can help the patient to recognize that his drinking is out of control, and encourage him to seek treatment. Once he himself becomes convinced that he can never take alcohol in any form, various types of treatment measures may prove valuable in the long-term management of his condition. These include psychotherapy, membership in organizations such as Alcoholics Anonymous (AA), and the use of certain drugs that help to deter the patient from drinking.

Disulfiram[+] (Antabuse) is the drug most commonly employed for this purpose. It acts to interfere with the activity of the enzyme acetaldehyde dehydrogenase, which catalyzes the second step in the metabolic degradation of ingested alcohol that has been absorbed into the bloodstream. The resulting accumulation of acetaldehyde is the cause of most of the discomforting symptoms described below. A similar enzymatic inhibition accounts for the unexpected adverse effects that sometimes occur when patients taking other drugs, such as the antiprotozoan agent metronidazole (Chap. 10) or the sulfonylurea-type drugs used in treating diabetes (Chap. 25), drink an alcoholic beverage.

When a patient who has taken the daily dose of disulfiram also takes an alcoholic drink, a typical reaction soon begins. Within a few minutes the patient's skin turns bright red and warm as a result of peripheral vasodilation. The vasodilation sets off a pounding vasodilator-type headache and, as the blood pressure drops, the patient feels faint, weak, and dizzy and becomes nauseated. Violent vomiting, heart palpitations, chest pains, and dyspnea may develop. Sometimes the cardiovascular complications have proved fatal to patients with myocardial disease or cerebral damage who have begun to drink while under treatment with disulfiram. Thus, disulfiram must never be given to an alcoholic without the patient having been fully informed about what to expect if a drink is taken.

Patients who backslide, drink, and become ill because of a reaction between the alcohol and residual disulfiram in the body may require no treatment if the effects are merely unpleasant. However, more severe reactions may be treated by intravenous administration of massive doses of ascorbic acid (vitamin C) and of an antihistaminic drug such as diphenhydramine HCl (Benadryl). It may be necessary to treat shock by infusing saline and dextrose solution and by administering an adrenergic vasopressor drug such as ephedrine. Inhalation of oxygen 95% and carbon dioxide 5% is also recommended.

The use of this deterrent drug in properly selected patients has proved desirable in various ways. The patient's willingness to take a daily tablet is itself an indication of a desire to stop drinking. Moreover, those who decide to take the drug each morning are relieved of the need to make countless decisions as to whether or not to take a drink that day. Then, as the days of abstinence lengthen into weeks and months, the patient realizes that he can, after all, get along without drinking. This often serves to reinforce his motivation and increases the likelihood of his profiting from concurrent psychotherapy.

A patient may sometimes stop taking disulfiram deliberately to be able to drink on a particular occasion. This can usually be done without experiencing discomfort after a week or less without the drug, although reactions to alcohol may occur as long as 2 weeks after the last dose. To avoid temptation of this type, some alcoholics who really want to stop drinking have consented to try a new experimental procedure: the subcutaneous implantation of disulfiram, which greatly slows its rate of absorption and lengthens its presence in the patient's blood. With this method of administration, a patient who begins drinking may not get very sick at first. However, heavy drinking cannot be continued for long, because the disulfiram–alcohol reaction becomes increasingly severe over a period of a few days. Patients on disulfiram must be cautioned to avoid alcohol in *all* forms, including certain desserts and candies, Irish and other types of liqueur-containing coffees, and certain over-the-counter drugs, many of which have appreciable alcohol content.

Pathologic effects of chronic alcoholism

Some alcoholics fail to respond to any known treatment program, including psychotherapy combined with the use of tranquilizing, antidepressant, and deterrent drugs.

Their continued heavy drinking leads almost inevitably to damage to various vital organs, including the liver and the central and peripheral nervous systems. Some of the tissue damage seen in chronic alcoholics is thought to be caused by the direct action of alcohol; other difficulties are caused by malnutrition. Some syndromes appear to be caused by a combination of both the direct and indirect effects of excessive drinking.

Some of the pathologic effects commonly seen in far-advanced alcoholics are described below, along with the types of treatment that are employed in efforts to alleviate such tissue damage.

Gastrointestinal tract. High concentrations of alcohol are directly irritating to the mucosal lining of the stomach. Thus, cases of acute and chronic gastritis are quite common in heavy drinkers of concentrated alcoholic beverages such as "straight" whiskey. The nausea and vomiting caused by this inflammatory reaction often prevent the drinker from satisfying the requirements of the physical dependence on alcohol, thus precipitating withdrawal symptoms.

Ordinarily, acute gastritis is relieved when the alcoholic stops drinking and begins to eat again. Meanwhile, the symptoms usually respond to treatment with antacids and antispasmodics, and to phenothiazine-type antiemetics (Chap. 46). Although alcohol has not been proved to cause peptic ulcer, it does stimulate gastric acid secretion and is thus undesirable in patients who already have ulcers. Gastric bleeding is common in alcoholic patients with ulcers.

Liver. Acute and chronic liver disease is commonly seen in people who have been drinking large amounts of alcohol for a long time. Acute alcoholic hepatitis, a condition resembling infectious hepatitis, sometimes develops during a drinking bout. It is characterized by anorexia, nausea, vomiting, abdominal pain, jaundice, and an enlarged liver. The incidence of chronic hepatic disorders such as fatty liver and cirrhosis, is much higher in chronic alcoholics than in the general population. However, not all heavy drinkers—and, indeed, only a small proportion of them—develop cirrhosis of the liver. (See Chapter 41 for a discussion of the management of the complications of cirrhosis and alcoholic hepatitis.)

Although the drinker's faulty dietary habits undoubtedly play an important part in his developing serious liver disease, there is evidence that alcohol itself has adverse effects on hepatic function when taken in immoderate amounts for prolonged periods. It has been found, for example, that even alcoholics who are eating an adequate diet sometimes develop an enlarged fatty liver when their intake of alcohol is also high. Apparently, alcohol promotes the accumulation of fat in the liver by affecting the functioning of some of its enzyme systems in a way that increases intrahepatic fat synthesis.

The metabolic links between alcoholic hepatitis, fatty liver, and development of cirrhotic scarring are still uncertain. However, if a patient with hepatic fat infiltration can be helped to stop drinking before fibrous connective tissue has proliferated too far, the liver's remarkable regenerative properties can come into play. Recovery is often rapid when the alcoholic begins to eat again. The patient should be encouraged to eat the prescribed diet, which is high in proteins, lipotropic substances such as choline and methionine, and B-complex vitamins such as folic acid and cyanocobalamin.

Nervous system. Previous sections have described in detail the progressive disturbance in neurologic function that occurs as a result of an episode of acute alcoholic intoxication, or drunkenness; they have also described the withdrawal of alcohol from a person who has been drinking heavily for some time and indicated that this may set off various nervous system disturbances including delirium and convulsions. Here, the neurologic complications that show up only after many months or even years of uncontrolled drinking will be described.

In some of these disorders, the damage is a result mainly of malnutrition rather than of the direct effects of alcohol. Such nutritional disorders include Wernicke's encephalopathy, Korsakoff's psychosis, and alcohol polyneuropathy.

Wernicke's disease. This disorder is marked by the sudden onset of clinical signs of three types—ocular muscle paralysis, ataxia, and mental confusion. Once the disease is recognized and treated with massive doses of *thiamine*, the ocular signs and muscular incoordination clear up quickly, and the patient becomes more alert and responsive.

Korsakoff's psychosis. Some patients continue to show mental symptoms even after they have recovered from the acute phase. These alcoholics are suffering from a peculiar type of intellectual impairment called Korsakoff's psychosis. This is characterized by a disturbance in memory, especially the memory of recent events, as well as by an inability to learn new material.

Even when the patient has improved after several months of hospitalization, he still has difficulty in putting past events into their proper sequence. Most victims of this amnesia-type psychosis are unable to function in society, and must be institutionalized. Apparently, in such cases, the severe thiamine deficiency has caused neuropathologic lesions in the thalamus that have gone too far to be corrected in the same manner as can the cerebellar lesions of Wernicke's disease.

Alcoholic polyneuropathy. Many patients show signs of damage to the motor and sensory fibers of peripheral nerves. Most complain of muscle weakness of the legs and arms, or numbness and tingling of the skin. A few suffer from burning pain in the feet or hands or deep aching of the legs. Such polyneuropathy is thought to be the result of a multiple vitamin deficiency resulting from a state of semistarvation.

Treatment mainly involves the daily administration of large doses of thiamine, pyridoxine, pantothenic acid, riboflavin, and other vitamins. These may have to be given by injection because of the patient's persistent vomiting or other GI complications. Salicylates, and occasionally codeine, may be ordered for relief of muscle pains during the long weeks of convalescence. The patient should be encouraged to consume the ordered diet, which is high in calories from protein and which is supplemented by multiple vitamins.

Cardiac complications. Ordinary doses of alcohol have few, if any, direct effects on the heart. As previously indicated, the sedative and analgesic actions of alcohol may even be beneficial for some patients with pain from coronary insufficiency. However, excessive drinking can adversely affect cardiac function in various ways. Acute intoxication may set off transient cardiac irregularities that can usually be relieved by sedation with a barbiturate or with a minor tranquilizer such as chlordiazepoxide or hydroxyzine, but that may require cardiac antiarrhythmic drugs such as propranolol. Chronic alcoholics sometimes suffer from heart muscle damage. Cardiomyopathy of this type may be a manifestation of beriberi, a disease resulting from a deficiency of vitamin B_1. As in the latter condition, alcoholic patients may develop congestive heart failure. In addition, prolonged excessive drinking may have a direct toxic effect to the myocardium that makes the heart susceptible to development of cardiac rhythm irregularities during bouts of acute alcoholic intoxication.

Respiratory tract infections. Before the advent of the antibiotic era, many alcoholics died of pneumonia, and even today alcoholics suffer frequent acute bronchopulmonary infections. There is evidence that the presence of alcohol in the blood, even in *non*alcoholics, may interfere with the migration of macrophages from the blood into tissues that are being invaded by infectious organisms. This effect of alcohol in inhibiting one of the body's main defense mechanisms against infection may account for the alcoholic's low resistance. In any case, the incidence of pulmonary tuberculosis among alcoholics is very much higher than in the general population, presumably because of self-neglect and the unsanitary conditions in which the alcoholic may be forced to live.

The incidence of acute and chronic bronchitis is also high in alcoholics. This may be because drinking reduces the production of the respiratory tract fluids that act as a natural protective covering to the mucosa, and mucous secretions tend to accumulate in the lungs during drinking bouts. Alcoholics may also be heavy smokers—and smoke more heavily when drinking—and commonly suffer from pulmonary fibrosis and emphysema. Finally, prolonged alcoholic stupor may lead to hypostatic pneumonia, and the alcoholic may aspirate vomitus while recovering consciousness.

Kidneys. Despite former claims that alcohol was a cause of nephritis, there seems to be no evidence that alcohol damages the kidneys or even that its use is harmful to patients who have nephritis. Drinking is, however, undesirable for patients with genitourinary tract infections. The increased urinary output induced by drinking alcoholic beverages may cause urgency and frequency in patients with enlargement of the prostate gland.

The diuretic effect of alcohol is related only in part to the fact that beer drinkers and others take in large quantities of fluid. A rising alcohol level in the blood, brain, and other tissues inhibits the secretion of the antidiuretic hormone (ADH) of the posterior pituitary gland. As indicated in Chapter 20, the resulting lack of ADH, a hormone that causes the renal tubules to reabsorb water filtered by the glomeruli, causes a greater proportion of the glomerular filtrate to leave the body and produce a larger volume of urine. The accompanying loss of electrolytes, including magnesium, may account for the irritability and tremors that occur during a hangover or as part of the alcohol withdrawal syndrome. A rebound retention of water and electrolytes during the later decrease in blood alcohol content may also be a cause of hangover and withdrawal discomfort.

Teratogenesis. It has been shown that women who drink alcohol to excess during pregnancy deliver babies who have a relatively high incidence of birth defects. The physical abnormalities of the fetuses and the developmental and behavioral difficulties that often occur during childhood follow a characteristic pattern called the *fetal alcohol syndrome.* The congenital abnormalities include microcephaly and facial anomalies, malformations of the hands—for example, permanently flexed fingers—and defects of the septum of the heart and of the genitalia. The IQs of affected children average 35 to 40 points below normal.

The risk and extent of teratogenesis seems to be related to the peak BAC reached on any one or more days during the first trimester. A definite risk develops when a woman drinks alcoholic beverages equal to 3 oz of absolute alcohol daily—for example, about six drinks of distilled spirits daily. Thus, even those women who are not chronic alcoholics should be warned not to drink in "binge" fashion, because fetal defects could develop from a single incident of heavy drinking on any day during the developmental period. More recent evidence indicates that even one or two drinks, and drinking *late* in pregnancy, may harm the fetus. Thus, women should be cautioned not to drink alcohol during pregnancy, and women with drinking problems should be advised to avoid becoming pregnant.

Additional clinical considerations: alcoholism

The nursing care of the alcoholic patient is a complex and difficult challenge. Because society accepts the use of alcohol within certain limits, many such people do not consider themselves as "alcoholics," and have a difficult time accepting medical intervention with their problem.

The total care of alcoholic patients should begin with teaching programs about the physiologic effects of the drug, as well as about the psychological problems that develop. The mass media and community programs have undertaken such teaching programs, often aimed, of necessity, at younger and younger audiences. National groups of Alcoholics Anonymous and similar support groups offer educational programs to help identify the person who has become an alcoholic, and to provide therapy for him and his family.

As mentioned previously, numerous systemic effects occur as a result of alcohol use. The nurse caring for a patient who is a known alcoholic must consider these changes and provide the appropriate comfort, nutritional, and safety measures that the patient will require. It is also important to remember that liver cells and thus liver function are altered by alcohol. Because most drugs are metabolized in the liver, the alcoholic patient may be unable to metabolize and detoxify standard drug dosages adequately. Most patient history forms contain some question(s) about the use of alcohol to alert the nurse to the possibility of systemic changes related to alcohol use, to the possibility of drug intolerances, and to the possibility of withdrawal.

The care of the chronic alcoholic who has numerous medical problems can be discouraging as well as challenging. Societal attitudes can easily influence the approach to the patient, and particular care must be taken to offer this patient the same opportunities for care, teaching, and support that other patients receive.

Methyl alcohol. The one-carbon monohydric alcohol methanol (wood alcohol) is a much weaker depressant of the CNS than the two-carbon alcohol ethanol. It is, however, a much more toxic substance, because it is oxidized by the body to the toxic metabolites *formaldehyde* and *formic acid.* The gradual buildup of formic acid can result in severe and often fatal acidosis and, in this acidic medium, formaldehyde damages the cells of the retina and causes blindness.

Poisoning. Ethyl alcohol sold for drinking purposes is sometimes adulterated with methyl alcohol. If this mixture is taken internally, the methanol adds little to the inebriating effect of the ethanol. However, when the effects of ethanol intoxication wear off, the effects of the much more slowly metabolized methanol begin to appear. Depending on the total amount of the mixture that was ingested, and on the relative amounts of each type of alcohol in it, signs and symptoms develop about 8 to 36 hours after ingestion.

The patient complains of severe headache, dizziness, blurred vision, nausea, vomiting, and severe abdominal pain. Later the patient's dilated pupils may fail to react to light, vision is blurred, and finally blindness ensues. In the more severe cases, delirium and then coma develop rapidly, and the patient dies of respiratory failure after a brief period of severe convulsive spasms. Most of these severe symptoms are the result of acidosis, pancreatitis, and the effects of formaldehyde on the cells of the retina.

Treatment requires prompt correction of the acidosis by the intravenous infusion of a solution of sodium bicarbonate and glucose or of sodium lactate solution. The results of treatment with these alkali solutions are often dramatic. However, the infusion is not stopped as soon as the symptoms vanish because the continued slow oxidation of the methanol results in the production of still more formic acid, which may cause a late relapse into the acidotic state. Thus, the alkali treatment is continued for several days, with frequent laboratory monitoring to avoid development of alkalosis, which can be equally dangerous. Unfortunately, permanent blindness may result despite quick correction of the acidosis by bicarbonate treatment and the use of such measures as keeping the patient's eyes covered.

Ethyl alcohol is also sometimes administered as an antidote in amounts calculated to maintain a blood level of about 100 mg%. The basis for this treatment is experimental evidence indicating that the presence of ethanol in the body delays the metabolism of methanol by inhibiting the enzymes responsible for converting it to its toxic metabolites. Thus, it has been recommended that small doses of ethanol be administered repeatedly to reduce the rate at which formaldehyde and formic acid are formed, and thus prevent blindness and other toxic effects of methanol.

Although poisoning sometimes occurs from drinking adulterated ethyl alcohol that is not known to contain methanol, most cases occur among those who drink paint remover or antifreeze fluid, despite the presence on the containers of a label indicating the danger of their methanol content when taken internally.

Volatile solvent abuse

Nurses are aware that many household products contain organic chemicals that can be hazardous when inhaled. These products should be used only after reading the directions on the label, which often advise that the substance be used only in a well-ventilated place to avoid accidental poisoning. Thus, it is astounding to find that teen-agers, college students, and others often sniff such organic solvents deliberately just for "kicks"—all the while unaware of the organic damage that these chemicals can cause.

Organ damage

The volatile solvents used in model airplane glues, plastic cements, and other commonly abused products may be any of many different chemical compounds (Table 53-4). Often these are substances known to cause damage to the liver, kidneys, and bone marrow under some circumstances. The people who sniff solvents to experience certain changes in consciousness may have no idea, of course,

1123

Table 53–4. Some volatile solvent chemicals in products sniffed for recreational purposes

Volatile solvents	Where found
Acetone	Used as a solvent for many organic substances
Benzene	In tube repair kits
Carbon tetrachloride	In spot removers
Ethylene dichloride	
Fluorocarbons (*e.g.*, trichlorofluoromethane, dichlorodifluoromethane)	In pressurized aerosol containers
Gasoline	
Isoamyl acetate (banana oil or pear oil)	In flavorings, solvents, perfuming agents, various manufacturing processes
Methyl cellosolve	
Trichlorethane	In spot removers and in pressurized aerosol containers
Trichloroethylene	In spot removers
Toluene	In model airplane glues and cements

that they may be subjecting themselves to such organ damage. However, some users have suffered blood dyscrasias and abnormalities in liver function that have resulted in jaundice, hepatic coma, and kidney failure.

The immediate effects sought by the sniffers of these chemicals, which are general depressants of the CNS, are similar to those that people often feel during the early induction phase of the stages of anesthesia (Chap. 52). These generally include a feeling of floating or dizziness, blurring and doubling of vision, noises and ringing in the ears, or even actual visual and auditory hallucinations. The user is often described as "acting drunk" because he may stagger and his speech may be slurred and his talk incoherent. When even larger amounts are inhaled, drowsiness, stupor, or even unconsciousness and coma may result.

Deaths have occurred as a result of respiratory failure. This may be the result of medullary respiratory center depression by such anesthetic drugs. Sometimes suffocation has resulted when plastic bags containing the chemicals were placed over the person's face, and then cut off his oxygen intake while he was unconscious. It has been found that many cases of sudden death were the result of cardiac arrest caused by the fluoromethane compounds used as carriers in many aerosol sprays. This

is similar to what happens occasionally when certain halogenated hydrocarbons cause heart irregularities in patients during induction of anesthesia.

Psychomotor stimulant abuse and dependence

Drugs that stimulate the CNS are very widely used without medical supervision. Millions of middle-class Americans, including housewives, business executives, truck drivers, and students, misuse such substances as the amphetamines, phenmetrazine HCl (Preludin), and related drugs for nonmedical purposes. There has also been a revival in abuse of the related stimulant cocaine. This drug is fashionable at present among people in show business and others wealthy enough to afford it.

Amphetamines

Effects

As indicated in more detail in Chapter 47, drugs such as *amphetamine sulfate* (Benzedrine), *dextroamphetamine sulfate* (Dexedrine) and *methamphetamine HCl* (Desoxyn) exert two main effects on the CNS:

1. They cause *increased alertness* and *wakefulness* and reduced awareness of fatigue.
2. They affect a person's *mood*, making him feel more *confident* and *outgoing* and willing to work.

Most medical uses of these and related psychomotor stimulants are based on the ability of small doses to produce one or both of these effects in many patients.

The amphetamines also have *sympathomimetic* actions (Chap. 17). Thus, they can cause such physical effects as heart palpitations, headache, high blood pressure, dry mouth, and dilated pupils, particularly when large doses are administered. The first medical use of amphetamine was as an inhalant for relief of nasal congestion, an effect brought about by its ability to constrict the dilated blood vessels of the mucosal lining of the nose. Amphetamine abuse began with prisoners who removed the drug-containing fillers of the inhalers and took their entire contents for the drug's systemic central effects rather than for its local peripheral effects.

Patterns of amphetamine misuse and abuse

People take stimulants for various reasons and in several different ways. Some patterns of misuse do not lead to psychological dependence but may result in undesired side-effects. Others abuse these drugs in ways that produce habituation and possibly degrees of psychological dependence that may lead to disruption of their usual family relations and life styles. A relatively small group of people becomes both psychologically and physically dependent on amphetamines to a degree that totally involves them in a type of drug-seeking and drug-taking behavior that can have disastrous and even fatal results.

Occasional use. The amphetamines are most commonly misused by people who are trying to improve their ability to perform various tasks. Thus, for instance, students cramming for exams, executives trying to complete a big job, truck drivers on long-distance hauls, and writers racing to meet a deadline may take amphetamines in small doses to ward off fatigue and sleepiness so that they can continue working. Athletes often take amphetamines in attempts to better their ordinary performance records. Long-distance cyclists, for instance, have said that these drugs increase their endurance, and professional football players often use amphetamines to "psyche" themselves up for the violent contacts of this game. (Such practices have increased in recent years to include the illegal use of drugs such as cocaine by many professional athletes.)

Occasional misusage of this type does not necessarily cause serious harm, but may do so in some circumstances. The student who stays awake all night to study by taking amphetamines may be no worse off than if he had drunk several cups of traditional caffeine-containing black coffee. In either case, however, his performance on the exam may not be good if he becomes fatigued from loss of a night's sleep. If he takes more amphetamines to fight fatigue during the exam and continues to do so for the whole exam period, he risks physical exhaustion and possible collapse. Bicycle race competitors have reportedly died of heart attacks while pushing themselves excessively with the aid of amphetamines. The point is that these drugs do not actually increase a person's energy nor eliminate the body's need for rest; they only mask feelings of fatigue.

Continued use. The most prevalent form of amphetamine abuse is that which occurs when dependence-prone persons discover that these drugs can produce a degree of mood elevation or euphoric elation that they find very desirable. This commonly happens among middle-class adults who may first have received the drug on a prescription. Thus, for example, a housewife with a weight problem takes the drug in prescribed dosage for suppressing her appetite. However, she may so enjoy the newfound feeling of well-being that she begins to self-administer the drug in larger doses and—as tolerance develops—at more frequent intervals. Because these large amounts make her feel irritable, tense, and jittery, she may then begin to take barbiturates or tranquilizers to reduce these disagreeable feelings. Before long, she may become so dependent on "uppers" and "downers" that she develops a degree of social and emotional deterioration that makes it difficult for her to care for her family or to carry out her other normal activities.

This common form of amphetamine abuse, with its serious consequences for the person and society, has led many to question whether the medical benefits of these drugs are so valuable as to warrant the risks involved in their being so readily available. Several rulings have had the effect of reducing the FDA-approved clinical indications for these drugs (see Chap. 47). Legislators have now called for the removal of amphetamines from the market entirely, particularly those products in which these stimulants are combined with barbiturates.

Spree-type abuse. The most dangerous form of abuse involves the continued administration of truly massive doses of amphetamines, usually by the intravenous route. Used in this way by so-called speed freaks or meth-heads—mainliners of *methamphetamine*—these drugs can cause severe psychological and physical damage. Although death from overdosage is rare, the life style of the long-term heavy user is extremely hazardous.

Psychological effects. The immediate effect of a rapid IV injection is the sudden onset of an intensely pleasurable feeling, called a "flash" or "rush." This is often followed by a sensation of extreme mental and physical power. The person in this state becomes very active and talkative and stays awake continuously, taking increasingly frequent doses and often going for days without food or rest. As tolerance develops—as it very rapidly does with these drugs—intake of a drug such as methamphetamine, which has a therapeutic dose of between 2, 5, and 15 mg daily, may rise to as much as 1000 mg every 2 or 3 hours!

A "run" of this type, during which the abuser stays continuously awake, usually lasts for 3 to 6 days. Groups of users gather together, talking incessantly and making less and less sense. Finally, however, the hypomanic user often falls into an exhausted sleep that lasts 12 to 18 hours and from which he cannot be readily aroused. Upon awakening from such a "fallout" or "crash," the person feels so depressed physically and mentally that he begins injecting large doses again to fight off fatigue, lethargy, and general malaise.

Physical dependence. This pattern of "runs" followed by "comedowns" of increasing length, from which the "speed freak" wakens with feelings of physical and mental misery, has led some physicians to call amphetamines "addicting" on the basis of their ability to produce a *withdrawal syndrome* when their use is discontinued. These physicians suggest that the semicomatose state that sometimes lasts 3 or 4 days and the following lethargy and fatigue that may go on for several weeks are evidence of more than merely the unmasking of a state of exhaustion. They believe that it is, instead, the result of physiologic and biochemical adaptations similar to those that occur with the chronic abuse of other drugs that cause physical dependence. Thus, the physical discomfort that follows the recovery sleep is said to reinforce the abuser's psychological craving and lead to the rapid return to amphetamine abuse. In any case, these drugs can correctly be classified as "addictive" solely on the basis of the strong psychological dependence that they produce in some people, who then become totally committed to a life style that revolves around seeking and "shooting" amphetamines.

Toxic psychosis. Those who continue to pursue this drug-taking pattern frequently suffer a psychosis that is indistinguishable from the paranoid type of schizophrenia (Chap. 46). The hypomanic user has visual and auditory hallucinations, and these in turn lead to terrifying delusions. Reacting to feelings of suspicion and unwarranted fear of imminent betrayal, the hostile hyperactive amphetamine (or cocaine) abuser can become violent. Assaults and murders have been committed by stimulant abusers in this mental state. Usually, however, the person's eccentric behavior results in his hospitalization before he harms anyone.

Treatment. Hospitalized patients who are permitted to withdraw from amphetamines in a sheltered environment tend to recover rather readily from the most disabling effects of this florid phase of the illness. The administration of the phenothiazine antipsychotic agent *chlorpromazine HCl* (Thorazine) is often quite effective for controlling the patient's hyperactivity, agitation, and fear, and for modifying the dangerously disorganized behavior that these emotions may trigger. Ordinarily, the toxic psychosis from amphetamine abuse dissipates in a few days. However, some patients may continue to have paranoid ideation and other residual effects for many months, and some who may have had latent prepsychotic traits may have to remain hospitalized for years as a result of the overt psychosis set off by these drugs.

Medical complications. Occasionally, a person who "over amps" (takes an IV overdose) may fall unconscious and awaken hours later temporarily paralyzed and unable to speak. This is thought to result from drug induced constriction of brain blood vessels, leading to transient cerebral ischemia that produces effects mimicking a stroke. Some people, in addition, show signs of organic brain damage—confusion, disorientation, and gaps in memory—that may be the result of amphetamine-induced cerebral ischemia. Other abusers sometimes suffer severe chest pains that are presumably the result of coronary vessel constriction. Deaths following high fever and circulatory collapse have also been reported.

More common, however, in the chronic heavy abuser of amphetamines, are signs of physical deterioration that stem from infection and malnutrition. Small skin injuries often fail to heal and become abscessed and ulcerated. Part of this skin damage is done by the patient, who often picks compulsively at his skin, perhaps because

he is hallucinating that insects are crawling under it, a condition called formication. As occurs with heroin "mainliners," hepatitis, tetanus, and bacterial endocarditis can develop as a result of infections by pathogenic microorganisms transmitted through the sharing of unsterilized needles.

Rehabilitation

Amphetamine abuse can lead to severe psychological and physical deterioration. However, some abusers seem able to make a complete recovery when their life situation is favorable for rehabilitation. Those who have a home and family and a job or profession are most likely to be able to abstain from further drug taking, and thus make a complete recovery.

On the other hand, prospects for recovery are poor for those persons—often suffering from severe personality disturbances, character disorders, or even borderline psychoses—who return to the drug-oriented subcultures of some large cities. These people not only fail to stop taking amphetamines but tend to become multiple drug users, involved with many other drugs in addition to "speed," including various hallucinogens, barbiturates, and heroin.

Cocaine

This central stimulant, which is employed in medicine legitimately only for its local anesthetic effects (Chap. 14), is essentially similar to the amphetamines in its ability to cause euphoria and, when used more than occasionally, psychological dependence. However, certain differences may lead to more serious physical consequences in some who develop a compulsive craving for cocaine. For one thing, this drug has a much shorter duration of action than the amphetamines. Thus, those who want to maintain a cocaine "high" have to inject the drug much more frequently, and they often build up gradually to very large daily doses that may cause physical dependence.

Toxicity

Unlike amphetamines, which rarely cause convulsions, cocaine can set off seizures (see Chapter 14 concerning the central and cardiovascular toxicity of local anesthetics). This drug may also damage the nasal mucosa of people who habitually take cocaine by sniffing it. Such use by "snorters" or "horners" can lead to local ulceration of the membranes and sometimes to erosion of the nasal septum. Thus, the current casual "recreational" use of cocaine by rock musicians, professional athletes, and others can be physically as well as psychologically harmful if the habit gets out of control.

Hallucinogenic drugs

Terminology

The psychotropic* (mind-affecting) drugs listed below have been widely publicized, mainly because they can

---

* This term applies to *any* drug that exerts an effect on mental functioning. Thus, all the drugs discussed in this chapter (and any others that can cause psychopharmacologic effects in some circumstances) can be said to be psychotropic agents.

produce dramatic changes in consciousness even when taken in small *nontoxic* amounts.

Some hallucinogenic or psychotomimetic drugs

Belladonna alkaloids (atropine, scopolamine)
Bufotenine (from certain toads and fungi)
Diethyltryptamine (DET)
Dimethyltryptamine (DMT)
Dimethoxymethylamphetamine (DOM; STP)
Ibogaine (from certain African shrubs)
Lysergic acid diethylamide (LSD; "acid")
Mescaline (from peyote)
Methoxymethylenedioxyamphetamine (MMDA)
Methylenedioxyamphetamine (MDA)
Morning glory seeds
Myristica (nutmeg)
Peyote (cactus buttons)
Phencyclidine (PCP; Sernylan)
Psilocybin and psilocyn (from Mexican mushrooms)

They are commonly called *hallucinogens, psychotomimetics,* and *psychedelics,* or are often given other names. None of these terms is entirely satisfactory for describing all that these agents may do, but a brief review of the terms may be useful for indicating their various possible actions.

Hallucinogen is a term that indicates the ability of these drugs to produce changes in perception. LSD and mescaline, for example, are particularly likely to cause visual hallucinations.

Psychotomimetic is a term that suggests the ability of these drugs to cause abnormal thinking, delusions, and behavior such as that which occurs in natural psychoses. However, these drugs rarely precipitate a true psychosis such as schizophrenia.

Psychedelic is a term that means "mind expanding." Its use is meant to imply that these drugs can open a person's mind to new insights and increase creativity. Actually, however, this type of euphoric effect is relatively rare.

Although no one term is adequately descriptive, in summary it may be said that these drugs can produce changes in perception, thought, mood, and behavior. In the following discussion of LSD, the prototype and most potent of these drugs, emphasis will be mainly on its subjective effects and on the nature of its adverse effects and their medical management.

Lysergic acid diethylamide (LSD)

This semisynthetic derivative of the ergot fungus (Chap. 23) is one of the most powerful of all substances known to produce effects on body function. Doses as low as 25 micrograms (μg) can cause detectable changes in the normal neurophysiology of the human brain. In addition to its subjective psychopharmacologic and behavioral effects, this drug produces pharmacodynamic alterations in autonomic functions. These are mainly sympathomimetic in nature (Chap. 17) and are marked by a rise in heart rate and in blood pressure, pupillary dilation, piloerection ("gooseflesh"), and an increase in body temperature and in perspiration.

Effects

Perception changes. Although the specific changes in sensory perception that an individual may report after taking LSD are unpredictable, such changes are quite reliably brought about within less than an hour after a person takes between 100 and 200 mg orally. Generally, the person who has ingested a dose of "acid" becomes aware that the things that he sees seem to begin changing in shape and color. Hearing may also seem to become more acute. Rarely, a person may report a crossing over of these and other senses, so that he "sees" sounds and "hears" or "tastes" or "feels" colors. This translation of sensory perceptions is called *synesthesia.*

These and the various bizarre visions sometimes reported are not usually true hallucinations, which by definition are false perceptions that have no basis in reality. They are instead sensory *illusions* or, at most, *pseudo*hallucinations. That is, an object that seems to change in shape or color actually exists, and music that is heard in distorted form is actually being played. Similarly, the person who sees flashes of brilliant color or unusual geometric patterns realizes that what he seems to be perceiving does not really exist in the external world but is actually going on inside his own head because of the effects of the LSD that he has taken. (People who are having true hallucinations are convinced that their altered perceptions are real, and they react accordingly.)

Subjective responses. The person who has taken LSD also responds in one way or another to the altered perceptions. That is, thinking and emotions are naturally affected by the illusions that are experienced. However, the response at any time cannot be predicted, because it depends not only on each person's underlying personality, but also on the *set* and the *setting*—that is, on the person's emotional and mental state and expectations at the time the drug is taken, and the total environment in which the LSD experience takes place, including the physical surroundings and the presence of other people.

In practice, all these factors combine to determine whether the person who "drops acid" has a "good trip" or a "bad trip." If, for example, the experience takes place in pleasant surroundings and in the presence of people who are friendly and trusted—that is, in a *positive setting*—and if the drug taker has a good idea of what to expect and is looking forward to it with anticipation (*positive set*), the LSD experience is likely to prove interesting and pleasurable.

If, on the other hand, a person doesn't know what to expect and is anxious or fearful of adverse drug effects, the perceptual changes brought about by the drug may well provoke anxiety, fear, and panic. Similarly, if he is surrounded by people whom he dislikes—police officers, for example—and if he is experiencing drug-induced sensory misperceptions in a locked ward or a jail cell, his thought processes may become paranoid and his behavior bizarre.

The psychedelic state. This relatively rare mental state sometimes develops in people who take LSD while in a highly positive set. The person feels that the unusual sensations that he is experiencing are profoundly meaningful and of great personal significance. Often, for example, the person tends to believe that, under the drug's influence, he has gained insight, not only into his own nature but into that of all humanity. He may, in fact, feel that he has found answers to the hidden secrets of the universe or that he has had a mystical experience revealing the true nature of existence and of God.

Some users of LSD claim that these drug-induced revelations have permanently altered their view of life. They claim that they have learned to love people and to relate to them better than ever before. Skeptics doubt that the insights gained while under the influence of LSD are likely to be carried over into a person's daily life. Still, some psychiatrists consider the drug to be a useful aid in psychotherapy, because some patients are then better able to bring their unconscious psychodynamics into conscious awareness.

Adverse psychotomimetic effects. LSD was originally used in research into the nature of schizophrenia, because it was felt that the drug's effects mimicked those of this illness. Most authorities now feel that the differences between LSD-induced mental states and natural, or spontaneous, schizophrenic states are too great for the drug to be really useful for such research. Nevertheless, those who are already psychologically disturbed may sometimes be precipitated into an overt psychosis as the result of an LSD experience.

The emotional effects of LSD are highly unpredictable. Sometimes a person may interpret the drug-induced sensory changes in ways that make him feel happy (a "good trip"). However, the next experience may be marked not by euphoria but by intensely disagreeable dysphoric feelings (a "bad trip"). The most common psychological disability is development of an *acute panic reaction,* an occurrence in which the person temporarily feels so frightened that he loses insight and emotional control.

It is difficult to determine what effects of LSD may make a person feel so threatened that he panics. It may be the drug's ability to break down barriers between reality and unreality. This may then lead to a loss of identity and to feelings of depersonalization. Thus, for example, a person may experience a distortion of body image and feel that his body is breaking up or about to disappear. The thought that he may "never be able to come back"—which he cannot properly evaluate because of a temporary loss of ability to test reality—may set off anxiety, apprehension and, finally, acute panic.

Management of panic. It is most important to prevent the patient who is in a drug-induced state of agitation from harming himself. Often, a friend is assigned to guide the "bum tripper" through the period of several hours in which the person remains in this state of fear and bewilderment, or he may have to be protected against injuring himself by leaping from a window, running into traffic, or other dangerous behavior.

Usually, friends succeed in "talking down" the panicky patient. Often, however, hospitalization is necessary for patients who are suffering from a relatively prolonged panic reaction. Here, the efforts of an authority figure such as a physician or nurse may be helpful in bringing the patient back to reality. As in the case of alcoholic patients suffering from delirium tremens and other confused, disoriented persons (described earlier in this chapter), the nurse repeatedly reassures the patient and talks in simple terms that help to define the real situation. Simply repeating his name and letting him know where he is can be reassuring. Telling him repeatedly that he is only having a drug reaction and that it will soon wear off also helps the patient to regain his insight and reassemble his own view of reality.

Pharmacotherapy. Occasionally, when a patient does not respond to interpersonal or verbal efforts to reassure him and help him to regain insight, the administration of sedative–antianxiety or antipsychotic agents may be employed to reduce the long-lasting agitation. Parenteral doses of *diazepam* (Valium) or *chlordiazepoxide* (Librium) help to control anxiety and panic. For patients who have been precipitated into a state of LSD-induced psychosis, *chlorpromazine HCl* (Thorazine) may have the most effective calming action. Occasionally, a patient who suffers a prolonged depressive reaction may do best when treated with the antidepressant drug *imipramine HCl* (Tofranil).

Chronic use. During the final years of the 1960s, LSD was widely used, not only for occasional experimentation by college students and others, but on a daily basis by people involved in the psychedelic drug culture. Such chronic use raised questions concerning the possible adverse long-term psychological and physiologic effects of LSD. These questions have never been clearly answered, despite continuing research. This is partly because different studies produced conflicting data, and partly because these data were often interpreted on the basis of the personal values of the observers rather than with scientific objectivity.

Long-term psychological effects. A small minority of chronic users of LSD, called "acid heads," have been described as having become psychologically dependent on this drug and as showing characteristic psychological changes. Actually, this drug does *not* seem to produce feelings that people find so desirable that they develop a craving for it and continue to engage in compulsive drug-seeking behavior to maintain their euphoria. In this sense, LSD does *not* cause the type of psychological dependence that is a characteristic of true addiction, nor does this drug produce physical dependence as might be manifested by signs and symptoms of withdrawal when its long-term use is abruptly discontinued.

However, some chronic users in the "hippie" movement have been called psychologically dependent in the sense that taking LSD and experiencing the mental effects that it produces became their main motivation. It is difficult to determine whether use of the drug in this way was a cause or an effect of the desire to "drop out" of society to live an offbeat life style. It is also uncertain whether such psychological changes as apathy, passivity, and lack of motivation to strive for success in our society were drug-induced, or whether the use of psychedelic drugs followed these persons' deliberate decisions not to compete for material success.

Some psychiatrists have described a form of psychosis that they attribute to the long-term abuse of LSD. This is marked *not* by the acute break with reality that sometimes occurs as described above, but by a gradual withdrawal akin to that seen in chronic undifferentiated schizophrenia. This diagnosis has been disputed by other psychiatrists, who feel that the chronic users of psychedelic drugs are, at most, eccentric, and that their passivity and flight from violence—if drug-induced at all—might be psychologically beneficial for many other people and for society as a whole.

Long-term physical effects. The question of whether LSD causes long-lasting physical damage also remains unsettled and a source of continuing controversy. It has, for example, been suggested that the drug might cause breaks in chromosomes. Such damage could result in two types of adverse effects:

1. Chromosomal translocation of the type that has been detected in white blood cells could lead to leukemia.
2. Damage to germ cells (sperm or ovum) or to the cells of the fetus directly could cause birth defects in the children of parents who took LSD before pregnancy, or in the infant of a mother who took the drug during pregnancy.

Scientists, at present, disagree as to whether LSD-induced genetic abnormalities and neoplastic changes have actually occurred in humans. Although the evidence is not conclusive at this time, these reports of rearrangements in genetic material have caused concern in both physicians and in former users of LSD. Nurses talking to youngsters about drugs should discuss the possibility of these adverse effects in a matter-of-fact manner, pointing out that the data are inconclusive in this area.

Rehabilitation

The psychological effects of LSD are apparently not so strong that chronic users find the drug difficult to give up. This is evident in the fact that many of those who once stopped working or studying and who dropped out of the larger society and into the drug-oriented subculture have been able to return rather readily to a more ordinary life style. Thus, the nurse who is involved in treating a patient who has suffered an acute panic reaction or acute psychotic break can often help to foster rehabilitation following recovery from the acute episode.

The nurse can, for example, try to help the patient recognize the adverse effects that continued drug-taking can have on his life, and put him in touch with clinics and people who can help with many of his problems. He can then often be convinced that the gap between his personal values and those of society is not so great, and that he can find fulfillment by other means than the drug experience. He may then voluntarily decide to give up the drug.

Other hallucinogens

Multiple drug use is a common characteristic of people who drop out of society and become part of the drug subculture. As a result, they are often hospitalized following intoxication by one or a combination of unknown drugs. Some of these agents, such as those of the belladonna–stramonium type, have been known for centuries; others are more recently synthesized chemicals, about which very little information is available. These drugs cannot be discussed in detail here, but a brief description of the effects of a few may serve as examples of the problems created by their abuse.

Centrally acting anticholinergics. *Belladonna, stramonium,* and other drugs of the "nightshade" family have long been known to cause disorientation, confusion, hallucinations, and delirium. Many synthetic drugs also exert central and peripheral effects similar to those of *atropine* and *scopolamine,* the main alkaloids of these plants. Because proprietary products of this type are being abused, nurses should recognize the typical signs and symptoms of *anticholinergic* drug toxicity as described in Chapter 16 and elsewhere in this text, and should be prepared to help handle such cases of acute behavioral toxicity.

Psychotomimetic amphetamines. Several psychoactive substances that are chemically related to both amphetamine and mescaline (see below) have reportedly caused bizarre mental effects when taken by drug users. These substances include DOM (also known as STP, initials said to stand for "serenity, tranquility and peace"), MDA ("mellow drug of America"), and MMDA, among others. These drugs produce mental effects similar to those of LSD and physical effects similar to those of the atropinelike anticholinergic drugs and adrenergic, or sympathomimetic drugs. DOM, a drug with a prolonged duration of action—16 to 24 hours compared to the 8- to 12-hour LSD trip—has caused acute panic reactions accompanied by tachycardia, blurred vision and photophobia, and dry mouth. Administration of chlorpromazine may ameliorate the patient's panic but worsen the physiologic side effects of this drug. Actually, "street" drugs are so often different from what they are claimed to be that it is difficult to be sure that the effects reported can actually be attributed to DOM alone.

Mescaline. This is the psychoactive alkaloid of the peyote cactus plant. Taken in capsule form or dissolved in a drink, the crystalline powder extracted from the crude cactus causes mainly visual hallucinations, spatial distortions, and intensified color patterns, particularly when the user keeps the eyes closed. This drug does not ordinarily induce disorientation and loss of insight. However, discomforting effects similar to those seen with an overdose of epinephrine or other sympathomimetic drugs often occur. These include anxiety, heart palpitations, sweating, and dilated pupils. Because mescaline is closely related chemically to epinephrine, these effects are no doubt those of this drug. However, much of what is sold on the street as "mescaline" proves on chemical analysis to be a mixture of other substances. *Psilocybin* and *psilocyn* are derivatives of certain Mexican mushrooms that, like peyote, have been used for centuries by American Indians in their religious rites.

Phencyclidine (PCP). This drug was introduced originally for use as an adjunct to anesthesia, with effects similar to those of ketamine (Chap. 52). However, because psychotoxicity occurred frequently during the clinical trials, it was never marketed for human use, and it was legally employed instead only in veterinary medicine under the trade name Sernylan. It is now no longer available legally. The white crystalline powder known as "angel dust" that circulates in the "street drug" trade comes mainly from illicit laboratories, where it is easily prepared at low cost.

Because of the frequency with which PCP causes "bad trips," it has never been a popular abuse drug, and there are few regular users. However, this cheap, readily available substance is often passed off as LSD, mescaline, and even cocaine. Thus, as is so often the case with illegal drugs purchased on the street, the buyer of a substance of unknown identity, purity, or potency who receives PCP instead of something else or as an additive or contaminant in it may suffer an unexpectedly severe reaction. For example, people smoking marihuana cigarettes into which PCP has been mixed have exhibited violent behavior and psychotic reactions such as are rarely seen with that relatively mild drug (see below).

Low doses of phencyclidine taken orally tend to cause symptoms similar to those of alcoholic intoxication, except for the additional development of nystagmus and other ocular signs. When inhaled in high doses or injected, the drug can cause a mental state marked by disordered thought processes difficult to distinguish from those of schizophrenia. (In rare cases, this progresses to a form of chronic schizophrenia that is very difficult to treat.) The patient's agitated behavior may be made more bizarre by rigid, jerky movements of the arms. This is probably an effect of the drug on subcortical extrapyramidal motor centers that may progress to even more acute dystonic reactions. These are marked by spasms of large muscle masses—for example, torticollis, opisthotonos (Chap. 47) and even potentially fatal status epilepticus (Chap. 50). Death from overdosage has occurred as a result of respiratory failure in comatose patients.

Although the overall use of PCP in the United States began to decline early in the 1980s, the use in large urban areas appears still to be increasing. Patients poisoned by PCP are best treated by being secluded in a quiet environment, because noise and other stimuli tend to increase their agitation. It is probably best not to "talk down" PCP patients while their behavior is still bizarre, because this may also make them more agitated. Diazepam (Valium) is the best drug for controlling both their excitement and muscle spasticity. It is preferred to phenothiazine-type tranquilizers and to other antipsychotic drugs such as haloperidol (Chap. 46), which can themselves set off acute dystonic reactions. Propranolol has also been used to control both the cardiovascular and CNS symptoms and signs. Psychiatric intervention should not be attempted until the patient's condition has stabilized and he is no longer hallucinating.

Marihuana and related cannabis derivatives

The cannabis controversy

The use of marihuana and related drugs for so-called recreational purposes has risen sharply in recent years. An estimated 40 million Americans have now tried smoking "pot" or taken hashish. Marihuana use is most widespread among adolescents and other young people. More than half of young adults between 18 and 25 years of age have tried the drug, and about half of all young people who have ever tried it continue to use it at least occasionally. A survey of high school seniors indicated that close to 10% report using marihuana more than 20 times each month.

The question of whether use of cannabis derivatives is hazardous to mental and physical health has created considerable controversy. No drug is, of course, ever safe in all the various circumstances in which it may be employed. Thus, questions of any drug's safety can be answered only on the basis of carefully collected scientific data and, even then, the answers to specific questions may have to be qualified because of an incomplete understanding of the drug's effects in many of the circumstances in which it is used.

Unfortunately, many people hold emotionally charged opinions about marihuana use that are not based on the now known facts about its psychopharmacologic and other effects. Instead, their views are usually conditioned by personal, cultural, or social values. Often they work to influence public policy by advocating the passage or the repeal of laws. This is, of course, desirable in a democratic society, provided that such policy is finally determined on the basis of scientific knowledge rather than by personal prejudices.

The nurse as an educator

The nurse has many opportunities to provide factual information concerning the psychological and physiologic effects of marihuana and other drugs. School and public health nurses are often called on to provide factual information to various age groups. The audience may need information related to its own use or potential use of the drug, the effects of the drug on family members, or the controversial medicolegal issues that surround the use of this drug.

The following discussion of cannabis derivatives will present information about the acute and chronic effects of the use of these drugs. There is now general agreement about the immediate effects of marihuana in various circumstances. However, many questions concerning the long-term effects of its chronic use remain unsettled. New information is continually being added to what is known about marihuana. The nurse who is responsible for teaching people about this drug and its use must remain informed about current research findings so as to present accurate information to those who receive much conflicting information through the mass media.

The plant and its products

One difficulty in discussing marihuana has been the fact that—unlike ethyl alcohol, for example—it is not a pure substance of known potency. Marihuana is made up of the leaves and flowering tops of the hemp plant, *Cannabis sativa*, a weed that grows in many parts of the world. The effects of smoking the dried plant parts, which are rolled loosely into cigarettes ("joints"; "sticks"), vary, depending on their concentration of psychoactive constituents. The weed that grows in this country has a relatively low level of the resinous material that contains the active ingredients. Marihuana from Mexico is somewhat stronger, and specially selected and cultivated plants grown in Jamaica—called ganja—are relatively rich in the resin, as are those from India, Egypt, Vietnam, and other warm, sunny, tropical countries.

The resinous secretion from the plant's flowers is also available as *hashish*, or charas, a product between five and ten times as potent as marihuana itself. This substance may be smoked in a pipe or mixed into candies, cookies, or drinks and eaten. "Hashish oil," a liquid concentrate extracted from the plant, has appeared in illicit channels. It may contain as much as 60% of the main active constituent *delta-9-tetrahydrocannabinol* (Δ^9-THC). This substance, which is now available in pure form from both natural and synthetic sources, has served as the basis for research studies on the true pharmacologic effects of all these plant products. However, the presence of other constituents of marihuana, such as cannabidiol, for example, may modify the effects of the major ingredient in ways that could account for the drug's variable effects when it is obtained from different sources.

Acute psychological and physical effects

All the various factors that influence the response to any drug (Chap. 4) may modify the effects of cannabis derivatives. Thus, for example, in addition to differences in potency of various products, the drug's manner of administration often affects what people feel. That is, the inhalation of a high concentration of THC from smoking a marihuana cigarette has a rapid and sometimes intense effect, while ingesting the same dose in food or drink has a slower, less strong, but more prolonged effect. In addition, of course, such nonpharmacologic factors as the set and the setting (see Chap. 4 and above) also influence the subjective responses to this and other psychoactive substances.

Sensory, mental, and emotional effects. Despite the variability with which different people respond to psychoactive drugs, the following broad generalizations can be made about marihuana and its major constituent:

1. Small doses of THC, equivalent to between one to four marihuana cigarettes, tend to produce effects somewhat similar to those of the general depressant drugs, such as alcohol and the barbiturates.
2. Much higher doses, equal to between five and ten smoked cigarettes, bring on perceptual changes similar to those caused by ingesting small doses of LSD.

The most commonly reported effect that a smoker first reports within 15 minutes of inhaling an adequate dose of THC is a feeling of floating and drowsiness. Most marihuana users find this pleasurably relaxing. The user also often claims to have a heightened sensitivity to external stimuli. Thus, the colors of a work of art may seem brighter and richer or the pattern of a rug more intricate, the sounds of music may seem more exciting or be better appreciated, and foods may seem tastier than usual. Studies also indicate that with moderate doses perception of time and distance may be distorted. Thus, time seems to pass very slowly and distances become difficult to judge correctly.

The marihuana smoker's emotional response to what he feels when "high" varies most markedly with whether or not others are present. Alone, he may simply obtain a quiet satisfaction from awareness of the drug-induced sensory changes, and his thoughts may turn inward if he happens to be inclined toward introspection. On the other hand, those who are part of a group of like-minded people may get gay and giddy when "blowing pot" together. In such a setting there may be a lot of silly giggling and sometimes uncontrollable laughter in response to aspects of the situation that seem hilariously funny. This is, of course, similar to what sometimes happens when people are drinking alcohol in a group. However, the loss of inhibitions with marihuana is mainly verbal rather than behavioral, and marihuana intoxication rarely results in aggressive or violent behavior, as is commonly the case with alcohol.

Psychomotor effects. Moderate amounts of marihuana—for example, the dose of THC taken in by smoking two cigarettes—tend to impair a person's ability to perform tasks requiring complex motor coordination, such as driving a car. It now seems clear, not only from results of laboratory studies of the smoker's responses in simulated driving situations but from actual driving performance and a statistical study of fatal highway accidents, that the effects of driving while intoxicated with marihuana are similar to those of alcoholic intoxication. That is, although some people may do reasonably well while "stoned," many may suffer a sufficient degree of impaired judgment and coordination to endanger themselves and others when driving. (Of course, the additive effects of the two drugs—and the two are now commonly taken together—may well be worse than those of either marihuana or alcohol alone.)

Other physical effects. The most commonly reported physiologic effect of marihuana is an increase in pulse rate. Tachycardia of this type is not serious in healthy young people. However, the extra workload of a rapid heart rate could be dangerous for people with cardiac abnormalities. People with coronary heart disease, for example, develop anginal chest pains sooner when they exercise after smoking marihuana. The drug also causes a bronchodilatory effect, which can facilitate smoking in patients with asthma or other obstructive pulmonary diseases. Other effects include hypotension, reddening of the eyes, a reduction in intraocular pressure, and an increase in appetite, particularly for sweets. Ordinarily, all the mental and physical effects of mild marihuana intoxication wear off in an hour or two, and occasional ex-

perimental use of one or two cigarettes seems to be harmless to health, at least in those who do not try to drive while intoxicated.

Adverse acute effects

Not all experimenters with marihuana find its effects pleasant. Some get only a dry, sore throat; others become nauseated and dizzy, and they may vomit. They may complain of feeling weak, "fuzzy," "doped," or "weird," and may find themselves distressed by the thought that they are losing control of their emotions, thinking, and behavior.

Acute panic reaction. This is the most common adverse psychological reaction to marihuana. It seems most likely to occur in an inexperienced user who is anxious and fearful to begin with. Becoming upset by the drug-induced perceptual changes, he may lose his perspective and feel that he is having a nervous breakdown or losing his mind. However, unusually high doses sometimes set off acute panic even in people experienced in the use of marihuana or hashish. As in the case of LSD, a person may become particularly alarmed by distorted perceptions of body image or by feelings of depersonalization.

Acute psychotic reaction. Rarely, a person who has taken a high dose or who has some pre-existing personality or mental problem may suffer an acute psychotic break. In addition to such symptoms of an acute brain syndrome as confusion, disorientation and memory impairment, the person may develop paranoid ideation, and his behavior may become violent. However, such reactions are almost always transient and are readily responsive to treatment, unlike the case in a paranoid schizophrenic reaction that occurs spontaneously.

Flashbacks. Some people have reported recurrences of the feelings that they had had when smoking marihuana on a previous occasion, at a time when they have none of the drug in their systems. Sometimes, also, individuals who had taken hallucinogens such as LSD or mescaline in the past have reported a spontaneous return to the hallucinogenic state upon smoking a single marihuana cigarette months later. Such so-called flashbacks may be startling and upsetting, but those who have experienced them have required little treatment.

Treatment. Managing adverse psychological reactions to marihuana is essentially similar to that employed when the cause of panic or psychosis is LSD or other hallucinogens (see above). That is, most reactions are best terminated by staying with the panicky person and repeatedly assuring him that the cause of the strange feelings is the drug that was taken, which will wear off before long. More agitated patients may require parenteral administration of an antipsychotic drug such as *chlorpromazine HCl* (Thorazine). The patient must, of course, be kept from harming himself or others while still disturbed or violent.

Long-term physical and psychological effects

Physical effects. *Tolerance and physical dependence* do not develop in people who use marihuana in the ordinary way—that is, small amounts taken for recreational purposes in social situations. However, it is evident from research done in hospital units that tolerance does develop in those who continue to take frequent large doses of THC and other cannabis derivatives in a pattern that is not typical of the way these drugs are commonly employed in this country. Similarly, when such experimental subjects are abruptly deprived of the drug that they had been getting in large doses, many show signs and symptoms similar in some respects to those of the withdrawal syndrome seen in abusers of sedative–hypnotics. These included the sudden onset, after 6 to 8 hours, of restlessness, irritability, tremor, nausea, vomiting, and diarrhea.

The only common physical effect of continued use of cannabis products is the cough that occurs in heavy marihuana smokers. This is no worse than that caused by smoking cigarettes made of tobacco. However, as with the smoking of ordinary cigarettes, heavy use of marihuana could lead to impairment of pulmonary function as a result of chronic bronchitis and emphysema. Even long-term use of large doses does not, however, seem to have the adverse effects on vital organs that often occur in chronic alcoholism, and no deaths have occurred as a direct effect of acute cannabis overdosage.

Further research will be necessary to determine whether some of the potentially serious effects of long-term marihuana use that have occasionally been reported in the literature are actually valid hazards. This drug has reportedly caused basic changes in cell metabolism, impairment of the body's immune responses, an increase in the number of abnormal chromosomes, and impaired endocrine gland function resulting particularly in changes in male sex hormone and growth hormone levels. However, much remains to be learned about whether chronic use of cannabis products can really have the hazardous effects suggested by such reports.

Psychological effects. The vast majority of marihuana users do not develop psychological dependence on this drug. That is, very few people have shown a compulsive need to continue the heavy use of marihuana or hashish. Nevertheless, considerable concern is often expressed about so-called potheads, people who become so overwhelmingly preoccupied with taking these and other drugs that they cannot function in ordinary society.

Some pediatric psychiatrists and other authorities are particularly concerned that adolescents who become habituated to the effects of marihuana may suffer impaired personality development. They feel that use of the drug during a time when youngsters are making the difficult transition to adult life may prevent them from working out their problems in ways that foster maturity. Heavy use of this drug, they suggest, may lead to a loss of motivation and to further attempts to escape reality through the use of "hard" drugs such as heroin.

It is, of course, always difficult to say whether involvement with any drug to the exclusion of interest in pursuing objectives that society values is caused by a person's exposure to the drug, or whether excessive drug taking reflects a prior personality disturbance. However, no study has ever produced evidence that cannabis is the cause of the so-called *amotivational syndrome* or of any specific drug-induced psychopathology. Similarly, there seems to be no *pharmacologic* evidence to support the view that the use of cannabis makes people more susceptible to opiate abuse and dependence. That is, the fact that some of those who experiment with marihuana go on to abuse barbiturates, amphetamines, LSD, and heroin does *not* mean that the drug has pharmacologic effects that somehow sensitize a user's system so that more dangerous drugs are then sought out and abused. However, the public's failure to differentiate between marihuana and "harder" drugs accounts in part for the harsh penalties imposed for possession of cannabis derivatives. People arrested and convicted for such offenses can obviously suffer social "side-effects" more serious than the known effects of the drug itself.

Social and legal aspects

The question of the place of marihuana in today's society has tended to polarize people. At one extreme are those who view the drug as such a threat to their social and cultural values that they advocate imprisonment for all those who are caught with even a small amount of marihuana for their personal use. Others feel that this drug should be at least as freely available as alcohol and tobacco—legal substances that are known to cause serious disabilities in those who abuse them. Beyond suggesting, as has already been done above, that putting people in prison for possession of marihuana does not seem desirable, no attempt will be made to settle the current question of whether the possession or use of cannabis products should be "decriminalized," a term that, in any case, tends to generate more heat than light.

The following facts can be useful in helping people to formulate an educated opinion about the controversy:

1. Marihuana in small doses is a mild intoxicant that is similar to alcohol in some respects.
2. Much larger doses may induce more marked perceptual changes, but these are weak compared to those caused by LSD and other hallucinogens.
3. Marihuana is not a narcotic, and its use does not induce an opiate-type dependence nor lead directly to heroin addiction.

4. Marihuana intoxication does not cause immoral, violent, or antisocial behavior, even though it can lead to injury or death as a result of a driving accident or some other mishap.

Therapeutic uses

Although the cannabis plant and its derivatives have been used in folk medicine for several millennia, marihuana and related drugs have until recently had no approved medical uses in this country. However, the availability of *pure* Δ^9-THC and other natural and synthetic constituents that could be studied by modern scientific methods has resulted in a revival of interest in possible therapeutic applications of their pharmacologic properties. Attention has focused on new properties that differ from the sedative–hypnotic and pain-relieving effects for which cannabis was once mainly used.

The *antiemetic effect* of THC has proved useful in cancer patients receiving chemotherapeutic agents that cause loss of appetite as well as nausea and vomiting that are not well controlled by standard antiemetic agents. The benefits for patients unable to tolerate these side-effects of cancer chemotherapy appear to outweigh such side-effects as drowsiness and the typical perceptual changes of the drug-induced "high." As indicated in Chapters 12 and 41, Δ^9-THC is available, under certain circumstances, from the National Cancer Institute for this use, and FDA approval for marketing several commercial preparations of chemicals related to Δ^9-THC is expected soon.

The *drop in intraocular pressure* produced when people with normal internal eye pressure smoke marihuana has led to investigations of the possible effectiveness of its constituents for bringing about a decrease in the elevated pressure of patients with glaucoma (Chap. 42). An eye drop preparation for topical application has proved effective in animals. However, its safety in humans and its efficacy in comparison to other available drug treatment has not been determined at this time.

The *bronchodilator effect* of inhaled THC may make it useful for treating asthmatic patients. Aerosolized THC does not have the irritating effect of smoked marihuana on the mucosa of the respiratory tract. It is said to produce a more persistent relief of bronchospasm and reduction in airway resistance than some standard medications (Chap. 40).

The status of most such potential products is uncertain at present and, in the current regulatory climate, some may never become clinical entities. That is, the development and testing of all new drugs is an expensive and time-consuming procedure today. In the case of cannabis products, the problems are compounded by the possibility of their being misused and abused. However, organic chemists may be able to synthesize chemical congeners of cannabis, constituents that would have one or another of the therapeutically desirable properties and yet be free of the various drawbacks of the natural cannabinoids, such as psychotoxicity, tachycardia, and tolerance development during prolonged use in the treatment of chronic disorders.

Additional clinical considerations: drug abuse

The most effective intervention for drug abuse and addiction is prevention. Intense national and local education programs have been developed in the 1980s to deal with the drug problem through problem identification and prevention. Schoolchildren, along with their parents, are receiving educational literature and programs as early as elementary school in widespread attempts to prevent drug problems from developing. Unfortunately, there is often strong peer pressure for youngsters to experiment with drugs at an early age, and drugs are available to those who wish to try them. A very important aspect of the nurse's role in public health matters is the continued support of such educational programs as well as case finding and interventions in the community.

Drug abuse, however, is not a clearly defined area of intervention. Society accepts and even promotes the use of drugs to relieve myriad problems. The distinction between drug use and drug abuse, therefore, involves society's mores and even politics. The nurse is in a key position, when doing patient and family teaching, to present factual information about the risks of abuse and signs to watch for. It is usually safe to say that any chemical, or drug, used in excess has the potential for abuse and for the physical problems that can result. People need to be educated about what constitutes a "drug," the importance of following the instructions on prescriptions, not combining several medications, and seeking assistance in finding nondrug solutions to their problems. All patients who receive patient teaching programs can benefit from the reiteration of this information.

Patients who become addicted to drugs need support and encouragement throughout their withdrawal process and in their attempts to alter their life style to accept a drug-free life. Patients may be frightened, hostile, or discouraged; they can generally be encouraged to share these feelings with the nurse, and often the nurse is therefore the most appropriate health-care professional to help patients learn to cope with the changes in life style that face them. As with other potentially emotional and judgmental issues that must frequently be dealt with, the nurse is best able to help the patient with a drug abuse problem when personal feelings, biases, and judgments have been confronted and taken care of. The nursing care of the patient with a drug addiction problem can be frustrating, discouraging, and challenging.

Summary of the therapeutic effects of ethyl alcohol (ethanol)

Local effects

1. Evaporation from the skin has a cooling effect that is desirable in sponge bathing of feverish patients.
2. Evaporation from the external ear has a desirable drying effect, helpful for preventing growth of microorganisms in the external ear canal and resulting "swimmer's ear."
3. Application to the unbroken skin has a disinfecting effect, useful in presurgical scrubbing and as an antiseptic for injection sites.
4. Astringent, cleansing, and skin conditioning effects help to prevent decubitus ulcers.
5. Rubefacient (skin-reddening) action makes it desirable for use in liniments and skin rubs.
6. Solvent effect is useful for removing phenol that has been spilled on the skin or for removing toxin-containing oil of the poison ivy plant.
7. Local injection close to nerve trunks and ganglia has been employed for pain relief and for producing local vasodilation.

Systemic effects

Central effects of small doses, including sedation, hypnosis, and analgesia, may be desirable for relief of tension and pain and for other purposes in some patients.*

1. In angina pectoris and peripheral vascular diseases, these central effects, rather than vasodilation, are responsible for any benefits of medicinal whiskey.
2. In cancer, alcohol has been used for pain relief, especially in combination with narcotic analgesics and phenothiazines.
3. In obstetrics, alcohol has been employed for preventing premature labor; selective β_2-adrenergic agonists are now generally considered to be safer and more efficacious.
4. The "digestant" or "stomachic" effects sought when alcoholic drinks are taken before meals are probably brought about by relief of tension and anxiety. (That is, the "appetizer" effect is really caused by sedation rather than by an increase in digestive secretions, even though concentrated alcoholic solutions act locally to stimulate gastric secretion in tests of stomach function.)
5. The diaphoretic (sweat-inducing) action of alcoholic drinks used by laymen for reducing fever (antipyretic) in "head colds" is a central effect.
6. The hypnotic (sleep-producing) effect may be useful as an occasional "nightcap" but is potentially harmful in people prone to abuse drugs.

* Alcohol in large amounts has been used in the past, together with opiates, to produce general anesthesia. However, its prolonged excitement stage and narrow safety margin make it unsuitable for this purpose in modern anesthesia.

Summary of drug abuse signs and symptoms

Opiates

Early effects. Face flushed; skin warm, moist and itchy; nausea and vomiting may occur; drifts in drowsy, dreamlike state—the "high"; restlessness and excitement sometimes occur, however; pupils constricted to "pinpoint" size.

Late effects. Overdose may cause coma, pulmonary edema, cardiovascular collapse, or respiratory failure; chronic cases have needle marks, scars ("tracks"), sores, and abscesses on skin; medical complications may include thrombophlebitis, hepatitis, endocarditis, and tetanus.

Barbiturates and other sedative–hypnotics and tranquilizers

Moderate intoxication. Understanding and judgment impaired; speech slurred, slow, and confused; difficulty in walking (may stagger); appearance often unkempt or untidy; irritable, easily upset—may be impulsive in behavior.

Severe intoxication. A period of confusion, excitement, and delirium may be followed by deep sleep, stupor, coma; breathing slow and shallow; blood pressure falls to shock levels.

Solvents (inhalation of glues, plastic cements, gasoline lighter fluids, aerosol mixtures, and other such substances)

Effects vary, depending on the actual chemical contents, but often resemble those of intoxication by alcohol: drowsiness, dizziness, confusion, combativeness, motor incoordination; possible perceptual changes and hallucinations; also possible is a brief period of excitement followed by sudden cardiac arrest.

Psychomotor stimulants (amphetamines, and others)

Small to moderate overdosage. Nervousness, restlessness, jitteriness, irritability, and insomnia, for all of which the abuser may self-administer barbiturates; also mouth dryness, dilated pupils, heart palpitations.

Spree-type, or chronic use of large overdoses. Intensely active, talkative, and hypomanic; increasingly confused and disorganized; frightened by perceptual changes and hallucinations; possible development of delusions and paranoid feeling, thinking, and behavior;

physical effects of failure to eat may include severe weight loss and failure of skin lesions to heal.

LSD, mescaline, and other hallucinogens

Psychopharmacologic effects. Vary considerably but may include perceptual changes, mostly visual; changes in sense of body in relation to environment; emotions ranging from elation to anxiety and fear; thinking confused and disorganized.

Physical effects. Face may be flushed or pale; may feel cold, have gooseflesh and shiver; pulse rate, blood pressure, and body temperature may all be raised; pupils may be dilated.

Marihuana and related cannabis products

Small amounts. Feeling of floating, drowsiness, and relaxation; thirst, coughing, nausea, and vomiting.

Moderate to high doses. Perceptual changes, particularly distortions in time and space and increased awareness of colors and sounds; possible visual hallucinations; occasionally, confusion, anxiety, and panic; rarely, acute psychosis.

Summary of treatment measures in acute alcoholic intoxication

Acute alcoholic excitement ("pathologic intoxication")

Sedation. Phenothiazine tranquilizers with sedative and antiemetic components, such as *promazine HCl* (Sparine) and *chlorpromazine HCl* (Thorazine), may be administered parenterally to control hyperexcitability, nausea, and vomiting. Patients should be kept lying down to avoid drug-induced postural hypotension. The antianxiety agents or minor tranquilizers—*chlordiazepoxide* (Librium), *diazepam* (Valium), and *hydroxyzine* (Atarax; Vistaril)—are sometimes preferred for this purpose, because they are not likely to cause either the postural hypotension that occurs with the phenothiazines or the excessive central depression (coma and respiratory paralysis) that may develop when barbiturates are administered to quiet intoxicated patients who have a BAC of 200 mg% or more.

Acute alcoholic stupor and coma

1. The patient's stomach is emptied by gastric lavage if it is thought that it still contains large amounts of unabsorbed alcohol. Care is taken, of course, to prevent aspiration of the gastric contents.

2. No drugs are needed to arouse the patient, but analeptics are occasionally employed parenterally to help respiration and to reduce the depth of depression. Caffeine sodium benzoate (0.5 g) may be administered parenterally.

3. Mechanical ventilation may be employed for maintaining respiratory exchange in respiratory paralysis. Inhalation of 5% carbon dioxide may increase the depth of shallow breathing.

4. Attempts may be made to hasten the rate of alcohol removal from the body by hemodialysis or by the administration of diuretics to increase urinary flow.

5. Injection of intravenous fluids for combating shock and overcoming the effects of dehydration and malnutrition is desirable. Various vitamins, minerals, and electrolytes are commonly added to dextrose solutions for intravenous infusion.

Summary of treatment measures in acute alcoholic withdrawal syndromes

Drug treatment

Sedation to counteract anxiety and tremulousness. *Chlordiazepoxide* (Librium) is preferred to other general depressant drugs such as barbiturates and paraldehyde for early treatment of tremulousness and anxiety in mild to moderate cases of withdrawal. *Diazepam* (Valium) may be employed to control convulsive seizures ("rum fits") that sometimes occur on the second day of withdrawal. Patients with a prior history of epileptic seizures may receive standard anticonvulsants such as *phenytoin* (Dilantin) and *phenobarbital*, at first parenterally, and later as oral maintenance therapy. Patients with delirium tremens may require large doses of such general depressants as *amobarbital* (Amytal) and *phenobarbital*, as well as the benzodiazepines already mentioned and the phenothiazines discussed below.

Antipsychotic agents to counteract alcoholic hallucinosis. Signs of toxic psychosis that sometimes appear on about the second or third day of withdrawal, including auditory hallucinations, confusion, disorientation, and agitation, are best counteracted with increased doses of phenothiazine-type tranquilizers. Some physicians prefer to raise the dosage of *promazine* and *chlorpromazine* (see above) to keep patients deeply sedated and to prevent development of delirium. Others employ phenothiazines such as *trifluoperazine* (Stelazine) and other less sedating antipsychotic agents such as *haloperidol* (Haldol).

Other measures

1. *Fluids and electrolytes* are administered parenterally to replace the patient's large fluid losses from fever, severe sweating, vomiting, and hyperventilation. A 5 or 10% dextrose in saline solution is infused, and potassium or sodium chloride or bicarbonate added as required, in accordance with the result of frequent checks of the patient's serum electrolyte levels. B-complex vitamins may also be administered IM, or by addition to the infusion fluid, to make up for the depletion of these nutrients during the period of drinking.

2. *Osmotic diuretics* such as urea or mannitol may be administered by intravenous drip to reduce intracranial pressure, if cerebral edema develops, or to counteract circulatory overload by parenteral fluids.

3. *Nursing care* should be sympathetic and understanding. Patients should not be restrained, if this can be avoided, and measures for increasing orientation to their surroundings should be employed. For example, concrete statements telling patients where they are should be made repeatedly and spoken slowly.

   The nurse should always carefully explain what is about to be done before undertaking any procedure, because the patient, reacting in fear to visual, auditory, and tactile hallucinations, may struggle against attempts to feed and bathe him as well as against potentially painful procedures, such as blood taking or spinal punctures.

   It is desirable to keep the room lighted at night and not to leave the patient unattended. The calm and reassuring presence of the nurse and a firm but gentle manner are most important for keeping the patient relatively quiet.

Summary of major drug withdrawal syndromes

Opiate abstinence signs and symptoms

Mild reaction. Running nose and eyes; sweating; yawning.

Moderate reaction. Loss of appetite; muscular contractions ("kicking the habit"); dilated pupils; gooseflesh ("cold turkey").

*Severe reaction.** Sleeplessness, or sleep marked by constant restlessness; shivering with cold, alternating with hot flashes and fever; nausea, retching, vomiting, diarrhea; rapid, irregular breathing; heart palpitations and high blood pressure.

General depressant abstinence signs and symptoms†

Minor manifestations. Restlessness, nervousness, anxiety, and insomnia; tremulousness, muscular twitching, weakness; abdominal cramps, nausea, and vomiting.

Major manifestations. Convulsive seizures of the grand mal type, or status epilepticus occasionally; confusion, disorientation, hallucinations; delusions and delirium; motor agitation, high fever; cardiovascular collapse.

* This is relatively rare today for two reasons: (1) heroin in the highly diluted form generally available does not ordinarily lead to high physical dependence and severe withdrawal sickness; and (2) methadone substitution and withdrawal results in a mild, although more prolonged, illness.
† Withdrawals of sedative–hypnotics and antianxiety drugs and alcohol (ethanol).

Case study

Presentation

SR, an active 22-year-old college student, became an inveterate licorice eater during his senior year in college. He was known to consume two to three bags of licorice a day. Toward the end of the semester he began to notice feelings of weakness, dizziness, and lethargy. Attributing these feelings to being out of shape, he decided to take up jogging with a 3-mile run around the campus. SR made it to the end of the course but, shortly after, he collapsed and was taken to the emergency department with complaints of lower limb paralysis, generalized weakness, and respiratory distress. Physical findings revealed BP 80/55; P 110, with occasional PVCs; R 32, labored and shallow; hyporeflexia throughout, and muscular weakness. His serum potassium level was found to be 2.9 mEq/liter.

What are the appropriate interventions for SR?

Discussion

SR's most immediate needs will be support of vital functions and reversal of the hypokalemia. Once his acute situation has been stabilized, the underlying cause of the problem should be determined and appropriate interventions should be instituted. In SR's case, it was determined that he was suffering from a form of substance abuse. Licorice contains glycyrrhizic acid, which when consumed in large amounts causes a renal tubule exchange of ions that results in a retention of sodium and an excretion of potassium—a pseudoaldosteronism. The signs and symptoms of hypokalemia and sodium retention are thus produced: edema, muscle weakness, lethargy, cardiac irritability, and respiratory distress. SR was probably aware of the slow development of a progressive, chronic hypokalemia. The stress of the sudden, severe exercise was enough to precipitate an acute hypokalemic episode.

SR will need thorough and accurate patient teaching about his problem. The experience can be used as an opportunity to explain the problems of drug use, misuse, and abuse, as well as to explore what drugs or other chemicals can cause problems when used in excess. SR will require some time to recover from his hypokalemia, and should be encouraged during this period to discuss the reasons for his compulsive licorice eating, as well as other ways to cope with frustration or anxiety. The staff nurses may also benefit from inservice classes, using SR's case as an example of "drug" misuse, to explore their understanding of and feelings about the use, misuse, and addiction to drugs. This is a very broad and often poorly understood area that is becoming increasingly more important in clinical practice.

Drug digest

Disulfiram (Antabuse)

Actions and indications. This drug is used as an aid to psychotherapy or to other supportive measures in the treatment of chronic alcoholism. It is not a cure for alcoholism but may help selected patients to stay sober. The patient knows that, if any alcohol is taken while this drug is still in his system, the Antabuse–alcohol reaction will be the result. This is marked by such discomfort as a throbbing headache, nausea and vomiting, breathing difficulty, and heart palpitations. **Adverse effects, cautions, and contraindications.** Disulfiram itself causes few ill effects other than skin rashes occasionally, or mild

drowsiness or headaches that disappear when treatment is continued with smaller doses. However, patients taking alcohol may then suffer severe reactions, including possibly fatal cardiovascular difficulties. The drug is contraindicated in patients with heart disease and in those who cannot understand and follow instructions, including psychotic alcoholics. It is never given without the patient's full knowledge or when he has been drinking.

Patients are cautioned not to take alcohol in any form, including cough mixtures or alcohol-containing foods, and alcohol should

even be avoided in products for external application, such as liniments and after shave lotions. Other drugs to be avoided are paraldehyde and metronidazole. Drug reactions between disulfiram and phenytoin, isoniazid, and coumarin-type anticoagulants may intensify the toxicity of these drugs. Thus, their dosage may have to be adjusted downward. **Dosage and administration.** Treatment is begun with a single daily dose of 0.5 g, usually taken in the morning. Later, after a week or two, the dose may be reduced to 0.25 or 0.125 g and maintained at that level for months or even years, if necessary.

References
Drug abuse

Adverse effects of cocaine abuse. Med Lett Drugs Ther 26:51, 1984

Detzer E et al: Detoxifying barbiturate addicts: Hints for psychiatric staff. Am J Nurs 76:1306, 1976

Diagnosis and management of acute drug abuse reactions. Med Lett Drugs Ther 25:85, 1983

DiPalma JR: Antagonists to the battle. RN 39:95, 1976

Doyle KM et al: Treating the drug abuser. Public Health Rev 10:77, 1982

Dupont RI et al (eds): Handbook of Drug Abuse. Washington, DC, U.S. Government Printing Office, National Institutes of Drug Abuse. 1979

Gay GR: Clinical management of acute and chronic cocaine poisoning. Ann Emerg Med 11:562, 1982

Gold MS et al: Opiate withdrawal using clonidine. JAMA 243:343, 1980

Jaffe JH: Drug addiction and drug abuse. In Gilman AG, Goodman LS, Gilman A (eds): Goodman & Gilman's The Pharmacological Basis of Therapeutics, 6th ed, pp 535–584. New York, Macmillan, 1980

Khantzion E, McKenna J: Acute toxic and withdrawal reactions associated with drug use and abuse. Ann Intern Med 90:361, 1979

Klonoff H: Marijuana and driving in real-life situations. Science 186:317, 1974

Krepick DS et al: Heroin addiction: A treatable disease. Nurs Clin North Am 8:41, 1973

Liden CB: Phencyclidine. Nine cases of poisoning. JAMA 234:513, 1975

Mendelson WB et al: The Use and Misuse of Sleeping Pills. New York, Plenum Press, 1980

Nicotine gum. Med Lett Drugs Ther 26:47, 1984

Redmond DE Jr, Krystal JH: Multiple mechanisms of withdrawal from opioid drugs. Ann Rev Neurosci 7:443, 1984

Resnick RB et al: Assessment of narcotic antagonists in the treatment of opioid dependence. Ann Rev Pharmacol Toxicol 20:463, 1980

Robinson GM, Sellers EZ: Diazepam withdrawal seizures. Can Med Assoc J 126:944, 1982

Valentine NM: Narcotic antagonists: Treatment tool for addiction. Nurs Clin North Am 11:541, 1976

Van Dyke C: Cocaine. Sci Am 246:128, 1982

Wilford BB: Drug Abuse: A Guide for the Primary Care Physician. Chicago, American Medical Association, 1981

Yowell S et al: Working with drug abuse patients in the ER. Am J Nurs 77:82, 1977

Alcohol and alcoholism

Clarren SK, Smith DW: Fetal alcohol syndrome. N Engl J Med 298:1063, 1978

Eneanya DI et al: The actions and metabolic fate of disulfiram. Ann Rev Pharmacol Toxicol 21:575, 1981

Finnegan LP: The effects of narcotics and alcohol on pregnancy and the newborn. Ann NY Acad Science 362:136, 1981

Jacob M, Sellers E: The role of drugs in chronic alcoholism. Drug Ther Bull 53, 1978

Knott D et al: Guidelines for diagnosis and alcohol detoxification. Drug Ther Bull 35, 1978

Koch–Weser J et al: Alcohol intoxication and withdrawal. N Engl J Med 294:757, 1976

Mendelson JH, Mello NK: Biologic concomitants of alcoholism. N Engl J Med 301:912, 1979

Ouellette E et al: Adverse effects on offspring of maternal alcohol abuse during pregnancy. N Engl J Med 297:528, 1977

Ritchie JM: The aliphatic alcohols. In Gilman AG, Goodman LS, Gilman A (eds): Goodman & Gilman's The Pharmacological Basis of Therapeutics, 6th ed, pp 376–390. New York, Macmillan, 1980

Sellers EM et al: Drugs to decrease alcohol consumption. N Engl J Med 305:1255, 1981

Sellers EM, Kalant H: Alcohol intoxication and withdrawal. N Engl J Med 294:757, 1976

Shaywitz BA: Fetal alcohol syndrome: An ancient problem rediscovered. Drug Ther Bull 95, 1978

Thompson WL et al: Diazepam and paraldehyde for treatment of delirium tremens. Ann Intern Med 82:175, 1975

Section 9

Miscellaneous therapeutic and diagnostic agents

9 Up to now, this text has dealt only with drugs. However, substances that are not classified as such because they do not possess pharmacologic actions useful in therapy are often used in the treatment and diagnosis of disease. This section will discuss several unrelated types of natural and synthetic substances that the nurse is often called on to administer, or about which the nurse may be called on to advise people.

There are four groups of therapeutic and diagnostic agents taken up in this final section:

1. Substances that correct body fluid disturbances
2. Vitamins and minerals
3. Immunologic agents
4. Drugs used for diagnosis, especially in roentgenography

The nurse who has occasion to make frequent use of these substances should, of course, also consult more specialized texts for the details of administration of these nonpharmacologic agents.

Chapter 54

Blood and body fluid replenishers and vitamins and minerals

54

Blood and its components

Nurses are often responsible for various aspects of the clinical use of blood and blood components—for example, when working with children being treated for acute leukemia, patients with bleeding disorders, accident victims, and other patients who need treatment with blood fractions. Nursing specialists in the field of transfusion are familiar with techniques for collecting and storing blood and are, of course, skilled in starting and maintaining transfusions. All nurses who administer blood should know the therapeutic purpose of each component that they administer and must be quick to recognize and deal with any adverse reactions that may develop during the infusion of this vital fluid and all of its fractions.

Blood and its components are physiologic substances rather than pharmacologic agents. Thus, this textbook will not offer detailed discussions of this form of *non*drug therapy. It will describe only a few topics of current clinical significance. The nurse who wants to specialize in this area will very likely have to undertake an intensive training program requiring several months of study and practice. Those who have not had such specialized courses, but whose practice requires them to make frequent use of blood and blood components, should consult other sources for more detailed information concerning these *non*pharmacologic therapeutic agents.

Whole blood

This tissue differs from others in that it is a fluid with properties that permit its being put into containers and treated in ways that facilitate its preservation, storage, and transport. It is a complex mixture of formed elements—red blood cells, platelets, and leukocytes—suspended in a solution of plasma proteins and salts (electrolytes) together with various other substances. Its actual composition varies, depending on the conditions in which

it is stored and the length of such storage, because the different constituents of freshly drawn blood tend to deteriorate at different rates.

Most authorities believe that there are now only a few indications for the administration of whole blood. They feel that most patients are better served by receiving the specific blood components they require. This is true for two reasons: component transfusion therapy is safer than whole blood transfusion, and blood is a resource that can be most efficiently employed by separating each donated unit into fractions that can be used in many different patients.

Indications

The most common of the current indications for whole blood is in the management of patients who are suffering from continued acute and massive hemorrhage. Some such patients may need many units of blood to maintain sufficient blood volume to prevent hemorrhagic shock and to keep the amounts of oxygen reaching the tissues at levels high enough to sustain the life of the cells. However, even in such critical situations, most patients can be adequately managed with red blood cell concentrates supplemented by solutions containing proteins or even noncolloidal (crystalloid) substances.

Whole blood may also be used in the exchange transfusion treatment of newborn infants suffering from erythroblastosis and occasionally in older children with Reye's syndrome, or in adults with acute fulminating hepatitis who have passed into hepatic coma. In erythroblastosis, removal of the baby's blood and replacement with whole blood can help to prevent brain damage from hyperbilirubinemia and to maintain oxygen flow to the tissues. Care is required to avoid overloading the circulation of these and other anemic newborn infants, who should continue to receive only small incremental amounts of blood rather than massive transfusions.

1142

Formerly, patients undergoing open heart surgery required many units of fresh, whole heparinized blood for priming the cardiopulmonary bypass machine oxygenator and for other purposes. Here, too, however, the current trend is toward the use of other fluids for priming purposes—for example, low-molecular-weight dextran or dextrose in saline solution (see below). Blood lost by the patient during the procedure can be adequately replaced by red cell concentrates combined with fresh frozen plasma.

In various other clinical situations in which patients require specific components such as platelets, granulocytes, and specific clotting factors, the former practice of transfusing whole blood is being abandoned. This is partly because whole blood is too dilute to furnish sufficient amounts of the required components without the risk of circulatory overload. In such situations, and in most others, it is now thought that the risks of administering whole blood outweigh its benefits.

Reactions to whole blood transfusion

Other hazards of whole blood transfusion, in addition to the previously mentioned danger of circulatory overload, include the possible occurrence of antigen–antibody reactions during or shortly after the transfusion of even a single unit of whole blood. The inadvertent administration of incompatible blood can, for example, cause rapid destruction of the patient's own red cells, with a resulting release of hemoglobin from the erythrocytes and subsequent hemoglobinuria and kidney failure. Common early signs of such a hemolytic reaction include chills and fever, headache, flushing of the face, chest and lower back pain, and the sudden development of a state of shock.

In recent years there has been increased evidence of risk of transmitting AIDS (acquired immune deficiency syndrome), hepatitis B, or hepatitis non-A non-B from a virus or some other unidentifiable factor transferred by blood transfusion.

Management. If signs and symptoms of a transfusion reaction occur, the transfusion must be immediately discontinued, because further infusion of blood increases the severity of such reactions. Usually, treatment is begun at once to prevent possible damage to the renal tubules. The osmotic diuretic mannitol may be administered intravenously in an effort to maintain adequate blood flow through the kidneys. Often, after diuresis develops, the patient's blood volume and electrolyte balance are maintained by continuous infusion of other intravenous fluids until there is no longer any danger of renal failure.

---

* Over 4,000 Americans die of hepatitis B annually from among the estimated 170,000 people per year who contract the disease. However, about 70,000 of such cases are *not* associated with transfusion and, consequently, the mortality rate from transfusion hepatitis represents ony a fraction of the total deaths. The incidence of the disease and of deaths from it can be expected to decline as a result of advances in screening and disease detection techniques.

If the patient fails to respond with a brisk diuresis, fluid intake may be restricted. A diet low in protein may also be prescribed to avoid accumulation of nitrogenous wastes, and the plasma potassium levels should be closely monitored. If blood urea nitrogen (BUN) and potassium levels rise (hyperkalemia) despite such medical and dietary management, the patient may require hemodialysis during the period of acute kidney shutdown.

Prevention. Measures to avoid incompatibility reactions begin with the processing of blood drawn from the donor in the blood center that collects, stores, and makes it available. One of the most important purposes of processing is to determine the donor's blood group and Rh type. After these and other laboratory tests are completed, the unit containing the donated blood must be labeled to indicate all the test results, and the label should also accurately identify the donor from whom the blood was drawn. Similarly, blood specimens taken from the patient who is to receive donated blood must be properly identified following tests to determine the blood's group and type and its serologic compatibility with donor blood.

The nurse does not ordinarily participate in such procedures, which are the responsibility of the technical staff. It is very difficult to prevent laboratory errors that result in the patient's receiving mismatched blood. However, before administering blood, a nurse should meticulously follow the hospital's routine for transfusions of blood. The single most important step in ensuring that blood is administered to the patient for whom it is intended is to identify both the donor blood and its recipient with the utmost accuracy. Compare the name on the patient's wristband with that on the unit container obtained from the blood bank to check that both names are identical. Many institutions require that two staff members check and sign for blood transfusions. The transfusion should be begun only after the appropriate identification checks have been made.

Risk of infection. A complication of blood transfusions that is actually more likely to occur than hemolytic immune reactions resulting from infusion of incompatible blood or allergic reactions is the result of transmission of viral hepatitis, hepatitis non-A non-B, or AIDS. Hepatitis B (serum) hepatitis can cause death, particularly among elderly patients, as a result of liver cell necrosis.* Because this form of the disease is associated with the presence of detectable hepatitis antigens and antibodies, blood banks are now required to test all donor blood for the presence of hepatitis B surface antigen (HB_sAg).

Unfortunately, despite the development of increasingly sensitive tests that are often expensive, complex, and time-consuming, only between one-half to two-thirds of hepatitis B carriers can currently be detected among prospective blood donors. Thus, it is desirable to exclude not only those with a positive test for HB_sAg, but also anyone with a history of hepatitis, including that associated with hepatitis A, or infectious hepatitis, which is known to be transmitted by injection as well as by the fecal–oral route.

Avoiding the use of blood obtained from commercial donors is another way to reduce the incidence of transfusional hepatitis B. The incidence of positive tests for HB$_s$Ag has been found to be at least ten times as high in blood obtained from paid donors and commercial blood banks as it is in blood from volunteer donors, a population in whom only about 1 in 1000 are carriers and that, in general, enjoys better health because of higher living standards. Unfortunately, there is a chronic shortage of voluntary donors, because only about 3 million people—3 or 4% of all those who could do so—donate their blood voluntarily.

Of course, even if the concept of a completely voluntary donor population were to be achieved, it would still be impossible to detect HB$_s$Ag-contaminated blood in all cases. There is, in addition, no practical way to screen for the presence of hepatitis A virus in donated blood. However, such infectious hepatitis has a low fatality rate, and it may be preventable by the administration of gamma globulin, a product that has *not* proved to be effective for preventing serum hepatitis. The use of hepatitis B vaccine in high-risk populations, as well as the availability of hepatitis B immune globulin, may well prevent much of the hepatitis B now caused by blood transfusions.

Other diseases that may be transmitted by transfusions of fresh whole blood include non-A, non-B hepatitis—a serious form of hepatitis associated with a history of several blood transfusions, but for which no viral cause has yet been identified; malaria; syphilis; possibly infectious mononucleosis; other viral infections; and AIDS, which many authorities believe is also caused by a virus. Malaria has rarely been reported, and blood that is serologically positive for syphilis can be safely transfused after being stored under refrigeration for at least 4 days.

Autologous transfusions. One almost certain way to avoid the risk of disease transmission, hemolytic immune reactions, and allergic reactions resulting from exposure to other foreign antigens is to transfuse with blood that was previously taken from the patient by phlebotomy. Patients who are thought likely to need blood or red cell transfusions in an elective surgical operation planned in the following 2 weeks may donate units of their own blood for use at that time. Because whole blood begins to deteriorate within 1 or 2 weeks and cannot be stored under ordinary conditions for more than 21 days, it may have to be frozen for use in the future. This is sometimes done for people with relatively rare blood types who want to be sure that their type of blood is available if needed at a later time.

There has been a reawakening of interest in the immediate autotransfusion of blood shed by a patient during a surgical procedure. Before World War II and the development of blood bank transfusional services, it was not uncommon for a surgeon to collect blood accumulating in the patient's peritoneal cavity and immediately reinject it into the ciculation—during an operation for ruptured spleen, for example—or to do so for a patient being surgically treated for a ruptured ectopic pregnancy. Because of certain potential serious complications, such retransfusions were largely abandoned in favor of the use of readily available blood from a homologous donor.

Intraoperative transfusions of this type are beginning to come back into favor in some centers because of the development of specially designed equipment and sophisticated procedures for collecting and reinfusing blood lost by the patient during surgery. Autotransfusion is now used mainly during vascular surgery, such as aortic reconstruction, aortic aneurysm management, and operations on obstructed or traumatized blood vessels. It has also been employed in patients with hepatic lacerations leading to persistent bleeding from liver tissue and in uremic patients who are planning to undergo a renal transplant, which might be rejected because of the presence of antigens in foreign blood.

Some authorities suggest that when certain mechanical problems that affect the quality of the shed blood are solved, the infusion of autologous blood in the above and many other clinical situations may markedly reduce the need for donated blood during and following surgery. At present, when shed blood is exposed to air and to tissues lining the cavities in which it is accumulating, it is changed in various ways that make it more coagulable. Similarly, during suctioning and collection of blood prior to its reinfusion, red blood cells are subject to hemolytic breakdown. Care is required during reinfusion to avoid possible air embolism.

Equipment is now available for reducing these drawbacks when blood is suctioned from the surgical field and drawn through microfilters for removal of debris and for reducing bubbling. The defoamed, defatted blood can then be more safely collected in reservoirs, treated with acid citrate dextrose (ACD) anticoagulant or with heparin, and returned to the patient by way of tubing leading to a vein and a needle centered in the vein. Once such equipment has been purchased, the cost of autotransfusion is said to be small, particularly when patients would otherwise require many units of expensive donor blood, which has had to be previously collected, stored, and distributed. The patient's own freshly shed and recycled blood is also of better quality than whole blood that has been stored for even a few days and has begun to lose its oxygen-carrying capacity.

Blood components

The availability of machines and methods that can separate whole blood into its several cellular components and make better use of the leftover plasma has resulted in a steady reduction in the clinical use of whole blood and in the replacement of whole blood transfusions by blood component therapy (Table 54-1). As indicated earlier, this is not only because each patient can be treated more effectively and safely with the specific component that is required in concentrated form, but also because blood centers can make more economical use of each unit of donated blood. That is, it is wasteful to transfuse whole blood when only one or two of its components are needed by a particular patient. Instead, it is more efficient to separate and administer the blood component that is needed, while saving the other components of the same donated unit for use in other patients.

Cellular components

Red blood cells are separated from the plasma of whole blood by centrifugation or sedimentation under sterile conditions. Under ordinary storage conditions, fresh packed red cells are useful for transfusion for only the same 21-day period as whole blood, and may even begin to lose their oxygen-carrying capacity within only a few days. This is thought to be because, even though the erythrocytes themselves survive several weeks of storage, they suffer a more rapid loss of a substance called *diphosphoglycerate* (DPG), which is required for the red blood cells to release oxygen into the tissues to which they have transported the gas from the lungs.

Frozen red blood cells, prepared by mixing the separated red cells with a solution containing glycerol, and then placing the glycerolized blood in a freezer at temperatures between −70° and −85°C, can be kept for several years without loss of viability. When needed, the frozen red cell unit is thawed, and the glycerol is removed by repeated machine washings with special solutions. The red cells are ready to use after being resuspended in normal saline solution.

Because washing also removes antigenic substances from the separated red cells, transfusion reactions are claimed to be less likely to occur when reconstituted frozen red cells are employed. Their use may also be preferred for renal (and other) transplant patients whose

Table 54–1. Blood components and plasma expanders*

Official or generic name	Trade name or synonym	Usual adult dosage and administration
Blood and blood components†		
Citrated whole human blood USP	—	500–1000 ml (1 or 2 U) IV
Normal human plasma USP	—	500–1500 ml IV
Normal human serum albumin USP 5%, 25%	Albuminar-5; Buminate 5%; Albuminar 25; Buminate 25%	500–1000 ml of 5% solution, IV 50–75 g/protein/day IV
Packed human blood cells USP	Packed red cells	Equivalent of 1 or 2 U of whole blood IV
Plasma, platelet-rich	Thrombocyte Concentrate	Equivalent of 1 or 2 U of whole blood IV
Plasma protein fraction, human USP	Plasmanate; Plasma-Plex	50–75 g protein IV (up to 1.5 liter of 5% solution)/day
Plasma extenders or expanders		
Dextran 40	Low molecular weight dextran; 10% LMD; Rheomacrodex; Gentran 40	10–20 ml/kg body weight of 10% solution IV
Dextran 70	High molecular weight dextran; Macrodex; Dextran 75; Gentran 75	500 ml of 6% solution IV, not more than 20 ml/kg body weight
Hetastarch	Hydroxyethyl starch; Hespan	500–1000 ml of a 6% solution IV

* See also Chapters 34 and 55.
† Mostly available through blood banks, rather than from commercial manufacturers.

tissues might be sensitized by the presence of antigens from residual plasma, platelets, granulocytes, and other debris ordinarily left on unwashed red cells.

Both packed and frozen red blood cells are useful for elevating the hematocrit of patients with acute and occasionally chronic anemia. Their use in patients who require only an increase in oxygen-carrying capacity is preferable to the use of whole blood, in which the unneeded fluid portion may overload the circulation of some patients and cause congestive heart failure. In general, red blood cells should now be used in almost all elective transfusions for which whole blood was formerly employed routinely.

Platelets can now also be obtained from donated whole blood for transfusion into patients with severe thrombocytopenia. Platelet transfusion is most commonly required by patients whose bone marrow cannot produce the precursors of circulating platelets—the megakaryocytes, which, when they mature, break up into these fragments that play such an important part in preventing bleeding (Chap. 34). Patients whose platelet counts have dropped below 40,000/mm³ are likely to begin bleeding spontaneously, unless they are transfused with products such as *platelet-rich plasma* or *platelet concentrates* prepared by removing most of the plasma as well as the red blood cells from whole blood soon after it is donated.

Patients with leukemia, lymphomas, and other neoplastic diseases often require platelet transfusions to control or prevent bleeding following bone marrow depression induced by drug or radiation therapy. Adult men usually require about 8 to 10 units of platelets to raise their counts to relatively safe levels after the count has fallen to about 10% of normal and bleeding has begun or threatens to do so. Lower daily doses may be effective for controlling bleeding in children with leukemia. However, huge doses are often needed during the course of a chronic illness, because platelets have a relatively short life span in the circulation—only 7 to 10 days at most and even less when infection, fever, and active bleeding are going on.

Fortunately, donors of platelets can contribute this blood component much more frequently than when whole blood has to be collected. Often, for example, a family member with compatible blood can donate large numbers of platelets every week for long periods without suffering thrombocytopenia or other ill effects. This has been made possible by *plateletpheresis,* a procedure by which the platelets from a unit of drawn whole blood are promptly separated by centrifugation, and the rest of the donor's blood is returned to the circulation. The process can be repeated immediately with a second unit of blood, and the same donor may make a similar donation of platelets later in the week, when red blood cells and plasma are again returned to the bloodstream within minutes of their withdrawal.

Granulocytes can also be separated from whole blood and transfused into patients with dangerously low white blood cell (WBC) counts. Unlike red cells and even platelets, which can be kept viable for a few days when properly collected and stored, granulocytes last only a few hours when removed from the bloodstream. Thus, they must be used immediately.

New procedures for *continuous leukopheresis* are being investigated for use in making leukocyte transfusions in leukemia and other cancer patients who are severely granulocytopenic and are suffering from septicemia. Because of the great numbers of granulocytes required to increase the cell count significantly, it was once common to use patients with chronic myelocytic leukemia as donors, whose white cell counts are two or three dozen times as high as those of normal people. Now, however, normal donors can make massive contributions of white cells by having their blood passed through a continuous flow cell separator containing a system of efficient filters. During a single day, 12 liters of a donor's blood can be processed for granulocytes while all the other components are being immediately returned to the blood.

Reports indicate that the recipients of granulocyte transfusions who are provided with enough white cells to raise their WBC counts by between 200 and 1000 cells/mm³ sometimes respond with marked clinical improvement. However, the incidence of serious tranfusion reactions to granulocytes is much higher than when other cellular components of whole blood—red cells and platelets—have been transfused. Bone marrow transplantation, in which a donor's bone marrow is infused intravenously into a carefully matched recipient, has become more common in recent years. This technique provides healthy stem cells, and the recipient's total blood picture often returns to normal rapidly.

Plasma products

Plasma, the cell-free fluid portion of uncoagulated whole blood, is now obtained in fresh form from single donors subjected to *plasmapheresis,* a process that permits immediate return of the red cells to the circulation. The freshly harvested plasma contains clotting factors that can be kept labile by promptly freezing the product. Both fresh and fresh-frozen plasma can be used in the management of patients with clotting deficiency disorders. Plasma can also be processed to obtain other derivatives or fractions, such as the concentrates employed in treating the hemophilias (Chap. 34) and the immune globulins used for preventing or treating various infections (Chap. 55).

Plasma can, of course, also be infused to expand the blood volume of shock patients and burn victims or others who are losing large amounts of fluid and blood proteins. However, because of the risk of hepatitis and other reactions, other safer substances are being increasingly employed for this purpose. These include both substances prepared by further fractionation of plasma and various artificial colloidal substances, which can be substituted for the natural proteins of plasma and its fractions.

Normal serum albumin, a concentrated fraction of the main component of plasma, has various advantages over the parent substance. Because it has been heat-treated to destroy the virus, there is no hepatitis hazard, and the lack of blood group antibodies makes reactions of the incompatibility type impossible. It remains stable when stored for long periods at room temperature and even longer when kept at somewhat lower temperatures.

This substance is available as 5 and 25% solutions, both of which can be employed to expand the blood volume of patients in shock following trauma, burns, blood loss, and infection. The 25% solution can also be used to treat patients with low plasma protein levels (hypoproteinemia).

Because of its low salt content, such so-called *salt-poor* albumin is best for patients suffering from nephrosis or from the ascites of hepatic cirrhosis. It has a desirable dehydrating effect in patients with cerebral edema. Because it can bind bilirubin in the circulation, normal serum albumin has been used as an adjunct to exchange transfusions in treating erythroblastosis fetalis. By helping to lower hyperbilirubinemia, the product can prevent kernicterus in the newborn infant.

Plasma protein fraction, the material remaining after removal of fibrinogen and globulin, is also free of hepatitis risk. The virus is killed or inactivated by treating this fraction with heat at a temperature that does not denature its protein content. Because blood antibodies are also removed, recipients of plasma protein fraction incur no risk of red cell damage. This fraction is used mainly for its albumin content, and is therefore indicated in most of the same clinical situations for which normal serum albumin is employed. Like the latter, it can be stored for several years at room temperature and cannot, of course, be used in treating patients with coagulation defect disorders.

Plasma expanders or extenders

Various substances obtained from sources other than blood can expand reduced plasma volume, because—like the plasma proteins—they exert a colloidal osmotic pressure, or oncotic, effect (Table 54-1). The most commonly used materials employed as plasma expanders in treating shock have various advantages over whole blood and plasma itself, including their relative cheapness and ready availability. They do not transmit the diseases associated with transfusions or cause incompatibility-type reactions. However, all the currently available colloidal plasma substitutes can cause allergic and anaphylactoid reactions.

(Although they are commonly called "plasma substitutes," these substances do not have all the properties of plasma.)

Solutions of two types of nonhuman macromolecules are available for use as adjuncts in the treatment and prevention of shock (Chap. 30) and for some other therapeutic purposes: (1) *hetastarch* (Hespan) was the first of a series of substances prepared by chemically modifying corn starch to be introduced for use in raising intravascular colloidal osmotic pressure; (2) *dextran* is a polysaccharide prepared by the action of a specific microorganism on a sucrose-containing medium. This bacterial action links glucose units into lengthy branched chain molecules of high molecular weight. For use as a plasma expander, the crude dextran is then treated chemically to break it up into smaller molecules. Two products with different average molecular weights are available.

Dextran 70 (Macrodex) has a molecular weight close to that of serum albumin—about 70,000. Thus, when a solution of this substance is injected intravenously, it shares many of the properties of the natural plasma proteins. For example, it can draw fluid from the extravascular spaces into the blood, thus expanding the plasma volume. Unlike saline and glucose solutions, dextran does not readily leak out of the vessels, so it affects osmotic pressure and vascular volume for long periods.

Although dextran—like plasma and serum albumin—is no substitute for whole blood when a large quantity of red cells has been lost, it does help to overcome hypovolemic shock, whether caused by hemorrhage or by trauma or burns. Because it is safer than plasma (no transfusion-related hazards) and cheaper than serum albumin, dextran solution is ofen used to prevent shock during surgery. Care must be taken to avoid overloading the circulation in kidney shutdown, because this could precipitate congestive heart failure and pulmonary edema.

Dextran may act as an allergen and occasionally causes antigen–antibody reactions of varying degrees of severity. Thus, the patient should be assessed for signs such as urticaria and wheezing during dextran administration so that the infusion can be stopped promptly, if necessary. Patients are also observed for any signs of bleeding tendencies, because a transient increase in bleeding time is sometimes seen several hours following dextran infusion.

A dextran of lower molecular weight—about 40,000—has been developed. Although more readily excreted and shorter in action, it has properties that make it superior in some situations. A 10% solution of this dextran 40 (Rheomacrodex; 10% LMD) has a low viscosity, which makes it advantageous as a priming fluid in heart–lung pump procedures (extracorporeal circulation). Used in this way as a hemodiluent, it tends to keep blood cells from sludging within small vessels. This action, which protects capillaries from being blocked by clumped red cells, may prove especially useful in traumatic shock.

However, when a dextran 40 solution is administered IV to a poorly hydrated patient, there is some danger that it may cause further dehydration by drawing water from the extravascular, or tissue, fluids into the plasma. Thus, to avoid this and possible renal failure, patients who show signs of dehydration should receive additional fluid—perhaps in the form of an infusion of an osmotic diuretic, such as mannitol (Chap. 27). The experimental use of dextran for the prevention of thromboembolic episodes in patients with deep vein thrombosis has been discussed in Chapter 34.

Blood substitutes

Scientists have been studying substances that might be able to perform the oxygen transporting function of red blood cells just as the substances discussed above can perform the oncotic function of the plasma proteins. They have, for example, developed certain synthetic chelating agents and perfluorocarbon derivatives that show considerable promise as vehicles for carrying oxygen to the tissues. In addition, free and modified forms of hemoglobin have been employed in animals to carry out both the oncotic and oxygen-carrying functions of blood.

Synthetic substitutes. Perfluorocarbon family chemicals have proved to be very effective carriers of oxygen when infused into the circulation of experimental animals that have had most of their own blood removed.* To be useful as a total substitute for blood, these chemicals must be emulsified and mixed with one of the plasma expanders discussed above: dextran, or a hydroxyethyl starch derivative. Rats that have had their own blood exchanged for such "artificial blood" have remained in excellent condition. Despite the fact that the perfused fluid lacks clotting factors or leukocytes and immune globulins, bleeding and infection have not been a problem. The perfluorocarbons stay in the circulation long enough for the animals' own hematopoietic mechanisms to begin functioning again.

Hemoglobin solutions. Investigators have long been interested in the possibility of transfusing solutions of free hemoglobin removed from red blood cells. This protein not only can bind oxygen, transport it to the tissues, and unload it there, but it can also serve to expand the blood volume because it has a molecular weight close to that of albumin, the plasma protein mainly responsible for oncotic activity. The main difficulty in earlier attempts to employ hemoglobin solutions as a plasma expander with oxygen-carrying capacity was the fact that free hemoglobin appeared to cause kidney damage.

It is now known that hemoglobin does not cause renal toxicity when certain constituents of the hemolyzed blood cells from which it was obtained are removed. Removal of lipids and the particulate matter that makes up the stroma or supporting tissues of the red cells results in production of hemoglobin solutions that can be safely injected. Continuous infusions of such stroma-free hemoglobin have kept bloodless experimental animals alive long enough to allow their own blood cells and proteins to regenerate and reach normal levels.

Because stroma-free hemoglobin is rapidly removed from the body, attempts have been made to modify the hemoglobin molecule to lengthen its stay in the circulation. Solutions in which hemoglobin has been made into complexes with other substances or altered by chemical treatment have helped to keep it in the circulation for longer periods after infusion. However, other problems still remain to be solved.

The ready availability of synthetic blood substitutes or of hemoglobin obtained from outdated human whole blood would help to solve many problems associated with present blood bank practices. Not only would such artificial substances help to spare blood supplies for those clinical situations in which their use is most essential, but they would offer many applications in areas of research, including studies of hematopoiesis itself.

The most important applications are clinical, particularly in accident emergencies in which large amounts of blood have been lost and there is no time for blood typing. Apparently, the use of hemoglobin preparations during emergency situations following severe trauma has already had extensive human clinical trials in Russia. Further research on modified hemoglobin, which can stay in the circulation for long periods following infusion, may lead to its use in such chronic blood disorders as sickle cell anemia and thalassemia, as well as in cancer patients with prolonged drug-induced aplastic anemia.

Additional clinical considerations

Although some do not consider the administration of blood and blood products to be part of drug therapy, their use has many of the same implications as the use of more traditional drugs. The patient who is to receive blood should be thoroughly assessed to provide baseline data from which the response to the blood can be evaluated. A history of previous transfusions and reactions to the transfusions should be noted. Any history of allergic reactions should also be noted, particularly if the patient has not received blood before. The patient and significant others need to be told why the blood is being given, how long the transfusion will take, and to expect frequent assessments during the procedure. The patient should also be advised to report any discomfort that may be experienced, including chills, back pain, or headache. Some people find the use of blood to be frightening, and they will need support and encouragement. The fear of

---

* Among the chemicals of this class employed experimentally are perfluorodecalin and perfluorotripropylamine, which have been made available for investigational purposes in a commercial product called Fluosol DA.

AIDS and hepatitis is very common and the patient will need to know what, if any, risks are involved in the situation. Some religious sects do not allow the transfusion of blood and, as is true with all medical procedures, the patient must have the opportunity to refuse the procedure. The nurse is often the health-care professional who is in the best position to facilitate the most appropriate and acceptable therapy for the patient.

There are several technical aspects of care that must be considered when administering blood and blood products. The blood can only be given intravenously, and must be given through a large-bore needle, 18-gauge or larger, to protect the fragile red blood cells and to permit the viscous fluid to flow freely. The tubing through which the blood will flow should first be primed with an isotonic fluid. Dextrose and other nonisotonic solutions can damage the blood during delivery, causing serious problems for the patient. Normal saline is the solution of choice. It is important to remember that no *drugs* should be run into the same line. Blood often needs to be warmed before it is administered; warming coils are available from most blood banks for this purpose.

As mentioned previously, proper identification of the patient and the blood is extremely important. The transfusion should be started slowly, at a rate no faster than 3 or 4 ml/min, and the patient should be monitored frequently, if not continually. After the first 50 ml have been infused, the rate of infusion can be increased if no adverse reaction has been noted. A unit of blood (510 ml) should be infused over approximately 2 hours. The patient's underlying medical condition and response to the blood will determine how much blood will be needed and how fast it can be given.

Once a blood product has been administered, the container is usually returned to the blood bank and appropriate documentation is taken care of. The patient should continue to be closely evaluated for adverse reactions for at least 2 hours after the transfusion has been completed.

The patient teaching guide summarizes key points to include when teaching a patient who is to receive blood. The guide to the nursing process summarizes the clinical aspects to include in the nursing care of these patients.

Patient teaching guide: blood and blood products

In teaching the patient about the specific problem and therapy, the following points should be included to explain the transfusion of blood or blood products:

1. The type of blood product being used

2. The reason this product is needed

3. Risks associated with the use of this product, including precautions that are taken to decrease such risks

4. How the product will be given (*e.g.,* IV), and what site will be used

5. How long the transfusion will take

6. The reason for frequent monitoring during the transfusion, and what monitoring to expect (*e.g.,* T, P, R, BP)

7. Signs and symptoms that should be reported:

   Headache
   Chills
   Back pain
   Fast heartbeat
   Difficulty in breathing
   Pain at the infusion site
   Flushing

Guide to the nursing process: blood and blood products

Assessment	Nursing diagnoses	Interventions	Evaluation
Past history (underlying medical conditions): Transfusions; reactions Allergies: reactions Medication history: any drug patient is currently taking	Potential alteration in comfort: pain during transfusion Knowledge deficit regarding therapy Potential alteration in cardiac output Fear Potential alteration in tissue perfusion	Safe and appropriate administration of blood: • Identity • Large-gauge needle • Isotonic solution • Rate regulation Comfort measures • Positioning of infusion site • Environmental control Patient teaching regarding procedure Support and encouragement to deal with therapy Life support and emergency measures in the event of transfusion reaction	Monitor therapeutic effect of blood Monitor for adverse reactions: • Chills, fever • Flank pain • Hematuria • ↑ R • ↑ P • Flushing • Delayed reactions: jaundice Evaluate effectiveness of comfort measures Evaluate effectiveness of teaching program Evaluate effectiveness of support and encouragement offered Monitor effectiveness of emergency and life support measures, as needed
Physical assessment Neurologic: orientation, affect, reflexes Cardiovascular: JVP, BP, P, perfusion Respiratory: R, adventitious sounds GI: abdominal exam Renal: urinalysis Other: T; type and cross match blood, if necessary			

Fluids and electrolytes

The proper functioning of every cell in the body depends on the composition of the fluids that surround it. If the volume and composition of this internal environment are drastically altered and allowed to remain that way, severe functional disturbances soon develop. Thus, when the body's defense mechanisms fail to maintain internal homeostasis, therapeutic measures must be taken.

Most important are measures that correct the primary causes of the homeostatic disorder—disease, trauma, and poisoning, for example. It is often necessary to correct the abnormality by supplying missing minerals, water, and nutrients. Some substances commonly employed to overcome fluid and electrolyte deficiencies are listed in Table 54-2.

Water, salt, and acid–base imbalances
Although a discussion of the fundamental principles of fluid and electrolyte therapy is beyond the scope of a pharmacology textbook, the different products available

for treating various types of water, salt, and acid–base imbalances will be briefly reviewed.

Simple dehydration, in which the patient has lost water and salt in equal proportion, is best counteracted by administration of an *isotonic solution of sodium chloride,* preferably by mouth. However, when fluid–electrolyte loss has been severe as a result of vomiting and diarrhea, an intravenous infusion may be more rapidly effective. In addition, because other electrolytes in addition to sodium may have been lost, fluids for replacement of several salts at once may be ordered.

Products that contain combinations of several electrolytes in proper isotonic balance include *Ringer's solution, lactated Ringer's solution,* and various commercial preparations of multiple salts in high, low, or intermediate electrolyte concentrations.

Other states of abnormal hydration include those in which relatively little electrolyte loss has occurred. In such cases of hypertonic dehydration, water alone is provided to make up the deficit caused by water loss. For this purpose, a *5% dextrose infusion* by vein is preferred for maintaining isotonicity. The dextrose also provides

Table 54–2. Fluid–electrolyte and nutritional replenishers

Agent	Comments
Treatment of abnormal hydration states	
Dehydration	
Dextrose injection (5% in H$_2$O) USP	IV as required
Dextrose and sodium chloride injection USP (various combinations available)	IV as required
Sodium chloride injection (isotonic, 0.9%)	IV as required
Sodium chloride injection (3%; 5%)	IV as required
Balanced electrolyte injection (Isolyte; Normosol; Plasmalyte)	IV as required
Other electrolyte depletion conditions	
Potassium chloride USP (Kaochlor; Kay Ciel; SK-Potassium Chloride)	Oral, 16–24 mEq of potassium daily; IV, up to 10 mEq/hr; or up to 100–200 mEq daily
Potassium gluconate (Kaon)	Oral, 20 mEq of potassium bid
Potassium bicarbonate; potassium citrate (in Potassium Triplex; K-Lyte)	Variable oral dosage
Calcium gluconate USP	Oral, 15 g daily
Magnesium sulfate USP	8–24 mEq magnesium/day
Ringer's injection USP	IV or SC, as required
Lactated Ringer's injection USP	IV or SC, as required
Acidosis treatment	
Citrate and citric acid solutions (Polycitra)	Oral; dose varies with patient
Sodium bicarbonate USP (tablets and injection)	Oral or IV, as required
Sodium acetate USP	IV, as required
Sodium lactate injection USP (1/6 molar solution)	IV, as required
Tromethamine (THAM)	IV, as required
Alkalosis treatment	
Ammonium chloride USP	Oral, 1–3 g bid or qid
Potassium chloride, sodium chloride, and others	See above
Nutritional deficiency treatment	
Amino acid injection (FreAmine III; Nephramine)	IV in various concentrations
Crystalline amino acid infusions (Travasol; FreAmine III)	Total parenteral nutrition; various dosages
Hypertonic dextrose injection USP	IV in various concentrations
Fructose (levulose) in water	IV, as required
Invert sugar injection (Travert)	IV, as required
High-calorie solution for injection (Hi-Cal 900; Isolyte H 900; Normosol-M 900)	IV, as required
Protein hydrolysate injection (Propac; PDP)	Oral, 1g/kg body weight/day
Intravenous fat emulsion (Intralipid; Travamulsion)	IV, up to 500 ml first day, up to 2.5 g/kg body weight/day

a source of energy but, because it is metabolized by the body in processes that require insulin, it is not administered to dehydrated patients who are in diabetic coma. The patient whose plasma has reached normal tonicity can be switched to an infusion of several isotonically balanced electrolytes to bring the extracellular fluid content back to normal.

In cases of dehydration that are marked by an excessive loss of *sodium (hyponatremia)*, higher concentrations of sodium chloride (3 or 5%) are employed to make up the deficit. This hypotonic type of dehydration is sometimes seen in patients with Addison's disease who should also receive adequate corticosteroid replacement therapy. Hyponatremia that develops during diuretic therapy requires adjustment of the diuretic drug dosage, in addition to rehydration with one of these hypertonic sodium solutions.

Other electrolytes are also often depleted during treatment with potent diuretics. Loss of *potassium* is the most serious result of such overtreatment, particularly in patients who are also receiving digitalis. *Hypopotassemia (hypokalemia)* is best treated by administration of potassium chloride in liquid form, preferably by mouth but also by carefully monitored intravenous infusion.

In other disorders marked by severe vomiting and diarrhea, hypokalemia may be accompanied by the loss of several other electrolytes. Thus, in this and other disorders, it is often also necessary to correct loss of cations such as calcium and magnesium and anions such as chloride and bicarbonate. Solutions of *magnesium sulfate, calcium gluconate, ammonium chloride,* and *sodium bicarbonate* are available for IV use in such cases (Table 54-2).

Acid–base imbalances are the result of a buildup or excessive loss of hydrogen ions. *Acidosis* is, of course, best counteracted by removing the underlying cause of the disorder. However several *systemic alkalinizers* are also available for oral or intravenous administration. Administration of *sodium bicarbonate solution* is the simplest and most effective way to treat metabolic acidosis, in which plasma bicarbonate has fallen to a relatively low level as compared to the high hydrogen and chloride ion concentrations—for example, in salicylate poisoning.

Another systemic alkalinizer, sometimes administered alone or combined with sodium and potassium chloride salts, is *tromethamine* (THAM). It has been used to correct the metabolic acidosis that develops during cardiac arrest and in the cardiac bypass procedures used in heart surgery. Its dosage must be very carefully regulated to avoid development of metabolic alkalosis.

Metabolic alkalosis has various causes that must be corrected. The human body can tolerate acidosis much better and for longer periods of time than it can tolerate alkalosis. This acid–base imbalance is not overcome by supplying hydrogen ions directly but by furnishing chloride ions. This is best done by administering *sodium chloride* or *potassium chloride* solutions by vein. *Ammonium chloride*

is sometimes employed to counteract alkalosis caused by certain poisons.

Parenteral nutrition

Patients who cannot take enough food or fluids by mouth to meet their nutritional needs may be fed following oral intubation or, with increasing frequency, by vein. Those who are still in a state of reasonably good nourishment or in an only moderately depleted state usually receive short-term infusions of dilute solutions of dextrose, amino acids, fat emulsions, and other nutrients by way of a large *peripheral* vein, usually one located in the arm. In more serious clinical situations, patients who require long-term parenteral nutrition receive solutions administered through a *central* venous catheter inserted by way of the subclavian vein, with its tip located in the superior vena cava. Such central venous nutrition, parenteral hyperalimentation, or total parenteral nutrition (TPN) requires skilled personnel who have had special education and training in the principles of hyperalimentation and in their application to various clinical situations. Although the technical details of these procedures cannot be covered here, some important aspects concerning such parenteral products and their proper administration will be reviewed.

Total parenteral nutrition (TPN). This procedure permits the infusion of large amounts of nutrients in relatively small amounts of fluid. It can offer complete nourishment for long periods to patients suffering from serious gastrointestinal tract disorders, cancer, or chronic kidney failure. However, TPN is a potentially hazardous procedure, which requires close monitoring of the patient's metabolic function to avoid possibly fatal fluid and electrolyte imbalances, and employment of careful aseptic techniques to prevent infection. Thus, its use is reserved for those patients in whom feeding by oral intubation or nutritional support by peripheral intravenous infusion is not enough for meeting their caloric needs or for overcoming their severely catabolic states.

Such patients include those unable to take food because of severe damage to some portion of the alimentary tract—for example, children with an esophageal stricture resulting from ingestion of lye, and those suffering from severe malnutrition as a result of malabsorption syndrome or chronic vomiting. People who may also profit from parenteral hyperalimentation also include not only those with chronic diarrhea or dysentery and gastrointestinal tract obstruction, anomalies, or diseases such as ulcerative colitis and diverticulitis, but also victims of extensive burns and others with markedly increased protein requirements. Such chronic patients are often sent home with TPN lines; they are taught to care for the line and to administer the nutritional solution in the home setting.

Among the basic nutrients administered by prolonged continuous infusion are the following: hypertonic dextrose solutions, concentrated carbohydrates that serve as the major source of calories; amino acids for counteracting negative nitrogen balance, the metabolic state that prevails when patients are eliminating more nitrogen than they are ingesting in the form of protein-containing foods; and vitamins, electrolytes, and minerals of various types. Some points to be considered in administering each of these nutrients are discussed below, but other sources should be consulted by nurses assigned to such clinical situations.

Hypertonic dextrose injections of various strengths are available to provide adequate calories in a minimal volume of water for patients suffering from extreme malnutrition or renal shutdown. The rate of infusion must be closely controlled to avoid administering more glucose than the kidney tubules can reabsorb. If the renal threshold for glucose is exceeded, and this sugar spills over into the urine (glycosuria), a situation similar to that which commonly occurs in diabetes mellitus may develop and lead to hyperosmotic nonketotic dehydration, the result of osmotic diuresis.

To avoid development of this syndrome and a resulting sequence of complications that could lead to diabetic-type coma and death, it is important to monitor the patient's urinary glucose levels daily and to measure the blood glucose level periodically. Occasionally, it becomes desirable to add insulin to the infusion, if the patient's own pancreas fails to compensate for hyperglycemia by increasing its secretion of the hormone. Because the simultaneously administered amino acids are reducing substances, their use can cause false positive results in tests with reagents that depend on the use of reducing substances. Thus, only products that detect urinary glucose specifically should be employed in this situation.*

Essential amino acids and lipids must also be infused in amounts that meet each patient's specific requirements and at an appropriately constant rate. Dosage must be conservative to avoid development of hyperammonemia, not only in patients with liver disease and in infants or children with genetic metabolic defects, but also in patients with no prior history of hepatic dysfunction. If symptoms develop, the further infusion of amino acids should be discontinued until the patient's condition has been re-evaluated. It is also important to infuse amino acids at a constant slow rate, rather than by periodic rapid injections, because too rapid infusion may result in their metabolic conversion to glucose (gluconeogenesis), instead of their being used to build new tissue protein.

Electrolytes and minerals such as potassium, phosphorus, and magnesium are particularly important in this type of nutritional therapy, as are the water soluble B-complex vitamins, which are required for proper utilization of the infused carbohydrates and proteins. Ascorbic acid may also be added to the infusion fluid but vitamin K should not be part of the same solution, because it can be inactivated by the presence of that reducing substance. Trace metals such as zinc, copper, cobalt, and similar elements required in only minute quantities need not be added routinely, but they can be employed as supplements to these solutions if definite evidence of a deficiency develops (see below).

Prevention of infection is, of course, crucial to the well-being of these often debilitated patients. To avoid possible septicemia caused by bacterial pathogens or by the fungus *Candida albicans*, the catheter and the site of injection must receive meticulous aseptic care. Daily changes of IV tubing are made employing aseptic techniques, and sterile dressings are also changed every few days after defatting the surrounding skin with ether or acetone and applying an anti-infective ointment. Finally, the patient's *psychological state* must be considered, including teaching needs about the procedure being used and emotional support to help the patient cope with dependency, a change in self-concept that may develop, and the altered nutritional status and the implications that has on his activities.

Vitamins and minerals

Vitamins

Physiologic functions. Vitamins are substances that the body requires for carrying out essential metabolic reactions. Because the body cannot biosynthesize enough of these compounds to meet all its needs, preformed vitamins must be obtained from vegetable and animal tissues taken in as foodstuffs (Table 54-3).

The body needs only small amounts of vitamins because they function mainly as *coenzymes*—substances that activate the protein portion of enzymes. Small quantities of enzymes catalyze a great deal of biochemical activity. Thus, tiny amounts of vitamins go a long way, and any excess of these nonprotein cofactors is either rapidly excreted by the kidneys or gradually broken down to inactive fragments after storage in the tissues.

Dietary deficiencies

Ordinarily, a person who eats a well-balanced diet takes in enough of these natural nutrients to meet the everyday needs of the body. In such circumstances there is no need to supplement the intake with purified vitamin concentrates in pharmaceutical form. To take vitamins in amounts that exceed the body's requirements is a needless expense and, occasionally, the ingestion of excessive amounts of vitamins may prove toxic.

There are, however, various situations in which supplemental vitamins may be valuable to avoid development of multiple deficiencies of these nutrients. Even people who are in good health and eat an adequate diet sometimes need extra nutrients, including vitamins, at

---

* *Clinitest* tablets are *not* desirable; products that will *not* give false positive tests include *Clinistix*, *Diastix*, and *Tes-Tape*.

Table 54–3. Vitamins and related substances

Official or generic name	Trade name or synonym	Recommended dietary allowance*	Usual adult therapeutic dose
Water-soluble vitamins			
Ascorbic acid USP	Vitamin C	60 mg, approximately	50–100 mg, oral; 50–250 mg, parenteral
Bioflavonoids	Vitamin P	None	No established use
Biotin	—	100–200 mg	5–10 mg/daily
Calcium pantothenate USP	Vitamin B_5; pantothenic acid	10 mg	20–100 mg, oral
Choline dihydrogen citrate, and other choline salts	Choline	Unknown	250 mg–1 g/daily
Cyanocobalamin USP	Vitamin B_{12}	3 µg, approximately	25–1000 µg, oral or parenteral
Folic acid USP	Folacin; pteroylglutamic acid; Folvite	0.4 mg	1 mg, oral or parenteral
Inositol	Inosite; hexahydrocyclo-hexane	Unknown	1–3 g, oral
Niacin USP	Nicotinic acid Vitamin B_3	13–18 mg	50–100 mg oral, up to 500 mg/day
Niacinamide USP	Nicotinamide, source of vitamin B_3	As above	500 mg oral or parenteral
Para-aminobenzoic acid	PABA	Unknown (associated with B vitamins)	12 g
Pyridoxine HCl USP	Vitamin B_6	2.0–2.2 mg	10–600 mg, oral or parenteral
Riboflavin USP	Vitamin B_2	1.2–1.6 mg	5–10 mg, oral; 50 mg, IM
Thiamine HCl USP	Vitamin B_1	1.0–1.4 mg	5–30 mg oral or 10–20 mg IM, tid
Fat-soluble vitamins			
Vitamin A USP	Aquasol	4,000–5,000 U	10,000–100,000 U, oral
Vitamin D preparations:			
Calcifediol USP	Calderol; 25-$(OH)D_3$; 25-hydroxycholecalciferol		300–350 µg/week
Calcitriol	Rocaltrol; $1\alpha,25$-$(OH)_2D_3$ $1\alpha,25$-dihydroxychole-calciferol		0.25 µg
Dihydrotachysterol	Hytakerol; DHT		0.75–2.5 mg/day
Ergocalciferol USP	Drisdol; vitamin D_2; Calciferol; vitamin D	200 U	50,000–500,000 U, oral
Vitamin E	α tocopherol; Aquasol; Eprolin Gelseals	12–15 U	100–1,000 U
Vitamin K		Not established; estimated at 0.03 µg/kg body weight for adults, 1–5 µg/kg body weight for neonates	

Table 54-3. Vitamins and related substances (continued)

Official or generic name	Trade name or synonym	Recommended dietary allowance*	Usual adult therapeutic dose
Phytonadione USP	Vitamin K$_1$; Mephyton; Aqua MEPHYTON; Konakion		5–25 mg, oral; 10–25 mg, parenteral†
Menadiol sodium diphosphate USP	Vitamin K$_4$; Synkayvite		5–10 mg, oral; 5–15 mg qd or bid, parenteral
Menadione USP	Vitamin K$_3$		5–10 mg, oral

* These adult allowances, which are set by the Food and Nutrition Board of The National Academy of Sciences–National Research Council, are amounts recommended for maintaining good nutrition in normal people under ordinary living conditions.
† Deaths have occurred during and after IV administration of Aqua MEPHYTON

certain periods of their lives. This is true, for example, of infants fed by formula, as well as women during pregnancy and lactation. Children often require some supplementation of their dietary vitamin intake during periods of rapid growth.

Vitamin supplementation is desirable for the many people who do not eat properly. Some have developed poor eating habits; others have never learned what foods are needed for a balanced diet containing adequate quantities of all the vitamins. Poverty prevents some people from purchasing enough of the foods needed for good nutrition.

However, many people who can well afford to purchase a full quota of nutritionally desirable foods often fail to do so. For example, alcoholics and other emotionally disturbed people are likely to eat foods that do not supply adequate amounts of vitamins. People who adhere to faddish diets may develop deficiencies of several vitamins found together in the foods that are absent from their diets. Occasionally, a person adheres too strictly to a religious code regulating diet.

In all such cases, patients should be helped to get adequate amounts of vitamins through better dietary planning or from supplementary vitamin concentrates. The physician or dietician often determines how the patient's diet should best be supplemented, while the nurse is in the best position to concentrate on helping the patient realize the need for a properly balanced diet and on teaching what should be known about proper eating. The dietary requirements should be developed with due consideration of religious beliefs, economic constraints, personal tastes, and the practices of the patient's ethnic group in regard to diet.

Patients with certain types of pathology are among those most likely to develop vitamin deficiencies. In various gastrointestinal disorders, for example, vitamins may not be absorbed from food. If parenteral feeding is necessary, vitamin supplementation is almost certainly required. During prolonged chronic illnesses most patients lose their appetites and become unwilling or unable to eat well. The nurse should encourage the patient to eat properly. Vitamins are often added to the patient's diet in amounts calculated to make up for those that are not obtained from food. High-potency pills—that is, *therapeutic* vitamin formulations are usually prescribed when deficiencies of one or more vitamins are evident or seem likely. The nurse should remain alert for signs of vitamin deficiency, such as glossitis (inflamed tongue) and fissures in the corners of the mouth, especially in elderly people and in those who follow a borderline diet, so that they can be referred to the appropriate health-care facility for evaluation.

Excess vitamins
Most people do not need therapeutic multivitamin formulations (megavitamins) and should be advised not to spend their money on such high-potency vitamins. If either the fat-soluble or some water-soluble vitamins are continually ingested in excess, toxicity may occur. The fat-soluble vitamins (Vitamins A, D, E, and K) are stored in the body and can accumulate; they have long been known to cause toxicity in overdosage. Until recently, overdosage of the water-soluble vitamins has been considered to be wasteful but not dangerous because these vitamins are promptly excreted in the urine. However, there is now evidence that prolonged intake of excessive amounts of Vitamin B$_6$ (pyridoxine), niacin, and Vitamin C (ascorbic acid) can cause serious adverse effects (see below). Thus, for persons in normal health who feel the need for nutritional insurance, products containing only low doses of vitamins are adequate. Provided the person does not overpay for what should be available at moderate

cost, such supplementation is harmless and, in view of the proved value of placebos in many medical situations, vitamins may even provide psychological benefits far beyond their actual physiologic effects for those who believe in their value. It is usually advisable not to recommend specific vitamin formulations; it is much more useful to teach people to eat a diet adequate in vitamin content. Determining whether a patient needs a vitamin supplement and, if so, which vitamins and in what amounts, is usually determined through consultation with the dietician and physician.

Allowances

Although it is advisable not to tell people what vitamins to purchase, if they feel that they need vitamins, they should be encouraged to look for the least expensive product that will meet their needs. People should be encouraged to read the labels to compare the formulas and prices of competing products, which sometimes vary considerably in cost. The Food and Drug Administration requires that the labels of all vitamin products indicate the amounts of each ingredient and the proportion of the *recommended dietary allowances* (RDA) represented. The RDA represents the highest daily allowance for each nutrient. By referring to the percentage of the RDA that various foods and supplements contain, people can determine the adequacy of their diet.

A vitamin supplement need not, of course, meet the RDA, because those who eat less than an adequate diet still fulfill many or most of their vitamin needs. People tend to think that if a little is good, more is that much better. Actually, it has never been shown that larger amounts of vitamins are ordinarily more beneficial and, in fact, high doses of some vitamins have been shown to be dangerous. Thus, products that are labeled to indicate relatively low RDAs are adequate, if priced proportionately low.

Patients who take more than one vitamin preparation may well be taking toxic levels of some vitamins. The FDA regulates the amount of vitamins A and D that can be found in any one product, an attempt to protect the public from the dangers of toxicity from these vitamins, but people who take more than one product can develop toxicity. The public needs to be educated about vitamins and their potential dangers. Special health food diets and megavitamins are recent fads that may be found together with physical fitness programs. People need to know the real impact of such programs. Products containing many times the RDA are best purchased only after consultation with a physician.

Water-soluble vitamins

Certain vitamins are commonly considered together because they are all water-soluble, and most are found in the same types of foods. They are subdivided into vitamin C and the B-complex group. The latter include thiamine, riboflavin, nicotinic acid, pyridoxine, pantothenic acid, folic acid, cyanocobalamin (B_{12}) and, possibly biotin, choline, inositol, and para-aminobenzoic acid (PABA). Two of these—folic acid and cyanocobalamin—have been discussed in Chapter 35 because they are best reserved for the treatment of macrocytic anemias resulting from deficiencies of one or another or both of these blood-building B vitamins.

Thiamine. Thiamine was the first of the B-complex vitamin group to be isolated and chemically identified. Thus, it is also known as *vitamin B,* and—because it counteracts the neurologic signs and symptoms of beriberi—as the *antineuritic* and *antiberiberi* vitamin. Its natural sources include meats, whole cereal grains, and yeast.

When ingested with foods that contain it, thiamine is converted to a coenzyme that is important in carbohydrate metabolism. A lack of thiamine results in a reduction in numerous biochemical reactions that are essential to the normal functioning of all living cells. However, overt symptoms of thiamine deficiency appear most commonly in the form of malfunctioning of nerve cells and as gastrointestinal (GI) and cardiovascular system disabilities.

The *neurologic difficulties*—seen today in this country mostly in alcoholic patients—are manifested mainly in complaints stemming from peripheral neuritis. These include sensory nerve signs such as tingling, burning, and aching, and motor nerve disabilities leading to muscle weakness and paralysis. Central nervous system (CNS) function is often disturbed by a lack of thiamine, as indicated by irritability, depression, inability to concentrate, and loss of memory.

Cardiovascular complications of thiamine deficiency include signs of congestive heart failure such as edema, dyspnea, and tachycardia, together with various cardiac irregularities. Adverse GI effects include loss of appetite, vomiting, and chronic diarrhea.

The RDA is approximately 1.2 mg, ranging from 1.0 to 1.4 mg. No more than 2 mg a day is ever needed as a vitamin supplement in normally healthy people who have an ordinary diet. However, patients with diagnosed thiamine deficiency may require as much as 30 mg, three times a day. This is best administered parenterally. Once the thiamine stores return to normal in this way, low oral doses are sufficient.

Thiamine replacement therapy usually produces prompt improvement in patients suffering from beriberi, alcoholic neuritis, and the neuritic and cardiovascular complications that sometimes occur in pregnant women and in others whose diets lack this vitamin. Patients with similar symptoms that, however, do not stem from a deficiency of thiamine cannot be expected to improve. Thiamine injections, though, were once often part of the management of trigeminal neuralgia and other types of neuritis. Improvements that followed such thiamine therapy were probably the result of a placebo reaction or were purely coincidental.

Riboflavin. This substance, vitamin B$_2$, gets its name from the sugar ribose and from its yellow color (Latin *flavus,* yellow). It is converted in the body to two coenzymes that work together with a wide variety of proteins to catalyze many of the cellular respiratory reactions from which the body derives its energy. Rich dietary sources of riboflavin include dairy products (milk and cheese), eggs, meats, green vegetables, beans, and whole cereal grains.

Deficiency of riboflavin does *not* result in a definite disease such as beriberi, but is accompanied by various typical lesions. Ocular symptoms include itching, burning, photophobia, and tearing. The cornea may show signs of invasion by tiny capillaries (vascularization). A typical lesion of the lips and angles of the mouth (cheilosis) is characterized by development of deep fissures in the mucous membranes and skin, together with inflammation of the tongue (glossitis).

The RDA for riboflavin is 1.2 to 1.6 mg. Riboflavin deficiency states may be treated with injections totaling up to 50 mg daily, followed by oral doses of 5 to 10 mg daily for maintenance, together with an adequate diet. Actually, ariboflavinosis rarely occurs alone, and patients who require treatment usually receive thiamine, niacin, and other B-complex vitamins simultaneously.

Niacin (nicotinic acid). Nicotinic acid has only a slight chemical resemblance to nicotine and none of that potent alkaloid's widespread pharmacologic actions. Thus the official name *niacin* is preferred; the term *niacinamide* is used for its amide derivative, which is equally effective in various essential metabolic reactions. Both dietary substances, as well as the essential amino acid *tryptophan,* which is derived from dietary protein, are converted into two coenzymes that play a vital role in many enzyme-catalyzed biochemical reactions.

The coenzymes into which niacin, niacinamide, and tryptophan are biosynthesized are nicotinamide adenine dinucleotide (NAD), formerly known as diphosphopyridine nucleotide (DPN), and nicotinamide adenine dinucleotide phosphate (NADP), once called triphosphopyridine nucleotide (TPN). These substances, the physiologically active forms of niacin, take part in many important cellular oxidation–reduction reactions. Specifically, they act as hydrogen acceptors for dehydrogenase enzymes in many steps of intermediary metabolism. When the hydrogen is transferred to flavin-containing enzymes, these pyridine nucleotides become available once more in oxidized form for further reactions.

A lack of these metabolically essential substances results finally in *pellagra,* a nutritional deficiency disorder affecting the skin, digestive tract, and nervous system. In its milder form, subclinical pellagra—as seen sometimes in chronic alcoholics, for example—is manifested by nervousness, insomnia, headache, itching–burning skin sensations, and GI upset. The full-blown pellagra syndrome, now relatively rare in this country as a result of niacin-enrichment of diets in endemic areas, includes the following characteristic changes: symmetric skin eruptions resembling sunburn—on the backs of both hands, for example—that tend to heal as darkened scars; a characteristically bright red swollen tongue, together with other oral lesions and heavy salivation; and mental disturbances, ranging from confusion, depression, and memory loss to psychosis marked by dementia, hallucinations, and delusions.

Pellagra occurs most commonly when diets are low not only in niacin but also in dietary protein containing tryptophan (of which 60 mg is equivalent to 1 mg of niacin). Thus, people whose protein comes mainly from cornmeal instead of from meat, milk, and eggs are especially susceptible to pellagra, because corn products are deficient in the amino acid tryptophan. Niacin itself is found in only low quantities in corn, whereas large amounts are present in lean meats, liver, peas, beans, potatoes, and fish.

Pellagra responds readily to high oral doses of niacin (50 mg up to ten times daily); much lower doses are adequate for maintenance therapy. Occasionally, psychotic patients and those suffering from GI malabsorption syndromes require parenteral therapy.

Niacin releases histamine and often causes flushing of the skin, and sometimes—especially following injections—a fall in blood pressure. The nurse should explain that the flushing is a natural reaction, so that the patient will not worry unnecessarily that an allergic reaction is occurring. Patients who complain of weakness or dizziness from niacin are advised to lie down until the discomfort passes and to report the reaction. Nicotinamide, which is the preferred form of the vitamin because it does not cause these local and systemic circulatory effects, may be substituted. Unlike niacin itself, however, this amide derivative cannot, of course, be used clinically as a vasodilator, nor is it effective for reducing serum cholesterol levels. People who ingest large amounts of niacin in foods* have also experienced flushing, skin rashes, pruritus, GI disturbances, and even the exacerbation of asthma, all presumably as a result of the release of histamine. Chronic ingestion of 3 g/day has caused uricosuria and precipitated gouty arthritis.

Pyridoxine. This substance and the related compounds pyridoxal and pyidoxamine make up the essential dietary factor called *vitamin B$_6$*. All are enzymatically converted in the body to the coenzyme pyridoxal phosphate.

---

* One recent report describes skin rashes and pruritus after pumpernickel bagels containing 190 mg of niacin were eaten.

This physiologically active form of the vitamin then combines with various proteins to catalyze many different types of metabolic reactions. It is necessary, for example, for the biosynthesis of NAD from tryptophan. In addition, this biologically active form of the vitamin plays an important part in amino acid metabolism, in certain fatty acid syntheses, and in the biosynthesis of many neurotransmitters.

Pyridoxine is found naturally in the same dietary sources as thiamine. The RDA is 2.2 mg, but more is probably required during pregnancy and when the intake of protein—and the subsequent rate of reactions involving amino acids—is unusually high. Although no specific disease is associated with pyridoxine deficiency, skin and mucosal lesions and convulsions have occurred in those deprived of the vitamin.

A syndrome resulting in convulsive seizures was once seen, for example, in some infants fed a modified milk formula deficient in pyridoxine. The peripheral neuritis that sometimes develops during isoniazid therapy in tuberculosis is believed to result because this drug can block the conversion of dietary pyridoxine to its biologically active form. To overcome this competitive blockade and to prevent the resulting peripheral neuritis, pyridoxine supplements are commonly administered for prophylaxis together with the daily dosage of the antituberculosis drug.

Pyridoxine is a prime example of the fact that vitamins may interact with drugs in ways that can alter the effectiveness of each type of agent. As previously indicated, parkinsonism patients taking the drug levodopa were deprived of its beneficial effects when they simultaneously took multivitamin products containing pyridoxine. On the other hand, women using oral contraceptives sometimes show reduced serum concentrations of pyridoxine (among other B-complex vitamins). Thus, they then require larger doses of not only pyridoxine but also of riboflavin and other vitamins that act together with vitamin B_6.

The continued ingestion of high doses of pyridoxine has recently been found to be associated with the development of severe peripheral neuropathies. Seven people who took several grams of pyridoxine a day for two or more months developed ataxia, loss of somatosensory and kinesthetic senses in their limbs, and perioral numbness, all of which improved greatly within several months of stopping pyridoxine, although recovery was incomplete.

Pantothenic acid. This organic acid is so widely distributed in natural foods that specific deficiencies are unlikely to occur. An ordinary American diet containing about 10 mg of pantothenic acid provides an adequate intake of this vitamin. Deficiencies produced experimentally by administration of an antivitamin compound are marked by GI disturbances, headache, and fatigue.

Pantothenic acid is converted in the body to the metabolically important coenzyme A, which takes part in various vital biochemical reactions. The acetylated form of this enzyme is involved in carbohydrate and fatty acid metabolism and in the formation of the neurotransmitter acetylcholine. A derivative, *dexpanthenol*, has been advocated for relief and prevention of paralytic ileus, on the apparent assumption that this substance increases biosynthesis of the neurotransmitter that helps to regulate the motility of the gut. There is no adequate evidence that postoperative paralytic ileus is related to a deficiency of pantothenic acid or to a resulting lack of acetylcholine.

Although the daily requirement for this vitamin is unknown, and no RDA has been established, it is considered to be an essential substance, and its salt, calcium pantothenate, is a common constituent of many multivitamin preparations.

Ascorbic acid. This essential dietary substance is water-soluble but is so different in its natural distribution in foods from the vitamin B complex group that it was given the separate designation *vitamin C.* The term *ascorbic acid* stems from its ability to prevent the deficiency disease scurvy (*i.e.,* it is the *antiscurvy* or *antiscorbutic vitamin*). It is found in fruits such as oranges, lemons, and limes and in vegetables, including cabbage, tomatoes, and potatoes.

Ascorbic acid plays an important part in biologic oxidation–reduction reactions. Unlike the B vitamins, it is not converted into a coenzyme that then combines with proteins to catalyze metabolic steps. Instead, vitamin C acts in various other ways to aid the activity of many different types of enzyme systems, including especially sulfhydryl systems, which it helps to keep in the activated reduced form.

Deficiency of vitamin C interferes with the formation of the connective tissue substance that cements cells together. Loss of collagenous fibers from this bed of intracellular connective tissues leads to development of widespread lesions. Local bleeding, for example, is believed to be the result of excessive fragility of the capillary walls. In scurvy, the gums become red and swollen and bleed readily. The teeth are loosened and bone is lost from the jaws. Joints and growing long bones are also subject to hemorrhages. All such symptoms of vitamin C deficiency are relieved in a few days by the administration of 50 to 250 mg of ascorbic acid daily, divided into several fractional doses. Once healing becomes apparent, dosage can be lowered gradually to 5 to 100 mg or less.

The RDA is normally 60 mg. An intake of such amounts ordinarily makes up for the amounts of the vitamin that the body uses each day. However, the rate of oxidation of vitamin C may markedly increase in cases of tuberculosis or other infectious diseases. The requirements of such patients may be met by raising the daily intake of ascorbic acid to about 120 mg. There is no evidence that this vitamin has any therapeutic value for patients not suffering from an overt deficiency of ascorbic acid, but its administration is advocated for treating a wide variety of clinical conditions, and it has wide popularity as a prophylactic agent against the common cold.

However, the ingestion of large doses (1 g or more) has caused diarrhea and uricosuria. Large doses have also caused hemolysis in patients with a deficiency of G-6-PD, and have predisposed some patients to the formation of oxalate stones in the urinary tract. In addition, high doses can decrease the efficacy of oral anticoagulants and increase estrogen levels. Women taking high doses during pregnancy have given birth to infants who developed scurvy when they no longer received enough ascorbic acid to maintain the high levels to which they were exposed *in utero*.

Miscellaneous water-soluble food factors

Several substances widely distributed in nature are believed to be important nutrients, but how much, if any, is required by humans is not established. These include biotin, para-aminobenzoic acid, inositol, and choline.

Choline. Choline is a lipotropic agent sometimes employed therapeutically to reduce the fat content of the liver in the treatment of Laennec's cirrhosis in chronic alcoholics and in other patients. However, it is doubtful whether supplementary choline is required by patients with hepatic cirrhosis who can eat a high-protein diet. Meat, milk, and eggs supply enough choline and the amino acid methionine (which can substitute for choline) to meet the needs for fat-transporting substances. Choline is also combined with acetylcoenzyme A in the enzymatically catalyzed biosynthesis of acetylcholine. However, there is no evidence that a lack of dietary choline ever leads to a deficiency of this important neurotransmitter.

There is evidence that the administration of choline in pharmacologic doses may be beneficial to some patients with certain neurologic and memory disorders. Supplementing the diets of these patients, whose conditions are *not* caused by a nutritional deficiency of choline, appears to have led to symptomatic improvement in some cases. This may be because choline is absorbed into the blood, passes the blood–brain barrier, and is quickly converted to acetylcholine, the neurotransmitter that may be present in insufficient quantities in the brain cells of these patients.

Among the disorders treated with choline supplements is the tardive dyskinesia of mental patients who have previously received phenothiazines and butyrophenone-type antipsychotic drugs for prolonged periods (Chap. 46). Reports of success in decreasing choreiform movements in a substantial proportion of these patients have led to trials of oral choline administration in manic patients and in the common form of presenile dementia called Alzheimer's disease. Results in these conditions

have not yet proved the usefulness of choline in such cases.

Although choline causes no serious side-effects, its chronic ingestion in large quantities causes some patients to develop a fishy body odor. For this reason *lecithin*, a dietary source of choline that does not impart a fishy odor, has been tried as an alternative treatment for tardive dyskinesia. The commercial preparations of lecithin available at present have only a low content of that substance. Thus, patients must consume very large quantities to achieve therapeutic dose levels. Efforts are being made to prepare pure lecithin for experimental use in these brain disorders.

Fat-soluble vitamins

Vitamins A, D, E, and K, the fat-soluble essential food factors, tend to stay in the body for much longer periods than the water-soluble B vitamins and ascorbic acid. Absorption of these vitamins requires the presence of adequate amounts of digestible fat and bile salts in the intestinal tract. Once absorbed, little is lost by way of the kidneys, and considerable amounts of these vitamins may be stored in body fat, muscles, and liver. Because small amounts may be released from such reservoirs as required to meet metabolic needs, symptoms of deficiency are slow to develop, even during long periods of inadequate dietary intake. On the other hand, the lack of efficient excretory mechanisms may lead to accumulation of some of the vitamins to toxic levels if excessive amounts are ingested.

Vitamin A. This essential dietary substance is found in the fat of milk, yolk of eggs, and liver. Although it does not occur as such in plants, vitamin A is formed in the body from carotene, the plant pigment responsible for the color of carrots and other deep yellow and dark green vegetables. When carotene rather than already formed vitamin A is the main dietary source of the vitamin, the daily requirement of 4000 to 5000 U of vitamin A may double.

Deficiency of vitamin A may develop as a result of a prolonged intake of an inadequate diet. More commonly, it occurs in patients with certain chronic digestive diseases that interfere with absorption of fats and the vitamins dissolved in them. Patients with obstructive biliary disease, hepatitis, cirrhosis, steatorrhea, and chronic diarrhea are most likely to develop this type of avitaminosis as a result of inadequate absorption, even when the diet contains adequate amounts of the vitamin.

Signs and symptoms of vitamin A deficiency. These are manifested mainly in changes in ocular structure and function and in other epithelial tissue abnormalities. Night blindness, a decreased ability to adapt to darkness or dim light, is an early deficiency symptom. Dryness and then deformity of the cornea may lead to permanent visual impairment if not quickly detected and corrected by administration of vitamin A. The skin may become dry and keratinized. Diarrhea may follow pathologic changes in the epithelial lining of the GI tract and, in the urinary tract, stones may form around pieces of shedding epithelium. Growth and development of infants and children is slowed by persistent, uncorrected dietary lack of vitamin A.

Treatment. Once diagnosed, a deficiency state is treated with high daily doses—10,000 to 100,000 U—of vitamin A. Even higher parenteral doses may be administered for a few days to correct corneal and other ocular lesions quickly. The daily dose is then reduced to that employed as a dietary supplement during pregnancy, lactation, and in infants—that is, about 5000 U daily.

People with vitamin A deficiencies are especially susceptible to infections of the eyes, skin, and respiratory tract. This does not mean, however, that administration of vitamin A supplements to those whose dietary intake is adequate will lessen susceptibility to infections. As is true with other vitamins, there is no evidence that intake of vitamin A in excess of ordinary requirements helps to prevent or relieve colds, speeds the healing of skin infections, or in any way overcomes symptoms that are similar to those seen in deficiency states but are not caused by a lack of the vitamin. Poisoning, characterized by headache, drowsiness, vomiting and papilledema, has occurred in adults who took a single dose of 1,500,000 U. Infants who are acutely poisoned show a bulging fontanel.

Chronic overdosage with vitamin A products has resulted in hypervitaminosis A, a toxic state marked mainly by bone and skin lesions. If the condition is correctly diagnosed and the vitamin withdrawn immediately, recovery usually occurs before long. An illness that results from eating polar bear liver is believed to be the result of its high vitamin A content. The manner in which excesses of this vitamin cause poisoning is not well understood.

Vitamin D. Vitamin D is actually two related substances with similar biologic activity: *ergocalciferol* (vitamin D_2), and *cholecalciferol* (vitamin D_3). (The original vitamin D, or D_1, was found to be a mixture of D_2 and D_3.) Ergocalciferol is obtained by irradiating the plant sterol ergosterol with ultraviolet rays. Similar irradiation of the skin sterol 7-dehydrocholesterol by sunlight results in its activation and formation of vitamin D_3. The latter is also obtained by irradiating other sterols of animal origin—those in milk fat, for example—and is also the form present in fish liver oils.

There is evidence that the biologically active form of vitamin D is actually a steroid hormone, which is produced by the kidneys in response to certain physiologic stimuli. In addition, it is now known that dietary vitamin D_3 must first be metabolically activated before it can perform its hormonal functions on its target tissues—the intestine and the bones of the skeleton. This vitamin undergoes enzymatic hydroxylation in the liver to a metabolite, which is carried to the kidneys by the blood. A renal enzyme system then converts this metabolite to $1\alpha,25$-dihydroxyvitamin D_3, an extremely potent hormone, also called *calcitriol*, and available as Rocaltrol for use in certain special clinical situations (see below).

Dietary sources of vitamin D are relatively limited. Egg yolk and milk contain small amounts, but other foods eaten by Americans do not adequately satisfy even minimal needs. (Eskimos meet their needs by eating fish livers rich in this vitamin.) A significant proportion of most people's need for vitamin D is met by exposing the skin to sunlight, because ultraviolet rays stimulate the synthesis of this vitamin from skin sterols. The main sources of this vitamin in the American diet are in milk and other foods that have been enriched by ultraviolet irradiation or by the addition of vitamin D concentrates. When such fortified products are unavailable, the diets of infants, rapidly growing children, and pregnant or lactating women are supplemented with 200 U of this vitamin daily, especially during the winter months in temperate zones.

The main action of vitamin D is to aid the absorption of ingested calcium from the GI tract. By raising the blood levels of calcium and of the phosphate that moves with it, vitamin D tends to facilitate the deposition of these minerals in bone. Thus, a deficiency of vitamin D in infants and children can quickly lead to rickets, and adults may develop osteomalacia. People who suffer from a lack of parathyroid hormone (hypoparathyroidism) are also treated with large doses of vitamin D—50,000 to 500,000 U daily. This helps to increase the intestinal absorption of dietary calcium and of any calcium supplements that the patient may require.

Once these metabolic bone disorders have developed, rapid administration of relatively high doses of vitamin D is required to heal the bone lesions and to prevent permanent deformity of skeletal structures. Infants with rickets may receive about ten times the daily prophylactic dose, or about 2000 to 4000 U, each day for several weeks or until bone x-rays reveal adequate mineralization; dosage is then reduced to 1000 or 2000 U daily and finally to the 200-U maintenance level. Adults with softening and malformation of the bones (resulting from lack of vitamin D and *not* caused by osteoporosis) may receive up to 50,000 U of this vitamin for a time.

Some patients fail to respond to ordinary or sometimes even massive doses of vitamin D. Among these are patients in chronic renal failure, and particularly those undergoing frequent renal dialysis. The resulting hypocalcemia leads to various skeletal structure abnormalities, which have been collectively termed *renal osteodystrophy.*

These bone diseases can be most effectively and safely treated with tiny doses of *calcitriol* (Rocaltrol), a substance so active that initial oral doses of only 0.25 μg a day usually provide a satisfactory response when supplemented by an adequate daily intake of a calcium supplement, usually about 1 g daily. This promotes prompt remineralization and healing of bone lesions. Usually within 1 week the patient's plasma shows an increased level of calcium and a reduction in the elevated parathyroid hormone level that had developed as a compensatory response to the previously low plasma calcium concentration.

Patients taking this extremely potent form of vitamin D metabolite must be closely monitored to avoid development of *hyper*calcemia. Fortunately, this condition is readily reversible by tapering the dosage of this drug, and the patient's excessively elevated serum calcium level returns to normal within a few days. This offers a significant advantage over the previously available treatments for such conditions as renal osteitis fibrosa cystica and osteomalacia, in which the administration of massive doses of ordinary vitamin D and high-calcium supplements sometimes led to long-sustained hypercalcemia and to the development of many metastatic calcification lesions.

Toxicity is, however, a definite threat when this vitamin is taken in excessive doses for more than a few weeks or months. Hypervitaminosis D, as this condition is called, results in the movement of calcium from bones to blood (hypercalcemia). This mineral may then be deposited in such tissues as the kidneys, heart, and blood vessels. Fatalities have resulted from impaired renal function. However, the condition is readily reversible if further administration of the vitamin is stopped, and the patient is put on a low-calcium–high-fluid regimen.

In summary, vitamin D supplementation requires more careful attention to dosage than any other nutrient. It is more difficult to get enough of this vitamin naturally than any other, and at the same time it is easy to get too much. Thus, infants receive vitamin D supplements promptly when artificial feeding is begun, yet care is required to keep the daily dosage at a safe level. Adults who have an adequate diet ordinarily need no vitamin supplementation, yet vitamin D deficiencies are likely to develop during prolonged periods of physiologic stress. Thus, the addition of 200 U of vitamin D daily is certainly desirable during pregnancy and lactation.

Vitamin E. Several natural substances called tocopherols possess biologic activity of the vitamin E type. Of these, α-tocopherol most potently counteracts the effects of vitamin E deficiency in experimental animals whose diet lacks this vitamin. This substance is available in synthetic form and in wheat germ oil, the main natural source. Fresh lettuce leaves and the fat of milk and eggs are other foods in which vitamin E is found.

Deficiency of this vitamin for long periods in several animal species results in effects that resemble certain clinical disorders in humans. For example, rats are rendered sterile, rabbits and guinea pigs develop skeletal muscular dystrophy, and several species suffer various types of cardiac muscle lesions.

In humans there is no reliable evidence that vitamin E therapy cures sterility, strengthens muscles in dystrophic patients, or is of benefit in cardiovascular disorders. There is, in fact, no proof at this time that humans require this vitamin and that its absence results in any clinical syndrome that is counteracted by tocopherol administration. Nevertheless, many products containing vitamin E are marketed and advocated for treating a number of conditions, including sterility, habitual abortion, skin disorders, muscular dystrophy, and peripheral vascular diseases. Although large doses have been taken for long periods of time without causing apparent toxicity, large doses have caused GI effects and can both antagonize Vitamin K and increase the efficacy of oral anticoagulants (see Chap. 34).

Multiple vitamin combinations

As mentioned, a deficiency of only one vitamin is rare. More likely to occur is a deficiency of combinations of vitamins that are found together in the same types of foods when the dietary intake of these foods is inadequate or when some GI disorder interferes with their absorption. Thus, it is customary to combine several of the B-complex vitamins, alone or with ascorbic acid, or the fat-soluble vitamins A, D, and K may be combined. For full supplementation both water-soluble and fat-soluble vitamins are often administered together.

Many multivitamin preparations contain only 50% of the RDA. These relatively low dosages adequately supplement the amounts of natural vitamins in a diet that is considered to be somewhat less than adequate. Other multivitamin products contain about 150% of the RDA. Such preparations are preferred if prolonged illness has resulted in a marked reduction in food intake, or if a therapeutic diet is not adequate in nutritional factors—in allergic states, for instance, or in chronic disease of some portion of the digestive tract. A third type of multivitamin product containing 300 to 500% of the RDA is for patients who require specific vitamin therapy or supportive therapy in pathologic conditions in which vitamin requirements are markedly increased.

Minerals and trace elements

The roles in body metabolism of such electolytes as sodium and potassium have been discussed, and it has been indicated how imbalances among these and various other cations and anions can lead to serious, potentially fatal malfunctioning of the heart and the neuromuscular system, among other vital organs. The importance of such substances as iodides and lithium has been indicated briefly, and a much fuller treatment was given to the topic of iron metabolism (Chap. 35). This chapter will conclude with a brief review of the element *calcium*, which plays a part in many physiologic functions, and certain other elements that the body requires in tiny amounts or traces. Two new drugs used in treating Paget's disease of bone are also discussed in this section.

Minerals

Calcium. In the form of its phosphate and carbonate salts, calcium makes up a major part of the skeletal system. It plays an important part in maintaining neuromuscular activity in a normal state, and in regulating the rhythm of the heart; it is an essential factor in the series of complex steps leading to blood coagulation. The body's stores of this mineral must be replenished through ingestion of foods that are high in calcium—for example, milk and milk products. Children and pregnant women need more dietary calcium than others, and their diets may have to be supplemented with calcium salts.

Calcium metabolism is regulated by the complexly related interactions of vitamin D and its metabolites (above) and the hormone produced by the parathyroid gland. Another hormone, called calcitonin, which is secreted by special cells of the thyroid gland, also plays a part in maintaining the balance of calcium between the blood plasma and the bones. Many factors can upset the relationships between these regulators of calcium homeostasis and thus lead to *hypo*calcemia or *hyper*calcemia, with resulting disorders of bone metabolism and malfunctioning of the cardiovascular and neuromuscular systems.

Hypocalcemia, a reduction in calcium levels of the blood below the normal 10 mg/100 ml, may occur as a result of a dietary deficiency of this mineral. A lack of vitamin D and of the parathyroid hormone, both of which help to regulate the body's complex calcium economy, may also lead to a drop in blood calcium levels. When these substances are lacking, dietary calcium is inadequately absorbed from the upper GI tract, and calcium tends to move from bone to the blood. This can cause rickets and osteomalacia.

Despite this drain of the calcium stored in bone, blood levels may finally fall so far below normal that signs of excessive neuromuscular excitability appear. This is manifested by muscular fibrillations, twitching, tetanic spasms, and finally exhausting convulsions. The main treatment of *hypocalcemic tetany*, no matter what the underlying cause, is to raise the blood level of the mineral back to normal. In an emergency this is best accomplished by a slow and careful intravenous injection of available soluble salts, such as *calcium chloride* or *calcium gluconate*.

These salts are injected slowly to avoid the adverse effects of high calcium concentrations on the heart. Care is required, especially with the acidic and highly irritating calcium chloride salt, to avoid leakage into extravascular tissues. Calcium gluconate injection may also cause abscess formation in infants when given intramuscularly. Both these drugs may be administered by mouth for milder states of tetany, but less irritating salts such as *calcium lactate* and *calcium levulinate* are often preferred for this purpose. When hypocalcemic tetany is the result of hypoparathyroidism, calcium injections may be supplemented by administering parathyroid hormone extracts parenterally.

During pregnancy and lactation, the demands of the fetus or infant may double the mother's daily requirement for calcium. Dietary calcium in milk is supplemented by preparations containing calcium salts alone or combined with vitamin D. The ordinary multivitamin and mineral supplements are relatively low in calcium. (A one-a-day capsule containing a dozen or more different vitamins and minerals but only about 250 mg of a calcium salt does not go very far toward satisfying a daily requirement of almost 2 g of elemental calcium.)

Because the bulky salts of calcium are not easily put into capsules or tablets convenient for swallowing, other dosage forms are often preferred. Unless the patient doesn't mind swallowing a dozen or so tablets a day containing *calcium carbonate* or *calcium phosphate*, the nurse may suggest that the powdered mineral be sprinkled on food or that an aqueous suspension prepared cheaply by a pharmacist be swallowed at each meal. Flavored wafers that contain a large amount of a calcium salt are also available. In any event, patients should be told that, as is the case with iron salts, adequate quantities of calcium are best obtained in cheaply prepared dosage forms containing a single ingredient rather than in expensive—and nutritionally inadequate—polypharmacal combinations. This applies also to elderly patients who may require calcium for osteoporosis and to families with several growing children, although their daily requirements are best satisfied by drinking a quart of vitamin D-enriched milk.

Hypercalcemia, an abnormal elevation of plasma calcium levels, has many different causes other than such rare situations as excessive calcium intake, or the milk-alkali syndrome discussed in Chapter 41. One of these—the ingestion of excessive amounts of vitamin D and its metabolites—has been discussed above. The development of this disorder in cancer patients, particularly when the neoplasm originates in the bones or metastasizes to them, was briefly taken up in Chapter 12, together with discussions of the employment of prednisone and other corticosteroids and of the use of the cytotoxic antibiotic mithramycin, in attempts to reduce the dangerously high plasma calcium levels and prevent the kidney damage that is likely to develop when hypercalcemia occurs as a complication of cancer.

Calcitonin, a hormone secreted in increased quantities by the thyroid gland when plasma calcium levels rise excessively, has also been tried in the management of hypercalcemic states. However, although the commercially available salmon calcitonin preparation Calcimar helps to decrease the plasma level of calcium and phosphorus for a time by favoring their entrance into bone, other measures that promote calcium excretion are preferred, including infusions of *sodium sulfate* and *sodium phosphate* solutions, or slow intravenous administration of the chelating agent *edetate disodium* (EDTA; Endrate).

Paget's disease. This bone-deforming disease, also known as osteitis deformans, responds to treatment with a synthetic form of salmon calcitonin, which has more potent calcium-regulating activity than the polypeptide hormone obtained from humans or other mammals. This substance seems to act in part by suppressing the overactivity of the osteoclasts (cells that act to remove osseous tissue). The synthetic polypeptide may also increase new bone formation by stimulating osteoblastic activity. Patients with moderate to severe Paget's disease symptoms have reported a reduction in bone pain, and those who had difficulty in moving about tend to become more active.

Although one drawback of this drug treatment is the need to make daily injections, side-effects are relatively infrequent and transient. These include inflammatory reactions at the injection site, flushing of the face, swelling or tenderness of the hands, and itching, as well as occasional nausea and vomiting and allergic hypersensitivity reactions. Some patients have relapsed following a period of initial improvement. This may be because of production of antibodies that neutralize the polypeptide hormone. Failure to maintain improvement may also stem from secondary hyperparathyroidism as a compensatory response to the calcitonin-induced hypocalcemia.

Etidronate disodium (Didronel) is also used for suppressing symptomatic Paget's disease of bone. Unlike calcitonin, it is not a hormone, but a substance similar in chemical structure to pyrophosphate, a compound important in control of bone mineralization. Administered orally in a 6-month treatment course, this drug is said to bring about improvement in about three out of five patients; apparently, it acts by decreasing the excessive rate at which bone is being broken down and built up.

Following the first course the drug is discontinued for at least 3 months while the patient's progress is observed by bone scan studies and by following such biochemical indices as serum alkaline phosphate levels and urinary excretion of hydroxyproline. If these biochemical indicators reveal an end of the initial remission, or if the patient's symptoms return, a second treatment course may be instituted.

This drug is said to be well tolerated, with minor GI symptoms being the only occasional complaint. However, daily dosage should be raised only gradually and should be carefully controlled, because the accumulation of this chemical in bony tissue may prevent it from retaining the minerals needed for the buildup of new bone. Demineralization marked by the appearance of pain in previously pain-free bone sites may appear as a result of overdosage; this can lead to fractures in patients with a severe form of Paget's disease.

Trace elements

The body also requires other elements in addition to calcium, phosphorus, iron, iodine, and others already discussed here and elsewhere in his book. Although these minerals are toxic when taken in large doses, many seem to be nutrients essential to normal cellular function. The roles of other trace elements in human nutrition are still uncertain. Here, brief summaries about some of what is known at present about these micronutrients will be presented.

Fluorine, in the form of fluorides, plays a part in the formation of tooth enamel and in the mineralization of bone. The best sources of this substance seem to be naturally occurring fluoridated water and plants grown in soil through which such water flows. The addition of this element to the water supplies of communities without naturally fluoridated water has proven to be effective in reducing the rate of dental caries. Despite vociferous protests by people and groups who oppose such measures because they believe fluorides to be poisonous, most toxicologists state that the presence of one part per million of the element in artificially fluoridated water is a safe and practical measure. Fluoride solutions, applied topically to the teeth of young children by dentists and dental hygienists, also appear to be an effective prophylactic measure against caries. Fluorides are also available as dietary supplements for this purpose and are also contained in most toothpastes.

Zinc is an element needed for the functioning of numerous enzymes essential in cellular metabolic processes involving tissue growth and repair. The government-established RDAs for zinc range from 3 mg daily for infants to 25 mg daily for lactating women, with most adults requiring about 15 mg daily. This substance is best obtained by eating animal protein foods, because its absorption from ingested grains is partially interfered with by the presence of phytates—salts of phytic acid that form complexes with this and other metals, including iron.

Zinc deficiency reduces the normal growth rate of children and has been shown to be associated with impairment of the sense of taste—a situation that could, of course, cause a child's appetite to be poor and thus affect growth and health. However, zinc supplements are expensive and rarely necessary because of the abundance of this element in meat, eggs, and other foodstuffs. Pharmacologic doses of zinc salts are employed experimentally to accelerate wound healing, in acne treatment, and in other medical disorders. Nausea and vomiting are a common side-effect of zinc-induced intestinal irritation.

Magnesium is also essential for the functioning of many enzyme systems, and a deficiency of this element can result in many types of malfunction leading to neuromuscular and mental abnormalities and cardiomyopathies. Adult RDAs for this element range between 330 and 350 mg daily, an amount readily obtainable from an ordinary diet. Actually, this substance is so abundant in both the diet and the body that it is not truly a trace element. That is, it comes closer to calcium in its place in the body economy than it does to the other substances discussed here.

Copper is required for the functioning of various

enzymes involved in cellular respiratory processes, including cytochrome oxidase. It is so readily available in both meats and plant foods in amounts far exceeding the body's needs that dietary deficiencies rarely if ever develop in humans. Thus, there seems to be no need for its addition to the dietary supplement products that list its presence on their labels. Its presence in products containing iron is, for example, unnecessary for the correction of iron deficiency anemia (Chap. 35).

Cobalt is also unnecessary as a supplementary adjunct to iron in the treatment of anemia. This element is, however, essential for formation of cyanocobalamin (vitamin B_{12}), which is required in minute amounts for prevention of certain other types of anemia. As indicated in Chapter 35, that vitamin is abundantly available in animal protein, and dietary cobalt is not itself required for formation of red blood cells. The need for cobalt in human nutrition has not been established. However, it has been employed experimentally by hematologists in pharmacologic doses in certain relatively rare refractory anemias. Accidental overdosage of cobalt salts has caused fatal poisoning.

Manganese and *molybdenum* are elements that serve as components of several enzyme systems. The tiny amounts needed for metabolic purposes are readily obtainable from various dietary sources. No known deficiency states have been reported in humans. Thus, their presence in dietary supplements seems to be unnecessary.

Other elements for which a need may exist in certain animal species include chromium, selenium, vanadium, nickel, and tin. There is some evidence of the possible occurrence of a chromium deficiency in some poorly nourished people, but no RDA has yet been established for this element or for any others in this group.

Additional clinical considerations

As indicated above, the role of vitamins and minerals in human functions is not as yet completely understood. The FDA has established RDAs for those elements whose functions are better understood, and for which a clinical deficiency syndrome occurs. Unfortunately, the FDA cannot control many aspects of vitamin preparations, and many are available over the counter (OTC); if used in combination, toxicity can result. Advertising is very influential in the buying habits of the general public and, in recent years, there has been increasing emphasis on health foods, vitamins, and youth in advertising. Many people, in efforts to be "healthy" and youthful, take supplemental vitamins—sometimes in place of meals, often in excess.

An important aspect of nursing care should include teaching patients about nutritional and vitamin needs. The initial patient medication history should include questions about the use of vitamins as OTC preparations. The patient should be taught the need for an adequate diet, and the patient who desires to take supplemental vitamins and minerals should understand the significance of RDAs, that fat-soluble vitamins need to be taken with food to be absorbed, and that these compounds are intended to be supplemental and cannot replace eating nutritious foods.

Patients who are known to have an inadequate diet should be assessed for the signs and symptoms of the various vitamin deficiencies. Patients who are institutionalized for long periods of time may develop various deficiencies, and this should be kept in mind if a patient develops mouth sores or skin lesions, or has difficulty in healing. Such deficiencies are easily treated, but are all too often missed.

Case study

Presentation

DD and FP, two white, female college juniors, came into the University Health Service, quite upset, with their chief complaint being "We think we have hepatitis—we're turning orange."

Their physical examinations and histories were very similar, and were significant for the following findings: Both young women had been experiencing progressive fatigue, malaise, joint pain, headache, and irritability. Both patients were taking oral contraceptives and several multivitamin preparations. They had both been on very rigid diets for 6 weeks: no breakfast, only green salads for lunch and dinner, and various multivitamin supplements. One girl noted that she had had no menses over the last few weeks, despite careful adherence to her oral contraceptive schedule.

Both patients had dry, scaling, somewhat orange skin, fissures in the lips and corners of the mouths, inflamed and dry oral mucosa, and dry and brittle hair with some hair loss. One patient had slight splenomegaly.

After several laboratory studies were done, the diagnosis of hypervitaminosis A was made. The patients were told to discontinue the vitamin supplements and were referred to the nurse for teaching about diet and nutrition. What nursing interventions are appropriate?

Discussion

DD and FP, first of all, will need support and encouragement, and will need reassurance that they do not have hepatitis. The signs and symptoms of hypervitaminosis A should be discussed with them—orange, dry, scaly skin; cracked lips and mouth; inflamed oral mucosa; dry, brittle hair and loss of hair; headache, fatigue, malaise, lethargy, anorexia, vomiting, amenorrhea; and splenomegaly. The patients can be assured that all these uncomfortable problems will resolve when the vitamin A levels return to normal.

Once DD and FP have been reassured, and they are less anxious and seem ready to learn, the nurse should begin to teach them about proper nutrition and diet. The problem with vitamin A was compounded in this case. The patients took several multivitamin preparations each day, far exceeding the RDA for vitamin A, they ate only large amounts of green and yellow vegetables—high sources of natural vitamin A, and they both took oral contraceptives, which tend to increase the absorption of vitamin A. The patients should be assured that they are not alone in having gotten themselves into this situation, and that many people do not understand the RDAs and the potential toxicity of certain vitamins and minerals. A dietician could be consulted for a safe, nutritious diet, and one that would lead to weight reduction, if appropriate. The RDAs should be explained, and the vitamins and minerals that can be toxic should be indicated. A single daily multivitamin preparation could be suggested, if the patients feel that they would like to take a vitamin. Ideally, the patients can be brought in for several teaching sessions to evaluate their understanding of diet and nutrition, and to monitor their progress in the resolution of the hypervitaminosis A. Such an incident also provides an excellent opportunity for preventative teaching sessions for staff, as well as for other patients in a similar age group.

References

Blood and its components

Aisner J: Platelet transfusion therapy. Med Clin North Am 6:1133, 1977

Geyer RP: Substitutes for blood and its components. In Jamieson GA, Greenwalts TJ (eds): Blood Substitutes and Plasma Expanders. New York, Allen R. Liss, 1978

Higby DJ, Burnett D: Granulocyte transfusions: Current status. Blood 55:2, 1980

Horoschak I: Autotransfusion. Promising alternative to donor blood. RN 38:33, 1975

Juliani LM: Precautions to take with dextrose and hypertonic saline. RN 44:66, 1981

Lang DJ: Hazards of blood transfusion. Adv Pediatr 24:311, 1977

Schwarz T: It's not artificial blood—but it can do the work of RBCs. RN 45:38, 1982

Vitamins, minerals and other nutrients

Chalmers TC: Effects of ascorbic acid on the common cold. Am J Med 58:532, 1975

Coburn JW et al: Advances in vitamin D metabolism as they pertain to chronic renal disease. Am J Clin Nutr 29:1283, 1976

Cohen EL, Wurtman RJ: Brain acetylcholine: Control by dietary choline. Science 191:561, 1976

Danford DE, Munro HN: The vitamins. Introduction. In Gilman AG, Goodman LS, Gilman A (eds): Goodman and Gilman's The Pharmacological Basis of Therapeutics, 6th ed, pp 1551–1559. New York, Macmillan, 1980

Danford DE, Munro HN: Water-soluble vitamins. In Gilman AG, Goodman LS, Gilman A (eds): Goodman and Gilman's The Pharmacological Basis of Therapeutics, 6th ed, pp 1560–1582. New York, Macmillan, 1980

DeLuca HF: Vitamin D endocrinology. Ann Intern Med 85:367, 1976

DeRose J et al: Response of Paget's disease to porcine and feline calcitonins. Am J Med 56:858, 1974

Haussler MR, Cordy PE: Metabolites and analogues of vitamin D: Which for what? JAMA 247:841, 1982

Kolata GB: Research news. Mental disorders: A new approach to treatment? Science 203:36, 1979

Mandel HG, Cohn VH: Fat-soluble vitamins. In Gilman AG, Goodman LS, Gilman A (eds): Goodman and Gilman's The Pharmacological Basis of Therapeutics, 6th ed, pp 1583–1601. New York, Macmillan, 1980

Rodman MJ: A fresh look at OTC drug interactions:

Effects you can't afford to overlook. Vitamins. RN 46:77, 1983

Scott ML: Advances in our understanding of vitamin E. Fed Proc 39:2736, 1980

Sturtridge WC, Wilson DR: Management of hypercalcemia. Drug Ther (Hosp) 7:102, 1982

Suttie JW: The metabolic role of vitamin K. Fed Proc 39:2730, 1980

Toxic effects of vitamin overdosage. Med Lett Drugs Ther 26:73, 1984

Chapter 55

Immunologic
agents

55

Active and passive immunity

Immunity is a state of relative resistance to disease that develops after exposure to the specific agent responsible for an infection. Some people or species are born with an innate ability to resist certain diseases. Most people, however, are not congenitally immune to the common infectious diseases. Instead, they *acquire* immunity in the process of fighting off the foreign microbial invaders.

Active immunity of this type is brought about by the body's response to proteins and polysaccharides in the invading viruses and bacteria. These chemicals foreign to the tissues act as an *antigen.* That is, they stimulate the gradual formation of immune *antibodies* by the plasma cells of activated B lymphocytes. These specifically structured protective protein molecules then circulate in the serum, particularly in its gamma globulin fraction. Then, whenever the same foreign substance enters the body in the future, the antibodies of the immune serum combine with the antigen, and an antigen–antibody reaction occurs (Chap. 36).

Passive immunity is the transfer of immune serum from an animal or a human who has been actively immunized to a person who has not been previously exposed to the pathogen, and who thus must borrow antibodies to combat or ward off an infection caused by that organism. These borrowed antibodies begin immediately to attack the invaders or to neutralize their toxins, exactly as would antibodies made by the patient's own tissues if there had been time enough for them to have been formed in adequate amounts. A drawback of passive immunity is that the supply of antibodies can be exhausted.

Actively or passively acquired antibodies act in the same ways. They may make bacteria clump together (agglutinate), precipitate, or break up, or they may help the body's inflammatory response to destroy the invader. Some antibodies (antitoxins) prevent the poisons produced by tetanus or diphtheria bacilli from becoming fixed to body tissues, thus forestalling the worst effects of infections by these pathogens.

Immunization

Active immunization can also be *artificially acquired* without the need to suffer an actual clinical or subclinical infection through exposure to the pathogens. That is, a person may be inoculated with products derived from microorganisms or their toxins, which have lost their pathogenic power but can still stimulate antibody production. The amount of antigen *primarily* produced in this way may not be great compared to that formed during a spontaneous infection. However, in artificially acquired active immunity, as in natural active immunity, later exposure to the same antigen somehow stimulates the rapid production of large quantities of antibody through the activation of the memory B cells that were formed with the initial exposure.

This so-called *secondary response* in an actively immunized person accounts, in part, for the relatively long duration of active immunity as compared to passive immunity. The latter lasts only a few weeks and then disappears as the borrowed antibody is broken down and removed from the body. Active immunity, on the other hand, may last a lifetime, especially if reinforced by periodic administration of booster inoculations to stimulate a rapid secondary rebound of antibody levels. Thus, passive immunity, although useful in an emergency because of the immediate protection it provides, is less desirable in the long run than the more slowly developing but longer lasting and reinforceable active immune state.

Immunoprophylaxis has been one of the most important medical advances that have lengthened life expectancy from about 35 to 70 years during the last 100 years. Children have been the chief beneficiaries, because infectious diseases killed two out of five born in this country late in the last century. Today, routine immunizations in infancy against diphtheria, tetanus, measles, mumps, rubella, and whooping cough have caused deaths from these diseases to drop to the vanishing point. Smallpox has virtually been wiped out worldwide.

Attempts to protect people by artificial immunization date back to ancient times. The Chinese tried to produce mild cases of smallpox by exposing people to material taken from patients with relatively light cases. They hoped in this way to prevent more serious infections during epidemics of more virulent forms of this potentially deadly disease. However, the use of fluids and scabs taken directly from smallpox patients had inherent dangers that limited the usefulness of this procedure. (Although usually mild, the contagious disease spread in this way may sometimes cause virulent smallpox.)

Thus, millions of people continued to die of smallpox even after the introduction of artificial inoculation into Europe about 1720. The first truly successful procedure was developed late in the same century following Dr. Edward Jenner's discovery that people could be protected against smallpox by infecting them with *cowpox,* a related but much milder bovine disease.

This procedure—called *vaccination* (from the Latin *vacca,* a cow, and *vaccinia,* the term for cowpox)—has completely eradicated smallpox since it has been universally practiced. Its widespread use in this country and in Europe during the last century seems to have wiped out this scourge that had killed hundreds of millions and blinded or disabled countless others. People inoculated with fluid harvested from cowpox vesicles usually develop only a localized lesion, but the antibodies induced by this antigenic stimulus can protect them completely against smallpox.

Immunization is now employed to prevent various other infections in addition to smallpox. In this country, infants are now commonly immunized against diphtheria, tetanus, and pertussis (whooping cough) with a "triple antigen" vaccine administered during their first 6 months. They are also inoculated against poliomyelitis. The introduction of Salk vaccine in 1955, followed by the Sabin oral polio vaccine, reduced the incidence of this crippling and frequently fatal disease from close to 60,000 cases in this country in 1952 to only 65 cases in 1966, but the disease is still prevalent in some tropical countries without widespread vaccination programs. Measles, mumps, and rubella vaccines have been introduced for protection against these very common and sometimes serious childhood diseases. Vaccination (the term is sometimes used for inoculations against other diseases in addition to smallpox) may also be employed in special circumstances against influenza, typhoid, hepatitis B, and other infections. Scientists are at present coming close to perfecting vaccines for syphilis, malaria, and other infectious diseases not previously preventable by biologic prophylactic measures.

Products for active immunity

Antigenic products employed for conferring active immunity artificially are mainly of two types: *vaccines* are made from the microorganisms—viruses, bacteria, and rickettsia—responsible for various diseases; *toxoids* are made from the toxins, or poisons, secreted by certain bacteria. It is the toxins that are responsible for the most devastating effects of diseases caused by these organisms, such as diphtheria and tetanus.

Vaccines. These may contain either the "killed" (or, more correctly, chemically inactivated) microorganisms, or live viruses or bacteria that have been treated to reduce their virulence. Both types of vaccines are safe, because special handling has destroyed their ability to cause disease without affecting their ability to stimulate production of antibodies. Vaccines made from bacteria grown in artificial media and then killed are said to be somewhat safer because they are relatively free of foreign protein that might cause allergic reactions.

Virus vaccines, on the other hand, cannot be washed free of the foreign protein of the living animal tissues in which viruses must be grown and made to reproduce. Thus, patients known to be sensitive to egg protein, for example, could suffer an allergic reaction when immunized with a vaccine that contains virus grown in chick embryos. Live virus vaccines are, however, no more dangerous than those containing "dead" virus, and viruses that are alive but weakened in pathogenic potency are claimed to produce immunity of longer duration. This is related to the greater amounts of antibody produced by introducing harmless virus particles that have retained some ability to reproduce in body tissues. Also, such so-called *live, attenuated virus vaccines* often produce immunity after a single dose, whereas killed virus vaccines usually require administration of several doses at properly spaced intervals. Both types of virus vaccines require the periodic administration of boosters in order to keep antibodies at high protective levels.

Toxoids. These are vaccines made by modifying the toxins secreted by certain bacteria so that they are no longer poisonous but can still stimulate production of antibodies by the tissues of the inoculated person. That is, careful treatment with heat or chemicals such as formaldehyde destroys their poisonous qualities without affecting their ability to act as antigens to stimulate B cells and to confer long-lasting immunity.

The duration of the immunizing effects of toxoids may be lengthened by precipitating or adsorbing the toxoids by various methods, in which chemicals such as alum, aluminum hydroxide, and aluminum phosphate are employed. Such adsorbed toxoids persist in the tissues for longer periods after injection, and thus stimulate production of greater quantities of protective antibodies. However, the relatively insoluble adsorbed toxoids also tend to cause more frequent local reactions, such as redness and swelling. These reactions may be more painful and disabling in older children and adults. Thus, adults are often started on even smaller immunizing doses of these products than are young children.

Products for passive immunity

Immune sera (antisera) are products obtained from the blood of animals (usually horses) or humans who have been exposed to infectious organisms or to their toxic secretions. These antisera may contain antitoxins, antivenins, and—today, only occasionally—antibacterial and antiviral antibodies. The character of the antibodies depends on the nature of the antigen with which the donor was naturally or artificially inoculated.

For example, horses may be hyperimmunized by being injected repeatedly with diphtheria or tetanus toxoids or with pit viper or black widow spider venom. At first, very small doses are administered, and the amount of antigen given is then gradually raised. After a period of weeks, when tests indicate that the toxin-neutralizing antibodies have reached a maximum level, the animals are bled. After removal of the red cells, the separated serum is purified and concentrated. This involves precipitation of the globulin fraction of the blood to rid it of other plasma proteins and of nonprotein impurities, leaving mainly the antibody-containing fraction.

Despite such purification procedures, these products obtained from animal blood may still cause allergic reactions in some people. That is, the animal protein may act as an allergen, a substance that causes *hypersensitization* (Chap. 39), the other of the two basic types of biologic immune reactions. This phenomenon differs from that which produces protective antibodies against infection. The patient is, instead, made prone to suffer allergic reactions.

Such serum sickness reactions may be delayed for several days, until the patient's tissues build up antibodies that react with the foreign protein still in the circulation. The delayed reaction may be marked by general discomfort, fever, hives, swollen glands, and joint pains. A patient previously sensitized to horse serum may suffer an immediate and more severe anaphylactoid reaction if re-exposed to horse serum.

Patients who require passive immunization must be closely questioned about possible previous exposures to horse serum or past allergic reactions. To avoid setting off serious serum reactions, the immune serum may be withheld from patients with a history of earlier allergic episodes, particularly when they show a strong positive reaction to skin or ophthalmic tests for sensitivity to horse serum. If the seriousness of the patient's infection warrants the risk of treatment with antisera, the emergency equipment for managing an acute allergic reaction must be kept readily available. This should include epinephrine, oxygen, corticosteroids, and antihistamines, and the equipment for administering these agents, as well as life support equipment.

Human blood serum. This also serves as a source of immune globulins containing antibodies against various bacterial and viral infections. Such homologous sera have the advantage of being free of the foreign allergenic proteins that are responsible for horse serum reactions. *Immune serum globulin*, a product obtained from the pooled plasma of human donors, contains antibodies against various common infectious diseases, including measles, German measles (rubella), poliomyelitis, and infectious hepatitis. It has been most frequently employed to prevent or modify the severity of measles and infectious hepatitis in those known to have been exposed to other persons with these infections. This product is sometimes also administered to women of childbearing age who have been exposed to the rubella virus of German measles. This virus can cause congenital malformations in infants exposed to it *in utero* during the first 12 weeks of pregnancy. Administration of immune globulin is recommended when tests indicate that a woman may be both pregnant and susceptible to rubella.

Other human immune globulin products containing antibodies against specific diseases are also now available. These products are especially prepared from the blood of patients who have recently recovered from a particular infection, such as measles, pertussis, polio, or hepatitis B. They may also be made from the plasma of hyperimmunized human volunteer donors in whom high counts of measles or tetanus antibodies have been built up from gradual administration of graded doses of the infectious agent or toxoid. Such products are especially useful when tests reveal that the patient is both susceptible to the pathogenic organism and highly sensitive to horse serum. Although the use of such homologous serum products in an emergency is safe and usually effective, such passive immunization is no substitute for active immunoprophylaxis employed long before exposure to disease.

Immunologic products in individual infections

The most important immunologic products currently employed in the prevention and treatment of disease will now be discussed in the context of the conditions against which they are used. That is, rather than discuss these agents in the traditional grouping as active or passive immunizing agents, the various infectious diseases in which these products are employed and the place of such products in the prevention and treatment of these diseases will be reviewed. (See also Table 55-1 for dosage and administration information for these products.)

Botulism

Botulism is a frequently fatal disease caused by eating canned foods contaminated by the rod-shaped bacillus

Table 55–1. Immunologic agents

Disease	Organism	Products employed	Dosage and administration
Botulism	*Clostridium botulinum*	Botulism equine antitoxin (ABE; passive immunity)	Available from CDC
Cholera	*Vibrio cholerae*	Cholera vaccine USP (active immunity)	SC or IM 0.5 ml, then 0.5 ml in 1 week to 1 mo; repeat booster of 0.5 ml every 6 mo
Diphtheria	*Corynebacterium diphtheriae*	Diphtheria antitoxin USP (passive immunity);	Prophylactic: 10,000 U IM or IV; therapeutic: 20,000–80,000 U IM or IV
		Diphtheria toxoid, adsorbed (active immunity)	SC or IM: two injections of 0.5 ml, 6–8 wk apart; booster dose, 12 months later
		Diphtheria toxin (Schick test)	Intracutaneous 0.1 ml
Hepatitis	Hepatitis B virus	Hepatitis B immune globulin, human (HBIG; passive immunity)	0.06 ml/kg body weight (usual adult dose 3–5 ml) within 7 days of exposure, IM, gluteal or deltoid region preferred; repeat 28–30 days later
		Hepatitis B vaccine (Hepatavax B; active immunity)	IM only: 1.0 ml initially, repeated at 1 mo and 6 mo
Influenza	Various strains of influenza virus	Influenza virus vaccine USP (Fluogen; active immunity)	0.5 ml, IM injection
Measles	Rubeola virus	Measles virus vaccine, live attenuated (Attenuvax; active immunity)	SC: 1000 $TCID_{50}$*
		Measles immune globulin (MIG; passive immunity)	Prophylactic: IM 0.22 ml/kg body weight
Meningitis	Several strains of meningococci	Meningococcal polysaccharide vaccine A, C, Y, and W (Menomune; active immunity)	0.5 ml, SC
Mumps	Various strains of parotitis virus	Mumps virus vaccine, live (Mumpsvax; active immunity)	SC: 5000 $TCID_{50}$*
Pertussis	*Bordetella pertussis*	See combination vaccines	
		Pertussis immune globulin (PIG; passive immunity)	1.25 ml IM, as soon after exposure as possible; repeat injection in 1–2 wk
Plague	*Pasteurella pestis*	Plague vaccine, USP (active immunity)	IM: three doses—1 ml, followed by 0.2 ml in 4 wk and 0.2 ml in 6 mo
Pneumonia	Various pneumococcal strains	Pneumococcal vaccine, polyvalent (Pneumovax; active immunity)	SC or IM, 0.5 ml
Poliomyelitis	Various strains of polio virus	Poliovirus vaccine, live, oral, trivalent (TOPV; Sabin; active immunity)	Two doses of 2 ml, PO, 6–8 wk apart; repeat booster dose in 6–12 mo

Table 55–1. Immunologic agents (continued)

Disease	Organism	Products employed	Dosage and administration
		Poliomyelitis vaccine, inactivated (IPU, Salk; active immunity)	SC: three doses of 1 ml each at 4–6-wk intervals; booster dose 6–12 mo later (vaccine of choice only in immunosuppressed patients)
Rabies	Various strains of rabies virus	Rabies vaccine, human diploid cell cultures (HDCV; Imovax; active immunity)	Six IM doses of 1.0 ml on days 0, 3, 7, 14, 30, and 90
		Rabies immune globulin (RIG; passive immunity)	IM: 0.133 ml/kg body weight, given with first dose of vaccine, one-half of dose infiltrated around the wound, remainder given IM
Rubella	Rubella virus	Rubella virus vaccine, live (Meruvax; active immunity)	SC: 1000 $TCID_{50}$ of rubella*
Smallpox	Variola virus	Smallpox vaccine (Dryvax; active immunity)	Multiple pressure site technique of administration
Tetanus	*Clostridium tetani*	Tetanus toxoid USP (active immunity)	SC: three injections of 0.5 ml, 4–8 wk apart
		Tetanus toxoid adsorbed USP (active immunity)	IM: two injections of 0.5 ml, 4–6 wk apart
		Tetanus antitoxin (passive immunity)	1500–5000 U IM or SC for prophylaxis; 50,000–100,000 U IV or IM for treatment
		Tetanus immune globulin (Homo-tet; Hyper-tet; passive immunity)	IM: 250 U for prophylaxis; IM: 3000–6000 U for therapeutic treatment
Tuberculosis	*Mycobacterium tuberculosis*	BCG vaccine USP (active immunity)	0.1 ml intradermal
		Old tuberculin tine test (diagnostic)	Puncture, intracutaneous
		Purified protein derivative of tuberculin USP (PPD; diagnostic)	5 tuberculin U, intracutaneous
Typhoid	*Salmonella typhosa*	Typhoid vaccine USP (active immunity)	SC: two doses of 0.5 ml, at least 4 wk apart
Yellow fever	Virus	Yellow fever vaccine USP (YF-Vax; active immunity)	SC: 0.5 ml

Combination vaccines

Disease	Organism	Products employed	Dosage and administration
Diphtheria and tetanus	See above	Diphtheria and tetanus toxoid (DT; active immunity)	IM; two doses of 0.5 ml at 4–8-wk intervals; booster dose of 0.5 ml in 6–12 mo
Diphtheria, tetanus, and pertussis	See above	Diphtheria and tetanus toxoid and pertussis vaccine (DPT; active immunity)	IM: three doses of 0.5 ml, at 4–8-wk intervals; booster dose of 0.5 ml in 1 yr

(continued)

Table 55–1. Immunologic agents (continued)

Disease	Organism	Products employed	Dosage and administration
Measles and rubella	See above	Measles and rubella virus vaccine, live (M-R-Vax II; active immunity)	SC: 1000 $TCID_{50}$ of measles virus, and 1000 $TCID_{50}$ of rubella*
Measles, mumps, and rubella	See above	Measles, mumps, and rubella virus vaccine, live (M-M-R-II; active immunity)	SC: 1000 $TCID_{50}$ of measles, 5000 $TCID_{50}$ of mumps, and 1000 $TCID_{50}$ of rubella*
Rubella and mumps	See above	Rubella and mumps virus vaccine, live (Biavax II; active immunity)	SC: 1000 $TCID_{50}$ of rubella, 5000 $TCID_{50}$ of mumps*
General passive immunity			
		Immune globulin (gamma globulin; ISG)	IM: 0.02 ml/kg body weight; dosage varies with indications

* $TCID_{50}$ means tissue culture infectious doses, a reference to the assay for vaccine activity.

Clostridium botulinus. This organism produces an exotoxin that has been called "the most poisonous poison" because of the minute amounts required to disrupt nerve impulse transmission to skeletal muscles and produce fatal respiratory failure.

Botulism antitoxin containing antitoxic antibodies, obtained from the serum of horses inoculated with the two most common strains of the organism, may be lifesaving if injected IV early enough. Once the ingested toxin has become fixed to the victim's tissues, it cannot be counteracted by even massive doses of antitoxin. However, in such cases, the antitoxin is given anyway to neutralize any still unbound toxin while the patient is receiving supportive treatment.

The antitoxin is most effective when administered to other people who have been exposed to the organisms, but who have not yet suffered any ill effects—perhaps because they ate less of the contaminated food than the others. The antitoxin may then prevent muscle paralysis or other severe effects of the infection from ever appearing in these people. This antitoxin is available from the Centers for Disease Control (CDC) in Atlanta.

Cholera

Cholera is an acute infectious disease caused by ingesting food and drink contaminated by fecal matter containing the bacillus *Vibrio cholerae.* Infection is characterized by the sudden onset of severe diarrhea and vomiting. Large volumes of fluid are rapidly lost in the frequent watery stools and through heavy vomiting. Extreme dehydration can cause death from circulatory collapse within a few hours after several days of anuria and uremia.

Cholera vaccine is recommended for travelers to India and the Middle and Far East. The vaccine produces only a relatively short partial immunity; therefore, booster vaccinations are advised every 4 to 6 months for people staying in areas where cholera is endemic. Other measures for preventing infection should, of course, not be neglected. In areas in which cholera is present and the quality of the water supply is uncertain, water should be boiled and chlorinated. Food should not be eaten raw and should be protected from flying insects.

Diphtheria

Diphtheria is an acute infectious disease caused by the airborne bacillus *Corynebacterium diphtheriae*, which produces and secretes a poisonous exotoxin. Damage to the tissues of the throat causes necrosis and an inflammatory reaction that often results in formation of a suffocating membrane. Death can occur from hypoxia unless a tracheotomy is performed. Congestive heart failure may follow toxic myocardial damage. Paralysis of cranial and peripheral nerves may occur as late complications of diphtheria.

Diphtheria antitoxin administered immediately and in adequate quantities is the most important immediate treatment measure. Injected IM or IV before the toxin has been bound to body cells, the antitoxic antibodies combine with it and prevent tissues from being injured by circulating toxin. Early treatment with antitoxin and with penicillin (to eradicate the toxin-secreting bacteria) has brought about a drop in the diphtheria mortality rate from the former 20 to 50% to only about 2%.

Although the antitoxin may also be employed to protect people who have been exposed to diphtheria, even if they are asymptomatic, the danger of inducing allergic reactions in those sensitive to horse serum limits its usefulness for prophylaxis. It may be preferable to keep the exposed person under close observation and to administer the antitoxin only at the appearance of early signs of illness. On the other hand, if passive prophylactic or therapeutic immunization seems essential, tests for horse serum sensitivity are employed and, if these are positive, the patient must first be desensitized by frequent subcutaneous injections of small doses before receiving larger amounts of antitoxin.

Diphtheria toxoid is the type of preparation preferred for long-term prophylactic immunization against diphtheria. It is available alone or combined with tetanus toxoid (DT) or with tetanus toxoid and pertussis vaccine (DPT), and all three (toxoid and combinations) are also available in the adsorbed forms, which cause longer stimulation of antibody formation by the body but tend also to produce more painful local reactions.

Diagnostic diphtheria toxin is employed in the Schick test of the degree of a person's immunity to diphtheria. Injection of a small amount of test toxin between layers of skin on the flexor surface of the forearm produces a red swollen area within a few days in susceptible people. A positive Schick test indicates the need for active immunoprophylaxis with diphtheria toxoid. If, on the other hand, an adult proves to be Schick-negative, the series of injections of the toxoid, which sometimes causes severe local and systemic reactions in people who have become allergic to the foreign protein in it, may be unnecessary.

Hepatitis

Hepatitis has long been an enigmatic disease, many aspects of which were poorly understood. Scientists have, however, succeeded in sorting out the differences and similarities in routes of transmission, clinical course, and prognosis between hepatitis A, B, and non-A, non-B, and have made advances in the detection of hepatitis B and in immunologic protective measures against this destructive viral liver disease.

Progress can be dated from the development of a test to detect the hepatitis B surface antigen (HB_sAg), which was at first known as the Australian antigen. This was followed by even more sensitive tests employing radioimmune assays (RIA) and methods for detecting HB_sAg antibody, HB_cAg (hepatitis B core antigen), and numerous other markers. These studies led to the introduction of *human hepatitis B immune globulin* (H-BIG), a product containing high levels of the HB_sAg antibody, which offers passive immunity protection to people exposed to the infective agent. This product is very expensive and is used only for those people who have definite clinical exposure to hepatitis B.

Hundreds of thousands of people annually contract hepatitis B in North America. After an incubation period of 6 to 24 weeks, depending on the route of exposure, people develop signs and symptoms such as anorexia, nausea, and vomiting; fever, jaundice, and malaise; abdominal discomfort in the upper right quadrant; and sometimes urticaria and joint pain. The initial infection is fatal in only a few cases, but some patients develop chronic hepatitis, cirrhosis, or even hepatocellular cancer. In most cases, people recover slowly after 1 or 2 months of weakness and disability.

More than two million people, including clinical and laboratory personnel, dentists, physicians, nurses, custodial workers, and homosexual men with many partners are thought to have a high risk of being exposed to hepatitis B. The disease can be transmitted in many ways in addition to the transfusion of contaminated blood: for example, accidental puncture by a bloody hypodermic needle; the splashing of contaminated material on mucous membranes; or the ingestion of even a drop of contaminated fluid while pipetting blood or fluid. These high-risk people are those who would best benefit from the recently developed hepatitis B vaccine (Heptavax B). This vaccine, it is hoped, will protect those who are at high risk for exposure to the virus by inducing antibody protection before live virus penetrates into the liver.

Administration of hepatitis B immune globulin as soon as possible after exposure—preferably within 7 days—followed by a second intramuscular injection about 1 month after exposure, taking care to avoid accidental intravenous injection, has proved helpful for protecting hospital personnel and others known to have been exposed to hepatitis B and who have not responded to hepatitis B vaccine with adequate antibody production. Pain and tenderness tend to occur commonly at the injection site, but serious systemic reactions are rare in people with no history of previous allergic reactions to any human immune globulin preparation. However, patients should be observed for development of hives or angioedema, and epinephrine should be available for emergency treatment of anaphylactic reactions.

Influenza

Influenza is one of the common viral respiratory infections that afflict hundreds of millions of people annually. Epidemics are frequent, and even pandemics have occurred at rare intervals. The influenza pandemic of 1918 and 1919 led to the deaths of an estimated 20 million people, mostly from secondary bacterial infections. Local death rates tend to rise during influenza epidemics as a result of such complicating infections in elderly and debilitated patients.

Influenza virus vaccine is considered to be desirable for administration to adults over 45 years old and to people of all ages with conditions that might make them more likely to suffer from influenza complications—patients with chronic cardiac, lung or kidney disease, for example, or diabetics. Despite the statements that are commonly made about their lack of effectiveness, influenza virus vaccines have proven to be frequently useful for short-term prophylaxis.

The main reason for failure of past influenza vaccines to protect against this infection is that the various viral strains tend to undergo frequent mutations. This means that the antibodies built up in a person by prior influenza vaccination may be unable to counteract the new strain of virus to which he is now being exposed. For this reason, scientists at the National Institutes of Health (NIH) try constantly to detect changes in the nature of prevailing influenza virus strains. The Division of Biologic Standards of NIH then determines the strains of virus that should go into any newly formulated influenza vaccine. The products licensed for distribution each year are best administered in the autumn. Many communities offer flu vaccine clinics each year to provide easy access to the vaccine for susceptible people. Influenza vaccines containing suitably selected strains of virus should then give good protection to most people during the winter months, when influenza infections most commonly occur.

Measles

Measles is mainly a childhood disease, but it can also develop in adults who have not been previously infected. Although uncomplicated measles is rarely serious, the disease is potentially fatal, especially for children under 5 years old and for elderly nonimmune patients. Otitis media and bronchopneumonia are among the most common complications. Encephalitis is another of the dangerous sequelae of measles that make prevention and treatment with modern immunologic agents so valuable.

Measles immune globulin (MIG), a product high in measles antibodies, is effective for *preventing* measles in susceptible people when administered soon after they have been exposed to the virus. Measles immune globulin is also used to *modify* an attack of measles so that the symptoms are relatively mild and the illness is rarely followed by complications. An advantage of such modification, which is carried out by administering doses of measles antibody products much smaller than those used for complete prevention, is that it permits the invading virus to make most people permanently immune to measles. On the other hand, those who have been completely, but temporarily, protected by passive immunization will require later vaccination.

Measles vaccine of the live attenuated virus type is now available. Every child who has not had measles

should be immunized with this vaccine. Such immunization is particularly important for children with chronic cardiac or bronchopulmonary diseases. Live virus attenuated measles vaccines of two types are now available. One contains the so-called *Edmonston B strain* of virus; the other contains the *Schwarz strain* in which the pathogenic potential of the virus has been still further reduced. Both are claimed to be effective for inducing long-lasting active immunity in about 99% of nonimmune children over 1 year of age. Younger infants do not respond as well because antibodies passively acquired from the mother *in utero* and still circulating in the child's blood may destroy the live virus before it can stimulate a satisfactory response by his own tissues.

The live virus vaccines can cause adverse reactions. The Edmonston B-strain virus sometimes produces high fever and rash. These measles signs can be reduced—especially when the vaccine is to be given to children with a history of convulsions—by also administering a dose of measles immune globulin too small to interfere with the desired antibody response. The Schwarz-strain vaccine is said not to require such supplementation ordinarily, because this more attenuated virus rarely causes febrile reactions or skin eruptions.

Children in whom the immune response has been depressed may be unable to respond to the virus vaccine. Live virus vaccines may expose such patients to infection. Thus, their use is contraindicated in children who are being treated with corticosteroid drugs or with antineoplastic agents or irradiation.

Mumps

Mumps is ordinarily a minor illness of childhood marked by fever of short duration and a distinctive puffing out of the cheeks and jaw as a result of parotid gland inflammation and swelling (parotitis). Complications are very rare in young children but occur in a higher proportion of people who contract the infection as adults. These include inflammation of the testes (orchitis), a painful condition that can occasionally result in some loss of fertility. More rarely, meningoencephalitis may complicate mumps.

A live attenuated *mumps virus vaccine* is available. A single injection can stimulate production of protective antibodies in most children and adults. The antibody pattern appears to be similar to that induced by a natural mumps infection. This vaccine is routinely used in all children over 12 months of age and in adults with no previous exposure to the mumps. The vaccine is recommended for use at 15 months or older, but can be given any time after 12 months of age. Infants younger than this still have maternal antibodies, which may interfere with the natural immune response. This is often given as a combination vaccine of measles, mumps, and rubella.

Pertussis

Pertussis (whooping cough) is a respiratory disease that occurs mainly in infants and other young children. Inadequately treated cases have a high mortality rate in infants under 6 months old. However, the death rate has been remarkably reduced since the advent of broad-spectrum antibiotic therapy.

Pertussis immune globulin of human origin may be employed to reduce the severity of pertussis and for passive prevention. Serum sickness from this product is highly unlikely, and no cases of transmission of serum hepatitis by administration of this product have been reported.

Pertussis vaccine is now part of the routine regimen of immunization in early infancy. The first injection is made at, or even before, 3 months of age; this is followed by at least two more monthly injections and by a booster, about 1 year after the last injection of the first series. Boosters may also be administered at ages 3 and 6 and at times of epidemics. Vaccination is withheld from children with diseases involving the nervous system because of their relative susceptibility to neurologic reactions. This is most often given in a combined vaccine containing diphtheria, tetanus, and pertussis. Despite the widespread use of pertussis vaccine, almost 2500 cases were reported in the United States in 1983.

Pneumonia

Pneumococcal infection is a leading cause of death worldwide and a major cause of not only pneumococcal pneumonia but also of otitis media and meningitis. The epidemiologic data, which come mainly from municipal hospitals where the incidence may be higher than in the general population, indicate that between 200,000 and one million cases of pneumococcal pneumonia occur annually in the United States and cause between 14,000 and 66,000 deaths.

About half of all children develop a pneumococcal illness during the first 10 years of life. Most commonly this is an otitis media, but in children under 5 years of age pneumococcal meningitis is a not uncommon complication. Despite the availability of effective antimicrobial therapy, morbidity and mortality caused by invasive pneumococcal disease remain high because these bacteria can cause irreversible physical damage during the first 5 days of the illness.

A *polyvalent pneumococcal vaccine* (Pneumovax) protects high-risk patients against lobar pneumonia and bacteremia caused by the 23 types of pneumococci that are believed to be responsible for most infections. The vaccine is indicated for people 50 years of age and over, those with chronic cardiac and respiratory diseases or with other chronic debilitating disorders, including patients in nursing homes or extended-care facilities, and those convalescing from severe illnesses.

Children under 2 years of age may not respond with production of a satisfactory level of antibodies against some of the types of pneumococci contained in the vaccine. Thus, it is not recommended for use in this group. Studies are ongoing, however, to determine the possible effectiveness of vaccination against pneumococcal otitis media in infants. Protection that the vaccine may offer against other pneumococcal diseases in addition to pneumonia, such as pneumococcal meningitis, is also under study. Some experimental studies in sickle cell anemia patients and in people who have impaired splenic function or who have undergone a splenectomy have reportedly shown this vaccine to be effective.

Vaccination causes no systemic reactions except for an occasional low-grade fever on the first day. Most people do complain, however, of soreness at the injection site, which is sometimes accompanied by redness and induration for a couple of days. Revaccination sooner than 3 years is not recommended, because antibodies produced by the initial protective injection are believed to persist much longer than that, and their presence may provoke much more severe local reactions. The vaccine is not recommended for use in pregnant women, because its possible effects on the fetus are unknown. It is not currently recommended for children under 2 years of age except in the experimental trials mentioned above.

Poliomyelitis

Poliomyelitis, or infantile paralysis, is an acute viral disease that, until a few years ago, occurred in this country as frequent sporadic epidemics. Damage to the gray matter of the spinal cord results in muscular paralysis; involvement of the medulla oblongata (bulbar polio) can cause rapidly progressive respiratory failure. Fortunately, the availability of vaccines for active immunization has remarkably reduced the incidence of this disease—until relatively recently common and dreaded.

Poliomyelitis vaccines are of two main types: an inactivated virus vaccine (Salk vaccine); and a live oral attenuated virus vaccine (Sabin vaccine). The Salk vaccine, introduced in 1953, was the first to be employed. Administered in a series of four injections, it stimulates antibodies against types I, II, and III polio virus and thus has proved to be highly successful for producing active immunity and protecting against paralysis. However, because this injected virus does not lead to significant resistance to growth of the virus in the intestine, it does not prevent spread of the disease by carriers. It is used now only for those patients with a compromised immune system.

The live oral vaccine, on the other hand, does induce resistance to viral growth in the intestine. Thus, because of this and its apparent ability to produce a longer-lasting immunity, the Sabin vaccine is preferred for immunizing children.

The three types of monovalent live oral vaccines may be given separately or together in trivalent form for the primary immunization of infants. Monovalent vaccines are given in three doses and trivalent vaccines in either two or three doses, beginning at about 2 months of age—that is, at the time of the first diphtheria–tetanus–pertussis inoculation. The primary series is completed with a dose of trivalent vaccine at 12 to 15 months, and an additional dose is commonly administered at the time the child enters school. The vaccine should not be used in patients with suppressed immune systems, and the dose should be deferred if a child has an active respiratory infection.

Rabies

Rabies (hydrophobia) is a virus infection of wild animals, including bats and skunks, that sometimes spreads to domestic animals, particularly dogs, which may then transmit the disease by attacking and biting humans. The disease has a relatively long incubation period, during which immunologic prophylaxis and therapy may be effective but, once symptoms appear, the disease is inevitably fatal, following convulsions and progressive muscular paralysis that finally affects the muscles of respiration.

Antirabies serum should be administered immediately to severely bitten persons, along with rabies vaccine. This antibody-containing passive immunization product—which provides immediate protection until the vaccine induced antibodies appear—is both injected intramuscularly and infiltrated around the bites in an effort to neutralize the virus locally before it begins to spread to the nervous system. Use of this agent is accompanied by local treatment with detergents, topical antiseptics, including alcohol 70%, and debridement, if necessary under local anesthesia. Suturing of bite wounds should, if possible, be delayed.

Rabies vaccine is used in two general ways: first, as a pre-exposure immunoprophylactic agent for persons who have *not* been bitten but who run a high risk of exposure to rabies because of their occupation (*e.g.,* dogcatchers, veterinarians) or their avocations (*e.g.,* spelunkers who investigate bat-infested caves). Second, the vaccine is administered to people who have been bitten by an animal suspected of being rabid. The vaccine series is usually preceded by injection of rabies immune globulin (RIG), which supplies preformed antibodies to deal with the virus before the vaccine can lead to the production of antibodies. Half of the immune globulin is injected into the area of the bite, and the remainder is given IM. Such postexposure immunoprophylaxis requires a course of daily injections under the skin of the abdomen for 14 to 21 days.

Rabies vaccine prepared from a virus grown in duck egg embryos and then inactivated was once preferred to older rabies vaccines that were made from viruses grown on rabbit nervous tissue. The latter caused a relatively high incidence of neurologic or neuroparalytic reactions. Because the duck embryo vaccine is free of the so-called paralytic factor found in mammalian nervous tissue, it can be given without fear that its use might result in a fatal reaction. A rabies vaccine made from human diploid cell cultures (HDCV) is presently used. The use of a human-based vaccine avoids many of the potential allergies of duck- or rabbit-based vaccines. This vaccine is given IM in the deltoid muscle or the buttocks. After exposure, the vaccine is given in six doses on days 0, 3, 7, 14, 30, and 90. The first dose is given concurrently with RIG (above). However, unnecessary use of rabies vaccine should be avoided, because the course of treatment is often painful and may result in severe local erythematous reactions and in abdominal distress, nausea, and vomiting.

Rubella

German measles, as indicated earlier, is a mild childhood disease, but it poses great risk for the developing fetus. A live attenuated *rubella virus vaccine* has proven successful in producing effective antibody levels against rubella for at least 6 years after vaccination. It is now recommended that all children over 12 months of age receive the vaccine, preferably at about 15 months of age, as well as adolescent and adult men who have no appreciable titers to rubella. Adolescent and adult women should be screened for susceptibility to rubella and, if they do not have appreciable antibody titers, may be vaccinated if they are not pregnant and agree not to become pregnant for at least 3 months. It is advisable to vaccinate and prevent clinical rubella from developing before a pregnancy occurs; the risk that the vaccine may pose to a developing fetus, however, has not been established.

There is no evidence that the vaccine will prevent illness if given after exposure to the virus. Some common side-effects to the vaccine include fever, arthralgia, transitory arthritis, rash, and headache. Anyone receiving the vaccine should be aware of the possibiiity of these side-effects, and should be instructed in ways to make these side effects more tolerable (*e.g.,* local application of heat and rest for the arthritis, aspirin for headache and fever).

It is common practice to give children over the age of 12 months a combination vaccine of measles, mumps, and rubella. This facilitates the immunization scheduling and decreases the number of injections that the child must have.

Smallpox

Smallpox, as indicated previously, was once one of the most widespread and deadly of acute infectious diseases. The World Health Organization (WHO) has declared that smallpox has been eradicated. *Smallpox vaccine* is no longer used routinely, but is reserved for use only for those who are at high risk for exposure to the virus—specifically, scientists and laboratory workers.

Tetanus

Tetanus (lockjaw) is a disease caused by contamination of wounds with the bacillus *Clostridium tetani*. This organism and its spores are found most commonly in fields fertilized with animal excreta. However, ordinary soil and even dust may carry the organism and it may even, in fact, sometimes be found on unsterilized surgical dressings to which it has been borne through the air on dust particles.

Once tetanus bacilli gain entrance to the tissues, they begin to multiply and produce their toxins. The danger is greatest when the organism is driven deep into tissues that have been traumatized and contaminated by debris. Gunshot wounds, compound fractures, and other injuries characterized by crushing and destruction of tissues offer favorable sites for the growth of tetanus bacilli. However, even relatively minor skin punctures may sometimes be the cause of tetanus infections.

The main symptoms of tetanus, which usually take several days and occasionally weeks to develop, involve the central nervous system. The continuing convulsions that can finally end in death are caused not by the bacilli but by the toxic products given off during their growth. When tetanus toxin reaches the central nervous system, it prevents the release of the inhibitory neurotransmitter, glycine, thus producing severe convulsive spasms (see Chap. 47).

Tetanus antitoxin obtained from horse serum was formerly the only product used to neutralize the bacterial toxins before they become fixed to nervous tissue. However, *tetanus immune globulin* prepared from human blood plasma is now preferred for passive immunization procedures, because it does not cause allergic reactions like those sometimes seen after administration of the antitoxin. Another advantage of administering gamma globulin from human serum is that the antibodies stay at effective levels for 3 weeks or more—which is several times the duration of availability of antitoxin-induced antibodies. This provides protection for the full incubation period of most tetanus cases. However, human globulin is no substitute for tetanus toxoid, which should be administered at the same time to produce active immunization.

Tetanus toxoid is a very valuable vaccine that provides good, prolonged protection when given prior to injury. It is administered in early infancy and reinforced periodically with booster shots at intervals of about 10 years and after injuries that might be contaminated with tetanus organisms. The series of three subcutaneous injections rarely causes reactions other than occasional local redness and swelling. The adsorbed tetanus toxoid is somewhat more likely to cause local reactions, but its longer duration of action permits active immunization with only two injections. Both the toxoid solution and the adsorbed toxoid suspension are available combined with diphtheria toxoid and pertussis vaccine in the triple antigen (DPT) combinations that, together with oral polio vaccine, constitutes the infant's earliest series of immunizations.

Tuberculosis

The nature of this disease and its treatment with tuberculostatic chemotherapeutic agents has been discussed in Chapter 8. Here only the use and status of certain diagnostic and immunoprophylactic agents will be discussed.

Old tuberculin USP and the *purified protein derivative of tuberculin USP* are preparations of the growth products of the tubercle bacillus that are used as aids in the diagnosis of tuberculosis. Injected intracutaneously, minute amounts produce positive reactions (*e.g.*, redness, edema) in those who are, or have ever been, infected with the tuberculosis organism. A negative reaction indicates that the person does not have tuberculosis—and also shows that no antibodies have been built up to defend against future invasion, in case of exposure to the risk of infection. Tuberculin tests are done routinely on children, health-care providers, and high-risk groups living in institutions. A change in tuberculin reactivity can be detected easily, and appropriate diagnostic and therapeutic action can then be taken.

BCG vaccine is an active immunizing product prepared from the living cells of the *bacillus Calmette Guerin*, an attenuated strain of an organism that causes bovine tuberculosis. Its value for immunoprophylaxis against tuberculosis is debatable, and most authorities agree that its routine use in large-scale public health tuberculosis control programs is unnecessary in this country. In fact, because its administration produces positive tuberculin test reactions and thus makes diagnosis more difficult, its widespread use is considered to be undesirable. Nevertheless, this immunizing agent *has* been administered to hundreds of millions of people living in high-risk areas elsewhere in the world, and its use here is recommended for tuberculin-negative people who are exposed to infection and who cannot be readily protected by other control measures (*e.g.*, migrant workers and others often living under crowded unsanitary conditions).

Typhoid fever

Typhoid is an acute systemic infection caused by a *Salmonella* organism that enters the GI tract through ingestion of contaminated food or water and then makes its way into the bloodstream. The disease, which is marked by malaise and the gradual development of a persistent fever and a rose-colored rash resembling that of typhus (hence the name, "typhoid"), may be relatively mild or rapidly fatal. Related paratyphoid-type *Salmonella* organisms cause less severe infections than *S. typhosa*, the pathogen of true typhoid fever.

Typhoid vaccine and *typhoid–paratyphoid vaccine* have been less important than advances in sanitation in reducing the incidence of typhoid fever in this country. Their efficacy as active immunoprophylactic products is certainly not great enough to warrant neglect of sanitation by vaccinated persons. However, even though protection offered by available typhoid and combination, or "triple," vaccine (containing three types of *Salmonella* organisms) is limited and short-lived, their use by travelers in areas where typhoid is endemic is recommended by some authorities. Vaccination against typhoid is also indicated for medical laboratory workers and others who might contact fecal matter containing typhoid bacteria. The procedure should not be performed while the person is ill with an infection or if he has diabetes or nephritis. Local and systemic reactions, although not severe, occur in a high proportion of those receiving the typhoid vaccines. Passive immunization is not employed in treating typhoid, but the broad-spectrum antibiotics, especially chloramphenicol, have proved to be highly effective.

Other diseases

Vaccines are also available for *yellow fever* and *plague.* Yellow fever vaccine is a live attenuated virus that is recommended for those traveling to a country that requires yellow fever vaccination because of an endemic disease problem. The vaccine is good for 10 years.

Plague vaccine is recommended for all people living in or traveling to a known plague area. Many foreign countries and several western states in the United States (*e.g.,* California, New Mexico, Utah, Nevada, Colorado, Arizona, Idaho, and Oregon) are known plague areas. The vaccine is given in two primary injections followed by a booster in 3 to 6 months. Repeated injections cause increased sensitivity, and patients with a sensitivity reaction to an initial dose may require a reduced booster dosage and careful evaluation after the injection.

Additional clinical considerations

There are many active and passive immunizing agents available for treating and preventing various acute infectious diseases. Because many of these infections, particularly those caused by viruses, cannot yet be effectively treated with pharmacologic agents, active immunoprophylaxis is very valuable in preventing these diseases. Children should be routinely immunized against the diseases that could be most harmful to them. Although immunizations are not required by law, most public school systems in the United States require routine immunizations as part of their admission standards. Children who receive their immunizations as part of routine well-baby care are protected from the potential complications of these diseases before being exposed to them. People traveling to other countries often must receive immunizations against diseases that are endemic to that area. These regulations should be checked before traveling abroad.

Whenever an immunization is required, the pa-tient should be evaluated for allergies, particularly to any of the vaccine culture media or animal sources of antibodies—for example, horse, chicken, egg, duck. If a known allergy exists and the patient requires the vaccine, divided doses are often used, or a series of desensitizing injections is given first. Emergency equipment should be readily available when the vaccine or toxoid is given to manage any acute reaction.

Immunization is contraindicated for any person who is immunosuppressed—whether from disease or from drug therapy (*e.g.,* cancer drugs, corticosteroids). Patients who are immunosuppressed usually cannot respond to the vaccine or toxoid and may become ill as a result of the altered immune response. In the same way, a patient with an acute infection should also avoid immunization, because his body may be unable to respond appropriately. Immunization during pregnancy is contraindicated, because the safety of vaccines during pregnancy has not been established.

Adverse effects often occur when a vaccine is given. These reactions range from local inflammation— pain, swelling, and redness—at the injection site to more systemic reactions that are typical of an active immune response—fever, arthralgia, myalgia, rash, malaise, weakness. In adults, such serum sickness may not occur for 6 to 12 days. The patient should be made aware of the possibilities of these reactions. Several comfort measures should also be suggested if these occur: aspirin or acetaminophen for fever and pain; aspirin and rest for the arthralgia and myalgia; decreased environmental stimuli; small frequent meals. Aspirin may be taken prophylactically following an immunization to avert these adverse reactions before they occur. The date of the immunization should be recorded by the patient for future reference.

The patient teaching guide summarizes points that should be included when teaching a patient about immunizations. The guide to the nursing process summarizes the clinical considerations that should be incorporated into the nursing care of a patient receiving an immunization.

Passive immunity is obtained by injecting the patient with preformed antibodies in gamma globulin or specifically sensitized gamma globulin. This type of immunization is usually reserved for the patient who has been exposed to an infectious disease. It is not unusual for an entire nursing staff to require gamma globulin after a previously undiagnosed patient is found to have one of these diseases. Patients who are acutely ill are also often given gamma globulin to help their body deal with the specific antigen until their own immune system can respond to it. Patients should know that injections of gamma globulin are usually quite painful; the injection site may be sore for several days. Warm soaks applied to the area may help, and aspirin may help to relieve the systemic discomforts that can occur.

Patient teaching guide: immunizations

The immunization you received today was for _____ . It would be a
good idea to write down the date and type of immunization that was given in a
ready reference place. A booster immunization should be given in _____
months. This immunization helps your body to develop antibodies to protect you
against _____ if you should be exposed to the disease.

Instructions:

1. The injection site may be sore or painful. Heat applied to the area may help this discomfort.

2. You may experience any of the following adverse effects:

   | Fever, muscle aches, joint aches, fatigue, malaise | Aspirin may help these discomforts. Rest, small meals, and quiet may also help. |

3. These side-effects should pass within 2 to 3 days. If they become very uncomfortable, or persist longer than a few days, notify your nurse or physician.

4. Booster immunizations are required for many immunizations. You should receive a booster immunization in _____ months (if appropriate).

Guide to the nursing process: immunizations

Assessment	Nursing diagnoses	Interventions	Evaluation
Past history (*contraindications*): Acute infection Immune deficiency disease Pregnancy Allergies: *Serum base for this preparation (e.g., egg, duck, horse, chicken); others; reactions* Medication history (*contraindications*): Corticosteroids Antineoplastic drugs **Physical assessment** Cardiovascular: P, BP, peripheral perfusion	Potential alteration in comfort: pain Knowledge deficit regarding drug therapy Potential alteration in tissue perfusion secondary to acute reaction	Proper preparation and administration of immunization Provision of comfort measures: Pain relief measures: • Aspirin • Heat Small meals Rest Quiet environment Patient teaching regarding drug therapy Support and encouragement to deal with discomfort Provision of emergency measures and life	Evaluate therapeutic effect, if appropriate: serum titers Monitor adverse effects to drug: • Pain • Discomfort • Serum sickness Evaluate effectiveness of comfort measures Evaluate effectiveness of patient teaching program Evaluate effectiveness of support and encouragement offered Evaluate effectiveness of emergency measures

(continued)

Assessment	Nursing diagnoses	Interventions	Evaluation
Respiratory: R, adventitious sounds Skin: lesions Musculoskeletal: joints, range of motion		support, if adverse reaction occurs	and life support, if indicated

Case study

Presentation

SD, a 25-year-old mother of one, brought her 2-month-old baby girl, B, into the well-baby clinic for a routine evaluation. B was found to be a healthy growing baby within the normal limits of all parameters for a baby her age. At the end of the well-baby visit, B was given her first DPT injection and trivalent oral polio vaccine.

What information should the nurse running the well-baby clinic give to SD before she leaves?

Discussion

Most babies in the United States receive routine immunizations based on the recommendations of the American Academy of Pediatics. The usual schedule is shown in Table 55-2. SD should be given information about the immunizations that her baby should receive and the reasoning behind the scheduling of the immunizations. She should be advised to record the immunizations and dates given for future reference. This information will be needed when B goes to school. The American Academy of Pediatrics often supplies an immunization record card for parents' use to record this information.

SD should be alerted to the possible adverse effects of the immunization. The baby may have a very sore injection site, may develop a fever, and may become fussy and irritable. SD can be advised to give the baby an appropriate dose of baby aspirin or baby acetaminophen when she gets home to avert these reactions and, if fever does develop, she can be advised of the appropriate intervals to remedicate the baby. SD should be asked to call the nurse if the baby has a prolonged or severe reaction. She should also be asked to make a note of the baby's reactions, because babies who have severe reactions may require divided doses of future immunizations.

Table 55–2. Immunization schedule for babies and children

Vaccine	Age					
	2 mo	4 mo	6 mo	15 mo	18 mo	4–6 yr
DPT (diphtheria, pertussis, tetanus)	✓	✓	✓		✓	✓
Trivalent polio	✓	✓	✓*		✓	✓
Measles				✓		
Mumps				✓		
Rubella				✓		

* Optional, depending on where the patient lives

When explaining the immunization schedule to SD, it is important to point out that it is possible to vary from this schedule, within limits, with no ill effects. If the baby has an acute infection at one of the prescribed times, the immunization will be deferred until the infection has resolved. It should also be pointed out that smallpox vaccines are no longer given in this country.

SD should be encouraged to ask any questions that she might have and should be assured that the temporary discomfort the baby experiences is more desirable than the potentially devastating complications of the diseases from which the immunizations protect the baby. Prophylactic immunizations are an important aspect of preventive health care, and should be encouraged for all patients.

References

American Academy of Pediatrics: Report of Committee on Infectious Diseases, 19th ed. Evanston, IL, American Academy of Pediatrics, 1982

Ammann AJ et al: Polyvalent pneumococcal polysaccharide immunization of patients with sickle cell anemia and patients with splenectomy. N Engl J Med 297:897, 1977

Arvin AM et al: Human leukocyte interferon for treatment of varicella in children with cancer. N Engl J Med 306:761, 1982

Bernard KW et al: Human diploid cell rabies vaccine. JAMA 247:1138, 1982

Grady GF: Hepatitis B immunoglobulin—prevention of hepatitis from accidental exposure among medical personnel. N Engl J Med 293:1067, 1975

Hepatitis B vaccine. Med Lett Drugs Ther 24:75, 1982

Krugman S, Katz SL: Childhood immunization procedures. JAMA 237:2228, 1977

Selekman J: Immunization: What's it all about? Am J Nurs 80:1440, 1980

Drugs are sometimes administered to diagnose disease rather than to treat it. The basis for the use of some drugs in diagnosing disease is the fact that diseased organs respond differently to these drugs than do normally functioning organs. For example, patients with myasthenia gravis respond to low doses of *edrophonium* (Tensilon) differently from patients in whom neuromuscular transmission is normal. This is the basis for the use of this drug to differentiate myasthenia gravis from other disorders marked by muscle weakness. This chapter will describe the diagnostic use of other drugs that evoke unusual responses in the presence of pathology.

This chapter will also describe drugs that are used to aid in visualizing internal organs by x-ray—radiographic agents (Table 56-3)—and it will mention briefly the general uses of radioactive isotopes for diagnosis (Table 56-2).

This chapter will not describe the various materials of biologic origin such as the skin test antigens used in testing for tuberculosis, diphtheria, and other infectious diseases, and for allergies. It will also omit reference to the various chemical reagents and aids used in measuring the amounts of such substances as sugar or acetone in blood, urine, or other body fluid samples. In this text the coverage of diagnostic agents is limited to those that are administered to the patient; agents that are added to test tubes containing body fluids are beyond the scope of a pharmacology textbook. The details of diagnostic tests of all types may best be found in various excellent books that deal with clinical laboratory tests and their interpretation.

Like the drugs used in therapy, the drugs used in diagnostic tests can produce adverse reactions. These are either extensions of the desired effect in the diagnostic test, or manifestations of effects on other organ systems, including allergic reactions. Table 56-1 lists some of the drugs that are used as diagnostic agents, with their uses, the most common adverse reactions, cautions, and con-

traindications. All these agents are contraindicated in patients who have previously experienced an allergic reaction to them. In addition, the safety of many of these agents in pregnant and nursing women and in young children has not been established. Because diagnostic agents are usually administered in a radiologic or specialized diagnostic laboratory by medical personnel with special training, and because the dosage of many of these agents depends on the particular use of the agent and often on the individual patient's response, information about the dosage and administration of these agents is not considered appropriate for a nursing pharmacology text. However, it is important that the nurse know what drugs and disease conditions can alter or invalidate the results of a diagnostic test that is proposed for a patient (see Chap. 2). Accordingly, the last column of Table 56-1 lists drugs and diseases that can interact with each test, and Table 56-4 provides this information for radiopaque agents.

Digestive system function tests

Gastric acid secretion
Drugs are sometimes employed to determine whether a patient's stomach has the ability to secrete gastric acid (see also Chap. 41). Patients with pernicious anemia lack this ability. Alcohol and caffeine are among the many chemicals that can provoke increased secretion of gastric acid. However, in the clinical setting, histamine, its analogue, betazole (Histalog), and pentagastrin (Peptavlon) are more commonly employed for this purpose.

Histamine phosphate strongly stimulates the gastric glands to secrete increased quantities of acid. If the stomach fails to respond to a subcutaneously administered dose of this drug, the presence of pernicious anemia or stomach cancer may be suspected. This must, of course, be confirmed by other types of diagnostic tests.

Table 56–1. Some drugs used in diagnostic tests*

Drug	Diagnostic use	Contraindications, cautions, and adverse effects	Drugs and diseases that can alter test results
Digestive system function tests			
Gastric acid secretion			
Histamine phosphate	To test gastric acid secretory ability in the diagnosis of pernicious anemia, gastric carcinoma, and atrophic gastritis	*Contraindicated* in asthma, hypo- or hypertension, and severe pulmonary, cardiac, or renal disease; have epinephrine on hand to treat adverse effects; may cause bronchoconstriction, asthma, hypo- or hypertension, tachycardia, hives, abdominal cramps, nausea, vomiting, circulatory collapse, shock	Cimetidine (Tagamet) and other histamine H_2-receptor blockers inhibit gastric acid secretion stimulated by histamine
Betazole hydrochloride (Histalog)	As for histamine	Use with caution in patients with history of allergy; have epinephrine on hand to treat adverse effects; causes fewer adverse effects than histamine; may cause headache, hypotension, flushing of the face, hives, asthma, weakness, and syncope	Cimetidine inhibits gastric acid secretion stimulated by betazole
Pentagastrin (Peptavlon)	As for histamine; also used in diagnosis of Zollinger–Ellison syndrome	Use with caution in patients with pancreatitis, liver, or gallbladder disease; excessive dosage may inhibit gastric acid secretion; causes fewer and less severe adverse effects than histamine or betazole; may cause headache, dizziness, abdominal pain, intestinal cramps, urge to defecate, nausea, vomiting, allergic reactions	Cimetidine inhibits gastric acid secretion stimulated by pentagastrin
Azuresin (Diagnex Blue)	Given orally to test gastric acid secretory ability without need for sampling gastric contents; urine is colored blue or green if gastric acid has liberated dye from resin	May cause allergic reactions; urine may be colored blue or green for several days	Preparations containing salts of calcium (Ca), magnesium (Mg), or aluminum (Al); (*e.g.*, antacids) may interfere with test results, as may salts of barium (Ba) (used in radiologic exam of upper gastrointestinal tract) and iron (Fe); vomiting, diarrhea, dehydration, severe liver or kidney disease, and gastrectomy may all cause inaccurate results

(continued)

Table 56–1. Some drugs used in diagnostic tests* (continued)

Drug	Diagnostic use	Contraindications, cautions, and adverse effects	Drugs and diseases that can alter test results
Liver function			
Sulfobromophthalein sodium (Bromsulphalein sodium; BSP)	Used in diagnosis of cirrhosis, liver carcinoma, and other liver disorders	Definitely *contraindicated* in newborns, who lack metabolizing enzymes for this drug; use with caution in patients with history of allergy; may cause allergic reactions, anaphylaxis, hypotension, nausea; urine and feces will be colored red	Steroids (androgens, estrogens, and oral contraceptives) interfere with BSP excretion and therefore with test results; narcotic analgesics and MAO inhibitors may also cause inaccurate results
Indocyanine green (Cardio-Green)	As for sulfobromophthalein	*Contraindicated*, because of iodide content, in patients allergic to iodides; appears to cause fewer adverse effects than BSP; radioiodide uptake studies should be delayed 1 wk after BSP test; may cause allergic reactions, including anaphylaxis	Probenecid may interfere with test results
Gallbladder function and pancreatic exocrine function			
Bentiromide (Chymex)	To test pancreatic exocrine function	*Contraindicated* in patients taking methotrexate; can cause nausea, vomiting, diarrhea, and headache	Many drugs may interfere with test results: acetaminophen, local anesthetics, chloramphenicol, sulfonamides, thiazides, and sunscreens and multivitamin preparations containing PABA
Ceruletide diethylamine (Tymtran)	To contract the gallbladder during radiologic examination of the gallbladder and bile ducts; to facilitate the collection of a sample of bile (for chemical and cytologic analyses) from the duodenum; to speed the transit of barium through the small intestine during radiologic examination	*Contraindicated* in patients with intestinal obstruction; may induce premature labor in pregnant women near term; possibly serious adverse effects in patients who have bile duct obstruction, gallbladder inflammation, appendicitis, peritonitis, bowel ulceration, acute pancreatitis, or acute abdomen of any cause; may increase insulin release during glucose tolerance test; may cause dizziness, hypotension, sweating, feeling of flushing, abdominal pain, nausea, diarrhea, urge to defecate	

Table 56–1. Some drugs used in diagnostic tests* (continued)

Drug	Diagnostic use	Contraindications, cautions, and adverse effects	Drugs and diseases that can alter test results
Cholecystokinin (CCK)	As for ceruletide; used with secretin to stimulate pancreatic secretion	Although not reported, CCK could theoretically cause the same adverse effects as ceruletide; therefore, the same cautions should be used as for ceruletide	
Secretin	To stimulate pancreatic secretion into the duodenum, when it is necessary to collect pancreatic juice for analysis in the diagnosis of pancreatic exocrine disease and pancreatic carcinoma (by exfoliative cytology); to stimulate the secretion of gastrin in the diagnosis of Zollinger–Ellison syndrome	*Contraindicated* in acute pancreatitis; use with caution, and then only after an IV test dose, in patients with a history of allergy or asthma	Patients who have inflammatory bowel disease, who have undergone vagotomy, or who are taking anticholinergic (atropinelike) drugs may show a lower-than-normal response to secretin; alcoholic patients and those with liver disease may show a greater-than-normal response
Sincalide (Kinevac)	As for ceruletide; used with secretin to simulate pancreatic secretion	As for ceruletide	

Cardiovascular system function tests

Diagnostic tests in hypertensive patients

Histamine phosphate	Provocative test used when intermittent hypertension is suspected to be caused by pheochromocytoma; allows correlation of urinary catecholamine levels with blood pressure	See Gastric acid secretion, above; this test is also *contraindicated* in the elderly and in patients with resting blood pressure > 150/110; have epinephrine at hand to treat severe hypotension, and phentolamine to treat severe hypertension	Antihypertensive drugs, sympathomimetics, narcotic analgesics, and sedatives should be withheld for 24 to 72 hr before the test
Phentolamine mesylate (Regitine)	To differentiate hypertension caused by pheochromocytoma from essential hypertension	*Contraindicated* in coronary heart disease; if marked hypotension occurs, myocardial infarction or cerebrovascular spasm may also occur	Antihypertensive drugs, sedatives, analgesics, and all nonessential drugs should be withheld for 24–72 hr before the test
Saralasin acetate (Sarenin)	To test for angiotensin II–dependent hypertension	Patient must be mildly sodium-depleted by furosemide or by low-sodium diet for test	Antihypertensive drugs should be withheld for 1–2 wk before the test

(continued)

Table 56–1. Some drugs used in diagnostic tests* (continued)

Drug	Diagnostic use	Contraindications, cautions, and adverse effects	Drugs and diseases that can alter test results
		to be safe and meaningful; may cause marked hypo- or marked hypertension, extrasystoles, headache, malaise, nausea, pain at injection site; rebound hypertension may occur up to 3 hr after the test; therefore, monitor blood pressure for at least 3 hours after the test	

Measurement of blood volume and cardiac output

Drug	Diagnostic use	Contraindications, cautions, and adverse effects	Drugs and diseases that can alter test results
Evans blue	To determine circulating blood volume	Skin and sclerae (whites of eyes) may be stained blue for several weeks	
Fluorescein sodium	To determine circulation time and patency of the circulation of the extremities	Use with caution in patients with history of allergy; may cause allergic reactions, nausea, vomiting, hypotension, shock; skin and urine fluoresce and are dyed yellow	
Indocyanine green (Cardio-Green)	To determine cardiac output	See Liver function, above	
Isosulfan blue (Lymphazurin 1%)	Adjunct to lymphography	Use with caution in patients with history of allergy; have facilities available to treat severe allergic reactions; urine will be colored blue for up to 24 hr	

Kidney function tests

Drug	Diagnostic use	Contraindications, cautions, and adverse effects	Drugs and diseases that can alter test results
Phenolsulfonphthalein (phenol red; PSP)	To determine renal blood flow and overall renal function	Use with caution in patients with history of allergy; may cause allergic reactions; urine will be colored red	Uricosuric drugs used to treat gout, penicillins, and cephalosporins may all compete with PSP for renal tubular secretory sites and give false test results; drugs that can alter urine color should be avoided for 24 hr before the test
Sodium aminohippurate (paraminohippuric acid; PAH)	To determine renal blood flow and tubular secretion	May cause nausea, vomiting, flushed feeling	Sulfonamides can interact with chemicals used to assay PAH; uricosuric drugs, probenecid, penicillins, and cephalosporins can give false test results, as with PSP

Table 56–1. Some drugs used in diagnostic tests* (continued)

Drug	Diagnostic use	Contraindications, cautions, and adverse effects	Drugs and diseases that can alter test results
Sodium indigotin disulfonate (indigo carmine)	To localize ureteral orifices during cystoscopy; to identify severed ureters; to test overall renal function	Test for allergy in patients with history of allergy to other antigens; may cause bronchoconstriction and allergic skin reactions	
Inulin	To determine glomerular filtration rate	High doses can raise plasma osmolality and cause osmotic diuresis; monitoring of fluid and electrolyte balance is important with these patients	
Mannitol	To determine glomerular filtration rate	*Contraindicated* in patients with edema, severe kidney impairment, or severe pulmonary congestion, and in dehydrated patients; may cause chills, chest pain, hypotension, osmotic diuresis, fluid and electrolyte imbalance, nausea, allergic skin reactions	

Diagnosis of myasthenia gravis

Drug	Diagnostic use	Contraindications, cautions, and adverse effects	Drugs and diseases that can alter test results
Edrophonium chloride (Tensilon)	Used in differential diagnosis of myasthenia; and to differentiate myasthenic from cholinergic crisis	*Contraindicated* in patients with obstruction of GI or urinary tracts; use with caution in patients with asthma or cardiac arrhythmias; have atropine at hand; may cause lacrimation, sweating, bronchoconstriction, increased secretions in airway, cardiac arrhythmias, urinary incontinence, diarrhea, nausea	

Neuroendocrine function tests (endocrine target organs, anterior pituitary, and endocrine hypothalamus)

Drug	Diagnostic use	Contraindications, cautions, and adverse effects	Drugs and diseases that can alter test results
Arginine HCl (R-Gene 10)	To test human growth hormone (HGH) release from anterior pituitary in diagnosis of such conditions as panhypopituitarism and pituitary dwarfism	*Contraindicated* in patients with history of allergy; have antihistamine at hand; may cause headache, flushing, numbness, nausea, vomiting	Pre- and postdrug levels of HGH are elevated in pregnancy and in patients taking oral contraceptives
Chorionic gonadotropin (HCG)	To test for Leydig cell function in diagnosing male primary hypogonadism	May cause headache, irritability, edema, pain at injection site	

(continued)

Table 56-1. Some drugs used in diagnostic tests* (continued)

Drug	Diagnostic use	Contraindications, cautions, and adverse effects	Drugs and diseases that can alter test results
Corticotropin (ACTH: Acthar)	To test adrenal cortical function in diagnosis of such conditions as Addison's disease	Administer skin test to patients allergic to pork before giving ACTH; before testing, consider all contraindications to chronic therapeutic use of ACTH—for example, systemic fungal infections, ocular herpes	
Cosyntropin (Cortrosyn)	This synthetic peptide with ACTH-like activity is considered to be a safer way to test adrenal function than using ACTH itself	May cause allergic reactions, but risk is less than with ACTH	
Gonadorelin HCl (Factrel); synthetic luteinizing hormone releasing hormone (LH-RH); gonadotropin releasing hormone (Gn-RH)	To test hypothalamic–pituitary gonadotropic function	May cause headache, nausea, abdominal discomfort, pain and itching at injection site	Estrogens, androgens, progestins, oral contraceptives, glucocorticoids, spironolactone, levodopa, digoxin, phenothiazines, and other dopamine antagonists may alter test results
Insulin	To test anterior pituitary ability to release HGH and ACTH, in diagnosis of such conditions as panhypopituitarism	May cause severe hypoglycemic reactions; patient should be carefully monitored	
Metyrapone (Metopirone)	To test hypothalamic-pituitary function; used especially in diagnosis of hypopituitarism	*Contraindicated* in adrenal cortical insufficiency; adrenal responsiveness to ACTH must be demonstrated before the test with metyrapone; may cause headache, dizziness, nausea, vomiting, allergic reactions	Phenytoin (diphenylhydantoin; Dilatin), estrogen therapy, and pregnancy can alter results
Parathyroid hormone (Parathyroid)	To diagnose hypoparathyroidism	*Contraindicated* in patients with elevated blood calcium levels; use with caution in presence of renal or cardiac disease; may cause diarrhea, weakness, vomiting, anorexia	
Protirelin (Thypinone; Relefact TRH)	To test anterior pituitary function; used in diagnosis of hypopituitarism; used in establishing etiology of hypothyroidism	Frequently causes changes in blood pressure; therefore, measure blood pressure before drug and frequently for 15 min after drug; may cause headache, nausea, abdominal discomfort, urge to urinate	Thyroid hormones, levodopa, and aspirin alter test results

Table 56–1. Some drugs used in diagnostic tests* (continued)

Drug	Diagnostic use	Contraindications, cautions, and adverse effects	Drugs and diseases that can alter test results
Radioactive iodine	To diagnose hyperthyroidism		Iodine, thyroid preparations, and antithyroid drugs, as well as iodinated radiographic contrast media, can alter test results
Thyrotropin (thyroid stimulating hormone; Thytropar)	To differentiate primary from secondary (pituitary) hypothyroidism	*Contraindicated* in coronary thrombosis and untreated Addison's disease; use with caution in patients with angina, cardiac failure, and allergy to beef proteins	
Tolbutamide sodium (Orinase Diagnostic)	To diagnose insulin-producing pancreatic islet cell adenoma (insulinoma)	*Contraindicated* in patients allergic to sulfonylurea drugs (*e.g.*, tolbutamide; chlorpropamide); use with caution in patients with severe liver or kidney disease; have carbohydrate and epinephrine at hand; may cause pain along vein used for injection	Many drugs potentiate the hypoglycemic response to tolbutamide and can therefore alter test results; these include dicumarol, salicylates, sulfonamides, phenylbutazone, probenecid, MAO inhibitors, β-adrenergic receptor blockers, and chloramphenicol

* These drugs are all contraindicated in patients who have previously shown an allergic reaction to them. The safety of most of these drugs has not been demonstrated in pregnant and nursing mothers or in young children.

The effects of histamine may not be limited to the gastric glands but can also affect the smooth muscle of blood vessels, the bronchioles, and other sites. Histamine is a good illustration of the principle that diagnostic agents can produce serious adverse reactions. With histamine, overdosage, accidental injection into a vein, or hypersensitivity, may result in severe headache, breathing difficulties, or cardiovascular collapse. The use of histamine is contraindicated in patients with a history of bronchial asthma or chronic obstructive pulmonary disease.

Betazole hydrochloride (Histalog) also stimulates gastric acid secretion and is used for the same purpose as histamine. However, it does not cause side-effects as often or as severe as those seen with histamine. Headache, urticarial skin reactions, and bronchoconstriction are relatively rare, but caution is still required in asthmatic patients and in others with a history of hypersensitivity. The most common side-effects experienced by the patient are sweating, flushing of the face, and a feeling of warmth.

Pentagastrin (Peptavlon) is a peptide that is related chemically to gastrin, the endogenous substance that normally stimulates gastric acid secretion. It has come into

use recently and has largely replaced histamine and betazole in tests of gastric acid secretion. It is also used to test for hypersecretion of hydrochloric acid in patients suspected of having Zollinger–Ellison syndrome. It causes fewer cardiovascular and respiratory side-effects than histamine or betazole, but still causes a significant incidence of adverse reactions, mostly related to the gastrointestinal tract: nausea, vomiting, abdominal pain, and the urge to defecate.

Azuresin (Diagnex Blue) is a substance also used for determining whether acid is present in the stomach or absent (achlorhydria). Its use eliminates the need to collect gastric acid with a stomach tube, as is the case when histamine, betazole, or pentagastrin are employed. Instead, the urine is examined for the presence of this dye exactly 2 hours after the oral administration of the granules. The presence of free hydrochloric acid in the stomach liberates a blue dye from the resin with which it is combined. This dye is then absorbed into the bloodstream and carried to the kidneys for excretion. The collected urine specimen is then examined visually and its color is compared with a standard. Side-effects rarely occur, but the results of this test are less accurate than those obtained by gastric intubation and direct collection of stomach acid following administration of a gastric acid stimulant. False results are most likely to occur in the presence of kidney disease, impaired gastrointestinal absorption, and other pathologic states.

Liver function

The ability of the liver to remove from the blood such dyes as *sulfobromophthalein sodium* (Bromsulphalein Sodium; BSP) and *indocyanine green* (Cardio-Green) is an index of the liver's functional capacity and of the extent to which it may have been reduced in such diseases as cirrhosis of the liver, or in hepatic and metastatic carcinoma. Healthy liver cells remove these dyes from the blood and excrete them into the bile soon after the dye is injected intravenously. The damaged liver does not do so as readily. As a result, the dye stays in the bloodstream at higher levels for a longer time after injection.

These tests of hepatic function do not always detect the presence of gross damage that may be seen in a biopsy sample. Liver function, as determined by these tests, may seem more or less normal despite the presence of gross pathology. Nevertheless, by the use of a battery of such tests, it is often possible to rule out some diseases or to determine the degree of their severity.

Adverse reactions to both of these dyes can occur. Allergic reactions have occurred to Bromsulphalein, especially when the drug has leaked out of the vein at the injection site. Patients who are allergic to iodides may show an allergic reaction to the iodide in indocyanine green; anaphylaxis has occurred. Tests of thyroid function using radioactive iodine uptake are invalid for at least 1 week after this dye has been used.

Rose bengal, radioactively labeled to facilitate its measurement in feces, is sometimes used as a liver and biliary duct test in infants. Thyroid uptake of the dye must first be blocked by Lugol's solution. Stools are colored red by the dye.

Gallbladder function

Drugs that stimulate the gallbladder to contract are sometimes given during radiologic examination of the gallbladder and its ducts to facilitate diagnostic visualization. These drugs are also given to facilitate the collection of a sample of bile from the duodenum.

The drugs used include *cholecystokinin* (CCK), the peptide hormone made by cells in the wall of the small intestine, which physiologically stimulates contraction of the gallbladder, and two smaller synthetic peptides that are related chemically and pharmacologically to cholecystokinin—*ceruletide diethylamine* (Tymtran) and *sincalide* (Kinevac). All three agents produce similar effects. In addition to stimulating the gallbladder to contract, they relax the sphincter of Oddi; increase the motility of the stomach and intestines; delay gastric emptying, in part

by producing pylorospasm; and stimulate the pancreas to secrete digestive enzymes into the duodenum.

Although fewer adverse reactions have been reported for cholecystokinin, the similarity of the digestive system effects produced by all three peptides strongly suggests that adverse reactions referrable to the digestive system could be produced by all three agents. Adverse reactions to ceruletide and sincalide are mainly manifestations of these effects on the digestive system (*i.e.*, nausea, vomiting, abdominal discomfort, and an urge to defecate). The sweating, hypotension, and dizziness reported with ceruletide may be secondary to the nausea and abdominal cramps. The contraindication of bowel obstruction and the precautions listed for ceruletide (Table 56-1) should also be considered when the administration of cholecystokinin or sincalide is contemplated.

Pancreatic exocrine function

Secretin is another hormone produced in cells of the wall of the small intestine. It stimulates the pancreas to secrete a large volume of fluid high in sodium bicarbonate. Cholecystokinin or sincalide are sometimes given with secretin to facilitate obtaining a duodenal aspirate, which can then be analyzed to assess pancreatic function or can be analyzed cytologically.

Secretin also stimulates the secretion of gastrin in patients with gastrinoma (Zollinger–Ellison syndrome); when given to diagnose this syndrome, blood levels of gastrin are measured.

No adverse reactions to secretin have been reported but, because of its effect on the pancreas, secretin should not be given in acute pancreatitis. Patients with a history of allergies should receive a small test dose first.

Bentiromide (Chymex), a substituted derivative of para-aminobenzoic acid (PABA), has recently been introduced as a diagnostic agent to test for pancreatic insufficiency. The drug is administered orally. PABA is cleaved from the drug molecule by the pancreatic enzyme chymotrypsin, and is then absorbed from the small intestine, conjugated in the liver, and excreted in the urine, from which it is assayed. The amount of PABA in the urine indicates the amount of chymotrypsin secreted by the pancreas. This test has the advantages of being noninvasive and causing few serious adverse effects (nausea, vomiting, diarrhea, and headache have been reported, and one patient developed a hypersensitivity reaction), but both false positive and false negative results have occurred. Because PABA displaces methotrexate from binding sites, bentiromide should not be given to patients taking methotrexate.

Intestinal absorption

D-Xylose (Xylo-Pfan) is administered orally to test the absorptive ability of the jejunum and upper small intestine. Urine or blood levels of the drug are measured.

To determine malabsorption of specific nutrients, test doses are sometimes given orally and the nutrients or metabolites are measured in the blood or as they are excreted in the urine. Substances measured in this way include *cyanocobalamin* (vitamin B_{12}) and *triglycerides*. Cyanocobalamin is administered with a radioactive cobalt (^{57}Co) label and urinary excretion of the agent is determined; ^{14}C-labeled triglycerides are given and the amount of $^{14}CO_2$ produced and exhaled is determined.

Lactase deficiency, a cause of diarrhea and other digestive disturbances, is very common (90% of Orientals, 75% of American blacks and Indians) and can be diagnosed by the oral administration of *lactose*. When lactase is deficient in the cells of the small intestine, the sugar molecule remains in the intestinal lumen, where it acts osmotically as a laxative. In lactase deficiency, the blood glucose level, which normally increases after the test dose is given, does not rise.

Stasis of the small intestine

Orally administered *glycocholic acid*, labeled with ^{14}C, is administered orally and the expired air is tested for $^{14}CO_2$. Normally little $^{14}CO_2$ would be produced but, in cases of intestinal stasis, intestinal bacteria proliferate and produce ^{14}C-glycine from the glycocholic acid. This in turn is absorbed and further metabolized to $^{14}CO_2$.

Cardiovascular system function tests

Establishment of the cause of hypertension

Pheochromocytoma, a tumor of the adrenal medulla and other chromaffin cell tissues, causes a form of secondary hypertension. The presence of this tumor may be detected by the patient's response to various diagnostic drugs. Injection of *histamine phosphate*, for example, stimulates chromaffin cell tumors to secrete a mixture of epinephrine and norepinephrine. This release of catecholamines in large quantities provokes a steep rise in blood pressure in patients with this tumor. Warnings concerning the administration of histamine, and adverse reactions caused by it, have been described above (see Gastric acid secretion). In general, histamine is considered too dangerous to be used in diagnosing pheochromocytoma.

Phentolamine mesylate (Regitine), an α-adrenergic receptor blocking agent, is considered to be safer in testing for pheochromocytoma. However, unlike histamine, it does not cause a rise in blood pressure. Instead, patients with this condition respond to administration of this drug with a drop in blood pressure.

In patients with essential hypertension, however, the high blood pressure fails to fall significantly following injection of phentolamine. Thus, this drug aids in differentiating between primary hypertension and high blood pressure that is the result of the presence of this tumor—a type of secondary hypertension.

Another form of hypertension is angiotensin II-dependent. Angiotensin II is the most potent pressor substance known. This endogenous hormone, formed by the action of the enzyme renin on a precursor substance, is released into the blood by the kidney (Chap. 26). The renin–angiotensin system has been implicated in some patients with hypertension.

Saralasin acetate (Sarenin), an analogue of angiotensin II, is given as a diagnostic agent to patients suspected of having angiotensin-dependent hypertension. Saralasin binds to angiotensin II receptors, where it acts as a weak agonist. When circulating levels of angiotensin are low, these weak agonist properties are evidenced by an increase in blood pressure; however, when circulating levels of angiotensin are high (*e.g.*, in angiotensin-dependent hypertension), saralasin acts as a competitive antagonist of angiotensin II, and blood pressure falls. When combined with other tests (*e.g.*, determination of circulating plasma renin activity), the saralasin test can help to diagnose hypertension that is dependent on the renin–angiotensin system. Both for patient safety and for meaningful test results, the test must be performed under well-controlled conditions (*i.e.*, sodium depletion, no antihypertensive drugs) in the hospital. Marked pressor and depressor responses are expected; rebound hypertension has occurred up to 3 hours after the drug was administered. Blood pressure must be carefully monitored.

Measurement of circulatory function: blood volume and cardiac output

Dyes and other drugs are sometimes injected directly into the bloodstream to help determine such aspects of circulatory function as blood volume and cardiac output. Their use sometimes produces data that aid in the management of shock and other disorders of circulatory function. Some of these drugs have caused serious adverse effects.

Evans blue is injected intravenously as a means of determining the plasma volume of patients who may be suffering from shock, heart failure, or other disorders leading to development of circulatory abnormalities. The degree to which the dye is diluted in the plasma is measured colorimetrically from a blood sample. The results of such studies are sometimes helpful in deciding on the treatment to be employed in cases of cardiovascular collapse, dehydration, and other disorders. This test may leave the patient's skin tinged blue for several weeks.

Indocyanine green (Cardio-Green) is a dye used mainly for determining cardiac output, but it is also used to determine blood flow through the liver and hepatic function (see above). A freshly prepared solution is injected intravenously, and the extent to which the dye is diluted in blood is measured in blood withdrawn from arteries. Adverse reactions and warnings about its use have been described above (under Liver Function).

Fluorescein and its salts are used to determine circulation time, the extent to which blood vessels are open or blocked, and for other purposes not involving circulatory function. The time required for the dye to move from the arm vein into which it is injected to various other blood vessels is measured by detecting fluorescence at the second site under ultraviolet light. This drug, which is excreted in the bile, is also used for outlining the bile ducts and gallbladder. Occasional nausea and vomiting are the only adverse effects. This dye is also used topically in the eye to detect defects in the conjunctival and corneal surfaces.

Another dye, *isosulfan blue* (Lymphazurin 1%), has recently been introduced as an adjunct to lymphography. Injected subcutaneously, it is taken up into the lymphatic vessels of the region, making these vessels a bright blue and facilitating their delineation. Adverse reactions, all of an allergic type, have occurred in 1.5% of patients; facilities to treat life-threatening allergic reactions should be available for ½ to 1 hour after administration. Local anesthetics should not be administered in the same syringe with this dye, because immediate precipitation occurs when the two agents are mixed.

Various radioactively labeled substances are used to measure blood or plasma volume—for example, ^{125}I- or ^{131}I-labeled serum albumin. ^{51}Cr-labeled sodium chromate is injected to measure red cell volume, red cell survival time, and gastrointestinal blood loss.

Kidney function tests

Phenolsulfonphthalein (phenol red) is the chemical most commonly employed in studies of renal function. It is excreted to some extent by glomerular filtration, but most of it is excreted by renal tubular secretion. Although the test gives only a rough measure of the extent to which kidney function is reduced, its simplicity makes it useful for quick screening to determine whether the patient's excretory function is severely impaired. Poor elimination of the dye indicates that serious renal insufficiency may be present.

The patient forces fluids for about an hour before the test and then empties the bladder just before the dye is injected intravenously or into a muscle. Urine samples are collected at specified intervals and the amount of dye that appears in each sample is measured colorimetrically. Occasional allergic reactions are the only adverse effects reported. Patients should be warned that their urine will be red. The concurrent administration of other weakly acidic drugs (penicillins) can interfere with test results because these drugs compete for tubular secretory sites.

Sodium aminohippurate (PAH), a substance secreted by the kidney tubules, is used to determine the ability of the tubules to perform their excretory function. It is also employed to measure plasma flow through the kidneys. The drug is administered by vein in doses intended to raise the amount in the plasma to certain predetermined levels. The infusion is made slowly to avoid various side-effects that occur when the plasma level rises too rapidly. These include a sudden sensation of skin warmth, nausea, or vomiting. The concurrent administration of sulfonamides can interfere with test results (sulfonamides interact with the reagents used to measure PAH), as can the administration of penicillin or drugs (probenecid, salicylates) that have a uricosuric effect. These drugs and uric acid can interfere with the renal tubular secretion of PAH.

Sodium indigotin disulfonate (indigo carmine) is a dye that is normally excreted by the kidneys rapidly after intravenous administration. It is used mainly to localize the ureteral orifices during cystoscopy. The appearance of the dye in the urine can also be used as an index of renal function. Bronchoconstriction and allergic skin reactions have occurred following the administration of this dye. Therefore, patients with a history of allergic reactions should be tested for allergy to this drug before it is injected for renal function tests.

Inulin and *mannitol* are infused intravenously and their urinary excretion measured as an index of the glomerular filtration rate. Both drugs can cause an osmotic diuresis in high doses. Mannitol should be infused slowly, and should not be given to patients with severe renal impairment or edema. It has caused a number of adverse effects.

^{131}I-labeled iodohippurate sodium and *chlormerodrin* labeled with either ^{197}Hg or ^{203}Hg have also been used in testing kidney function. Chlormerodrin is a mercurial diuretic, which, like other organic mercury compounds, may cause mouth irritation, stomach upsets, skin eruptions, fever, and dizziness in patients who are allergic to mercurials.

Use of edrophonium in the diagnosis of myasthenia gravis

The use of *edrophonium chloride* (Tensilon) in diagnosing myasthenia gravis, and in differentiating myasthenic from cholinergic crisis, have both been described in detail in Chapter 15, and will not be repeated here.

Neuroendocrine dysfunction tests

Drugs of various types are employed to test the functioning of the endocrine hypothalamus, and such endocrine glands as the anterior pituitary, pancreas, thyroid, parathyroid, and the adrenal cortex (see also Section 4, Endocrine Drugs). Some of these drugs also have therapeutic uses, which have been described earlier in this text. When used in conjunction with the patient's signs and symptoms, and with other laboratory diagnostic tests,

tests using these drugs can often pinpoint quite precisely the cause of hypo- or hyperfunction of endocrine glands, and provide the basis for rational therapy (*e.g.,* hormone replacement therapy, surgery, or suppression of a hyperactive gland by drugs).

The diagnostic use of many of these drugs is based on an understanding of the physiologic and biochemical complexities of neuroendocrine function, including the role of hypothalamic releasing factors in the control of the anterior pituitary, the role of anterior pituitary tropic hormones in the control of secretion by endocrine target organs, and the negative feedback role of hormones from endocrine target organs (Chap. 20). The fundamental premise of all these tests is that hypo- and hyperfunctioning endocrine organs will differ from normal endocrine organs in their response to the diagnostic drug.

Drugs that are or act like anterior pituitary tropic hormones

Some of these drugs are themselves anterior pituitary tropic hormones, or they are drugs that act like anterior pituitary tropic hormones and cause endocrine target organs to synthesize and release more hormone.

Corticotropin (adrenocorticotropic hormone; ACTH), prepared from porcine anterior pituitary, and *cosyntropin,* a synthetic fragment of the corticotropin molecule, stimulate the production and release of corticosteroids from the normal adrenal cortex. Cosyntropin is less likely than ACTH to cause allergic reactions. Normally, the injection of either of these drugs is followed by a marked increase in the blood and urine levels of adrenal corticosteroids. These levels can be measured. The increase does not occur in patients with adrenal insufficiency (Addison's disease).

Thyrotropin (thyroid-stimulating hormone; TSH), prepared from bovine anterior pituitaries, ordinarily acts like endogenous human TSH and stimulates the thyroid gland to take up more iodine and to synthesize and release more thyroid hormone. Allergic reactions to this bovine preparation of thyrotropin are not uncommon. Thyrotropin has been used to distinguish between primary hypothyroidism (caused by a deficiency in the thyroid gland itself) and secondary hypothyroidism (caused by a deficiency in the production of TSH by the anterior pituitary). In this test, radioactive iodine uptake by the thyroid gland is determined before and after TSH administration. In primary hypothyroidism iodine uptake is not increased by TSH; in secondary hypothyroidism iodine uptake is markedly increased. The recent introduction of a test that measures circulating TSH levels has largely made this diagnostic test obsolete.

Chorionic gonadotropin (human chorionic gonadotropin; HCG) is produced by the human placenta, but its actions are identical to those of pituitary luteinizing hormone (LH). Like LH, HCG stimulates the Leydig cells of the testes to secrete testosterone, which can be assayed in blood samples. HCG is used diagnostically in testing gonadal function in suspected cases of hypogonadism.

Drugs that are or act like hypothalamic releasing factors

Another group of drugs are hypothalamic releasing factors, or they are drugs that act like hypothalamic releasing factors. They stimulate the release of hormones from the anterior pituitary.

Protirelin (thyrotropin releasing hormone; TRH) is a synthetic tripeptide believed to be identical to natural TRH produced by the hypothalamus. It stimulates the anterior pituitary to release TSH, which can be measured in the serum. It is used diagnostically in distinguishing between primary and secondary hypothyroidism, in tests of anterior pituitary function—for example, when panhypopituitarism (deficient secretion of all anterior pituitary hormones) is suspected, and in determining the adequacy of thyroid hormone replacement therapy.

Gonadorelin (synthetic luteinizing hormone releasing hormone, LH-RH; also called synthetic gonadotropin releasing hormone, Gn-RH) releases gonadotropins from the anterior pituitary. The increase in circulating LH is measured and compared to that of normal control samples to diagnose gonadotropin deficiency.

Clomiphene is a weak estrogen agonist. Its therapeutic use in treating female infertility has already been described (Chap. 23). It is used diagnostically, in men only, as a test for gonadotropin release from the anterior pituitary. Like gonadorelin, clomiphene normally releases gonadotropins from the pituitary.

Arginine HCl (an amino acid), *insulin* (a pancreatic hormone), and *levodopa* (a drug used to treat Parkinson's disease) are three diverse drugs that cause the anterior pituitary to release growth hormone, which can be measured in the plasma. They are used diagnostically in evaluating pituitary dwarfism, acromegaly, gigantism, and panhypopituitarism.

Other drugs

The use of other drugs in diagnostic tests of neuroendocrine function is based on various drug actions.

Dexamethasone, a synthetic corticosteroid (Chap. 21), is used to test the function of the anterior pituitary–adrenal axis, for example, in diagnosing adrenal cortical hyperfunction and Cushing's disease. Normally, the administration of dexamethasone decreases the amount of ACTH produced by the anterior pituitary, and the plasma ACTH levels and urinary steroid levels fall. However, in Cushing's disease, ACTH secretion is relatively unaffected by plasma levels of glucocorticoid hormones and drugs such as dexamethasone that normally inhibit its secretion.

Metyrapone (Metopirone) is employed to test pituitary gland function. Ordinarily, when a person is subjected to stress, the anterior pituitary gland responds by increasing its output of the hormone corticotropin. This, in turn, stimulates the adrenal cortex to secrete cortisol. Before metyrapone is administered, adrenal responsiveness to corticotropin must be established. In people with a normally functioning pituitary gland, metyrapone impedes cortisol production and secretion, resulting in an outpouring of corticotropin by the pituitary gland. The increase in corticotropin stimulates the accumulation of cortisol precursors, whose metabolites can be assayed in the urine. In patients with poor pituitary gland function, this response to the administration of metyrapone is markedly reduced, leading to a diagnosis of hypopituitarism.

Radioactive iodine, labeled with ^{131}I, is sometimes administered to test thyroid gland function. The radioactive label facilitates measurement of the iodine uptake by the thyroid, and this is then compared to the uptake by normally functioning glands.

Parathyroid hormone (PTH; parathyroid) is administered to diagnose idiopathic and postoperative hypoparathyroidism. Urine phosphorus levels are measured before and after the drug is given. PTH increases the urinary excretion of phosphorus in both normal patients and in those with hypoparathyroidism, but the increase is much greater in patients with hypoparathyroidism.

Tolbutamide is a drug that causes the release of insulin from the pancreas. Its use in treating adult-onset diabetes has already been described (Chap. 25). It is used diagnostically in patients suspected of having an insulinoma, an insulin-secreting tumor of the pancreatic islet cells. After tolbutamide is given, a patient with an insulinoma shows a more marked fall in the blood glucose level that is of longer duration than normal because of an excessive release of insulin.

Diagnostic agents that are radioactive isotopes

Radioactive isotopes are often given for diagnostic purposes because of the ease of detecting them, even when widely distributed throughout the body. Even extremely low concentrations of isotopically labeled chemicals can be detected externally by instruments that pick up γ (gamma) rays emitted from organs in which the isotope is concentrated. For example, radioactive iodine is used to diagnose thyroid gland disorders, and radioactive phosphorus is similarly employed for localizing brain tumors.

Other isotopes are sometimes used to trace the absorption of vitamin B_{12} and nutrients, to measure blood flow through the heart, kidneys, and elsewhere, and to visualize internal organs by holding a scintillation scanner over the body and determining the distribution of γ ray-

emitting radioisotopes. However, x-rays are often preferred for this, because they give clearer pictures of organ contours and motility and because the use of radiopharmaceuticals for diagnosis poses many pharmaceutical problems, and requires considerable care to avoid exposure of patients and personnel to radiation.

Table 56-2 shows some radioactively labeled drugs that are used in diagnostic tests. Although the amount of radioactivity in doses of these agents used for diagnostic purposes is low, irradiation of organs that concentrate a radioactive agent may be of concern. Unless the thyroid is being tested, Lugol's solution is often administered prior to testing with a radioactive iodine-tagged compound to inhibit the thyroid uptake and concentration of the radioactive iodine. When isotopes are used diagnostically in women of childbearing age, they should be given in the first few days of the menstrual period to minimize the risk of fetal exposure. Lactating mothers should bottle feed their child for a few days after these diagnostic tests because isotopes may pass into the breast milk.

Radiopaque media for radiographic diagnosis

Radiopaque substances are chemicals that cannot be penetrated by x-rays. They are employed as contrast media to make visible various internal structures, including the gallbladder and gastrointestinal tract, kidneys, lungs, and other organs. There are two classes of contrast media: suspensions of barium sulfate and iodinated organic chemicals. Barium is administered only by mouth or rectally for radiographic examination of the upper or lower gastrointestinal tracts, respectively. A very few of the iodinated compounds are taken by mouth either for local radiopaque effects in the intestinal tract or for their radiopaque effects after they are absorbed and excreted into organs such as the gallbladder. Sometimes contrast media are instilled directly into the organ that is to be visualized—the uterus, or intrathecal space, for example—or they are injected intravenously or intra-arterially. Table 56-3 shows some of these radiopaque agents, along with their primary diagnostic uses. Some of the more common brand names are given along with the generic names. Note the similarity in brand names for different concentrations of an agent, and even for different agents.

Table 56-4 lists contraindications, warnings, drug interactions, and adverse reactions for barium and for the iodinated agents. Life-threatening adverse reactions have occurred, especially with use of the iodinated agents. Thus, it is important to watch the patient closely for early signs of drug reactions so that treatment measures may be instituted immediately. The patient is also observed for delayed reactions after returning to the unit. If treated in a clinic or a physician's office, it is important to ask the patient to wait in the reception area for immediate

Table 56–2. Some radioactively labeled drugs used in diagnostic tests

Drug	Diagnostic use
Tracer drugs used in function tests	
Cyanocobalamin ^{57}Co	To test vitamin B_{12} absorption
^{14}C-labeled triglycerides	To test triglyceride absorption
^{14}C-labeled glycocholic acid	To diagnose stasis of upper small bowel
^{131}I-rose bengal	Liver function test
^{125}I-serum albumin	To measure blood or plasma volume
^{131}I-serum albumin	To measure blood or plasma volume
Sodium chromate ^{51}Cr ^{51}Cr-labeled red blood cells	To measure red cell volume and survival time; to measure gastrointestinal blood loss
^{197}Hg- or ^{203}Hg-chlormerodrin	To assess anatomy and function of kidneys
Iodohippurate sodium ^{131}I	To measure kidney function
Na^{125}I Na^{131}I	To measure thyroid function
Radiolabeled substances used to delineate tumors or structural abnormalities	
Na^{131}I	To diagnose thyroid abnormalities
Sodium pertechnetate ^{99m}Tc ^{32}P-sodium phosphate	To localize brain tumors
^{31}P	Potential use with nuclear magnetic resonance to delineate extent of tissue damage after myocardial infarct or stroke

observation following the test. Often, such an observation period can be combined with an offer of a beverage, which is usually most welcome to the patient who has arrived in a fasting state for the diagnostic tests. The waiting period and offer of light refreshment also serve to lessen the anxiety usually engendered by such tests before the patient resumes normal activity, such as driving a car.

Barium sulfate

Barium sulfate is the most commonly used substance for outlining the viscera of the gastrointestinal tract. It is administered orally as a thick paste for esophageal studies or as a dilute suspension prior to searching for peptic ulcerations or upper gastrointestinal tract lesions. Lower bowel lesions are looked for following a cleansing enema and instillation of a large amount of a warmed barium sulfate retention enema.

Barium that is not completely expelled from the gastrointestinal tract may be constipating. Thus, a cleansing enema after the procedure may assist the evacuation of the barium. In any case, it is important to note the state of bowel motility. Other than its tendency to cause constipation, barium sulfate itself is an entirely safe pharmacologic substance. It does not irritate the gastrointestinal mucosa and is not absorbed into the systemic circulation.

Iodinated radiopaque agents

Cholecystography, a procedure used in the diagnosis of gallbladder disease, is carried out with two types of radiopaque compounds: those administered by mouth and those given intravenously.

The oral iodinated contrast media include *iopanoic acid* and the calcium and sodium salts of *ipodate*, which act quite quickly to make the gallbladder opaque to x-rays. These substances are taken 1 or 2 hours after a fat-free evening meal. Nothing other than small amounts of water is taken by mouth before the x-ray examination on the next morning.

The intravenously administered substances, such as *iodipamide meglumine*, are used for better visualization of the gallbladder and bile ducts of patients in whom results were poor with the orally taken agents. Adverse

Table 56–3. Some radiopaque agents used in radiology

Agent	Primary diagnostic uses
Barium salts	
Barium sulfate	Given only orally or rectally for visualization of upper and lower gastrointestinal tracts
Iodinated contrast media	
Aqueous injectable agents	
Diatrizoate meglumine (Cardiografin; Cystografin; Gastrografin; Hypaque Meglumine†; Reno M 30)	Gastrointestinal radiography, angiography, intravenous and retrograde urography
Diatrizoate sodium (Hypaque Sodium; Hypaque†)	
Iodamide meglumine (Renovue-65)	Intravenous and retrograde urography
Iodipamide meglumine (Cholografin Meglumine)	Intravenous cholangiography
Iodoxamate meglumine (Cholovue)	Intravenous cholecystocholangiography
Iothalamate meglumine (Cysto-Conray; Conray†)	Angiography
Iothalamate sodium (Angio-Conray; Conray†)	
Methiodal sodium (Skiodan Sodium)	Intravenous and retrograde urography
Metrizamide (Amipaque)	Myelography; computerized tomography of intracranial subarachnoid space
Oil for lymphography or hysterosalpingography	
Ethiodized Oil (ethiodol)	For lymphography or hystero-salpingography; *not* for intravenous, intra-arterial, or intrathecal use
Oral preparations used only for oral cholecystography	
Iocetamic acid (Cholebrine)	Only use is oral cholecystography
Iopanoic acid (Telepaque)	
Ipodate calcium (Oragrafin Calcium)	
Ipodate sodium (Oragrafin Sodium)	
Tyropanoate sodium (Bilopaque)	

* Concentration and dose vary with the diagnostic test.
† These drug names contain various suffixes, depending on the individual preparation's contents and concentration.

reactions are much more likely to occur with drugs that are administered by this route.

These adverse effects are especially likely in patients with liver and kidney disease, because these organs do not readily excrete the injected dose of the drug when damaged by disease. Thus, procedures employing iodinated radiopaque compounds are contraindicated in pa-tients with a history of hepatic or renal insufficiency resulting from acute injury of these organs. Patients whose history reveals hypersensitivity to iodine are also not good candidates for diagnostic procedures employing these agents.

During the first 15 to 30 minutes after injection of an iodinated diagnostic agent, the patient should be

Table 56—4. Contraindications, warnings, drug interactions and adverse reactions to barium salts and iodinated radiopaque agents

	Iodinated agents	Barium salts
Contraindications Warnings	Allergy to iodine Use with caution and careful monitoring in patients with the following conditions: Pheochromocytoma: agents may cause hypertensive crises Sickle cell anemia: agents promote sickling in patients homozygous for this disease Hepatic or renal disease: agents may be cleared more slowly than normal; therefore, these patients are at added risk of adverse effects After intravascular injection, life-threatening adverse effects (see below) may occur; monitor patient closely for 1 hr PBI and ^{131}I uptake tests may be altered for 1 wk–2 yr IV urographic agents may alter urinalysis; collect urine sample before or 3 days after test	Given *only* orally or rectally
Adverse effects	Anaphylactic reactions: allergic reactions to iodine, hives, sneezing, wheezing, laryngospasm, angioneurotic edema, anaphylactic shock; cardiovascular reactions: hypotension, shock, coronary insufficiency, cardiac arrhythmias, fibrillation, or arrest, sensation of warmth, flushing, vasodilation; fever; extravasation will cause burning pain; symptoms that may be attributable to anxiety or to requirements for the test procedure such as fasting or dehydration: trembling, headache, chest tightness, awareness of heartbeat, nausea	Constipation; after rectal administration, perforation of bowel and peritonitis have occurred rarely; stools colored white; unless contraindicated, consider administration of a laxative to assist expulsion of barium
Drug–drug interactions	Metrizamide may cause seizures in patients taking CNS stimulants or psychotropic drugs (*e.g.,* phenothiazines, butyrophenones, tricyclic antidepressants, MAO inhibitors); these drugs lower seizure threshold and should not be given 48 hr pre- to 24 hr post-test	High doses of calcium carbonate (taken by some peptic ulcer patients as antacid) may cause cementlike fecal impactions

carefully watched for signs of histamine-release reactions and other possible ill effects. Sneezing, wheezing, and skin swellings may be the first indications of even more severe anaphylactoid reactions. Thus, the drugs and equipment for dealing with this dangerous emergency should always be readily available during radiographic procedures employing parenterally administered radiographic drugs.

Some patients seem to be especially susceptible to cardiovascular effects that do not occur in most people who receive ordinary injectable diagnostic doses. These reactions are often manifested by a fall in blood pressure and reflex tachycardia. Thus, it is desirable to check the patient's blood pressure periodically. Failure to detect and treat severe hypotension has been followed by myocardial infarction, renal failure, and other complications.

Urography—x-ray visualization of the urinary tract—is carried out shortly after intravenous injection of one of the water-soluble organic iodine contrast media, such as *diatrizoate meglumine* or *diatrizoate sodium*. Soon after these materials are slowly infused, they are carried to the kidneys and begin to appear in the urine. Serial x-rays are taken beginning about 5 minutes after the contrast medium has been injected completely, when dense shadows develop in the urinary collecting system.

In *retrograde urography* the contrast medium is instilled into the kidneys through catheters placed by cystoscopy. Thus, the kidneys and the urinary collecting system are outlined without spreading the chemical throughout the body by way of the circulation. In both this and the above procedures, it is customary to administer a laxative about 12 hours before the administration of the contrast medium. This, and the subsequent withholding of food, empties the bowel and thus minimizes development of abdominal shadows that might make it difficult to interpret the urographic roentgenograms.

Renal arteriography delivers the contrast medium solution directly into the renal arteries through rapid injection into the abdominal aorta. Although this procedure often reveals defects in the renal circulation better than any other test, it is relatively hazardous. Two newer agents, *iothalamate meglumine* and *iothalamate sodium*, are said to be safer than earlier contrast media for carrying out this test and other angiographic procedures such as cardiac, aortic, and cerebral circulatory x-ray studies. In these studies, the solutions are injected swiftly into the vessels of the organ that is to be visualized. For example, dilute solutions are injected directly into the carotid and vertebral arteries before x-rays of the brain–blood circulation are taken.

Instillation of oily or viscous iodized contrast media directly into hollow organs, rather than by way of the blood, is often employed for visualizing certain areas. For example, the uterine cavity and fallopian tubes are visualized by introducing *ethiodized oil* (Ethiodol), or one of the water-soluble iodine preparations made suitably viscous by the addition of a thickening agent. This procedure, *hysterosalpingography,* is used in sterility studies to determine the patency of the tubes and in the diagnosis of other gynecologic conditions.

Myelography, visualization of the spinal cord, is carried out by instillation of an iodinated contrast medium into the subarachnoid space. This procedure is widely used for finding evidence of herniated intervertebral disks and other sources of spinal cord compression. After the fluoroscopic or roentgenographic examination, the contrast agent is aspirated from the spinal fluid.

Additional clinical considerations

Patient safety

This must be a major consideration when performing an invasive test for diagnostic purposes. The benefit-to-risk ratio of the test should be evaluated carefully. If the patient's underlying medical condition might invalidate the results of the test and put the patient at risk unnec-essarily, or if the patient's medical condition predisposes him to dangerous side-effects, serious consideration should be given to the real need for the information provided by this particular test. In many cases there is another way to obtain the same information, or there are data already available to provide the same answers. The nurse, in assessing the total patient situation, is often in the position to present such an issue to the health-care team for consideration.

Patient teaching

This is an essential aspect of any diagnostic test (see Patient teaching guide: diagnostic tests). In most situations there is an element of fear and anxiety associated with diagnostic procedures. Patients fear the unknown—What will happen to me during this procedure?—and are anxious about the results of the test—What will they find? To allay some fears, the patient should know what will be done, any discomfort involved, any signs or symptoms to anticipate during or after the procedure (*e.g.,* feeling flushed, sweating, having feces or skin of abnormal color), what the procedure will feel like, and how long after the test the results will be known. The patient will also need to know what preparatory measures to take, and why. These measures include cleansing enemas, laxatives, fasting, and stopping certain medications. If the test is being done on an outpatient basis, the patient's understanding of and cooperation with the preparatory protocol will determine the accuracy of the test. A written set of directions is often essential.

The results of the test will introduce a whole new area of patient teaching. If the tests are negative some patients may be reassured, while other patients will find such a report a source of more anxiety. This is especially likely if the signs and symptoms that resulted in this test still persist. In such instances, negative test results leave the patient with the same fears and unanswered questions. If the results are positive, the patient will need teaching about the disease that has been diagnosed.

All patients will need support and encouragement before, after, and during these diagnostic tests. It is important to remember that, to the patient involved, no test is "just routine." To the patient, the test is a frightening life experience that will have to be dealt with. The nurse is usually the member of the health-care team who can best help the patient and family to cope with and adapt to this experience.

Technical considerations

Many solutions that are used for diagnostic purposes are inherently quite unstable, and therefore must be prepared just before injection. The manufacturer's directions should be checked for information about the stability and preparation of such agents.

Care must be taken when administering these agents intravenously or intra-arterially to maintain sterility of the area and to prevent extravasation of the drug into the tissues. Many of these drugs are very irritating to the tissues; several, including the dyes and chlormerodrin, are directly tissue-toxic and can cause local necrosis.

It is also important to monitor the exposure of the patient to radioactive substances. If a patient undergoes repeated diagnostic tests involving the use of radio-active tracers and repeated x-rays, the amount of radiation exposure could be a concern. Knowing the total patient situation will help to avoid inadvertent overexposure to radioactivity.

The guide to the nursing process for drugs used for diagnosis provides a summary of the clinical considerations that apply to these drugs.

Patient teaching guide: diagnostic tests

Preparatory measures:

These include such measures as diet, enemas, and fluids.

Procedure:
1. What it will feel like
2. Discomfort that may occur
3. Signs and symptoms to anticipate (*e.g.*, sweating; flushing; urine, feces, skin turning colors)
4. How long after the test the results will be known

Results:
1. Disease and its implications
2. Need for more tests
3. Support and encouragement

Guide to the nursing process: drugs used for diagnosis

Assessment	Nursing diagnoses	Interventions	Evaluation
Past history (underlying medical conditions): Allergies Previous exposure to drug: reaction Last meal Medication history: Drugs being taken Last dose **Physical assessment** Neurologic: orientation, reflexes Cardiovascular: blood pressure, pulse, cardiac output Respiratory: rate, adventitious sounds	Potential alteration in comfort Potential alteration in bowel elimination Potential alteration in cardiac output Potential alteration in respiratory function Fear related to test and to possible results Knowledge deficit regarding test and results	Pretest preparation as per protocol for the test (*e.g.*, fasting, enemas) Patient teaching and preparation: What it will feel like Signs and symptoms to anticipate Results and implications Preparation and safe administration of drug Support and encouragement Provision of comfort measures: pain relief, positioning,	Monitor response to drug Monitor for adverse effects of drug Monitor for exacerbation of medical conditions Evaluate effectiveness of teaching plan Evaluate effectiveness of support measures

(continued)

Assessment	Nursing diagnoses	Interventions	Evaluation
Gastrointestinal: bowel sounds, output Renal: urinary output, electrolyte status Skin: lesions, temperature, sweating		environment control Provision of life support measures, if necessary	

Case study

Presentation

MC is a 40-year-old man with a 3-month history of epigastric pain, which is most severe 2 to 3 hours after eating. An upper GI x-ray series has been ordered to rule out a duodenal ulcer. The test will be done in 2 days as an outpatient procedure. As the nurse responsible for his care, what do you need to do now?

Discussion

The nurse responsible for MC's care will need to do some preliminary assessment. A past history of gastrointestinal problems, particularly obstruction, paralytic ileus, or fistulas, would contraindicate the use of barium in this procedure. MC's current gastrointestinal status should be evaluated by assessing bowel sounds, and by asking about frequency of bowel movements. MC will need to know that he should fast the day of the test; that if barium is given, he will be asked to drink a thick, chalky substance that might be unpleasant; that he may be asked to change position frequently while the x-rays are being taken; that some preliminary results will be available immediately but that his physician will receive the results within a few days; that, following the test, fluids should be pushed and measures should be taken to avoid the constipation that often comes with barium ingestion; and that, until the barium has completely passed out of the body, his stools will be light and clay-colored. MC should be encouraged to ask questions and to express any concerns that he might have now, or later in a phone call. He should be told to let you know when his stools have returned to normal. A card with the major teaching points listed for reference would be most helpful to many patients.

References

Bentiromide—a test of pancreatic insufficiency. Med Lett Drugs Ther 26:50, 1984

Crocker D, Vandam LD: Untoward reactions to radiopaque contrast media. Clin Pharmacol Ther 4:654, 1963

Elking MP, Kabat HF: Drug-induced modification of laboratory test values. Am J Hosp Pharm 25:485, 1968

Hoppe JO: Some pharmacological aspects of radiopaque compounds. Ann NY Acad Sci 78:727, 1959

Oldendorf WH: NMR imaging: Its potential clinical impact. Hosp Pract 17:114, Sept 1982

Pentagastrin. Med Lett Drugs Ther 17:60, 1975

Saralasin for diagnosis of renovascular hypertension. Med Lett Drugs Ther 24:3, 1982

Schmidt RM, Margolin S: Harper's Handbook of Therapeutic Pharmacology, Philadelphia, Harper & Row, 1981

Sincalide for cholecystography. Med Lett Drugs Ther 19:36, 1977

Synthetic LH–RH. Med Lett Drugs Ther 25:106, 1983

Appendix

Practice problems in dosage and solutions

Answer the following questions using the formulas and conversions outlined in Chapter 3. The correct answers are found after the problems.

Problems

1. Change to equivalents within the system:

    a. 100 mg = _____ g
    b. 1500 g = _____ kg
    c. 0.1 liter = _____ ml
    d. 500 ml = _____ liter

2. Convert to units in the metric system:

    a. 150 gr = _____ g
    b. ¼ gr = _____ mg
    c. 45 minims = _____ ml
    d. 2 quarts = _____ liter

3. Convert to units in the household system:

    a. 4 or 5 ml = _____ tsp
    b. 30 ml = _____ tbsp

4. Convert the weights in the following problems:

    a. Your patient weighs 170 lb. What is his weight in kilograms? 170 lb = _____ kg
    b. Your patient weighs 3200 g. What is his weight in pounds? 3200 g = _____ lb

5. *Ordered:* Robitussin cough syrup 225 mg
   Available: Robitussin 600 mg in 1 oz

   You will give _____ ml.

6. *Ordered:* Ferrous sulfate 240 mg
   Available: Ferrous sulfate 40 mg = 1 ml

   You will give _____ ml.

7. *Ordered:* Elixir acetaminophen gr v
   Available: Elixir acetaminophen 120 mg = 5 ml

   You will give _____ ml.

8. *Ordered:* Codeine ¼ gr q 4 hr prn for pain

   Each dose will contain _____ mg.

9. *Ordered:* Chloramphenicol 0.5 g PO q 6 hr
   Available: Chloramphenicol 250 mg per capsule

    a. How many capsules will you give at each dose?
       _____ capsules
    b. How many *milligrams* of chloramphenicol will your patient receive at each dose?
       _____ mg

10. *Ordered:* Mellaril 0.1 g PO q 8 hr
    Available: Mellaril 30 mg. = 1 ml

    You will give _____ ml.

11. *Ordered:* Orinase tablets 1 g after breakfast and 0.5 g after lunch
    Available: Orinase 500-mg tablets

    a. How many tablets would you give your patient after:
       breakfast? _____
       lunch? _____
    b. How many milligrams of Orinase will your patient receive each day?
       _____ mg

12. *Ordered:* Lanoxin 0.25 mg PO qd
    Available: Lanoxin 0.5 mg = 2 ml

    You will give _____ ml; this equals
    _____ minims.

13. The physician has ordered penicillin G 200,000 U
    for your patient. You have available a multidose
    vial labeled 300,000 U/ml. How many milliliters
    would you prepare to give your patient?

    _____ ml

14. The physician has ordered 800 U of heparin for
    your patient. You have available a 5-ml vial
    labeled 10,000 U/ml.

    You will give _____ ml.

15. You have an order for ampicillin 300 mg IV. The
    vial reads "Ampicillin 500 mg/vial; add 1.8 ml
    diluent to obtain 250 mg/ml." Calculate the
    amount in milliliters that you need to give.

    _____ ml

16. You have an order to add 20 mg of KCl per liter
    to your IV. You need to add the proper amount
    of KCl to a 500-ml bottle. The KCl bottle reads
    60 mg/30 ml. How many ml of KCl should you
    add to the 500-ml IV bottle?

    _____ ml

17. You have an order for Tylenol (acetaminophen)
    60 mg PO for temperature elevation of 38.5°C.
    Acetaminophen Elixir bottle reads: "120 mg/5
    ml." Calculate the amount in milliliters that you
    need to give.

    _____ ml

18. *Ordered:* 6.5 mg
    Label: 10 mg/ml

    You would give _____ ml.

19. *Ordered:* 0.35 mg
    Label: 1.2 mg/2 ml

    You would give _____ ml.

20. *Ordered:* 80 mg
    Label: 50 mg/ml

    You would give _____ ml.

21. *Ordered:* 150,000 U
    Label: 400,000 U/5 ml

    You would give _____ ml.

22. *Ordered:* 75,000 U
    Label: 500,000 U/10 ml

    You would give _____ ml.

23. *Ordered:* 1.5 g
    Label: 500 mg/ml

    You would give _____ ml.

24. *Ordered:* 1200 mg
    Label: 2.5 g/5 ml

    You would give _____ ml.

25. *Ordered:* 100 mg aminophylline IV piggyback, stat
    Available: 500 mg/2.5 ml

    You would give _____ ml.

26. Digoxin 0.125 mg PO is ordered for a patient
    who has difficulty in swallowing. The bottle of
    elixir is labeled 0.5 mg/2 ml. How much would
    you give?

    _____ ml

27. Ampicillin 700 mg PO is ordered. The drug is
    supplied as 1 g/3.5 ml. How much drug should be
    given?

    _____ ml

28. 0.05 g of Aldactone PO is ordered. The tablets
    available contain 25 mg/tablet. How many tablets
    should be given?

    _____ tablets

29. Tetracycline 0.75 g PO is ordered. The drug is
    supplied in 250-mg tablets. How many tablets
    should be given?

    _____ tablets

30. From 25.0 mg of drug in powder form you need
    to prepare a solution containing 2.0 mg of drug/
    ml. You will add diluent until you have how many
    milliliters of solution?

    _____ ml

31. You need to prepare 8 oz of normal saline
    solution (0.9%). How many milligrams of salt
    would you need to add to 8 oz of water?

    _____ mg

32. A vial of penicillin G is labeled as 3,000,000 U of
    dry drug. How much solution containing 400,000
    U/ml can you make?

    _____ ml

33. The standard adult dose of meperidine is 75.0 mg. What dose would be appropriate for a 10-month-old infant?

———————— mg

34. The standard adult dose of tetracycline is 250.0 mg qid. What would be the safe dose for a child weighing 30 lb?

———————— mg

35. The usual adult dose of morphine sulfate is gr $^1/_6$. What would be the safe dose for an infant 6 months old?

———————— gr

36. The usual adult dose of Benadryl is 50.0 mg. What would be the safe dose for a child weighing 27 lb?

———————— mg

37. The usual adult dose of penicillin is 500,000 U/dose. What would be the safe dose for a child weighing 75 lb?

———————— U

38. 3 g of sulfasuxidine PO qid is ordered for a patient who weighs 110 lb. The usual adult dose is 60 mg/kg qid. How much drug is this patient receiving?

———————— mg/kg

Is this a safe dose?

————————

39. *Ordered:* Caffeine sodium benzoate gr vii ss
Available: Caffeine sodium benzoate 0.5 g in 2.0 ml

How much would you give?
———————— ml

40. *Ordered:* Atropine sulfate 0.3 mg
Available: Atropine sulfate gr $^1/_{150}$/ml

How much would you give?
———————— ml

41. *Ordered:* 500 ml D-5-W over 4 hr
Available: IV set with drop factor of 10

What is the flow rate?

a. ———————— ml/hr
b. ———————— drops/min

42. *Ordered:* 100 ml D-10-W over 4 hr
Available: IV set with drop factor of 60

What is the flow rate?

a. ———————— ml/hr
b. ———————— drops/min

43. *Ordered:* 250 ml packed cells to run over 2 hr
Available: IV blood set with drop factor of 6

What is the flow rate?

a. ———————— ml/hr
b. ———————— drops/min

44. *Ordered:* 1000 ml normal saline to run over 10 hr
Available: IV set with drop factor of 15.

What is the flow rate?

a. ———————— ml/hr
b. ———————— drops/min

45. You have 50 ml of a 2% solution of lidocaine. How many mg of lidocaine do you have?

———————— mg

Answers

1. a. 0.1 g
   b. 1.5 kg
   c. 100 ml
   d. 0.5 liter
2. a. 9 g
   b. 15 mg
   c. 3 ml
   d. 2 liter
3. a. 1 tsp
   b. 2 tbsp
4. a. 77 kg
   b. 7 lb
5. 11.25 ml
6. 6 ml
7. 12.5 ml
8. 15 mg
9. a. Two capsules
   b. 500 mg
10. 3.3 ml
11. a. breakfast: two
       lunch: one
    b. 1500 mg
12. 1 ml; 15 or 16 minims
13. 0.66 (0.7) ml
14. 0.08 ml
15. 1.2 ml
16. 5 ml
17. 2.5 ml
18. 0.65 ml
19. 0.58 (0.6) ml
20. 1.6 ml
21. 1.9 ml
22. 1.5 ml
23. 3 ml
24. 2.4 ml
25. 0.5 ml
26. 0.5 ml
27. 2.45 ml
28. Two tablets
29. Three tablets
30. 12.5 ml
31. 2160 mg
32. 7.5 ml
33. 5.0 mg
34. 50.0 mg
35. $\frac{1}{150}$ gr
36. 9.0 mg

37. 250,000 U
38. 60 mg/kg or
    3000 mg qid;
    yes
39. 1.8 ml
40. 0.75 ml
41. a. 125 ml/hr
    b. 21 drops/min
42. a. 25 ml/hr
    b. 25 drops/min
43. a. 125 ml/hr
    b. 13 drops/min
44. a. 100 ml/hr
    b. 25 drops/min
45. 1000 mg

Indexes

Drug digest index

General index

Page numbers followed by f *indicates an illustration;* t *following a page number indicates tabular material.*

General index

American Journal of Nursing, 19
American Nurses' Association nursing diagnoses, 30
Amicar (aminocaproic acid), 721–722
Amidate (etomidate), 1094
amikacin, 180
amiloride (Midamor), 568
amino acids in parenteral nutrition, 1153
τ-aminobutyric acid, 298
aminocaproic acid (Amicar), 721–722
aminoglutethimide (Cytadren), 277
aminoglycosides, 179, 180t. *See also specific drugs*
  adverse effects of, 181–182
  antibacterial spectrum of, 180
  in hepatic encephalopathy, 871
  interaction with penicillin, 158
  nursing process guide, 182–183
  patient teaching guide, 182–183
  pharmacokinetics of, 180–181
  uses of, 181
aminophylline, 818
  in angina pectoris, 655
  in pulmonary edema, 672
  in status asthmaticus, 823–824
aminopyrine, 762
  leukopenia and, 93
amitriptyline (Elavil), 310, 980
ammonia in blood, 871–872
ammoniated mercury, 909
ammonium chloride, 1152
amnesia
  from barbiturates, 939
  during labor, 955
amoxapine (Asendin), 980
amoxicillin (Amoxil; Larotid), 154
Amoxil (amoxicillin), 154
amphetamines, 363, 1000
  abuse of, 1124–1126
  action of, 310
  clinical indications for, 1001–1002
  pharmacology of, 1000–1001
  psychotomimetic, 1129–1130
amphotericin B, 209
ampicillin (Amcill; Omnipen), 148, 154–155
  in respiratory disease, 817
amrinone (Inocur), 621
amyl nitrite, 653
anabolic agents, 510t–511t, 513–514. *See also androgens*
analeptics, 1005
analgesia, 1084
analgesic-antipyretics
  abuse of, 754–755
  dosage of, 755t
  effectiveness of, 754
  nonsalicylate, 760–762
    toxicity of, 761–762
  salicylate, 756
  self-medication with, 755
analgesics, 1062. *See also opiates and specific drug*
analogue, 8
Ananase (bromelains), 697
anaphylactic reaction, 89–90, 795
  prevention of, 799
  treatment of, 799–800
anaplasia, 253
anasarca, 613
Ancef (cefazolin sodium), 162
Ancobon (flucytosine), 207–208
androgens. *See also anabolic agents and testosterone*
  adverse effects of, 512–513, 518
  clinical considerations in, 514–515
  drug interactions with, 515
  function of, 508–509
  laboratory test interactions with, 515
  nursing process guide, 516–517
  patient teaching guide, 515–516
  secretion of, 418, 507–508, 507f
  therapeutic uses of, 509, 511–512, 517–518
    in cancer, 276
    in women, 513
Anectine (succinylcholine), 394
anemia, 731
  anabolic agents in, 514
  androgen therapy in, 513
  clinical considerations in, 739–740
  drug-induced, 91–93

  aplastic, 93–94, 176
  hemolytic, 92–92, 762
  folic acid deficiency, 738–739
  iron deficiency, 731–732
  iron fortification of food and, 735
  iron poisoning in, 735
  iron supplements in, 732–733, 733t
  iron therapy for, 733–735
  megaloblastic, 735–736
    Vitamin B$_{12}$ deficiency, 736–738
  pernicious, 736
  self-medication in, 739
anesthesia and anesthetics. *See also pain and specific drug*
  action of, 63–65
  balanced, 1083–1084
  basal, 1084, 1092–1093
  caudal, 314
  dissociative, 1093
  epidural, 314, 320, 322
  field (ring), 314
  fluorinated, 1091–1092
  general, 1083, 1089t–1090t. *See also anesthesia and anesthetics, inhalation*
    neuromuscular junction blocking drugs with, 399–400
    objectives of, 1084
    patient teaching and, 1094–1097
    postanesthesia measures in, 1006, 1096
    premedication for, 1094–1095
    types of, 1084
  infiltration, 313–314
  inhalation, 1097. *See also anesthesia and anesthetics, general*
    anesthetic syndrome and, 1085–1088, 1086f
    pharmacokinetics of, 1084–1085
  local, 316t. *See also nerve block*
    action of, 312, 213f
    administration of, 313–315, 314f
    clinical applications of, 317–318
    contraindications for, 323
    interactions of, 322–323
    nursing process guide, 324–325
    patient safety and, 322
    patient teaching guide, 324
    pharmacokinetics of, 312–313
    toxic reactions to, 320–322, 323t
  in ocular surgery, 885, 885t
  regional, 1095. *See also anesthesia and anesthetics, local*
    intravenous, 314
  nonbarbiturate, 1093–1094
  spinal, 314, 314f, 319–320
    adrenergic drugs and, 372–373
  topical, 313
  in vomiting, 865
Anesthesin (benzocaine), 317
anesthetic syndrome, 1097–1098
angel dust, 1130
angina pectoris, 650–651. *See also antianginal agents*
  β-adrenergic blocking drugs in, 381
angioneurotic edema, 798–799
angiotensin (Hypertensin). *See also renin-angiotensin system*
  in hypertension test, 1191
  in hypotension, 372
ankylosing spondylitis, 772
anorectal lesions, laxatives in, 853–854
anoretic drugs, 1001–1002, 1002t
anorexia in chemotherapy, 279
anovulation, 483
  progesterone therapy in, 485–486
Antabuse (disulfiram), 1120
antacids
  adverse effect of, 846–847
  in peptic ulcer, 833, 834t, 835–837
    clinical considerations in, 838–839
    patient teaching guide, 839–340
    self-medication in, 838–839
antagonism, drug, 61, 63, 79. *See also specific drug*
anthralin, 909
anthraquinone, 851
antianginal agents, 651–652, 652t
  β-adrenergic receptor blocking drugs, 656–657
  calcium channel blockers, 657–658

  clinical considerations in, 658
  nitrate-type, 652–655
    adverse effects of, 661
  nonnitrate-type, 655–656
  nursing process guide, 661
  patient teaching guide, 659–660
antianxiety agents. *See tranquilizers*
antiarrhythmic drugs, 630, 631t–632t. *See also cardiac arrhythmia and specific drug*
  adverse effect of, 646
  clinical considerations in, 642
  clinical indications for, 645–646
  diet interaction with, 643
  drug interaction with, 642–643
  nursing process guide, 644–645
  patient teaching guide, 643–644
antibacterial drugs, action of, 62
antibiotics, 116. *See also specific drug and disease, e.g., penicillins, tetracyclines*
  in acne, 911
  in diarrhea, 859–860
  in eye infection, 887–888
  in hepatic encephalopathy, 871
  in respiratory obstructive disease, 817
  in skin infection, 917–918
antibody, 89–90, 90f, 1167
  antiviral, 131
  production in allergy, 794
anticholinergic drugs, 342–344, 344t. *See also mydriatic-cycloplegic agents*
  clinical considerations in, 348–349
  in diarrhea, 861
  nursing process guide, 352
  patient teaching guide, 350–351
  pharmacology of, 344, 349t–350t
    cardiovascular, 345–346
    central nervous system, 347–348
    exocrine gland, 346–347
    eye, 347
    gastrointestinal, 344–345
    respiratory, 346
    urinary, 345
  in parkinsonism, 1029–1031, 1030t
  in peptic ulcer, 840–841
  poisoning by, 348
  in urinary tract infection, 187
  in vomiting, 866–867
anticholinesterase agents, 307, 328, 330. *See also miotic drugs*
  skeletal muscle effects of, 332
anticlotting factors, 704
anticoagulants, 706, 713t. *See also specific drug and disorder*
  clinical considerations in, 722–723
  contraindications for, 710
  drug interaction of, 82–83, 83t, 714–715, 714t
  indications for, 710–711, 726
  in myocardial infarction, 664–665
  nursing process guide, 725
  patient teaching guide, 723–724
anticonvulsants. *See antiepileptic drugs*
antidepressants. *See also depression and stimulants*
  monoamine oxidase inhibitors, 983–984
  in psychotic depression, 988–989
  side effects of, 994
  tricyclic, 980, 981t
    adverse effects of, 980, 982
    in alcoholic patient, 1120
    clinical indications for, 980
    nursing process guide, 991–992
    patient teaching guide, 990–991
    treatment of toxicity, 982
antidiuretic hormone, 559–560. *See also vasopressin*
  synthesis of, 410–411
antidopaminergic drugs in vomiting, 865–866
antidote, 63, 101, 102t–103t, 103–105
antiemetics, 862, 863t–864t, 864
  in cancer chemotherapy, 255
  centrally acting, 865–867
  clinical considerations in, 867
  delta-9-tetrahydrocannabinol, 1134
  locally acting, 864–865
  phenothiazines, 967
antiepileptic drugs, 934, 1041–1043, 1043t. *See also epilepsy*